HEART TRANSPLANTATION

HEART TRANSPLANTATION

James K. Kirklin, M.D.
Professor of Surgery
Director of Cardiothoracic Transplantation
UAB Endowed Professor of Cardiovascular Surgical Research
Division of Cardiothoracic Surgery
University of Alabama at Birmingham Medical Center
Birmingham, Alabama

James B. Young, M.D.
Medical Director, Kauffman Center for Heart Failure
Head, Section of Heart Failure and Cardiac Transplant Medicine
Department of Cardiology
Cleveland Clinic Foundation
Cleveland, Ohio

David C. McGiffin, M.D.
Professor of Surgery
Division of Cardiothoracic Surgery
Department of Surgery
University of Alabama at Birmingham Medical Center
Birmingham, Alabama

Foreword by Norman E. Shumway, M.D.

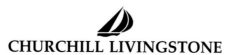

CHURCHILL LIVINGSTONE
An Imprint of Elsevier Science
New York   Edinburgh   London   Philadelphia

CHURCHILL LIVINGSTONE
An Imprint of Elsevier Science

The Curtis Center
Independence Square West
Philadelphia, Pennsylvania 19106

Library of Congress Cataloging-in-Publication Data

Kirklin, James K.
   Cardiac transplantation / James K. Kirklin, David McGiffin, James B.
Young.
      p. ; cm.
   ISBN 0–443–07655–3
   1. Heart—Transplantation.
      [DNLM: 1. Heart Transplantation.   WG 169 K589c 2002]   I.
McGiffin, David.   II. Young, James B.   III. Title.
   RD598.35.T7 K55 2002
   617.4'120592—dc21

                                                                      2001028605

Publishing Director: Richard Lampert
Editorial Assistant: Susan Klumb
Production Manager: Donna L. Morrissey

HEART TRANSPLANTATION   ISBN 0–443–07655–3

Printed in the United States of America.

Last digit is the print number: 9   8   7   6   5   4   3   2   1

This book is dedicated to the physicians, surgeons, and researchers who have committed their lives to the quest for successful transplantation of the human heart; to the patients who have gained and lost their lives in pursuit of or after receiving the gift of transplantation; to the organ donors and their families who have provided that gift; and to our families, who have provided unconditional love, tolerance, and support throughout this project.

Collaborators

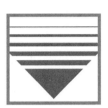

ROBIN K. AVERY, M.D.
Staff Physician, Department of Infectious Disease and Transplant Center, Cleveland Clinic Foundation, Cleveland, Ohio
Infections After Heart (and Heart/Lung) Transplantation

RAYMOND L. BENZA, M.D.
Assistant Professor of Medicine, Division of Cardiovascular Diseases, University of Alabama at Birmingham, Birmingham, Alabama
Cardiac Allograft Vasculopathy (Chronic Rejection)

ROBERT C. BOURGE, M.D.
Professor and Director, Division of Cardiovascular Disease, University of Alabama at Birmingham, Birmingham, Alabama
Cardiac Allograft Rejection

ROBERT N. BROWN, B.S., Ch.E.
Division of Cardiothoracic Surgery, University of Alabama at Birmingham, Birmingham, Alabama
Survival After Heart Transplantation

RICHARD E. CHINNOCK, M.D.
Professor and Vice Chair, Loma Linda Children's Pediatric Hospital, Loma Linda University Medical Center, Loma Linda, California
Pediatric Heart Transplantation

JAMES F. GEORGE, Ph.D.
Associate Professor of Surgery, Medicine, Microbiology, Division of Cardiothoracic Surgery, University of Alabama at Birmingham, Birmingham, Alabama
History of Cardiac Transplantation; Immunology in Relation to Cardiac Transplantation; Pretransplant Immunologic Evaluation and Management; Immunosuppressive Modalities; Xenotransplantation

WALTER K. GRAHAM, J.D.
United Network for Organ Sharing, Richmond, Virginia
Resource Allocation in Heart Transplantation

WILLIAM L. HOLMAN, M.D.
Professor of Surgery, Division of Cardiothoracic Surgery, University of Alabama at Birmingham, Birmingham, Alabama
Mechanical Support of the Failing Heart

ROBERT L. KORMOS, M.D.
Professor of Surgery, Director of Thoracic Transplantation and Artificial Heart Program, University of Pittsburgh Medical Center, Pittsburgh, Pennsylvania
Mechanical Support of the Failing Heart

DAVID C. NAFTEL, Ph.D.
Professor of Surgery, Division of Cardiothoracic Surgery, University of
Alabama at Birmingham, Birmingham, Alabama
*Methodology for Clinical Research in Cardiac Transplantation; Survival After
Heart Transplantation*

PETER G. PAPPAS, M.D.
Professor of Medicine, Department of Medicine, Division of Infectious
Disease, University of Alabama at Birmingham, Birmingham, Alabama
Infections After Heart (and Heart/Lung) Transplantation

F. BENNETT PEARCE, M.D.
Associate Professor of Pediatrics, LM Bargeron, Jr. Division of Pediatric
Cardiology, UAB School Medicine, Birmingham, Alabama
Pediatric Heart Transplantation

BARRY K. RAYBURN, M.D.
Associate Professor of Medicine, Medical Director, Cardiac
Transplantation, University of Alabama at Birmingham, Birmingham,
Alabama
Other Long-Term Complications

E. RENE RODRIGUEZ, M.D.
Associate Professor of Pathology, Director, Clinical Services
Cardiovascular Pathology, The Johns Hopkins University School of
Medicine, Baltimore, Maryland
Cardiac Allograft Rejection

JOSE TALLAJ, M.D.
Fellow, Division of Cardiovascular Diseases, University of Alabama at
Birmingham, Birmingham, Alabama
Cardiac Allograft Vasculopathy (Chronic Rejection)

CARMELA D. TAN, M.D.
Senior Lecturer, The Johns Hopkins University School of Medicine,
Baltimore, Maryland
Cardiac Allograft Rejection

CONNIE WHITE-WILLIAMS, R.N., M.S.N.
Cardiothoracic Transplant Coordinator, University of Alabama at
Birmingham, Birmingham, Alabama
Quality of Life After Heart Transplantation

Foreword

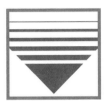

This is a book for the ages. It is comprehensive. It is beautifully written. It is the culmination of a most remarkable dedication to the science and art of heart transplantation by the authors. The completeness with which this subject is treated is reminiscent of bygone days when scribes would withdraw from the mundane world to create an oeuvre that would defy the passage of time.

Those of us who grew up with open heart surgery are well acquainted with the elder Kirklin, John W. His industry and attention to detail characterized a brilliant career that started in Minnesota at the Mayo Clinic and then to Birmingham, the University of Alabama. John's remarkable textbook on cardiac surgery must have been an inspiration for this book. The genetic link is indeed obvious, especially in regard to its intellectual peptides.

This book is authored, not edited. A few outstanding collaborators have joined the authors to provide specific information for some chapters. The book, therefore, exhibits a constancy not possible in edited textbooks. From the history of transplantation to the potential of xenografts, each chapter is a full treatise in itself.

Orthotopic transplantation of the heart in the laboratory is nearing the half century mark. Clinical application also is now very much grown up. The ancient adage that any cardiac surgical procedure successful in the dog is less difficult in the human proved to be quite correct. Societal changes resulting from the brain death definition of death opened the door for the extension of transplantation to include the heart and heart lungs. The influence of Sir Peter Medawar, who is truly the father of transplantation, is fully appreciated by the authors. Medawar was not only a brilliant basic scientist/Nobel Laureate but also a great friend and even admirer of the clinician. He in fact trained several fortunate surgeons in his laboratories. Severely challenged physically he remained incredibly productive until his death in 1987. Finally, a word in praise of James Young is very much in order. With Starzl-like industry Jim Young and his surgical colleagues at the Cleveland Clinic have made that institution a destination for heart failure patients from all over the world.

Oscar Wilde once remarked after hearing a particularly erudite and witty statement, "I wish I had said that." To which the author of the epigram replied, "You will, Oscar, you will!" Well, I wish I had written a textbook like this of Kirklin, Young and McGiffin, but there is no way I ever could! You will join me in being delighted that the authors have gone to such great extremes to do so.

Norman E. Shumway, M.D.
Professor of Cardiothoracic Surgery
Stanford University School of Medicine
Stanford, California

Preface

This textbook is designed to provide comprehensive information about all aspects of cardiac transplantation, such that contained in one text is most of the relevant information which forms the basis for clinical and basic research in cardiac transplantation and for the comprehensive care of heart transplant patients prior to transplantation, during the transplant procedure, and for the remainder of their transplant lives. This book is intended for all persons with an interest in the subject of heart transplantation, including the most expert heart transplant physicians and surgeons; basic, clinical, and social scientists interested in this field; physicians, surgeons, and students in training; other medical professionals participating in the care of heart transplant patients; and non-medical persons who wish to use this as a resource for detailed information on all aspects of this complex field.

The three authors of this textbook bring a wealth of personal experience to this effort, with a combined experience in heart transplantation exceeding 50 man-years. Two of the three authors (JKK and DCM) are heart transplant surgeons and one (JBY) is a heart failure specialist and transplant cardiologist. The two heart transplant surgeons (JKK and DCM) have, between them, personally performed over one thousand thoracic transplant operations (heart, heart/lung, and lung transplantation), a vast experience encompassing all aspects of heart transplantation from neonates to adults. These authors also have an extensive personal experience with mechanical circulatory support devices and alternative surgical procedures for advanced heart failure. The other author (JBY) has a huge experience in all medical aspects of heart failure and heart transplantation at two institutions, currently directing medical care for this complex group of patients in one of the highest volume heart transplant centers (Cleveland Clinic) in the United States. All three authors have held or currently hold director positions in cardiac transplantation and/or heart failure programs. As further evidence of their combined expertise, one author (JKK) is currently Editor of the *Journal of Heart and Lung Transplantation* and another (JBY) is the current President of the International Society for Heart and Lung Transplantation. These comments are intended only to indicate the level of experience and expertise brought to bear on this subject by the three authors and the depth of coverage that the reader should expect.

The decision to produce an *authored text* rather than an edited one deserves special comment. It is the authors' belief that most edited textbooks suffer to some degree from variability in commitment, depth of coverage, and overlapping content of individual chapters written by separate contributing authors. In contrast, the three authors, working together to provide a finished product reflective of their combined views, expertise, and experience, wrote the final versions of all chapters in this textbook. We hope this approach provides a comprehensive yet cohesive resource on the current state of heart transplantation. We are indebted to a small group of collaborators who are recognized experts in their field and agreed to provide specific and sometimes comprehensive information about particular aspects of certain chapters. However, the final writing of every chapter was the responsibility of the three authors.

Of necessity, many of the experiences and views of the authors reflect the practices of cardiac transplantation at the authors' home institutions; namely, the Cleveland Clinic and the University of Alabama at Birmingham. However, the entire field of cardiac transplantation has been researched for this text, and we have made intense efforts to include special viewpoints of other institutions through some of our collaborators, through our many interactions with other experts in the field, and through their writings.

Several comments about the organization of the book should be helpful to the reader. The 24 chapters of the textbook encompass all major areas of heart transplantation. The first section, *Background of Heart Transplantation,* includes chapters on history, immunology, and clinical research methodology. The second section includes five chapters relevant to *The Patient Before Transplantation,* including the clinical and physiologic basis of heart failure, medical and nontransplant surgical heart failure therapies, the selection of patients for transplantation, special aspects of pretransplant immunologic evaluation, and mechanical support as a bridge to transplantation. The third section, *The Transplanted Heart,* includes three chapters which cover organ donation and the donor heart, the heart transplant operations, and physiology of the transplanted heart. The fourth section, *Management of the Transplant Patient,* includes four chapters dealing with early postoperative management of the transplant recipient, immunosuppressive drugs and other modalities, detailed information on all aspects of cardiac allograft rejection, and a comprehensive discussion of infectious complications after heart transplantation. The fifth section includes four chapters which focus on *Long-Term Outcome After Heart Transplantation,* including extensive analyses of short- and long-term survival, the vexing problem of chronic rejection (allograft coronary artery disease), numerous other long-term complications, and an extensive discussion of quality of life after heart transplantation. The final section includes five chapters which discuss *Special Situations in Heart Transplantation,* including detailed coverage of pediatric heart transplantation, the experience and results of heart/lung and other transplants combining hearts with other organs, cardiac retransplantation, the basic foundations and current expectations of xenotransplantation, and allocation of resources in the field of heart transplantation.

Each chapter outline inclues the primary (bolded in box form) and secondary headings within the chapter. When necessary for clarity, secondary headings within the text also are subdivided by tertiary (bolded heading in italics) and quaternary (non-bolded, freehanging) headings. Key words are bolded for easy reference. An important additional feature of the book is the liberal use of "boxes" to designate more technical information which may be of interest to some readers but can be omitted without interrupting the natural flow of the text. When a phrase within the text is followed by the notation (see Box), this alerts the reader that this phrase will be the title of more detailed information contained in a subsequent box. The reference list for each chapter is organized alphabetically to facilitate the identification of specific references. All 24 chapters were updated with current references during the final year of the project (2000) prior to the forwarding of chapters to the publisher.

One of the major drawbacks in writing a comprehensive textbook about such a rapidly evolving field as heart transplantation is the risk that major portions of the book are already outdated within a short time after publication. While acknowledging that risk, it is our hope that this book will convey the essential aspects of the state of heart transplantation today, and that it will provide the reader with a sound foundation which will facilitate the acquisition and interpretation of future information about this fascinating and life-extending therapy for advanced heart failure.

James K. Kirklin
James B. Young
David C. McGiffin

Acknowledgments

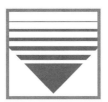

A comprehensive work of this type requires the help of numerous colleagues to "make it happen." Through the six years of research and writing (and several earlier years of dreaming), countless individuals have contributed their time, knowledge, and energy to this process. We are particularly indebted to the *collaborators*, all of whom provided special expertise in specific areas. Without their input, the final product would have been far less than it is. However, two of our collaborators made special ongoing contributions; Dr. Jim George and Dr. David Naftel, our close colleagues in heart transplantation research at UAB. They provided the bulk of information on Chapter 2 (JFG) and Chapter 3 (DCN), spending countless hours interacting with the authors to produce these chapters which are comprehensive with respect to research and immunology, yet designed to be readable and easily digested. A special tribute also goes to Ms. Peggy Holmes, the Publications Manager for JKK, who throughout the years of this project single-handedly provided the clerical support for the final chapter manuscripts, was a colleague and confidant for many difficult decisions during the process, and committed a major portion of her life to this effort.

At the University of Alabama at Birmingham, our medical and surgical colleagues in heart failure and transplantation, including Dr. Robert C. Bourge, Dr. Barry K. Rayburn, Dr. Raymond L. Benza, Dr. Brian A. Foley, Dr. Mark F. Aaron, Dr. William L. Holman, and Dr. George L. Zorn, Jr. provided the intellectual and patient-care environment in the management of patients with advanced heart failure and heart transplantation from which we have gained much of our experience and viewpoints. Dr. Arnold G. Diethelm provided the leadership in overall transplantation and Dr. Albert D. Pacifico the leadership in Cardiothoracic Surgery which fostered a successful heart transplant program. Other colleagues provided valuable assistance in reviewing specific chapters, including Dr. John Stevenson Bynon, Jr., Director of Liver Transplantation, Dr. William Lell, formerly Director of Cardiac Anesthesia, and Dr. Craig Hoesley, Division of Infectious Disease. Our knowledge and techniques of organ procurement were aided in a major way by the individuals providing leadership in the Alabama Organ Bank, including Dr. Arnold G. Diethelm, Dr. Mark H. Deierhoi, Mr. Michael G. Phillips, and Mr. Charles Patrick along with all of their colleagues.

At the Cleveland Clinic Foundation, we are equally indebted to our medical and surgical colleagues. The heart failure and cardiac transplant medicine section includes Drs. Corinne Bott-Silverman, Gary Francis, Donald Hammer, Robert Hobbs, Karen James, Suzanne Lutton, Roger Mills, Gustavo Rincon, Randall Starling, David Taylor, and Mohamed Yamani. Drs. Michael Banbury, Patrick McCarthy, Nicholas Smedira, and Jose Navia provide superb surgical services. The huge volume of patients cared for by this team and the outstanding clinical results are a testimonial to the collective expertise, which contributed immeasurable to the attitudes and therapeutic strategies expressed in this book.

Many of the analyses presented in this textbook were based on two large multi-institutional databases, the Cardiac Transplant Research Database (CTRD) and the Pediatric Heart Transplant Study (PHTS), for which UAB was the data analysis center. We are greatly indebted to the member institutions of both databases for their generous participation, long hours of data collection, and their profound intellectual contributions to the many presentations and publications based on these analyses. In the CTRD, we acknowledge the generous participation of the following institutions: Abbott Northwestern Hospital, Albuquerque Presbyterian Hospital, Hahnemann University Hospital, Bowman Gray School of Medicine, Brigham and Women's Hospital, Cleveland Clinic Foundation, Columbia Presbyterian, Downstate Heart Transplant Center, Emory University, University of Florida, Shands Hospital, Henry Ford Hospital, Hershey Medical Center, Indiana University Hospital, Johns Hopkins Hospital, Loyola University Medical Center, St. Luke's Hospital, Medical College of Virginia, Massachusetts General Hospital, Methodist Hospital of Indiana, St. Mary's Hospital, Mayo Clinic, Northwestern University, Ochsner Clinic Transplant Program, Ohio State University, Cardiology, Rush Presbyterian-St. Luke's Medical Center, Medical University of South Carolina, Charleston, Sharp Memorial, St. Joseph's Hospital, St. Luke's Episcopal Hospital, Sentara Norfolk Hospital, St. Louis University, Tampa General Hospital, Baylor College of Medicine/The Methodist Hospital, Temple University School of Medicine, Tulane University, University of Alabama at Birmingham, University Hospitals of Cleveland, University of California, LA, University of Cincinnati Medical Center, University of Louisville, Jewish Hospital, University of Iowa, University of Michigan Medical Center, University of Minnesota, University of Utah Health Sciences Center, University of Texas SW Medical Center, University of Washington Medical Center, Hunter Holmes McGuire VA Medical Center, Vanderbilt University, Washington University Medical Center, and Yale University School of Medicine. In the PHTS, we acknowledge the generous participation of the following institutions: Arkansas Children's Hospital, Albuquerque Presbyterian Hospital, Cleveland Clinic Foundation, Children's Hospital Medical Center, Cardinal Glennon Children's Hospital, Children's Hospital of Michigan, Children's Hospital of Pittsburgh, Children's Memorial Hospital, University of Texas SW Medical School/Children's Medical Center, Children's National Medical Center, Children's Hospital of Philadelphia, Columbia University–Babies Hospital, University of Florida/ Shands Hospital. The Hospital for Sick Children, Indiana University Medical Center, Loma Linda University Medical Center, Loyola University Medical Center, Mayo Clinic, Medical College of Virginia, Minneapolis Heart Institute, Mount Sinai Medical Center, Oregon Health Sciences University, Ohio

State University Medical Center, Primary Childrens' Medical Center, Rainbow Babies and Children's Hospital, Rush Children's Heart Center, St. Louis Children's Hospital, St. Francis Medical Center, Stanford University Medical Center, Texas Children's Hospital, University of Alabama at Birmingham, University of California at Los Angeles, University of Colorado/The Children's Hospital-Denver, University of Michigan Transplant, University of South Florida/All Children's Hospital, Vanderbilt University Medical Center, Children's Hospital of the King's Children/Eastern Virginia Medical School, Children's Hospital, and Engleston Children's Hospital.

Most of the surgical illustrations were provided by Sam and Amy Collins, who spent many hours working with the authors to create accurate depictions of the transplant operations.

A book of this size requires tremendous support in the generation of text, tables, and graphics. At UAB this invaluable service was provided by Ms. Jane Owenby, Ms. Apryl Crosswy, Ms. Mary Lynn Clark, Mr. Robert Brown, and Mr. Todd Weiss; and at Cleveland Clinic by Ms. Lisa Paciorek.

Throughout this process, we had the incredibly good fortune to deal with two outstanding publishing companies, and their editors, namely, Allan Ross at Churchill Livingstone and Richard Lampert at W. B. Saunders. Their encouragement, sage advice, and at times intense stimulation was pivotal in moving the project forward.

It is almost unbelievable to calculate the literally thousands of man-hours put in by the authors on this project. With this time commitment, in the midst of busy professional careers in cardiac surgery, heart failure, and transplantation, the toll on the authors' families was excessive. Yet, they remained loving, tolerant, and for the most part cheerful supporters of this undertaking, although at times renamed the book with certain expletives. We would, therefore, like to lovingly acknowledge the support of our spouses, Terry Kirklin, Claire Young, Alison McGiffin, and George Holmes (husband of Peggy Holmes); and our children, Kimberly and Adam Kirklin, Brad Vernon, Ben and Peter McGiffin, and Joseph, James, Rebecca, and Christine Young.

A special tribute must also be paid to Dr. John W. Kirklin, who provided continuous moral support to the project, and whose legendary textbook, *Cardiac Surgery*, was the inspiration for this effort.

Finally, with deep humility, we would like to acknowledge the unselfish and continuous efforts of the United Network of Organ Sharing in their efforts to make transplantation possible, and to the International Society for Heart and Lung Transplantation, whose commitment to scientific advancements in thoracic transplantation provided the forum for much of the information contained in this text.

James K. Kirklin
James B. Young
David C. McGiffin

Contents

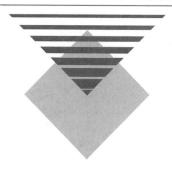

Background of
Heart Transplantation

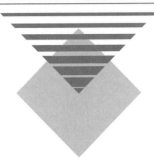

CHAPTER ONE

History of Cardiac Transplantation

with the collaboration of
JAMES F. GEORGE, Ph.D.

Development of Surgical Techniques for Heart and
Heart–Lung Transplantation
Development of the Immunologic Basis of
Transplantation
Development of Clinical Cardiac and Cardiopulmonary
Transplantation
Evolution of a System for Organ Allocation and
Distribution and a Mechanism for Reporting the Results
of Transplantation

The evolution of scientific advancements that paved the way for clinical cardiac transplantation spans the era of the twentieth century. For the successful widespread application of clinical heart transplantation, four areas of scientific and logistic development were required: (1) development of surgical techniques and organ preservation for cardiac transplantation, (2) elucidation of the immunologic basis of transplantation, (3) demonstration that clinical cardiac transplantation is feasible, and (4) development of a system for the identification and allocation of organs for transplantation.

The history of cardiac transplantation reveals a medical and public fascination with the prospect of transplanting the heart from one dead human to another living but dying human. The development of appropriate techniques allowed an initial foray into cardiac transplantation before there was adequate development of critical knowledge in other areas. The transformation of cardiac transplantation into an effective therapy for end-stage heart disease would await the evolution of appropriate knowledge.

It is important to remember that heart transplantation did not develop in a clinical vacuum. Rather, this operation followed developments in kidney transplantation and paralleled advances in other solid organ transplantation. Particularly important was development of new immunosuppressive strategies based on greater insight

gathered from clinically focused basic research in the field of immunology. In addition to perfecting cardiac transplant operative techniques, the development of satisfactory methods of organ preservation, first with hypothermia and subsequently with special infusates, set the stage for widespread organ sharing and allocation in organ transplantation. Finally, the ability to perform clinical histocompatibility matching drove success rates for kidney transplantation higher and allowed clinicians to better understand the nuances of allograft rejection.

DEVELOPMENT OF SURGICAL TECHNIQUES FOR HEART AND HEART–LUNG TRANSPLANTATION

Although earlier isolated experiments made reference to transplantation of the heart, organized experimental studies in heart transplantation began with the work of Carrel and Guthrie at the beginning of the twentieth century (Table 1–1).

Alexis Carrel (see Box) was the dominant early pioneer in the development of surgical techniques of experimental transplantation. He reported the first experimental heterotopic heart transplant in a dog model in 1905.[15] Carrel's pioneering experiments in vascular surgery and organ transplantation culminated in his being awarded the Nobel Prize in Physiology and Medicine in 1912 (Fig. 1–1).

Charles Claude Guthrie (see Box) (Fig. 1–2), working in collaboration with Alexis Carrel and later independently, developed and refined surgical techniques for transplantation of the heart, heart and lungs, and other organs.[32]

Frank C. Mann and **James T. Priestly,** at the Mayo Clinic, extended the work of Carrel to further investigate mammalian kidney and heart transplantation. In 1933, using a canine model, the authors observed survival of the heterotopically transplanted heart for up to 8 days.[49] Although not identifying it as such, the authors pro-

TABLE 1-1	Landmark Events in the Evolution of Cardiac Transplantation
1905	Carrel and Guthrie transplant hearts and other organs into dogs
1908	Metchnikoff relates inflammation to immunity
1912	Shone sets forth the concepts of transplantation immunology
1933	Mann and Priestly suggest that biologic events (ultimately understood as allograft rejection) limit canine cardiac heterotopic transplant experimentation
1940–1950s	Demikhov experiments with heart and heart–lung transplant models in Russia
1944	Medawar suggests that allograft rejection is an immunologic process
1945	Owen reports that cell chimeras in cattle display tolerance
1951	Marcus, Wong, and Luisada speculate on therapeutic potential of heart transplantation
1953	Downie reproducibly demonstrates canine heterotopic heart transplant success
1957	Webb uses hypothermic cardiac preservation for heart transplant experiments
1958	Goldberg, Berman, and Akman perform first orthotopic canine heart transplant using cardiopulmonary bypass support
1959	Cass and Brock refine experimental orthotopic surgical technique
1960s	Lower and Shumway report rejection to be the main challenge in canine heart transplant and suggest that long-term survival could be achieved with immunosuppression
1962	Reemstma reports prolonged survival after canine orthotopic heart transplantation
1964	Hardy performs first human xenograft (chimpanzee) heart transplant
1965	Kondo and Kantrowitz suggest newborn puppies are immunologically privileged
1967	Barnard performs first human-to-human heart transplant
1968–1971	100 to 200 heart transplants performed worldwide with limited success; moratorium established
1974	Caves develops technique of graft surveillance with endomyocardial biopsy
1980	Cyclosporine is introduced into clinical transplant arena with center proliferation

vided insight into the phenomenon of unmodified rejection, noting that the explanted hearts were infiltrated with lymphocytes, mononuclear cells, and neutrophils, often with associated edema. They speculated correctly that "failure of the homotransplanted heart to survive is not due to the technique of transplantation but to some biologic factor which is probably identical to that which prevents survival of homotransplanted tissues and organs."[49]

Vladimir P. Demikhov, working in Russia between the 1940s and early 1960s, performed a large number of ingenious surgical experiments in transplantation, including multiple technical variations of heterotopic heart transplantation (with maximum canine survival of 32 days), successful combined heart–lung transplantation, studies on methods of maintaining heart and lung function during procurement and implantation, and studies of artificial circulatory support. He may have been the first to implant an auxiliary heart within the thorax and to replace the heart. His published book

on his transplantation experiments was translated into English in 1962.[23]

Emanuel Marcus, along with **Wong** and **Luisada** at the Chicago Medical School, refined the techniques of experimental heterotopic cardiac transplantation in the dog and speculated, as had Mann and Priestly, about the immunobiologic barriers to clinical application of heart transplantation for the treatment of end-stage heart disease (1951–1953).[50, 51]

W. B. Neptune and colleagues at Hahneman Medical college transplanted the heart and lungs from one animal to another using hypothermia (1953).[54]

H. G. Downie at the Ontario Veterinary College demonstrated reproducible successful canine heterotopic transplantation with average graft survival of 129 hours (1953).[25]

Watts R. Webb and colleagues at the University of Mississippi demonstrated that heterotopically transplanted canine hearts could function after preservation for 6 to 8 hours if stored at 4°C in nutrient solution after flushing blood elements (1957).[73] They also had several publications between 1957 and 1961[72, 74] on combined heart–lung transplantation, in which they emphasized the problem of posttransplant pulmonary insufficiency.

Mauricio Goldberg, along with **Berman** and **Akman** at the University of Maryland, developed an experimental technique for canine orthotopic transplantation using a cuff of recipient left atrium (1958).[27]

Gumersindo Blanco and colleagues from the University of Puerto Rico reported a study on heart–lung transplantation in which two of eight animals had return of normal respirations after discontinuation of cardiopulmonary bypass (CPB) (1958).[12]

M. H. Cass and **Sir Russell Brock,** in London, reported a technique of orthotopic cardiac transplantation combining pulmonary venous and caval anastomoses into two atrial anastomoses (1959).[17]

Keith Reemstma and colleagues at Tulane University demonstrated prolonged survival after canine orthotopic transplantation (1962)[57, 59] and the ability of a heterotopically transplanted heart to temporarily support the circulation (1966).[52]

Yoshio Kondo, Adrian Kantrowitz, and colleagues at Downstate Medical Center in Brooklyn, New York, studied extended preservation up to 24 hours with immature canine hearts (1965), and demonstrated prolonged survival (maximum >112 days) after heart transplantation in puppies without immunosuppressive therapy.[41] These studies suggested the potential for immunologic "privilege" in the newborn, and encouraged Kantrowitz to later attempt infant cardiac transplantation.

Norman Shumway (see Box) (Fig. 1–3) and **Richard Lower,** working at Stanford University, established a focused cardiac transplantation research program in the 1960s aimed at bringing cardiac transplantation to clinical fruition. Richard Lower subsequently became Chief of Cardiac Surgery at the Medical College of Virginia and developed a highly successful cardiac transplant program. In heart–lung transplantation, Lower and Shumway had canine survivors for up to 4 days with spontaneous respiration, and the Stanford group em-

Alexis Carrel

Alexis Carrel provided the early experimental ground work for vascular surgery and cardiac transplantation. During his internship in Lyon, France, in 1894, the President of the French Republic, Sadi Carnot, was assassinated with a fatal knife wound that severed the portal vein, and expert surgeons were not able to control the bleeding. Carrel hypothesized that surgical techniques to repair or reattach blood vessels could be lifesaving in such situations.

He later dropped out of clinical medicine (1901) to pursue a career in experimental vascular surgery.[60] Between 1904 and 1906, Carrel collaborated with Charles C. Guthrie at the University of Chicago to produce a number of classic experimental surgical studies involving reimplantation or transplantation of arteries, veins, kidneys, thyroid glands, transplantation of a puppy's heart into the neck of an adult dog, and transplantation of the heart and both lungs.[15, 16] In a 1907 publication reviewing a series of vascular experiments performed in collaboration with Guthrie,[15] Carrel described the technique of heart transplantation in a dog, noting that following transplantation of the heart into the neck of a larger dog, "strong fibrillar contractions soon occurred. Afterward contractions of the auricles appeared, and, about an hour after the operation, effective contractions of the ventricles began. The transplanted heart beat at the rate of 88 per minute, while the rate of the normal heart was 100 per minute."

Thus, Carrel had demonstrated that not only transplantation of the heart was technically feasible, but also that complete removal and reimplantation of the heart could result in organized spontaneous cardiac contractions.[15, 29]

In 1912, Carrel was awarded the Nobel Prize in Physiology and Medicine, honoring his contributions in experimental studies in vascular surgery and transplantation. His interests later expanded to problems of organ preservation and perfusion techniques, and he collaborated with aviator Charles Lindbergh on projects of organ perfusion and preservation at Rockefeller University in the 1930s.[60]

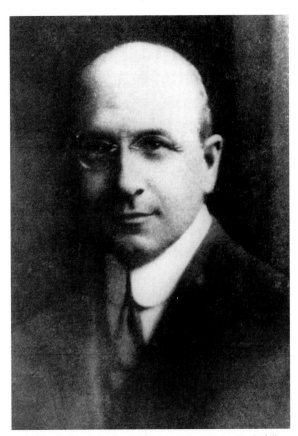

FIGURE **1–1.** Alexis Carrel (1872–1944), Associate, Rockefeller Institute. (From Shumacker HB Jr: The Evolution of Cardiac Surgery. Bloomington: Indiana University Press, 1992, with permission.)

phasized the importance of phrenic nerve preservation in 1961.[66]

Aldo Castaneda and colleagues at the University of Minnesota reported long-term survival after autotransplantation of the heart and both lungs in baboons.[18, 19]

Bruce Reitz and co-workers at Stanford developed an extensive primate experience in heart–lung transplantation and autotransplantation[61] in preparation for the first successful human heart–lung transplant.

DEVELOPMENT OF THE IMMUNOLOGIC BASIS OF TRANSPLANTATION

Modern immunologic concepts relating to transplantation emerged at the beginning of the twentieth century with the evolution of immunologic concepts of host de-

fense. It is remarkable to note the parallel historical development of the immunologic concepts and the surgical techniques necessary for transplantation.

Elie Metchnikoff (see Box), a Russian embryologist and zoologist, is generally credited with the notion of **immunity.** He recognized the role of phagocytic cells in inflammation and host defense. He was awarded the Nobel Prize in Medicine for this work in 1908.[21]

Karl Landsteiner began a series of experiments in 1901 that demonstrated that humans could be grouped according to the tendency of their sera to agglutinate erythrocytes from other individuals.[10, 42] This work ultimately led to the ABO system of blood typing. This was one of the first schemes based on the assumption that the ability to accept tissue or cells from another individual (i.e., compatibility) was dependent on measurable genetic factors, thereby opening the door to a rational, scientific approach to histocompatibility.

George Shone summarized prevailing views about the basic phenomena of transplantation in 1912 in his book entitled *Heteroplastic and Homoplastic Transplantation*.[63, 68] The basic rules of "transplantation immunity," as stated by Shone were:

1) Transplantation into a foreign species (heteroplastic = xenogeneic; xenogeneic means "derived or obtained from an organism of a different species") invariably fails.

Charles Claude Guthrie

Charles Claude Guthrie was an instructor in physiology at the University of Chicago when Alexis Carrel came to Chicago in 1905. Dr. G. N. Stewart, Chairman of the Department of Physiology, introduced Carrel to Guthrie and suggested the two work together. According to a letter written by Guthrie, they "agreed to full mutual collaboration in all phases of the work, including publications."[32] The two scientists actually only worked together for two brief periods: June to late August 1905, and January to late March 1906. It was a time of great productivity, yielding 21 joint publications. Carrel left Chicago in 1906 to take a position at the Rockefeller Institute, but the two men continued an active correspondence until about 1908. At about the same time, Guthrie was named Head of the Department of Physiology and Pharmacology at Washington University in St. Louis. Guthrie's interest and work in transplantation continued, and he performed many successful experimental transplants of the heart, combined heart and lungs, kidneys, thyroid, ovaries, and entire limbs.[32] He recorded his experimental observations in a book entitled *Blood Vessel Surgery and Its Applications*, published in 1912.[31] Ironically, this was the same year Carrel was awarded the Nobel Prize.

From a collection of letters between Carrel and Guthrie, analyzed by Samuel Harbison, it appears likely that Carrel failed to give proper acknowledgment of Guthrie's critical contributions to Carrel's success in the early years of experimental surgery and transplantation. For example, it was Guthrie who suggested to Carrel the importance of including all three vessel wall layers in the vascular anastomosis.[32] Furthermore, it appears from their mutual correspondence that Guthrie enjoyed greater initial success with his transplant experiments than did Carrel. In one instance, Guthrie wrote to Carrel of his objections and subsequently published an article in *Science*[30] about Carrel's failure to give Guthrie proper credit in a presentation Carrel gave to Johns Hopkins Medical Society in 1906.[14]

In retrospect, it appears to be an injustice that no credit was given to Guthrie when Carrel was awarded the Nobel Prize in 1912.

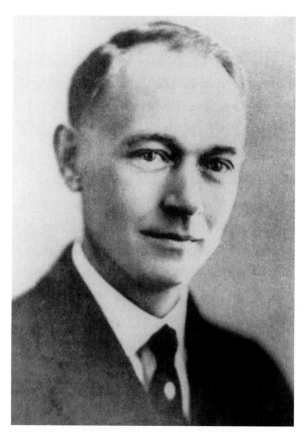

FIGURE 1–2. Charles Claude Guthrie (1880–1958), Professor of Pharmacology and Physiology, University of Pittsburgh. (From Shumacker HB Jr: The Evolution of Cardiac Surgery. Bloomington: Indiana University Press, 1992, with permission.)

define the loci that apparently controlled tumor rejection or histocompatibility.[68] In 1924, Little founded the Jackson Memorial Laboratory at Bar Harbor, Maine, devoted to cancer research through studies of genetically homogeneous animals. At the Jackson Laboratories, George Snell discovered a genetic locus related to the phenomenon of tumor rejection, the H-2 locus, which we now know as the major histocompatibility locus in the mouse.[69]

In 1924, **Emile Holman** characterized the immune response as having the features of specificity and exhibiting memory.[37] Such responses are not usually instantaneous, are directed only toward the particular antigen to which an individual is exposed; and upon second exposure to the antigen, responses are quicker, stronger, and longer lasting. The relevance of these observation to the potential transplantation of tissues and organs was not truly appreciated for another 20 years.

K. Landsteiner and **W. M. Chase** demonstrated in 1942 that delayed hypersensitivity could be transferred to another animal using intact cells from a sensitized animal.[43]

F. MacFarlane Burnet and **F. Fenner** in the late 1940s proposed the clonal selection theory (a theoretical concept of antibody formation by a cell and/or its genetically identical descendent) to explain the phenomenon of the "amnestic" antibody response in which subse-

2) Transplantation into unrelated members of the same species (homoplastic = allogeneic; allogeneic means "genetically different but belonging to or obtained from the same species") usually fails.
3) Autografts (grafts from and to the same individual of any species) almost invariably succeed.
4) There is a primary take and delayed rejection of the first graft in the allogeneic recipient.
5) There is an accelerated rejection of a second graft in a recipient that had previously rejected a graft from the same donor.
6) The closer the "blood relationship" between donor and recipient, the more likely the graft success.

Geneticists **Clarence C. Little** and **George Snell** developed inbred strains of mice that could be used to

Norman Shumway

Norman Shumway is generally considered the father of clinical cardiac transplantation. After completing medical school at Vanderbilt University and surgical training at the University of Minnesota, he became the Chairman of the Department of Cardiac Surgery at Stanford. During the 1960s, Shumway coalesced the experimental efforts of his predecessors and developed a research team that paved the way for clinical cardiac transplantation. They studied the effects of selective hypothermia in cardiac preservation[48, 64, 65] and reported a simplified technique of orthotopic cardiac transplantation that would later become the standard clinical method.[43] Using immunosuppression to prolong graft survival, Lower, Dong, and Shumway demonstrated the utility of electrocardiographic monitoring as a guide to antirejection therapy.[46, 48] In 1965, Shumway wrote these prophetic comments: "In the laboratory, the beating heart of the donor animal is removed and preserved while the beating heart of the host is excised and discarded. For successful homotransplantation in man, it would be necessary legally to deprive of life both the donor, a hopeless brain injury for example, and the host whose own heart has not yet stopped beating. Considerable social, moral, and legal reformation must preceed any serious clinical application of a challenging laboratory experiment. The use of heterologous donors does not importantly diminish the problem. Evolution of a perfect subhuman species of organ donors appears remote. Perhaps the cardiac surgeon should pause while society becomes accustomed to resurrection of the mythological chimera."[66] In preparation for clinical cardiac transplantation, Shumway's team demonstrated survival for 230 days following canine transplantation.[45, 46]

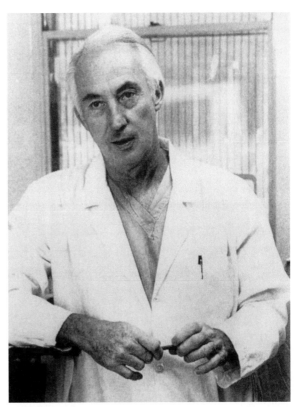

FIGURE 1-3. Norman Edward Shumway (1923–), Professor of Surgery, Stanford University (From Shumacker HB Jr: The Evolution of Cardiac Surgery. Bloomington: Indiana University Press, 1992, with permission.)

quent exposure to an antigen resulted in a greater antibody response.[13]

Ray D. Owen reported in 1945 that dizygotic (genetically nonidentical) twin cattle that shared blood circulation in utero were red cell chimeras (containing cells from the other twin)[56] and therefore each was tolerant to antigens from the other.

During World War II, **Peter Medawar** (see Box) began a series of observations with **T. Gibson** which generated their hypothesis in 1943 that graft rejection was mediated by "active immunization."[26] Medawar elucidated the characteristics of first-set and second-set rejection using rabbit skin grafts,[53] noting the important role of the lymphocyte. In 1960, Medawar and Burnet received the Nobel Prize in Medicine for the discovery of acquired immunologic tolerance.

Thus, the first half of the twentieth century was marked by a large conceptual shift in the perceptions of the major mechanisms of immunity (the cellular mechanisms) as they relate to transplant rejection. During the second half of the twentieth century, there was an explosion of information regarding the mechanisms of cellular immunity that result in induction of the immune response and activation of the antigraft effector response. Furthermore, this knowledge allowed development of potent and effective, though imperfect, immunosuppressants which made successful solid organ transplantation possible.

DEVELOPMENT OF CLINICAL CARDIAC AND CARDIOPULMONARY TRANSPLANTATION

In 1964, **James Hardy** and colleagues performed the first heart transplant into a human, using a chimpanzee heart.[33, 35] Hardy's team had pursued laboratory investigations in cardiac transplantation for the previous 8 years.[34, 36, 40, 44, 73] They had planned to use a human donor, but the selected recipient (a 68-year-old man in shock from end-stage ischemic cardiomyopathy with respiratory failure, obtundation, and a freshly amputated gangrenous leg) was too close to death to await a donor. Thus, Hardy and his team elected to use a chimpanzee donor (as a xenotransplant, a graft from an individual of a different species than the recipient), based on studies of chimpanzee renal transplants in humans.[35] The xenotransplanted heart contracted well on cardiopulmonary bypass but was apparently too small to support the circulation unassisted. The patient died approximately 1½ hours after discontinuation of cardiopulmonary bypass.

Elie Metchnikoff

Elie Metchnikoff (1845–1916) was at the center of the debate concerning cellular versus humoral (antibody-mediated) immunity. Metchnikoff's hypothesis about cellular immunity stemmed from the observations he made while conducting research in Messina using starfish larvae that were transparent, thus allowing him to observe events that occurred internally. In his description of the experiment in his Nobel Lecture, he was to say, "Sharp splinters were introduced into the bodies of Bipinnaria and the next day I could see a mass of moving cells surrounding the foreign bodies to form a thick layer. The analogy between this phenomenon and what happens when a human has a splinter that causes inflammation and suppuration is extraordinary."[1] The concept that this mechanism could be generally applied to host defense in high organisms was quickly attacked,[71] primarily because many pathologists at the time viewed inflammation as a deleterious response rather than a beneficial one.[67] Thus, there came to be two schools of thought on the cellular and humoral basis of immunity. This debate raged for the next 30 years and ultimately resulted in the lack of acceptance of Metchnikoff's assertions despite the fact that Metchnikoff and his group produced a large number of papers showing that antibody alone could not account for all forms of an apparent immune response. Although he received the Nobel Prize for his work in 1908, the humoral view of immunity remained the predominant paradigm well into the twentieth century. The concept of cellular immunity (by which it is meant that the "immune response" is mediated by cells, with or without noncellular elements) was not revived in any significant way until the 1940s. As a result, immunologists did not become involved in transplantation research until the renaissance of transplantation that began with Peter Medawar's experiments during World War II (see below).

Peter Medawar

Peter Medawar (1915–1987) was trained in pathology and zoology in Oxford. His insightful observations and elegant experiments in transplant immunology provided the foundations for the modern idea that transplant rejection is a product of the immune response, and that immunologic tolerance could be induced in situations in which a cellular immune response usually developed. His critical observations began with the study of burn patients during World War II. There were very few tools available for the treatment of such patients, so Peter Medawar began careful observations of the results of treatments for burns as they were currently practiced. Medawar and his colleagues noted the fate of skin grafts placed on a woman who had been severely burned by an incendiary device. The burns encompassed a large area, so there was a need to provide a covering over the burns that would at least provide temporary protection. This was done using "pinch grafts" in which a pinch of skin on an undamaged portion of the burn victim's body would be pinched, and the top of the pinch would be cut off and placed on the burn. In this case the burns were so extensive that they were unable to obtain a sufficient number of pinch grafts, so they supplemented them with pinch grafts from her brother. For clinical reasons, they obtained a second set of grafts from her brother about 2 weeks later. They carefully observed the fate of the grafts from two different sources and found that the fate and timing of rejection of the grafts were different. The autologous grafts continued to grow and eventually formed a layer of tissue that covered the area of the burn near the graft, but the grafts from the brother were rejected more quickly. Medawar and Gibson concluded that the graft rejection was mediated by "active immunization."[26] Medawar was able to define the characteristics of this type of antigraft response using rabbits in which he carefully characterized the timing, specificity, and effect of dose (graft size) on graft rejection upon second exposure to the antigen.[53] Medawar speculated that "the inflammation that accompanied the homograft reaction was probably of the anaphylactic type and that the reaction was atypical in that the lymphocyte played a prominent role."[53] (It must be remembered that, at the time the previous quote was written, no one had yet identified the lymphocyte as an important cell in this process.)

About 10 years after he published the landmark paper describing the characteristics of graft rejection, he published a critically important paper entitled "Actively Acquired Tolerance of Foreign Cells,"[11] which described a means by which an individual (in this case, a mouse) could be rendered tolerant to histoincompatible grafts. He summarized the experiments in the introduction to the paper in which he writes, "If, for example, a foetal mouse of one inbred strain (say, CBA) is inoculated in utero with a suspension of living cells from an adult mouse of another strain (say, A), then, when it grows up, the CBA mouse will be found to be partly or completely tolerant of skin grafts transplanted from any mouse belonging to the same strain as the original donor."

This phenomenon is the exact inverse of "actively acquired immunity," and he proposed to describe it as "actively acquired tolerance." By 1953, Medawar had developed a method by which a mouse could be rendered "tolerant" (tolerance is a situation in which an immune response fails to develop, either then or in the future, in spite of the presence of a stimulating antigen, as was the case with Owen's cattle) to histoincompatible grafts[11] (the grafts were still histoincompatible, but there was no response to them). In essence, he accomplished this by inducing in mice a repetition of what Owen had described in cattle. Medawar apparently appreciated many of the details in these phenomena, but he was in this regard unique to the field of transplantation at the time. Many of the details have been accepted as the basis for "tolerance" and for "self-tolerance." The immune response is a process in which the body sets in motion a specific response (i.e., localized to that antigen) by (1) producing antibodies and/or (2) an infiltration of the area by leukocytes.

Christiaan Barnard

Christiaan Barnard completed his surgical and postgraduate training at the University of Minnesota under Wangensteen and Varco. Barnard was mesmerized by the possibility of heart transplantation. After returning to Cape Town, South Africa, he took a 3-month sabbatical in 1966 to study with Dr. David Hume and Richard Lower at the Medical College of Virginia, learning about renal transplantation in preparation for his vision of human heart transplantation.[8] When he returned to Cape Town, he assembled a nucleus of specialists in tissue compatibility, bacteriology, biochemical support, cardiology, and nursing care for human heart transplantation. He developed a protocol in which none of the doctors involved in the transplant could make a determination of brain death in a potential donor. He developed an experience in renal transplantation, and performed 48 experimental heart transplants in dogs prior to the first human heart transplant experiment. In the first week of November 1967, Louis Washkansky was selected to be the first transplant recipient. Washkansky was a 53-year-old ex-boxer with great psychological strength who was dying from end-stage ischemic cardiomyopathy following multiple heart attacks. He had developed severe biventricular failure with refractory peripheral edema, hepatic insufficiency, renal insufficiency, and diabetes. He waited 1 month before receiving his heart transplant. On December 3, a donor was identified. A young woman named Denise Darvall and her mother had been hit by an oncoming speeding car while crossing a busy street. The mother was instantly killed and her daughter suffered irreversible brain injury. Denise was determined to be brain dead hours later, and the transplant operation was planned. As soon as she was pronounced dead and her heart stopped, cardiopulmonary bypass was rapidly initiated and hypothermia induced. The transplant was performed with a donor ischemic time of approximately 30 minutes.

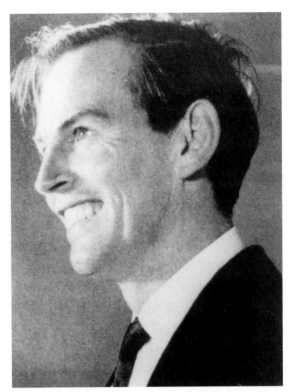

FIGURE **1-4.** Christiaan Barnard (1922–2001), Professor of Cardiac and Thoracic Surgery, University of Cape Town. (From Shumacker HB Jr: The Evolution of Cardiac Surgery. Bloomington: Indiana University Press, 1992, with permission.)

The first human-to-human heart transplant (allograft) was performed in Cape Town, South Africa, by **Christiaan Barnard** (see Box) on December 3, 1967[4] (Fig. 1–4). The recipient was Louis Washkansky, a 53-year-old patient with end-stage ischemic cadiomyopathy.

The immunosuppression protocol included local irradiation to the transplanted heart, hydrocortisone, azathioprine, and prednisone. Actinomycin C for antirejection prophylaxis was administered for 3 days.[5] Unfortunately, after an apparently satisfactory early recovery, he developed pneumonia on the 12th day and succumbed to *Pseudomonas* and *Klebsiella* pneumonia 18 days after his transplant. Following Barnard's historic first human-to-human heart transplant, the event received massive media attention, probably more publicity than any single medical event in this century (Fig. 1–5).

Three days after the Cape Town operation, **Adrian Kantrowitz** performed the second human heart transplant (on December 6, 1967) in Brooklyn.[38] The recipient was an 18-day-old infant with Ebstein's malformation, refractory congestive heart failure, and previous aortopulmonary shunt for severe cyanosis. The patient received the heart of an anencephalic infant, but died 5 hours later of cardiac failure and refractory acidosis.

On January 2, 1968, Barnard performed the third human heart transplant on Dr. Philip Blaiberg, a 46-year-old dental surgeon with refractory congestive heart failure, severe coronary artery disease, and a large left ventricular aneurysm. He became the first long-term survivor, living for 18 months following his heart transplant procedure.

Norman Shumway performed the fourth heart transplant 4 days later on January 6, 1968, and this patient died 2 weeks later. After this, other heart transplants followed rapidly in a number of institutions. By the end of 1968, cardiac transplantation had been performed in 102 patients in 50 different institutions in 17 countries. The results were generally miserable, with 60% mortality by the eighth postoperative day and a mean survival of only 29 days.[22]

By 1970, the medical community and the general public had become disenchanted with the premature experiment of human cardiac transplantation. Thus, during the 1970s, only a few institutions continued clinical cardiac transplantation, the major thrust being concentrated at Stanford University under the direction of Dr. Shumway.[70] During that decade, the 1-year survival after transplantation at Stanford gradually increased from 22% to 65%.[28]

A technique for serial sampling of the myocardium for rejection surveillance through the use of a bioptome

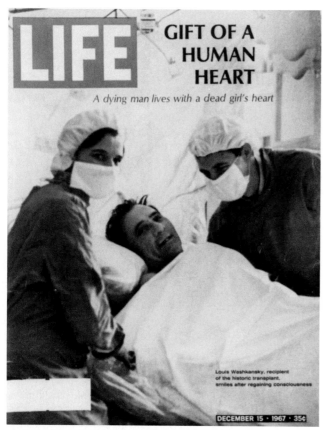

LIFE

GIFT OF A HUMAN HEART

A dying man lives with a dead girl's heart

Louis Washkansky, recipient of the historic transplant, smiles after regaining consciousness

DECEMBER 15 · 1967 · 35¢

FIGURE **1–5.** The world's first human-to-human heart transplant, featured as the cover story in *Life Magazine* on December 15, 1967. (From TimePix. New York: Time Inc., with permission.)

was developed by **Philip Caves** (an English surgeon working at Stanford),[20] and **Margaret Billingham** (at Stanford) described a histologic system for grading cardiac allograft rejection.

With the introduction of **cyclosporine immunotherapy** in the early 1980s, the success of cardiac transplantation improved, resulting in a rapid proliferation of cardiac transplant activities and programs.

Heterotopic heart transplantation (transplantation of the heart into an abnormal position while leaving the native heart intact) was first performed by Barnard and colleagues in the early 1970s, and in 1981 they reported their experience with 30 such operations with 1-year survival just over 60%.[6, 7]

After Hardy's early unsuccessful attempt at **xenotransplantation** in 1964, there were scattered unsuccessful xenotransplant attempts after Barnard's first human-to-human transplant in 1967. Cooley, for example, reported a fatal heart transplant early in his experience with a sheep as the donor.[66]

Perhaps the most notable adventure into xenotransplantation was the "Baby Fae" experiment in which **Leonard Bailey** and colleagues at Loma Linda transplanted a baboon heart into a newborn infant with hypoplastic left heart syndrome on October 26, 1984. The baby survived 20 days, and death was possibly related to an ABO-mismatch.[2, 3] This single experience renewed intense scientific interest in the possibility of xenotransplantation, but also aroused intense public debate over

the issue of primate donors for human transplantation. Ironically, the Baby Fae experience did not lead to another cardiac xenotransplant procedure in the coming decade, but it did highlight the emergence of neonatal heart transplantation as an option for end-stage neonatal heart disease. Over the following decade, the Loma Linda group would generate a landmark experience with superb survival after infant cardiac transplantation.

The first **combined heart–lung transplant** procedure was performed by **Denton Cooley** on September 15, 1969, in a 2-month-old infant who survived only 14 hours. **C. Walton Lillehei** performed the same procedure in an adult patient in New York 3 months later, and that patient survived 8 days. After a sustained experimental investigation of heart–lung transplantation, **Bruce Reitz** and colleagues at Stanford performed the first successful combined heart–lung transplantation in 1981. Long-term survival was possible with the availability of cyclosporine, and the first successful series of patients undergoing heart–lung transplantation was published by Reitz and colleagues the following year.[62]

EVOLUTION OF A SYSTEM FOR ORGAN ALLOCATION AND DISTRIBUTION AND A MECHANISM FOR REPORTING THE RESULTS OF TRANSPLANTATION

The identification of morally and ethically suitable sources of nonliving donor organs was critical to the evolution of heart transplantation. The definiton and determination of death (after which organ donation would be ethically acceptable) were subjects of considerable debate during the initial foray into transplantation (Table 1–2). During the early experience with kidney

TABLE 1–2	**Evolution of the Concept of Brain Death**
1954	Kidney transplant with identical twin as donor
1962	Kidney for transplant procured after failed open heart surgery when patient still on cardiopulmonary bypass support
1964	"Heart-beating" kidney donor used at Karolinska Institute
1964	Hardy performs xenograft (chimpanzee) human heart transplant because of inability to procure satisfactory human donor heart
1965	Concept of "cerebral death" formulated by Frykholm in Sweden
1967	Starzl performs liver transplants using donors satisfying "neurologic death" concept (but organs removed after withdrawal of care leads to cessation of heart beat)
1967	Barnard performs first heart transplant using donor satisfying "brain death" criteria (but organ removed after withdrawal of care leads to cessation of heart beat)
1967	Kantrowitz transplants heart of anencephalic infant into 18-day-old neonate dying of congenital heart disease
1968	Wada indicted for murder in Japan after heart transplant using "brain dead" donor
1968	"Harvard Criteria" for brain death developed
1980s	President's Commission develops "Guidelines for Determination of Brain Death" with dissemination of Uniform Death Act in the United States

transplantation, there were attempts at using heart-beating organ donors who were "about to die" in the operating room because the patient could not be separated from cardiopulmonary bypass support after open heart surgery. These situations were rare, but the first such kidney procurement took place in 1962.[24] Since these organ donors were certain to die when cardiopulmonary bypass support was discontinued, kidneys were removed before death, albeit with permission of next of kin.

Another source of heart-beating donors was patients whose brain function had ceased but mechanical support systems were in place while physicians awaited the occurrence of asystole (generally in an intensive care unit). When the concept of brain death evolved, patients without brain function who were mechanically ventilated and artificially stabilized with parenteral administrations were able to have these heroic measures abruptly withdrawn. Cessation of heart beat would obviously occur quickly after withdrawal of care. This new concept of brain death was revolutionary and created considerable debate.

The first organ procurement from an individual with a beating heart but cessation of brain function occurred in Sweden in 1964. This operation sparked acrimonious debate that delayed identification of suitable organ donors in Sweden for many years. Frykholm, a neurosurgeon in Stockholm, presented a proposal in 1965 requesting codification of a new concept of death he referred to as "cerebral death." A specific request was made to permit use of organs from these individuals once "death" had been certified, even though the heart would continue to beat. Cerebral death was a less strict definition of "brain death" because it allowed for some midbrain function to persist. In 1967, Starzl performed the first successful liver transplant and Barnard performed the first heart transplant using donors meeting "neurologic death" criteria that was based essentially on the total brain death criteria employed today. Importantly, however, both surgeons removed life support, which precipitated cardiac arrest and a pulseless state prior to donor organ removal. The difficulty in accepting equivalency of "brain death" with cessation of heart beat and death by traditional diagnosis was most apparent in 1968 in Japan when physicians and surgeons involved with procurement of organs for transplant from a brain-dead drowning victim were censured and publicly vilified. The cardiac surgeon Wada Jura was even indicted for murder.[39]

Because of the controversy surrounding both withdrawal of heroic care in the futile or seemingly dead (except for a heart beat) critical care unit patient and the dilemma of donor organ sources, a committee was charged at Harvard University in 1968 to consider the **definition of brain death** further and determine what characteristics inevitably described irreversible coma. The goal was to describe the clinical characteristics of coma from which individuals would never recover and was ultimately associated with cessation of cardiac function.[9] This set the stage for developing criteria for the declaration of brain death (absence of brain function) with a heart-beating donor which would allow for the

ethical retrieval of organs for transplantation. Subsequent minor modifications of this criteria were formulated in the **Uniform Determination of Death Act** in the United States in 1980.

In order for organ transplantation to make an impact in the treatment of end-stage organ diseases, it rapidly became apparent that organized national systems must be established for the procurement and equitable distribution of organs harvested for transplantation. When the safety of long-distance transport of organs in kidney and later heart transplantation became evident, the need for such a system intensified. In the United States, the evolution of an organized and fair system for organ distribution resulted in the formation of the **United Network of Organ Sharing** (UNOS) (see Box), the current vehicle for organ sharing in the United States.[53]

Mr. Gene Pierce became the first executive director of UNOS and held that position from 1984 through October 1995. During his tenure and under his guidance, UNOS involved dedicated members of the transplant community in the evolution and maintenance of an effective, efficient, and fair system of organ allocation and distribution. It became a national and international resource for transplant patient–related information and education, and it was a model for the subsequent development of international organ procurement agencies. The stated goals of UNOS are to: (1) establish a national organ procurement and transplantation network under the Public Health Services Act; (2) improve the effectiveness of the nation's renal and extrarenal organ procurement, distribution, and transplantation systems by increasing the availability of and access to donor organs for patients

---

United Network of Organ Sharing

The historical development of the United Network of Organ Sharing dates back to the mid-1960s. Stimulated by the knowledge that graft survival after cadaveric kidney transplantation was improved with more closely genetically matched donors and recipients, the kidney disease and control agency of the United States Public Health Service awarded seven contracts to transplant centers for the purpose of transporting kidneys for transplantation. On June 27, 1969, the Southeastern Regional Organ Procurement Program was awarded one of these contracts. In 1975, the Southeastern Organ Procurement Foundation (SEOPF) was incorporated with 18 institutions in a six-state area in response to increased activity in organ transplantation. The UNOS was established in January 1977 for the purpose of developing a computerized system for improved matching of kidneys nationally. In 1984, an "Organ Center" was developed within UNOS to provide 24-hour-a-day service for the matching of organs with recipients throughout the United States. The National Organ Transplant Act, passed in 1984, provided for a national organ procurement and distribution network to improve the quantity, quality, and equity of organ transplantation throughout the United States. In 1986, UNOS was awarded the federal contract to operate the National Organ Procurement and Transplantation Network.

with end-stage organ failure; (3) develop, implement, and maintain quality assurance activities; and (4) systematically gather and analyze data and regularly publish the results of the national experience in organ procurement and preservation, tissue typing, and clinical organ transplantation.[55]

With the emergence of cardiac transplantation as a viable therapeutic option for end-stage heart disease, a clear need existed for a forum through which scientific information could be shared. To serve this need, the **International Society for Heart Transplantation** (later renamed the International Society for Heart and Lung Transplantation) was founded in 1981.

References

1. Anonymous: The Nobel lectures in immunology. The Nobel prize for physiology or medicine, 1908, awarded to Elie Metchnikoff & Paul Ehrlich "in recognition of their work on immunity." Scand J Immunol 1989;30:383–398.
2. Bailey LL: Role of cardiac replacement in the neonate. Heart Transplant 1985;IV:506–509.
3. Bailey LL, Nehisen-Cannarella SL, Concepcion W, Jolley WB: Baboon-to-human cardiac xenotransplantation in a neonate. JAMA 1985;54:3321–3329.
4. Barnard CN: A human cardiac transplant: an interim report of a successful operation performed at Groote Schuur Hospital, Cape Town. S Afr Med J 1967;41:1271–1274.
5. Barnard CN: Human cardiac transplantation: An evaluation of the first two operations performed at the Groote Schuur Hospital, Cape Town. Am J Cardiol 1968;22:584–596.
6. Barnard CN, Barnard MS, Cooper DKC, Curico CA, Hassoulas J, Novitsky D, Wolpowitz A: The present status of heterotopic cardiac transplantation. J Thorac Cardiovasc Surg 1981;81:433–439.
7. Barnard CN, Losman JG, Curcio CA, Sanchez HE, Wolpowitz A, Barnard MS: The advantage of heterotopic cardiac transplantation over orthotopic cardiac transplantation in the managment of severe acute rejection. J Thorac Cardiovasc Surg 1977;74:918–924.
8. Barnard CN, Pepper CB: One Life. New York: Macmillan, 1969.
9. Beecher HK, Adams RD, Barger AC, and the Ad Hoc Committee of the Harvard Medical School: Report of the ad hoc committee of the Harvard Medical School to examine the definition of brain death. A definition of irreversible coma. JAMA 1968;205:85–88.
10. Bibel DJ: Milestones in Immunology. A Historical Exploration. Madison: Science Tech Publishers, 1988.
11. Billingham RE, Brent L, Medawar PB: 'Actively acquired tolerance' of foreign cells. Nature 1953;172:603–606.
12. Blanco G, Adam A, Rodriguez-Peres D, Fernandez A: Complete homotransplantation of canine heart and lungs. Arch Surg 1958;76:20–24.
13. Burnet FM, Fenner F: The Production of Antibodies. 2nd ed. New York: Macmillan, 1949.
14. Carrel A: Surgery of the blood vessels and its application to changes in circulation and transplantation of organs. Johns Hopkins Hosp Bull 1906;17:26.
15. Carrel A: The surgery of blood vessels. Johns Hopkins Hosp Bull 1907;18:18.
16. Carrel A, Guthrie CC: The transplantation of veins and organs. Am Med 1905;10:1101–1102.
17. Cass MH, Brock R: Heart excision and replacement. Guys Hosp Rep 1959;108:285.
18. Castaneda AR, Arner A, Schmidt-Habelman P, Muller JH, Zamora R: Cardiopulmonary autotransplantation in primates. J Thorac Cardiovasc Surg 1972;37:523–531.
19. Castaneda AR, Zamora R, Schmidt-Habelmann P, Horning J, Murphy W, Ponto D, Muller JH: Cardiopulmonary autotransplantation in primates (baboons): Late functional results. Surgery 1972;72:1064–1070.
20. Caves PK, Billingham ME, Stinson EB, Shumway NE: Serial transvenous biopsy of the transplanted human heart. Improved management of acute rejection episodes. Lancet May 4th, 1974; 821–826.
21. Chernyak L, Tauber AI: The birth of immunology: Metchnikoff, the embryologist. Cell Immunol 1988;117:218–233.
22. Cooley DA, Bloodwell RD, Hallman GL, Nora JJ, Harrison GM, Leachman RD: Organ transplanation for advanced cardiopulmonary disease. Ann Thorac Surg 1969;8:30–46.
23. Demikhov VP: Experimental Transplantation of Vital Organs. New York, Consultants Bureau, 1962.
24. DeVita MA, Snyder JV, Grenvik A: History of organ donoation by patients with cardiac death. Kennedy Inst Ethics J 1993;3:113–129.
25. Downie HG: Homotransplantation of the dog heart. Arch Surg 1953;66:624–636.
26. Gibson T, Medawar PB: The fate of skin homografts in man. J Anat 1945;77:299–314.
27. Goldberg M, Berman EF, Akman LC: Homologous transplantation of the canine heart. J Int Coll Surg 1958;30:575–586.
28. Griepp RB: A decade of human heart transplantation. Transplant Proc 1979;11:285–292.
29. Griepp RB, Ergin MA: The history of experimental heart transplantation. Heart Transplant 1984;3:145–151.
30. Guthrie CC: On misleading statements. Science 1909;XXIX:29.
31. Guthrie CC: Blood Vessel Surgery and Its Applications. London: Edward Arnold; New York: Longmans, Green & Co, 1912.
32. Harbison SP: Origins of vascular surgery: The Carrel-Guthrie letters. Surgery 1962;52:406–418.
33. Hardy JD, Chavez CM: The first heart transplant in man. Am J Cardiol 1968;22:772–781.
34. Hardy JD, Chavez CM, Eraslan S, Adkins JR, Williams RD: Heart transplantation in dogs. Procedures, physiologic problems and results in 142 experiments. Surgery 1966;60:361.
35. Hardy JD, Chavez CM, Kurrus FD, Neely WA, Eraslan S, Turner MD, Fabian LW, Labecki TD: Heart transplantation in man. Developmental studies and report of a case. JAMA 1964;188:1132–1140.
36. Hardy JD, Kurrus FD, Chavez CM, Webb WR: Heart transplantation in infant calves; evaluation of coronary perfusion to preserve organs during transfer. Ann NY Acad Sci 1964;120:766.
37. Holman E: Protein sensitization in isoskin grafting. Is the latter of practical value? Surg Gynecol Obstet 1924;38:100.
38. Kantrowitz A, Huller JD, Joos H, Cerruti MM, Carstensen HE: Transplantation of the heart in an infant and an adult. Am J Cardiol 1968;22:782–790.
39. Kimura R: Japan's dilemma with the definition of death. Kennedy Inst Ethics J 1991;1:123–131.
40. Kurrus F, Hardy JD, Chaves CM, Elliott RL: Heart transplantation. Fed Proc 1964;23:201.
41. Kondo Y, Gridel F, Kantrowitz A: Heart transplantation in puppies: Long term survival without immunosuppressive therapy. Circulation 1965;31, 32(suppl 1):181.
42. Landsteiner K: Ueber agglutination-serscheinungen normalen menschliechen blutes. Wien Klin Wochenenschr 1901;14:1132–1134.
43. Landsteiner K, Chase MW: Experiments on transfer of cutaneous sensitivity to simple compounds. Proc Soc Exp Biol Med 1942;49:688–690.
44. Lee SS, Webb WR: Cardiac metabolism as influenced by ischemia, refrigeration and enzyme precursors. Am Surg 1959;25:776.
45. Lower RR, Dong E, Shumway NE: Long-term survival of cardiac homografts. Surgery 1965;58:110.
46. Lower RR, Dong E, Shumway NE: Suppression of rejection crises in the cardiac homograft. Ann Thorac Surg 1965;1:645.
47. Lower RR, Shumway NE: Studies on the orthotopic homotransplantation of the canine heart. Surg Forum 1960;11:18.
48. Lower RR, Stofer RC, Shumway NE: Homovital transplantation of the heart. J Thorac Cardiovasc Surg 1961;41:196–204.
49. Mann FC, Priestly JT, Markowitz J, Yater WM: Transplantation of the intact mammalian heart. Arch Surg 1933;26:219–224.
50. Marcus E, Wong SNT, Luisada AA: Homologeous heart grafts: Transplantation of the heart in dogs. Surg Forum 1951;2:212.
51. Marcus E, Wong SNT, Luisada AA: Homologous heart grafts. I. Technique of interim parabiotic perfusion II. Transplantation of the heart in dogs. Arch Surg 1953;66:179–191.
52. McGough EC, Brewer PL, Reemtsma K: The parallel heart: Studies of intrathoracic auxiliary cardiac transplants. Surgery 1966;60:153–158.
53. Medawar PB: The behavior and fate of skin autografts and skin homografts in rabbits. J Anat 1944;78:176–199.

54. Neptune WB, Cookson BA, Bailey CP, Appler R, Rajkowski F: Complete homologous heart transplantation. Arch Surg 1953; 66:174.
55. Phillips MG (ed): Organ Procurement, Preservation and Distribution in Transplantation. Richmond: UNOS, 1991.
56. Owen RD: Immunogenetic consequences of vascular anastomoses between bovine twins. Science 1945;102:400–401.
57. Reemtsma K: The heart as a test organ in transplantation studies. Ann N Y Acad Sci 1964;120:778–785.
58. Reemstma K, McCracken BH, Schlegel JU, Pearl MA, Pearce CW, DeWitt CW, Smith PE, Hewitt RL, Flinner RL, Creech O Jr: Renal heterotransplantation in man. Ann Surg 1964;160:384.
59. Reemstma K, Williamson WE, Iglesias F, Pena E, Sayegh SF, Creech O Jr: Studies in homologous canine heart transplantation: Prolongation of survival with a folic acid antagonist. Surgery 1962;52:127.
60. Reitz BA: In Baumgartner WA, Reits BA, Achuff SA (eds): Heart and Heart-Lung Transplantation. Philadelphia: WB Saunders Company, 1990.
61. Reitz BA, Burton NA, Jamison SW, Bieber CP, Pennock JL, Stinson EB, Shumway NE: Heart and lung transplantation. Autotransplantation in primates with extended survival. J Thorac Cardiovasc Surg 1980;80:360–372.
62. Reitz BA, Wallwork JL, Hunt SA, et al: Heart-lung transplantation: Successful therapy for patients with pulmonary vascular disease. N Engl J Med 1982;306:557–564.
63. Schöne G: Die Heteroplastiche und Homöoplastiche Transplantation. Berlin: Springer-Verlag, 1912.
64. Shumway NE, Lower RR, Stofer RC: Selective hypothermia of the heart in anoxic cardiac arrest. Surg Gynecol Obstet 1959; 109:750–754.
65. Shumway NE, Lower RR: Special problems in transplanation of the heart. Ann NY Acad Sci 1964;120:773–777.
66. Shumacker HB Jr: The Evolution of Cardiac Surgery. Bloomington: Indiana University Press, 1992.
67. Silverstein AM: The history of immunology. In Paul WE (ed): Fundamental Immunology. 2nd ed. New York: Raven Press, 1993.
68. Silverstein AM: A History of Immunology. San Diego: Academic Press, 1989.
69. Snell GD: Methods for the study of histocompatibity genes. J Genet 1948;49:87–108.
70. Stinson EB, Dong E Jr, Schroeder JS, Harrison DC, Shumway NE: Initial clinical experience with heart transplantation. Am J Cardiol 1968;22:791–803.
71. Tauber AI, Chernyak L: The birth of immunology. II. Metchnikoff and his critics. Cell Immunol 1989;121:447–473.
72. Webb WR, Howard HS: Cardiopulmonary transplantation. Surg Forum 1957;8:313–317.
73. Webb WR, Howard HS: Restoration of function of the refrigerated heart. Forum Am Coll Surg 1957;8:302.
74. Webb WR, de Guzman V, Hooper JE: Cardiopulmonary transplantation: Experimental study of current problems. Am Surg 1961;27:236–241.

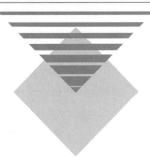

CHAPTER TWO

Immunology in Relation to Cardiac Transplantation

with the collaboration of
JAMES F. GEORGE, Ph.D.

THE IMMUNOLOGIC RESPONSE

WHAT IS THE FUNCTION OF THE IMMUNE SYSTEM?

An organism, such as a human being, can be defined as an integrated collection of living cells that behave in a concerted fashion and maintain a distinct identity relative to other organisms. In order to exist, a living thing must have mechanisms that enable it to maintain its structure and its distinctness relative to all that surrounds it. In the biological world as we know it, the smallest component with this ability (excluding viruses, prions, and certain other microorganisms) is the **cell,** which is a collection of molecules (multiatomic structures that make up the smallest unit of a given substance) that constitute the smallest possible component of a living thing that still retains the properties of life. (One could debate about the fundamental properties of that which we call life, but most will agree that living things have common properties, such as growth, response to stimulation, and reproduction. For our purposes, this definition should suffice.) To maintain this identity, the organism must prevent the permanent intermingling of its cells with other organisms, and it must prevent its basic structure from being destroyed by other things that surround it, including other organisms. Thus, to any organism, there is an entity called "**self,**" which constitutes the group of cells that maintains a distinctive identity relative to the rest of the universe, and "**nonself**" which is everything else. Note that this definition of nonself also includes other members of the same species.

Organisms exist in a relentlessly competitive environment in which they compete for food (molecules from which energy can be generated and molecules that can be used as components for the maintenance of physical structure, metabolism, and reproduction) and space in which to exist. In general, food molecules can be acquired at the lowest energy cost if another organism has already converted the molecules into usable form. Therefore, most organisms will gain more by the acquisition of food from other organisms. Bacteria are an example of organisms that exist in this fashion. Organisms that invade the body do so in the quest for food and space in which to grow. Disease is caused when those activities disrupt homeostasis in the host organism. Therefore, in order to maintain self-integrity, complex organisms such as humans must have a means by which they can exclude entry of other organisms into the body and remove such organisms if they gain entry. Otherwise they will be rapidly consumed as food by the life around them (decay is an example of this process). Thus, most multicellular organisms possess an **immune system,** which functions to detect the entry of nonself into the body, to eliminate it if possible, and to isolate it if not.

In terms of organ transplantation, the events that are normally seen following transplantation of a heart from one human to another are a function of the immune system as defined above. A heart from another person constitutes **nonself** and therefore will be the target of the immune system, which has evolved over time to be highly selective in the identification of nonself and highly effective at the elimination or isolation of nonself introduced into the body.

There are certain features of a system (the immune system) that can effectively defend the body from invasion by other organisms. First, it must have a means by which it can **detect the presence of nonself.** Second, there must be **a means to isolate or eliminate the nonself invader** (such as a transplanted organ, which to the immune system is just another nonself "thing" that must be eliminated). Third, it must accomplish the first two objectives **without causing irreparable damage to the rest of the body.** As the reader will see further in this chapter, the systems that accomplish these objectives do so by means of specialized organs, cells, and molecules.

HOW IS NONSELF DETECTED BY THE IMMUNE SYSTEM?

The central question in the detection of nonself is this: How can one tell if cells or molecules originating from another organism are different? At the macro level, one can distinguish members of the same species by small differences in appearance, such as facial features. By the pattern of features on the outside of an individual, one can recognize specific individuals or groups of individuals. At the cellular level, a similar process of pattern recognition must also occur in which nonself is distinguished from cells that belong to the body. This pattern recognition can occur at the cellular level because each cell has on its surface a very large number of different molecules, each with their individual patterns of three-dimensional structure, charge, and spatial distribution on the cell membrane. For the purposes of recognition, these surface molecules serve as markers for different cell types and for cells from different individuals. An example of **cell surface molecules** that can distinguish

different individuals or groups of individuals is blood group antigens (Fig. 2–1).

Thus, variation between individuals occurs at the macro level, at the cellular level, and at the molecular level. One might expect that molecules that perform the same function in two different individuals of the same species, who are otherwise identical, might be absolutely identical in structure. For many molecules, this statement appears to be true. But analysis of the structure of **proteins** and the **genes** that code for them reveals that some molecules can be variable in different individuals. (Genes are the information repository for the amino acid sequence of proteins in the form of deoxyribonucleotide triplets, the sequence of which determines the amino acid sequence of a protein.) Variation in the nucleotide sequence of genes often results in a change in the amino acid sequence. This, in turn, results in an alteration of the three-dimensional structure and charge of the protein.

From the perspective of clinical transplantation, it is the variation in the **peptide components** (which are themselves composed of amino acids) of proteins that allows the immune system to distinguish cells originating from other individuals. Let X represent a protein with the amino acid sequence BYWAYWY from one individual, and Z represent a protein with the amino acid sequence BYIAYWY that performs the same function in another individual of the same species. The specific amino acids represented by the letters are not important here. Note that the first occurrence of the amino acid W in protein X has been replaced by the amino acid I in protein Z. This change in amino acid sequence may or may not alter the function of that protein (e.g., the efficiency of enzyme catalysis), but it is highly likely

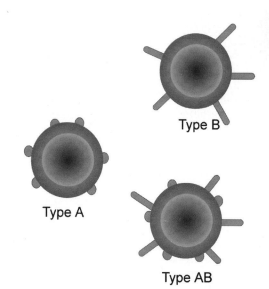

FIGURE **2–1.** A schematic representation of the differing surface features of erythrocytes from individuals with different blood types. Cells from type A individuals are recognized by natural antibodies in type B and type O individuals that bind to N-acetyl-galactosamine residues (semicircle) attached to a series of residues collectively called H-substance. Cells from type B individuals bear galactosamine residues (elongated oval) recognized by natural antibodies in type A and type O individuals. In each case, erythrocytes can be differentiated on the basis of specific molecular features on the cell surface that, on a population basis, can be used to delineate broad groups of people.

that the three-dimensional structure of the protein, which is partly determined by the amino acid sequence, will be altered. Molecules that vary in this fashion from individual to individual are said to be **polymorphic.** It is this polymorphism that serves as the basis by which nonself can be detected. (Note that polymorphisms among proteins is not the only thing by which self can be distinguished from nonself. However, in clinical transplantation, protein polymorphism is by far the predominant feature that drives rejection.)

WHICH COMPONENTS OF THE IMMUNE SYSTEM ELIMINATE NONSELF?

Obviously, the immune system did not evolve for the purpose of rejecting transplanted allografts. The **effector mechanisms** (methods by which cells of the immune system eliminate nonself) that are observed during **allograft rejection** are the result of systems developed for the purpose of defending the body from invasion by infectious agents or toxins. One can categorize the responses to nonself into two major divisions: the adaptive immune system and the innate immune system.

The **adaptive immune system,** whose responses are mediated by T-lymphocytes (T-cells) and B-lymphocytes (B-cells), requires an interval after first being exposed to nonself before its destructive effects are manifest. **Cytotoxic T-lymphocytes** (CTLs) are particularly adept at this task. These cells can proliferate extensively in the presence of nonself and directly kill those cells using a variety of mechanisms, which are discussed later in this chapter.

If we accept that nonself is distinguished on the basis of **polymorphic cell surface proteins,** then we must infer that there is something on the surface of cells of the immune system that can distinguish between different versions of a polymorphic molecule. In the mammalian immune system, **lymphocytes** express (make available on the cell surface) protein molecules called **antigen receptors** that can bind to nonself (polymorphic) proteins. They are named such because nonself molecules (peptides) that can be detected by the immune system are called **antigens.** The distinguishing feature of antigen receptors is that the end of the receptor that is exposed to the world outside the cells can bind to antigens. Therefore, when an antigen receptor binds to an antigen, another portion of the molecule that is inside the cell initiates a series of biochemical reactions that "activate" (to be defined in detail later) the lymphocyte, ultimately culminating in an immune response. In this way, the presence of nonself is detected. **T-lymphocytes** are the cells that can specifically detect the presence of **nonself peptides,** and the **antigen receptors** are the apparatus by which they effect this function.

Activation of **B-lymphocytes** by nonself results in the formation of **antibodies,** which are molecules specifically targeted by the organism against **nonself peptides, cells, or portions of cells.** In heart transplantation, this mechanism of eliminating nonself is the basis of **humoral rejection.** Antibodies can also serve as markers and can aid in the attachment of cytotoxic T-cells to their target. Antibodies also serve as points of attachment for phagocytic cells, which have receptors that bind to a non–antigen-binding portion of the antibody molecule.

The **innate immune system** includes more immediate, less specific responses that are not dependent on antigen receptors on T- and B-lymphocytes. This differs from the adaptive immune system, in that the destructive response occurs rapidly and does not have the latent period necessary for lymphocyte activation and antibody formation. The innate (nonadaptive) response to nonself relies on the process of **inflammation** and elements of the **humoral amplification system** (complement, coagulation, fibrinolytic, and kallikrein cascades). Through secretion of soluble factors (cytokines), phagocytes can be recruited to the site of infection or injury, which is also accompanied by migration of cells involved in the specific immune responses.

Following cardiac transplantation, both types of immune responses are likely present, beginning with the nonadaptive inflammatory response during initial reperfusion following a period of donor organ ischemia. Antigens present in the transplanted organ then stimulate the adaptive immune system, with T-cell and B-cell activation.

IS THERE SPECIFICITY OF ANTIGEN RECEPTORS FOR CERTAIN PEPTIDES OR PROTEINS (ANTIGENS)?

This question is important because the number of different proteins to which an organism could be exposed is extremely large. Previous experiences with other biological receptors have shown that they tend to bind only one thing very well. If this is true, then one must also assume that antigen receptors are highly variable in structure in order to bind so many different things. Structural analysis has shown that all antigen receptors have a **variable region** that binds to antigens, and a constant region that serves as an interface with other cell surface molecules and also communicates information into the interior of the cell. Later in this chapter, we discuss in detail what specific features of an antigen are recognized, the molecular basis of binding by an antigen receptor, and the means by which a cell creates a variable region using a minimum of genetic information.

Considerable scientific evidence indicates that each lymphocyte carries **only one type** of antigen receptor on its surface, each of which is specific for a single antigen (peptide). Thus, if a T-lymphocyte contains, on average, about 100,000 antigen receptors on its surface, all of them will be identical and will bind to only one specific antigen. Given the huge number of foreign antigens that an organism (or individual) may encounter, how does an individual produce enough T-cells to account for all of them? The answer is likely in part evolutionary in that species with an inadequate variety (repertoire) of lymphocyte antigen receptors would succumb to foreign invasion (infections) and not survive to propagate themselves. A branch of theoretical immunology deals with other explanations for this phenomenon.

HOW DOES THE ANTIGEN RECEPTOR "KNOW" THAT A BOUND PROTEIN (OR PEPTIDE) IS NONSELF?

We have shown that the components necessary for self/ nonself discrimination are present in the body in the form of antigen receptors, and in the form of polymorphic proteins on the surface of cells from another organism. However, these features do not indicate how a particular receptor would discriminate between a self protein or a protein from another organism. The answer to this question, in short, is that a particular receptor does not discriminate between self and nonself. Instead, self/nonself discrimination is a function of a population of lymphocytes that contains a large number of antigen receptors. Each lymphocyte has a unique antigen receptor with a unique specificity (i.e., the ability to bind a particular antigen and no other). The production of a large number of lymphocytes, each with its own antigen receptor that can bind to a single unique antigen, ensures that most of the items that would be encountered can be detected by the immune system. Note that some lymphocytes can be found with antigen receptors that will bind to more than one antigen. Such lymphocytes are said to be **cross-reactive.** Self/nonself discrimination is introduced into this system by a process of selection, in which potentially harmful lymphocytes that could react with self antigen are eliminated. This process of selection takes place among T-cells while they develop in the thymus. Except in disease states, self antigens do not bind (and therefore activate) T-cells. Thus, if the lymphocyte antigen receptor binds to anything, it is "assumed" that the bound thing is nonself.

WHAT ABOUT THE SPECIAL SITUATION OF PREGNANCY?

A mother can successfully and repeatedly bear children even though they are histoincompatible (because they bear polymorphic molecules derived from the father). This has been a difficult question for immunologists because the prevention of rejection of the fetus is normal, and it is difficult to study a mechanism of preventing rejection when that rejection almost never occurs. However, careful observations have indicated that the mechanism of fetal acceptance is probably not passive. The mechanism most often postulated is that fetal antigens are sequestered within the separate blood supply of the fetus, and therefore the mother's immune system never "sees" the fetal antigens. In fact, most mothers make antibodies specific for fetal antigens, indicating that the placenta does not completely prevent antigens from entering the maternal circulation. However, the placenta does prevent the mother's T-cells from crossing to the fetal circulation. The interface layer of cells between the mother and the fetus is the trophoblast, which does not express classical major histocompatibility complex (MHC) antigens, but does express HLA-G (a class Ib MHC molecule), which has been shown to inhibit lysis by natural killer (NK) cells, an element of the innate immune system. It is certain that maintenance of the fetus is a multifactorial process involving the differential expression of surface antigens, secretion of soluble factors, and sequestration of antigens, the active suppression of the mother's immune response towards the fetus and partial isolation of the fetus from the response that does result.

Other sites that are known to be immunologically privileged, such as the eye, have a number of immunologic mechanisms that have been implicated in the suppression of host responses towards donor tissue. These mechanisms involve antigenic stimulation (in the anterior chamber of the eye) of immune cells which travel systemically and appear to actively suppress the immune response in the eye. This is extremely important in preventing the sequelae of acute inflammation within the eye, which could lead to blindness.

GENERAL TERMINOLOGY OF THE IMMUNE RESPONSE

The discussion of the mechanism of complex systems is best begun with a detailed discussion of what such a system does and the parts from which it is made. With a clear understanding of the components of the immune system, we can then proceed with a discussion of the mechanisms that give rise to the functional features that have been observed. In this respect, however, we will largely confine our discussion to those aspects of the immune system as they relate to solid organ transplantation in general, and the heart in particular.

The immunologic response is an integrated bodily response, meaning that various components of the immune system, while located in different regions of the body, are coordinately regulated and are often redundant. Much of this chapter is devoted to the details of this integration. It is customary for immunologists to classify parts of an immunologic response as "cellular" or "noncellular" (the latter also is often called "humoral"). These terms most often refer to the component that directly produces the observed effect. In a **cellular immunologic response,** one would observe host cells being recruited to the site of the response, and in a humoral or noncellular response, antibodies and/or complement can be found at the site of action and in the circulation. Therefore, in the "immunologic response" to a transplanted heart, we are referring to a multifaceted phenomenon.

Inherent in most discussions of the immunologic response are a number of words; these include **antigen** (usually, but not always a peptide, which may be on a cell surface, within a cell, or may be a soluble substance in the noncellular portions of the patient's blood and/ or body fluids and which stimulates some activity by the immune system), **antibody** (a soluble substance which can kill cells and perhaps tissues without the direct aid of another cell usually through activation of complement or with the aid of another cell that binds to the antibody), **immunity** (the result of an immunologic process by which an individual is able to resist a particular disease or condition), **chimera** (an individual who/

which contains, without evident damage, cellular components, or intact cells, originating in another individual), **induction** (a process of generating something), **immunologic tolerance** (a condition in which the immune system fails to react to a specific antigen(s) and yet remains otherwise active without immunosuppression), **processing** (breaking antigens into smaller pieces and then displaying them on the cell surface), **presenting** (a process of making something available to something else, usually in the context of displaying antigens on the cell surface), **allograft** (a graft from another individual of the same species as the graft recipient), **xenograft** (a graft from another individual of a different species from the graft recipient), **signal** (the transmission of information across the plasma (cell) membrane), **expression** (to make something available on the cell surface or to secrete something into the surrounding environment), and **cytokines** (soluble proteins produced by cells that alter the behavior of other cells).

KEY COMPONENTS OF THE IMMUNE SYSTEM IN TRANSPLANTATION

The major **cellular** components of the immune system are T-lymphocytes, B-lymphocytes, NK cells, antigen-presenting cells (APCs), and granulocytes. The major **molecular** components of the immune system are the MHC molecules, cytokines, adhesion molecules, antigen receptors, immunoglobulins, and complement. **Lymphocytes** are a subgroup of leukocytes (which are relatively easily identified) that play a major role in the immune response. Leukocytes also include granulocytes (neutrophils, eosinophils, and basophils) and plasma cells (derived from B-lymphocytes), as well as lymphocytes. Lymphocytes are named such because of their relative abundance in the lymph and lymph nodes. They are the cells that confer the immune response with specificity by virtue of antigen receptors on their surfaces.

MHC MOLECULES

The proteins primarily responsible for the immune response to organ transplantation are called **MHC** (major histocompatibility complex) antigens. To understand the central role of MHC molecules, it is important to understand that T-cells only recognize antigenic peptides which are contained within the MHC-binding groove on the surfaces of antigen-presenting cells. To appreciate the advantage of the evolution of such a system, recall that there are a number of barriers that *restrict* the ability of an organism to gain entry into the host. There are physical barriers, such as the skin, and there are nonspecific cellular and humoral defenses (such as the complement system). If an organism evades these modes of defense, then B- and T-cell–mediated responses must be targeted at accessible and vulnerable phases of the organism's life cycle. B-cell–mediated responses in the form of secreted antibodies can target organisms such as viruses while they are in free solution in blood or bodily fluids. This is particularly useful in preventing the spread or the expansion of populations of invading organisms, and once immunized, it can present a further barrier to reinfection. However, this mode of defense is largely ineffective against pathogens that can exist within a host cell and are therefore shielded against antibodies in solution. Thus, unless molecules unique to the invading pathogen are on the surface of the cell, there is no way to determine which cells harbor the organism. The pathways for antigen presentation provide a solution to this problem. In these pathways, both cytosolic and exogenous proteins are processed into peptides and presented on the surface of the cell. Unique peptides from an intracellular pathogen can be captured by the MHC molecules and transported to the surface of the cell. The cell can then be recognized as bearing foreign antigens and targeted for destruction before it can be used for reproduction by a pathogenic organism.

In each species, MHC antigens have been given different names. In the mouse they are called H-2 antigens. In the human, the MHC antigens are termed **human leukocyte antigens** (HLA). The major histocompatibility complex is called a complex because it consists of a group of **genes** on the short arm of chromosome 6 that code for a number of proteins that are expressed on the cell surface. (Fig. 2–2). The principal important feature of these genes is that they are **polymorphic,** meaning that there are small variations among individuals in the nucleotide sequence of the genes (and therefore the amino acid sequence of the resulting protein product), but the same overall structure is retained. Therefore, for any given MHC gene, there are likely to be multiple variations (also called **alleles**) of that gene distributed among a group of individuals. Since there are as many as 30 to 50 genes within the MHC complex, each of which may have multiple variations in a given population, the number of different combinations of MHC variations is

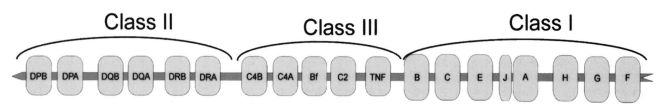

FIGURE **2–2.** A simplified map of the human major histocompatibility complex. Class I (E, H, G, and F), II, and III. The A, B, C, and DR genes are most often routinely typed at most transplant centers. The genes for tumor necrosis factor (TNF) and complement components can be found in the class III region.

large.[40, 161, 212] It is the **polymorphism** (variation) in the genetic sequences of MHC molecules that is the **ultimate basis for graft rejection.** Because MHC molecules are highly polymorphic, it is very unusual for a randomly selected donor to have MHC molecules that are identical to the recipient. The variability of the MHC provides protection for a population against destruction by a single pathogenic virus or other organism. The reason for this is that the MHC molecules serve as structures that contain antigen for presentation to T-cells. Since they are polymorphic, the same peptide presented by MHC molecules from different individuals will appear to have a different three-dimensional shape to T-cells. Therefore, a peptide from a virus that could escape immune recognition in one individual (perhaps because it resembles a self-antigen), might not escape recognition in another.

Note that in any discussion regarding the role of MHC molecules in transplantation, one must distinguish between the donor and recipient MHC molecules. In the "normal" mode of antigen presentation, such as that found with viral antigens or some other foreign protein, the *donor* MHC molecules can be considered as nothing more than a source of antigen. The *donor* MHC molecules are ingested by the *recipient* antigen-presenting cells and processed into peptides, which are subsequently loaded into *recipient* MHC molecules for presentation to recipient T cells. The most relevant feature of donor MHC molecules is the extent that they differ from recipient MHC and are therefore nonself. The more extensive the difference in amino acid sequence, the more likely it is that the donor MHC molecule will be broken into peptides that appear to be nonself. At the level of antigen presentation, the immune system does not "know" the source of a peptide, but examines it to determine whether it is self or nonself, which is a function of the amino acid sequence of the peptide. In the special case of *direct antigen presentation* (see later section), intact *donor* class II MHC molecules on *donor* antigen-presenting cells or donor endothelial cells may play an important role in T-cell activation.

MHC antigens can be divided into major and minor categories. There is a specific MHC nomenclature (see Box) which describes these antigens.

Structure

The functions of MHC molecules are closely related to their three-dimensional structure and their high degree of polymorphism. Figure 2–3 shows two different views of an MHC molecule in which there is a distinct groove formed by two α-helices that lie on top of a β-pleated sheet.[38] This groove constitutes the region in which processed peptides reside when they are presented to a T-cell by an APC. It is important to note that a T-cell will only respond to an antigen (peptide) which is contained in the MHC peptide-binding groove of an APC. This MHC groove may contain nonself peptides or self peptides (from normal cellular breakdown), but the groove is never empty. The polymorphic region of the MHC molecule lies in and around the peptide-binding groove, thus the exact shape of the peptide–MHC protein complex as seen by a T-cell will vary in different individuals

MHC Nomenclature

The nomenclature of the MHC antigens and genes is closely tied to the manner in which the MHC antigens were discovered. The MHC loci in the mouse were discovered first through a program of inbreeding and observation of tumor graft rejection. The advent of solid organ transplantation in humans provided a motivation to define the MHC locus in humans. This process began when Jean Dausset and others observed in 1958 that sera from patients who received kidneys or blood transfusions contained antibodies that would react to leukocytes from the organ or blood donor.[56] Sera from these individuals were called *antisera*, and since the sera were reactive to leukocytes, the antigens that were bound by the antisera were called *human leukocyte antigens*, or HLA. These antigens were named A, B, and C in order of their discovery. A fourth antigen, called HLA-D, was first identified using mixed lymphocyte cultures. Antibodies were found that reacted to antigens that appeared to be in, or closely proximal to, the HLA-D locus. These antigens were called HLA-D related, or HLA-DR. Other gene products were identified and named HLA-DQ and HLA-DP with the letters Q and P chosen simply due to their proximity to R in the English alphabet.

because different side groups may project into and out of the groove due to polymorphism of MHC polypeptides.

Classes

The proteins of the MHC complex are broadly subdivided into groups called class I (the Roman numeral I), class Ib, class II, and class III. Class I and class II proteins are most commonly referred to in the context of transplantation and have similar overall three-dimensional shapes (i.e., both classes form a peptide-binding groove), but differ in terms of the composition of the polypeptide chains that constitute the MHC molecule, their distribution on different cells and tissues in the body, and the biochemical pathways that result in the loading of an antigenic peptide into the groove (Table 2–1).

Class I

The classic human **MHC class I** molecules that are routinely typed for solid organ allografts are called A, B, and C. Class I molecules are expressed on the surface of virtually all nucleated cells, although the level of expression can vary significantly among different cell types. The highest surface density is generally found on lymphocytes on the order of 1 to 5×10^5 molecules per cell. Somatic cells, such as fibroblasts, muscle cells and endothelial cells can have much lower levels of expression, but some can be induced to express much higher levels by cytokines such as interferon-γ (IFN-γ). This inducibility is probably a significant factor in the initiation and perpetuation of a rejection episode. As more inflammatory factors are generated during a rejection episode, it would also be expected that the level of MHC

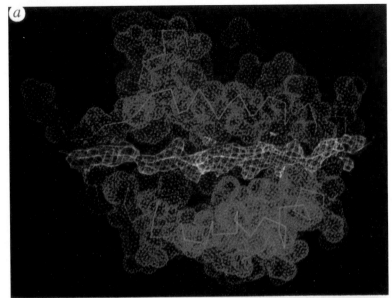

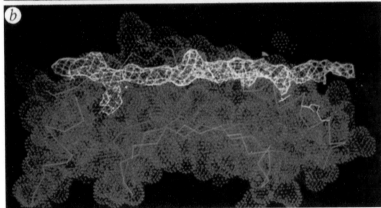

FIGURE **2–3.** The three-dimensional structure of the extracellular portion of HLA-DR1 as determined by x-ray diffraction. The van der Waals surface of DR1 is shown in blue, and the peptide surface is shown in orange/red. *A,* Top view of the peptide-binding groove as it would appear to a T-cell receptor. This view clearly shows the walls formed by the α-helical portions of the chains that form the walls of the peptide binding groove. *B,* Side view with the β1 domain helix removed for clarity. This view clearly shows the side chains of the peptide residing in the groove. (From Brown JH, Jardetzky TS, Gorga JC, et al: Three-dimensional structure of the human class II histocompatibility antigen HLA-DR1. Nature 1993;364:33–39. Copyright 1993 Macmillan Magazines Limited, with permission.)

expression on donor vascular endothelial cells and muscle cells would increase, further increasing the antigenicity of the cells.[61, 63, 178, 179, 206]

The HLA-A gene includes more than 50 possible alleles, the HLA-B gene includes more than 75 alleles, and HLA-C gene more than 30 alleles.[40] They are composed of two chains: a larger highly polymorphic heavy α-chain coded by a gene in the MHC complex on chromosome 6, and a smaller nonpolymorphic β-chain called $β_2$-microglobulin that is coded by a gene located outside

the MHC on chromosome 15[176, 177] (Fig. 2–4). The larger chain, called the α-chain, is composed of five protein domains designated $α_1, α_2, α_3,$ a transmembrane domain, and a cytoplasmic domain. The polymorphic part of the chain that constitutes the peptide binding region primarily encompasses the $α_1$ and $α_2$ regions. The $α_1$ and $α_2$ domains form a peptide-binding region in which they interact three-dimensionally to form a platform of eight antiparallel strands forming a β-pleated sheet that is flanked by two long α-helical regions that form the floor

TABLE 2-1	**Properties of Class I and Class II MHC Molecules**	
PROPERTY	CLASS I (A, B, AND C)	CLASS II (DR, DP, AND DQ)
Protein structure	44-kDa α chain—highly polymorphic; 12-kDa $β_2$-microglobulin β chain	33- to 35-kDa α chain; 26- to 28-kDa β chain—highly polymorphic
Tissue distribution	Ubiquitous	Mostly B cells, macrophages, and dendritic cells (often called "professional antigen-presenting cells"), may be expressed on endothelial cells
Method of antigen processing	Endogenous	Exogenous
Predominant T-cell subtype that interacts with the MHC molecule	$CD8^+$ T-cells	$CD4^+$ T-cells

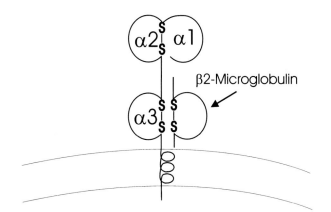

FIGURE **2–4.** Schematic of an MHC class I molecule. An MHC class I molecule consists of two polypeptide chains. The α-chain has three immunoglobulin-like domains designated α_1, α_2, and α_3. The latter domain also serves as the binding site for the CD8 molecule. The α chain has an α-helical transmembrane portion that connects to the signal transduction machinery in the interior of the cell. β_2-Microglobulin is noncovalently linked to the α chain, and is required for expression of the MHC molecule on the cell surface.

and walls of the peptide-binding groove, respectively. Within this region, peptide fragments eight or nine amino acids in length are presented in the peptide-binding groove. The α_3 domain is highly constant in sequence among class I MHC molecules. This domain interacts extensively with β_2-microglobulin, and this association appears to be necessary to maintain the correct conformation of the MHC molecule for cell-surface stability. The α_3 domain interacts with the **CD8 molecule** on the surface of T cells,[75, 76] thus usually restricting the recognition of antigen displayed in the groove of class I HLA molecules to CD8+ T cells. The CD nomenclature (see Box) designates surface molecules based on their reactivity with monoclonal antibodies.

Nomenclature of CD Cell Surface Molecules

Functional studies of the immune system have shown that distinct subpopulations of leukocytes exist in nearly all cellular compartments of the body. In an attempt to identify and isolate such subpopulations, immunologists have raised monoclonal antibodies that are reactive with distinctive antigens on the cell surface. By observing the pattern of reactivity with these antibodies, leukocytes with unique developmental and functional properties can be distinguished. Analysis of the cell surface proteins that constitute the targets for these monoclonal antibodies have shown that many of these antigens have similar structure and function in different species. Most of the antigens were named after the antibody that was used to identify them, leading to considerable confusion. To resolve this problem, a uniform nomenclature was established for human antigens, which is now applied to several other species. Since some monoclonal antibodies reacted with the same cell surface protein that often identified a particular stage of differentiation, such antibodies were said to define a *cluster of differentiation*, which is abbreviated CD. Each cluster of differentiation or CD antigen, is assigned a unique number.

Class Ib

Class Ib molecules are similar to the classical class I molecules and are able to associate with β_2-microglobulin, but are less polymorphic and smaller in size.[195] Many of these molecules were first identified by molecular mapping rather than through functional or serologic assays; therefore, their function is unknown. Only HLA-A, HLA-B, and HLA-C MHC class I molecules have been shown to influence rejection of allografts. However, some class Ib molecules have been shown to present antigen.[195] These molecules include HLA-E, HLA-F, and HLA-G.[33, 35, 66, 98] Further analysis has more recently shown that some exhibit a restricted distribution. HLA-G, for example, is expressed in human embryos prior to implantation.[110, 129] HLA-E and HLA-G are also expressed in amnionic epithelium suggesting that they may play a role in the maintenance of maternal–fetal tolerance during pregnancy.[98, 129] Genetic analysis has shown that HLA-H and HLA-J are pseudogenes; therefore, they are not expressed.

Class II

The primary class II molecules relevant to human solid organ transplantation are called HLA-DR, HLA-DP, and HLA-DQ. These molecules are composed of a 33 to 35-kDa α-chain and a 26- to 28-kDa β-chain that are noncovalently associated (Fig. 2–5). Each of these chains contain two domains designated α_1 and α_2, and β_1 and β_2, respectively, and are expressed as transmembrane proteins. The α_1 and α_2 domains form the structure of the antigenic peptide-binding cleft. The β_2 domain interacts with **CD4 molecules,** which restricts the presentation of antigen in the groove of class II MHC molecules to CD4+ T-cells. Furthermore, the antigenic peptides displayed in the groove are derived from the exogenous processing pathway (see next section). The three-dimensional structure of an HLA-DR molecule was determined using x-ray crystallography (Fig. 2–3).[103] The peptide cleft of class II is very similar to class I except that the ends of the cleft are open so that longer peptides can be accommodated.

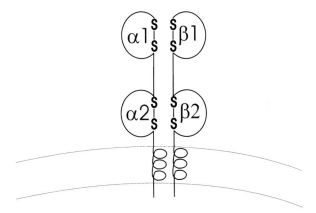

FIGURE **2–5.** Schematic of an MHC class II molecule composed of an α and β chain, each with two immunoglobulin-like domains designated α_1, α_2, and β_1, β_2, respectively. The majority of polymorphism in MHC class II molecules is in the β chain. The α chain is nearly invariant.

One of the key differences between class I and class II MHC molecules is that class I molecules are expressed on most nucleated cells in the body, whereas class II molecules are expressed on a restricted range of cell types that are generally involved in antigen processing and presentation such as macrophages/monocytes, dendritic cells, and B cells. Like class I molecules, the expression of class II molecules is inducible. Exposure of vascular endothelial cells to IFN-γ will up-regulate the surface expression of class II MHC molecules.[1, 11, 20, 165, 239] Other cells such as granulocytes, fibroblasts, and T-cells will also express class II MHC molecules following exposure to specific cytokines or when they are in the vicinity of an inflammatory process.[88]

Class III

Class III molecules have no known involvement in antigen presentation, although some are involved in antigen processing. Class III gene products are functionally and structurally diverse, and include complement components (C4b, C4a, C2, and factor B), the cytokine tumor necrosis factor-α (TNF-α), and heat shock proteins.[40]

Cell Processing of Antigens

Two basic pathways exist for cell processing of antigen which subsequently are displayed on the cell surface in the peptide-binding groove of an MHC molecule: the exogenous and the endogenous pathways.

Exogenous Pathway

Proteins originating from outside the cell and presented with MHC class II molecules are processed via the **exogenous pathway**[21, 149] (Fig. 2–6). **This is the principal pathway for processing and presenting alloantigens following organ transplantation.** The process is initiated when the antigen binds to the surface of the APC. The protein is internalized via receptor-mediated endocytosis or by phagocytosis and is retained in a vesicle. Alternatively, proteins in solution can be internalized by fluid-phase endocytosis to form endosomes. The proteins are subsequently broken down into peptides of 13 to 18 amino acids in length.[48, 102, 182, 193] The degradation of the protein into peptides takes place through several acidic compartments, each containing hydrolytic enzymes.

In the model illustrated in Figure 2–6 (not all components have been experimentally verified) the MHC class II molecule is synthesized in the endoplasmic reticulum. The molecule then noncovalently associates with an invariant chain in the groove (having the same basic amino acid sequence in all individuals) that is believed to serve at least two functions. The first is that it blocks the peptide-binding cleft in the MHC molecule in which an antigenic peptide would normally reside, presumably to prevent endogenous peptides from occupying the site before loading by a peptide processed via the endocytic pathway. The second function is that the amino-terminal end of the invariant chain guides the MHC molecule from the endoplasmic reticulum to the Golgi apparatus, and ultimately to the endocytic vesicles that contain the peptide fragments. Another class II–like molecule, called HLA-DM, catalyzes the removal of the invariant chain and the loading of a peptide in the peptide-binding groove. Although HLA-DM consists of α and β chains that closely resemble other class II molecules, it is not expressed at the cell surface but is found predominantly in vesicles in the cytoplasm. Following loading of the peptide (which in the case of transplantation, may be either donor MHC class I or II) into the binding cleft of

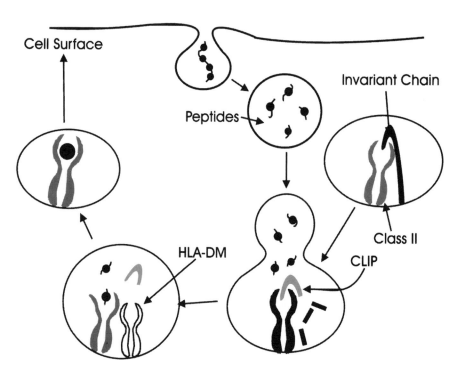

Cell Surface

Peptides

HLA-DM

Invariant Chain

Class II

CLIP

FIGURE **2–6.** Major histocompatibility complex class II molecule synthesis and processing of exogenous antigens. An exogenous antigen can be phagocytized or endocytosed (either receptor-mediated endocytosis or pinocytosis) by an antigen-presenting cell. Once internalized, the antigen is degraded in a series of acidic compartments (including lysosomes) to produce peptides that are 13 to 18 amino acids long, which can then be situated in the peptide-binding groove of a class II MHC molecule. At the same time, newly synthesized class II molecules are assembled and associated with the invariant chain in the endoplasmic reticulum. When the complex enters the endosomal compartment, the invariant chain is degraded, leaving a fragment called class II associated invariant chain peptide (CLIP) that occupies the peptide-binding groove of the class II molecule. The class II–like molecule, HLA-DM, catalyzes the release of CLIP and the loading of the antigenic peptide into the peptide-binding groove of the class II molecule.

the class II molecule, it is then transported to the cell surface for presentation to T-cells.[84]

Any protein from the donor organ can serve as an antigen. This includes donor MHC molecules that can be "eaten" via phagocytosis of shed donor cells, and cellular fragments or by fluid-phase endocytosis. The proteins are then broken down into peptides presumably via the exogenous pathway and presented within the binding groove of self-MHC molecules. Although the exogenous pathway is generally associated with MHC class II molecules, exogenous peptides can, under certain conditions, also be processed and presented with class I molecules.[41, 204] Thus, recipient APCs will have self-MHC molecules (usually class II, but also class I) containing peptides from MHC molecules originating from the donor.

Endogenous Pathway

Proteins originating from *inside* the cell are processed via the **endogenous pathway**,[43, 192] complexed with MHC class I molecules, and presented to T-cells[92, 99, 149] (Fig. 2–7). This pathway is distinctly different from the exogenous pathway discussed above and likely does not play a major role in transplant rejection. It is important to note that presumably any cell (not just APCs) uses this pathway in the presentation of internal peptides on MHC class I molecules. In the current model of this pathway, the endogenous proteins are degraded in the cytoplasm by a large protease complex called a proteosome. The resulting peptides are transported into the endoplasmic reticulum by a transporter protein in the membrane of the endoplasmic reticulum called the TAP transporter (*t*ransporter *a*ssociated with antigen *p*rocessing). Class I MHC molecules are synthesized in the endoplasmic reticulum, and loaded with a processed peptide. The resulting MHC–peptide complex is then transported via the Golgi apparatus to the surface,

TABLE 2–2	T-Cell Facts

- The thymus is required for T-cell development.
- When mature, all T-cells express CD3 surface molecules.
- Peripheral T-cells express CD4 or CD8 molecules, but not both.
- CD4 and CD8 surface markers identify T-cell populations with different immunologic capabilities (see Table 2–3).
- T-cells regulate antiviral and antifungal cellular immune responses
- T-cells regulate activation and differentiation of B-cells and switching of antibody secretion from IgM to other classes.

where it serves as a recognition site for cytotoxic CD8+ T-cells (which were previously stimulated by CD4+ [T-helper] cells which in turn had been activated by the same antigenic peptides processed by APCs through the exogenous pathway.) This pathway is typically utilized in the body's defense against intracellular pathogens such as viruses, whose proteins can be degraded and presented on the cell surface, resulting in the cell's destruction by cytotoxic CD8+ T-cells. It is important to note that, although endogenous processing is generally associated with class I MHC molecules, this pathway can also provide peptides which are presented with class II MHC molecules.[137]

T-LYMPHOCYTES

T-lymphocytes represent the most important part of the response of the transplant patient to the alloantigens from the transplanted heart (or other organ).[184, 187] T-lymphocytes are, by definition, lymphocytes with CD3 molecules (part of the T-cell antigen receptor) on their surface, and (usually) with either CD4 or CD8 molecules on their surface (Table 2–2). There are two basic subtypes of T-lymphocytes, similar in their morphology but varied in their functions. The **helper T-**

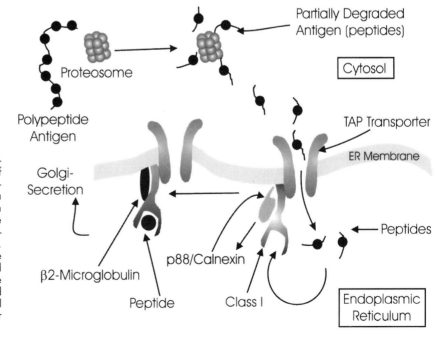

FIGURE **2–7.** Synthesis of major histocompatibility complex class I molecules and processing of endogenous antigens. Class I molecules are assembled in the endoplasmic reticulum with calnexin, a membrane-bound protein. β₂-Microglobulin is then substituted for calnexin and the class I molecule binds to the TAP transporter. Proteins in the cytoplasm are degraded to peptides by proteosomes. The peptides are transported into the lumen of the endoplasmic reticulum by the TAP transporter, and a peptide is loaded into the peptide-binding groove of the class I molecule. The molecule is then released from the TAP transporter and exported to the cell surface via the Golgi complex. TAP, transporter associated with antigen processing.

lymphocyte expresses CD4 molecules on its surface and functions primarily to detect nonself antigens by virtue of its T-cell receptors. Once activated, it can also recruit other cells (CD8$^+$ T-cells, other CD4$^+$ T-cells, B cells, phagocytes, neutrophils, and other inflammatory cells) into the immune response. The other type is called the **cytotoxic T-lymphocyte,** which differs from the helper T-lymphocyte in that it has CD8 molecules on its surface (Table 2–3). It functions primarily as an effector cell which kills target cells (cells which express nonself antigen in the groove of a class I MHC molecule) and, under special circumstances, may suppress other cells (prevent them from being activated) (see later section, Tolerance in Transplantation).

The Thymus Gland and T-Lymphocytes

T-lymphocytes gained their name from the discovery that the **thymus** gland is required for the maturation and subsequent appearance of T-lymphocytes in the peripheral circulation. The precursor cells that will eventually develop into T-lymphocytes originate in the bone marrow. T-cell precursors migrate to the thymus where they first appear in the subcapsular cortex. At this point, they have not yet "expressed" (produced and moved to the cell surface) CD3, CD4, or CD8 molecules. However, they soon begin to do so, resulting in many T-lymphocytes having both CD4 and CD8 molecules present on their surfaces.

During the process of thymic development, T-lymphocytes acquire a T-cell receptor, which confers the ability to bind a processed form of an antigen. All the T-cell receptors on a given cell are the same, but the T-cell receptors on each cell are unique with respect to T-cell receptors on other cells. As a T-cell multiplies, each of its progeny will bear the same T-cell receptor. Therefore, each T-cell with a unique receptor is called a "clone," and therefore a group of cells derived from the same parent (and therefore bearing identical receptors) are said to be derived from a single clone. Because of the genetic mechanism by which this diverse array of T-cell receptors are produced, the specificity of each clone (i.e., the antigen to which the receptor is capable of binding) is not predetermined to be helpful to the host. A critical part of the development of the immune system is the elimination of certain T-cells that are harmful to an individual's chance of survival.[124] For example, T-cells that bind to self-antigens can attack components of one's own body (seen as autoimmune diseases). Other T-cells are ineffective at binding to self-MHC molecules (required for T-cell activation) and are therefore useless to the immune system. These undesirable cells are selectively identified and destroyed in the thymus in a process called **selection.** During the selective process, the cells migrate from the thymic cortex to the medulla from which they migrate to the periphery.

T-Cell Receptor

In order for a T-lymphocyte to detect the presence of a nonself antigen, it must have an antigen receptor. The **T-cell receptor** confers to T-lymphocytes the capability of binding to antigen and MHC molecules in a specific manner, a characteristic acquired by T-lymphocytes as they undergo the selection process in the thymus. This receptor is the primary structure that is used for the detection of nonself antigens, including nonself MHC antigens present on the transplanted heart. Each T-lymphocyte clone has a T-cell receptor that is unique with respect to the receptors of other T-cell clones and therefore also has a unique T-cell genetic sequence compared to other T-cell clones.

Functional analyses of T-cell populations have shown that the number of antigens to which an individual can respond is very large. Estimates of the number of possible different T-cell receptor genes are as high as 10^{15}. Thus, in each individual, there is a pool of T-cells, each bearing a unique T-cell receptor variable region sequence. This pool of unique T-cells constitutes the so called T-cell repertoire producing greater than 10^{12} unique T-cell receptors in a given individual.

In order to code for the large array of different T-cell receptors using a reasonable amount of genetic material, the genes for the T-cell receptor are assembled from segments that can be assembled in a combinatorial fashion (the gene segments are combined, each having multiple possible amino acid sequences). Although it was known that T-cell–mediated responses were antigen specific and that T-cells must possess some type of antigen receptor, the T-cell receptor molecule was not identified until the early 1980s, when the tools, in the form of clone-specific monoclonal antibodies and nucleic acid probes generated from subtractive cDNA libraries, became available.[49, 50, 91, 126, 136, 253, 254]

TABLE 2–3	T-Cell Types	
	CD4$^+$ (HELPER)	CD8$^+$ (CYTOTOXIC)
Specificity	Recognize antigen in association with class II MHC molecules expressed on antigen-presenting cells	Recognize antigen in association with class I MHC molecules
Function	Undergo activation by antigen-presenting cells and proliferate. Facilitate the activation, proliferation, and differentiation of cytotoxic T-cells. Provide "help" for the activation and differentiation of B-cells, and regulate antibody class switching. Facilitate inflammation by secretion of cytokines.	Can kill virus-infected cells and cells expressing nonself antigens.
Proportion of peripheral T-cell population	Two thirds	One third
Subtypes	TH1 and TH2, possibly others	Type 1 and Type 2

Given the specificity of T-cell responses and the ability to respond to a wide array of different antigens, it is not surprising that the genetic structure of T-cell receptor genes is organized in a manner that is similar to immunoglobulins (see later section B-Lymphocytes). The T-cell receptor belongs to a diverse group of proteins in the immunoglobulin superfamily (a superfamily is a group of related proteins that have some degree of amino acid sequence homology). All proteins in the immunoglobulin superfamily have one or more immunoglobulin domains, which are regions of 70 to 110 amino acids that bear homology with the immunoglobulin variable or constant region domains. Each domain usually contains cysteine residues that connect a disulfide bonded loop of 55 to 75 amino acids.

The portion of the T-cell receptor that contacts the antigenic peptide–MHC complex is a heterodimer of two covalently linked polypeptide chains designated α and β (note that there is a smaller T-cell population that bears different T-cell receptor chains called γ and δ). The α chain is 40 to 60 kDa and the β chain is 40 to 50 kDa (Fig. 2–8).[89] The α and β chains each have a variable region (V-region) that forms a series of loops that typically contains an extremely variable amino acid sequence that arises from the combinatorial joining of the gene segments that make up the variable portion of the gene.[24, 245, 253] The complex rearrangement of T-cell variable region gene segments (see Box) makes possible the huge array of unique T-cell receptors in each individual (Fig. 2–9).

The α and β chains are associated with a complex of membrane-bound proteins designated the **CD3 complex**.[173] The CD3 complex is formed from five invariant polypeptide chains in which the T-cell receptor heterodimer is associated with the CD3 complex. The CD3 complex is required for the expression of the T-cell receptor on the cell surface and is responsible for the transduction of a transmembrane signal when the T-cell receptor complex is perturbed by antigen or cross-linked by other molecules.[247] One of the most vivid demonstrations of this fact is the "cytokine syndrome," which occurs after administration of OKT3 (see Chapter 13).

Rearrangement of Variable Region Gene Segments in the T-Cell Receptor

The portion of the genes that code for the V-region of the T-cell receptor is composed of a series of gene segments called **variable** (V), **diversity** (D—found only in the β and δ chains), and **joining** (J) (Fig. 2–9).[245] In the human T-cell receptor β-locus, there are at least 63 different variable regions that have been expressed.[175, 200, 240] There are also two diversity gene segments and 13 functional J-segments.[12, 16, 52, 197, 198, 228] Functional T-cell receptor genes are assembled through a process of rearrangement of the genomic DNA in which the intervening DNA between the two gene segments (e.g., a diversity gene segment and a joining gene segment) is spliced out. Given that any diversity gene segment could combine with any joining gene segment which, in turn, could combine with any variable gene segment, the number of possible combinations is large. The results of this recombination is made even more variable by the presence of mechanisms that make the joining process itself highly variable. For example, the diversity and joining gene segments can join with each other in a variety of different places due to the "nibbling" of nucleotides from the end of the gene segment. There is also random addition of bases to the gene segment ends, which increases the variability even further.

Perturbation of the CD3 complex triggers a transmembrane signal in the T-cell and causes the release of factors that promote cytokine production. These cytokines (particularly TNF-α) generate the symptoms that can be observed following administration of OKT3.[44–46, 82, 227]

Antigen Recognition by T-Lymphocytes

In the context of the immunologic response, the term "recognition" refers to the ability of a lymphocyte to respond to the presence of a specific antigen. For this event to occur, an antigen receptor on the surface of a

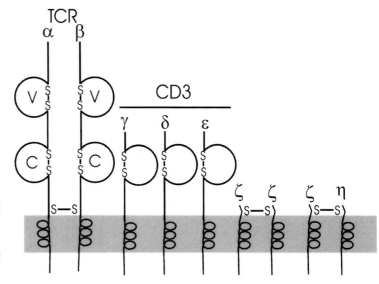

FIGURE **2–8.** The T-cell receptor is a multichain complex. The T-cell receptor complex consists of a heterodimer which, in the majority of T-cells, consists of an α and β chain each of which has immunoglobulin-like domains, as indicated by the loops held together by disulfide (S-S) bonds. These chains constitute the portion of the molecule that binds the antigen–MHC complex on the surface of an antigen-presenting cell. The α and β chains are noncovalently linked to the CD3 complex, that consists of chains called γ, δ and ε. The two additional chains can be either of two pairs composed of two ζ-chains, or of a ζ-chain and a η-chain. The CD3 complex transmits a signal through the plasma membrane (shaded in gray) into the interior of the cell.

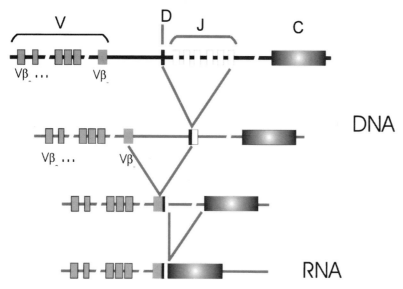

FIGURE **2–9.** T-cell receptor gene arrangement. Diversity in the number of distinct T-cell receptor molecules, each having distinct specificities for antigenic peptides in conjunction with an MHC molecule, is generated by assembling the gene from a series of interchangeable gene segments that can be assembled in different combinations in a process called gene rearrangement. In this example, the T-cell receptor β-chain gene rearrangement begins with the juxtaposition of a diversity (D) segment with one of the several possible joining (J) gene segments. The intervening DNA between the gene segments is removed. This is followed by rearrangement of the subsequent DJ rearrangement with one of many different variable (V) gene segments to form a fully rearranged β-chain gene. This gene can then be transcribed into RNA, and is then spliced to a constant region C. This RNA transcript is then translated to the protein that is subsequently expressed on the surface of the cell.

T-cell must bind to the antigenic molecule and transmit a signal to the interior of the cell. The unique aspect of immunologic recognition is that it is highly specific, meaning that only one particular antigen will be detected by a single T-cell clone despite the presence of a large and diverse array of other antigens.

T cells recognize antigen only in the presence of self-MHC. In the case of helper T-cells, which initiate the cellular (in contrast to antibody mediated) response to transplant antigens, the antigen must be associated with an MHC complex on the cell surface through a process called **antigen presentation.** This presentation can be performed by a limited array of cell types collectively called **antigen-presenting cells.** Before a T-cell reacts to an antigen, the antigen must be internalized within the APC, in which it is broken down into polypeptides approximately 7 to 13 amino acids in length. The peptides are then physically associated with MHC molecules and exported to the cell surface as a complex. As noted previously, MHC molecules are said to be class I, class II, or class III, based on their structure, tissue distribution, and genetic location. The most important functional difference between class I and class II MHC molecules for the purposes of this discussion is that "helper T-cells" (i.e., T-cells which have on their surface CD4 molecules) respond only to those other cells that have **class II MHC**

molecules on their surfaces. Cytotoxic T-cells (CD8⁺) cells respond to those cells that have **class I MHC** molecules on their surfaces. A number of other T-cell surface molecules have been identified which participate in the immune response (Table 2–4).

ANTIGEN-PRESENTING CELLS

Since T-cells recognize antigens only on the surface of other cells, a functionally distinct class of cells exists that present antigens to T-lymphocytes. These cells process antigen by breaking them down into individual peptides, inserting the peptides into the peptide-binding groove of MHC molecules, and transporting them to the cell surface (Table 2–5).

Cells that serve as APCs are **dendritic cells, macrophages,** and **B cells.** Of the three, dendritic cells are considered to be the most important because they can present antigen to T-lymphocytes very efficiently. Dendritic cells have a very large surface area, therefore increasing the probability of contact with T-lymphocytes as they migrate through areas where the dendritic cells reside. Dendritic cells can be found scattered throughout most lymphoid and nonlymphoid tissues, and they possess a distinctive phenotype that includes an increased

TABLE 2–4	**Major T-Cell Markers**	
NAME	SYNONYMS*	FUNCTIONS
CD2	T11, LFA-2, sheep red blood cell receptor	Adhesion (CD58) molecule. Binds LFA-3 (CD58). Can trigger T-cell activation.
CD3	T3	T-cell receptor complex bearing the subunits used in transmembrane signaling.
CD4	T4	Adhesion. Acts as a co-receptor for the T-cell receptor by binding to MHC class II. Also a receptor for human immunodeficiency virus.
CD7		Function unknown. One of the earliest markers to appear during thymic development. Also expressed on pluripotent hematopoietic stem cells.
CD8	T8	Adhesion. Acts as co-receptor.
CD28	Tp44	Co-stimulatory receptor (binds to B7.1 and B7.2).
CD45	T200, leukocyte common antigen	Expressed in several different isoforms due to alternative RNA splicing. Contains tyrosine phosphatase activity.
CD69	Activation inducer molecule (AIM)	Unknown. Expressed on activated T-cells, and on other lineages.

*Often no longer used.

TABLE 2-5	**Antigen-Presenting Cells (APCs)**

- Derived from bone marrow
- Process peptides and present antigen to T-cells
- Transport foreign antigens to lymph nodes for interaction with T-cells
- Express adhesion molecules that facilitate TCR binding to the peptide–MHC complex
- Provides co-stimulatory "second signals" to activate the T-cell

density of surface MHC class II molecules relative to other APCs such as macrophages and B cells. Dendritic cells isolated from lymphoid tissue are often called lymphoid dendritic cells. These cells are particularly adept at triggering T-lymphocyte responses in vitro.

Antigen presenting cells also provide a **second signal** that is necessary for T-cell activation. The second signal is the binding of another molecule on the surface of the T-cell in addition to the binding of the T-cell receptor by an antigen–MHC complex. Some of the molecules that increase adhesion of T cells to APCs during T-cell activation are listed in Table 2–6.

B-LYMPHOCYTES

B-lymphocytes are so named because they were originally described to arise from the **Bursa of Fabricius** in the chicken. There is no such organ in humans, and human B-lymphocytes have been subsequently shown to arise from the bone marrow. Unlike T-lymphocytes, B-lymphocytes have neither CD4 nor CD8 molecules on their surfaces, use surface immunoglobulins rather than T-cell receptors for the detection of antigen, and do not travel through the thymus during development. In contrast to T-lymphocytes, the end product of B-cell activation is the differentiation of B-cells into antibody-secreting plasma cells and memory B-cells (B-cells that are retained following the end of an immune response that are called upon when there is a subsequent exposure to the same antigen).

Antigen Recognition by B-Lymphocytes

Membrane-bound (surface) **immunoglobulins** serve as the antigen-binding portion of the antigen receptor for

B-lymphocytes. Like the T-cell receptor, surface immunoglobulins must bind to a large array of antigens, with the exception that immunoglobulins can bind to antigens in solution, and not antigenic peptides complexed with MHC molecules as T-cell receptor molecules do. They are also assembled from gene segments such that a large number of different immunoglobulin molecules can be assembled using a minimum of genetic material. In general, B-lymphocytes, like T-lymphocytes, do not normally mount a response against self antigens. However, not all antibody interactions with self molecules are harmful. The anti-idiotypic (antiself) response[105] refers to antibodies which have a specificity for certain autologous immunoglobulins as part of normal immune regulation. Theoretically, an ongoing humoral immune response may be beneficially inhibited by the production of these anti-idiotypic antibodies.

Antibody Structure

Immunoglobulins (antibodies) are produced in quantity by B-cells that have differentiated into plasma cells. They consist of four polypeptide chains in two pairs. Each pair of chains is identical to the other, consisting of a heavy chain and a shorter light chain, and each pair is linked to the other to form the complete antibody molecule shown in Figure 2–10.[64, 65, 73] The end of the molecule in which the light chain is paired to the heavy chain forms the antigen-binding portion of the molecule, which is approximately 107 to 115 amino acids long. This end of the molecule is called the variable region because the genes that code for the heavy and light chains are composed of segments that join together im-

TABLE 2-6	**Molecules that Increase Adhesion of T-Cell/APC Interactions during T-Cell Activation**

T-CELL SURFACE MOLECULE	LIGAND ON APC
LFA-1	ICAM-1
	ICAM-2
	ICAM-3
CD2	LFA-3(CD58)
CD5	CD72
CD28	B7.1 (CD80), B7.2 (CD86), CTLA-4
CD4	MHC class II
CD8	MHC class I

APC, antigen-presenting cell; LFA, leukocyte function associated; ICAM, intercellular adhesion molecule; MHC, major histocompatibility complex.

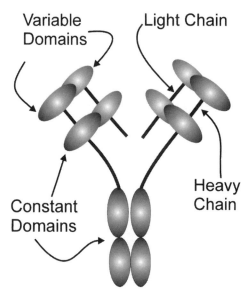

FIGURE **2–10.** A schematic of the structure of an immunoglobulin molecule. An individual antibody molecule consists of two heavy and two light chains. Each heavy chain and light chain combine to form a single antigen-binding region for a total of two antigenic binding sites. Both the heavy and light chains contain a series of sequence motifs about 100 amino acids in length that can fold into globular forms, which are called immunoglobulin domains. The two constant region domains in each heavy chain that are furthest from the variable domains constitute the Fc receptor and complement-binding portions of the molecule. The variable domains constitute the antigen-binding site.

precisely. The other end of the heavy chain, consisting of a single gene segment, is called the constant region, consisting of approximately 107 to 110 amino acids for the light chain and 310 to 330 amino acids for the heavy chain.[94] The constant region contains sites for a number of biologically important activities, such as the activation of complement. In order for the immune system to contend with the vast universe of different antigens, the antigen-binding portion of the molecule must be extremely heterogeneous. Special features of immunoglobulin antigen receptors and gene rearrangement (see Box) account for this heterogeneity.

The heavy chain constant regions form the basis of the classification of immunoglobulin (Ig) molecules into groups (also called isotypes) named (in relative decreasing order of abundance in the peripheral circulation) IgG, IgA, IgM, IgD, and IgE. IgG can be further subdivided into subclasses consisting of IgG1 through IgG4,

---

Immunoglobulin Antigen Receptors and Gene Rearrangement

If the genes for these molecules were constructed in the fashion in which most other genes are constructed (i.e., one gene = one protein), the number of structural genes that would code for antibody molecules would require most of the genome. Characterization of the immunoglobulin genes has established that the polypeptide chains are coded by genes that are assembled from multiple gene segments. During B-cell development, one of 30 diversity (D) gene segments is joined to one of 6 joining (J) segments by removal of the intervening genomic DNA in a process called gene rearrangement. To form the complete gene, the rearranged DJ segment is joined to one of 50 variable (V) region gene segments. Light chains are assembled in a similar fashion except that only variable (V) and joining (J) gene segments are used.[190, 225, 226] Thus, each B-cell potentially produces a unique immunoglobulin molecule. The potential diversity of gene rearrangement is further enhanced by the fact that the joining of gene segments is imprecise, such that individual nucleotides at the end of the gene segments can be removed during the joining process,[132, 133] and individual nucleotides can be randomly added to the ends of a gene segment.[8, 58] This results in a potential repertoire of immunoglobulin molecules that is extremely large, potentially with more than 10^{14} different antigen receptors.

Unlike the T-cell receptor, which is also assembled from individual gene segments, rearranged immunoglobulin V-regions can mutate. This process of somatic mutation is the basis for a phenomenon called "affinity maturation" where, as a humoral response proceeds, the affinity of the antibodies that are specific for an antigen increases with time.[25, 117] As the genes that code for an antigen-specific immunoglobulin mutate, an individual base change due to mutation can either increase the binding affinity, decrease the binding affinity, or change the specificity of an antibody molecule entirely. B-cells that lose the ability to bind antigen are allowed to die through the induction of apoptosis. Thus, through a process that resembles positive selection of thymocytes, B cells that bind antigen with higher affinity tend to accumulate.

---

and IgA can be divided into IgA1 and IgA2.[158] The constant regions of light chains are classified into two groups called κ and λ chains. The constant region portion of the molecule is that portion that mediates effector responses that can serve to accelerate the clearance of antigen or the destruction of microorganisms. The antigen-binding portion of the molecule separated from the constant region is called the F(ab') region or F(ab')$_2$ fragment depending on whether the fragment is monovalent or divalent, respectively. The remaining constant region fragment is called the Fc region.

Isotype Switching

When a unique antigen is encountered for the first time, the first antibody produced in response to that antigen is IgM. These IgM antibodies tend to be of lower affinity but are a strong activator of complement. Later responses are dominated by IgG as *isotype switching* occurs, in which the same variable region is joined to a different constant region by a process called *switch recombination,* resulting in a change in the effector functions of the antibody (Fig. 2–11). Isotype switching is directed by CD4$^+$ T cells through a series of surface interactions with B cells, which requires T-cell engagement with CD40 on B cells. Switching begins about 6 days following B-cell activation *in vivo,* and at about the same time that somatic mutation begins to occur in the variable region of the immunoglobulin gene.[205] IgG becomes the dominant isotype in the circulation and in the extracellular fluids, whereas IgA dominates in the mucosa. The pattern of cytokines present, in large part, determines what kind of switch will take place.

NATURAL KILLER CELLS

Morphologically, NK cells strongly resemble T- and B-lymphocytes, but they have an entirely different function. NK cells are not antigen specific and do not express either a T-cell receptor or immunoglobulins.[112] In 1975, two groups demonstrated that there was a population of lymphoid cells that could spontaneously lyse tumor cells and cell lines *in vitro.*[93, 116] These cells were called *natural killer cells,* or NK cells,[239] because the ability to lyse the target cells did not require prior immunization and was not restricted by the major histocompatibility complex like normal T-cell receptor–mediated lysis, and in fact, could also lyse cell targets that lacked the surface expression of MHC molecules. Subsequent experiments have indicated that an oversimplified but useful concept is that "T-lymphocytes kill what they *recognize* and NK cells kill what they *do not recognize.*"

It was learned relatively early that NK cells could kill (lyse) the target cells (or antigen) regardless of the presence or absence of the major MHC molecule complexes; in other words, they were unlike T-lymphocytes in that they could "kill" cells, even though the NK cells lacked on their surface MHC molecules. Natural killer cells tend to represent, in the peripheral blood, approximately 15% of lymphoid cells.

More recently, a class of surface receptors on NK cells has been described that bind to MHC molecules. These

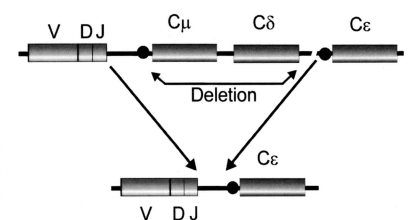

FIGURE **2-11.** A model of immunoglobulin isotype switching. Isotype switching occurs through a process called switch recombination. The rearranged VDJ gene segments that code for the variable region of the molecule recombine to a constant region gene segment that is further downstream, resulting in the deletion of the intervening DNA.

receptors, called killer-cell inhibitory receptors, inhibit killing by NK cells if they are bound to MHC molecules. Therefore, NK cells will kill cells having no MHC molecules or a nonself MHC molecule.

CYTOKINES

Many important soluble **molecules** play a role in the immunologic response. This group includes **cytokines,** which are secreted proteins that alter the behavior or properties of cells, and facilitate the recruitment of cells from other locations. Unlike hormones, most cytokines act locally and are not usually found in the circulation in large quantities because of their short half-life. Simple categorization of cytokine function is difficult because their activities often depend on the target cell type and the presence of other cytokines, whose activities may be similar (Table 2–7). The nomenclature of cytokines (see Box) is also confusing. In the context of transplanta-

TABLE 2-7	**Important Cytokines in Transplant Immunology**	
	SOURCE	RELEVANT FUNCTIONAL ACTIVITIES
IL-1	Monocytes, macrophages, endothelium, mesangial cells, fibroblasts, keratinocytes, most nucleated cells in response to injury	Inflammation, migration of neutrophils and macrophages; T-cell proliferation up-regulation of IL-2R; B-cell differentiation
IL-2	Activated T-cells, NK cells	Activation, growth, and differentiation of activated T-cells and thymocytes; increased NK activity; B-cell differentiation and proliferation
IL-4	Activated T-cells, mast cells	Cofactor in B-cell activation, growth, and differentiation; immunoglobulin class switching; activation, growth, and differentiation of T-cells, especially cytotoxic T-cells; proliferation of mast cell lines; inhibition of IL-2 action on B-cells and NK cells
IL-5	Activated T-cells, mast cells, eosinophils	Growth and differentiation of eosinophils
IL-6	Probably most nucleated cells	B-cell proliferation and antibody secretion; T-cell activation, growth, and differentiation; induction of acute phase proteins
IL-7	Bone marrow stromal cells, thymus	Stimuation of T- and B-cell precursors; T-cell maturation in the thymus; proliferation of mature T-cells; activation of NK cells
IL-8 and other chemokines	Activated T-cells, monocytes, endothelial cells, hepatocytes, fibroblasts, epithelial cells, chondrocytes, keratinocytes, neutrophils	Neutrophil activation, migration, and adhesion to activated endothelium; inflammation
IL-10	Activated T-cells, B-cells, monocytes and macrophages, mast cell lines, keratinocytes	Inhibition of synthesis of cytokines (mainly IFN-γ) by TH1 cells through inhibition of macrophage IL-12 synthesis
IL-12	Activated macrophages, activated B-cells, dendritic cells, keratinocytes	Induction IFN-γ production by NK cells; essential for TH1 cell differentiation and proliferation
IL-13	Activated T-cells	Inhibition of production of inflammatory cytokines
IFN-γ	Activated T-cells, NK cells	Activation of macrophages and monocytes; induction of MHC class I and class II; increase in NK activity; inhibits TH2 cell proliferation; inhibition of IL-4 induced B-cell activation
TNF-α	Monocytes, macrophages, T-cell, NK cells, Kupffer cells, microglia, B-cells	Inflammation; mediator of cachexia
TNF-β	Activated T-cells and B-cells	Cytotoxic for cells, particularly tumor cells; proinflammatory mediator
TGF-β	Platelets, activated macrophages, bone	Cell growth control; recruitment and activation of mononuclear cells in inflammation and wound healing

---

Nomenclature of Cytokines

Each new cytokine is usually named after the activity it supports, such as T-cell growth factor, or macrophage-activating factor. These names tend to be confusing because the activity of a cytokine can change depending on the target cell type. As a result, it is not unusual for two groups to identify the same molecule while using completely different experimental systems and names. Some immunologists will also use the term "lymphokine" to denote cytokines secreted by lymphocytes and "monokines" to denote cytokines produced by monocytes/macrophages. A naming convention has been established in which a cytokine is designated by the name interleukin followed by a number. For example, the cytokine formerly known as T-cell growth factor is called interleukin-2 (IL-2).

---

tion, the cytokines that have received most attention are those involved in inflammatory processes and in the regulation of T-cell–mediated responses. Cytokine production is one of the hallmarks of T-cell activation, and many research groups have attempted to use measurements of cytokine protein levels in the peripheral blood for immunologic monitoring.[72, 77, 114, 187, 227] Unfortunately, studies have thus far failed to convincingly correlate such levels with occurrence of rejection events in a clinically useful manner. In part, this could relate to the role of cytokines as largely local mediators, and levels in the periphery may not reflect local events.

Interleukin-2

One of the best characterized cytokines is IL-2, which is a key growth factor that is required for the expansion of T-cells during a T-cell–mediated response. The receptor for IL-2 (IL-2R) is composed of three subunits, designated α, β, and γ. Following stimulation, the cell begins to make the α chain of the T-cell receptor, which complexes with the remaining chains to form the high-affinity IL-2 receptor.[78, 209, 213] Stimulated cells begin to make IL-2, and also respond to IL-2 via the IL-2 receptor in an autocrine fashion. If the cell receives a co-stimulatory signal at the time of ligation (binding) of the T-cell receptor, it will begin to proliferate, and within a few days the progeny of the originally stimulated clone can increase by several orders of magnitude.

IL-2 is regulated at the transcriptional level.[106] Examination of the promotor region shows that transcription is regulated by transcription factors that bind to regulatory elements coded by the IL-2 gene. Some of these factors are regulated by co-stimulatory signals such as those through CD28, which can also affect the rate of IL-2 mRNA degradation.

Interleukin-6

Interleukin-6 was originally described by several different groups as interferon-$\beta2$,[241] IL-1 inducible 26-kDa protein, and as a factor that induced B-cells to differentiate

into plasma cells.[171] However, cloning of the factors that mediated these activities showed that they were from the same molecule.[189] This feature, in which a single molecule mediates a variety of activities, is a hallmark of many cytokines which act on a variety of cells. A number of laboratories have measured plasma or serum IL-6 levels following transplantation and have found no consistent specific correlation with rejection, because this cytokine can also be induced by infections and by surgical trauma alone. IL-6, like TNF and IL-1, is released during an "acute phase response" in which a global response is made to bacterial endotoxins. Like TNF, IL-6 has been implicated in cachexia.

Tumor Necrosis Factor

The ability of TNF to kill tumor cells led to its discovery and the reason for its name. It was originally described as a serum factor in mice treated with endotoxin and possessed the ability to induce hemorrhagic necrosis of sarcomas.[37] Further characterization has shown that it is secreted by activated macrophages, lymphocytes, mast cells, neutrophils, keratinocytes, astrocytes, microglial cells, smooth muscle cells, and tumor cells.[17] TNF has been identified as a primary inducer of cachexia,[29] and its primary activities *in vivo* are proinflammatory and cytotoxic. It is induced by other proinflammatory mediators such as IL-1, granulocyte-monocyte colony stimulating factor, TNF-α (an autocrine response), and by phorbol esters.[202, 229] The proinflammatory activity is stimulated through the activation of neutrophils, which then show increased phagocytic activity, degranulation, oxidative burst, and adherence to endothelium.[14, 15, 119, 194] Similar effects on macrophages are also observed. TNF and the TNF-related genes are all located within the MHC locus.

In its biologically active form, TNF exists as a 52-kDa trimer of three identical 17-kDa chains.[17, 62, 107, 201] TNF is the prototypical form of the eight-member TNF-ligand superfamily, which consists of type II membrane proteins (C-terminus extracellular, N-terminus intracellular, and a single transmembrane component).

Interferon-γ

IFN-γ was originally identified as a factor produced by T-cells that inhibited viral replication in vitro.[241] This cytokine is capable of regulating specific immune responses because of direct effects on T-cells in which the differentiation of T-cells involved in cellular immunity are augmented (called TH1 cells, see below) and differentiation into cells involved in humoral immunity (called TH2 cells) are inhibited. IFN-γ can also directly stimulate NK cells and cytotoxic T-cells. One of its most potent proinflammatory activities is as an activator of macrophages and monocytes. IFN-γ induces increased production of reactive oxygen and nitrogen intermediates including peroxynitrites, hydrogen peroxide, and nitric oxide.

IFN-γ has also been found to up-regulate the expression of HLA class I and HLA class II molecules on endothelial cells *in vitro* and therefore may serve to make these cells capable of presenting antigen and facilitate an immune response against donor tissue.[20, 159, 237, 239]

Pattern of Cytokine Release by T-Cell Clones (The TH1/TH2 Paradigm)

Characterization of the function of immune responses shows that antigenic stimulation can result in either a cellular or humoral response. Mossman and colleagues showed that subpopulations of T-cells could be identified that secrete specific cytokines[47, 150] (Fig. 2–12). Historically, the TH1 and TH2 designation referred to subsets of T-helper cells.[208] A more appropriate designation is type 1 and type 2 cells, since both CD4[+] and CD8[+] cells are capable of restrictive cytokine production.

Type 1 cells participate in *cellular responses* such as those directed towards mycobacterial antigens, and elaborate the proinflammatory cytokines IL-2 (a growth and differentiation factor for cytotoxic T-lymphocyte precursors) and IFN-γ (a potent macrophage activation factor). *Type 2 cells* primarily secrete IL-4, IL-5, IL-10, and IL-13, and are associated with *humoral immunity* against extracellular pathogens.[100, 150, 183, 252] IL-4 plays a special role in promoting B-cell proliferation and differentiation into antibody-producing cells. Type 0 cells do not appear to show a restricted pattern of cytokine production, and could either be precursors of the type 1 and type 2 subsets, or they could be a distinct subset.[55, 151]

A current model of immune regulation indicates that during T-cell activation, the APC and other "bystander" cells provide signals which direct the T cell toward type 1 or type 2 cytokine patterns. Apparently, the longer the immune stimulus persists, the more polarized the cytokine production, resulting in differing manifestations of the immune response.[151]

The type 1 and type 2 cell types are counterregulatory, and the balance between IL-12 and IL-4 determines their predominance.[167, 230, 231] The presence of IL-12, produced by dendritic cells and macrophages, promotes the development of TH1 cells and inhibits the appearance of TH2 cell activity.[3, 100, 118, 144] Conversely, IL-4, inhibits the development of TH1 cells by suppressing IL-12 production by monocytes.[54, 57] The source of IL-4 (and other cytokines which promote the TH2 response) is currently unclear, since these cytokines are both the primers and the products of TH2 cells. Basophils, mast cells, and other T-cell subsets have been implicated in the production of IL-4. Specific co-stimulatory signals during T-cell activation may also promote TH1 or TH2 predominance (see later section, Activation of T-Lymphocytes).[115, 186]

The TH1/TH2 paradigm has led to a model in which TH1 cells (proinflammatory) or TH2 cells (neutral or suppressive) can predominate in the control of the immune response in a clonally specific fashion,[55, 108, 139, 160, 208] but this may be an oversimplification of the pathogenesis of rejection.

ADHESION MOLECULES

Adhesion molecules are protein molecules which are formed within cells and then "secreted" into the environment of the cells which create them. They function to maintain structural integrity and position of body cells and promote adhesion of leukocytes to surrounding structures. These adhesion molecules include **integrins, selectins,** and **Ig superfamily adhesion molecules** (Table 2–8).

Cytokines, adhesion molecules, and similar molecules play a highly important supportive role in all immuno-

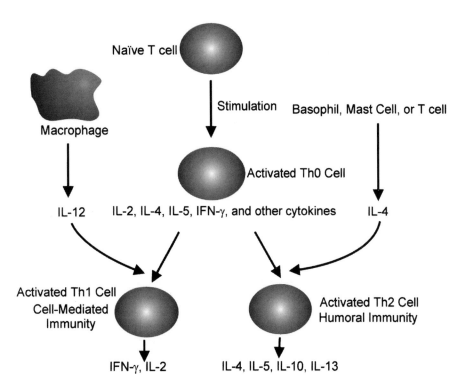

FIGURE **2–12.** Differentiation and cytokine secretion patterns of TH1 and TH2 cells. T cells can be divided into subsets based on their pattern of cytokine secretion. The differentiation of T cells into either TH1 and TH2 types is strongly influenced by the array of cytokines in the T-cell microenvironment. Interleukin-12 facilitates the development of TH1 cells, and IL-4 facilitates the development of TH2 cells. The differentiated cells, in turn, themselves secrete various cytokines that can influence the outcome of immune responses in which the T cells participate.

TABLE 2-8	Adhesion Molecules
CLASSIFICATION	NAME
β_1 Integrins	VLA-1
	VLA-2
	VLA-3
	VLA-4
	VLA-5
	VLA-6
β_2 Integrins	LFA-1 (CD11a/CD18)
	MAC-1 CD11b/CD18)
	CR4 (P150,95) (CD11c/CD18)
Selectins	P-selectin (CD62P)
	E-selectin (CD62E)
	L-selectin (CD62L)
Ig Superfamily	VCAM
	ICAM
	PECAM
	LFA-2 (CD2)
	LFA-3 (CD58)

logic responses, including rejection. Leukocytes adhere and localize to particular locations or microenvironments based on the pattern of molecular signals (from cytokines, adhesion molecules, and other molecules) on the surface of endothelial cells that line vessel walls. They may be up-regulated (caused to increase their numbers) by injury to the transplanted heart (or other organ) and by any sort of immune response.

Adhesion Molecules and Cellular Trafficking

A critical part of the immune response is the aggregation and transport of leukocytes into areas targeted for immunologic attack. Adhesion molecules mediate the initial interaction of T-cells with antigens, their migration, and their retention within a transplanted organ. Similarly, the activation of T-cells in the peripheral lymphoid organs such as the lymph nodes and spleen is also dependent on adhesion molecules. These molecules regulate the manner in which leukocytes home to various tissues and are retained following encounters with inflammatory molecules or antigens on the surfaces of other cells. In general, **integrins** act as cellular "glue," holding cells in position by anchoring to the extracellular matrix; cell-to-cell adhesion is usually the role of **selectins** and **immunoglobulin superfamily** molecules. Up-regulation (see Box) of immunoglobulin superfamily

Up-Regulation/Down-Regulation

Immunologists differentiate subpopulations of cells based on the pattern and density of cell surface molecules on the cells in question. Therefore, it is common to see or hear discussion of a cell population in which cell surface molecules begin to increase (are up-regulated) or decrease (down-regulated) in density based on time relative to some event or location. The density of cell surface molecules is typically determined using flow cytometry or immunofluorescence microscopy, with the brightness of the stained cell directly proportional to the density of the labeled molecules on the cell surface.

molecules along the vessel wall causes the leukocytes to stop rolling, stick to the wall, and migrate through it in a process called diapedesis (Fig. 2–13).[203]

It should be noted that, although initial graft reperfusion following implantation causes host leukocytes to enter the graft, it also allows leukocytes and other cell types in the donor organ to be flushed into the host. This material can travel through the blood and lymph to the peripheral lymphoid organs, particularly the spleen and lymph nodes, which are primary sites of the initiation of specific T-cell–mediated immune responses (Fig. 2–14). Thus, adhesion molecules play a major role in the pattern of lymphocyte traffic (see Box). T cells that are circulating through the blood and lymph can encounter donor antigens in the cortex of the lymph node (Fig. 2–15) or the white pulp of the spleen where they are retained, activated, and expand in numbers.[125] Otherwise, they pass through the cortex of the lymph node to the medulla, into the efferent lymphatics, and subsequently into the blood.

Integrins

The integrins are adhesion molecules that maintain cells in position by attaching one end of the integrin to the cytoskeleton of the cell and the other end to molecules of the extracellular matrix. Integrins also transmit signals from the extracellular matrix into the cell.[97] These surface molecules (named "integrins" in recognition of their importance to the structural integrity of the cell and surrounding tissue) mediate adhesion of cells during normal developmental processes, inflammation, and normal immune responses.

The integrins are heterodimers that contain two separate chains, each of which constitutes a determinant that reacts with monoclonal antibodies, hence they have two CD designations. Each integrin molecule consists of a noncovalently linked heterodimer of one α chain and one β chain, and they are divided into families based on the specific combination of α and β chains that are used. The β_1 family of integrins functions primarily in cell-matrix adhesion. In immune and inflammatory responses, most of the significant integrins belong to the β_2 family that uses a common β_2 chain, but different α chains.

Integrins play a critical role in reperfusion and rejection injury by facilitating the attachment of leukocytes to the vascular endothelial lining. Tight binding of the leukocyte depends on the integrin called **leukocyte function associated antigen** (LFA-1, also called CD11a/CD18) and **Mac-1** (also called CD11b/CD18), which are located on the leukocyte and bind to a molecule from the Ig superfamily, intercellular adhesion molecule-1 (ICAM-1 or CD54), which lies on the endothelial cell surface and can be up-regulated by inflammatory-type soluble mediators.[19, 28, 96] The integrins fix the cell on the endothelium, setting the stage for the migration of the leukocytes through the vessel wall (diapedesis).[142] LFA-1 on cytotoxic T cells can bind to ICAM-1 on target cells.

Selectins

Selectins are adhesion molecules which mediate rolling of leukocytes along the vascular endothelium[39, 169,

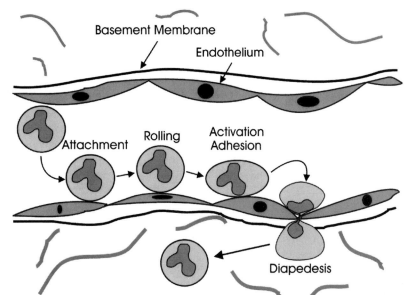

FIGURE **2–13.** Leukocyte attachment and diapedesis. The movement of leukocytes from the blood into other cellular compartments begins with the reversible attachment of leukocytes to the vascular endothelium via carbohydrate moieties on the vessel wall. This causes the leukocytes to roll along the vascular endothelium as the attachment points break and then reattach. As the leukocyte rolls, it may encounter chemokines or cytokines that up-regulate the expression of adhesion molecules such that the binding to the vessel wall is increased to the point that the cells stop rolling. The leukocytes can then squeeze between the endothelial cells and migrate through the vessel wall. (From Springer TA: Traffic signals on endothelium for lymphocyte recirculation and leukocyte emigration. Annu Rev Physiol 1995;57:827–872. ©1995 by Annual Reviews www.AnnualReviews.org, with permission.)

[180, 203, 207] by binding to carbohydrate moieties which are expressed by endothelial cells or other leukocytes. The selectin family includes P-selectin, E-selectin, and L-selectin. **P-selectin** (so named because it is found in storage granules of platelets) is also stored inside granules in endothelial cells called *Weibel-Palade bodies*,[236] and it is translocated to the plasma membrane within seconds following exposure to an "alarm" stimulus, such as IL-1, TNF, or IFN-γ.[141] IL-1 and TNF can be released by macrophages that have been activated by contact with infectious agents and IFN-γ can be released by T-cells that have encountered a specific antigen or have been activated by an encounter with an alloantigen from a solid organ allograft. Another selectin, **E-selectin** (so named because it is expressed by activated endothelial

cells) can appear within a few hours after exposure to TNF-α or lipopolysaccharide.[120, 121, 141] Both selectins bind to carbohydrate moieties of leukocyte glycoproteins, allowing the leukocytes to reversibly stick to the vessel wall and roll in the direction of blood flow, thus creating a situation in which the wall of the vessel is effectively "scanned" by leukocytes continuously rolling along the surface. Any stimulus that causes an up-regulation of the selectins along the vessel wall will cause the leukocytes to stick more tightly, inhibiting the rolling action, and causing them to accumulate in the area of the stimulus, setting the stage for tight binding and subsequent diapedesis through the vessel wall (Fig. 2–13). **L-selectins** (CD62L) (so named because they are primarily found on lymphocytes) control lymphocyte "homing"

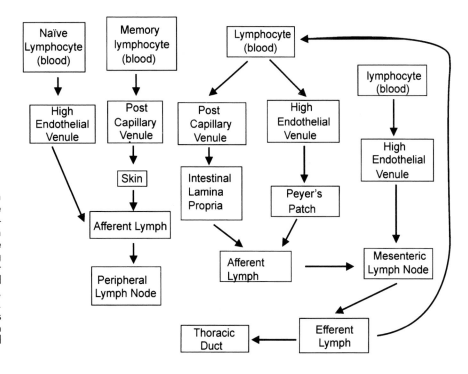

FIGURE **2–14.** Lymphocyte recirculation through the blood and lymph vasculature. The pattern of lymphocyte traffic through the vasculature and primary lymphoid organs results in the delivery of lymphocytes to areas where they are likely to encounter antigen-presenting cells. Antigen-presenting cells that encounter an antigen in the periphery are also delivered to these same areas. Note that, in this scheme, the spleen is part of the blood compartment. (Adapted from Springer TA: Traffic signals on endothelium for lymphocyte recirculation and leukocyte emigration. Annu Rev Physiol 1995;57:827–872.)

Patterns of Lymphocyte Circulation

Leukocytes adhere and localize to particular locations or microenvironments based on the pattern of molecular signals on the surface of endothelial cells that line vessel walls. The molecular signals are coded by the pattern and conformation of several different protein families that can change in their distribution and ability to mediate transmembrane signals based on events in the surrounding milieu, such as the presence of inflammation or cellular damage. Lymphocytes that have not encountered antigen for which they are specific normally circulate among an array of different cellular compartments. T-cell progenitors that arise in the bone marrow during adult life enter the thymic cortex and undergo a series of developmental steps that culminate in the release of mature T cells that are specific for antigen in combination with self-MHC molecules.[123, 168, 174] These cells then enter the peripheral blood and travel to the peripheral lymphoid organs, which include the lymph nodes, spleen, and gut-associated lymphoid tissue. Specialized endothelial cells in the lymph nodes express CD34 or other ligands for L-selectin on the lymphocytes.[28, 32] Thus, cells can enter the lymph nodes via the postcapillary venules or through the afferent lymphatic vessels.[111] The cells then enter the paracortex, a region that is populated by T-cells, macrophages, and interdigitating dendritic cells. It is in this microenvironment that circulating lymphocytes are likely to encounter antigen. The lymph node is an extremely efficient filtering device for antigen, trapping up to 90% of the antigens that enter the lymphatics in the form of free antigen, antigen–antibody complexes, and antigen retained within macrophages or dendritic cells. The interdigitating dendritic cells express a large amount of MHC class II antigens on the surface, and have long cytoplasmic processes that can contact up to 200 T-cells at a time. If the lymphocytes encounter antigen for which they are specific, they will be activated, and begin to proliferate within the paracortex.[4, 85, 180, 232]

The T-cells will then interact with B-cells, inducing the initial stages of B-cell activation. The T-cells and B-cells then migrate to the primary follicles in the cortex. The primary follicle then develops into a secondary follicle that has a central region of proliferating B-cells called a germinal center. The germinal center is the region in which B-cells progress in differentiation into a plasma cell, which produces and excretes large amounts of antibodies.

If a given T-cell does not encounter antigen, then instead of being retained in the lymph node, it will leave via the efferent lymphatic vessels in the medulla and reenter the blood via the thoracic duct or proceed to another lymph node.

This general model of lymphocyte recirculation operates for cells that have encountered nominal antigen as well as those that have been previously exposed to the antigen (memory T-cells). In transplant recipients, it is certain that cells and debris that are shed from the graft following transplantation immediately begin to accumulate in the secondary lymphoid organs where they are phagocytized by macrophages and dendritic cells and presented to T-cells. These sites also serve as reservoirs of alloantigen where T-cells that are reactive to the antigen can be activated as they circulate through the lymph node.

to lymph nodes by binding to endothelial cells of lymph node vessels.

Ig Superfamily Adhesion Molecules

The Ig superfamily adhesion molecules include the intercellular adhesion molecules (ICAMs), vascular cell adhesion molecules (VCAMs), platelet endothelial cell adhesion molecules (PECAMs), lymphocyte function associated antigen-2 (LFA-2) (CD2), and LFA-3 (CD58). This family of adhesion molecules **facilitates the movement of leukocytes through the vascular endothelial layer** (diapedesis) (Fig. 2–13).

ICAM is expressed on multiple cell types, including dendritic and endothelial cells. It binds to the integrin LFA-1. Thus, LFA-1 on cytotoxic T-lymphocytes can bind to ICAM-1 on target cells (such as donor vascular endothelial cells).

VCAM is expressed on activated endothelial cells, dendritic cells, tissue macrophages, bone marrow fibroblasts, and myoblasts. VCAM binds to the integrin VLA-4, promotes adhesion of lymphocytes, eosinophils, and monocytes to activated endothelium, and thereby plays an important role in the recruitment of leukocytes to sites of inflammation.

PECAM is expressed on platelets, leukocytes, and at the junctions between endothelial cells, and facilitates the migration of the leukocyte through the vessel wall.

LFA-2 is expressed on the surface of T-cells, thymocytes, and NK cells and participates in their activation. It participates in the activation of T-cells by binding CD58 (LFA-3).

Once through the vessel wall, leukocytes will move toward a site of inflammation or a specific immune response under the guidance of chemoattractant molecules. These processes will also occur in the tissues of solid organ allografts. Graft injury during harvest, storage, and reperfusion can induce a significant up-regulation of adhesion molecules on the vascular endothelium. Similarly, rejection episodes can also result in the production of cytokines that have been shown to cause substantial increases in the density of adhesion molecule expression on the cell surface.[181, 211] Thus, the adhesive interactions that play a normal role in defense against pathogens can play a significant role in allograft rejection as well. During early reperfusion of the allograft following implantation, the inflammatory response initiated by ischemic and reperfusion injury facilitates the adhesion and diapedesis of leukocytes into the graft. Thus, it is likely that the process of infiltration of the graft by leukocytes begins immediately following revascularization.

COMPLEMENT

Complement is the name of a group of proteins; the members of this group are also enzymes (an enzyme, without itself being changed, catalyzes chemical reactions). The elements of complement which form the familiar "complement cascade" are present in all humans. Although in descriptions it may seem as if new members

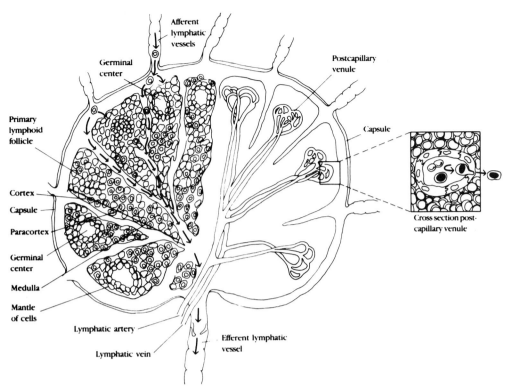

FIGURE **2–15.** The morphology of a lymph node. The lymph node, like the thymus, can be divided into regions called the cortex and medulla. Cells enter the cortex of the node via the afferent lymphatic vessels or the high endothelial venules. Cells can leave via the efferent lymphatic vessel and reenter the blood circulation via the thoracic duct. B-cells that encounter antigen will form primary lymphoid follicles and then migrate to form germinal centers. Plasma cells can remain in the node or leave via the efferent lymphatic vessel and migrate to the bone marrow. (From Immunology by Janis Kuby © 1992, 1994, 1997, 2000 by WH Freeman and Company. Used with permission.)

of the cascade are formed, they are actually preformed and have been present in the individual for a long time.

Most discussions regarding the immune response concentrate on those aspects in which lymphocytes play a key role. Lymphocyte-directed responses can be characterized as highly specific and, upon second exposure to the antigen, capable of providing a more effective defense through increasingly higher avidity for a specific antigen, a quicker response time, and longer lasting effector reactions. However, a time lag of days to weeks can occur before the appearance of effective cell-mediated immunity or the secretion of sufficient amounts of specific antibody. Therefore, other subsystems of the **immune response** (sometimes called *innate immunity*) have evolved which are capable of discriminating self from nonself and have response times of seconds to minutes.

Complement is one such system. It has features that facilitate a fast response and provide strong amplification; thus, activation of a few molecules at the beginning of the pathway results, during or at the end of the activation, in a significant biological response. The proteins that compose the complement system are constitutively ("by nature") present in the circulating plasma in relatively large quantities, so there is no time required for protein synthesis. Components of the complement pathway (see Box) are sequentially activated, and each molecule can activate the production of multiple molecules that are later in the sequence, resulting in enormous

amplification (Fig. 2–16). These characteristics mean that complement can provide a first line of defense against the accidental introduction of bacteria or other foreign cells into the body.

Obviously, tissue allografts constitute foreign cells and, under the proper conditions, can activate complement. **Hyperacute rejection** is one of the most spectacular manifestations of the speed and potency of complement activation by preformed antibody directed against a transplanted organ.

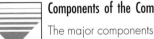

Components of the Complement Pathway

The major components of the complement pathway are named in a specific manner, using the letter C followed by a number. Other components of the complement system called factors are named by an isolated and capitalized letter (other than C), followed by a number. Proteolytically cleaved fragments of these factors are distinguished by adding a lower case suffix, using "a" for the smaller fragment and "b" for the larger one. Other proteins which are considered to be part of the complement regulatory and receptor system are designated by their binding specificity (that to which the complement fragment specifically binds, such as "C4 binding protein"), this "binding specificity" being a separate numbering system, or the number of an attached CD fragment.

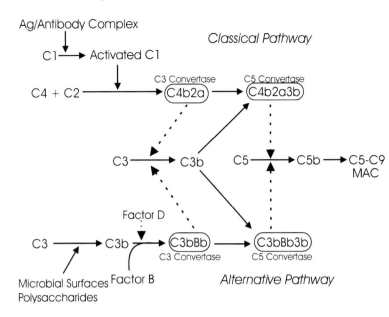

FIGURE **2-16.** The initiation of the classical and alternative pathways of complement activation. Note that the pathways converge at the formation of the C3 convertase and therefore use a common pathway for the formation of the membrane attack complex (MAC). See text for details.

Pathways for Complement Activation

There are two pathways for complement activation (see Box): the classical pathway (usually activated when antigen is engaged by antibody), and the alternative pathway (activated by lipopolysaccharide components of foreign cell surfaces such as bacteria, fungi, and certain tumor cells) (Fig. 2–16).

Mechanism of Direct Cell Lysis by Complement

Direct cell killing by complement is facilitated by the **membrane attack complex.** The formation of the membrane attack complex results from the formation of C5a and C5b by the convertases generated via the classical or alternative complement pathways. The C5b fragment then binds C6 and C7 in succession. C7 causes the complex that was hydrophilic to become hydrophobic, which confers the complex with the capability to insert itself into the lipid bilayer. C8 and C9 then sequentially bind to form the lytic complex. C9 forms into a polymeric complex, with multiple C9 monomers forming a pore in the plasma membrane that results in a loss of membrane integrity and subsequent cell lysis.[30, 59, 60, 153, 191, 196]

Complement Regulatory Proteins

Obviously, the formation and breakdown of C3 convertases must be regulated, or a single activation event could deplete all of the complement components and precipitate a system-wide inflammatory response. In addition, mechanisms must exist to protect host cells from the effects of complement activation. Usually, complement components are bound to the surface of the target cell and therefore do not threaten host cells. However, there is some spontaneous activation of complement components in the plasma, and these proteins have the potential to destroy any cells that contact them. Activa-

tion of the alternative pathway is prevented by soluble factors H and I, which degrade C3b. Endothelial cells contain specific inhibitors of complement activation, including decay accelerating factor (DAF), which inhibits C3 convertase. CD59 and homologous restriction factor (HRF) inhibit the formation of the membrane attack complex.

The Role of Complement in Phagocytosis

In addition to direct cell killing, complement also facilitates the discrimination of self from nonself by phagocytes and other inflammatory cells by marking cells with complement components through a process called **opsonization.** For example, the activation of C3 near a foreign surface results in the deposition and covalent linkage of a proportion of C3b molecules on the cell surface. Neutrophils bearing the CR1 complement receptor are then able to bind to the cells and eliminate them.

The Role of Anaphylatoxins

Two complement fragments, C3a and C5a, are called anaphylatoxins because they mediate a wide range of effects including chemotaxis and granule exocytosis by mast cells and basophils, resulting in the release of histamine and leukotrienes.[80, 242] This results in the contraction of smooth muscle cells and increased vascular permeability, which facilitates diapedesis and migration of neutrophils, monocytes, basophils, and mast cells. C5a is the most potent anaphylatoxin, with the ability to act on all myeloid lineages, including neutrophils, basophils, eosinophils, macrophages, and monocytes. In addition, anaphylatoxins have the ability to act directly on vascular endothelial cells, stimulating P-selectin (therefore increasing the ability of neutrophils to bind) and causing increased vascular permeability.[242]

Pathways for Complement Activation

The **classical pathway** is called such because it was the first to be discovered in the late nineteenth century, when the observation was made that the addition of serum and antibody to a mixture containing bacteria resulted in lysis of the bacteria within a short time.[161, 212] Classical pathway activation occurs when *antigen is engaged by antibody*, either in the form of a multimeric IgM molecule or several adjacent IgG molecules (IgG1, IgG2, IgG3, but not IgG4). This results in a conformational change in the Fc region of the immunoglobulin, exposing sites capable of binding the first component of complement. **C1**, which is composed of three subunits called C1q, C1r, and C1s, will bind to the immunoglobulin Fc region via two of six globular heads of the C1q subunit. The C1r subunit is a serine protease that subsequently becomes activated and in turn cleaves the serine protease proenzyme C1s subunit such that the active site becomes exposed. C1s then cleaves **C4**, the second component of complement to be activated (and activated only by the classical pathway).[13, 109, 188, 196, 255] The proteolysis of C4 results in the production of two fragments, C4a and a larger C4b fragment. C4b contains an intrachain thiolester group that can react with H_2O or form covalent linkages with proteins in solution or on the cell surface. C4b binds to C2 and the **C2** component of the resulting complex is cleaved into C2a and C2b, forming a C4bC2a complex (note that C2 is an exception to the rule of nomenclature in which the larger fragment is given the "b" suffix; for this reason, some texts have reversed the suffix nomenclature).[23, 152] This complex is also called a **C3 convertase** because it is highly active in cleaving **C3** into C3a and C3b. C3b contains an exposed intrachain thiolester bond like C4b that mediates the attachment of the C3b fragment to the C4bC2a complex. This thiolester bond can also facilitate the attachment of C3b to the cell surface, providing a marker and attachment point for phagocytic cells. The C4bC2aC3b complex binds to **C5** via the C3b component and the C2a component proteolytically splits the C5 molecule into C5a and C5b. C5b can go on to catalyze formation of the membrane attack complex.[140, 243]

The **alternative pathway** is an ancient system that does not require the presence of immune complexes, as this pathway can be activated directly by foreign surfaces, especially bacteria and fungi. The ultimate goal of complement activation is the formation of convertases leading to generation of anaphylatoxins and activation of the membrane attack complex. The convergence point for both pathways, as shown in Figure 2–16, is the formation of the C3 convertase. The intact thiolester bond in **C3** can be spontaneously hydrolyzed to $C3(H_2O)$ in a process called "C3 tickover." $C3(H_2O)$ binds soluble factor B (the analog of C2 in the classical pathway), forming a $C3(OH)B$ complex that is permissive to proteolysis by factor D, which results in formation of $C3(OH)Bb$,[147] the C3 convertase of the alternative pathway.[51, 67] If not degraded via regulatory pathways, it can cleave more C3 molecules. The C3Bb complex tends to dissociate relatively rapidly, a process that is inhibited by properdin.[70, 199] The ultimate fate of C3b depends on the surface upon which it has been deposited. If the surface is nonactivating, (e.g., self), the C3b preferentially associates with factor H, a cofactor for factor I–mediated cleavage of C3b into iC3b. iC3b is further cleaved into C3c and then released into the fluid phase. Activator surfaces, such as lipopolysaccharides, fungi, or certain tumor cells, confer C3b with a higher affinity for factor B than for H, resulting in the formation of the C3 convertase.[18, 154]

ACTIVATION OF THE IMMUNE SYSTEM FOLLOWING HEART TRANSPLANTATION

THE INCITING EVENT

The inciting event to the "immunologic response" referred to above is the insertion into the patient of most of the heart removed from another human being. When the circulation is restored to the transplanted heart, the innate immune system generates an inflammatory response induced by reperfusion of the transplanted heart after the period of ischemia inflicted by harvesting and transport of the heart. When the donor heart is perfused by the recipient's blood, nonself components (cells, debris, and soluble proteins) are carried from the donor heart to other parts of the body. The recipient's blood also carries self components, some of which are generated by or are parts of the immune system, into the donor heart. These events set in motion a series of molecular and cellular mechanisms that, if left unchecked, will compromise cardiac function and eventually result in the destruction of the donor heart through a process called **allograft rejection.** The pathological events initiated by the rejection process, the identification of this process, and its control by the administration of immunosuppressive drugs and other modalities form the critical areas of scientific development which have culminated in prolonged survival of organs transplanted into another individual, which is otherwise a hostile (to the transplanted organ) immunologic environment. These important aspects of the rejection process are discussed in Chapter 14.

DETECTION OF THE TRANSPLANTED HEART BY THE IMMUNE SYSTEM

As noted above, the inciting event is the transfer of the donor heart into the recipient, and the subsequent removal of the cross-clamp once the appropriate vascular connections are made. It is at that point that the immune system becomes "aware" of the presence of nonself tissue. At the moment of cross-clamp removal, the residual preservation solution is flushed from the heart, and it is then perfused by recipient blood. This mixture immediately carries out of the donor heart a large number of donor cells, proteins (some of which will be soluble MHC molecules), and cellular fragments. Many of these cells and cellular fragments have donor MHC molecules on their surfaces that are different from those of the host, and are therefore marked as nonself. Within minutes, the blood carries the donor materials to the spleen and lymph nodes and these same materials are also carried to the draining lymph nodes via the lymphatics. Lymph nodes are extremely efficient filtering devices for antigen, trapping up to 90% of free (soluble) antigen, antigen–antibody complexes, and antigen retained within macrophages and dendritic cells. In a similar fashion, APCs within the spleen are capable of trapping large amounts of antigen. T cells travel to the lymph nodes, spleen, and lymphoid tissues associated with the gut through the peripheral blood and through afferent lymphatic vessels.[111] The cells enter the paracortex of the lymph node, a region that is populated by T-cells, macrophages, interdigitating dendritic cells (so named because they have long cytoplasmic arms that extend into the lymph node and can contact up to 200 T-cells at a time). If the T-cells have a T-cell receptor capable of binding to MHC molecules containing a particular peptide, they will be activated (a process in which the T-cell changes its morphology, its behavior, and begins to proliferate). The T-cells will then interact with B-cells, inducing the initial stages of B-cell activation. The T-cells and B-cells then migrate to the regions of the lymph node cortex called primary follicles. The primary follicle then develops into a secondary follicle that has a central region of proliferating B-cells called a germinal center. The germinal center is the region in which B-cells progress in differentiation into a plasma cell, which produces and excretes large amounts of antibodies. If a given T-cell does not encounter antigen, then instead of being retained in the lymph node, it will leave via the efferent lymphatic vessels in the medulla and reenter the blood via the thoracic duct or proceed to another lymph node.

Another route by which the immune system becomes aware of the transplanted heart is through the migration of **donor** APCs from the heart. In mice, APCs have been observed to migrate rapidly out of the transplanted heart into the recipient spleen.[128] Presumably, such cells would also migrate via the lymph and blood to lymph nodes where they can also encounter the T-cells that circulate through the lymphoid tissues.

PRESENTATION OF DONOR ANTIGEN TO T-LYMPHOCYTES

The presentation of antigen in the presence of a solid organ allograft is more complex because there is also a source of **donor APCs** that can present antigen to the recipient T-cells. In addition, the donor MHC molecules are the most immunogenic of alloantigens and can also be broken down into peptides, complexed with intact MHC molecules via antigen processing, and presented to T-cells. Such alloantigens, containing foreign MHC complex molecules, can be presented to the recipient T cells in two ways: indirect presentation and direct presentation (Table 2–9).

Direct Recognition of Donor Antigens by T-Lymphocytes

When the recipient T-cell receptor engages directly with a **donor antigen-presenting cell** (also called "passenger

TABLE 2–9	Characteristics of Responses to Alloantigens Presented via the Direct and Indirect Pathways	
	DIRECT	INDIRECT
Antigen processing required	No	Yes
Proportion of primary T-cell responders	1–5%	1/10,000
Source of antigen-presenting cells	Donor	Recipient only unless there is a class II match between donor and recipient

lymphocytes") carried into the recipient by the donor organ and containing intact MHC molecules, this is termed **direct allorecognition** (Fig. 2–17A). These donor MHC molecules will typically differ from recipient MHC molecules in primary amino acid sequence, but the overall three-dimensional structure will be quite similar. Thus, to recipient T-cells, the donor MHC molecules can strongly resemble recipient MHC molecules that contain a foreign peptide in the binding cleft. In other words, a recipient T-cell that may be specific for a viral peptide complexed with a recipient MHC molecule can cross-react with a donor MHC molecule. In *direct* allorecognition, either CD4+ or CD8+ T-lymphocytes can interact directly with the donor APC, since both donor MHC class I and class II molecules will be expressed, leading to the subsequent activation phase and effector phase of rejection. In direct allorecognition, it is therefore the **intact donor MHC complex** that is the stimulus for binding to the recipient T-cell, having recognized it as nonself. The specific antigen presented in the groove of this complex is often unimportant.

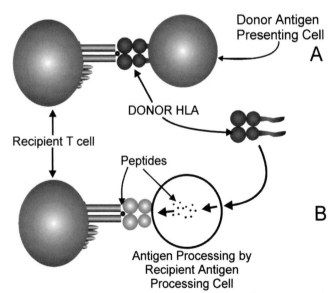

FIGURE **2–17.** Comparison of direct and indirect allorecognition. *A,* Direct presentation, where the unprocessed form of the donor antigen is recognized by an alloreactive T-cell. *B,* In indirect recognition, the donor HLA molecule is taken into the interior of a *recipient* antigen-presenting cell, broken into small peptides (i.e., processed), and the peptides placed into the groove of a *recipient* HLA molecule.

Indirect Recognition of Donor Antigens by T-Lymphocytes

When shed MHC molecules from the donor organ are processed and presented by *recipient* APCs to recipient T-cells in the manner discussed above, this process is called **indirect allorecognition** (Fig. 2–17B).[2, 22, 63, 130, 135, 238] Donor peptides typically undergo processing via a specific mechanism called the **exogenous pathway** and are then presented on the surface of antigen-presenting cells with recipient MHC class II molecules. It is important to note that these peptides might come from either donor MHC class I or class II molecules. CD4[+] T-helper cells bind to this complex via the T-cell receptor, initiating activation of CD4[+] T-helper cells, which then secrete cytokines and initiate the effector phase of the rejection response

Contributions of Direct and Indirect Pathways in Allograft Rejection

The relative contributions of the direct and indirect pathways of allorecognition in allograft rejection have not yet been clearly established, but both play a role (Table 2–9). *In vitro* studies of antigen presentation in short-term mixed lymphocyte cultures have shown that cells that recognize the alloantigen via the direct pathway are at least two orders of magnitude more prevalent than cells that respond to antigen via the indirect pathway,[9, 135] such that 2–10% of T-cells will react to antigens presented within a *donor* MHC complex (direct presentation) versus 1 in 10,000 that typically react to alloantigens or other antigens presented within a self-MHC complex (a host APC in the indirect pathway).[9, 135, 238] An unproven assertion states that early acute allograft rejection is predominately mediated by the direct pathway, since the grafts may carry a significant number of "passenger-leukocyte" APCs. During transplantation, the associated inflammatory response may up-regulate expression of MHC molecules on endothelial and other donor cell surfaces, promoting the direct pathway. As donor APCs die and donor cell MHC expression is presumably less predominant, it has been hypothesized that later rejection is predominately mediated by the indirect pathway. However, donor endothelial cells may express class II MHC molecules to variable degrees following transplantation and allow some ongoing allorecognition via the direct pathway.

ACTIVATION OF T-LYMPHOCYTES

The detection of the presence of nonself involves the transport of antigen to various lymphoid organs, and the presentation of that antigen to T-lymphocytes. This results in T-cell activation, which is usually observed as a change in the expression of various cell surface molecules, the secretion of soluble factors, a change in the morphology of the cell, and proliferation.

When discussing T-cell activation in the sections that follow, we are referring primarily to activation of a naive (meaning that it has never before encountered this antigen) **helper (CD4[+]) T-lymphocyte.** Once activated, the helper T-cell clone goes on to proliferate and releases cytokines or dies. Since new helper T-cells are being generated after passage through the thymus, this process can theoretically occur throughout the life of the graft.

The activation of helper T-lymphocytes which encounter donor antigen can be divided into three phases: the recognition phase, the activation phase, and the effector phase.

Recognition Phase (Signal 1)

The initial step in activation of the T-helper cell by alloantigen is the binding of the T-cell receptor (TCR) to the antigen–MHC complex. This is often termed "**signal 1**" (Table 2–10). However, the actual binding affinity of the TCR to antigenic peptide–MHC complex is too low to create stable adhesion and activation.

The Activation Phase (Second and Third Signals that Commit the T-Lymphocyte to Activation)

The binding of the T-cell receptor by antigen–MHC on the cell surface of the antigen-presenting cell results in the generation of a transmembrane signal. This signal alone, while necessary, is insufficient for T-cell activation and subsequent clonal expansion. A second simultaneous co-stimulatory signal must be provided by the same antigen-presenting cell on which the antigen–MHC complex is encountered (Fig. 2–18).[7, 34, 86, 134] This is called "**signal 2.**"

The role of accessory molecules (see Box) is critical to the process of T-cell activation. The most completely described co-stimulatory molecules are the B7.1 and B7.2 molecules, which are structurally similar glycoproteins (proteins containing sugar residues) that belong to the immunoglobulin superfamily and are generally thought to be specific for antigen-presenting cells (Fig. 2–18). Binding of the B7 molecules by the CD28 molecule on the T-cell in combination with a signal via the T-cell receptor results in increased transcription of cytokine genes. Cytokine genes that are most affected are those promoting IL-2 production and expression of the IL-2 receptor (Table 2–7).

When the TCR is engaged by the antigenic peptide–MHC complex in the presence of co-stimulatory pro-

TABLE 2–10	**Signals Necessary for Helper T-Cell Activation**

Signal 1
  Contact signal between T-cell receptor and MHC–peptide complex on antigen-presenting cell (APC) in combination with T-cell CD4 or CD8 surface molecule

Signal 2
  Co-stimulating signal from B7.1 and B7.2 molecules on APC after ligation by CD28 molecule on T-cell

Signal 3
  Up-regulation of cytokine gene expression; increased secretion of IL-2

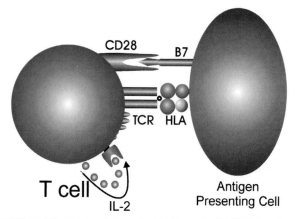

FIGURE 2-18. Co-stimulation of a T-cell via the B7/CD28 pathway. The presentation of an antigen–MHC complex to a T-cell is the primary activation signal, and is also the one that confers specificity to the interaction. However, the primary signal is insufficient to trigger a T-cell. The T-cell must receive an additional signal that can be transmitted via the binding of the CD28 molecule by the B7 molecule on the antigen-presenting cell. The T-cell will then begin producing IL-2, which can bind to IL-2 receptors in an autocrine fashion as shown here, but can also stimulate and assist in the recruitment of other T-cells.

teins, the next steps in T-cell activation occur within the cytoplasm (Fig. 2–19). A cascade of cytoplasmic reactions, initiated primarily by protein tyrosine kinases, constitute the cytoplasmic signaling pathways which lead to activation of nuclear transcription factors. One

The Role of Accessory Molecules and Adhesion Molecules in T-cell Activation

Antigen presentation requires cell–cell contact between a T-lymphocyte and an APC, a process that occurs in a milieu in which there is mechanical movement and shear forces (such as in the blood stream). T-lymphocytes are clearly not sessile, and are therefore in nearly constant motion as they travel through the body "scanning" surfaces for MHC complexes containing the appropriate peptide. At some point, this event will occur and the T-lymphocyte will "stick" momentarily in the area in which the antigen–MHC complex is expressed. However, there is considerable evidence that, by itself, the binding of the T-cell receptor is not enough to result in the activation of T-cell or to ensure that the T-lymphocyte remains in the same general location long enough to do anything. Other molecules, which have been called accessory molecules, also assist in the T-cell receptor/antigen interaction (see Table 2–6). The CD4 and CD8 molecules are important in this regard, and serve to increase the total affinity of the interaction between the T-lymphocyte and the APC. Both CD4 and CD8 bind to nonpolymorphic regions of the MHC class II and class I molecules, respectively. Other molecules, aptly named *adhesion molecules,* also serve to increase the affinity of the interaction between T-lymphocytes and the APCs bearing the appropriate antigen. The net effect of all these interactions is that the T-lymphocyte and the APC stick together and begin to exchange signals in the form of surface receptor–ligand interactions and the secretion of soluble mediators such as cytokines.

of the substrates of tyrosine phosphorylation is ZAP-70, a tyrosine phosphoprotein that associates with the CD3-zeta subunit, and is thought to augment IL-2 production via the CD28 co-stimulatory pathway. Fyn is a tyrosine kinase coupled to the T-cell receptor that, when activated, leads to the phosphorylation of phospholipase Cγ1 (PLCγ). This phospholipase hydrolyzes a phosphodiester bond of phosphatidylinositol 4,5-biphosphate (PIP$_2$), a membrane lipid. The hydrolysis produces inositol 1,4,5-triphosphate (IP$_3$) and diacylglycerol (DAG) which act as second messengers. DAG activates the protein kinase C pathway for activation of nuclear transcription factors. IP$_3$ binds to a specific intracellular receptor that results in release of an intracytoplasmic store of calcium in the endoplasmic reticulum and also opens calcium channels, allowing influx of calcium into the cell. The increase in calcium concentration leads to an increase in the activity of **calcineurin,** a calmodulin (CaM)-dependent serine/threonine phosphatase. Calcineurin dephosphorylates a subunit of nuclear factor of activated T cells called NF-Atp, which is a constitutive nuclear transcription factor present in the cytoplasm. The dephosphorylated NF-Atp is translocated into the nucleus where it binds to another subunit called NF-Atn. The fully assembled NF-AT molecule can then mediate gene transcription through promotors such as IL-2 promotor, that contain NF-AT binding sites. This is followed by transcription and IL-2 protein synthesis. IL-2 is a cytokine that, when secreted, can act in an autocrine fashion in which the T cell that secretes the IL-2 is stimulated via its own IL-2 receptors, which, in turn, can be stimulated to make more IL-2. IL-2 can also act in a paracrine fashion and stimulate the activation and differentiation of other T cells.

The transmembrane signal induced by the binding of IL-2 with the IL-2 receptor (CD25) is termed **signal 3.** Intracellular pathways relay signals from the IL-2 receptor (IL-2R) to induce progression of the cell cycle from G$_1$ to S (proliferation). The exact mechanisms that relay these signals are unknown, but may involve cyclins (proteins which activate crucial protein kinases that control stages of the cell cycle) and proteins that promote cell cycling by binding to and activating cyclin-dependent kinases. The mammalian target of rapamycin protein (mTOR) likely lies along this pathway, but the exact details are unknown.

Following T-cell activation, expression of an additional molecule called CTLA-4, that closely resembles the CD28 molecule in sequence and binds to the B7 molecules with higher affinity than CD28, also increases. However, binding via the CTLA-4 molecule results in a negative signal, thus rendering the activated T-cells less sensitive to subsequent stimulation.[5, 131] This decreased responsiveness may have the beneficial effect of down-regulating the immune response when it is no longer needed. The most important implication of the requirement for co-stimulation is that only professional APCs (such as dendritic cells and macrophages) can produce the B7 molecules and therefore activate T-cells. It is likely that this is a mechanism that results in protection from the activation of autoreactive T-cells.

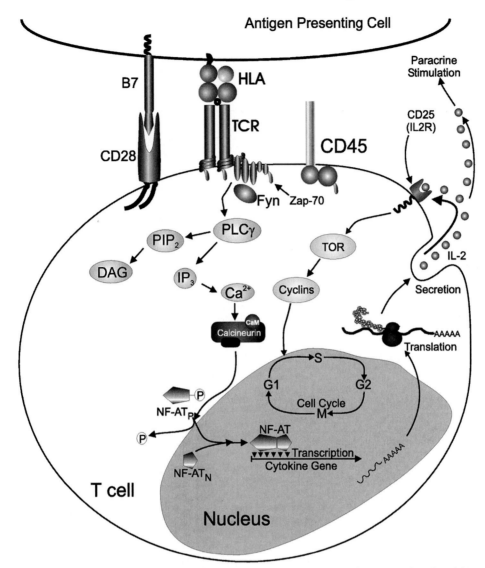

FIGURE 2-19. Binding of the T-cell receptor to antigen–MHC results in a transmembrane signal mediated by a cascade of proteins. *Fyn* is a tyrosine kinase coupled to the T-cell receptor that, when activated, leads to the phosphorylation of phospholipase $C\gamma 1$ (PLCγ). The phospholipase hydrolyzes a phosphodiester bond of phosphatidylinositol 4,5-triphosphate (PIP$_2$), a membrane lipid. The hydrolysis produces inositol 1,4,5-triphosphate (IP$_3$) and diacyglycerol, which act as second messengers. IP$_3$ binds to a specific intracellular receptor that results in release of an intracytoplasmic store of calcium in the endoplasmic reticulum and also opens calcium channels, allowing influx of calcium into the cell. The increase in calcium concentration leads to an increase in the activity of calcineurin, a calmodulin-dependent serine/threonine phosphatase. Calcineurin dephosphorylates NF-Atp, a constitutive nuclear factor present in the cytoplasm. The dephosphorylated NF-Atp is translocated into the nucleus where it binds to NF-Atn. The fully assembled molecule can then mediate transcription through promoters that contain NF-AT binding sites, including IL-2 stimulated via its own IL-2 receptors, which, in turn, can stimulate it to make more IL-2. IL-2 can also act in a paracrine fashion and stimulate the activation and differentiation of other T cells. The binding of the IL-2 receptor (CD25) by IL-2 results in a transmembrane signal that ultimately results in entry into the cell cycle.

ACTIVATION OF B-LYMPHOCYTES

B-cell activation begins in a sequential fashion with the capture of antigen by immunoglobulin molecules on the B-cell surface. The antigen is then internalized, degraded, processed into peptides, loaded into the groove of MHC class II molecules, and delivered to the cell surface. A primed T-cell specific for that antigen–MHC complex then binds to the presented antigen on the B cell and begins a process of mutual activation.[166]

The end product of B-cell activation is the differentiation of B-cells into antibody-secreting plasma cells and

the production of memory B-cells. B-cell activation begins in a sequential fashion that is similar to that described for T-cells (Fig. 2–20).

Signal 1—Binding of Antigen to the Antigen Receptor

The first signal begins with the capture of antigen (nonself) by antigen receptors (immunoglobulin molecules) on the B-cell surface. The antigen is then transported to the interior of the cell and processed in the same manner that is done by antigen-presenting cells (for a B-cell is,

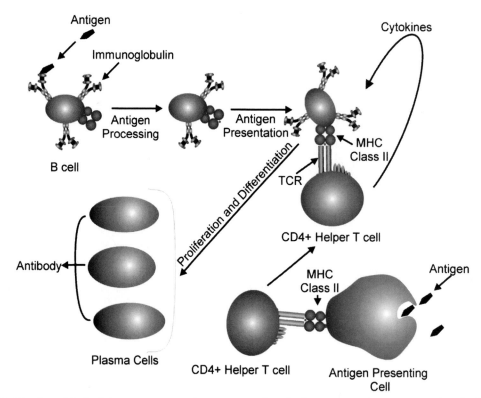

FIGURE **2–20.** A model of cellular cooperation in the generation of antibody responses. The generation of antibody requires the cooperation of T-cells and B-cells, both of which bind to antigen via different molecular mechanisms. A CD4⁺ helper T-cell is activated when it encounters antigen in the presence of co-stimulation on an antigen-presenting cell. That cell then binds to processed antigen on the surface of the appropriate B-cell, secretes cytokines, and expresses CD40, which together serve to activate the B-cell, causing it to proliferate and differentiate into antibody-secreting plasma cells. Note that the contact between the T-cell and B-cell is mediated by processed antigen, thus assuring that the B-cell is activated by the appropriate T-cell clone. TCR, T-cell receptor.

in fact, also classified as an antigen-presenting cell).[67] The resulting antigenic peptides are loaded into the groove of MHC class II molecules and delivered to the cell surface.

Signal 2—Encounter with an Antigen-Specific T-Cell and Subsequent Signaling via CD40/CD40 Ligand

When a B cell enters a lymph node (or spleen) it may encounter a CD4⁺ T-cell that has the appropriate T-cell antigen receptor that can bind to the nonself-peptide–MHC complexes on the B-cell surface. The two cells then engage in a process that has been called "mutual activation."[166]

T-Cell Role in Antibody Production

In order to differentiate into immunoglobulin-producing plasma cells, B-cells must first receive antigen-specific signals through immunoglobulin (also called the B-cell receptor) expressed on the cell surface, and receive antigen-specific T-cell help in the form of a co-stimulatory signal and cytokine stimulation. Surface immunoglobulin can bind to antigen and deliver it into the interior of the cell, where it is processed and

returned to the cell surface as peptides complexed with MHC class II molecules. This processed antigen on the B-cell serves as the attachment point for the proper T-cell clone to bind to the B-cell and provide the appropriate signals.[166] Earlier in this chapter, it was noted that T-cells do not bind to soluble antigen, but to antigenic peptides placed in a groove in an MHC molecule on a cell capable of processing antigen, such as B-cells, dendritic cells, and macrophages. When professional antigen presenting cells, such as dendritic cells, encounter antigen, they process it and migrate to the T-cell zones of lymph nodes. Naive T-cells pass by these cells in the lymph node, and the ones that can bind to a particular MHC–peptide complex will be retained in the lymph node. At the same time, antigen-specific B cells are also trapped in the nodes, and can come into contact with the T-cells that have been presented antigen. The B-cell triggers the T-cell by contact with the T-cell receptor via the MHC–peptide complex and by secretion of cytokines. The T-cell, in turn, secretes cytokines and synthesizes the CD40 ligand molecule. CD40 ligand (also called gp39) binds to the CD40 molecule on the B cell. The B cell, in turn, up-regulates the co-stimulatory molecules B7.1 and B7.2. The T-cell then receives a co-stimulatory signal via the CD28 molecule that binds to B7.1 and

B7.2. The CD40/CD40–ligand interaction also plays a key role in secondary humoral responses, isotype switching, and the maintenance of germinal centers.

ACTIONS TAKEN AGAINST THE TRANSPLANTED HEART BY THE IMMUNE SYSTEM

Following detection by the immune system and activation of the systems that initiate and control effector mechanisms, a number of other systems will be mobilized with the "intent" of elimination or isolation of the transplanted heart. However, it should be noted that, although the general qualities and morphology of **immunologic effector mechanisms** are well characterized, the precise contribution they make to clinical cardiac allograft rejection remains incompletely understood.

ROLE OF CYTOTOXIC T-LYMPHOCYTES (CELLULAR REJECTION)

All of the regulatory mechanisms (antigen presentation, T-cell activation via multiple signals) discussed in the previous sections are oriented toward the control of effector cells that perform the physical task of killing or isolating nonself and toward the prevention of responses to self. Effector cells that have a nonspecific mechanism of action include monocytes/macrophages, mast cells, eosinophils, and granulocytes. Lymphoid effector cells are specifically directed toward antigen-bearing target cells via antigen receptors and are therefore less likely to injure cells that are in close proximity to the target cell.

There is evidence that **cytotoxic T lymphocytes** (CTLs) play an important role in the effector phase leading to acute rejection. First, CD8+ CTLs specific for graft antigens are enriched in the cellular infiltrate. Second, the ability to reject a graft with memory response kinetics can be adoptively transferred from one animal to another using CD8+ T-cells. Third, one can isolate CTLs from the cellular infiltrate that can lyse graft parenchymal cells. CTLs can be found in large numbers among graft-infiltrating cells, although a minority of such cells are actually graft-specific.[61, 90, 135]

Like most T-cells, precursors develop within the thymus, but are largely selected for reactivity to antigen in conjunction with MHC class I molecules. The CD8 molecule is expressed on the vast majority of CTLs and acts as an accessory molecule to the T-cell receptor by binding to the α_3 domain of an MHC class I molecule. It also participates in a transmembrane signal during the process of T-cell activation. Cytotoxic T-cells that have not encountered antigen are called CTL precursors (CTLPs). In order to drive the cells to differentiate into full-blown CTLs, they must receive multiple signals (Table 2–11). Like T-helper cells, cytotoxic T-cells cannot be activated with a single signal, but require the binding of multiple surface molecules that transmit additional signals though the cell membrane. The T-cell receptor

TABLE 2–11	Signals Necessary to Differentiate CTL Precursors into Cytoxic T Cells

Engagement by allogenic MHC class I molecule or peptide–MHC complex
Co-stimulation via molecule such as CD28
Expression of high-affinity receptors for IL-2 on CTL percursor
IL-2 from CD4+ cells

---

must be engaged by allogeneic MHC molecules or by an antigenic peptide–MHC complex, and there must be an additional signal via a co-stimulatory molecule such as CD28. This serves to activate the CTLPs such that they can proliferate and differentiate into CTLs in response to IL-2 through increased expression of the high-affinity receptor for IL-2 (Fig. 2–21).

Once a CTL receives the appropriate signals, it will administer a "lethal hit" to the target cell that results in the destruction of that cell through two separate molecular pathways[10, 26, 170]: one involving the **exocytosis** of molecules that form pores in the target cell membrane allowing the entry of other effector molecules,[138] and the other occurring through **ligand-mediated triggering of apoptosis**. The initiation of the events that lead to target cell death occur within a very short time. Programming of the target cell to die can occur within 5 minutes, although several hours may pass before visible effects become apparent.

Exocytosis-Mediated Cytolysis

One of the most striking characteristics of the lethal hit is that it is a directional phenomenon. "Bystander" cells that reside in close proximity to the CTL/target conjugate are not affected. This is a result of the highly directional release of the granules that store two classes of molecules called perforin and granzymes. Shortly following the conjugation of the CTL and target cell, the CTL reorients the secretory apparatus and focuses the release of granules toward the target cell (Fig. 2–22).[26, 27] Isolation and characterization of the molecules contained within the granules have shown that they contain **perforin**, a calcium-dependent lytic protein that bears a resemblance to the C9 component of complement, but unlike C9, it can by itself mediate the calcium-dependent lysis of target cells. Upon contact with the target cell membrane, perforin polymerizes to form a protein-lined hole that spans the cell membrane and looks like a ring in electron micrographs. These holes apparently destroy the integrity of the cell membrane and allow the entry of other molecules released from the granules into the cytoplasm of the target cell. Other molecules released from the granules are proteoglycans, lysosomal enzymes, and several serine proteases called **granzymes.** Although it has been shown that isolated granules can mediate the lysis of target cells, the precise molecular mechanisms by which they cause lysis are not well understood. The addition of granzymes by themselves will not mediate lysis without the addition of perforin, suggesting that perforin allows the molecules to enter the cell, where they subsequently begin to degrade intracel-

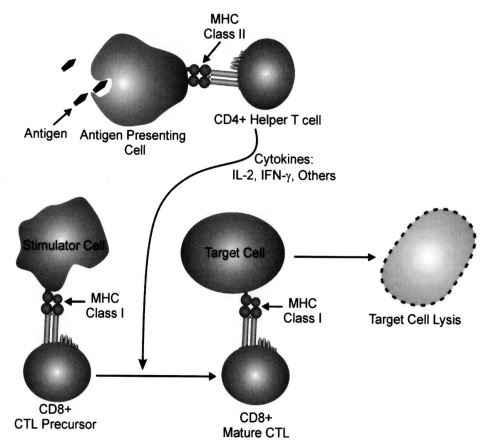

FIGURE **2–21.** Activation and differentiation of cytolytic T-lymphocyte precursors (CTLp) via cooperation with TH cells and through binding of multiple ligands on the cell surface. CTLp generation requires the cooperation of CD4+ helper cells, which are activated by antigen presented in the context of MHC class two by antigen-presenting cells. The stimulator cells, which can be cells bearing a viral antigen or an alloantigen, initiate the process of CTL generation by binding to the CTLp via an MHC class I molecule. Cytokines generated by the CD4 helper T-cells drive the maturation of CTLp into mature cytotoxic T-lymphocytes. The cytotoxic T-lymphocyte can then administer a "lethal hit" to the target cell resulting in the target cell lysis.

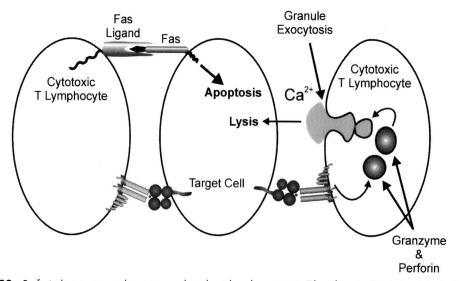

FIGURE **2–22.** Perforin/granzyme and receptor-mediated cytolysis by cytotoxic T-lymphocytes (CTL). A cytotoxic T-lymphocyte can cause the lysis of a target cell through two nonmutually exclusive pathways. The contact of the Fas molecule on the surface of the target cell by Fas-ligand on the CTL can result in the initiation of apoptosis. Release of perforin and granzymes by exocytosis can cause the formation of pores in the target cell membrane. (Modified from Berke G: Cytotoxic T cells and mechanisms of tissue injury. *In* Tilney NL, Strom TB, Paul LC [eds]: Transplantation Biology: Cellular and Molecular Aspects. Philadelphia: Lippincott-Raven Publishers, 1996, pp 435–455, with permission.)

lular proteins, and possibly indirectly trigger apoptosis, which results in the fragmentation of cellular DNA.

Receptor Ligand Mediated Apoptosis

The second major pathway for induction of cell death by the CTL is through receptor-mediated apoptosis and lysis. Two lines of evidence support the role of this pathway. The first is through *in vitro* studies that show that perforin-mediated lysis is calcium dependent, yet the addition of a calcium-chelating agent does not completely abolish lysis.[224] Second, mice in which the perforin gene has been inactivated are still able to generate CTLs capable of killing target cells.[138]

Like exocytosis-mediated lysis, the process of apoptosis begins with the recognition of the target cell via the T-cell receptor and its associated accessory molecules followed by the induction of a protein called **Fas ligand** (FasL or CD95 ligand) in the cytolytic T-cell.[26] The FasL molecule binds a molecule called **Fas** (CD95) on the target cell, which subsequently transmits a signal through the target cell membrane that results in the induction of apoptosis (see Box) also termed "pro-

grammed cell death," which is a different process than cell necrosis.

ROLE OF ANTIBODIES (HUMORAL REJECTION)

The term humoral rejection refers to the production of antibodies and/or the activation of complement in response to exposure to an antigen. The response is mediated by B-lymphocytes. Unlike T-cells, which only react to antigens on the surface of other cells, antibodies can react with antigens in solution or on the cell surface. Considerable evidence suggests that antibodies can play a significant role in rejection, particularly those antibodies that are specific for donor MHC antigens. The effector mechanisms are largely mediated by the constant region, which ultimately is the region that confers functional specialization of the various antibody classes (also known as isotypes). IgA, for example, is largely associated with mucosal immunity and is abundant throughout the body, although its role in antigraft responses is largely undescribed. The antibodies mostly associated with humoral rejection have been **IgM** and **IgG**. Four types of effector mechanisms have been associated with humoral responses as discussed below.

Neutralization

Many molecules mediate their effects via an active site or through binding to a receptor. Antibodies can directly interfere with these activities by blocking the relevant sites through steric hindrance (i.e., physically blocking the site). Beneficial effects against bacterial toxins can be mediated this way, but the role of this mechanism in transplantation is unknown. One could speculate that antibodies could interfere with polymorphic receptors and therefore block the action of molecules that are important to cardiac function.

Opsonization

Antibodies can also facilitate nonself recognition by acting as a "tag" that can be recognized by phagocytic cells in a process called **opsonization** (facilitation of phagocytosis through the coating of cells or particles with immune complexes). Inclusion of antibody in assays of phagocytosis has been shown to increase the rate of phagocytosis by 4,000-fold.

CD16 is a cell surface molecule that can be found on NK cells, macrophages, neutrophils, and myeloid precursors. This molecule, also called the FcγIII receptor, binds to IgG molecules that have complexed with antigen and mediates a transmembrane signal upon binding that results in the secretion of proinflammatory and cytotoxic soluble factors such as cytokines that can kill the donor cell bound to the antibody. This mechanism is also called **antibody-dependent cellular cytotoxicity (ADCC)**.

Complement Activation

Certain subclasses of IgG and IgM can bind to C1q of the classical complement pathway, triggering the com-

Apoptosis

The morphology of programmed cell death, called apoptosis,[157, 246] is distinct from that of necrosis. Necrosis is characterized by cytoplasmic changes in which the mitochondria swell, the cell loses the ability to make adenosine triphosphate (ATP), and loss of regulation of the osmotic gradient across the plasma membrane results in the lysis of the cell. Apoptosis (pronounced ap-o-TO-sis, with a short *a* as in attic)[53] is characterized by relatively intact cellular organelles, but the nucleus exhibits striking changes in the form of margination of chromatin and the breakup of the nucleus into "beads" of dense chromatin surrounded by a membrane.[53] Cytoplasmic membrane-bound vesicles are released, and the net result is the destruction of the cell without the elicitation of an inflammatory response that usually accompanies necrosis.

The induction of apoptosis can occur through a number of different molecular pathways. The Fas protein (CD95, also called APO-1) is a 48-kDa transmembrane glycoprotein that belongs to the TNF family of molecules and is expressed on a variety of tissue types that include lymphoid cells. When this molecule is bound by its ligand, called Fas-ligand, a transmembrane signal is initiated that results in the activation of the apoptotic pathway.[74, 157, 244]

One of the most striking features of apoptosis is that it is dependent on biochemical mechanisms of the apoptotic cell and is therefore considered a form of cellular suicide. Further study of the phenomenon has shown that apoptosis is a means by which cells are eliminated in the normal course of tissue differentiation and in the regulation of immune responses. In the latter case, self-reactive T-cells and B-cells are induced to undergo apoptosis and are therefore eliminated as potentially facilitating autoimmune disease. In the last few years, there has been increasing interest in the role of apoptosis regarding its role in the normal regulation of immune function, in cell differentiation, and possibly in certain disease states.[42, 223]

plement cascade, which is associated with a number of activities that can be highly deleterious to the transplanted organ. One of the most spectacular manifestations of this mechanism can be found in the phenomenon of hyperacute rejection, which is now seldom observed in clinical transplantation. **Hyperacute rejection** is mediated by preexisting (i.e., are present prior to transplantation) antibodies which, upon cross-clamp removal, enter the vasculature and bind to the vascular endothelium. They then fix complement, which causes direct lysis of endothelial cells, and the elaboration of complement components causes a massive infiltration of granulocytes. In extreme cases, the organ can be destroyed within minutes after reperfusion. In the case of clinical transplantation, it is suspected that low levels of antibody can trigger complement activation which, with its proinflammatory properties, can potentiate inflammation and cell injury.

IMMUNOLOGIC TOLERANCE

In the current era, the morbidity and imperfect prevention of rejection associated with the use of immunosuppressive drugs has resulted in a continuation of the effort to artificially produce immunologic tolerance in humans undergoing organ transplantation. However, even more than 50 years following Medawar's classic experiments (see Chapter 1), complete agreement has not been reached on what constitutes immunologic tolerance. Some have favored the term "operational tolerance," which names a state in which a histoincompatible allograft is accepted with the use of continuous immunosuppression. Others have added the stipulation that tolerance must be specific, meaning that an allograft remains functional even when an unrelated third-party graft on the same host is rejected. This stipulation is of great importance, since ideally one would be able to establish permanent graft survival without impairing the ability to respond to infectious agents. For our purposes, we will use the term tolerance to mean specific acceptance of a histoincompatible allograft while maintaining reactivity to third-party graft antigens.

Tolerance, as defined above, does not normally occur in recipients of transplanted allogeneic solid organs, but does occur naturally during embryonic life when the fetal immune system learns to distinguish self from nonself, and during pregnancy when the allogeneic fetus develops in a female that would normally react to paternal antigens. Examination of the mechanisms of the induction of tolerance in these situations has been instructive, and suggests that some or all of such mechanisms could operate in individuals in which tolerance has been artificially induced.

In addition, the data generated from numerous experimental studies clearly show that there are a number of distinct pathways by which an immune response directed towards a cardiac allograft can be turned off or inhibited.

MECHANISMS OF SELF-TOLERANCE

The immune response can be highly specific, and one of the hallmarks of this specificity is that a strong reaction can be elicited towards nonself antigens, whereas responses toward antigens that constitute self are suppressed or absent. This specificity is acquired through multiple mechanisms that act on lymphocytes as they mature and after they have seeded to various locations in the periphery.

Thymic Selection

Since the specificity of a cellular immune response is a function of specific recognition of antigen by T-lymphocytes, the structures on these T-cells that mediate recognition constitute a central control point. Therefore, the repertoire of antigens to which a population of lymphocytes can respond is a function of their ability to recognize antigenic peptides in the peptide-binding grooves of MHC class I and class II molecules.

Positive Selection

Positive selection (selection of the useful) occurs in the thymic cortex, in which the majority of thymocytes (T-cell progenitors) express both the CD4 and CD8 accessory molecules (Fig. 2–23). Only those T-cells that react to self-MHC molecules expressed by a given individual are allowed to survive (Fig. 2–24). Current evidence suggests that such cells are programmed to die, but are rescued when they receive a signal through the T-cell receptor when it binds to an MHC molecule.

Negative Selection

A process of negative selection occurs when progenitor cells have a high affinity receptor for self-MHC molecules alone or react to self-MHC and peptides from self-antigens. This process results in the destruction of approximately 95% of the T-cell progenitors that arise in the cortical region of the thymus (Fig. 2–24). Throughout this process, there are surface molecules that are expressed in a stage-specific fashion. Receptor engagement is also accompanied by engagement of the CD4 or CD8 molecules by a monomorphic portion of the MHC class II or class I molecules, respectively. The CD4 and CD8 molecules apparently increase the affinity of cell–cell contact by the immature T-cells. The T-cell progenitor then down-regulates either the CD4 or CD8 molecules to produce $CD4^+/CD8^-$ T-cells specific for antigenic peptides in the context of class II MHC, or $CD4^-/CD8^+$ T-cells specific for peptides in the context of MHC class I. Cells directly reactive to any self-antigens that develop in the thymus are deleted. The remaining cells are reactive to foreign antigens in the context of self-MHC class I or class II molecules and are exported to the periphery.

Peripheral Tolerance

One can readily see that thymic deletion of self-antigen reactive cells could not constitute the sole mechanism

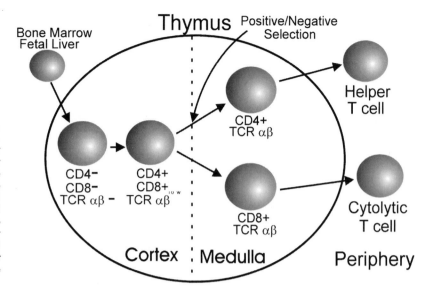

FIGURE **2-23.** The ontogeny of T-cells in the thymus. The thymus is the primary site of T-cell development. Precursor cells from the bone marrow (and the fetal liver during embryonic life) enter the thymic cortex initially expressing few or no antigens associated with mature T-cells. The cells will then simultaneously express the CD4 and CD8 antigens early in their development and soon express low levels of the T-cell receptor on the cell surface. As the cells move from the thymic cortex to the medulla, they increase their level of T-cell receptor expression, stop expressing either CD4 or CD8, and are subject to positive and negative selection. Cells that survive this selection process eventually move to the medulla, and are exported to the periphery.

of tolerance towards self-antigens, since many such antigens never reach the thymus, or are not produced during embryonic development in which there are few mature T-cells. In addition, some self reactive T-cells do escape thymic deletion. Therefore, there must be a form of peripheral tolerance in which mature T-cells that escape thymic deletion are prevented from reacting to self-antigens.[124, 221, 249]

Deletion

Deletion is a process by which potentially reactive T-cells are physically destroyed through lysis or induction of apoptosis. Deletion, then, is the peripheral equivalent of negative selection in the thymus, although the signals that result in this destruction are undoubtedly different. This process occurs when antigen-presenting cells or

cells bearing MHC class I antigens bind to antigen-specific T cells via the T-cell receptor, but instead of delivering a signal that results in activation, a signal results in the induction of apoptosis in that T-cell. This phenomenon was initially described by Richard Miller and colleagues,[71, 95, 156, 215] who called these deletional antigen presenting cells **veto cells** and formally defined them as cells that specifically inactivate clones of precursor cells that interact with them. Later evidence has supported the notion that this process is deletional.[185, 221]

Anergy

In a situation in which a specific immune response is initiated, a CD4[+] T-cell encounters antigen presented on the surface of an antigen-presenting cell. However, if the antigen-presenting cell fails to generate a second

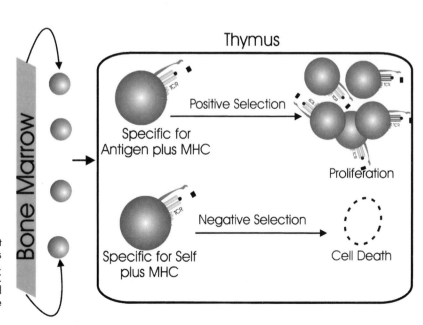

FIGURE **2-24.** Thymic selection. Selection of cells that can react with antigen–MHC occurs in the thymus through a process of positive and negative selection. Harmful cells that react with self-antigens or self–MHC alone are negatively selected. Those cells that are useful (those that react with self-MHC and an antigen) are rescued from programmed cell death.

signal (e.g., in the form of B7 binding to CD28 on the T-cell), the T-cell is rendered anergic, a state in which the T-cell fails to respond to antigen even when antigen is later presented by antigen-presenting cells that are capable of transmitting a second signal. Anergic T-cells fail to produce IL-2, suggesting that the anergic state is at least partially due to the failure of nuclear transcription factors to bind to regulatory portions of the IL-2 gene promoter. Anergic T-cells can remain intact for extended periods, and the anergic state can be broken with the addition of IL-2 *in vitro*.[68, 104, 127] Experimentally, anergy can be induced by presenting antigen on lipid membranes or by presenting T-cells with antigen in the presence of antibodies that block the CD28/B7 interaction.[83]

Suppression

Multiple experiments in the 1960s and 1970s revealed that certain immunization protocols (such as administration of large doses of aqueous antigens) would result in a state of tolerance in the immunized animal. If lymphocytes were adoptively transferred from the injected animal to a naive recipient, that recipient also became tolerant to the antigen used to immunize the first animal, despite the fact that the animal could respond to other antigens.[81] Therefore, it was postulated that this effect was mediated by a distinct subpopulation of T-cells called suppressor T-cells. However, attempts to isolate clones or generate T-cell hybridomas of suppressor cells have been largely unsuccessful. Therefore, the biology of such T-cells remains largely unresolved and the study of these cells has fallen into disfavor. More recently, the data have been reinterpreted in the context of the theory discussed in the next section, which postulates that suppression results from secretion of inhibitory cytokines in response to antigenic stimulation.

Immune Deviation

As noted earlier in this chapter, CD4$^+$ cells and probably CD8$^+$ cells can be divided into subpopulations based on the differential expression of cytokines. Immune deviation refers to the TH1/TH2 paradigm (see earlier section, Cytokines) in the context of tolerance induction. The type 1 cells (also called TH1 cells for helper T cells) secrete IL-2 and IFN-γ and provide regulation/stimulation of cellular responses. Type 2 cells (also called TH2 cells for helper cells) secrete IL-4, IL-5, IL-10, and IL-13, and provide help for B-cell responses and isotype switching. The immune deviation theory postulates that tolerance can result from the deviation of an immune response toward one type or the other. Since TH1 and TH2 responses are counterregulatory, a preponderance of available T-cells toward a type 2 response would result in the lack of cellular responses towards the immunizing antigen. The role of immune deviation is still controversial. Some maintain that, whereas this phenomenon has been demonstrated in select circum-

stances, it may be an oversimplification of events that occur *in vivo*.

TOLERANCE IN TRANSPLANTATION

Donor-Specific Blood Transfusion

History

The use of blood transfusions has always been associated with the risk of sensitization of the recipients such that they can develop strong antidonor antibody responses that could result in hyperacute rejection of a subsequently transplanted organ. However, as early as the 1960s, it was observed that kidney allograft recipients who had received previous blood transfusions could have a significantly higher mean graft survival than individuals who did not receive transfusions.[6, 69, 87, 145, 146, 163] A large retrospective study of pretransplant blood transfusion in clinical renal allograft recipients showed an apparent benefit in graft survival.[163, 164] Therefore, many centers began to routinely use pretransplant blood transfusions as a means of improving graft survival. This practice was abandoned in the late 1980s following the realization that the benefit was minimal following the introduction of cyclosporine and the realization of the small but real hazard from human immunodeficiency virus, hepatitis B, and cytomegalovirus in the blood supply.

Mechanism

The mechanisms of extended graft survival or tolerance induction by donor-specific blood transfusion have been controversial. In general, donor-specific blood transfusion is conceptually similar to bone marrow administration in that each technique involves the introduction of cells from the donor, which is followed by the induction of tolerance or the extension of graft survival. Van Twuyver has shown that, like bone marrow–induced tolerance, administration of cells results in the disappearance of donor specific cells from the peripheral circulation.[36, 113, 234, 235] The effect is facilitated by sharing of one MHC class II antigen between donor and recipient,[113, 155] a result that mirrors results obtained from the rhesus monkey bone marrow–induced tolerance model.[222] Such results argue strongly for a veto mechanism, the hallmark of which is the selective deletion of donor-specific T-cell precursors dependent on the administration of donor cells.

An alternative view is that the tolerance induction via blood transfusion is not an active process mediated by the infused cells, but is the result of the mere presence of the antigen on the donor cells. This idea is supported by experiments in which recipient strain fibroblasts are transfected with the genes for MHC antigens from the donor strain, and infused into a naive recipient prior to transplantation.[143, 248, 249] Animals treated in this fashion exhibit extended graft survival, with the magnitude of the extension of survival dependent on the dose of transfected cells.

Clinical Relevance

Following the introduction of cyclosporine, the apparent advantage from pretransplant blood transfusions was much smaller.[162] In addition, it was found that the risk of sensitization was high relative to the potential benefit in survival. Some investigators suggested that preoperative blood transfusion was, in fact, a screening mechanism in which individuals who tended to develop antidonor antibodies were identified and excluded from transplantation, resulting in higher overall graft survival.[163] Given the modest benefit and higher risk of presensitization, the majority of renal transplant centers do not use this protocol. Since the majority of cardiac transplantation centers began following the introduction of cyclosporine, blood transfusion was never used as a routine clinical practice in heart transplantation, although occasional reports still appear regarding its use or efficacy.[210, 233]

Donor Bone Marrow–Induced Tolerance

History

Although Medawar's results[31] showed that tolerance can be induced in immature animals, Monaco and Wood later showed that lasting, stable tolerance can be induced in *adult* mice by administration of rabbit antilymphocyte serum just before and just after transplantation followed by intravenous injection of donor bone marrow cells at 1 week after-transplantation (Fig. 2–25).[148, 250] It should be noted that this is not a bone marrow transplantation protocol. The cytoablative therapy does not completely ablate sessile T-cell populations and does not result in

the establishment of a large donor bone marrow population. This protocol was derived empirically using a mouse strain combination that differed at a single locus of the major histocompatibility complex.

This mouse model of tolerance has been adapted to a rhesus monkey model in order to determine the immunologic mechanisms of tolerance induction in primates, with the intention of facilitating its future application to clinical transplantation.[214, 217, 219, 221]

Mechanism

The postulated mechanism by which the bone marrow cells delete donor-specific cells begins with the initial interaction of the T-cell receptor on the recipient's donor-specific T-cells with the allogeneic MHC molecules present on the bone marrow cells (Fig. 2–26). It is this interaction which confers the specificity of the eventual deletion of donor-reactive T cells. At the same time, the CD8 molecules stabilize the T-cell receptor/MHC molecule interaction by binding to the α_3 domain of the MHC class I molecules of the opposing cells. Engagement of the CD8 molecule on the bone marrow cell results in the transmission of a signal through the plasma membrane resulting in an increase in the transcription of mRNA from the genes that code for the TGF-β and Fas-ligand molecules. These molecules are secreted or expressed, respectively, on the surface of the cell. Studies in the mouse model suggest that the interaction of the veto cells with graft-specific T cells results in the induction of apoptosis via the Fas/Fas-ligand pathway. Use of bone marrow cells from a strain of mice that do not have functional Fas-ligand molecules results in the failure to induce tolerance.[79]

Measurements of the frequency of donor-specific precursor cytotoxic T-lymphocytes in transplant recipients who have received donor bone marrow indicate that the frequency of donor-specific cytotoxic T-lymphocyte precursor cells becomes undetectable following the infusion of donor bone marrow cells, suggesting that the precursors are deleted by the bone marrow cells.[218, 251] Donor-specific deletion in this manner is a hallmark of a veto mechanism, which was originally described by Miller as a functional subpopulation of cells that specifically inactivate or delete clones of precursor T-cells that interact with them.[71, 95, 156, 215] *In vitro* studies show that the veto activity in monkeys is radiation sensitive, requires cell–cell contact, and is dependent on the presence of cells bearing CD2, CD8, and CD16.[216, 218]

Ablation of T-cells in this model was first done using rabbit antithymocyte globulin (RATG). RATG is produced by immunizing rabbits with human thymocytes. The resulting rabbit serum is fractionated such that the IgG component of the serum remains (hence, the name antithymocyte globulin). RATG is a polyclonal antibody preparation and therefore contains antibodies that are specific for a number of cell surface molecules, including CD3, CD4, CD8, and a variety of non–T-cell-specific specificities.[172] Treatment with RATG results in a profound decrease in the proportion of lymphocytes in the peripheral circulation that can last for several weeks. If kidney transplant recipients are infused with bone

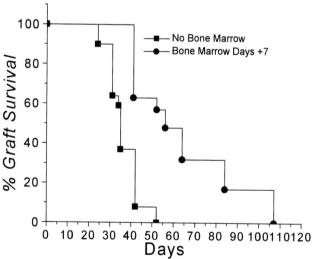

FIGURE **2–25.** Skin allograft survival in mice treated with antilymphocyte serum and donor bone marrow. In these experiments (C57BL/6xA/J), F1 mice were given an intraperitoneal injection of rabbit antilymphocyte serum at days −1 and +2 relative to transplantation of C3H strain skin at day 0. At day +7, mice were given C3H strain bone marrow cells intravenously. Note that extension of graft survival was conferred only when donor bone marrow was administered. (Modified from Monaco AP, Gozzo JJ, Wood ML, Liegeois A: Use of low doses of homozygous allogeneic bone marrow cells to induce tolerance with antilymphocyte serum [ALS]: Tolerance by intraorgan injection. Transplant Proc 1971;3:680–683.)

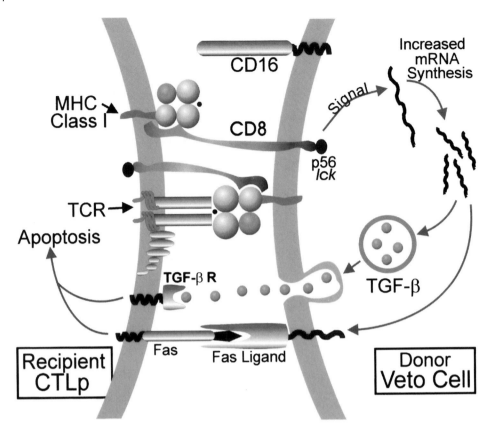

FIGURE **2–26.** A model of the molecular interactions involved in veto-mediated tolerance. Tolerance induced by donor bone marrow requires cell-to-cell contact between the veto cells and the recipient cytotoxic T-lymphocytes. Antigen specificity is conferred by contact between the T-cell receptor on the cytotoxic T-lymphocyte and the MHC antigens on the surface of the veto cell. The CD8 molecule can bind to the α_3 domain on the MHC class I molecules of the recipient cells, and, in turn, the CD8 molecule on the recipient's cell can bind to the α_3 domain of the MHC class I molecule of the veto cells. Current data suggest that the veto effect is caused by the induction of apoptosis in the recipient cytotoxic T-lymphocytes. Apoptosis can be induced by Fas-ligand or TGF-β.

marrow cells from the donor, there is a significant increase in median graft survival. If the bone marrow cells are fractionated by removal of DR$^+$ (MHC class II–positive cells, and therefore most antigen-presenting cells and activated T-cells) cells, the efficiency of tolerance induction is increased, with a median graft survival of 4.5 months and a 30% 1-year graft survival. Analysis of the frequency of T-cells in the peripheral blood using limiting dilution analysis shows that the bone marrow infusion results in the apparent alloantigen-specific deletion of donor-specific cytotoxic T-cell precursors in the circulation.[216, 218, 221]

Clinical Relevance

In the rhesus monkey model, a preclinical tolerance induction protocol has been established in which monkeys receive a perioperative dose of an anti-CD3 immunotoxin consisting of an anti-CD3 antibody covalently coupled to an engineered form of diphtheria toxin in which the protein domain conferring specificity has been altered so that the toxin can bind to a cell only via the anti-CD3 antibody.[122, 220] As is required for the induction of tolerance using donor bone marrow, the immunotoxin ablates the resident T-cells, so that when the bone marrow is administered, a small population of bone marrow cells can establish residence in the host, a state

that is often called **microchimerism.** When repopulation of the T-cells begins, it occurs in an environment in which newly arisen donor-specific T-cells are deleted by bone marrow cells that act as veto cells. Using this protocol in monkeys with either RATG or immunotoxin as a cytoablative drug has resulted in the longest recorded survival times for kidney allografts without immunosuppression.[101, 220, 222] The primary limitation in this model has been that the tolerance appears to be "split," meaning that cellular responses are inhibited, but the ability to generate antidonor antibodies remains. As a consequence, a significant proportion of the tolerant recipients eventually lose their grafts to chronic rejection, a scenario that strongly resembles that of long-term allograft recipients receiving conventional therapy. However, further manipulation of the recipient, particularly in a way that would inhibit the indirect pathway of alloantigenic presentation, could possibly ameliorate this problem.

At the time of this writing, bone marrow–induced tolerance appears to be the tolerance induction protocol closest to clinical application because it can be performed with little to no preconditioning.

References

1. Adams PW, Lee HS, Waldman WJ, Sedmak DD, Morgan CJ, Ward JS, Orosz CG: Alloantigenicity of human endothelial cells.

1. Frequency and phenotype of human T helper lymphocytes that can react to allogeneic endothelial cells. J Immunol 1992;148:3753–3760.

2. Adams PW, Lee HS, Waldman WJ, Sedmak DD, Orosz CG: Allo-antigenicity of human endothelial cells. III. Quantitated indirect presentation of endothelial alloantigens to human helper T lymphocytes. Transplantation 1994;58:476–483.

3. Afonso LC, Scharton TM, Vieira LQ, Wysocka M, Trinchieri G, Scott P: The adjuvant effect of interleukin-12 in a vaccine against Leishmania major. Science 1994;263:235–237.

4. Ager A: Regulation of lymphocyte migration into lymph nodes by high endothelial venules [review]. Biochem Soc Trans 1997; 25:421–428.

5. Akalin E, Chandraker A, Sayegh M, Turka LA: Role of the CD28:B7 costimulatory interaction in alloimmune responses [review]. Kidney Int Suppl 1997;58:S8–S10.

6. Alexander JW, Babcock GF, First MR, Davies CB, Madden RL, Munda R, Penn I, Fidler JP, Cofer R, Stephens G, Schroeder TJ, Hariharin S, Cardi M, Manzler A, Cohen L, Mendoza N, Clyne D, Giese F: The induction of immunologic hyporesponsiveness by preoperative donor-specific transfusions and cyclosporine in human cadevaric transplants. A preliminary trial. Transplantation 1992;53:423–427.

7. Allison JP: CD28-B7 interactions in T-cell activation [review]. Curr Opin Immunol 1994;6:414–419.

8. Alt FW, Baltimore D: Joining of immunoglobulin heavy chain gene segments: implications from a chromosome with evidence of three D-JH fusions. Proc Natl Acad Sci U S A 1982;79:4118–4122.

9. Ansari AA, Wang YC, Kanter K, Naucke N, Sell KW: Indirect presentation of donor histocompatibility antigens contributes to the allogeneic response against human cardiac myocytes. J Heart Lung Transplant 1992;11:467–477.

10. Apasov S, Redegeld F, Sitkovsky M: Cell-mediated cytotoxicity: contact and secreted factors [review]. Curr Opin Immunol 1993;5:404–410.

11. Araake M, Uchiyama T, Imanishi K, Yan XJ: Activation of human vascular endothelial cells by IFN-gamma: acquisition of HLA class II expression, TSST-1-binding activity and accessory activity in T cell activation by the toxin. Int Arch Allergy Appl Immunol 1991;96:55–61.

12. Arden B, Klotz JL, Siu G, Hood LE: Diversity and structure of genes of the alpha family of mouse T-cell antigen receptor. Nature 1985;316:783–787.

13. Arlaud GJ, Colomb MG, Gagnon J: A functional model of the human C1 complex. Immunol Today 1987;8:106–111.

14. Atkinson YH, Marasco WA, Lopez AF, Vadas MA: Recombinant human tumor necrosis factor-alpha. Regulation of N-formylmethionylleucylphenylalanine receptor affinity and function on human neutrophils. J Clin Invest 1988;81:759–765.

15. Atkinson YH, Murray AW, Krilis S, Vadas, MA, Lopez AF: Human tumour necrosis factor-alpha (TNF-alpha) directly stimulates arachidonic acid release in human neutrophils. Immunology 1990;70:82–87.

16. Baer R, Lefranc MP, Minowada J, Forster A, Stinson MA, Rabbitts TH: Organization of the T-cell receptor alpha-chain gene and rearrangement in human T-cell leukaemias. Mol Biol Med 1986;3:265–277.

17. Barbara JA, Van ostade X, Lopez A: Tumour necrosis factor-alpha (TNF-alpha): the good, the bad and potentially very effective [review]. Immunol Cell Biol 1996;74:434–443.

18. Barnum SR, Volanakis JE: Structure and function of C3. In Cruse JM, Lewis RE (eds): The Year in Immunology 1989–90. Molecules and Cells of Immunity. Basel: Karger, 1990, pp 208–228.

19. Bates PA, Berendt A, Bennett R, Cabanas C, Craig A, Harvey J, McDowall A, Hogg N: Leukocyte integrin activation [review]. Pathol Biol 1992;40:785–788.

20. Batten P, Yacoub MH, Rose ML: Effect of human cytokines (IFN-gamma, TNF-alpha, IL-1 beta, IL-4) on porcine endothelial cells: induction of MHC and adhesion molecules and functional significance of these changes. Immunology 1996;87:127–133.

21. Benham A, Tulp A, Neefjes J: Synthesis and assembly of MHC-peptide complexes [review]. Immunol Today 1995;16:359–362.

22. Benichou G, Fedoseyeva E, Lehmann PV, Olson CA, Geysen HM, McMillan M, Sercarz EE: Limited T cell response to donor MHC peptides during allograft rejection. Implications for selective immune therapy in transplantation. J Immunol 1994;153:938–945.

23. Bentley DR: Primary structure of human complement component C2. Homology to two unrelated protein families. Biochem J 1986;239:339–345.

24. Bentley GA, Mariuzza RA: The structure of the T cell antigen receptor [review] Annu Rev Immunol 1996;14:563–590.

25. Berek C, Milstein C: Mutation drift and repertoire shift in the maturation of the immune response. [review]. Immunol Rev 1987;96:23–41.

26. Berke G: The CTL's kiss of death [review]. Cell 1995;81:9–12.

27. Berke G: Cytotoxic T cells and mechanisms of tissue injury. In Tilney NL, Strom TB, Paul LC (eds): Transplantation Biology: Cellular and Molecular Aspects. Philadelphia: Lippincott-Raven, 1996, pp 435–455.

28. Berlin C, Bargatze RF, Campbell JJ, von Andrian UH, Szabo MC, Hasslen, SR, Nelson RD, Berg EL, Erlandsen SL, Butcher EC: Alpha 4 integrins mediate lymphocyte attachment and rolling under physiologic flow. Cell 1995;80:413–422.

29. Beutler B, Mahoney J, Le Trang N, Pekala P, Cerami A: Purification of cachectin, a lipoprotein lipase-suppressing hormone secreted by endotoxin-induced RAW 264.7 cells. J Exp Med 1985; 161:984–995.

30. Bhakdi S, Tranum-Jensen J: Complement lysis: a hole is a hole. Immunol Today 1991;12:9:318–320.

31. Billingham RE, Brent L, Medawar PB: 'Actively acquired tolerance' of foreign cells. Nature 1953;172:603–606.

32. Bishop DK, Jutila MA, Sedmak DD, Beattie MS, Orosz CG: Lymphocyte entry into inflammatory tissues in vivo. Qualitative differences of high endothelial venule-like vessels in sponge matrix allografts vs isografts. J Immunol 1989;142:4219–4224.

33. Boucraut J, Guillaudeux T, Alizadeh M, Boretto J, Chimini G, Malecaze F, Semana G, Fauchet R, Pontarotti P, Le Bouteiller P: HLA-E is the only class I gene that escapes CpG methylation and is transcriptionally active in the trophoblast-derived human cell line JAR. Immunogenetics 1993;38:117–130.

34. Boussiotis VA, Gribben JG, Freeman GJ, Nadler LM: Blockade of the CD28 co-stimulatory pathway: a means to induce tolerance [review]. Curr Opin Immunol 1994;6:797–807.

35. Boyson JE, McAdam SN, Gallimore A, Golos TG, Liu X, Gotch FM, Hughes AL, Watkins DI: The MHC E locus in macaques is polymorphic and is conserved between macaques and humans. Immunogenetics 1995;41:59–68.

36. Breur-Vriesendorp BS, Vingerhoed J, van Twuyver E, de Waal LP, Ivanyi P: Frequency analysis of HLA-specific cytotoxic T lymphocyte precursors in humans. Transplantation 1991;51: 1096–1103.

37. Brouckaert P, Libert C, Everaerdt B, Takahashi N, Cauwels A, Fiers W: Tumor necrosis factor, its receptors and the connection with interleukin 1 and interleukin 6 [review]. Immunobiology 1993;187:317–329.

38. Brown JH, Jardetzky TS, Gorga JC, Stern LJ, Urban RG, Strominger JL, Wiley DC: Three-dimensional structure of the human class II histocompatibility antigen HLA-DR1. Nature 1993;364:33–39.

39. Butcher EC: Leukocyte-endothelial cell recognition: three (or more) steps to specificity and diversity [review]. Cell 1991;67: 1033–1036.

40. Campbell RD, Trowsdale J: Map of the human MHC. Immunol Today 1993;14:349–352.

41. Carbone FR, Bevan MJ: Class-I-restricted processing and presentation of exogenous cell-associated antigen in vivo. J Exp Med 1990;171:377–387.

42. Carson DA, Ribeiro JM: Apoptosis and disease [review]. Lancet 1993;341:1251–1254.

43. Ceman S, Rudersdorf RA, Petersen JM, DeMars R: DMA and DMB are the only genes in the class II region of the human MHC needed for class II-associated antigen processing. J Immunol 1995;154:2545–2556.

44. Charpentier B, Hiesse C, Ferran C, Lantz O, Fries D, Bach JF, Chatenoud L: Acute clinical syndrome associated with OKT3 administration. Prevention by single injection of an anti-human TNF monoclonal antibody [in French]. Presse Med 1991;20:2009–2011.

45. Chatenoud L, Bach JF: T lymphocyte activation induced by monoclonal anti-CD3 antibodies: Physiopathology of cytokine release [in French]. C R Seances Soc Biol Fil 1991;185:268–277.

46. Chatenoud L, Ferran C, Bach JF: The anti-CD3-induced syndrome: a consequence of massive in vivo cell activation [review]. Curr Top Microbiol Immunol 1991;174:121–134.

47. Cher DJ, Mosmann TR: Two types of murine helper T cell clone. II. Delayed-type hypersensitivity is mediated by TH1 clones. J Immunol 1987;138:3688–3694.

48. Chicz RM, Urban RG, Lane WS, Gorga JC, Stern LJ, Vignali DASJL: Predominant naturally processed peptides bound to HLA-DR1 are derived from MHC-related molecules and are heterogeneous in size. Nature 1992;358:764–768.

49. Chien Y-H, Becker DM, Lindsten T, Okamura M, Cohen DI, Davis MM: A third type of murine T-cell receptor gene. Nature 1984;312:31–35.

50. Chien Y, Iwashima M, Kaplan KB, Elliott JF, Davis MM: A new T-cell receptor gene located within the alpha locus and expressed early in T-cell differentiation. Nature 1987;327:677–682.

51. Christie DL, Gagnon J: Amino acid sequence of the Bb fragment from complement Factor B. Sequence of the major cyanogen bromide-cleavage peptide (CB-II) and completion of the sequence of the Bb fragment. Biochem J 1983;209:61–70.

52. Clark SP, Yoshikai Y, Taylor S, Siu G, Hood L, Mak TW: Identification of a diversity segment of human T-cell receptor beta-chain, and comparison with the analogous murine element. Nature 1984;311:387–389.

53. Cohen JJ: Programmed cell death in the immune system. Adv Immunol 1991;50:55–85.

54. D'Andrea A, Aste-Amezaga M, Valiante NM, Ma X, Kubin M, Trinchieri G: Interleukin 10 (IL-10) inhibits human lymphocyte interferon gamma-production by suppressing natural killer cell stimulatory factor/IL-12 synthesis in accessory cells. J Exp Med 1993;178:1041–1048.

55. Dallman MJ: Cytokines and transplantation: Th1/Th1 regulation of the immune response to solid organ transplantation in the adult. Curr Opin Immunol 1995;7:632–638.

56. Dausset J: The Nobel Lectures in Immunology. The Nobel Prize for Physiology or Medicine, 1980. The major histocompatibility complex in man. Past, present, and future concepts. Scand J Immunol 1992;36:145–157.

57. De Waal Malefyt R, Figdor CG, Huijbens R, Mohan-Peterson S, Bennett B, Culpepper J, Dang W, Zurawski G, de Vries JE: Effects of IL-13 on phenotype, cytokine production, and cytotoxic function of human monocytes. Comparison with IL-4 and modulation by IFN-gamma or IL-10. J Immunol 1993;151:6370–6381.

58. Desiderio SV, Yancopoulos GD, Paskind M, Thomas E, Boss MA, Landau N, Alt FW, Baltimore D: Insertion of N regions into heavy-chain genes is correlated with expression of terminal deoxytransferase in B cells. Nature 1984;311:752–755.

59. DiScipio RG: The relationship between polymerization of complement component C9 and membrane channel formation. J Immunol 1991;147:4239–4247.

60. DiScipio RG: The size, shape and stability of complement component C9. Mol Immunol 1993;30:1097–1106.

61. Duquesnoy RJ, Demetris AJ: Immunopathology of cardiac transplant rejection [review]. Curr Opin Cardiol 1995;10:193–206.

62. Eck MJ, Sprang SR: The structure of tumor necrosis factor-alpha at 2.6 A resolution. Implications for receptor binding. J Biol Chem 1989;264:17595–17605.

63. Eckels DD: Alloreactivity: allogeneic presentation of endogenous peptide or direct recognition of MHC polymorphism? A review [review]. Tissue Antigens 1990;35:49–55.

64. Edelman GM, Cunningham BA, Gall WE, Gottlieb PD, Rutishauser U, Waxdal MJ: The covalent structure of an entire gamma G immunoglobulin molecule. Proc Natl Acad Sci U S A 1969;63:78–85.

65. Edelman GM, Gall WE, Waxdal MJ, Konigsberg WH: The covalent structure of a human gamma G-immunoglobulin. I. Isolation and characterization of the whole molecule, the polypeptide chains, and the tryptic fragments. Biochemistry 1968;7:1950–1958.

66. el Kahloun A, Vernet C, Jouanolle AM, Boretto J, Mauvieux V, Le Gal, JY, David V, Pontarotti P: A continuous restriction map from HLA-E to HLA-F. Structural comparison between different HLA-A haplotypes. Immunogenetics 1992;35:183–189.

67. Engers HD, Unanue ER: The fate of anti-Ig-surface Ig complexes on B lymphocytes. J Immunol 1973;110:465–475.

68. Essery G, Feldmann M, Lamb JR: Interleukin-2 can prevent and reverse antigen-induced unresponsiveness in cloned human T lymphocytes. Immunology 1988;64:413–417.

69. Fabre JW, Morris PJ: The effect of donor strain blood pretreatment on renal allograft rejection in rats. Transplantation 1972;14:608–617.

70. Fearon DT, Austen KF: Properdin: binding to C3b and stabilization of the C3b-dependent C3 convertase. J Exp Med 1975;142:856–863.

71. Fink PJ, Shimenkovitz RP, Bevan MJ: Veto cells. Annu Rev Immunol 1988;6:115–137.

72. Fisher PE, Suciu-Foca N, Ho E, Michler RE, Rose EA, Mancini D: Additive value of immunologic monitoring to histologic grading of heart allograft biopsy specimens: implications for therapy. J Heart Lung Transplant 1995;14:1156–1161.

73. Fleischman JB, Pain RH, Porter RR: Reduction of gammaglobulins. Arch Biochem Biophys Suppl 1962;1:174.

74. Fournel S, Genestier L, Robinet E, Flacher M, Revillard JP: Human T cells require IL-2 but not G1/S transition to acquire susceptibility to Fas-mediated apoptosis. J Immunol 1996;157:4309–4315.

75. Gao GF, Tormo J, Gerth UC, Wyer JR, McMichael AJ, Stuart DI, Bell JI, Jones EY, Jakobsen BK: Crystal structure of the complex between human CD8alpha(alpha) and HLA-A2. Nature 1997;387:630–634.

76. Garboczi DN, Ghosh P, Utz U, Fan QR, Biddison WE, Wiley DC: Structure of the complex between human T-cell receptor, viral peptide and HLA-A2 [comment]. Nature 1996;384:134–141.

77. Gaston RS: Cytokines and transplantation: a clinical perspective [review] Transplant Sci 1994;(Suppl 1):S9–S19.

78. Gaulton GN, Williamson P: Interleukin-2 and the interleukin-2 receptor complex [review]. Chem Immunol 1994;59:91–114.

79. George JF, Sweeney SD, Goldstein DR, Kirklin JK, Thomas JM: An essential role for fas-ligand in transplantation tolerance. Nat Med 1998;4:333–335.

80. Gerard C, Gerard NP: C5A anaphylatoxin and its seven transmembrane-segment receptor [review]. Annu Rev Immunol 1994;12:775–808.

81. Gershon RK, Cohen P, Hencin R, Liebhaber SA: Suppressor T cells. J Immunol 1972;108:586–590.

82. Goumy L, Ferran C, Merite S, Bach JF, Chatenoud L: In vivo anti-CD3-driven cell activation. Cellular source of induced tumor necrosis factor, interleukin-1 beta, and interleukin-6. Transplantation 1996;61:83–87.

83. Green D, Flood P, Gershon RK: Immunoregulatory T-cell pathways. Annu Rev Immunol 1983;1:439–464.

84. Green JM, DeMars R, Xu X, Pierce SK: The intracellular transport of MHC class II molecules in the absence of HLA-DM. J Immunol 1995;155:3759–3768.

85. Gretz JE, Kaldjian EP, Anderson AO, Shaw S: Sophisticated strategies for information encounter in the lymph node: the reticular network as a conduit of soluble information and a highway for cell traffic [review]. J Immunol 1996;157:495–499.

86. Guinan EC, Gribben JG, Boussiotis VA, Freeman GJ, Nadler LM: Pivotal role of the B7:CD28 pathway in transplantation tolerance and tumor immunity [review]. Blood 1994;84:3261–3282.

87. Halasz NA, Orloff MJ, Hirose F: Increased survival of renal homografts in dogs after injection of graft donor blood. Transplantation 1964;2:453–458.

88. Halloran PF, Autenried P, Ramassar V, Urmson J, Cockfield S: Local T cell responses induce widespread MHC expression. Evidence that IFN-gamma induces its own expression in remote sites. J Immunol 1992;148:3837–3846.

89. Haskins K, Kubo R, White J, Pigeon M, Kappler J, Marrack P: The major histocompatibility complex-restricted antigen receptor on T cells. I. Isolation with a monoclonal antibody. J Exp Med 1983;157:1149–1169.

90. Hayry P, Leszczynski D, Nemlander A, Ferry B, Renkonen R, von Willebrand E, Halttunen J: Donor-directed cytotoxic T cells and other inflammatory components of acute allograft rejection. Ann N Y Acad Sci 1988;532:86–105.

91. Hedrick SM, Cohen DI, Nielsen EA, Davis MM: Isolation of cDNA clones encoding T cell-specific membrane-associated proteins. Nature 1984;308:149–153.

92. Heemels MT, Ploegh H: Generation, translocation, and presentation of MHC class I-restricted peptides [review]. Annu Rev Biochem 1995;64:463–491.

93. Herberman R, Nunn M, Holden H, Lavrin D: Natural cytotoxic reactivity of mouse lymphoid cells against syngeneic and allogeneic tumors. II. Characterization of effector cells. Int J Cancer 1975;16:230–239.

94. Hilschmann N, Craig LC: Amino acid sequence studies with Bence-Jones proteins. Proc Natl Acad Sci U S A 1965;53:1403–1409.

95. Hiruma K, Nakamura H, Henkart PA, Gress RE: Clonal deletion of postthymic T cells: veto cells kill precursor cytotoxic T lymphocytes. J Exp Med 1992;175:863–868.

96. Hogg N, Landis RC: Adhesion molecules in cell interactions [review]. Curr Opin Immunol 1993;5:383–390.

97. Horwitz AF: Integrins and health. Sci Am 1997;276:68–75.

98. Houlihan JM, Biro PA, Harper HM, Jenkinson HJ, Holmes CH: The human amnion is a site of MHC class Ib expression: evidence for the expression of HLA-E and HLA-G. J Immunol 1995;154:5665–5674.

99. Howard JC: Supply and transport of peptides presented by class I MHC molecules [review]. Curr Opin Immunol 1995;7:69–76.

100. Hsieh CS, Macatonia SE, Tripp CS, Wolf SF, O'Garra A, Murphy KM: Development of TH1 CD4+ T cells through IL-12 produced by Listeria-induced macrophages. Science 1993;260:547–549.

101. Hubbard WJ, Thomas JM: Cytoablation and cytoreduction strategies in transplant tolerance. Curr Opin Organ Transplant 1997;2:36–46.

102. Hunt DF, Michel H, Dickinson TA, Shabanowitz J, Cox AL, Sakaguchi KAE, Grey HM, Sette A: Peptides presented to the immune system by the murine class II major histocompatibility complex molecule I-Ad. Science 1992;256:1817–1820.

103. Jardetzky TS, Brown JH, Gorga JC, Stern LJ, Urban RG, Chi Y-I, Stauffacher C, Strominger JL, Wiley DC: Three-dimensional structure of a human class II histocompatibility molecule complexed with superantigen. Nature 1994;368:711–718.

104. Jenkins MK, Schwartz RH: Antigen presentation by chemically modified splenocytes induces antigen-specific T cell unresponsiveness in vitro and in vivo. J Exp Med 1987;165:302–319.

105. Jerne NK: Idiotypic networks and other preconcieved ideas. Immunol Rev 1984;79:5–24.

106. Johnston JA, Bacon CM, Riedy MC, O'Shea JJ: Signaling by IL-2 and related cytokines: JAKs, STATs, and relationship to immunodeficiency [review]. J Leukoc Biol 1996;60:441–452.

107. Jones EY, Stuart DI, Walker NP: Structure of tumour necrosis factor. Nature 1989;338:225–228.

108. Joseph JV, Guy SP, Brenchley PE, Parrott NR, Short CD, Johnson RW, Hutchinson IV: Th1 and Th2 cytokine gene expression in human renal allografts. Transplant Proc 1995;27:915–916.

109. Journet A, Tosi M: Cloning and sequencing of full-length cDNA encoding the precursor of human complement component C1r. Biochem J 1986;240:783–787.

110. Jurisicova A, Casper RF, MacLusky NJ, Mills GB, Librach CL: HLA-G expression during preimplantation human embryo development. Proc Natl Acad Sci U S A 1996;93:161–165.

111. Jutila MA: Function and regulation of leukocyte homing receptors [review]. J Leukoc Biol 1994;55:133–140.

112. Kaminsky SG, Nakamura I, Cudkowicz G: Genetic control of the natural killer cell activity in SJL and other strains of mice. J Immunol 1985;135:665–671.

113. Kast WM, van Twuyver E, Mooijaart RJ, Verveld M, Kamphuis AG, Melief CJ, de Waal LP: Mechanism of skin allograft enhancement across an H-2 class I mutant difference. Evidence for involvement of veto cells. Eur J Immunol 1988;18:2105–2108.

114. Keever-Taylor CA, Witt PL, Truitt RL, Ramanujam S, Borden EC, Ritch PS: Hematologic and immunologic evaluation of recombinant human interleukin-6 in patients with advanced malignant disease: evidence for monocyte activation. J Immunother Emphasis Tumor Immunol 1996;19:231–243.

115. Khoury SJ, Akalin E, Chandraker A, Turka LA, Linsley PS, Sayegh MH, Hancock WW: CD28-B7 costimulatory blockade by CTLA4lg prevents actively induced experimental autoimmune encephalomyelitis and inhibits Th1 but spares Th2 cytokines in the central nervous system. J Immunol 1995;155:4521–4524.

116. Kiessling R, Petranyi G, Klein G, Wigzell H: Genetic variation of in vitro cytolytic activity and in vivo rejection potential of non-immunized semi-syngeneic mice against a mouse lymphoma line. Int J Cancer 1975;15:933–940.

117. Kim S, Davis M, Sinn E, Patten P, Hood L: Antibody diversity: somatic hypermutation of rearranged VH genes. Cell 1981;27:573–581.

118. Kiniwa M, Gately M, Gubler U, Chizzonite R, Fargeas C, Delespesse G: Recombinant interleukin-12 suppresses the synthesis of immunoglobulin E by interleukin-4 stimulated human lymphocytes. J Clin Invest 1992;90:262–266.

119. Klebanoff SJ, Vadas MA, Harlan JM, Sparks LH, Gamble JR, Agosti JM, Waltersdorph AM: Stimulation of neutrophils by tumor necrosis factor. J Immunol 1986;136:4220–4225.

120. Klein CL, Bittinger F, Kohler H, Wagner M, Otto M, Hermanns I, Kirkpatrick CJ: Comparative studies on vascular endothelium in vitro. 3. Effects of cytokines on the expression of E-selectin, ICAM-1 and VCAM-1 by cultured human endothelial cells obtained from different passages. Pathobiology 1995;63:83–92.

121. Klein CL, Kohler H, Bittinger F, Wagner M, Hermanns I, Grant K, Lewis JC, Kirkpatrick CJ: Comparative studies on vascular endothelium in vitro. I. Cytokine effects on the expression of adhesion molecules by human umbilical vein, saphenous vein and femoral artery endothelial cells. Pathobiology 1994;62:199–208.

122. Knechtle SJ, Vargo D, Fechner J, Zhai Y, Wang J, Hanaway MJ, Scharff J, Hu H, Knapp L, Watkins D, Neville DM Jr: FN18-CRM9 immunotoxin promotes tolerance in primate renal allografts. Transplantation 1997;63:1–6.

123. Kruisbeek AM: Development of alpha beta T cells [review]. Curr Opin Immunol 1993;5:227–234.

124. Kruisbeek AM, Amsen D: Mechanisms underlying T cell tolerance. Curr Opin Immunol 1996;8:233–244.

125. Kuby J: Immunology. New York: WH Freeman and Co, 1992.

126. Labarrere CA, Pitts D, Halbrook H, Faulk WP: Tissue plasminogen activator, plasminogen activator inhibitor-1, and fibrin as indexes of clinical course in cardiac allograft recipients. An immunocytochemical study. Circulation 1994;89:1599–1608.

127. Lamb JR, Skidmore BJ, Green N, Chiller JM: Induction of tolerance in influenza virus-immune T lymphocyte clones with synthetic peptides of influenza hemagglutinin. J Exp Med 1983;157:1434–1447.

128. Larsen CP, Morris PJ, Austyn JM: Migration of dendritic leukocytes from cardiac allografts into host spleens. A novel pathway for initiation of rejection. J Exp Med 1990;171:307–314.

129. Le Bouteiller P: Regulation of the expression of HLA class I genes in human trophoblasts [review; in French]. Pathol Biol 1995;43:628–635.

130. Lechler R, Lombardi G: Structural aspects of allorecognition. Curr Opin Immunol 1991;3:715–721.

131. Lenschow DJ, Walunas TL, Bluestone JA: CD28/B7 system of T cell costimulation [review]. Annu Rev Immunol 1996;14:233–258.

132. Lieber MR: Site-specific recombination in the immune system [review]. FASEB J 1991;5:2934–2944.

133. Lieber MR, Chang CP, Gallo M, Gauss G, Gerstein R, Islas A: The mechanism of V(D)J recombination: site-specificity, reaction fidelity and immunologic diversity [review]. Semin Immunol 1994;6:143–153.

134. Linsley PS, Ledbetter JA: The role of the CD28 receptor during T cell responses to antigen [review]. Annu Rev Immunol 1993;11:191–212.

135. Liu Z, Sun YK, Xi YP, Maffei A, Reed E, Harris P, Suciu-Foca N: Contribution of direct and indirect recognition pathways to T cell alloreactivity. J Exp Med 1993;177:1643–1650.

136. Loh EY, Lanier LL, Turck CW, Littman DR, Davis MM, Chien YH, Weiss A: Identification and sequence of a fourth human T cell antigen receptor chain. Nature 1987;330:569–572.

137. Long EO: Antigen processing for presentation to CD4+ cells. New Biol 1992;4:274–282.

138. Lowin B, Beermann F, Schmidt A, Tschopp J: A null mutation in the perforin gene impairs cytolytic T lymphocyte- and natural killer cell-mediated cytotoxicity. Proc Natl Acad Sci U S A 1994;91:11571–11575.

139. Lowry RP: The relationship of IL-4, IL-10 and other cytokines to transplantation tolerance. Transplant Sci 1993;3:104–112.

140. Lundwall AB, Wetsel RA, Kristensen T, Whitehead AS, Woods DE, Ogden RC, Colten HR, Tack BF: Isolation and sequence analysis of a cDNA clone encoding the fifth complement component. J Biol Chem 1985;260:2108–2112.

141. Luscinskas FW, Ding H, Lichtman AH: P-selectin and vascular cell adhesion molecule 1 mediate rolling and arrest, respectively, of CD4+ T lymphocytes on tumor necrosis factor alpha-activated vascular endothelium under flow. J Exp Med 1995;181:1179–1186.

142. Luscinskas FW, Kansas GS, Ding H, Pizcueta P, Schleiffenbaum BE, Tedder TF, Gimbrone MA Jr: Monocyte rolling, arrest and spreading on IL-4-activated vascular endothelium under flow is mediated via sequential action of L-selectin, beta 1-integrins, and beta 2-integrins. J Cell Biol 1994;125:1417–1427.

143. Madsen JC, Superina RA, Wood KJ, Morris PJ: Immunological unresponsiveness induced by recipient cells transfected with donor MHC genes. Nature 1988;332:161–164.

144. Manetti R, Parronchi P, Giudizi MG, Piccinni MP, Maggi E, Trinchieri G, Romagnani S: Natural killer cell stimulatory factor (interleukin 12 [IL-12]) induces T helper type 1 (Th1)-specific immune responses and inhibits the development of IL-4-producing Th cells. J Exp Med 1993;177:1199–1204.

145. Marquet RL, Heystek GA, Tinbergen WJ: Specific inhibition of organ allograft rejection by donor blood. Transplant Proc 1971; 3:708–710.

146. Medawar PB: Immunity to homologous grafted skin. II. The relationship between the antigens of blood and skin. Br J Exp Pathol 1945;27:15–24.

147. Mole JE, Anderson JK, Davison EA, Woods DE: Complete primary structure for the zymogen of human complement factor B. J Biol Chem 1984;259:3407–3412.

148. Monaco AP, Gozzo JJ, Wood ML, Liegeois A: Use of low doses of homozygous allogeneic bone marrow cells to induce tolerance with antilymphocyte serum (ALS): tolerance by intraorgan injection. Transplant Proc 1971;3:680–683.

149. Monaco JJ: Pathways for the processing and presentation of antigens to T cells [review]. J Leukoc Biol 1995;57:543–547.

150. Mosmann TR, Coffman RL: TH1 and TH2 cells: different patterns of lymphokine secretion lead to different functional properties. Annu Rev Immunol 1989;7:145–173.

151. Mosmann TR, Sad S: The expanding universe of T-cell subsets: Th1, Th2 and more [review]. Immunol Today 1996;17:138–146.

152. Muller-Eberhard HJ: Molecular organization and function of the complement system. Annu Rev Biochem 1988;57:321–347.

153. Muller-Eberhard HJ: Molecular organization and function of the complement system [review]. Annu Rev Biochem 1988; 57:321–347.

154. Muller-Eberhard HJ, Schreiber RD: Molecular biology and chemistry of the alternative pathway of complement [review]. Adv Immunol 1980;29:1–53.

155. Munson JL, van Twuyver E, Mooijaart RJ, Roux E, ten Berge IJ, de Waal LP: Missing T-cell receptor V beta families following blood transfusion. The role of HLA in development of immunization and tolerance. Hum Immunol 1995;42:43–53.

156. Muraoka S, Miller RG: Cells in bone marrow and in T cell colonies grown from bone marrow can suppress generation of cytotoxic T lymphocytes directed against their self antigens. J Exp Med 1980;152:54–71.

157. Musci MA, Latinis KM, Koretzky GA: Signaling events in T lymphocytes leading to cellular activation or programmed cell death [review]. Clin Immunol Immunopathol 1997;83:205–222.

158. Natvig JB, Kunkel HG: Human immunoglobulins: classes, subclasses, genetic variants, and idiotypes [review]. Adv Immunol 1973;16:1–59.

159. Newton-Nash DK, Eckels DD: Effects of localized HLA class II beta chain polymorphism on binding of antigenic peptide and stimulation of T cells. Hum Immunol 1992;33:213–223.

160. Nickerson P, Steiger J, Zheng XX, Steele AW, Steurer W, Roy-Chaudhury P, Strom TB: Manipulation of cytokine networks in transplantation: false hope or realistic opportunity for tolerance? [review]. Transplantation 1997;63:489–494.

161. O'Leary JJ, Chetty R, Graham AK, McGee JO: In situ PCR: pathologist's dream or nightmare? [review]. J Pathol 1996;178:11–20.

162. Opelz G: Improved kidney graft survival in nontransfused recipients. Transplant Proc 1987;19:149–152.

163. Opelz G, Sengar DPS, Mickey MR, Terasaki PI: Effect of blood transfusions on subsequent kidney transplants. Transplant Proc 1973;5:253–259.

164. Opelz G, Terasaki PI: Improvement of kidney-graft survival with increased numbers of blood transfusion. N Engl J Med 1978; 299:799–803.

165. Otsuka A, Hanafusa T, Kono N, Tarui S: Lipopolysaccharide augments HLA-A,B,C molecule expression but inhibits interferon-gamma-induced HLA-DR molecule expression on cultured human endothelial cells. Immunology 1991;73:428–432.

166. Parker DC: T cell-dependent B cell activation [review]. Annu Rev Immunol 1993;11:331–360.

167. Paul WE, Seder RA: Lymphocyte responses and cytokines [review]. Cell 1994;76:241–251.

168. Pawlowski TJ, Staerz UD: Thymic education—T cells do it for themselves [review]. Immunol Today 1994;15:205–209.

169. Pizcueta P, Luscinskas FW: Monoclonal antibody blockade of L-selectin inhibits mononuclear leukocyte recruitment to inflammatory sites in vivo. Am J Pathol 1994;145:461–469.

170. Podack ER: Execution and suicide: cytotoxic lymphocytes enforce Draconian laws through separate molecular pathways [review]. Curr Opin Immunol 1995;7:11–16.

171. Poupart P, Vandenabeele P, Cayphas S, Van Snick J, Haegeman G, Kruys V, Fiers W, Content J: B cell growth modulating and differentiating activity of recombinant human 26-kd protein (BSF-2, HuIFN-beta 2, HPGF). EMBO J 1987;6:1219–1224.

172. Rebellato LM, Gross U, Verbanac KM, Thomas JM: A comprehensive definition of the major antibody specificities in polyclonal rabbit antithymocyte globulin. Transplantation 1994;57:685–694.

173. Reinherz EL, Meuer S, Fitzgerald KA, Hussey RE, Levine H, Schlossman SF: Antigen recognition by human T lymphocytes is linked to surface expression of the T3 molecular complex. Cell 1982;300:735–743.

174. Robey E, Fowlkes BJ: Selective events in T cell development [review]. Annu Rev Immunol 1994;12:675–705.

175. Robinson MA, Mitchell MP, Wei S, Day CE, Zhao TM, Concannon P: Organization of human T-cell receptor beta-chain genes: clusters of Vbeta genes are present on chromosomes 7 and 9. Proc Natl Acad Sci U S A 1993;90:2433–2437.

176. Robinson PJ, Graf L, Sege K: Two allelic forms of mouse beta 2-microglobulin. Proc Natl Acad Sci U S A 1981;78:1167–1170.

177. Robinson PJ, Lundin L, Sege K, Graf L, Wigzell H, Peterson PA: Location of the mouse beta 2-microglobulin gene B2m determined by linkage analysis. Immunogenetics 1981;14:449–452.

178. Rose ML, Coles MI, Griffin RJ, Pomerance A, Yacoub MH: Expression of class I and class II major histocompatibility antigens in normal and transplanted human heart. Transplantation 1986; 41:776–780.

179. Rose ML, Navarette C, Yacoub MH, Festenstein H: Persistence of donor-specific class II antigens in allografted human heart two years after transplantation. Hum Immunol 1988;23:179–190.

180. Rosen SD, Hwang ST, Giblin PA, Singer MS: High-endothelial-venule ligands for L-selectin: identification and functions [review]. Biochem Soc Trans 1997;25:428–433.

181. Ruan XM, Qiao JH, Trento A, Czer LS, Blanche C, Fishbein MC: Cytokine expression and endothelial cell and lymphocyte activation in human cardiac allograft rejection: an immunohistochemical study of endomyocardial biopsy samples. J Heart Lung Transplant 1992;11:1110–1115.

182. Rudensky AY, Preston-Hurlburt P, Hong S-C, Barlow A, Janeway CA: Sequence analysis of peptides bound to MHC class II molecules. Nature 1991;353:622–627.

183. Salgame P, Abrams JS, Clayberger C, Goldstein H, Convit J, Modlin RL, Bloom BR: Differing lymphokine profiles of functional subsets of human CD4 and CD8 T cell clones. Science 1991;254:279–282.

184. Salter MM, Kirklin JK, Bourge RC, Naftel DC, White-Williams C, Tarkka M, Waits E, Bucy RP: Total lymphoid irradiation in the treatment of early or recurrent heart rejection. J Heart Lung Transplant 1992;11:902–912.

185. Sambhara SR, Miller RG: Programmed cell death of T cells signaled by the T cell receptor and the alpha 3 domain of class I MHC. Science 1991;252:1424–1427.

186. Sayegh MH, Akalin E, Hancock WW, Russell ME, Carpenter CB, Linsley PS, Turka LA: CD28-B7 blockade after alloantigenic challenge in vivo inhibits Th1 cytokines but spares Th2. J Exp Med 1995;181:1869–1874.

187. Schulman LL, Ho EK, Reed EF, McGregor C, Smith CR, Rose EA, Suciu-Foca N: Immunologic monitoring in lung allograft recipients. Transplantation 1996;61:252–257.

188. Schumaker VN, Zavodszky P, Poon PH: Activation of the first component of complement [review]. Annu Rev Immunol 1987; 5:21–42.

189. Sehgal PB, May LT, Tamm I, Vilcek J: Human beta 2 interferon and B-cell differentiation factor BSF-2 are identical. Science 1987;235:731–732.

190. Seidman JG, Leder A, Edgell MH, Polsky F, Tilghman SM, Tiemeier DC, Leder P: Multiple related immunoglobulin variable-region genes identified by cloning and sequence analysis. Proc Natl Acad Sci U S A 1978;75:3881–3885.

191. Setien F, Alvarez V, Coto E, DiScipio RG, Lopez-Larrea C: A physical map of the human complement component C6, C7, and C9 genes. Immunogenetics 1993;38:341–344.

192. Sette A, DeMars R, Grey HM, Oseroff C, Southwood S, Appella E, Kubo RT, Hunt DF: Isolation and characterization of naturally processed peptides bound by class II molecules and peptides presented by normal and mutant antigen-presenting cells. Chem Immunol 1993;57:152–165.

193. Sette A, Grey HM: Chemistry of peptide interactions with MHC proteins [review]. Curr Opin Immunol 1992;4:79–86.

194. Shalaby MR, Aggarwal BB, Rinderknecht E, Svedersky LP, Finkle BS, Palladino MA Jr: Activation of human polymorphonuclear neutrophil functions by interferon-gamma and tumor necrosis factors. J Immunol 1985;135:2069–2073.

195. Shawar SM, Vyas JM, Rodgers JR, Rich RR: Antigen presentation by major histocompatibility complex class I- B molecules [review]. Annu Rev Immunol 1994;12:839–880.

196. Sim RB, Reid KB: C1: molecular interactions with activating systems [review]. Immunol Today 1991;12:307–311.

197. Siu G, Clark SP, Yoshikai Y, Malissen M, Yanagi Y, Strauss E, Mak TW, Hood L: The human T cell antigen receptor is encoded by variable, diversity, and joining gene segments that rearrange to generate a complete V gene. Cell 1984;37:393–401.

198. Siu G, Kronenberg M, Strauss E, Haars R, Mak TW, Hood L: The structure, rearrangement and expression of D beta gene segments of the murine T-cell antigen receptor. Nature 1984;311:344–350.

199. Smith CA, Pangburn MK, Vogel CW, Muller-Eberhard HJ: Molecular architecture of human properdin, a positive regulator of the alternative pathway of complement. J Biol Chem 1984;259:4582–4588.

200. Sorger SB, Hedrick SM: Highly conserved T-cell receptor junctional regions. Evidence for selection at the protein and the DNA level. Immunogenetics 1990;31:118–122.

201. Spies T, Morton CC, Nedospasov SA, Fiers W, Pious D, Strominger JL: Genes for the tumor necrosis factors alpha and beta are linked to the human major histocompatibility complex. Proc Natl Acad Sci U S A 1986;83:8699–8702.

202. Spriggs DR, Deutsch S, Kufe DW: Genomic structure, induction, and production of TNF-alpha [review]. Immunol Ser 1992;56:3–34.

203. Springer TA: Traffic signals on endothelium for lymphocyte recirculation and leukocyte emigration [review]. Annu Rev Physiol 1995;57:827–872.

204. Staerz UD, Karasuyama H, Garner AM: Cytotoxic T lymphocytes against a soluble protein. Nature 1987;329:449–451.

205. Stavnezer J: Immunoglobulin class switching. Curr Opin Immunol 1996;8:199–205.

206. Steinhoff G, Wonigeit K, Schafers HJ, Haverich A: Sequential analysis of monomorphic and polymorphic major histocompatibility complex antigen expression in human heart allograft biopsy specimens. J Heart Transplant 1989;8:360–370.

207. Stewart M, Thiel M, Hogg N: Leukocyte integrins [review]. Curr Opin Cell Biol 1995;7:690–696.

208. Strom TB, Roy-Chaudhury P, Manfro R, Zheng XX, Nickerson PW, Wood K, Bushell A: The Th1/Th2 paradigm and the allograft response [review]. Curr Opin Immunol 1996;8:688–693.

209. Sugamura K, Asao H, Kondo M, Tanaka N, Ishii N, Ohbo K, Nakamura M, Takeshita T: The interleukin-2 receptor gamma chain: its role in the multiple cytokine receptor complexes and T cell development in XSCID [review]. Annu Rev Immunol 1996;14:179–205.

210. Tassani P, Otto D, Szekely A, Meiser B, Uberfuhr P, Pfeiffer M, Jaenicke U: Transfusion of platelet-rich plasma from the organ donor during cardiac transplantation. J Clin Anesth 1997;9:409–414.

211. Taylor PM, Rose ML, Yacoub MH, Pigott R: Induction of vascular adhesion molecules during rejection of human cardiac allografts. Transplantation 1992;54:451–457.

212. Teo IA, Shaunak S: Polymerase chain reaction in situ: an appraisal of an emerging technique [review]. Histochem J 1995;27:647–659.

213. Theze J, Alzari PM, Bertoglio J: Interleukin 2 and its receptors: recent advances and new immunological functions [review]. Immunol Today 1996;17:481–486.

214. Thomas JM, Carver FM, Burnett CM, Thomas FT: Enhanced allograft survival in rhesus monkeys treated with anti- human thymocyte globulin and donor lymphoid cells. Transplant Proc 1981;13:599–602.

215. Thomas JM, Carver FM, Cunningham P, Olsen L, Thomas FT: Veto cells induce long-term kidney allograft tolerance in primates without chronic immunosuppression. Transplant Proc 1991;23: 11–13.

216. Thomas JM, Carver FM, Cunningham PR, Olson LC, Thomas FT: Kidney allograft tolerance in primates without chronic immunosuppression—the role of veto cells. Transplantation 1991; 51:198–207.

217. Thomas JM, Carver FM, Foil MB, Hall WR, Adams C, Fahrenbruch GB, Thomas FT: Renal allograft tolerance induced with ATG and donor bone marrow in outbred rhesus monkeys. Transplantation 1983;36:104–106.

218. Thomas JM, Carver FM, Kasten-Jolly J, Haisch CE, Rebellato LM, Gross U, Vore SJ, Thomas FT: Further studies of veto activity in rhesus monkey bone marrow in relation to allograft tolerance and chimerism. Transplantation 1994;57:101–115.

219. Thomas JM, Carver FM, Thomas FT: Enhanced allograft survival in rhesus monkeys treated with anti- human thymocyte globulin and donor lymphoid cells. Surg Forum 1979;30:282–283.

220. Thomas JM, Neville DM, Contreras JL, Eckhoff DE, Meng G, Lobashevsky AL, Wang PX, Huang ZQ, Verbanac KM, Haisch CE, Thomas FT: Preclinical studies of allograft tolerance in rhesus monkeys: a novel anti-CD3-immunotoxin given peritransplant with donor bone marrow induces operational tolerance to kidney allografts. Transplantation 1997;64:124–135.

221. Thomas JM, Verbance KM, Carver FM, Kasten-Jolly J, Haisch CE, Gross U, Smith JP: Veto cells in transplantation tolerance. Clin Transplant 1994;8:195–203.

222. Thomas JM, Verbanac KM, Smith JP, Kasten-Jolly J, Gross U, Rebellato LM, Haisch CE, Carver FM, Thomas FT: The facilitating effect of one-DR antigen sharing in renal allograft tolerance induced by donor bone marrow in rhesus monkeys. Transplantation 1995;59:245–255.

223. Thompson CB: Apoptosis in the pathogenesis and treatment of disease [review]. Science 1995;267:1456–1462.

224. Tirosh R, Berke G: T lymphocyte-mediated cytolysis as an excitatory process of the target. I. Evidence that the target may be the site of Ca^{2+} action. Cell Immunol 1985;95:113–123.

225. Tomlinson IM, Cook GP, Carter NP, Elaswarapu R, Smith S, Walter G, Buluwela L, Rabbitts TH, Winter G: Human immunoglobulin VH and D segments on chromosomes 15q11.2 and 16p11.2. Hum Mol Genet 1994;3:853–860.

226. Tomlinson IM, Cook GP, Walter G, Carter NP, Riethman H, Buluwela L, Rabbitts TH, Winter G: A complete map of the human immunoglobulin VH locus [review]. Ann N Y Acad Sci 1995;764:43–46.

227. Toyoda M, Galfayan K, Wachs K, Czer L, Jordan SC: Immunologic monitoring of OKT3 induction therapy in cardiac allograft recipients. Clin Transplant 1995;9:472–480.

228. Toyonaga B, Yoshikai Y, Vadasz V, Chin B, Mak TW: Organization and sequences of the diversity, joining, and constant region genes of the human T-cell receptor beta chain. Proc Natl Acad Sci U S A 1985;82:8624–8628.

229. Tracey KJ, Cerami A: Tumor necrosis factor: a pleiotropic cytokine and therapeutic target [review]. Annu Rev Med 1994; 45:491–503.

230. Trinchieri G: Interleukin-12: a proinflammatory cytokine with immunoregulatory functions that bridge innate resistance and antigen-specific adaptive immunity [review]. Annu Rev Immunol 1995;13:251–276.

231. Trinchieri G: Function and clinical use of interleukin-12 [review]. Curr Opin Hematol 1997;4:59–66.

232. Van den Berg TK, Yoshida K, Dijkstra CD: Mechanism of immune complex trapping by follicular dendritic cells [review]. Curr Top Microbiol Immunol 1995;201:49–67.

233. van der Mast BJ, Balk AH: Effect of HLA-DR-shared blood transfusion on the clinical outcome of heart transplantation. Transplantation 1997;63:1514–1519.

234. van Twuyver E, Kast WM, Mooijaart RJ, Melief CJM, de Waal LP: Transfusion-induced skin allograft enhancement across an H-2 class I mismatch is caused by a clonal deletion of donor-specific cytotoxic T-lymphocyte precursors within the allograft. Transplant Proc 1989;21:1169–1170.

235. van Twuyver E, Kast WM, Mooijaart RJ, Wilmink JM, Melief CJM, de Waal LP: Allograft tolerance induction in adult mice associated with functional deletion of specific CTL precursors. Transplantation 1989;48:844–847.

236. Wagner DD: The Weibel-Palade body: the storage granule for von Willebrand factor and P-selectin [review]. Thromb Haemost 1993;70:105–110.

237. Waldman WJ, Knight DA, Adams PW, Orosz CG, Sedmak DD: In vitro induction of endothelial HLA class II antigen expression by cytomegalovirus-activated CD4+ T cells. Transplantation 1993;56:1504–1512.

238. Watschinger B, Gallon L, Carpenter CB, Sayegh MH: Mechanisms of allo-recognition. Recognition by in vivo-primed T cells of specific major histocompatibility complex polymorphisms presented as peptides by responder antigen-presenting cells. Transplantation 1994;57:572–576.

239. Watson CA, Petzelbauer P, Zhou J, Pardi R, Bender JR: Contact-dependent endothelial class II HLA gene activation induced by NK cells is mediated by IFN-gamma-dependent and -independent mechanisms. J Immunol 1995;154:3222–3233.

240. Wei S, Charmley P, Robinson MA, Concannon P: The extent of the human T-cell receptor V beta gene segment repertoire. Immunogenetics 1994;40:27–36.

241. Weissenbach J, Chernajovsky Y, Zeevi M, Shulman L, Soreq H, Nir U, Wallach D, Perricaudet M, Tiollais P, Revel M: Two interferon mRNAs in human fibroblasts: in vitro translation and Escherichia coli cloning studies. Proc Natl Acad Sci U S A 1980; 77:7152–7156.

242. Wetsel RA: Structure, function and cellular expression of complement anaphylatoxin receptors [review]. Curr Opin Immunol 1995;7:48–53.

243. Wetsel RA, Ogata RT, Tack BF: Primary structure of the fifth component of murine complement. Biochemistry 1987;26: 737–743.

244. Winoto A: Cell death in the regulation of immune responses [review]. Curr Opin Immunol 1997;9:365–370.

245. Winoto A, Mjolsness S, Hood L: Genomic organization of the genes encoding mouse T-cell receptor alpha-chain. Nature 1985;316:832–836.

246. Wong B, Choi Y: Pathways leading to cell death in T cells [review]. Curr Opin Immunol 1997;9:358–364.

247. Wong B, Park CG, Choi Y: Identifying the molecular control of T-cell death; on the hunt for killer genes [review]. Semin Immunol 1997;9:7–16.

248. Wood KJ: Antigen induced tolerance. In Ildstad KJ (ed): Chimerism and Tolerance. Austin: RG Landes, 1995, pp 15–29.

249. Wood KJ: New concepts in tolerance [review]. Clin Transplant 1996;10:93–99.

250. Wood ML, Monaco AP, Gozzo JJ: Use of homozygous allogeneic bone marrow for induction of tolerance with antilymphocyte serum: dose and timing. Transplant Proc 1971;3:676–676.

251. Wood ML, Orosz CG, Gottschalk R, Monaco AP: The effect of injection of donor bone marrow on the frequency of donor-reactive CTL in antilymphocyte serum-treated, grafted mice. Transplantation 1992;54:665–671.

252. Yamamura M, Uyemura K, Deans RJ, Weinberg K, Rea TH, Bloom BR, Modlin RL: Defining protective responses to pathogens: cytokine profiles in leprosy lesions. Science 1991;254:277–279.

253. Yanagi Y, Yoshikai Y, Leggett K, Clark SP, Aleksander I, Mak TW: A human T cell-specific cDNA clone encodes a protein having extensive homology to immunoglobulin chains. Nature 1984; 308:145–149.

254. Yoshikai Y, Anatoniou D, Clark SP, Yanagi Y, Sangster R, Van den Elsen P, Terhorst C, Mak TW: Sequence and expression of transcripts of the human T-cell receptor beta-chain genes. Nature 1984;312:521–524.

255. Ziccardi RJ, Cooper NR: The subunit composition and sedimentation properties of human C1. J Immunol 1977;118:2047–2052.

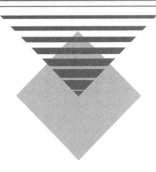

Methodology for Clinical Research in Cardiac Transplantation

with the collaboration of
DAVID C. NAFTEL, Ph.D.

OVERVIEW OF CLINICAL RESEARCH IN CARDIAC TRANSPLANTATION

Clinical research is the formal application of hypothesis development and testing, study design, data collection and analysis, and generation of inferences from studies that involve **patients.** This chapter focuses on methodology for clinical research; it does *not* discuss research methodology for animal or laboratory experimentation. Human cardiac transplantation research spans a number of scientific disciplines and, in many respects, is a model for clinical research. The complexities of the scientific basis for cardiac transplantation and the inherent uncertainties in short- and long-term patient care following transplantation provide many opportunities for creating and implementing strategies for improving patient outcome. The generation of useful and accurate information in this complex, dynamic field is facilitated by a **highly structured scientific approach** to clinical research. This chapter is intended to provide a scientific foundation and pragmatic approach to data collection, analysis, and interpretation.

The basic ingredient of effective clinical research in cardiac transplantation is an individual with specific expertise in the area of investigation. In the current era of emphasis on outcomes research, it is increasingly important to also have the participation of an individual with special skills in statistical methodology and analysis. **Statistics** is the science of creating, developing, and applying techniques such that the uncertainty of inductive inferences can be evaluated.[67] Additional personnel are usually necessary for data collection, computer data entry, and patient follow-up. Although not necessary for excellent clinical studies, it is useful for some transplant programs to organize research efforts within a specialized cardiac transplant research unit, in which specific personnel are identified and frequent formal meetings occur for the planning and implementation of clinical research.

As in any research endeavor, each study in cardiac transplantation should have clear goals and detailed plans and methods to reach these goals. The ultimate aim of most such studies is to improve results after cardiac transplantation, particularly in terms of duration of survival, quality of life, and freedom from morbid events. Although many studies add critical fundamental knowledge to the field, another major focus is the prediction of and improvement in outcome for *individual patients* so that the most effective utilization can be made of the scarce resource of donor organs. For the large population of patients with end-stage heart disease for whom cardiac transplantation is not advisable or is unavailable, the same study methods can be applied to alternative therapies. All such studies require special methods of analysis, which will be discussed in this chapter. The general term for such patient-specific oriented research is outcomes research.

Outcomes Research is the study of specific events (outcomes) in a patient's life after a specific diagnosis or intervention (e.g., heart transplantation). Interest is focused on the predictors and time-related probabilities of the outcome events. The goal is to quantify the likelihood of various events in order to facilitate complex medical decisions.

Although outcomes research is a recent term, it describes research activities that have been conducted during the entire twentieth century and before. The field of outcomes research became a focused effort in the late 1980s as governmental agencies, insurance companies, and patients demanded more useful information on clinical outcomes and costs after specific diseases and interventions. This included the ability to compare interventions, physicians, and hospitals. Length of hospital stay, patterns of referrals, mortality, and morbidity all became targets for "outcomes research." In the United States, the Agency for Health Care Research and Quality became a major nation-wide influence as a sponsor for research that answered the question "which intervention is best for a specific patient" instead of merely "which intervention is better." During the 1990s, the movement gained momentum worldwide as the demand increased for evidence-based medical practice.

The numerical examples in this chapter will, for the most part, come from two multi-institutional studies[54] as well as the experience at the University of Alabama at Birmingham (UAB). The **Cardiac Transplant Research Database** (CTRD) was established in 1990 by the Working Group of Transplant Cardiologists and the Divisions of Cardiothoracic Surgery and Cardiology at UAB. The data collection and analysis center for this multi-institutional database currently resides in the Department of Surgery at UAB. The CTRD has grown to include a wide variety of transplant professionals from 43 institutions. At the end of 1999, 7,000 transplanted patients with current follow-up were in the database. In addition to detailed information on recipient, donor, and initial immunosuppression, the database also collects information on important posttransplant events, including death, retransplantation, infections, rejections, allograft vasculopathy, and malignancies. The **Pediatric Heart Transplant Study** (PHTS), a multi-institutional database for pediatric heart transplantation, was established in 1993 by a group of pediatric transplant professionals and the Department of Surgery at UAB. It was modeled after the CTRD and includes all patients listed for cardiac transplantation at each institution. At the end of 1999, 23 participating institutions had 1,400 listed pediatric patients and 1,000 transplanted patients.

BASIC CONCEPTS AND DEFINITIONS

STATISTICAL FOUNDATIONS OF RESEARCH

The field of statistics is based on the following premises: (1) quantifiable laws, relations, "truths," or constants (i.e., parameters) exist for a given situation or group of patients; (2) there is an element of individual variability within these truths; (3) these truths are usually unknown or incompletely quantified; (4) the truths must be estimated from a limited collection (sample) of the data; (5) the estimates will have uncertainty associated with them; and (6) the uncertainty of the estimates is a function of the individual variability and the size of the sample.

A **parameter** is a constant in a statistical equation. *Parameters* are also values (constants) that describe specific distributions (see later section, Parametric Estimation). For example, values for the mean and standard deviation of a given normal distribution are parameters of that distribution. Thus, in a pure statistical context, the term "parameter" is always a **numerical value** which is a constant in a mathematical equation describing a distribution. In most statistical models (equations), the parameters are actually unknown and must be either assumed (based on theoretical or statistical considerations) or estimated (by a statistical calculation derived from a specific data set). It is important to distinguish the statistical use of the term parameter from its use in a nonstatistical sense. *Webster's New World Dictionary, Third College Edition,* defines parameter as "a factor or characteristic." Many investigators have used the term parameter in this manner, describing characteristics of a population or a study (which really implies the variables under examination). This use of the term parameter is often confusing since it is not consistent with its statistical meaning.

Variables are characteristics of the subject under investigation. Age, gender, height, and marital status of a transplant patient are all examples of variables. Variables are classified according to their possible values. For example, gender is a **discrete** variable because it has only two discrete possibilities: male or female. Other examples of discrete variables are race, blood type, and type of insurance. If a discrete variable has an order to its possible values, then it is called an **ordinal** variable. New York Heart Association Functional Class is an example of an ordinal variable because it has four possible values and they are ordered: 1, 2, 3, and 4. **Continuous** variables have values which can be any number within some range. For example, patient height can be any value within a biologically plausible range. The actual number of possible values is only limited by the gradation of the measuring device. Sometimes a continuous variable is transformed into a discrete or an ordinal variable. For example, the continuous variable age could be changed into a new variable "pediatric patient: yes/no" according to a definition of pediatric age. Age can be transformed into a decade variable, which would be an ordinal variable.

Each variable has a distribution of its possible values. A **distribution** is an equation that relates a value of a variable with the probability that it will occur. A distribution has a specific function form, and it has constants known as *parameters*. For example the normal distribution (see Box) is a specific function form and it has parameters μ (mean) and σ (standard deviation) that determine the location and spread of the distribution (Fig. 3–1, see Box). The term **parametric** refers to a **distribution** (equation) with its specific statistical parameters (values for mean, standard deviation, etc.). Parametric

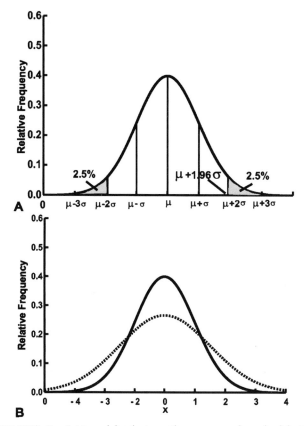

FIGURE **3–1.** *A*, Normal distribution with mean, μ, and standard deviation, σ. The total area under the curve is 1. The area of each shaded portion is 0.025 or 2.5% of the total. *B*, Two normal distributions. The solid curve is a normal distribution with $\mu = 0$ and $\sigma = 1$. The dashed curve is a normal distribution with $\mu = 0$ and $\sigma = 1.5$.

The Normal Distribution

Suppose *x* is a continuous random variable. This means that *x* is a characteristic of a subject, for example, age; and *x* can take on any value within some reasonable range. If one had many values of *x* then the density or relative frequency of these values could be displayed by a histogram and described by an equation or model. One such density that has been found to occur frequently in nature is the **normal distribution** (Fig. 3–1). This basic distribution has also been termed gaussian or bell-shaped. If *x* has a normal distribution, then the density of *x* is defined by Equation 1 (see Appendix).

The random variable, *x*, can theoretically have any value from minus infinity to plus infinity, although in practice this does not happen. For a normal distribution, certain probability statements can be made about the variable *x*. If *x* is chosen at random, then the probability that *x* will be greater than μ is 0.5, the probability that *x* will be in the interval $\mu - \sigma$ to $\mu + \sigma$ is 0.685, the probability that *x* will be in the interval $\mu - 2\sigma$ to $\mu + 2\sigma$ is 0.954, and the probability that *x* will be greater than $\mu + 1.96\sigma$ or less than $\mu - 1.96\sigma$ is 0.05.

In reality, the form of the density and the values of the parameters are rarely known. If the researcher is willing to assume a normal distribution, then μ and σ can be estimated from a finite sample of observed *x*'s. An estimate for μ is the mean of the *x*'s and an estimate for σ is the standard deviation of the *x*'s. (Other estimates for these parameters are possible. For example, the sample median is also an estimate for μ.) Just as *x* has a distribution, these estimates also have distributions of possible values.

---

may also describe the relation between two variables, which can be expressed by an **equation.**

Many continuous variables have a normal distribution; however, this is only one of an infinite number of possible distributions. The actual distribution is usually unknown because it is the distribution for the entire population. Its shape can be visually estimated by a histogram of sample values. In performing parametric analysis, statisticians often refer to *modeling* a data set. This means that an equation has been generated that is directly based on a specific distribution which is assumed to approximate the distribution of the data set. As will be seen in subsequent sections, the ability of the equation to "fit" (describe) the data can be directly examined by plotting the lines or curves generated by the equation (distribution) superimposed on a depiction of the data points. This may be a scattergram or another descripton of the data which does not assume a specific distribution (nonparametric), such as a cumulative distribution frequency (see subsequent sections) for non–time-related variables or the Kaplan-Meier method for depicting time-related survival (see later section, Comparison of Survival Curves).

There are an infinite variety of distributions, and a major portion of the field of statistics is concerned with identifying useful distributions, determining the form of the parameter estimates, and quantifying the uncertainty of these estimates. In general, non-time-related data are most often (though sometimes incorrectly) approximated by the normal distribution, whereas time-related data are better approximated by other distributions, such as hazard-based functions (see later section, Survival Curves). Thus, when using the term **parametric** in statistical analyses, it is synonymous with *described by an equation, described by a model,* or *described by an assumed distribution.* Similarly, parametric tests of significance require an assumption about the data distribution. Tests of significance that do not require specification of a distribution are called **nonparametric tests** of significance.[37] Usually a parametric test is better able to detect differences if the assumed distribution is correct.

Descriptive Statistics

Traditionally, there are two main branches of statistics: descriptive and inferential. Descriptive statistics are numerical summary descriptors of a collection or sample of numbers. Their purpose is to reduce a collection of observed values of a variable into a few numbers (statistics) that describe the values. Quantities of information will be lost in this process, but the loss is offset by the gain in reducing the information contained in the values to a few easily interpreted numbers. Descriptive statistics are divided into measures of central tendency and measures of variability. Measures of **central tendency** include mean, median, and mode. The arithmetic **mean** $\bar{x}$ of n sample values is expressed by Equation 2 (see Appendix). The **median** of a sample is the midvalue, such that half the values in the sample exceed it and half the values are below it. The **mode** is the sample value that occurs most frequently.

Measures of **variability** (dispersion) for a sample include range, standard deviation, variance, skewness, and kurtosis. The **range** is the interval between the lowest and highest values of the variable under examination. The sample **standard deviation (SD)** is a measure of the amount of variation among the individual values of x (see Equation 3 in Appendix).

The sample **variance** is the square of the sample standard deviation. **Skewness** is a measure of the deviation of the distribution of values in a sample from a normal symmetric distribution. **Kurtosis** is a measure of dispersion that can be used to measure departure from normality for a sample.

Inferential Statistics

Inferential statistics is the branch of statistics that uses information from a sample to learn (infer) about a population. The process is inherently uncertain because a sample contains incomplete information about a population. The two components of inferential statistics are (1) estimation of population numerical characteristics (parameters) based on the information available from the sample and (2) quantifying the uncertainty of the estimates.

The initial step in the process of inferential statistics is the specification of a research question or hypothesis (the notion of "truth" that is being investigated). Sup-

pose, for example, a researcher is interested in knowing the proportion of residents in the state of Alabama who have medical insurance, but resources do not exist to canvass all residents. A sample of residents could be queried and their results could be used to estimate the proportion for the entire state population. In this case the population is easy to define.

Sometimes the population is not so obvious. Consider a surgical intervention such as cardiac transplantation performed at a specific hospital. Suppose an investigator desires to know the 30-day mortality for cardiac transplantation at that hospital. Using descriptive statistics, the 30-day mortality for the last calendar year could be calculated. This would be the hospital's observed 30-day mortality (for that year) and there would be no element of uncertainty. But one could think of the hospital as having a true 30-day mortality that can only be estimated by last year's cases. In fact, the true proportion would only be known with certainty if a very large number of patients were transplanted. Statisticians think of the actual transplants as a sample of a very large, but not actually identifiable, population of patients. The observed mortality from the sample becomes an estimate of the true proportion. The **uncertainty** (see next section) of this estimate can be calculated and, therefore, the likelihood that it reflects "truth" about the population.

MEASURES OF THE DEGREE OF UNCERTAINTY

The use of statistics in science and medicine stems from the desire to estimate the likelihood of a given observation occurring again or being representative of an entire "population" of things, animals, or people. In the seventeenth century, Galileo formalized the laws of chance (now known as the theory of probability) in response to gamblers' questions about the "odds" of winning or losing.[23] Over the centuries it has become increasingly accepted that things in the physical and biologic worlds behave according to laws of probability.[27]

Point Estimates (Parameter Estimation)

The value of a parameter estimated by a sample of the population is termed a point estimate. An observed hospital mortality of 10% is a "point estimate" of the "true" mortality for the overall population being considered. The mean ischemic time in a heart transplant experience is a point estimate. A survival curve generated by an estimated parametric equation is a continuous point estimate. Thus, based on information obtained from the sample, a parameter (or point) estimate is calculated. Selection of the **sample** is crucial for valid estimates. A sample that is not representative of the population will not produce reliable estimates and may introduce bias (an effect that deprives a statistical estimate from being representative by systematically distorting it) into the analysis. In clinical studies it is often not possible to randomly select a sample from all possible members of a population. However, a proper protocol for selecting the patients within the population will increase the likelihood that the sample is representative of the population, realizing that the specific value of the estimate would almost certainly change if another sample were drawn. For many forms of estimates, statistical theory has produced a method for quantifying the **uncertainty of an estimate.**

Standard Error

In contrast to standard deviation, which is a measure of the variability of individual values, the **standard error** is a measure of the variability of the **estimate.** In estimating the true proportion in a population, such as the true 30-day mortality (number of patients who died/total number transplanted) following cardiac transplantation, probability statements can be made using the estimate and the standard error. For an estimated proportion, the equation for the standard error is the square root of $p(1 - p)/n$, where p is the sample proportion and n is the number of subjects in the sample.

Confidence Limits

The confidence limits (CLs), also called confidence intervals, may be calculated directly from the standard error (SE) or the standard deviation (SD).[60] For continuous variables that have a symmetric distribution, the standard deviation can be used to create approximate **confidence intervals for an individual.** The interval from the mean − 1 SD to the mean + 1 SD will contain approximately 70% (actually 68.3%) of the individual values. This 70% confidence interval for an individual can also be used to predict that the value for the next individual has a 70% chance of falling in the interval. Other CLs can be calculated depending on the width of the interval. For example, a 95% confidence limit is created by the mean ± 2 SD (see Equation 4 in Appendix). The SE for continuous variables can be used in a similar manner to create **confidence limits for the mean.** Thus, the interval from the sample mean − 1 SE to the sample mean + 1 SE has an approximately 70% chance of containing the population mean.

The SE for proportions can also be used to calculate confidence intervals. The interval calculated from 1 SE below the estimate to 1 SE above the estimate has approximately a 70% chance of containing the true proportion. It should be noted that although the calculation of CL from the SE is commonly performed, it is an approximation and holds true only if n is large (greater than about 100). Thus, in instances where n is smaller, a more tedious calculation is necessary, and the resultant CLs are asymmetric about the estimate.

Confidence limits can be displayed in tables or plotted, and their interpretation can be understood intuitively. Notice that the width of the CL is a function of the sample size (Table 3–1 and Fig. 3–2). As the sample size increases, the width of the CLs decreases, a more precise estimate is obtained, and there is less uncertainty where the population parameter lies (i.e., what the "truth" is). From the proper calculations, any CL can be derived, such as 50%, 70%, 90%, and 95%. As noted

| TABLE 3-1 | Influence of Sample Size on Confidence Limits and p Values* |

GROUP	n	N	%	70% CL (%)	p VALUE
A	10	5	50	30–70	.36
B	10	3	30	14–51	
A	30	15	50	39–61	.11
B	30	9	30	21–41	
A	50	25	50	42–58	.04
B	50	15	30	23–38	
A	100	50	50	44–56	.004
B	100	30	30	25–35	

CL, confidence limits.
* This table compares hospital death for two groups of patients. Each comparison has the same difference in mortality but the sample size changes.

above, the 70% CLs (actually 68.3%) are equivalent to 1 SE above and below the point estimate and 95% CLs enclose 2 SE's on either side of the estimate. When 70% CLs for two estimates just touch, this is approximately equivalent to a p value of .08 to .1. (Nonoverlapping 70% CLs indicate p < .08, and overlapping 70% CLs indicate $p > .1$). When 95% CLs just touch, then the p value is approximately .01.

Sample Size

When planning a study, a key question is that of necessary sample size (see Box) (Table 3–2). The time table of a study and the necessary financial and personnel resources are all functions of sample size. If the major purpose of a study is to estimate a single parameter (such as the true proportion of hospital death or the true mean ejection fraction) then the sample size depends on how "confident" one wishes to be in the estimate. If the purpose of a study is to compare two groups then the

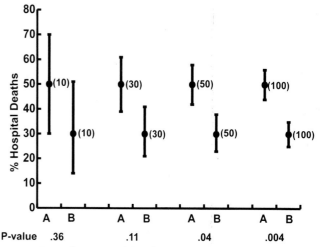

FIGURE 3-2. Illustration of the effect of sample size on p values and confidence limits for four comparisons of hospital death. The numbers in parentheses are sample sizes for the groups. The estimates, confidence limits, and p values are all presented in Table 3-1.

TABLE 3-2	**Sample Size for Comparing Two Proportions**				
p_1	p_2	p_2-p_1	α	POWER	n
.3	.5	.2	.05	.8	74
.4	.5	.1	.05	.8	305
.45	.5	.05	.05	.8	1,233
.3	.5	.2	.05	.9	102
.4	.5	.1	.05	.9	423
.45	.5	.05	.05	.9	1,708
.3	.5	.2	.01	.8	119
.4	.5	.1	.01	.8	496
.45	.5	.05	.01	.8	2,001
.3	.5	.2	.01	.9	154
.4	.5	.1	.01	.9	643
.45	.5	.05	.01	.9	2,595

p_1, estimated proportion in group 1; p_2, estimated proportion in group 2; p_2-p_1, difference to be detected; α, significance level (1 tail); power, probability of detecting difference if it exists; n, sample size required in each group.

sample size is a function of the difference that the researcher wishes to detect and the power he desires to detect the difference. Usually sample size calculations are based on the major endpoint of an example and the simplest possible formulation of the null and the alternative hypothesis.[32]

p *Values*

The *p* value is an integral part of modern inferential statistics. It is a numerical quantification of the evidence (observed data) for a research hypothesis. The "*p*" in *p* value stands for probability. Thus, the history of the *p* value is a history of probability and its role in inferential statistics. During the seventeenth century, several French mathematicians became interested in probability as it applied to games of chance.[19] Probability models such as the binomial distribution were formulated for the probability of *x* successes out of *n* attempts. The role of the normal distribution in statistics became established by the central limit theorem, which states that the mean of *n* observations tends to a normal distribution as *n* becomes large. Early twentieth century statisticians incorporated the *p* value as a measure of evidence for or against a hypothesis. Sir Ronald Fisher (who is often credited with suggesting the .05 "significance rule") stated that "no scientific worker has a fixed level of significance at which from year to year, and in all circumstances, he rejects hypotheses; he rather gives his mind to each particular case in the light of his evidence and his ideas."[26]

The *p* value is the most commonly encountered measure of uncertainty. It is the probability of obtaining a result as extreme or more extreme than the one observed if, in fact, the distribution (characteristics) of the test sample are the same as the comparison population. All methods for calculation of a *p* value have in common a comparison of 1 or more point estimates, a measure of the variability of each estimate, and an estimate of the variability of the comparison. In general, a *p* value asks, "if the null hypothesis is true (i.e., there is no difference

between the parameters), then what is the likelihood that the observed difference between two (or more) point estimates is due to chance alone?" For example, when the *p* value is .05, there are 5 chances out of 100 that the observed difference was due to chance alone (if, in fact, there is no real difference between the parameters). When the *p* value is less than about .05, it is commonly concluded in experimental and clinical research that the observed (or greater) differences would occur so rarely (5 out of 100 times) by chance alone that it is appropriate to conclude that the actual parameters are, in fact, different. Such differences are said to be "statistically significant."

In formal statistical terms, the basic hypothesis underlying the *p* value is the **null hypothesis,** which assumes that there is no difference between the two parameters (which could represent two mortality rates, results of differing treatments, results of experimental protocols, etc.). Assume that the researcher is employing a .05 "level of significance." If the *p* value is <.05, then the chances of this, or a more extreme, observed difference if the null hypothesis is true (i.e., there is really no difference in the parameters being estimated) are less than 5 out of 100, and the null hypothesis is rejected. If, in fact,

Sample Size

Sample Size for a Single Proportion

Suppose a study is being planned to estimate the proportion of patients who are working at 5 years after transplant. The researcher wants to be 95% confident that the estimate is within .10 of the true proportion. From previous work, the proportion is expected to be approximately .4. The equation for a confidence interval for a proportion can be rearranged to solve for n. A 95% confidence interval is approximately equal to 2 SE about the estimated proportion and is described by the expression in Equation 4 (see Appendix).

Sample Size for Comparing Two Proportions

Estimating the sample size necessary for a study to compare two proportions requires specification of several numerical components:

1. Estimate both proportions to be compared based on past studies or experience (p_1, p_2).
2. Specify the difference (p_1-p_2) to be detected if it exists.
3. Specify the power (probability) of detecting the difference if it exists. The power $(1 - \beta)$ is equal to 1 minus the type II error.
4. Decide the desired significance level (type I error) of the study. This is the probability (α) of rejecting the null hypothesis of no difference when the null hypothesis is true.

The formula for the necessary sample size for each group is shown in Equation 5[67] (see Appendix). Table 3-2 gives sample size calculations for a few combinations of α, power $(1-\beta)$, p_1 and p_2. The sample size increases as the difference to be detected decreases, the α decreases, or the power increases.

the null hypothesis is true, there is .05 probability that it will be incorrectly rejected. This is known as a **type I error** (i.e., the chance of concluding that a real difference exists when in fact it does not). Thus, the standard p value is α in Table 3–3 (probability of type I error). There is another possibility. The alternative hypothesis may be true (and the null hypothesis false), so that the parameters may, in fact, be different. But, by chance the observations generate 2 point estimates that are close enough so that the test of significance yields a p value greater than .05. The researcher would not reject the null hypothesis (and would conclude incorrectly that there is no difference in the point estimates). This is known as a **type II error** (Table 3–3).

The p value is a direct function of the observed difference and the sample size. It is a convenient summary statistic that simultaneously examines and reduces these two components into one number. Just as every p value should be judged in light of the hypothesis that is being tested and the assumptions for the test statistic, it should also be viewed in light of observed difference and the sample size. Table 3–1 contains several comparisons of proportions that illustrate the effect of sample size and observed difference on the p value.

The phrases "one-tailed p value" and "two-tailed p value" are commonly encountered. Which one is used depends on the research hypothesis being tested. When the hypothesis relates to differences in either direction, then a "two-tailed p value" is used. When the research hypothesis relates to differences in only one direction ("less than," for example), then a one-tailed p value is used. A two-tailed p value is always equal to or greater than a one-tailed p value. In most cases, the two-tailed p value is twice as large as the one-tailed p value. In this book, all p values are two-tailed unless specifically noted to be one-tailed.

All p values are the result of tests of significance applied to data in order to examine a specific hypothesis. A number of "test statistics" are available to examine such hypotheses, depending on the types of point estimates compared and the fit of the data to the assumptions underlying the test. These are discussed in more detail in the later section, Initial Examination of Variables.

Power

The power of a test is its ability to correctly accept specific alternative hypotheses. As seen in Table 3–3, power is the probability $(1 - \beta)$ of correctly concluding that the null hypothesis is false. Power is the complement of type II error in that the sum of their probabilities is 1.

In Table 3–1 the upper two p values indicate no statistical differences, thus forcing the acceptance of the null hypothesis that there is no difference in the underlying mortality between the two groups. The technical statistical statement is "there is insufficient evidence to reject the null hypothesis and therefore the null hypothesis is accepted." Some investigators may find this conclusion hard to accept when the observed proportions are quite different. The question then becomes "if a certain difference truly exists, what is the probability of detecting the difference by rejecting the null hypothesis?" This probability is the **power** of a study. A low-powered study can only detect very large differences, and conversely a high-powered study can detect small differences. Increased power for a specified difference to be detected is a function of increased sample size or decreased variability of the outcome under investigation or a combination of the two. Any test of significance can theoretically have an associated power calculation if both the null and a specific alternative hypothesis are given.

Power can be specified as part of the design of a study and is a key component of the sample size calculation. Power can also be calculated after data is collected to check the ability of a study to detect specific alternative hypotheses. Table 3–2 shows the important influence of the desired significance level, the expected or observed difference between the proportions in the two groups, and the desired power on the required sample size in each group.

MEASURES OF UNCERTAINTY AND MEDICAL DECISIONS

The statistical foundations of research play an important role in facilitating medical decisions in the face of uncertainty (as reflected by the p value in an analysis). When interpreting a p value, a number of assumptions have been made; namely, that the study was conducted properly, the data are correct, and the test of significance is appropriate. (Remember, there is no way to statistically correct deficits in a study).

An understanding of the interplay between statistical significance and **clinical significance** is necessary for the effective use of statistics. Consider two studies to compare the 30-day mortality of interventions A and B (Table 3–4). The first study resulted in a large difference in the mortality rates but was based on a small number of patients. The second study has a large number of patients but a much smaller difference in mortality rates. Thus, a study with a large number of patients requires

TABLE 3–3	Study Conclusions and the Associated Probabilities		
	TRUE SITUATION	INVESTIGATOR'S CONCLUSION	
		H_0 True	H_0 False
Correct and erroneous conclusions	H_0 true	Correct conclusion	False positive (type I error)
	H_0 false	False negative (type II error)	Correct conclusion
Probabilities of correct and erroneous conclusions	H_0 true	$1-\alpha$	α
	H_0 false	β	$1-\beta$ (power)

H_0, null hypothesis.

TABLE 3-4	Clinical versus Statistical Significance				
		DEATHS			
GROUP	n	N	%	70% CL (%)	p Value
A	25	15	60	48–71	.047
B	25	8	32	21–44	
A	1,000	600	60	58–62	.046
B	1,000	556	56	54–57	

only a small observed difference in order to reach statistical significance. The small observed difference may not be clinically important and, therefore, it may be statistically significant but not clinically significant.

When using p values to facilitate complex medical decisions, it is often helpful to know the actual p value, rather than simply reporting the p value as either "$p < .05$" or "$p > .05$." Particularly when considering a change in therapy based on the results of a study, the p value (statistical significance) must be viewed in the context of the clinical consequences of making such a change. For example, suppose a novel immunosuppressive regimen is easier to administer, less toxic, and less expensive than the standard regimen. A study is made comparing rejection frequency with each treatment regimen. The novel immunosuppressive regimen generates a rejection frequency that is less than that with standard therapy, but the p value is .08. Despite the finding of a p value ">.05," knowledge of its specific value (.08) informs the investigators that the p value was actually quite close to .05 (and the likelihood of a type I error is 8% rather than 5%). In this situation, if there were other potential advantages of the novel therapy, a p value of .08 may be sufficient to justify a change in immunosuppressive protocol.

Another important issue relates to **statistical significance** versus **clinical truth**. A single study that yields a "significant" p value does not prove that a true difference exists. Rather, it indicates the probability that the observed (or more extreme) difference was due to chance alone. However, if multiple additional studies from reliable investigators examine the same issue and find similar "significant" differences, then the medical community may elect to accept these differences (demonstrated by multiple studies) as "truth."

ADDITIONAL STATISTICAL CONCEPTS FOR RESEARCH

Continuity of Nature

The application of statistical equations to biological phenomena requires a basic assumption; that the behavior of biological systems is generally continuous between small measurable points, rather than demonstrating sharp "cut-offs." For example, nature does not make only tall people and short people. Within some unknown range, people can have a nearly infinite number of different heights. The only limitation is the gradation of the measuring device. Similarly, the principle of continuity can be applied to making inferences at the extremes (upper and lower ends) of data sets. For example, if a risk factor analysis indicates that longer ischemic times of the donor heart are associated with increased mortality, and if the highest observed ischemic time was 5 hours, then one would logically infer that an ischemic time of 7 hours would carry an even higher risk (even though no specific observations were made at that particular ischemic time). The confidence of such an inference is affected by a number of factors, such as the number of observations at the extremes, the width of the confidence limits, and the p value for the variable examined.

Preservation of Information

A direct consequence of the continuity-of-nature concept is the value of preserving information. Since many clinical studies examine (and analyze) small samples and/or uncommon events, there is a potential advantage in utilizing all possible information from the study. Thus, strategies that systematically discard certain pieces of data (that were otherwise accurately and rigorously collected) and analytic techniques that transform continuous variables to dichotomous or discrete groups may lose information and potentially obscure an important relationship.

Time Zero

The concept of "time zero" is an important component of clinical research. Factors at or before time zero are the independent variables, and variables after time zero are the dependent or outcome variables. This concept is totally connected to the detailed statement of the research hypothesis. For example, if the research purpose is to identify risk factors for death after transplantation, then a more detailed statement might be "at the moment that the transplant operation is completed, what factors about the recipient and the donor are associated with posttransplant survival?" Such a hypothesis would preclude examination of intensive care unit (ICU) variables as potential risk factors because these variables are not known at the completion of the operation. In fact, the ICU variables could be outcome variables in such a study. Time zero is the moment the operation ends, and potential risk factors are only those variables known at that instant. Time until the outcome variable is measured from the time zero. Depending on the purpose of the study, time zero may be the time of listing, the end of the operation, time of hospital discharge, 1 year after transplant, the end of a rejection episode, and so forth.

Cause and Effect Versus Association

Statistical significance can be an indication of cause and effect under certain carefully designed experimental conditions, such that a change in one variable *causes* a change in another variable. For example, lowering the temperature of water below 32°F will cause the water to turn to ice. Increasing the dose of insecticide will increase the proportion of dead mosquitoes. (Even this cause-and-effect relationship does not specify the actual biologic mechanism whereby increasing the dosage causes death).

However, in most clinical studies, other than randomized trials, statistical significance is only an indication of **association.** Change in one variable tends to coincide with change in another variable. The outcome variable in a clinical study is called the **dependent variable.** A variable being examined for its effect upon the outcome variable is called an **independent variable.** Independent variables are measured before or at time zero, and dependent or outcome variables occur after time zero.

Risk Factors

Risk factors are independent variables that are associated with an outcome variable. A change in a risk factor is associated with a change in the probability of the outcome variable. If the outcome variable is time-related, such as death after transplantation, then a change in the risk factor is associated with a shift in the time-related probability of the outcome. In specifying a risk factor, it is necessary to give the direction of the increased risk. For example, specifying age as a risk factor for death is not very informative. Specifying "younger age" as a risk factor is more useful.

Some risk factors can be manipulated for a future patient in an attempt to reduce the risk. For example, in survival after transplant, there are identifiable donor risk factors which can potentially be modified by donor selection. Other risk factors (such as patient demographic risk factors) cannot be manipulated for an individual, but can serve to identify patients who are at high risk for some event.

Interaction

An interaction between two risk factors in a multivariable analysis exists when the effect of one independent variable (risk factor) on an outcome is dependent on the value of a second independent variable (risk factor). For example, the increased risk of long donor ischemic time may be very pronounced in an older recipient and very small for a younger recipient. This would constitute an interaction between ischemic time and recipient age. The statistical significance of an interaction can be explicitly tested in a multivariable analysis.

Risk-Adjusted Estimates

Sometimes a comparison of two groups of patients for an outcome (e.g., hospital death) seems unfair because one group of patients is "riskier" than the others. Risk adjustment is a way of statistically adjusting the estimates so that the differential risk is eliminated.

Suppose hospital death after transplant is being compared between two hospitals. The results are shown in Table 3–5. These estimates of hospital death are not risk adjusted. However, Hospital B has a higher proportion of urgent status patients than does Hospital A (Table 3–6). A single risk-adjusted estimate for each hospital can be calculated by recalculating the estimate assuming

TABLE 3-5	Risk-Unadjusted Mortality			
		HOSPITAL DEATH		
HOSPITAL	n	N	%	70% CL (%)
A	100	18	18	14–23
B	100	30	30	25–35
p value (χ^2)			.047	

the two hospitals had the same proportion (prevalence) of each status.

The combined proportion of urgent status patients is $[(20 + 50)/200] = .35$ and the proportion of non-urgent status patients is .65. These proportions can be used to weight the corresponding proportion dead within each hospital.

Hospital A: (.35) (.60) + (.65) (.08) = .26

Hospital B: (.35) (.50) + (.65) (.10) = .24

Therefore the **risk-adjusted** hospital mortality for hospital A is .26 or 26%, for hospital B, 24%. These risk-adjusted estimates are much closer than the original unadjusted estimates. The .p value for hospital effect after adjustment for status is .8 (from a logistic analysis).

Predictions

Predictions are numerical assertions about a future outcome usually based on analyses of groups of patients, and almost always involve a degree of uncertainty. For many, these predictions are the key reason for the analysis of patient data by a collaborative team of the statistician and medical investigators. Predictions are by-products of the quantitative understanding of a study, usually expressed in a model (equation) that relates the variables of interest. These patient-specific predictions can be used to facilitate medical decisions and to improve the informed consent of a patient selecting one treatment over another.

Bayesian Inference

Although a parameter of a population is a constant, it is usually unknown. The process of drawing inferences about parameters based on a sample of a population has several different theoretical foundations within the field of statistics. The preceding discussion is a description of the classical approach. Bayesian inference, named for Thomas Bayes, assumes that a parameter is a varying

TABLE 3-6	Risk-Stratified Mortality				
			HOSPITAL DEATH		
HOSPITAL	STATUS	n	N	%	70% CL (%)
A	Urgent	20	12	60	46–73
	Nonurgent	80	6	8	4–12
B	Urgent	50	25	50	42–58
	Nonurgent	50	5	10	6–16

quantity that has a distribution of possible values. Before the investigator conducts a study, he attempts to quantify this distribution based on past results or theoretical considerations or both. Then the investigator uses the data from a new study to modify the distribution of the parameter. Usually the modification is to make the distribution tighter (have a smaller variance). The end result of an analysis is a new distribution for a parameter. This distribution can then be modified by a subsequent study.[3]

DESIGN OF CLINICAL RESEARCH STUDIES

As stated previously, clinical research embodies the variety of formal (involving a specific prestudy design intended to generate new information) studies which involve patients. Such studies provide the foundation of **evidence-based** clinical practice, which is the scientific demonstration of treatment efficacy with provision of data that will allow reasoned determination of risk and benefit associated with any treatment. Great strides in clinical medicine were made when a shift occurred from simply collecting and recording observations to generating hypotheses that were then rigorously tested and objectively evaluated. An important difference exists between decisions based on experience and observations as opposed to properly designed and analyzed clinical studies. Ideally, clinical observations and practices should be supported, refined, or refuted by formal clinical studies.

The variety of types of clinical studies complicates simple categorization, since many categories are not mutually exclusive, nor is there uniform agreement about their precise definition. The classification presented here is intended to identify the most common study designs which would be applicable to cardiac transplantation (and to most other clinical endeavors). The variety of formal clinical studies can be generally divided into those which are considered *experimental* and those which are *observational* (Table 3–7).

EXPERIMENTAL STUDIES

An experiment involving patients generally takes the form of a **randomized clinical trial.** Proper randomization (as originally conceived by Fisher[26]) is the hallmark of a clinical experiment, performed in a setting in which replications of the experiment can be performed under similar conditions. A randomized clinical trial, then, is a prospective clinical experiment in which patients are randomly assigned to two or more groups in order to compare a scientific outcome. The groups generally include a specific type of new or alternative therapy which is compared with either placebo (no treatment) or another therapy. This form of study is generally regarded as the most rigorous method of testing a clinical hypothesis.

Advantages of Randomized Clinical Trials

The randomized clinical trial or experiment is the purest method of approximating a controlled laboratory experiment in which only one factor is varied that is relevant to the outcome. If the set of circumstances are nearly identical in the study groups, conclusions regarding cause and effect may be warranted. Because of the public and scientific perception that a proper randomized trial is most likely to be "definitive," such trials potentially have the greatest impact on medical decision-making. Prestigious peer-reviewed medical and scientific journals usually give priority to randomized, prospective clinical trials compared with observational studies. Furthermore, the Food and Drug Administration in the United States and similar agencies in other countries usually require appropriate randomized trials before releasing final approval of most drugs (such as immunosuppressive agents).

Limitations of Randomized Clinical Trials

Despite the huge value of proper randomized trials, there are distinct potential limitations. Randomized trials are frequently expensive and time-consuming, depending on requirements of sample size and study budget. Because of the critical importance of maximizing

TABLE 3–7	Types of Clinical Studies		
Study Type	Advantage	Disadvantage
Clinical experiment (randomized clinical trial)	"Gold standard" Mimics a laboratory experiment Given the most credence by the scientific and lay community	Expensive Inferences about patients with characteristics differing from the study population must be made with caution Results may not be applicable to patients in a different treatment or time era Inability to recruit patients due to physician practice or ethical issues
Observational studies	Can include wide spectrum of patients Only alternative when randomization is inappropriate or impossible Can be cost-effective Can be faster	Cannot establish cause and effect Sometimes lacks the scientific and study control rigor of a randomized trial Investigation of an important risk factor may be handicapped by either low prevalence or correlation with other risk factors

the uniformity of patient populations, disease type and severity, and additional therapies (other than the specific treatment under investigation), it is difficult to avoid subtle introduction of bias or study group differences which could importantly impact results (Table 3–8).

Another major limitation is the potential for generation of inferences which exceed the study population. Unless appropriate multivariable analysis (see later sections) is utilized in the study analysis, extending inferences beyond the specific study population is often inappropriate. The scientific community, news media, and lay population have often been guilty of inappropriately extending inferences from randomized trials to populations which were not specifically examined in the study. Because of the constant evolution of therapies which might constitute the "control" group, changing populations, and possibly altered natural history of disease states, the reliability of applying conclusions from clinical experiments to future medical practice must always be made with caution.

Finally, the ethics of a randomized trial must be critically evaluated prior to its implementation. In general, a true clinical experiment (or randomized clinical trial) is only justified if the participating physicians and health care providers truly "do not know" which therapy (under investigation) is superior. If they believe that the therapy under study (or its alternative) is superior, then it becomes unethical to enroll a patient in a randomized trial (in which some patients will not receive a therapy which the physician believes is superior). Thus, in many instances in which clinical experience or previous nonrandomized studies clearly indicate the value of a given treatment modality, true randomized clinical studies in that context would be unethical.

Since the primary responsibility of a clinical investigator is to provide the patient with superior therapy if it is available, an ethical dilemma may occur if the investigators conclude that the study drug is superior or inferior to its alternatives during the course of a trial. If this conclusion is reached, the trial should be stopped. **Formal stopping rules** are therefore necessary for discontinuation of a trial. One method to avoid premature conclusions based on *accumulating evidence* is to form an external monitoring committee which has sole access to the data as they are accrued, and results are not communicated to the investigators unless specific ethical stopping criteria are met. Although periodic examination of the data set to determine a specific overall sig-

nificance level is a common method, the likelihood of finding a "positive" result (by chance) on at least one occasion becomes quite high as the number of "looks" increases. In practice, the decision to terminate a study is generally made jointly between statisticians and clinical investigators using a more informal process.

OBSERVATIONAL STUDIES

The vast majority of clinical research studies do not fulfill the criteria of a formal experiment and are termed **observational.** Specifically, such studies do not include randomization as part of the study design. Because of the inability to strictly control study conditions and restrict important variability to the variable under examination, such studies can generally *not* draw conclusions regarding *cause* and *effect.* Instead, using the methodology presented in this chapter, *statistically significant associations* between independent and dependent (outcome) variables are sought. Cause-and-effect relationships can only be concluded after additional studies or laboratory experiments.

Although some have criticized the lack of "purity" of observational studies, multiple statistical methods (as discussed in this chapter) have been effectively utilized in *properly designed studies* to draw meaningful inferences which have profoundly impacted medical decision-making. **Prospective studies** are designed to examine a future time period that occurs after the planning and design of the study. Information (data) is collected "as it happens." **Retrospective** studies are designed to examine events which occurred before the onset of the actual study. This study design is particularly useful in the epidemiology of chronic diseases or conditions, for which introduction of the potential cause and observation of an effect may take years or decades. Such studies can also be a cost-efficient method of performing preliminary investigations that can provide a rational basis for more extensive (and costly) experimental studies. Univariable and multivariable techniques for risk factor identification (as discussed in this chapter) can be applied to either prospective or retrospective studies.

A variety of observational study designs have been described, many of which are not mutually exclusive.

Cohort Studies

A cohort or "follow-up" study identifies two or more groups of patients that are free of the event under study at the initiation of follow-up. These studies are usually prospective.

Longitudinal Studies

Longitudinal studies describe changes or events in a population sample over time, usually without predetermined groups for analysis. The length of follow-up differs among patients, and the study design may be either prospective or retrospective.

TABLE 3-8	**Issues to Consider When Planning a Randomized Clinical Trial**

Is the hypothesis clearly stated and understood?
Have patient selection criteria been precisely defined?
Are sample size calculations reasonable?
Will characterizations of patients not studied affect the study inferences?
Are therapeutic and ancillary treatment regimens well defined?
Has randomization been ensured?
Are endpoints appropriate and well characterized?
Have α and β error levels been prestated?
What are the procedures for handling patient dropouts and those lost to follow-up?

Case-Controlled Studies

In case-controlled studies, each individual patient in a study group is linked to another patient with similar clinical characteristics. This study design is usually retrospective and intended to reduce or eliminate differences in the values for all variables except those few which are being specifically examined for their impact on outcome. Case-controlled studies are often a method of accounting for other variables without using multivariable analytic techniques. In general, however, they are less likely to reveal truth than either proper randomized studies or multivariable analysis.

Cross-Sectional Studies

A study that includes all patients in a population sample at the time of investigation is termed a cross-sectional study. Such retrospective studies do not have a time-related component and indicate a prevalence of an event in an overall population at a given time.

Multi-Institutional

Multi-institutional studies involve two or more institutions with similar study patient populations. Such studies have the advantage of a large n. Large numbers of patients can be accumulated in a short amount of time, thus minimizing time-related changes in clinical therapies. For rare conditions, multi-institutional studies may be the only practical way to accumulate sufficient patients to draw appropriate inferences. Another advantage is the ability to overcome possible unusual center-specific results (bias) that might arise from single-institution studies. Valuable intellectual collaboration usually results from multi-institutional endeavors, drawing upon the unique expertise of individuals at multiple institutions.

The disadvantages of multi-institutional studies include decreased study control related to data acquisition, patient enrollment, and patient follow-up; variability in the inclusion of all eligible patients at each institution; increased time, expense, and human resources required to perform an effective study; and a potential sacrifice in quality of conclusions due to imperfect or incomplete data.[54]

Registries

Registries typically collect data from multiple institutions for purposes other than pure research, such as for governmental agencies, societies, and insurance purposes. They frequently tend not to have detailed outcome data, and the standards for data quality may not be as rigorous as for databases designed specifically for research.

Laboratory-Based

This rather nonspecific term indicates a specific type of study in which a patient variable (usually based on laboratory examination of human specimens from tissues, blood, or other body fluids) is analyzed over time in relationship to specific interventions or as a possible predictor of future events. The patient's pretreatment value is compared with values within the same patient following treatment, intervention, or an event.

META-ANALYSIS

A formalized review of the literature (usually from multiple institutions) which identifies and summarizes the available published information on a specific topic is termed a meta-analysis. Statistical techniques of data analysis are applied to the summary statistics of individual studies which have been combined into a common dataset. The basic process of meta-analysis is analogous to the methods of analyzing data in primary clinical research. A major disadvantage of such analyses is that they do not reveal patient-specific predictors, as can be generated from multivariable analysis of single or multi-institutional studies. An *effect size* is calculated for each reported study, which is the number of standard deviations by which a control group could have been benefited or harmed by exposure to the therapy under investigation. Effect sizes are summarized to produce a global test for the effect of a drug (or intervention). Proper meta-analysis involves statement of a formal hypothesis, identification of primary and related fields of knowledge, identification and gathering of appropriate studies for evaluation, development of criteria for study quality, construction of a code book for data entry, data analysis and determination of effect size, and reporting of results.

COMPONENTS OF A CLINICAL RESEARCH PROJECT

Generation of a Research Hypothesis

The research hypothesis is a formal translation of an informal belief or observation into a statement that can be tested by experimentation and/or a properly designed clinical study. The research hypothesis provides the central theme of the research project.[41]

Selection of Study Design

The study design is the specific structure of the study in terms of the method of patient selection or enrollment. The selection of a specific design is influenced by the size of the potential study population, the ethics and practicality of randomized versus observational data generation, the number of patients available for study, the desired duration of study, and available study budget. A study design should also be selected based on its likelihood of providing definite support or rejection of the study hypothesis.

Patient Selection

There must be a clear basis and criteria for patient inclusion and exclusion, based on sampling the patient population with greatest relevance to the study hypothesis.

Timetable

Each study should have a predetermined duration, either in terms of number of patients enrolled or calendar dates for starting and stopping patient enrollment.

Budget

A specific list of expenses for the study is generated and compared with the financial resources available. The budget is heavily influenced by the sample size.

Sample Size

Sample size is one of the most important elements of study design. Without a sample size large enough to detect useful clinical differences, a study is doomed before it is ever begun. Although the question of sample size usually comes up during the early stages of planning a study, there actually must first be many elements firmly established. These include (1) statement of the research hypothesis, (2) specification of a primary endpoint, (3) estimate of the standard deviation of the primary endpoint, (4) specification of allowable type I error and type II error, and (5) statement of the clinical difference that the study should have the power to detect.

Institutional Review Boards

All clinical research projects and experimental studies involving human subjects should be submitted to the local institutional review board for approval. This includes studies that only involve collection of existing data from the patient medical record.

Planned Statistical Analyses

During the planning stages of a study, all of the planned statistical analyses should be carefully laid out. These analyses will focus on the patient endpoints or outcomes as they relate to the research hypothesis. Generation of anticipated tables and figures is a useful exercise which may uncover inadequacies of study design, sample size, and variables to be collected.

Expected Results

A formal written discussion of expected results is recommended in order to gauge the impact of the study on basic knowledge and patient-specific decision-making. This offers another opportunity to evaluate the appropriateness of the hypothesis, the study design, and the collected variables.

Data Collection and Management

Before the study begins, all data collection forms must be generated and tested. The data collection process must be continually monitored and summarized. (This step is discussed in detail later as a separate section.)

Patient Follow-Up

Patient follow-up is part of most studies with time-related outcomes. For example, a study that examines survival should have a specific follow-up protocol that attempts to provide secure data on survival for each patient. Although some patients may be difficult to contact, the goal should be 100% follow-up. In outcomes research in heart transplantation, follow-up should be available in 95% of patients.

Statistical Analysis

Once the data are ready for examination, the statistical analysis can begin. The majority of this chapter is devoted to the analysis of data, especially time-related outcomes. Conceptually, the statistical analysis can be broken into two distinct components: formal planned analyses and data-driven analyses. The formal planned analyses are specified during the planning of the study. The data-driven analyses are a less formal process of examining the data. Hypotheses are not prespecified. Plots, group comparisons, and even multivariable analyses are used to find and estimate relationships among variables. In this setting, the investigator must remember that when testing at a .05 level of significance there will be approximately 5% of the p values that will be significant by chance alone. This process of analysis can be very useful in detecting unexpected relationships or in generating new hypotheses for future formal studies.

Presentation of Results

The presentation of results in a clear manner that is relevant to the research hypothesis enhances the audience's ability to comprehend and judge the value of the work. Proper use of figures and tables is a critical part of this process.

Implications for Patient Treatment

The report of a clinical study should include a section describing the relevance of the results to future patient treatment. This could include speculation if clearly labeled.

Formulation of New Hypotheses

Rarely does a research study provide complete definitive information on a topic. More often, during the course of study, new avenues for research become apparent or even necessary. Explicit formulation of these new hypotheses will help guide future research.

Validation with Future Studies

Due to the nature of the scientific method, most research results and inferences will have uncertainty. Depending on the importance of the research, future studies may be necessary to determine the reproducibility of the study finding.

DATA COLLECTION AND MANAGEMENT

The goal of data collection is the creation of a research data set that is suitable for statistical analysis. Ideally, this data set should have undergone appropriate scrutiny so as to provide accurate data on the variables relevant to the study hypothesis. This goal is best accomplished by utilizing a formal protocol of data collection and checking, regardless of the type of study (retrospective, prospective, randomized clinical trial, etc.) and the data source (paper medical record, computerized medical record, laboratory files, questionnaire, etc.).

The process of data collection requires a documented detailed protocol that should include the following steps:

1) The **necessary information (variables)** to be collected is determined. The most important aspect of the data collection relates to the selection of variables to be examined. This process occurs during the initial design of the study, and requires a balance between examination of all relevant and meaningful variables (in relationship to the hypothesis) and avoiding inclusion of numerous extraneous variables that do not pertain to the stated hypothesis and may (as a result of the additional labor required for their collection) compromise the accuracy of more relevant variables. The selection of variables is more complex in multi-institutional studies with many participating investigators. The situation is particularly complex in research-oriented databases in which selection of variables for ongoing data collection must anticipate future hypotheses that have not yet been generated.

2) The actual **sources of data** are identified. Will the data be contained in the patient medical record or will newly generated data be captured? Within practical limits, we recommend obtaining copies of all original documents and maintaining notebooks with a section for each patient's documents.

3) Once the variables to be collected have been specified and the sources of data determined, then a **form for recording the data** is constructed. (For some studies, data can be entered into a computer directly from source documents so that special computer "screens" rather than data collection forms are constructed.) The design of the form should simultaneously allow for ease of recording data and for ease of entering the data into a computer. Both the medical investigator and the statistician should contribute to the form design. The medical investigator will assist in form layout (according to source documents and logical grouping of variables) and specification of the possible values for each variable. The statistician examines each variable for its ability to be statistically analyzed.[21] The data collection form is further refined by the person who will be completing the form and by the data entry personnel.

4) The **collection of the data** should follow a set timetable with periodic progress evaluation by the investigators. Ideally this process should be as time-compacted as possible.

5) **Data entry** is best accomplished by dedicated personnel when possible. Questions which arise during data entry can be resolved through communication between data entry personnel, data collectors, and project investigators.

6) **Data entry software** has evolved greatly during recent years. Computer screens that mimic the data collection forms can be created which provide menu selection lists for data values, recognize and flag impossible or inconsistent values, and improve the overall data quality.

7) Even with good data entry software, **checking of all data** is necessary. The data for a patient can be printed and compared with the original data collection forms and source documents.

8) Large studies may require dedicated personnel for **managing the data** within the computer. The tasks include merging data from different sources, writing computer code for data entry, internal coding of data, creation of derived variables, managing computer resources, and arranging data sets according to the statistical techniques employed.

INITIAL EXAMINATION AND COMPARISON OF VARIABLES

When the data have been collected and checked, each variable should be summarized by one or more formal statistical techniques prior to formal multivariable analyses. This initial description of individual variables allows the investigators to become familiar with the data, check for missing data, check for unusual or impossible data, determine if a variable contains enough information for analysis, produce summary statistics, and help determine the appropriate coding of a variable for input into a multivariable analysis. A summary of test statistics is provided in Table 3–9.

TABLE 3-9	*Statistical Methods for Hypothesis Testing (Generation of p Values)*	
PURPOSE	STATISTICAL METHOD	ASSUMED DISTRIBUTION
Comparison of two variables		
Both discrete	χ^2 test*	Binomial
	Fisher's exact test* (small sample size)	Multinomial
One discrete, one continuous	t test*	Normal
	Wilcoxon	None
Both continuous	Pearson correlation (r)*	Bivariate normal
Comparison of survival curves	Log rank	Proportional hazards
	Gehan-Wilcoxon	None
	Parametric (likelihood ratio test)*	Hazard based

* Parametric tests.

TABLE 3-10	One-Way Frequency Table	
RECIPIENT BLOOD TYPE	n	%
A	115	42
B	34	13
AB	16	6
O	107	39
Total	272	100
Unknown*	15	

* When there are unknown data, the percentages for levels of a variable should be calculated based on the total patients with data.

TABLE 3-11	Contingency Table of Discrete Variables			
			DEAD	
GROUP	n	N	%	70% CL (%)
A	48	25	52	44–60
B	227	24	11	8–21
Total	275	49	18	15–21
p value (χ^2)			<.0001	

CL, confidence limits.

ONE VARIABLE: DISCRETE OR CONTINUOUS

A one-way (examining a single variable) frequency distribution of each variable, discrete or continuous, is the first step. This will provide a summary of the data (e.g., the percent of transplant recipients who are blood type O), will identify any impossible values, and indicate the amount of missing data (Table 3–10).

A frequency of a continuous variable will also identify missing and unusual values. It will give the minimum, maximum, and median values as well as the percentiles of the distribution of the variable. If the number of observations is large, then a graphical representation of the percentiles may be used instead of the tabular frequencies (Fig. 3–3). This is called a cumulative distribution frequency (CDF). For example, the 90th percentile of the CDF indicates that 90% of patients (or data points) have that or a smaller value. Once the frequencies have been examined, then descriptive statistics can be calculated for the central tendency (mean, median, mode) and the variability (variance, standard deviation, standard error, range, percentiles) of the data.

TWO VARIABLES: BOTH DISCRETE

A two-way table that summarizes the frequencies of each combination of discrete variables is known as a

contingency table. The outcome event death can be initially examined as a discrete non time-related variable (e.g., total deaths or 30-day mortality) (Table 3–11). A useful test of significance can be performed by visual examination of the **70% confidence limits.** If the confidence limits do not overlap, then the p value for comparing the proportions is less than approximately .10. The formal test statistic for comparison of proportions is the χ^2 test of significance.[46, 72] If either the total events for the table are small (< about 5) or if one of the variables has a very low frequency, then a **Fisher's exact test** is more appropriate (Table 3–12).[26] Fisher's exact test is usually given as a one-tail test and the χ^2 test is usually a two-tail test.

TWO VARIABLES: ONE DISCRETE AND ONE CONTINUOUS

The most common example of this situation is a discrete variable that is a group identifier and a continuous variable that describes individuals within the group. Table 3–13 contains a comparison of mean heights (continuous variable) for male and female transplant recipients (discrete variable). If the distribution of heights within each gender is approximately normally distributed, then a two-sample t test (a parametric test) is appropriate for **comparing the means.** The data and the comparison can be illustrated in two ways. Figure 3–4 A contains a

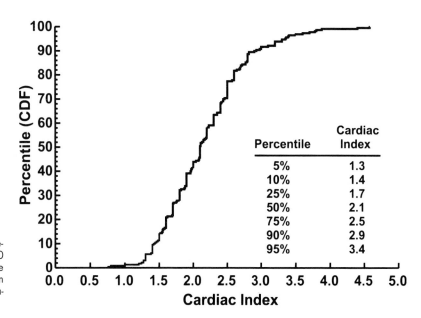

Percentile	Cardiac Index
5%	1.3
10%	1.4
25%	1.7
50%	2.1
75%	2.5
90%	2.9
95%	3.4

FIGURE **3–3.** Percentiles (or cumulative distribution frequency) of cardiac index (liters/minute/meter^2) for 230 patients listed for transplantation. For this sample, the mean = 2.2, median = 2.1, minimum = 0.8, maximum = 4.6, and the standard deviation = 0.62. CDF, cumulative distribution frequency.

TABLE 3-12	Contingency Table of Discrete Variables for Small Numbers

			HOSPITAL DEATHS		
GROUP	n	N	%	70 CL (%)	
A	20	7	35	23–49	
B	15	1	7	0.9–21	
p value (Fisher's)			.055		
p value (χ^2)			.048		

TABLE 3-13	Comparison of Discrete and Continuous Variables

RECIPIENT GENDER	n	HEIGHT (x ± SE, in cm)
Male	205	177 ± 0.5
Female	40	163 ± 1.1
p value (t test)		<.0001

SE, standard error; x, mean.

histogram for each group with a superimposed estimated normal distribution. Figure 3–4B is a comparison of the nonparametric CDF and the estimated CDF normal distribution, which is a different display of the same normal distribution as in Figure 3–4 A.

If the distribution does not appear to be normal, then there are two options. First, a mathematical transformation of the variable may yield a new variable that is normally distributed, and a t test can be employed on the new variable. For example, blood loss during cardiac surgery has a distribution that clusters near zero but has a "tail" that extends to larger values. A logarithmic transformation of such a variable will often be normally distributed. A second option is to abandon the parametric approach and instead utilize a test of significance that does not require specification of the underlying distribution. There are several such nonparametric tests,

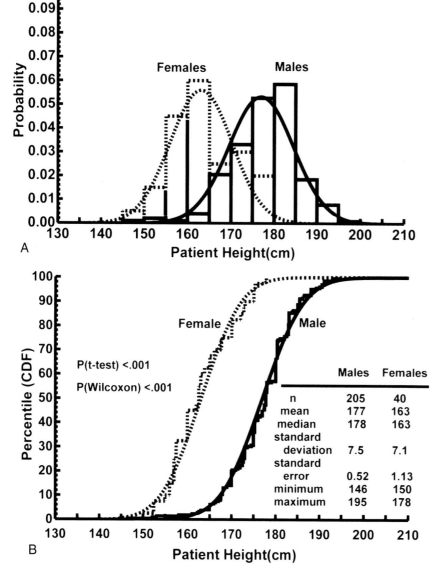

FIGURE 3-4. A, A histogram of patient heights for females (n = 40) and males (n = 205). The curved lines are the corresponding estimated normal distributions. The normal distributions are estimated by replacing the parameters, μ and σ, by their estimates, X̄ and SD. B, Cumulative distribution frequency (CDF) for height in females (n = 40) and males (n = 205). The jagged lines are the observed (nonparametric) CDFs and the smooth lines are the estimated normal (parametric) CDFs (which can be directly computed from the normal distribution curve in A).

but the most common one is the **Wilcoxon test,** which **compares the medians.** It is important to note that the Wilcoxon text assumes that, although the distribution of the variable within each group is not known, the distributions are identical except for the shift in location.

TWO VARIABLES: BOTH CONTINUOUS

The initial step in examining the relationship between two continuous variables is to plot the data in a scattergram (Fig. 3–5). The shape of the relationship, the existence of outliers, and the range of the two variables can be visualized. A statistic that is commonly used to assess the relationship between two continuous variables is the **Pearson correlation coefficient (r)** (see Equation 6 in Appendix). The correlation coefficient measures the linear relationship between the two variables. In the scattergram of points, the "thinness" of the ellipse of points reflects the absolute size of r, with a thinner ellipse (closer to truly linear) indicated by a larger absolute value of r and a wider ellipse (further from truly linear) indicated by a smaller absolute value of r. The inclination of the axis upward (both variables are increasing together, a positive correlation) or downward (one variable decreases as the other increases, a negative correla-

tion) determines the sign of r. The value of r always lies between -1 and $+1$. A value of $+1$ indicates a perfect positive correlation and a value of -1 indicates a perfect negative or inverse correlation. The associated p value indicates the probability that the observed linear relationship occurred by chance. The r value and the p value for the correlation both examine the closeness of fit of the scattergram to a linear relationship. The p value is determined by the r value and the sample size; the larger the r value, the smaller the p value.

MISSING DATA

A major function of the initial examination of collected data is the assessment of missing data, which may be unavailable or available but not collected. There is nothing to be done in the first case, but in the second case an extra effort to collect the data is warranted. Once as much of the missing data have been captured as possible, one must decide how to handle missing data in the statistical analysis. Most statistical software packages for multivariable analyses look at all of the variables specified in the model and then only include patients in the analysis who have data for all of the variables. This approach can drastically reduce the number of pa-

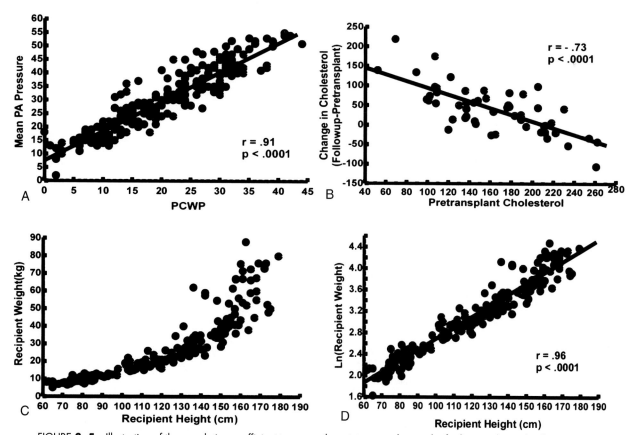

FIGURE 3–5. Illustration of the correlation coefficient to assess the existence and strength of a linear relationship between two continuous variables. A, Plot of mean pulmonary artery pressure and pulmonary capillary wedge pressure (PCWP) in mm Hg among 261 patients before transplantation. The positive value of r that is near 1.0 indicates a strong positive linear relation. B, Example of a less strong negative relation. The variables illustrated are change in cholesterol (mg/dL) from pretransplant to follow-up in 55 patients. C, Plot of pretransplant weight and height in 230 school-age children. The relation is positive but not linear. D, Logarithmic transformation of weight, which is linearly related to height.

tients who are included in an analysis. There are several approaches to minimize the effect of missing data: (1) eliminate the variable from consideration in the multivariable analysis because the data are just too incomplete (although no statistical rules exist for deciding how much missing data are too much); (2) replace the missing value with the mean (or median) of the variable for the patients who have data (which will allow the patient with missing data to be part of the analysis but will not allow the patient to contribute to the assessment of the variable as a risk factor); or (3) estimate the missing value by regression techniques.

The investigators must realize that missing data is often not a random event. Patients who are missing a variable may be different from other patients, and it is possible to test for this and make an adjustment. For example, patients who are missing quality-of-life data at the time of follow-up after transplant may have been too sick to complete the questionnaire and thus actually represent the poorest quality of life (rather than random missing data).

SURVIVAL CURVES (AND OTHER TIME-RELATED EVENTS)

Survival analysis is the branch of statistical methodology that is applied to outcomes that are time related.[1] The historical basis of survival analysis (see Box) stems from an interest in examining the effect of disease states on human survival. However, the methods are applicable to any event (or outcome) that is associated with time.

UNIQUE FEATURES

There are four aspects of the analysis of time-related events that require a special statistical methodology:

1) The data are usually incomplete and must be analyzed before all patients have experienced the event. A given patient may still be alive at the time of analysis so that his time until death is unknown. However, it is known that his time until death is greater than the time he has been observed. Survival analysis makes use of this incomplete (censored) information rather than disregard it.

2) The time-related shape of the probabilities of the event is often of clinical and scientific interest. For example, what is the probability that a patient will survive for 1 year, or 2, or 10? What is the period of highest risk? Is the risk decreasing or increasing over time?

3) It is often desirable to identify risk factors that are associated with increased risk of the event.

4) Specific statistical methods are needed to make time-related predictions of event probabilities that are specific to a patient and his or her particular risk factors.

Historical Basis of Survival Analysis

The roots of survival analyses can be traced to John Graunt in 1662, who developed rudimentary life tables for survival in London during the era of the bubonic plague.[4, 17, 31, 34] He emphasized the concepts of comparisons among life tables and identification of incremental risk factors, which led to a series of recommendations regarding ways to limit the spread of the bubonic plague. Graunt also introduced the "hazard function," which he defined as the "peril or danger of the occurrence of various calamities over a specified interval of time." William Lerry, a colleague of Graunt, introduced the notion of the hazard function changing over time.[53] The modern application of survival statistics to clinical experiences began with Berkson at the Mayo Clinic in the 1940s.[7] Kaplan (working at Bell Telephone Laboratories investigating the life history of vacuum tubes in telephone cables buried in the ocean) and Meier (working in biostatistical analyses at Johns Hopkins University) refined the application of survival statistics for small sample size.[39] Feigel and Zelen applied multivariable risk factor analysis to *time-related* death after acute myelogenous leukemia in which they assumed a constant hazard across time.[25] In 1972, Cox developed a semiparametric method which provided the general template for multivariable analysis of time-related events.[15, 16] This pivotal contribution stimulated much of the subsequent research and development of parametric methods for multivariable analysis in the hazard function domain, which are discussed in this chapter.

Despite the tremendous conceptual advance of Cox's methods, the assumption of *proportional hazards* (with an unknown underlying hazard function) was a disadvantage in attempting to define risk factors for time periods in which the hazards did not remain proportional. Furthermore, this method did not allow the ability to plot patient-specific depictions of outcome events. Subsequently, parametric models of hazard functions which varied over time were developed. In 1986, Blackstone, Naftel, and Turner developed a system of parametric survival analysis (three-phase hazard function model), which provided a general, mathematically robust system of parametric survival distribution equations which could be applied to a wide range of survival distribution shapes.[11]

MATHEMATICAL FUNCTIONS THAT DESCRIBE SURVIVAL

Before proceeding to estimation of time-related event probabilities, the definitions of mathematical functions that describe survival must be established. The **death density function,** $f(t)$, is the probability that an individual dies in the interval t to $t + \Delta t$. The **cumulative density function,** $F(t)$, is the probability that an individual dies in the interval 0 to t. The **survivorship function,** $S(t)$, is the probability that an individual survives to time t. The **hazard function,** $\lambda(t)$, is the probability that an individual who is alive at time t will die in the interval t to $t + \Delta t$. The hazard function is also known as the hazard rate, failure rate, instantaneous death rate, instantaneous failure rate, intensity function, and force of mortality. **The units of the hazard function (risk) are events per unit of time.** Therefore it is a rate. The **cumulative hazard function** $\Lambda(t)$, is the integral from 0 to t of the hazard function. Mathematically, all of these functions are related so that specification of any one of them automatically specifies all of the others. The relations are:

$$F(t) = \int_0^t f(t)$$

$$S(t) = 1 - F(t)$$

$$\lambda(t) = f(t)/S(t)$$

$$\Lambda(t) = -\ln[S(t)]$$

$$f(t) = -S'(t)$$

Each of these survival functions can be estimated using either **parametric** (based on a mathematical equation) or **nonparametric** methods. In practice, the distribution forms are not known. Nonparametric estimation makes no assumptions about the mathematical equation (model or distribution) that describes the functions. Parametric estimation assumes a model (distribution) and then estimates the parameters (see later section, Parametric Estimation).

CENSORING

If the exact times until the event under study were known for each patient in a study, then the standard statistical methods of summarizing and analyzing a continuous variable could be used. However, in most clinical research some patients have unknown time until the event. This incomplete data is called **censored data,** which is the incomplete observation of time to the event (Fig. 3–6).

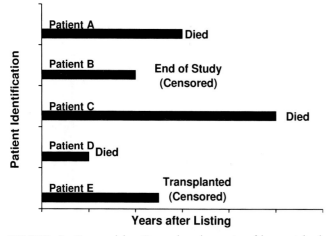

FIGURE **3–6.** Censored data (incomplete observation of the event death after listing) for patients listed for transplantation. Patients A, C, and D died during the study period without receiving a transplant. Patient B was alive and awaiting transplant at the end of the study and is censored at that time. Patient E underwent transplantation and is censored at that time.

In **right censored data** "time 0" is known for the patient, but the time of death is unknown. The time of censoring is the date that the patient is last known to be alive (or event free). Therefore, an interval can be calculated so that the actual, but unknown, time of death is longer than the known interval. The known interval is incomplete data regarding time until death. This is called right-censored data. There are at least three ways that right-censored data can exist. The most common situation is that the patient is still alive at the closing date of the study. The second situation occurs when a patient is lost to follow-up so that after a known date the patient can no longer be followed. This would include patients who move away and no longer can be found or an administrative decision that is made to no longer follow patients who are not receiving care at the study hospital. Censored data arising from this second situation should be minimized. The third situation occurs when a patient is no longer at risk for the event of interest, such as a patient who dies while waiting and thus is no longer "at risk" for a transplant. The date of death will become his or her date of censoring for the event transplantation.

In **left-censored data,** the date of death is known but the date of "time 0" is unknown. This would occur in a transplant patient when his or her date of death is known but the date of transplant is unknown. Although this situation is rare in transplant research, it often occurs in natural history of disease studies where the date of death is known but the date of acquiring the disease is unknown.

In **interval-censored data,** it is known that the patient has died, but the exact date of death is unknown. This could occur in transplant studies with annual follow-up when a patient is known to be alive at one follow-up and dead at the next, but the actual date of death is unknown.

Each of these types of censoring has different implications regarding nonparametric and parametric survival estimation. Most discussions of censoring refer to right-censored data. The fact that a patient is censored should have no connection to the likelihood of that patient experiencing the event being studied (noninformative censoring). Ideally, censoring would be an event that occurs by a random process or at least a process that is independent of the outcome event. If censored events are *not* completely independent of the event under study, the censoring process is called **informative censoring** because the act of censoring actually contains information about the event being studied.

NONPARAMETRIC ESTIMATION

The nonparametric estimation (*not* described by a mathematical equation or a specific distribution) of time-related events includes three basic methods: **actual** survival estimates, **life table methods,** and the **Kaplan-Meier method.** Although statisticians have argued this point, the life table method and Kaplan-Meier method have been termed **actuarial** (in contrast to actual) estimates because, unlike actual estimates, the actuarial method allows individuals whose follow-up is incomplete (due to either length of follow-up or censoring) to be included in the survival estimate. Estimation of the various functions that describe survival (or any other event) can be accomplished using nonparametric techniques where no **equation** (model or distribution) is assumed for the distribution of survival times.

If there is **no censoring,** then the methods are relatively simple. The **density function,** $f(t)$, is estimated by a histogram of death times. The number of intervals and the number of observations both affect the usefulness of this estimation. The population **cumulative density function,** $F(t)$, is estimated by the CDF of the sample. The **survivorship function,** $S(t)$, is estimated by 1 minus the CDF. Using the relation between cumulative hazard and survivorship function, $\Lambda(t)$ can be estimated by $-\ln [1 - F(t)]$. The hazard function, $\lambda(t)$, can be estimated by dividing time into intervals, just as with a histogram, and counting the number of patients alive at the beginning of an interval and the number who die during the interval. The hazard function for the interval is estimated by the proportion of patients who die during the interval among those who were alive at the beginning of the interval. The hazard function can also be visually estimated by differentiating the cumulative hazard with respect to time. In other words, the hazard is equal to the slope of the cumulative hazard.

When there is censoring, then all of these estimation strategies must change. Estimating the density and the hazard function is complex. Estimating the survivorship function has been a focus of statisticians and actuaries since the seventeenth century.

Actual Survival

When examining time-related outcomes such as survival, freedom from rejection, or freedom from infection, the simplest estimation method is an arithmetic counting of events among the subset of patients with a specific duration of follow-up. In survival analysis, this has been termed actual survival. A major disadvantage of this method is that only those patients with at least the prescribed follow-up period can be included in the survival calculation. Thus, if one wishes to examine 5- and 10-year survival among 100 patients undergoing cardiac transplant, we must know how many patients actually had potential follow-up of 5 and 10 years. For example, consider the calculation if 30 patients had potential follow-up of 5 years (at which time 25 were alive and 5 had died) and only 15 patients had potential follow-up of 10 years (at which time 10 were alive and 5 had died). In this example, the actual mortality at 5 years would be the 5 patients who died in the numerator and in the dominator the 5 deaths plus the 25 surviving patients, giving a 5-year mortality of 5/30 = 16.7%. The survival would be 100% minus 16.7% or 83.3%. Similarly, the 10-year mortality would be 5/15 = 33.3% and a 10-year survival of 66.7%. A major disadvantage of this technique is that 5-year survival is calculated solely on the basis of 30 of the 100 patients and 10-year survival solely on the basis of 15 of the 100 patients. The other patients had varying durations of survival.

Life Table Methods

Life table methods were originally created for large sample sizes and are designed to calculate survival probabilities at selected, usually equally spaced, time intervals. There are a variety of life table methods but the calculations all follow the same general pattern.[28, 45] The calculations center around the number of patients at risk for the event at the beginning of a particular time interval and how many of these patients experience the event during the interval. From this information, the probability of surviving the interval can be calculated (Fig. 3–7A). These interval probabilities can be used to estimate the survivorship function, the death density function, and the hazard function (Fig. 3–7B). Censoring is accommodated by including a patient in all calculations based on intervals before or including their censoring time and excluding them in all calculations based on intervals after their censoring time.

There are several **limitations** to life table methods. The choice of the time intervals is arbitrary and does affect the value of the estimates. If the intervals are too wide, then the shape of the survival estimates is unknown during the intervals. Finally, life table methods are not well suited to small sample sizes.

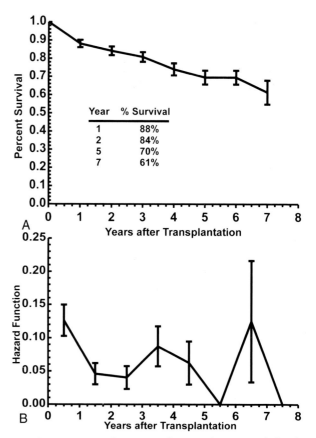

FIGURE **3–7.** _A,_ Survival estimates after transplantation calculated annually according to the life table method. The bars about the estimates are 70% confidence limits. _B,_ Corresponding hazard function estimates. The y-axis is the probability of dying during the yearly interval if the patient is alive at the beginning of the interval. The bars represent 70% confidence limits.

Product Limit Estimation

The process of generating a Kaplan-Meier actuarial curve by the product limit method is best illustrated by example. Consider 10 patients, 7 of whom die with the following survival times: 2, 6, 6, 10, 10, 13, and 13 years. Among the remaining three, the duration of follow-up (point of censoring) is 7, 11, and 14 years. For the first 2 years, there is no censoring, so S(t) (the survival function) is estimated by the proportion of patients alive at each death time. This is also 1−CDF. At 2 years there is one death, so that .10 of the patients have died and .90 are alive. S(2) equals .90. The survival at 6 years can be calculated using conditional probabilities.[28] Just before 6 years, .9 of the patients are alive. Then two patients of the remaining nine patients die, leaving 7/9 of the 9/10 being alive at the end of the interval (6 years). Multiplication is used for conditional probabilities so that S(6) = 9/10 · 7/9 = 0.7. At 7 years, one patient is censored because 7 years is the duration of his follow-up. At 10 years, the next two patients die. Just before 10 years, there are six patients still being followed. At the end of that interval (10 years), the conditional survival S(10) = 9/10 · 7/9 · 4/6 = 0.47. Note that the numerator and denominator for the last interval are reduced by 1 because of the patient censored at year 7 (Fig. 3–8).

Kaplan-Meier Method

The Kaplan-Meier actuarial method of estimating survival (or freedom from any event) estimates percentage survival at the time of each event[39] and is the standard technique utilized in most clinical studies that examine survival over time. Each estimate (a proportion) incorporates the number of patients who have experienced an event since the last estimate and the number of patients at risk, taking into account censoring. The Kaplan-Meier estimation is known as product limit estimation[39] (see Box) because of the form of its calculations (Fig. 3–8). This method of estimating survival probability is

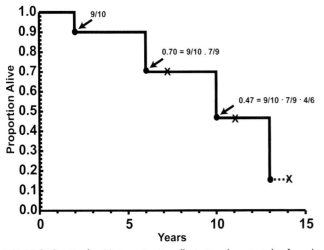

FIGURE **3–8.** Kaplan-Meier estimation illustrating the principle of conditional probabilities. The closed circles represent deaths and the x's represent censored observations. The details of the calculations are given in the text.

well suited to smaller samples and can give a more continuous representation of survival than life table methods. S(t) is reestimated each time that an event occurs. Therefore, the shape of S(t) can be better visualized throughout the timespan. This is valuable in the analysis of many events where the shape is changing quickly during the early time period (Fig. 3–9).

A basic premise in the Kaplan-Meier method is the presence of "noninformative censoring," which means that the unit (or patient) censored at any specific time has the same probability of the event under study as units (or patients) that run beyond that time. When using this methodology to estimate survival for a group such as patients listed for (and awaiting) transplantation, patients are censored at the time of transplantation and at the time of last follow-up if they are alive. When a Kaplan-Meier depiction of patients awaiting transplantation is examined, there is a natural tendency to assume that such an actuarial estimate approximates the natural history of the disease process treated medically without transplantation. In other words, it is assumed that patients censored at the time of transplantation have the same probability of subsequent death (without transplantation) as other patients with the same duration of follow-up. This is often not the case, since many patients are selected for transplantation because their health care providers believe they are "about to die" or become seriously ill. Thus, this type of censoring is *not* always noninformative, and the resulting actuarial curve provides the most optimistic (and likely false) estimate of survival without transplantation.

In Figure 3–10, we have illustrated two actuarial curves for patients with hypoplastic left heart syndrome after listing for cardiac transplantation. The upper curve looks at the event "death" in which a patient is censored at the time of transplantation and as stated above, provides the most optimistic survival estimate. The lower curve is the "worse case" scenario, in which the event examined is death or transplantation. If this is used as the estimate of survival after listing, it is assumed that all patients who are transplanted are selected because they are just about to "die" without transplantation. Clearly, this provides an unfairly low estimate of survival without transplantation. The truth lies somewhere in between, and its exact details cannot be determined by the Kaplan-Meier method.

PARAMETRIC ESTIMATION

As stated previously, parametric estimation utilizes an **equation** (i.e., assumes a distribution) to approximate (estimate) the survival function. The hazard function is particularly useful for indicating the immediate "risk" attached to an individual known to be alive at time t, and comparisons of the instantaneous risk for groups of individuals are facilitated.[16] If a model (equation) for S(t), and therefore λ(t), can be reasonably assumed and the parameters of the model can be estimated from data, then the many advantages of parametric survival analysis can be exploited, including a better understanding of the risk of an event over time, the generation of contin-

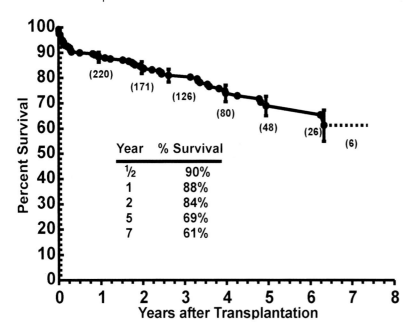

FIGURE **3-9.** Kaplan-Meier survival estimates for a group of 271 transplanted patients. Each death is represented by a circle that is positioned along the x-axis at the time of death and along the y-axis at the estimate of survival (or freedom from the event death) as calculated by conditional probabilities. The bars represent 70% confidence limits. The numbers in parentheses are the number of patients at risk at that time. The dotted line indicates the maximum follow-up.

uous lines to estimate event probabilities between actual events, and a powerful mechanism for identification of risk factors.[36] The selection of a model for a particular set of data is the most crucial step in the generation of inferences based on parametric analysis. The actual selection process is based on past analyses, medical experiences, and/or the data itself. The goal is selection of a simple model (containing few parameters) that fits the data well and approximates the time-related distribution of the outcome.

Constant Hazard Model

There are many models that have been investigated for survival analysis. The most commonly used and the simplest is the **negative exponential**. This model is also

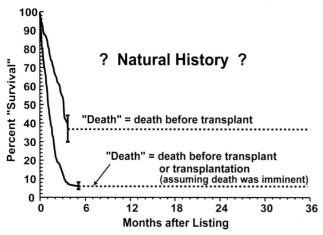

FIGURE **3-10.** Two depictions of the survival of pediatric patients listed for transplantation using different definitions of "death." The top curve analyzes the event death while waiting for transplant. Patients who are transplanted are censored at time of transplant. It is assumed that transplantation is not an indication of imminent death. The bottom curve analyzes the composite event of death before transplant or transplant. The assumption is that transplantation is an indicator of imminent death.

known as the **constant hazard model** because the **hazard is not a function of time.** The forms of the constant hazard model are:

Hazard function: $\lambda(t) = \mu$

Cumulative hazard: $\Lambda(t) = \mu t$

Survivorship function: $S(t) = e^{-\mu t}$

Death density function: $f(t) = \mu e^{-\mu t}$

Cumulative density function: $F(t) = 1 - e^{-\mu t}$

Figure 3–11 illustrates these distributions. This is called the exponential survivorship model because $S(t)$ is a negative exponential function. It is also called an exponential decay model (see Box). In this model, the instantaneous risk of the event is constant over time. This model contains one parameter, μ, which is the constant hazard. Notice that the higher $\lambda(t)$ is, the more quickly patients die as displayed by $S(t)$. Figure 3–12 depicts a data set which was modeled by a constant hazard function.

Models with a Varying Hazard

In most situations, time-related events do not occur with an equal risk over time. In transplant-related events such as infection and rejection, the risk is higher early after transplantation, whereas the risk of allograft vasculopathy increases late after transplantation. Since the hazard function represents the instantaneous risk of an event over time, models which assume a constant hazard would be a poor approximation of reality after transplantation. Models that are more flexible (i.e., do not assume a constant hazard) can be conceptualized in the hazard domain.[58] Some of the more common models are listed in Table 3–14. The hazard function (instantaneous risk of an event) can be increasing, decreasing, or U shaped.[2, 13, 30, 43]

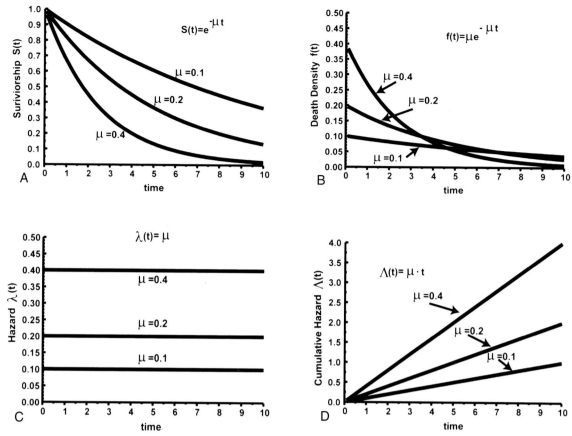

FIGURE 3–11. Functional forms of the negative exponential distribution (constant hazard). *A,* Survivorship function for three different values of μ (the hazard function). It displays the probability of freedom from the event. *B,* Death density function, which is the relative frequency of death. *C,* Hazard function for the negative exponential distribution. It is a constant across time. *D,* Cumulative hazard function, which is the integral of the hazard function from 0 to *t.*

Blackstone, Naftel, and Turner[11] took this a step further by creating a **three phase hazard model** that decomposes the hazard into as many as three additive phases: early, constant, and late (Fig. 3–13). The ability to model (generate an equation) and display rapidly increasing or decreasing risk is a major advantage of the hazard function domain in the analysis of events after transplantation.

The general forms of the hazard and cumulative hazard functions are

$$\lambda(t, \Theta) = \sum_{j=1}^{3} \mu_j g_j (t, \Theta_j)$$

and

$$\Lambda(t_1 \Theta) = \sum_{j=1}^{3} \mu_j G_j (t_j \Theta_j)$$

where μ_j is a scaling (or proportionality) parameter for the jth phase, g_j is a generic shaping function for the jth phase, Θ_j is a vector of shaping parameters associated with g_j, G_j is the integral of g_j, and t is time until the event. Scaling parameters adjust the hazard function along the y-axis, and shaping parameters determine the shape of the hazard function within each phase.

This model belongs to the class of parametric survival models known as mixture distributions or competing risks models. Each phase consists of a parametric shaping distribution function (an equation which determines the shape of the hazard curve). These shaping distributions are generic functions that give rise to a set of sub-

Exponential Decay Model

The parameter μ has several mathematical properties that make it useful in describing survival.

First, the inverse of μ is equal to the mean survival time. Second, μ is the rate of deaths per unit time. This is also known as the decay rate. For example, if $\mu = 0.10$ and time is measured in years, then deaths are occurring at the rate of 0.10 per year. From this, the survival at one year can be calculated: $S(1) = e^{-\mu \cdot 1} = e^{-0.1} = 0.905$.

If one is willing to assume a constant hazard for a given survival situation, then the next step is to estimate μ based on observed data. If there is no censoring, then the estimate of μ, denoted by $\hat{\mu}$ described by Equation 7 (see Appendix).

Notice $\hat{\mu}$ is the inverse of the sample mean. If there is right-censoring, then the estimate of $\hat{\mu}$ is described by Equation 8 (see Appendix).

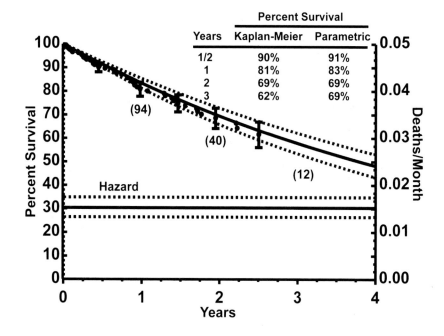

FIGURE **3–12.** Parametric survival estimates for a constant hazard model which provides a good fit (agreement) to the Kaplan-Meier estimates. The data set is a group of nonurgent, nonhospitalized patients listed for cardiac transplantation in the Cardiac Transplant Research Database. The estimate for μ (hazard) and its 70% confidence limits (CLs) is indicated by the lower solid line and the surrounding dashed lines. The closed circles represent individual events in the Kaplan-Meier analysis. The error bars indicate $\pm$ 1 standard error and the dashed lines the 70% CL. The numbers in parentheses indicate the number of patients followed at that time. The horizontal axis is years after listing.

models than can accommodate a wide range of possible distribution shapes and contain a complex system of equations. A few of the shapes for early-phase and late-phase hazards (see Box) are illustrated in Figure 3–14.

Since most transplant survival experiences are poorly approximated with a constant hazard (Fig. 3–15), a model providing an early plus a constant phase of hazard provides much closer agreement between the parametric and nonparametric survival estimates (Fig. 3–16). The resultant hazard illustrates the early elevated risk of death (early phase), which gradually merges with the constant hazard. The shape of the early phase is determined by the parameter estimates, which in turn are a function of the data.

Except for the constant hazard function, the actual computations for the hazard parameter estimates do not have a single closed form equation for the calculation. Instead, a computer-based iterative stepwise process of refining the estimate process is employed using a numerical approach to obtain "maximum likelihood estimates."[20, 38] Estimates are numerically adjusted until parametric estimates are found that provide the best fit (i.e., provide the maximum likelihood) with the observed data. The theory of maximum likelihood includes a process for the calculation of standard errors for the parameter estimates. In actual practice, we use the SAS estimation programs[10] for the three-phase model to compute the complex mathematics of the multiple phase

hazard function for a given data set of time-related events.

COMPARISON OF SURVIVAL CURVES (TIME-RELATED OUTCOME)

The earlier section, Initial Examination of Variables, has already covered univariable analysis when the outcome variable does not have an associated time component. This section covers the case when the outcome variable is a **time-related event.**

NONPARAMETRIC COMPARISONS OF SURVIVAL CURVES

No Censoring

The general approach is to calculate separate survival estimates (curves) for groups of patients (defined by the variable of interest) and then compare the curves. The phrase "compare the curves" deserves special comment. If there is **no censoring,** so that each patient died and a time of death was recorded, then the survival of the two groups could be compared by a *t* test for comparison of "mean" survival (as discussed in the previous section,

TABLE 3–14	Hazard Functions	
DISTRIBUTION	ASSUMPTION ABOUT THE HAZARD FUNCTION	HAZARD FUNCTION
Exponential	Constant hazard	μ_1
Rayleigh	Increasing	$\mu_1 + \mu_2 2t$
Weibull	Increasing or decreasing hazard	$\mu_3 \eta t^{-1}$
Gompertz	Early component of increased risk	$\mu_3 e^{(t/\eta)/\tau}$
Makeham-Gompertz	Early component of increased risk that reduces to a constant phase of risk	$\mu_2 + \mu_3 e^{(t/\eta)/\tau}$
Three-phase hazard model	Maximum of three additive phases: early, constant, and late	$\lambda_1(t) + \lambda_2(t) + \lambda_3(t)$

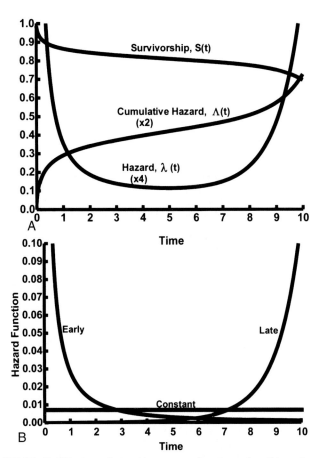

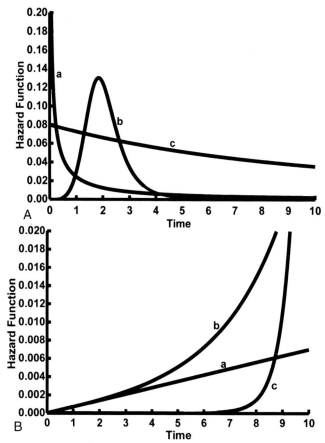

FIGURE **3-13.** Interrelationship among functions describing time-related events. *A*, Relationship between the three-phase hazard function, the survivorship function, and the cumulative hazard function. The hazard function is infinite at time zero, rapidly falls to a low level, then rises steeply. *B*, Decomposition of the hazard function into separate but overlapping phases of hazard that, when added, constitute the hazard function depicted in *A*. Its phases are labeled early, constant, and late to denote the times at which the influence of each is dominant.

FIGURE **3-14.** *A*, Typical forms of hazard function $[\lambda(t)]$ generated by the early-phase generic equation. μ_1 is the scaling parameter; and δ, ρ, m, and ν are shaping parameters. In all cases $\delta = 0$ and $m = 1$. In a $\rho = 2$, $\nu = 2$, and $\mu_1 = .2$; in b $\rho = 2$, $\nu = 0.2$ and $\mu_1 = 0.2$; in c $\rho = 20$, $\nu = 1$, and $\mu_1 = 1.6$. Notice that $\lambda(t)$ may approach infinity as time approaches 0 as in a $(m \; \nu > 1)$; it may begin at 0, slowly rise, then peak and fall as in b $(m \; \nu < 1)$; or it may begin at a finite value and fail as in c $(m \; \nu = 1)$. *B*, Typical forms of hazard function $[\lambda(t)]$ generated by the late-phase generic equation. μ_3 is the scaling parameter; and τ, α, γ, and η are shaping parameters. In a, $\alpha = 1$, $\tau = 1$, $\gamma = 1$, $\eta = 2$ and $\mu_3 = 0.00035$; in b, $\alpha = 0$, $\tau = 8$, $\gamma = 2$, $\eta = 1$, and $\mu_3 = 0.022$; in c, $\alpha = 0$, $\tau = 3$, $\gamma = 2$, $\eta = 1$, and $\mu_3 = 6.8 \times 10^{-7}$. Notice that $\lambda(t)$ may increase linearly as in a Rayleigh (a), it may curve sharply upward after a prolonged period of imperceptible rise (c), or it may take on an intermediate form (b).

Early Phase and Late Phase Hazards

The form of the early phase cumulative hazard function is shown in Equation 9 (see Appendix).

The full complexity of the early phase is rarely used. Special cases, usually found by setting one or more parameters to 0 or 1, greatly reduce the complexity. Figure 3–14A illustrates a few of the possible hazard shapes from the early phase model.

The form of the constant phase cumulative hazard function is $\Lambda_2(t) = \mu_2 t$ where μ_2 is the constant hazard and t is time. This is just the constant hazard for the negative exponential.

The form of the late phase cumulative hazard function is as in Equation 10 (see Appendix). The full complexity of the late phase is also rarely used. Figure 3–14B illustrates a few of the late phase shapes. For example, if $\gamma = 2$, $\alpha = 0$, and $\eta = 1$, then the late phase reduces to Equation 11 (see Appendix), which is a linearly increasing hazard.

Two Variables: One Discrete and One Continuous.) The *t* test compares the mean survival times for the two groups assuming a normal distribution of death times. This comparison may not be appropriate if the distribution of survival times does not have a normal distribution. The median survival time can be compared with a **Wilcoxon nonparametric test.**

Censoring

The presence of **censoring** complicates the matter. When the actual time of death is not known for all patients, then the mean time to death cannot be calculated. For this reason, mean survival times are rarely discussed or compared except when certain parametric distributions are assumed. Nonparametric estimates are better suited for estimating medians and other percentiles. Univariable analysis of time-related outcomes are usually com-

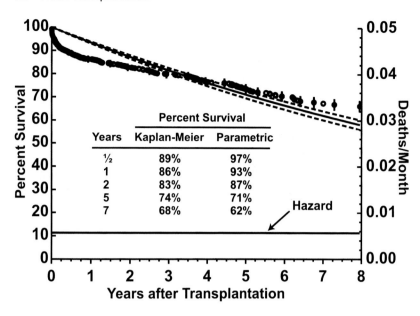

FIGURE **3–15.** Comparison of Kaplan-Meier non-parametric and constant hazard parametric models for estimation of survival after transplantation in 1,000 patients. Here, the constant hazard model provides a *poor* approximation of the Kaplan-Meier. The circles are Kaplan-Meier nonparametric estimates and the bars are 70% confidence limits. The top solid line is a parametric estimate assuming a negative exponential model. The lower solid line is the resultant parametric constant hazard function. The dashed lines enclose 70% confidence limits.

parisons of nonparametric survival curves. The first step in comparison of nonparametric survival curves for two or more groups is visual inspection and comparison of the Kaplan-Meier curves. This comparison is enhanced if 70% confidence limits are plotted. Places where the 70% confidence limits do not overlap may be viewed as an informal indication of difference.

The **log rank test** is the most commonly used test to compare nonparametric survival curves. The log rank test is designed to detect a difference between survival curves when the survival rate in one group is consistently higher than the other group and the ratio of the two hazard rates is constant over time (Fig. 3–17).[49] All deaths are weighted equally. The log rank test is Cox proportional hazard regression for a single discrete variable. It assumes proportional hazards for the two groups and therefore examines an average hazard across time.

Although it is always a valid test of the null hypothesis that the survival functions of two populations are the same, the log rank test may not be able to detect a true difference if the ratio of hazard rates is not constant over time.

An alternative nonparametric test of survival curves is the generalized Wilcoxon test,[71] the most common being the **Gehan-Wilcoxon test,**[29] which is a test of medians and detects differences more readily if the hazards are not proportional. The Gehan-Wilcoxon test attaches more weight to early deaths than later ones (Fig. 3–18), whereas the **log rank test** gives equal weight to all deaths.

Direct examination of the Kaplan-Meier plot is crucial to the interpretation of nonparametric survival tests. Without graphical display of the survival, these nonparametric tests are of limited value.

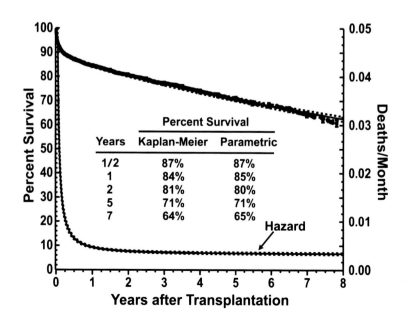

FIGURE **3–16.** Same Kaplan-Meier depiction as in Figure 3–15, but modeled with a two-phase hazard model that consists of an early and a constant phase. This provides a much better fit to the Kaplan-Meier than the constant hazard in Figure 3–15. The circles are Kaplan-Meier nonparametric estimates and the bars are 70% confidence limits. The lower solid line is the resultant parametric hazard function. The dashed lines enclose 70% confidence limits.

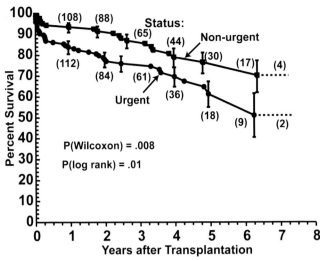

FIGURE 3-17. Two Kaplan-Meier depictions for survival after transplantation, stratified by urgency of status. Both nonparametric tests are significant. According to the figure, the difference in survival develops during the first 6 months. The more significant Gehan-Wilcoxon test, which weighs early events more, reflects this fact. The nonoverlapping 70% confidence limits also visually aid in assessing differences.

PARAMETRIC COMPARISONS OF SURVIVAL CURVES

Parametric comparisons can provide additional insight because the estimated hazard functions can be visually compared (Fig. 3–19). *P* values can be calculated by **likelihood ratio tests** if the two individual models are contained within a more general model. The hazard functions can also be compared by examining the confidence limits around the **hazard estimates.** The hazard ratio is a specific method for examining relative risks (the risk or probability of an event in one curve or group

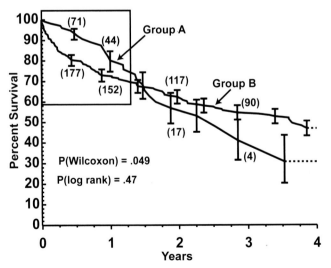

FIGURE 3-18. Two Kaplan-Meier depictions showing different patterns of survival. Nonparametric tests are not well suited to this situation. The log rank test assumes proportional hazards for the two groups and therefore examines an average hazard across time. It is not significant because the differing early and late effects cancel each other out. The significance of the Gehan-Wilcoxon test is a reflection of the early difference between the two groups (indicated by the box).

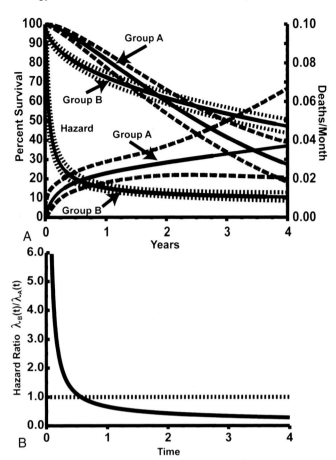

FIGURE 3-19. *A*, Parametric survival and hazard estimates for two groups of patients with differing patterns of survival. Figure 3–17 contains the nonparametric estimates. Group A has a delayed early phase of hazard combined with a linearly increasing phase. Group B has a high early phase that declines to a constant phase of hazard. *B*, Hazard ratio (hazard B/hazard A) for the two parametric hazard functions in *A*. A ratio of 1 indicates no difference in hazard. A ratio greater than 1 indicates an increased risk for group B. A ratio less than 1 indicates an increased risk for group A.

compared with another) and is obtained by dividing, point by point, one hazard function by the other. A *p* value can be calculated for various portions of the survival curves depending on the shapes of the hazard functions. The likelihood that differences between the survival curves are due to chance can also be examined by comparing the **confidence limits** of the hazard functions.

MULTIVARIABLE ANALYSIS

THE GENERAL STRATEGY OF MULTIVARIABLE ANALYSIS

The exact future timing of an outcome event for a specific patient can rarely, if ever, be determined. Conversely, a time-related outcome is rarely a totally random occurrence. The timing of an outcome is a function of many factors including patient-specific, treatment-specific, and perhaps institution-specific variables. Although a perfect cause-and-effect profile may be impossible to determine, **risk factors** can usually be identified which, known at time zero, are **associated with** an increased likelihood of the outcome. It is important to remember that "association" in the statistical sense does not necessarily imply causality. **Multivariable analysis** refers to the process of generating an equation which relates the independent variables, or risk factors (with their associated coefficients, standard errors, and p values), to the dependent (outcome) variable. The **coefficients** (β) are parameters (constants) for the risk factors in the equation and are estimated from the data. These risk factors have also been called incremental risk factors, covariates, predictive variables, correlates, and explanatory variables.

The mathematical model that generates a multivariable analysis generally has two basic features. First, it is an **iterative process,** which means that a series of mathematical steps are directed by a systematic algorithm, or plan, to find the value of a coefficient and its p value by starting at the extremes and working toward a central value. Second, this mathematical process requires simultaneous computations of all potential independent variables. Because of the computational load and complexity, computers are required for this process.

Risk factors identified by this process should be considered in light of medical judgment. However, if medical judgment disagrees considerably with the statistical estimate, it is likely that one or more key variables have been left out of the model-building process. Once again, the vital interaction between medicine and statistics is emphasized.[48, 55]

Thus, the **goal of a multivariable analysis** is to produce a set of risk factors that are associated with the outcome. Ideally, these risk factors would be predictive of the outcome in future patients and would give insight into cause-and-effect relations. There are a number of statistical methods for multivariable risk factor analysis (Table 3–15). The proper method depends on the form of the outcome variable and its mathematical relation to the risk factors.

Once an appropriate method is selected, the strategy for reducing a set of potential risk factors into a group of significant risk factors is similar for all methods. The steps for producing a final set of risk factors are listed below.

1) The investigator produces a **list of potential risk factors** to be evaluated, including possible interactions among variables. The potential list of risk factors may be generated in part by preliminary univariable (risk "unadjusted") analyses.

2) **Numerical coding** of each qualitative variable and each specified interaction allows computer programs to accept numeric variables. Recipient gender might be coded in the computer as F for female and M for male. This would be transformed into a new variable, perhaps called "male," where 1 = male and 0 = female. Other variables may not be so obvious. Pretransplant diagnosis may have many variations coded as numbers or letters in the computer. The frequencies and medical relevance of these diagnoses must be examined in order to group them into numerical values which would make medical sense. Part of the coding process is the creation of transformed variables. For certain variables, a mathematical function (transformation) of a continuous variable may be more significant than the original variable.

3) Each potential risk factor should be examined **univariably** for association with the outcome. Familiarization with the data is facilitated and variables are identified that are not suited for further consideration, including variables that have too many missing values, or too few events in a level. Consider a retrospective study of a center's transplant experience where there have been 100 transplants. Donor gender may have been specified by the researcher as an important potential risk factor for death, but the univariable analysis may reveal that out of the 100 donors in the study only 3 were female. In this case, there is not enough information to estimate the effect of donor gender.

4) A common strategy for decreasing the list of potential risk factors for inclusion in a multivariable analysis is to include only those variables that are significant univariably. We disagree with this strategy, since it ignores the key feature of risk adjustment that comes from a multivariable analysis. The significance of a risk factor after adjustment for other risk factors in the model is produced by a multivariable analysis; that is, the significance of a risk factor is determined after the other risk factors are accounted for. This adjusted p value can be either larger or smaller than the unadjusted (univariable) p value. Therefore, a variable that is not significant univariably may become significant after adjustment for the other risk factors.

5) There are differing statistical approaches to correlated variables. If two variables are highly correlated, then both will not be in the final model. There may also be combinations of variables that are correlated with a single variable, such as height

TABLE 3–15	Statistical Techniques for Multivariable Analysis	
PURPOSE OF MULTIVARIABLE ANALYSIS	STATISTICAL METHOD	ASSUMED DISTRIBUTION
Risk factors for yes/no outcomes	Logistic regression	Logistic
Risk factors for time-related outcomes	Cox proportional hazards regression	Proportional
	Logistic regression and Cox regression	Logistic/proportional
	Parametric regression in the hazard function domain	Hazard
Risk factors (predictors) for continuous outcomes	Multiple regression analysis (linear or nonlinear)	Normal around a linear function

and weight with body surface area. The statistician must be aware of these correlations to avoid a strange model in which one variable is counteracting another correlated variable. In many cases, a medical expert in the area of study can guide the examination of correlated variables.

6) The actual mathematical process of selecting the final set of risk factors has numerous methodological possibilities.[22] **Forward stepwise selection** is a common statistical and computer intensive method for identifying the risk factors. First, a significance level for entering the model and a significance level for remaining in the model is specified. These significance levels are type I errors, but they do not have to be equal. Each of the potential risk factors is examined as if it is the only variable in the model. The risk factor with the lowest (most significant) p value is selected for entry into the model. Next, p values are recomputed for all variables not in the model after adjustment for the one variable that has already been entered into the model. The variable with the lowest adjusted p value is entered into the model as the second variable. Now the p value for the first variable in the model is recomputed, adjusted for the second variable. It is possible that the first variable will no longer be significant according to the level specified for remaining in the model. If this happens, then the first variable is removed from the model and the p value for the remaining variable is recomputed. This circumstance would happen if the first and second variable were correlated. This process of examining variables not in the model after adjustment for variables in the model is continued. Each time a new variable is entered, p values for variables already in the model are recomputed after adjustment for the new variable and all of the other variables in the model. A variable that has become nonsignificant is removed. This entire process is continued until none of the variables not in the model meet the significance level for entry into the model. Although this is the general process, there are a number of modifications that are possible, depending on the actual software package used. For example, many packages allow the forcing of a variable into the model, regardless of its p value. Other packages allow a variable to never enter the model, but the p value for entry is recomputed for each step of the model-building process.

7) Once the computer has produced a final set of risk factors, the univariable p value for each risk factor is again examined. Any variable that is significant after adjustment for other risk factors but is not significant univariably should be closely examined to determine what adjustment caused the significance. Conversely, a variable that was significant univariably but is not significant after adjustment for other factors should also be examined.

8) The final model should be carefully scrutinized by the investigator for medical consistency. He or she may elect to try substitution of one variable for another possibly correlated variable or a variable

that makes better medical sense. The final model is usually the result of a close collaboration between the medical investigator and the statistician. Different researchers will produce different models from the same data because of the many opportunities for subjectivity, or perhaps more accurately the many opportunities for experience and knowledge to influence the direction of the analysis.[55] Thus, multivariable analysis should never be viewed as an "automated" process. Rather, there must be expert input from the investigators at each step.

MULTIVARIABLE ANALYSIS OF YES/NO OUTCOMES

Many important clinical outcome events either do not have a time element or time can be removed. Insertion of a balloon pump during surgery is an outcome that has no time element. Death occurring within a certain time period, such as 30-day death or hospital death, is an outcome where time has been removed. The earlier section Initial Examination of Variables discusses the univariable analysis of binary (yes/no or success/failure) outcomes.

Multivariable analysis of binary outcomes can be initially approximated by multiple subsets of univariable analyses. For example, a comparison of hospital death according to urgency status could be examined separately for each recipient gender, which would convey information about the effect of status on death while "adjusting" for gender. It would also allow an examination of an interaction which answers the question, "Is the effect of status on hospital death the same for both gender groups?" Although this strategy for identifying risk factors provides important insights about potential risk factors, it quickly breaks down as the number of subsets increases.

Logistic regression is the recommended method of multivariable analysis for identifying risk factors for a binary outcome. An event that can have **two possible outcomes and does not have a time-related component** is a candidate for logistic regression.[63] The goal is identification of risk factors that are associated with an increase in the probability of the event. A model (equation) for probability must have two major constraints: it must be bounded by 0 at the lower end and by 1 at the upper end. The logistic equation is a mathematical function that meets these constraints (Fig. 3–20).[5]

The logistic regression model was apparently first described by Verhulst in 1838 (to describe French and Belgian population behavior),[69] reported by Pearl and Reed from Johns Hopkins University in 1920 (to describe the pattern of autocatalytic reactions),[61] and later by Berkson in the same decade (to describe reaction between enzymes and substrate).[6, 8] Walker and Duncan applied the logistic method to risk factor analysis for non-time-related events in the Framingham Study.[70] In 1979, Blackstone and Kirklin applied the logistic equation to risk factor identification for events after cardiac surgery.[40]

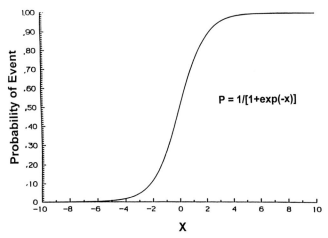

FIGURE **3-20.** The logistic equation for modeling probability of an event. The general form of the equation is $p(\text{event}) = 1/[1 + \exp(-\alpha - \beta x)]$, where $p(\text{event})$ is probability of event, α is a location parameter, β is a slope parameter and x is a risk factor. The depicted equation is for $\alpha = 0$ and $\beta = 1$.

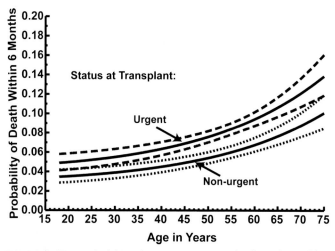

FIGURE **3-21.** Probability solutions (nomograms) for the multivariable logistic analysis presented in Table 3–16. The figure illustrates the effect of recipient age on the probability of dying within 6 months of transplant. The additional risk factors in the equations were set such that ventilator = no, donor age = 35 years, and ischemic time = 200 minutes. The two solid lines are the estimates according to patient urgency status. The dotted lines are 70% confidence limits.

The mathematical basis of the logistic model can be illustrated by considering the possible relationship between a variable x and the event hospital death. $p_i = 1 + \exp(-\beta_0 - \beta_1 x_{1j})$, where p is the probability of the event, x_{1j} is the value for the risk factor x_1 for the jth patient, and β_0 and β_1 are regression coefficients (parameters). The model can be linearized by the logit transformation $\ln[(1 - p)/p] = -(\beta_0 + \beta_1 x_1)$, where ln is the natural log transformation.

In this form, the model resembles a linear regression problem. The intercept β_0 controls the shift, and β_1 controls the steepness. The β's are estimated from the data. When there are multiple independent variables, analogous strategies to multiple linear regression can be employed. Estimation of the regression coefficients (parameters) requires an iterative process by computer.

The predicted probability calculated from the logistic model can be used to illustrate the effects of the risk factors on the probability of an event. The result is a visual depiction of the effect of one or more risk factors on the probability of an event (Table 3–16 and Fig. 3–21).

The odds ratio is a convenient technique for depicting the effect of risk factors in a logistic regression analysis. A modified depiction of the odds ratio can be used for continuous risk factors (Table 3–16). Odds ratio and relative risk (see Box) are often used interchangeably (in error), but the actual calculation of each is different. In multivariable analysis, calculation of odds ratio and relative risk is a computer-based iterative process. However, the calculations for a single risk factor are simpler and intuitive. The **odds ratio** is calculated by the odds of an event (dead) divided by the odds of nonevent (alive). The odds ratio is produced by dividing this proportion in one group by the proportion in another group. The **relative risk** is the risk (or probability) of an event in one group divided by (compared to) the risk of that event in another group. The interpretation of relative risk is more intuitive than odds ratio. For example, a relative risk of 3 indicates that a patient with treatment

TABLE 3–16	Risk Factors (Logistic) for Death within 6 Months of Heart Transplant*		
RISK FACTOR	COEFFICIENT ± SE	ODDS RATIO	*p* VALUE
Recipient			
Age (yr) (younger)	0.0215 ± 0.0061	1.27	.0004
Urgent status at tx	0.361 ± 0.133	1.44	.006
Ventilator at tx	1.65 ± 0.26	5.23	<.0001
Donor			
Age (yr) (older)	0.0312 ± 0.0064	1.32	<.0001
Ischemic time (min) (longer)	0.0431 ± 0.0078	1.61	<.0001
Intercept (β_0)	−4.26 ± 0.24		

tx, transplant.
* Both recipient and donor age (yr) have been divided by 10 and squared. Therefore, the odds ratio depends on the specific values of ages being compared. The odds ratio in the table for recipient age compares the effects of the ages 50 and 60 years. The odds ratio for donor age compares the effects of the ages 40 and 50 years. Ischemic time (min) has been divided by 60 and squared. The odds ratio compares ischemic times of 300 and 360 minutes. Note that odds ratio is not equivalent to relative risk (see text). The coefficient (β) is multiplied by the value of the variable or, for a dichotomous variable, by 0 or 1.

Odds Ratio and Relative Risk

Odds ratio and relative risk are two statistical calculations for estimating the univariable effect of a risk factor. An algebraic representation of the association between a dichotomous risk factor and death is:

TREATMENT	DEAD	ALIVE	TOTAL
A	a	b	$a + b$
B	c	d	$c + d$
Total	$a + c$	$b + d$	$a + b + c + d$

The odds of death for a treatment is defined as the number dead divided by the number alive so that

$$odds_A = a/b$$

$$odds_B = c/d$$

The risk (or probability of death) for a treatment is defined as the number dead divided by the total number for the treatment, so that

$$risk_A = a/(a + b)$$

$$risk_B = c/(c + d)$$

The **odds ratio** is the ratio of the odds.

$$Odds\ ratio = \frac{odds_A}{odds_B} = \frac{a/b}{c/d} = \frac{ad}{bc}$$

The **relative risk** is the ratio of the risk in group A to that in group B.

$$Relative\ risks = \frac{risk_A}{risk_B} = \frac{a/(a + b)}{c/(c + d)}$$

An example of these calculations follows:

TREATMENT	DEAD	ALIVE	TOTAL
A	50	150	200
B	10	90	100
Total	60	240	300

$$odds_A = \frac{50}{150} = .33 \qquad risk_A = \frac{50}{200} = .25$$

$$odds_B = \frac{10}{90} = .11 \qquad risk_B = \frac{10}{100} = .10$$

$$odds\ ratio = \frac{.33}{.11} = 3.0; \quad relative\ risk = \frac{.25}{.10} = 2.5$$

The odds ratio can range from zero to infinity. A ratio of 1.0 indicates equivalent estimated odds in the two groups. A ratio greater than 1 indicates increased odds with treatment A. A ratio of less than 1 indicates increased odds with treatment B.

Although these measures are useful in estimating the effect of a single risk factor, their utility is increased if the risk of death is given for both groups. Consider a study where the risk of death in treatment A is .50 and in treatment B is .25. The relative risk (.50/.25) is 2.0. Consider another study where the risk of death in treatment A is .10 and in treatment B is .05. The relative risk (.10/.05) is also 2.0. Although the relative risks are equal, the individual estimated risks are necessary for a complete description of the impact of the treatment. If the probabilities of death in each group are either very low or very high, then the odds ratio and the relative risk produce similar numbers.

A is estimated to be three times more likely to die than a patient with treatment B.

MULTIVARIABLE ANALYSIS OF TIME-RELATED OUTCOMES

Cox Proportional Hazards Regression

In 1972, D. R. Cox published the methodology for semiparametric identification of multiple risk factors. This general regression model is best described in the hazard domain where levels of a risk factor adjust an unspecified hazard function proportionately across time.[15] The driving assumption of Cox regression is that of **proportional hazards.**[14] Any two hazard functions that are defined by two different levels of a single risk factor are proportional across all time (Table 3–17). The **hazard ratio** is the calculation of **relative risk** applied to hazard functions. For a dichotomous variable, the hazard ratio indicates the factor by which the risk factor increases the hazard (if the other risk factors are unchanged). For continuous variables, the hazard ratio must be calculated for two specific values of the risk factor.

The fact that the hazard function is unspecified in the Cox proportional hazards model (see Box) provides a major advantage in the ease of mathematical computations. Indeed, this critical contribution of Cox and his colleagues provided the impetus for other investigators to focus on the application of survival statistics to the understanding of risk factors for time-related events. As brilliant as Cox's contributions are, Cox himself realized the limitations of the "proportional hazards" method in examining risk factors (which may be different or at least not proportional) for early and late events[15] (such as death after transplantation). If Kaplan-Meier curves have been stratified according to levels of a risk factor and these curves cross, then the hazard functions are not proportional. Alternatively, the stratified cumulative hazard functions can be examined for proportionate

TABLE 3-17	Risk Factor Analysis (Cox Regression) for Death after Transplantation*		
RISK FACTOR	COEFFICIENT ± SD	HAZARD RATIO	p VALUE
Recipient			
Age (yr) (younger)	−0.33 ± 0.11	0.74	.003
VAD at time of tx	1.01 ± 0.39	2.74	.01
Creatinine	0.75 ± 0.42	2.13	.07
Donor			
Ischemic time (min) (longer)	0.027 ± 0.013	1.35	.04

VAD, ventricular assist device; tx, transplant.

* The hazard ratio is the relative risk associated with a specific risk factor. The coefficients are the parametric estimates which are multiplied by the value of each risk factor (in the case of dichotomous variables, by either 0 if absent or 1 if present). See text for further details. The hazard ratio for age compares the effect of ages 1 month and 1 year. The hazard ratio for creatinine compares the effects of creatinines of 1 and 2 and the hazard ratio for ischemic time compares times of 300 and 360 minutes.

Cox Proportional Hazards Model

The general form of the model is given in the hazard domain, where the hazard function for a specific individual with his or her specific values of risk factors is given by:

$$\lambda_i(t) = \lambda_o(t) \exp(\beta_o + \beta_1 x_{1i} + \beta_2 x_{2i} + \ldots + \beta_k x_{ki}),$$

where $\lambda_o(t)$ is the underlying or baseline hazard function, $x_1, \ldots, x_k$ are risk factors, and $\beta_1, \ldots, \beta_k$ are coefficients (parameters) for the risk factors.

The function, $\exp(\beta_o + \beta_1 x_{1i} + \beta_2 x_{2i} + \ldots + \beta_k x_{ki})$, produces a single number for the patient. This number modifies $\lambda_o(t)$ proportionately across time to produce a hazard and therefore a survivorship curve that is unique to the patient and his or her risk factors.

For a single dichotomous risk factor the model reduces to a simple form. For example, let x represent the risk factor gender, where $x = 1$ if the patient is male and $x = 0$ if the patient is female. The hazard function for a female is: $\lambda_f(t) = \lambda_0(t)e^{\beta \cdot 0} = \lambda_0(t)$. The hazard function for a male patient is $\lambda_m(t) = \lambda_0(t)e^{\beta \cdot 1} = k\lambda_0(t)$, where $k = e^{-\beta}$. The ratio of the hazards is

$$\frac{\lambda_m(t)}{\lambda_f(t)} \frac{k \cdot \lambda_0(t)}{\lambda_0(t)} = k$$

Due to the relationship between $S(t)$, $\Lambda(t)$, and $\lambda(t)$, the following relation holds when hazards are proportional: $S_m(t) = [S_f(t)]^k$. For a single continuous risk factor, the hazard function for a specific patient is $\lambda_i(t) = k_i\lambda_0(t)$, where $k_i = \exp(\beta x_i)$ and x_i is a specific value of the continuous risk factor. There is no specific hazard ratio associated with the risk factor x. Instead, a hazard ratio can be calculated for two specific values of the risk factor x.

Using this proportional hazards model, Cox developed an estimation procedure that estimates the risk factor coefficients without specifying the form of $\lambda_0(t)$ or estimating the parameters associated with $\lambda_0(t)$. The coefficients can be easily transformed into estimated hazard ratios by exponentiation. His method is based on maximum likelihood estimation.

slopes across time which that result from proportional hazards. The assumption of proportional hazard would not be true for a risk factor if the effect of risk was different between the early period and a later period.[16] Other methods to address this situation are discussed in subsequent sections.

Logistic Regression and Cox Regression

When a major surgical intervention such as heart transplantation has occurred, it is often desirable to investigate the existence of one set of risk factors for early outcomes and another set of risk factors for outcomes after the perioperative period. One statistical approach utilizes a combination of logistic regression and Cox regression. Logistic regression is used to identify risk for events that occur during a specific time period, such as the first 30 days, thereby removing the time-related element. Cox regression is then used for events after 30 days, with time to the event included in the analysis. Therefore, only 30-day survivors are included in this analysis and time zero occurs at 30 days after surgery (Table 3–18). The selection of 30 days as the break point between the logistic and Cox analysis is arbitrary. Examination of the Kaplan-Meier curve may provide insight in choosing a dividing point between early and late risk.

Parametric Survival Regression

Parametric survival regression in the **hazard function domain** is a method for identifying variables that are associated with increased risk, where risk is defined as a specified function of time. The mathematical foundation of parametric survival regression is analogous to a t test for comparing two groups, in which the investigator assumes that the data arise from a normal distribution. The t test, with its resultant p value, allows the researcher to decide if the data came from a single normal distribution or from two different normal distributions as defined by a parameter shift in the mean. This is a parametric analysis.

Parametric survival regression operates in a similar manner when investigating a single dichotomous variable. The investigator assumes that the data arise from a specified distribution. Parametric survival regression,

TABLE 3-18	**Risk Factors for Death after Heart Transplantation***					
	LOGISTIC (DEATH WITHIN 1 MONTH)			COX (ALL DEATHS AFTER 1 MONTH)		
RISK FACTOR	Coefficient ± SE	Odds Ratio	p Value	Coefficient ± SE	Hazard Ratio	p Value
Age (younger)	−0.418 ± 0.094	0.680	<.0001			
VAD at time of tx	2.00 ± 0.61	7.41	.001			
IV inotropes at time of tx				0.69 ± 0.34	1.99	.05
Ischemic time (longer)				0.037 ± 0.017	1.50	.03

VAD, ventricular assist device; tx, transplant.
* See text for difference between odds ratio and hazard ratio (relative risk). The odds ratio for age compares the effect of ages 1 month and 1 year. The odds ratio for ischemic time compares times of 300 and 360 minutes. The data set for this example is the same as for Table 3–17.

with its resultant p value, allows the researcher to decide if the data come from a single distribution or from two different distributions as defined by a shift in a parameter. Thus, unlike the Cox regression model, the hazard function (distribution) is defined in parametric survival analysis. The mathematical basis for the parametric multivariable survival analysis was developed by Feigl and Zelen in 1965.[25] They developed a model for a constant hazard, in which the underlying survival distribution is the negative exponential. They let the parameter μ be a linear function of risk factors so that each patient has their own specific survival and hazard functions that are dependent on their values of the risk factors.

As discussed in the earlier section, Parametric Comparison of Survival Curves, the three-hazard model allows identification of up to three separate but overlapping phases of hazard.[11] The effect of risk factors is estimated by proportional hazards regression within each phase of hazard. This allows the common situation where a risk factor is important only during a specific phase of hazard (e.g., the early period of increased risk after an operation): $\lambda(t) = \mu_1 g_1(t,x) + \mu_2 g_2(t,x) = \mu_3 g_3(t,x)$, where each μ is a log linear function of the risk factors that scales the hazard phase; g_1, g_2, and g_3 are the "shaping" functions; t is time to event, and x represents the risk factors, $\mu = \exp(\beta_0 + \beta_1 x_1 + \ldots \beta_k x_k)$. The individual β's (coefficients) can be exponentiated to produce risk factor hazard ratios for a specific hazard phase.

Stepwise selection of the risk factors is accomplished in the same manner as all multivariable models with one generalization. Instead of a single list of potential risk factors to be examined, there is a list for each phase of the model that has been identified. The basic steps for parametric hazard regression are:

1) Select an underlying, medically reasonable model (see earlier section, Survival Curves).
2) Estimate the parameters of the model and therefore determine the phases of risk.
3) Choose the potential risk factors.
4) Examine each potential risk factor univariably.
5) Trim the list based on medical and statistical considerations.
6) Perform the stepwise selection of the risk factors.

Thus, the unique advantages of parametric multivariable analysis in the hazard function domain lies in the ability to closely model the actual changing risk (hazard) over time and to generate tabular displays of the risk factors in each phase (Table 3–19) and visual representations (nomograms) based on the solutions to the multivariable equations (Figs. 3–22 and 3–23).

MULTIVARIABLE ANALYSIS OF CONTINUOUS OUTCOMES

The two preceding sections have covered binary outcomes (e.g., death) either with or without an associated time to the outcome. This section covers outcomes that are continuous variables, excluding outcomes that are measured continuously or serially across time. The technique of **multiple regression analysis** is the primary multivariable method for identifying risk factors for continuous outcome variables without a time component. Examples include cardiac output early after transplantation, total number of rejection episodes during the first year after transplantation, and hospital costs. In each case, the investigator may want to identify variables (risk factors) that are associated with changes in the outcome.

The standard terminology for multiple regression variables is **dependent variable** for the outcome variable and **independent variables** for the risk factors or "predictors." The **linear model** is $y_i = \beta_0 + \beta_1 x_{1i} + \beta_2 x_{2i} + \ldots + \beta_k x_{ki} + \varepsilon_i$, where y_i is the outcome for the ith individual, β_0 is the intercept, x_{ji} is the value of the jth risk factor for the ith individual, β_j is the coefficient (parameter) for the jth risk factor, and ε_i is a random component (error) for the ith individual.

The risk factors can be continuous, ordinal, or dichotomous. If a risk factor is continuous or ordinal, then a linear relation between y and x is assumed, where β is the slope. If a risk factor is dichotomous, then the two values for x correspond to a mean change in y equal to β. Interactions between two risk factors can be incorporated into the model.

p Values for the risk factors are based on tests of null hypotheses, where the β's are equal to zero. The required assumption is that individual deviations about the line have a normal distribution. Estimation of the β's is a closed form (noniterative) process. Several measures of the adequacy of the model have been developed. The key measure is r^2, which calculates the percentage of the total variation of y that is explained by the risk factors. Adequacy of the linear relationship can be examined by plots.

TABLE 3-19   **Risk Factors (Parametric Hazard Analysis) for Death after Heart Transplantation**

	EARLY HAZARD PHASE			CONSTANT HAZARD PHASE		
	Coefficient ± SE	Hazard Ratio	p Value	Coefficient ± SE	Hazard Ratio	p Value
Demographic						
Black race				0.843 ± 0.273	2.32	.002
Clinical						
Ventilator at transplant	1.29 ± 0.23	3.62	<.0001			
Previous sternotomy	0.433 ± 0.116	1.54	.0002			
PVR (higher)	0.0761 ± 0.0322	1.08	.02			
Insulin-dependent diabetes				1.11 ± 0.31	3.04	.0004
HLA-DR mismatch	0.244 ± 0.113	1.28	.03			
Donor						
Age (older)	0.0383 ± 0.0062	1.04	<.0001			
Body surface area (smaller)	−0.799 ± 0.254	0.45	.002			
Diabetes	1.24 ± 0.36	3.46	.0005			
Diffuse wall motion abnormalities	0.967 ± 0.329	2.63	.003			
Ischemic time (higher)	0.0282 ± 0.0086	1.03	.001			

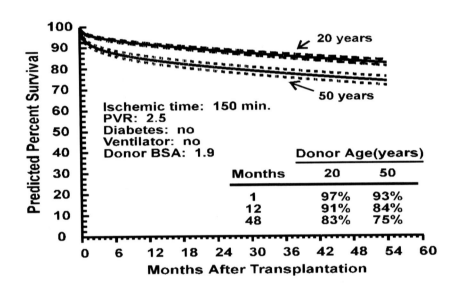

FIGURE **3-22.** Predicted survival after transplant for a specific patient according to two donors; one donor who is age 20 years and the other donor who is age 50 years. The predictions are solutions of parametric multivariable analysis presented in Table 3-19 for white race, no previous sternotomy, and no wall motion abnormalities. The dashed lines are 70% confidence limits.

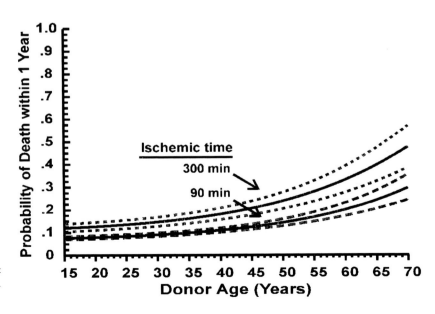

FIGURE **3-23.** Illustration of the effect of donor age and ischemic time on the probability of death within 1 year of transplant. The estimates are solutions of the parametric multivariable analysis presented in Table 3-19.

TABLE 3-20	Multivariable Nonlinear Regression Analysis for Prediction of Polyclonal Level as a Function of Monoclonal Specific Cyclosporine Level*		
VARIABLE	COEFFICIENT ± SE		p VALUE
Monoclonal specific (log)	0.714 ± 0.047		<.0001
SGOT	0.00327 ± 0.0010		<.0001

SGOT, serum glutamic oxaloacetic transaminase.
* Intercept = 2.38; R^2 = .66.

If the relation between the outcome and the risk factors is not linear, then there are two alternatives. One is **nonlinear regression,** which is considerably more complex than linear regression. The other approach is to mathematically transform either the y's or the x's so the result is a linear relationship.[22]

A visual depiction of the impact of a risk factor can be derived from the regression model. This is accomplished by calculating a new prediction, as the value of a specific risk factor is incrementally changed and all other risk factors are held at a constant value. A nonlinear multiple regression analysis with risk factors and a nomogram is presented in Table 3–20 and Figures 3–24 and 3–25.[12]

COMPETING OUTCOMES

In most research involving a time-related event, interest is focused on a single event, such as death after transplantation. Each patient is observed until the event occurs or until the patient is removed from risk due to censoring. The censoring occurs usually because the patient is alive at the end of the study, lost to follow-up, or withdrawn alive. However, there are situations where several mutually exclusive events are possible for each patient, and interest is focused on the simultaneous time-related probabilities of these events. The usual single-event analysis can partially analyze this situation by examining only one event at a time while censoring patients who experience one of the other events. This approach implies a strong assumption about independence of the events which may not be true, and it cannot provide simultaneous time-related probability estimates of the several events. **Competing outcomes** (usually called competing risks in the statistical literature)[18, 62] methodology can provide these estimates. Competing outcomes analysis is defined as the simultaneous probability estimation of the time course of multiple mutually exclusive events. At any point in time, these probability estimates will sum to 1.

HISTORY OF COMPETING OUTCOMES

Methodology for competing risks has been evolving since the eighteenth century, when Daniel Bernoulli presented a solution to the following question: If smallpox were eliminated as a cause of death, what would be the effect on mortality from all other causes for various age groups?[9] Bernoulli constructed tables to answer this question under the assumption that a patient saved from smallpox was at the same risk of death from other causes as the rest of the population. This would not be true if smallpox tended to prey upon the weak who were at increased risk of death from other causes. Actuaries began constructing multiple tables during the nineteenth century to sort out the proportion of insured clients who actually died or became permanently disabled or let their policies lapse.

Competing risk analysis, particularly in the parametric domain, has only recently been applied to cardiac surgical experience. Grunkemeier and colleagues[33] have proposed the terms "actuarial" and "actual" to describe the Kaplan-Meier estimates and competing outcome estimates, respectively. Other terms that describe the "actual" probability include cumulative incidence function[38] and cause-specific failure probability.[28] We have recently applied the competing outcomes method to the

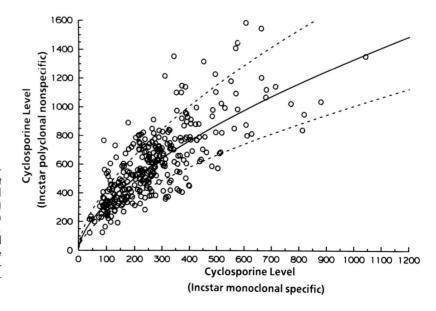

FIGURE **3–24.** Scattergram and nonlinear regression analysis of cyclosporine levels using two different assays. The solid line is the estimated relation and the dotted lines are 70% confidence limits (± 1 SD) for individual predictions. (From Bourge RC, Kirklin JK, Ketchum C, Naftel DC, Mason DA, Siegel AL, Scott JW, White-Williams C: Cyclosporine blood monitoring after heart transplantation: A prospective comparison of monoclonal and polyclonal radioimmunoassays. J Heart Lung Transplant 1992;11:522–529.)

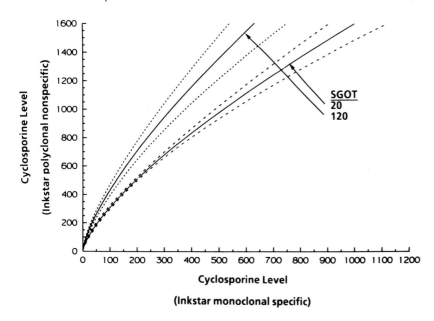

FIGURE **3-25.** Nomogram from the solution of the multivariable analysis for the data displayed in Figure 3–24. The nonlinear regression analysis presented in Table 3–20 is solved for two different levels of SGOT. The dotted lines are 70% confidence limits for the prediction of the mean. (From Bourge RC, Kirklin JK, Ketchum C, Naftel DC, Mason DA, Siegel AL, Scott JW, White-Williams C: Cyclosporine blood monitoring after heart transplantation: A prospective comparison of monoclonal and polyclonal radioimmunoassays. J Heart Lung Transplant 1992;11:522–529.)

analysis of possible outcome events after listing for cardiac transplantation[51] and following transplantation.[50]

SITUATIONS IN WHICH COMPETING OUTCOMES ANALYSIS IS USEFUL

Competing outcomes analysis may be applied if a patient has an event that defines a starting point or a time zero and subsequently continues to be followed until he or she experiences any one of a number of mutually exclusive outcome events. For example, consider a patient who is listed for cardiac transplantation, which defines his or her personal starting point. There are multiple mutually exclusive outcome possibilities for this patient: the patient may die while waiting for a transplant, the patient may receive a transplant, or may be removed from the transplant list because of changing clinical condition (too ill or too well) (Fig. 3–26). Initially, a group of patients are in a pool of patients who are waiting for an event to happen. As time passes, patients

experience one of the events and therefore "flow" into an event "bucket."

In this situation of multiple possible outcomes events, the competing outcomes analysis provides the most accurate estimate of the probability of each mutually exclusive outcome event. At any point in time, estimates are produced of the proportion of patients who have experienced each of the mutually exclusive events and the proportion of patients who have yet to experience an event. These proportions are the probability estimates. The sum of these probability estimates is 1.0 at each point in time. A similar analysis can be applied to outcome events after transplantation.

LIMITATIONS OF COMPETING OUTCOMES METHODS

The use of the competing outcomes method relies on the assumption that all events are mutually exclusive, which is not always the case. For example, outcome

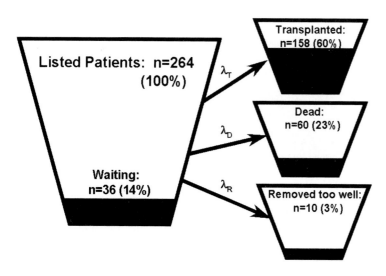

FIGURE **3-26.** Competing outcomes depiction for patients awaiting heart transplantation (data from the Pediatric Heart Transplant Study for patients listed for heart transplantation between January 1993 and January 1995). The large "bucket" includes the total pool of listed patients, each of whom is followed over time to one of three mutually exclusive endpoints, indicated by the three smaller "buckets." At the end of 6 months, the remaining patients waiting (without experiencing an endpoint) are shown at the bottom of the large bucket. The γ's are rates of "flow" from the large bucket to a small bucket. They are analogous to hazard rates for the end points.

TABLE 3-21	Competing Outcomes Analyses by the Counting Method*									
	MONTHS AFTER LISTING									
	0		.5		1		3		6	
OUTCOME	N	%	N	%	N	%	N	%	N	%
Alive: waiting	264	100	182	69	135	51	55	21	36	14
Alive: removed (too well)	0	—	3	1	6	2	8	3	10	3
Death: waiting	0		24	9	34	13	53	20	60	23
Transplanted	0	—	25	21	89	34	148	56	158	60
Total	264	100	264	100	264	100	264	100	264	100

* All patients have at least 6 months of follow-up.
Adapted from McGiffin DC, Naftel DC, Kirklin JK, Morrow WR, Towbin J, Shaddy R, Alejos J, Rossi A, and the Pediatric Heart Transplant Study Group: Predicting outcome after listing for heart transplantation in children: Comparison of Kaplan-Meier and parametric competing risk analysis. J Heart Lung Transplant 1997;16:713–722.

events after cardiac transplantation may include "death from infection" and "death from rejection." Identification of which category to assign a given patient may be difficult if, for example, the patient received augmented immunosuppression for severe rejection and subsequently developed fatal infection. In that instance, assignment of "death from rejection" or "death from infection" may be difficult, since *both* contributed to the fatal outcome.

COMPETING OUTCOMES ANALYSIS

Two general methods are available for providing the estimates of the probabilities for each outcome event: nonparametric and parametric methods.

Nonparametric Methods

Counting Tables

Counting tables provides a tabulation of the proportion of patients with each outcome at a specific time point.

All patients must have a minimal length of follow-up that is greater than the last entry in the table. This is the easiest method to calculate and understand, but it cannot handle intermediate censoring. At selected time points, patients are divided into mutually exclusive event categories according to whether or not the patient has experienced the event. If the patient has not yet experienced any event, he or she remains in the group of patients designated as "waiting." Proportions are then calculated which estimate the proportion of patients who will actually experience each event by the selected time point or will still be waiting for an event to occur (Table 3–21).[51]

Adaptation of Kaplan-Meier

The Kaplan-Meier method can be adapted to provide the time-related estimates of the proportion of patients experiencing each of the mutually exclusive events (Fig. 3–27). The steps are:

1) Construct an "event" variable for each patient that is "yes" if a patient experiences any one of the

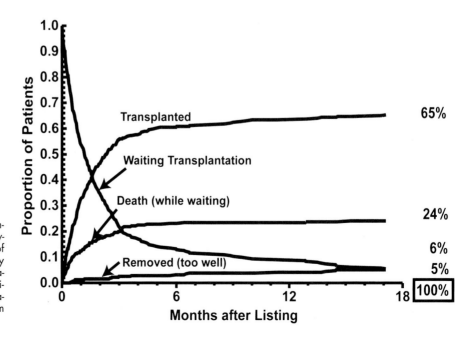

FIGURE **3-27.** Adaptation of the Kaplan-Meier method for competing outcomes analysis illustrating the time-related proportion of patients experiencing each of three mutually exclusive outcomes after listing for transplantation. The solid lines are nonparametric estimates from an adapted Kaplan-Meier calculation. At each point in time, the estimates sum to 1.00 (or 100%).

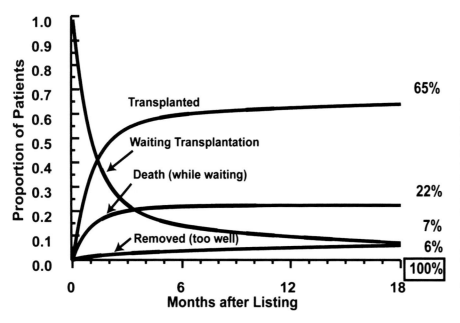

FIGURE **3-28.** Parametric competing outcomes analysis illustrating the time-related proportion of patients experiencing each of three mutually exclusive outcomes after listing for transplantation. The solid lines are parametric estimates based on hazard function analysis of each individual event. At each point in time, the estimates sum to 1.00 (or 100%). There is close agreement between these estimates and the nonparametric estimates in Figure 3–27. (From McGiffin DC, Naftel DC, Kirklin JK, Morrow WR, Towbin J, Shaddy R, Alejos J, Rossi A, and the Pediatric Heart Transplant Study Group: Predicting outcome after listing for heart transplantation in children: Comparison of Kaplan-Meier and parametric competing risk analysis. J Heart Lung Transplant 1997;16:713–722.)

multiple events. The sum of these "yeses" will be the sum of all the mutually exclusive events.

2) Calculate the usual Kaplan-Meier curve for this combined event. This curve will form the basis of the competing outcomes depiction. It is the time-related proportion of patients in the waiting bucket.

3) Each time an event occurs, the overall Kaplan-Meier curve "drops" to a new estimate of freedom from the combined event. The amount of this drop is now added to the appropriate bucket for the kind of event that actually occurred. This time-related accumulation is the estimate of the actual proportion who experience the particular event.

Parametric Method and Risk Factor Identification

The parametric method uses event-specific hazard rates to estimate the accumulation of probability (or proportions of patients) into event categories. The analysis begins with the calculation of the hazard function (or instantaneous risk) of each event. The estimate of the hazard is determined independently for each event, censoring for other events. The competing outcomes depiction is derived from the hazard for each event and can

be conceptualized as simply counting what actually happens to each patient as they are "siphoned" into each of the possible events. The estimated hazard function for each event is used to simultaneously deplete the proportion of patients at risk at each point in time. While the patients are being removed from risk, they are being accumulated into an actual proportion experiencing each event. At each point in time the sum of the proportion of patients at risk and the proportions experiencing each event is equal to 1 (Fig. 3–28).[51]

A parametric competing outcomes depiction for a patient, accounting for his or her specific risk factors, is accomplished by the same hazard approach (Table 3–22). Risk factors for each event are identified in the manner for single event-hazard analysis. Using a patient's values for the risk factors, a patient-specific hazard for each event is estimated, which can then generate the estimated probability of each time-related outcome event (Fig. 3–29).[51]

Competing Outcomes (Actual) Versus Kaplan-Meier (Actuarial) for Multiple Outcome Events

The Kaplan-Meier and competing outcomes methods provide different probability estimates when examining

TABLE 3-22	**Risk Factors for Outcomes after Listing**				
LONGER TIME TO TRANSPLANT		DEATH WHILE WAITING		REMOVED (TOO WELL)	
Infants	Children	Infants	Children	Infants	Children
Smaller size	Status II	Inotropic support	Status I	None identified	
Blood type O	Blood type O	Smaller size	Ventilator		
Younger age	CMV positive	Blood type O			

CMV positive, positive cytomegalovirus serology.
Adapted from McGiffin DC, Naftel DC, Kirklin JK, Morrow WR, Towbin J, Shaddy R, Alejos J, Rossi A, and the Pediatric Heart Transplant Study Group: Predicting outcome after listing for heart transplantation in children: Comparison of Kaplan-Meier and parametric competing risk analysis. J Heart Lung Transplant 1997;16:713–722.

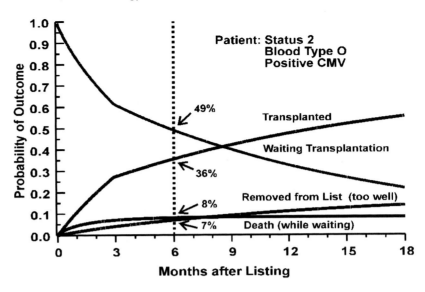

FIGURE **3–29.** Predicted time-related probability of outcome after listing for a specific child. The estimates are based on the patient's predicted hazards from the multivariable analysis of each outcome (see Table 3–21). At each point in time, the estimates add to 1.0. For example, by 6 months after listing, this patient has a .36 chance of being transplanted, .07 chance of being removed (too well) from the list, an .08 chance of dying while waiting and a .49 chance of being alive and still waiting. (From McGiffin DC, Naftel DC, Kirklin JK, Morrow WR, Towbin J, Shaddy R, Alejos J, Rossi A, and the Pediatric Heart Transplant Study Group: Predicting outcome after listing for heart transplantation in children: Comparison of Kaplan-Meier and parametric competing risk analysis. J Heart Lung Transplant 1997;16:713–722.)

multiple outcome events. The Kaplan-Meier method was originally devised to portray a single time-related event but is now often used to depict a single event in the setting of multiple competing events. It has not been generally appreciated by clinical users of this method that the necessary censoring process in the setting of multiple competing events may lead to an inaccurate estimate of the proportion of patients *actually* experiencing the event under study. When multiple events are possible, these estimates become "conditional" estimates. The condition is "provided that the patient experiences none of the other events." In other words, the estimates have removed the effect of the other events (Fig. 3–30A).[51] Thus, when multiple outcomes exist, the usual Kaplan-Meier analysis *does not* estimate the actual proportion of patients who will experience a given outcome. Competing outcomes analysis *does* estimate the actual proportion of patients who will experience each event (Fig. 3–30B).[51]

REPEATED EVENTS

Most time-related outcome analyses examine single (or terminal) outcome events, such as death, transplantation, first rejection, first infection, and so forth. However, time-related events that can occur *more than once* in a single patient are an everyday reality for heart transplantation patients. Rejection of the donor heart can occur at any time, regardless of the number of previous rejection episodes and the elapsed time since transplant. The same is true for infections. Even transplantation itself becomes a repeated event for some patients as they receive a second or even a third transplant. Thus, repeating events are events that can occur more than once in a single patient, and each occurrence has an associated unique time. Characterization of the pattern (distribution) of these repeated events and identification of the associated risk factors are necessary steps in the process to understand and then reduce or even eliminate these events. There are a number of approaches to such

a statistical analysis, each with its own assumptions, advantages, and limitations.

Repeating events are similar to the usual type of events that are analyzed by survival methods (i.e., there is an interval of time from a definite beginning point until a definite endpoint, which is the time of the event under investigation). For some patients, the time of the event is unknown, such that censoring occurs. The many analytic methods for repeating events are all useful to describe or answer some aspect of the time-related distribution of the events and the identification of risk factors. Estimation of the time-related accrual of a repeating event is the most complete description for repeating events because it can be used to estimate the number of events during any time interval of interest.

LINEARIZED RATES USING ALL EVENTS

The most common way to analyze repeated events is the calculation of a linearized rate of events per time unit.[47] Grunkemeier et al.[33] have made extensive use of linearized rates in summarizing the medical literature on morbid events such as thromboembolism after human heart valve replacement with a biological or mechanical prosthetic heart valve.[32, 33] The necessary information for this approach is the number of events for each patient and the length of follow-up time for each patient. Its chief advantage is that it is easy to calculate and it can accommodate multiple occurrences of a morbid event in a single patient. The **disadvantage** of this approach is that the **assumption of a constant hazard rate** is almost surely false for most events after heart transplantation.

PIECEWISE LINEARIZED RATES

Rather than estimate a single constant rate across the entire follow-up interval, one can calculate **separate constant rates for different specified time intervals**. This method overcomes some of the problems associated

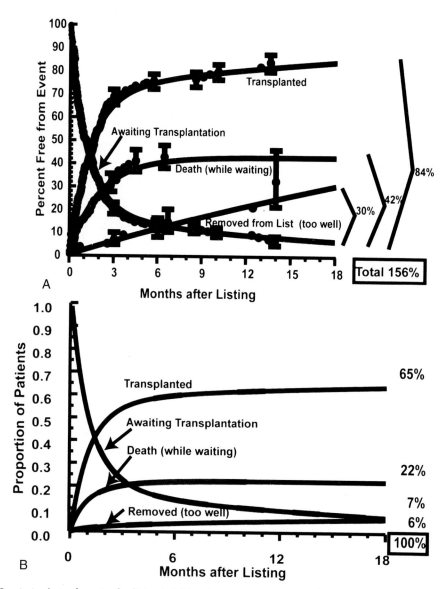

FIGURE **3–30.** *A,* Analysis of events after listing in 264 pediatric patients using Kaplan-Meier methods. The closed circles are the actuarial estimates and the solid lines are parametric estimates. The "awaiting transplantation" curve is the estimated freedom from all of the events. The other curves are the time-related percent of patients experiencing the event *assuming* that they experience no other event. For example, the transplanted curve is the percent chance (or probability) of obtaining a transplant assuming that the patient does not die and is not removed from the list. These conditional estimates do not add to 100%. *B,* Competing outcomes analysis of events (transplant, death, removal from transplant list, and waiting) after listing for transplant. The curves are parametric estimates of the mutually exclusive outcomes based on the hazard analysis of each individual outcome. At each point in time, the estimates add to 100%.

with the assumption of a constant hazard by examining an assumed constant rate for various arbitrarily defined time intervals. Time varying hazards can be approximated by this approach, in which the event can be either the first event or all events.

This approach is a good way to investigate the shape of the hazard for repeating events, and it can also be used to calculate a cumulative number of events at any point in time for a given patient (Fig. 3–31). However, there are important disadvantages. It is subject to the arbitrary division of the time scale, and in order to approximate a smooth function, this method requires a large amount of follow-up time in many patients who must also have many events. Thus, this approach does not work well for any low-frequency event.

Risk factors can be initially examined through stratification. If there are sufficient data, this is an excellent way to investigate the existence of differing hazard patterns in different patient risk subsets. However, the necessity for many events and a large amount of follow-up time limits the process.

CUMULATIVE NUMBER OF EVENTS ACROSS TIME

Many times it is the accrual **rate** of repeating morbid events that is of greatest interest. Questions to be answered include: How many rejection episodes will a patient have during the first year? How many episodes

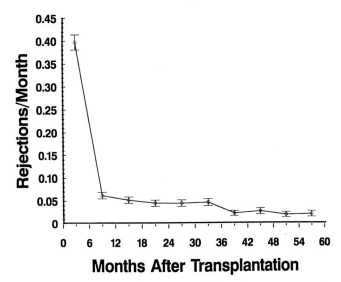

FIGURE 3-31. Depicton of rejection episodes per patient per month. A linearized rate is calculated for each 6-month interval following transplantation. Multiple events for a single patient are included. The calculations are made for 6-month intervals by dividing the total number of episodes for all patients in the interval by the total amount of follow-up during the interval. This graph can be used to crudely estimate the accrual rate of rejection episodes for a single patient.

can the patient expect during the second year? These questions can only be answered by a method that estimates the accrual of events in a continuous time-related manner. The nonparametric method developed by Nelson[59] allows examination of changing rate of accrual of events and estimation of the expected number of events during any defined time interval (Fig. 3–32). The slope of the curve can be used to evaluate the possibility of increasing or decreasing rates. If the rate is indeed constant, then the cumulative function is a straight line with slope equal to the rate of accrual of the event. **Risk factors** can be univariately evaluated through stratified curves combined with confidence intervals. Multivari-

able analysis for risk factors can be generated by multiple linear or nonlinear regression techniques (see previous sections).

RISK FACTOR IDENTIFICATION WITH REENTRY AT THE TIME OF AN EVENT

Another method that is especially useful for risk factor analysis is the reentry method. It is constructed in the following manner. Each time a patient experiences an event, he or she is reentered with a new time zero that is equal to the time of the current rejection episode. This creates an observation for each event and each censored time. Therefore, the number of observations is greater than the number of patients, but the total follow-up (exposure) time is the sum of the individual patient exposure times. Risk unadjusted depictions can be generated by a modification of the Kaplan-Meier analysis (nonparametric). Risk factor analysis can be identified from Cox proportional hazards or parametric hazards analysis as discussed in the sections on multivarible analyses for time-related events. The unique feature of this approach is that potential risk factors can include any variable that is known at each new time zero.

This method of analysis is particularly suited to the identification of risk factors for repeating events such as rejection after cardiac transplantation.[42, 44] The key feature of this complex analysis is the understanding that "time zero" is the time of transplant for the first rejection episode, but for all subsequent rejection episodes (the repeating event) time zero must be reset. Each rejection episode becomes the new time zero, and risk factors are identified for time until the subsequent rejection event. Any variable (pretransplant characteristics, time since transplant, number of prior rejection or infection episodes, etc.) whose value can be determined from data acquired before transplant or after transplant but

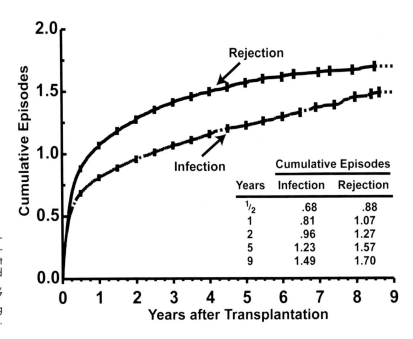

FIGURE 3-32. Estimated time-related cumulative episodes of rejection and infection based on 4,245 transplant patients. The y-axis is the number of episodes that a single patient is predicted to accumulate by the stated number of years. For example, at 5 years after transplant, a patient is estimated to have 1.23 infection and 1.57 rejection episodes. The accumulation rate is high during the first year and slows to an approximate constant rate.

Years	Cumulative Episodes	
	Infection	Rejection
1/2	.68	.88
1	.81	1.07
2	.96	1.27
5	1.23	1.57
9	1.49	1.70

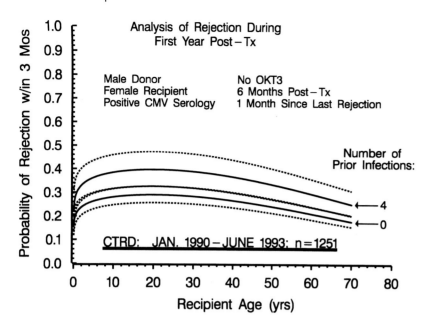

FIGURE **3–33.** A nomogram from the solution of the multivariable equation for recurrent rejection during the first posttransplant year. The risk factors are presented in Table 3–23. The nomogram is stratified according to number of prior infection episodes. The dashed lines represent the 70% confidence limits. (From Kubo SH, Naftel DC, Mills RM Jr, O'Donnell J, Rodeheffer RJ, Cintron GB, Kenzora JL, Bourge RC, Kirklin JK, and the Cardiac Transplant Research Database Group: Risk factors for late recurrent rejection after heart transplantation: A multiinstitutional, multivariable analysis. J Heart Lung Transplant 1995;14:409–418.)

before each rejection episode can be used in the risk factor analysis (Fig. 3–33 and Table 3–23).[44]

PATIENT-SPECIFIC AND GROUP-SPECIFIC PREDICTIONS

One of the most powerful applications of parametric multivariable analysis is the depiction of the probabilities of outcome events for individual patients with known characteristics.[56, 66] Since in parametric analysis the equations for probability of an outcome are completely specified with all parameters being estimated, specific solutions of the multivariable equations can be readily plotted along with confidence intervals. These

TABLE 3-23	Risk Factors for Recurrent Rejection During First Year after Transplantation
RISK FACTOR	p VALUE
Recipient	
Female	.03
Younger age (except infants)	<.0001
Clinical	
Positive CMV serology (Pre-tx)	.0005
Donor	
Female	.03
Induction therapy	
Use of OKT3	<.0001
Time related factors	
Fewer months since transplantation	<.0001
Fewer months since last rejection	.0004
Greater number of previous infections	.05

CMV, cytomegalovirous; Pre-tx, pretransplantation.
Adapted from Kubo SH, Naftel DC, Mills RM Jr, O'Donnell J, Rodeheffer RJ, Cintron GB, Kenzora JL, Bourge RC, Kirklin JK, and the Cardiac Transplant Research Database Group: Risk factors for late recurrent rejection after heart transplantation: A multiinstitutional, multivariable analysis. J Heart Lung Transplant 1995;14;409–418.

depictions are called **nomograms.** A variety of depictions can be selected to illustrate the effect of one or multiple risk factors. The predicted outcome for an **individual patient** is generated by inserting his or her specific values for the risk factors and solving the multivariable equation. Such predictions provide the statistical information to facilitate **patient-specific decisions** and informed consent for interventions based on individual predicted outcome. Similarly, the predicted outcome for a **group of patients** in a **risk-adjusted** manner can be generated from a parametric multivariable model for another group and compared to observed outcome. The actual process for calculating these depictions is different for each type of parametric multivariable analysis.

In **multiple linear regression,** the relation between a continuous outcome is completely numerically specified once the coefficients have been estimated. The outcome for a specific patient can be predicted by inserting his or her values for the risk factors and calculating the outcome. The standard errors of the coefficients are used in calculation of a confidence interval for the predicted outcome. For patients in the sample, the predicted outcome can be compared with the patient's actual outcome. Large differences between the two in many patients suggest that the model may be inadequate.

In a similar manner, patient-specific outcomes can be predicted by a **logistic regression** analysis. Specific values from the patient for each risk factor variable can be inserted into the logistic equation to produce a probability of that patient experiencing the outcome event.

Parametric hazard function modeling is a particularly useful tool for predicting patient-specific time-related outcomes.[52] The basic assumptions when producing predictions are (1) the form of the model is appropriate, (2) the estimates are based on good data, (3) the final set of risk factors are the result of intense professional collaboration, and (4) the predictions are tempered, as strongly as necessary, by clinical judgment. The use of hazard function analysis to provide group-specific predictions is illustrated in Figure 3–34.[68]

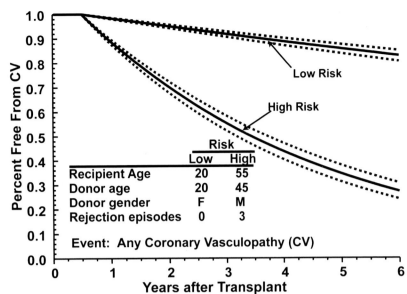

	Risk	
	Low	High
Recipient Age	20	55
Donor age	20	45
Donor gender	F	M
Rejection episodes	0	3

Event: Any Coronary Vasculopathy (CV)

FIGURE **3–34.** Group-specific predicted freedom from coronary vasculopathy based on multivariable analysis of 2,880 patients. The event is any detectable disease by angiography after 6 months following transplant. Risk factors examined included pretransplant variables and rejection history during the first 6 months after transplant. The solid lines with their 70% confidence limits depict high-risk and low-risk groups for development of allograft vasculopathy.

VALIDATION

The statistical analysis of data involves uncertainty, assumptions, and inferences from limited information. After the inferences of a study have been generated, the analysis and inferences should undergo a process called **validation,** which provides evidence that the conclusions (inferences) of a scientific investigation are generalizable to other institutions and experiences and that the inferences can be applied to future patients. The validation process determines if the study is free from bias and otherwise conforms to its stated purpose.

GENERAL STEPS FOR VALIDATION

1) Purpose: Is the purpose of the study clearly stated and is it relevant?
2) Design of the study: Is the design adequate to meet the purpose? Does the study have a sufficient sample size (and therefore power) to detect clinically important effects? Is the follow-up of patients conducted properly and is there a high completion proportion (i.e., >95%)?
3) Date: Have the correct variables been collected to address the purpose? Are the data of high quality? Are missing data a problem?
4) Statistical analysis: Each statistical analysis (t test, χ^2 test, Kaplan-Meier estimation, parametric survival analysis, Cox regression, logistic regression, etc.) requires a specific unique set of assumptions. Have the assumptions been examined and formally tested when possible? Are multivariable results reproducible?
5) Visual comparison with Kaplan-Meier estimates: The best way to judge a parametric survival model is to compare the resultant survival plot with the Kaplan-Meier nonparametric estimates. Systematic differences can quickly be detected.

6) Nested models: Many parametric models can be derived from more general mathematical models. This feature allows statistical testing of the necessity to include additional phases of hazard, for example, to more closely approximate time-related data.
7) Divide the data: The patients can be randomly divided into two groups. Choose a model and estimate the parameters for one of the groups of patients and then check the adequacy of the model for the other group of patients. This can be done by comparing the parametric survival plot (from the first group) with the Kaplan-Meier plot of the second group. Similarity of the plots would be evidence that the parametric model is a reflection of reality.
8) Outside data sources: For some researchers, validation can only be accomplished by applying an analysis to an independent collection of data. This is accomplished in the same manner as described in the preceding paragraph. The independent source of data would be either from another institution or later data from the same institution.

VALIDATION OF MULTIVARIABLE MODELS

The first check for a final multivariable model is to examine the list of risk factors for clinical reasonableness. This would include a check of the believability of the risk factor effects as illustrated by nomograms. Often, there is a potential risk factor that is important clinically and also univariately but is not in the final risk factor model. Estimated survival according to levels of the potential risk factor can be calculated by averaging the predicted survival of each patient in the different levels. The individual predictions are calculated from the parametric risk factor equation. The calculated average survival for each level should resemble the Kaplan-Meier survival curves stratified by the same levels of the potential risk factor.

TABLE 3-24		Decile-Predicted Analysis for 6-Month Death after Transplantation According to Logistic Multivariable Risk Factors	
DECILE*	N	EXPECTED DEATHS†	OBSERVED DEATHS
1	421	12.9	13
2	422	16.6	19
3	422	19.0	17
4	421	21.4	12
5	422	24.0	30
6	422	26.9	18
7	421	30.5	38
8	422	35.4	44
9	422	43.4	44
10	421	78.9	74
Total	4,216	309.0	309
p value (χ^2)		.07	

* The 10 deciles are generated by dividing the group into 10 nearly equal subsets stratified by the likelihood of death according to the multivariable analysis.
† Number of deaths predicted by a solution of the multivariable analysis.

Another approach is to randomly divide the patients into two groups and analyze each group separately. The final two models can be compared for similarities and differences. In some cases, differences may be explained by variables that are correlated. For example, weight may be in one model and body surface area in the other.

Validation can also be accomplished by applying the parametric risk factor equation to a new group of patients and comparing the predictions with the actual outcomes.[64] This comparison of predicted to actual outcome can be examined by a measure of **goodness of fit of the logistic model** and the identified risk factors. One way to do this is to calculate the probability for each patient and then divide the patients into 10 groups according to level of the predicted probability. Within each of the ten groups, the sum of the probabilities is the predicted number of events for that group. This predicted sum can be compared with the observed number of deaths in the group by a χ^2 test of significance. A significant p value indicates that the model is not predicting well (Table 3–24).

COMPUTER PROGRAMS TO FACILITATE OUTCOMES RESEARCH

There are many software packages for the entry, management, analysis, and presentation of data. Three of the most comprehensive are SPSS (Statistical Package for the Social Sciences), BMDP (Biomedical Computer Programs),[24] and SAS.[10, 35, 57, 65] The following discussion is specific to SAS, but the general functions exist in most large packages.

SAS is a complete system of computer programs for all aspects of data handling and analysis. Developed originally at North Carolina State University in the early 1970s, SAS is now a large software company. Most universities and many businesses use SAS.

TABLE 3-25	SAS Procedures For Statistical Analysis
STATISTICAL FUNCTION	SAS PROCEDURE
One variable	
Mean, range, standard deviation, standard error	PROC MEANS
Percentiles, frequencies, skewness, kurtosis	PROC UNIVARIATE
Two variables	
Scattergram	PROC PLOT
Correlation	PROC CORR
Contingency table	PROC FREQ
χ^2 test of properties	PROC FREQ
Fisher's exact test	PROC FREQ
t test	PROC TTEST
nonparametric (Wilcoxon, etc.)	PROC NPAR1WAY
Time-related estimates of event probabilities	
Kaplan-Meier estimate	PROC LIFETEST
Life table estimates	PROC LIFETEST
Parametric estimates	PROC LIFEREG, PROC HAZARD*
Three-phase hazard estimate	PROC HAZARD
Comparisons of survival curves	
Nonparametric	PROC LIFETEST
Parametric	PROC LIFEREG, PROC HAZARD*
Three-phase hazard	PROC HAZARD
Multivariable analysis	
Multiple linear regression	PROC REG
Logistic regression	PROC LOGISTIC
Cox proportional hazards	PROC PHREG
Parametric	PROC LIFEREG, PROC HAZARD*
Three-phase hazard	PROC HAZARD
Competing outcomes	
Nonparametric	PROC LIFETEST†
Parametric	PROC LIFEREG,† PROC HAZARD*†
Three-phase hazard	PROC HAZARD†

* Not currently commercially available; available through Internet access.
† Requires additional user programming.

SAS can accept data in almost any electronic form including data from other statistical packages and spreadsheet programs. SAS also has its own ability for data entry. User-created data entry screens can mimic paper forms. Menus for value selection for a variable can be inserted. Built-in data checks can be incorporated to increase the quality of the data.

Complete data management capabilities exist within SAS. Data sets can be merged, subsetted, and updated. There are transformation functions and arithmetic functions to create new variables from inputed variables. Figures can be created from a flexible (and complex) graphing portion of SAS. The software packages available from SAS for various statistical functions are summarized in Table 3–25.

References

1. Austin MA, Berreyesa S, Elliott JL, Wallace RB, Barret-Connor E: Methods for determining long-term survival in a population based study. Am J Epidemiol 1979;110:747.
2. Bailey RC: Some uses of a modified Makeham model to evaluate medical practice. J Wash Acad Sci 1988;78:339–353.
3. Barnett V: Comparative Statistical Inference. New York: John Wiley & Sons, 1973, pp 164–198.
4. Benjamin B: In Kruskal WH, Tanur JM (eds): International Encyclopedia of Statistics. Vol 1. New York: The Free Press, 1978, pp 435–437.
5. Berkson J: Why I prefer logits to probits. Biometrics 1951;7:327.
6. Berkson J, Flexner LB: On the rate of reaction between enzyme and substrate. J Gen Phys 1928;11:433.
7. Berkson J, Gage RP: Calculation of survival rates for cancer. Proceedings of the Staff Meetings of the Mayo Clinic 1950;25:270–286.
8. Berkson J, Hollander F: Chemistry—on the equation for the reaction between invertase and sucrose. J Wash Acad Sci 1930;20:157.
9. Bernouli D: Essai d'une nouvelle analyse de la mortalite causee par la petite verole, et des avantages de l'inoculation pour le prevenir: Historie vec les memoirs. Paris: Academie Royale des Sciences, 1760, pp 1–45.
10. Blackstone EH, Naftel DC: SAS Institute Inc. Changes and enhancements to the SAS system: Release 5.18 under OS and CMS (SAS Technical Report P-175). Cary, NC: SAS Institute, Inc., 1988.
11. Blackstone EH, Naftel DC, Turner ME Jr: The decomposition of time-varying hazard into phases, each incorporating a separate stream of concomitant information. J Am Stat Assoc 1986; 81:615–624.
12. Bourge RC, Kirklin JK, Ketchum C, Naftel DC, Mason DA, Siegel AL, Scott JW, White-Williams C: Cyclosporine blood monitoring after heart transplantation: A prospective comparison of monoclonal and polyclonal radioimmunoassays. J Heart Lung Transplant 1992;11:522–529.
13. Bradley DH, Bradley EL, Naftel DC: A generalized Gompertz-Rayleigh model as a survival distribution. Math Biosc 1984; 70:195–202.
14. Breslow NE: Analysis of survival data under the proportional hazards model. Int Stat Rev 1975;43:45.
15. Cox DR: Regression models and life tables. J R Stat Soc 1972;34:187-220.
16. Cox DR, Oakes D, Silverman BW: Analysis of Survival Data. New York: Chapman & Hall, Ltd, 1984.
17. David FN: Bills of mortality. In Games, Gods, and Gambling. A history of probability and statistical ideas. London: Griffin & Co, 1962, pp 98–109.
18. David HA, Moeschberger ML: The Theory of Competing Risks. New York: Macmillan, 1978.
19. DeMoivre A: The Doctrine of Chances. 1756. Reprint, 3rd ed. New York: Chelsea, 1967.
20. Dennis JE Jr, Schnabel RB: Numerical Methods for Unconstrained Optimization and Nonlinear Equations. Englewood Cliffs, NJ: Prentice-Hall, Inc, 1983.
21. Dillman DA: Mail and Telephone Surveys. New York: John Wiley & Sons, 1978.
22. Draper NR, Smith H: Applied Regression Analysis. New York: John Wiley & Sons, 1996.
23. Eisenhart C: Expression of the uncertainties of final results. Science 1968;160:1201.
24. Engleman L: Stepwise Logistic Regression. In Dixon WJ, Brown MB (eds): BMDP Biomedical Computer Programs P-series, 1979. Los Angeles: University of California, 1979, pp 517.1–517.3.
25. Feigel P, Zelen M: Estimation of exponential survival probabilities with concomitant information. Biometrika 1965;21:826–838.
26. Fisher RA: Statistical Methods and Scientific Inference. 3rd ed. New York: Hafner Press, 1973.
27. Galilei G: Sopra le scoperte dei dadi, as summarized. In Langley R (ed): Practical Statistics Simply Explained. New York: Dover, 1970.
28. Gaynor JJ, Feuer EJ, Tann CC: On the use of cause-specific failure and conditional failure probabilities: Examples from clinical oncology data. J Am Stat Assoc 1993;48:324–330.
29. Gehan EA: A generalized Wilcoxon test for comparing arbitrarily singly-censored samples. Biometrika 1965;52:203–222.
30. Gompertz B: On the nature of the function expressive of the law of human mortality. Philos Trans R Soc Lond 1825;115:513.
31. Graunt J: Natural and political observations made upon the Bills of Mortality. 1662. Reprinted. Baltimore: Johns Hopkins Press, 1939.
32. Grunkemeier GL, Johnson DM, Naftel DC: Sample size requirements for evaluating heart valves with constant risk events. J Heart Valve Dis 1994;3:53–58.
33. Grunkemeier GL, Thomas BR, Star A: Statistical considerations in the analysis and reporting of time-related events: Application to analysis of prosthetic valve-related thromboembolism and pacemaker failure. Am J Cardiol 1977;39:257.
34. Hacking I: Political arithmetic. In The Emergence of Probability. Cambridge: Cambridge University Press, 1975, pp 102–110.
35. Harrell F: The LOGIST procedure. In SAS Supplemental Library User's Guide. Cary, NC: SAS Institute, 1980, pp 83–102.
36. Hazelrig JB, Turner ME Jr, Blackstone EH: Parametric survival analysis combining longitudinal and cross-sectional-censored and interval-censored data with concomitant information. Biometrics 1982;39:1–15.
37. Hollander M, Wolfe DA: Nonparametric Statistical Methods. New York: John Wiley & Sons, 1973.
38. Kalbfleisch JD, Prentice RL: The Statistical Analysis of Failure Time Data. New York: John Wiley & Sons, 1980, pp 168–171.
39. Kaplan EL, Meier P: Nonparametric estimation from incomplete observations. J Am Stat Assoc 1958;53:457.
40. Kirklin JW: A letter to Helen. J Thorac Cardiovasc Surg 1979;78:543.
41. Kirklin JW, Blackstone EH, Naftel DC, Turner ME: Influence of study goals on study design and execution. Control Clin Trials 1997;18:488–493.
42. Kirklin JK, Naftel DC, Bourge RC, White-Williams C, Caulfield JB, Tarkka MR, Holman WL, Zorn GL: Rejection after cardiac transplantation. A time-related risk factor analysis. Circulation 1992;86:(suppl II):II-236.
43. Kodlin D: A new response time distribution. Biometrics 1967; 23:227–239.
44. Kubo SH, Naftel DC, Mills RM Jr, O'Donnell J, Rodeheffer RJ, Cintron GB, Kenzora JL, Bourge RC, Kirklin JK, and the Cardiac Transplant Research Database Group: Risk factors for late recurrent rejection after heart transplantation: A multiinstitutional, multivariable analysis. J Heart Lung Transplant 1995;14:409–418.
45. Kuzma J: A comparison of two life table methods. Biometrics 1967;23:51.
46. Larntz K: Small-sample comparisons of exact levels for chi-square goodness-of-fit statistics. J Am Stat Assoc 1978;73:253.
47. Lee ET: Statistical Methods for Survival Data Analysis. Belmont, CA: Lifetime Learning Publications, 1980.
48. Lew RA, Day CL Jr, Harrist TJ, Wood WC, Mihm MC Jr: Multivariate analysis: Some guidelines for physicians. JAMA 1983; 249:641.
49. Mantel N: Evaluation of survival data and two new rank order statistics arising in its consideration. Cancer Chemotherapy Rep 1966;50:163.
50. McGiffin DC, Kirklin JK, Naftel DC, Bourge RC: Competing outcomes after heart transplantation: A comparison of eras and outcomes. J Heart Lung Transplant 1997;16:190–198.
51. McGiffin DC, Naftel DC, Kirklin JK, Morrow WR, Towbin J, Shaddy R, Alejos J, Rossi A, and the Pediatric Heart Transplant

Study Group: Predicting outcome after listing for heart transplantation in children: Comparison of Kaplan-Meier and parametric competing risk analysis. J Heart Lung Transplant 1997;16: 713–722.

52. Meijler FL: Contribution of the risk factor concept to patient care in coronary heart disease. J Am Coll Cardiol 1983;1:3–19.

53. Moriyama IM, Gustavus SO: Cohort mortality and survivorship: United States Death-Registration Studies, 1900–1968. *In* Vital and Health Statistics, Analytical Studies. Series 3, No. 16. Rockville, MD: U.S. Department of Health, Education, and Welfare.

54. Naftel DC: Editorial Comment. Do multi-institutional studies represent a higher level of research than single institution studies? J Heart Lung Transplant 1996;15:124–135.

55. Naftel DC: Letter to the Editor: Do different investigators sometimes produce different multivariable equations from the same data? J Thorac Cardiovasc Surg 1994;107:1528–1529.

56. Naftel DC: Survival analysis methods for treatment effectiveness research. Medical Effectiveness Research Data Methods AHCPR Pub. No. 92-0056:137-150, July 1992.

57. Naftel DC, Blackstone EH: The analysis of survival data with concomitant information using parametric models: PROC HAZARD and PROC HAZPRED. SAS Users' Group International Twelfth Annual Conference Proceedings. Dallas, TX: SAS Institute, 1987, pp 1116–1171.

58. Naftel DC, Bradely EL: A review and comparison of eight two-parameter generalizations of the negative exponential distribution. Biometrics 1983;39:808.

59. Nelson W: Graphical analysis of system repair data. J Qual Technol 1988;20:24–35.

60. Neyman J: On the problem of confidence intervals. Ann Math Stat 1935;6:111.

61. Pearl R, Reed LT: On the rate of growth of the population of the United States since 1790 and its mathematical representation. Proc Natl Acad Sci U S A 1920;6:275.

62. Prentice RL, Kalbfleisch JD, Peterson AV Jr, Flournoy N, Farewell VT, Breslow NE: The analysis of failure times in the presence of competing risks. Biometrics 1978;34:541.

63. Reed LJ, Berkson J: The application of the logistic function to experimental data. J Phys Chem 1929;33:760.

64. Rodeheffer RJ, Naftel DC, Stevenson LW, Porter CB, Young JB, Miller LW, Kenzora JL, Haas GJ, Kirklin JK, Bourge RC, and the Cardiac Transplant Research Database Group: Secular trends in cardiac transplant recipient and donor management in the United States 1990 to 1994—a multi-Institutional study. Circulation 1996; 94:2883–2889.

65. SAS Institute: Technical Report: P-175. Cary, NC: SAS Institute, 1988, pp 192–265.

66. Spiegelhalter DJ: Probabilistic prediction in patient management and clinical trials. Stat Med 1986;5:421–433.

67. Steel RGD, Torrie JH: Principles and Procedures of Statistics: A Biometrical Approach. 2nd ed. New York: McGraw-Hill, 1980.

68. Ventura H, Kirklin J, Eisen H, Michler R, Clemson B, O'Donnell J, Dumas-Hicks D, Porter C, Naftel D, McGiffin D, and the Cardiac Transplant Research Database (CTRD): The combined impact of pretransplant risk factors and rejection frequency and severity on the prevalence of post transplant coronary vasculopathy [abstract]. J Heart Lung Transplant 1997;16:66.

69. Verhurlst PF: Notice sur la loi que la population suit dans son accroissment. Math Phys 1838;10:113.

70. Walker SH, Duncan DB: Estimation of the probability of an event as a function of several independent variables. Biometrika 1967;54:167–179.

71. Wilcoxon F: Individual comparison by ranking methods. Biomet Bull 1947;1:80.

72. Yates F: Contingency tables involving small numbers and the χ^2 (squared) test. J R Stat Soc 1934;1(suppl):217.

Appendix

EQUATION 1

$$f(x) = \frac{1}{\sigma\sqrt{2\pi}} e^{-\frac{(x-\mu)^2}{2\sigma^2}}$$

where $f(x)$ is the normal density function of the continuous variable x. The mean, μ, and standard deviation, σ, are constants (parameters) that determine the location and the spread, respectively, of the density. π is the number 3.1416 and e is the number 2.7183.

EQUATION 2

$$\bar{x} = \frac{\sum\limits_{i=1}^{n} x_i}{n}$$

where $\bar{x}$ is the arithimetric mean of n sample values, and x_i is the specific value of x for a patient.

EQUATION 3

$$SD = \frac{\sum\limits_{i=1}^{n} (x_i - \bar{x})^2}{n-1}$$

where SD is the standard deviation of the sample, $\bar{x}$ is the sample mean, and n is the sample size.

EQUATION 4

$$95\% \text{ CL} = \hat{p} \pm 2 \times \sqrt{\hat{p}(1-\hat{p})/n}$$
$$d = 2 \times \sqrt{\hat{p}(1-\hat{p})/n}$$
$$n = \frac{4\,\hat{p}(1-\hat{p})}{d^2}$$

where 95% CL is the 95% confidence limits for a single proportion. $\hat{p}$ is the estimated proportion (assumed before the actual study), n is the unknown sample size, and

d is ½ the width of the 95% CL (the desired "precision" of the study).

EQUATION 5

$$n = 0.5 \left(\frac{(Z_\alpha + Z_\beta)}{\arcsin\sqrt{p_1} - \arcsin\sqrt{p_2}}\right)^2$$

where n is the necessary sample size (see Table 3–2). Z_α is the number of standard deviations that encompass the proportion $1 - \alpha$ of the distribution. Z_β is the number of standard deviations for $1 - \beta$ (see Table 3–3). Arcsin is a trigonometric function.

EQUATION 6

$$r = \frac{\sum\limits_{i=1}^{n} (x_i - \bar{x})(y_i - \bar{y})}{\sqrt{\sum\limits_{i=1}^{n} (x_i - \bar{x})^2 \sum\limits_{i=1}^{n} (y_i - \bar{y})^2}}$$

where r is the correlation coefficient and x_i and y_i are individual data points.

EQUATION 7

$$\hat{\mu} = (\bar{t})^{-1} = \frac{n}{\sum\limits_{i=1}^{n} t_i}$$

where $\hat{\mu}$ is the sample value for μ (the constant hazard) and t is the time to an event.

EQUATION 8

$$\hat{\mu} = \frac{d}{\sum\limits_{i=1}^{d} t_i + \sum\limits_{j=1}^{n-d} T_i}$$

where $\hat{\mu}$ is the sample value for μ (as in Equation 10) in the presence of right censoring, d is the number of deaths, Σt_i is the sum of survival times for patients who died, and ΣT_i is the sum of censored times.

EQUATION 9

$$\Lambda_1(t) = \mu \left[\frac{|\nu|-\nu}{2|\nu|} + \frac{\nu}{|\nu|} \left[1 + \frac{m}{|m|} \left(\frac{|m|-m}{2|m|} + \frac{B(t)}{\rho} \right)^{-1/\nu} \right]^{-1/m} \right]$$

$$B(t) = \frac{e^{-\delta t}-1}{\delta}$$

where $\Lambda_1(t)$ is the early phase cumulative hazard function; μ is the scaling parameter; ν, m, δ, and ρ are shaping parameters; and $t > 0, -1 < \delta < 1$, $\rho > 0$, ν and m unbounded.

EQUATION 10

$$\Lambda_3(t) = \mu_3 \left[\left(1 + \left(\frac{t}{\tau} \right)^\gamma \right)^{1/\alpha} - 1 \right]^\eta$$

where $\Lambda_3(t)$ is the late-phase cumulative hazard function; μ_3 is the scaling parameter; and τ, α γ, and η are shaping parameters.

EQUATION 11

$$\Lambda_3(t) = \mu_3 t^2 \qquad \lambda_3(t) = \mu_3 2t$$

where $\Lambda_3(t)$ is the late-phase cumulative hazard function and μ_3 is a scaling parameter. This function is the linearly increasing component of the Rayleigh hazard function.

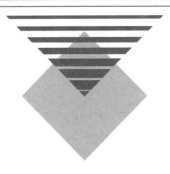

The Patient
Before Transplantation

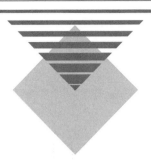

CHAPTER FOUR

Pathophysiology and Clinical Features of Heart Failure

HISTORICAL PERSPECTIVES

It is likely that the "heart failure syndrome" has been recognized and treated for millennia.[81] This conclusion is supported by the accumulation and preservation of medical knowledge about "dropsical conditions" in ancient medical history, long before an understanding emerged of the state's relationship to heart failure (Table 4–1).[58, 61]

DROPSY IN ANCIENT MEDICAL HISTORY

Reference to dropsy (the pathologic accumulation of diluted lymph in body tissues and cavities) possibly caused by cardiac decompensation can be found in relics of ancient civilizations.[50] However, making the link between heart failure and cardiac dropsy by understanding cardiovascular anatomy, myocyte and circulatory physiology, and cell biology took two millennia. Egyptian writing, as well as more contemporary study of mummified cadavers, suggests that cardiovascular disease was present in ancient civilizations, and it is recorded that the Egyptians felt that abnormalities in the pulse reflected cardiovascular disease. An early clinical description of a patient with heart failure can be found in the Ebers papyrus, which dates from 1600 BC, indicating that dropsical conditions were present at that time.[58, 61] Of course, dropsy can be caused by many noncardiac conditions such as cirrhosis, nephrotic syndrome, and myxedema, so that it is challenging, even in the contemporary practice of medicine, to differentiate cardiovascular conditions that can precipitate fluid retention from other system failure.[128, 130, 131] Predating Christ by some three centuries, ancient Greeks seemed to struggle with rudimentary knowledge of the pulse. Hippocrates possibly alluded to the end stages of heart failure when he described cachexia and fluid retention, stating "the flesh is consumed and becomes water . . . the shoulders, clavicles, chest, and thighs melt away. This illness is fatal."[58] One of the more dramatic references to a possible case of heart failure in ancient times was the miraculous cure of a "dropsical" patient by Jesus Christ that Luke the Evangelist (and physician) described in the New Testament.

In order to link deranged cardiovascular physiology to heart failure, it was necessary to understand the integrated function of the heart and peripheral circulation. Galen's (131–201 AD) belief that the heart's primary function was to generate and distribute heat throughout the body[50] was the dominant medical view of the heart

TABLE 4-1	Heart Failure Through the Ages: Historical Developments and Therapies	
HISTORIC PERIOD/INNOVATOR	YEAR/PERIOD	DEVELOPMENT
Ebers Papyrus	1600 BC	Dropsy in ancients
Hippocrates	300 BC	Detailed cachexia with dropsy
Jesus Christ	33 AD	Cures dropsy
Bartoletti	1576–1630	Described dyspnea producing sudden death
Sydenham	1680	Bleeding, purges, emesis for dropsy
Withering	1785	Text: *On Dropsy*
Corvisart	1812–1860	Leeches, purges, bleeding, squill, nitrates, calomel diuretics; subcutaneous morphine sulfate
Karrell	1866	Skim milk diet
Flint	1873	Digitalis, ether, opiates
Southey	1877	Lymphatic drainage tubes
Osler	1892	Pathophysiology of heart failure
Einthoven	1901	Electrocardiography
McKenzie	1910	Amyl nitrate for pulmonary edema
Herrick	1912	ECG changes of cardiac ischemia
Ringer	1915	Electromechanical properties of cardiac contraction
Starling and Frank	1918	"Law of the heart"
	1930	Quinidine and digoxin for atrial fibrillation
Cutler	1930s	Thyroidectomy for heart failure
Burch	1960s	Bed rest for cardiomyopathy; thiazides, furosemide, ethacrynic acid introduced
Moulopolis	1966	Intra-aortic balloon counterpulsation
Barnard, Shumway and others	1967	Human heart transplant
Braunwald, Mason, Sonnenblick, Cohn	1970s	"Vasodilators" in heart failure
Pfeffer, Yusuf, Cohn	1980s	"ACE inhibitors" in heart failure
Waagstein, Hjalmarson, Swedburg, Bristow, Packer	1990s	"Beta blockers" in heart failure
Cooley, Debakey, Dor, Carpentier and numerous other cardiac surgeons	1990s	Surgical procedures and mechanical devices for the treatment of advanced heart failure
Prediction	2010	Prevention and molecular guided therapy

until the seventeenth century. Although he described many features of the heart, including the basic function of heart valves and arterial pulsations, Galen failed to realize that the heart is a pump.[61]

It was not until the Italian Renaissance that Realdo Columbo (1516–1559) and Girolamo Fabrizio d'Acquapedente (1533–1619) set the stage for William Harvey (1578–1657) to describe the circulation of blood.[59, 92] Harvey's observations, published in 1628, the year of Shakespeare's death, were based on publications by Andreus Vesalio (1514–1564), professor of anatomy at the University of Padua, who had published the first great anatomic text.[118] Harvey cited a mathematical model to support his theory that blood "is driven round a circuit with an unceasing, circular sort of movement."[61, 92]

Following the publication of Harvey's description of the physiology of the circulation, several subsequent depictions of congestive heart failure can be found. For example, Bartoletti (1576–1630) detailed case histories of patients with a peculiar dyspnea associated with "sudden death." He reported that these patients suffered for significant periods from respiratory difficulties with walking that were relieved with rest, and he characterized these patients as having intermittent "suffocation."

SEVENTEENTH AND EIGHTEENTH CENTURY PERSPECTIVES

Therapeutic approaches to dropsical conditions were primitive for centuries. As recently as the late seventeeth

century, Thomas Sydenham suggested bleeding, purges, vomiting, blistering, garlic, and wine or good ale as therapies for dropsical conditions.[117] These approaches characterized the severe limitations of physicians in the seventeeth century, but many of these seemingly rudimentary ministrations persisted in one fashion or another through to the twentieth century. It was Withering's seminal publication in 1785 that changed the clinician's approach to dropsy by advocating careful prescription of foxglove tea, now well known to contain a cardiac glycoside, to select individuals with congestive states.[128] Withering knew the implications of giving foxglove preparations to the wrong patient or in improper dosages. Indeed, when criticized by contemporaries who had failed while trying to use this prescription, Withering pointed out that the critic's use of the herbal remedy and their patient selection did not follow his detailed instructions. He suggested that imprudent administration of excessively potent foxglove tea could precipitate a disturbing spectrum of nausea, vomiting, visual disturbance, and cardiovascular collapse we now know is digitalis intoxication. Furthermore, Withering noted that responders to his therapy had, at the outset, "weak and thready pulse" coupled with a "pale countenance." Though Withering never directly connected the condition of dropsy with cardiac and cardiovascular insufficiency, his description is likely of dropsical patients with severe congestive heart failure and atrial fibrillation. Dropsical patients with nephrotic syndrome, tuberculous peritonitis, myxedema, or hepatic cirrhosis, all common conditions in the late eighteenth century, would be more likely to exhibit "robust and regular

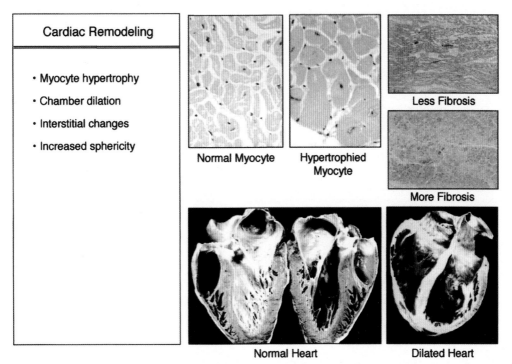

Cardiac Remodeling

- Myocyte hypertrophy
- Chamber dilation
- Interstitial changes
- Increased sphericity

Normal Myocyte

Hypertrophied Myocyte

Less Fibrosis

More Fibrosis

Normal Heart

Dilated Heart

FIGURE **4-4.** The facets of heart failure; anatomic and morphologic responses (cardiac ''remodeling''). Cardiac remodeling is the anatomic hallmark of heart failure. It is characterized by myocyte hypertrophy, cardiac chamber dilation, and interstitial matrix changes, all of which lead to an enlarged and more spherical heart that contracts and relaxes inefficiently. Shown in this figure are hypertrophied myocytes, fibrosed interstitium, and cardiac dilation compared with more normal specimens.

pulses with ruddy complexion" and these were the individuals not expected by Withering to diurese after foxglove tea.

PHYSIOLOGIC PERSPECTIVES

Despite increasing insight into the relationship of cardiovascular pathophysiology to dropsical conditions in the eighteenth and nineteenth centuries, progress with respect to therapies was still slow. Corvisart, in 1812, continued to suggest purges, bleeding, leeches, physical removal of ascites and pleural effusions, as well as direct puncture of edematous legs; but he also suggested drugs such as squill (a cardiac glycoside) and nitrated drinks.[24] More aggressive use of diuretics, although most being toxic and weak, can be noted in the mid nineteenth century with prescription of mercurial preparations (largely calomel) and potassium bitartrate. Subcutaneous morphine sulfate injection was used in the 1860s to ameliorate dyspnea, and the Karrell diet, which was primarily low-sodium-content skim milk, was proposed in 1866. Austin Flint, in 1883, suggested that digitalis, ether, and opiates could be helpful to relieve the dropsical conditions he observed and correctly linked the signs and symptoms to decompensated ventricular hypertrophy.[36] Flint was one of the first to suggest that the heart went through a long period of quiescent compensated hypertrophy in settings of valvular insufficiency or stenosis before decompensating to the congestive heart failure syndrome.[48, 54, 103] Indeed, Flint may have first coined the term "heart failure" in its modern context, though he still suggested that dry cupping, paracentesis, thoracentesis, and leg incisions could be helpful in treating dropsy. Southey promoted direct insertion of tubes into leg lymphatics to treat edema in 1877, and bromides were used with increasing frequency for sedation of dyspneic patients. Diuretics prescribed for this condition in the late nineteenth century included theophylline, theobromine, and urea salts.

At the turn of the last century, catharsis and blood letting were common treatments. Supplemental oxygen was used in early 1900, and Sir James McKenzie in 1910 suggested that amyl nitrate was useful as well as digitalis, oxygen, purgatives, and venisection.[73] Mercurial diuretics were prescribed with increasing frequency in the 1920s and 1930s, and during this period of time, thyroidectomy was even employed to treat more severe cases of congestive heart failure (even when not due to thyrotoxicosis). The cardiac chair was introduced about this time, and diet therapies began to focus on water and salt restriction, with bed rest virtually always a component of congestive heart failure treatment. Indeed, this recommendation, which had been generally prescribed through the decades, culminated in the 1960s when George Burch recommended complete and compulsive long-term bed rest after the diagnosis of cardiomyopathy was made.[130]

It was in the late eighteenth and early nineteenth centuries that modern-day insight into heart and circulatory physiology developed. Understanding the pathophysiology better set the stage for contemporary heart failure

treatment. William Osler contributed greatly to the understanding of heart failure in his writings of 1892,[91] which described the transition from cardiac hypertrophy as an adaptive mechanism to a pathologic process when the enlarged heart muscle degenerates. Characterization of the electrocardiogram by Einthoven in 1901 led to great insight and understanding of pulse abnormalities and ultimately allowed James B. Herrick's description in 1912 of the electrocardiographic patterns of myocardial infarction, which led to understanding the relationship of ischemic syndromes to heart failure and death.[130] Mechanical characteristics of the heart and cardiovascular system were initially elucidated in the early 1900s by the renowned physiologists Frank and Starling, and this paved the way for understanding circulatory changes resulting from abnormalities of heart function.[34, 60, 127] Elegant studies performed by Ringer led to more accurate characterization of the electromechanical properties necessary for cardiac contraction, particularly the importance of calcium as a contractile substrate.[58]

TOWARD GREATER INSIGHTS

A better understanding of the condition of atrial fibrillation led to recommendations in the 1930s that atrial flutter and atrial fibrillation associated with congestive heart failure should be treated with quinidine and digitalis. More potent diuretics, such as the carbonic anhydrase inhibitor diamox, were introduced in 1950. The potent alpha blocking antihypertensive drug hexamethonium was introduced in 1956. Still, as late as the middle part of the twentieth century, mechanical interventions such as ligation of the inferior vena cava, thyroidectomy, and radioactive iodine thyroid gland ablation were used as therapies. Intra-aortic balloon counterpulsation for hemodynamic collapse secondary to severe heart failure was first proposed in 1966, with surgical treatment of left ventricular aneurysm performed in 1962. The late 1950s and early 1960s were also the eras when cardiac valvular surgery as treatment for heart failure due to valvular disease began in earnest, driven by the development of cardiopulmonary bypass to temporarily support cardiopulmonary circulation during open heart surgical procedures performed with the heart arrested.[43] Thiazide diuretics were introduced in 1962, furosemide in 1965, and ethacrynic acid in 1966. Though the first human heart transplant actually occurred in 1963 (a primate heart was used), the first human-to-human cardiac transplant was performed in December 1967 (see Chapter 1).

Prior to the 1970s the pharmacologic management of heart failure consisted largely of cardiac glycoside preparations and diuretics.[12] However, the 1970s brought the realization of the value of vasodilating drugs (nitroprusside becoming available in 1976 and hydralazine in 1977) and intravenous inotropic agents.[19] Dopamine became available in 1972 with dobutamine following in 1975. These sympathomimetic drugs were useful when given parenterally to patients with severe cardiovascular compromise, but the hope that suitable oral inotropic agents could be developed has been repeatedly dashed by observations demonstrating that chronic inotropic medications are generally associated with increased mortality rather than significant attenuation of symptomatic heart failure. J. Willis Hurst's 1978 textbook on cardiovascular diseases[55] recommended treating heart failure by decreasing physical and emotional stress, low salt diet, digitalis, diuretics (including thiazide, furosemide, ethacrynic acid, spironolactone, and mercurial agents), and vasodilators (including nitroprusside, isosorbide dinitrate, and hydralazine).

The decade of the 1980s became the era of angiotensin-converting enzyme inhibitor therapy for heart failure. Captopril became available in 1980 with enalapril following in 1984, and though initially used because of their vasodilating effects, it subsequently became evident that these drugs beneficially alter the humoral milieu that is now known to be characteristic of heart failure. Exactly why these drugs work so well in heart failure remains a mystery. The interest in agents which block neurohormonal abnormalities in heart failure was supported by many landmark clinical trials performed in the late 1970s.[19] The contemporary era of heart failure therapy has been characterized by numerous important clinical trials which have better defined the role of angiotension-converting enzyme inhibitors, digitalis, beta blocking drugs, calcium channel blocking drugs (not particularly beneficial), and antiarrhythmic drugs (generally found to be harmful in the face of left ventricular dysfunction).[130, 131]

With an increased professional and public awareness of the potentially devastating outcome of advanced heart failure, new diagnosis and treatment strategies have been proposed that focus more on asymptomatic patients with left ventricular dysfunction. An understanding has emerged that heart failure is not always associated with a "congested" state, but is, rather, a complicated spectrum of cardiac dysfunction noted in patients who can be entirely asymptomatic as well as those manifesting intractable congestive states, pulmonary edema, or cardiogenic shock. Considerable emphasis has recently focused on attenuation of adrenergic cascades known important in perpetuating the heart failure syndrome and more frequent use of agents that modify inflammatory components of the syndrome. The spectrum of approaches to treat heart failure patients has broadened dramatically, with medical therapeutics interdigitating intimately with a variety of procedures, including the application of conventional cardiac operations such as repair of mitral valve disease, coronary revascularization, and ventricular remodeling in patients with severe systolic dysfunction. In addition, the last decade has been marked by a dramatic rise in the use of mechanical left and right ventricular assist devices which have repeatedly demonstrated their ability to be effective and lifesaving options in seriously ill patients with cardiogenic shock. These remarkable machines are most often today used to "bridge" patients to cardiac transplantation (see Chapter 8), but have also served as temporizing devices "bridging" patients to recovery such that removal of the pumps has sometimes been possible. Protocols are now underway to evaluate use of these assist devices as long-term treatment options for end-stage heart failure as an alternative to cardiac transplantation.

KATZ'S SIX "PARADIGMS" OF UNDERSTANDING HEART FAILURE

Table 4–2 lists the six paradigms which Arnold Katz put forth as the essence of biologic insight into the modern understanding of heart failure.[62] One can see the progression from clinical observation to syndrome codification to anatomic correlation with perturbed circulatory physiology to understanding cell biochemistry and molecular biodynamics associated with heart failure. This evolution of the modern understanding of heart failure has set the stage for developing additional therapies and even, possibly, finding a cure for heart failure.

DEFINITON AND OVERVIEW OF THE HEART FAILURE SYNDROME

Heart failure is a complex syndrome (Fig. 4–1) that is caused by a specific cardiac muscle injury, which may be primarily in the right ventricle, the left ventricle, or both, and may result in primary systolic or diastolic dysfunction.[131] The resulting cardiac derangement induces a cascade of abnormal events including cardiac molecular biodynamic (the molecular basis of myocyte growth and repair as it relates to cardiac function) changes which result in cardiac pump dysfunction, perturbation of circulatory homeostasis, and physiologic responses that attempt to maintain adequate organ perfusion (Table 4–3). The body's attempts at compensating for the abnormal pump function include stimulation of myocyte growth, neurohormonal responses and defensive circulatory and inflammatory reactions.[62] The effect of this intertwining network of events is the clinical manifestations of heart failure, which can range from asymptomatic patients to those with chronic congestive heart failure, acute pulmonary edema and cardiogenic shock, or sudden cardiac death syndrome.[130, 131]

Although the syndrome is caused by many diseases, the **pathophysiology of heart failure** is rooted primarily

TABLE 4-2	Katz's Six "Paradigms" of Understanding the Syndrome of Heart Failure

1. Clinical observations leading to syndrome codification (dropsical conditions described)
2. Anatomic findings correlated to clinical observations (cardiac remodeling and congestive states)
3. Understanding circulatory physiology (peripheral organ flow regulation)
4. Insight into cardiac hemodynamics (Starling and Frank "law of the heart")
5. Demonstration of perturbed cell biochemistry and bioenergetics (abnormal myocyte contraction, relaxation, and energetics)
6. Clarification of molecular biodynamics (insight into molecular mediated cardiac growth abnormalities)

Modified from Katz AM: Heart Failure. Philadelphia: Lippincott Williams & Wilkins, 2000, with permission.

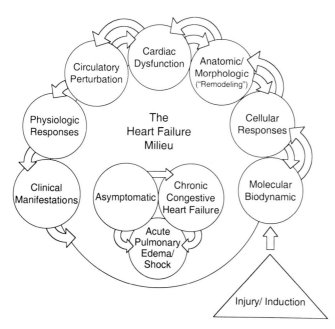

"Failure is the inability to measure up to certain normal standards"
Webster's Dictionary

FIGURE **4-1.** The facets of heart failure; complexity of the syndrome. When considering definitions of heart failure, one must remember that failure, generally speaking, is the inability to measure up to certain normal standards. Heart failure is, then, a complex syndrome that is caused by a specific injury to the heart which induces a wide-ranging cascade of abnormal events including molecular biodynamic changes, cellular responses, and anatomic/morphologic changes which result in cardiac dysfunction, circulatory system perturbation, and physiologic responses which attempt to maintain adequate organ perfusion. The net effect of this cascading but intertwining network of events is the clinical manifestations of heart failure, which can range from asymptomatic patients to those with chronic congestive heart failure, acute pulmonary edema, and cardiogenic shock.

in altered cellular protein and organelle repair, replacement, and maintenance. The physiologic disturbances of the myocyte cell membrane, cellular organelles, and interstitial matrix (which contains the capillary network, lymphatic vessels, adrenergic endings, collagen matrix, fibrous tissue, and macrophages) produce abnormalities

TABLE 4-3	**Pathophysiologic Definition of Heart Failure: Issues**

- Myocardial injury causes acute or chronic myocyte dysfunction (systolic and/or diastolic; right and/or left ventricular)
- Myocyte passive tension and work load increases
- Myocyte interstitial matrix stiffens
- Peripheral vascular bed blood flow is altered (initially decreased in subtle fashion)
- Subsequent mechanical, humoral, neurohormonal, and inflammatory responses appear in an attempt to create systemic organ flow compensation
- Compensatory mechanisms ultimately produce a maladaptive circulatory state characterized by myocyte hypertrophy, cardiac dilatation, and interstitial cardiac matrix changes (the components of remodeling)
- Patients may present without symptoms or suffer from a variety of fatigue, dyspnea, or dropsical states that fluctuate in severity based on treatment protocols, diet, physical conditioning, and diseases precipitating the heart failure syndrome

of excitation–contraction and repolarization–relaxation. **The hallmark of heart failure is myocyte hypertrophy with or without cardiac chamber dilatation.**

The stimuli which cause myocyte injury induce a return to the fetal phenotype of myocyte gene products and growth factors (Fig. 4–2),[62, 105] in an apparent effort to power up the contractile capabilities of these units. Resultant hypertrophied cells do not, however, contract with as much force and efficiency as do normal myocytes.

The initial compensatory response to myocyte injury and subsequent deleterious effects of these events results in certain cellular responses (Fig. 4–3). Downregulation of beta-adrenergic receptors can be noted in the myocardium of patients with heart failure. Though both beta$_1$- and beta$_2$-adrenergic receptor subtypes are seen in the myocardium, it is only the beta$_1$ receptor which is significantly altered (Fig. 4–3).[8, 9, 122]

The long-term sequelae of increased myocardial wall stress from volume or pressure overload and the perturbed neurohumoral environment characterizing heart failure is **cardiac "remodeling"** (Fig. 4–4). This is the anatomic, morphologic, and conformational shape change that is the consequence of myocyte hypertrophy, cardiac chamber dilation, and interstitial matrix changes (resulting in increased myocardial stiffness), which all combine to create a more spherical ventricle.

The hypertrophied, dilated, spherical heart contracts inefficiently, with systolic and diastolic cardiac dysfunction ensuing (Fig. 4–5). Systolic abnormalities result because the degree of cardiac chamber emptying with any one heart beat is diminished, and this attenuates normal forward flow and systemic tissue perfusion. In those with primarily systolic dysfunction, load-independent contractility is reduced and end-diastolic pressure increased while stroke volume falls. On the other hand, patients with primarily diastolic dysfunction have relatively preserved contractility but a much stiffer heart that is difficult to fill. This results in relatively maintained stroke volume but a shift in the diastolic component of the pressure–volume loop upward, reflecting abnormalities during ventricular filling. In reality, most patients have a combination of systolic and diastolic cardiac dysfunction, with one component becoming the dominant abnormality.

As a result of cardiac injury, myocyte passive tension and workload in more normally functioning cells increase when damaged cells can no longer normally bear the burden of circulatory demands. As stroke volume and cardiac output decrease, the distribution of blood to peripheral organs is diminished (though initially the changes may be subtle). Baroreceptor dysfunction occurs with cardiac output modulation triggered by systemic nervous system activation and adrenergic hormone outpouring. Tachycardia develops as cardiac output is determined, to a large extent, by the the relationship of heart rate to stroke volume. Autoregulation of systemic organ blood flow and local regulatory efforts act to initially preserve cardiac and central nervous system perfusion at adequate levels (Fig. 4–6). These feedback mechanisms are rooted in sympathetic nervous activation, renin-angiotensin-aldosterone release, in-

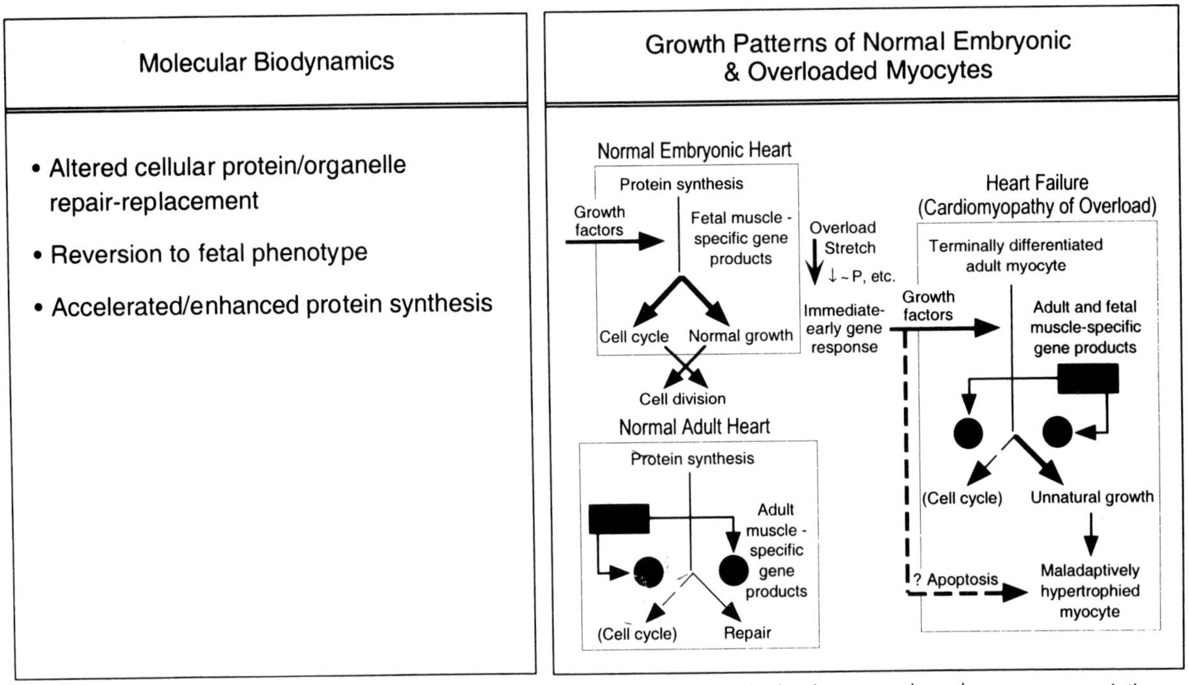

Molecular Biodynamics	Growth Patterns of Normal Embryonic & Overloaded Myocytes
• Altered cellular protein/organelle repair-replacement • Reversion to fetal phenotype • Accelerated/enhanced protein synthesis	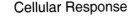

FIGURE **4–2.** The facets of heart failure; molecular biodynamics. Cardiac muscle development is based on gene transcription during embryonic and postnatal development. This process entails determination (creation of cardiac muscle phenotype in pluripotent stem cells of the lateral plate mesoderm) and differentiation (sequential induction of developmentally regulated, tissue restricted proteins that have regional specification). Adaptation of the myocyte to physiologic and pathologic stresses is related to plasticity of differential gene expression in response to certain endogenous and exogenous signals.

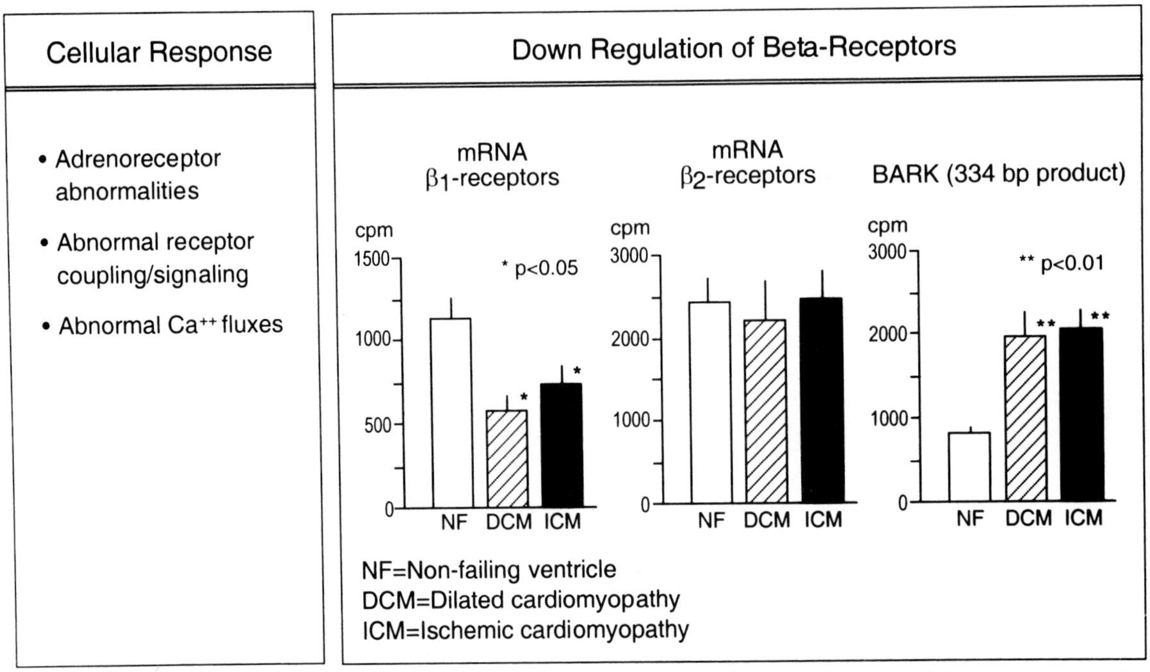

Cellular Response	Down Regulation of Beta-Receptors
• Adrenoreceptor abnormalities • Abnormal receptor coupling/signaling • Abnormal Ca^{++} fluxes	mRNA β_1-receptors mRNA β_2-receptors BARK (334 bp product) NF=Non-failing ventricle DCM=Dilated cardiomyopathy ICM=Ischemic cardiomyopathy

FIGURE **4–3.** The facets of heart failure; cellular response. Many myocyte and interstitial matrix cellular responses occur in the heart failure milieu. Adrenoreceptor abnormalities can be observed with down-regulation of the beta$_1$-adrenergic receptor in both dilated and ischemic cardiomyopathy patients as reflected by messenger RNA (mRNA). There is also up-regulation of beta-adrenergic receptor kinase (BARK), which phosphorylates beta-adrenergic receptors and thereby contributes to their uncoupling from the G-protein–cyclase complex.

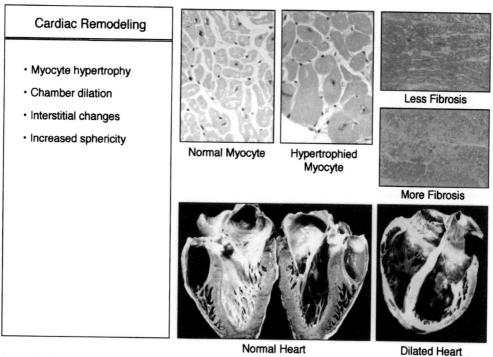

FIGURE 4–4. The facets of heart failure; anatomic and morphologic responses (cardiac "remodeling"). Cardiac remodeling is the anatomic hallmark of heart failure. It is characterized by myocyte hypertrophy, cardiac chamber dilation, and interstitial matrix changes, all of which lead to an enlarged and more spherical heart that contracts and relaxes inefficiently. Shown in this figure are hypertrophied myocytes, fibrosed interstitium, and cardiac dilation compared with more normal specimens.

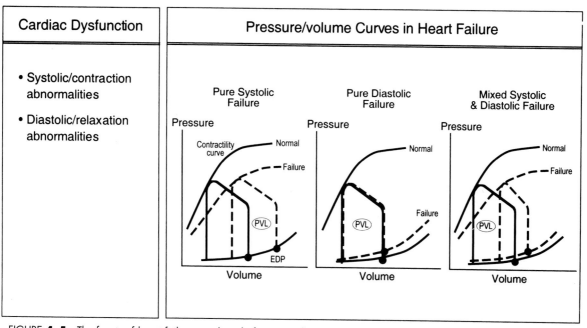

FIGURE 4–5. The facets of heart failure; cardiac dysfunction. Abnormalities of ventricular systolic and diastolic function are best characterized by pressure–volume curves that demonstrate that in systolic dysfunction the primary problem is reduction of contractility with a shift of the loop to the right such that cardiac ejection is driven by higher end-diastolic pressures, with stroke volume, and therefore cardiac output, being less than normal. In patients with diastolic dysfunction primarily, contractility may be normal (or even supranormal), but the operational end-diastolic filling pressure is greatly elevated when compared with any given volume in more normal patients. In reality, most patients with heart failure have a combination of systolic and diastolic dysfunction, but with each to highly variable degrees and one generally being the predominant problem.

Circulatory Perturbation	Autoregulation in Heart Failure	Regulation of Cardiac Output
• Baroreceptor dysfunction • Systemic flow decrement • Autoregulatory system failure (NO, prostacycline, endothelin changes)	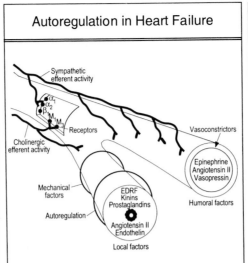	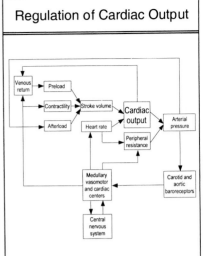

FIGURE **4-6.** The facets of heart failure; circulatory perturbation. The result of decrement in stroke volume and cardiac output is baroreceptor dysfunction and reduced systemic organ perfusion. A variety of mechanisms are in place to regulate cardiac output and peripheral blood flow. The sympathetic nervous system and adrenergic stimulation of the heart and systemic organs cause cardiac output increase, to a certain extent, with autoregulation of blood flow systemically attempting to protect vital organs. NO, nitric oxide; EDRF, endothelium-derived relaxing factor (also called nitric oxide).

flammatory cytokine induction, and changes in local organ blood vessel flow regulation (Fig. 4–7). The cardiac and circulatory changes are initially **adaptive** and compensatory but ultimately produce a maladaptive circulatory state (**deadaptation**) characterized by myocyte hypertrophy, cardiac dilatation, and cardiac interstitial matrix stiffening (the hallmarks of remodeling) (Fig. 4–4). As the condition worsens, the heart may become incapable of supplying adequate nutrition to peripheral organs, and removal of cellular metabolic waste products becomes impaired. When this occurs, symptoms and physical findings manifest. **Thus, the initially effective homeostatic circulatory compensatory mechanisms themselves exacerbate the remodeling process.**

Depending on the degree of cardiac dysfunction and circulatory perturbation, patients may be asymptomatic or suffer from a variety of symptoms such as fatigue, dyspnea, or dropsy that fluctuates in severity based on treatment protocols, diet, physical conditioning, diseases precipitating the heart failure syndrome, and a variety of environmental factors, such as exposure to alcohol, nicotine, or other known cardiotoxic compounds. If treatment is either absent or not effective, symptoms progress to a combination of congestive heart failure and low cardiac output. The most severe manifestation of heart failure is cardiogenic shock (Fig. 4–8).

In summary, cardiac failure is the clinical manifestation of the heart's inability to appropriately orchestrate the symphonic interaction of myocyte contractile elements, which results in perturbation of cardiac pump performance and circulatory homeostasis. Although the syndrome is caused by many diseases, the myocardial hallmark of heart failure is myocyte hypertrophy and cardiac chamber dilation. Excitation–contraction and repolarization–relaxation abnormalities must be understood in the context of myocyte cell membrane, cellular organelle, and interstitial matrix physiology. The cardiac interstitium, importantly, cannot be ignored, as it contains the capillary network, lymphatic vessels, adrenergic endings, collagen matrix, fibrous tissue, fibroblasts, and macrophages. All of these elements contribute to abnormal contraction/relaxation patterns in heart failure. Pump and circulatory perturbation precipitate a host of autoregulatory, neurohormonal, and inflammatory system responses designed initially to maintain reasonable organ perfusion, but which eventually contribute to cardiac remodeling, further perturbing normal function. Diagnosis of the problem is based on correlation of symptoms (or lack thereof) to systolic and diastolic properties characteristic of the heart failure syndrome. Treatment follows after an appropriate diagnosis is made and the severity of the syndrome staged.

SCOPE OF THE HEART FAILURE PROBLEM

Recent estimates suggest that 4 million Americans have heart failure, with 15 million patients affected worldwide (Table 4–4). This is an underestimation of the problem because it focuses on those individuals with symptomatic congestive heart failure. Still, in 1990 in the United States alone, there were 700,000 hospital discharges with a primary diagnosis of congestive heart failure, representing a fourfold increase from 1971.[131] Deaths in the United States in 1990 believed to be primarily due to heart failure were estimated to be 280,000. The prevalence of heart failure increases with the aging population of the United States and most other industrial countries. Indeed, it is predicted that the prevalence of heart failure in the United States will be almost 6 million individuals by the year 2030. Using Framingham Study cohorts, mortality in symptomatic males with congestive heart failure has been reported to be 50% at 24 months. Congestive heart failure is the United States

Physiologic Responses

- Sympathetic nervous system upregulation

- Renin-angiotensin-aldosterone release

- Inflammation (IL$_1$, IL$_6$, TNFα)

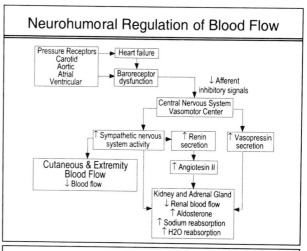

Neurohumoral Regulation of Blood Flow

Plasma TNFα Levels in Patients with NYHA Class I-IV Heart Failure*

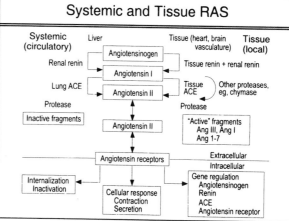

Systemic and Tissue RAS

FIGURE **4–7.** The facets of heart failure; physiologic responses. Several important and intertwining physiologic responses to heart failure are now known important in perpetuating the syndrome. Sympathetic nervous system up-regulation can increase cardiac afterload, decrease perfusion of the kidneys, and increase the heart rate. Reduced renal blood flow triggers more adrenergic outpouring, and increased systemic levels of renin, angiotensin II, and aldosterone can be noted and related to increased renal sodium and fluid retention. These hormones also likely adversely affect the myocyte and interstitial matrix of the heart. Inflammatory cytokines also contribute to cardiac remodeling and perpetuation of the syndrome. RAS, renin-angiotensin system; TNF, tumor necrosis factor; ACE, angiotensin-converting enzyme.

Health Care and Financing Administration's largest and most expensive burden. Estimates of direct annual expenditures for the treatment of heart failure range from $10 to $40 billion. Each heart failure hospitalization costs approximately $6,000–$12,000, with a 20% to 30% readmission rate.

SETTING THE STAGE FOR HEART FAILURE

Understanding the pathogenic responses of the myocardium to injury which result in heart failure requires insight into cellular molecular dynamics and the biochemical interplay of energy substrates which account for both normal and abnormal myocardial development, growth, and function.[3] Furthermore, it is important to relate cardiac morphogenesis to contractile abnormalities and pump dysfunction. Though we will initially focus on the myocyte, the myocardium has several different cellular lines and interstitial matrix substances which are all critically important to effect normal cardiac

contraction and relaxation.[5] Generally, the heart is composed of 50% myocytes, with the remaining cellular matrix being nonmuscular cells including fibroblasts and endothelial cells. Myocytes are, from a volume perspective, much larger, however, making up more than 80% of the total volume of the heart. During human embryonic development, differentiation, commitment, and morphogenesis of the cells occur in an organized fashion that is controlled by a variety of regulating genes and gene products. These systems generally become quiescent postpartum but are now known to be recruited in some fashion or another when the heart is injured acutely or chronically (Fig. 4–2). This process has been termed "reversion to fetal phenotype" (the term *phenotype* here refers to the overall behavior of a cell, including differentiation, development, growth, and cell functions).

MORPHOLOGIC DEVELOPMENT OF THE HEART

The morphologic progression from the embryonic cardiogenic plate to the development of a linear heart tube

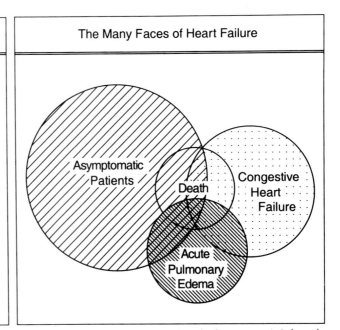

Clinical Manifestations	The Many Faces of Heart Failure
• Asymptomatic LVD • Congestive state • Low output state • Cardiogenic shock • Combinations	Asymptomatic Patients · Death · Congestive Heart Failure · Acute Pulmonary Edema

FIGURE **4-8.** The facets of heart failure; clinical manifestations. The pathophysiologic events described in Figures 4–1 through 4–7 are the underpinnings of the clinical heart failure syndrome. Clinical manifestations can range from asymptomatic or minimally symptomatic left ventricular dysfunction to congestive and low-output states of varying degrees and severity. Cardiogenic shock represents the most severe form of heart failure. More generally, a combination of symptoms due to congestion and low cardiac output is noted.

structure with subsequent looping, chamber and outflow tract septation, and formation of the cardiac valves is stimulated by a specific signaling cascade which orchestrates highly specific cell growth, division, and differentiation. The embryonic endocardium and myocardium are separated by an extracellular matrix substance called the cardiac jelly, and mesenchymal cells which colonize this acellular matrix substance give rise to the cardiac valves. Specific precursor cells for both endocardium and myocardium have been identified in the lateral mesoderm, and neurocrest cells play an important role in the proper differentiation of the cardiac structures. A class of genes called *homeobox* genes plays a critical role in regulating the synthesis of proteins involved in organogenesis.[62] Several homeobox gene products have been detected in the developing as well as the adult human heart. Abnormal expression of homeobox genes and cardiac growth factors may account for some of the developmental abnormalities of the heart that have been observed.

EXPRESSION OF CARDIAC MUSCLE GENES

During development of cardiac muscle, there are many genes transcribed to encode the proteins necessary for specialized functions of the mature heart,[16] including essential components of the contractile apparatus such as myosin heavy and light chains, alpha-cardiac actin, troponin-I, troponin-C, troponin-T, tropomyosin, structural proteins that comprise the sarcomere, membrane proteins involved in excitation–contraction coupling, and enzymes controlling adenosine triphosphate regeneration. Many of the same genes activated during differentiation of cardiac myocytes are also expressed in differentiated striated muscle cells, whereas others are quite specific to the myocardium. There are also regional patterns of gene expression within the heart that are highly specific and evolve during different embryonic stages. For example, atrial natriuretic factor and atrial myosin light chain-I (*MLC1A*) are restricted with respect to their activity in the adult heart to the atria, but during embryonic development these genes are expressed by ventricular tissue. Alpha-myosin heavy chain (MHC) and beta-MHC messenger RNA are both expressed at high levels in the cardiac tube by day 8 of mouse embryogenesis, a time when contractile activity can be detected. When septation occurs with formation of atrial and ventricular chambers, these myosin transcripts be-

TABLE 4-4	**The Scope of the Heart Failure Problem**

- Four million Americans have symptomatic heart failure
- 15 million patients affected worldwide
- 700,000 hospital discharges in 1990 with primary diagnosis of heart failure (four fold increase from 1971)
- 280,000 deaths in 1990 primarily due to heart failure
- 50% of heart failure patients over 65 years (prevalence of syndrome increases from 3/1,000 males aged 50–59 to 27/1,000 males 80–89 years)
- With aging United States population heart failure prevalence estimated to be almost six million by 2030
- Mortality overall in symptomatic males is 50% at 24 months in Framingham cohorts
- Congestive heart failure is United States Health Care Financing Administration (HCFA) largest and most expensive diagnosis-related group (DRG)
- Each heart failure hospitalization costs $6,000–$12,000 (U.S. dollars)
- Three-month readmission rates for heart failure can be 20–30%

come modulated such that alpha MHC expression is restricted to the atrium and beta MHC to the ventricle of the neonatal heart. In the postnatal environment, alpha MHC again increases in the ventricle and the beta MHC disappears.

Some overlap occurs between the expression of muscle-specific genes in skeletal and cardiac muscle, suggesting that a few common regulatory pathways exist to control muscle-specific transcription. Although mechanisms that control cardiac muscle transcription are poorly characterized (since cell culture lines which can reproduce the events involved in determination and differentiation of cardiac specific muscle cells are unavailable), a partial understanding has been gained from studying control mechanisms for skeletal muscle embryogenesis. Differentiation of skeletal muscle is controlled by a group of muscle-specific proteins referred to as the MyoD family which, when activated, initiates a cascade of events culminating in myoblastic differentiation.[100] MyoD is a member of the family of transcription factors called basic helix-loop-helix (bHLH) proteins, which regulate cell proliferation and differentiation in a wide spectrum of organisms.[16, 62, 88] However, *MyoD* genes have not been identified in cardiac myocytes, and undifferentiated cardiac myocytes have not been isolated. Thus, the bHLH factors that control cardiac myocyte differentiation are likely more complex than those involved in skeletal myoblast differentiation. These observations help explain the difficulty encountered when trying to gain insight into myocardial molecular dynamics by studying skeletal muscle models.

CARDIAC GROWTH FACTORS AND THEIR RECEPTORS

As noted, abnormal myocyte growth is one of the maladaptive responses to the abnormal pump function which characterizes heart failure. A cascade of gene activation occurs when cardiac myocytes are exposed to stresses such as ischemia, stretch, or increased developed tension.[62] Some genes are activated rapidly by stress, which if prolonged, leads to the synthesis of transcription factors for *late-response* genes. Some of the important gene products which promote cardiac remodeling are peptide growth factors. These factors constitute a series of regulatory protein families exhibiting both positive and negative effects on cell growth and differentiation. These proteins appear to trigger signal transduction cascades important during cardiac organogenesis.[105] Many of the proteins involved in normal growth factor signal transduction are products of cellular genes called proto-oncogenes (genes which are rapidly activated in response to stress). These proteins include growth factors themselves, growth factor receptors, membrane-associated and cytosolic-coupling proteins, and growth factor–induced transcription factors.

Peptide growth factors operate in paracrine (exerting their effect on local cells), autocrine (exerting effects on the cell that produces it), and intracrine (exerting its effects on intracellular membranes such as the sarcolemmal receptor) fashion. The most thoroughly studied cardiac growth factors are heparin-binding **fibroblast growth factors** (FGFs) and **transforming growth factors** (TGFs). Adult myocardium contains high levels of the prototypic acidic and basic FGF as well as FGF-6. Development of the heart is associated with a complex portfolio of growth factor expression as might be expected by the requirement to form cardiac valves, induce septation, create the ventricular outflow tracts, and establish the cardiac muscle cells themselves. TGF-β appears important during early skeletal muscle formation and is likely of critical importance in regulating cardiac morphogenesis.

Several classes of growth factors (in particular, platelet-derived growth factor [PDGF], epidermal growth factor [EGF], insulin-like growth factor [IGF] and FGF) induce biochemical signals by protein-tyrosine chymase activity. Ligand binding causes receptor dimers to form, and this activates receptors by juxtaposing chymase domains such that they can phosphorylate one another. Subsequent recruitment of specific signaling enzymes such as phosphatidylinositol-3-chymase with phosphotyrosines occurs in the systolic domain of the activated receptor. Several genes encode FGF receptors, and during cardiac embryogenesis transcripts can be found in the endocardial cushion and valve primordia with other subtypes being detected in cardiac muscle. Receptors for TGF-β and for activin (which is a member of the TGF-β superfamily), lack tyrosine chymase activity and, instead, possess an intrinsic serine-threonine chymase domain.

GROWTH FACTOR–INDUCIBLE TRANSCRIPTION FACTORS

The cascade of events involving membrane-associated and cytoplasmic signaling molecules activated by growth factors in turn causes the immediate upregulation of a battery of transcription factors that are believed to couple growth factor ligand binding to long-term structural and functional responses.[105] Growth factor–induced nuclear proteins include products of many proto-oncogenes, such as c-*myc*, c-*fos*, and c-*jun*.[15, 16] The expression of these proto-oncogenes in cardiac cells appears also to be triggered by other trophic signals such as adrenergic agonists, mechanical stretch, and mechanical load. The promoters for several cardiac genes, including atrial natriuretic factor, contain binding sites for c-*fos* and c-*jun* proteins. Under usual circumstances, cardiac expression of c-*myc* down-regulates rapidly in late-gestation embryos.

SETTING THE STAGE FOR ADAPTATION–DEADAPTATION

Figure 4–9 recapitulates in different perspective the concepts initially elaborated in Figure 4–2. In summary, the program of cardiac gene transcription during embryonic and postnatal development includes a process called **determination,** which is the establishment of the cardiac muscle phenotype in pluripotent stem cells of the lateral

Molecular Biodynamics	Adaptation - Deadaptation*
• Altered cellular protein/organelle repair-replacement • Reversion to fetal phenotype • Accelerated/enhanced protein synthesis	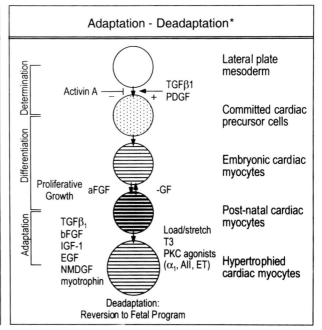

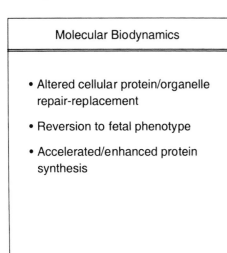

FIGURE **4–9.** The facets of heart failure; molecular biodynamics: myocyte determination, differentiation, and adaptation. Adaptation and deadaptation of myocytes accounts for their ability to hypertrophy after injury or during physiologic stress. A variety of growth factors liberated in response to myocardial pressure and volume overload states induces postnatal cardiac cells to hypertrophy by reverting to a fetal protein program that produces myocyte contractile elements that resemble those noted in utero more than in the adult. These cells do not contract with the same efficiency and power as do adult myocytes. *Deadaptation refers to reversion to fetal patterns of cardiac gene products. TGF, transforming growth factor; FGF, fibroblast growth factor; IGF, insulin-like growth factor; EGF, epidermal growth factor; PDGF, platelet-derived growth factor.

plate mesoderm and is thought to be triggered by TGF-β and PDGF. **Differentiation** is the sequential induction of developmentally regulated tissue-restricted proteins that have regional specification. **Adaptation** of the cell occurs in response to physiologic and pharmacologic stimulation and accounts for postnatal cardiac myocyte growth and development. Certain stimuli such as load and stretch or growth factors cause cell enlargement or hypertrophy with reactivation of the fetal genotypic program. This results in hypertrophied cardiac cells.

THE PHYSIOLOGY OF CARDIAC CONTRACTION AND RELAXATION

Table 4–5 summarizes the cardiac elements which are essential for normal excitation–contraction and repolarization–relaxation of the heart. These players, when in harmony, produce the fine symphony of cardiac contraction. Dissonance results in heart failure. Contraction and relaxation of the heart is a complex process that requires cellular contractile units, with the release of calcium from cisternal stores when ion-mediated electrical potentials cross the sarcolemmal membrane. This process induces thick and thin filament contractile proteins to interdigitate. This is an energy-dependent process requiring oxygen and specific metabolic substrates for success. It is vulnerable to disruption at several points, and this will cause varying degrees of systolic and diastolic dysfunction.

CARDIAC CONTRACTILE PROTEINS

From an anatomic standpoint, myocytes are arranged in an orderly fashion within the fibrous skeleton of the heart, which includes the cardiac valves.[89] The central element producing contractile force is the **cardiac sarcomere.** Striated cardiac muscle is banded together such that change in sarcomere shape produces synergistic shortening. Sarcomeres are joined end to end and aligned across the breadth of the cell. This results in the characteristic striated appearance of the myocyte when viewed under the light microscope. Electron microscopy reveals that the sarcomere contains two types of filaments interdigitating during contraction: a **thick fila-**

TABLE 4-5	The Symphonic Elements of Cardiac Contraction: Excitation–Contraction and Repolarization–Relaxation

MYOCYTE	CARDIAC INTERSTITIUM
Cell membrane	Capillary network
Receptors	Lymphatic network
Channels	Adrenergic nerve endings
Cell organelles	Basement membrane
Nucleus	Collagen matrix
Mitochondria	Fibrous tissue
Sarcolemma	Fibroblasts
Sarcoplasmic reticulum	Macrophages
Cytoplasmic matrix	
Regulatory complexes	
Myofilaments	

ment consisting of myosin, and a **thin filament** made of actin. The ultrastructure of a working myocardial cell is detailed in Figure 4–10.[90]

The interaction between proteins found amongst the thick and thin filaments of the sarcomere accounts for contraction. These proteins are myosin, actin, tropomyosin, troponin-C, troponin-I, and troponin-T. The **A band** represents the region of the sarcomere occupied by the thick filaments into which thin filaments extend from either side. **Myosin** creates the thick filament and hydrolyzes adenosine triphosphate (ATP) while interacting with actin. **Actin, tropomyosin,** and the **troponin** proteins (C, I, and T) create the thin filament. Actin activates myosin adenosine triphosphatase (ATPase) and interacts with myosin. Tropomyosin modulates the actin–myosin interaction. Troponin-C binds calcium, and troponin-I inhibits actin–myosin interactions and troponin-T binds troponin complex to tropomyosin. From an ultrastructural viewpoint, the **I band** is the region of the sarcomere occupied only by thin filaments, with these extending toward the center of the sarcomere from the Z lines which bisect each I band. The **sarcoplas-**

mic reticulum is a membrane network that surrounds the contractile proteins and consists of the sarcotubular network at the center of the sarcomere and cisternae which abut on the T tubules and sarcolemma. The **transverse tubule system** is lined by a membrane that extends from the sarcolemma and carries the extracellular space into the myocardial cell. Mitochondria can be seen richly dispersed throughout the cardiac cell.

CONTRACTILE PROTEIN RESPONSE TO CALCIUM

When calcium concentrations rise intracellularly, a series of events is triggered which induces conformational change of the thick and thin filaments such that sarcomere shortening occurs.[89] Figure 4–11 diagrams the key structures and major calcium fluxes occurring during myocyte excitation–contraction coupling.[90] Calcium enters the cell from the extracellular fluid via membrane calcium channels. Most of this calcium triggers subsequent calcium release from the sarcoplasmic reticulum, but a small

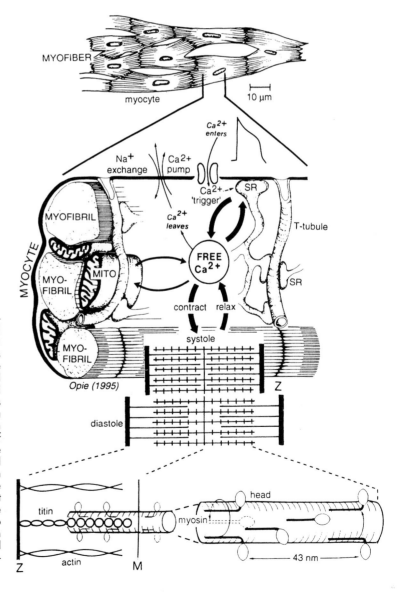

FIGURE **4–10.** Ultrastructure of the myocyte. Contractile proteins are arranged in bundled, linear fashion, the thick and thin filaments interdigitating. The sarcoplasmic reticulum (SR) is a membrane network that surrounds the contractile proteins and consists of the sarcotubular network at the center of the sarcomere and the cisternae, which abut on the T-tubules and the sarcolemma. The transverse tubule system (T-tubule) is lined by a membrane that extends from the sarcolemma and carries the extracellular space into the myocardial cell. Mitochondria (MITO), the essential site for energy production, are shown in the central sarcomere. Cardiac contraction occurs because of changing concentrations of calcium in the myocyte. At the molecular level, myocyte movement or contraction is caused by the interaction of actin with myosin, a process that is driven by calcium ion presentation to the contractile proteins. It is the myosin heads projecting from the thick myosin bodies that provides the movement for the thin filament. Titin is a large molecule that supports the myosin molecules by anchoring to the Z line. Titin also provides elasticity to the myocyte. (From Opie LH: The Heart. Physiology, from Cell to Circulation. 3rd ed. Philadelphia: Lippincott-Raven Publishers, 1998, with permission.)

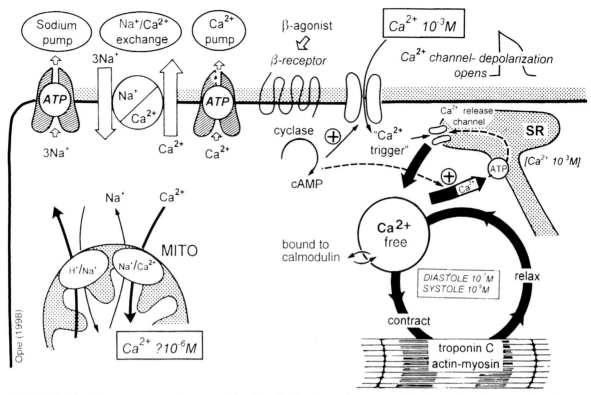

FIGURE 4-11. Myocyte structure related to calcium flux. Calcium flux in the myocyte is both passive and energy dependent. Calcium enters the cell from the extracellular fluid via plasma membrane calcium channels. Although most of this calcium triggers calcium release from the sarcoplasmic reticulum, a small protein directly activates the contractile proteins. Calcium transport back into the extracellular fluid involves two plasma membrane systems: sodium-calcium exchange and the plasma membrane energy-dependent calcium pump. Movements of calcium into and out of mitochondria (MITO) buffer cytosolic calcium concentrations. See text for details. (From Opie LH: The Heart. Physiology, from Cell to Circulation. 3rd ed. Philadelphia: Lippincott-Raven Publishers, 1998, with permission.)

amount directly activates the contractile proteins. Calcium transport back into the extracellular fluid involves two plasma membrane systems; the sodium–calcium exchange pump and the plasma membrane-calcium exchange pump. The sarcoplasmic reticulum membrane regulates two calcium fluxes including calcium release from the subsarcolemma cisternae and active calcium uptake by the calcium pump of the sarcotubular network. Calcium diffuses within the sarcoplasmic reticulum in a third calcium flux, returning to the subsarcolemma cisternae where it is stored in complex with calsequestrin and other calcium-binding proteins. Binding with and dissociation of calcium from the high-affinity calcium-binding sites of troponin-C account for the contractile protein interaction. It should be noted that presentation of activating calcium to the contractile proteins involves passive ion fluxes, but relaxation requires the active transport of calcium upward against a concentration gradient. The passive diffusion of calcium is extremely rapid and occurs at a rate 100,000 times faster than that of active calcium transport engineered by the ATP-dependent calcium pumps. Cardiac systole, therefore, is much faster than relaxation. The fact that diastole is longer than systole helps maintain a steady state in which calcium influx during excitation–contraction coupling does not cause excessive systolic calcium accumulation, since calcium is a cytotoxic cation.

EXCITATION–CONTRACTION COUPLING

Binding of calcium to troponin-C weakens the bond connecting troponin-I to actin and this causes a rearrangement of the proteins of the thin filament which shifts the tropomyosin molecules toward the center of the groove between the two actin strands. It is the movement of tropomyosin away from its blocking position that enables myosin cross-bridges to interact with active sites on actin causing systole. The heart returns to its diastolic or relaxed state when calcium removal from troponin-C returns tropomyosin to its inhibitory position in the thin filament. It is the transmembrane extracellular-to-intracellular-to-extracellular ionic shifts which characterize depolarization of the cell surface membrane, making calcium, the final contraction signal mediator, available to contractile proteins. Excitation–contraction coupling and relaxation are, therefore, controlled by an interdigitated system of calcium channels and pumps. Finely regulated control of these membrane systems enables the heart to adjust its systolic force and diastolic properties to wide-ranging physiologic, pharmacologic, and pathophysiologic environments; **attenuation of these contractile force and relaxation properties is the hallmark of heart failure.**[47]

CARDIAC CELLULAR ELECTROPHYSIOLOGY

Calcium flux and mechanical activity in the heart are triggered by a phase of regenerative and propagated tissue depolarization which starts in systole. The systolic action potential emanates from the diastolic resting potential. When the myocardial cell is at rest, its internal cell membrane is negatively charged compared with the outside, whereas during the action potential the inside of the membrane becomes transiently positively charged compared with the outside (ranging from −80 mv to +20–30 mv) (Fig. 4–12). These values correspond to the resting potential at the peak of the action potential. The resting potential results from dominant background membrane conductance for potassium ions, with conductance being the electrical result of ionic permeability. If the resting membrane is impermeable or almost impermeable to any ion other than potassium, the resting potential is equal or very close to the equilibrium potential for potassium ions. The cardiac cellular action potential is triggered either by a diastolic phase of slow depolarization or pacemaker potential, large enough to act in its final phase as a biologic stimulus (spontaneous activity), or by the action potential upstroke of neighboring cells playing a similar but much faster stimulating role (propagated activity). The cardiac action potential, for example, can result from the opening of two membrane ionic conductances, a fast and brief conductance for sodium ions, and a slower, smaller, and much more prolonged conductance for calcium ions. The termination of the action potential results from the opening of a delayed conductance for potassium ions.

Recordings of action potentials from various parts of the heart demonstrate significant differences in shape, amplitude, and duration of the electrical waveform. However, they all are characteristically made up of a fast upstroke followed by a long-lasting plateau. The upstroke, or rapid phase of depolarization, is highest and fastest in Purkinje fibers, with the plateau being highest in ventricular myocardium. It is the synergistic activation and propagation of the electrical impulse which creates cardiac rhythm and regulates calcium-dependent contractile forces.

MYOCARDIAL METABOLISM

In order to provide power for energy-dependent systolic and diastolic cardiac activities, the heart must consume and provide adenosine triphosphate (ATP) and adenosine diphosphate (ADP). It is the conversion of chemical energy into physical energy which allows the heart to contract, allowing distribution of metabolic substrates and oxygen to the peripheral organs. The heart, however, does not store large quantities of ATP, which is the chemical energy substrate required. ATP must be continuously resynthesized from its breakdown products of ADP and phosphate. Obviously, the greater the work of the heart, the higher the ATP turnover rate, rate of oxygen consumption, rate of substrate utilization, and rate of metabolic waste product production (carbon dioxide and lactic acid). When the heart cannot convert chemical potential energy sources into mechanical energy expenditure, functional and metabolic abnormalities will ensue, and this is one of the fundamental problems in failing ventricles. At a very basic level heart failure can be considered the systemic expression of impaired energy transfer within the heart. Because the heart meets the vast proportion of its energy demands by oxidative phosphorylation of ADP, it is not surprising that the capillary density in heart muscle is greater than in other organs and cardiac cells are packed with mitochondria, the cell organelle possessing the enzymes required for oxidative metabolism. Indeed, a close correlation exists between mitochondria volume fraction, heart rate, and total body oxygen consumption.

Figure 4–13 outlines the stages of energy transfer in heart muscle and the substrates utilized to create Krebs cycle intermediates and ATP, the ultimate source of energy from a biochemical standpoint. The heart's energy needs can be met by five different substrates, including glucose, lactate, fatty acids, ketone bodies, and amino acids, with the relative contribution of each of these substances changing moment to moment and being dependent upon plasma concentration or availability, hormonal homeostatic fluxes, organ perfusion, and cardiac workload demands. Three stages of energy transfer occur in the heart muscle, including the Krebs citric acid

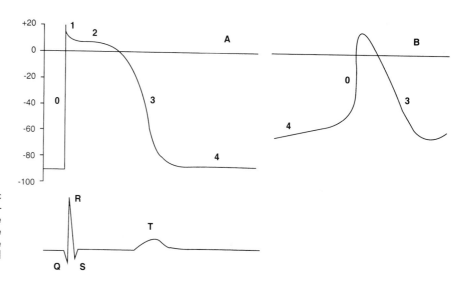

FIGURE **4–12.** Development of the cardiac action potential. The action potential of a non-pacemaker myocyte is shown with its five phases (0 to 4) in A and is contrasted to the action potential in a pacemaker cell in B. The transmembrane voltage changes are correlated to an electrocardiogram below A.

Energy Transfer in Heart Muscle

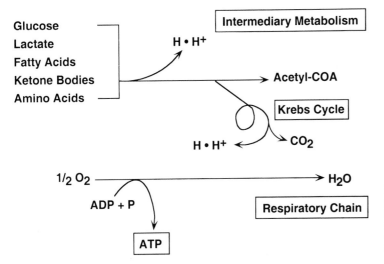

FIGURE **4-13.** Energy transfer in heart muscle. There are three stages of energy transfer in cardiac muscle, which consist of intermediary metabolism, the Krebs citric acid cycle, and the respiratory chain. The aim of intermediary metabolism is the production of acetyl-CoA for oxidation in the Krebs citric acid cycle and, ultimately, ATP synthesis.

cycle, the respiratory chain, and intermediary metabolism (which is responsible for production of acetyl-coenzyme A that is required for oxidation in the Krebs citric acid cycle). Basic by-products of cellular respiration include carbon dioxide and water. Changes in substrate utilization by the normal heart have been well characterized, with varying contributions made depending on different physiologic stress states. A relative consistency of the contribution of glucose, however, is noted throughout a wide range of workloads. The heart, then, utilizes a wide range of metabolic substrate to meet its energy needs with oxidative phosphorylation of ADP. It is important to note that it is ATP-ADP turnover, not ATP content of the cells, that determines workload capabilities of the myocardium and, therefore, the functional state of the heart. Unlike skeletal muscle, the heart is virtually incapable of anaerobic respiration. Myocardial metabolism with reference to donor heart ischemia is further discussed in Chapter 9.

MECHANISMS OF CARDIAC INJURY

Different diseases cause myocardial injury in different fashions (Table 4–6). Heritable disorders, for example, produce molecular genetic perturbation at the outset, with contractile protein production abnormalities be-

coming evident. Indeed, it is not uncommon for patients with myotonic or Duchenne's muscular dystrophy to die of an arrhythmia or heart failure rather than from the peripheral muscle disease. Patients with hypertrophic cardiomyopathy have now been demonstrated to have heritable disorders of troponin production that leads to ventricular hypertrophy and cardiac failure. Volume or pressure overload produced by valvular insufficiency or stenosis and hypertension induce abnormal molecular responses that cause myocyte production to become more representative of the fetal than adult phenotype. The return to the fetal phenotype with subsequent myocyte contractile and relaxation abnormalities which ultimately impair systemic perfusion and cause metabolic disturbances is characteristic of heart failure.[94]

Diseases such as myocardial infarction, lymphocytic myocarditis, or anthracycline poisoning attack the myocyte itself, causing premature cell death. Sometimes, injury is very acute, as would be the case with anoxia from acute coronary thrombosis. At other times, cellular injury and loss occur more slowly, with steady but inexorable myocyte demise occurring after up-regulating the normal apoptosis program. Table 4–7 is an extensive, but not necessarily all-inclusive, list of the many diseases which can precipitate the heart failure syndrome. This presentation adheres to the classification of cardiomyopathies most recently proffered by the World Health Organization and International Federation of Cardiology

TABLE 4–6	The Heart Failure Milieu: Routes of Myocardial Injury	
SITE	MECHANISM	EXAMPLE
Nucleolar DNA	Heritable disorder	Muscular dystrophy
Myocyte organelle	Perturbation in contractile protein production	Volume overload (MR, AI) Pressure overload (HTN, AS)
Myocardial cell	Necrosis and apoptosis	Myocardial infarction Anthracycline toxicity Alcoholic cardiomyopathy

MR, mitral regurgitation; AI, aortic insufficiency; HTN, hypertension; AS, aortic stenosis; DNA, deoxyribonucleic acid.

| **TABLE 4–7** | **Classification of Heart Failure Etiologies** |

Dilated cardiomyopathy
 Idiopathic
Hypertrophic cardiomyopathy
 Idiopathic hypertrophic subaortic stenosis (IHSS)
 Hypertrophic obliterative cardiomyopathy (HOCM)
 Hypertrophic nonobstructive cardiomyopathy
Restrictive cardiomyopathy
 Specific infiltrating diseases
 Idiopathic
Arrhythmogenic right ventricular cardiomyopathy
 Idiopathic right ventricular outflow tract tachycardia
 Arrhythmogenic right ventricular dysplasia
Unclassifiable cardiomyopathies
 Atypical presentation
  Fibroelastosis
  Systolic dysfunction without dilation
  Mitochondrial cardiomyopathy
 Mixed presentation (dilated/hypertrophic/restrictive)
  Amyloidosis (see "metabolic" section)
  Hypertension
Specific cardiomyopathies
 Ischemic
 Valvular obstruction/insufficiency
 Hypertensive
 Inflammatory
  Myocarditis
  Idiopathic lymphocytic
  Giant cell
  Autoimmune
  Infectious
   Coxsackievirus
   HIV
   Enterovirus
   Adenovirus
   Cytomegalovirus
   Bacterial (endocarditis/myocarditis)
   Chagas disease
Metabolic
 Endocrine
  Thyrotoxicosis
  Hypothyroidism
  Adrenal cortical insufficiency
  Pheochromocytoma
  Acromegaly
  Diabetes mellitus
	Familial storage disease/infiltration
	  Hemochromatosis
	  Glycogen storage disease
	  Hurler's syndrome
	  Refsum's syndrome
	  Niemann-Pick disease
	  Hand-Schüler-Christian disease
	  Fabry-Anderson disease
	  Morquio-Ullrich disease
	 Deficiency syndromes
	  Potassium metabolism disturbances (hypokalemia)
	  Magnesium deficiency
	 Nutritional disorders
	  Kwashiorkor
	  Anemia
	   Beri-beri
	   Selenium deficiency
	   Nonspecific malabsorption or starvation
	 Amyloid (primary, secondary, familial, hereditary, senile)
	 Familial Mediterranean fever
	General System Disease
	 Connective tissue disorders
	  Systemic lupus erythematosus
	  Polyarteritis nodosa
	  Rheumatoid arthritis
	  Scleroderma
	  Dermatomyositis
	  Nonspecific infiltrations and granulomas
	  Sarcoidosis
	  Leukemia
	 Muscular dystrophies
	  Duchenne's
	  Becker's
	  Myotonic
	 Neuromuscular disorders
	  Friedreich's ataxia
	  Noonan's syndrome
	  Lentiginosis
	 Sensitivity and toxic reactions
	  Alcohol
	  Catecholamines
	  Anthracyclines
	  Irradiation
	Peripartum cardiomyopathy (a heterogeneous group)

HIV, human immunodeficiency virus.

Task Force on the Definition and Classification of Cardiomyopathies.[99] This scheme is grouped mainly into cardiomyopathies having certain anatomic characteristics (such as dilated, hypertrophic, or restrictive elements) or addresses heart failure etiologies that result after specific injury such as that seen with ischemic heart disease. It is important to consider the etiologic spectrum when evaluating patients with heart failure because many diseases resulting in cardiomyopathy can be treated with complete resolution of the heart failure syndrome (such as heart failure due to thyrotoxicosis or myxedema).

Dilated cardiomyopathy is characterized by multichamber cardiac enlargement, whereas hypertrophic cardiomyopathy patients have small left ventricular cavity dimensions with marked muscle hypertrophy that can cause left ventricular outflow tract obstruction or actual cavity obliteration.[18] **Restrictive cardiomyopathy** is characterized by more normal chamber size (at least with respect to the ventricles), but impaired relaxation

or diastolic dysfunction is present that is not primarily due to muscular hypertrophy (in the classic sense).

Cardiomyopathies should be labeled by their etiologic component as well as anatomic and physiologic correlates. Therefore, a patient with prior myocardial infarction, active ischemic heart disease, and substantive congestion with a dilated left ventricle would correctly be labeled as having an ischemic dilated cardiomyopathy resulting in congestive heart failure. Obviously, multiple diseases can contribute to the cardiomyopathic process in an individual patient, and it is not particularly unusual to have a combination of ischemic heart disease, valvular heart disease (particularly mitral regurgitation in a setting of lateral wall myocardial infarction), or a combination of coronary heart disease, hypertension, and diabetes mellitus. The determination of which disease process is primary and characterization of additional comorbid conditions which can produce further myocardial injury is essential for the selection of proper heart failure therapies.

When epidemiologic information and clinical trial data are reviewed, ischemic heart disease appears to account for the preponderance of patients with both asymptomatic left ventricular systolic dysfunction and congestive heart failure. Hypertension is a frequent comorbidity. Valvular heart disease, diabetic cardiomyopathy, and idiopathic dilated cardiomyopathy represent, in most epidemiologic and clinical trial evaluations, about one third of the heart failure population. Active myocarditis or so-called viral cardiomyopathy is, in actuality, rarely diagnosed with certainty. Whether or not patients with idiopathic dilated cardiomyopathy have had, as the etiologic problem, preceding viral infection or inflammatory disease is contentious.

PATHOPHYSIOLOGY OF HEART FAILURE IN DETAIL

In order to gain further insight into the difficulty of heart failure and set the stage for proper therapeutics, including radical interventions such as cardiac transplantation, it is important to consider the pathophysiologic responses of the circulatory system in more detail. Particularly important will be linking knowledge of heart failure's pathophysiology to drug and surgical therapies designed to interrupt perturbations of the system.

MYOCARDIAL RESPONSES TO INJURY

In the face of normal loading conditions and normal myocyte systolic and diastolic function, reparative protein turnover is orderly and productive of adult cardiac muscle-specific gene products that will replenish or repair contractile elements during the normal stresses of daily contraction and relaxation (an event that occurs over 100,000 times each 24 hours). Many of the contractile protein and cell organelle structures regenerate every 30–90 days; and therefore, genetic plasticity of the cardiomyocyte with responses directed by varying stimuli is important in the normal and pathologic response to injury. It is also highly significant that terminally differentiated postnatal cardiomyocytes are likely not

TABLE 4-8	Myocyte Cell Membrane Receptor Sites Likely Important in Heart Failure Remodeling

Growth hormone
Angiotensin II
Norepinephrine/epinephrine
Tumor necrosis factor
Interleukin-1, -5, and -6
Tissue-derived growth factors
Endothelium-derived growth factors
Platelet-derived growth factors
Arginine vasopressin
Nitric oxide
Atrial natriuretic peptide

TABLE 4-9	Myocyte Necrosis Versus Apoptosis

CHARACTERISTICS

Necrosis
  Cellular dropsy
  Mitochondrial swelling
  Membrane integrity lost
  Random DNA degradation
  Inflammatory healing response
Apoptosis
  Cellular involution (shrinkage)
  No mitochondrial swelling
  Membranes intact initially
  Organized degradation of DNA (multiples of 180 base pair units)
  Little inflammatory response

DNA, deoxyribonucleic acid.

capable of significant cell division and, therefore, when myocyte death occurs, it is an irreplaceable loss.

HYPERTROPHY, DILATION, NECROSIS, AND APOPTOSIS

When specific diseases cause alteration in individual or grouped myocyte load, myocyte membrane receptors are activated by the increased load (passive mechanical stretch or pressure) and stimulation of humoral receptor sites.[66] This results in the shifting of protein synthesis to the previously described prenatal pattern (Figs. 4–2 and 4–9).[72] Both the quantity of myocyte proteins, particularly contractile proteins, as well as the quality of these peptides are affected by this immature phenotypic expression.[28] It is the **increased production of myocellular organelle elements and proteins, particularly contractile proteins, that leads to cellular hypertrophy and subsequent chamber dilation,** the clinical hallmarks of cardiac remodeling and the essence of heart failure pathophysiology.[71] Importantly, **pathologically hypertrophied myocytes do not contract or relax normally.** Cell membrane receptors that play an important role in the remodeling process are listed in Table 4–8. Activation of these receptors precipitates intracellular second messengers (substances that carry signals from one place to another when they diffuse through the cytoplasm or along the cytosolic surface of the plasma membrane) such as cyclic adenosine monophosphate and inositoltrisphosphate to induce a variety of intracellular enzyme mediators which then up-regulate genomic expression of excessive adult and fetal muscle cell–specific gene products. Unnatural growth of the cells follows which, collectively, results in myocardial hypertrophy and subsequent systolic and diastolic dysfunction.

A growing compendium of evidence suggests that both cell necrosis and apoptosis are important in the life–death cycle of the cardiac myocyte.[84] **Apoptosis** (Table 4–9) specifically refers to cell death from the process of myocyte condensation without disruption of the cell membrane but eventual fragmentation with pinocytosis of cell content and phagocytosis by neighboring cells. (The word *apoptosis* itself is a Greek term characterizing the slow but steady falling away of petals from a flower pistil.) **Myocyte necrosis,** on the other hand, is marked by cell surface membrane disruption, inflammation, and fibrotic replacement of myocyte tissue lost (Table 4–9). Whereas cell necrosis is commonly due to myocardial infarction, viral or bacterial infections, and exposure to toxins such as adriamycin or alcohol, triggering factors for apoptosis are less well characterized and likely mediated by multiple mechanisms including superoxide exposure, cytokines such as tumor necrosis factor, and mechanical alteration of myocyte geometry (seen as excessive individual myocyte load prompted by myocyte stretch).

Apoptosis may be triggered when a terminally differentiated adult myocyte is excessively stimulated by the multiple growth hormones essential for normal myocyte regulatory homeostasis and up-regulated in a setting of myocardial failure.[22, 51, 87] The induction of hypertrophy, therefore, likely leads to cell loss via apoptosis which, in turn, begins the self-perpetuating downward spiral of remodeling, clinical heart failure, humoral milieu perturbation, molecular biodynamic alteration, and further cell loss. Obviously, acutely injurious events resulting in sudden cell necrosis are also important and can be superimposed upon this chronic more insidious and subtle programmed cell death. Myocyte loss with subsequent load shifts to remaining contractile cells further perpetuates the cycle by leading to greater myocyte depletion and more cell death.

CARDIAC REMODELING

The hallmarks of cardiac remodeling (Fig. 4–4) are myocyte hypertrophy and cardiac dilation with increased interstitial matrix formation, which begins as a compensatory mechanism to maintain contractile power and preserve wall stress.[41] As myocardial degeneration progresses, this process becomes maladaptive and contributes to worsening heart failure.[38, 45]

From a morphologic standpoint, myocardial hypertrophy is caused by increased numbers of myofibrils and mitochondria as well as by enlargement of existing mitochondria and the cell nucleus. Increases in intracellular disorganization can be noted and characterized by loss of contractile elements, disruption of Z bands, interruption of the parallel arrangement of sarcomeres, and fibrous tissue infiltration. Depending upon the type of stimulus, ventricular remodeling can occur in two general fashions best characterized by the differences seen in the myocardium of patients with heart failure due to pressure overload compared with that of patients with volume overload states. Parallel sarcomere development and hypertrophy create concentric ventricular remodeling, with mass increasing greater than volume. Sarcomere hypertrophy in series leads to eccentric remodeling, with volume change greater than mass increase. In both situations, however, compensatory hypertrophy develops in an attempt to maintain wall stress within normal calculated levels. Thus, heart failure seen in a setting of hypertension (pressure overload) is characterized by a small left ventricular chamber dimension with significant left ventricular muscle growth and hypertrophy in which diastolic dysfunction or left ventricular cavity filling abnormalities predominate over reduced systolic performance. Eccentric left ventricular hypertrophy characterizes volume overload states seen with significant mitral insufficiency or aortic regurgitation where ventricular dilation is the predominant observation. Myocardial hypertrophy and dilation increase wall stress significantly. Since wall stress is the major determinant of myocardial oxygen demand, cell energetics is affected and gradually impaired. Indeed, ventricular hypertrophy in itself will contribute to myocardial blood flow diminution.

THE CARDIAC INTERSTITIUM

Though it is important to focus on the myocyte during cardiac injury and development of failure, the cardiac interstitium is also extraordinarily sensitive to the same mechanical, inflammatory, neurohumoral, and hormonal mediators of myocyte growth described above.[10, 126] Furthermore, cardiac interstitial matrix changes will affect both systolic and diastolic properties of the heart (Fig. 4–4). The interstitium is composed primarily of collagen, elastin, glycoproteins, adrenergic nerve endings, blood and lymph vessels, mesenchymal cells, fibroblasts, pericytes, macrophages, and fluid that is an ultrafiltrate of plasma. Fibroblasts appear in the cardiac interstitium more intensely during wound healing and precipitate fibrogenesis and remodeling of noncellular matrix. A low-grade ongoing interstitial inflammatory process is likely constant in the heart and reflects a process of normal cardiac repair and maintenance. By its very nature, the myocardial interstitial matrix is resistant to stretch during diastole and therefore contributes to limitations with respect to ventricular dilatation, and this effect is responsible for pathologic stiffness associated with diastolic dysfunction. Reciprocal regulation of collagen turnover in cardiovascular tissue exists with **stimulators of fibrosis,** including angiotensin II, TGF-β, and endothelin-1 and -3. **Inhibitors of fibrosis** include bradykinin, prostaglandins, and nitric oxide. When stimulated, the interstitial matrix response is to increase collagen synthesis, reduce collagenase activity, and stiffen the entire matrix, leading to pathologic degrees of dysfunction.

MYOCYTE MEMBRANE RECEPTOR RESPONSES

Membrane receptors responsible for modulating intracellular calcium release and uptake include adrenergic receptor systems made up of alpha and beta units. As part of the cardiac response to injury, membrane receptors likely are significantly altered in both concentration and function (Fig. 4–3).[9] Like any of the other cellular elements, membrane receptors both internally and externally are regulated with respect to density and function by cellular molecular events. Adrenergic receptors elicit intracellular activities that are either antagonistic or additive to the activity of other receptors. Furthermore, the effects of alpha- and beta-adrenergic receptors are such that they must be reviewed in conjunction with their effects on the peripheral circulation, which will be discussed subsequently.

Alpha-Adrenergic Receptors

The autonomic nervous system alters the contractile state of the heart by stimulating specific receptors, which produce alterations in the influx of calcium and other ions. Although present in cardiac tissue, alpha-adrenergic receptors play a greater role in regulating vascular tone through alterations in calcium flux in vascular smooth muscle. In cardiac myocytes, alpha-adrenergic receptors stimulated by norepinephrine induce growth of cardiac myocytes[101] and the reappearance of fetal isoforms of contractile proteins.[89] Though there are several categories of alpha-adrenergic receptors, only alpha₁-receptors demonstrate significant myocardial density. These receptors modulate change in intracellular cytoplasmic calcium concentration that affects several important functions. Stimulation of alpha-1-adrenergic receptor pathways modulates heart rate (intrinsic rate of electrical depolarization), myocardial contractility, passive and active wall tension, as well as peripheral vascular resistance. The density of alpha-1 receptors increases modestly in settings of heart failure, and it has been hypothesized that this eventually leads to greater myocardial hypertrophy and growth. Stimulation of alpha-1-receptors also can increase cardiac dysrhythmias.

Beta-Adrenergic Receptors

Cardiac beta-adrenergic receptors may be of subtype beta₁ or beta₂, but the majority are beta₁. Beta₁ receptors constitute about 80% of the beta receptors in the left ventricle and about 60% in the atria.[9] In the peripheral circulation, most noncardiac receptors are beta₂ subtype. When a beta-adrenergic receptor is occupied by an agonist (such as norepinephrine or epinephrine), a G-protein complex, is required to convert the neurostimulus to the intracellular changes necessary for augmented contractility (a process referred to as signal transduction).[5, 85] G proteins consist of a superfamily of proteins that bind to guanine triphosphate, which is necessary for the activation of adenylyl cyclase in the sarcolemma.[35, 85] The combination of the beta receptor, the G-protein complex and adenylyl cyclase is called the beta-adrenergic system.[114] Adenylyl cyclase produces cyclic adenosine monophosphate (cAMP) which acts through a messenger protein called kinase-A to increase inward movement of calcium through the sarcolemma of the T-tubule. The beta-adrenergic system plays a critical role in modulating inotropic, chronotropic, and lusitropic (diastolic relaxation) activities. It appears that in the heart failure setting, selective down-regulation (decrease in beta receptor density) of beta₁-adrenergic receptor subtypes is noted without much change in beta₂ subtypes. This down-regulation of beta₁-adrenergic receptors alters the beta₁ and beta₂ subtype population, which may have implications with respect to drug selec-

tion (e.g., selective vs. nonselective beta-adrenergic receptor blocking drugs) when treating patients with heart failure.[37] Another mechanism of decreased beta-adrenergic responsiveness may result from increased expression of beta-adrenergic receptor kinase (BARK), an enzyme that phosphorylates beta-adrenergic receptors and thereby contributes to their uncoupling from the G-protein–cyclase complex[122] (Fig. 4–3).

CIRCULATORY RESPONSE TO HEART FAILURE

Myocardial injury with compensatory remodeling alters ventricular function by impairing contractility and relaxation (Figs. 4–4 and 4–5). The systemic circulatory response to heart failure occurs primarily as a result of inadequate cardiac output and elevated atrial pressures. This can range from subtle perturbation to dramatic and clinically overt low-stroke-volume and low-output states with subsequent systemic congestion. A wide range of mitigating circumstances will influence each individual's presentation, depending on the principal location of injury, predominance of diastolic versus systolic dysfunction, circulatory system integrity, aerobic cardiovascular conditioning, and treatment used. Whatever the mode of presentation, an essential element of the heart failure syndrome is the reduction in stroke volume which triggers subsequent peripheral flow derangement (Fig. 4–6). It is the **peripheral flow derangement** which is largely responsible for altering normal neurohormonal circulatory homeostasis. When flows are altered, tissue perfusion homeostasis is maintained by a variety of vasodilating and vasoconstrictor responses. A complicated positive- and negative-feedback loop interaction occurs between peripheral baroreceptors in the vascular network, the central nervous system, and solid organs such as the kidney. The autonomic nervous system is largely responsible for much of this flow control. Autonomic balance is coordinated by afferent nervous system signaling from peripheral baroreceptors located in the heart, lungs, and great vessels.

CHEMORECEPTOR AND BARORECEPTOR RESPONSES

Chemoreceptors located in the carotid bodies, in the skeletal muscle, as well as in the skin and other visceral organs sense oxygen saturation, carbon dioxide levels, and acid–base balance; and contribute to afferent signaling. Cardiopulmonary baroreceptors in heart and pulmonary vasculature as well as in the aortic arch and carotid sinus produce afferent neurosignaling to the central nervous system via the vagus and glossopharyngeal nerves. Normally, activation of these systems signals the sympathetic outpouring to be decreased and parasympathetic central nervous system efferent activity increased (Fig. 4–6).

It is this baroreceptor activity that principally modulates nervous system tone during changes in intravascular volume or pressure. When volume depletion or hypotension is sensed by these receptors, decreased receptor stimulation effected by reduced arterial wall stretch reduces afferent signaling, thereby decreasing parasympathetic activity and increasing sympathetic stimulation. This is associated with an increase in epinephrine and norepinephrine release with subsequent vasoconstriction and positive inotropic and chronotropic effects.

When the circulatory derangements of heart failure persist, the baroreceptor response becomes dysfunctional, accounting for the increased sympathetic and reduced parasympathetic nervous system activity, which is exacerbated by a decrease in efferent inhibitory input. This is manifested by increased venous and arterial tone, higher systemic vascular resistances, increased resting heart rates, and decreased electrocardiographic R-R interval variability (a surrogate marker of parasympathetic tone). Baroreceptor function also stimulates midbrain vasopressin release, with its subsequent stimulation of renal renin secretion.

NEUROHORMONAL CONTRIBUTIONS TO CIRCULATORY DYSFUNCTION

The term *neurohormonal* reflects previous observations that many molecules identified in the heart failure syndrome were elaborated by the neuroendocrine system and acted on the heart in an endocrine fashion.[75] However, it is now known that certain of the neurohomonal factors such as norepinephrine and angiotensin II are also synthesized within the heart and act in an autocrine or paracrine fashion. In addition, molecules such as angiotensin II and endothelin are peptide growth factors which are also produced directly by myocytes. Though peripheral blood flow is largely determined by interactions between sympathethic efferent nerve signaling, several autoregulatory systems are also active and important in the peripheral circulation. The vasoconstricting systems which can increase afterload include the sympathetic nervous system, the renin-angiotensin-aldosterone system, arginine vasopressin, and endothelin. Vasodilating systems are stimulated by atrial natriuretic factors, kallikrein-kinin systems, vasodilating prostaglandin, and endothelial-derived relaxing factor (Table 4–10). These various feedback loops are stimulated or inhibited by varying degrees of vasoconstriction or vasodilation sensed locally. The important concept of the neurohormonal contribution to heart failure is that many humoral factors may interact with one another in a variety of positive and negative feedback loops which begins long before clinical heart failure symptoms are present as a compensatory mechanism to support organ perfusion in the presence of cardiac dysfunction. Eventually, these compensatory adaptations become maladaptive, promoting progression of the heart failure syndrome.

Sympathetic Nervous System

Systemic circulatory regulation is largely the result of the sympathetic nerve terminal with neurotransmitter release occurring at the sympathetic neuroeffector junction. This is modulated by a variety of hormones and other substances acting on receptors located at the presynaptic nerve ending. Prostanoids, purines, histamines, 5-hydroxytryptamine, atrial natriuretic factor, dopamine, and acetylcholine inhibit norepinephrine release, whereas epinephrine and angiotensin II increase norepinephrine release from the neuroeffector junction.

Though the "intent" of activation of the sympathetic nervous system is maintenance of vital organ perfusion, the ultimate result is worsening of cardiac pump performance and deterioration of the circulatory state. Activation of the sympathetic nervous system is intertwined with multiple other components of the neurohormonal system. Elevated levels of norepinephrine reduce the sensitivity of arterial and cardiopulmonary baroreceptors (which normally act to counterregulate increased sympathetic tone).

As heart failure develops, there is a general increase in sympathetic activation and decrease in parasympathetic activation.[21, 119, 124] During the initial stages of heart failure, stimulation of the sympathetic limb of the autonomic system and activation of the renin-angiotensin system (see below) is compensatory in nature, acting to

---

TABLE 4–10   Humoral Factors in Heart Failure Important in Regulation of Vascular Circulation

VASOCONSTRICTING/VASODILATING FACTORS

Vasoconstricting factors (primarily antinatriuretic and may stimulate/accelerate myocyte growth/hypertrophy)
    Renin-angiotensin-aldosterone
    Epinephrine-norepinephrine
    Neuropeptide Y
    Vasopressin
    Endothelin
    Thromboxane
Vasodilating factors (largely natriuretic and may inhibit/reverse myocyte growth/hypertrophy)
    Prostaglandin
    Natriuretic peptides
    Kinins
    Nitric oxide (endothelium-derived relaxing factor)
    Vasoactive intestinal peptide
    Calcitonin gene-related peptide
    Substance P
    Endorphins

increase perfusion pressure to vital organs and expand the generally inadequate arterial blood volume. Eventually, these **"compensatory" mechanisms become deleterious** and exacerbate the heart failure syndrome by promoting vasoconstriction, increasing cardiac afterload, decreasing arrhythmia threshold, promoting retention of salt and water, and inducing electrolyte abnormalities.

Plasma norepinephrine concentration generally reflects the activity of the sympathetic nervous system and is generally significantly elevated in patients with heart failure, even when left ventricular dysfunction is asymptomatic.[20, 23, 39] Plasma norepinephrine levels may be two to three times higher than in normal subjects,[13, 40, 119, 124] and the degree of norepinephrine level elevation correlates with the severity of heart failure as judged by ejection fraction,[119] depression of cardiac index,[40, 124] elevation of pulmonary capillary wedge pressure,[40, 124] and cardiac mortality.[21]

Prolonged stimulation of the sympathetic nervous system (with excessive norepinephrine levels) is associated with (or may induce) a progressive decrease in the density of myocardial beta-adrenergic receptors, rendering the myocardium less sensitive to adrenergic hormone stimulation.

In contrast to circulating norepinephrine levels, the concentration of norepinephrine in cardiac tissue is much lower than normal in advanced heart failure.[13, 14, 106] This may represent a depletion in norepinephrine stores in cardiac adrenergic nerve endings, perhaps due to prolonged cardiac adrenergic activation during heart failure.[25, 95]

Renin-Angiotensin-Aldosterone System

Circulating renin is primarily released from the juxtaglomerular apparatus of the kidney, which is composed of juxtaglomerular cells in the media of preglomerular afferent arterioles and the macula densa, a modified region of the tubular epithelium of the distal tubule, lying adjacent to the juxtaglomerular cells. The release of renin from the juxtaglomerular cells is responsible for the conversion of angiotensinogen to the inactive peptide angiotensin I. Angiotensin I is subsequently converted to angiotensin II by the angiotensin-converting enzyme (ACE). This reaction occurs primarily in the lungs, but systemic tissue conversion pathways are also apparent where proteases such as chymase appear responsible for producing angiotensin II in a system distinct from the angiotensin-converting enzyme dependent pathways (Fig. 4–7). Most (>90%) of angiotensin-converting enzyme in the body is actually found in tissues (including blood vessel walls, heart, and kidney) and less than 10% in the circulation.[29, 31] This tissue-renin-angiotensin system may be activated during heart failure, with increased expression of myocardial ACE.[53, 101, 111]

A number of factors are known to trigger renin release from the renal juxtaglomerular cells. These include increased renal sympathetic nervous system efferent nerve activity, decreased sodium delivery to the macula densa of the distal tubules, reduced renal perfusion pressure, and diuretic therapy. Atrial natriuretic factor, on the other hand, appears to inhibit the release of renin.

The physiologic effects of renin are mediated through angiotensin II, which is a powerful vasoconstricting agent (Table 4–11) and promotes tubular reabsorption of sodium by inducing aldosterone secretion as well as directly promoting reabsorption of salt. Angiotensin II also stimulates water intake by increasing thirst and further facilitates the release of norepinephrine by stimulating sympathetic nerve endings which, in addition to the direct vasoconstrictor action of angiotensin II, contribute to the arterial vasoconstriction of the renin-angiotensin system.

In cardiac tissue, angiotensin II induces cellular proliferation of cardiac fibroblasts in vitro that may contribute to the fibrosis that is characteristic of some forms of cardiomyopathy.[26, 78, 108] Hypertrophy of neonatal ven-

---

TABLE 4–11   Renal Effects of Neurohormonal Activation in Heart Failure

Vasoconstrictor activities
  Angiotensin II
    Efferent greater than afferent arteriolar constriction
    Enhanced sodium reabsorption in proximal tubule
    Stimulates adrenal aldosterone synthesis and release
  Aldosterone
    Enhanced sodium reabsorption with potassium secretion in collecting duct
  Arginine vasopressin
    Increased water reabsorption in medullary collecting duct
    Increased sodium chloride reabsorption in medullary ascending limb of Henle's loop

Vasodilator activities
  Natriuretic peptides
    Increase glomerular filtration rate
    Promote diminished sodium reabsorption in collecting duct
    Suppress renin activity
    Inhibit aldosterone synthesis and release
    Inhibit vasopressin release
  Renal prostaglandins
    Promote renal vasodilation
    Decrease tubular sodium reabsorption in ascending limb of Henle's loop
    Inhibit vasopressin action in collecting duct

tricular myocytes in vitro is induced by angiotensin II, possibly acting through release of norepinephrine (known to induce mild hypertrophy through stimulation of alpha-adrenergic receptors).[112, 125] In the kidney, angiotensin II induces constriction of the efferent postglomerular arterioles, which promotes an increase in filtration fraction and increased tubular solute and water reabsorption. Stimulation of the renin-angiotensin system is an early and sustained phenomenon in the development of heart failure, which acts in concert with the adrenergic neurohormonal system to maintain arterial pressure in states of reduced peripherial perfusion. In addition to plasma norepinephrine levels, renin, vasopressin, natriuretic peptide, and epinephrine levels are increased in chronic heart failure, even in relatively asymptomatic patients; and the magnitude of increase roughly correlates with the severity of heart failure.[39] Activation of the renin-angiotensin-aldosterone system is associated with hyponatremia, an unfavorable prognostic indicator in the heart failure syndrome.[29, 69]

Prostaglandin System

The heart failure syndrome also causes the kidneys to release prostacyclin and prostaglandin E_2, which are potent vasodilators (Table 4–11). With renin-angiotensin system activation, prostaglandins are also synthesized within the kidneys,[27, 83, 115] and induce vasodilatation of afferent renal arterioles.[86] This acts to increase glomerular filtration pressure and filtration fraction.[107] Other effects of prostaglandins important in heart failure include peripheral inhibition of the vasoconstrictor actions of angiotensin II,[30] inhibition of renal tubular sodium reabsorption,[16] and inhibition of vasopressin release and action in the renal collecting ducts.[4, 33] Thus, renal prostaglandins are important in the attenuation of adverse renal effects of the renin-angiotensin system.

Atrial Natriuretic Peptide Family

Atrial natriuretic peptides (ANPs) induce natriuresis (excretion of sodium), vasodilation, inhibition of renin and aldostrone, and inhibition of vascular smooth muscle proliferation (antimitogenic effects).[7] This atrial-derived peptide is a 28-residue C-terminal peptide derived from a 126-amino-acid precursor.[6] ANP interacts with two receptors, atrial natriuretic peptide receptor-A (the biologically active receptor) and atrial natriuretic peptide receptor-C (which inactivates atrial natriuretic peptide).[1, 64] Experimental studies indicate that atrial stretch is a major stimulus for secretion of ANP.[32] Another important natriuretic peptide in heart failure may be brain or B-type natriuretic peptide, which is found in atrial as well as ventricular tissue, and may be released in response to ventricular stretch.[131] A third natriuretic peptide, C-type natriuretic peptide, appears to be released from endothelial cells and causes vasodilatation and inhibits endothelin,[65] but does not induce natriuresis or attenuate activation of the renin-angiotensin system.[131] Atrial natriuretic peptides are apparently activated early in the heart failure syndrome, but once severe and chronic congestive heart failure is present the kidney appears less responsive to ANP,[17, 42, 76, 97, 113] possibly related to peptide receptor down-regulation and increased enzymatic degradation.[11, 104]

Vasopressin

Arginine vasopressin (AVP) is a potent vasoactive hormone formed by neuronal cells of the hypothalamic nuclei and stored in the posterior lobe of the pituitary gland. Its primary actions in congestive heart failure are peripheral vasoconstriction and renal water retention. The main osmotic stimulus for vasopressin release is hyponatremia. Nonosmotic stimuli include excessive diuresis, hypotension, angiotensin II, and certain baroreceptor mechanisms.[109, 110] Also called *antidiuretic hormone*, AVP plasma levels are usually elevated in patients with congestive heart failure, and the elevated levels correlate in general with clinical and hemodynamic severity of heart failure and the serum sodium level.[46, 96, 98] The physiologic effects of vasopressin are primarily mediated through vascular endothelial receptors (type 1) and renal receptors (type 2).

Endothelin

Endothelin includes a family of peptides (ET-1, ET-2, and ET-3) that possess potent vasoconstrictor properties.[56] Plasma endothelin levels are significantly elevated in patients with congestive heart failure, and higher levels have been correlated with high pulmonary pressures, elevated right atrial pressure, high pulmonary vascular resistance, worse New York Heart Association Classification, and lower left ventricular ejection fraction.[52, 77] It is likely that elevated endothelin levels represents a biologic marker for vascular damage, and endothelin itself may directly contribute to the vasoconstrictor state of heart failure. Increased plasma endothelin levels have been identified in patients with primary pulmonary hypertension, and it is a likely mediator of renal vasoconstriction. In addition, endothelin may further promote adverse effects of the heart failure syndrome by promoting smooth muscle cell growth and myocardial remodeling.

Endothelium-Derived Relaxing Factor

Endothelium-derived relaxing factor (EDRF) potentiates vasodilation via a short-acting mediator, **nitric oxide,** which induces production of cyclic guanosine monophosphate. Nitric oxide, prostaglandin E_2, and prostacyclin are major endogenous vasodilators synthesized by vascular endothelial cells, whereas endothelin and angiotensin II are major vasoconstrictors produced by vascular endothelial cells. Therefore, both nitric oxide and endothelin have a major role in the control of peripheral vasoconstriction and vasodilation. In the heart failure syndrome, regulation of endothelial-dependent vasodilatation and constriction may be altered and actually contribute to the vasoconstricted state. The actual endothelium-derived relaxant factor is nitric oxide, which is synthesized by nitric oxide synthases from the amino acid L-arginine. Nitric oxide acts to modulate the activity of endogenous vasoconstrictors, and endothelial release of nitric oxide is stimulated by the interaction of norepinephrine, vasopressin, thrombin, and endothelin with specific endothelial surface receptors.[68, 93]

Endorphins

β-Endorphin, an opiate compound primarily released from the pituitary gland, is a vasodilating factor (see Table 4–10) that is elevated in patients with congestive heart failure.[63] Opiate antagonists have been shown in animal studies to improve heart failure hemodynamics.[67, 102]

Other Peptides

Calcitonin gene-related peptides have been identified in the myocardium and vasculature as well as the peripheral nervous system.[82, 121] These peptides have been shown to induce arteriolar vasodilation, tachycardia, and exert positive inotropic effects. Levels of these peptides, however, have correlated poorly with heart failure severity.[2]

Substance P has been identified with calcitonin gene-related peptide and may also induce tachycardia and vasodilation.[44, 79]

Vasoactive intestinal peptide also possesses vasodilatory, positive chronotopic, and inotropic effects,[57] though its role in heart failure remains speculative.

PROINFLAMMATORY CYTOKINES

Recently, proinflammatory cytokines (interleukin-1, interleukin-6, and tumor necrosis factor-α [TNF-α]) have been discovered to play a significant role in patients with heart failure, particularly those with more advanced syndromes (Fig. 4–7). As congestive heart failure worsens, high systemic levels of TNF-α are common and correlate with diminished survival.[49] Furthermore, a relationship exists between other perturbed neurohormonal systems and the level of proinflammatory cytokines noted. TNF-α is a potent negative inotropic cytokine in some animal models, and it is actually produced by the myocardium as a response to increased afterload. Though initially believed important only in cardiac cachexia, it appears that cytokines play a much broader role in the pathophysiology and perpetuation of the heart failure syndrome.[70, 120]

PULMONARY RESPONSES TO HEART FAILURE

The circulatory impairment induced by heart failure produces a multitude of pulmonary abnormalities. The congestive state (chronic elevation of left atrial pressure) induces bronchial submucosal edema and reduction in small-airway caliber, producing obstructive abnormalities noted on pulmonary function testing,[129] particularly reduction in peak expiratory flow rates and forced expiratory volumes. Reduction in lung volume secondary to cardiomegaly likely produces a moderate restrictive defect with reduced vital capacity.[129] Reduction in pulmonary diffusion capacity for carbon monoxide is contributed to by alveolor and interstial edema as well as inherent membrane diffusion abnormalities which have not been completely characterized. Acute bronchospasm, sometimes called cardiac asthma, can complicate acute pulmonary edema. Abnormalities in intrinsic pulmonary gas exchange are exacerbated further by deficiencies observed in respiratory skeletal muscle function.[74] Respiratory muscle strength is reduced in patients with severely symptomatic congestive heart failure, and this correlates somewhat with their complaints of dyspnea as well as a reduction in peak exercise oxygen uptake. Furthermore, deoxygenation of respiratory muscles has been observed to occur during exercise even when significant arterial desaturation is absent, and contributes to the dyspnea and fatigue of chronic congestive heart failure. The reasons for this muscle performance–circulatory system uncoupling are not well understood. Thus, there is a multitude of intertwined abnormalities such as increased pulmonary artery and venous pressure, pulmonary vasculature edema, airway luminal narrowing, diminished lung volumes, impaired gas transfer, and respiratory muscle inadequacy that contribute to symptoms in heart failure. Further complicating these issues are pulmonary comorbid conditions such as chronic obstructive pulmonary disease, interstitial fibrosis, and pulmonary infections.

CLINICAL MANIFESTATIONS OF HEART FAILURE

The clinical manifestations of heart failure are directly linked to the degree of decompensation that occurs in the circulatory system, ultimately reflected by fluid retention and congestion and decreased cardiac output with compromised systemic organ perfusion. Fluid retention causes varying degrees of dyspnea and edema, whereas flow aberrations contribute to weakness, fatigue, and exercise limitation. Of course, no symptom should be considered in isolation. They are all interconnected and can sometimes be difficult to sort through with respect to significance and etiology. Furthermore, not all symptoms and physical findings classically associated with heart failure (e.g., dyspnea, cough, and leg edema) are always due to heart failure.

EXERCISE INTOLERANCE

Exercise places additional demands on the circulatory system, as metabolic energy requirements peripherally increase. During exercise, cardiac output demands can rise to levels 5 or 10 times those present in resting subjects. Normal subjects have a well-integrated oxygen delivery pathway which moves the substrate from the ambient air to skeletal muscle mitochondrial oxidative systems, returning quickly and efficiently carbon dioxide and acid by-products of cellular respiration to expired air or urine. The reduced exercise tolerance is primarily related to the inability of the heart to pump an adequate amount of blood peripherally; however, skeletal muscle energy substrate utilization is now known to be important as well. These peripheral systems are perturbed in patients with heart failure, and therefore it is not solely a limitation in the maximal cardiac output capacity of the heart which causes exercise intolerance in individuals with heart failure.

Additional factors contributing to exercise limitation in the heart failure patient include perturbation of respiratory muscle function, diminished oxygen diffusing capacity across the alveolar membrane, peripheral vascular changes which impair delivery of oxygenated blood to muscle, attenuated oxygen extraction by skeletal muscle, reduction in oxidative capacity of muscle mitochondria, altered extraction of lactate and carbon dioxide, as well as the general inability of patients to tolerate dyspnea signals. In stable heart failure patients there may be an uncoupling between the various measurements which are correlated with severity of heart failure (such as left ventricular ejection fraction, left ventricular dimension, and hemodynamics) and maximal oxygen uptake ($\dot{V}O_2$max). For example, some patients can achieve quite satisfactory $\dot{V}O_2$max levels despite having very low ejection fraction.

THE CONGESTIVE STATE OF HEART FAILURE

Although heart failure has usually meant congestive heart failure (accumulation of peripheral and pulmonary interstitial fluid secondary to elevated right and left atrial pressure), the heart failure syndrome is a broad spectrum ranging from patients without significant symptomatology, to those with dyspnea and fatigue, to those with cardiogenic shock and circulatory collapse. Most heart failure patients do not spend a majority of their days significantly volume overloaded. However, when volume overload does occur, it contributes to pulmonary vascular and skeletal muscle aberrations noted in more advanced syndromes. Congestion develops because the renal response to circulatory, neurohormonal, and hormonal changes triggered by heart failure signals

the kidney to retain salt and water (Table 4–11, Fig. 4–7). Both extrarenal and intrarenal mechanisms affect the kidney's ability to maintain body fluid composition and volume within tolerable ranges. Increased tubular sodium and water reabsorption and/or decreased excretion result in the salt and water retention states of severe heart failure. Vasoconstrictive neurohormonal activation processes signal the kidney to retain salt and water, and this appears to be mediated by cardiac and vascular baroreceptors with stimulation of the sympathetic nervous system, which in turn leads to activation of the renin-angiotensin-aldosterone cascade and release of vasopressin as a response to dimishing organ perfusion and blood pressure. Vasodilator actions of prostaglandins and various natriuretic peptides are responsible for ameliorating some of these adverse effects. Administration of diuretics, vasodilating drugs, and neurohormonal blocking agents will all affect the degree of salt and water retention occurring at any given time in any specific patient. In the more advanced stages of heart failure, the renal effects of neurohormonal activation ultimately result in hypervolemia; hyponatremia; and disordered magnesium, potassium, and chloride handling.

PROGRESSION TO ADVANCED OR END-STAGE HEART FAILURE

Figure 4–14 plots linearized mortality event curves for placebo groups in several mortality endpoint clinical trials. They demonstrate that different cohorts of heart failure patients have vastly different prognoses. This is important in understanding the characteristics which delineate more advanced stages of heart failure (Fig. 4–8). Individuals with refractory heart failure are those in whom the syndrome has relentlessly progressed with worsening symptoms rooted in congestive or low-cardiac-output states that require multiple and frequently prolonged hospitalization for management of symptomatology and organ dysfunction. The clinical diagnosis of this stage of heart failure should be made only after aggressive and appropriate heart failure therapies have been begun, and particularly only in patients adequately treated with what has now become standard

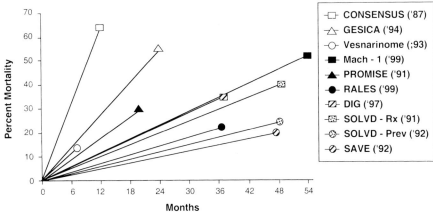

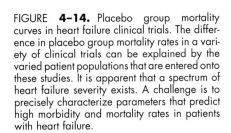

FIGURE **4-14.** Placebo group mortality curves in heart failure clinical trials. The difference in placebo group mortality rates in a variety of clinical trials can be explained by the varied patient populations that are entered onto these studies. It is apparent that a spectrum of heart failure severity exists. A challenge is to precisely characterize parameters that predict high morbidity and mortality rates in patients with heart failure.

triple therapy for congestive heart failure as detailed in Chapter 5. Mortality rates for this severely ill group are generally in the range of 50–75% at 1 year and in excess of 80–90% at 2 years.

Generally, the patient with refractory heart failure has experienced symptoms for many years and often has many comorbid conditions. As alluded to, symptoms are those characteristic of congestion with dyspnea predominating and low-output states manifest by weakness or fatigue during minimal exertion or even at rest. These individuals frequently cannot dress or shower without assistance or stopping to rest periodically. This patient population frequently is cachectic or, at the least, undernourished and has very low ejection fraction (generally <0.25), high ventricular filling pressures (resting pulmonary capillary wedge pressure generally >18 mm Hg), and cardiac index frequently less than 2 L/min/m² despite aggressive oral medication therapies. Clinical signs of congestion include elevated jugular venous pressure, pulmonary rales, positive hepatojugular reflex, peripheral edema, and ascites. Metabolic abnormalities often include hyponatremia, prerenal azotemia, or renal insufficiency, hypo- or hyperkalemia, alkalosis, and hyperuricemia. Anemia and low-grade fever not due to an obvious infection, but possibly related to cytokine production, can also be noted in these very ill patients. Chest radiography often shows profound cardiomegaly, and commonly the lung fields are congested with pleural effusions or fluid in fissures. The electrocardiogram is frequently characterized by low voltage, multiple Q waves, interventricular conduction disorders, and atrial or ventricular arrhythmias. Metabolic exercise testing, if it can be performed, rarely results in $\dot{V}O_2$max greater than 10 or 12 mL O_2/kg/min after the patient has reached anaerobic threshold (see further discussion in Chapter 6). Chronotropic incompetence (the inability to increase heart rate with exercise) and lack of a normal rise in blood pressure with exercise are also frequently noted.

DEATH OF PATIENTS WITH HEART FAILURE

Patients with heart failure die, most often, of progressive multiorgan failure that develops because of the relative energy starvation in peripheral vital organs. The circulatory system's inability to maintain appropriate energy supply is the primary cause of renal insufficiency and failure. Organ congestion impairs normal cellular respiration and function as well. Intercurrent events, such as new myocardial infarction, stroke, or peripheral embolism (both to the pulmonary and central arterial circuits) can cause death. As the heart failure syndrome progresses and worsens, these events are more likely to occur.

On the other hand, patients with heart failure also frequently die suddenly, presumably due to ventricular tachycardia or ventricular fibrillation. In addition to the morphologic remodeling characteristic of heart failure, "electrical remodeling" occurs as well. This predisposes the heart to malignant arrhythmias. Interestingly, the proportion of patients dying of sudden cardiac death is greater when compensated congestive heart failure is present. Importantly, data suggest that a substantial number of, but not all, sudden deaths result from ventricular tachycardia/fibrillation. There are other causes of sudden cardiac death (electromechanical dissociation, sinus bracycardia, atrioventricular heart block, ruptured aortic aneurysm, massive pulmonary embolus, intracranial hemorrhage or embolus), but malignant ventricular arrhythmias likely account for the majority of episodes. Little is actually known about the factors that destabilize repolarization in heart failure patients, setting the stage for malignant ventricular arrhythmias, but certainly abnormalities developing in the membrane ion channels, potassium currents, sodium-potassium exchange systems, and the sarcoplasmic uptake mechanism for calcium are at play. Other factors are also likely important, including those associated with dilation and stretch of the myocardium and interstitial fibrosis. Additionally, hypokalemia due to diuretics, hypomagnesemia, digoxin toxicity, and proarrhythmic effects of antiarrhythmic agents can all set the stage for arrhythmia and sudden death in patients with heart failure.

DIAGNOSIS AND EVALUATION OF PATIENTS WITH HEART FAILURE

As mentioned above, individuals with heart failure can have a wide spectrum of presentations that are largely based on the predominance of systolic and/or diastolic dysfunction and selective cardiac chamber enlargement which may induce or be caused by cardiac valve dysfunction. Diagnostic evaluation must consider the individual diseases that precipitate abnormal chamber filling or emptying. The heart failure severity must be assessed and factors identified that precipitate clinical decompensation, which is usually manifest by fluid retention and volume overload. These principles are particularly important in the patient with more advanced heart failure, especially in those considered for more aggressive therapy such as cardiac transplantation. Still, it is important to remember that not all dropsical patients have heart failure, and complaints of dyspnea should not automatically point towards cardiac dysfunction. These issues can be distilled into several critical questions to ask whenever the diagnosis of heart failure is considered: (1) Is myocardial or circulatory failure actually present? (2) What caused the problem in the first place? (3) What precipitated the exacerbation of the present symptoms? (4) What is the patient's prognosis? (5) Can symptoms be ameliorated or eliminated? (6) What can be done to address the underlying etiology? (7) Can progression of the syndrome be halted? Selection of patients for cardiac transplantation (as well as all therapeutic options) is intimately linked to answers to these questions.

The Agency for Health Care Policy and Research (AHCPR) diagnostic algorithm for evaluating heart failure patients, the first consensus report emerging regarding heart failure, focuses on symptomatic patients with stable, generally compensated, congestive heart failure not requiring hospitalization, but it provides the essential elements of heart failure diagnosis and some reasonable recommendations regarding treatment, though new data have subsequently emerged regarding several important strategies. The AHCPR diagnostic algorithm (Fig. 4–15) suggests specific and objective evaluation of all patients with complaints that could possibly relate to congestive heart failure such as paroxysmal nocturnal dyspnea, orthopnea, dyspnea on exertion, lower extremity edema, decreased exercise tolerance, unexplained

confusion, altered mental status, nonspecific fatigue in an elderly patient, and gastrointestinal symptoms that might relate to mesenteric congestion (nausea, abdominal pain, bloating, and ascites).[130, 131]

Important physical findings that suggest cardiomegaly and central vascular volume overload include an elevated jugular venous pressure, positive abdominal jugular reflex, a third heart sound, a laterally displaced apical cardiac impulse, pulmonary rales not clearing

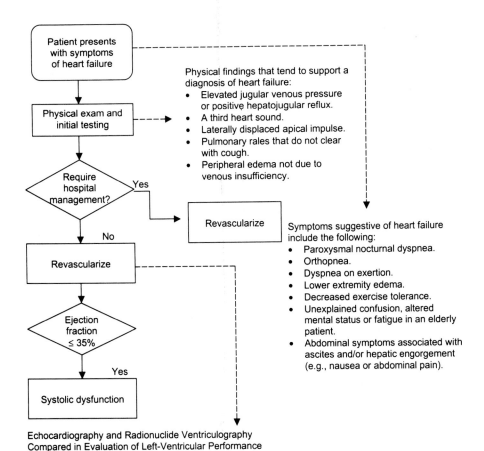

Echocardiography and Radionuclide Ventriculography Compared in Evaluation of Left-Ventricular Performance

Test	Advantages	Disadvantages
Echocardiogram	Permits concomitant assessment of valvular disease, left-ventricular hypertrophy, and left-atrial size Less expensive than radionuclide ventriculography in most areas Able to detect pericardial effusion and ventricular thrombus More generally available	Difficult to perform in patients with lung disease Usually only semi-quantitative estimate of ejection fraction provided Technically inadequate in up to 18% of patients under optimal circumstances
Radionuclide ventriculogram	More precise and reliable measurement of ejection fraction Better assessment of right-ventricular function	Requires venipuncture and radiation exposure Limited assessment of valvular heart disease and left-ventricular hypertrophy

FIGURE 4–15. Agency for Health Care Policy and Research (AHCPR) guideline for the diagnosis of heart failure. The AHCPR guideline for the diagnosis and treatment of heart failure was the first consensus document to emerge regarding this malady and stressed the importance of relating symptoms of dyspnea, weakness, and fatigue to left ventricular dysfunction. The guideline focused on stable outpatients with heart failure due to systolic left ventricular dysfunction. The diagnosis algorithm stressed the importance of determining the ejection fraction in heart failure patients and attempting to identify treatable ischemic heart conditions.

with cough, and peripheral edema not due to venous insufficiency. Findings suggestive of congestive heart failure should prompt determination of left ventricular function (usually by echocardiographic or radionuclide ventriculographic study) in order to quantify the degree of systolic left ventricular dysfunction and differentiate between diastolic and systolic components of the syndrome. Echocardiography is advantageous because it allows concomitant assessment of valvular heart disease, ventricular hypertrophy, and cardiac chamber dimension, as well as giving insight into diastolic dysfunction (abnormal ventricular filling patterns), particularly when Doppler echocardiographic techniques are utilized. Echocardiography is also generally less expensive, less complex to perform, and more readily available than radionuclide ventriculography. Ancillary studies that should be done include electrocardiography, a complete blood count, serum electrolytes, urinalysis, characterization of hepatic and renal function, serum albumin, and thyroid function tests.

Though there is not a consensus, it is likely prudent to perform echocardiography in every patient suffering an acute myocardial infarction or with a history of prior myocardial infarction. Additionally, elderly patients with chronic hypertension, prior coronary bypass graft surgery, or percutaneous coronary interventions, particularly in the setting of comorbid conditions such as diabetes mellitus or peripheral vascular disease, should have echocardiography performed at some intermittent screening interval. This approach is quite different than prior methods of diagnosing heart failure, which related

complaints of dyspnea, orthopnea, and paroxysmal nocturnal dyspnea to a history of edema and to physical findings of pulmonary rales, a third heart sound, jugular venous distention, and pedal edema. Table 4–12 delineates diagnostic criteria used in the Framingham Heart Study, The Study of Men Born in 1913, and the Boston Heart Failure Scale, which all employed, to a greater or lesser extent, these more traditional heart failure signs and symptoms as criteria to diagnose congestive heart failure.[80] Patients with these complaints and findings will often have congestive heart failure, but these criteria miss the larger cohort of individuals with asymptomatic, or minimally symptomatic, ventricular dysfunction who are euvolemic. Indeed, the positive predictive value of paroxysmal nocturnal dyspnea, orthopnea, or history of edema with respect to a diagnosis of heart failure defined as a left ventricular ejection fraction below 0.50 is quite low.

There are certain ancillary putative prognostic factors that help diagnose and characterize the condition. Particularly important are factors predicting higher morbidity and mortality.[80] Findings associated with more severe forms of heart failure are listed in Table 4–13. However, by utilizing the current operational definition of heart failure, which is vastly more encompassing than the congestive state characterized by the three scales listed in Table 4–12, we can better couple treatment recommendations to appropriate clinical cohorts. Still, it is important to focus on the more advanced stages of congestive heart failure when considering cardiac transplantation as therapy.

TABLE 4–12   Criteria for Diagnosing Heart Failure in Early Studies

THE FRAMINGHAM HEART STUDY	THE STUDY OF MEN BORN IN 1913	THE "BOSTON SCALE" CRITERIA
Major criteria	**Cardiac scores**	**Category I: history**
• Paroxysmal nocturnal dyspnea	• Heart disease	• Rest dyspnea (4 points)
• Neck vein distention	• Angina pectoris	• Orthopnea (4 points)
• Rales	• Swollen legs (evenings)	• Paroxysmal nocturnal dyspnea (3 points)
• Cardiomegaly	• Dyspnea at night	• Dyspnea on walking on level (2 points)
• Acute pulmonary edema	• Rales	• Dyspnea on climbing (1 point)
• S3 gallop	• Atrial fibrillation	**Category II: physical examination**
• Increased venous pressure (≥16 cm H₂O)	**Pulmonary scores**	• Heart rate: 91–110 (1 point); >110 (2 points)
• Circulation time ≥ 25 sec	• Bronchitis/asthma	• Jugular venous pressure elevation (if > 6 cm H₂O, 2 points; if > 6 cm H₂O plus hepatomegaly or leg edema, 3 points).
• Hepatojugular reflux positive	• Cough, phlegm, wheezing	• Lung rales—basilar (1 point); more than basilar (2 points)
Minor criteria	• Rhonchi	• Wheezing (3 points)
• Ankle edema	**Stages of CHF**	• Third heart sounds (3 points)
• Night cough	1. Cardiac score only	**Category III: chest radiography**
• Hepatomegaly	2. Cardiac score and dyspnea or cardiac score and treatment for CHF	• Alveolar pulmonary edema (4 points)
• Pleural effusion	3. Cardiac score, dyspnea, and treatment for CHF	• Interstitial pulmonary edema (3 points)
• Vital capacity reduced by 1/3 from predicted		• Bilateral pleural effusion (3 points)
• Tachycardia (≥120)		• Cardiothoracic ratio ≥ (3 points)
• Weight loss of more than 4.5 kg over 5 days in response to treatment with diuretic		• Upper zone flow redistribution (2 points) (Point value within parentheses and no more than 4 points from each category allowed. Hence a maximum possible of 12 points).
Definite CHF: 2 major criteria or 1 major and 2 minor criteria		"Definite" CHF: 8–12 points "Possible" CHF: 5–7 points

From Mills RM, Young JB: Practical Approaches to the Treatment of Heart Failure. Baltimore: Williams & Wilkins, 1998, with permission.

TABLE 4–13	Putative Prognostic Factors in Heart Failure: Predicting Adverse Events (Observations)

Demographic
  Male sex
  Older age
  Black race
Etiology
  Coronary artery disease
  Multiple prior myocardial infarctions
History/symptoms
  NYHA Class III/IV
  Length of symptoms
  Comorbid diseases such as diabetes and COPD
  Syncope
  Permanent pacer need
Physical Exam
  Resting tachycardia
  Persistent S3
  Hypotension
  Insidious/subtle signs of shock
  Refracting volume overload
  Ascites
  Cachexia
Elevated proinflammatory crystallines
  Tumor necrosis factor
  Interleukin-1 and -6
Hemodynamics
  Elevated right atrial, pulmonary artery, pulmonary wedge, left ventricular end-diastolic pressures
  Low cardiac output/index
  Reduced left ventricular stroke-work index
  Flat cardiac output despite elevated filling pressure with exercise
  Inappropriate tachycardia
  Fall of systolic blood pressure during exercise
  Exercise-induced arrhythmias

Chest Radiograph
  Cardiothoracic ratio
  Persistent pleural effusion
  Obstructive pulmonary disease
Electrocardiography
  Atrial fibrillation
  LBBB/IVCD
  Sustained/nonsustained ventricular tachycardia
  Trifascicular heart block
  Low QRS voltage
  Electrical alternans
  Extensive Q-wave formation
  Late SAECG depolarizations
Biochemistry profile
  Hyponatremia
  Azotemia
  Elevated serum creatinine
  Hypomagnesemia
Elevated neurohormones
  Renin
  Norepinephrine
  Epinephrine
  Aldosterone
  Natriuretic peptides
Echocardiogram/radionuclide ventriculogram
  Increased diastolic volume
  Ventricular hypertrophy
  Segmental wall motion abnormalities
  Severity of mitral regurgitation
  Left and right ventricular ejection fraction
  Abnormal left ventricular filling dynamics
Cardiopulmonary exercise testing
  Peak $\dot{V}O_2$ below 15 mL O_2/kg/min
  Peak $\dot{V}O_2$ less than 50% predicted
  Chronotropic incompetence

COPD, chronic obstructive pulmonary disease; LBBB, left bundle branch block; IVCD, interventricular conduction delay; SAECG, signal average electrocardiogram.

References

1. Almeida FA, Suszuki M, Scarborough RM, Lewicki JA, Maack T: Clearance function of type C receptors of atrial natriuretic factor in rats. Am J Physiol 1989;256:R469–R475.

2. Anand IS, Gardner J, Wander GS, O'Gara P, Harding SE, Ferrari R, Cornacchiari A, Panzall A, Wahi PL, Poole-Wilson PA: Cardiovascular and hormonal effects of calcitonin gene-related peptide in congestive heart failure. J Am Coll Cardiol 1991;17:208–217.

3. Beltrami CA, Finato M, Rocco M, Geruglio GA, Puricelli C, Cigola E, Sonnenblick EH, Olivetti G, Anversa P: The cellular basis of dilated cardiomyopathy in humans. J Mol Cell Cardiol 1995; 27:291–305.

4. Berl T, Raz A, Wald H, Horowitz J, Czaczkes W: Prostaglandin synthesis inhibition and the action of vasopressin: studies in man and rat. Am J Physiol 1977;232:F529–F537.

5. Berridge MJ: Inositol trisphosphate and calcium signalling. Nature 1993;361:315–325.

6. Bloch KD, Zisfein JB, Margolies MN, Homcy CJ, Seidman JG, Graham RM: A serum protease cleaves proANF into a 14-kilodalton peptide and ANF. Am J Physiol 1987;252:E147–E151.

7. Brandt RR, Wright RS, Redfield MM, Burnett JC: Atrial natriuretic peptide in heart failure. J Am Coll Cardiol 1993;22:86A–92A.

8. Bristow MR: Changes in myocardial and vascular receptors in heart failure. J Am Coll Cardiol 1993;22(supppl A):61A–71A.

9. Bristow MR, Hershberger RE, Port JD, Rasmussen R: Beta$_1$ and beta$_2$ adrenergic receptor-mediated adenylate cyclase stimulation in nonfailing and failing human ventricular myocardium. Mol Pharmacol 1989;35:295–303.

10. Brooks W, Bing OHL, Robinson KG, Slawsky MT, Chaletsky DM, Conrad CH: The effect of angiotensin-converting enzyme inhibition on myocardial fibrosis and function and hypertrophy to the failing myocardium from the spontaneously hypertensive rat. Circulation 1997;96:4002–4010.

11. Cavero PG, Margulies KB, Winaver J, Seymour AA, Deameu MG, Birmett KC: Cardiorenal actions of neutral endopeptidase inhibition in experimental congestive heart failure. Circulation 1990;82:196–201.

12. Chatterjee K: Heart failure therapy and evolution. Circulation 1996;94:2689–2693.

13. Chidsey CA, Braunwald E, Morrow AG: Catecholamine cretion and cardiac stores of norepinephrine in congestive heart failure. Am J Med 1965;39:442.

14. Chidsey CA, Sonnenblick EH, Morrow AG, Braunwald E: Norepinephrine stores and contractile force of papillary muscle from the failing human heart. Circulation 1966;33:34.

15. Chien KR, Knowlton KU, Zhu H, Chien S: Regulation of cardiac gene during myocardial growth and hypertrophy: molecular studies of an adaptaive physiologic response. FASEB J 1991; 5:3037–3046.

16. Chien KR, Zhu H, Knowlton KU, Miller-Hance W, van-Blisen M, O'Brien TX, Evans SM: Transcriptional regulation during cardiac growth and development. Annu Rev Physiol 1993;55:77–95.

17. Cody RJ, Atlas SA, Laragh JH, Kubo SH, Covit AB, Ryman KS, Shaknovich A, Pondolfino K, Clark M, Camargo MJF, Scaraborough RM, Lewicki JA: Atrial natriuretic factor in normal subjects and heart failure patients. Plasma levels and renal, hormonal, and hemodynamic responses to peptide infusion. J Clin Invest 1986;78:1362–1374.

18. Cohn JN: Structural basis for heart failure: ventricular remodeling and its pharmacological inhibition. Circulation 1995;91:2504–2507.

19. Cohn JN: The management of chronic heart failure. N Engl J Med 1996;335:490–498.

20. Cohn JN, Johnson G, Ziesche S, Cobb F, Francis G, Tristani F, Smith R, Dunkman WB, Loeb H, Wong M, Bhat G, Goldman S, Fletcher RD, Doherty J, Hughes CV, Carson P, Cintron G, Shabetai

R, Haakenson C: A comparison of enalapril with hydralazine-isosorbide dinitrate in the treatment of chronic congestive heart failure. N Engl J Med 1991;325:303–310.

21. Cohn JN, Levine TB, Olivari MT, Garberg V, Lura D, Francis GS, Simon AB, Rector T: Plasma norepinephrine as a guide to prognosis in patients with chronic congestive heart failure. N Engl J Med 1984;311:819.

22. Colucci WS: Apoptosis in the heart. N Engl J Med 1996;335:1224–1226.

23. CONSENSUS Trial Study Group: Effects of enalapril on mortality in severe congestive heart failure. N Engl J Med 1987;316:1429–1435.

24. Corvisart-Desmartes JN: Essay on the Organic Diseases of the Heart. Paris: N.P., 1812.

25. Covell JW, Chidsey CA, Braunwald E: Reduction of the cardiac response to postganglionic sympathetic nerve stimulation in perimental heart failure. Circ Res 1966;19:51.

26. Crabos M, Roth M, Hahn AWA, Erne P: Characterization tensin II receptors in cultured adult rat cardiac fibroblasts: co-signaling systems and gene expression. J Clin Invest 1994;93:2372.

27. DeForrest JH, David JO, Freeman RH, Seymour AA, Rowe BP, Williams GM, Davis TP: Effects of indomethacin and meclofenamate on renin release and renal hemodynamic function during chronic sodium depletion in conscious dogs. Circ Res 1980;47:99–107.

28. Drexler H, Hasenfuss G, Holubarsch C: Signaling pathways in failing human heart muscle cells. Trends Cardiovasc Med 1997;77:151–160.

29. Dzau VJ: Tissue renin-angiotensin system in myocardial hypertrophy and failure. Arch Intern Med 1993;153:937.

30. Dzau VJ, Packer M, Lilly LS, Swartz SL, Hollenberg NK, Williams GH: Parostaglandins in severe congestive heart failure: relation to activation of the renin-angiotensin system and hyponatremia. N Engl J Med 1984;310:347–352.

31. Dzau VJ, Re R: Tissue angiotensin system in cardiovascular medicine. A paradigm shift? Circulation 1994;89:493.

32. Edwards BS, Zimmerman RS, Schwab TR, Heublein DM, Burnett JC Jr: Atrial stretch, not pressure, is the principal determinant controlling the acute release of atrial natriuretic factor. Circ Res 1988;62:191–195.

33. Fejes-Toth G, Magyar A, Walter J: Renal response to vasopressin after inhibition of prostaglandin synthesis. Am J Physiol 1977;232:F416–F423.

34. Fishberg A: Heart Disease. Philadelphia: Lea & Febiger, 1937.

35. Fleming JW, Wisler PL, Watanabe AM: Signal transduction by G-proteins in cardiac tissues. Circulation 1992;85:420–433.

36. Flint A: A Treatise on the Principles and Practice of Medicine. 4th ed. Philadelphia: Lea, 1873.

37. Fowler MD, Laser JA, Hopkins GL, Minobe W, Bristow MR: Assessment of the beta adrenergic receptor pathway of the intact failing human heart: progressive receptor downregulation and sub-sensitivity to agonist response. Circulation 1986;74:1290–1302.

38. Francis GS: Changing the remodeling process in heart failure: basic mechanisms and laboratory results. Curr Opin Cardiol 1998;13:156–161.

39. Francis GS, Benedict C, Johnstone DE, Kirlin PC, Nicklas J, Liang C, Kubo SH, Rudin-Toretsky E, Yusuf S, SOLVD Investigators: Comparison of neuroendocrine activation in patients with left ventriculr dysfunction with and without congestive heart failure. A substudy of the studies left ventricular dysfunction (SOLVD). Circulation 1990;82:1724.

40. Francis GS, Goldsmith SR, Levine TB, Olivari MT, Cohn JN: The neurohumoral axis in congestive heart failure. Ann Intern Med 1984;101:370.

41. Francis GS, McDonald KM: Left ventricular hypertrophy: an initial response to myocardial injury. Am J Cardiol 1992;69:3G–9G.

42. Freeman RH, Davis JO, Vari RC: Renal response to atrial natriuretic factor in conscious dogs with caval constriction. Am J Physiol 1985;248:R495–R500.

43. Friedberg CK: Diseases of the Heart. 2nd ed. Philadelphia: WB Saunders Company, 1956.

44. Fuller RW, Maxwell DL, Dixon DMS, McGregor GP, Barnes VF, Bloom SR, Barnes PJ: The effect of substance P on cardiovascular and respiratory function in normal subjects. J Appl Physiol 1987;62:1473–1481.

45. Gerdes AM, Kellerman SE, Moore JA, Muffly KE, Clark LC, Reaves PY, Malec KB, McKeown PP, Schocken DD: Structural remodeling of cardiac myocytes in patients with cardiac ischemic heart disease. Circulation 1992;86:426–430.

46. Goldsmith SR, Francis GS, Cowley AW Jr: Arginine vasopressin and the renal response to water loading in congestive heart failure. Am J Cardiol 1986;58:295–299.

47. Gomez AM, Valdivia HH, Cheng H, Lederer MR, Santan LF, Cannel MB, McCune SA, Altschue RA, Lederer WJ: Defective excitation-contraction coupling and experimental cardiac hypertrophy in heart failure. Science 1997;276:800–896.

48. Grossman W, Jones D, McLaurin LP: Wall stress and patterns of hypertrophy in the human left ventricle. J Clin Invest 1975;56:56–64.

49. Guillermo TA, Kapadia S, Benedict C, Oral H, Young JB, Mann DL: Proinflammatory cytokine levels in patients with depressed left ventricular ejection fraction: a report from the studies of left ventricular dysfunction (SOLVD). J Am Coll Cardiol 1996;27:1201–1206.

50. Harris CRS: The Heart and Vascular System in Ancient Greek Medicine. Oxford: University Press, 1973.

51. Hetts SW: To die or not to die? An overview of apoptosis and its role in disease. JAMA 1998;279:300–307.

52. Hiroe M, Hirata Y, Fujita N, Umezawa S, Ito H, Tsujino M, Koike A, Nogami A, Takamoto T, Marumo F: Plasma endothelin levels in idiopathic dilated cardiomyopathy. Am J Cardiol 1991;68:1114–1115.

53. Hirsch AT, Talsness CE, Schunkert H, Paul M, Dzau VJ: Tissue-specific activation of cardiac angiotensin converting enzyme in experimental heart failure. Circ Res 1991;6:475.

54. Hood WP Jr, Rackley CE, Rolett EL: Wall stress in the normal and hypertrophied human left ventricle. Am J Cardiol 1968;22:5550–5558.

55. Hurst JW, Logue RB: In Hurst WJ, Logue RB, Schlant RC, Wenger NK (eds): The Heart, Arteries, and Veins. 4th ed. New York: McGraw-Hill, 1978.

56. Inoue A, Yanagisawa M, Kumura S, Kasuya Y, Miyauchi T, Goto K, Masaki T: The human endothelin family: three structurally and pharmacologically distinct isopeptides predicted by three separate genes. Proc Natl Acad Sci U S A 1989;86:2863–2867.

57. Karasawa Y, Furikawa Y, Ren LM, Takei M, Murakami M, Naritra M, Chiba S: Cardiac response to VIP and VIPogic-cholinergic interaction in isolated dog heart preparations. Eur J Pharm 1990;187:9–17.

58. Katz AM: Evolving concepts of heart failure: cooling furnace, malfunctioning pump, enlarging muscle: part I. J Card Fail 1997;3:319–334.

59. Katz AM: Evolving concepts of heart failure: cooling furnace, malfunctioning pump, enlarging muscle: part II. J Card Fail 1998;4:67–81.

60. Katz AM: Heart Failure. Philadelphia: Lippincott Williams & Wilkins, 2000.

61. Katz AM: Is heart failure an abnormality of myocardial cell growth? Cardiology 1990;77:346–56.

62. Katz AM: Knowledge of the circulation before William Harvey. Circulation 1957;15:726–734.

63. Kawashima S, Fukutake N, Nishian K, Asakuma S, Iwasaki T: Elevated plasma beta-endorphin levels in patients with congestive heart failure. J Am Coll Cardiol 1991;17:53–58.

64. Koller KJ, Lowe DG, Bennett GL, Minamino N, Kangawa K, Matsuo H, Goeddel DV: Selective activation of the B natriuretic peptide receptor by C-type natriuretic peptide (CNP). Science 1991;252:120–1123.

65. Kohno M, Horio T, Yokokawa K, Kurihara N, Takeda T: C-type natriuretic peptide inhibits thrombin- and angiotensin II-stimulated endothelin release via cyclic guanosine 3',5'-monophosphate. Hypertension 1992;19:320–325.

66. Komuro I, Yazaki Y: Intracellular signaling pathways and cardiac myocytes induced by mechanical stress. Trends Cardiovasc Med 1994;4:117–121.

67. Liang CS, Imai N, Stone CK, Woolf PD, Kawashima S, Tuttle RR: The role of endogenous opioids in congestive heart failure:

effects of nalmefene on systemic and regional hemodynamics in dogs. Circulation 1987;75:443–451.

68. Lamas S, Marsden PA, Li GK, Tempst P, Michel T: Endothelial nitric oxide synthase: molecular cloning and characterization of a distinct constitutive enzyme isoform. Proc Natl Acad Sci U S A 1992;89:6348–6352.

69. Lee WH, Packer M: Prognostic importance of serum sodium concentration and its modification by converting-enzyme inhibition in patients with severe chronic heart failure. Circulation 1986;73:257–267.

70. Levine B, Kalman J, Mayer L, Fillit HM, Packer M: Elevated circulating levels of tumor necrosis factor in severe chronic heart failure. N Engl J Med 1990;323:236–241.

71. Lovell BH: Transition from hypertrophy to failure. Circulation 1997;96:3825–3827.

72. Lowes BD, Minobe W, Abraham WT, Rizeq MN, Bohlmeyer TJ, Quaife RA, Roden RL, Dutcher DL, Robertson AD, Voelkel NF, Badesch DB, Groves BM, Gilbert EM, Bristow MR: Changes in gene expression in the intact human heart: down-regulation of alpha myocine heavy chain and hypertrophy, failing ventricular myocardium. J Clin Invest 1997;100:2315–2324.

73. MacKenzie J: Disease of the Heart. London: N.P., 1910.

74. Mancini DM, Henson D, LaManca J, Donchez L, Levine S: Benefit of selective respiratory muscle training on exercise capacity in patients with chronic congestive heart failure. Circulation 1995;91:320–329.

75. Mann DL: Mechanisms and models in heart failure. Circulation 1999;100:999–1008.

76. Margulies KB, Heublein DM, Perrella MA, Burnett JC Jr: ANF-mediated renal cGMP generation in congestive heart failure. Am J Physiol 1991;260:F562–F568.

77. Margulies KB, Hildebrand FL, Lerman A, Perrella MA, Burnett JC: Increased endothelin in experimental heart failure. Circulation 1990;82:2226–2230.

78. Matsubara H, Kanasaki M, Murasawa S, Tsukaguchi Y, Nio Y, Inada M: Different expression and regulation of angiotensin II receptor subtype cardiac fibroblasts and cardiomyocytes in culture. J Clin 1994;93:1592.

79. McEwan JR, Merjanin N, Larkin S, Fuller RW, Dollery CT, MacIntyre I: Vasodilation by calcitonin gene-related peptide and substance P: a comparison of their effects on resistance and capitance vessels of human forearms. Circulation 1988;77:1072–1080.

80. Mills RM, Young JB: Practical Approaches to the Treatment of Heart Failure. Baltimore: Williams & Wilkins, 1998.

81. Morely-Davies A, Nolan J: Heart failure: a historical context. In McMurray JJV, Cleland JGF (eds): Heart Failure in Clinical Practice. St Louis: Mosby, 1996.

82. Mulderry PK, Ghatei MA, Rodrigo J, Allen JM, Rosenfeld MG, Polak JM, Bloom SR: Calcitonin gene-related peptide in cardiovascular tissues of the rat. Neuroscience 1985;14:947–954.

83. Muther RS, Potter DM, Bennett WM: Aspirin-induced depression of glomerular filtration rate in normal humans: role of sodium balance. Ann Intern Med 1981;94:317–321.

84. Narula J, Haider N, Virmani R, DiSalvo TG, Kolodgie FD, Hajjar RJ, Schmidt U, Semigran MJ, Dec GW, Khaw BA: Apoptosis and myocytes in end stage heart failure. N Engl J Med 1996;335:1182–1189.

85. Neer EJ, Clapham DE: Signal transduction through G-proteins in the cardiac myocyte. Trends Cardiovasc Med 1992;2:6–11.

86. Oliver JA, Sciacca RR, Pinto J, Cannon PJ: Participation of prostaglandins in the control of renal blood flow during acute reduction of cardiac output in the dog. J Clin Invest 1981;67:229–237.

87. Olivetti G, Abbi R, Quaini F, Kajstura J, Cheng W, Nitahara JA, Quaini E, DiLoreto C, Beltrami CA, Krajewski S, Reed JC, Anversa P: Apoptosis of the failing human heart. N Engl J Med 1997; 336:1131–1141.

88. Olson EN: Regulation of muscle transcription by the MyoD family. The heart of the matter. Circ Res 1993;72:1–6.

89. Opie LH: The Heart: Physiology and Metabolism. 2nd ed. New York: Raven Press, 1991, pp 67–126, 147–175.

90. Opie LH: The Heart. Physiology, from Cell to Circulation. 3rd ed. Philadelphia: Lippincott-Raven Publishers, 1998.

91. Osler W: The Principles and Practice of Medicine. New York: Appleton, 1892.

92. Pagel W: New light on William Harvey. Basel: Karger, 1976.

93. Palmer RM, Ashton DS, Moncada S: Vascular endothelial cells synthesize nitric oxide from L-arginine. Nature 1988;333:664–666.

94. Pfeffer MA, Braunwald E: Ventricular remodeling after myocardial infarction: experimental observations and clinical implications. Circulation 1990;81:1161–1172.

95. Pool PE, Covell JW, Levit M, Gibb J, Braunwald E: Reduction of cardiac tyros hydroxylase activity in experimental congestive heart failure. Its role depletion of cardiac norepinephrine stores. Circ Res 1967;20:349.

96. Pruszczynski W, Vahanian A, Ardailou R, Acar J: Role of antidiuretic hormone in impaired water excretion of patients with congestive heart failure. J Clin Endocrinol Metab 1984;58: 599–603.

97. Redfield MM, Edwards BS, Heublein DM, Burnett JC Jr: Restoration of renal response to atrial natriuretic factor in experimental low-output heart failure. Am J Physiol 1989;257:R917–R923.

98. Riegger GAJ, Liebau G, Koschiek K: Antidiuretic hormone in congestive heart failure. Am J Med 1982;72:49–55.

99. Rodkey SM, Ratliff NB, Young JB: Cardiomyopathy and myocardial failure. In Topol EJ (ed): Textbook of Cardiovascular Medicine. Philadelphia: Lippincott-Raven, 1998.

100. Rubin SA: The molecular and cellular biology of cardiac failure. In Hosenpud JD, Greenberg BH (eds): Congestive Heart Failure. 2nd ed. Philadelphia: Lippincott Williams & Wilkins, 2000.

101. Sadoshima J, Xu Y, Slayter HS, Izumo S: Autocrine release of angiotensin-II mediates stretch-induced hypertrophy of cardiac myocytes in vitro. Cell 1993;75:977–984.

102. Sakamoto S, Stone CK, Woolf PD, Liang C: Opiate receptor antagonist in right-sided congestive heart failure: naloxone exerts salutary hemodynamic effects through its action on the central nervous system. Circ Res 1989;65:103–114.

103. Sandler H, Dodge HT: Left ventricular tension and stress in man. Circ Res 1963;13:91–104.

104. Schiffrin EL: Decreased density of binding sites for atrial natriuretic peptide on platelets of patients with severe congestive heart failure. Clin Sci 1988;74:213–218.

105. Schneider MD, Roberts R, Parker TG: Modulation of cardiac genes by mechanical stress: the oncogene signaling hypothesis. Mol Biol Med 1991;8:167–183.

106. Schoffer J, Tews A, Langes K, Bleifeld W, Reimitz PE, Mathey DG: Relationship between myocardial norepinephrine content and left ventricular function—an endomyocardial biopsy study. Eur Heart J 1987;8:748.

107. Schor N, Ichikawa I, Brenner BM: Mechanisms of action of various hormones and vasoactive substances on glomerular ultrafiltration in the rat. Kidney Int 1981;20:442–451.

108. Schorb W, Peeler TC, Madigan NN, Conrad KM, Baker KM: Angiotensin induced protein tyrosine phosphorylation in neonatal rat cardioblasts. J Biol Chem 1994;269:19626.

109. Schrier RW: Pathogenesis of sodium and water retention in high-output and low-output cardiac failure, nephritic syndrome, cirrhosis and pregnancy. N Engl J Med 1988;319:1058–2264 (p1) and 1127–1134 (p2).

110. Schrier RW, Berl T, Anderson RJ: Osmotic and nonosmotic control of vasopressin release. Am J Physiol 1979;236:F321–F332.

111. Schunkert H, Dzau VJ, Tang SS, Hirsch AT, Apstein CS, Lorell BH: Increased rat cardiac angiotensin converting enzyme activity and mRNA expression in pressure overload left ventricular hypertrophy. Effects on coronary resistance, contractility, and relaxation. J Clin Invest 1990;86:1913.

112. Schunkert H, Sadoshima JI, Cornelius T, Kagaya Y, Weinberg EO, Izumo S, Riegger G, Lorell BH: Angiotensin induced growth responses in isolated adult rat hearts. Evidence load-independent induction of cardiac protein synthesis of angiotensin II. Circ Res 1995;76:489.

113. Scriven TA, Burnett JC Jr: Effects of synthetic atrial natriuretic peptide on renal function and renin release in acute experimental heart failure. Circulation 1985;72:892–897.

114. Spinale FG, Tempel GE, Mukherjee R, Eble DM, Brown R, Vacchiano CA, Zile MR: Cellular and molecular alterations in the B-adrenergic system with cardiomyopathy induced by tachycardia. Cardiovasc Res 1994;28:1243–1250.

115. Stahl RA, Attallah AA, Bloch DL, Lee JB: Stimulation of rabbit renal PGE$_2$ biosynthesis by dietary sodium restriction. Am J Physiol 1979;237:F344–F349.

116. Stokes JB, Kokko JP: Inhibition of sodium transport by prostaglandin E_2 across the isolated perfused rabbit collecting tubule. J Clin Invest 1977;59:1099–1104.

117. Sydenham T: A treatise of the gout and dropsy. *In* The Works of Thomas Sydenham, M.D.: On Acute and Chronic Diseases. Vol 2. London: Robinson, Otridge, Hayes, and Newbery, 1683.

118. Thiene G: The discovery of circulation and the origin of modern medicine during the Italian Renaissance. Cardiovasc Pathol 1997;6:79–88.

119. Thomas JA, Marks BH: Plasma norepinephrine in congested heart failure. Am J Cardiol 1978;41:233.

120. Torre-Amione G, Kapadia S, Lee J, Durand JB, Bies RD, Young JB, Mann DL: Tumor necrosis factor alpha and tumor necrosis factor reception in the failing human heart. Circulation 1996; 93:704–711.

121. Tschopp FA, Tobler PH, Fischer JA: Calcitonin gene-related peptide in the human thyroid, pituitary and brain. Mol Coll Endocrinol 1984;36:53–57.

122. Ungerer M, Bohm M, Elce JS, Erdmann E, Lohse MJ: Altered expression of β_1-adrenergic receptors in the failing human heart. Circulation 1993;87:454.

123. Ungerer M, Parruti G, Bohm M, Puzicha M, DeBlasi A, Erdmann E, Lohse MJ: Expression of β-arrestins and β-adrenergic receptor kinases in the failing human heart. Circ Res 1994;74:206–213.

124. Viquerat CE, Daly P, Swedberg K, Evers C, Curran D, Parmley WW, Chatterjee K: Endogenous catecholamine levels in chronic heart failure: relation to the severity of dynamic abnormalities. Am J Med 1985;78:455.

125. Waspe LE, Ordahl CP, Simpson PC: The cardiac heavy chain isogene is induced selectively in a-adrenergic stimulated hypertrophy of cultured rat heart myocytes. J Clin 1990;85:1206.

126. Weber KT: Extracellular matrix remodeling in heart failure: a role for de novo angiotensin II generation. Circulation 1997; 96:4065–4082.

127. Wiggers CJ: Physiology in Health and Disease. Dynamics of Valvular Lesions. 5th ed. Philadelphia: Lea & Febiger, 1949, pp 786–801.

128. Withering W: An Account of the Fox glove and Some of Its Medical Uses: Practical Remarks on Dropsy and other Diseases. London: Robinson and Paternoster-Row, 1785.

129. Wright RS, Levine MS, Bellamy PE, Simmons MS, Batra P, Stevenson LW, Walden JA, Laks H, Tashkin DP: Ventilatory and diffusion abnormalities in potential heart transplant recipients. Chest 1990;98:816–820.

130. Young JB: Chronic heart failure management. *In* Topol EJ (ed): Textbook of Cardiovascular Medicine. Philadelphia: Lippincott-Raven 1998.

131. Young JB, Pratt CM: Hemodynamic and hormonal alterations in patients with heart failure: toward a contemporary definition of heart failure. Semin Nephrol 1994;14:427–440.

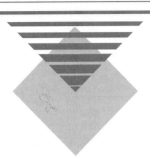

CHAPTER FIVE

Medical and Nontransplant Surgical Therapy of Heart Failure

CHRONIC HEART FAILURE TREATMENT STRATEGY

OVERVIEW

When considering transplant therapeutics in any specific patient, assessment of more conventional treatments is mandatory. Of particular importance is the optimization of medical therapy and consideration of surgical alternatives to heart transplant.[3, 6, 10, 113, 204, 270] Treating patients with heart failure no longer consists simply of prescribing diuretics and digitalis to patients with dropsy. Rather, a wide range of therapeutic options are available which are targeted against the various components of the heart failure syndrome (Table 5–1). The elements of the definition of heart failure as discussed in Chapter 4 can be related to an overall strategy to ameliorate its severity and prevent its progression (Table 5–2). Formulation of the specific therapeutic protocols for such patients is a challenging task that must be rooted in the concepts of evidence-based medical practice. Whenever heart failure treatment strategies are proposed, clinicians must recognize that cost and patient compliance with recommendations will affect one's ability to successfully intervene. Furthermore, therapeutic recommendations depend upon clinicians' ability to make the proper diagnosis, stage the syndrome severity and time-related prognosis appropriately, and then select drug and procedural interventions that are likely to diminish morbidity and decrease heart failure's high mortality rate. It is important to distinguish between therapeutic approaches relevant to those patients with asymptomatic or minimally symptomatic left ventricular dysfunction, those with chronic (usually congestive) symptomatic heart failure, those with acute decompensation and cardiogenic shock, and those with intractable advanced or so-called end-stage states. Each of these patient groups presents varying diagnostic and therapeutic challenges. Cardiac transplantation is reserved for patients with either intractable acute cardiogenic shock or chronic heart failure not responding satisfactorily to more conservative medical and surgical approaches.

TABLE 5-1	Evolving Insight into Heart Failure and its Therapies

Heart failure is a dropsical condition
- Lymphatic drainage tubes
- Primitive diuretic therapies
- "Foxglove" tea

Heart failure is central cardiac pump inadequacy
- Cardiac glycoside preparations
- Alternative inotropic therapies
- Cardiac transplantation
- Mechanical ventricular assist devices/total artificial hearts

Heart failure is caused by decompensated ventricular hypertrophy
- Antihypertensive therapy
- Surgical repair of valvular defects

Heart failure is circulatory dysfunction
- Vasodilator therapy

Heart failure is an endocrinopathy
- ACE-I therapy
- A-II receptor blockade
- Beta-blocker therapy

Heart failure is a fever
- Cytokine modulating agents

Heart failure is a complicated milieu of pump dysfunction, myocardial remodeling, humoral perturbation, and subsequent circulatory insufficiency
- ACE-I therapy
- Digoxin therapy
- Diuretic therapy
- Beta-blocker therapy
- Surgical therapies (revascularization, remodeling, valve repair, transplantation)

ACE-I, Angiotensin converting enzyme inhibitor; A-II, angiotensin-II.

Pharmacotherapeutic and operative strategies for heart failure have undergone dramatic evolution over the past four decades.[67, 212, 232] Focus originally had been upon diuretics and cardiac glycosides with intense search for alternative inotropic agents, driven by the philosophy that diminished contractility was the single most significant pathophysiologic aberration in heart failure. Indeed, direct-acting vasodilators were first used with some frequency only in the 1970s after insight grew into the importance of humoral factors associated with the disparate and complex systolic and diastolic dysfunction issues. Angiotensin-converting enzyme (ACE) inhibitors and beta-adrenergic receptor blocking drugs have subsequently assumed more prominent roles. Interestingly, the therapeutic focus today has clearly shifted toward prescription of agents which inhibit adrenergic stimulation of the heart.[168] Currently, study of specific angiotensin-II receptor blocking compounds, centrally acting alpha-adrenergic blocking agents, calcium channel blockers, neutral endopeptidase inhibitors, natriuretic peptides, and drugs which attenuate endothelial perturbations common in heart failure is ongoing. Equally important has been clarification of therapeutic strategies that have proven to be detrimental to heart failure patients. For example, many inotropic drugs have proven disappointing because of their association with higher mortality rates when evaluated in carefully designed mortality endpoint clinical trials (e.g., oral milrinone, vesnarinone, and ibopamine). Furthermore, most antiarrhythmic agents and calcium channel blockers evaluated in patients with heart failure have been associated with greater harm than benefit. Today,

much can be done to attenuate the poor natural history of advanced heart failure, but much more is necessary. It is particularly important to focus on the subset of patients with devastating end-stage heart failure, because their suffering is great and outcome without transplantation is dismal.

BASIC TREATMENT PHILOSOPHY

Strategies should be developed so that both asymptomatic and symptomatic patients, particularly those with advanced heart failure, are receiving tailored therapy (Fig. 5–1). A tremendous menu of therapies exists, and the best approach to the patient with asymptomatic systolic left ventricular dysfunction differs from that for symptomatic individuals. Besides allowing amelioration of symptoms with pharmacologic or surgical therapy, the early identification of individuals with insidious hemodynamic and humoral perturbation is necessary to prevent the development of congestive states or other symptoms. These "preventive strategies" are designed to limit ongoing harmful cardiac remodeling (see Chapter 4). Treatment strategies are designed to ameliorate symptoms, when present, while maintaining functional capacity at maximal levels in order to keep patients out of the hospital. Both prevention and treatment strategies should focus on reversing remodeling and reducing mortality (Fig. 5–2).

RELATIONSHIPS BETWEEN VARIOUS TREATMENT STRATEGIES AND PATHOPHYSIOLOGY

An important basic tenet is that diseases known to be injurious to the heart should be treated primarily so that

TABLE 5-2	A Contemporary Definition of Heart Failure Related to Therapies

IMPORTANT CONSIDERATIONS

Myocardial injury causes acute or chronic myocyte dysfunction (systolic and/or diastolic)
- Prevent injury to the heart

Myocyte passive tension and work loads increase
- Use preload and afterload reduction techniques

Myocyte interstitial matrix stiffens
- Prevent inflammation and fibrosis

Peripheral vascular bed blood flow is altered
- Increase cardiac output and organ perfusion

Subsequent mechanical, humoral, neurohormonal, and inflammatory responses appear in an attempt to create systemic organ flow compensation
- Block adverse humoral factors

Compensatory mechanisms ultimately produce a maladaptive circulatory state
- Reverse the remodeling of the heart/vascular network

Patients may present without symptoms or suffer from a variety of fatigue, dyspnea, or dropsical states that fluctuate in severity based on treatment protocols, diet, physical conditioning, and diseases precipitating the heart failure syndrome
- Design therapies based on syndrome stage
- Institute therapy for asymptomatic ventricular dysfunction
- Make patient envolemic
- Optimize hemodynamics

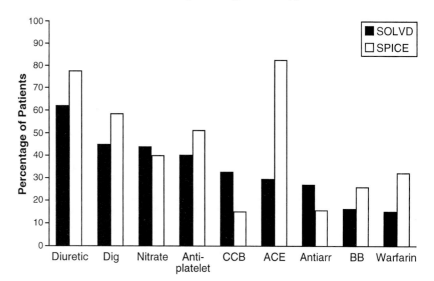

FIGURE **5-1.** Prescription practice in patients with heart failure: comparison of the SOLVD (Study of Left Ventricular Dysfunction) and SPICE (Study of Patients Intolerant Converting Enzyme) registries.

continued myocardial injury can be averted. Examples of this strategy include antibiotic prophylaxis for acute rheumatic fever, antihypertensive therapy, and intervention in patients with obstructive coronary artery disease. When myocyte injury has occurred, both passive tension and workload increase, and this may be prevented by preload and afterload reduction with drugs that have these effects. The myocardial interstitial matrix stiffens substantially in patients with heart failure as collagen and fibrous tissue are laid down aggressively. Though prevention of inflammation and fibrosis intuitively seems important, precise treatment strategies to accomplish this are not yet defined. Alteration in peripheral flow (which is generally decreased) should be addressed with techniques that optimize cardiac output and organ perfusion. These endpoints are generally accomplished by manipulating vascular resistance. The abnormal humoral and neurohormonal response characteristic of heart failure can be blocked by a variety of drugs including ACE inhibitors, angiotensin-II receptor site blockers, and alpha- and beta-adrenergic receptor site blockers. Additional new therapies are needed to alter the regressive genetic processes apparent in heart failure, as detailed in Chapter 4.

INTEGRATION OF DIAGNOSTIC EVALUATION AND MANAGEMENT STRATEGY

Important questions to ask when contemplating treatments for chronic heart failure patients are summarized in Table 5–3.[6] Of prime importance is whether or not the patient actually suffers from heart failure and if symptoms presented or physical findings noted are, in reality, related to a failing cardiovascular system. Not all patients with weakness, fatigue, dyspnea, and dropsical states have heart failure. Also important is the fact that patients with heart failure can present with these symptoms and physical findings, and have them more related to comorbid diseases than to their cardiac dysfunction. Next, the clinician should determine the etiology of the heart failure syndrome. It is particularly important to identify diseases that can be treated and cured, or at the least ameliorated, so that progression of remodeling and the heart failure syndrome can be prevented. It is then imperative to perform an evaluation and to confirm the diagnosis and stage the syndrome's severity. Specific factors are sought which may have precipitated the patient's deterioration. Medication noncompliance, exces-

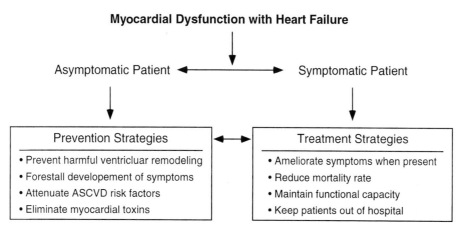

FIGURE **5-2.** Philosophy of heart failure treatment; the juxtaposition of "prevention" and "treatment" options.

TABLE 5-3	**Integration of Diagnostic Evaluation into a Management Strategy**

QUESTIONS TO ASK WHEN DESIGNING THERAPEUTIC PROTOCOLS FOR CHRONIC HEART FAILURE PATIENTS

- Does the patient actually suffer from heart failure and are presenting symptoms or physical findings related to this diagnosis?
- What is the etiology of the syndrome?
- What evaluation is needed to confirm diagnosis, clarify etiology, and stage syndrome severity?
- What precipitated the patient's deterioration?
- How severe is the heart failure syndrome and what is the patient's short- and long-term prognosis?
- Is the patient on medications that are potentially detrimental in the heart failure milieu?
- How should the patient be treated acutely?
- How should the patient be treated chronically?
- Can the precipitating disease process be cured or can the state of heart failure be ameliorated?
- What social factors played a role in morbidity and what social support mechanisms should be considered as adjunctive therapeutic measures?
- How should follow-up be planned?

sive sodium or fluid consumption, worsening ischemic syndromes, new atrial and ventricular arrhythmias, intercurrent infection, uncontrolled chronic obstructive pulmonary disease, diabetes mellitus, and hypertension trigger pathophysiologic responses that ultimately produce symptomatic congestive heart failure.

Staging the syndrome's severity is not only critical to proper design of treatment but also helps predict the short- and long-term prognosis. An often unasked question is whether individual patients are consuming medications that can be detrimental in the setting of heart failure, such as nonsteroidal anti-inflammatory drugs, certain calcium channel blockers, and Vaughn Williams Class I antiarrhythmic agents. Unfortunately, social factors that play a significant role in morbidity are often neglected, and it is important to consider important lifestyle change issues (e.g., low-sodium diet, cigarette smoking cessation, and medication compliance) that will enhance any heart failure treatment regimen. Finally, appropriate plans for long-term follow-up will be necessary to ensure optimization of treatments, monitor for drug toxicities and side effects, discover developing disease, and pick up intercurrent events.

PATIENT AND FAMILY EDUCATION

The Agency for Health Care Policy and Research (AHCPR)[159] guidelines for topics to cover during patient, family, and caregiver education and counseling are summarized in Table 5–4.[6] Patients with heart failure should not be simply given a medication prescription or operated upon. It is critically important to explain to the patient the nature and cause of the heart failure and reasons for symptoms if the patient is symptomatic. Also important is detailing symptoms that herald worsening heart failure and strategies to pursue if symptoms do appear or progress. Instruction with regard to monitoring daily weights, blood pressure, pulse rate, and blood sugar for diabetics is helpful. Findings might guide the appropriately educated patient to alter daily medications (increasing diuretics for short periods of time when evidence of worsening congestion is noted). Careful explanation of treatment and care plans is important if one wishes to gain acceptance of therapeutic strategies. This will promote compliance and may help to reduce

or prevent hospital admission or readmission. It is important to discuss specific patient responsibilities with regard to cessation of tobacco and alcohol use, salt restriction, and fluid intake reduction. The important role

TABLE 5-4	**Suggested Topics for Patient, Family, and Caregiver Education and Counseling**

General Counseling
- Explanation of heart failure and the reason for symptoms
- Cause or probable cause of heart failure
- Expected symptoms
- Symptoms of worsening heart failure
- What to do if symptoms worsen
- Self-monitoring with daily weights, blood pressure, pulse rate, blood sugar (in diabetics)
- Explanation of treatment/care plan
- Clarification of patient's responsibilities
- Importance of cessation of tobacco use
- Role of family members or other caregivers in the treatment/care plan
- Availability and value of qualified local support group
- Importance of obtaining vaccinations against influenza and pneumococcal disease

Prognosis
- Life expectancy
- Advance directives
- Advice for family members in the event of cardiac arrest

Activity recommendations
- Cardiac rehabilitation programs with supervised exercise protocols
- Recreation, leisure, and work activity
- Exercise
- Sex, sexual dysfunction, and coping strategies

Dietary recommendations
- Sodium restriction
- Avoidance of excessive fluid intake
- Alcohol restriction if appropriate
- Low animal fat diet if appropriate

Medications
- Effects of medications on qualify of life and survival
- Dosing of drugs
- Likely side efffects and what to do if they occur
- Coping mechanisms for complicated medical regimens

Importance of compliance with treatment/care plan
- Methods to ensure medications taken timely
- Provision of forms to record medications taken
- Pulse rate, blood pressure, weight charts

Modified from Konstam M, Dracup K, Baker D: Heart failure: evaluation and care of patients with left ventricular systolic dysfunction. Clinical practice guideline. AHCPR Publication No. 94-0612. Rockville, MD: Agency for Health Care Policy and Research, U.S. Department of Health and Human Services, June 1994.

of a family member or other caregiver in the treatment plan should be stressed. Attenuation of atherosclerosis risk factors in order to prevent progression of coronary artery disease with subsequent cardiac events might prevent or delay deterioration. Obtaining vaccinations at appropriate intervals against influenza and pneumococcal disease could prevent a serious hemodynamic problem resulting from an episode of infectious disease.

The patient's prognosis should be frankly discussed and advanced directives elicited; this is particularly important for those patients suffering from the end-stage ravages of advanced heart failure syndromes. Advice should be given to family members regarding resuscitation efforts if this is deemed appropriate.

Activity recommendations need to focus on the benefits of aerobic exercise. Recreational, leisure, work, and exercise activities should be addressed, and patients should be encouraged to perform aerobic activities that are symptom limited. Exercise should not be prohibited in patients with heart failure and, in fact, aerobic activities should be strongly encouraged, although patients with more advanced stages of heart failure will have to limit their activity. These recommendations to patients are embodied in the statement "do what you can, and don't do what you can't."

Dietary recommendations are essential and focus on restriction of salt and excess fluid intake. Alcohol might be prohibited in certain situations, such as when patients are diagnosed as having dilated cardiomyopathy or, obviously, alcoholic cardiomyopathy. Whether or not alcohol should be prohibited in individuals with ischemic cardiomyopathy is a contentious issue at the present time.

The effects of medication on quality of life and survival should be reviewed with schemes designed to optimize treatment compliance. One must emphasize the necessity of taking drugs in a timely fashion, and it is good practice to provide forms to record medication consumption, pulse rate, blood pressure, and daily weights, so that the patient can take an active part in his or her therapeutic program.

INSIGHTS GAINED FROM REGISTRIES AND CLINICAL TRIALS

In the management of complex clinical conditions such as heart failure, therapeutic practices are more likely to yield predictable results when based on inferences derived from formal clinical studies (evidence-based practice of medicine) rather than anecdotal experiences. The implementation of an evidence-based approach to the pharmacotherapy of heart failure is facilitated by the knowledge gained from large clinical trials.[3] As a technique of clinical investigation, the **clinical trial** (involving randomization between defined therapies or therapy vs. placebo for a specified patient population) has become the "gold standard" for defining the appropriate appliction of many medical therapies. The role of

clinical trials in heart failure therapy (see Box) is apparent (Table 5–5) when reviewing current heart failure treatment guidelines, particularly with reference to specific pharmacologic therapies.

Beginning in 1994 with publications from the AHCPR,[6] American College of Cardiology (ACC)/ American Heart Association (AHA),[10, 270] European Society of Cardiology,[112] ACTION-Heart Failure group,[204] and most recently from the Heart Failure Society of America (HFSA),[4] new diagnosis and treatment protocols have been rooted in a compendium of clinical trials giving insight into heart failure therapies (both old and newly emerging). Each has advanced new concepts when appropriate (such as beta-blocker therapies addressed in the ACTION-Heart Failure and HFSA guidelines), pointed out bona fide controversy (such as routine use of anticoagulants addressed in ACC/AHA and HFSA guidelines), and cautioned against therapies which at one time were routine because of their intuitive "logic" but subsequently determined to be detrimental (such as antiarrhythmic therapy with Vaughn Williams class I agents discussed in ACTION-Heart Failure and HSFA guidelines).

Though anecdotal reports and small case series have contributed to our insight regarding heart failure treatment, it has been the larger, randomized, well-controlled, multicenter clinical trial (usually with mortality endpoints) which has given the greatest insight into best management strategies for these patients. By mimicking practices reported in clinical trials, treatment protocols can be established that are generalizable, safe, and effective. Table 5–5 summarizes a large group of randomized clinical trials that have influenced the design of heart failure therapeutic algorithms. These particular experiences have been selected because they provide important insight into treatment of a broad spectrum of heart failure patients. They are listed in Table 5–5 alphabetically according to their trial acronym rather than being presented in historic sequence. Throughout the ensuing discussion of heart failure treatment paradigms, reference will be made to these clinical projects. These landmark clinical studies began in the late 1970s and generally focused on pharmaceutical strategies, but a few have evaluated surgical interventions (primarily coronary artery bypass graft surgery). Clinical heart failure trials emerging in the 1980s and 1990s are generally characterized by evaluation of heart failure treatment practices that seemed intuitive with respect to benefit, but proved harmful when put to the test of mortality endpoints. Several inotropic agents with varying degrees of vasodilating properties improved heart failure symptoms but at the cost of greater mortality. The 1990s have been marked by better clarification of the role of digitalis and adrenergic blocking drugs. It should, however, be noted that these guidelines are, for the most part, applicable to reasonably stable outpatients with mild to moderate symptomatic congestive heart failure due to left ventricular systolic dysfunction. As heart failure severity worsens, and particularly when hospitalization is required, high-quality clinical trial

The Role of Clinical Trials in Heart Failure Therapy

Clinical trials have played a key role in the refinement of heart failure therapy by providing objective information regarding benefits and detriments of medical management strategies. Clearly, clinical trials are appropriate for a limited number of clinical situations guided by the medical/scientific question posed and ethical considerations. The concept of clinical equipoise must be fulfilled in the design of any clinical trial, indicating that a clear doubt exists within the medical community and among the participating physicians about the efficacy or superiority of one drug (or therapy) versus another in a defined medical situation.[122] In addition, the design of clinical trials may be flawed by inherent design features such as patient entry bias (see Chapter 3). For example, there is commonly an important attrition of patients between screening for clinical studies and final trial entry/randomization. It is not unusual to see a 10 or 20:1 ratio between patients screened and those ultimately included. Despite these and other limitations, properly designed clinical trials have provided important information and greatly influenced the practice of medicine for many complex conditions, including heart failure.

Ideally, there should be an intimate link between everyday clinical patient encounters raising questions regarding therapeutic challenges and performance of clinical trials. After testing hypotheses in properly designed studies, treatment strategies based on therapeutic algorithms used in the trials emerge. Subsequent to that, caregivers should be educated with respect to the strategies likely to produce benefit as opposed to those associated with adverse or neutral outcomes. Furthermore, clinical trials can be used to determine both cost of intervention and cost savings generated by specific strategies. Clinical trials, thus, are one of the best, though certainly not the only, means to create care standards. Unfortunately, clinical trials involving drugs are often driven by the desire to test new therapies with potential for commercial viability, and emerging drugs may be put to the test only if there exists potential for substantial investment return. Thus, our desire to practice evidence-based medicine is hampered greatly by this dilemma (contemporary reality is that many important heart failure treatment questions will not be tested because funding is unavailable). It is important to note that situations where clinical expertise does not exist, acute life-threatening settings, and circumstances where clinical practice has become well defined using alternative evaluation techniques are not generally subjected to randomized clinical trials. Interestingly, most routinely performed surgical procedures, including cardiac transplantation, have not been evaluated using formal randomized clinical trial protocols, but the role of transplantation in the therapy of advanced heart failure is clear because the preponderance of information from other types of outcomes research (see Chapter 3) has established its efficacy compared with other therapies for certain patient subsets with advanced heart failure.

When evaluating results reported from emerging clinical trials, several important tenets must be remembered. The study must have a specific hypothesis that has been clearly stated with patient selection criteria precisely characterized. Investigators should be specific about why patients did not enter into the trial. One weakness of most clinical trials is the underrepresentation of women, children, the aged, and minority races. Furthermore, individuals with many comorbid conditions, a situation so often encountered in ordinary daily clinical practice, are generally excluded from participation in clinical trials. Sample size calculations must be appropriate, concomitant therapeutic and ancillary treatments well defined, bias control appropriate, and randomization successful so that comparison groups are similar. Study endpoints must be chosen carefully so that they are appropriate to the condition being studied, consistent, well defined, and have clinical relevance. The use of surrogate endpoints (e.g., reduction of premature ventricular contractions as a substitute for mortality in myocardial infarction patients with left ventricular systolic dysfunction) often generates misleading inferences, as many trials have demonstrated. Clinical trials should have acceptable statistical power to answer the specific questions asked and confidence limits of observations known and understood (see Chapter 3). Finally, appropriate procedures are required for handling clinical trial dropouts and patients lost to follow-up.

---

data become scanty and consensus regarding best treatment practices difficult to reach.

The evolution of common practice patterns in drug therapy for heart failure is documented in major registries which collected data on heart failure therapies. The **Studies of Left Ventricular Dysfunction** (SOLVD) registry analyzed cardiovascular drug usage in almost 6,000 patients identified as having heart failure due to both systolic and diastolic dysfunction in 1988.[274] A broad spectrum of patients with heart failure were examined, including some with predominately diastolic dysfunction. Drug use was determined in a population cross-sectional manner at the time patients were identified as having "heart failure." The clinical diagnosis of heart failure, rather than specific ejection fraction, allowed inclusion in the registry. Approximately three quarters of the participants were evaluated during a hospitalization, and this was usually for treatment of congestive heart failure. The median number of cardiovascular drugs used per patient was four, with diuretics taken by 62%, digoxin 45%, ACE inhibitors 32%, calcium channel blockers 36%, antiarrhythmic agents (not amiodarone) 22%, and beta-adrenergic blocking drugs 18%. At that time, only 18% of patients were on the combination of ACE inhibitor, diuretic, and digoxin. Data from the SOLVD registry indicate that in 1988, "triple drug" therapy for heart failure (ACE inhibitor, diuretic, and digoxin) was common only when heart failure was ad-

Text continued on page 150

TABLE 5-5	Select Heart Failure Clinical Trials (Listed Alphabetically According to Acronym)

ACRONYM	FULL TITLE	STUDY DESIGN	FINDINGS	THERAPEUTIC IMPLICATIONS
AIRE	Acute infarction Ramipril Evaluation	Effect of ramipril on morbidity and mortality of survivors of acute myocardial infarction with clinical evidence of heart failure	Significant reduction in mortality noted with ramipril; findings complement SAVE, SMILE, TRACE, GISSI-III, ISIS-IV	ACE-I therapy should be routinely started post-infarct when CHF or left ventricular dysfunction present
ATLAS	Assessment of Treatment with Lisinopril and Survival	Survival study of high- vs. low-dose lisinopril in moderate to severe CHF	Study launched in 1992 with a target of 3,000 patients	Will address question of "low"-dose ACE-I benefits in CHF patients
BEST	Beta-Blocker Evaluation Survival	Patients receiving standard treatment randomized to placebo or bucindolol to determine a mortality benefit in moderate to severe heart failure	No benefit noted in Class III, IV CHF patients with bucindolol	Either bucindolol is a beta blocker not associated with benefit in heart failure or population studied was resistant to benefit
CAMIAT	Canadien Myocardial Infarction Amiodarone Trial	Patient (n = 120) 6–45 days postinfarction without EF entry criteria but ECG ventricular arrhythmia followed for combined endpoint of arrhythmic death or resuscitated ventricular fibrillation; all-cause mortality and cardiac mortality secondary endpoint	Primary endpoint benefited with amiodarone but toxicity great (42.3% of treatment group stopped amiodarone by 2 years), all-cause mortality not reduced	Though not a heart failure trial per se, some patients obviously had LV dysfunction; amiodarone may benefit select post-MI patients, but difficult to tolerate
CARVEDILOL PROGRAM	The Effect of Carvedilol on Morbidity and Mortality in Patients with Chronic Heart Failure	Combined analysis of four distinct studies with varied patient enrollment criteria and outcome measures analyzing safety data regarding mortality events (n = 1,094)	Carvedilol reduced mortality from 7.8% to 3.2% ($p < .001$); findings and analysis controversial because this was not a prospective mortality endpoint trial, rather, a pooled analysis	More data supporting use of beta blocker (this one with alpha-blocking properties as well) in CHF; there may be important differences between selective and nonselective beta blockers in CHF
CASS	Coronary Artery Surgery Study	Survival Endpoint Randomized Study of CABG vs. "best" medical therapy of ischemic heart disease with 10-year follow-up (n = 780) performed over a decade ago	CABG did not prolong life or prevent infarcts compared to medical therapy except when EF < 0.50	One of several studies to suggest that coronary revascularization is important in patients with heart failure and ischemia
CAST	Cardiac Arrhythmia Suppression Trial	Mortality endpoint trial of Encainide and Flecainide post-MI in patients with PVCs and, generally, LV dysfunction.	Potent class I antiarrhythmic agents increase mortality in MI patients with LVD	Avoid Vaughn Williams Class I antiarrhythmics in CHF if possible
CHARM	Candesartan Cilexitil in Heart Failure Assessment of Reduction in Mortality and Morbidity	Placebo-controlled, blinded mortality endpoint trial of the angiotensin-II receptor blocker candesartan in 3 types of heart failure patients: those with EF > 0.40, those with EF < 0.40 and ACEI intolerance, and those with EF < 0.40 and on ACEI (add-on therapy)	Trial ongoing	Will help clarify role of an A-II blocker in a wide spectrum of heart failure patients
CHF-STAT	Congestive Heart Failure–Survival Trial of Antiarrhythmic Therapy	Survival study of amiodarone vs. placebo in CHF patients with 10 PVCs/hr	Amiodarone overall did not improve survival compared to placebo	Did not support hypothesis that amiodarone was helpful generally in CHF
CIBIS	Cardiac Insufficiency Bisoprolol Study	Bisoprolol (a selective beta blocker) added to diuretics/vasodilator with mortality endpoint	Trend toward morbidity reduction without statistically significant reduction in mortality	Added to portfolio suggesting beta blockers beneficial in some CHF patients

Table continued on following page

TABLE 5-5 Select Heart Failure Clinical Trials (Listed Alphabetically According to Acronym) (*Continued*)

ACRONYM	FULL TITLE	STUDY DESIGN	FINDINGS	THERAPEUTIC IMPLICATIONS
CIBIS-II	Cardiac Insufficiency Bisoprolol Study-II	Placebo-controlled mortality endpoint trial of 2,647 patients given bisoprolol for 16 months	Significant reduction in mortality	Longer trial than CIBIS-I with more ill population and higher dose of bisoprolol; 34% reduction in mortality, particularly sudden death
COMET	Comparison of Metoprolol/ Carvedilol Trial	Active drug control design with metoprolol compared to carvedilol in 4,000 stable CHF patients	Trial ongoing	Study will give important insight into possible superiority of nonselective, vasodilating beta blocker in mild–moderate CHF
CONSENSUS	Cooperative North Scandanavian Enalapril Survival Study	Enalapril added to digoxin and diuretic in severe heart failure (NYHA Class IV)	Dramatic reduction in mortality at 6 months	ACE-I a very important addition in CHF
COPERNICUS	Carvedilol Prospective Randomized Cumulative Survival Trial	Carvedilol vs. placebo in 1,800 NYHA Class IIIB, IV CHF with mortality endpoint	Trial ongoing	An evaluation of beta-blocker therapy in more advanced heart failure
C-SMART	Cardiomyoplasty-Skeletal Muscle Assist Trial	Randomized cardiomyoplasty trial in 100 NYHA Class III heart failure patients	Equivalent survival with improved exercise tolerance and quality of life in surgery group	Trial stopped early because of patient enrollment problems, cardiomyostimulator device now unavailable
DIG	Digoxin Investigation Group	Survival evaluation to assess the mortality effect of digoxin vs. placebo in stable CHF when used with ACE-I and diuretics (n > 7,000)	No survival benefit with digoxin but morbidity (CHF hospitalizations) reduced	Digoxin is an important agent in CHF to reduce morbidity but likely has no mortality impact
ELITE	Evaluation of Losartan in the Elderly	Tolerability and morbidity/ mortality study of 722 patients over age 65 with Class II, III, IV CHF assigned to either losartan or captopril	Losartan better tolerated and had lower mortality than captopril	The A-II receptor blocker losartan may be a reasonable substitute for ACE-I in CHF
ELITE-II	Evaluation of Losartan in the Elderly-II	Comparison of losartan to captopril with mortality endpoint in 3,152 NYHA Class III, IV CHF with EF < 0.40 and age > 0.60.	No mortality difference between ACE-I and A-II blocker in this trial; however, trial not powered to demonstrate equivalence	Role of A-II blockers in CHF still not clear. One should not substitute an A-II blocker for an ACE-I routinely
EMIAT	European Myocardial Infarction Amiodarone Trial	Patients 5–21 days post-MI EF < 40% randomized (n = 1,486) with mortality primary endpoint	Primary endpoint, death, not reduced by amiodarone but combined endpoint of arrhythmic death/ resuscitated cardiac arrest reduced slightly	No definite benefit with amiodarone in post-MI LV dysfunction and toxicity of drug significant in this study
FACET	Flosequinan ACE-Inhibition Trial	Exercise and quality of life endpoint trial with flosequinan 100 mg of 75 mg added to digoxin, diuretic, and ACE-I	100-mg dose improved patients clinically	Subsequent mortality trial demonstrated increase in death rates, drug may make patient feel better but at a cost of higher mortality
FIRST	Flolan International Randomized Survival Trial	Mortality study of conventional therapy vs. continuous IV epoprostenol (prostacycline) in end-stage congestive heart failure	This study was terminated prematurely due to increased mortality and clinical deterioration in the epoprostenol group	Prostacyclin not an option for chronic parenteral infusion in heart failure; mortality is increased
GESICA	Group Study of Heart Failure Argentina	Placebo-controlled study of amiodarone in moderate to severe CHF assessing mortality as a primary endpoint	Mortality was significantly reduced with amiodarone (42%) compared to placebo (53%)	Suggested amiodarone can be used in some CHF patients

Table continued on opposite page

TABLE 5-5 Select Heart Failure Clinical Trials (Listed Alphabetically According to Acronym) (*Continued*)

ACRONYM	FULL TITLE	STUDY DESIGN	FINDINGS	THERAPEUTIC IMPLICATIONS
HOPE	Heart Outcomes Prevention Trial	Randomized 2 × 2 factorial design of ramapril and vitamin E in approximately 9,500 patients at high risk of CV events including development of CHF	Impressive reductions in CV events including development of CHF, particularly in diabetics with ACE-I but not vitamin E	ACE-I (ramapril) are powerful agents when given early to patients at risk of CV events with benefit not entirely due to BP reduction
IMAC	Intervention in Myocarditis and Acute Cardiomyopathy with IV Immunoglobulin	Randomized, double blind, multicenter trial in 61 patients with new-onset cardiomyopathy who received intravenous IVIG or placebo	No differences in outcomes with LVEF being primary endpoint	IVIG likely plays no role in benefiting patients with new-onset cardiomyopathy presumed to be inflammatory in etiology
LIDO	Levosimendan Infusion vs. Dobutamine	Randomized, double blind, multicenter comparison of the efficacy and safety of 24-hr levosimendan infusion vs. dobutamine in severely decompensated CHF patients (N ~ 200)	Both drugs hemodynamically active with fewer deaths in group exposed to levosimendan at 180-day follow-up (concomitant medications not specified/controlled)	Study raises the important question of long-term effects of short-term vasoactive drug infusion
MACH-I	Mortality Assessment in Congestive Heart Failure	Mibefradil, a T-type calcium channel blocker compared to placebo in 2,390 patients with NYHA Class II, III CHF on ACE-I, diuretics, digoxin	Mibefradil increased mortality compared to placebo by 11%	Calcium channel blockers remain concerning in CHF, with mibefradil likely adversely interacting with drugs that prolong the QT interval
MADIT	Multicenter Automatic Defibrillator Implantation Trial	Randomized trial of AICD vs. conventional therapy in post-MI patients with EF ≤ 0.35, NSVT, and nonsuppressible VT on EP study	AICD leads to better survival in this high-risk ASCVD population with heart failure; beta blockers and amiodarone did not appear to have significant impact on hazard ratio	Provides an alternative strategy for treatment of select patients with heart failure and life-threatening ventricular arrhythmias
MDC	Metoprolol in Dilated Cardiomyopathy	Effect of metoprolol vs. placebo on survival in dilated cardiomyopathy	Compared to placebo, metoprolol patients had improved symptoms and cardiac function; 34% fewer primary endpoints of death or transplant listing with metoprolol	Provided some support for beta-blocker use in CHF patients but study design criticized
MERIT-HF	Metoprolol CR/XL Randomized Intervention Trial in Heart Failure	Tested efficacy of adding beta blocker metoprolol to standard therapy in NYHA Class II, III CHF (n ~ 4,000), morbidity/mortality endpoints	Highly significant (35%) decrease in mortality with metoprolol; Trial stopped early	Additional evidence supporting beta-blocker use in mid–moderate CHF; metoprolol properties different from carvedilol and bisoprolol
MIRACLE	Multicenter, Randomized, Cardiac Resynchronization Trial	Randomized, exercise/QOL endpoint clinical trial of atrial-biventricular pacing in NYHA Class III, IV CHF patients with wide QRS but no indications for a pacemaker	Trial ongoing	Study may justify mechanical approach to CHF that will improve efficiency of cardiac contraction resynchronization and decrease mitral regurgitation
MIRACE-ICD	Multicenter, Randomized, Cardiac Resynchronization Trial–Defibrillator	Randomized, exercise/QOL endpoint clinical trial of atrial-biventricular pacing with device having ICD capabilities in patients with indication for ICD but not a pacemaker	Trial ongoing	Extends concepts being evaluated in MIRACLE, but CHF patient applicability being broadened by coupling ICD capabilities to cardiac resynchronization
MOXCON	Moxonidine in Congestive Heart Failure	Mortality endpoint trial planned for ~4,000 NYHA Class III, IV CHF patients with EF < 0.40	Study terminated early because moxonidine associated with increase in mortality	Reasons for adverse outcomes not clear; concept of central alpha blockade in heart failure deserves more scrutiny

Table continued on following page

TABLE 5–5	Select Heart Failure Clinical Trials (Listed Alphabetically According to Acronym) (Continued)			
ACRONYM	FULL TITLE	STUDY DESIGN	FINDINGS	THERAPEUTIC IMPLICATIONS
OPTIME	Optimal Management of Decompensated Heart Failure	Randomized milrinone vs. dobutamine study where patients (n = 950) admitted for CHF management, but not decompensation to the point of requiring inotropes, were studied to see if LOS could be shortened	No impact on LOS outcomes; more adverse events with milrinone	Routinely prescribed inotropes in CHF patients generally likely not beneficial and could be associated with an increase in adverse events (new atrial fibrillation and sustained hypotension, $p < .05$)
PRAISE	Prospective Randomized Amlodipine Survival Evaluation	Effect of amlodipine, a long-acting calcium antagonist, vs. placebo on survival against background of digoxin, diuretic, ACE-I	Benefits seemed confined to dilated cardiomyopathy group; overall drug seemingly well tolerated	Suggested at least one calcium channel blocker might be safe and possibly advantageous in select nonischemic CHF patients
PRAISE-II	Prospective Randomized Amlodipine Survival Evaluation-II	Randomized, multicenter, placebo-controlled add on amlodipine therapy in 1,800 patients with dilated, nonischemic cardiomyopathy with mortality primary endpoint	No harm or benefit detected with amlodipine therapy	In a properly powered mortality endpoint clinical trial, the calcium channel blocker amlodipine did not confer benefit and negated suggestion on benefit in PRAISE-I
PRECISE/MOCHA	Prospective Randomized Evaluation of Carvedilol on Symptoms and Exercise/ Multicenter Oral Carvedilol Heart Failure Assessment	Patients randomized to placebo vs. carvedilol in three distinct subgroups to accommodate mild, moderate, or severe CHF; ascending carvedilol dose as tolerated (PRECISE) vs. fixed-dose carvedilol (MOCHA)	Trials combined with two others to suggest mortality reduction; effects on exercise tolerance minimal; clinical CHF improved	Carvedilol may be first beta bocker (with alpha-blocking properties) to be given regulatory approval for heart failure therapeutics
PRIME-II	Prospective Randomized Studies of Ibopamine on Mortality and Efficacy	Placebo-controlled mortality endpoint trial of a novel dopaminergic-1 active agent in 2,200 advanced CHF patients	Trial stopped prematurely after 1,906 patients because of excessive treatment group mortality	Though drug has primary effects of peripheral and renal vasodilation without significant inotropic or proarrhythmia, there was a negative mortality impact; drug will likely not be developed
PROFILE	Prospective Randomized Flosequinan Longevity Evaluation	Effect of flosequinan vs. placebo on survival, against background of digoxin, diuretic, ACE-I	A higher mortality rate in the flosequinan group (100 mg/day) was observed compared to placebo	Forced withdrawal of flosequinan from the market in May 1993
PROMISE	Prospective Randomized Milrinone Survival Evaluation	Survival evaluation of milrinone vs. placebo against digoxin, diuretic, ACE-I background	Milrinone produced decreased survival and increased side effects compared to placebo	Phosphodiesterase inhibitors used chronically in heart failure likely to improve symptoms at the risk of higher mortality
PROVED	Prospective Randomized Study of Ventricular Failure and the Efficacy of Digoxin	Efficacy evaluation in patients with stable heart failure, on digoxin and diuretics, randomized to continued digoxin or withdrawal onto placebo (same design as PROVED)	Digoxin withdrawal group demonstrated significant deterioration of exercise and increased treatment failure	Small trial support for digoxin use in CHF (and caution against stopping drug)
RADIANCE	Randomized Digoxin and Inhibitor of Angiotensin Converting Enzyme Inhibitor	Patients with moderate to severe heart failure were randomized to remain on digoxin or be withdrawn on placebo	Patients withdrawn to placebo had deterioration of exercise performance, and worsening symptoms compared to individuals maintained on digoxin	"Triple" therapy with ACE-I, diuretic, digoxin likely is best baseline approach to CHF treatment

Table continued on opposite page

TABLE 5–5	Select Heart Failure Clinical Trials (Listed Alphabetically According to Acronym) (Continued)

ACRONYM	FULL TITLE	STUDY DESIGN	FINDINGS	THERAPEUTIC IMPLICATIONS
RALES	Randomized Aldactone Evaluation Study	Randomized, multicenter, placebo-controlled mortality endpoint trial in 1,663 NYHA Class III, IV CHF patients over the age of 60	30% reduction in risk of death ($p < .001$) with low doses of aldactone	Older patients with more advanced CHF may benefit with aldactone added on to other agents to more completely block the adverse neurohormonal milieu associated with heart failure. Hyperkalemia could be a problem.
RENAISSANCE	Randomized Etamercept North American Strategy to Study Antagonism of Cytokines	Randomized, composite endpoint placebo controlled, multi-center trial with twice-weekly injections of TNF modulator added on to standard therapies in NYHA Class III, IV CHF patients with EF < 30%	Trial ongoing	Results will give insight into the role of cytokines in heart failure
RESOLVD	Candesartan Cilexetil in Heart Failure Assessment of Reduction in Mortality and Morbidity	Randomized, placebo-controlled, international, multicenter mortality endpoint trial of candesartan in 6,500 patients with NYHA Class III, IV CHF; three groups assessed: ACE-I intolerant, EF > 0.40, EF < 0.40, and on ACE-I	Trial ongoing	Tests A-II blocker across the broad spectrum of CHF; only ongoing trial evaluating this strategy in ACE-I intolerant and "diastolic dysfunction" patients
SAVE	Survival and Ventricular Enlargement	Effect of placebo vs. captopril on survival and ventricular enlargement in LV dysfunction patients post-MI	Captopril improved survival, functional status, and reduced repeat myocardial infarction compared to placebo	Even in asymptomatic ventricular dysfunction postinfarct ACE-I beneficial
SOLVD (Treatment and Prevention Trials)	Studies of Left Ventricular Dysfunction Trial	Patients with symptomatic heart failure and decreased ejection fraction (treatment trial) or asymptomatic LV dysfunction (prevention trial) were randomized to placebo vs. enalapril	Enalapril improved survival and symptoms in the treatment trial and delayed onset or progression of heart failure in the prevention trial	Taken together, trials established concept that ACE-I first-line therapy in all heart failure patients (not just CHF)
SPICE	Studies of Patients Intolerant of Converting Enzyme Inhibitors	Registry to determine true incidence of ACE-I intolerance in CHF patients with EF < 0.40 and randomized, double-blind, placebo-controlled, pilot study of 75 ACE-I patients	In registry of about 10,000 patients, 80% successfully up-titrated on ACE-I; true intolerance noted in a little over 10% with cough being greatest problem; candesartan well tolerated in ACE-I intolerant patients	Reasonable to say 80% of CHF patients with low EF can be on ACE-I, and the A-II blocker candesartan was well tolerated when ACE-I were not
SWORD	Effect of d-Sotalol on Mortality in Patients with Left Ventricular Dysfunction after Recent and Remote Myocardial Infarction	Randomized, placebo-controlled, multicenter trial in patients with EF below 0.40 and recent (6–42 days) or remove (> 42 days) infarction (n = 3,121)	Study stopped prematurely because of excess treatment mortality (5% vs. 3% death rate, $p < .008$) in Sotolol group	Even an antiarrhythmic agent with only pure K^+ channel blocking effects has adverse outcome in heart failure patients
VEST	Vesnarinone Survival Trial	Large-scale mortality endpoint trial of 60-mg and 30-mg doses in NYHA Class III, IV patients on digoxin, diuretic, and ACE-I	Increased mortality noted in contrast to prior study that suggested dramatic benefit	Role of vesnarinone in CHF now in question; certain subgroups may benefit but this is yet to be determined

Table continued on following page

TABLE 5–5 **Select Heart Failure Clinical Trials (Listed Alphabetically According to Acronym)** *(Continued)*

ACRONYM	FULL TITLE	STUDY DESIGN	FINDINGS	THERAPEUTIC IMPLICATIONS
V-HeFT-I	Veterans Administration Cooperative Vasodilator Heart Failure Trial I	Parallel study of the effects of placebo, prazosin, and hydralazine on survival	Hydralazine and isosorbide dinitrate improved survival; prazosin was no different than placebo	First study to confirm that vasodilators could save lives in CHF
V-HeFT-II	Veterans Administration Cooperative Vasodilator Heart Failure Trial II	Parallel study of enalapril vs. hydralazine/ isosorbide dinitrate on survival in moderate heart failure	Enalapril significantly improved survival; hydralazine/isosorbide dinitrate improved EF and exercise	First to demonstrate incremental benefit of vasodilators with endocrinologic effects
V-HeFT-III	Veterans Administration Cooperative Vasodilator Heart Failure Trial III	2 × 2 factorial design study evaluating the efficacy of felodipine, digoxin, and placebo	No mortality reduction noted; felodipine seemingly well tolerated	Felodipine possibly another calcium channel blocking drug that can be used safely in CHF, though not beneficial
VMAC	Vasodilator Management of Congestive Heart Failure	Randomized, multicenter, NTG-controlled, symptom/hemodynamic endpoint, clinical trial (n = 500) of natrecor (BNP) infusion in severe CHF in patients	Trial ongoing	Vasodilating efficacy of BNP in severe CHF demonstrated; VMAC designed to evaluate safety of different infusion strategies, including those not utilizing ICU/PAP pressure monitoring
WATCH	Warfain Anticoagulation Trial in CHF	Multicenter, randomized, placebo-controlled trial of anticoagulation vs. platelet inhibition to reduce CHF morbidity/ mortality	Trial ongoing	Study will clarify wisdom of routine anticoagulation strategies in CHF patients
XAMOTEROL	Xamoterol in Severe Heart Failure	Survival endpoint evaluation in 516 CHF patients; placebo-controlled, multicenter, European	Xamoterol associated with higher mortality at 90-day point	Inotropic agents with beta-agonist effects increase mortality in CHF patients

CHF, congestive heart failure; EF, ejection fraction; ECG, electrocardiogram; LV, left ventricular; MI, myocardial infarction; CABG, coronary artery bypass grafting; PVC, premature ventricular contraction; LVD, left ventricular dysfunction; ACE-I, angiotensin-converting enzyme inhibitors; A-II, angiotensin-II; IV, intravenous; CV, cardiovascular; BP, blood pressure; IVIG, intravenous immunoglobulin; AICD, automatic implantable cardioverter defibrillator; NSVT, nonsustained ventricular tachycardia; EP, electrophysiology; ASCVD, atherosclerotic cardiovascular disease; QOL, quality of life; LOS, length of stay; TNF, tumor necrosis factor; NTG, nitroglycerin; BNP, brain natriuretic peptide; ICU, intensive care unit; PAP, pulmonary artery pressure.

vanced (ejection fraction < 0.20 and several concomitant signs and symptoms of heart failure present).

In a study performed by the Clinical Quality Improvement Network Investigators, an audit of 460,000 hospitalized patient charts between 1992 and 1993 demonstrated that diuretics were used in 86% of heart failure patients, ACE inhibitors in 53%, digoxin in 46%, calcium channel antagonists in 20%, and beta-adrenergic blockers in 15%.

The **Study of Patients Intolerant to Converting Enzyme Inhibitors** (SPICE) registry (which included international centers with heart failure experience and expertise) gathered similar data in 1997 from 10,000 patients with systolic left ventricular dysfunction, of which 81% of the patient population was currently on ACE inhibitors, with 57% taking digoxin, 78% on diuretics, 16% on calcium channel antagonists, 14% on antiarrhythmic drugs, and 26% on beta-adrenergic blocking agents.[16]

Both the SOLVD registry and the SPICE registry demonstrated the preponderance of ischemic heart disease as the cause of heart failure.

These registries documented evolution toward nearly routine use of ACE inhibitors and diuretics in the therapy of heart failure, the increased utilization of beta-adrenergic blocking agents, and less frequent use of calcium channel antagonists and nonamiodarone antiarrhythmic drugs (Fig. 5–1). In the future, a major emphasis will shift to earlier diagnosis of asymptomatic ventricular dysfunction, and this will allow implementation of strategies known to be effective in attenuating ventricular dysfunction by preventing the cardiac remodeling processes characteristic of heart failure. Finally, greater understanding of the molecular biodynamics, humoral perturbation, and circulatory derangements of heart failure, as detailed in Chapter 4, will likely lead to new heart failure treatment strategies aimed at alteration of the regressive genetic processes apparent in heart failure.

PHARMACOLOGIC THERAPY OF CHRONIC HEART FAILURE

RECOMMENDED TREATMENT ALGORITHMS

The medications commonly used in heart failure treatment protocols are listed in Table 5–6 and the AHCPR

algorithm for pharmacologic management of patients with heart failure is outlined in Figure 5–3. This scheme focuses largely on symptomatic out-of-hospital patients with suspected congestive heart failure and was published before recommendations regarding beta-blocker use were developed. For patients with mild dyspnea on exertion but no clinical evidence of volume overload, it is recommended that therapy be initiated with an ACE inhibitor and that the drug chosen be titrated to appropriate doses. Proper dose is defined as that used in clinical drug trials demonstrating morbidity and mortality reduction (Table 5–6). If symptoms do not resolve,

TABLE 5-6	**Medications Commonly Used for Heart Failure**			
DRUG	INITIAL DOSE (MG)	TARGET DOSE (MG)	RECOMMENDED MAXIMAL DOSE (MG)	MAJOR ADVERSE REACTIONS
Thiazide diuretics				
Hydrochlorothiazide (Hydrodiuril)	25 qd	As needed	50 qd	Postural hypotension, hypokalemia, hyperglycemia, hypomagnesia, rash, rare severe reactions (pancreatitis, bone marrow suppression, and anaphylaxis)
Chlorthalidone (Hygroton)	25 qd	As needed	50 qd	
Thiazide-related				
Metolazone (Zaroxolyn)	2.5 qd	As needed	10 qd	Same as thiazide diuretics
Loop diuretics				
Furosemide (Lasix)	20–80 qd	As needed	240 bid	Same as thiazide diuretics
Torsemide (Demadex)	10 qd	As needed	200 qd	
Bumetanide (Bumex)	0.5–1.0 qd	As needed	10 qd	
Ethacrynic acid (Edacrin)	50 qd	As needed	200 bid	
IV diuretic				
Furosemide (Lasix)	10–40 bolus	As needed	1,000 qd	Same as thiazide diuretics
Chlorothiazide (Diuril)	250 bolus	As needed	1 g bid	
Potassium-sparing diuretics				
Spironolactone (Aldactone)	25 qd	As needed	100 bid	Hypotension, especially if administered with ACE inhibitor, rash, gynecomastia (spironolactone only)
Triamterene (Maxzide)	50 qd	As needed	100 bid	Little info regarding use in heart failure
Amiloride (Midamor)	5 qd	As needed	20 bid	Little info regarding use in heart failure
ACE inhibitors				
Enalapril (Vasotec)	2.5 bid	10 bid	20 bid	
Captopril (Captopen)	6.25–12.5 tid	50 tid	100 tid	Hypotension, hyperkalemia, renal insufficiency, cough, skin rash, angioedema, neutropenia
Lisinopril (Prinivil, Zestril)	5 qd	20 qd	40 qd	
Quinapril (Accupril)	5 qd	20 qd	20 qd	
Ramipril (Altace)*	1.25 bid	10 bid	10 bid	
Fosinopril (Monopril)	2.5 or 5 bid	20 bid	20 bid	
Benazepril (Lotensin)†	2.5 or 5 bid	20 bid	20 bid	
Trandolapril (Mavik)†	1.0 qd	4 qd	4 qd	
Moexipril (Univasc)†	7.5 qd	30 qd	30 qd	
Digoxin				
(Digoxin, Lanoxin)	0.25 qd	As needed	As needed	Cardiotoxicity, confusion, nausea, anorexia, visual disturbances
Hydralazine (Apresoline)	10–25 tid	75 tid	100 tid	Headache, nausea, dizziness, tachycardia, lupus-like syndrome
Isosorbide dinitrate (Isodril, Sorbitrate)	10 tid	40 tid	80 tid	Headache, hypotension, flushing
Beta blockers				
Carvedilol (Coreg)	3.125 bid	25 bid (≤85 kg) 50 bid (≤85 kg)	25 bid (≤85 kg) 50 bid (≤85 kg)	Bradycardia, hypotension, AV block, worsening CHF, bronchospasm, dyspnea
Metoprolol (Toprol XL)	25 qd	50 qd	100 qd	
Metoprolol (Lopressor)	25 bid	50 bid	100 bid	
Bisoprolol (Zebeta)	1.25 bid	5 qd (≤ 85 kg) 10 qd (≤ 85 kg)	20 qd	

* FDA labeled for heart failure following acute MI.
† Not FDA labeled for heart failure therapy.

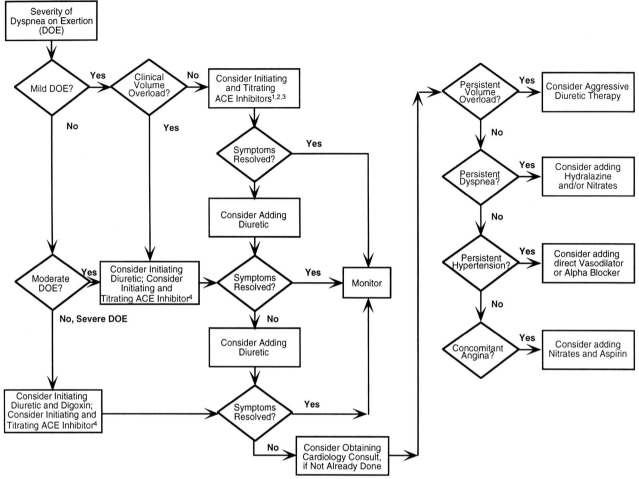

FIGURE 5-3. AHCPR (Agency for Health Care Policy and Research) algorithm for pharmacologic management of heart failure patients.

consideration should be given to adding diuretic therapy, and if symptoms still persist, digitalization is suggested. In patients with mild dyspnea on exertion and clinical volume overload evident on examination, it is recommended that both diuretics and ACE inhibitors be initiated.

According to the AHCPR algorithm, patients presenting with moderate dyspnea on exertion are best served by initiating diuretic, digoxin, and an ACE inhibitor together. In those patients whose symptoms do not resolve readily despite initiation of triple therapy, acceleration of diuretic protocol is suggested. As an alternative or in conjunction with this, addition of hydralazine or long-acting nitrates or both are appropriate. It is important to use long-acting nitrates and aspirin in individuals with concomitant angina pectoris.

Persistent hypertension despite adequate diuretic and ACE inhibitor therapy must be addressed aggressively. The AHCPR recommended several agents other than diuretics, beta-adrenergic blocking drugs, and ACE inhibitors that could be considered options to treat hypertension or high normal blood pressure in patients with heart failure (Table 5–7). It is important to consider these alternative drugs because, with the exception of amlodipine and felodipine, calcium channel blocking drugs

are likely best avoided in heart failure settings. The direct-acting vasodilators, peripherally acting alpha-adrenergic blockers, centrally acting alpha-adrenergic blockers, and angiotensin-II receptor blockers provide attractive alternatives. The AHCPR suggestions must be combined with subsequent recommendations published regarding beta-blocker use in heart failure.

ANGIOTENSIN-CONVERTING ENZYME INHIBITORS

ACE inhibitors are first-line agents in patients with all forms of heart failure. Their salutary effects result from a blockade of the renin-angiotensin-aldosterone system and balanced arterial and venous vasodilation. Additional effects of ACE inhibitors can be predicted from the knowledge of the physiologic effects of the renin-angiotensin system[173] (see Chapter 4). As a consequence of the beneficial effect of ACE inhibitors on reducing afterload and preload, the ventricular wall stress and myocardial oxygen demands are reduced. Inhibition of angiotensin-II–induced aldosterone stimulation results in reduced sodium and water retention and reduction in intravascular volume. Since angiotensin-II stimulates

TABLE 5-7	Medications Other than Diuretics, Beta Blockers, and ACE Inhibitiors to Treat Hypertension or High-Normal Blood Pressure in Patients with Heart Failure		
DRUG	INITIAL DOSE (MG)	MAXIMUM DOSE (MG)	MAJOR ADVERSE REACTIONS
Direct vasodilators			
Minoxidil (Loniten)	2.5 tid	80 qd	Fluid retention, hair growth, thrombocytopenia, leukopenia
Peripheral alpha-Adrenergic blockers			
Doxazosin (Cardura)	1 qd	16 qd	Postural hypotension, dizziness, syncope, headache
Terazosin (Hytrin)	1 qd	20 qd	Similar to doxazosin
Prazosin (Minipres)	1 tid	10 qd	Similar to doxazosin
Centrally acting alpha blockers			
Clonidine tablets (Catapres)	0.1 bid	0.6 bid	Sedation, dry mouth, blurry vision headache, bradycardia
Clonidine patch (TTS-1)	0.1 weekly	0.3 weekly	Same as clonidine; contact dermatitis
Guanabenz (Wytensin)	4 bid	64 bid	Similar to clonidine
Guanfacine (Tenex)	1 qd	3 qd	Similar to clonidine
Angiotensin-II receptor blockers			
Losartan (Cozaar)	25 qd	50 qd	Major effects: hypotension, renal insufficiency, dizziness
Valsartan (Diovan)	80 qd	320 qd	Same as losartan, plus hyperkalemia, edema, neutropenia
Irbesartan (Avapro)	150 qd	300 qd	Same as losartan
Candesartan (Atacand)	16 qd	32 qd	Same as losartan, plus headache and upper respiratory tract infection
Telmisartan (Micardis)	40 qd	80 qd	Same as losartan

the sympathetic nervous system through local release of norepinephrine, ACE inhibitors theoretically could reduce arrhythmogenic tendencies in infarcted or cardiomyopathic muscle.[24] ACE inhibitors may also retard interstitial collagen deposition in the heart through inhibition of norepinephrine-induced alpha-adrenergic stimulation.[266]

Table 5–6 lists selective ACE inhibitors that have been evaluated extensively with mortality endpoint trials so that proper target doses can be defined. A broad spectrum of heart failure patients have been studied with ACE inhibitors (Table 5–5). The Cooperative North Scandinavian Enalapril Survival Study (CONSENSUS)[72, 173, 252] was the first large mortality endpoint clinical trial evaluating an ACE inhibitor in this setting. This study demonstrated profound mortality reduction in severely ill congestive heart failure patients with an ACE inhibitor compared with placebo therapy (6-month mortality, 26% vs. 41%; $p = .002$). The dramatic CONSENSUS results promoted the neurohumoral blocking hypothesis in heart failure, which opined that mortality reduction could be achieved by blocking certain aspects of neurohormonal up-regulation characteristic of heart failure and, specifically, the renin-angiotensin-aldosterone cascade.

Subsequently, the second Veterans Administration Cooperative Vasodilator Heart Failure Trial (V-HeFT-II)[69, 70] compared the combination of hydralazine and isosorbide dinitrate to the ACE inhibitor enalapril in New York Class II and Class III patients and demonstrated that enalapril effected greater mortality reduction than did the direct-acting vasodilator combination. V-HeFT-I had compared hydralazine–isosorbide dinitrate combination with placebo and prazosin in moderately symptomatic heart failure patients and was the first clinical trial to demonstrate that some direct-acting vasodilators were likely effective in heart failure patients.[66] V-HeFT-I further suggested that not all vasodilators producing hemodynamic benefit were alike. Prazosin did not attenuate mortality. V-HeFT-II explored

this concept further by raising the question of whether agents primarily blocking humoral factors were better in heart failure than those with only hemodynamic actions. Enalapril was associated with greater mortality reduction than the direct-acting vasodilator combination (hydralazine–isosorbide dinitrate).

The SOLVD program[247] evaluated enalapril in asymptomatic or minimally symptomatic patients (and therefore extended the spectrum of heart failure into patients with only left ventricular systolic dysfunction, i.e., ejection fraction < 0.35). This "prevention trial" studied enalapril as first-line treatment in patients with early functional manifestations of heart failure and demonstrated significant reduction in the combined endpoint of congestive heart failure morbidity (hospital admission for heart failure) and mortality. This trial was the first mortality endpoint randomized clinical trial to suggest that early ("preventive strategy") administration of ACE inhibitors could attenuate progression toward clinically manifest heart failure when used as a first-line drug in asymptomatic or minimally symptomatic patients with left ventricular systolic dysfunction. In patients with symptomatic congestive heart failure in the SOLVD "treatment trial" (1991), enalapril significantly reduced mortality, morbidity, and major ischemic events such as acute myocardial infarction. Substudy evaluation demonstrated that in both the prevention and treatment trials, enalapril significantly attenuated myocardial remodeling by blocking ventricular dilation and cardiac mass increase. Observations from SOLVD shifted the heart failure therapeutic paradigm from simply a diuretic and digoxin prescription begun when patients developed congestive heart failure to **instituting ACE inhibitor therapy first and early in the disease course, even in noncongested, asymptomatic or minimally symptomatic patients.**

The issue of ACE inhibitor use routinely after myocardial infarction in patients with heart failure also has added credence to the fact that these drugs are critically important in those with ventricular dysfunction. The

Survival and Ventricular Enlargement (SAVE)[218] trial demonstrated that captopril improved survival and functional status and reduced subsequent myocardial infarctions compared with placebo when this ACE inhibitor was begun soon after acute myocardial infarction and left ventricular systolic dysfunction (ejection fraction < 0.40) was noted, even in the absence of substantive congestive heart failure. Several other clinical trials after acute myocardial infarction have confirmed that ACE inhibitors begun shortly after the event were associated with significant benefit when either asymptomatic systolic left ventricular dysfunction or mild clinical congestive heart failure was present. These trials included the Acute Infarction Evaluation (AIRE) study[251] evaluating ramipril, the SMILE trial evaluating zofenopril, and the TRACE[157] trial evaluating trandolapril. Thus captopril, ramipril, zofenopril, and trandolapril trials indicated long-term benefit when ACE inhibitors are employed routinely after myocardial infarction if heart failure or left ventricular dysfunction is present.

Several large trials of ACE inhibitors after myocardial infarction suggest that the routine maintenance administration of these agents early after the event (i.e., irrespective of presence or absence of left ventricular systolic dysfunction or symptomatic congestive heart failure) produces short-term reduction in mortality rates. The International Study of Infarct Survival-IV (ISIS-IV) and Gruppo Italiano per lo Studio Della Streptochinasi Nell Infarto Miocardico III (GISSI-III)[128] included patients with a wide spectrum of ejection fractions. Their positive findings suggest that early administration of ACE inhibitors following myocardial infarction would translate into short- and long-term survival benefit. The CONSENSUS-II study, which also randomized post infarction patients in unselected fashion to therapy with an ACE inhibitor or placebo, did not demonstrate significant reduction in mortality or morbidity. This trial, however, randomized only 6,000 patients in comparison with the much larger "mega" trials, ISIS-IV and GISSI-III. Despite the results of this one trial, the compendium of data supports **use of angiotensin-converting enzyme inhibitors after myocardial infarction when heart failure is clinically manifest or left ventricular systolic dysfunction is apparent.**

As a group, these drugs appear to retard or prevent the development of symptomatic congestive heart failure when prescribed early in the course of a patient's disease,[127] and should be considered first-line drug therapy, even as monotherapy. Though the beneficial effects of ACE inhibitors are likely related to common properties of these drugs, regulatory labeling has been based on the type of clinical trial performed. For example, some agents have been suggested useful in the postinfarct setting, such as captopril, and others have been given labeling approbation for claims of morbidity as well as mortality reduction (such as enalapril). No matter which agent is chosen, the prescription of these drugs in dosages similar to those employed during clinical trial performance and in similar patient populations is important. It has been suggested that underdosing of captopril is common. This may be fueled by fear of causing unacceptable reduction in blood pressure or

worsening renal function. Precise definition of optimal blood pressure in patients with ventricular dysfunction and heart failure has become a contentious issue, with no precise target pressure easily identifiable. It seems, however, that the lowest blood pressure a patient can tolerate (in the absence of cardiac ischemia) without significant orthostatic symptoms, obtundation, or renal dysfunction is the best blood pressure in any specific clinical setting.

Additional important observations regarding ACE inhibitor benefits were made in the Heart Outcomes Prevention Trial (HOPE) trial. This study tested the hypothesis that routine prescription of ramipril in almost 10,000 patients without heart failure but with high risk of having an atherosclerotic event would reduce morbidity and mortality. This concept was proven when routine prescription of ramipril resulted in a dramatic reduction in subsequent development of heart failure over a 4.5-year period of time. This reinforces the argument that ACE inhibitors (and ramipril in this particular case) should be used early to prevent manifest ventricular dysfunction in patients at risk of developing heart failure. Interestingly, vitamin E, which was also evaluated in this trial, had no effects whatsoever on the prestated endpoints.

Table 5–8 is a scheme utilized for initiating ACE inhibitor therapy in patients hospitalized with congestive states who have not previously been on these drugs. The algorithm is based on using the shorter acting agent captopril acutely, avoiding its concomitant administration during aggressive diuretic use, with a transition to the longer acting agents (which might be better tolerated from a patient compliance standpoint). Reasonable daily target doses for these drugs are 150 mg for captopril, 20 mg for enalapril, and 20 mg for lisinopril.

Patients who are at risk of developing orthostatic hypotension after ACE inhibitor exposure include those

---

TABLE 5–8 Initiating ACE Inhibitor Therapy in Hospitalized Patients

Captopril incremental increase:
- 6.25 mg → 12.5 mg → 25 mg → 50 mg
- Hold diuretic 1 hr before and 1 hr after initial dose if concerned about low BP
- Begin 12.5 mg orally (6.25 mg in labile* patient)
- After 2 hr increase dose (if tolerated) to 25 mg orally
- After 6 hr increase dose (if tolerated) to 50 mg tid
- Target dose is 100–150 mg/day

Enalapril incremental increase:
- 2.5 mg → 5 mg → 10 mg
- Hold diuretic 1 hr before and 1 hr after initial doses if concerned about low BP
- Begin 5 mg orally (2.5 mg in labile patient)
- After 6 hr increase dose (if tolerated) to 10 mg orally
- After 12 hr increase dose (if tolerated) to 10 mg bid
- Target dose is 20 mg/day

Chronic maintenance ACE-I targets:†
- Captopril 50 mg tid
- Enalapril 10 mg bid
- Lisinopril 20 mg qd

* Labile patients are those with hyponatremia, azotemia, volume depletion, and orthostatic or relative hypotension.
† Other ACE-I have labeling approval for heart failure therapy, but those selected are representative short, medium, and long-term agents and representative of the ACE-I group.

with hyponatremia, azotemia, volume depletion (particularly after acute and aggressive diuretic administration), and orthostatic dizziness or syncope. These problems can frequently be avoided with reduction of the ACE inhibitor dose, utilization of a shorter acting agent, diminution of diuretic doses or, indeed, elimination of diuretics completely when a patient is no longer congested. It is very important to remember that ACE inhibitors are likely more important than diuretics in the heart failure patient with respect to prevention of detrimental remodeling and mortality. In general, when congestive states are relieved, it is more appropriate to sacrifice diuretic administration so that ACE inhibitors can be commenced (or maintained) rather than continuing high diuretic doses to the exclusion of ACE inhibitor use.

The administration of ACE inhibitors can be challenging. In the SOLVD program, an analysis of adverse effects of enalapril in 6,797 patients (double blind and placebo controlled) followed over a 40-month average period noted that 28% of patients randomized to drug compared with 16% randomized to placebo experienced side effects. Most of the excess side effects were mild. Still, enalapril use compared with placebo was associated with a higher rate of orthostatic hypotension (15% vs. 7%), azotemia (4% vs. 2%), cough (5% vs. 2%), fatigue (6% vs. 4%), and hyperkalemia (1.2% vs. 0.4%). Side effects resulted in discontinuation of therapy in 15% of the treatment group compared to 9% of the placebo group.

The SPICE registry and trial gives more insight into issues of so-called **ACE inhibitor intolerance.** Of the 8,485 patients in this registry of heart failure patients with systolic dysfunction exposed to an ACE inhibitor, 9% were deemed intolerant. The majority of patients were said to be intolerant of the ACE inhibitor because of intractable cough and, indeed, this represented approximately two thirds of the intolerant group. Renal insufficiency and symptomatic hypotension accounted for approximately one quarter of the intolerant group. In the 158 patients found not to have received an ACE inhibitor because of perceived high risk, the majority had renal insufficiency. It is important, however, to put the benefits of ACE inhibitors into perspective when utilizing these agents in heart failure patients. Drug discontinuation for a mild cough might not be in the best long-term interest of the heart failure patient. An explanation of the rationale behind using these agents will often motivate patients to keep taking them despite minor side effects. Also, cough is frequent in heart failure patients anyway. One should make certain that this complaint is not due to congestion, which could be relieved by diuretic intensification, or secondary to primary pulmonary abnormalities such as chronic obstructive pulmonary disease.

Special caution is advisable in the **administration of ACE inhibitors in the presence of renal dysfunction.**[219] Exacerbation of renal dysfunction is a known potential complication of ACE inhibitors in heart failure therapy.[206] Because angiotensin-II affects postglomerular arterial tone, **ACE inhibitors have a selective renal effect on the glomerular efferent arterioles.** ACE inhibitors limit renal autoregulatory ability to preserve glomerular filtration rate by increasing efferent arterial tone. The deleterious renal effects of ACE inhibitors may be especially pronounced in patients with marginal cardiac output (and therefore renal perfusion) or low blood pressure. This tendency is aggravated with aggressive diuretic therapy, which may further decrease circulating plasma volume. These potentially deleterious effects must be balanced against the beneficial effects of ACE inhibitors on cardiac performance, which may improve overall renal perfusion. Factors associated with worsening of renal dysfunction during ACE inhibitor administration include low cardiac output or poor renal perfusion, preexisting renal dysfunction (elevated creatinine and elevated urea/creatinine ratio), mean arterial pressure less than 80 mm Hg, and large doses of diuretics. Factors which portend an improvement in renal function with ACE inhibitors include improvement in cardiac output, mean arterial pressure greater than 80 mm Hg, increase of sodium intake, and reduction in diuretic dosage. **In general, if the serum creatinine doubles during ACE inhibitor therapy, strong consideration should be given to dose reduction or discontinuation of the ACE inhibitor.** In the CONSENSUS I (CONSENSUS 1991) trial (enalapril compared to placebo in patients with class III or IV congestive heart failure), a doubling of creatinine was experienced in 11% of the enalapril group versus 3% in the placebo group, and the serum creatinine was actually reduced in 24% of the enalapril group, illustrating the trade-off between favorable hemodynamic effects and potentially deleterious renal vascular effects on renal function.[174]

DIURETICS

Because heart failure has traditionally been associated with dropsical conditions, diuretics have previously been the mainstay of treatment.[32] Their main utility, however, must be placed in proper perspective. Diuretics should continue to play an important role in treating patients with heart failure, but primarily those with congestive states.[63] Diuretics have never been studied in large-scale heart failure mortality endpoint trials with the exception of aldactone in the Randomized Aldactone Evaluation Study (RALES) trial,[233] and the drug was not given in diuretic strength nor was the observed benefit due to diuresis.[219] Furthermore, there are few data to support the contention that diuretics in general prevent adverse remodeling. Of concern is the fact that diuretics have been demonstrated to increase many of the neurohumoral factors felt detrimental in the heart failure setting (particularly when patients are excessively diuresed). Studies that do provide support for use of thiazide diuretics to prevent heart failure progression are limited to clinical hypertensive trials where diuretics faired well with respect to diminution of morbidity and mortality.[160, 244, 260] When thiazide diuretics are used in hypertensive patients, cardiovascular event rates including development of congestive heart failure are dramatically reduced. Furthermore, there is no question that diuretics are essential agents to relieve volume overload states sometimes associated with heart failure. However, congestion is not always present in patients with heart failure, and patients may develop congestive states that quickly resolve with pulsed or intermittent diuretic therapy. Attention to low-sodium diet seems particularly important in the therapeutic strategy.

Common problems associated with chronic diuretic therapy include hyponatremia, hypokalemia, hyperkalemia (with potassium-sparing agents), metabolic alkalosis, and increased uric acid levels, all of which set the stage for worsening renal function (Table 5–9).[32] Furthermore, carbohydrate metabolism can be frequently disturbed during chronic diuretic administration, which may result in hyperglycemia, insulin resistance, decreased insulin secretion, and a nonketotic hyperosmolar state. Lipid perturbation is also reported after diuretic therapy, but its significance is not well understood. Diuretic-specific side effects include the ototoxicity of furosemide, gynecomastia and galactosuria of spironolactone, metabolic acidosis caused by carbonic anhydrase inhibitors, and hyperkalemia caused by potassium-sparing diuretics such as spironolactone.

If diuretics are felt important to treat congestive states, generally the least potent and toxic drug (thiazides such as hydrochlorothiazide or chlorthalidone) is prescribed in the lowest dose necessary to induce effective diuresis (see Table 5–6 for dosage suggestions). As the congestive state worsens, longer acting and more potent loop diuretics such as furosemide, bumetanide, or torsemide are prescribed. In refractory edematous states, combinations of diuretic classes may be necessary.[110] It should be emphasized that failure to mobilize salt and water is often due to inadequate sodium and fluid restriction, particularly in individuals recently diuresed and at risk of sodium retention. **Ensuring low sodium consumption is therefore essential to success when using diuretic agents.** Acute diuretic resistance is generally overcome with an increased single diuretic dose. Chronic resistance can be addressed with a coadministration of a thiazide or potassium-sparing diuretic with a loop diuretic. Using combinations of agents active at different

nephron sites is essential. It does not make clinical or pharmacologic sense to use two agents acting at the same point (such as combining furosemide with torsemide). Altered bioavailability may account for some aspects of diuretic resistance, and differing absorption kinetics have been reported with furosemide, bumetanide, and torsemide.[33, 215] Sometimes switching among these oral loop diuretics proves helpful. Alternatively, giving diuretics intravenously in high dose pulses or even with a continuous infusion can be effective in overcoming diuretic resistance.

Diuretics reduce blood volume and lower cardiac filling pressures with subsequent reduction in myocardial wall stress, pulmonary edema, and peripheral congestion—all advantageous effects in a patient with congestive heart failure. However, reduction in plasma volume, particularly to an excessive point, might activate the renin-angiotensin-aldosterone axis and stimulate up-regulation of the sympathetic nervous system. This will paradoxically promote further sodium and fluid retention while increasing impedance to left ventricular ejection and could contribute to the progression of detrimental heart failure remodeling. For this reason, diuretic therapy alone is not justified during heart failure treatment, and one might even consider discontinuing these agents in patients without congestive states or in whom the congestive state is easily resolved with intensification of sodium restriction or intermittent pulsed diuretic administration.

The best method for initiating diuretic therapy is controversial. Some patients may respond to transient oral pulses of diuretics with resolution of the congestive state occurring quite dramatically and rapidly. Institution or reemphasis of the importance of a low-salt diet in many patients will prevent fluid reaccumulation, and these individuals do not necessarily require long-term maintenance diuretic therapy. On the other hand, some patients might need intermittent but regular oral pulses of diuretics, whereas others will undoubtedly require continuous administration of diuretics in large doses or combinations. Stopping diuretics entirely or creating intervals of "drug holiday" should be considered in patients who have been on diuretics for chronic congestive heart failure, but have resolved their fluid retention state. Patients requiring less than 40 mg of furosemide daily or its equivalent with no clinically detectable volume overload and well-controlled blood pressure can frequently have diuretics stopped.[134] When diuretics are given long-term, one must consider concomitant administration of potassium and magnesium supplements. Magnesium can be important in maintaining adequate potassium levels. On the other hand, because of the effects of ACE inhibitors, serum potassium levels can rise in some patients, setting the stage for hyperkalemia when potassium supplementation is administered. Proper electrolyte surveillance is mandatory.

It is also important to consider the potassium-sparing aldosterone antagonist and diuretic **spironolactone** in congestive heart failure patients. The RALES trial (Table 5–5) evaluated the effect of spironolactone on morbidity and mortality in 1,663 New York Heart Association (NYHA) Class IIIB or IV congestive heart failure patients

---

TABLE 5–9 Common Problems with Diuretics

Electrolyte disturbances
- Hyponatremia
- Hypokalemia (hyperkalemia with K^+-sparing agents)
- Hypomagnesemia
- Hypocalciuria
- Hyperuricemia
- Metabolic alkalosis

Carbohydrate metabolism perturbation
- Hyperglycemia
- Insulin resistance
- Decreased insulin secretion
- Nonketotic hyperosmolar state

Lipid abnormalities
- Increased low-density lipoprotein
- Increased very-low-density lipoprotein
- Increased total cholesterol
- Increased triglycerides

Diuretic-specific side effects
- Furosemide—ototoxicity
- Spironolactone—gynecomastia and galactorrhea
- Acetazolamide—metabolic acidosis
- Potassium-sparing diuretics—hyperkalemia

with depressed ejection fraction.[222] It is important to note that the population had severe congestive heart failure and were aged greater than 60 years. Patients randomized to 25 mg/day of spironolactone (many were only on 15 mg/day and a few were on 50 mg/day) had a 30% reduction in death ($p < .001$), a 30% reduction in hospitalization for cardiac causes, a 32% reduction in death or hospitalization for cardiac causes, and a 35% reduction in progression of heart failure. Hyperkalemia was uncommon in this trial (though still concerning), and spironolactone had to be stopped in about 10% of males because of the development of painful gynecomastia. As mentioned, spironolactone's beneficial effects were not related to diuresis. This drug can be considered an important adjunctive therapy in NYHA Class III/IV congestive heart failure patients who are already taking digoxin, other more potent diuretics, ACE inhibitors, and even beta blockers, although clinicians should still be wary of hyperkalemia.

DIGOXIN

After two centuries of use, controversy still persists regarding administration of cardiac glycosides such as digoxin in patients with heart failure. Actions that make digoxin attractive include positive inotropy, negative chronotropy, and digoxin's ability to favorably modulate neurohumoral factors in heart failure. By increasing baroreceptor sensitivity, digoxin appears to attenuate sympathetic nervous system tone, decrease plasma norepinephrine concentration, and diminish renin and angiotensin levels. The controversy about using digoxin has centered around patient selection, dosing, and whether or not beneficial effects with respect to morbidity and mortality could be expected. Little debate exists regarding digoxin's utility in congestive heart failure patients with atrial fibrillation. However, in this situation it is not clear whether digoxin is more helpful because of its ability to control heart rate or by precipitating other beneficial effects listed above. Digoxin benefits may have little to do with positive inotropic effects.

Some insight has been gained into the contemporary role of digoxin in patients with heart failure and normal sinus rhythm. The Prospective Randomized Study of Ventricular Failure and the Effect of Digoxin (PROVED)[259] and the Randomized Assessment of Digoxin on Inhibitors of the Angiotensin-Converting Enzyme (RADIANCE)[207] assessed the contribution of digoxin therapy to a patient's clinical status when used in a setting of either diuretic (PROVED) or combination diuretic and ACE inhibitor therapy (RADIANCE). These trials are particularly important because they clarify the role of "triple" heart failure therapy in patients with congestive heart failure. Among patients with left ventricular ejection fraction less than 0.35, withdrawal of digoxin in stable congestive heart failure patients increased the probability of worsening heart failure, particularly that requiring hospital admission. Patients remaining on digoxin exercised longer and had an increase in their ejection fraction. The lowest probability of treatment failure was seen in patients treated with the triple

drug combination of digoxin, diuretic, and ACE inhibitor. Although the combination of digoxin and a diuretic was far better than a diuretic alone, the combination of diuretic and ACE inhibitor produced results similar to the digoxin and diuretic combination. Thus, withdrawal of digoxin in stable congestive heart failure patients is associated with higher adverse event rates, and stopping digoxin should be avoided.

The effect of cardiac glycosides on survival has been more difficult to ascertain. Moss and colleagues[192] in 1981 evaluated the effect of digitalis therapy on 4-month postdischarge cardiac mortality after an acute myocardial infarction and demonstrated an insignificant difference in mortality among treatment cohorts except in the group with combined ventricular dysfunction and arrhythmias, in which digitalis was associated with increased mortality. By multivariable analysis, however, digoxin therapy was not identified as an independent predictor of mortality following myocardial infarction.[21]

In a large multicenter trial to evaluate the impact of digoxin on mortality in heart failure, the Digoxin Investigation Group (DIG)[90] evaluated nearly 8,000 patients with digoxin added to a background of ACE inhibitors and diuretic therapy. Results of this trial at the 4-year follow-up point demonstrated that digoxin had no effect on mortality. However, digoxin reduced hospitalization and favorably affected the combined endpoint of death or hospitalization due to worsening congestive heart failure. Of note, those having digoxin withdrawn had congestive heart failure endpoints much earlier and more frequently than the remaining placebo-treated patients. A trend toward increased death due to arrhythmic events in certain subgroups has led some to urge caution in the use of digoxin. However, the most appropriate interpretation of the study results is that digoxin in this trial has been shown safe with substantive reduction in clinically significant morbid events and that benefit is additional to ACE inhibitor and diuretic therapy in patients with congestive heart failure.[4, 202, 271] Analysis of the diastolic dysfunction subset demonstrated exactly the same beneficial outcome with respect to reduction in congestive heart failure endpoints. No mortality benefit was seen in this group either. Though digoxin appears effective in patients with congestive heart failure and normal left ventricular systolic function, its routine prescription in this group of patients is still a contentious subject.

The relationship between digoxin dosage and/or plasma levels and the likelihood of adverse outcome is debated.[2, 4] A subset analysis of the DIG trial suggests that the proportion of patients with very high digoxin levels obtained during routine surveillance are more likely to suffer an adverse outcome. The diagnosis of digoxin toxicity is related to elevated plasma levels of the drug and symptoms. In reality, few data are available concerning the precise relationship of plasma levels to digoxin's physiologic effects. Redfors[236] first explored in 1972 the relationship between plasma digoxin concentration and clinical effects of this drug using the reduction in heart rate in patients with atrial fibrillation as an endpoint. Observations of systolic ejection time intervals suggested that higher digoxin doses and levels produced greater inotropic impact. However, a more detailed analysis of the pooled PROVED and RADIANCE trial database showed a progressive increase in exercise time in patients with baseline digoxin levels of 0.9–1.2 ng/mL and levels greater than 1.2 ng/ml when compared to placebo. Thus, even at lower serum concentration, digoxin was effective. A similar observation was made in the PROVED/RADIANCE[272] pooled analysis when the percentage of patients developing clinical congestive heart failure was determined. Low doses and levels of digoxin were just as effective in preventing the development of heart failure compared with higher doses and serum levels. In these trials, digoxin was superior to placebo regardless of plasma concentration and dose. It is likely, then, that high doses of digoxin are unnecessary to achieve benefit in congestive heart failure patients.

NEWER ORAL INOTROPIC AGENTS

Although decreased contractility clearly is one hallmark of heart failure, much has been learned about humoral factors precipitating and perpetuating detrimental cardiac remodeling, which is the primary deleterious event occurring in these patients. Few inotropic agents have met the challenge of being able to reduce both morbidity and mortality. Although some (such as vesnarinone, milrinone, and flosequinan) appear to improve congestive heart failure symptomatology, increased mortality is common.[205, 211] It is important to distinguish chronic therapy with these oral drugs from the use of inotropic agents parenterally (such as dobutamine and milrinone), which can be life-sustaining when acute heart failure appears or as a last ditch attempt to control the patient's symptomatology, particularly when heart failure is advanced.

Milrinone (a phosphodiesterase inhibitor) given orally was associated with significant mortality in the Prospective Randomized Milrinone Survival Study (PROMISE) trial,[209] and this led to discontinuation of efforts to pursue this compound as an orally active heart failure agent. Most of the excessive death risk in this study was due to sudden cardiac death syndrome. Parenteral milrinone is still available for patients with cardiogenic shock or severe congestive heart failure decompensation with marginal hemodynamics. Recently, milrinone's use in patients admitted to the hospital for a severe congested state but with hemodynamics not warranting parenteral inotropes was studied. The concept was to shorten hospital length of stay and subsequent hospital readmission rates. The Optimal Management of Decompensated Heart Failure (OPTIME) trial randomized 950 patients admitted for congestive heart failure to receive either 48 hours of milrinone or placebo. There were no differences noted in major endpoints when parenteral milrinone was added on top of basic therapies (mostly parenteral diuretics). On the other hand, milrinone infusion was associated with more sustained hypotension and new-onset atrial fibrillation ($p < .05$) in this trial. Though more ill patients as characterized by lower serum sodium at admission had fewer

subsequent readmissions after milrinone, routine use of this drug in hospitalized heart failure patients could not be supported by this trial.[79]

Vesnarinone is an orally active quinolinone preparation that exerts its positive inotropic effect not only by inhibiting phosphodiesterase enzyme but also by decreasing the delayed outward and inward potassium current, increasing intracellular sodium concentration by prolonging opening of sodium channels, and prolonging the action potential in a rate-dependent fashion. The initial vesnarinone mortality endpoint clinical trial consisted of nearly 500 patients with left ventricular ejection fraction less than 0.30 who were treated with digoxin and an ACE inhibitor.[115] There was a remarkable 62% reduction in risk of all causes of mortality and a 50% reduction in combined morbidity and mortality with a 60-mg dose of the drug. These results were highly significant but should be balanced against the fact that the dose of 120 mg/day increased mortality such that this arm of the randomized (and blinded) study was stopped early into the trial. Furthermore, vesnarinone sometimes causes neutropenia. Clinical trials suggested that the incidence of this complication was 1–5% and may relate to the drug's attenuation of certain aspects of cytokine activation. Also confusing is the fact that vesnarinone in some experiences produced clinical benefit at doses that did not produce positive inotropic actions *in vitro*.

The encouraging observations noted in the first vesnarinone mortality trial have been tempered by the recently completed Vesnarinone Survival Trial (VEST), which was a much larger scale, placebo-controlled, multicenter mortality endpoint clinical trial. VEST demonstrated excess mortality in the 60-mg dose group compared with placebo, which was contrary to the findings in the previous vesnarinone study.[68] Particularly disturbing was the fact that the 60-mg dose was associated with an increase in sudden cardiac death without favorable impact on secondary endpoints such as quality of life, hospitalization frequency, or worsening heart failure. There has been a recent suggestion that the increased mortality caused by vesnarinone in VEST was related to a subgroup of patients with a particularly noxious circulating metabolite and that in the subset without this substance, mortality and morbidity reduction was noted. Also important was the observation that withdrawal of vesnarinone did not seem to cause patient deterioration. Thus, the role of vesnarinone in the chronic therapy of heart failure remains doubtful.

Ibopamine is an oral inotropic agent once considered promising in congestive heart failure because of its dopaminergic activity, with stimulation of dopamine-1 and dopamine-2 receptors as well as beta$_1$– and beta$_2$–adrenergic receptors.[262] A dose-related hemodynamic and inotropic response has been noted with this drug. Patients with heart failure have increased cardiac output with reduced ventricular filling pressures and increased renal blood flow at low doses. Though several trials suggested a beneficial effect on exercise performance, the multicenter Prospective Randomized Studies of Ibopamine on Mortality and Efficacy (PRIME-II) trial was prematurely stopped because of increased mortality noted with this inotropic agent.[136] Subgroup analysis revealed that the increased mortality was associated with concomitant use of amiodarone.

Explanation of the rather dismal performance of oral inotropic agents in heart failure mortality endpoint clinical trials remains elusive, but may relate to the likely proarrhythmic effect of agents which increase systolic intracellular calcium concentration. Furthermore, agents which do not attenuate adverse neurohumoral factors associated with heart failure may lack efficacy, especially if they actually increase humors such as epinephrine, norepinephrine, renin-angiotensin, and aldosterone. Still, however, at least one new inotropic drug, **levosimendan,** is undergoing clinical evaluation.[138] Levosimendan has experimentally demonstrated an anti-ischemic effect and has actions independent of traditional cyclic adenosine monophosphate activating pathways. It appears to sensitize the downstream sarcolemmal network to intracellular calcium. Most studies have used the parenteral agent in hospitalized patients with decompensated congestive heart failure. It is a powerful vasodilator in this setting. There is some suggestion that long-term morbidity is reduced after exposure to the drug, but this remains controversial.

DIRECT-ACTING VASODILATORS

It is now generally accepted that reduction of preload and afterload in congestive heart failure patients with direct-acting vasodilators reduces morbidity and mortality when specific agents are prescribed.[53, 66] Relaxation of the venous capacitance vessels diminishes preload, which will improve congestive symptomatology, whereas peripheral arteriolar dilation causes afterload to fall, with subsequent reduction of impedance to ventricular emptying. However, excessive afterload reduction might reflexly activate the sympathetic nervous system and renin-angiotensin-aldosterone axes with subsequent adverse effects on the kidney and cardiovascular network in general. Venous capacitance vessels can be dilated by nitrates such as nitroglyerin, nitroprusside, and isosorbide dinitrate and mononitrate preparations. Hydralazine primarily dilates arterial resistance vessels. Table 5–7 summarizes medications other than diuretics, beta blockers, and ACE inhibitors useful to treat hypertension or high normal blood pressure in patients with heart failure. Combination of arterial and venous dilation occurs with ACE inhibitors and some alpha-adrenergic blockers (e.g., guanabenz and clonidine). Calcium channel blocking drugs are arteriolar dilators as well, but the absence of concomitant venous dilatation is a disadvantage.

Sudden dyspnea can be alleviated with acute administration of short-acting sublingual nitroglycerin, but secure evidence is lacking for long-term attenuation of detrimental mechanical responses seen in the failing ventricle.[119, 120] Though isolated use of long-acting **oral nitrates** in congestive heart failure patients is useful at times, the development of nitrate tolerance may occur, and no preparation currently has regulatory labeling indication for this use. Still, nitrate preparations as a group are theoretically quite beneficial, inducing nitric oxide release within vascular smooth muscle cells. Nitric oxide results in guanylate cyclase activation, which increases cyclic guanosine monophosphate with subsequent muscle cell relaxation and vasodilation. Particularly in the setting of atherosclerosis, endothelial dysfunction is associated with decreased nitric oxide availability, and the nitrate supplies exogenous nitric oxide to the vascular wall, reducing vessel tone. Some evidence also suggests that nitrates have antiplatelet effects that might be important to patients with ischemic heart disease.

Nitrate tolerance develops when blood levels are constantly elevated, and hemodynamic effects are generally lost with chronic exposure. Enhancement of vascular superoxide production secondary to exposure to nitrates may be a mechanism in the development of tolerance. *In vitro* studies suggest that **hydralazine,** which has an antioxidant effect, prevents the nitrate-mediated formation of vascular superoxide and thus retards nitrate tolerance. This observation may provide an explanation for benefits seen in Ve-HeFT-I with the combination of isosorbide dinitrate and hydralazine.

By virtue of its capability to become a sulfhydryl donor, **captopril** is another drug that might combat nitrate tolerance.[18] Alternatively, nitrate tolerance can be reversed after a drug washout period of 10–12 hours. Isosorbide mononitrate preparations given once daily (such as Imdur) or in asymmetric twice daily fashion (Ismo) can obviate tolerance. When nitroglycerin patches are used (an efficient way to deliver nitrates) they should be limited to 8- or 12-hour administration periods, either at night to combat nocturnal dyspnea or during the day to treat exercise intolerance and dyspnea. These patches must not be left in place for 24 hours if nitrate tolerance is to be avoided.

In patients whose symptomatology results from high ventricular filling pressures, pulmonary edema, and low cardiac output usually in the face of elevated systemic vascular resistance, symptoms are usually improved with the combination of diuretics, digoxin, and ACE inhibitors (triple drug heart failure therapy). Utilizing hemodynamic monitoring to optimize intracardiac pressures and flow seemingly translates into attenuated morbidity and mortality. This "tailored" approach to heart failure management is based on the use of combination vasodilating agents.

Although hydralazine has proven beneficial in heart failure regimens, some arteriolar vasodilating compounds have failed to provide demonstrable survival benefit. Prasozin, for example, is a peripheral alpha-adrenergic blocking drug useful in treating hypertension and was one of the first agents to demonstrate hemodynamic efficacy when studied in heart failure patients undergoing cardiac catheterization. Its actions when taken orally appeared to mimic the effects of parenteral nitroprusside. In Ve-HeFT-I, however, prazosin was no better than placebo.[66]

Flolan (prostacyclin) was associated with excessive mortality when given to end-stage heart failure patients ill enough to justify insertion of a permanent central venous catheter infusion system with parenteral drug administration. Results of the Flolan International Randomized Survival Trial (FIRST) trial[42] were not encouraging and again emphasized that vasodilating effects cannot always be translated into tangible clinical benefit.

Brain natriuretic peptide (nesiritide) is a powerful preload- and afterload-reducing agent because of its vasodilating capabilities.[186] Whether or not the renal effects of natriuretic peptides given parenterally in the clinical setting are evident and beneficial is not clear. Nesiritide has been demonstrated efficacious from a hemodynamic and symptomatic standpoint when given intravenously, and hemodynamics have also improved after longer term intermittent subcutaneous administration. Also, nesiritide is much less likely to cause important arrhythmias than dobutamine or dopamine during infusion. Best contemporary nesiritide administration practices have been defined by the ongoing Vasodilator Management of Congestive Heart Failure (VMAC) trial (Table 5–5). Severely congested patients with blood pressure ≥ 90 mm Hg seem to generally respond to a 2 ng/kg bolus followed by a 0.01 ng/kg/min continuous infusion.

CALCIUM CHANNEL BLOCKING AGENTS

Calcium channel antagonists are vasodilating agents that are quite effective in reducing blood pressure and systemic vascular resistance, but they generally have negative inotropic activity and are associated with baroreflex-mediated increases in sympathetic tone. As clinical trials have demonstrated either a worsening of mortality or no effect of calcium channel blockers in the treatment of heart failure,[201] their use has steadily declined (SPICE registry). Interestingly, in the late 1980s, more patients in the SOLVED registry were on calcium channel blockers than on angiotensin-converting enzyme inhibitors, with almost one third of heart failure patients receiving a calcium channel antagonist. The SPICE registry, which collected data a decade later, demonstrated that calcium channel antagonist use in congestive heart failure populations had fallen to about 15%. It is currently recommended that for individuals with heart failure and hypertension, blood pressure might better be reduced with more aggressive prescription of ACE inhibitors, diuretics, beta-adrenergic blockers, angiotensin-II receptor blocking agents, or other vasodilating antihypertensive compounds (Table 5–7). Likewise, in the patient with heart failure, coronary artery disease, and angina pectoris, more aggressive nitrate prescription should be considered rather than treatment with calcium channel blockers. For individuals who have had acute myocardial infarction complicated by left ventricular systolic dysfunction, calcium channel blockers more often than not have proved detrimental, with greater likelihood of adverse events noted in randomized trials studying drugs such as nifedipine and diltiazem.

Amlodipine and **felodipine** have been the only two calcium antagonists studied to date that have demonstrated possible efficacy or at least neutral effects[70, 208] in heart failure therapy. In the Prospective Randomized Amlodipine Survival Evaluation (PRAISE) trial (Table 5–5), amlodipine reduced the combined risk of fatal and nonfatal events by 31% ($p = .04$) and the risk of death by 46% ($p < .001$) in nonischemic cardiomyopathy, but had no effect on ischemic cardiomyopathy. The survival benefit with amlodipine in dilated cardiomyopathy was only present when it was combined with digoxin and an ACE inhibitor.

This observation was not confirmed in the PRAISE-II trial, which randomized about 1,800 patients with nonischemic heart failure and NYHA Class III or IV symptoms to amlodipine or placebo with background ACE inhibitors, diuretics, and digoxin in a fashion similar to PRAISE-I. No beneficial effect of amlodipine was noted on morbidity or mortality. When PRAISE-I and -II results are combined there is a 34% event rate (morbidity and mortality) with placebo and 33% with amlodipine ($p = .81$). Thus, it appears that amlodipine plays no role in the primary treatment of heart failure. Use of this drug in this population seems not to be associated with detrimental effects.

Data from the Ve-HeFT-III trial (Table 5–5) indicate that felodipine prescribed on top of ACE inhibitors in patients with mild to moderate heart failure improves left ventricular function, exercise tolerance, and certain hormonal factors, but does not reduce long-term mortality or morbidity.[70] It also appears to be a safe agent for treatment of patients with mild to moderate heart failure but, as with amlodipine, should not be used as primary therapy of heart failure.

Mibefradil is a newer non–voltage-regulated T-channel calcium blocker. The drug was clinically available as an antihypertensive and antianginal agent but withdrawn from the market after the Mortality Assessment in Congestive Heart Failure (MACH-I) trial.[23, 171, 172, 194] This drug differs substantially from available calcium channel blockers with respect to its structure and mechanism of action. Mibefradil is a potent peripheral and coronary vasodilating drug without negative inotropic effects. This latter pharmacologic activity is likely due to the paucity of T-channel receptors in the ventricular myocardium. Mibefradil also has effects on sinoatrial nodal activity similar to other calcium channel blockers which effect slowing of the heart rate and increased atrioventricular conduction time. Mibefradil has been shown to reduce sudden death in experimental animal studies and its vasodilating properties could be beneficial in patients with heart failure. The drug has a long half-life and is suitable to be given once daily. In MACH-I, 2,390 NYHA Class II to IV patients were randomized to either placebo or mibefradil[170] on top of standard "triple" heart failure therapy and followed an average of 26 months. Unfortunately, mibefradil increased mortality by 11% and largely so when patients were also given agents likely to prolong electrocardiographic QT interval.

Unlike ACE inhibitors as a class of drugs, calcium channel blocker use in patients with heart failure has not reliably shown significant benefit when given as primary therapy, and harm has occasionally been demonstrated.[129, 200] If one feels compelled to use a calcium channel blocker in patients with left ventricular dysfunction, amlodipine and felodipine are the only two reasonable options.

ANGIOTENSIN-II RECEPTOR BLOCKERS

Angiotensin-II receptor blocking drugs have some similar endpoint activity as ACE inhibitors but lack bradykinin-potentiating activity, which is linked to the cyclooxygenase pathways potentiated by ACE inhibitors (which have also been called kininases or bradykinin-potentiating factors).[101, 126] They represent an attractive option in heart failure when considered both as an alternative to ACE inhibitors and as agents that might be combined with this drug class. Drugs capable of specific blockade at angiotensin-II receptor sites theoretically might induce similar benefits when compared with ACE inhibitors but without some of the troublesome side effects sometimes noted with these agents.

As detailed in Chapter 4, angiotensin-II is believed responsible for many of the adverse effects of the altered humoral milieu characteristic of the heart failure state.[275] Stimulation of the angiotensin-II receptor site (AT1 specifically) appears to mediate vasoconstriction, sodium retention, myocyte hypertrophy, endothelin secretion, and interstitial fibrosis. It is important to note that an AT2 receptor site is also present and likely biologically active in patients with heart failure. AT2 receptor stimulation (increased in heart failure) likely provides an important counterregulatory influence to the detrimental effects of AT1 stimulation by angiotensin-II.

Rather than inhibiting the production of angiotensin-II by blockade of ACE, angiotensin receptor blockers inhibit receptor activation. Currently available angiotensin receptor blockers are selective for the AT1 receptor. Theoretic benefit of these drugs include blocking receptor interaction of angiotensin produced by enzymes other than ACE and increasing angiotensin-II levels in comparison with ACE inhibitors, allowing maintained or increased stimulation of AT2 receptors. On the other hand, theoretical concerns about angiotensin receptor blockers include the potential deleterious effects of increased angiotensin-II levels systemically and AT2 receptor mediated enhancement of apoptosis. Furthermore, whether or not angiotensin receptor blockers beneficially attenuate coronary heart disease events, ameliorate diabetic nephropathy, and prevent the development of heart failure is not known. Also unclear is the importance of no bradykinin effects, which rise with ACE inhibitor therapy and possibly contribute to ACE inhibitor benefit, but can be blocked with aspirin.[135, 195, 196, 199]

Data from small clinical trials suggests that the hemodynamic actions of angiotensin receptor blockers are similar to ACE inhibitors with respect to blood pressure lowering in hypertensive patients and systemic vascular resistance reduction in patients with heart failure.[78, 88, 130, 132, 137] Furthermore, these drugs seem to have a modest effect on improvement in exercise capacity similar to that expected with ACE inhibitors and have a comparable magnitude of norepinephrine level reduction in heart failure.

Recent experience with the first commercially available angiotensin-II receptor blocking drug, **losartan,** in symptomatic heart failure demonstrates beneficial hemodynamic effects acutely as well as after 12 weeks of therapy.[78] There was a dose-related response up to 50 mg daily of losartan. Higher doses did not seemingly achieve additive effects. Losartan reduces preload and afterload with subsequent increase in cardiac output, but the hemodynamic action may not be as dramatic as ACE inhibitors. In addition to the favorable hemodynamic effects of losartan, animal models suggest that the drug can induce regression of ventricular hypertrophy.

The first larger scale clinical trial that gave some insight into morbidity and mortality after use of angiotensin II receptor blocking drugs in heart failure was the Evaluation of Losartan in the Elderly (ELITE)[220, 221] study, a multicenter, international, prospective, double-blind, randomized trial specifically designed to assess whether or not losartan was better tolerated than captopril with respect to development of renal dysfunction. The incidence of persistent renal dysfunction was the same in both losartan and captopril cohorts (10.5%). Losartan overall, however, appeared to be better tolerated than captopril, with no reports of cough, rash, or angioneurotic edema (common with captopril). Interestingly, losartan was also associated with less mortality (though this was not a primary endpoint), both early and throughout the 48-week observation period, mainly accounted for by a lower sudden cardiac death rate in the losartan group. Survival benefits of losartan were observed throughout all subgroups except women.

ELITE-I was not designed, however, to be a mortality endpoint trial and only randomized about 700 patients. The follow-up ELITE-II trial was a properly powered mortality endpoint study with over 3,000 patients randomized. ELITE-II did not confirm observations and inferences made in ELITE-I. There was no comparative benefit for losartan and a trend toward better outcomes with fewer sudden deaths with captopril.[220, 265]

The Randomized Evaluation of Strategies for Left Ventricular Dysfunction (RESOLVD) pilot study was a two-stage randomized trial of candesartan (an angiotensin-II receptor blocker), enalapril, and metoprolol in patients with congestive heart failure.[185] The combination of ACE inhibitor and candesartan provided greater improvement in some neurohumoral markers of significant heart failure and ventricular function (ejection fraction and cardiac volumes) than candesartan or ACE inhibitor alone. Addition of the beta blocker metoprolol appeared to further improve outcome with respect to these endpoints. Most importantly, RESOLVD demonstrated that patients could be titrated onto an aggressive medication protocol that included, diuretic, digoxin, ACE inhibitor, angiotensin receptor blocker, and beta blocker.

The SPICE program,[132] in addition to supporting a heart failure registry, was also a pilot study evaluating candesartan in patients deemed intolerant to ACE inhibitors (who were then randomized to receive either candesartan or placebo). Patients previously intolerant to ACE inhibitors were found for the most part to tolerate angiotensin-II receptor blocking agents no worse than placebo (about 85% of the time).

At the present time, ACE inhibitors remain the therapy of choice in patients with heart failure due to systolic left ventricular dysfunction to inhibit the renin-angiotensin system.[117] Currently, one should not initiate angiotensin receptor blocking agents in patients with new-onset heart failure or switch to these drugs from a tolerated ACE inhibitor program. It may be reasonable to use angiotensin receptor blockers in patients with ACE inhibitor intolerance; however, the combination of hydralazine and isosorbide dinitrate has more evidence to suggest benefit *de novo* in congestive heart failure patients. Several ongoing trials (Table 5–5) will give greater insight into the issue of angiotensin receptor blockade in a wide spectrum of heart failure, including their use as add-on therapy or in ACE inhibitor–intolerant patients.

ALDOSTERONE ANTAGONISTS

Increased renin and angiotensin levels stimulate aldosterone secretion in patients with heart failure, and elevation of this hormone enhances sodium retention, increases sympathetic activation and parasympathetic inhibition, while promoting myocardial remodeling by increasing collagen synthesis and stiffening the interstitial matrix. ACE inhibitors in heart failure only transiently decrease aldosterone levels. Some concern has existed about using aldosterone antagonists in conjunction with ACE inhibitors because of the potential for developing hyperkalemia. The RALES trial (Table 5–5) was designed to determine if low doses of spironolactone (generally 15–25 mg daily) in addition to digoxin, diuretic, and ACE inhibitor would decrease mortality and morbidity in patients with NYHA Class III and IV congestive heart failure.[222] The 1,663 patients randomized were quite ill, as evidenced by the 46% placebo group mortality rate at the 35-month follow-up point. Important to note is the fact that RALES excluded patients with potassium levels greater than 5.0 mmol/L or creatinine greater than 2.5 mg/dL. Only about 10% of the population were on beta blockers. The relative risk of death in the spironolactone group was .70, with 95% confidence intervals (CI) of .60–.82 ($p < .001$). Risk of death from both progressive heart failure and sudden cardiac death was reduced, as was the frequency of hospitalization for heart failure. Mortality reduction was not associated with diuresis, and it is believed that the morbidity and mortality reduction noted was solely due to reversal of perturbed neurohormone systems. In this trial, hyperkalemia necessitating drug withdrawal was unusual, but painful gynecomastia was reported in 10% of males in the study.

Recommendations, then, call for administration of **spironolactone at low, nondiuretic, doses (25 mg or less daily) in addition to standard "triple" therapy in patients with more severe congestive heart failure syndromes** (NYHA Class III and IV) who have **a creatinine less than 2.5 mg/dL and serum potassium below 5.0 mmol/L while on an ACE inhibitor.** ACE inhibitor administration should not be sacrificed if hyperkalemia develops. Rather, potassium supplements should be decreased or eliminated, or if problems persist the spironolactone should be stopped.

BETA-ADRENERGIC BLOCKING DRUGS

Beta blockers can generally be categorized according to their ability to block the different beta- and alpha-adrenergic receptors as well as other pharmacologic effects[12] (Table 5–10). Some agents are relatively beta$_1$ selective (e.g., metoprolol), but others are non-specific beta blockers (blocking both beta$_1$ and beta$_2$ receptors; e.g., propranolol). Additionally, some beta-adrenergic blocking drugs actually have intrinsic sympathomimetic activity. Finally, some agents, such as the recently studied drug carvedilol, combine beta$_1$ and beta$_2$-adrenergic receptor blocking activity with alpha-blocking capabilities (Table 5–10). The beneficial effect of beta-adrenergic antagonist seems paradoxical in view of their negative inotropic effect. However, the potentially favorable effect of chronic beta blocker administration on cardiac function may relate to alterations at multiple levels of cardiac activity. A reduction of heart rate, reduction in peak left ventricular end-systolic pressure, and reduction in ventricular afterload are usually observed, with only a slight decrease in myocardial oxygen consumption and improved cardiac metabolic efficiency.[103, 106, 140] Chronic heart failure is known to induce down-regulation of beta-adrenergic receptors, and this may theoretically be reversed with chronic beta-blocker therapy, which induces up-regulation of myocardial beta-receptors (see Chapter 4). Beta blockade theoretically could reduce the incidence of sudden death due to ventricular arrhythmias (as of yet unproven).

The use of beta-adrenergic blocking drugs in heart failure today is now accepted as being essential in patients with mild to moderate congestive heart failure due to systolic left ventricular dysfunction. Several clinical trials, including Cardic Insufficiency Bisoprolol Study (CIBIS)-I and -II,[60, 61] Prospective Randomized Evaluation of Carvedilol on Symptoms and Exercise (PRE-CISE)[210] and Multicenter Oral Carvedilol Heart Failure Assessment (MOCHA), the Carvedilol in Heart Failure Program in general,[203] Metoprolol CR/XL Randomized Intervention Trial in Heart Failure (MERIT-HF),[176] and Beta-Blocker Evaluation Survival (BEST)[37] (Table 5–5) have evaluated a variety of heart failure subsets, generally supporting the concept that beta-adrenergic blocking drugs are useful in select and stable patients. Even older trials, including the Beta Blocker Heart Attack Trial (BHAT)[20] and the Timolol Post-infarction Trial (1981) both demonstrated substantive benefit when beta blockers were prescribed early after myocardial infarction, particularly in the subset with significant clinical peri-infarct congestive heart failure. However, in the 15 years since BHAT results were reported, it has been difficult to clarify the issues regarding beta-adrenergic blocker benefits in patients with left ventricular systolic dysfunction. Aggressive, high-dose, rapid up-titration of beta blockers has often been associated with worsening of heart failure.[104]

TABLE 5-10 Pharmacodynamic Properties of Beta-Adrenergic Antagonists

GENERIC NAME	PROPRIETARY NAME	ADRENERGIC RECEPTOR SELECTIVITY	PARTIAL AGONISM (ISA)	INVERSE AGONISM†	LIPID SOLUBILITY	VASODILATOR ACTIVITY	OTHER ACTIONS
Acebutol	Sectral	Beta-1	+		+	+	
Atenolol	Tenormin	Beta-1	0		0	0	
Betaxolol	Kerlone	Beta-1	0		0		
Bevantolol*		Beta-1	0		++	+	
Bisoprolol	Zebeta	Beta-1	0		+	0	
Bucindolol*		Beta-1, beta-2	0		0	++	"Direct vasodilator"
Carteolol	Cartrol	Beta-1, beta-2	++		0	0	
Carvedilol	Coreg	Beta-1, beta-2 alpha-1	0	+	+	++	
Celiprolol*		Beta-1	+	+	+	++	
Esmolol	Brevibloc	Beta-1		0	0	+	
Labetalol	Trandate Normodyne	Beta-1, beta-2, alpha-1	+		++	++	
Metoprolol	Lopressor	Beta-1	0	++	++	0	
Nadolol	Corgard	Beta-1, beta-2	0		0	0	
Nebivelol*		Beta-1	0		0	+	"Direct vasodilator"
Oxprenolol*	Trasico	Beta-1, beta-2	++		+	0	
Penbutolol	Levatol	Beta-1, beta-2	++		+++	0	
Pindolol	Visken	Beta-1, beta-2	++		0		
Propranolol	Inderal	Beta-1, beta-2	0	++	+++	0	
Sotalol	Betapace	Beta-1, beta-2	0		0	0	Class III antiarrhythmic
Timolol	Blocadren	Beta-1, beta-2	0	***	0	0	

ISA, intrinsic sympathomimetic activity; +, mild effect; ++, moderate effect; ***, marked effect.
* Not approved by the U.S. Food and Drug Administration at the time of this writing.
† Inverse agonism—the ability to bind and stabilize the inactive conformation of G protein–linked receptors—has not been well defined for beta-adrenergic antagonists to date in the context of human cardiovascular pharmacology.
Adapted from Antman EM, Kelly RA: Pharmacology therapy of cardiac arrhythmias. In Antman EM, Ruitherford JD (eds): Coronary Care Medicine: A Practical Approach. Norwell, MA: Kluwer Academic Press, 1996.

In the more recently completed series of **carvedilol** clinical heart failure trials, new and important insight into beta blocker therapy has been gained.[203] A pooled analysis of four randomized, placebo-controlled, multicenter clinical trials demonstrated a 33% risk reduction for death in patients with mild to moderate congestive heart failure treated with carvedilol. Exercise tolerance was *not* generally improved with carvedilol therapy, but congestive heart failure symptomatology, NYHA functional classification, and general patient well-being were beneficially affected. Carvedilol has also been said to have potent antioxidant properties that might provide additional and favorable pharmacologic effects in the heart failure milieu.

Metoprolol has also been extensively evaluated in patients with heart failure. The Metoprolol in Dilated Cardiomyopathy (MDC) trial was an early study which randomized 383 patients with NYHA Class II or III congestive heart failure due to nonischemic dilated cardiomyopathy with left ventricular systolic dysfunction. There was a 34% reduction in adverse outcomes in the metoprolol group, but this was entirely due to a reduction in cardiac transplantation in the metoprolol group and the p value was only .058. Indeed, there were actually more deaths in the metoprolol group, but this was not statistically significant (23 vs. 19; p = .69).

Longer acting, sustained-release metoprolol (Toprol-XL) was used in the 3,991-patient MERIT-HF trial,[176] which was a mortality endpoint study including NYHA Class II to IV patients (though 96% were Class II or III). There was a 34% reduction in mortality in the metoprolol group, for a relative risk reduction of .66 (95% CL, .53–.81; p < .006). The annual mortality rate was 11% in the placebo group and 7.2% in the metoprolol arm (Table 5–5).

The CIBIS-I study (1994) evaluated **bisoprolol** in 641 patients with ischemia or nonischemic NYHA Class III and IV congestive heart failure patients with primary endpoint all-cause mortality (Table 5–5). Overall, there was no significant reduction in total mortality, and hospitalizations were reduced by 28% (p < .01). This led to a larger more robustly powered study, CIBIS-II, which evaluated bisoprolol in 2,647 patients followed an average of 1.3 years with 80% of patients NYHA Class III (1999). Also, CIBIS-II up-titrated the beta blocker to a higher dose than was used in CIBIS-I (10 mg vs. 5 mg), though starting doses were the same (1.25 mg daily), with up-titration slow and controlled. CIBIS-II was prematurely terminated because this beta blocker reduced annual mortality rate by 34% (risk reduction, .66; 95% CL, .59–.81; p < .0001). Hospitalizations for worsening heart failure were decreased by 32%, and this was also highly significant (p < .0001). Importantly, despite a post hoc analysis of CIBIS-I suggesting that bisoprolol benefit might be related only to patients without coronary disease, CIBIS-II demonstrated mortality reduction in ischemic and nonischemic groups of patients entered into the trial.

The BEST beta-blocker trial (Table 5–5) has been the only recent large-scale mortality endpoint clinical trial to not demonstrate benefit with a beta blocker in heart failure patients (though no harm was noted).[105] **Bucindolol** was randomly given to 2,700 NYHA Class III or IV heart failure patients with ejection fraction less than 0.35 and followed an average of 18 months. Mortality was not significantly decreased with bucindolol, though a favorable trend was noted overall except in African Americans and NYHA Class IV patients. This trial recruited a population that was seemingly more ill and more racially and gender diverse than other beta-blocker heart failure studies, and whether or not this accounts for the observed lack of benefit is not clear. Also possible is that bucindolol and other beta blockers not yet studied in heart failure populations behave differently than carvedilol, metoprolol, and bisoprolol.

Based on these observations it is suggested that **beta-blocker therapy with either carvedilol, metoprolol, or bisoprolol be routinely used in NYHA class II or III heart failure patients with left ventricular systolic dysfunction who are on baseline "triple" therapy including, generally, an ACE inhibitor, digoxin, and diuretic to control fluid retention.**[166] It is also appropriate to consider beta-blocker therapy in patients with left ventricular systolic dysfunction who are asymptomatic (NYHA Class I) and on an ACE inhibitor, but the data are less secure for this group. In order to increase the likelihood of successful beta-blocker up-titration, a period of clinical stability on standard triple therapy is suggested before initiation of beta-blocker therapy. When these agents are begun, initial doses should be low with conservative intervals (every 2 weeks or so) chosen for up-titration evaluation visits. When substantive congestion occurs or new problems develop during beta-blocker up-titration, adjustment of concomitant medications may be all that is necessary (such as increasing the intensity of diuretic dose).

To reemphasize, the role of beta-blocker therapy in patients with NYHA Class IV clinical symptomatology is controversial.[67] Patients exhibiting this degree of heart failure frequently have beta-adrenergic blocking drugs down-titrated or discontinued on presentation to determine if a relationship exists between beta-adrenergic blocking drug activity and congestive heart failure decompensation. However, preliminary reports have suggested that NYHA Class IV congestive heart failure patients can experience benefit when carvedilol is cautiously up-titrated. Indeed, the Carvedilol Prospective Randomized Cumulative Survival Trial (COPERNICUS) trial was recently prematurely stopped because of benefits noted in the carvedilol-treated group. This study randomized the most ill congestive heart failure patients to date. It appears that when rendered euvolemic, very advanced heart failure patients have substantial benefit with carvedilol. Irrespective of the severity of the syndrome, **when beta-adrenergic blocking drugs are given to patients with heart failure they should be started at low doses.** With carvedilol, initial doses as low as 3.125 mg twice daily are recommended

with gradual up-titration to target doses of 25 or 50 mg twice daily.

MANAGEMENT OF VENTRICULAR ARRHYTHMIAS

One of the most challenging issues in patients with heart failure is cardiac arrhythmias.[154] The incidence of atrial and ventricular arrhythmias in this group is likely related to the underlying myocardial substrate. The initial treatment of ventricular arrhythmias in the heart failure milieu is effective relief of the congestive state and optimization of ventricular performance with vasodilators, diuretics, and ACE inhibitors. Correction of fluid balance and electrolyte disorders is also essential. Atrial fibrillation should be converted to normal sinus rhythm whenever possible. With persistent atrial fibrillation, proper anticoagulation is important to minimize the risk of thromboembolism.

Vaughn Williams Class I antiarrhythmic agents carry important risks when clinical congestive heart failure is present, particularly after an acute myocardial infarction. The Cardiac Arrhythmia Suppression Trial (CAST)[102] and Effect of D-Sotol on Mortality in Patients with Left Ventricular Dysfunction after Recent and Remote Myocardial Infarction (SWORD) trials (Table 5–5) indicated that encainide, flecainide, morizicine, and D-sotalol increased mortality when used in the patients at highest risk of arrhythmia-induced sudden cardiac death, perhaps because such patients are also at highest risk of having proarrhythmic events associated with antiarrhythmic agents. A direct relationship exists between lower ejection fraction and increased likelihood of antiarrhythmic drug toxicity and failure to control malignant ventricular arrhythmias.[131, 227] The one exception to this observation may be beta-adrenergic blocking drugs and amiodarone.[133]

The role of **amiodarone** in heart failure patients "at increased risk" for arrhythmic events remains controversial, largely because of disparate results and differing study design in the numerous clinical trials which have examined amiodarone efficacy. The Group Study of Heart Failure Argentina (GESICA) study[96] demonstrated a survival benefit of amiodarone in patients with moderate to severe congestive heart failure, but the study was unblinded and the drug was discontinued frequently because of intolerance. However, in the Congestive Heart Failure–Survival Trial of Antiarrhythmic Therapy (CHF-STAT) trial[181] (Table 5–5) (a placebo-controlled trial in patients with congestive heart failure who had 10 or more premature ventricular contractions per hour on ambulatory monitoring), amiodarone failed to improve overall survival when compared to placebo.

The European Myocardial Infarction Amiodarone Trial (EMIAT)[146] and the Canadian Myocardial Infarction Amiodarone Trial (CAMIAT)[41] (Table 5–5) examined the benefit of amioclarone following acute myocardial infarction. Amiodarone reduced the incidence of ventricular fibrillation or presumed arrhythmic death (CAMIAT) and the incidence of presumed arrhythmic death and resuscitated cardiac arrest (EMIAT) in survivors of acute myocardial infarction, but the frequency of drug discontinuation due to intolerance was high.

In an analysis of pooled clinical trial data (The Amiodarone Trials Analysis Investigators),[11] amiodarone appeared to have a beneficial effect on the reduction of sudden cardiac death/presumed arrhythmic death, but no effect on nonarrhythmic deaths. There was no difference in treatment effect between postmyocardial infarction and congestive heart failure patients, and the best single predictor of arrhythmic/sudden cardiac death among all patients was symptomatic congestive heart failure. These investigators concluded that prophylactic amiodarone reduces the rate of sudden cardiac death/presumed arrhythmic death in high-risk patients with recent myocardial infarction or congestive heart failure, and this effect results in an overall reduction of total mortality by 10–20%. A second amiodarone trial meta-analysis reached similar conclusions.

The compendium of amiodarone trials suggests that the agent does not worsen morbidity or increase mortality in heart failure patients (in contradistinction to other antiarrhythmic drugs), and seems an appropriate choice when heart failure patients require an antiarrhythmic agent for treatment of problematic atrial or ventricular dysrhythmias. The combination of beta-adrenergic blockers and amiodarone is also likely beneficial. Unfortunately, amiodarone is expensive and often poorly tolerated with toxicities that include pulmonary fibrosis, thyroid function disorders, photosensitization syndromes, and neuropathy. Low-dose amiodarone (50 or 100 mg daily) may be better tolerated while still having some effects.

In heart failure patients with significant sustained ventricular arrhythmias, insertion of **automatic implantable defibrillating devices** (AICDs) is an attractive alternative to chronic antiarrhythmic drugs. The Multicenter Automatic Defibrillator Implantation Trial (MADIT) study[155] (Table 5–5) studied the prophylactic use of an implantable defibrillation device compared to conventional medical therapy in individuals after myocardial infarction considered at high risk for ventricular arrhythmias (left ventricular ejection fraction of 0.35 or less in patients who were asymptomatic from nonsustained ventricular tachycardia with nonsuppressible arrhythmia elicited during electrophysiologic study). Mortality was significantly reduced when the defibrillating device was implanted compared to the use of conventional antiarrhythmics. There was no suggestion that amiodarone, beta blockers, or any other antiarrhythmic drug combination produced a significant survival increment when used in conjunction with the implantable defibrillator. In a more general population with life-threatening ventricular arrhythmias, the antiarrhythmics vs. implantable defibrillators (AVID) trial demonstrated 25% reduction in mortality over 3 years in patients who received a defibrillator compared to those randomized to receive antiarrhythmic drug therapy,[14] which was usually amiodarone. Although this trial was not a heart failure trial per se, patients with important ventricular dysfunction were common. Thus, the AICD appears to be first-line choice for the specific high-risk groups identified by the criteria employed in the AVID[14] and MADIT trials. AICD insertion also represents an alternative strategy to antiarrhythmic drug prescription in patients with acute myocardial infarction or significant heart failure who are at high risk of sudden cardiac death as suggested by the presence of significant ventricular arrhythmias.

The prophylactic use of implantable cardiac defibrillators at the time of coronary artery bypass graft surgery in patients at high risk for ventricular arrhythmias has been evaluated in the Coronary Artery Bypass Graft Patch (CABG-Patch) trial.[25] This trial found no evidence of improved survival among patients with coronary heart disease, depressed left ventricular systolic function, and an abnormal signal average electrocardiogram when a defibrillator was implanted prophylactically at the time of elective coronary artery bypass surgery.

ACC/AHA guidelines regarding heart failure therapeutics (1996) caution against aggressive pharmacologic or mechanical treatment of asymptomatic ventricular arrhythmias, particularly those that are unsustained. To consider either a drug treatment strategy or implantation of an arrhythmia termination device, patients should have significantly symptomatic ventricular tachycardia (not simply palpitations or premature ventricular contractions, couplets, or nonsustained ventricular tachycardia detected during routine surveillance monitoring) or an episode of syncope or sudden cardiac death syndrome related to ventricular dysrhythmia.

In summary, studies of pharmacologic therapy in heart failure suggest that the greatest benefit from antiarrhythmic drugs in preventing presumed arrhythmogenic sudden cardiac death occurs in patients with left ventricular systolic dysfunction and only mild to moderate symptoms. As functional impairment increases and ejection fraction falls, drug therapies become less effective in preventing sudden cardiac death in heart failure groups. Angiotensin-converting enzyme inhibitors are important but provide only modest, if any, protection against sudden cardiac death; whereas beta-adrenergic blockers and amiodarone may decrease the risk somewhat more. Because of the known adverse outcome of heart failure patients treated with Vaughn Williams Class I antiarrhythmic drugs, quinidine and procainamide should be avoided in the treatment of ventricular arrhythmias of heart failure.[7, 59, 62, 99, 100, 114, 228] Cardioverter defibrillating devices, either surgically implanted or transvenous devices, may be effective in high-risk populations.[44] **Implantable defibrillators should be considered first-line treatment options for heart failure patients with a history of sustained rapid ventricular tachycardias or at least one episode of cardiac arrest.** On the other hand, patients with ischemic heart disease, signal averaged electrocardiographic abnormalities, and low ejection fraction undergoing elective coronary artery bypass surgery do not seem candidates for prophylactic insertion of a defibrillator.

ANTICOAGULATION

Controversy exists regarding the benefit of routine anticoagulation in patients with heart failure, since clear benefit has not been demonstrated in well-designed, prospective, placebo-controlled clinical trials. Some studies have suggested a lower incidence of pulmonary and peripheral emboli in patients anticoagulated, so it may be prudent to anticoagulate heart failure patients with a history of systemic or pulmonary embolism or when left or right ventricular thrombi are noted on echocardiography. In the SOLVD trial,[8] patients anticoagulated had fewer cardiac events than those not anticoagulated, but the analysis was post hoc.[98] Clear indication for aggressive anticoagulation is the presence of atrial fibrillation. Another group likely to benefit, at least with short-term anticoagulation, is patients with acute anterior wall myocardial infarction and ventricular dysfunction. Patients receiving anticoagulant therapy should be carefully monitored with a goal of achieving an international normalized ratio for prothrombin time between 2 and 4.[15]

COMMON PITFALLS IN HEART FAILURE THERAPY

Table 5–11 summarizes many common pitfalls that challenge clinicians during evaluation and treatment of heart failure patients. This is particularly important in patients with more advanced heart failure and those being considered for transplantation. Possibly the most important pitfall is inadequate recognition of the syndrome! Frequently, patients will present with symptoms related to ventricular dysfunction and heart failure, yet their complaints are attributed to other causes such as anxiety, hyperventilation, or functional bowel disorders. Initiation of therapy late in the patient's disease course compromises the likelihood of reducing long-term morbidity and mortality.

Early recognition of underlying disease states in the heart failure milieu is essential if preventive therapies are to be effective. For example, when reversible myocardial ischemia is present, coronary revascularization can dramatically improve clinical outcomes in the face of ventricular dysfunction. It is important to recognize the patient who will benefit from procedures such as valve repair or replacement and left ventricular remodeling. Unrecognized hyperthyroidism, hypothyroidism, poorly controlled diabetes mellitus, and inadequate control of hypertension will contribute to worsening of the heart failure state. Atrial arrhythmias are deleterious, and every attempt should be made to keep patients in normal sinus rhythm. Bradyarrhythmias may respond

---

TABLE 5-11   Common Pitfalls in the Treatment of Heart Failure: Factors Predisposing To Heart Failure Decompensation

Inadequate syndrome recognition
• Symptoms unrelated to cardiac dysfunction
• Treating late in the course of the illness
Ignoring underlying disease state
• Not correcting areas of reversible myocardial ischemia
• Not considering patients for standard (though higher risk) surgical procedures such as valve repair/replacement or aneurysmectomy
• Unrecognized hypo-/hyperthyroidism
• Poorly controlled diabetes mellitus
• Inadequate control of hypertension
• Not treating dyslipidemia
• Not treating chronic obstructive pulmonary disease
• Not considering possibility of cardiac metastasis in malignancies
Not recognizing/treating certain comorbidities
• Intercurrent infections
• Hypoventilation–sleep apnea syndromes
Patient-related factors
• Poor compliance with drug treatment protocols
• Inadequate salt and water restriction
• Excessive alcohol consumption
• Cigarette smoking
• Obesity
• Cardiovascular deconditioning
Pharmacotherapeutic issues
• Inadequate ACE-I therapy (or drug not begun)
• Suboptimal doses of vasodilators
• Ineffective diuretic use
• Excessive diuresis
• Discontinuation of digoxin in stable CHF patients
• Down-titration of ACE-I instead of diuretics for hypotension or azotemia
• Concomitant use of potentially harmful medications (certain antiarrhythmics, nonsteroidal anti-inflammatory drugs, beta blockers, or calcium channel antagonists in certain circumstances)
Other treatment concerns/pitfalls
• Administration of anthracyclines
• Not evaluating/correcting-controlling atrial fibrillation
• Inappropriate drug treatment of certain ventricular arrhythmias
• Not considering pacemaker therapies for chronotropic incompetence
• Not preventing/treating hypokalemia, hypomagnesemia, hyponatremia
• Salt/fluid administration parenterally for orthostatic hypotension or hyponatremia
• Failure to use hemodynamic monitoring to resolve confusion or challenging situations

ACE-I, angiotensin converting enzyme inhibitor; CHF, congestive heart failure.

to pacemaker therapy. Atrioventricular nodal ablation may rarely be advisable when atrial fibrillation causes rapid ventricular responses that cannot be controlled with medications.

Because of the cytokine storm often associated with infections, not recognizing or appropriately treating underlying infections may precipitate worsening congestive states. Finally, hypoventilation/sleep apnea syndromes worsen heart failure, but when treated with theophylline preparations or nocturnal positive-pressure breathing devices the heart failure symptoms can sometimes dramatically improve. Poorly compliant patients present difficult situations, but aggressive counseling, cardiac rehabilitation, and streamlining of therapeutic protocols are often helpful.

Inadequate salt and water restriction sets the stage for hyponatremia, hypokalemia, and substantive edema despite aggressive diuretic use. Excess alcohol consumption, particularly in patients with normal coronary arteries and cardiomyopathy, is likely harmful and can contribute to worsening congestive states. Concomitant use of potentially harmful medications such as nonsteroidal anti-inflammatory agents might precipitate fluid retention, and their use should be discouraged.

Excessive intravascular volume depletion with diuretics can be counterproductive by producing orthostatic symptoms and further activating adverse neurohumoral factors that could contribute to worsening ventricular dysfunction and more detrimental cardiac remodeling. On the other hand, diuretic doses that are too low, diuretic combinations that are not rational (such as combining two loop diuretics), and failure to switch from oral to parenteral diuretic administration when necessary all act to promote persistent fluid retention.

ACE inhibitor therapy should be started and then titrated to appropriate doses (doses that were used and deemed effective in clinical trials) rather than sacrificing the ACE inhibitor in an aggressively diuresed patient. Individuals becoming hypotensive after ACE inhibitor therapy who are concomitantly taking high doses of diuretics or multiple diuretic classes should have the diuretic dose or dosing combinations reduced rather than compromising ACE inhibitor therapy.

Administration of a parenteral salt solution for orthostatic hypotension or hyponatremia should be avoided, since it perpetuates a cycle of aggressive diuretic administration, subsequent hypotension, parenteral fluid administration, then congestion and hyponatremia developing after volume expansion. Only patients with shock and clear-cut intravascular volume depletion should have volume-expanding agents administered. It is usually best to allow hyponatremia to correct gradually with salt and water restriction and, possibly, concomitant parenteral loop diuretic administration. Orthostatic hypotension generally responds to bed rest with reduction in diuretics or sometimes concomitant vasodilator reduction. When situations become confusing and volume status is clinically difficult to assess, direct hemodynamic monitoring is indicated to assist therapeutic decisions.

STRATEGIES TO CONSIDER WHEN CONGESTION PERSISTS DESPITE OPTIMIZED MEDICAL THERAPY

Table 5–12 lists several strategies that can be helpful when there is persistent congestion despite aggressive oral diuretic administration in dropsical outpatients. First, one should review the pitfalls listed in Table 5–11 to identify issues that might account for decompensation and deterioration. One can then institute strategies to address and ameliorate these problems. Naturally, many patients simply have progression of their disease with persistence or worsening of the congestive state despite optimized medical therapies. In these individuals, placing pulmonary artery catheters and objectively measuring hemodynamics is important to clarify confusing and complex heart failure situations. Administration of parenteral vasodilator and/or inotropic therapy often provides dramatic and prompt benefit, improving renal perfusion and aiding delivery of diuretics to their sites of action in the nephron. Nitroglycerin, nitroprusside, dobutamine, or milrinone infusions can set the stage for effective transition to chronic oral vasodilating and diuretic preparations. Continuous diuretic infusions, usually with a loop diuretic such as furosemide or bumetanide, are potential alternatives in patients with refractory congestive heart failure and dropsy. Though controversial, infusion of so-called renal doses of dopamine (< 5 μg/kg/min) might be helpful in patients refractory to diuretics in the setting of worsening renal function. When significant volume overload and fluid retention persist despite all of these strategies, hemofiltration, ultrafiltration, continuous venovenous hemodialysis, or possibly peritoneal dialysis can remove substantial volume and improve congestive symptoms dramatically.

TABLE 5–12	**Strategies to Consider when Congestion Persists Despite Optimized Digoxin, Diuretic, and ACE-I or Vasodilator Therapy: Considerations**

Placement of pulmonary artery catheter with capabilities of measuring capillary occlusive pressure (cardiac output determination and oximetric mixed venous saturation measurement capabilities also helpful)
Arterial line placement to help guide vasodilator therapy
Hemodynamically guided
  Parenteral vasodilator therapy (nitroglycerin, nitroprusside)
  Parenteral inotrope therapy (dobutamine, milrinone)
Continuous parenteral loop diuretic
Infusion of "dopaminergic" or "renal" doses of dopamine (< 5 μg/kg/min)
Hemofiltration/ultrafiltration
Peritoneal dialysis

TABLE 5-13	Major Causes of Acute Heart Failure

Acute myocardial ischemia-infarction
Complications of myocardial infarction
  Acute mitral regurgitation (papillary muscle rupture)
  Ventricular septal rupture
  Cardiac free wall rupture with pericardial tamponade
Acute valvular catastrophe (mitral or aortic insufficiency)
Severe, poorly controlled hypertension
Myocarditis
Sustained cardiac arrhythmias (particularly those with rapid
  ventricular response)
Acute pulmonary embolism
Decompensation of chronic heart failure
Acute aortic dissection with myocardial ischemia-infarction or
  cardiac tamponade from pericardial effusion

PHARMACOLOGIC THERAPY FOR ACUTE HEART FAILURE DECOMPENSATION

Acute heart failure management requires both rapid identification of the underlying factors precipitating the low-output state and interventions designed to improve circulatory dynamics. Acute intervention can range from therapy with intravenous nitrates and diuretics to more aggressive pharmacologic support with combinations of parenteral inotropic, vasodilating, and vasopressor agents. In complicated situations, hemodynamic monitoring is essential. In circumstances where a surgically repairable cardiac lesion has been identified or where cardiac transplantation is considered an option, mechanical circulatory support options are available that can maintain the patient until definitive treatments can be instituted. These include placement of intra-aortic counterpulsation balloon pumps, extracorporeal membrane oxygenation systems, and left ventricular assist devices (see Chapter 8).

Because of the complexity and diverse nature of the acute heart failure syndrome, treatment must be individ-

ualized with options tailored to each individual circumstance. The ultimate success of acute heart failure management weighs heavily on the rapid institution of effective pharmacologic support to relieve symptoms and reverse hemodynamic derangement while simultaneously pursuing definitive diagnostic studies. The inability to identify and correct underlying lesions causing acute heart failure decompensation is generally associated with high mortality. Table 5–13 lists many conditions which can cause acute heart failure. Many of these problems can be definitively treated with a favorable impact on short- and intermediate-term prognosis. Although the majority of patients presenting with acute heart failure suffer from some degree of myocardial systolic dysfunction, diastolic heart failure with preserved left ventricular ejection fraction may also occur in some patients with underlying restrictive or hypertrophic myocardial abnormalities. When **acute pulmonary edema** is the presenting problem, consideration must be given to multiple cardiac and noncardiac etiologies. One major cause of acute heart failure is myocardial infarction, particularly when complications such as papillary muscle rupture with sudden and voluminous mitral regurgitation and ventricular septal or cardiac free wall rupture with pericardial effusion and cardiac tamponade are seen. Other causes of acute heart failure include sudden valvular insufficiency due to bacterial endocarditis or aortic root dissection and rupture of a mitral valve chordae tendineae. Severe and poorly controlled hypertension can lead to acute heart failure decompensation, as can sudden onset of myocarditis, sustained cardiac arrhythmias (particularly tachyarrhythmias), and acute pulmonary embolism.

Table 5–14[168] summarizes some of the important differences between acute and chronic heart failure syndromes. Patients with decompensated chronic heart failure generally present with low cardiac output and worsening pulmonary and peripheral edema or congestion. Factors precipitating acute heart failure decompensation in a patient with chronic ventricular dysfunction and heart failure are often subtle. Prominent symptoms

TABLE 5-14	Comparisons of Acute, Decompensated, and Stable Chronic Heart Failure		
FEATURE	ACUTE HEART FAILURE	DECOMPENSATED CHRONIC HEART FAILURE	STABLE CHRONIC HEART FAILURE
Symptom severity	Marked	Marked	Mild to moderate
Pulmonary edema	Frequent	Frequent	Rare
Peripheral edema	Rare	Frequent	Frequent
Weight gain	None to mild	Marked	Frequent
Total body volume	No change or mild increase	Markedly increased	Increased
Cardiomegaly	Uncommon	Usual	Common
LV systolic function	Variably depressed (diastolic dysfunction important)	Reduced	Markedly reduced
Wall stress	Elevated	Markedly elevated	Mild to marked
Activation of sympathetic nervous system	Marked	Marked	Mild to marked
Activation of RAAS	Acutely abnormal	Marked	Mild to marked
Acute ischemia	Common	Occasionally	Rare
Hypertensive crisis	Common	Occasionally	Rare
Reparable lesions*	Common	Occasional	Occasional

LV, left ventricle; RAAS, renin-angiotensin-aldosterone system.
*Coronary thrombosis, acute mitral regurgitation, etc.
Adapted from Leier CV: Unstable heart failure. *In* Braunwald E (ed): (Colucci WS). Atlas of Heart Disease. 1995;4:9.2–9.15.

are exertional dyspnea (often even at rest), orthopnea, paroxysmal nocturnal dyspnea, and profound fatigue. The physical examination generally reveals peripheral edema and central venous congestion. Pulmonary rales may be present but are certainly not necessary to diagnose acutely decompensated heart failure. Indeed, pulmonary findings may be relatively unremarkable in a decompensated chronic heart failure patient even when marked elevation of cardiac filling pressures is documented during cardiac catheterization. A gallop rhythm and murmur of mitral regurgitation are common auscultatory findings with cardiomegaly detected clinically. This contrasts with the findings of acute heart failure with pulmonary edema where cardiac size is usually normal and mitral regurgitation generally not audible even when mitral regurgitation is severe (due to equilibration of pressures between the left ventricle and normally sized left atrium). A broad range of presenting features exists, and specific physical findings are often dependent on the underlying lesion and duration of cardiac dysfunction.

Table 5–15 summarizes several of the hemodynamic patterns characteristic of low cardiac output states and acute heart failure. Although usually unnecessary in the uncomplicated patient with acute pulmonary edema, **hemodynamic monitoring** with a flow-directed thermodilution pulmonary artery catheter provides essential information for management of the patient that does not respond initially to standard therapy (usually nitroglycerin and diuretics) and is vital in managing those patients with persistent hypotension and shock syndromes. Patients with cardiogenic shock will have evidence of hypoperfusion on examination that includes a narrow pulse pressure, cool skin, reduced urine output, and mental status changes. Frequent assessment of cardiac output and ventricular filling pressure are essential to appropriately guide pharmacotherapeutic intervention, as well as making decisions about the need for mechanical circulatory support. Other indications for hemodynamic monitoring include patients with acute heart failure where volume status is in question and in cases of pulmonary edema without a clear cardiac etiology. Hemodynamic monitoring will help quantify the severity of hemodynamic compromise resulting from specific valvular heart lesions or conditions such as pericardial tamponade, right ventricular infarction,

ventricular septal rupture, or circulatory collapse secondary to various shock syndromes (see Table 5–15).

During hemodynamic monitoring, cardiac output, pulmonary capillary wedge pressure, pulmonary artery pressure, right atrial pressure, systemic arterial pressure, heart rate, heart rhythm and calculated systemic vascular resistance, as well as pulmonary vascular resistance are essential observations. Additionally, the measurement of mixed venous oxygen saturation can be important, particularly when thermodilution cardiac output may not be reliable (as in the setting of significant tricuspid regurgitation). Repeated assessment of these parameters can guide pharmacologic therapies such that optimal hemodynamics for each individual patient can be achieved.

The immediate goals of acute heart failure management are to relieve symptoms, reverse hemodynamic derangements, preserve myocardial blood flow and energetics, and maintain clinical and hemodynamic stability while pursuing a definitive diagnosis of the problem. Table 5–16 presents a strategy for using hemodynamic measurements to direct therapy for decompensated heart failure patients. Initial therapeutic decisions are strongly influenced by systemic arterial pressure; however, optimal arterial pressures for each patient are quite variable. Generally, the lower the blood pressure the better, as long as the patient is not suffering from severe orthostatic hypotensive symptoms and has preserved renal function. Important hypotension is usually classified as an arterial systolic blood pressure less than 80 mm Hg when there is concomitant evidence of organ hypoperfusion (such as altered central nervous system activity or renal insufficiency). When these findings become apparent in a setting of hypotension, it is important to augment arterial pressure to a level where myocardial and systemic organ perfusion and function are not jeopardized.

Generally, hemodynamic goals include maintenance of the cardiac index above 2.2 L/min/m², pulmonary capillary wedge pressure below 20 mm Hg (< 17 mm Hg in the patient with chronic heart failure), systemic vascular resistance at 1,000–1,200 dynes/sec · cm⁻⁵, and right atrial pressure less than 12 mm Hg. Goals may vary greatly from patient to patient depending on the cause and acuteness of cardiac dysfunction. Optimal pulmonary capillary wedge pressure can thus be defined as the lowest pressure that can be maintained

TABLE 5-15	**Common Hemodynamic Patterns in Low Cardiac Output States**					
	CO	RAP	PAP	PCWP	SVR	SVO₂
Acute pulmonary edema	Variable	→	Variable	Variable	Variable	Variable
Cardiogenic shock	↓	↑	↑→	↑→	↑↑	↓↓
Decompensated heart failure	↓	↑	↑↑	↑↑	↑	↓
Acute right ventricular failure	↓	↑↑	→↓	→↓	↑	↓
Massive pulmonary embolism	↓	↑	↑	→	↑	↓
Acute aortic/mitral valve insufficiency	↓	→	↑	↑↑	↑	↓
Cardiac tamponade	↓	↑*	↑*	↑*	↑	↓
Hypovolemic shock	↓	↓	↓	↓	↑	↓

CO, cardiac output; RAP, right atrial pressure; PAP, pulmonary artery pressure; PCWP, pulmonary capillary wedge pressure; SVR, systemic vascular resistance; ↑, increased; →, normal; ↓, decreased; ↑↑, markedly increased.
*Equalization of pressures is characteristic.

TABLE 5-16   Hemodynamic-Directed Protocol for Decompensated Heart Failure

A. General hemodynamic goals
1. RAP ≤ 12 mm Hg
2. PCWP ≤17 mm Hg
3. SVR 1,000–1200 dyne/sec/cm^5 (12–15 Wood units)
4. CI > 2.5 L/min/m^2
5. "Optimum" systolic or mean BP is the lowest pressure that adequately supports renal function and central nervous system activity without significant orthostatic symptoms (systolic BP generally > 85–90 mm Hg)

B. Patient-specific hemodynamic goals
1. "Optimum filling pressure" (PCWP): lowest pulmonary capillary wedge pressure that can be maintained without preload-related decline in systolic BP and/or CI. A higher PCWP (18–20 mm Hg) is usually required in acute myocardial injury.
2. "Optimum afterload" (SVR): lowest SVR that leads to reasonable cardiac index while maintaining adequate systolic BP (generally > 80 mm Hg) and renal perfusion (urine output > 0.5 mL/kg/hr).

C. Specific intravenous pharmacologic therapy
1. Nitroprusside: begin when combined pre- and afterload reduction is most important hemodynamic goal
   • Start at 0.1–0.2 μg/kg/min
   • Titrate upward by 0.2 μg/kg/min at 3- to 5-minute intervals
   • Target hemodynamics (Section A)
   • Hemodynamic effects resolve rapidly when infusion stopped
2. Nitroglycerin: begin when preload reduction is primarily desired
   • Start at 0.2–0.3 μg/kg/min
   • Titrate at 3- to 5-minute intervals
   • Be aware of tolerance
   • Target hemodynamics (Section A)
   • Effects resolve rapidly when infusion stopped
3. Dobutamine: begin when both inotropic and vasodilating effects desired
   • Start at 2.5 μg/kg/min
   • Attempt to keep dose < 15 μg/kg/min; avoid significant tachycardia
   • Consider adding low-dose dopamine or milrinone to assist with augmenting renal perfusion and/or achieving hemodynamic endpoints
   • Hemodynamic effects resolve over minutes to hours when infusion stopped, but benefits occasionally persist longer
4. Milrinone: begin when vasodilating more than inotropic effects are desired
   • Dose range is 0.3–0.8 μg/kg/min (usual is 0.5 μg/kg/min)
   • Target hemodynamics (Section A)
   • Excessive hypotension with loading dose; would avoid loading in acute heart failure
   • Prolonged hemodynamic effects after drug is stopped

RAP, right atrial pressure; PCWP, pulmonary capillary wedge pressure; SVR, systemic vascular resistance; CI, cardiac index; BP, blood pressure.

without a preload-related decline in systolic arterial pressure or cardiac index. Dilated cardiomyopathy patients with severe systolic left ventricular dysfunction usually have stroke volumes which are primarily afterload dependent. Therefore, relatively normal pulmonary capillary wedge pressure can be targeted in these chronic patients during episodes of decompensation.

As with left heart filling pressure, the optimal systemic vascular resistance is the lowest one that can be achieved while maintaining adequate systemic perfusion, utilizing parameters mentioned previously. When significant systemic hypotension is present, however, therapy with vasopressor doses of **dopamine** (> 5 μg/kg/min) should be used. Failure to achieve an acceptable blood pressure response with higher doses of dopamine warrants consideration of switching to more potent alpha-adrenergic stimulating drugs such as epinephrine or norepinephrine. When perfusion remains inadequate despite aggressive adrenergic drug infusion, preparations should be made for proceeding to mechanical assistance, if that is an appropriate option when considering long-term strategies. In refractory hypotension and shock, mortality is extremely high if a surgically correctable lesion is not identified or if mechanical support is not instituted early.

Decompensated congestive heart failure with low cardiac output but acceptable, or, particularly, elevated arterial pressure may initially be treated with nitroprusside to augment forward stroke volume and reduce mitral valve regurgitation. If cardiac output increases appropriately with nitroprusside but left ventricular filling pressure remains elevated, then nitroglycerin can be added for further preload reduction. If both cardiac output and pulmonary capillary wedge pressure remain unacceptable, consideration of changing to or adding milrinone is appropriate. Dobutamine is another excellent drug choice in this situation. It has vasodilating properties and is a potent inotrope. Other therapeutic considerations would include the addition of "low-dose" dopamine to augment renal blood flow. Frequent assessment of volume status is important to assist with decisions regarding intravenous diuretic administration and/or an upward dose titration of parenteral nitroglycerin or nitroprusside when hemodynamic tolerance to these drugs becomes manifest.

Thus, the approach to the pharmacologic support of the patient with cardiogenic shock or severely decompensated heart failure must be individualized and guided by objective hemodynamic measurements. Evaluation of multiple clinical parameters including urine output, hepatic, and renal function measurements is necessary for appropriate drug selection and dose titration. Table 5–17 summarizes the pharmacologic effects of various vasodilating, inotropic, and "inodilator" medications. Further details of intravenous inotropic and vaso-

TABLE 5-17   Properties of Beta-Stimulants, Inotropic Vasodilators (Inodilators), and Nitrates

	ALPHA > BETA	BETA1-STIMULATION	BETA1 > BETA2	MIXED BETA1 AND BETA2 EFFECTS	PDE INHIBITORS	DOPAMINERGIC	NITRATES
Drug examples	NE	Dobutamine (also some beta$_2$)	Isoproternol	Epinephrine (also some alpha)	Amrinone, milrinone	Dopamine	Nitroglycerin, nitroprusside
Inotropic effect	++	++	+++	+++	+	++	0
Arteriolar vasodilation	0	+	+	+	++	+	++
Vasoconstriction	+++	0	0	++	0	+	0
Chronotropic effect	+	+	+++	++	+	+	0
Increase in blood pressure	+++	0/+	+	++	0/−	0/+ (high-dose dopamine)	−
Direct diuretic effect	0	0	0	0	0	++	0
Arrhythmia risk	+	+	+++	+++	+/++	+	0
Use in CHF	+	++	0	0	++	++	++
Use in resuscitation	+	++	+/0	+	0	++	0

NE, norepinephrine; CHF, congestive heart failure; PDE, phosphodiesterase;+, increase; 0, no effect; −negative effect.

dilator therapy are provided in Chapter 12. The major hemodynamic effect of **nitrates** is to evoke a reduction in ventricular filling pressure and volume by increasing venous capacitance through venodilation. Nitroglycerin is a more potent venodilator than is nitroprusside. **Nitroprusside,** on the other hand, is a more effective arteriolar vasodilating agent which reduces afterload more than preload. Intravenous nitroglycerin at a typical starting dose of 0.2 μg/kg/min may be rapidly uptitrated by 0.1–0.2 μg/kg/min increments to improve symptoms and reduce pulmonary and systemic venous pressures. Pharmacodynamic tolerance occurs during chronic infusion of both intravenous nitroglycerin and nitroprusside, but this is generally overcome by increasing doses. Chronic infusion of nitroprusside is complicated by thiocyanate toxicity, which must be considered when prolonged infused is required. Nitroprusside is administered intravenously with an infusion pump like nitroglycerin and usually started at a dose of 0.10–0.20 μg/kg/min with titration to the desired hemodynamic endpoint. Both drugs can cause hypotension, but this is rapidly reversed with discontinuation of the infusion.

An alternative vasodilator is nesiritide (natrecor), which is a genetically engineered β-type human natriuretic peptide recently approved for intravenous administration in acutely decompensated congestive heart failure patients. This drug may also have beneficial natriuretic and diuretic effects and may actually be better tolerated and more effective than intravenous nitroglycerin when given as a 2 ng/kg bolus followed by a 0.01 ng/kg/min continuous infusion. Nesiritide has also been given in combination with dopamine and dobutamine and prescribed in a wide range of acutely decompensated heart failure states, including those with acute coronary syndromes and renal insufficiency.

Dobutamine is a synthetic catecholamine acting primarily via beta$_1$–adrenergic stimulation. It is a potent inotropic drug with significant arteriolar vasodilating properties. **Isoproterenol** also has potent inotropic effects and is a beta$_1$- and beta$_2$-adrenergic receptor stimulating drug with beta$_1$ effects greater than beta$_2$ effects. Chronotropic effects of isoproterenol can be profound. Arrhythmia risk is therefore high with this agent, but it is very effective in patients with sinus bradycardia. **Epinephrine** has mixed beta$_1$- and beta$_2$-adrenergic effects with positive inotropy, significant vasoconstriction, and substantial chronotropic action. As already mentioned, **dopamine** has both inotropic and renal arteriolar vasodilating effects. Lower doses of dopamine are more effective for increasing renal perfusion with higher doses of dopamine being primarily alpha-adrenergic stimulating doses. Norepinephrine is a potent natural catecholamine with both alpha-adrenergic and beta$_1$-adrenergic properties. Although it has marked positive inotropic effects, the predominant action is dose-related vasoconstriction.[65, 167, 193] When used as an isolated agent, the resultant marked increase in afterload and contractility severely increases myocardial oxygen consumption. Although it is an effective agent in supporting blood pressure in shock-like states when dopamine and dobutamine are not successful, patients with acute decompensation of heart failure who require norepinephrine for support should be considered for mechanical circulatory assistance (see Chapter 8). Phosphodiesterase inhibitors are represented by amrinone and **milrinone.** Amrinone is rarely used today because of induced thrombocytopenia. Milrinone has rather profound arteriolar vasodilating actions but still is a positive inotropic agent.

Sometimes diuretic resistance can be overcome with chronic infusion of a loop diuretic in parenteral fashion. Diuretics, angiotensin-converting enzyme inhibitors, and digoxin are all given simultaneously with parenteral inotropic drugs. Combinations of pharmacologic agents can be helpful to achieve desired hemodynamic endpoints. The use of multiple agents to support the failing circulation may provide advantages over single drug infusion, since acute hemodynamic decompensation is associated with many different abnormalities that cannot always be effectively addressed by a single agent. Administration of an inotropic agent will ameliorate systolic dysfunction by improving contractility and stroke volume, but cardiac filling pressures and systemic vascular resistance (with its associated mitral valve regurgitation) may not be beneficially affected. On the other hand, a pure vasodilator alone may be insufficient to support the circulation and, in fact, can produce excessive hypotension when myocardial contractility is severely diminished and systemic blood pressure already low. Using only a vasopressor to raise blood pressure in a patient with hypotension will increase afterload, filling pressures, and wall stress, all of which will subsequently reduce cardiac output and potentiate myocardial ischemia.

Several combinations of intravenous drug infusions are theoretically appealing in the setting of severe acute heart failure. The simultaneous administration of dobutamine, for example, and a vasodilator such as nitroglycerin or nitroprusside will augment stroke volume and lower cardiac filling pressures more effectively than any of these agents alone. This combination can be particularly useful in patients with cardiogenic shock resulting from a complication of myocardial infarction such as ventricular septal or papillary muscle rupture. Also, the phosphodiesterase inhibitor milrinone offers the advantage of being a potent vasodilator and positive inotropic agent. There are some advantages to combining dobutamine (a beta antagonist) and milrinone (a phosphodiesterase inhibitor) simultaneously. The rationale behind this approach is based on the fact that each drug has different but complementary actions which increase contractility by elevating cyclic adenosine monophosphate levels in cardiac myocytes, and there is often an additive effect of combination therapy on major hemodynamic parameters.

Dobutamine and low-dose dopamine is also a commonly used combination. The rationale behind this approach is to achieve the inotropic effect of dobutamine with concomitant renal vasodilation that can result from low-dose dopamine infusion while minimizing the chronotropic effects of each drug. This combination is usually considered in the patient exhibiting marginal urine output and poor responsiveness to diuretics despite seemingly adequate central hemodynamics and systemic blood pressure.

Combination pharmacologic therapy is generally reserved for conditions associated with severe hemodynamic derangement such as cardiogenic shock or severely decompensated chronic heart failure. It is rarely indicated in acute pulmonary congestion by itself where a diuretic and vasodilator or inotropic compound alone will generally suffice. Combination infusion therapeutics would be indicated for a more immediate and prolonged circulatory stabilization while definitive therapy is pursued. Another potential advantage of combination parenteral therapy is to enable the use of lower doses of drugs so that significant untoward effects may be avoided. Again, the success of this approach, as with any treatment of acute and chronic heart failure, is highly dependent on the etiology and potential for myocardial recovery. In the patient where combination therapy is

deemed useful, hemodynamic monitoring should always be employed at some point to guide treatment endpoints.

Mechanical circulatory support should be considered in both acute and chronic heart failure patients when decompensation reaches the point where peripheral organ function (particularly renal and hepatic function) is disturbed to the extent that significant and potentially irreversible abnormalities become manifest. Nuances of acute and chronic circulatory support are considered in Chapter 8. One must remember, however, that the principles of acute and chronic heart failure therapeutics must be employed prior to institution of this aggressive treatment of refractory heart failure.

ADDITIONAL STRATEGIES TO CONSIDER DURING TREATMENT OF ADVANCED OR REFRACTORY HEART FAILURE

Table 5–18 summarizes the approach to patients with progressive and steadily worsening heart failure despite maximal oral therapy. In these patients the number of therapeutic options are reduced, but many still exist. When all attempts fail to create an adequate pharmacotherapeutic program that is successful in keeping patients symptom-free over the long term, consideration of more radical surgical interventions (see next section) or cardiac transplantation is appropriate. Alternative drug treatment strategies include long-term parenteral drug infusion protocols generally using dobutamine, milrinone, dopamine, or combinations of these drugs. In the refractory heart failure patient, chronic parenteral

---

TABLE 5–18 **Refractory Heart Failure and Treatment Options***

Higher risk standard operative procedures
- Coronary revascularization
- Valve repair/replacement
- Aneurysmectomy
- Endoventricular circular patch plasty
- Transmyocardial laser revascularization

Chronic/intermittent parenteral drug infusion
- Dobutamine
- Milrinone

Dialysis
- Hemofiltration
- Ultrafiltration
- Continuous venovenous hemodialysis
- Peritoneal dialysis

Cardiac transplantation

Developing operative procedures
- Dynamic cardiomyopathy
- Ventricular assist devices
- Volume reduction surgery
- Pacemaker therapeutics ("cardiac resynchronization")

"Hospice" care
- Eliminate pain and suffering
- Alternative dyspnea
- Psychological/spiritual support

---

*Assuming patients are aggressively managed with "triple" therapy and ancillary medical difficulties have adequately been administered.

infusion of inotropic agents or "inodilators" can dramatically reduce symptoms albeit at the risk of increasing mortality. One must weigh carefully the risks and benefits of this approach. It may be an entirely acceptable trade-off in the truly end-stage patient suffering greatly from refractory congestive states particularly when cardiac transplantation is no longer an option. The necessity of indwelling central venous catheter access in these patients creates many additional challenges and generally prompts the necessity of providing skilled home nursing caregivers in order to ensure that infections and other catheter complications are minimized. Whether or not chronic infusion of inotropic drugs is necessary, or if they can be given in pulsed parenteral fashion once weekly or monthly over shorter periods of time (6–12 hours), is not known. Also unknown is the best approach to attempt long-term drug weaning. Finally, the role of biventricular cardiac resynchronizing pacemaker insertion for congestive heart failure patients with wide QRS intervals on the electrocardiogram is being actively explored.

SURGICAL THERAPY (NONTRANSPLANT) FOR ADVANCED HEART FAILURE

It is readily apparent that the demand for cardiac transplantation will never be satisfied by the current supply of suitable donor hearts. Consequently, a number of surgical therapies for the treatment of cardiac failure have evolved, including coronary bypass surgery for patients with ischemic heart disease and poor ventricular function, cardiomyoplasty, left ventricular restoration procedures for regional left ventricular dysfunction, partial left ventricular resection, mitral valve repair for cardiomyopathy, and implantation of chronic mechanical circulatory support devices. It is not only the supply and demand imbalance of donor hearts that has fueled the search for surgical alternatives to transplantation, but also the possibility that some of these procedures may produce results as good as those currently offered by cardiac transplantation, particularly for the less advanced stages of heart failure. Furthermore, these procedures have an important role in patients who have contraindications to cardiac transplantation. One of the important challenges for the future is to determine the respective roles of each of these therapies in the spectrum of heart failure, including surgery in the earlier stages of heart failure, surgery as a bridge to cardiac transplantation, and definitive alternatives to heart transplant. In the same way as patients with complex congenital heart disease may find themselves on a pathway leading to, for example, a Fontan operation and ultimately to cardiac transplantation, so may patients with end-stage ischemic heart disease follow a similar pathway. This may involve bridging therapy such as coronary bypass surgery or a left ventricular restoration procedure ultimately leading to cardiac transplantation (the goal being to provide the patient with the best long-term survival and quality of life). It is through the development of patient-specific equations (see Chapter 3) that the best decisions for the advisability of one procedure versus another will likely be made.

CORONARY ARTERY BYPASS SURGERY FOR ISCHEMIC HEART FAILURE

Ischemic heart disease remains the most important cause of congestive cardiac failure in the United States.[142, 253] Heart failure as a result of coronary artery disease may be due to (1) chronic ischemia-related left ventricular dysfunction; (2) acute reversible left ventricular systolic and/or diastolic dysfunction; (3) mechanical complication of acute myocardial infarction including acute or chronic mitral regurgitation, ruptured ventricular septum, and left ventricular aneurysm; and (4) any combination of the above. It is in the context of considering cardiac transplantation versus coronary artery bypass grafting (CABG) that the entity of chronic ischemia-related left ventricular dysfunction becomes important.

The pathology of ischemic cardiomyopathy is a complicated mixture of reversible as well as irreversible ischemic injury with areas of scar occurring as a result of myocyte necrosis together with the secondary phenomena of infarct expansion and remodeling. An important component of ischemic left ventricular dysfunction is the loss of coronary flow reserve[269] (the ability to increase coronary blood flow in response to increasing myocardial metabolic demand) due to obstructive coronary artery disease. This loss of coronary flow reserve results in inadequate myocardial perfusion and myofiber hypoxia with the production of myocardial dysfunction (Fig. 5–4).[187] A major component of chronic left ventricular dysfunction due to coronary artery disease that has important therapeutic implications is the phenomenon of **stunning** and **hibernation.** Both these terms arose out of the recognition that even though there may be failure of the contractile process with ischemia, myocytes may still be viable and under certain circumstances subsequently recover function. Stunning[27, 34, 116, 141] is a process of depressed systolic and diastolic myocardial function secondary to short-term total or near total reduction of coronary blood flow followed by restoration of blood flow, and recovery of myocardial function. Under the circumstances of repetitive ischemic episodes in which the myocytes are unable to completely recover, myocyte function may continue to be depressed (repetitive stunning). The hallmarks of stunning are normal or near normal coronary blood flow with acutely depressed ventricular function (mismatch of coronary blood flow and function). Stunning may be seen together with acute ischemic syndromes, hibernation, or myocardial infarction.

The physiology of hibernation[35, 232, 238] centers on the down-regulation of myocardial function to match the reduced oxygen supply due to impaired coronary blood flow. By matching function to reduced blood flow, the myocardium is protected against persistent ischemia and cell viability is maintained. This state of hibernation is maintained as long as there is hypoperfusion, but when normal coronary blood flow is restored, myocar-

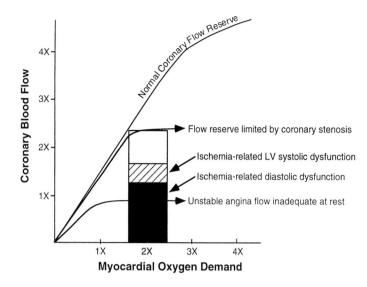

FIGURE **5–4.** Decrease in coronary flow reserve with progressive coronary obstruction. (From Mills RM, Pepine CJ: Heart failure secondary to coronary artery disease. *In* Hospenpud JD, Greenberg BH [eds]: Congestive Heart Failure. New York: Springer-Verlag, 1994.)

dial dysfunction in the area of hibernation may be returned to normal, although the time course of recovery may take up to 12 months.[230, 231] It is the phenomena of hibernation and stunning which underpins the potential reversibility of chronic left ventricular dysfunction in coronary artery disease (Fig. 5–5).[229]

Currently, a growing body of clinical evidence supports the concept of recovery of function of hibernating myocardium after revascularization[9, 54, 237, 255, 257] and percutaneous transluminal coronary angioplasty (PTCA).[45, 64, 261, 267] Areas of abnormal segmental wall motion in the presence of coronary artery disease without demonstrable hibernating myocardium generally show little or no contractile improvement following revascularization.[266] Thus, identification of hibernating myocardium (Table 5–19) plays a central role in the identification of patients who would likely benefit from revascularization procedures.[50] There are a number of approaches to the identification of hibernating myocardium (see Box), but the method that is probably the most reliable (and perhaps the "gold standard") is positron emission tomography (PET) combining evaluation of metabolic activity and myocardial perfusion (Fig. 5–6).[30]

The time course of recovery of contractile function after revascularization in patients with hibernating myocardium is quite variable and almost certainly reflects the complex substrate involved in myocardial dysfunction (a mixture of hibernating muscle, normal muscle, and irreversibly damaged muscle) and the complex recovery process, which includes both restoration of biochemical processes and possible remanufacture of components of the contractile apparatus. The concept of variable recovery of hibernating myocardium (Fig. 5–7) has clinical and experimental support.[229] The acute recovery of hibernating myocardium[257] likely occurs in patients where the myocardium is essentially normal. Subacute recovery (recovery taking days to weeks) has been described after coronary bypass surgery[180] and percutaneous transluminal coronary angioplasty.[197] A study by Nienaber and colleagues[197] demonstrated that after PTCA there was recovery of perfusion, but persistence of abnormal metabolic and contractile function which had normalized on follow-up an average of 2–3 months after angioplasty. These findings are consistent with delayed improvement in left ventricular function in experimental models[152, 156, 182, 243, 264] and in patients after angioplasty.[80, 152] There is evidence that in clinically hi-

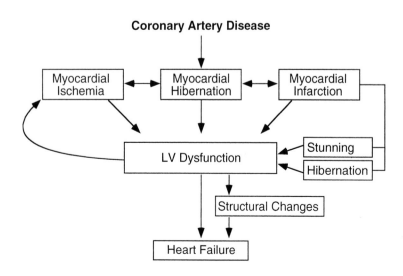

FIGURE **5–5.** Coronary artery disease may result in myocardial ischemia, hibernation, or infarction, all of which are associated with left ventricular dysfunction. Stunning may be superimposed on ischemia or hibernating myocardium on reperfusion. Except for infarcted myocardial tissue, all other states are potentially reversible with appropriate timely treatment. (From Rahimtoola SH: From coronary artery disease to heart failure: role of the hibernating myocardium. Am J Cardiol 1995;75:16E.)

TABLE 5-19	Approaches to Identifying Viability in Hibernating Myocardium

A. Assessment of regional myocardial function using radionuclide methods, echocardiography, or magnetic resonance imaging during or after:
  1. Nitroglycerin
  2. Postextrasystolic potentiation
  3. Catecholamine infusion (dobutamine)
  4. Exercise
  5. Synchronized diastolic coronary venous retroperfusion
B. Assessment of perfusion, membrane integrity, and metabolism:
  1. Thallium-201 scintigraphy, rest and exercise redistribution
  2. Technetium-99m sestamibi
  3. Positron emission tomography
       Flow: rubidium-82
       Metabolism: fluorine-18-fluorodeoxyglucose, carbon-11-acetate
  4. Magnetic resonance spectroscopy

Adapted from Castro PF, Bourge RC, Foster RE: Evaluation of hibernating myocardium in patients with ischemic heart disease. Am J Med 1998;104:69.

bernating myocardium recovery may take many months (chronic recovery). Morphologic myocyte injury (characterized by loss of contractile material and increased myocyte glycogen content) has been identified in biopsies from left ventricles with known hibernating myocardium, which suggests that recovery of con-

Identification of Hibernating Myocardium

The methods of accurate identification of viable myocardium can be grouped into two categories: (1) assessment of regional myocardial functional reserve after provocation, and (2) assessment of perfusion membrane integrity and metabolism[50] (Table 5-19). Noninvasive identification of hibernating myocardium has become a complex technological area and clearly not free of controversy. Provocation testing to demonstrate systolic wall thickening (contractile reserve) during dobutamine infusion with imaging by either echocardiography or magnetic resonance imaging is a commonly used method. The biphasic response (augmentation of systolic function followed by deterioration in function) appears to have the highest predictive value for hibernating myocardium.[30] However, this response is probably very dependent on dobutamine dose and the ratio of hibernating muscle to infarcted or scarred muscle. Perfusion imaging using tracers such as thallium-201 and technetium-99 sestamibi may overestimate the potential for improvement in regional function after revascularization.

PET determines viability by matching metabolism and myocardial blood flow. In the presence of myocardial ischemia there is a switch from fatty acid to glucose utilization and hence the tracer ^{18}F-deoxyglucose (FDG) will be taken up by viable myocardium. If an area of myocardium has high FDG uptake relative to myocardial blood flow (MBF), this FDG:MBF mismatch is indicative of ischemic, stunned, or hibernating myocardium, whereas an FDG:MBF match is likely to represent an area of scar or infarcted muscle.

It would be unrealistic to expect complete concordance between these methods of identifying hibernating myocardium, as different markers of hibernation are being measured. However, there appears to be reasonable concordance between these methods.[30]

tractile function may require a considerable period of time.[13, 246, 263]

The survival of patients with ischemic heart disease and heart failure is generally poor, with an annual mortality of approximately 30–50%.[121, 213] Survival of patients undergoing medical therapy for coronary artery disease and severe left ventricular dysfunction is considerably decreased in those patients who have evidence of hibernating myocardium[87] (Fig. 5–8), presumably reflecting the vulnerability of these patients to ischemic events. With the demonstration that left ventricular function may improve with revascularization by coronary bypass surgery or percutaneous transluminal coronary angioplasty, considerable interest developed in the use of revascularization for patients with ischemic heart disease and heart failure. This was a logical extension from the known beneficial effect on survival of coronary bypass surgery in patients with three-vessel coronary artery disease and impaired left ventricular function from the Coronary Artery Surgery Study (CASS) and the European Coronary Surgery Study.[49, 112]

Numerous studies[109, 149, 162, 163, 175, 245, 248] have shown that coronary artery bypass surgery in high-risk patients with severely impaired left ventricular function can be performed with low operative mortality. An informal comparison with cardiac transplantation indicates that survival of these patients is comparable to or better than that of transplantation. Obviously, this is not an appropriate comparison, since many of these patients did not have heart failure severe enough to warrant cardiac transplantation. However, it does suggest that coronary bypass surgery should be considered, under certain circumstances, before cardiac transplantation in patients with an ischemic cardiomyopathy. In deciding between coronary bypass surgery (or PTCA) and cardiac transplanation for patients with advanced ischemic cardiomyopathy, criteria which indicate the potential for myocaradial improvement must be weighed against important risk factors for surgical mortality, including left ventricular dilatation, elevated left ventricular end-diastolic pressure, mitral regurgitation (moderate or severe), reoperative coronary bypass surgery, pulmonary hypertension, and impaired right ventricular function.

The criteria which favor revascularization rather than cardiac transplantation for ischemic cardiomyopathy

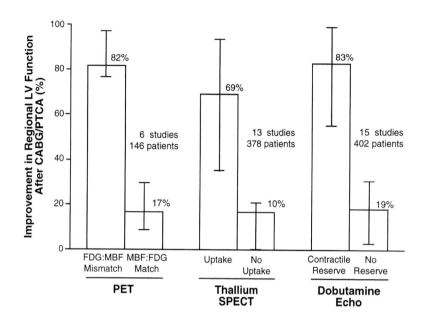

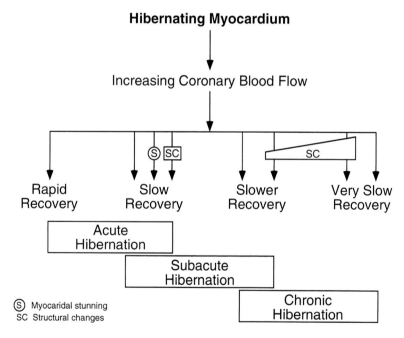

FIGURE **5-6.** Likelihood of improved regional LV function after revascularization based on noninvasive methods to detect viable myocardium. Data are summarized from six studies using PET, involving 146 patients, in which enhanced ^{18}F-fluorodeoxyglucose (FDG) uptake relative to myocardial blood flow (MBF) was used as a marker of myocardial viability. These PET data are compared with 13 studies using thallium SPECT involving 378 patients, and 15 studies using dobutamine echocardiography involving 402 patients. The range of values reported from the individual studies is indicated by the horizontal bars connected by vertical lines. The shaded bars represent the positive predictive value, and the open bars represent the inverse of the negative predictive value. CABG, coronary artery bypass graft surgery; PTCA, percutaneous transluminal coronary angioplasty. (From Bonow RO: Identification of viable myocardium. Circulation 1996;94:2674.)

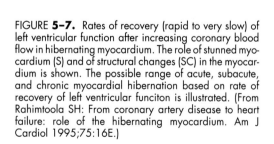

FIGURE **5-7.** Rates of recovery (rapid to very slow) of left ventricular function after increasing coronary blood flow in hibernating myocardium. The role of stunned myocardium (S) and of structural changes (SC) in the myocardium is shown. The possible range of acute, subacute, and chronic myocardial hibernation based on rate of recovery of left ventricular funciton is illustrated. (From Rahimtoola SH: From coronary artery disease to heart failure: role of the hibernating myocardium. Am J Cardiol 1995;75:16E.)

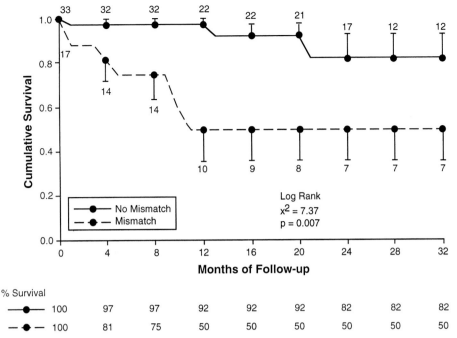

FIGURE **5-8.** Cumulative survival of the 50 patients receiving medical therapy for ischemic heart disease and severe left ventricular dysfunction. Patients are subgrouped according to the presence (n = 17) or absence (n = 33) of positron emission tomographic mismatch. (From DiCarli MF, Davidson M, Little R, Khanna S, Mody FV, Brunken RC, Czernin J, Rokhsar S, Stevenson LW, Laks H, Hawkins R, Schelbert HR, Phelps ME, Maddahi J: Value of metabolic imaging with position emission tomography for evaluating prognosis in patients with coronary artery disease and left ventricular dysfunction. Am J Cardiol 1994;73:527.)

include three-vessel coronary artery disease (severe proximal stenoses with good distal target vessels) and evidence of hibernating myocardium. Obviously, important risk factors, particularly left ventricular dilatation and other traditional risk factors for death after coronary artery surgery, including age and comorbidity, are incorporated into the decision-making process. The importance of hibernating myocardium in patients undergoing revascularization is evident from the study of DiCarli,[86] who reported a substantial survival benefit in patients with left ventricular dysfunction (with or without heart failure) undergoing coronary bypass surgery versus medical therapy, but this benefit only occurred in patients with PET mismatch (Fig. 5–9). Furthermore, the survival benefit in patients with a PET mismatch was independent of the severity of symptoms. (Fig. 5–10). Patients with heart failure as their predominant symptom clearly may experience considerable improvement both in symptoms[87, 212] and in left ventricular systolic function. In fact, the number of hibernating left ventricular segments appears directly related to the degree of improvement in left ventricular systolic function following revascularization[212] (Fig. 5–11).

The importance of hibernating myocardium for survival benefit following revascularization has been indirectly challenged by the finding that failure of global left ventricular systolic function to improve after coronary bypass surgery (the implication being that important hibernating myocardium was absent) may still be associated with improvement in heart failure symptoms and a survival benefit that is similar to that of patients who

experience improvement in global left ventricular systolic function after revascularization.[242] This underscores the complexity of the physiologic response to revascularization in this condition and points to additional mechanisms which may be operative, such as improvement in diastolic function, reduction in dynamic mitral regurgitation, reduction in left ventricular remodeling, and restoration of coronary flow reserve. Survival benefit in the absence of improved systolic left ventricular function may also relate to greater protection from subsequent myocardial infarctions. The problem of ischemic mitral regurgitation in patients with an ischemic cardiomyopathy is also vexing, but our current approach is to repair mitral regurgitation at the time of surgical revascularization only in patients where it is echocardiographically moderate or severe.

Not surprisingly, there are many individual approaches to coronary bypass surgery in these high-risk patients with many different opinions regarding myocardial protection, preoperative use of intra-aortic balloon pump counterpulsation, use of metabolic support with triiodothyronine and glucose-insulin potassium solution, arterial versus venous conduits, and total versus incomplete revascularization. Nevertheless, the results suggest that despite all these controversies in surgical strategy, revascularization in selected patients with ischemic cardiomyopathy may produce improvement in symptoms of heart failure, improve left ventricular systolic function, and result in intermediate term survival that may be at least as good as that achieved by cardiac transplantation. Therefore, in all patients with an isch-

With PET Mismatch

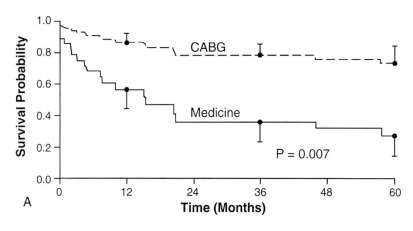

A

Without PET Mismatch

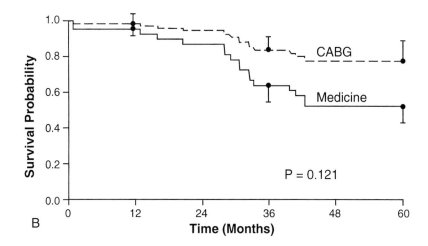

B

FIGURE **5-9.** Plot shows adjusted Kaplan-Meier estimated survival probability for patients with left ventricular dysfunction treated medically and with CABG by (A) presence or (B) absence of PET mismatch. (From DiCarli MF, Maddahi J, Rokhsar S, Schelbert HR, Biano-Batlles D, Brunken RC, Fromm B: Long-term survival of patients with coronary artery disease and left ventricular dysfunction: implications for the role of myocardial viability assessment in management decisions. J Thorac Cardiovasc Surg 1998;116:997.)

emic cardiomyopathy, revascularization should be examined as an option before cardiac transplantation is advised.

DYNAMIC CARDIOMYOPLASTY

Clinical dynamic cardiomyoplasty developed as a result of the convergence of two trains of investigation—the use of skeletal muscle to replace or augment cardiac muscle and the discovery that fatigable fast-twitch muscle fibers could be transformed to fatigue-resistant slow-twitch fibers. The earliest use of skeletal muscle in cardiac surgery was as a means of repairing or reinforcing lost cardiac muscle. DeJesus in 1931 used skeletal muscle to repair a traumatic ventricular injury,[81] and skeletal muscle was subsequently used both experimentally and clinically to repair myocardial defects[58,169,216] and increase myocardial vascularization.[19] A number of experimental attempts were made to use skeletal muscle dynamically to assist cardiac function,[83,147,177] but the problem of skeletal muscle fatigue prevented its application for long-term cardiac assistance. Salmons and Stréter demonstrated that skeletal muscle could be transformed from fatigable fast-twitch fibers into fatigue resistant slow-

twitch fibers by electrical stimulation.[240] These developments resulted in the first clinical application of skeletal muscle assist in 1985[46] and the subsequent widespread application of this technique.

The biochemistry of transformation involves changes not only in the energy-producing pathways, but also in muscle phenotype and muscle mechanics. Skeletal muscle fibers are either slow-twitch type I fibers or fast-twitch type II fibers,[22] and for the latissimus dorsi muscle fibers to be fatigue-resistant the protocol of electrical stimulation must transform the predominant type II muscle fibers to type I fibers.[217,240] The transformation process involves changes in metabolic pathways for generation of ATP. Maintaining fast-twitch is expensive in energy terms, and the change to slow-twitch fibers, which results in greater energy economy for the production of ATP, involves a switch from glycolytic pathways to oxidative phosphorylation, with an associated increase in mitochondrial volume[107] and capillary density.[38] Transformation also involves changes in calcium flux with reduced uptake of calcium by the sarcoplasmic reticulum,[241] the slow-twitch muscle requiring less speed of cross-bridge formation.[77] Parallel with these metabolic changes is a conversion of the myosin heavy and light chain isoforms that are typical of the fast-twitch type to

With Severe Angina

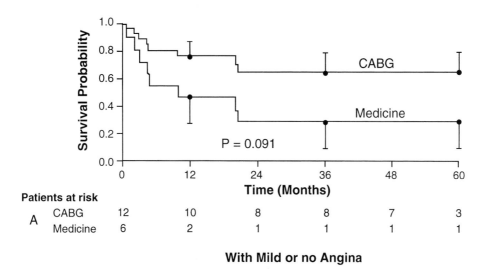

Patients at risk

		0	12	24	36	48	60
A	CABG	12	10	8	8	7	3
	Medicine	6	2	1	1	1	1

With Mild or no Angina

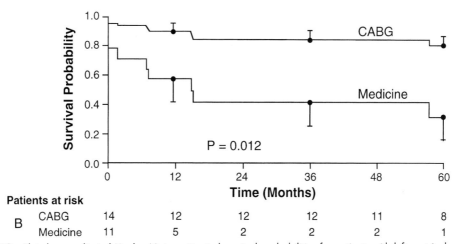

Patients at risk

		0	12	24	36	48	60
B	CABG	14	12	12	12	11	8
	Medicine	11	5	2	2	2	1

FIGURE **5–10.** Plot shows adjusted Kaplan-Meier estimated survival probabilities for patients with left ventricular dysfunction and a PET mismatch treated medically and with CABG among patients with (A) severe angina or (B) mild or no angina. (From DiCarli MF, Maddahi J, Rokhsar S, Schelbert HR, Biano-Batlles D, Brunken RC, Fromm B: Long-term survival of patients with coronary artery disease and left ventricular dysfunction: implications for the role of myocardial viability assessment in management decisions. J Thorac Cardiovasc Surg 1998;116:997.)

FIGURE **5–11.** Correlation between the number of viable dysfunctional LV segments and the absolute changes in LVEF (δEF) following revascularization. The equation for this relationship is $Y = 1.2X + -3.97$. (From Pagano D, Townend JN, Littler WA, Horton R, Camici PG, Bonser RS: Coronary artery bypass surgery as treatment for ischemic heart failure: the predictive value of viability assessment with quantitative positron emission tomography for symptomatic and functional outcome. J Thorac Cardiovasc Surg 1998;115:791.)

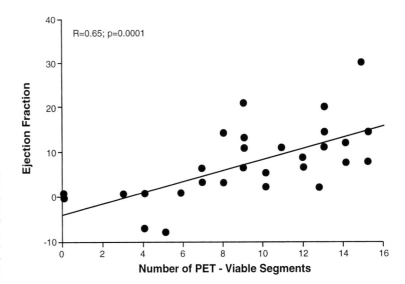

those of the slow-twitch type.[39] All of these changes are reflected in the demonstration[1] that the oxygen consumption of chronically stimulated experimental skeletal muscles is less than control muscles.

The surgical technique involves mobilization of the entire latissimus dorsi muscle with severing of all the attachments, including the humeral tendon, while preserving the neurovascular pedicle (Fig. 5–12).[47] The intramuscular stimulation leads are then attached to the latissimus dorsi muscle flap (Fig. 5–13).[47] A section of the second rib is removed to create a window through which the muscle flap is passed into the left pleural space together with the stimulation electrodes, and the humeral tendon is sutured to the periosteum of the third rib (Fig. 5–14).[47] The latissimus dorsi mobilization incision is then closed. The patient is then placed supine, and through a median sternotomy the pericardial cavity is opened and the epicardial sensing electrodes are attached to the right ventricle. The latissimus dorsi muscle is then passed posterior to the heart and the edge of the muscle is anchored to the pericardium adjacent to the right atrium and pulmonary artery (Fig. 5–15).[47] The base of the flap is passed anteriorly to cover as much of the right ventricle as possible. The diaphragmatic edge and lateral side of the flap are sutured to each other snugly but without causing any compression of the heart (Fig. 5–16).[47] The myocardial sensing leads and

the stimulator leads are attached to the cardiomyostimulator, which is placed in the abdominal pocket. Cardiopulmonary bypass is usually not required for the procedure.

The muscle conditioning process does not commence for 2 weeks to allow the latissimus dorsi muscle, which frequently is ischemic at the end distal to the neurovascular pedicle, to recover and to allow fusion of the wrap to the epicardium. The electrical stimulation protocol to produce muscle transformation was proposed by Carpentier[51] and involves delivery of a single pulse with every other cardiac cycle for 2 weeks. Following this, two pulses are delivered every other cardiac cycle and this is increased every 1–2 weeks up to 12 weeks after cardiomyoplasty so that pulse trains that are able to stimulate full contraction of the muscle wrap are delivered. The R-wave is the trigger for delivery of the muscle stimulation, and the time delay from R-wave to muscle stimulation is adjusted using echocardiography to ensure that the stimulation of the muscle wrap occurs after mitral valve closure. The cardiomyostimulator has a cardiac channel which senses the R-wave, counts the programmed synchronization ratio, and triggers the stimulation burst to the wrap following a programmed synchronized delay. The cardiomyostimulator has a muscle channel which is connected to the wrap. The synchronization ratio, pulse entrained duration, pulse amplitude, and sensing threshold can all be adjusted.

The clinical benefit of dynamic cardiomyoplasty for patients suffering from advanced heart failure was originally reputed to be **systolic** augmentation of the failing left (and possibly right) ventricle. Some studies have demonstrated an increase in left ventricular ejection fraction with the stimulator "on" versus "off,"[144] and beat-to-beat increase in load-independent indices of contractility (canine cardiomyopathy model).[214] Unfortunately, despite the demonstration of improvement in clinical symptoms, multiple clinical studies have failed to show consistent and sustained improvement in systolic ventricular function.[46, 57, 82, 144, 165, 178, 191] Multiple explanations for this observation have been suggested, including the relative devascularization of the lower third of the muscle which results from the single stage harvest procedure. Experimental and clinical studies have documented atrophy and fibrosis in the latissimus wrap 1 or more years after the procedure, possibly related to ischemia.[188] Other explanations have focused on the relative inefficiency of skeletal muscle compared to cardiac muscle. Skeletal muscle, which works by linear shortening, is very inefficient at producing radial shortening, when wrapped around the heart, and 90% of the power producing linear shortening is wasted.[239] Furthermore, the skeletal muscle wrap is quite inefficient in producing systolic augmentation for large cardiac volumes within the time span of the cardiac cycle.[139]

Another explanation for the clinical improvement is the notion that cardiomyoplasty acts as an elastic constraint preventing ventricular dilation and promoting reverse remodeling of the left ventricle. This concept, also called the **girdling effect,** has both clinical[148] and experimental[43] support. The study by Kass and colleagues[148] demonstrated that after cardiomyoplasty in

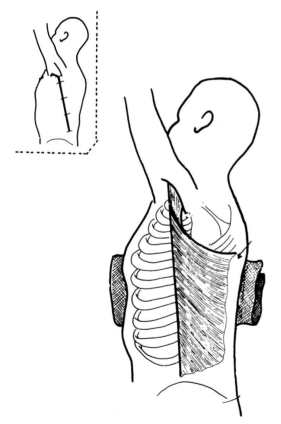

FIGURE **5–12.** Cardiomyoplasty: detachment of latissimus dorsi muscle. (From Carpentier A, Chachques JC: Cardiomyoplasty: surgical technique. *In* Carpentier A, Chachques JC, Grandjean P [eds]: Cardiomyoplasty. Mount Kisco, NY: Futura Publishing Company, 1991, with permission.)

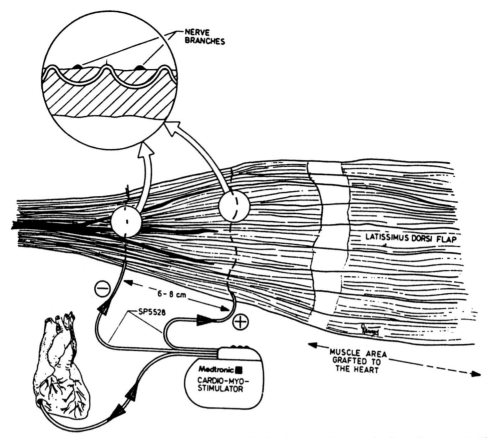

FIGURE **5-13.** Cardiomyoplasty: placement of myostimulating leads in latissimus dorsi muscle. (From Carpentier A, Chachques JC: Cardiomyoplasty: surgical technique. *In* Carpentier A, Chachques JC, Grandjean P [eds]: Cardiomyoplasty. Mount Kisco, NY: Futura Publishing Company, 1991, with permission.)

three patients there was a leftward shift in the end-systolic pressure–volume relationship as well as a reduction in left ventricular volume at 12 months after operation (Fig. 5–17). Another postulated mechanism of action of dynamic cardiomyoplasty is a reduction in ventricular wall stress because of the increased thickness due to the wrap,[96, 198] which may translate into reduced myocardial oxygen consumption.[189] Thus, the proposed explanation for the clinical benefit of the latissimus dorsi muscle wrap involves elements of muscle **transformation** (systolic assist) and **conformation** (girdling effect).

A lack of demonstrated survival advantage with cardiomyoplasty over medical treatment has been an important factor in hindering widespread acceptance of this procedure. A multicenter trial[125] of cardiomyoplasty showed no survival advantage when compared to a matched reference group of heart failure patients (Fig. 5–18). Important risk factors predicting poor survival after cardiomyoplasty include NYHA Class IV, atrial fibrillation, severe mitral regurgitation, extremely low left ventricular ejection fraction (< about 0.12–0.15), severe left ventricular dilatation (end-diastolic dimension > about 7–7.5 cm), marked elevation of resting pulmonary capillary wedge pressure (> about 25 mm Hg), multivessel coronary artery disease, severe reduction in exercise performance (especially with peak oxygen consumption < about 10 mL/kg/min), and the need for an intra-aortic balloon pump.[48, 52, 108, 124, 235] The high

early mortality for cardiomyoplasty in patients with very advanced forms of heart failure (as indicated by these risk factors) is not unexpected given the lack of hemodynamic benefit for at least 8–12 weeks (during the obligatory period of muscle training). These considerations lead to the refinement of patient selection criteria. It is now clear that **cardiomyoplasty should only be considered** in patients with persistent symptoms of heart failure who are in **NYHA Class III** (and not in Class IV) **without important valvular regurgitation, coronary artery disease, or cardiac dysrhythmias**

The only multi-institutional randomized trial between cardiomyoplasty and medical therapy was initiated in 1994. The Cardiomyoplasty-Skeletal Muscle Assist Trial (C-SMART), included patients in NYHA Class III with heart failure treatment optimized with medical therapy, adequate noncardiac organ system function, left ventricular ejection fraction less than 0.40, left ventricular end-diastolic pressure less than 35 mm Hg, and peak oxygen consumption 10–22 mL/kg/min.[31, 154, 273] Between 1994 and 1999, 103 patients were randomized to medical or surgical therapy (the trial was terminated early because of slow patient enrollment). The 6-month results of the C-SMART trial demonstrated a low hospital mortality (4%) and significant improvement in symptomatic status, exercise tolerance, and quality of life in patients undergoing cardiomyoplasty compared to medical therapy.

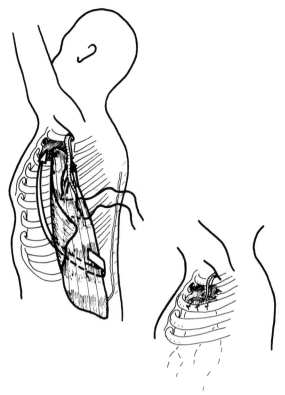

FIGURE **5-14.** Cardiomyoplasty: rotation of latissimus dorsi muscle into the chest (see text for further details). (From Carpentier A, Chachques JC: Cardiomyoplasty: surgical technique. *In* Carpentier A, Chachques JC, Grandjean R [eds]: Cardiomyoplasty. Mount Kisco, NY: Futura Publishing Company, 1991, with permission.)

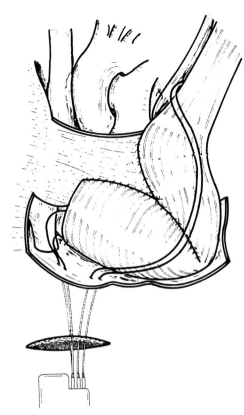

FIGURE **5-16.** Cardiomyoplasty: final appearance. (From Carpentier A, Chachques JC: Cardiomyoplasty: surgical technique. *In* Carpentier A, Chachques JC, Grandjean P [eds]: Cardiomyoplasty. Mount Kisco, NY: Futura Publishing Company, 1991, with permission.)

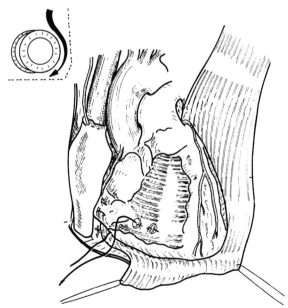

FIGURE **5-15.** Cardiomyoplasty: wrapping the heart with latissimus dorsi muscle. (From Carpentier A, Chachques JC: Cardiomyoplasty: surgical technique. *In* Carpentier A, Chachques JC, Grandjean P [eds]: Cardiomyoplasty. Mount Kisco, NY: Futura Publishing Company, 1991, with permission.)

The Medtronic Corporation no longer manufactures the cardiomyostimulator, which has currently eliminated this procedure from consideration in the United States. However, other myostimulator devices are under development, such as the LD PACE II pulse generator, which provides variable synchronization ratios that allow the muscle to rest at night when the patient is asleep (and potentially reduce muscle fatigue of the wrap).[55] Other means of using skeletal muscle assist are under investigation including skeletal muscle ventricles[36, 254] and aortomyoplasty (sketal muscle providing arterial counterpulsation either in the ascending or descending thoracic aorta), a procedure that has been performed clinically with hemodynamic and symptomatic benefits.[258]

The girdling effect of cardiomyoplasty has stimulated the development of volume constraining devices designed to prevent further left ventricular enlargement in patients with cardiomyopathy. By the Laplace relationship, wall stress is proportional to intraventricular pressure and ventricular radius and inversely proportional to wall thickness. Thus, larger ventricles with a larger radius develop increased wall stress, which in turn leads to increased myofibril tension, greater ATP requirement for myofibril contraction, and increased myocardial oxygen consumption. Mechanical devices have been designed to favorably affect wall stress by retarding left ventricular dilatation without adversely affecting myocardial compliance (diastolic function).

Baseline

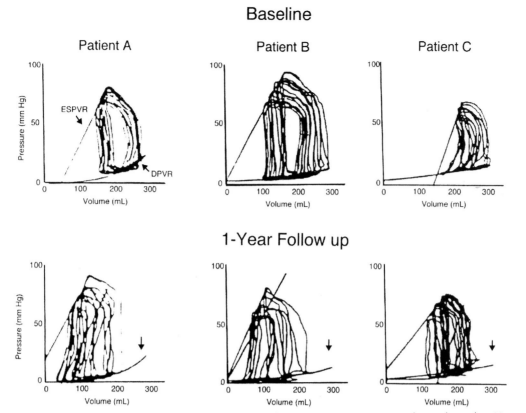

FIGURE **5-17.** Long-term effects of cardiomyoplasty on cardiac function as seen in pressure–volume relationship. Ventricular pressure–volume loops and relations are shown for each patient at baseline (before cardiomyoplasty) and 1 year after operation. All patients demonstrated a reduction in chamber volume. Vertical arrows show initial end-diastolic volume. DPVR, diastolic pressure–volume relationship; ESPVR, end-systolic pressure–volume relationship. (From Kass DA, Baughman KL, Pak PH, Cho PW, Levin HR, Gardner TJ, Halperin HR, Tsitlik JE, Acker MA: Reverse remodeling from cardiomyoplasty in human heart failure: external constraint versus active assist. Circulation 1995;91:2314.)

The advantages of such devices include (1) simplicity, (2) absence of a blood contact surface, (3) relatively low cost compared to other mechanical therapies for advanced heart failure, (4) low surgical risk, and (5) the potential for retarding the development of advanced heart failure in NYHA Class III patients. Clinical studies of such devices are in their initial phase.[226]

LEFT VENTRICULAR RESTORATION PROCEDURES

Left ventricular dilatation, whatever the cause, is characterized geometrically by an increased radius of curvature of the left ventricular wall and an abnormal volume/mass relationship. The procedure of partial left

FIGURE **5-18.** Actuarial survival in phase II multicenter clinical trial for dynamic cardiomyoplasty (DCMP): comparison between patients having DCMP and matched reference group. (From Furnary AP, Jessup FM, Moreira LF: Multicenter trial of dynamic cardiomyoplasty for chronic heart failure. The American Cardiomyoplasty Group. J Am Coll Cardiol 1996;28:1175.)

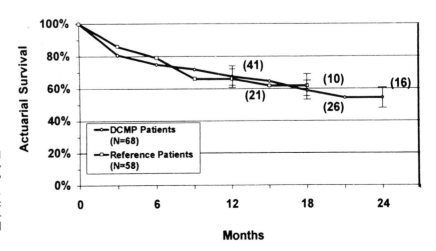

ventricular resection (PLVR) or Batista procedure was designed to specifically restore the volume/mass relationship of the ventricle toward normal. The infarct excluding endoventricular circular patch plasty (EVCPP) or Dor procedure and mitral valve repair for mitral regurgitation associated with a cardiomyopathy can also be considered left ventricular restoration procedures.

EVCPP or Dor Procedure for Postinfarction Left Ventricular Scar

Following an acute transmural myocardial infarction, the necrotic muscle cicatrizes, thins, and attenuates. In order to maintain forward output, a series of secondary changes occur, principally in the remaining contractile portion of the ventricle, a process known as remodeling (see Chapter 4). The resultant ventricular dilatation is accompanied by an increase in wall tension due to an increased radius of curvature of the ventricle. This requires increased myocardial oxygen consumption and provides a stimulus for further remodeling, setting the stage for heart failure as described in Chapter 4. The end result of scar formation and thinning in an area of infarcted left ventricular free wall and/or septum may range from a small area of akinesis with nearly normal overall ventricular systolic function, to larger areas of akinesis with ventricular enlargement and depressed global systolic function, to actual dyskinesis (left ventricular aneurysm) of a major wall segment.

The surgical treatment of left ventricular scar evolved from the resection of left ventricular aneurysms (a term which implies a large dyskinetic scar with significant paradoxical movement on an imaging study) for the relief of heart failure. The original technique for left ventricular aneurysm resection, first reported by Cooley and colleagues in 1958,[75] involved resection of the aneurysm and linear closure of the resulting defect. The reduction in heart size and improvement in heart failure symptoms were dramatic if the left ventricular volume was returned toward normal and the nonaneurysmal portions of the ventricle had nearly normal contractility (also a major determinant of survival).[40]

Despite the acceptance of left ventricular aneurysm resection as a standard cardiac surgical procedure, it was often associated with marked distortion of left ventricular geometry with potentially important effects on left ventricular function.[123] Subsequent techniques focused on the restoration of left ventricular geometry. The technique of Jatene[143] involved circular reduction of the neck of the aneurysm to restore more normal left ventricular geometry. Contemporaneously, Cooley[74] and Dor[92] described an almost identical procedure which involves placement of a patch within the ventricle at the border zone between the scar and contractile portion of the ventricle so that the nonfunctioning portion of the ventricle is excluded. This procedure restores more normal ventricular geometry, can improve ventricular systolic function, and may reverse the unfavorable process of remodeling.

As experience increased with surgical removal of dyskinetic areas of scar, interest developed in extending these surgical concepts to large areas of akinetic scar,

which are invariably associated with depressed function of the contractile area of the left ventricle. Application of EVCPP to akinetic scar was initially impeded by the notion that resection of akinetic areas of infarcted muscle is associated with a higher operative mortality and a lower likelihood of improvement in left ventricular function compared to patients with dyskinesis. However, EVCPP has been applied by Dor and colleagues[94] to akinetic left ventricular scar, akinesia and dyskinesia being regarded as part of the same pathological process of scar formation after acute myocardial infarction and associated with the same consequences with regard to remodeling of the residual ventricular muscle.[76, 179]

EVCPP requires the usual methods of cardiopulmonary bypass and can be performed with or without cardioplegia (at the University of Alabama at Birmingham [UAB] the procedure is performed on the beating heart). In the case of anteroseptoapical scars with akinesis or dyskinesis, the scar is opened, mural thrombi removed, and a pursestring suture is placed around the base of the aneurysm at the junction of scar and the contractile portion of the ventricle (Fig. 5–19).[91, 118] This suture creates a neck when tightened down, and the degree to which it is tightened is determined by a visual assessment of the size of the ventricular chamber. A Dacron patch is then fashioned to the size of the opening in the ventricle, and the patch is then sutured to the "neck" at the level of the circumferential pursestring suture (Fig. 5–20) excluding the nonfunctional apical portion of the septum (Fig. 5–21).[92] The ventriculotomy is usually closed with a simple running suture,[73] although an alternative method involves application of resorcin formol glue to the suture line and suturing of the edges of the excluded scar to the patch for hemostasis.[91] At this stage, cardioplegia is administered (if the EVCPP has been performed on the beating heart) and ancillary procedures such as coronary bypass surgery or mitral valve surgery performed. For posteroinferior left ventricular areas of transmural scar, the procedure is similar but the patch to repair the defect has a triangular shape, the base of the triangle being sutured to the posterior mitral annulus. If mitral valve replacement is required, this can be performed through a transventricular approach. If ventricular tachycardia is associated with a left ventricular aneurysm, then cryoablation of the border zone is performed in association with EVCPP.[95]

After EVCPP for an anterior aneurysm, salutary effects are seen on ventricular shape, regional wall motion, and hemodynamics.[224] Prior to EVCPP, regional left ventricular wall curvature (the reciprocal of the radius of the circle that best fits the region of interest) is quite abnormal, particularly in the anterobasal and inferoapical regions corresponding to the contractile wall adjacent to the aneurysms. After EVCPP, the inward curvature of the inferoapical border is replaced by a more normal outward curvature both in systole and in diastole.[93] End-diastolic and end-systolic left ventricular volumes are reduced. Global ejection fraction is increased, and this is largely accounted for by improved systolic shortening of the inferior wall.[93] The restoration of a more normal geometry after EVCPP is associated with improved regional myocardial performance of the left

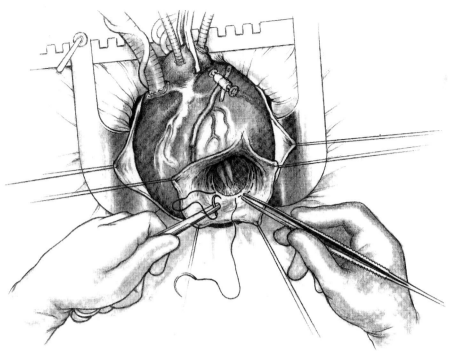

FIGURE **5-19.** The initial step in reconstruction of the left ventricle is the placement of a circumferential pursestring suture around the entire base of the aneurysm at the junction of endocardial scar and normal myocardium. When tied down at the proper tension, this suture restores the normal orientation of the uninvolved muscle fibers of the ventricle exclusive of the aneurysm. (From Dor V: Left ventricular aneurysms: the endoventricular circular patch plasty. Semin Thorac Cardiovasc Surg 1997;9:123, with permission.)

ventricular wall remote from the anterior wall of the aneurysm, and these areas of abnormal geometry are potentially areas of high local wall stress.[224] In fact, preoperatively abnormal left ventricular wall geometry may be a prerequisite for improvement in regional wall

motion after EVCPP.[85] Di Donato and colleagues reported similar hemodynamic improvement in patients with large akinetic scars as in those with dyskinesis.[85]

Survival after EVCPP in the Dor series[84] is indicated in Figure 5–22. The cause of in-hospital death in all cases was low cardiac output, and late deaths were from heart failure or sudden death. There was a substantial im-

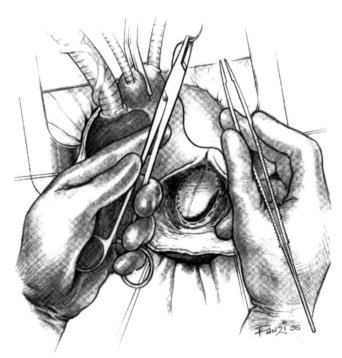

FIGURE **5-20.** The endocardial patch is anchored at the level of the circumferential pursestring suture to complete the closure of the left ventricle.

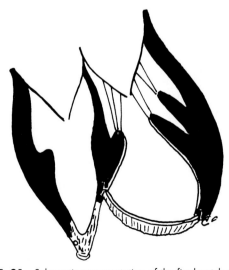

FIGURE **5-21.** Schematic representation of the final patch placement at the level of the junction between scar and contractile portion of the ventricle, excluding the nonfunctional apical septum. (From Dor V, Sabatier M, Di Donato M, Montiglio F, Toso A, Maioli M: Efficacy of endoventricular patch plasty in large postinfarction akinetic scar and severe left ventricular dysfunction: comparison with a series of large dyskinetic scars. J Thorac Cardiovasc Surg 1998;116:50–59, with permission.)

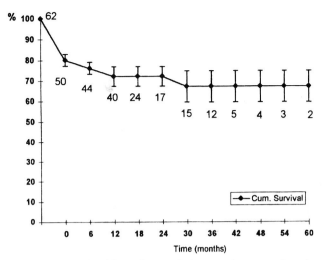

FIGURE **5–22.** Life table analysis, including operative mortality, after aneurysmectomy with patch repair in patients with postinfarction left ventricular aneurysm and severely depressed pump function. Numbers superimposed on graph indicate number of patients available at the beginning of the interval. Cum, cumulative. (From Di Donato M, Sabatier M, Montiglio F, Maioli M, Toso A, Fantini F, Dor V: Outcome of left ventricular aneurysmectomy with patch repair in patients with severely depressed pump function. Am J Cardiol 1995;76:557.)

provement in NYHA class. The survival curves of two groups of patients undergoing EVCPP, one with akinetic scar and one with dyskinetic scar, is presented in Figure 5–23.[94] However, it should be mentioned that although it has been reported that survival in patients undergoing EVCPP for large akinetic scars is no different from that of patients undergoing the procedure of dyskinetic scars based on Figure 5–23 where a global *p* value was said to be "not significant,"[92] visual inspection of the survival curves does suggest that with increasing time from operation there is an evident difference, with the long-term survival of patients with akinetic scars having inferior survival, with a 5-year survival of less than 50% in that report.

The current indications for EVCPP are primarily for patients with large dyskinetic or akinetic scars with good function of the contractile portion of the ventricle and heart failure, angina, or ventricular arrhythmias. A more controversial indication is extension of EVCPP to pa-

tients who are either asymptomatic or minimally symptomatic and who have akinetic or dyskinetic scars with good function of the contractile portion, since performance of this procedure may have significant long-term hemodynamic benefits in preventing remodeling and subsequent deterioration of function of the contractile regions. Even more controversial is the extension of this procedure to patients with severe heart failure, large akinetic scars, and poor function of the contractile regions, a situation where cardiac transplantation is frequently considered. Although it has been claimed[94] that survival of these patients is similar to that of patients undergoing this procedure for more traditional indications, the late survival of these patients may not prove to be as good. There are unanswered questions regarding the longer term outcome in such patients with akinetic scars and whether this procedure will reverse the unfavorable remodeling of the contractile portion of the ventricle. However, the procedure in this setting may find a place as perhaps a bridge to cardiac transplantation, and patients with large ventricular akinetic scars should at least be considered for EVCPP before a decision is made to proceed with cardiac transplantation.

Partial Left Ventricular Resection

PLVR arose from the efforts of Dr. Randas Batista[17] in the unlikely setting of a provincial hospital in Brazil as an alternative procedure for patients with medically refractory heart failure and dilated ventricles for whom no other option (particularly cardiac transplantation) was available. In contrast to EVCPP, which resects nonviable myocardium in an area of myocardial infarction, the PLVR procedure involves resection of viable myocardium, usually in patients with nonischemic dilated cardiomyopathy. The operation (and to some extent the surgeon) appeared on the surgical scene as a phenomenon that had unusual appeal, and the operation was uncharacteristically embraced by many surgeons without the rigorous follow-up that is usually necessary. The purpose of the operation was to restore the volume/mass ratio toward normal and hence reduce left ventricular volume, reduce left ventricular wall stress, improve systolic function, and ameliorate the symptoms of heart

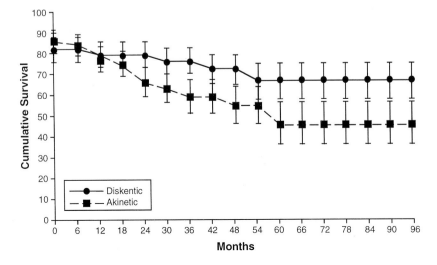

FIGURE **5–23.** Life table analysis of survival after EVCPP stratified into those patients with a dyskinetic scar and those with an akinetic scar. Although the Wilcoxon statistic indicated that there was not a significant difference between the two groups, visual inspection and the nonoverlapping measures of uncertainty do suggest that with increasing time there is inferior survival in the akinetic group. (From Dor V, Sabatier M, Di Donato M, Montiglio F, Toso A, Maioli M: Efficacy of endoventricular patch plasty in large postinfarction akinetic scar and severe left ventricular dysfunction: comparison with a series of large dyskinetic scars. J Thorac Cardiovasc Surg 1998;116:50–59.)

failure. The optimal left ventricular diameter (and therefore the extent of resection) following the procedure is based on assumptions from the law of Laplace (see previous discussion).

The operation is performed using cardiopulmonary bypass on either the beating heart or with the usual methods of myocardial preservation, and left ventricular volume is reduced by removing a slice of posterolateral wall between the anterolateral and posteromedial papillary muscles. The circumference of left ventricular muscle that is removed is determined by the known relationship between circumference and diameter, such that approximately for every 3 cm of left ventricular circumference that is removed, left ventricular end-diastolic dimension is reduced by approximately 1 cm (Fig. 5–24).[190] Mitral regurgitation is corrected through either an annuloplasty or mitral valve replacement and the ventriculotomy is closed. A number of hemodynamic benefits have been reported to occur after PLVR, including reduction in end-diastolic and end-systolic left ventricular volume,[150, 184, 223] increase in ejection fraction,[190] increase in cardiac index,[190] and increase in stroke volume.[225] The hemodynamic benefits (or detriments) are likely to be considerably more complicated than a simple laplacian reduction in wall stress. Mathematical models have been used to determine explanations for these hemodynamic benefits, and perhaps not surprisingly these models have confirmed the heterogeneous nature of the clinical changes. Pressure volume and stress strain analyses[89] predicted an improvement in ejection fraction, systolic elastance, and preload recruitable stroke work and decrease in left ventricular wall stress. However, these benefits were due to the geometric changes, and the Frank-Starling relationship predicted depression of pump function. A finite element model[234] predicted a mixed effect on ventricular function with an increase in the slope of preload recruitable stroke work, but a decrease in diastolic compliance causing a small decrease in the Starling relationship. Another model suggested that the residual wall stress/strain state of the myocardium (the persistence of residual strain and stress in the zero pressure situation) may be an important component of the pathophysiology of ventricular dilatation, and the model predicted that PLVR may establish more favorable diastolic filling conditions.[161]

When the spectacular anecdotes were replaced by rigorous examination of the results of the procedure, the findings were disappointing.[164] The result of Dowling and colleagues[97] indicated that the 12-month freedom from death or the need for relisting for cardiac transplantation was only 56%, which is similar to the findings of Stolf and colleagues,[250] most of the deaths being due to heart failure or sudden death. These findings are supported by the extensive experience and analysis of McCarthy and colleagues from the Cleveland Clinic (McCarthy P, Meeting of the American Association of Thoracic Surgeons, May 2000). Thus, survival after this procedure is clearly inferior to cardiac transplantation (see Chapter 18), and it may even be inferior to that of medical treatment for dilated cardiomyopathy. Therefore, this procedure would only seem appropriate in countries where no option exists for cardiac transplantation.

Mitral Reconstruction in Cardiomyopathy

The notion of mitral valve repair for severe mitral regurgitation in patients with dilated cardiomyopathy or isch-

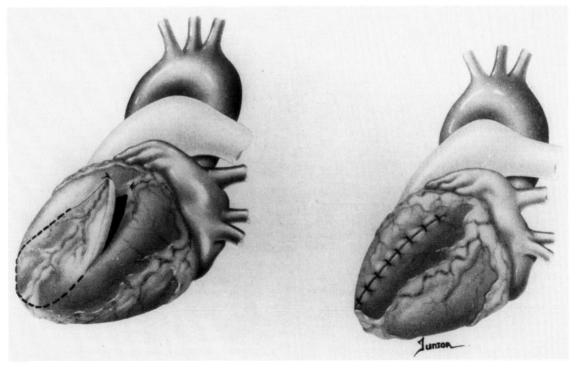

FIGURE **5–24.** Schematic representation of partial left ventriculectomy. (From Moreira LFP, Stolf NAG, Bocchi EA, Bacal F, Giorgi MCP, Parga JR, Jatene AD: Partial left ventriculectomy with mitral valve preservation in the treatment of patients with dilated cardiomyopathy. J Thorac Cardiovasc Surg 1998;115:800, with permission.)

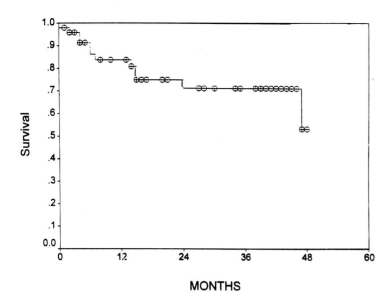

FIGURE **5–25.** Kaplan-Meier depiction of survival after mitral valve reconstruction for patients with cardiomyopathy. (From Bolling SF, Pagani FD, Deeb GM, Bach DS: Intermediate-term outcome of mitral reconstruction in cardiomyopathy. J Thorac Cardiovasc Surg 1998;115:381.)

emic cardiomyopathy is, at first glance counterintuitive. In patients undergoing mitral valve replacement for mitral valve disease with left ventricular dysfunction, left ventricular function is invariably initially worse after the operation and constitutes an important risk factor for mitral valve replacement. However, the initial experience with mitral valve repair for secondary mitral regurgitation due to a dilated cardiomyopathy appears to result in symptomatic and hemodynamic benefits, and this approach should probably be considered as a ventricular restoration procedure, which returns the quite abnormal left ventricular mass/volume ratio toward normal. The mechanism of secondary mitral regurgitation in dilated cardiomyopathy is related to dilatation of the mitral annulus[29] and alterations in ventricular geometry.[158] Mitral regurgitation in ischemic cardiomyopathy, like dilated cardiomyopathy, has a component of dilatation of the mitral annulus, but there is an additional component of discoordination of the subvalvar apparatus (which includes the chordae, papillary muscles, and the left ventricular wall from which they arise) and is more complex than simple papillary muscle dysfunction.[151] This is a self-perpetuating process progressively increasing the volume load on an already dilated and poorly functioning ventricle. The survival of patients with dilated cardiomyopathy and heart failure who develop mitral regurgitation is known to be poor.[26, 145, 249]

The study by Bolling and colleagues[28] is really the seminal study of this approach and involved mitral valve repair in 48 patients with advanced dilated cardiomyopathy, severe left ventricular dysfunction (left ventricular ejection fraction ranging from 0.08–0.25), severe mitral regurgitation, and NYHA Class III or IV congestive heart failure. All patients underwent a flexible mitral ring annuloplasty, and the important postoperative findings were significant improvements in heart failure symptoms and left ventricular ejection fraction, reduced left ventricular end-diastolic and end-systolic volumes, and marked reduction in sphericity of the left ventricle. The actuarial survival (Fig. 5–25) appears to be superior

TABLE 5-20	Summary of Approach to Heart Failure Therapeutics

1. Make appropriate diagnosis
- Dyspnea, edema, and rales are not always congestive heart failure

2. Stage syndrome severity
- Discover asymptomatic left ventricular systolic dysfunction
- Heart failure does not always mean congestive heart failure
- Therapeutics of heart failure varies with severity of syndrome

3. Treat underlying diseases
- Address etiology of heart failure syndrome
- Eliminate exacerbating factors

4. Stop potentially harmful drugs or those of unproved benefit
- Antiarrhythmic agents (particularly Vaughn Williams Class I drugs)
- Calcium channel blockers
- Nonsteroidal anti-inflammatory agents
- Tricyclic antidepressants
- Nasal decongestants/antihistamines
- Beta blockers on occasion
- Anticoagulants (?)

5. Begin therapeutic regimens with proven efficacy
- Drugs to prevent functional deterioration
  ACE inhibitors
  Beta blockers
- Drugs to reduce mortality
  ACE inhibitors
  Beta blockers
  Hydralazine/isosorbide dinitrate
  Spironolactone

6. Drugs to controls symptoms
- Diuretics
- Digoxin
- ACE inhibitors
- Hydralazine/isosorbide dinitrate

7. Prescribe rational polypharmacy
- Aim for fewest side effects possible
- Program designed to ensure compliance
- Consider cost of drugs employed

8. Consider surgical options
- Coronary revascularization
- Valve repair/replacement
- Ventricular remodeling procedures

9. Encourage regular aerobic exercise activity
- "You can do what you can do but can't do what you can't"
- Avoid sedentary lifestyle

to that of the natural history of the disease process and informal comparison of mitral reconstruction in this condition with the results of cardiac transplantation would suggest that the results are similar (at least over the first 3 years). At least some of the late deaths in this series have resulted from heart failure and sudden death, suggesting that in some patients the disordered structure and function of the heart may have progressed. The mechanism of the efficacy of this procedure has been hypothesized to be in part due to restoration of the mass/volume relationship of the left ventricle more toward normal.[28] Bolling and colleagues have also suggested that placing an undersized mitral annuloplasty ring reestablishes an ellipsoid shape to the base of the left ventricular cavity.[28] Similar results have also been reported by McCarthy and colleagues.[183] The role of this

procedure is yet to be established and it may eventually find a place either as an intermediate procedure to delay the need for transplantation or as an alternative procedure in patients for whom cardiac transplantation is contraindicated.

SUMMARY OF HEART FAILURE THERAPEUTICS

Tailored therapeutic protocols in heart failure are based on the progression of a patient's heart failure syndrome from insidious to symptomatic to advanced or refractory settings (Table 5–20 and Fig. 5–26). The most appropriate strategies incorporate the philosophy of "preven-

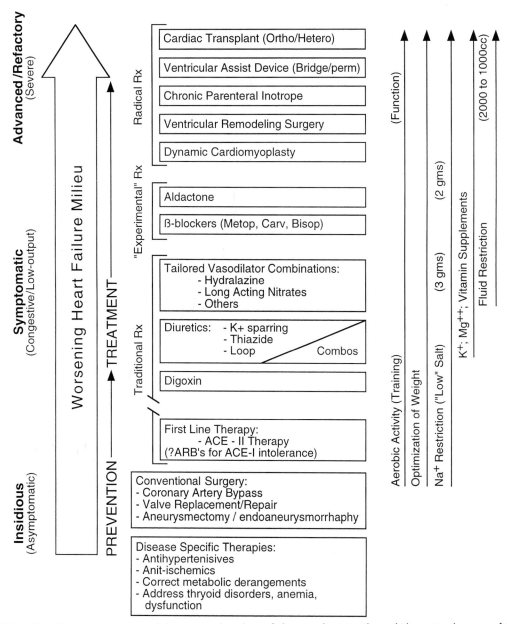

FIGURE **5–26.** Schematic summary of the approach to heart failure emphasizing the multidimensional nature of lifestyle modification, primary disease treatment, pharmacologic management, and surgical therapies.

tion" maneuvers as well as "treatment" strategies. Also important is the coupling of efforts to address underlying diseases with medication prescriptions or surgical interventions that are appropriate and lifestyle changes including increased aerobic activity; optimization of weight status; modification of diet, sodium, fluid and alcohol consumption; and appropriate vitamin and electrolyte supplementation. Making an appropriate diagnosis is of paramount importance as is staging the heart failure syndrome severity. Knowing the stage of heart failure for any specific patient will dictate the aggressiveness of therapeutic protocols. Drugs with potentially detrimental effects or unproven benefit should be considered for discontinuation. It is important early in the disease course to begin appropriate therapeutic protocols demonstrated to prevent functional deterioration, reduce mortality, and control symptoms if necessary. Underlying this practice is the principal of "rational polypharmacy." Because patients are often on multiple drugs and drug combinations, the clinician must review carefully appropriateness of any prescription in order to simplify the overall regimen whenever possible. Drugs, furthermore, should be dispensed in such a fashion that the fewest side effects appear, helping ensure patient compliance. Finally, chronic bed rest is no longer an important component of heart failure therapy. Medications used today have largely supplanted archaic bed rest prescriptions. We now know it is quite important that all patients, except those with the most severe end stages of heart failure, attempt to exercise aerobically. Indeed, patients with heart failure should be referred to supervised cardiac rehabilitation programs if at all possible to become schooled in aerobic training practices.

Included in the current armamentarium of heart failure therapy are a number of surgical options for improving coronary perfusion, treating valvular insufficiency, and reducing ventricular volume. Assessment of the potential risks and long-term benefits of these procedures for the individual patient is a vital component of tailored therapy.

The treatment of patients with heart failure is, then, no longer simply the prescription of diuretics and digoxin to a dropsical individual. Confirmation of the diagnosis is essential, staging the syndrome is mandatory, and consideration of the wide spectrum of available options, including both pharmacologic and surgical therapies, is necessary if optimal outcome is to be expected. If the principles and tactics delineated in this chapter are followed, it is likely that many patients with heart failure will experience substantial improvements in symptomatology and prognosis. Only after more standard aggressive strategies are pursued, and have been demonstrated to be inadequate, should candidacy for cardiac transplantation be considered.

References

1. Acker M, Anderson WA, Hammond RL, DiMeo F, McCullum J, Statum M, Velchik M, Brown WE, Gale D, Salmons S, Stephenson LW: Oxygen consumption of chronically stimulated skeletal muscle. J Thorac Cardiovasc Surg 1987;94:702.

2. Adams KF, Gheorghiade M, Uretsky BF, Patterson JH, Schwartz TA, Young JB: Clinical benefits of low serum digoxin concentrations in heart failure [abstract]. J Am Coll Cardiol 1999;33:185A.

3. Adams KF Jr, Baughman KL, Dec WG: Heart Failure Society of America: Guidelines for management of patients with heart failure caused by left ventricular systolic dysfunction-pharmacological approaches. J Card Fail 1999;5:357–382.

4. Adams KF Jr, Gheorghiade M, Uretsky BF, Young JB, Ahmed S, Tomasko L, Packer M: Patients with mild heart failure worsen during withdrawal from digoxin therapy. J Am Coll Cardiol 1997;30:42–48.

5. Afridi I, Kleiman NS, Raizner AE, Zoghbi WA: Dobutamine echocardiography in myocardial hibernation. Optimal dose in predicting recovery of left ventricular function after coronary angioplasty. Circulation 1995;91:663.

6. Agency for Healthcare Policy and Research: Heart failure guideline panel. Heart failure: evaluation and care of patients with left ventricular systolic dysfunction. Rockville, MD: US Dept of Health and Human Services, 1994. Clinical Practice Guideline 11. AHCPR Publication 94–0612.

7. Al-Khadra AS, Salem DN, Rand WM, Udelson JE, Smith JJ, Konstam MA: Warfarin anticoagulation and survival: a cohort analysis from the Studies of Left Ventricular Dysfunction (SOLVD). J Am Coll Cardiol 1998;31:749–753.

8. Al-Khadra AS, Salem DN, Rand WM, Udelson JE, Smith JJ, Konstam MA: Antiplatelet agents and survival: a cohort analysis from the Studies of Left Ventricular Dysfunction (SOLVD) trial. J Am Coll Cardiol 1998;31:419–425.

9. Alderman EL, Fisher LD, Litwin P, Kaiser GC, Myers WO, Maynard C, Levine F, Schloss M: Results of coronary artery surgery in patients with poor left ventricular function (CASS). Circulation 1983;68:785.

10. American College of Cardiology/American Heart Association Task Force on Practice Guidelines: Guidelines for the evaluation and management of heart failure. Circulation 1995;92:2267–2784.

11. Amiodarone Trials Meta-Analysis Investigators: Effect of prophylactic amiodarone on mortality after acute myocardial infarction and in congestive heart failure: meta analysis of individual data from 6,500 patients in randomised trials. Lancet 1997;350:1417–1424.

12. Antman EM, Kelly RA: Pharmacological therapy of cardiac arrhythmias. In Antman EM, Ruitherford JD (eds): Coronary Care Medicine: A Practical Approach. Norwell, MA: Kluwer Academic Press, 1996.

13. Ausma J, Furst D, Thoné F, Shivalkar B, Flameng W, Weber K, Ramaekers F, Borgers M: Molecular changes of titin in left ventricular dysfunction as a result of chronic hibernation. J Mol Cell Cardiol 1995;27:1203.

14. AVID Investigators: A comparison of antiarrhythmic drug therapy with implantable defibrillators in patients resuscitated from near-fatal ventricular arrhythmias. N Engl J Med 1997;337:1576–1583.

15. Baker DW, Wright RF: Management of heart failure IV. Anticoagulation for patients with heart failure due to left ventricular systolic dysfunction. JAMA 1994;272:1614–1618.

16. Bart BA, Ertl G, Held P, Maggioni AP, McMurray J, Michelson EL, Rouleau JL, Stevenson LW, Swedberg K, Young JB, Yusuf S, Sellers MA, Granger CB, Califf RM, Pfeffer MA, SPICE Investigators: Contemporary management of patients with left ventricular dysfunction. Results from the Study of Patients Intolerant of Converting Enzyme Inhibitors (SPICE) Registry. Eur Heart J 1999;20:1182–1190.

17. Batista RJV, Santos JLV, Takeshita N, Bocchino L, Lima PN, Cunha MA: Partial left ventriculectomy to improve left ventricular function in end-stage heart disease. J Card Surg 1996;11:96.

18. Bauer JA, Fung HL: Concurrent hydralazine administration prevents nitroglycerin-induced hemodynamic tolerance in experimental heart failure. Circulation 1991;84:35–39.

19. Beck CS: The development of a new blood supply to the heart by operation. Ann Surg 1935;102:801.

20. BHAT: A randomized trial of propranolol in patients with acute myocardial infarction I. Mortality results. JAMA 1982;247:1707–1714.

21. Bigger JT Jr, Fleiss JL, Rolnitzsky LM, Merab JP, Ferrick KJ: Effect of digitalis treatment on survival after acute myocardial infarction. Am J Cardiol 1985;55:623–630.

22. Billeter R, Weber H, Lutz L, Howald H, Eppenberger HM, Jenny E: Myosin types in human skeletal muscle fibers. Histochemistry 1980;65:249.

23. Billups SJ, Carter BL: Mibefradil withdrawn from the market [letter]. Ann Pharmacother 1998;32:841.

24. Binkley PF, Haas GJ, Starling RC, Nunziata E, Hatton PA, Leier CV, Cody RJ: Sustained augmentation of parasympathetic tone with angiotensin converting enzyme inhibition in patients with congestive heart failure. J Am Coll Cardiol 1993;21:655.

25. Block M, Breithardt G: The implantable cardioverter defibrillator and primary prevention of sudden death: the Multi-center Automatic Defibrillator Implantation Trial (MADIT) and the Coronary Artery Bypass Graft Patch (CABG-Patch) Trial. Am J Cardiol 1999;83:7478.

26. Blondheim DS, Jacobs LE, Kotler MN, Costacurta GA, Parry WR: Dilated cardiomyopathy with mitral regurgitation: decreased survival despite a low frequency of left ventricular thrombus. Am Heart J 1991;112(3 pt 1):763.

27. Bolli R: Mechanism of myocardial "stunning." Circulation 1990;82:723.

28. Bolling SF, Pagani FD, Deeb GM, Bach DS: Intermediate-term outcome of mitral reconstruction in cardiomyopathy. J Thorac Cardiovasc Surg 1998;115:381.

29. Boltwood CM, Tei C, Wong M, Shah PM: Quantitative echocardiography of the mitral complex in dilated cardiomyopathy: the mechanism of functional mitral regurgitation. Circulation 1983;68:498.

30. Bonow RO: Indentification of viable myocardium. Circulation 1996;94:2674.

31. Bourge RC, Young JB, Kirklin JK, McGiffin DC: Dynamic cardiomyoplasty: patient selection considerations as applied in the C-SMART study to reduce hospital mortality [abstract]. Basic Appl Myol 2000;10:59.

32. Brater DC: Diuretic therapy. N Engl J Med 1998;339:387–395.

33. Brater DC, Chennavasin P, Sweiwell R: Furosemide in patients with heart failure: shift in dose-response curves. Clin Pharmacol Ther 1980;28:182–186.

34. Braunwald E, Kloner RA: The stunned myocardium: prolonged, postischemic ventricular dysfunction. Circulation 1982;66:1146.

35. Braunwald E, Rutherford JD: Reversible ischemic left ventricular dysfunction: evidence for the "hibernating myocardium." J Am Coll Cardiol 1986;8:1467.

36. Bridges CR Jr, Stephenson LW: Skeletal muscle-powered cardiac assist devices. In Chiu R, Bourgeois J (eds): Transformed Muscle for Cardiac Assist and Repair. Mount Kisco, NY: Futura Publishing Company, Inc, 1990.

37. Bristow MR, Gilbert EM, Abraham WT, Robertson AD: Carvedilol produces dose-related improvements in left ventricular function and survival in subjects with chronic heart failure. MOCHA Investigators. Circulation 1996;94:2807–2816. Comment in: Circulation 1996;94:2793–2799, 2800-2806, 2807–2816; Circulation 1997; 96:2743–2744.

38. Brown MD, Cotter MA, Hudlická O, Vrbová G: The effects of different patterns of muscle activity on capillary density, mechanical properties and structure of slow and fast rabbit muscles. Pflugers Arch 1976;361:241.

39. Brown WE, Salmons S, Whalen RG: The sequential replacement of myosin subunit isoforms during muscle type transformation induced by long-term electrical stimulation. J Biol Chem 1983; 258:14686.

40. Burton NA, Stinson EB, Oyer PE, Shumway NE: Left ventricular aneurysm. J Thorac Cardiovasc Surg 1979;77:65–75.

41. Cairns JA, Connolly SJ, Robert R, Gent M: Randomized trial of outcome after myocardial infarction in patients with frequent or repetitive ventricular premature depolarisations: CAMIAT. Canadian Amiodarone Myocardial Infarction Arrhythmia Trial Investigators [published erratum appears in Lancet 1997; 349:1776]. Lancet 1997;349:675–682. Comment in: Lancet 1997; 349:662-663. Comment in: Lancet 1997;349:1767. Comment in ACP J Club 1997;127:30–31.

42. Califf RM, Adams K, McKenna WJ, Gheorgiade M, Uretsky BF, McNulty SE, Darius H, Schulman K, Zannad F, Handberg-Thurkmond E, Harrell FE Jr, Wheeler W, Soler-Soler J, Swedberg K: A randomized controlled trial of epoprostenol therapy for

severe congestive heart failure: the Flolan International Randomized Survival Trial (FIRST). Am Heart J 1997;134:44–54.

43. Capouya ER, Gerber RS, Drinkwater DC, Pearl JM, Sack JB, Aharon AS, Barthel SW, Kaczer EM, Chang PA, Laks H: Girdling effect of nonstimulated cardiomyoplasty on left ventricular function. Ann Thorac Surg 1993;56:867.

44. Cappato R: Secondary prevention of sudden death: the Dutch Study, the Antiarrhythmics Versus Implantable Defibrillator Trial, the Cardiac Arrest Study Hamburg, and the Canadian Implantable Defibrillator Study [review]. Am J Cardiol 1999; 83:68D-73D.

45. Carlson EB, Cowley MJ, Wolfgang TC, Vetrovec GW: Acute changes in global and regional rest left ventricular function after successful coronary angioplasty: comparative results in stable and unstable angina. J Am Coll Cardiol 1989;13:1262.

46. Carpentier A, Chachques JC: Myocardial substitution with a stimulated skeletal muscle: first successful clinical case. Lancet 1985;8440:1267.

47. Carpentier A, Chachques JC: Cardiomyoplasty: surgical technique. In Carpentier A, Chachques JC, Grandjean P (eds): Cardiomyoplasty. Mount Kisco, NY: Futura Publishing Company, 1991.

48. Carpentier A, Chachques JC, Acar C, Relland J, Mihaileanu S, Bensasson D, Kieffer JP, Guilbour P, Tournay D, Roussin I, Grandjean PA: Dynamic cardiomyoplasty at seven years. J Thorac Cardiovasc Surg 1993;106:42.

49. CASS principal investigators and their associates: Coronary artery surgery study (CASS): a randomized trial of coronary artery bypass surgery. Circulation 1983;68:939.

50. Castro PF, Bourge RC, Foster RE: Evaluation of hibernating myocardium in patients with ischemic heart disease. Am J Med 1998; 104:69.

51. Chachques JC, Grandjean PA, Pfeffer TA, Perier P, Dreyfus G, Jebara V, Acar C, Levy M, Bourgeois I, Fabiani JN, Deloche A, Carpentier A: Cardiac assistance by atrial or ventricular cardiomyoplasty. J Heart Transplant 1990;9:239.

52. Chachques JC, Grandjean PA, Schwartz K, Mihaileanu S, Fardeau M, Swynghedauw B, Fontaliran F, Romero N, Wisnewsky C, Perier P, Chauvaud S, Bourgeois I, Carpentier A: Effect of latissimus dorsi dynamic cardiomyoplasty on ventricular function. Circulation 1988;78(suppl III):III-203.

53. Chatterjee K, Parmley WW, Massie B, Greenberg B, Werner J, Klausner S, Norman A: Oral hydralazine therapy for chronic refractory heart failure. Circulation 1976;54:879–883.

54. Chatterjee K, Swan HJC, Parmley WW, Sustaita H, Marcus HS, Matloff J: Influence of direct myocardial revascularization on left ventricular asynergy and function in patients with coronary heart disease with and without previous myocardial infarction. Circulation 1973;47:276.

55. Chekanov VS, Chachques JC, Carraro U, Chi RCJ, Stephenson LW: Novel functions (work-rest and day-night regimens) in a new cardiomyostimulator for cardiac bioassist. Basic Appl Myol 2000;10:39–48.

56. Chen FY, DeGuzman BJ, Aklog L, Lautz DB, Ahmad RM, Laurence RG, Couper GS, Cohn LH, McMahon TA: Decreased myocardial oxygen consumption indices in dynamic cardiomyoplasty. Circulation 1996;94(suppl):239.

57. Chiu RCJ, Odim JNK, Burgess JH, and the McGill Cardiomyoplasty Group: Responses to dynamic cardiomyoplasty for idiopathic dilated cardiomyopathy. Am J Cardiol 1993;72:475.

58. Christ JE, Spira M: Application of latissimus dorsi muscle to the heart. Ann Plast Surg 1982;8:118.

59. Ciaccherie M, Castelli G, Cecchi F, Nannini M, Santoro G, Troiani V, Zuppiroli A, Dolara A: Lack of correlation between intracavitary thrombosis detected by cross-sectional echocardiography and systemic emboli in patients with dilated cardiomyopathy. Br Heart J 1989;62:26–29.

60. CIBIS Investigators: A randomized trial of beta-blockade in heart failure: the Cardiac Insufficiency Bisoprolol Study (CIBIS). Circulation 1994;90:1765–1773.

61. CIBIS Investigators: The Cardiac Insufficiency Bisoprolol Study (CIBIS-II): a randomized trial. Lancet 1999;353:9–13.

62. Cioffi G, Pozzoli M, Forni G, Franchini M, Opasich C, Cobelli F, Tavazzi L, Rossi D: Systemic thromboembolism in chronic heart failure. A prospective study in 406 patients. Eur Heart J 1996; 17:1381–1389.

63. Cody RJ, Kubo SH, Pickworth KK: Diuretic treatment for the sodium retention of congestive heart failure [review]. Arch Intern Med 1994;154:1905–1914.

64. Cohen M, Charney R, Hershman R, Fuster V, Gorlin R, Francis X: Reversal of chronic ischemic myocardial dysfunction after transluminal coronary angioplasty. J Am Coll Cardiol 1988; 12:1193.

65. Cohn JN: Comparative cardiovascular effects of tyramine, ephedrine, and norepinephrine in man. Circ Res 1965;16:174.

66. Cohn JN, Archibald DG, Ziesche S, Franciosa JA, Harston WE, Tristani FE, Dunkman WB, Jacobs W, Francis GS, Flohr KH, Goldman S, Cobb FR, Shah PM, Saunders R, Fletcher RD, Loeb HS, Hughes VC, Baker B: Effect of vasodilator therapy on mortality in chronic congestive heart failure. Results of a Veterans Administration Cooperative Study. N Engl J Med 1986;314:1547–1552.

67. Cohn JN, Fowler MB, Bristow MR, Colucci WS, Gilbert EM, Kinhal V, Krueger SK, Lejemtel T, Narahara KA, Packer M, Young ST, Holcslaw TL, Lukas MA: Safety and efficacy of carvedilol in severe heart failure. The U.S. Carvedilol Heart Failure Study Group. J Card Fail 1997;3:173–179.

68. Cohn JN, Goldstein SO, Greenberg BH, Lorell BH, Bourge RC, Jaski BE, Gottlieb SO, McGrew F, DeMets DL, White BG: A dose-dependent increase in mortality with vesnarinone among patients with severe heart failure. Vesnarinone Trial Investigators. N Engl J Med, 1998;339:1810–1816. Comment in: N Engl J Med 1998;339:1848–1850. Comment in: N Engl J Med 1999; 340:1511; discussion 1512.

69. Cohn JN, Johnson G, Ziesche S, Cobb F, Francis G, Tristani F, Smith R, Dunkman WB, Loeb H, Wong M, Bhat G, Goldman S, Fletcher RD, Doherty J, Hughes CV, Carson P, Cintron G, Shabetai R, Haakenson C: A comparison of enalapril with hydralazine-isosorbide dinitrate in the treatment of chronic congestive heart failure. N Engl J Med 1991;325:303–310. Comment in: N Engl J Med 1991;1;325:351–353.

70. Cohn JN, Ziesche S, Smith R, Anand I, Dunkman WB, Loeb H, Cintron G, Boden W, Baruch L, Rochin P, Loss L: Effect of the calcium antagonist felodipine as supplementary vasodilator therapy in patients with chronic heart failure treated with enalapril: V-HeFT III. Vasodilator-Heart Failure Trial (V-HeFT) Study Group. Circulation 1997;96:856–863.

71. Colucci WS, Packer M, Bristow MR, Gilbert EM, Cohn JN, Fowler MB, Kruegger SK, Hershberger R, Uretsky BF, Bowers JA, Sackner-Bernstein JD, Young ST, Holcslaw TL, Lukas MA, for the US Carvedilol Herat Failure Study Group: Carvedilol inhibits clinical progression in patients with mild symptoms of heart failure. Circulation 1996;94:2800–2806.

72. CONSENSUS Trial Study Group: Effects of enalapril on mortality and severe congestive heart failure: results of the Cooperative North Scandinavian Enalapril Study. N Engl J Med 1987;316: 1429–1435.

73. Cooley DA: Ventricular endoaneurysmorrhaphy: a simplified repair for extensive postinfarction aneurysm. J Card Surg 1989; 4:200.

74. Cooley DA: Ventricular endoaneurysmorrhaphy: results of an improved method of repair. Tex Heart Inst J 1989;16:72.

75. Cooley DA, Collins HA, Morris GC Jr, Chapman DW: Ventricular aneurysm after myocardial infarction: surgical excision with use of temporary cardiopulmonary bypass. JAMA 1958;167:557.

76. Couper GS, Bunton RW, Birjiniuk V, DiSesa VJ, Fallon MP, Collins JJ, Cohn LH: Relative risks of left ventricular aneurysmectomy in patients with akinetic scars versus true dyskinetic aneurysms. Circulation 1990;82(suppl IV):IV-248–IV-256.

77. Crow MT, Kushmerick MJ: Chemical energetics of slow- and fast-twitch muscles of the mouse. J Gen Physiol 1982;79:147.

78. Crozier I, Ikram H, Awan N, Cleland J, Stephen N, Dickstein K, Frey M, Young J, Klinger G, Makris L: Losartan in heart failure. Hemodynamic effects and tolerability. Losartan Hemodynamic Study Group. Circulation 1995;91:691–697.

79. Cuffe MS, Califf RM, Adams KF, Bourge RC, Colucci W, Massie B, O'Connor CM, Pina I, Quigg R, Silver M, Robinson LA, Leimberger JD, Gheorghiade M: Rationale and design of the OPTIME CHF trial: outcomes of a prospective intravenous milrinone for exacerbations of chronic heart failure. Am Heart J 2000;139:15–22.

80. deFeyter PJ, Suryapranata H, Serruys PW, Beatt K, Van Den Brand M, Hugenholtz PG: Effects of successful percutaneous transluminal coronary angioplasty on global and regional left ventricular function in unstable angina pectoris. Am J Cardiol 1987;60:993.

81. DeJesus FR: Breves consideraciones sobre un caso de herida penetrante del corazon. Bol Assoc Med P R 1931;23:380.

82. DeLahaye F, Jegaden O, Montagna P, Desseigne P, Blanc P, Vedrinne C, Touboul P, Saint-Pierre A, Perinetti M, Rossi R, Itti R, Mikaeloff P: Latissimus dorsi cardiomyoplasty in severe congestive heart failure: the Lyon experience. J Card Surg 1991;6:106.

83. Dewar ML, Drinkwater DC, Wittnich C, Chiu RC-J: Synchronously stimulated skeletal muscle graft for myocardial repair. J Thorac Cardiovasc Surg 1984;87:325.

84. Di Donato M, Sabatier M, Montiglio F, Maioli M, Toso A, Fantini F, Dor V: Outcome of left ventricular aneurysmectomy with patch repair in patients with severely depressed pump function. Am J Cardiol 1995;76:557.

85. Di Donato M, Sabatier M, Toso A, Barletta G, Baroni M, Dor V, Fantini F: Regional myocardial performance of non-ischaemic zones remote from anterior wall left ventricular aneurysm. Effects of aneurysmectomy. Eur Heart J 1995;16:1285.

86. DiCarli MF, Davidson M, Little R, Khanna S, Mody FV, Brunken RC, Czernin J, Rokhsar S, Stevenson LW, Laks H, Hawkins R, Schelbert HR, Phelps ME, Maddahi J: Value of metabolic imaging with positron emission tomography for evaluating prognosis in patients with coronary artery disease and left ventricular dysfunction. Am J Cardiol 1994;73:527.

87. DiCarli MF, Maddahi J, Rokhsar S, Schelbert HR, Bianco-Batlles D, Brunken RC, Fromm B: Long-term survival of patients with coronary artery disease and left ventricular dysfunction: implications for the role of myocardial viability assessment in management decisions. J Thorac Cardiovasc Surg 1998;116:997.

88. Dickstein K, Chang P, Willenheimer R, Haunso S, Remes J, Hall C, Kjekshus J: Comparison of the effects of losartan and enalapril on clinical status and exercise performance in patients with moderate or severe chronic heart failure. J Am Coll Cardiol 1995; 26:438–445.

89. Dickstein ML, Spotnitz HM, Rose EA, Burkhoff D: Heart reduction surgery: an analysis of the impact on cardiac function. J Thorac Cardiovasc Surg 1997;113:1032.

90. Digitalis Investigation Group: The effect of digoxin on mortality and morbidity in patients with heart failure. N Engl J Med 1997;336:525–533.

91. Dor V: Left ventricular aneurysms: the endoventricular circular patch plasty. Semin Thorac Cardiovasc Surg 1997;9:123.

92. Dor V, Saab M, Coste P, Kornaszewska M, Montiglio F: Left ventricular aneurysm: a new surgical approach. Thorac Cardiovasc Surg 1998;37:11.

93. Dor V, Montiglio F, Sabatier M, Coste P, Barletta G, DiDonato M, Toso A, Baroni M, Fantini F: Left ventricular shape changes induced by aneurysmectomy with endoventricular circular patch plasty reconstruction. Eur Heart J 1994;15:1063.

94. Dor V, Sabatier M, Di Donato M, Montiglio F, Toso A, Maioli M: Efficacy of endoventricular patch plasty in large postinfarction akinetic scar and severe left ventricular dysfunction: comparison with a series of large dyskinetic scars. J Thorac Cardiovasc Surg 1998;116:50–59.

95. Dor V, Sabatier M, Montiglio F, Rossi P, Toso A, Di Donato M: Results of nonguided subtotal endocardiectomy associated with left ventricular reconstruction in patients with ischemic ventricular arrhythmias. J Thorac Cardiovasc Surg 1994;107:1301.

96. Doval HC, Nul DR, Grencelli HO, Perrone SV, Bortman GR, Curiel R, for the GESICA Investigators: Randomized trial of low-dose amiodarone in severe congestive heart failure. Lancet 1994;344:493–498.

97. Dowling RD, Koeni S, Laureano MA, Cerrito P, Gray LA: Results of partial left ventriculectomy in patients with end-stage idiopathic dilated cardiomyopathy. J Heart Lung Transplant 1998; 17:1208.

98. Dries DL, Rosenberg YD, Waclawiw MA, Domanski MJ: Ejection fraction and risk of thromboembolic events in patients with systolic dysfunction and sinus rhythm: evidence for gender differences in the studies of left ventricular dysfunction trials [pub-

lished erratum appears in J Am Coll Cardiol 1998;32:555]. J Am Coll Cardiol 1997;29:1074–1080.

99. Dunkman WB: Thromboembolism and antithrombotic therapy in congestive heart failure. [review]. J Cardiovasc Risk 1995; 2:107–117.

100. Dunkman WB, Johnson GR, Carson PE, Bhat G, Farrell L, Cohn JN: Incidence of thromboembolic events in congestive heart failure. The V-HeFT VA Cooperative Studies Group. Circulation 1993;87(suppl VI):VI-94–VI-101.

101. Dzau VJ, Lilly LS, Swartz SL, Hollenberg NK, Williams GH: Prostaglandins in severe congestive heart failure: relation to activation of the renin-angiotensin system and hyponatremia. N Engl J Med 1984;310:347–352.

102. Echt DS, Liebson PR, Mitchell B, Peters RW, Obias-Manno D, Barker AH, Arensberg D, Baker A, Friedman L, Greene HL, Huther ML, Richardson DW: Mortality and morbidity in patients receiving encainide, flecainide, or placebo. The Cardiac Arrhythmia Suppression Trial. N Engl J Med 1991;324:781–788. Comment in: N Engl J Med 1991;325:584–585. Comment in: N Engl J Med 1992;327:1818.

103. Eichhorn EJ: Medical therapy can improve the biological properties of the chronically failing heart: a new era in the treatment of heart failure. Circulation 1996;94:2285–2296.

104. Eichhorn EJ: Practical guidelines for initiation of beta-adrenergic blockade in patients with chronic heart failure. Am J Cardiol 1997;79:794–798.

105. Eiechhorn EJ: Experience with beta blockers in heart failure mortality trials [review]. Clin Cardiol 1999;(suppl V):V-21–V-9.

106. Eichhorn EJ, Heesch CM, Barnett JH, Alvarez LG, Fass SM, Grayburn PA, Hatfield BA, Marcoux LG, Malloy CR: Effect of metoprolol on myocardial function and energetics in patients with nonischemic dilated cardiomyopathy: a randomized, double-blind, placebo-controlled study. J Am Coll Cardiol 1994;23:1310.

107. Eisenberg BR, Salmons S: The reorganization of subcellular structure in muscle undergoing fast-to-slow type transformation: a stereological study. Cell Tiss Res 1981;220:449.

108. El Oakley RM, Jarfis JC: Cardiomyoplasty: a critical review of experimental and clinical results. Circulation 1994;90:2085.

109. Elefteriades JA, Morales DLS, Gradel C, Tollis G, Levi E, Zaret BL: Results of coronary artery bypass grafting by a single surgeon in patients with left ventricular ejection fractions ≤30%. Am J Cardiol 1997;79:1573.

110. Epstein M, Lepp BA, Hoffman DS, Levinson R. Potentiation of furosemide by metolazone in reffractory edema. Curr Ther Res 1977;21:656–667.

111. Erick A, Jaques AK, Mejira LD: Quantitative evaluation of regional and global left ventricular shape, volume, and function using three- and two-dimensional echocardiography after ventricular remodeling surgery (Batista operation) for end-stage heart failure due to idiopathic dilated cardiomyopathy. Circulation 1997;96:1344.

112. European Coronary Surgery Study Group: Long term results of prospective randomized study of coronary artery bypass surgery in stable angina pectoris. Lancet 1982;2:1173.

113. European Society of Cardiology: Task force of the working group on heart failure. The treatment of heart failure. Eur Heart J 1997;18:736–753.

114. Falk RH: A plea for a clinical trial of anticoagulation in dilated cardiomyopathy. Am J Cardiol 1990;65:914–915.

115. Feldman AM, Bristow MR, Parmley WW, Carson PE, Pepine CJ, Gilbert EM, Strobeck JE, Hendrix GH, Powers ER, Bain RP, White BG: Effects of vesnarinone on morbidity and mortality in patients with heart failure. Vesnarinone Study Group. N Engl J Med 1993;329:149–155. Comment in: N Engl J Med 1993;329:201–202. Comment in: ACP J Club 1994;120(suppl 1):2.

116. Ferrari R, Visioli O: Stunning: damaging or protective to the myocardium? Cardiovasc Drugs Ther 1991;5:939.

117. Flather MD, Yusuf S, Kober L, Pfeffer M, Hall A, Murray G, Torp-Pedersen C, Ball S, Pogue J, Moye L, Braunwald E: Long-term ACE-inhibitor therapy in patients with heart failure or left-ventricular dysfunction: a systematic overview of data from individual patients. Lancet 2000;355:1575–1581. Comment in: Lancet 2000;355:1568–1569.

118. Fontan F: Transplantation of knowledge. J Thorac Cardiovasc Surg 1990;99:113.

119. Franciosa JA, Cohn JN: Contrasting immediate and long-term effects of isosorbide dinitrate on exercise capacity in congestive heart failure. Am J Med 1980;69:559–566.

120. Franciosa JA, Cohn JN, Jose E, Fabie A: Hemodynamic effects of orally administered isosorbide dinitrate in patients with congestive heart failure. Circulation 1974;50:1020–1024.

121. Franciosa JA, Wilen M, Ziesche S, Cohn JN: Survival in men with severe chronic left ventricular failure due to either coronary heart disease or idiopathic dilated cardiomyopathy. Am J Cardiol 1983;51:831.

122. Freedman B: Equipoise and the ethics of clinical research. N Engl J Med 1987;317:141–145.

123. Froehlich RT, Falsetti HL, Doty DB, Marcus ML: Prospective study of surgery post left ventricular aneurysm. Am J Cardiol 1980;45:923.

124. Furnary AP, Chachques JC, Moreira LF, Grunkemeier GL, Swanson JS, Stolf N, Haydar S, Acar C, Starr A, Jatene AD, Carpentier AF: Long-term outcome, survival analysis, and risk stratification of dynamic cardiomyoplasty. J Thorac Cardiovasc Surg 1996; 112:1640.

125. Furnary AP, Jessup FM, Moreira LF: Multicenter trial of dynamic cardiomyoplasty for chronic heart failure. The American Cardiomyoplasty Group. J Am Coll Cardiol 1996;28:1175.

126. Gainer JV, Morrow JD, Loveland A, King DJ, Brown NJ: Effect of bradykinin-receptor blockade on the response to angiotensin-converting enzyme inhibitor in normotensive and hypertensive subjects. N Engl J Med 1998;339:1285–1292.

127. Garg R, Yusuf S: Overview of randomized trials of angiotensin-converting enzyme inhibitors on mortality and morbidity in patients with heart failure. JAMA 1995;273:1450–1456.

128. GISSI Investigators: Effects of lisinopril and transdermal glyceryl trinitrate singly and together on 6-week mortality and ventricular function after acute myocardial infarction. Lancet 1994;343:1115–1122.

129. Goldstein RE, Boccuzzi SJ, Cruess D, Nattel S: Diltiazem increases late-onset congestive heart failure in postinfarction patients with early reduction in ejection fraction. The Adverse Experience Committee; and the Multicenter Diltiazem Postinfarction Research Group. Circulation 1991;83:52–60. Comment in: Circulation 1991;83:336–338.

130. Gottlieb SS, Dickstein K, Fleck E, Kostis J, Levine TB, LeJemtel T, DeKock M: Hemodynamic and neurohormonal effects of the angiotensin II antagonist losartan in patients with congestive heart failure. Circulation 1993;88(4 pt 1):1602–1609.

131. Gottlieb SS, Kukin ML, Medina N, Yushak M, Packer M: Comparative hemodynamic effects of procainamide, tocainide, and encainide in severe chronic heart failure. Circulation 1990;81:860–864. Comment in: Circulation 1990;81:1151–1153.

132. Granger CB, Kuch J, McMurray J, Rouleau JL, Swedberg K, Young JB, Yusuf S, Held P, Pfeffer MA, on behalf of the SPICE Investigators: A randomized trial evaluating tolerance to candesartan cilexitil in patients with congestive heart failure and intolerance to angiotensin-converting enzyme inhibitors [abstract]. J Am Coll Cardiol 1999;33:189A.

133. Greene HL, Graham EL, Werner JA, Sears GK, Gross BW, Gorham JP, Kudenchuk PJ, Trobaugh GB: Toxic and therapeutic effects of amiodarone in the treatment of cardiac arrhythmias. J Am Coll Cardiol 1983;2:1114–1128.

134. Grinstead WC, Francis MJ, Marks GF, Tawa CB, Zoghbi WA, Young JB: Discontinuation of chronic diuretic therapy in stable congestive heart failure secondary to coronary artery disease or to idiopathic dilated cardiomyopathy. Am J Cardiol 1994;73: 881–886.

135. Hall D, Zeitler H, Rudolph W: Counteraction of the vasodilator effects of enalapril by aspirin in severe heart failure. J Am Coll Cardiol 1992;20:1549–1555.

136. Hampton JR, Kleber FX, Cowley AJ, Ardia A, Block P, Cortina A, Cserhalmi L, Follath F, Jensen G, Kayanakis J, Lie KI, Mancia G, Skene AM, for the Second Prospective Randomised Study of Ibopamine on Mortality and Efficacy (PRIME II) Investigators: Randomized study of effect of ibopamine on survival in patients with advanced severe heart failure. Lancet 1997;349:971–977.

137. Hamroff G, Latz SD, Mancini D, Blaufarb I, Bijou R, Patel R, Jondeau G, Olivari MT, Thomas S, Jemtel THL: Addition of angiotensin II receptor blockade to maximal angiotensin-converting

enzyme inhibition improves exercise capacity in patients with severe congestive heart failure. Circulation 1999;99:990–992.

138. Hasenfuss G, Pieske B, Castell M, Kreschmann B, Maier LS, Just H: Influence of the novel inotropic agent levosimendan on isometric tension and calcium cycling in failing human myocardium. Circulation 1998;98:2141–2147.

139. Hayward MP: Dynamic cardiomyoplasty: time to wrap it up? Heart 1999;82:263.

140. Heesch CM, Marcoux L, Hatfield B, Eichhorn EJ: Hemodynamic and energetic comparison of bucindolol and metoprolol for the treatment of congestive heart failure. Am J Cardiol 1995;75:360.

141. Heyndrickx GR, Millard RW, McRitchie RJ, Maroko PR, Vatner SF: Regional myocardial functional and electrophysiological alterations after brief coronary occlusion in conscious dogs. J Clin Invest 1975;56:978.

142. Ho KKL, Pinsky JL, Kannel WB, Levy D: The epidemiology of heart failure: the Framingham Study. J Am Coll Cardiol 1993; 22(suppl A):6A.

143. Jatene AD: Left ventricular aneurysmectomy. J Thorac Cardiovasc Surg 1985;89:321–331.

144. Jatene AD, Moreira LFP, Stolf NA, Bocchi EA, Seferian P, Fernandes PMP, Abensur H: Left ventricular function changes after cardiomyoplasty in patients with dilated cardiomyopathy. J Thorac Cardiovasc Surg 1991;102:132.

145. Juilliere Y, Danchin A, Briancon S, Khalife K, Ethevenot G, Balaud A, Gilgenkrantz JM, Pernot C, Cherrier F: Dilated cardiomyopathy: long-term follow-up and predictors of survival. Int J Cardiol 1988;21:269.

146. Julian DG, Camm AJ, Frangin G, Janse MJ, Munoz A, Schwartz PJ, Simon P: Randomised trial of effect of amiodarone on mortality in patients with left-ventricular dysfunction after recent myocardial infarction: EMIAT. European Myocardial Infarct Amiodarone Trial Investigators [published errata appear in Lancet 1997; 349:1180 and 1997;349:1776]. Lancet 1997;349:667–6674. Comment in: Lancet 1997;349:662–663. Comment in: Lancet 1997; 349:1767, 1768, 1768–1769; discussion 1769–1770. Comment in: ACP J Club 1997;127:31.

147. Kantrowitz A, McKinnon W: The experimental use of the diaphragm as an auxilliary myocardium. Surg Forum 1959;9:266.

148. Kass DA, Baughman KL, Pak PH, Cho PW, Levin HR, Gardner TJ, Halperin HR, Tsitlik JE, Acker MA: Reverse remodeling from cardiomyoplasty in human heart failure: external constraint versus active assist. Circulation 1995;91:2314.

149. Kaul TK, Agnihotri AK, Fields BL, Riggins LS, Wyatt DA, Jones CR: Coronary artery bypass grafting in patients with an ejection fraction of twenty percent or less. J Thorac Cardiovasc Surg 1996;111:1001.

150. Kawaguchi AT, Sugimachi M, Sunagawa K, Takeshita N, Koide S, Verde JL, Batista RJV: Intraoperative left ventricular pressure-volume relationships in patients undergoing left ventricular diameter reduction. Circulation 1997;96:I-198.

151. Kay GL, Kay JH, Zubiate P, Yokoyama T, Mendez M: Mitral valve repair for mitral regurgitation secondary to coronary artery disease. Circulation 1986;74:I-88.

152. Kent KM, Bonow RO, Rosing DR, Ewels CJ, Lipson LC, McIntosh CL, Bacharach S, Green M, Epstein SE: Improved myocardial function during exercise after successful percutaneous transluminal coronary angioplasty. N Engl J Med 1982;306:441.

153. Kirklin JK, Young JB, Bourge RC, Silver M: Cardiomyoplasty skeletal muscle assist randomized Trial (C-SMART) 6 month results [abstract]. Basic Appl Myol 2000;10:74.

154. Kjekshus J: Arrhythmias and mortality in congestive heart failure [review]. Am J Cardiol 1990;65:421–481.

155. Klein H, Auricchio A, Reek S, Geller C: New primary prevention trials of sudden cardiac death in patients with left ventricular dysfunction: SCD-HEFT and MADIT-II [review]. Am J Cardiol 1999;83:91D–97D.

156. Kloner RA, DeBoer LWV, Darsee JR, Ingwall JS, Hale S, Tumas J, Braunwald E: Prolonged abnormalities of myocardium salvaged by reperfusion. Am J Physiol 1981;241:H591.

157. Kober L, Torp-Pederson C, Carlsen JE, Bagger H, Eliasen P, Lyngborg K, Videbaek J, Cole DS, Auclert L, Pauly ZNC, Aliot E, Persson S, Camm JA: A clinical trial of the angiotensin-converting enzyme inhibitor trandolapril in patients with left ventricular dysfunction after myocardial infarction. Trandolapril Cardiac

Evaluation (TRACE) Study Group. N Engl J Med 1995;333:1670–1676. Comment in: ACP J Club 1996;124:61. Comment in: N Engl J Med 1996;334:1546.

158. Kono T, Sabbah HN, Rosman H, Alam M, Jafri S, Goldstein S: Left ventricular shape is the primary determinant of functional mitral regurgitation in heart failure. J Am Coll Cardiol 1992; 20:1594.

159. Konstam M, Dracup K, Baker D: Heart failure: evaluation and care of patients with left ventricular systolic dysfunction. Clinical practice guideline. AHCPR Publication No. 94-0612. Rockville, MD; Agency for Health Care Policy and Research, U.S. Department of Health and Human Services. June 1994.

160. Kostis JB, Davis BR, Cutler J, Grimm RH, Berge KG, Cohen JD, Lacy CR, Perry HM, Blaufox MD, Wassertheil-Smoller S, Black HR, Schron E, Berkson DM, Curb JD, Smith WM, McDonald R, Applegate WB: Prevention of heart failure by antihypertensive drug treatment in older persons with isolated systolic hypertension. SHEP Cooperative Research Group. JAMA 1997;278: 212–216.

161. Kresh JY, Wechsler AS: Heart reduction surgery can reconstitute the residual stress-strain state of the left ventricle. J Thorac Cardiovasc Surg 1998;116:1084.

162. Kron IL, Cope JT, Baker LD, Spotnitz HM: The risks of reoperative coronary artery bypass in chronic ischemic cardiomyopathy: results of the CABG Patch Trial. Circulation 1997;96(suppl II):II-21.

163. Kron IL, Flanagan TL, Blackbourne LH, Schroeder RA, Nolan SP: Coronary revascularization rather than cardiac transplantation for chronic ischemic cardiomyopathy. Ann Surg 1989; 210:348.

164. Laks H, Marelli D: The current role of left ventricular reduction for treatment of heart failure. J Am Coll Cardiol 1998;32:1809.

165. Lange R, Sack FU, Voss B, DeSimone R, Thielmann M, Nair A, Brachmann J, Haussmann R, Fleischer F, Hagl S: Treatment of dilated cardiomyopathy with dynamic cardiomyoplasty: the Heidelberg experience. Ann Thorac Surg 1995;60:1219.

166. Lechat P, Packer M, Chalon S, Cucherat M, Arab T, Boissel JP: Clinical effects of beta-adrenergic blockade in chronic heart failure: a meta-analysis of double-blind, placebo-controlled, randomized trials. Circulation 1998;98:1184–1191.

167. Leier CV: Acute inotropic support: intravenously administered positive inotropic drugs. In Leier CV (ed): Cardiotonic Drugs: A Clinical Review. New York: Marcel Dekker, Inc, 1991, pp 63–105.

168. Leier CV: Unstable heart failure. In Braunwald E (ed): (Colucci WS). Atlas of Heart Disease. Philadelphia: Blackwell Sciences, 1995;4:9.2–9.15.

169. Leriche R: Essai Experimental de traitement de certains infarctus du myocarde et de l'anevrysme du coeur par une greffe de muscle strie. Bull Soc Nat Chir 1933;59:229.

170. Levin TB: The Design of Mortality Assessment in Congestive Heart Failure Trial (MACH-1, mibefradil). Clin Cardiol 1997; 20:320-326.

171. Levine TB: The design of the Mortality Assessment in Congestive Heart Failure Trial (MACH-1, mibefradil). Clin Cardiol 1997; 20:320–326.

172. Levine TB, Bernink PJ, Caspi A, Elkayam U, Geltman EM, Greenberg B, McKenna WJ, Ghali JK, Giles TD, Marmor A, Reisin LH, Ammon S, Lindberg E: Effect of mibefradil, a T-type calcium channel blocker, on morbidity and moderate to severe congestive heart failure: the MACH-1 study. Mortality Assessment in Congestive Heart Failure Trial. Circulation 2000;7:758–764.

173. Ljungman S: Renal function, sodium excretion and the renin-angiotension-aldosterone system in relation to blood pressure. An epidemiological and physiological study. Acta Med Scand Suppl 1982;663:108.

174. Ljungman S, Kjerkshus J, Swedberg K, for the CONSENSUS Group: Renal function in severe congestive heart failure during treatment with enalapril (the Cooperative North Scandinavian Enalapril Survival Study (CONSENSUS) Trial. Am J Cardiol 1992;70:479–487.

175. Louie HW, Laks H, Milgalter E, Drinkwater DC, Hamilton MA, Brunken RC: Ischemic cardiomyopathy: criteria for coronary revascularization and cardiac transplantation. Circulation 1991; 84(suppl III):III-290.

176. M-HS Group: Effect of metoprolol CR/XL in chronic heart failure: metoprolol CR/XL randomized intervention trial in congestive heart failure (MERIT-HF). Lancet 1999;353:2001–2007.

177. Macoviak JA, Stephenson LW, Spielman S, Greenspan A, Likoff M, Sutton MSJ, Reichek N, Rashkind WJ, Edmunds LH: Replacement of ventricular myocardium with diaphragmatic skeletal muscle. Short-term studies. J Thorac Cardiovasc Surg 1981; 81:519.

178. Magovern JA, Magovern GJ Sr, Maher TD, Benckart DH, Park SB, Christlieb IY, Magovern GJ: Operation for congestive heart failure: transplantation, coronary artery bypass, and cardiomyoplasty. Ann Thorac Surg 1993;56:418.

179. Mangschav A: Akinetic versus dyskinetic left ventricular aneurysms diagnosed by gated scintigraphy: difference in surgical outcome. Ann Thorac Surg 1989;47:746.

180. Marwick TH, MacIntyre WJ, Lafont A, Nemee JJ, Salcedo EE: Metabolic responses of hibernating and infarcted myocardium to revascularization: a follow-up study of regional perfusion, function, and metabolism. Circulation 1992;85:1347.

181. Massie BM, Fisher SG, Deedwania PC, Singh BN, Fletcher RD, Singh SN: Effect of amiodarone on clinical status and left ventricular function in patients with congestive heart failure. CHF-STAT Investigators [published erratum appears in Circulation 1996;94:2668]. Circulation 1996;93:2128–2134.

182. Matsuzaki M, Gallagher KP, Kemper WS, White F, Ross J Jr: Sustained regional dysfunction produced by prolonged coronary stenosis: gradual recovery after reperfusion. Circulation 1983; 68:170.

183. McCarthy PM, Bishay EB, Hoercher KJ: Mitral valve surgery for cardiomyopathy: late outcomes and effect on rehospitalization for congestive heart failure. Circulation 1999;100(suppl I):I-514.

184. McCarthy PM, Starling RC, Wong J, Scalia GM, Buda T, Vargo RL, Goormastic M, Thomas JD, Smedira NG, Young JB: Early results with partial left ventriculectomy. J Thorac Cardiovasc Surg 1997;114:755.

185. McKelvie R, Pericak D, Held P: Comparison of candesartan, enalapril, and their combination in congestive heart failure: Randomized Evaluation of Strategies for Left Ventricular Dysfunction (RESOLVD pilot study) [abstract]. Eur Heart J 1998;19(suppl):133.

186. Mills RM, LeJemtel TH, Horton DP, Liang C, Liang R, Silver MA, Liu C, Chatterjee K: Sustained hemodynamic effects of nesiritide (human 6-type natriuretic peptide) in heart failure: A randomized, double-blind, placebod controlled clinical trial. Natrecor Study Group. J Am Coll Cardiol 1999;34:155–162.

187. Mills RM, Pepine CJ: Heart failure secondary to coronary artery disease. In Hosenpud JD, Greenberg BH (eds): Congestive Heart Failure. New York: Springer-Verlag, 1994.

188. Misawa Y, Mott BD, Lough JO, Chiu RCJ: Pathologic findings of latissimus dorsi muscle graft in dynamic cardiomyoplasty: clinical implications. J Heart Lung Transplant 1997;16:585–595.

189. Monnet E, Orton EC: Myocardial oxygen consumption is affected by dynamic cardiomyoplasty in dogs with adriamycin-induced cardiomyopathy. J Card Surg 1998;13:475.

190. Moreira LFP, Stolf NAG, Bocchi EA, Bacal F, Giorgi MCP, Parga JR, Jatene AD: Partial left ventriculectomy with mitral valve preservation in the treatment of patients with dilated cardiomyopathy. J Thorac Cardiovasc Surg 1998;115:800.

191. Moreira LFP, Stolf NAG, Bocchi EA, Pereora-Barretto AC, Meneghetti JC, Giorgi MCP, Moraes AV, Leite JJ, da Luz PL, Jatene AD: Latissimus dorsi cardiomyoplasty in the treatment of patients with dilated cardiomyopathy. Circulation 1990;82(suppl IV):IV-257.

192. Moss AJ, Davis HT, Conrad DL, DeCamilla JJ, Odoroff CL: Digitalis-associated cardic mortality after myocardial infarction. Circulation 1981;64:1150–1156.

193. Mueller H, Ayres SM, Gianneli S, Conklin EF, Mazzara JT, Grace WJ: Effect of isoproterenol, L-norepinephrine, and intra-aortic counterpulsation on hemodynamics, and myocardial metabolism in shock following acute myocardial infarction. Circulation 1972;45:335–351.

194. Mullins ME, Linden DH, Smith GW, Norton RL, Stump J: Life-threatening interaction of mibefradil and beta-blockers with dihydropyridine calcium channel blockers. JAMA 1998;280:157–158.

195. Nawarskas JJ, Spinler SA: Does aspirin interfere with the therapeutic efficacy of angiotensin-converting enzyme inhibitors in hypertension or congestive heart failure? [review]. Pharmacotherapy 1998;18:1041–1052.

196. Nguyen KN, Aursnes I, Kjekshus J: Interaction between enalapril and aspirin on mortality after acute myocardial infarction: subgroup analysis of the Cooperative New Scandinavian Enalapril Survival Study II (CONSENSUS II). Comment in: Am J Cardiol 1997;80:1122. Am J Cardiol 1997;79:115–119.

197. Nienaber CA, Brunken RC, Sherman CT, Yeatman LA, Gambhir SS, Krivokapich J, Demer LL, Ratib O, Child JS, Phelps ME, Schelbert HR: Metabolic and functional recovery of ischemic human myocardium after coronary angioplasty. J Am Coll Cardiol 1991;18:966.

198. Oh JH, Badhwar V, Chiu RC: Mechanism of dynamic cardiomyoplasty. J Card Surg 1996;11:194.

199. Oosterga M, Anthonio RL, deKam PJ, Kingma JH, Crijns HJ, van Gilst WH: Effects of aspirin on angiotensin-converting enzyme inhibition and left ventricular dilation one year after acute myocardial infarction. Comment in: Am J Cardiol 1999;83:641. Am J Cardiol 1998;81:1178–1181.

200. Packer M: Calcium channel blockers in chronic heart failure. The risks of physiologically rational therapy. Circulation 1990;82: 2254–2257.

201. Packer M: Pathophysiological mechanisms underlying the adverse effects of calcium channel-blocking drugs in patients with chronic heart failure. Circulation,1989;80(suppl IV):IV-54–IV-67.

202. Packer M: End of the oldest controversy in medicine. Are we ready to conclude the debate on digitalis? [editorial; comment]. Comment in: N Engl J Med 1997;336:525–533. N Engl J Med 1997;336:575–576.

203. Packer M, Bristow MR, Cohn JN, Colucci WS, Fowler MB, Gilbert EM, Shusterman NH: The effect of carvedilol on morbidity and mortality in patients with chronic heart failure. U.S. Carvedilol Heart Failure Study Group. N Engl J Med 1996;334:1349–1355. Comment in: N Engl J Med 1996;334:1396–1397. Comment in: N Engl J Med 1996;335:1318; discussion 1319–1320. Comment in: ACP J Club 1996;125:61.

204. Packer M, Cohn JN: Consensus recommendations for the management of heart failure. Am J Cardiol 1999;83:1–38.

205. Packer M, Elkayam U, Sullivan JM, Pearle DL, Massie BM, Creager MA, and the Principal Investigators of the REFLECT Study: Double-blind, placebo-controlled study of the efficacy of flosequinan in patients with chronic heart failure. J Am Coll Cardiol 1993;22:65–72.

206. Packer M, Gottlieb SS: Adverse effects of converting-enzyme inhibition in patients with severe congestive heart failure: pathophysiology and management. Postgrad Med J 1986;62(suppl 1):179–182.

207. Packer M, Gheorghiade M, Young JB, Costantini PJ, Adams KF, Cody RJ, Smith LK, Van Voorhees L, Gourley LA, Jolly MK: Withdrawal of digoxin from patients with chronic heart failure treated with angiotensin converting enzyme inhibitors. RADIANCE Study. N Engl J Med 1993;329:1–7. Comment in: N Engl J Med 1993;329:51–53. Comment in: N Engl J Med 1993;329:1819–1820. Comment in ACP J Club 1994;120 (suppl 1):1.

208. Packer M, O'Connor CM, Ghali JK, Pressler ML, Carson PE, Belkin RN, Miller AB, Neuberg GW, Frid D, Wertheimer JH, Cropp AB, DeMets DL: Effect of amlodipine on morbidity and mortality in severe chronic heart failure. Prospective Randomized Amlodipine Survival Evaluation Study Group. N Engl J Med 1996;335:1107–1114. Comment in: ACP J Club 1996;126:30. Comment in: N Engl J Med 1997;336:1023; discussion 1024.

209. Packer M, Rodeheffer RJ, Ivanhoe RJ, DiBianco R, Zeldis SM, Hendrix GH, Bommer WJ, Elkayam U, Kukin ML, Mallis GI, Sollano JA, Shannon J, Tandon PK, DeMets DL, for the PROMISE Study Research Group: Effect of oral milrinone on mortality in severe chronic heart failure. N Engl J Med 1991;325:1468–1475.

210. Packer M, Sackner-Bernstein JD, Liang C, Goldscher DA, Freeman I, Kukin ML, Kinhal V, Udelson JE, Klapholz M, Gottlieb SS, Perle D, Cody RJ, Gregory JJ, Kantrowitz NE, LeJemtel TH, Young ST, Lukas MA, Shusterman NH, for the PRECISE Study Group: Double-blind, placebo-controlled study of the effects of carvedilol in patients with moderate to severe heart failure. Circulation 1996;94:2793–2799.

211. Packer M, Swedberg K, Pitt B, Fisher L, Klepper M, and the PROFILE Investigators and Coordinators: Effect of flosequinan on survival in chronic heart failure: preliminary results of the PROFILE study. Circulation 1993;88(suppl I):301.

212. Pagano D, Townend JN, Littler WA, Horton R, Camici PG, Bonser RS: Coronary artery bypass surgery as treatment for ischemic heart failure: the predictive value of viability assessment with quantitative positron emission tomography for symptomatic and functional outcome. J Thorac Cardiovasc Surg 1998;115:791.

213. Parmley WW: Pathophysiology and current therapy of congestive heart failure. J Am Coll Cardiol 1989;13:771.

214. Patel HJ, Polidori DJ, Pilla JJ, Plappert T, Kass D, Sutton MSJ, Lankford EB, Acker MA: Stabilization of chronic remodeling by asynchronous cardiomyoplasty in dilated cardiomyopathy: effects of a conditioned muscle wrap. Circulation 1997;96:3665.

215. Patterson JH, Adams KF, Applefeld MM, Corder CN, Massie BR, for the Torsemide Investigators Group: Oral torsemide in patients with chronic congestive heart failure: effects on body weight, edema, and electrolyte excretion. Pharmacotherapy 1994;14:514–521.

216. Petrovsky BV: Surgical treatment of cardiac aneurysms. J Cardiovasc Surg 1966;7:87.

217. Pette D, Smith ME, Staudte HW, Vrbová G: Effects of long-term electrical stimulation on some contractile and metabolic characteristics of fast rabbit muscles. Pflugers Arch 1973;338:257.

218. Pfeffer MA, Braunwald E, Moye LA, Basta L, Brown EJ, Cuddy TE, Davis BR, Geltman EM, Goldman S, Flaker GC, Klein M, Lamas GA, Packer M, Rouleau J, Rouleau JL, Rutherford J, Wertheimer JH, Hawkins CM: Effect of captopril on mortality and morbidity in patients with left ventricular dysfunction after myocardial infarction. Results of the Survival and Ventricular Enlargement trial. The SAVE Investigators. N Engl J Med 1992;327:669–677. Comment in: N Engl J Med 1992;327:725–727. Comment in: N Engl J Med 1993;328:966–967; discussion 968–969. Comment in: N Engl J Med 1993;329:1204–1206.

219. Pitt B: Randomised trial of losartan versus captopril in patients over 65 with heart failure (Evaluation of Losartan in the Elderly Study, ELITE) Lancet 1997;349:747–752. Comment in: Lancet 1997;349:1473; discussion 1475. Comment in: Lancet 1997;349:1474; discussion 1475. Comment in: ACP J Club 1997;127:29.

220. Pitt B, Poole-Wilson PA, Segal R, Martinez FA, Dickstein K, Camm AJ, Konstam MA, Riegger G, Klinger GH, Neaton J, Sharma D, Thivagarajan B: Effect of losartan compared with captopril on mortality in patients with symptomatic heart failure: randomised trial—the Losartan Heart Failure Survival Study ELITE II. Lancet 2000;355:1582–1587. Comment in: Lancet 2000;355:1568–1569.

221. Pitt B, Poole-Wilson P, Segal R, Martinez FA, Dickstein K, Camm AJ, Konstam MA, Riegger G, Klinger GH, Neaton J, Sharma D, Thiyagarajan B: Effects of losartan versus captopril on mortality in patients with symptomatic heart failure: rationale, design, and baseline characterstics of patients in the Losartan Heart Failure Survival Study—ELITE II. Comment in: J Card Fail 1999;5:77. J Card Fail 1999;5:146–154.

222. Pitt B, Zannad F, Remme WJ, Cody R, Castaigne A, Perez A, Palensky J, Wittes J: The effect of spironolactone on morbiditiy and mortality in patients with severe heart failure. Randomized Aldactone Evaluation Study Investigators. N Engl J Med 1999;341:709–717. Comment in: N Engl J Med 1999;341:753–755.

223. Popovic Z, Miric M, Gradinac S, Neskovic AN, Jovovic L, Vuk L, Bojic M, Popovic AD: Effects of partial left ventriculectomy on left ventricular performance in patients with nonischemic dilated cardiomyopathy. J Am Coll Cardiol 1998;32:1801.

224. Pouleur H, Rousseau MF, van Eyll C, Charlier AA: Assessment of regional left ventricular relaxation in patients with coronary artery disease: importance of geometric factors and changes in wall thickness. Circulation 1984;69:696–702.

225. Powell K, Bernhard S, Ding X, McCarthy P, White R: Demonstration of improved ventricular function in dilated cardiomyopathy (DM) by surgical left-ventricular remodeling (LVR) using dynamic cardiac MRI. Circulation 1997;96:I-464.

226. Power JM, Raman J, Dornom A, Farish SJ, Burrell LM, Tonkin AM, Buxton B, Alferness CA: Passive ventricular constraint amends the course of heart failure: a study in an ovine model of dilated cardiomyopathy. Cardiovasc Res 1999;44:549–555.

227. Pratt CM, Eaton T, Francis M, Woolbert S, Mahmarian J, Roberts R, Young JB: The inverse relationship between baseline left ventricular ejection fraction and outcome of antiarrhythmic therapy: a dangerous imbalance in the risk-benefit ratio. Am Heart J 1989;118:433–440.

228. Rahimtoola SH: The pharmacologic treatment of chronic congestive heart failure. Circulation 1989;80:693–699.

229. Rahimtoola SH: From coronary artery disease to heart failure: role of the hibernating myocardium. Am J Cardiol 1995;75:16E.

230. Rahimtoola SH: A perspective on the three large multi-center randomized clinical trials of coronary bypass surgery for chronic stable angina. Circulation 1985;72(suppl V):V-123.

231. Rahimtoola SH: The hibernating myocardium in ischemia and congestive heart failure. Eur Heart J 1993;14(suppl A):22.

232. Rahimtoola SH: The hibernating myocardium. Am Heart J 1989;117:211.

233. RALES Investigators: Effectiveness of spironolactone added to an angiotensin-converting enzyme inhibitor and a loop diuretic for severe chronic congestive heart failure (The Randomized Aldactone Evaluation Study [RALES]). Am J Cardiol 1996;78:902–907.

234. Ratcliffe MB, Hong J, Salahieh A, Ruch S, Wallace AW: The effect of ventricular volume reduction surgery in the dilated, poorly contractile left ventricle: a simple finite element analysis. J Thorac Cardiovasc Surg 1998;116:566.

235. Rector TS, Benditt D, Chachques JC, Chiu RCJ, Delahaye F, Jessup M, Kirkorian G, Thiene G, Titus J: Retrospective risk analysis for early heart-related death after cardiomyoplasty. J Heart Lung Transplant 1997;16:1018–1025.

236. Redfors A: Plasma digoxin concentration—its relation to digoxin dosage and clinical patients with atrial fibrillation. Br Heart J 1972;4:383–389.

237. Rees G, Bristow JD, Kremkau EL, Green GS, Herr R, Griswold HE, Starr A: Influence of aortocoronary bypass surgery on left ventricular performance. N Engl J Med 1971;284:1116.

238. Ross J Jr: Myocardial perfusion-contraction matching: implications for coronary heart disease and hibernation. Circulation 1991;83:1076.

239. Salmons S, Jarvis JC: Cardiomyoplasty: a look at the fundamentals. In Carpentier A, Chachques JC, Grandjean P (eds): Cardiomyoplasty. New York: Futura Publishing Co, 1991, p 35.

240. Salmons S, Stréter FA: Significance of impulse activity in the transformation of skeletal muscle type. Nature 1976;263:30.

241. Salmons S, Vrbová G: The influence of activity on some contractile characteristics of mammalian fast and slow muscles. J Physiol 1969;201:535.

242. Samady H, Elefteriades JA, Abbott BG, Mattera JA, McPherson CA, Wackers FJT: Failure to improve left ventricular function after coronary revascularization for ischemic cardiomyopathy is not associated with worse outcome. Circulation 1999;100:1298.

243. Schwaiger M, Schelbert HR, Ellison D, Hansen H, Yeatman L, Vinten-Johansen J, Selin C, Barrio J, Phelps ME: Sustained regional abnormalities in cardiac metabolism after transient ischemia in the chronic dog model. J Am Coll Cardiol 1985;6:336.

244. SCR Group: Prevention of stroke by antihypertensive drug treatment in older persons with isolated systolic hypertension: final results of the Systolic Hypertension in the Elderly Program (SHEP). JAMA 1991;265:3255–3264.

245. Shapira I, Isakov A, Yakirevich V, Topilsky M: Long-term results of coronary artery bypass surgery in patients with severely depressed left ventricular dysfunction. Chest 1995;108:1546.

246. Shivalkar B, Maes A, Borgers M, Ausma J, Scheys I, Nuyts J, Mortelmans L, Flameng W: Only hibernating myocardium invariably shows early recovery after coronary revascularization. Circulation 1996;94:308.

247. SOLVD Investigators: Effect of enalapril on survival in patients with reduced left ventricular ejection fractions and congestive heart failure. N Engl J Med 1991;325:293–303.

248. Spencer FC: In discussion of: Kron IL, Flanagan TL, Blackbourne LH, Schroeder RA, Nolan SP: Coronary revascularization rather than cardiac transplantation for chronic ischemic cardiomyopathy. Ann Surg 1989;210:348.

249. Stevenson LW, Fowler MB, Schroeder JS, Stevenson WG, Dracup KA, Fond V: Poor survival of patients with idiopathic cardiomyopathy considered too well for transplantation. Am J Med 1987;83:871.

250. Stolf NA, Moreira LFP, Bocchi EA, Higuchi ML, Bacal F, Bellotti G, Jatene AD: Determinants of midterm outcome of partial left

ventriculectomy in dilated cardiomyopathy. Ann Thorac Surg 1998;66:1585.

251. TAIREAS Investigators: Effect of ramipril on mortality and morbidity of survivors of acute myocardial infarction with clinical evidence of heart failure. Lancet 1993;342:821–828.

252. TCTS Group: Effects of enalapril on mortality in severe congestive heart failure: results of the Cooperative North Scandinavian Enalapril Survival Study (CONSENSUS). N Engl J Med 1987; 316:1429–1435.

253. Teerlink JR, Goldhaber SZ, Pfeffer MA: An overview of contemporary etiologies of congestive heart failure. Am J Cardiol 1991;121:1852.

254. Thomas GA, Baciewicz FA, Hammond RL, Greer KA, Lu H, Bastion S, Jindal P, Stephenson LW: Power output of pericardium-lined skeletal muscle ventricles, left ventricular apex to aorta configuration: up to eight months in circulation. J Thorac Cardiovasc Surg 1998;116:1029.

255. Tillisch J, Brunken R, Marshall R, Schwaiger M, Mandelkern M, Phelps M, Schelbert H: Reversibility of cardiac wall motion abnormalities predicted by positron tomography. N Engl J Med 1986;314:884.

256. Timolol Post Myocardial Infarction Group: Timolol-induced reduction in mortality and reinfarction in patients surviving acute myocardial infarction. N Engl J Med 1981;304:801–807.

257. Topol EJ, Weiss JL, Cuzman PA, Dorsey-Lima S, Blanck TJJ, Humphrey LS, Baumgartner WA, Flaherty JT, Reitz BA: Immediate improvement of dysfunctional myocardial segments after coronary revascularization: detection by intraoperative transesophageal echocardiography. J Am Coll Cardiol 1984;4:1123.

258. Trainini J, Barisani JC, Fischer EIC, Chada S, Christen AI, Elencwajg B: Chronic aortic counterpulsation with latissimus dorsi in heart failure: clinical follow-up. J Heart Lung Transplant 1999;18:1120.

259. Uretsky BF, Young JB, Shahidi FE, Yellen LG, Harrison MC, Jolly MK: Randomized study assessing the effect of digoxin withdrawal in patients with mild to moderate chronic congestive heart failure: results of the PROVED trial. PROVED Investigative Group. J Am Coll Cardiol 1993;22:955–962. Comment in: J Am Coll Cardiol 1994;24:578–579.

260. VACSGOA Agents: Effects of treatment on morbidity in hypertension II. Results in patients with diastolic blood pressure averaging 90 through 114 mm Hg. JAMA 1970;213:1143–1152.

261. van den Berg EK, Popma JJ, Dehmer GJ, Snow FR, Lewis SA, Vetrovec GW, Nixon JV: Reversible segmental left ventricular dysfunction after coronary angioplasty. Circulation 1990;81:1210.

262. Van Veldhuisen DJ, Veld AJM, Dunselman PHJM, Lok DJA, Dohmen HJM, Poortermans JC, Withagen AJAM, Pasteuning WH, Brouwer J, Lie KI: Double-blind placebo-controlled study of ibopamine and digoxin in patients with mild to moderate heart failure: results of the Dutch Ibopamine Multicenter Trial (DIMT). J Am Coll Cardiol 1993;22:1564–1573.

263. Vanoverschelde J-LJ, Wijns W, Depre C, Essamri B, Heyndrickx GR, Borgers M, Bol A, Melin JA: Mechanisms of chronic regional postischemic dysfunction in humans: new insights from the study of noninfarcted collateral-dependent myocardium. Circulation 1993;2:237.

264. Vatner SF: Correlation between acute reductions in myocardial blood flow and function in conscious dogs. Circ Res 1980;47:201.

267. Velazquez EJ, Califf RM: All that glitters is not gold. Lancet 2000;355:1568-1569.

266. vom Dahl J, Altehoefer C, Sheehan FH, Buechin P, Uebis R, Messmer BJ, Buell U, Hanrath P: Recovery of regional left ventricular dysfunction after coronary revascularization: impact of myocardial viability assessed by nuclear imaging and vessel patency at follow-up angiography. J Am Coll Cardiol 1996;28:948.

267. vom Dahl J, Uebis R, Sheehan FH, Hood R, Nase-Hueppmeier S, Doerr R, Hanrath P: Factors influencing outcome of regional wall motion following percutaneous transluminal coronary angioplasty. Coron Artery Dis 1992;3:489.

268. Weber KT, Brilla CG: Pathological hypertrophy and interstitium. Circulation 1991;83:1849.

269. Winniford MD, Rossen JD, Marcus MC: Clinical importance of coronary flow reserve measurements in humans. Mod Concepts Cardiovasc Dis 1989;58:25.

270. World Health Organization Council on Geriatric Cardiology: Task Force on Heart Failure Education: Concise guide to the management of heart failure. J Card Fail 1996;2:153–158.

271. Young JB: Chronic heart failure management In Topol EJ (ed): Textbook of Cardiovascular Medicine. Philadelphia: Lippincott-Raven Publishers, 1998.

272. Young JB, Gheorghiade M, Uretsky BF, Patterson JH, Adams KF: Superiority of "triple" drug therapy in heart failure: insights from the PROVED and RADIANCE trials. Prospective Randomized Study of Ventricular Function and Efficacy of Digoxin. Randomized Assessment of Digoxin and Inhibitors of Angiotensin-Converting Enzyme. J Am Coll Cardiol 1998;32:686–692. Comment in: J Am Coll Cardiol 1998;32:693–694.

273. Young JB, Kirklin JK: Cardiomyoplasty-skeletal muscle assist randomized trial (C-SMART): 6 month results. Presented at the American Heart Association, Atlanta, GA, November 1999. Circulation 1999 (suppl I) 100:I-514.

274. Young JB, Weiner DH, Yusuf S, Pratt CM, Kostis JB, Weiss MB, Schroeder E, Guillote M: Patterns of medication use in patients with heart failure: a report from the Registry of Studies of Left Ventricular Dysfunction (SOLVD). South Med J 1994;88:514–523.

275. Zhou G, Tyagi SC, Katwa LC, Weber KT: Effects of angiotensin II and aldosterone on collagen gene expression and protein turnover in cardiac fibroblasts. Mol Cell Biochem 1996;154:171–178.

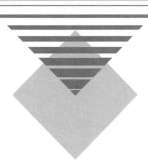

CHAPTER SIX

Recipient Evaluation and Selection

GENERAL CONSIDERATIONS

Advanced heart failure is the principal cause of death in over 40,000 patients yearly in the United States and a major contributing factor in 250,000 others.[8] In the United States alone, over $34 billion per year are spent on the care of patients with advanced heart failure.[157]

Historically, because of the unknown late outcome and the limited available donors, heart transplantation was offered only to those patients with less than 50% likelihood of 1-year survival with available medical or surgical therapy. However, as the survival and quality of life following cardiac transplantation have progressively improved (see Chapter 16), this therapy has been offered to patients in whom a survival benefit of transplantation is present after 1 year, but most pronounced after 2–3 years, particularly in the presence of marked symptoms of congestive heart failure, cardiac ischemia, or low cardiac output. Given the intense shortage of (and competition for) organs for transplantation, it is not surprising that uniform agreement has not been achieved among transplant centers and countries regarding the precise indications for, contraindications to, and timing of listing for transplantation. The decision-making process is further confounded by the paucity of secure information regarding risk-adjusted (and therefore patient-specific) time-related survival estimates for patients suffering from advanced forms of heart disease with no effective long-term medical or surgical therapy. The interpretation of available studies on the prognosis of patient subsets with advanced heart failure must also be tempered by the continuing evolution of available therapies. The balance between life-threatening forms of heart failure, on the one hand, and noncardiac conditions that may decrease patient and graft survival, on the other, forms the basis of the difficult decision-making process in allocating this scarce resource (Fig. 6–1).[202]

Because of ongoing controversies, experts in the field have periodically convened to promote standardization of selection criteria.[49, 146, 156] There is general agreement that cardiac transplantation should be reserved for those patients most likely to benefit in terms of both **life expec-**

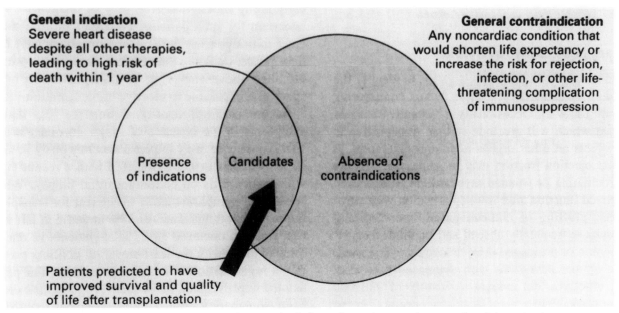

General indication
Severe heart disease despite all other therapies, leading to high risk of death within 1 year

General contraindication
Any noncardiac condition that would shorten life expectancy or increase the risk for rejection, infection, or other life-threatening complication of immunosuppression

Presence of indications

Candidates

Absence of contraindications

Patients predicted to have improved survival and quality of life after transplantation

FIGURE **6-1.** Intersecting circles demonstrate the principle of selection for cardiac transplantation of candidates who demonstrate indications without serious contraindications. As results of transplantation have improved, the indications broaden and the contraindications become less strict. (From Stevenson L, Couper G, Natterson B, Fonarow GC, Hamilton MA, Woo M, Creaser JW: Target heart failure populations for newer therapies. Circulation 1995;92[suppl II]:II-174–II-181, with permission.)

tancy and **quality of life.** The general approach to patients referred for consideration of cardiac transplantation is listed in Table 6–1. When applying a scarce resource such as cardiac transplantation, a balance must be achieved between appropriate utilization of the resource (donor hearts) to maximize graft survival and maximizing patient survival in those with the poorest expected outcome with other available therapies.

LIFE EXPECTANCY

If patients could be selected primarily on the basis of highest expected survival and quality of life at 1, 5, and 10 years, this would favor transplantation of less ill patients with acceptable expected survival with medical or nontransplant surgical therapy. Alternatively, if transplantation is reserved only for those patients closest to death from end-stage heart disease, the associated noncardiac organ dysfunction will drastically reduce the short and intermediate patient and graft survival, compromising effective utilization of organs. Thus an

TABLE 6-1	Approach to the Potential Candidate for Heart Transplantation

- Address potentially reversible causes and components of heart failure
- Evaluate severity of heart failure and functional capacity
- Tailor medical therapy to improve symptoms and reduce mortality
- Assess risks of deterioration or sudden death
- Identify indications for transplantation
- Exclude contraindications to transplantation
- Determine candidacy for transplantation
- Continue heart failure management with periodic reevaluation

inherent conflict exists between the concept of **maximal utilization** of donor organs (in terms of **organ survival**) and the **survival benefit** to the recipient. If sufficient patient-specific outcome information was available for patients with advanced heart failure, the survival benefit to an individual patient with transplantation could be estimated. We have used the term **survival benefit margin** (see Chapter 9) to quantify the expected benefit to a given patient. Benefit margin is calculated at any given point in time after transplantation by calculating the expected patient-specific survival with transplantation minus the expected survival without transplantation during the same time period. Thus, a patient with only 50% expected 1-year survival after transplant but with a 10% expected 1-year survival without transplantation would have an expected survival benefit margin of 40%. In contrast, a Class II middle-aged patient with advanced heart failure but well compensated and without other organ dysfunction might have an estimated survival of 95% at 1 year following transplantation versus 80% without transplantation. Such a patient would have a significantly lower survival benefit margin, namely, 15%. Obviously, some balance must be achieved between these two extremes, since transplantation should not be offered to a patient with an expected 1-year survival of 80% or more, but transplantation should also not be offered to a patient who is so sick that the anticipated 1-year survival with transplantation is only 50%. These principles in general apply to cardiac disease and its impact on other organ system function.

Thus, even if the time-related survival for individual patients with advanced heart failure could be accurately predicted (which currently is often not possible), and if the patient-specific survival of a potential recipient after transplantation (see Chapter 16) could be clearly established (which currently is not possible), there would continue to be philosophical differences regarding the appropriateness of allocating a scarce resource such as donor hearts primarily based on expected *graft survival* or *recipient survival benefit margin*. In addition to the severity and impact of heart failure on other organ systems, other **comorbid conditions** (disease or dysfunction of other organs unrelated to heart failure which independently reduce duration and/or quality of life) must also be included in the calculation of expected survival with and without transplantation (see later section). In practice, highly responsible physicians (medical and surgical) and other health care workers involved in cardiac transplantation strive to evolve a system which combines both priorities (with some differences among physicians, programs, and countries) to develop a "fair" method of selecting recipients for cardiac transplantation.

QUALITY OF LIFE

The definition, characterization, and quantification of quality of life after transplantation compared to that of the underlying cardiac condition has been difficult to elucidate, and the inability to apply rigorous tests of uncertainty has frustrated transplant professionals since the inception of transplantation. Despite these complexities (which are discussed in detail in Chapter 19), a formal part of the recipient selection involves identification of conditions present in the recipient or his environment which (although not necessarily immutable) would likely adversely affect his or her quality of life after (and therefore the benefit of) transplantation. Such potential factors, when identified, are evaluated in detail as part of the recipient selection process (see later section).

RISK FACTORS FOR MORTALITY IN PATIENTS WITH ADVANCED HEART FAILURE

There is general consensus that the prognosis for survival and quality of life of patients with New York Heart Association (NYHA) Class IV symptoms of heart failure who do not improve with medical/surgical therapy is sufficiently poor that consideration for cardiac transplantation is advisable. The major dilemma in decision-making involves those patients who are Class III at presentation or are promptly converted from Class IV to Class III/II with institution of appropriate medical therapy. Within this large group of patients, many studies have examined factors which predict a better or worse survival and impact the decision regarding listing for transplantation. The decision-making process for this large group of patients is critically important since (1) the available supply of organs is grossly inadequate to provide even a small fraction of these patients with transplantation; (2) allocation of a donor heart to a patient with a relatively better prognosis would deprive

a more seriously ill patient with a very short life expectancy (but preserved noncardiac organ function) the opportunity for transplantation at a time when his or her benefit would still be maximal; and (3) cardiac transplantation is not curative, is associated with its own chronic morbidity and survival limitation, and should therefore not be offered to patients with intermediate or long-term survival which approaches that of transplantation.

Identification of factors which predict mortality in ambulatory patients with advanced heart failure has been hampered by the complexity and variability of the heart failure syndrome, the evolving nature of medical treatment for heart failure, the retrospective nature of most studies, often small patient sample size, the infrequent application of appropriate multivariable analysis, and the almost uniform lack of patient-specific predictive models. These and other factors[207] which contribute to this difficult dilemma are listed in Table 6–2. Nevertheless, numerous risk factors[23] have been identified which are associated with adverse outcome in ambulatory patients with advanced heart failure (Table 6–3).

Thus, the complexity of selecting the appropriate time for listing is underscored by two important considerations. First, given the nature of transplantation, the waiting time is unpredictable after the decision is made to list. Second, despite numerous clinical studies in heart failure, few variables *consistently* predict duration of survival (or freedom from rapid deterioration) in advanced heart failure.

ETIOLOGY OF HEART DISEASE

Ischemic Cardiomyopathy

Although there is not uniform agreement,[232] most studies have concluded that patients with ischemic heart disease as the etiology for heart failure have a worse prognosis than patients with nonischemic cardiomyopathy.[43, 73, 94, 124, 190, 206] This notion is further supported by studies examining survival prior to transplantation of patients on the waiting list (see later section). Thus, if other clinical and hemodynamic variables are similar,

TABLE 6–2	Reasons for Inconsistency when Attempting to Identify Specific Prognostic Factors in Heart Failure Populations

- Small sample size in study populations
- Etiologic heterogeneity of study populations
- Varying stages of syndrome in populations studied
- Bias of inclusion/exclusion criteria in clinical trials
- Selective acquisition of clinical information (hemodynamic or exercise data not always obtained)
- Effect of patients entering and withdrawing from study protocol difficult to account for
- Duration of follow-up different
- Measurements frequently have high variability
- Relationship of variables assessed to acute therapy not accounted for
- Analysis techniques flawed from mathematical/statistical point of view

TABLE 6-3	Factors Correlating with Mortality Rates in Patients with Congestive Heart Failure

Clinical
Heart disease etiology
Heart disease duration
History of syncope
Hemodynamic
Left ventricular ejection fraction
Right ventricular ejection fraction
Pulmonary capillary wedge pressure
Right atrial pressure
Stroke work index
Cardiac index
Inotropic support required
Functional capacity
New York Heart Association Functional Class
Oxygen consumption at peak exercise (Vo$_2$max)
Distance covered during 6-minute walk
Neurohumoral/metabolic
Plasma norepinephrine
Plasma renin activity
Atrial natriuretic peptide
Leukocytosis
Serum sodium
Arrhythmias

patients with ischemic cardiomyopathy should be listed earlier in their disease course than patients with other forms of dilated cardiomyopathy.

Revascularization Versus Transplantation

Patients with ischemic cardiomyopathy without prior coronary bypass surgery should be evaluated for reversible ischemia, since bypass surgery in some cases may be an effective alternative to transplantation.

The primary indications for surgical coronary revascularization instead of transplantation for ischemic cardiomyopathy are discussed in detail in Chapter 5. The presence of severe left ventricular dysfunction and heart failure in patients with advanced ischemic heart disease accounts for about 50% of heart transplant procedures.[173] Therefore, decisions regarding transplantation versus alternative therapies to maximize survival, quality of life, and utilization of donors is particularly important in this disease entity. Due to ethical and other considerations, a prospective trial comparing the outcome of coronary revascularization versus heart transplantation in patients with severe left ventricular dysfunction (ejection fraction < about 0.20) has not been and likely never will be performed. Therefore, the decision in individual patients is based on an analysis of survival and quality of life of patients following cardiac transplantation, and in particular those transplanted for ischemic cardiomyopathy, compared to other surgical therapies for patients with advanced ischemic cardiomyopathy, using appropriate multivariable, risk-adjusted analyses. In general, cardiac transplantation is reserved for those patients with a high expected hospital mortality (> about 15%) with surgical revascularization. Since the 2-year survival following transplantation for such patients is generally about 80% (see Chapter 16), operative mortality exceeding about 15% would likely give an importantly inferior likelihood of 2-year survival compared to heart transplantation.[73]

The reported mortality after surgical therapy for patients with coronary artery disease and extremely poor left ventricular function (ejection fraction < about 0.20) is highly variable.[223] One study reported a hospital mortality of greater than 30% and 3-year survival of only 15% in such patients.[95] However, this experience was reported before the era of detailed studies of reversible ischemia and identification of viable myocardium. Another more recent publication reported 3-year survivals as high as 83% with ejection fraction less than 0.20 without prominent anginal symptoms.[114] Since most studies include a small number of patients, firm guidelines cannot be established with certainty. However, as detailed in Chapter 5, the primary objectives in considering patients for primary coronary artery bypass grafting with an ejection fraction less than about 0.20 are suitability of distal vessels for revascularization and indentification of viable myocardium (see Box) with reversible ischemia in the distribution of target vessels.[19, 63, 178, 187, 223]

Thus, **primary coronary artery bypass grafting** should be considered for patients with an ejection fraction greater than 0.15, left ventricular end-diastolic dimension less than about 65 mm, distal vessels suitable for bypass, and evidence of reversible ischemia in two or more (or isolated anterior) areas in which bypassable vessels are available.[93] Cardiac transplantation is generally considered the therapy of choice when patients with advanced heart failure and ischemic heart disease have extremely poor ventricular function (left ventricular ejection fraction less than about 0.15), symptoms primarily of heart failure with little or no angina, diffuse coronary artery disease with poor distal targets for revascularization, marked cardiomegaly, absence of documented reversible ischemia in viable myocardium, and/or accompanying poor right ventricular function (ejection fraction < 0.35). In the Coronary Artery Surgery Study (CASS), among patients with an ejection fraction less than 0.26, surgical therapy was effective in relieving anginal symptoms, but not heart failure symptoms.[7]

Although the risk of **reoperative surgery** with poor ventricular function is not clearly defined, the risk is considerably higher than for primary coronary bypass surgery for patients with severely depressed left ventricular function. We generally recommend that patients with ejection fraction less than about 0.25 and prior coronary surgery should not be considered for repeat bypass surgery unless angina is the primary symptom and there is strong evidence of reversible ischemia in the distribution of good target vessels. Ongoing clinical trials with emerging surgical and percutaneous revascularization techniques (transmyocardial laser revascularization and surgical revascularization coupled to ventricular remodeling procedures) will give greater insight into newer approaches.

Nonischemic Dilated Cardiomyopathy

In patients with dilated cardiomyopathy who are referred for transplant evaluation, transplantation can usually be safely deferred if there is prompt response to aggressive heart failure management. Dilated cardiomyopathy encompasses a variety of etiologies, all of

Identification of Viable Myocardium

The central issue in predicting improvement of severely depressed ventricular function following revascularization is the identification of myocardium in which contractile dysfunction is secondary to chronic hypoperfusion, so-called myocardial hibernation, in which myocyte contractile function (and thus energy requirement) is reduced in the setting of reduced oxygen supply.[187] The general options available for identification of viable myocardium in patients with ischemic cardiomyopathy are listed in Table 5–19. The "gold standard" for the assessment of cardiac muscle viability is the positron emission tomography (PET) (see discussion in Chapter 5), but this technique carries the disadvantages of higher cost and lack of widespread availability. In addition, conventional PET imaging does not provide information about regional wall motion.[34]

The most widely available technique for identification of viable myocardium is single photon emission computed tomography (SPECT) imaging with **thallium-201** (Tl-201). Regional myocardial concentration of Tl-201 is dependent on regional blood flow, entry into the myocyte (primarily by active transport), and myocyte clearance. The intracellular extraction of Tl-201 from blood is approximately 85%, even in hypoperfused myocardium unless there is irreversible injury to the sarcolemmal membrane, indicating necrotic myocardium. In viable myocardium, Tl-201 is continuously exchanged between myocardium and blood, the rate of exchange being proportional to the differences in concentration, and the resultant myocardial concentration being greatest in areas of highest myocardial blood flow. Over time, there is gradual "redistribution" of thallium concentration toward areas of ischemic but viable myocardium, indicated by a perfusion defect which reverses hours later. Standard clinical protocols for Tl-201 imaging typically include a second set of "redistribution" images 3–4 hours later, followed by either reinjection of a smaller dose with delayed imaging or reimaging 24 hours later. Tl-201 imaging is considered a very sensitive technique for the identification of viable myocardium, but it is less specific than other methods.[151, 167, 176, 197] Thus, if Tl-201 studies do not reveal viable myocardium, revascularization is unlikely to result in improvement in left ventricular function. However, evidence of viable myocardium by Tl-201 has less specificity than other techniques, such as dobutamine echocardiography and PET scanning.

Technetium-99m sestamibi is another useful imaging technique in which a lipophilic cation is initially distributed in the myocardium according to blood flow, with uptake primarily secondary to diffusion. Retention of the cation is dependent upon not only perfusion but also membrane integrity (and therefore viability).[16, 186] Although somewhat less sensitive than Tl-201, the sestamibi yields additional data on left ventricular function such as ejection fraction and ventricular volume.[197]

Magnetic resonance spectroscopy (MRS) is used to assess myocardial viability by the evaluation of metabolic activity in the myocardium. Phosphorus MRS detects changes in high-energy phosphate metabolism in myocardial cells resulting from ischemia or infarction,[172, 181, 182] but the abnormalities in adenosine triphosphate (ATP) and phosphocreatine are not specific for ischemia or absence of viability.[228]

which have in common the absence of important coronary artery disease and the presence of marked left (and often right) ventricular dilatation and severe systolic dysfunction (see Chapter 4). Most cases of cardiomyopathy in adults are "idiopathic" (etiology unknown). In these patients, the clinical, functional, and hemodynamic indices discussed in the remainder of this chapter determine the prognosis and therefore the need for cardiac transplantation. However, certain types of dilated cardiomyopathy are associated with *reversible* ventricular dysfunction and require special comment. Since spontaneous remission of these conditions may occur, a period of observation during aggressive medical therapy is advisable prior to listing, with the expectation that improvement may occur to a degree that transplantation is not necessary. In particular, lymphocytic myocarditis, peripartum cardiomyopathy, hypertensive cardiomyopathy, and alcoholic cardiomyopathy may undergo spontaneous remissions[69, 158] (see later sections). Since specific clinical, hemodynamic, or pathologic features which predict remission have not yet been identified, close follow-up is mandatory to identify deterioration and the need for listing.

EFFECT OF GENDER

Although several large heart failure trials[109, 125, 170, 208] suggest that angiotensin-converting enzyme (ACE) inhibitor therapy may be less effective in females than in males with advanced heart failure, it is currently unknown whether gender has an important influence on the rapidity of progression of heart failure. Therefore, gender per se does not influence current decisions regarding timing of listing for transplantation.

DURATION OF ILLNESS

A shorter duration of advanced heart failure symptoms is, in general, associated with a greater likelihood of remission. Several studies suggest that patients with important symptoms of less than 6–12 months' duration are more likely to respond to intensive medical therapy.[108, 204] However, such patients require close surveillance, since it is known that mortality and deterioration are most likely early after referral for heart failure management.[46, 205]

HEMODYNAMIC PERFORMANCE

Left Ventricular Systolic Function

Because of the known important impact of left ventricular dysfunction on survival, the measurement of left ventricular function and its reporting take a central role in determining the outcome of therapy for heart failure. The "common currency" of ventricular function is ejection fraction, which is the end-diastolic volume minus the end-systolic volume divided by the end-diastolic volume. Left ventricular ejection fraction is used in a variety of important ways: as an index of the severity of ventricular systolic dysfunction, as one means of determining the effectiveness of therapy for heart failure (including surgical therapy), in determining prognosis of patients with heart failure, to determine the advisability of an operation, and for comparing the results of one therapy (medical or surgical) versus another. Low ejection fraction (< 0.20) has been identified in multiple heart failure studies[124] as a risk factor for mortality. Yet it is important that the shortcomings of this measurement be recognized. A ventricle with an ejection fraction of 0.20 or less is consistent with varying degrees of cardiac dysfunction, since at that level of ejection fraction some patients could be very functional, others symptomatic with heart failure requiring intensive medical therapy, and others so ill that a ventricular assist device is required for survival. This undoubtedly results from the number of factors that interact to influence ejection fraction, including heart rate, preload, afterload, ventricular compliance, and inotropic state[17] (see Chapter 4). In addition to ejection fraction, which describes the global shortening performance of the ventricle, other important descriptors of ventricular performance include force generation, size of the ventricle, functional capacity of the patient, maximum oxygen consumption under stress, cardiac index, and filling pressures.[223] However, as an index of contractile function, ejection fraction does have the advantage that it can be easily measured by a number of techniques in nearly any patient situation. Nonetheless, one must realize that there is great technique-to-technique, interobserver, and intraobserver variability of ejection fraction measurement.

Initial assessment of resting hemodynamics in patients with heart failure generally includes measurement of left and right ventricular ejection fraction by one of a variety of techniques, most commonly echocardiography. Systolic left ventricular function (ejection fraction) has consistently been a powerful independent predictor of morbidity and mortality in patients with congestive heart failure. For example, an ejection fraction of less than 0.25 predicts major adverse events when compared with an ejection fraction of more than 0.35.[41] Since ejection fraction by echocardiography can be rapidly and noninvasively determined, this is one of the important initial studies to categorize the severity of ventricular dysfunction and therefore the likelihood for needing evaluation for transplantation. In the absence of diastolic dysfunction, it is rare for patients with dilated cardiomyopathy and an ejection fraction greater than 0.25 to require cardiac transplantation.[143] However, low ejection fraction (< 0.25) as an isolated variable in a group of patients with severe heart failure is poorly predictive of short- or intermediate-term mortality. Other hemodynamic and exercise studies are needed to further refine prognosis (see below).

Also important may be the serial assessment of ejection fraction, since progressive decrease in ejection fraction despite medical therapy is a poor prognostic sign. For example, a decrease in ejection fraction of more than 5% yearly has been associated with nearly twice the mortality of an ejection fraction which increases more than 5%.[40]

Right Ventricular Systolic Function

In patients with dilated or ischemic cardiomyopathy, right ventricular function (and therefore presumably right ventricular reserves) further refines risk stratification. Left ventricular failure is often associated with marked pulmonary hypertension, and associated right ventricular dysfunction aggravates tricuspid insufficiency and hepatic and other organ congestion. When severe right ventricular dysfunction accompanies left ventricular failure, organ congestion worsens as right atrial pressure rises.[57] Depressed right ventricular function and reserves may also prevent the normal increase in right ventricular output with exercise or exertion, further compromising already depressed left ventricular output.

Poor right ventricular function is a major predictor of intermediate mortality when it accompanies poor left ventricular function in the setting of heart failure. It is, however, more difficult to accurately determine right ventricular ejection fraction. In a study of patients with advanced heart failure, DiSalvo and colleagues identified, by multivariable analysis, right ventricular ejection fraction less than 0.35 at rest and exercise as the most significant predictor of death or deterioration to in-hospital mechanical or inotropic support.[60] In their study, the prognostic value of right ventricular ejection fraction was not dependent on the etiology or duration of heart failure (Fig. 6–2). Among patients with poor left ventricular function and advanced heart failure symptoms (Class III or IV), the 2-year mortality with right ventricular ejection fraction less than 0.35 was 70% in one study compared to 23% when the right ventricular ejection fraction exceeded 0.35. In this study, resting or exercise right ventricular ejection fraction greater than 0.35 was more predictive of survival in patients with NYHA Class III or IV symptoms than was oxygen consumption at peak exercise.[60]

Other Hemodynamic Indices

Resting hemodynamic measurements accurately reflect the state of cardiac performance at rest, but in themselves are poorly predictive of outcome.[211, 224, 230] By multivariable analysis, higher right atrial[145, 200, 211] pulmonary artery diastolic,[189] pulmonary systolic,[112, 183] pulmonary capillary wedge pressures,[2, 32, 108] and lower resting cardiac output have all been associated with increased mortality. Hemodynamic studies are more predictive when combined with exercise data (see below). For example, Rickenbacher and colleagues documented that a cardiac index of under 2 L/min/m^2 and a peak oxygen consumption of less than 12 mL/kg/min have a particularly poor prognosis.[183]

Hemodynamic measurements are most important as a guide to response to medical therapy. Improved hemodynamics after heart failure medical therapy predict a more favorable outcome. One study documented that a fall in pulmonary artery wedge pressure to less than 16 mm Hg on vasodilator therapy was associated with twice the 1-year survival compared to those patients who did not have such a response (83% vs. 38%, p = .0001).[206]

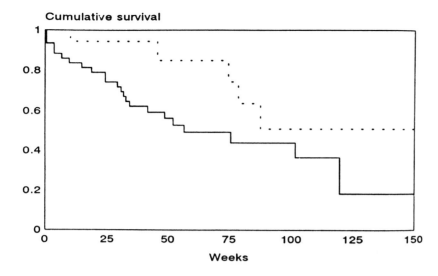

FIGURE **6–2.** Effect of right ventricular ejection fraction on event-free survival in patients with advanced heart failure. Nonfatal events included hospitalization for inotropic or mechanical support as a bridge to cardiac transplantation. The dotted line represents patients with a right ventricular ejection fraction ≥ 0.35. The solid line represents patients with a right ventricular ejection fraction < 0.35. (From DiSalvo TG, Mathier M, Semigran MJ, Dec WG: Preserved right ventricular ejection fraction predicts exercise capacity and survival in advanced heart failure. J Am Coll Cardiol 1995;25:1143–1151.)

Lower calculated stroke work index (the product of stroke volume and mean arterial pressure, normalized to body surface area), particularly during exercise, also predicts increased mortality. In one study, a stroke work index less than 20 g/m^2 at peak exercise predicted a 1-year mortality in excess of 60% compared to 13% when the peak exercise stroke work index exceeded this value.[86]

Although these and other studies which examine hemodynamic profiles as well as systolic function offer useful information about higher and lower risk groups, they are of limited value (except at the extremes) as isolated variables in predicting the appropriate time of listing for cardiac transplantation.

FUNCTIONAL CAPACITY

The New York Heart Association classification has been the standard method of subjectively classifying the functional capacity of patients with heart failure. One of the clearest indications for considering heart transplantation is the presence of Class IV heart failure (symptoms at rest or with any physical activity) despite optimal medical therapy. In most studies, the 1-year mortality in this setting ranges from 50–80%.[49, 53] The general mortality quoted for persistent Class III symptoms is 10–45% per year and for Class II patients 3–25% per year.[49] The prediction of mortality is further refined by other studies discussed below.

The **6-minute walk test** measures the distance an individual can walk during a single 6-minute test period. This is a useful test for following patients with mild or moderate heart failure, and a very short distance walked is associated with more frequent hospitalization and heart failure death.[199] However, quantitative cardiopulmonary testing (see below) is more useful in the patient with advanced heart failure.

CARDIOPULMONARY EXERCISE TESTING

Since Weber's initial description of the measurement of oxygen consumption in heart failure patients,[36, 90, 221] numerous studies have demonstrated that oxygen consumption at peak exercise (Vo$_2$max) provides valuable prognostic information in heart failure patients. This physiologic measurement is of particular relevance in heart failure, since the basic physiologic abnormality in the failing heart is the *inability to provide oxygen to peripheral tissues* at a rate sufficient to meet their aerobic requirements.

Physiologic Background

The heart, lungs, and blood hemoglobin (which in large part determines the blood's ability to take up and unload oxygen) are the primary vehicles which provide continuous oxygen availability to metabolizing tissues. Similarly, they are responsible for eliminating the carbon dioxide (CO$_2$) formed during oxidative metabolism and generated by the buffering of lactic acid by the bicarbonate system, which results in increased CO$_2$ production when lactate production is increased during anaerobic metabolism. The development of rapid response analyzers for determination of oxygen and carbon dioxide levels in expired gas has made it possible to determine oxygen uptake (Vo$_2$) and carbon dioxide production (Vco$_2$) during exercise. The term **cardiopulmonary exercise testing** has been applied to the monitoring, quantification, and interpretation of these and other parameters of respiration during graded levels of muscular work.

Maximal Oxygen Consumption

Cardiopulmonary exercise testing is performed in an incremental fashion, designed to identify when the patient reaches his or her **aerobic capacity** (plateau in oxygen uptake), which defines the maximal oxygen consumption. It follows from the Fick principle (Vo$_2$ = cardiac output × arterial–venous oxygen content difference) that maximal **whole body oxygen uptake** (Vo$_2$-max) is determined by maximal cardiac output and maximal tissue oxygen extraction (maximal arterial–venous O$_2$ difference). Vo$_2$max is usually a reliable and reproducible measure of overall aerobic capacity. A reduction in V_{O_2}max below normal levels is most commonly caused by the inability of the heart to appropriately increase cardiac output. Less common causes of reduced oxygen consumption are reduced ability to provide oxygen through the lungs (primary pulmonary insufficiency) and, rarely, the inability of tissues to appropriately extract oxygen. Since a reduction in V_{O_2} is usually caused by a reduction in maximal cardiac output, the degree of reduction in V_{O_2}max is considered a reliable indicator of the severity of heart failure.

Using breath-by-breath analysis of respiratory gas exchange, V_{O_2}max has been defined as a change in V_{O_2} of less than 1 mL/min/kg that is preferably maintained for 2 minutes (but at a minimum for 30 seconds). Since the use of V_{O_2} to predict mortality is based on *maximal* V_{O_2} during exercise, it is important to prove that oxygen consumption was truly maximal by documenting that the anerobic threshold was achieved at approximately 60–70% of V_{O_2}max.

Ventilatory Response

Minute ventilation (V_E) can be directly measured, as can V_{CO_2}. During aerobic work, V_E increases in proportion to both V_{O_2} and V_{CO_2}. During exercise, the increment in V_E is derived primarily from an increase in both tidal volume and respiratory rate. When cardiac performance is unable to keep up with the production of carbon dioxide, V_{CO_2} increases more rapidly than V_{O_2}. The respiratory exchange ratio (RER) (also called the respiratory quotient) is defined as V_{CO_2}/V_{O_2}. As discussed below, this ratio has relevance for determination of the anaerobic threshold.

Anaerobic Threshold

The **anaerobic threshold** is defined as that point during exercise when oxygen delivery (and therefore cardiac output) to exercising muscles is inadequate to sustain oxidative metabolism, and anaerobic pathways are utilized to a greater extent (identified by increased lactate production). In general, the more severe the impairment in exercise cardiac output (thus indicating worse heart failure), the earlier the onset of anaerobic metabolism. When monitoring mixed venous lactate levels during exercise, a rapid rise in mixed venous lactate levels (above about 12 mg/dL) occurs when anaerobic threshold has been reached.[218] The progressive increase in venous lactate (indicating a major shift toward anaerobic metabolism) is highly correlated with the onset of dyspnea in these patients.[220] The increased production of CO_2 during anaerobic metabolism promotes a reflex further increase in ventilatory drive. Thus, minute ventilation during exercise is most closely related to exercise V_{CO_2} (Fig. 6–3).

When measured clinically in the evaluation of patients with heart failure, the gas exchange anaerobic threshold (ATge) is approximated by the point at which the rate of CO_2 production (V_{CO_2}) abruptly increases (V-slope method) and by the point at which the V_{O_2} and V_{CO_2} slopes intersect (Fig. 6–4). With the increase in V_E associated with the increase in CO_2 production, the ratio of

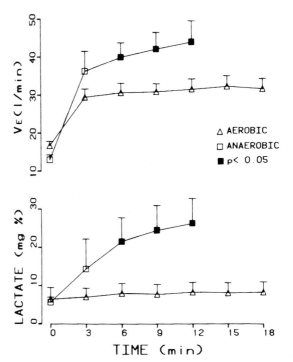

FIGURE **6-3.** The response of mixed venous lactate concentration and minute ventilation (V_E) during submaximal aerobic and anaerobic endurance exercise. Note the rise in serum lactate and progressive increase in V_E with the onset of anaerobic metabolism. (From Weber K, Janicki JS: Lactate production during maximal and submaximal exercise in patients with chronic heart failure. J Am Coll Cardiol 1985;6:717–724.)

V_E/V_{O_2} begins to progressively increase.[36] When the RER (see above) exceeds 1.0, CO_2 production is greater than the amount of oxygen able to be consumed, indicating the anaerobic threshold. Since anaerobic threshold typically occurs at approximately 60–70% of V_{O_2}max in heart failure patients,[219] it provides another indicator of the reliability of measured V_{O_2}max.

Differentiation Between Heart Failure and Primary Lung Disease as a Cause of Exertional Dyspnea

In patients with normal ventilatory reserves, the maximal V_E attained at V_{O_2}max is less than 50% of the ventilatory reserve as measured by maximal minute ventilatory volume (MVV).[222] In patients with interstitial lung disease, for example, the V_E is a higher proportion of MVV, and levels of V_E greater than 50% of MVV cannot be sustained for periods needed to achieve V_{O_2}max (Table 6–4). In addition, patients with primary pulmonary disease often develop hypoxemia with exercise and rarely reach anaerobic threshold or V_{O_2}max.[90] Furthermore, patients with primary limitation of exercise capacity due to problems other than those of a cardiac nature rarely achieve a RER greater than 1.10. This measurement should be included in every cardiopulmonary exercise test report to help determine accurately the cause and extent of a given patient's exercise disability.[90] Particularly challenging is sorting out the contributions of comorbid conditions to the patient with underlying heart

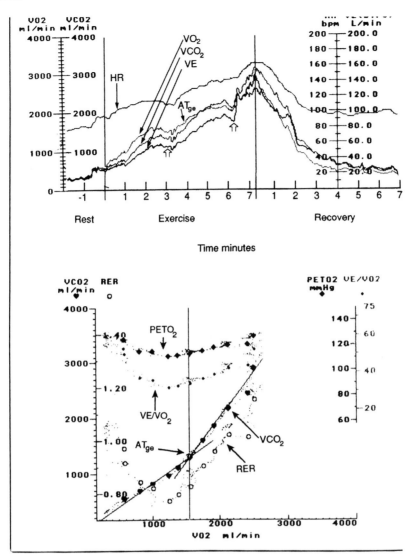

FIGURE 6-4. Cardiopulmonary exercise test in a healthy man using the Bruce protocol. The progressive linear increase in work output, heart rate, and oxygen consumption (V_{O_2}) is noted with steady-state conditions reached after 2 minutes in each of the first two stages (top panel). Open arrows indicate the beginning of each new 3-minute stage. The subject completed 7 minutes and 10 seconds of exercise, and peak V_{O_2} was 3.08 L/min. The anaerobic threshold (AT_{ge}), determined by the V-slope method is the point at which the slope of the rate of increase in V_{CO_2} relative to V_{O_2} changes, and occurred at a V_{O_2} of 1.3 L/min, or 42% of peak V_{O_2} within predicted values for a normal sedentary population (bottom panel). The AT_{ge} determined by the point at which the V_{O_2} and V_{CO_2} slopes intersect (1.8 L/min) (top panel) is slightly greater than the AT_{ge} determined by the V-slope method (bottom panel). The V-slope method usually provides a more reproducible estimate of AT_{ge}. PET_{O_2}, end-tidal pressure of oxygen; RER, respiratory exchange ratio; V_E/V_{O_2}, ratio of ventilation to oxygen uptake. (From Chaitman BR: Exercise stress tesing. *In* Braunwald E [ed]: Heart Disease. Philadelphia: WB Saunders, 1980, pp 153–176.)

failure, but obviously this situation is quite important when making a decision regarding the advisability of heart transplantation. Cardiac transplantation likely would not improve morbidity and symptoms when both significant heart and lung disease are present.

Other Determinants of V_{O_2}max

Age, gender, and muscle mass (or obesity) are known to affect V_{O_2}max in normal individuals.[217,219] These relations are partially described in regression equations based on age, gender, and height.[11, 27, 104, 217] Other factors which may influence V_{O_2}max include conditioning status, skeletal muscle structure,[59] pulmonary function, hemoglobin level, and patient motivation.[104, 216] However, in patients

with severe heart failure, the V_{O_2}max normalized to body weight (mL/kg/min) is less affected by these other variables than in the normal population.[1]

Judging Severity of Heart Failure by Exercise Testing

Since V_{O_2}max is generally a reflection of cardiac output during peak exercise, a reduction in V_{O_2}max at an RER greater than 1.10 is interpreted as a reduction in cardiac reserves and, therefore, an index of the severity of heart failure. Anaerobic threshold is also an indicator of the severity of heart failure, since its onset indicates the level of exercise at which oxygen supply is inadequate. The classification of severity of heart failure according to

TABLE 6-4	Distinguishing Between Cardiac and Ventilatory Causes of Exertional Dyspnea	
	CARDIAC	VENTILATORY
Vo_2max	Achieved, but reduced from normal	Not achieved
AT	Achieved, but reduced	Rarely achieved
$V_E$max	Value does not exceed 50% MVV	Value exceeds 50% MVV
Sao_2	Does not fall below 90%	Hypoxemia often appears

Vo_2max, maximal O_2 uptake; AT, anaerobic threshold; $V_E$max, maximal minute ventilation to incremental exercise; MVV, maximal voluntary ventilation obtained with pulmonary function testing; Sao_2, arterial O_2 saturation.
Adapted from Weber KT, Janicki JS, McElroy PA, Reddy HA: Concepts and applications of cardiopulmonary exercise testing. Chest 1988;93:843–847.

Vo_2max and anaerobic threshold is summarized in Table 6–5.

Predictive Value of Exercise Testing in Heart Failure Survival

Many studies have correlated Vo_2max with survival in heart failure patients.[41, 42, 124, 130, 131, 198, 202, 203] A consistent finding has been the very poor short-term survival ($\leq$30% 1-year survival) when Vo_2max is less than about 10 mL/kg/min, somewhat improved (30–80%) survival between about 10–18, and greater than 80% 1-year survival when Vo_2max exceeds about 18.

The study by Mancini and colleagues in 1991 focused attention on the application of peak oxygen consumption during maximal exercise testing for the selection of patients for cardiac transplantation.[131] Based on their analysis, these authors recommended that cardiac transplantation could be safely deferred in most patients with a Vo_2max greater than 14 mL/kg/min (Fig. 6–5).[222]

Others have suggested that V_E/Vco_2 and heart rate responses to exercise are more predictive of adverse outcome in heart failure patients than peak Vo_2 alone.[184] Compared with controls, heart failure patients had markedly abnormal ventilatory indices (V_E/Vco_2), chronotropic index (heart rate indexed for age), resting heart rate, functional capacity, and response to exercise. A

TABLE 6-5	Functional Impairment in Aerobic Capacity and Anaerobic Threshold as Measured During Incremental Treadmill Exercise		
SEVERITY	Vo_2MAX (ML/MIN/KG)	AT (ML/MIN/KG)	CI MAX (L/MIN/M² PREDICTED)
Mild to none	>20	>14	>8
Mild to moderate	16–20	11–14	6–8
Moderate to severe	10–16	8–11	4–6
Severe	6–10	5–8	2–4
Very severe	<6	<5	<2

Vo_2max, maximal O_2 uptake; AT, anaerobic threshold of Vo_2; CI max, maximal exercise cardiac index.
Adapted from Weber KT, Janicki JS, McElroy PA, Reddy HA: Concepts and applications of cardiopulmonary exercise testing. Chest 1988;93:843–847.

univariate analysis indicated that high V_E/Vco_2 (> 44) and low chronotropic index (< 0.50) were predictors of death.

Some studies have suggested that percentage of predicted maximal Vo_2 (derived from healthy individuals and normalized for gender, age, height, and weight) may provide greater prognostic information than peak Vo_2 normalized to body weight,[11, 27, 104, 217] particularly in women.[1] This may be especially relevant in estimating severity and prognosis of the heart failure syndrome in young and elderly patients. For example, the value of 14 mL/kg/min for Vo_2 (often quoted as the level above which transplantation can be safely deferred) represents approximately 60% of predicted Vo_2max for a 60-year-old man, but only 30% of predicted Vo_2max for a 20-year-old male. Several studies have suggested that a peak Vo_2 of **less than 50% of predicted** is a significant predictor of cardiac death within 1–3 years.[164]

However, not all studies have supported the predictive value of Vo_2max.[111] For example, an important study by DiSalvo and colleagues[60] performed extensive univariate and multivariable analyses on a group of patients with advanced heart failure, in which Vo_2max failed to identify patients with a more favorable prognosis (Fig. 6–6).

In refining the role of Vo_2max in predicting mortality in heart failure patients (and thus the timing of listing for transplantation), few studies have examined Vo_2max as a continuous variable by appropriate multivariable analysis for the prediction of mortality. Most studies have examined Vo_2 by stratified univariable depictions using somewhat arbitrary "cut-off" levels. One analysis of over 600 patients[149] identified peak Vo_2 as the significant predictor of mortality in heart failure patients, but the authors additionally examined the impact of selecting several arbitrary "cut-offs." Not surprisingly, they found a significant and important difference in mortality with cut-offs of 12, 14, and 16 mL/kg/min. Thus, it seems unfortunate that the somewhat arbitrary level of 14 has been selected by some clinicians as a functionally important dividing line between patients who can safely be treated medically and those who require listing for transplantation. How much "safer" is it to defer transplantation with at Vo_2max of 15 versus 14, or 16 versus 15? More desirable analyses would employ logistic or hazard function analyses (see Chapter 3), for example, in which peak Vo_2 was examined in a continuous fashion and combined with other variables in a multivariable analysis to identify predictors of 1-year or 2-year mortality. In that way, the use of a specific value of peak Vo_2 could be combined with other significant variables in a patient-specific prediction of survival, which could be more accurately compared with expected survival following transplantation.

METABOLIC FACTORS

Serum sodium is an important marker of prognosis in heart failure. Hyponatremia may reflect the effects of neurohumoral activation (see Chapter 4) and the intensity of diuretic therapy. Serum sodium decreases as

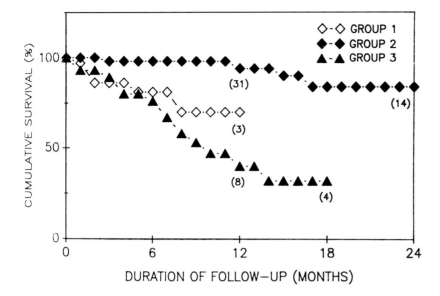

FIGURE **6-5.** Predictive value (risk unadjusted) of VO₂max in survival with advanced heart failure. *Group 1* had a VO₂ ≤ 14 mL/kg/min and were listed for transplantation. Patients were censored at the time of transplantation. *Group 2* had a VO₂max >14 mL/kg/min. *Group 3* had a VO₂max ≤ 14 ml/kg/min, but were not considered suitable for transplantation. (From Mancini D, Eisen H, Kussmaul W, Mull R, Edmunds L, Wilson J: Value of peak exercise oxygen consumption for optimal timing of cardiac transplantation in ambulatory patients with heart failure. Circulation 1991;83:778–786.)

vasopressin concentration and plasma renin activity increase. By univariate analysis, a serum sodium concentration of less than 130 mEq/L has been correlated with a survival rate of less than 20% at 1-year.[120]

NEUROHORMONAL ACTIVATION

As discussed in Chapter 4, activation of the renin-angiotensin and sympathetic nervous systems are part of the physiologic response to progressive heart failure. By univariate analysis, markers of neurohumoral activation during heart failure, such as plasma norepinephrine levels, plasma renin activity, and atrial natriuretic peptide correlate with survival.[20, 41, 42, 54, 124] Progressive elevation of plasma norepinephrine levels predicts poor outcome in patients with advanced heart failure.[74] Although there usually is wide variability of plasma norepinephrine levels, one study noted an 80% mortality at 2 years with norepinephrine levels of 1,200 pg/mL compared to 50%

in patients with levels of 200 pg/mL.[44] Leukocytosis and lymphocytosis have also correlated with higher mortality in patients awaiting cardiac transplantation, perhaps indicating greater neurohormonal activation.[180]

REFINEMENTS IN PREDICTING RESPONSE TO THERAPY

A great need exists for the development and prospective testing of algorithms which employ clinical, hemodynamic, exercise, and metabolic variables for the determination of prognosis in ambulatory heart failure patients. Currently, there is wide variability among institutions about the precise time in the course of heart failure at which response to therapy is deemed inadequate and cardiac transplantation is considered. However, from available studies, some indices indicating response to therapy and algorithms combining risk factors have been examined. Most patients who experience improve-

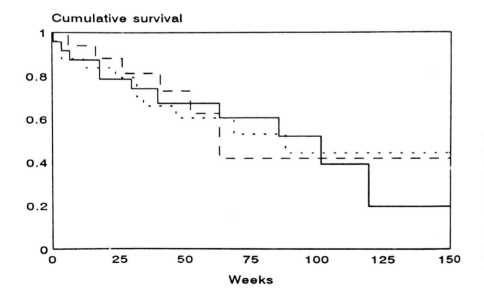

FIGURE **6-6.** Event-free survival (event = death or deterioration to inotropic or mechanical bridge to transplantation) in 67 advanced heart failure patients, stratified by peak VO₂. Solid line represents <10 mL/kg/min; dotted line represents VO₂ 10–14 mL/kg/min; dashed line represents VO₂ ≥ 14 mL/kg/min. (From DiSalvo TG, Mathier D, Semigran MJ, Dec WG: Preserved right ventricular ejection fraction predicts exercise capacity and survival in advanced heart failure. J Am Coll Cardiol 1995;25: 1143–1151.)

ment in left ventricular function after initiation of heart failure therapy survive with improved heart failure symptoms.[200] Improvement in ejection fraction typically occurs within 6–8 months, but it may occasionally take longer. Survival is also predicted by lower pulmonary capillary wedge pressure, lower right atrial pressure, and higher serum sodium levels during treatment. In contrast, worsening left ventricular function, low serum sodium, and high atrial pressures during therapy are poor prognostic signs. Among patients with symptoms of less than 6 months' duration at time of referral for evaluation, the subsequent failure of improvement in ejection fraction in the coming 6–12 months identifies a group at high risk for subsequent deterioration or death (Fig. 6–7).[200]

An integrated profile of left ventricular ejection fraction, clinical symptoms, etiology of heart failure, peak Vo₂, resting heart rate, QRS duration (especially if > 0.2 second) mean resting blood pressure, serum sodium, and hemodynamic data generates a clinical estimate of prognosis, modified by response to therapy, as noted above. Attempts to quantify the variables in an algorithm by Aaronson[2] (Table 6–6) and others are major steps toward standardizing the assessment of prognosis in the heart failure syndrome and decision-making regarding timing of transplant listing.

EVALUATION OF COMORBID CONDITIONS

When other noncardiac conditions exist which may adversely affect longevity and/or quality of life after trans-

plantation, they are generally called "comorbid conditions," defined as those disease processes which have a primary effect on noncardiac organ function and are not directly caused by cardiac failure or decompensation. Such conditions are of obvious importance, since they may reduce expected survival after cardiac transplantation, irrespective of or as a complex interaction with graft function. Also, comorbid conditions may actually be accounting for much of the perceived disability in some heart failure patients. Of particular interest is the impact of chronic immunosuppression on the natural history of these comorbid conditions. For many such conditions there is a paucity of secure information available to make rational decisions about so called "relative contraindications" because of small numbers of patients available for analysis and the reluctance to allocate a limited resource to patients whose comorbid conditions are considered "pushing the envelope." The lack of uniform agreement about the appropriateness of cardiac transplantation in the presence of certain comorbid conditions and systemic diseases is indicated in Table 6–7.[143]

AGE

There is not uniform agreement about the upper age limit for cardiac transplantation. In the absence of other life-limiting noncardiac conditions, the definition of an upper age limit becomes an ethical rather than medical decision. In properly selected patients, recipients over 60 years of age have a survival similar to younger patients.[15] Nonetheless, some programs limit heart transplantation to patients younger than 65 years of age. Older patients may rarely be selected if their noncardiac organ systems

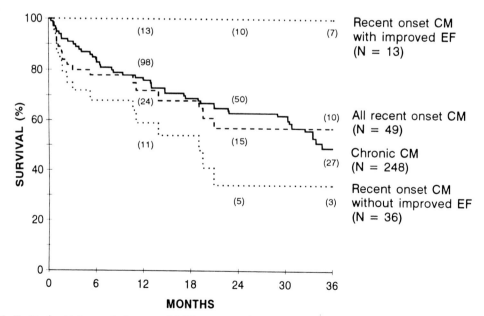

FIGURE **6–7.** Kaplan-Meier survival curves of 297 patients with primary dilated cardiomyopathy (CM) and advanced heart failure evaluated for cardiac transplantation. Survival was worse for patients with recent onset CM without improvement in ejection fraction (EF) with therapy (p = .03 vs. others). Survival for patients with recent onset cardiomyopathy and improvement was better than either survival for patients without improvement (p = .0009) or survival for patients with chronic cardiomyopathy (p = .0075, all p values by Mantel-Cox statistic). (From Steimle AE, Stevenson LW, Fonarow GC, Hamilton MA, Moriguchl JD: Prediction of Improvement in recent onset cardiomyopathy after referral for heart transplantation. J Am Coll Cardiol 1994;23:553–559.)

TABLE 6-6	A Model of Predictors of Mortality in Advanced Heart Failure			
VARIABLE	MODEL COEFFICIENT	ADJUSTED HAZARD RATIO (95% CI)*	WALD χ^2	p VALUE
Noninvasive model ($n = 268$)				
Ischemic cardiomyopathy	0.6931	2.00 (1.35, 2.97)	11.71	.0006
Resting heart rate (bpm)	0.0216	1.02 (1.01, 1.04)	11.45	.0007
LVEF (%)	−0.0464	0.96 (0.93, 0.98)	10.65	.0011
Mean blood pressure (mm Hg)	−0.0255	0.98 (0.96, 0.99)	8.94	.0028
IVCD	0.6083	1.84 (1.22, 2.76)	8.55	.0035
Peak V_{O_2} (mL/kg/min)	−0.0546	0.95 (0.91, 0.99)	6.76	.0093
Serum sodium (mmol/L)	−0.0470	0.95 (0.92, 1.00)	4.76	.0292
Invasive model				
Mean blood pressure (mm Hg)	−0.0289	0.97 (0.96, 0.99)	10.51	.0012
Resting heart rate (bpm)	0.0218	1.02 (1.01, 1.04)	9.32	.0023
IVCD	0.5931	1.81 (1.17, 2.80)	7.12	.0076
Peak V_{O_2} (mL/kg/min)	−0.0621	0.94 (0.90, 0.99)	6.81	.0091
Ischemic cardiomyopathy	0.5654	1.76 (1.15, 2.70)	6.75	.0094
LVEF (0%)	−0.0396	0.96 (0.93, 0.99)	6.70	.0096
Mean PCWP (mm Hg)	0.0285	1.03 (1.01, 1.05)	5.77	.0163
Serum sodium (mmol/L)	−0.0462	0.96 (0.91, 0.997)	4.32	.0376

LVEF, left ventricular ejection fraction; IVCD, interventricular conduction delay; PCWP, pulmonary capillary wedge pressure.

*Adjusted hazard ratio is the relative increase in the risk of an outcome event for patients with vs. patients without the characteristic for dichotomous variables or per unit increase in the variable for continuous variables. Note that Wald χ^2 associated with each variable cannot be validly compared between models because the sample sizes used to construct the models differed.

Adapted from Aaronson KD, Schwartz JS, Chen T, Wong K, Goin JE, Mancini DM: Development and perspective validation of a clinical index to predict survival in ambulatory patients referred for cardiac transplantation. Circulation 1997;95:2660–2667.

are normal, their cognitive function is totally intact, they have a strong will to live, their family support system is well-developed, and they have the potential for a good quality of life if normal cardiac function is restored. A few programs have addressed this issue by allocating

only older donor hearts (>50 years) to such elderly recipients.

PULMONARY VASCULAR RESISTANCE

As detailed in Chapter 20, the critical feature of elevated pulmonary vascular resistance (PVR) is the actual pulmonary systolic pressure at the completion of cardiopulmonary bypass in the transplant operation. The donor right ventricle generally tolerates poorly a systolic afterload over about 50 mm Hg and overt right ventricular dysfunction usually occurs above a pulmonary systolic pressure of 55–60 mm Hg, potentially resulting in acute right ventricular failure and death. The tolerance of the donor right ventricle to elevated afterload conditions (secondary to increased pulmonary vascular resistance) is partly a function of donor right ventricular reserves, ischemic/reperfusion injury, and possibly donor/recipient size ratio.

The vast majority of adult patients with advanced heart failure secondary to ischemic or dilated cardiomyopathy have a **reactive** component of elevated PVR which is directly responsive to the left atrial (or pulmonary capillary wedge) pressure. When elevated PVR is primarily reactive, the resistance falls rapidly following transplantation. If the donor heart left atrial pressure is normal, pulmonary artery systolic pressure, transpulmonary gradient, and pulmonary vascular resistance return to near normal levels within 1 week of transplant, with little further change during the coming year.[22]

It is generally recognized that there is a progressive increase in operative risk as PVR rises (see Chapter 16). Other risk factors interact with PVR to create a higher

TABLE 6-7	Heart Transplant Decisions: Are Certain Disease States Contraindications?	
	PROPORTION RESPONDING	
DISEASES	Yes (%)	Yes or Maybe (%)
Amyloidosis	58	85
Obesity (>125–150% ideal weight)	55	90
Scleroderma	51	95
Duchenne's muscular dystrophy	46	85
Sarcoidosis (pulmonary)	45	67
Active peptic ulcer disease	43	75
Systemic lupus erythematosus	35	88
COPD (FEV$_1$ <50% predicted)	32	82
Hypercoagulable state	28	84
Becker's muscular dystrophy	26	74
Giant cell myocarditis	23	55
Sarcoidosis (cardiac)	21	85
Rheumatoid arthritis	13	64
Poliomyelitis	13	58
Adriamycin cardiomyopathy	10	45
Alcohol cardiomyopathy	3	62
Adult congenital heart disease	3	15
Diabetes mellitus (noninsulin)	3	15
Diabetes mellitus (insulin)	3	32
Gallstones	0	8
Inactive peptic ulcer disease	0	0

COPD, chronic obstructive pulmonary disease; FEV$_1$, forced expiratory volume in 1 second.

Adapted from Miller LW, Kubo SH, Young JB, Stevenson LW, Loh E, Costanzo MR: Report of the consensus conference on candidate selection for heart transplantation—1993. J Heart Lung Transplant 1995;14:562–571.

or lower risk for a given level of resistance. In general terms, a PVR greater than about 5 Wood units (WU) which is unresponsive to pulmonary vasodilators and inotropic agents used to test reversibility of pulmonary vascular hypertension is a major contraindication to orthotopic cardiac transplantation.[146, 156] In order to define the reactive component of any elevation of pulmonary vascular resistance, a standard part of the cardiac transplant evaluation is performance of a right heart catheterization to document cardiac and pulmonary pressures (and resistance) (Fig. 6–8).[38] Clearly, the sustained hemodynamic response of pulmonary pressures to vasodilator therapy, such as milrinone, prostaglandin E_1,[76] nitroprusside,[50] nitroglycerin, or nitric oxide is a greater indicator of risk than absolute pulmonary vascular resistance. In one study, patients with a pulmonary vascular resistance which could not be lowered below 2.5 WU with vasodilators or accomplished only at the expense of systemic hypotension had an important increase in posttransplant mortality.[50] In patients with elevated pulmonary artery pressure (>50 mm Hg) and resistance with little reactivity (largely fixed), the risk of early mortality from acute cardiac failure rises dramatically.[38]

The **transpulmonary gradient** represents the pressure gradient across the pulmonary vascular bed (mean pulmonary artery pressure minus mean pulmonary capillary wedge pressure) and is independent of blood flow. When this gradient exceeds about 14 mm Hg, there is usually severe elevation of pulmonary vascular resistance. This parameter may be more useful than pulmonary vascular resistance (which requires calculation of cardiac output) in states of severe reduction of cardiac output. Some believe that a pulmonary artery diastolic pressure minus mean pulmonary artery capillary wedge pressure gradient more than 5 to 10 mm Hg predicts fixed elevation of pulmonary vascular resistance after transplant. More recent studies (unpublished data from Cardiac Transplant Research Database) indicate that the **pulmonary artery systolic gradient** (pulmonary systolic pressure minus mean pulmonary capillary wedge pressure) may also be a strong predictor of mortality from acute graft failure.

When pulmonary pressures remain severely elevated (>60 mm Hg) despite medical therapy, the pulmonary capillary wedge pressure (and therefore the transpulmonary gradient) is critical to the decision-making process. If the wedge pressure can be reduced with medical ther-

apy to about 20 mm Hg or less with little reduction in pulmonary artery pressure, a major fixed component is likely, and cardiac transplantation is very hazardous unless the heterotopic technique is employed. However, if medical therapy (sometimes over days to several weeks in an intensive care unit setting) fails to reduce pulmonary capillary wedge pressure to about 25 mm Hg or less and elevation of pulmonary artery systolic pressure higher than 60 mm Hg persists, secure conclusions about pulmonary reactivity cannot be made. In that instance, implantation of a left ventricular assist device may be warranted to force reduction of left atrial pressure and promote reversal of the reactive component.

PULMONARY DISEASE

The assessment of pulmonary function in patients being evaluated for cardiac transplantation is essential because of the possibility of coexistent lung disease (in particular, smoking-related emphysema and amiodarone-induced pulmonary fibrosis), but the assessment may be confounded by the effect of heart failure on pulmonary function testing.

Pathophysiology of Heart Failure–Induced Pulmonary Dysfunction

A number of pathologic mechanisms are involved in pulmonary dysfunction in patients with heart failure, each with functional consequences that may become evident on pulmonary function tests (Fig. 6–9).[67] **Pulmonary venous hypertension** results in distention of the pulmonary venous system, and with increasing hydrostatic pressure there is transudation of fluid into the interstitium surrounding the bronchioles, arterioles, and venules, producing a reduction in the diameter of the small airways. When the lymphatic vessels are no longer able to meet the drainage demands, the alveolar-capillary septae accumulate fluid and when the alveolar pressure is exceeded, fluid fills the alveolar spaces. In acute heart failure, there is evidence of both obstructive and restrictive ventilatory dysfunction with normal carbon monoxide diffusion capacity, with rapid improvement after treatment of heart failure.[123] **Pulmonary arterial hypertension** results in ventilation–perfusion

---

$$\text{Pulmonary vascular resistance (PVR, Wood Units (WU))}$$
$$\text{PVR} = \frac{(\text{PA mean} - \text{PCW})}{\text{CO}}$$

$$\text{Pulmonary vascular resistance index (PVRI, Wood Units} \cdot m^2)$$
$$\text{PVRI} = \frac{(\text{PA mean} - \text{PCW})}{\text{CI}} = \text{PVR} \cdot \text{BSA}$$

$$\text{Transpulmonary gradient (TPG, mm Hg.)}$$
$$\text{TPG} = \text{PA mean} - \text{PCW}$$

FIGURE **6–8.** Equations for the calculation of pulmonary vascular resistance indices. PA, pulmonary artery pressure; PCW, mean pulmonary capillary wedge pressure. (From Chen JM, Michler RE: The problem of pulmonary hypertension in the potential cardiac transplant recipient. In Cooper D, Miller L, Patterson G [eds]: The Transplantation and Replacement of Thoracic Organs. Lancaster: Kluwer Academic Publisher, 1996, pp 177-183.)

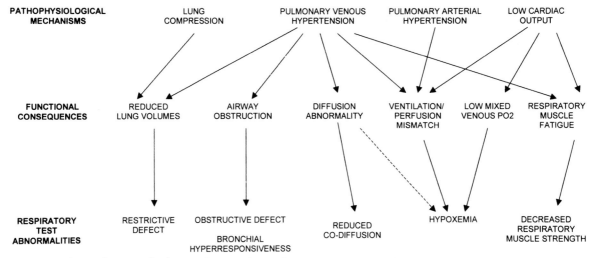

FIGURE **6–9.** Mechanisms of pulmonary function abnormalities in congestive heart failure. (From Faggiano P: Abnormalities of pulmonary function in congestive heart failure. Int J Cardiol 1994;44:1–8.)

mismatch contributing to hypoxemia. **Low cardiac output** contributes to hypoxemia through ventilation–perfusion mismatch. **Lung compression** due to pleural effusions and massive cardiomegaly may reduce lung volume. All of these effects can contribute to altered central nervous system control of respiration which causes periodic breathing patterns and further perturbs pulmonary and cardiac dynamics.[102]

Pulmonary Function Tests

A number of ventilatory abnormalities detected by pulmonary function testing may be found in isolation or in combination in patients with heart failure. An **obstructive ventilatory defect** may result from compression of the small airways by interstitial fluid, loss of elasticity of interstitial tissue holding the small airways open, bronchial wall edema, and bronchial mucosal plexus congestion increasing small airway resistance.[227] This increased airway resistance is reflected in the reduction of both forced expiratory volume in one second (FEV$_1$) and measures of mid-expiratory airflow. A **restrictive ventilatory defect** is quite common in patients with heart failure[98, 227] and is associated with a reduction in total lung capacity and forced vital capacity, which is probably the result of compression of gas-containing alveoli by interstitial and alveolar edema. **Impaired diffusion capacity (DL$_{CO}$)** is a common ventilatory abnormality in heart failure, and in a series of patients with chronic heart failure[227] 31% had an isolated diffusion impairment. In that study, the second most common ventilatory abnormality was a combined diffusion impairment and restrictive ventilatory abnormality. Other studies[152, 175, 193] confirm the frequent occurrence of impaired diffusion capacity in heart failure. Knowledge of the measurement of diffusion capacity (see Box) by the Roughton and Forster method[188] is key to understanding the effect of heart failure on diffusion capacity.

It is the reduction in the alveolar-capillary membrane diffusion capacity (D$_M$) that appears to be the most important determinant of diffusion capacity in heart fail-

ure.[174] Although a reduction in V$_C$ may be important[6] in patients with severe heart failure, V$_C$ is determined by two factors acting in opposite directions: increased pulmonary venous pressure tending to increase V$_C$, and pulmonary edema and pulmonary arterial hypertension tending to decrease V$_C$. The reduction in D$_M$ probably reflects an intrinsic abnormality of the alveolar-capillary membrane as well as a ventilation–perfusion mismatch reducing the effective surface area for gas exchange. Despite these derangements in heart failure, lung diffusion capacity (DL$_{CO}$) usually remains greater than 50% of normal.[29, 75, 141, 152]

Bronchial hyperresponsiveness to nonallergic stimuli has been demonstrated in patients with heart failure,[31, 65] presumably as a result of distention of submucosal bronchial vessels. This has been demonstrated clinically using methacholine inhalation, producing a

---

Measurement of Diffusion Capacity

The Roughton and Forster method of measuring pulmonary diffusion capacity for carbon monoxide (DL$_{CO}$) partitions DL$_{CO}$ into two components: D$_M$, which is the molecular diffusion of carbon monoxide across the alveolar-capillary membrane and θV$_C$, where θ is the rate of chemical reaction of carbon monoxide (which is dependent on the alveolar oxygen tension and hemoglobin concentration) and V$_C$ is the pulmonary capillary blood volume available for gas transfer. The Roughton and Forster equation

$$\frac{1}{DL_{CO}} = \frac{1}{D_M} + \frac{1}{\theta V_C}$$

separates the two component resistances—the diffusion resistance of the alveolar-capillary membrane ($\frac{1}{D_M}$) and the reactive resistance due to pulmonary capillary blood ($\frac{1}{\theta V_C}$).[174]

significant reduction in airflow. **Respiratory muscle weakness** has been described in patients with heart failure,[89] measured by maximum inspiratory and expiratory effort. The use of underperfused, weak respiratory muscles may contribute to the sensation of dyspnea.[132]

Alterations in Central Nervous System Control of Respiration

Central sleep apnea is often seen in patients with heart failure. Such patients often have daytime sleepiness, fatigue, somnolence, paroxysmal nocturnal dyspnea, orthopnea, and diminished cognitive function. The apneic episodes are associated with hypoxia and carbon dioxide retention which exacerbates the heart failure milieu. Though the most recognized respiratory pattern is intermittent Cheyne-Stokes respirations, a variety of "periodic breathing patterns" can be seen. The pathophysiology of periodic breathing is not completely understood but involves a complex neural feedback mechanism that is altered by central and peripheral chemo- and baroreceptors. The pattern of periodic breathing seems to be a consequence of the body's response to alterations in arterial carbon dioxide level that occur in patients with congestive heart failure. Pulmonary venous congestion leads to pulmonary vagal afferent stimulation and, therefore, hyperpnea. This is mediated through the J-receptors located in the pulmonary network. Hyperventilation lowers the arterial concentration of carbon dioxide below the apneic threshold and precipitates cessation of respiration from a central stimulatory standpoint. Periodic respirations in heart failure have been demonstrated to be a poor prognostic indicator, with patients having this finding demonstrating increased morbidity and mortality.[9]

Pulmonary Function Before and After Heart Transplantation

Following heart transplantation in patients with longstanding congestive heart failure, there is usually significant improvement in lung volumes and airflow.[3, 29, 154, 179] However, DL_{CO} may not improve[30, 141, 154, 179] (and may actually decrease)[5, 161] after cardiac transplantation, suggesting some permanent morphologic changes in the alveolar-capillary membrane. With normalization of pulmonary hemodynamics after transplant, V_C would be expected to decrease and D_M increase, but if V_C fell disproportionately it may contribute to a fall in DL_{CO} after transplantation. This persistence of abnormal diffusion capacity after cardiac transplantation may contribute to the observed exercise-induced hypoxemia in some recipients.[24] Improvement in diffusion capacity has been reported[101] after cardiac transplantation, and this does suggest that some remodeling of the abnormal alveolar-capillary membrane may occur.

Intrinsic Lung Disease

Severe chronic obstructive pulmonary disease (COPD) or severe bronchitis may predispose to recurrent pulmonary infections. Reduction in general pulmonary reserves in the presence of severe COPD may complicate weaning from a ventilator following cardiac transplantation, particularly in the presence of prior sternotomies if injury to the phrenic nerve occurs during dissection at the time of transplantation.

Pulmonary Dysfunction which Contraindicates Transplantation

When there is severe intrinsic lung disease with radiographic and clinical evidence of severity supported by pulmonary function tests, the likelihood of severe dyspnea and poor quality of life after cardiac transplantation is high. Although secure data are not available, cardiac transplantation may be considered ill advised if the FEV_1 is less than 40% of predicted, FVC is less than 50% of normal, and DL_{CO} is less than 40% of predicted in the presence of emphysema or pulmonary fibrosis. In the absence of identifiable intrinsic lung disease, a level of pulmonary function abnormality that precludes cardiac transplantation has not been defined. In the study by Bussieres,[29] no relationship was found between the degree of impairment of lung volume, airflow and diffusion capacity, and posttransplant survival, even in patients with an FEV_1 as low as 30% of predicted. Therefore, in patients with severe heart failure without known intrinsic lung disease who have impairment of lung volumes and airflow (FVC and FEV_1) as low as 30% of predicted and DL_{CO} 40% or greater of predicted, cardiac transplantation does not appear to be contraindicated.

Pulmonary Infarction

Recent pulmonary infarction should be considered a relative contraindication to cardiac transplantation because of the risk of recurrent emboli (from the original source) and possible abscess formation in the area of pulmonary infarction.[49, 231] In unusual situations, successful cardiac transplantation has been reported with pulmonary lobectomy at the time of transplantation.[129] Perhaps more important than the pulmonary infarction itself is an extensive evaluation of possible sources of the embolus prior to cardiac transplantation. Extracardiac sources of deep vein thrombosis should be identified and completely treated prior to cardiac transplantation due to the obvious risk of recurrent emboli following the transplant procedure. Anticoagulation and/or placement of an inferior vena caval filter is advisable for identified thrombus in the inferior vena cava or deep leg veins. Therapy for 4–6 weeks is advisable prior to transplantation to allow resolution of the deep vein thrombosis and scar formation in the area of pulmonary infarction.

RENAL DYSFUNCTION

Multiple studies have shown that preexisting renal dysfunction is a major risk factor for mortality after cardiac transplantation. A serum creatinine of 2 mg/dL and a creatinine clearance less than 50 mL/min portend a worse prognosis in adult patients following cardiac transplantation, particularly because of the necessity of cyclosporine or tacrolimus immunosuppression with their associated nephrotoxic effects. A major dilemma often exists in estimating the likelihood that renal dysfunction is secondary to severe low cardiac output and aggressive diuretic therapy or whether it is secondary to intrinsic renal disease. There is no specific level of serum creatinine or creatinine clearance which differentiates between intrinsic renal disease and normal kidneys with severely reduced cardiac output. Not surprisingly, when serum creatinine has been evaluated as a continuous variable, no specific level has been identified above which the risk abruptly increases.

The effective renal plasma flow (ERPF) (see Box), obtained by nuclear medicine techniques, is a useful adjunct to creatinine clearance. Although this technique has not been extensively studied in cardiac transplantation, an ERPF less than 200 mL/min is generally indicative of important underlying intrinsic renal disease affecting the distribution of renal blood flow, and in our opinion would represent a major risk factor for cardiac transplantation. Our approach to this problem is to obtain an ERPF study if the serum creatinine is 1.8 mg/dL or higher or if the creatinine clearance is less than 50 mg/min. If the ERPF is less than 200 mL/min in this setting, cardiac transplantation is not advisable unless combined heart/kidney transplant can be performed (see Chapter 21).

HEPATIC DYSFUNCTION

Hepatic dysfunction secondary to congestion (right heart failure) generally normalizes within the first sev-

---

Effective Renal Plasma Flow

One of the tests used to determine renal function and its adequacy for cardiac transplantation is effective renal plasma flow. This measurement is dependent on clearance of a radioactive tracer from the blood. To measure renal plasma flow the radioactive tracer must be metabolically inert, not cleared by any other organ other than the kidneys and completely excreted by the kidneys. The tracer currently used is a synthetic technetium compound ^{99m}Tc-MAG$_3$. Approximately 60% of this tracer is excreted (therefore, it is called *effective* renal plasma flow). The test involves a single injection of an accurately assayed quantity of tracer (defines volume of distribution) and at 44 minutes following injection, plasma is collected and assayed, which defines the volume excreted. It is not necessary to assay the tracer in the urine. The calculation of effective renal plasma flow is generated from an empirically derived formula and is generally accurate and reproducible. In patients with heart failure with considerable edema where the third space volume may be large (and may exceed the plasma volume), multiple plasma samples are drawn instead of a single 44-minute sample. One of the problems of ERPF in patients with heart failure is that the ERPF falls in parallel to decreases in cardiac output (and also recovers in parallel to increases in cardiac output) and, therefore, ERPF should not be used in isolation for determining candidacy for heart versus heart/kidney transplantation.

---

eral weeks following cardiac transplantation and is consistent with good long-term survival. However, if serum transaminase levels and bilirubin are more than twice normal value and/or are associated with anticoagulation abnormalities, underlying hepatic disease must be evaluated before listing for cardiac transplantation. The absence of hepatic cirrhosis and other progressive diseases must be documented with percutaneous or transjugular liver biopsy, since these conditions are associated with poor survival following (and therefore contraindicate) cardiac transplantation.

CEREBROVASCULAR AND PERIPHERAL VASCULAR DISEASE

Severe peripheral vascular disease is a risk factor for decreased late survival following cardiac transplantation. Even among patients accepted for cardiac transplantation, the presence of peripheral vascular disease was identified as a risk factor for late mortality in the Cardiac Transplant Research Database (unpublished data). The requirement for chronic prednisone therapy may promote progression of atherosclerotic vascular disease. Similarly, cerebrovascular disease increases the likelihood of stroke complications following cardiac transplantation. If cerebrovascular disease consists only of isolated, surgically correctable carotid artery stenosis, carotid endarterectomy may be performed prior to cardiac transplantation to minimize the risk of postoperative neurologic events. Thus, because of the associated increased risk of morbid events and late mortality, peripheral vascular disease and cerebrovascular disease should be considered relative contraindications to cardiac transplantation.

PEPTIC ULCER DISEASE

Active peptic ulcer disease may lead to gastrointestinal hemorrhage or perforation following cardiac transplantation and thus is a relative contraindication to cardiac transplantation until complete healing has been demonstrated endoscopically. In the recipient awaiting cardiac transplantation, aggressive medical therapy is advisable whenever peptic ulcer disease is identified. The routine use of prophylactic H$_2$ blocking agents is standard in many centers following transplantation.

ACTIVE SYSTEMIC DISEASE

Diseases which may or may not contribute to the heart failure syndrome through direct cardiac effects but also have systemic involvement should be individually evaluated for their potential impact on reducing posttransplant life expectancy and/or quality of life. Such systemic conditions are discussed separately in the later section, Special Conditions.

DIABETES

The presence of diabetes is no longer considered a contraindication to cardiac transplantation, but it does represent a risk factor for late morbidity and mortality. It is important, however, to exclude diabetic patients from transplantation if they have evidence of end-organ damage such as nephropathy, neuropathy, or retinopathy.[117, 148] Brittle diabetics with a large insulin requirement (even without end-organ damage) should be selected for cardiac transplantation with caution. Because of the likelihood of marked exacerbation of diabetes with steroids, such patients should be optimal candidates in other regards if they are selected for cardiac transplantation.

OBESITY

Marked obesity (140% or more of ideal body weight [IBW]) is a clear risk factor for morbid events and mortality in the intermediate term,[82] and therefore is a relative contraindication to cardiac transplantation. (IBW for men = 106 pounds for the first 5 feet of height + 6 pounds for each additional inch, and IBW for women = 100 pounds for the first 5 feet of height + 5 pounds for each additional inch).[156] Maintenance steroids aggravate obesity, which itself predisposes to diabetes, complications of osteoporosis, deconditioning, and possibly atherogenesis.[156] An analysis of patients in the Cardiac Transplant Research Database[82] identified percent of ideal body weight exceeding 140% as a risk factor for death and infection following cardiac transplantation (see Chapter 16). Therefore, patients who are greater than 140% of ideal body weight should be placed on a strict weight reduction program with a target weight to be achieved prior to proceeding with transplantation.

OSTEOPOROSIS

Although osteoporosis is likely not a specific risk factor for premature mortality, the presence of severe osteoporosis, particularly in an elderly patient, may be greatly aggravated by chronic steroid therapy. Osteoporosis should be considered along with other potential risk factors in deciding whether transplantation is advisable in an elderly patient.

INFECTION

The presence of active infection is a traditional absolute contraindication to cardiac transplantation if the infection is life-threatening and not readily reversible with antibiotic therapy. Clearly, cardiac transplantation would be ill advised in the presence of an important pneumonia, CNS infection, intra-abdominal sepsis, or active blood stream septicemia, since the likelihood of these infectious conditions progressing to a life-threatening state following the immunosuppression of transplantation would be high. However, certain infections, such as mediastinitis following implantation of a ventricular assist device, drive line infections, or, in some cases, partially treated endocarditis[61] are consistent with good outcome following cardiac transplantation (see Chapter 15), albeit at a higher risk of posttransplant mediastinal infection.

PRIOR MALIGNANCY

All patients should be screened appropriately for malignancies by a chest radiograph, mammogram, prostate-specific antigen, abdominal ultrasound, and complete physical examination. A history of prior malignancy increases the risk of a subsequent fatal malignancy following cardiac transplantation.[58] However, if there is no evidence of residual, recurrent, or metastatic disease for a sufficient period to consider the malignancy "cured," then cardiac transplantation may be considered. Although the suitable time period differs among malignancies, in general a malignancy-free interval of 5 years is considered suitable in order to proceed with cardiac transplantation. Rarely, patients with malignant tumors of the heart may undergo successful transplantation if there is no evidence of metastases or extension of the tumor beyond the surgical resection areas necessary for transplantation. This is, however, a contentious subject because malignant cardiac neoplasms can metastasize during the waiting period for organ allocation.

Squamous cell or basal cell carcinoma of the skin represents a curable condition with a low probability of metastatic lesions if completely excised. Thus, this malignancy, if completely excised, does not require an extended wait prior to cardiac transplantation.

NEUROCOGNITIVE AND PSYCHOSOCIAL FACTORS

The neuropsychological and social evaluation of patients considered for cardiac transplantation focuses on three specific areas. **Compliance** is the neurobehavioral capacity to adhere to a complex lifelong medical regimen.[119] **Comprehension** is the neurocognitive ability to give informed consent to the transplant procedure, to understand explanations and instructions about pre- and posttransplant care, and to understand the specific medical and follow-up instructions during the short- and long-term periods following transplantation. **Quality of life** assessment evaluates factors which are associated with the psychological perception following transplantation of happiness, well-being, and the desire for long-term survival. Thus, the primary goal of neuropsychological and social evaluation is to identify areas where patients may need additional support or behavioral modification and to eliminate patients from transplantation who, because of their neuropsychological traits or social environment, are at risk for poor survival or appear unlikely to enjoy an improved quality of life following cardiac transplantation.

Neurocognitive testing typically examines four domains of adjustment: cognitive, personality, coping, and affect measures.[83] In the cognitive domain, severe retardation and dementia are generally considered important contraindications to cardiac transplantation because of the need to comprehend a complex medical regimen. The **psychosocial evaluation** focuses on issues of compliance, coping skills, psychological hardiness, and family and social support systems. The goal of this evaluation is to identify patients who are emotionally stable, highly motivated to resume an active lifestyle following transplantation, compliant with medical advice, and have a supportive family or companions who are willing to make long-term commitments for the patient's well-being. Behavioral characteristics associated with poor compliance, such as ongoing or repeated substance abuse and alcoholism, should also be regarded as contraindications to cardiac transplantation.

The **psychiatric component** of the evaluation focuses on identification of active psychiatric disease. Severe depression which appears greater than would be appropriate for the level of heart failure, particularly if associated with current suicidal ideation, and active psychiatric disorders such as schizophrenia or severe paranoid ideations are absolute contraindications to successful cardiac transplantation.[122, 162, 171] These recommendations are supported by several studies which have concluded that certain more complicated psychiatric diagnoses are independent predictors of poor outcome.[35, 91, 92]

It is well known that the failure to adhere rigorously to the complex medical and follow-up regimen following cardiac transplantation, including compliance with medications, biopsy schedules, and informing the transplant center with symptoms of rejection or infection, constitutes a major risk factor for death and morbidity after transplantation. Unfortunately, there are few pretransplant psychosocial and sociodemographic factors which have been proven to predict poor compliance or adverse outcome after transplantation.[56, 134] Not surprisingly, considerable differences exist among institutions regarding precise neurocognitive and psychosocial factors which exclude patients from consideration for transplantation (Table 6–8).[143] Patients with a history of

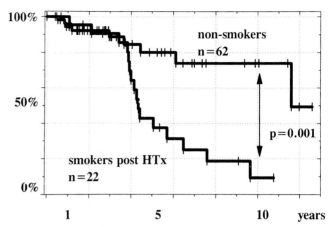

FIGURE 6–10. Kaplan-Meier analysis of the survival of patients who resume smoking during the first 6 months after transplant ($n = 22$) versus nonsmokers ($n = 62$) after orthotopic heart transplantation. Time 0 in the depiction is 6 months after heart transplant (HTx). (From Nagele H, Kalmar P, Rodiger W, Stubbe HM: Smoking after heart transplantation: an underestimated hazard? Eur J Cardiothorac Surg 1997;12:70–74.)

noncompliance or psychosocial risk factors for noncompliance should be reevaluated over time while participating in an intense outpatient heart failure program. Ability to keep appointments and adhere strictly to the medical, dietary, and lifestyle requirements of their heart failure management provides an opportunity to further assess the likelihood of patient compliance following cardiac transplantation.

TOBACCO AND ALCOHOL ABUSE

A history of smoking within the 6 months prior to cardiac transplantation is a known risk factor for intermediate-term mortality, partly related to poor patient compliance and partly related to the damaging effects of continued smoking after transplantation on allograft vasculopathy, progression of peripheral vascular disease, lung cancer, and general atherosclerosis.[229] One study indicated that resumption of smoking after cardiac transplantation was associated with decreased survival which became apparent 4 years after transplantation (Fig. 6–10).[150] Smokers had a higher incidence of transplant vasculopathy and malignancies (particularly lung cancer) compared to nonsmokers. Compliance with smoking cessation during heart failure treatment may be monitored with periodic unscheduled urinary nicotine levels. A history of alcoholism or drug abuse in the recent past are absolute contraindications to transplantation because of the known associated lack of compliance in such patients.

TABLE 6-8	Heart Transplant Decisions: Are Certain Circumstances Contraindications?

DISEASES	PROPORTION RESPONDING	
	Yes (%)	Yes or Maybe (%)
Current alcohol abuse	93	93
Current intravenous cocaine use	88	96
Current smoker	80	95
Current incarceration	78	91
Noncompliant with therapy	70	98
Current nasal cocaine use	70	98
Axis II psychiatric disorder	65	95
Mental retardation (IQ < 50)	65	90
Alcohol abuse < 6 months	62	88
No permanent address	53	90
Conviction of drug use	38	86
No social support systems	38	81
Current marijuana use	31	65
No medical insurance	28	67
History of felony incarceration	28	83
No phone	24	74
Language barrier	13	68
Mental retardation (IQ 51–80)	13	80
Alcohol abuse > 6 months	5	43
History of nonfelony incarceration	5	55
Not retired/does not want to work	5	23
Medicaid insurance only	5	8
Medicare insurance only	3	3
Axis I psychiatric disorder	3	41

Adapted from Miller LW, Kubo SH, Young JB, Stevenson LW, Loh E, Costanzo MR: Report of the consensus conference on candidate selection for heart transplantation—1993. J Heart Lung Transplant 1995;14:562-571.

INDICATIONS FOR CARDIAC TRANSPLANTATION

Cardiac transplantation should be reserved for those patients with advanced heart failure who are most

TABLE 6-9	**General Indications for Cardiac Transplantation**

Criteria for Consideration of Heart Transplantation in Advanced Heart Failure
- Significant functional limitation (NYHA Class III–IV heart failure) despite maximum medical therapy which includes digitalis, diuretics, and vasodilators, preferably angiotensin-converting enzyme inhibitors, at maximum tolerated doses
- Refractory angina or refractory life-threatening arrhythmia
- Exclusion of all surgical alternatives to transplantation such as the following:
  1. Revascularization for significant reversible ischemia
  2. Valve replacement for severe aortic valve disease
  3. Valve replacement or repair for severe mitral regurgitation
  4. Appropriate ventricular remodeling procedures

Indications for Cardiac Transplantation Determined by Severity of Heart Failure Despite Optimal Therapy
- Definite indications
  1. VO_2max <10 mL/kg/min
  2. NYHA Class IV
  3. History of recurrent hospitalization for congestive heart failure
  4. Refractory ischemia with inoperable coronary artery disease and left ventricular ejection fraction < 0.20
  5. Recurrent symptomatic ventricular arrhythmias
- Probable indications
  1. VO_2max <14 mg/kg/min (or higher with multiple other risk factors)
  2. NYHA class III–IV
  3. Recent hospitalizations for congestive heart failure
  4. Unstable angina not amenable to coronary artery bypass grafting, percutaneous transluminal coronary angioplasty with left ventricular ejection fraction < 0.25

NYHA, New York Heart Association.

likely to benefit in terms of improved quality of life and life expectancy. Patients with NYHA Class IV symptoms of heart failure, despite optimal medical therapy, have greater than 50% 1-year mortality and thus should be considered for cardiac transplantation. This includes patients who are dependent on intravenous inotropic support. In general, patients selected for cardiac transplantation should have a predicted 2-year survival less than about 60% with medical therapy.[155] Patients with advanced NYHA Class III symptoms of heart failure have a 1-year mortality which frequently exceeds 30%, and should be evaluated for cardiac transplantation. A final decision regarding appropriate therapy is based on assessment of the risk factors discussed above for mortality in advanced heart failure. General recommendations regarding indications and contraindications to cardiac transplantation as recommended by the International Society of Heart and Lung Transplantation in 1995 are summarized in Table 6–9.[143]

CONTRAINDICATIONS TO CARDIAC TRANSPLANTATION

General and specific contraindications to cardiac transplantation are based on assessment of comorbid conditions as discussed in the previous section. Standard

contraindications to cardiac transplantation are listed in Table 6–10. As discussed in prior sections, there are some conditions which represent "absolute" contraindictions to transplantation, but most (depending on severity and associated risk factors) are considered "relative" contraindications. These relative contraindications are, for the most part, comorbid conditions of varying degrees of severity. In making a final decision regarding the advisability of transplantation, the benefit margin of transplantation compared to other therapies must be considered along with the decrement in survival or quality of life conferred by any comorbid conditions (relative contraindications). In view of the paucity of data indicating the exact impact of many of these comorbid conditions, there is a considerable variability among transplant centers regarding the importance of specific contraindications (Tables 6–7 and 6–8).

TABLE 6-10	**Contraindications to Cardiac Transplantation**

General Contraindications
  Presence of any noncardiac condition that would itself shorten life expectancy or increase the risk of death from rejection or complications of immunosuppression
Specific Contraindications*
  Older age (> about 65 years) (program variability)
  Active infection
  Active peptic ulcer disease
  Severe diabetes mellitus with end-organ damage
  Severe peripheral vascular or cerebrovascular disease
  Coexisting active neoplasm
  Morbid obesity (> 140% predicted ideal body weight)
  Creatinine clearance <40–50 mL/min, ERPF < 200 mL/min†
  Bilirubin >2.5 mg/dL (when not due to reversible hepatic congestion), transaminases >2 × normal‡
  Severe pulmonary dysfunction with FVC and FEV_1 < about 40% of predicted, especially with intrinsic lung disease
  Pulmonary artery systolic pressure >60 mm Hg, mean transpulmonary gradient >15 mm Hg, and/or pulmonary vascular resistance >5 Wood units§
  Acute pulmonary thromboembolism
  Active diverticulitis
  History of smoking within last 6 months
  High risk of life-threatening noncompliance
    Inability to make strong commitment to transplantation
    Cognitive impairment severe enough to limit comprehension of medical regimen
    Psychiatric instability severe enough to jeopardize incentive for adherence to medical regimen
    History of recurring alcohol or drug abuse
    Failure of established stable address or telephone number
    Previous demonstration of repeated noncompliance with medication or follow-up
    Lack of independent family or social support system
    History of marked depression or emotional instability

ERPF, effective renal plasma flow.
* May be relative or absolute, depending on severity or program philosophy.
†May be suitable for cardiac transplantation if inotropic support and hemodynamic management produce a creatinine <2 mg/dL and creatinine clearance >50 mL/min. Transplantation may also be advisable as combined heart–kidney transplant.
‡Requires liver biopsy to exclude cirrhosis or other intrinsic liver disease.
§These apply only if the increased resistance is largely nonreactive (fixed). See text for details.

EVALUATION OF POTENTIAL CANDIDATES

The evaluation process for cardiac transplantation focuses on determination of the medical need for cardiac transplantation (indications for cardiac transplantation), identification and evaluation of comorbid conditions which could be contraindications to transplantation (see again Fig. 6–1), and the immunologic status of the recipient (necessary for proper recipient-donor matching). A standard evaluation protocol is listed in Table 6–11.[21]

An evaluation of social support and financial resources is of critical importance before accepting a patient for transplantation. A proper social support system is necessary to provide reinforcement for patient compliance with the complex medical regimen, to provide transportation to the transplant center should complications develop, and to maximize quality of life following transplantation. Cardiac transplantation is an expensive therapy, with requirements for costly follow-up procedures, medications, and follow-up medical care. Assessment of insurance coverage, both for the transplant procedure and the follow-up care, is of critical importance so that any financial obligations not covered by insurance can be reviewed with the patient and his or her family. Such information may play a critical role in the patient's decision to accept or reject cardiac transplantation therapy.

SPECIAL CONDITIONS

AMYLOIDOSIS

Amyloidosis is a systemic condition in which a variety of fibrillar amyloid proteins are deposited intracellularly in vital organs. In *primary* amyloidosis (including those forms associated with multiple myeloma), the amyloid protein is derived from immunoglobulin light chain.[99] *Secondary* amyloidosis includes forms associated with chronic inflammation, in which the amyloid protein is derived from acute phase proteins.[80] Amyloid deposition commonly occurs in kidney, liver, gastrointestinal tract, tongue, heart, adrenal glands, spleen, skeletal muscle, nerves, and tendon sheaths. When amyloid is deposited in the heart, it can be identified within myocardial cells and capillaries. The cells are gradually replaced by the amyloid fibrils,[45] resulting in a severe restrictive process.

Diagnosis

Systemic amyloidosis can be identified with special stains on rectal, gingival, bone marrow, liver, and myocardial biopsies. Typical pathologic features of amyloid can be identified by electron microscopy. A monoclonal gammopathy is associated with amyloidosis,[100, 116] and serum immunoelectrophoresis and urine protein elec-

TABLE 6–11	Evaluation Protocol for Cardiac Transplantation

General
  Complete history and physical examination
  Nutritional status evaluation*
  Blood chemistries including liver and renal profiles (bilirubin, SGOT[AST], alkaline phosphatase, BUN, creatinine, calcium, phosphorus, magnesium)
  Hematology and coagulation profile (complete blood cell count, differential, platelet count, prothrombin time [or international normalized ratio], partial thromboplastin time, fibrinogen)
  Serum electrolytes
  Lipid profile*
  Urinalysis
  24-hour urine for creatinine clearance (and protein if diabetic or urinalysis positive for protein)*
  Nuclear renal scan with measurement of effective renal plasma flow (ERPF)*
  Pulmonary function testing with arterial blood gases
  Ventilation–perfusion scan*
  Stool for heme ($\times$ 3)
  Mammography*
  Prostate-specific antigen (PSA)*
  Abdominal ultrasound study (liver, pancreas, gallbladder, and kidney evaluation)
  Carotid ultrasound
  Social evaluation
  Psychiatric evaluation
  Neuropsychiatric evaluation (neurocognitive evaluation)*
  Dental evaluation
  Sinus films*
Cardiovascular
  Electrocardiogram
  Chest x-ray (PA and lateral)
  Two-dimensional echocardiogram with Doppler study
  Exercise test with oxygen consumption (peak V_{O_2})
  Right heart catheterization with detailed hemodynamic evaluation
  Shunt series*
  Left heart catheterization with coronary angiography*
  Myocardial biopsy*
  Radionuclide angiogram (gated blood pool study)*
  Nuclear imaging study for myocardial viability (thallium-201 or positron emission tomography)*
  Holter monitor for arrhythmias (if ischemic cardiomyopathy)*
Immunology
  ABO blood type and antibody screen
  Panel reactive antibody (PRA) screen
  Human leukocyte antigen (HLA) typing (if to be listed for transplantation)
Infectious Disease Screening
  Serologies for: hepatitis A, B†, and C; herpes virus, human immunodeficiency virus (HIV), cytomegalovirus (CMV), toxoplasmosis, varicella, rubella, Epstein-Barr virus, venereal disease research laboratory (VDRL), Lyme titers*, histoplasmosis, and coccidioidomycosis complement fixing antibodies*
  Throat swab for viral cultures (CMV, adenovirus, herpes simplex virus)*
  Urine culture and sensitivity*
  Stool for ova and parasites*
  PPD (purified protein derivative) skin test with controls (i.e., mumps, dermatophytin, histoplasmosis, and coccidioidomycosis)*

*Only performed if appropriate or indicated.
†See also Chapter 15.

trophoresis may show evidence of monoclonal light chain proteins of the lambda type.[55]

In the heart, endomyocardial biopsy usually detects myocardial involvement, and supplemental electron microscopy typically shows dense intracellular collections of small fibers with a "matted hair" appearance.[45] In patients presenting with heart failure secondary to restrictive cardiomyopathy, cardiac biopsies should be obtained. If amyloid is suspected, a bone marrow aspirate should be performed to look for multiple myeloma and other plasma cell dyscrasias which are present in about 45% of patients with cardiac amyloidosis.[96] Additional biopsies should include oral mucosa, rectum, and tongue.[99] The classic Bence Jones protein in the urine is not a universal finding. Because of the frequency of hepatic involvement, a liver biopsy should also be considered.

Treatment

Therapy is generally ineffective in retarding the course of the disease, although chemotherapeutic regimens, particularly with melphalan and prednisone, may promote temporary disease regression.[196] Stem cell and bone marrow transplantation after chemical and whole body irradiation may eliminate the monoclonal plasma cell population in amyloidosis.[28]

Prognosis

It is estimated that over 90% of patients with primary amyloidosis will have myocardial involvement, of which about 65% develop cardiac symptoms prior to death. The major clinical manifestation is severe restrictive physiology with marked diastolic dysfunction and eventually systolic dysfunction and arrhythmias. Although there is great variability in individual modes of presentation and rapidity of progression, renal and cardiac failure are frequent causes of death. Once symptoms have developed, the median survival from the onset of cardiac symptoms to death is less than 6 months, with more than 90% dead within 2 years.[51, 81, 96]

Survival Following Transplantation

A limited experience exists with transplantation for amyloidosis, but available outcome studies suggests that virtually all surviving patients will show evidence of major organ system involvement and dysfunction and recurrence of amyloidosis in the transplanted heart.[55, 64, 166] The rate of amyloid progression in the transplanted heart is highly variable, and many patients remain asymptomatic for several years.[213] In a multicenter survey, 50% of patients had developed systemic organ dysfunction with amyloid involvement by 24 months, and 4-year survival was 40%.[97] Although isolated reports have suggested that cardiac function after transplantation can remain good for 4 years or more in some patients,[64, 88, 99] longer term follow-up has demonstrated progressive cardiac and noncardiac involvement in most cases.[64, 97] The major cause of death is progressive systemic or cardiac amyloidosis. The reported experience

at the Mayo Clinic offers a less pessimistic outlook, in that a small number of patients undergoing transplantation had an actuarial 5-year survival of 71% despite recurrence of cardiac amyloid in most patients. Another reported patient treated with cardiac transplantation and early aggressive chemotherapy survived more than 9 years following transplantation.[88]

Recommendation

Given the intense shortage of donor organs, amyloidosis should currently be considered a relative contraindication to cardiac transplantation until more effective forms of adjunctive therapy are available to arrest the progression of the systemic disease following transplantation. In a consensus conference on cardiac transplant selection in 1993, the majority of transplant cardiologists and surgeons regarded amyloidosis as a contraindication to cardiac transplantation.[143]

Patients with end-stage cardiac amyloid disease should be considered for transplantation only if they have advanced cardiac dysfunction, few other risk factors, and minimal evidence of systemic amyloid disease. Specifically, renal and hepatic function should be normal, myeloma and extensive bowel involvement excluded, and there should be no more than minor extracardiac involvement.

AMIODARONE

The use of chronic amiodarone therapy prior to transplantation had previously been considered an important risk factor for death after cardiac transplantation based on the reported incidence (about 15%) of fatal pulmonary complications in patients undergoing cardiac and general surgical procedures in the presence of acute[142] and chronic amiodarone therapy. Pulmonary decompensation was manifested by hypoxemia, pulmonary infiltrates, and pulmonary edema with low left atrial pressure.[84, 106] Since that time, however, considerable experimental evidence has implicated oxygen free radicals in the pathophysiology of postoperative lung toxicity (see further discussion in Chapter 12). Experimental studies suggest that the lung injury may be, in part, dose-related.[214]

In the current era, however, most programs employ a protocol of strict reduction of intra- and postoperative oxygen to an inspired oxygen concentration of 50% or less, theoretically reducing the production of oxygen free radicals.[62, 137, 214] With the frequency of amiodarone therapy in advanced heart failure, approximately 25–30% of patients currently coming to transplantation are on chronic amiodarone.

With strict maintenance of inspired oxygen concentrations less than 50% in the perioperative period and exclusion of patients with severe pretransplant pulmonary dysfunction, chronic amiodarone therapy is not a risk factor for posttransplant hospital mortality, but may be associated with a lower heart rate posttransplant and longer duration of hospital stay.[37]

Therefore, amiodarone should *not* be a contraindication to transplantation unless evidence of pulmonary fibrosis and/or severe pulmonary dysfunction are present. Once the patient is listed for transplantation, every effort should be made to reduce the dose of amiodarone to 200–400 mg/day (adult). Prior to and following operation, clear communication with anesthesia and nursing personnel should emphasize the importance of maintaining inspired oxygen concentration less than 50% as long as arterial oxygen saturation is 90% or higher. Close observation of pulmonary function and maintenance of low left atrial pressure are of importance during the first 5 or 6 days after transplantation.

SARCOIDOSIS

Sarcoidosis is a multisystem granulomatous disorder for which no cause is known. The hallmark of the disease is noncaseating granulomas that can occur in a number of different tissues. Sarcoidosis involves the myocardium in 20–30% of patients,[127, 195] and there are a number of pathologic manifestations of cardiac sarcoidosis. Involvement of the myocardium (which may be diffuse or focal) causes fibrosis which may result in global ventricular dysfunction in the case of diffuse involvement or localized scars in the case of focal involvement. Both the right and left ventricle may be involved, and the inflammatory and fibrotic process results in systolic and diastolic dysfunction,[72, 121, 185] although pure left ventricular diastolic dysfunction in the presence of normal systolic function has been described.[210] One manifestation of the fibrotic process is ventricular aneurysm formation.[4, 39, 121, 185] These aneurysms may range in size from small, relatively discrete lesions to ones that may involve a substantial portion of the ventricular wall, and both the left and right ventricle may be affected.[191] Pericardial involvement is common in association with myocardial sarcoidosis.[72, 78, 215] Valvular heart disease is uncommon, although mitral regurgitation may occur secondary to papillary muscle infiltration.[72, 177, 233] Rarely, involvement of the aortic,[70, 79] pulmonary,[185] and tricuspid[201] valves has been described.

Clinical manifestations of myocardial sarcoidosis are heart failure, conduction abnormalities (complete heart block being the most common) due to granulomatous or fibrous infiltration of the conduction system, constrictive pericarditis or pericardial effusions due to pericardial involvement, ventricular arrhythmias[70, 185] (which probably reflect widespread cardiac granulomatous or fibrous involvement or ventricular aneurysm formation), and atrial arrhythmias.

Diagnosis

Cardiac sarcoidosis is usually diagnosed by endomyocardial biopsy,[70, 128, 212] although a negative biopsy does not exclude the diagnosis. Extracardiac involvement may be sought using chest radiography, gallium-67 imaging (particularly with the use of SPECT),[165] serum angiotensin-converting enzyme tests (there is a general association between increased ACE levels and greater degrees of granulomatous inflammation), and biopsy of any lymphadenopathy.

Prognosis

Mortality associated with pulmonary sarcoidosis is low (5% of patients with pulmonary sarcoidosis die of respiratory failure).[194] Myocardial involvement with sarcoidosis appears to be more lethal than pulmonary sarcoidosis, but determination of precise survival statistics is complicated by the fact that the process may be clinically evident in only 40–50% of patients prior to death.[195] Based on autopsy studies, cardiac involvement is the cause of death in about 50% of patients. Average survival from the onset of symptoms of cardiac sarcoidosis is generally 1–3 years,[138, 168] although prolonged survival for up to 20 years has been described.[71]

Survival After Cardiac Transplantation

The major limitation of transplantation for this disease is the possible appearance of the process in other organs and/or recurrence in the graft.[229] There is, however, increasing experience with heart, lung, liver, and renal transplantation in patients with sarcoidosis. The use of immunosuppressive drugs following transplantation has not prevented disease recurrence or progression. Recurrence of noncaseating granulomas has been reported on endomyocardial biopsy after cardiac transplantation,[163] in the graft after liver transplantation,[169] in transplanted lungs (although not clinically apparent),[13, 18, 33, 103, 107, 135, 147] and after renal transplantation.[26, 192] A patient has been described undergoing liver transplantation[12] for hepatic sarcoidosis who died of progressive pulmonary sarcoidosis 9 months after liver transplantation. Despite recurrence or progression of disease, the intermediate-term survival of patients after cardiac, lung, liver, and kidney transplantation for sarcoidosis (although the numbers are small and follow-up short) appears similar to that of patients undergoing transplantation for other diseases.[14]

Recommendations

Despite the possibility of recurrence of sarcoidosis in the graft and/or the appearance of progressive extracardiac sarcoidosis, clinical symptoms may not appear for a prolonged period (years), and may be partially controlled with augmented steroid therapy. Therefore, despite uncertainty within the transplant community (Table 6–7), we believe the available evidence supports transplantation for cardiac sarcoidosis in patients with extensive cardiac involvement and symptoms of advanced heart failure (usually from restrictive cardiomyopathy) as long as there is minimal extracardiac involvements.

PERIPARTUM CARDIOMYOPATHY

Peripartum cardiomyopathy is defined as the onset of left ventricular dysfunction and congestive heart failure during the third trimester of pregnancy or in the first 6 months postpartum.[105, 158] The etiology of peripartum cardiomyopathy is unknown, but some have hypothesized an increased susceptibility of pregnant women to viral myocarditis.[158] Acute myocarditis can often (about 30% of patients) be demonstrated on myocardial biopsy, especially if biopsy is performed within 1 week of the onset of symptoms.[158] The course of heart failure is somewhat different in peripartum cardiomyopathy than in many other forms of cardiomyopathy, in that about half the patients experience prompt improvement in symptoms within 6 weeks, and the remainder develop progressive heart failure. The rapid recovery of many patients would be consistent with the known tendency for immunologic function (which may be depressed during pregnancy) to normalize soon after delivery, potentially enhancing viral clearance. The tendency for a large subset of patients to progressively deteriorate and die warrants close surveillance of their response to heart failure therapy. If heart failure progresses despite medical therapy, the poor prognosis warrants early consideration for cardiac transplantation.[158]

ACUTE MYOCARDITIS

Etiologies

Knowledge of the etiology, natural history, and treatment of acute myocarditis is incomplete, and all of these aspects impact on the advisability and timing of listing for cardiac transplantation. From a histological standpoint, myocarditis has been defined by the Dallas Criteria as "an inflammatory infiltrate of the myocardium with necrosis and/or degeneration of adjacent myocytes, not typical of the ischemic damage associated with coronary artery disease."[10] A wide variety of infectious (bacterial, fungal, rickettsial, viral, and spirochetal)[133] and noninfectious (drug-induced hypersensitivity,[68, 209] collagen vascular disease including polymyositis and dermatomyositis, Still's disease, eosinophilic myocarditis, and giant cell myocarditis) causes of acute myocarditis have been identified. After the rare noninfectious causes have been excluded, an infectious agent is rarely identified, and it is usually assumed that a virus is the etiological agent. "Lymphocytic myocarditis," "viral myocarditis," "idiopathic myocarditis," and "interstitial myocarditis" are terms that are usually regarded as synonymous.[66]

A number of cardiotropic enteroviruses, particularly coxsackie B virus, have been implicated in viral myocarditis, with experimental support from murine models of myocarditis. It remains unresolved whether the inflammatory process of myocarditis results from persistence of virus, an autoimmune response induced by the virus, or both. Several potential mechanisms may participate in the immune process, including sharing of antigenic determinants common to the infecting virus and myocytes, the development of autoantibodies, and/or the production of autoimmune cytotoxic T lymphocytes.[126, 226]

Management of Myocarditis

Information regarding the efficacy of anti-inflammatory and immunosuppression therapy for active myocarditis is incomplete, but it appears that only about 50% of patients demonstrate any improvement using a variety of immunosuppressive drugs including corticosteroids, azathioprine, cyclosporine, antithymocyte globulin, and OKT3.[160] Thus, the results of immunosuppressive therapy for acute myocarditis have been disappointing. A multicenter clinical trial of immunosuppressive therapy for biopsy-proven myocarditis showed no benefit of immunosuppression in terms of improvement in left ventricular function or survival.[136]

Prognosis

The natural history of myocarditis is uncertain, but probably most patients recover spontaneously. A small (and currently uncertain) proportion will progress either early or late to chronic inflammation, necrosis, and fibrosis resulting in a dilated cardiomyopathy and potentially refractory heart failure. Among patients with dilated cardiomyopathy referred for heart failure evaluation, a small proportion have biopsy-proven lymphocytic myocarditis.[87, 136] A study by Grogan and colleagues[87] found no difference in survival at 5 years between patients with and without lymphocytic myocarditis on biopsy. The overall mortality in a multi-institutional study was 20% at 1 year and 56% at 4 years, so close surveillance is required for signs of worsening heart failure and the potential need for cardiac transplantation.[136]

Survival After Cardiac Transplantation

Patients with acute myocarditis who proceed to profound circulatory failure may require continuous inotropic support or circulatory support with an intra-aortic balloon pump or left ventricular assist device. The timing of listing such patients for (or proceeding with) cardiac transplantation is problematic, since the survival of patients with active lymphocytic myocarditis following cardiac transplantation is generally less good than the survival of patients undergoing cardiac transplantation for other reasons (Fig. 6–11).[159] The inferior survival in

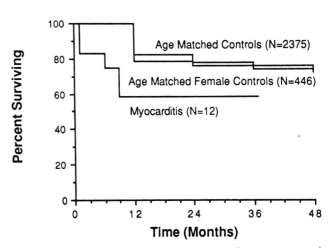

FIGURE **6-11.** Actuarial survival in heart transplant recipients with lymphocytic myocarditis compared with patients undergoing cardiac transplantation for other reasons (controls) ($p = .0014$). (From O'Connell JB, Dec W, Goldenberg IF, Starling RC, Madge GH, Augustine SM, Costanzo-Nordin MR, Hess ML, Hosenpud JD, Icenogl TB, Menlove RL, Billingham ME: Results of heart transplantation for active lymphocyte myocarditis. J Heart Lung Transplant 1990;9:351.)

patients with myocarditis is partly explained by a higher probability of acute cardiac rejection compared to other transplant patients. Furthermore, recovery of native ventricular function may occur after a period of circulatory support, without the need for transplantation.

Recommendations

In patients with suspected acute myocarditis who progress to circulatory failure, endomyocardial biopsy should be performed. If active myocarditis is found, a trial of immunosuppressive therapy appears warranted. In patients who require mechanical assistance for profound circulatory failure, cardiac transplantation in these patients should probably be delayed until there is endomyocardial biopsy proven inactivity of the inflammatory process. Furthermore, there is still the small possibility that ventricular function may improve and the assist device could subsequently be removed.

GIANT CELL MYOCARDITIS

Giant cell myocarditis (GCM) is a particularly lethal form of active myocarditis, typically affecting young adults between the ages of 20 and 45 years. The histopathological hallmarks are diffuse myocardial necrosis and an intramyocardial inflammatory infiltrate which contains multinucleated giant cells.[225] A number of systemic disorders may rarely be associated with giant cell myocarditis, including autoimmune diseases, granulomatous diseases (such as sarcoidosis and Wegener's granulomatosis), infectious diseases (such as tuberculosis, cryptococcosis, syphilis, and leprosy), tumors (thymoma and lymphoma), and hypersensitivity reactions.[47] In most cases, an underlying systemic disorder is never identified. Some studies suggest an autoimmune etiology mediated by $CD4^+$ T-cells.[48] The myocardium is infiltrated by T-cells and histocytes, but there is usually no other evidence of autoimmune disease.

Clinical Course, Therapy, and Prognosis

The clinical presentation appears to be of two general types: (1) patients with stable heart failure and dilated cardiomyopathy and (2) patients who present with sudden-onset heart failure and rapid decompensation, frequently with cardiogenic shock. The overall clinical course of patients with GCM appears to be significantly worse than that associated with viral myocarditis, with the development of rapid hemodynamic deterioration, ventricular arrhythmias and high-degree atrioventricular block, and sudden death.[47, 52] With rare exceptions,[139] the disease is poorly responsive to immunosuppression.[47, 140] However, in one multicenter study, the combination of cyclosporine, azathioprine, and steroids was associated with an improvement in median survival from 3.0 months (without therapy) to 12 months (with therapy).[48] Still, the prognosis is particularly poor with giant cell myocarditis, with only about 25% of patients surviving 1 year, compared to about 75% in the more common lymphocytic myocarditis.[48, 110]

Results of Cardiac Transplantation

The reported survival after cardiac transplantation is limited by small numbers,[25, 47, 85, 113, 153] but in a multi-institutional study of 34 patients, 30-day survival was 85% with 3-year survival of 70%,[48] similar to survival after cardiac transplantation for other conditions. It has been established that recurrence of giant cell myocarditis can be demonstrated in the transplanted heart (by endomyocardial biopsy) in about 25% of patients, can occasionally be associated with cardiac decompensation, but usually improves with augmented immunosuppression. It remains unresolved whether giant cell myocarditis is associated with greater rejection frequency following transplantation, or whether recurrence of myocarditis in the transplanted heart is reduced by administration of immunosuppressive therapy from the time of diagnosis (prior to transplantation).

Recommendation

Because of the lethal nature of giant cell myocarditis, cardiac transplantation is advisable for this entity in the presence of acute cardiac decompensation (often with ventricular assist support) and if severe heart failure persists after initial stabilization.

HEPATITIS C

The natural history of hepatitis C virus (HCV) infection in cardiac transplant recipients is largely unknown (see discussion in Chapter 15), but it does appear that in the majority of heart transplant recipients who are hepatitis C positive the likelihood of subsequent liver disease is relatively low, with a latent period usually greater than 5 years. Given the variability in response to therapy, depending on genotype and viral load (see Chapter 15), additional studies are required to characterize patient subsets who have a favorable outcome after cardiac transplantation.

Therapy in the Presence of Heart Failure

Currently, the most effective therapy for hepatitis C is a combination of ribovirin and interferon. Unfortunately, in patients with advanced heart failure awaiting transplantation, ribovirin may not be safe, since it is known to cause important hemolytic anemia and occasionally bone marrow suppression. The fall in hematocrit, which may frequently be 10 points or more, could induce an important worsening of heart failure symptoms. Interferon is known to generally stimulate the immune system and following transplantation may induce acute rejection.

Outcome After Transplantation

The Cardiac Transplant Research Database[118] examined the outcome of HCV-positive recipients who underwent cardiac transplantation. Among 3,084 patients undergoing cardiac transplantation between 1993 and 1997, only

52 (1.7%) were HCV-positive. HCV-positive serology was identified by multivariable analysis ($p = .03$) for both urgent and stable recipients to be a risk factor for a death within the first 4 years following transplantation. Survival at 6 months was 76% in HCV-positive recipients versus 89% for HCV-negative recipients ($p = .02$). The most common cause of death was infection, raising the possibility that HCV may have an adverse effect on resistance to infection in the presence of immunosuppression. However, no information is available from that analysis about patient subsets with a more favorable prognosis; for example, those patients with more favorable genotypes and/or low viral load.

More relevant current information may be derived from the experience in liver transplantation. Gane and colleagues examined the long-term outcome of hepatitis C infection after liver transplantation in a multi-institutional study.[77] Viremia after transplantation persisted in greater than 95% of patients, and it is likely that the same would be true following heart transplantation. When survival was compared between patients with and without evidence of HCV infection following liver transplantation, there was no difference in survival out to 5 years. However, there was a suggestion that a survival decrement may occur between 5 and 10 years, often related to progressive cirrhosis. Of importance, patients with genotype 1B were more likely to develop progressive cirrhosis, documented in greater than 50% of such patients. The authors also noted that every attempt should be made to minimize high-dose and chronic steroids following transplantation in hepatitis C patients, since steroids are known to markedly increase viral load.

Recommendations

Many cardiac transplant programs consider hepatitis C a relative contraindication to transplantation because of its known propensity to progressively induce inflammatory changes within the liver which ultimately progress to extensive fibrosis, cirrhosis, and death. The time course is usually measured in terms of decades, but may be greatly accelerated in the presence of chronic immunosuppression. However, based on studies in liver transplantation, we believe that selected patients positive for hepatitis C could be selected for cardiac transplantation.

A positive hepatitis C serology indicates only the presence of circulating antiviral antibody (which does not confer immunity against hepatitis C infection). Such patients being evaluated for heart transplantation should have a quantitative HCV determination by polymerase chain reaction (PCR) to detect presence and level of circulating virus. If no virus is detected and if liver function tests are normal with minimal or no inflammation by liver biopsy, such patients may either be "cured" or have minimal active disease. In this setting, a positive hepatitis C serology should *not* be considered a contraindication to transplantation, and the expected survival following cardiac transplantation should be similar to that of other patients. Because of the effect of chronic steroids on viral replication, an effort should be made to utilize minimal steroids or steroid-free immunosuppressive protocols.

Patients with positive serology and documented circulating viral levels (typically greater than 1 million copies/mL) have active disease. All such patients should have close examination of liver function tests and a liver biopsy to document the degree of hepatic involvement. If there is no evidence of fibrosis indicating early cirrhosis, such patients should be considered for cardiac transplantation (with an expected 5-year survival similar or somewhat less than other patients). In this setting, hepatitis C should be considered a "risk factor" for decreased late survival, but we believe that such patients should be selected for transplantation if no other comorbid conditions exist that would further decrease survival and if the potential benefit in terms of survival and quality of life is sufficiently high. In this situation, the genotype should also be considered, in that genotype 1 will likely have considerably worse response to therapy and possibly worse survival than genotype 2, and this should be considered in the decision-making process.

However, if the presence of circulating virus is accompanied by abnormal liver function tests which cannot be fully explained on the basis of heart failure and/or there is evidence of cirrhosis on liver biopsy, the intermediate term outcome following cardiac transplantation would likely be poor, and cardiac transplantation is contraindicated.

DECISION AND LISTING PROCESS

In most institutions, the complex evaluation process culminates in a final review of relevant information at regularly scheduled meetings of the heart transplant team, which includes transplant and heart failure cardiologists, transplant surgeons, other physicians involved in the patient's care, transplant coordinators, and social service personnel. A final decision is made by this team regarding the appropriateness of transplantation for a given patient. If a decision is made in favor of transplantation, a donor search is initiated. Patients are "listed" for transplantation by being placed on a national computerized waiting list, which in the United States is maintained by the United Network of Organ Sharing. Listing information includes patient name, weight, weight range of acceptable donors, blood group, and whether a prospective crossmatch will be needed at the time of final donor selection. In addition, the medical urgency ("status") of the recipient is indicated for further prioritization of recipients during the selection process. The urgency status codes in the United States are listed in Chapter 9.

MANAGEMENT OF PATIENTS AWAITING TRANSPLANTATION

During the waiting period, patients should be frequently reevaluated for the stability of their heart failure symp-

TABLE 6-12	**Criteria for Reevaluation of Waiting Candidates**

Clinical criteria
- Stable fluid balance without orthopnea, elevated jugular venous pressures, or other evidence of congestion
- Stable blood pressure with systolic at least 80 mm Hg
- Stable serum sodium (usually >133 mEq/L)
- Stable renal function (blood urea nitrogen usually <50 mg/dL, creatinine <2 mg/dL)
- Absence of symptomatic ventricular arrhythmias
- Absence of frequent angina
- Absence of severe drug side effects
- Stable or improving activity level without dyspnea during self-care or 1 block exertion
- Increasing ejection fraction by echocardiogram

Exercise criteria (if initial peak oxygen consumption <14 mL/kg/min)
- Improvement in peak oxygen consumption of ≥2 mg/kg/min
- Peak oxygen consumption of ≥14 mg/kg/min

Adapted from Stevenson L, Couper G, Natterson B, Fonarow GC, Hamilton MA, Woo M, Creaser JW: Target heart failure populations for newer therapies. Circulation 1995;92(suppl II):II-174–II-181.

toms, hemodynamic performance, and exercise capacity (Table 6–12).[202] The period of highest risk for outpatients occurs during the first several months following listing,[115] and close medical surveillance is necessary during that time. Signs of worsening heart failure or heart failure complications should prompt hospital admission for intense evaluation and therapy (Table 6–13). The seriousness of the heart failure condition in such patients is underscored by the fact that in most countries 10–30% of listed patients will die on the waiting list prior to cardiac transplantation.

Among stable patients waiting out of hospital, the greatest risk appears to be a sudden unexpected fatal event, usually cardiac in origin.[207] In a study of stable patients awaiting transplantation in the Cardiac Transplant Research Database (CTRD), death prior to transplantation was caused by a sudden out-of-hospital event

TABLE 6-13	**Frequent Indications for Admission of Waiting Candidates**

General Considerations
  To prevent death at home
  To prevent conditions which jeopardize perioperative outcome
Specific Considerations
  Unstable angina
  Syncope
  Frequent implantable cardioverter defibrillatory discharges
  Suspected embolic event
  Congestion refractory (Class IV) despite good compliance to increased diuretics, which:
    (a) renders patients bedridden
    (b) causes marked hepatic congestion
    (c) may worsen borderline pulmonary hypertension
  Systolic blood pressure persistently <80 mm Hg
  Pulse pressure <12 mm Hg, particularly with cool extremities
  Creatinine >2.0 mg/dL
  Clinical evidence of severe or progressive low cardiac output
  Clinical or catheterization evidence of severe pulmonary hypertension (pulmonary artery systolic >60 mm Hg)

Modified from Stevenson L, Couper G, Natterson B, Fonarow GC, Hamilton MA, Woo M, Creaser JW: Target heart failure populations for newer therapies. Circulation 1995;92(suppl II):II-174–II-181.

in 64% of deaths, of which nearly 90% were attributed to a cardiac event.[144] Patients with ischemic cardiomyopathy, higher right atrial pressure (more severe right ventricular failure), and lower ejection fraction were at greater risk for sudden cardiac death. For example, a patient with ischemic cardiomyopathy, ejection fraction less than 0.15, and right atrial pressure greater than 18 mm Hg at listing had greater than 50% chance of sudden unexpected death within a year of listing without transplantation[144] (Fig. 6–12). In a related analysis from the CTRD, patients listed for cardiac transplantation as stable outpatients (Status II) had a greater risk of death or deterioration to urgent status while waiting if they had one or more of the following risk factors: NYHA Class IV and/or inotropic support at listing, higher capillary wedge pressure, higher creatinine, or a diagnosis of ischemic cardiomyopathy.[115] The multivariable model predicted a 50% chance of deterioration or death within 1 year (without transplantation) if the patient at listing had ischemic cardiomyopathy with a wedge pressure more than 25 mm Hg and serum creatinine greater than 1.5 mg/dL. If the patient subset described above was on inotropic support at listing, the risk of deterioration or death within 1 year increased to 90%. The relationship between these risk factors is depicted in Figures 6–13 and 6–14. These subsets of patients merit close surveillance and a low threshold for hospitalization while waiting. For patients with a history of arrhythmic events, an implantable cardioverter defibrillator reduces the risk of sudden death[23] and should be considered for such patients at the time of listing.

Of course, patients also can improve significantly while awaiting cardiac transplantation and receiving medical therapy. Repeat echocardiography, metabolic

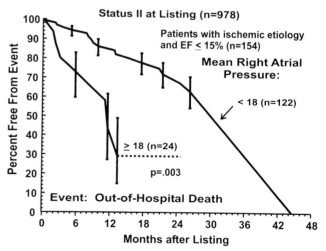

FIGURE **6–12.** Stratified actuarial of freedom from sudden unexpected death in nonurgent (Status II) patients awaiting cardiac transplantation (n = 978) between 1/1/92 and 6/30/94 in the Cardiac Transplant Research Database. Among the 154 patients with ischemic etiology and ejection fraction (EF) <0.15 (high-risk indicators by multivariable analysis), further risk was stratified by right atrial pressure at listing. (From Moriguchi J, Kirklin JK, Stevenson L, Boehmer J, Mullen G, Smart F, Rodeheffer R: Risk factors for sudden unexpected death in non-urgent [status II] patients awaiting cardiac transplantation [abstract]. J Heart Lung Transplant 1997;16:42.)

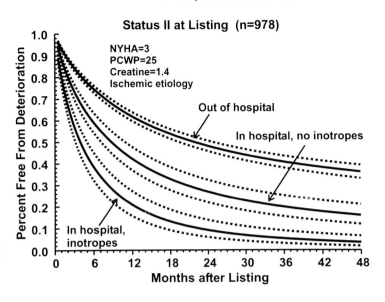

FIGURE **6-13.** Solution (nomogram) of the multivariable analysis for death or deterioration to urgent status in 978 patients listed as nonurgent (Status II) status in the Cardiac Transplant Research Database between 1/1/92 and 6/30/94. The plot depicts freedom from death or deterioration over time (since listing) for patients out of hospital at time of listing, those in-hospital on no inotropes, and those in-hospital on inotropes. The dashed lines indicate the 70% confidence limits. Other risk factors from the multivariable equation have been assigned a value as indicated on the plot. (From Kubo S, Stevenson L, Miller L, Kobashigawa J, Kenzora J, Torre G, Tolman D, Naftel D, Bourge R, Kirklin J, and the Cardiac Transplant Research Databsae (CTRD): Outcomes in non-urgent patients [status II] awaiging transplantation: risk factors for death or deterioration to stauts I urgent status [abstract]. J Heart Lung Transplant 1997;16:42.)

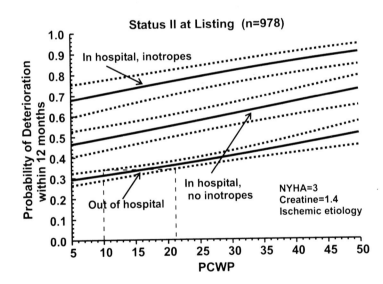

FIGURE **6-14.** Nomogram from the multivariable analysis described in Figure 6–13, in which the vertical axis is the probability of death or deterioration within 12 months, and the horizontal axis is the pulmonary capillary wedge pressure (PCWP) at listing. The vertical dashed lines indicate the value for PCWP at which a significant increase in risk occurred compared to a PCWP of 10 at listing for out-of-hospital patients.

exercise testing, and, probably, right heart catheterization are warranted every 6 months while waiting in the outpatient category. If substantive improvement occurs and a patient no longer meets the aforementioned criteria for heart transplantation, he or she should be placed in the deactivated status, but still followed compulsively.

References

1. Aaronson KD, Mancini D: Is percentage of predicted maximal exercise oxygen consumption a better predictor of survival than peak exercise oxygen consumption for patients with severe heart failure? J Heart Lung Transplant 1995;14:981–989.
2. Aaronson KD, Schwartz JS, Chen T, Wong K, Goin JE, Mancini DM: Development and prospective validation of a clinical index to predict survival in ambulatory patients referred for cardiac transplantation. Circulation 1997;95:2660–2667.
3. Adams A: Pulmonary function in the mechanically ventilated patient. Respir Care Clin North Am 1997;3:309–331.
4. Ahmed SS, Rozefort R, Taclob LT, Brancato RW: Development of ventricular aneurysm in cardiac sarcoidosis. Angiology 1977; 28:323.
5. Al-Rawas OA, Carter R, Stevenson RD, Naik SK, Wheatley DJ: The time course of pulmonary transfer factor changes following heart transplantation [abstract]. Eur Cardiothorac Surg 1997; 12:471–479.
6. Al-Rawas OA, Carter R, Stevenson RD, Naik SK, Wheatley DJ: The alveolar-capillary membrane diffusing capacity and the pulmonary capillary blood volume in heart transplant candidates. Heart 2000;83:156–160.
7. Alderman EL, Fisher LD, Litwin P, Kaiser GC, Myers WO, Maynard C, Levine F, Schloss M: Results of coronary artery surgery in patients with poor left ventricular function (CASS). Circulation 1983;68:785–795.
8. American Heart Association. Heart and Stroke Facts: 1996 Statistical Supplement. Statistical Supplement 1996.
9. Andreas S, Hagenah G, Moller C, Werner GS, Kreuzer H: Cheyne-Stokes respiration and prognosis in congestive heart failure. Am J Cardiol 1996;78:1260–1264.
10. Aretz HT, Billingham ME, Edwards WD: Myocarditis—a histopathologic definition and classification. Am J Cardiovasc Pathol 1986;1:3.
11. Astrand P: Human physical fitness with special reference to sex and age. Physiol Rev 1956;36(suppl):307–335.
12. Bain VG, Kneteman N, Brown NE: Sarcoidosis, liver transplantation and cyclosporine. Ann Intern Med 1993;119:1148.
13. Barbers RG: Lung transplantation in interstitial lung disease. Curr Opin Pulm Med 1995;1:401.
14. Barbers RG: Role of transplantation (lung, liver and heart) in sarcoidosis. Clin Chest Med 1997;18:865.
15. Baron O, Trochu JN, Treilhaud M, alHabash O, Remadi JP, Petit T, Duveau D, Despins P, Michaud JL: Cardiac transplantation in patients over 60 years of age [abstract]. Transplant Proc 1999; 31:75–78.
16. Beanlands RS, Dawood F, Wen WH, McLaughlin PR, Butany J, D'Amati G: Are the kinetics of technetium-99m methoxyisobutyl isonitrile affected by cell metabolism and viability? Circulation 1990;82:1802–1814.
17. Behrendt DM: Use and misuse of the ejection fraction. Ann Thorac Surg 1995;60:1166–1168.
18. Bjortuft O, Foerster A: Single lung transplantation as treatment for end-stage pulmonary sarcoidosis: recurrence of sarcoidosis in two different lung allografts in one patient. J Heart Lung Transplant 1994;13:24.
19. Bonow RO, Dilsizian V, Cuocolo A, Bacharach SL: Identification of viable myocardium in patients with chronic coronary artery disease and left ventricular dysfunction: comparison of thallium scintigraphy with reinjection and PET imaging with 18F-fluorodeoxyglucose. Circulation 1991;83:26–37.
20. Bourassa M, Guerne O, Bangdiwala S: Natural history and patterns of current practice in heart failure. J Am Coll Cardiol 1993;22(suppl A):14A–19A.
21. Bourge RC: Cardiac transplantation. In Bennett JC, Plum F (eds): Cecil Textbook of Medicine. Philadelphia: WB Saunders, 1996, pp 1–26.
22. Bourge RC, Kirklin JK, Naftel D, White C, Mason DA, Epstein AE: Analysis and predictors of pulmonary vascular resistance after cardiac transplantation. J Thorac Cardiovasc Surg 1991; 101:432–445.
23. Bourge RC, Stevenson L, Naftel D, Hobbs RE, Boehmer J, Hamilton MA, Kubo S, Kenzora JL, Smart F, Kirklin JK: Death awaiting cardiac transplantation: impact of the implantable cardioverter defibrillator [abstract]. J Heart Lung Transplant 1998;17:61.
24. Braith RW, Limacher MR, Mills RM, Leggett SH, Polock ML, Staples ED: Exercise-induced hypoxemia in heart transplant recipients [abstract]. J Am Coll Cardiol 1993;22:768–776.
25. Briganti E, Esmore DS, Fedeerman J, Bergin P: Successful heart transplantation in a patient with histopathologically proven giant cell myocarditis. J Heart Lung Transplant 1993;12:880.
26. Brown JH, Newstead CG, Jos V: Sarcoid-like granulomata in a renal transplant. Nephrol Dial Transplant 1992;7:173.
27. Bruce R, Kusumi F, Hosmer D: Maximal oxygen intake and nomographic assessment of functional aerobic impairment in cardiovascular disease. Am Heart J 1973;85:546–562.
28. Buren van M, Hene RJ, Verdonck LF, Verzijibergen FJ, Lokhorst HM: Clinical remission after syngeneic bone marrow transplantation in a patient with AL amyloidosis. Ann Intern Med 1995; 122:508–510.
29. Bussieres LM, Cardella CJ, Daly PA, David TE, Feindel CM, Rebuck AS: Relationship between preoperative pulmonary status and outcome after heart transplantation. J Heart Lung Transplant 1990;9:124–128.
30. Bussieres LM, Pflugfelder PW, Ahmad D, Taylor AW, Kostuk WJ: Evolution of resting lung function in the first year after cardiac transplantation [abstract]. Eur Respir J 1995;8:959–962.
31. Cabanes LR, Weber SN, Matran R, Regnard J, Richard MO, Degeorges ME, Lockart A: Bronchial hyperresponsiveness to methacholine in patients with impaired left ventricular function [abstract]. N Engl J Med 1989;320:1318–1322.
32. Campana C, Gavazzi A, Berzuini C: Predictors of prognosis in patients awaiting heart transplantation. J Heart Lung Transplant 1993;12:756–765.
33. Carre P, Rouquett I, Durand D: Recurrence of sarcoidosis in a human lung allograft. Transplant Proc 1995;27:1686.
34. Castro PF, Bourge RC, Foster RE: Evaluation of hibernating myocardium in patients with ischemic heart disease. Am J Med 1998;104:69–77.
35. Chacko RC, Harper RG, Gotto J, Young J: Psychiatric interview and psychometric predictors of cardiac transplant survival. Am J Psychiatry 1996;153:1607–1612.
36. Chaitman BR: Exercise stress testing. In Braunwald E (ed): Heart Disease. Philadelphia: WB Saunders, 1980, pp 153–176.
37. Chelimsky-Fallick C, Middlekauff HR, Stevenson WG, Brownfield ED, Hamilton MA, Drinkwater D, Laks H, Stevenson LW: Amiodarone therapy does not compromise subsequent heart transplantation. J Am Coll Cardiol 1992;29:1556–1561.
38. Chen JM, Michler RE: The problem of pulmonary hypertension in the potential cardiac transplant recipient. In Cooper D, Miller L, Patterson G (eds): The Transplantation and Replacement of Thoracic Organs. Lancaster: Kluwer Academic Publisher, 1996, pp 177–183.
39. Chun SK, Andy JJ, Jilly P, Curry C: Ventricular aneurysm in sarcoidosis. Chest 1975;68:392.
40. Cintron G, Johnson G, Francis G: Prognostic significance of serial changes in left ventricular ejection fraction in patients with congestive heart failure. Circulation 1993;87:17–22.
41. Cohn J, Johnson G, Shebetai R, Loeb H, Tristani F, Rector T, Smith R, Fletcher R: Ejection fraction, peak exercise oxygen consumption, cardiothoracic ratio, ventricular arrhythmias, and plasma norepinephrine as determinants of prognosis in heart failure. Circulation 1993;87(suppl VI):VI-5–VI-16.
42. Cohn J, Rector T: Prognosis of congestive heart failure and predictors of mortality. Am J Cardiol 1988;62:25A–30A.
43. Cohn JN, Archibald DG, Francis GS, Ziesch S, Franciosa JA, Harston WE, Tristani FE, Dunkman WB, Jacobs W, Flohr KH, Goldman S, Cobb FR, Shah PM, Saunders R, Fletcher RD, Loeb H, Hughes V, Baker B: Veterans Administration Cooperative

Study on Vasodilator Therapy of Heart Failure: influence of pre-randomization variables on the reduction of mortality by treatment with hydralazine and isosorbide dinitrate. Circulation 1987;75(suppl 4, pt 2):IV-49–IV-54.

44. Cohn JN, Levine TB, Olivari MT, Garberg V, Lura M, Francis GS, Simon RB, Simon ABM: Plasma norepinephrine as a guide to prognosis in patients with chronic congestive heart failure. N Engl J Med 1984;311:819–823.

45. Conner R, Hosenpud JD, Norman DJ, Pantely GA, Cobanoglu MA, Starr A: Heart transplantation for cardiac amyloidosis: successful one-year outcome despite recurrence of the disease. J Heart Lung Transplant 1988;7:165.

46. Consensus. The consensus Trial Study Group. Effects of enalapril on mortality in severe congestive heart failure: results of the Cooperative North Scandanavian Enalapril Survival Study. N Engl J Med 1987;316:1429–1435.

47. Cooper LT, Berry GJ, Rizeq M, Schroeder JS: Giant cell myocarditis. Transplant 1995;14:394.

48. Cooper LT, Berry GJ, Shabetai R, Multicenter Giant Cell Myocarditis Study Group Investigators: Idiopathic Giant-cell myocarditis—natural history and treatment. N Engl J Med 1997;336:1860–1866.

49. Costanzo MR, Augustine S, Bourge RC, Bristow M, O'Connell JB, Driscoll DJ, Rose EA: Selection and treatment of candidates for heart transplantation. Circulation 1995;92:3593–3612.

50. Costard-Jackle A, Schroeder JS, Folwer MB: The influence of preoperative patient characteristics on early and late survival following cardiac transplantation. Circulation 1991;84 (suppl 3):III-329–III-337.

51. Cueto-Garcia L, Reeder GS, Kyle RA, Wood DL, Seward JB, Naessens J, Offord KP, Greipp PR, Edwards WD, Tajik AJ: Echocardiographic findings in systemic amyloidosis: spectrum of cardiac involvement and relation to survival. J Am Coll Cardiol 1985;6:737–743.

52. Davidoff R, Palacios I, Southern J, Fallon JT, Newell J, Dec GW: Giant cell versus lymphocytic myocarditis. Circulation 1991;83: 953–961.

53. Dec GW, Fifer MA, Herrmann HC, Coca-Spofford D, Semigran MJ: Long-term outcome of enoximone therapy in patients with refractory heart failure. Am Heart J 1993;125:423–429.

54. deGroote P, Millaire A, Pigny P, Nugue O, Racadot A, Ducloux G: Plasma levels of atrial natriuretic peptide at peak exercise: A prognostic marker of cardiovascular-related death and heart transplantation in patients with moderate congestive heart failure. J Heart Lung Transplant 1997;16:956–963.

55. Deng M, Parjk JW, Roy-Chowdury R, Knieriem HJ, Reinhard U, Heinrich KW: Heart transplantation for restrictive cardiomyopathy: development of cardiac amyloidosis in preexisting monoclonal gammopathy. J Heart Lung Transplant 1992;11:139–141.

56. Dew MA, Roth LH, Thompson ME, Kormos RL, Griffith BP: Medical compliance and its predictors in the first year after heart transplantation. J Heart Lung Transplant 1996;15,631.

57. DiSalvo T, Mathier M, Semigran M, Dec G: Right ventricular ejection fraction is superior to maximum oxygen consumption in predicting event-free survival in advanced heart failure. J Am Coll Cardiol 1995;25:1143–1153.

58. DiSalvo T, Naftel D, Kasper EK, Rayburn B, Leier CV, Massin EK, Cishek MB, Yancy CW, Keck S, Aaronson KD, Kirklin J: The differing hazard of lymphoma vs. other malignancies in the curent era—a multiinstitutional study [abstract]. J Heart Lung Transplant 1998;17:70.

59. DiSalvo TG, Koelling TM, Muller-Ehmsen J, Schmidt U, Semigram MJ, Dec GW: Sex and left ventricular volume predict survival in heart transplant candidates with peak oxygen uptake between ten and fourteen milliliters per kilogram per minute. J Heart Lung Transplant 1997;16:869–877.

60. DiSalvo TG, Mathier M, Semigran MJ, Dec WG: Preserved right ventricular ejection fraction predicts exercise capacity and survival in advanced heart failure. J Am Coll Cardiol 1995;25:1143–1151.

61. DiSesa VJ, Sloss LJ, Cohn LH: Heart transplantation for intractable prosthetic valve endocarditis. J Heart Lung Transplant 1990; 9:142–143.

62. Donica SK, Paulsen AW, Simpson BR, Ramsay MA, Saunders CT, Swygert TH, Tappe J: Danger of amiodarone therapy and elevated inspired oxygen concentrations in mice. Am J Cardiol 1996;77:109–110.

63. Dreyfus GD, Duboc D, Blasco A, Vigoni F, Dubois C, Broadaty D, deLetdecker P, Bachet J, Goudot B, Guilmet D: Myocardial viability assessment in ischemic cardiomyopathy: benefits of coronary revascularization. Ann Thorac Surg 1994;57:1402–1408.

64. Dubrey S, Simms RW, Skinner M, Falk RH: Recurrence of primary (AL) amyloidosis in a transplanted heart with four year survival. Am J Cardiol 1995;76:739.

65. Eichacker PQ, Seidelman MI, Rothstein MS, Lejmtel T: Methacholine bronchial reactivity testing in patients with chronic congestive heart failure [abstract]. Chest 1988;93:336–338.

66. Ensley RD, Renlund DG: Myocarditis. *In* Willerson JT, Cohn N (eds): Cardiovascular Medicine. New York: Churchill Livingstone, 1995, p 894.

67. Faggiano P: Abnormalities of pulmonary function in congestive heart failure. Int J Cardiol 1994;44:1–8.

68. Fenoglio JJ, McAllister HA, Mullick FG: Drug related myocarditis I. Hypersensitivity myocarditis. Hum Pathol 1981;12:900.

69. Figulla HR, Rahlf G, Nieger M, Luig H, Kreuzer H: Spontaneous hemodynamic improvement or stablilization and associated biopsy findings in patients with congestive cardiomyopathy. Circulation 1985;71:1095–1104.

70. Fleming HA: Sarcoid heart disease. Br Heart J 1974;36:54.

71. Fleming HA: Cardiac sarcoidosis. Clin Dermatol 1986;4:143.

72. Fleming HA, Bailey SM: Sarcoid heart disease [abstract]. J R Coll Physicians Lond 1981;15:245–246.

73. Franclosa JA, Wilen M, Ziesche S, Cohn JN: Survival in men with severe chronic left ventricular failure due to either coronary heart disease or idiopathic dilated cardiomyopathy. Am J Cardiol 1983;51:831–836.

74. Francis GS, Cohn J, Johnson G, Rector TS, Goldman S, Simon A: Plasma norepinephrine, plasma renin activity, and congestive heart failure: relations to survival and the effects of therapy in V-HeFT II: the V-HeFT VA Cooperative Studies Group. Circulation 1993;87(suppl 6):VI-40–VI-48.

75. Franco-Cereceda A, Holm P, Brodin LA, Liska J, Larsen FF: ET-1 infusion increases systemic vascular resistance and depresses cardiac output in patients with chronic hypoxaemia and pulmonary hypertension. Scand Cardiovasc J 1999;33:151–156.

76. Frey B, Zuckerman A, Koller-Strametz J, Rodler S, Hulsmann M, Stanek B, Grimm M, Laufer G, Pacher R: Effects of continuous, long-term therapy with prostaglandin E1 preoperatively on outcome after heart transplantation [abstract]. Transplant Proc 1999;31:80–81.

77. Gane EJ, Portmann BC, Naoumov NV, Smith HM, Underhill JA, Donaldson PT, Maertens G, Williams R: Long-term outcome of hepatitis C infection after liver transplantation [abstract]. N Engl J Med 1996;334:815–20.

78. Garrett J, O'Neill H, Blake S: Constrictive pericarditis associated with sarcoidosis. Am Heart J 1984;107:394.

79. Ghosh P, Fleming HA, Gresham GA, Stovin PGI: Myocardial sarcoidosis. Br Heart J 1972;34:769.

80. Glenner GG: Amyloid deposits and amyloidosis [abstract]. N Engl J Med 1980;302:1283–1292.

81. Goodwin JF: Restrictive cardiomyopathy. *In* Willerson JT, Cohn N (eds): Cardiovascular Medicine. New York: Churchill Livingstone, 1995, p 871.

82. Grady KL, White Williams C, Naftel D, Costanzo MR, Pitts D, Rayburn B, VanBakel A, Jaski B, Bourge R, Kirklin J, and the Cardiac Transplant Research Database (CTRD): Are preoperative obesity and cachexia risk factors for post heart transplant morbidity and mortality: a multi-institutional study of preoperatiave weight-height indices [abstract]. J Heart Lung Transplant 1999; 18:750-763.

83. Greene AF, Sears SF: Psychometric assessment of cardiac transplantation candidates. J Clini Psychology Med Settings 1994;1: 135–147.

84. Greenspon AJ, Kidwell GA, Hurley W, Mannion J: Amiodarone-related postoperative adult respiratory distress syndrome [abstract]. Circulation 1991;84:407-415.

85. Gries W, Farkas D, Winters GL, Costanzo-Nordin MR: Giant cell myocarditis: first report of disease recurrence in the transplanted heart. J Heart Lung Transplant 1992;11:370.

86. Griffin BP, Shah PK, Ferguson J, Rubin SA: Incremental prognostic value of exercise hemodynamic variables in chronic congestive heart failure secondary to coronary artery disease or to dilated cardiomyopathy. Am J Cardiol 1991;67:848–853.

87. Grogan M, Redfield MM, Bailey KR: Long-term outcome of patients with biopsy proved myocarditis. Comparison with idiopathic dilated cardiomyopathy. J Am Coll Cardiol 1995;26:804–815.

88. Hall R, Hawkins PN: Cardiac transplantation for AL amyloidosis. BMJ 1994;309:1135.

89. Hammond MD, Bauer KA, Sharp JT, Rocha RD: Respiratory muscle strength in congestive heart failure. Chest 1990;98:1091–1094.

90. Hansen JE: Exercise instruments, schemes, and protocols for evaluating the dyspneic patient. Am Rev Respir Dis 1984;129:525–527.

91. Harper RG, Chacko RC, Kotik-Harper D, Young JB, Gotto J: Detection of a psychiatric diagnosis in heart transplant candidates with the Millon Behavioral Health Inventory. J Clin Psychol Med Settings 1998;5:187–197.

92. Harper RG, Chacko RC, Kotik-Harper D, Young JB, Gotto J: Self-report evaluation of health behavior, stress vulnerability, and medical outcome of heart transplant recipients. Psychosomat Med 1998;60:563–569.

93. Henry W, Laks H, Milgalter E, Drinkwater DC, Hamilton MA, Brunken RC, Stevenson LW: Ischemic cardiomyopathy. Circulation 1991;84:290–295.

94. Ho K, Anderson K, Grossman WK, Levy W: Survival after the onset of congestive heart failure in Framingham Heart Study subjects. Circulation 1993;20:301–306.

95. Hochberg MS, Parsonnet V, Gielchinsky I, Hussain SM: Coronary artery bypass grafting in patients with ejection fractions below forty percent: early and late results in 466 patients. J Thorac Cardiovasc Surg 1983;86:519–527.

96. Hosenpud JD: Restrictive cardiomyopathy. In Zpies DP, Rowlands DJ (eds): Progress in Cardiology. Philadelphia: Lea & Febiger, 1989.

97. Hosenpud JD, DeMarco T, Frazier OH, Griffith BP, Uretsky BF, Menkis AH, O'Connell JB, Olivari MT, Valantine HA: Progression of systemic disease and reduced long-term survival in patients with cardiac amyloidosis undergoing heart transplantation: followup results of a multicenter survey. Circulation 1991;84:338.

98. Hosenpud JD, Stibolt TA, Atwal K, Shelley D: Abnormal pulmonary function specifically related to congestive heart failure: comparison of patients before and after cardiac transplantation. Am J Med 1990;88:493–496.

99. Hosenpud JD, Uretsky BF, Griffith BP, O'Connell JB, Olivari MT, Valantine HA: Successful intermediate-term outcome for patients with cardiac amyloidosis undergoing heart transplantation: results of a multicenter survey. J Heart Lung Transplant 1990;9:346.

100. Isobe T, Osserman EF: Patterns of amyloidosis and their association with plasma cell dyscrasia, monoclonal immunoglobulins and Bence-Jones proteins. N Engl J Med 1974;290:473–477.

101. Jahnke AW, Leyh R, Gbuha M, Sievers HH, Bernhard A: Time course of lung function and exercise performance after heart transplantation. J Heart Lung Transplant 1994;13:412–417.

102. Javaheri S: A mechanism of central sleep apnea in patients with heart failure. N Engl J Med 1999;341:949–954.

103. Johnson BA, Duncan SR, Ohori NP, Paradis IL, Yousem SA, Grgurich WF, Dauber JH, Griffith BP: Recurrence of sarcoidosis in pulmonary allograft. Am Rev Respir Dis 1993;148:1373.

104. Jones N: Clinical Exercise Testing. Philadelphia: WB Saunders, 1988.

105. Julian DG, Szekely P: Peripartum cardiomyopathy. Prog Cardiovasc Dis 1985;27:223–240.

106. Kay GN, Epstein AE, Kirklin JK, Diethelm AG, Graybar G, Plumb VJ: Fatal postoperative amiodarone pulmonary toxicity. Am J Cardiol 1988;62:490–492.

107. Kazerooni EA, Jackson C, Cascade PN: Sarcoidosis: recurrence of primary disease in transplanted lungs. Radiology 1994;192:461.

108. Keogh AM, Baron DW, Hickie JB: Prognostic guides in patients with idiopathic or chronic dilated cardiomyopathy assessed for cardiac transplantation. Am J Cardiol 1990;65:903–908.

109. Kimmelstiel C, Goldberg RJ: Congestive heart failure in women: focus on heart failure due to coronary artery disease and diabetes. Cardiology 1990;77:71–79.

110. Kodama M, Matsumoto Y, Fujiwara M, Zhang S, Hanawa H, Itoh E, Tsuda T, Izumi T, Shibata A: Characteristics of giant cells and factors related to the formation of giant cells in myocarditis. Circ Res 1991;69:1042–1050.

111. Koelling TM, Semigran MJ, Mijller-Ehmsen J, Schmidt U, Mathier MA, Dec GW, DiSalvo TG: Left ventricular end-diastolic volume index, age, and maximum heart rate at peak exercise predict survival in patients referred for heart transplantation. J Heart Lung Transplant 1998;17:278–287.

112. Komajda M, Jais JP, Reeves B: Factors predicting mortality and idiopathic dilated cardiomyopathy. Eur Heart J 1990;11:824–831.

113. Kong G, Madden B, Spyrou N, Pomerance A, Mitchell A, Yacoub M: Response of recurrent giant cell myocarditis in a transplanted heart to intensive immunosuppression. Eur Heart J 1991;12:554.

114. Kron IL: When does one replace the heart in ischemic cardiomyopathy? Ann Thorac Surg 1993;55:581.

115. Kubo S, Stevenson L, Miller L, Kobashigawa J, Kenzora J, Torre G, Tolman D, Naftel D, Bourge R, Kirklin J, and the Cadiac Transplant Research Database (CTRD): Outcomes in non-urgent patients (status II) awaiting transplantation: risk factors for death or deterioration to status I (urgent status) [abstract]. J Heart Lung Transplant 1997;16:42.

116. Kyle RA, Greipp PR: Amyloidosis (AL) clinical and laboratory features in 229 cases. Mayo Clin Proc 1983;58:665–683.

117. Ladowski JS, Kormos RL, Uretsky BF, Griffith BP, Armitage JM, Hardesty RL: Heart transplantation in diabetic recipients. Transplantation 1992;49:303–305.

118. Lake KD, Smith CI, Pritzker MR, Renlond DE, Heilman JK, Smith AL, Miller LW, Weiss LT, Kirklin JK, Bourge RC, and the Cardiac Transplant Research Database (CTRD): Outcomes with hepatitis C following cardiac transplantation—a multi-institutional study [abstract]. J Heart Lung Transplant 1999;18:81.

119. LaMarache JA, Boll TJ: The neuropsychological evaluation of organ transplant patients: a review. Adv Med Psychother 1995;8:79–100.

120. Lee WH, Packer M: Prognostic importance of serum sodium concentration and its modification by converting enzyme inhibition in patients with severe chronic heart failure. Circulation 1986;73:257–267.

121. Lemery R, McGoon MD, Edwards WD: Cardiac sarcoidosis: a potentially treatable form of myocarditis. Mayo Clin Proc 1985;60:549.

122. Levenson JL, Olbrisch ME: Psychosocial evaluation of organ transplant candidates. A comparative survey of process, criteria, and outcomes in heart, liver, and kidney transplantation. Psychosomatics 1993;34:314–323.

123. Light RW, George RB: Serial pulmonary function in patients with acute heart failure. Arch Intern Med 1983;143:429–433.

124. Likoff MJ, Chandler SL, Kay HR: Clinical determinants of mortality in chronic congestive heart failure secondary to idiopathic dilated or to ischemic cardiomyopathy. Am J Cardiol 1987;59:634–638.

125. Limacher MC, Yusuf S, SOLVD: Gender differences in presentation, morbidity and mortality in the studies of left ventricular dysfunction (SOLVD): a preliminary report. In Wenger N, Sporoff L, Packard B (eds): Cardiovascular Health and Disease in Women. Greenwich: Le Jocq Communications, 1993, pp 345–348.

126. Limas CJ, Goldenberg JF, Limas C: Autoantibodies against β-adrenoceptors in human idiopathic dilated cardiomyopathy. Circ Res 1989;64:97–103.

127. Longcope WT, Freiman DG: A study of sarcoidosis: based on a combined investigation of 160 cases including 30 autopsies from the Johns Hopkins Hospital and Massachusetts General Hospital. Medicine 1952;31:1.

128. Lorell B, Alderman EL, Mason JW: Cardiac sarcoidosis. Diagnosis with endomyocardial biopsy and treatment with corticosteroids. Am J Cardiol 1978;42:143.

129. Loria KM, Salinger MH, Frohlich TG, Arentzen CE, Alexander JCJ, Anderson RW, Aaronson KD: Right lower lobectomy for pulmonary infarction before orthotopic heart transplantation. J Heart Lung Transplant 1991;10:325–328.

130. Mancini D, Coyle E, Coggan A, Beltz J, Ferraro N, Montain S, Wilson JR: Contribution of intrinsic skeletal muscle changes 31PNMR skeletal muscle metabolic abnormalities in patients with chronic heart failure. Circulation 1989;80:1338–1346.

131. Mancini D, Eisen H, Kussmaul W, Mull R, Edmunds L, Wilson J: Value of peak exercise oxygen consumption for optimal timing of cardiac transplantation in ambulatory patients with heart failure. Circulation 1991;83:778–786.

132. Mancini DM, Lamanca J, Henson D: The relation of respiratory muscle function to dyspnea in patients with heart failure. Heart Failure 1992;8:183–189.

133. Marboe CC, Fenoglio JJ: Pathology and natural history of human myocarditis. Pathol Immunopathol Res 1988;7:226.

134. Maricle RA, Hosenpud JD, Norman DJ, Pantely GA, Cobanoglu MA, Starr A: The lack of predictive value of preoperative psychologic distress for postoperative medical outcome in heart transplant recipients. J Heart Lung Transplant 1991;10:942–947.

135. Martinez FJ, Orens JB, Deeb M: Recurrence of sarcoidosis following bilateral allogeneic lung transplantation. Chest 1994;106:1597.

136. Mason JW, O'Connel JB, Herskowitz A: Clinical trial of immunosuppressive therapy for myocarditis. The Myocarditis Treatment Trial. N Engl J Med 1995;333:269–275.

137. Massey TE, Leeder RG, Rafeiro E, Brien JF: The 1994 Veylien Henderson Award of the Society of Toxicology of Canada. Can J Physiol Pharmacol 1995;73:1685.

138. Matsui Y, Iwai K, Tachibana T, Fruie T, Shigematsu N, Izumi T, Homma AH, Mikami R, Hongo O, Hiraga Y, Yamamoto M: Clinicopathological study on fatal myocardial sarcoidosis. Ann N Y Acad Sci 1976;76:251–304.

139. McFalls EO, Hosenpud JD, McAnulty JH, Kron J, Niles NR: Granulomatous myocarditis: diagnosis by endomyocardial biopsy and response to corticosteroids in two patients. Chest 1986;89:509.

140. McKeon J, Haagsman B, Bett JHN, Boyle CM: Fatal giant cell myocarditis after colectomy for ulcerative colitis. Am Heart J 1986;111:1208.

141. Mettauer B, Lampert E, Charloux A, Zhao QM, Epailly E, Oswald M, Frans A, Piquard F, Lonsdorfer J: Lung membrane diffusing capacity, heart failure, and heart transplantation. Am J Cardiol 1999;83:62–67.

142. Mieghem WV, Coolen L, Malysse I, Lacquet LM, Deneffe GJD, Demedts MGP: Amiodarone and the development of ARDS after lung surgery. Chest 1994;105:1645.

143. Miller LW, Kubo SH, Young JB, Stevenson LW, Loh E, Costanzo MR: Report of the consensus conference on candidate selection for heart transplantation—1993. J Heart Lung Transplant 1995;14:562–571.

144. Moriguchi J, Kirklin JK, Stevenson L, Boehmer J, Mullen G, Smart F, Rodeheffer R: Risk factors for sudden unexpected death in non-urgent (status II) patients awaiting cardiac transplantation [abstract]. J Heart Lung Transplant 1997;16:42.

145. Morley D, Brozena SC: Assessing risk by hemodynamic profile in patients awaiting cardiac transplantation. Am J Cardiol 1994;73:379–383.

146. Mudge GH, Goldstein S, Addonizio LJ, Caplan A, Mancini D, Levine TB, Ritsch MEJ, Stevenson LW: Twenty-fourth Bethesda conference: cardiac transplantation: task force 3: recipient guidelines/prioritization. J Am Coll Cardiol 1993;22:21–31.

147. Muller C, Briegel J, Haller M, Vogelmeier C, Bittman I, Welz A, Furst H, Dienemann H: Sarcoidosis recurrence following lung transplantation. Transplantation 1996;61:1117.

148. Munoz E, Longquist JLRB, Baldwin RT, Fort S, Duncan JM, Frazier OH: Long-term results in diabetic patients undergoing heart transplantation. J Heart Lung Transplant 1991;11:943–949.

149. Myers J, Gullestad L, Vagelos R, Do D, Bellin D, Ross H, Fowler MB: Clinical, hemodynamic, and cardiopulmonary exercise test determinants of survival in patients referred for evaluation of heart failure. Ann Intern Med 1998;129:286–293.

150. Nagele H, Kalmar P, Rodiger W, Stubbe HM: Smoking after heart transplantation: an underestimated hazard? Eur J Cardiothorac Surg 1997;12:70–74.

151. Nagueh SF, Vaduganathan P, Ali N, Blaustein A, Verani MS, Winters WL: Identification of hibernating myocardium: comparative accuracy of myocardial contrast echocardiography, rest-redistribution thallium-201 tomography and dobutamine echocardiography. J Am Coll Cardiol 1997;29:985–993.

152. Naum CC, Sciurba FC, Rogers RM: Pulmonary function abnormalities in chronic severe cardiomyopathy preceding cardiac transplantation. Am Rev Respir Dis 1992;145:1334–1338.

153. Nieminen MS, Salminen US, Taskinen E, Heikkila P, Partanen J: Treatment of serious heart failure by transplantation in giant cell myocarditis diagnosed by endomyocardial biopsy. J Heart Lung Transplant 1994;13:543.

154. Niset G, Sciurba FC, Rogers RB: Pulmonary function abnormalities in chronic severe cardiomyopathy preceding cardiac transplantation. Eur Respir J 1993;6:1197–1201.

155. O'Connell JAB, Gunnar RM, Evans RW, Fricker FJ: Task force 1: organization of heart transplantation in the U.S. J Am Coll Cardiol 1993;22:8.

156. O'Connell JB, Bourge RC, Costanzo-Nordin MR, Driscoll DJ, Morgan JP, Rose EA, Uretsky BF: Cardiac transplantation: recipient selection, donor procurement, and medical followup; a statement for health professionals from the Committee on Cardiac Transplantation of the Council on Clinical Cardiology. Circulation 1992;86:1061–1079.

157. O'Connell JB, Bristow MR: Economic impact of heart failure in the United States: time for a different approach. J Heart Lung Transplant 1994;13(suppl):S107–S112.

158. O'Connell JB, Costanzo-Nordin MR, Subramanian R, Robinson JA, Wallis DE, Scanlon PJ, Gunnar RM: Peripartum cardiomyopathy: clinical; hemodynamic, histologic and prognostic characteristics. J Am Coll Cardiol 1986;8:52–56.

159. O'Connell JB, Dec W, Goldenberg IF, Starling RC, Mudge GH, Augustine SG, Costanzo-Nordin MR, Hess ML, Hosenpud JD, Icenogl TB, Menlove RL, Billingham ME: Results of heart transplantation for active lymphocytic myocarditis. J Heart Lung Transplant 1990;9:351.

160. O'Connell JB, Mason JW: Immunosuppressive therapy in experimental and clinical myocarditis. Pathol Immunopathol Res 1988;7:292.

161. Ohar J, Osterloh J, Ahmed N, Miller L: Diffusing capacity decreases after heart transplantation. Chest 1993;103:861.

162. Olbrisch ME, Levenson JL: Psychosocial evaluation of cardiac transplant candidates: an international survey of process, criteria and outcomes [abstract]. J Heart Lung Transplant 1991;10:948–955.

163. Oni AA, Hershberger RE, Norman DJ: Recurrence of sarcoidosis in a cardiac allograft. Control with augmented corticosteroids. J Heart Lung Transplant 1992;11:367.

164. Osada N, Chaitman BR, Miller LW, Yip D, Cishek MB, Wolford TL, Donohue TJ: Cardiopulmonary exercise testing identifies low risk patients with heart failure and severely impaired exercise capacity considered for heart transplantation. J Am Coll Cardiol 1998;31:577–582.

165. Palevsky HI, Alavi A: Gallium-67-citrate scanning in the assessment of disease activity in sarcoidosis. J Nucl Med 1992;33:751.

166. Pelosi F, Capehart J, Roberts WC: Effectiveness of cardiac transplantation for primary (AL) cardiac amyloidosis. Am J Cardiol 1997;79:532.

167. Perrone-Filardi P, Pace L, Prastaro M, Squame F, Betocchi S, Soricelli A: Assessment of myocardial viability in patients with chronic coronary artery disease. Circulation 1996;94:2712–2719.

168. Perry A, Vuitch F: Causes of death in patients with sarcoidosis. A morphologic study of 38 autopsies with clinicopathologic correlations. Arch Pathol Lab Med 1995;119:167.

169. Pescovitz MD, Jones HM, Cummings OW, Lumeng L, Leapman SB, Filo RS: Diffuse retroperitoneal lymphadenopathy following liver transplantation—a case of recurrent sarcoidosis. Transplantation 1995;60:393.

170. Pfeffer MA, Braunwald E, Moye LA, Basta L, Brown EJJ: Effect of captopril on mortality and morbidity in patients with left ventricular dysfunction after myocardial infarction: results of the survival and ventricular enlargement trial: the SAVE Investigators. N Engl J Med 1992;327:669–677.

171. Phipps L: Psychiatric aspects of heart transplantation. Can J Psychiatry 1991;36:563–568.

172. Pohost G: Is 31P-NMR spectroscopic imaging a viable approach to assess myocardial viability? Circulation 1995;92:9–10.

173. Primo G, Le Clerc JL, Goldstein JP, De Sme JM, Joris MP: Cardiac transplantation for the treatment of endstage ischemic cardiomyopathy. Adv Cardiol 1988;36:293–297.

174. Puri S, Baker B, Dutka DP, Oakley CM, Hughes JMB, Cleland JGF: Reduced-alveolar-capillary membrane diffusing capacity in

chronic heart failure: its pathophysiological relevance and relationship to exercise performance. Circulation 1995;91:2769–2774.

175. Puri S, Baker B, Oakley CM, Hughes JMB: Increased alveolar/capillary membrane resistance to gas transfer in patients with chronic heart failure. Br Heart J 1994;72:140–144.

176. Qureshi U, Nagueh SF, Afridi I, Vaduganathan P: Dobutamine echocardiography and quantitatiave rest-redistribution 201Tl tomography in myocadial hibernation. Relation of contractile reserve to 201Tl uptake and comparative prediction of recovery of function. Circulation 1997;95:626–635.

177. Raftery EB, Oakley CM, Goodwin JF: Acute subvalvar mitral incompetence. Lancet 1966;2:393.

178. Ragosta M, Beller GA, Watson DD, Kaul S, Gimple LW: Quantitative planar rest-redistribution TI-201 imaging in detection of myocardial viability and prediction of improvement in left ventricular function after coronary bypass surgery in patients with severely depressed left ventricular function. Circulation 1993;87:1630–1641.

179. Ravenscraft SA, Gross CR, Kubo SP: Pulmonary function after successful heart transplantation: one year follow-up. Chest 1993;103:54–58.

180. Rayburn BK, Rodeheffer RJ, Young JB, Mullen GM, Torre G, Tolman DE, Gibbons RJ, Brown RN, Bourge RC, Kirklin JK, and the Cardiac Transplant Research Database (CTRD): Prognostic value of the relative lymphocyte concentration and white blood cell count in heart failure [abstract]. J Heart Lung Transplant 1999;18:47.

181. Rehr RB, Tatum JL, Hirsch JI: Effective separation of normal, acutely ischemic, and reperfused myocardium with P-31 MR spectroscopy. Radiology 1988;168:81–89.

182. Rehr RB, Tatum JL, Hirsch JI: Reperfused viable and reperfused-infarcted myocardium: differentiation with in vivo P-31 MR spectroscopy. Radiology 1989;172:53–58.

183. Rickenbacher PR, Trindade PT, Haywood JA: Transplant candidates with severe left ventricular dysfunction managed with medical treatment: characteristics and survival. J Am Coll Cardiol 1996;27:1192–1197.

184. Robbins M, Francis G, Pashkow FJ, Snader CE, Hoercher K, Young JB, Lauer MS: Ventilatory and heart rate responses to exercise. Better predictors of heart failure mortality and peak oxygen consumption. Circulation 1999;100:2411–2417.

185. Roberts WC, McAllister HAJ, Ferrans VJ: Sarcoidosis of the heart. Am J Med 1977;63:86.

186. Rocco TP, Dilsizian V, Strauss HW, Boucher CA: Technetium-99m isonitrile myocardial uptake at rest II. Relation to clinical markers of potential viability. J Am Coll Cardiol 1989;14:1678–1684.

187. Ross J: Myocardial perfusion-contraction matching, implications for coronary heart disease and hibernation. Circulation 1991;83:1076–1083.

188. Roughton FJW, Forster FE: Relative importance of diffusion and chemical reaction rates in determining rate of exchange of gases in human lung, with special reference to true diffusing capacity of pulmonary membrane and volume of blood in the lung capillaries. J Appl Physiol 1957;11:290.

189. Saxon LA, Stevenson WG, Middlekauf HR: Predicting death from progressive heart failure secondary to ischemic or idiopathic dilated cardiomyopathy. Am J Cardiol 1993;72:62–65.

190. Schocken D, Arrieta M, Leaverton P, Ross E: Prevalence and mortality rate of congestive heart failure in the United States. J Am Coll Cardiol 1992;20:301–306.

191. Scully RF, Galdabini JJ, McNeely BU: Case records of the Massachusetts General Hospital: weekly clinicopathological exercises. N Engl J Med 1975;29:1138.

192. Shen SY, Hall-Craggs MH, Posner JN, Shabazz B: Recurrent sarcoid granulomatous nephritis and reactive tuberculin skin test in a renal transplant recipient. Am J Med 1986;80:699.

193. Siegel JL, Miller A, Brown LK, DeLuca A: Pulmonary diffusing capacity in left ventricular dysfunction. Chest 1990;98:550–553.

194. Siltzbach LE, James DG, Neville E, Turiaf J, Battesti JP, Sharma OP, Hosoda Y, Mikami R, Odaka M: Course and prognosis of sarcoidosis around the world. Am J Med 1974;57:847.

195. Silverman KJ, Hutchins GM, Bulkley BH: Cardiac sarcoid: a clinicopathologic study of 84 unselected patients with systemic sarcoidosis. Circulation 1978;58:1204.

196. Skinner M, Anderson J, Wang M, Simms R, Falk R, Jones L, Cohen A: Treatment of patients with primary amyloidosis. In Kisilevsky R, Benson MD, Frangione B, Gauldie J, Muckle TJ, Young ID (eds): Amyloid and Amyloidosis. New York: Parthenon, 1994, pp 232–234.

197. Skoufis E, McGhie AL: Radionuclide techniques for the assessment of myocardial viability. Tex Heart Inst J 1998;25:272–277.

198. Slazchic J, Massie B, Kramer B, Topic N, Tubau J: Correlates and prognostic implication of exercise capacity in chronic congestive heart failure. Am J Cardiol 1985;55:42.

199. SOLVD I: Effect of enalapril on mortality and the development of heart failure in asymptomatic patients with reduced left ventricular ejection fractions. N Engl J Med 1992;327:685–691.

200. Steimle AE, Stevenson LW, Fonarow GC, Hamilton MA, Moriguchi JD: Prediction of improvement in recent onset cardiomyopathy after referral for heart transplantation. J Am Coll Cardiol 1994;23:553–559.

201. Stein MH, Gross JM, Shulman H: A case of cardiac sarcoidosis manifested by uncontrollable ventricular tachycardia. Am J Cardiol 1962;10:864.

202. Stevenson L, Couper G, Natterson B, Fonarow GC, Hamilton MA, Woo M, Creaser JW: Target heart failure populations for newer therapies. Circulation 1995;92(suppl II):II-174–II-181.

203. Stevenson L, Steimle A, Chelimsky-Fallick C, et al: Outcomes predicted by peak oxygen consumption during evaluation of 333 patients with advanced heart failure [abstract]. Circulation 1993;88(4 pt 2):94A.

204. Stevenson LW, Fowler MB, Schroeder JS, Stevenson WG, Dracup KA: Poor survival of patients with idiopathic cardiomyopathy considered too well for transplantation. Am J Med 1987;83:871–876.

205. Stevenson LW, Fowler MB, Schroeder JS, Stevenson WG, Dracup KA, Fond V: Poor survival of patients with idiopathic cardiomyopathy considered too well for transplantation. Am J Med 1991;18:919–925.

206. Stevenson LW, Tillisch JH, Hamilton M: Importance of hemodynamic response to therapy in predicting survival with ejection less than 20% secondary to ischemic or nonischemic cardiomyopathy. Am J Cardiol 1990;66:1348–1354.

207. Stevenson WG, Middlekauff HR, Stevenson LW, Saxon LA, Woo MA, Moser D: Significance of aborted cardiac arrest and sustained ventricular tachycardia in patients referred for treatment therapy of advanced heart failure. Am Heart J 1992;124:123–130.

208. Swedberg K, Held P, Kjekshus J, Rasmussen K, Ryden L, Wedel H: Effects of the early administration of enalapril on mortality in patients with acute myocardial infarction: results of the Cooperative New Scandinavian Enalapril Survival Study II (CONSENSUS II). N Engl J Med 1992;327:678.

209. Taliercio CP, Olney BA, Lie JT: Myocarditis related to drug hypersensitivity. Mayo Clin Proc 1985;60:463.

210. Tan LB, Dickie S, McKenna WJ: Left ventricular diastolic characteristics of cardiac sarcoidosis. Am J Cardiol 1986;58:1126.

211. Unverferth DE, Majorien RD, Moeschberger ML: Factors influencing one year mortality of dilated cardiomyopathy. Am J Cardiol 1984;54:147–156.

212. Valantine HA, Tazelaar HD, Macoviak J: Cardiac sarcoidosis: response to steroids and transplantation. J Heart Lung Transplant 1987;6:244.

213. Valantine HA, Billingham ME: Recurrence of amyloid in a cardiac allograft four months after transplantation. J Heart Lung Transplant 1989;8:337.

214. Vereckei A, Blazovics A, Gyorgy I, Feher E, Toth M, Szenasi G, Zsinka A, Foldiak G, Feher J: The role of free radicals in the pathogenesis of amiodarone toxicity. J Cardiovasc Electrophysiol 1993;4:161–177.

215. Verkleeren JL, Clover MU, Bloor C, Joswig BC: Cardiac tamponade secondary to sarcoidosis. Am Heart J 1983;106:601.

216. Wasserman K, Beaver W, Whipp B: Gas exchange theory and the lactic acidosis (anaerobic) threshold. Circulation 1990;81 (suppl)II-4–II-30.

217. Wasserman K, Hansen J, Sue D, Whipp BJ: Principles of Exercise Testing and Interpretation. Philadelphia: Lea & Febiger, 1986.

218. Wasserman K, McIlroy MB: Detecting the threshold of anaerobic metabolism in cardiac patients during exercise. Am J Cardiol 1964;14:844–852.

219. Weber KT, Janicki JS: Cardiopulmonary Exercise Testing: Physiologic Principles and Clinical Applications. Philadelphia: WB Saunders, 1986.

220. Weber K, Janicki JS: Lactate production during maximal and submaximal exercise in patients with chronic heart failure. J Am Coll Cardiol 1985;6:717–724.

221. Weber K, Kinasewitz G, Janicki J, Fishman A: Oxygen utilization and ventilation during exercise in patients with congestive heart failure. Circulation 1982;65:1213–1223.

222. Weber KT, Janicki JS, McElroy PA, Reddy HA: Concepts and applications of cardiopulmonary exercise testing. Chest 1988;93:843–847.

223. Wechsler AS: Coronary artery bypass grafting in patients with an ejection fraction of twenty percent or less. J Thorac Cardiovasc Surg 1996;111:998–1000.

224. Wilson JR, Schwartz S, Sutton MJ: Prognosis in severe heart failure: relation to hemodynamic measurement and ventricular ectopic activity. J Am Coll Cardiol 1983;2:1403–1410.

225. Wilson MS, Barth RF, Baker PB, Unverferth DV, Kolibash AJ: Giant cell myocarditis. Am J Med 1985;79:647.

226. Wolff P, Kuhl U, Schultheiss HP: Laminin distribution and autoantibodies to laminin in dilated cardiomyopathy and myocarditis. Am Heart J 1989;117:1303–1309.

227. Wright RS, Levine MS, Bellamy PE: Ventilatory and diffusion abnormalities in potential heart transplant recipients. Chest 1990;98:816–820.

228. Yabe T, Mitsunami K, Inubushi T, Kinoshita M: Quantitative measurements of cardiac phosphorus metabolites in coronary artery disease by 31P magnetic resonance spectroscopy. Circulation 1995;92:23.

229. Young JB: Redevelopment of disease in cardiac allografts. Graft 1999;2:S54–S59.

230. Young JB: Prognosis in heart failure. In Hosenpud JD (ed): Congestive Heart Failure. Philadelphia: Lippincott Williams & Wilkins, 2000, pp 655–671.

231. Young JN, Yazbeck J, Esposito G, Mankad P, Townsend E, Yacoub M: The influence of acute preoperative pulmonary infarction on the results of heart transplantation. J Heart Transplant 1986;5:20–22.

232. Yusuf S: Effect of enalapril and survival in patients with reduced left ventricular ejection fraction and congestive heart failure. N Engl J Med 1991;325:293–302.

233. Zoneraich S, Gupta M, Mehta J, Zoneraich O, Wessely Z: Myocardial sarcoidosis. Chest 1974;66:452.

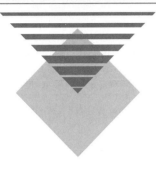

CHAPTER SEVEN

Pretransplant Immunologic Evaluation and Management

with the collaboration of
JAMES F. GEORGE, Ph.D.

The primary goals of immunologic evaluation prior to cardiac transplantation are the identification of individual potential recipients who have circulating anti-HLA antibodies and identification and avoidance of donor–recipient combinations which would carry an important risk of hyperacute or accelerated acute rejection. In this chapter we will review the immunologic basis for donor selection, the techniques involved in immunologic pretransplant evaluation, and the interpretation of these immunologic tests.

HISTORICAL NOTES

Experiments with tumor transplantation in the 1920s had clearly shown that there is a genetic basis for the acceptance and rejection of transplanted tumors in mice.[75, 81] When Sir Peter Medawar showed that allograft rejection was due to an immunologic response, the relationship between the genetic locus that controlled tumor rejection and the rejection of allografts was established.[26, 49] The observations of Terasaki[85] and Kismeyer-Nielson[41] in the early 1960s established that the single most important piece of information predicting early graft loss from rejection is the lymphocytotoxic crossmatch obtained at the time of transplantation.

ABO COMPATIBILITY

The ABO blood group antigens are carbohydrate structures carried on glycoprotein and glycolipid components of cell surfaces and tissues throughout the body and, most notably, on the surface of erythrocytes. In the human heart, blood group antigens are confined to the vascular endothelium and mesothelial cells on the surface of the epicardium.[87] In individuals who lack one or more of the ABO antigens, natural antibodies against the absent antigen appear during the first 6 months of life and are present permanently thereafter.[19]

An accepted requirement for successful cardiac transplantation is identical or compatible blood groups between donor and recipient (Table 7–1). If an allograft containing A or B blood antigens on its endothelial surfaces is transplanted into a recipient who has naturally occurring anti-A or anti-B antibody, hyperacute rejection or accelerated aggressive acute rejection will likely occur. When a donor and recipient display such **ABO incompatibility,** circulating antidonor hemagglutinins

TABLE 7-1	Blood Group Combinations Suitable for Cardiac Transplantation

SUITABLE COMBINATIONS	
Recipient	
A	Can receive an O or A heart
B	Can receive an O or B heart
O	Can receive only an O heart
AB	Can receive an A, B, O, or AB heart
Donor	
A*	Can go to A or AB recipient
B	Can go to B or AB recipient
O	Can go to O, A, B, or AB recipient
AB	Can go only to AB recipient

* An unproven possibility is that A_2 donors may be less likely to produce hyperacute rejection in an ABO-incompatible recipient (see text for discussion).

rapidly bind to endothelial cells and promote platelet deposition, granulocyte activation, and thrombosis, resulting in hyperacute rejection. Although transplantation in the presence of ABO incompatibility (donor heart A into recipient blood group B or O, B into A or O, AB into A, B, or O) would be expected to produce universal hyperacute rejection, there have been some exceptions. There is considerable variability among individuals in the level of blood group antigen expression in tissues, such as on cardiac endothelium. There also may be organ-specific differences in survival after transplantation against ABO compatibility, in that the results of liver transplantation appear somewhat more favorable than other organs.[21, 44, 64, 84] In heart transplantation, a multi-institutional survey reported hyperacute rejection in four (all within 24 hours) of eight patients transplanted with ABO-incompatible donor hearts (most of which were errors in blood type reporting). Of note, two of three long-term survivors had donor blood group A in which the subtype (A_1 or A_2) was not indicated.[14]

A specific exception to ABO incompatibility in transplantation may be donors of A_2 blood group. Blood group A contains subgroups A_1 and A_2. Subgroup A_1 acts like blood group A in its propensity for producing hyperacute rejection when transplanted into an ABO-incompatible recipient. However, donor subgroup A_2 may be less prone to producing hyperacute rejection, since the A_2 antigen is not readily displayed on the endothelial surfaces of the heart. Skin grafts from A_2 donors are not hyperacutely rejected when transplanted into B or O recipients.[9] A clinical trial of A_2 kidneys transplanted into O recipients produced graft outcome similar to ABO-compatible transplants.[5, 6] The mechanism may relate in part to the two different galactosaminyl-transferases produced by A_1 and A_2 genes,[72] resulting in a qualitative difference in the type of core saccharide-based A antigens.[90]

Heart transplant recipients receiving a heart from an ABO-compatible but not identical (O into A or B or AB, A into AB or B into AB) donor have similar survival to hearts from ABO-identical donors,[31] although some studies suggest somewhat better survival with identical blood groups.

Rh GROUP

The Rh antigens are present on erythrocytes but are not significant antigens in other tissues. Although some evidence suggests that Rh-positive renal transplant recipients have a somewhat greater allograft survival than Rh negative recipients,[60] studies in heart transplantation do not support an adverse effect of transplanting against Rh compatibility.[16]

TISSUE TYPING

RATIONALE

HLA antigens play a central role in the immune response, and the HLA genes are the most polymorphic known in the human genome (see also Chapter 2). **Haplotype** refers to the set of genes on any one chromosome. Every individual has two haplotypes (one from each parent) for the genes on the short arm of chromosome 6 which code for the MHC complex. Each haplotype contains antigens determined by the HLA-A, HLA-B, HLA-C, HLA-DR, and other loci. The two haplotypes for an individual make up the HLA phenotype, which is the complete list of HLA antigens possessed by that individual.[53] Studies of kidney graft survival in the early 1970s showed that, even with the crude serological typing methods in use at that time, a substantial survival benefit could be obtained when the HLA antigens were matched between donor and recipient. These results were confirmed by progressively larger studies in Europe and the United States.[57, 59, 61] Some benefit has also been demonstrated for heart transplantation, in which the time to first rejection, and possibly the probability of rejection-related death or retransplantation, is related to the number of HLA mismatches.[32]

Some studies suggest a higher incidence of rejection with HLA-DR[17, 23, 32, 38] and HLA-DQ mismatching[92] in heart transplantation. HLA class II mismatching may worsen survival after heart–lung transplantation.[22] However, because of the time limitations imposed by the current state of cardiac preservation during organ procurement, donor hearts for transplantation are currently not selected on the basis of prospective histocompatibility testing (with its obligatory time requirement).

NOMENCLATURE

The nomenclature for HLA typing is a reflection of the large amount of polymorphism (i.e., variation in the genetic sequence of individual genes in different individuals) found in the HLA locus. For most of the era of transplantation, the expression of HLA antigens in an individual has been determined by **serologic** testing, most commonly using sera from multiparous women, in whom pregnancy-induced antibody responses are used to identify single-antigen HLA groups and their subdivisions, known as "splits" (Table 7–2), which refer to further serologically based subdivisions of a "broad" serologic specificity. Monoclonal antibodies have been produced which define splits of various HLA alleles. In such a case, two or more distinct typing sera are found to react with cells bearing a "broad" specificity.

The names of the individual alleles of the HLA locus are assigned by the World Health Organization (WHO) Nomenclature Committee for Factors of the HLA System.[4] Newly reported alleles are updated in monthly nomenclature reports in the journals *Tissue Antigens, Human Immunology,* and the *European Journal of Immunogenetics.* The appearance of the name of an HLA antigen is dependent on the method by which it is identified. Using the **cytotoxicity** method discussed below, serologically defined HLA antigens are named according to the locus (e.g., A, B, C, DR, and DQ) followed by a number (an exception is the C locus, which uses the designation Cw to avoid confusion with complement components). Therefore, each allele will bear names such as A3, A29, B44, or DR13. A standard six-antigen HLA type for a recipient could be reported as A3,29 B44,49 DR13,14. Since each individual has two alleles of each gene and each gene is codominantly expressed, they must have two antigens named for each gene. In cases where there is only one allele detectable, the patient either has an allele that cannot be detected by the panel of antisera used or both alleles are the same in each haplotype and therefore cannot be distinguished.

Since an increasing number of tissue typing laboratories are implementing **DNA-typing** methods, the transplant clinician will observe a different nomenclature. Alleles detected by molecular typing are indicated by an asterisk following the name of the locus (e.g., DRB1*0101, although the asterisk is frequently omitted in tissue typing reports). In general, the name of the individual allele is a reflection of the fact that groups of alleles defined on the basis of DNA types are grouped within a single determinant detected by serologic reagents. Therefore, the numbers following the asterisk will consist of four or more digits, in which the first two digits indicate the name of the serologically defined antigen under which the DNA type is grouped. The third and fourth digits denote the individual allele. A fifth digit denotes a structurally identical mutant of an already existing allele. Another digit may indicate a polymorphism in an intron (reflected only in the genomic DNA, but not in the expressed protein product).[53] An optional "N" is introduced to indicate an allele that is not expressed ("nonexpressed" or "null") and an "L" indicates unusual (very high or very low) levels of expression. HLA class II molecules are structurally more complicated than class I molecules. Differences in HLA-DR alleles are almost entirely determined by variations in the DR β chain (the DR α chain is nearly constant).

TABLE 7–2	Known HLA Antigens by Serologic Testing				
HLA-A	**HLA-B**		**HLA-C**	**HLA-D**	**HLA-DQ**
A1	B5	B49 (21)	Cw1	DR1	DQ1
A2	B7	B50 (21)	Cw2	DR103	DQ2
A203	B703	B51 (5)	Cw3	DR2	DQ3
A210	B8	B5102	Cw4	DR3	DQ4
A3	B12	B5103	Cw5	DR4	DQ5 (1)
A9	B13	B52 (5)	Cw6	DR5	DQ6 (1)
A10	B14	B53	Cw7	DR6	DQ7 (3)
A11	B15	B54 (22)	Cw8	DR7	DQ8 (3)
A19	B16	B55 (22)	Cw9 (w3)	DR8	DQ9 (3)
A23 (9)*	B17	B56 (22)	Cw10 (w3)	DR9	
A24 (9)	B18	B57 (17)		DR10	
A2403	B21	B58 (17)		DR11 (5)	
A25 (10)	B22	B59		DR12 (5)	
A26 (10)	B27	B60 (40)		DR13 (6)	
A28	B35	B61 (40)		DR14 (6)	
A29 (19)	B37	B62 (15)		DR1403	
A30 (19)	B38 (16)	B63 (15)		DR1404	
A31 (19)	B39 (16)	B64 (14)		DR15 (2)	
A32 (19)	B3901	B65 (14)		DR16 (2)	
A33 (19)	B3902	B67		DR17 (3)	
A34 (10)	B40	B70		DR18 (3)	
A36	B4005	B71 (70)			
A43	B41	B72 (70)		DR51	
A66 (10)	B42	B73		DR52	
A68 (28)	Bw44 (12)	B75 (15)		DR53	
A69 (28)	Bw45 (12)	B76 (15)			
A74 (19)	B46	B77 (15)			
	B47	B7801			
	B48	Bw4			
		Bw6			

* A "split" is a serologic subdivision of a specificity. In such a case, two or more distinct typing sera are found to react with cells bearing a broad specificity. Many antigens have no splits. When a split is present, the broad specificity from which it is derived is indicated in parentheses.

TABLE 7-3	**Tissue Typing by Cytotoxicity (Serologic Testing)**

- Allo-antisera (containing anti-HLA antibodies) obtained from multiparous women or other highly sensitized individuals
- Recipient lymphocytes from peripheral blood, separated into T-cells and B-cells
- Complement-dependent antibody-mediated cytotoxicity (microlymphocytotoxicity techniques) used to serologically define HLA-A, -B, -C, -DR antigens
- HLA-A, -B, -C antigen types determined from T-cells, and HLA-DR antigens determined from B-cells

Therefore, all DR alleles identified by DNA typing are labeled DRB followed by four or more digits, as noted above, indicating variations in the β chain.

DETECTION OF HLA ANTIGENS BY CYTOTOXICITY (SEROLOGIC TESTING)

The requirements of a busy transplant service dictate that the determination of HLA type be accomplished quickly and at a reasonable cost. In most solid organ transplant centers, **tissue typing is performed routinely by cytotoxicity** (Table 7–3). More complex methods (such as DNA typing) are utilized primarily for identification of HLA class II antigens when they cannot be identified by serologic testing. Microlymphocytotoxicity, or **complement-dependent cytotoxicity** (CDC) is a test originally introduced by Terasaki and McClelland[2, 50, 86] that was devised to be simple, reproducible, and require small amounts of reagents. Cells to be typed are incubated with the typing antibodies and then complement is added. If the antibodies bind to the cells, the complement will be activated, resulting in cell death, which can be measured by using a vital dye. Cells that are dead begin to lose membrane integrity, so indicator

dyes that leak into cells (trypan blue or eosin) or out of cells (carboxymethyl fluorescein diacetate) can be used to identify dead cells under a microscope. This procedure is done with a panel of antisera, containing antibodies against a wide variety of HLA antigens (typically utilizing 72 wells, each with antibodies from a different individual). The pattern of reactivity with the various antisera allows assignment of the HLA type of the cells (Fig. 7–1). Since its introduction, this test has been modified in some laboratories in order to increase the convenience, sensitivity, and specificity of the assay. This often consists of using different incubation periods, wash steps, or temperatures. Some laboratories use a second antibody (often called antiglobulin) that is specific for human antibodies.[24, 34, 54] The addition of this reagent allows the use of antisera that do not fix complement. Ultimately, the quality of the test relies on the quality of the antisera, often derived from multiparous women or other highly sensitized patients, and the complement, which is usually derived from rabbit sera. The primary disadvantages of this method are: (1) some alleles will not be identified because the relevant antisera were not included in the test, and (2) the antisera that bind more than one HLA antigen complicate the interpretation of the results, sometimes leading to interlaboratory variation.

The cross-reactivity of many antisera has been characterized, leading to their classification into crossreacting antigen groups (CREGs).[66] In contrast to monospecific antisera, which bind to **private** antigenic epitopes (antigenic structures produced by a single HLA allele and defined by reactivity with an antibody that does not react with any other member of the same CREG), crossreactive antisera are believed to bind to **public** epitopes (antigenic structures shared by each member of the CREG). These public epitopes have been grouped by various schemes; one that is commonly used is presented in Table 7–4.[67]

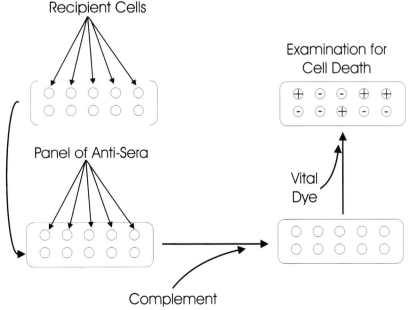

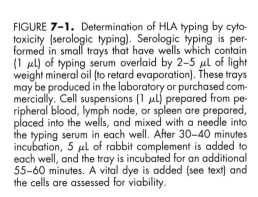

FIGURE **7–1.** Determination of HLA typing by cytotoxicity (serologic typing). Serologic typing is performed in small trays that have wells which contain (1 μL) of typing serum overlaid by 2–5 μL of light weight mineral oil (to retard evaporation). These trays may be produced in the laboratory or purchased commercially. Cell suspensions (1 μL) prepared from peripheral blood, lymph node, or spleen are prepared, placed into the wells, and mixed with a needle into the typing serum in each well. After 30–40 minutes incubation, 5 μL of rabbit complement is added to each well, and the tray is incubated for an additional 55–60 minutes. A vital dye is added (see text) and the cells are assessed for viability.

Recipient Cells

Examination for Cell Death

Panel of Anti-Sera

Vital Dye

Complement

TABLE 7-4	Frequencies and Composition of Cross-Reacting Groups (CREGS)	

CREG	ASSOCIATED PRIVATE* EPITOPES
1C	A1, 3, 36, 23, 24, 25, 26, 11, 28, 29, 30, 31, 32, 33, 34
2C	A2, 28, 23, 24, B57, 58
5C	B51, 52, 62, 63, 57, 58, 18, 35, 53, 71, 72
7C	B7, 13, 27, 54, 55, 56, 60, 61, 41, 42, 47, 48
8C	B8, 63, 64, 18, 38, 39
12C	B44, 45, 49, 50, 13, 60, 61, 41
4C (Bw4)	A23, 24, 25, 32, B13, 27, 37, 38, 44, 47, 49, 51, 52, 53, 57, 58, 59, 63, 77
6C	B7, 8, 18, 35, 39, 41, 42, 45, 46, 48, 50, 54, 55, 56, 60, 61, 62, 64, 65, 71, 72, 73, Cw1, w3, w7

* See text for definition. Splits of broader antigens are included. The broader antigens are not listed in this table, but are indicated in Table 7–2.

DNA TYPING

The advent of polymerase chain reaction (PCR) (see Box) technology as a routine technique has revolutionized tissue typing because it allows the identification of HLA alleles based on the nucleotide sequence of the genes in a relatively simple and reproducible fashion, without the need to clone and sequence individual genes. DNA typing can provide the highest level of accuracy and resolution because the genetic sequence is the ultimate determinant of expression of the HLA antigen on the cell surface. While commonly used in bone marrow transplantation, this technique has not yet become standard practice in solid organ transplantation. Instead, it is generally reserved for patients in whom determination of class II antigens is not possible by serologic methods. The polymerase chain reaction, as shown in Figure 7–2, is a technique in which a specific sequence of DNA can be amplified (increased in quantity by multiple orders of magnitude) from as little as a single cell to quantities amenable to analysis with standard molecular biology techniques.[52, 71] The exquisite specificity of PCR allows its use as a means of identification of alleles present in a given preparation of DNA. DNA typing can be done with low resolution in which the first two digits of an allele are assigned and is the equivalent of a high-quality serologic typing. High-resolution typing can assign all four digits of an allele and will distinguish greater than 90% of alleles.

This technology has been highly useful in situations where the amount of template is very small, such as endomyocardial biopsy specimens, or when a high degree of specificity is necessary, such as the evaluation of the presence of genetic polymorphisms that result from point mutations. The latter characteristic has proven to be particularly useful for DNA typing, which can require the identification of small sections of DNA that vary by only one or a few base pairs. The other advantage is that PCR is relatively simple to perform once the appropriate amplification conditions are determined. When the appropriate controls are used and precautions are taken, PCR can be relatively inexpensive and highly reproducible.

The standard method of PCR for HLA typing is **sequence specific PCR (PCR-SSP)**. This system is based

The Polymerase Chain Reaction (PCR)

The PCR is a technique that revolutionized molecular biology during the late 1980s.[52, 71] With this technique, a specific DNA sequence can be identified and amplified, cheaply and easily, in numbers by six or more orders of magnitude. The routine performance of PCR requires a thermostable (able to withstand high temperatures) DNA polymerase that catalyzes the extension of a new DNA strand that was begun by hybridization of a primer (small strands of artificially synthesized DNA ranging in length from approximately 12–30 base pairs) to the template DNA. This makes it possible to perform PCR without destroying the enzyme each time the temperature is raised to denature the two strands of DNA. The widespread clinical application of PCR is dependent on the adaptation of thermostable DNA-polymerases, like Taq-polymerase, and the development of programmable thermocyclers that can cycle the temperatures in the reactions automatically. Taq-polymerase was originally isolated from a thermophilic species of bacteria called *Thermis aquaticus* (hence the name Taq), first isolated from natural hot springs. A PCR cycle begins with template, which can be DNA isolated from a patient sample in quantities ranging from one molecule to several micrograms. The DNA is heated until the two strands dissociate, thereby providing a substrate that can be used for the synthesis of new strands of DNA (denaturation). The specific genetic sequence is identified by primers. Two primers bear sequences that are complementary to two regions of the gene (spaced by a convenient distance). The temperature is then lowered to provide conditions (which can be determined theoretically and then tested empirically) that are optimal for the hybridization of the primers to the complementary sequences on the template DNA. Following hybridization, the temperature is raised again, usually to 72°C.[10, 36, 42] During the extension process, new bases are added to the end of the primers, extending the DNA as far as the template allows. This completes a cycle that results in the doubling of the amount of DNA from a specific area of the original template DNA. To double the amount of DNA again, one only needs to repeat the cycle. Repeating the cycle is simple because a thermostable DNA polymerase is used to synthesize the new DNA and it is therefore not necessary to add more enzymes at the end of each cycle. In the second cycle, the new DNA strands are separated from the old ones by denaturation. The temperature is lowered so that the primers can hybridize to the template once again. Thus, in the ideal case, the amount of template DNA is increased by 2^n, where n is the number of cycles that the PCR is run. Therefore, assuming 100% efficiency, every 10 cycles results in an increase in the amount of DNA by 3 orders of magnitude.

on the fact that PCR can be highly specific. Amplification of a given stretch of DNA will only occur if the primers contained in the reaction mix can hybridize to the template DNA from the recipient. The tendency of the primers to hybridize to a specific sequence is a function of reaction conditions (especially temperature), the concentration of magnesium ions, primer concentration, and time. By adjustment of the conditions of the reactions and the sequences of the oligonucleotides, it is possible

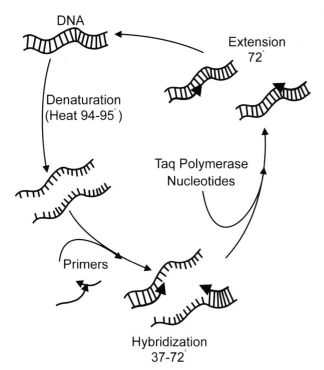

FIGURE **7-2.** The polymerase chain reaction (PCR) is a cyclic process that is usually carried out in an automatic heat block that can change temperatures according to a predefined programmable sequence. A typical PCR test begins with denaturation (separation of the two strands) of DNA at a temperature of 94°–95°C. After 30 seconds to 1 minute, the temperature is lowered to a point at which the primers can specifically bind to the complementary sequence on the template DNA strand (hybridization). After 30 seconds to 2 minutes, the temperature is raised to 72°C, which is an optimal temperature for extension of the DNA strand by *Taq* DNA polymerase. At this point, the strands are dissociated for another round by raising the temperature back to 94°C. Note that the time and temperatures given here can be highly variable.

to design a panel of PCR reactions in which a product is produced only when a particular allele is present in the test DNA. Therefore, by using a panel of reactions, each containing separate sets of primers, one can determine the presence and absence of given sets of alleles.[27,][70] A second set of primers, specific for a "housekeeping" gene that will be present in all individuals, is added at lower concentration to the reaction mix to serve as a positive control. This ensures that the absence of a product is not due to a problem in the reaction mixture (Fig. 7–3). To determine whether products were produced in the individual PCR reactions, the reaction products are separated using agarose gel electrophoresis. Visualization of a product in addition to the positive control indicates the presence of the particular allele for which the primers were specific. An additional method of PCR-based DNA typing which is less often used in clinical transplantation involves typing by sequence-specific oligonucleotide probes (PCR-SSOP), in which generic primers are used that will amplify as many different alleles as possible, and the products are detected with allele-specific oligonucleotide probes. Another method, called sequence-based typing (SBT), is a definitive method for the determination of HLA alleles because it generates the nucleotide sequence of the HLA genes.[68,][69,][73,][89] Although it is too laborious and expensive for

routine use in all clinical typing laboratories, advances in technology and instrumentation have made possible its use for individual cases where high-resolution typing is necessary, such as in bone marrow transplantation.

MIXED LYMPHOCYTE CULTURE

The mixed lymphocyte culture (MLC) is a unique *in vitro* assay because it is one of the strongest functional responses that can be elicited from unprimed T-lymphocytes in primary culture. The MLC response tests for the ability of T-cells to recognize and proliferate in response to leukocytes from another histoincompatible individual. Therefore, it is a functional measure of the cellular immune response that one individual might have for the histocompatibility antigens of another. The primary antigens that elicit the proliferative response are the HLA class II antigens, and the responder cells are CD4$^+$ T-cells (some CD8$^+$ class I specific cells can also respond). This characteristic enables the use of the MLC for class II typing. This is often done using homozygous typing cells, which are lymphoblastoid cell lines that have been immortalized by Epstein-Barr virus. These cell lines are derived from individuals who are homozygous at one or more of the class II loci. With the advent of DNA typing for HLA class II antigens, the MLC method is currently rarely used in clinical transplantation.

PANEL REACTIVE ANTIBODIES

In addition to HLA typing, another important part of the transplantation evaluation process is the routine examination of serum from a prospective transplant recipient for the presence of circulating anti-HLA antibodies, also called humoral sensitization. Sensitization is established by documenting the presence of circulating anti-HLA antibodies by the panel reactive antibody (PRA) test. The most common cause of sensitization is pregnancy.[78] Other common causes include prior blood transfusion, prior transplantation, or insertion of a ventricular assist device (see Chapter 8). Occasionally, a patient will demonstrate a positive PRA with anti-HLA antibodies and no obvious sensitizing event. These antibodies may represent cross-reactivity between bacterial or viral epitopes and HLA antigens.

CYTOTOXIC DETERMINATION OF PRA

In the cytotoxic test for PRA, the degree of humoral sensitization is estimated by the "% PRA," which is the percent of a cell panel of lymphocytes (representing the most common HLA antigens) against which the patient's serum reacts. Usually, 30–60 wells (each containing lymphocytes from a different individual) are used to represent a wide variety of HLA antigens.

To perform the cytotoxic test for PRA, the patient serum is incubated with a panel of cells of known HLA types (Fig. 7–4). Complement is added to the serum,

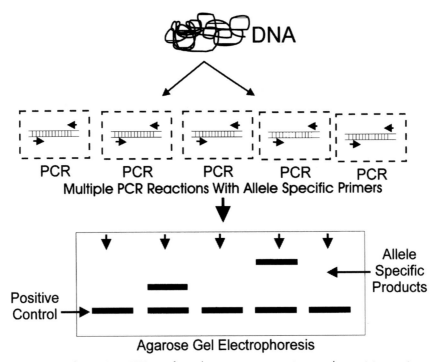

FIGURE 7–3. Sequence-specific PCR (PCR-SSP) is performed using separate reactions, each containing a unique set of oligonucleotide primers that are specific for a single allele or group of alleles. Based on the presence or absence of product after the reactions are run, one can determine the presence or absence of a given allele. In such reactions, two products, resulting from the specific allele and the positive control, are present. To separate them, the reaction products are loaded onto an agarose gel in which the products can be separated by their migration (induced by application of an electrical field) through an agarose matrix.

which, if there are antibodies reactive with the cells in the panel, will cause them to lyse. Lysis of each of the panel members is assessed using a vital dye, such as a combination of fluorescein diacetate and propidium iodide, which causes dead cells to fluoresce in a red color and live cells to fluoresce in a green color when observed under a fluorescence microscope. The PRA value is expressed as a percentage of the cell panel members (wells) that do not survive the complement treatment (i.e., the proportion of wells that are scored as "positive"). In some cases, since the HLA-type of the panel members are known, the pattern of reactivity with the cell panel members can be used to deduce the probable specificity of the panel reactive antibodies. There are several variations of the standard cytotoxic PRA. In an effort to increase the sensitivity, many laboratories add an additional antibody (anti-human globulin [AHG]) that will react with antibody from the patient serum that is bound to the test cells. This "second layer" of antibody has the effect of increasing the sensitivity of the assay in two ways. First, antihuman globulin can bind to antibodies bound to test cells and cause lysis by complement regardless of whether the antibody in the patient serum is capable of binding complement. Second, multiple anti-human globulin antibody molecules can bind a single patient anti-HLA antibody molecule, therefore increasing the likelihood of detection of the presumptive anti-HLA antibodies.

In order to determine whether the panel-reactive antibodies are primarily **IgM or IgG,** the patient serum can

be treated such that IgM is selectively degraded. The most common method of degradation is the use of reducing agents such as dithiothreitol (DTT) or dithioerythritol (DTE), which can dissociate IgM molecules selectively. An alternative method is heat inactivation, which takes advantage of the fact that IgM is more sensitive to heat denaturation than IgG. Thus, when a positive PRA is detected, the patient serum is usually treated with DTT or DTE. If the PRA value does not fall to zero, then the remaining activity can be attributed to IgG antibodies. Additional information can also be generated by using different cell subpopulations for the PRA cell panel. Many centers use purified T-cells and B-cells for cell panels.

A PRA greater than 10% is generally considered a **"positive" PRA,** in which case a prospective crossmatch is advisable at the time of transplantation. When a positive PRA is reported on a potential recipient, two additional pieces of information are critical: First, the **possibility of an autoantibody** should be excluded, and second, the **specificity of the HLA antigens** against which the patient's sera is reacting should be determined as completely as possible. Patients that show reactivity against a high percentage of the panel (high PRA) without evidence of HLA specificity are particularly likely to have autoantibodies. In the cytotoxic PRA method, autoantibodies are characterized by reactivity against the patient's own cells and are usually of the IgM isotype. Autoantibodies can be detected by performing a crossmatch against the patient's own T-cells, revealing a positive autocrossmatch. In addition, the PRA test is repeated after

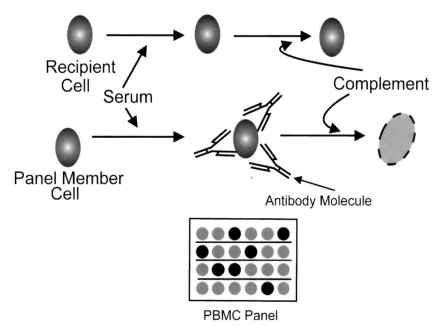

PBMC Panel

FIGURE 7–4. Panel reactive antibody testing. Serum from the recipient is incubated with autologous cells (for detection of autoantibodies and as a negative control) and with cells from a panel of donors. Cells from each cell donor are placed into separate wells, incubated with the patient serum and complement. Those wells in which lysis takes place (indicated by the dashed ring) indicate the presence of antibodies capable of binding to the cells and fixing complement. The percentage of panel members that are positive is reported as the "percent PRA." In some cases, the pattern of reactivity permits the deduction of the specificity of the antibodies detected in the PRA test. PBMC, peripheral blood mononuclear cells.

removal of IgM antibodies. The DTE-treated PRA (indicating presence of IgG antibodies only) is likely more reflective of actual anti-HLA antibody within the patient's serum[25] (Fig. 7–5). If this value is 0%, a prospective crossmatch at the time of transplantation is usually unnecessary.

The impact of sensitization (PRA > 10%) on posttransplant rejection is controversial, but several studies suggest that the presence of reactive antibodies (particularly if PRA exceeds about 25%) before transplant increases the incidence of posttransplant rejection.[45, 92]

In practice, the requirement for a prospective crossmatch at the time of transplant usually eliminates the option of long-distance procurement because of the difficulty in transporting donor blood or lymph nodes to the transplant center prior to organ harvesting. In general, transplantation is undertaken with caution in the setting of recipient anti-HLA antibodies directed against one or more HLA antigens in a donor, irrespective of the crossmatch, since persistence of antidonor antibodies after transplant predicts more severe rejection and poorer survival.[25]

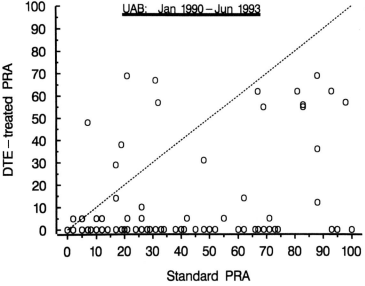

FIGURE 7–5. Scattergram of comparison between the standard panel-reactive antibody (PRA) and dithioerythritol-treated (DTE) PRA (indicating immunoglobulin G) for individual blood samples. Ninety-three percent of positive standard PRA values are zero after DTE treatment. The dashed line is the line of identity. The correlation coefficient is .43 and the p value is < .0001. (From George JF, Kirklin JK, Shroyer TW, Naftel DC, Bourge RC, McGiffin DC, White-Williams C, Noreull T: Utility of post-transplantation panel-reactive antibody measurements for the prediction of rejection frequency and survival of heart transplant recipients. J Heart Lung Transplant 1995;14:856.)

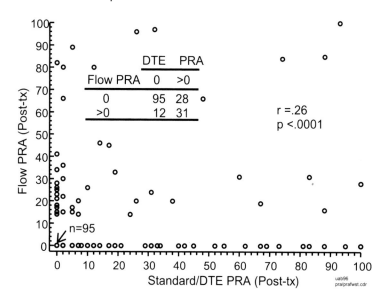

	DTE	PRA
Flow PRA	0	>0
0	95	28
>0	12	31

r =.26
p <.0001

n=95

FIGURE **7-6.** Scattergram of the relationship between flow-PRA and standard lymphocytotoxic DTE (dithioerythritol) PRA. (Unpublished data from University of Alabama at Birmingham, Division of Cardiothoracic Surgery, Birmingham, AL.)

FLOW CYTOMETRY DETERMINATION OF PRA

The lymphocytotoxic PRA is known to be less sensitive than several other more recently developed assays. Flow cytometry is an exquisitely sensitive method of de-termining PRA and is currently the preferred technique in many transplant centers. Because of the marked dif-ferences between lymphocytotoxic techniques and the methodology of flow cytometry (see Box), the correla-tion between the two methods in heart transplantation has been poor (Fig. 7–6).

 ### Methodology of Flow Cytometry

All immunofluorescence methods for the identifica-tion of cell surface antigens begin with the incuba-tion of the cells with an antibody, monoclonal or polyclonal, that is specific for the antigen of interest. This antibody may be directly conjugated to a fluorochrome, which emits light of a specific wavelength range when excited by light at another wavelength range and emits light of a specific color (usually green, yellow, or red). The presence of the antibody on the cell surface can be detected by a directly conjugated antibody that is specific for the primary antibody (Fig. 7–7).

There are a number of different methods that can be used to illuminate a cell and to detect the fluorescence that results from the presence of a fluorochrome. A standard immunofluorescence microscope illuminates the specimen with a xenon lamp. Such lamps emit light at frequencies that are optimal for the excitation of several fluorochromes, including fluorescein and rhodamine. Immunofluorescence is particularly suited for the examination of patterns of antibody binding to specific cells, since a flow cyto-meter can quantitatively measure the brightness of fluorescence of individual cells. Figure 7–8 shows a schematic of a flow cytometer with a single laser light source.

The flow cytometer can examine fluorescence at several differ-ent wavelength ranges simultaneously, and can also generate information regarding the size and internal complexity of individ-ual cells. An argon ion laser that emits blue-green light at a wave-length of 488 nm provides the excitation signal in most single-laser instruments. The light passes through a series of lenses that focus the beam through a flow cell. Cells are injected into the flow cell in a sample stream that is sheathed in fluid. As the cell passes through the flow cell, the laser beam impinges on it and

excites fluorochromes that may be present on or in the cell. At the same time, the passage of the cell in front of the laser causes the beam to scatter. Photomultiplier tubes (PMTs), which detect

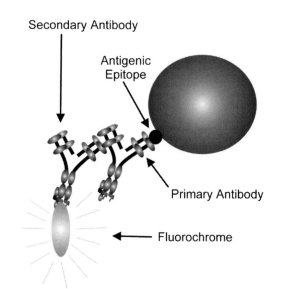

FIGURE **7-7.** Indirect immunofluorescence. Detection of an anti-genic epitope on the cell surface can be accomplished by first tagging it with an antibody (the primary antibody) that will specifically bind to the epitope. The presence of the primary antibody can be detected by another antibody that is specific for immunoglobulin light chains and is conjugated to a fluorochrome such as fluorescein, which will emit light at a wavelength of 519 nm when illuminated by an argon ion laser that emits light at 488 nm.

and amplify signals generated by individual photons (amplified light detectors), are mounted in front of and at 90 degrees relative to the path of the laser. The scattering of the light in front of the cell (called forward scatter) and to the side (called 90 degree light scatter or side scatter) can be detected by these PMTs (Fig. 7–9). The forward scatter gives an indication of cell size and the side scatter is an indication of the internal complexity or "granularity" of the cell passing through the laser beam. The light is also directed to a series of PMTs which are mounted behind light filters that selectively allow certain wavelength ranges of light to reach the PMTs. Therefore, one can easily use three or more fluorochromes if they can be excited by a single laser and each emit light at different wavelengths. Such analyses are called "three-color" or "four-color" analyses.

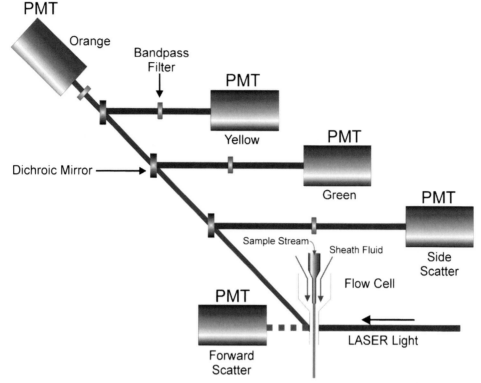

FIGURE 7–8. Schematic of the light path and major components of a flow cytometer. Cells to be analyzed are introduced into a flat sided quartz (internal dimensions are typically 100–400 μm) flow cell designed to surround the sample stream with a sheath of fluid. The sample stream proceeds through the flow cell and passes in front of a laser that illuminates the cell (e.g., lymphocyte) that is to be analyzed. Light emitted from the cell is passed through dichroic mirrors (interference filters that, in this case, allow longer wavelengths to pass, but reflect shorter wavelengths) that reflect a portion of the light to a photomultiplier tube (PMT). Band pass filters that allow through a wavelength range of light further narrow the range of the light impinging upon the PMT. In most cytometers, PMT filters are set to allow individual PMTs to detect green (510–540 nm), yellow (560–580 nm), orange (605–635 nm), and red (650 nm and above). The PMTs generate an electrical pulse that is roughly proportional to the number of photons that enters them. These pulses can be quantified in number and intensity by a computer.

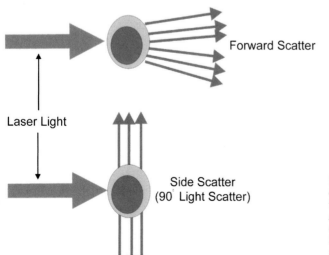

FIGURE 7–9. Forward scatter and side scatter detection in a flow cytometer. The laser light passes through the sample stream and the passage of a cell through the beam causes the light to scatter. A PMT mounted behind a mask (also called a beam stop) that lies directly in the path of the laser detects the scattered light. Another PMT, mounted at a 90-degree angle relative to the laser, detects light scattered by granular or opaque structures within the cell passing through the beam.

Although flow cytometry greatly increases the sensitivity of the PRA, this occurs at the cost of more work if a complete characterization of the specificity is required. Patient serum is incubated with a panel of test cells, which are then treated with a second antibody that is conjugated to a fluorochrome and is specific for human IgG. Performed in this fashion, a flow-cytometry PRA determination is a labor-intensive and expensive process because of the large number of samples (one for each of the panel members) which must be separately analyzed. To address this problem, many centers use a small panel of cells from 6–10 individuals and place them in a single tube containing patient serum.[11, 29, 80] This assay takes advantage of the fact that many HLA reactive antibodies possess specificities that react with a broad spectrum of CREGs (see again Table 7–4). The single tube flow cytometry PRA assay assumes that an antibody that binds to one member of a given CREG will bind to all other antigens that are a part of that same CREG. Thus, antibody that binds to HLA-A2, for example, will also bind to A28 because these two antigens belong to the same cross-reacting group.

In the past several years, the use of flow cytometry for PRA determination has been improved in convenience and consistency through the utilization of **beads coated with HLA antigens.** This has the advantage of reducing interlaboratory variation due to differences in the composition of the cell panel when live cells from individual humans are used. The test reagent consists of a pool of approximately 30 different beads, each of which is coated with purified HLA class I antigens isolated from lymphoblastoid cell lines bearing a known HLA type. Patient serum is incubated with the HLA-coated pooled beads. After they are washed, the beads are then treated with goat anti-human IgG antibody conjugated to a fluorochrome such as fluorescein. If there are anti-HLA antibodies in the patient sera that bind to beads bearing HLA antigens, the fluorescent beads will be detected by the flow cytometer. Theoretically, each 3.3% shift to the right of the negative control on a single parameter histogram represents binding to 1 of the 30 different bead preparations that have been combined into the one tube. In practice, many haplotypes are represented more than once in the panel of beads; therefore, the proportion of positive beads will often be larger for a single specificity. Note that, in the case of flow cytometry PRA, the term "percent PRA" has a somewhat different meaning than in the cytotoxic PRA. In this case, the percent PRA refers to the percentage of cells or beads that fluoresce brighter than the negative controls. How much this parameter will change when a single panel member is positive depends on the total number of panel members used in the assay. Determinations of the precise anti-HLA specificity of antibodies is made using a second set of bead preparations. These preparations consist of four groups of beads with each group containing eight different bead preparations of known HLA types. Each of the eight different beads in a group can be distinguished from other members of the group on the basis of fluorescence with a second fluorochrome. Therefore, reactivity with a specific member of a group can be identified. As in cytotoxic

PRA determinations, the specificity can then be determined by observation of the pattern of reactivity with individual panel members.

ENZYME-LINKED IMMUNOSORBENT ASSAY

The enzyme-linked immunosorbent assay (ELISA) technique is specific for IgG anti-HLA antibodies, and is based on the binding of serum immunoglobulin to specific soluble HLA class I antigens which coat the bottom of the wells of a plastic tray. As many as 96 wells may be available for examining reactivity to a large variety of anti-HLA class I antigens. This technique has the advantage over cytotoxic methods that it does not require the use of viable target cells. It is generally more sensitive than the cytotoxicity PRA and slightly less sensitive than flow cytometry. In addition, it requires less specialized equipment and is less labor intensive than flow cytometry. The interpretation of the result is less subjective than flow cytometry. A current disadvantage is that the choice of HLA antigens examined is determined by the kit rather than by expected prevalence in the anticipated donor population.

UTILIZATION OF PRA IN THE PATIENT AWAITING TRANSPLANTATION

Each patient listed for cardiac transplantation should undergo testing for PRA as a screening test for the presence of circulating anti-HLA antibodies (Table 7–5). If the PRA is 0% (no anti-HLA antibodies detected) and the patient has had no events likely to cause sensitization (development of anti-HLA antibodies), then a positive crossmatch is very unlikely. However, if there is a his-

TABLE 7–5	Management of Pretransplant PRA*	
VALUE	FURTHER TESTING	TREATMENT
0%	• Repeat PRA every 3 mo (every 1–2 mo if risk factors for sensitization)[†] • No crossmatch at transplant unless at risk for sensitization	None
>0%	• Determine IgG vs. IgM • Exclude autoantibodies or other non-HLA antibodies • Determine specificity of anti-HLA antibodies • Repeat every 1–2 mo • Crossmatch at time of transplant if anti-HLA antibodies present	None
>25%	• All of above	Consider PRA reduction therapy[†]

PRA, panel reactive antibody.
* Based on flow cytometry PRA.
† See text for details.

tory of pregnancy, prior blood transfusion, prior surgery, prior transplantation, or insertion of a mechanical assist device, PRA determinations are advisable every 1–2 months while awaiting transplantation. If a patient awaiting transplant receives a blood transfusion, the PRA should be repeated at monthly intervals for the next 6 months.

If the PRA is positive, and especially if greater than 10%, then specific tests for the presence of autoantibodies, either by cytotoxic or flow cytometry methods, are advisable. If anti-HLA antibodies are suspected, particularly if the PRA is high (> about 25%), specific lymphocytotoxic or flow cytometric methods are advisable to identify specific HLA antigens or CREGs against which antibodies are present. This may be important in decision-making regarding specific donors if the donor contains those HLA types. It is our practice to obtain formal prospective crossmatching in any patient who has a PRA exceeding 10% prior to transplantation.

MANAGEMENT OF THE SENSITIZED PATIENT

From the large experience in renal transplantation as well as heart transplantation, patients with an elevated PRA (sensitized) due to circulating anti-HLA antibodies have a greater likelihood of experiencing a positive crossmatch with a given donor than does a nonsensitized patient. The time to transplantation because of positive crossmatches becomes particularly prolonged when the PRA rises to 30–50% or higher, especially in the setting of prior pregnancies or an indwelling left ventricular assist device (see Chapter 8). Although their efficacy has not been proven, multiple modalities have been utilized prior to renal and cardiac transplantation to reduce the PRA and increase the probability of a negative crossmatch.

Multiple studies have shown that intravenous immunoglobulin (IVIG) can reduce anti-HLA alloreactivity (PRA) in patients awaiting cardiac transplantation,[30, 33, 35] including those supported with a left ventricular assist device (LVAD).[18, 33, 48] Intravenous immunoglobulin has been combined with plasmapheresis[62, 65] or cyclophosphamide.[33] In patients awaiting transplantation on LVAD support with elevated PRAs, we have utilized the protocol recommended by John and colleagues[33] in which IVIG (500 mg/kg) is administered daily for 4 days at 3-week intervals and intravenous cyclophosphamide (dose 500 mg/m^2) is administered 1 week later, also at 3-week intervals (while observing peripheral leukocyte counts). The mechanism proposed for the efficacy of cyclophosphamide is the reduction of B-cell–induced antibody production. IVIG is known to contain natural antibodies directed against interferon-γ which inhibit lymphocyte proliferation and tumor necrosis factor-α (TNF-α) secretion. It has also been postulated that the IVIG preparation may contain anti-idiotypic antibodies directed against idiotypic determinants on the anti-HLA antibodies.[28] John and colleagues[33] reported a 33% reduction in PRA within 1 week of IVIG/cyclophosphamide

therapy, though we have found the response to be highly variable among patients. We currently recommend discontinuation of this therapy if a sustained reduction in PRA is not achieved within three cycles.

Others have reported success with mycophenolate mofetil in reducing pretransplant PRA levels.[40, 74] In the report by Kimball and colleagues,[40] mycophenolate was effective in reducing human IgG anti-ATGAM in renal transplant recipients. We have found mycophenolate mofetil at a dose of 2–3 g/day in adults to be effective in reducing the PRA in some patients.

It is important to note that drawing therapeutic inferences from these studies is difficult because of the great variability in the PRA response between individuals and within the same individual from month to month, and the known tendency for the PRA to gradually decrease with time in many patients.

CROSSMATCHING

The crossmatch at the time of transplantation is typically the final test of immunologic compatibility between donor and recipient prior to making the decision to transplant. The goal of the "crossmatch" is the prevention of hyperacute rejection at the time of transplantation and accelerated severe acute rejection during the first 5–7 days after transplantation. With current crossmatch techniques, hyperacute rejection is extremely rare. The crossmatch tests the reactivity of recipient sera (with its potential anti-HLA antibodies) against donor lymphocytes obtained from peripheral blood or lymph node. In practice, a pretransplant "prospective" crossmatch is often omitted when a recent PRA is 0% because of the very low probability of hyperacute or accelerated acute rejection in that setting and because of the additional time prior to transplantation needed to obtain a crossmatch. In that instance a "retrospective" crossmatch is usually obtained in the hours following transplantation to make a final determination of the presence of antidonor antibodies. Some institutions require a crossmatch irrespective of the PRA in certain situations where sensitization is likely, such as in multiparous females,[78] patients on ventricular assist support, patients with multiple prior blood transfusions, and patients with prior transplantation. A positive complement-dependent lymphocytotoxic T-cell and B-cell crossmatch is a strong predictor of hyperacute or severe accelerated acute rejection. However, the presence of a negative cytotoxic crossmatch does not guarantee protection against hyperacute or severe early rejection. It has been hypothesized that *minimal clonal expansion* of TH1 and TH2 subsets of T-cells (see Chapter 2) plus B-cells is sufficient to produce a brief IgM (or IgM followed by IgG) response that is promptly "down-regulated," and detectable levels of IgG may not be present (thus producing a negative crossmatch).[55, 76, 77] However, with sustained stimulation following transplantation, B-cell clones expand and express increased affinity for the HLA antigen. *Significant clonal expansion* then occurs with TH1, TH2, and B-cell proliferation and the production of antibody. Serum anti-HLA antibodies become predominately IgG with sustained levels, and further antibody response is readily inducible with reexposure to even small amounts of these HLA antigens.[20]

COMPLEMENT-DEPENDENT LYMPHOCYTOTOXIC CROSSMATCH (CDC)

In the standard NIH CDC, donor lymphocytes from peripheral blood or lymph node are incubated with the patient's serum. Complement is added, and the test is read in the same manner as in cytotoxic panel reactivity assays. A rough measure of the degree of positivity is given by the percentage of donor cells killed following addition of the patient serum and complement. A crossmatch is considered positive when there is an increase in the percentage of dead cells in the test well (containing donor cells) compared to the control well. After correction for the control, 0–10% cell death is considered negative, 11–20% doubtful negative, 21–50% weakly positive, 51–80% positive, and 81–100% strongly positive. The interpretation also depends on the preparation of the donor cells. Unfractionated cell populations from peripheral blood can be used for the identification of anti-class I antibodies because T-cells (which comprise 75–85% of peripheral blood lymphocytes) express class I HLA but little class II. However, unpurified cell preparations may produce only a weakly positive reaction even in the presence of anti-class II antibodies because B-cells, which are HLA class I and class II positive, only constitute 15% of peripheral blood lymphocytes and 25% of lymph node lymphocytes. Many laboratories have avoided such complications by isolating T-cells and B-cells prior to conducting the crossmatch. A variety of isolation techniques are used, including density gradients, nylon wool columns, magnetic beads, erythrocyte rosettes, or affinity columns.

As with PRA determinations, the isotype of the antibodies causing the reaction can be determined. The lymphocytoxicity assay detects only complement fixing antibodies, either of IgM class or IgG subclasses IgG1 and IgG3. IgG subclasses IgG2 and IgG4 as well as IgA antibodies are not complement binding and therefore are not detected by this assay. IgM antibodies (less likely to be anti-HLA than the IgG antibodies) may be removed by treating the patients sera with either DTT or DTE.

A major weakness of the standard NIH CDC technique is that anti-HLA antibodies against the donor may not be detected if their concentration in peripheral blood is too low to fix enough complement to lyse the target cell membrane. Several additional methods have been utilized to increase the sensitivity of the standard NIH CDC method. The extended incubation method extends the incubation time of cells and serum from 30 minutes to 60 minutes and the incubation time for complement from 60 to 120 minutes, which increases the avidity of antibody binding and increases complement fixation. While increasing the sensitivity (ability to detect lower titers of anti-HLA antibodies), this method also increases the likelihood of a false-positive crossmatch secondary to non-HLA–mediated cytotoxicity.

The **Amos modification** increases the sensitivity of the lymphocytoxicity assay by including additional steps in which the donor-target cells are washed with cell culture media that acts to remove various anticomplementary factors from the serum and eliminate weakly bound autoantibodies,[19] both of which may contribute to a "false-negative" result with the NIH method.

The **anti-human globulin method** is a standard technique for increasing crossmatch sensitivity by a dilutional factor of 2 to 3 by adding a polyclonal anti-human immunoglobulin reagent (which itself can induce cell lysis in the presence of complement) such as anti-human kappa light chain, which crosslinks antibodies that have anti-HLA activity but are unable to fix complement.[37, 39] Thus, the AHG method detects additional anti-HLA antibodies that are present in too low concentration to be detected by the standard NIH CDC or are of a non–complement-binding isotype. Non–complement-binding anti-HLA antibodies do not induce target cell lysis through complement (but rather cause target cell death through the binding of a killer cell effector to the Fc fragment of IgG).

Autoantibodies may be detected by standard CDC crossmatch and can produce a "false-positive" crossmatch, since they do not represent anti-HLA antibodies. It is important to exclude autoantibodies as the cause of a positive crossmatch, since they are not damaging to the cardiac allograft and are not predictive of hyperacute rejection. They typically result from certain medications (such as hydralazine and procainamide), exposure to certain viral diseases, and from autoimmune diseases (such as systemic lupus erythematosis or rheumatoid arthritis). Autoantibodies are usually IgM and can therefore be removed from the patient's serum by DTT or DTE treatment. Less commonly, they may be IgG or IgA immunoglobulins. The definitive test for autoantibodies is the autocrossmatch, in which patient lymphocytes and serum are incubated together. Cell lysis indicates the presence of autoantibodies.

Since human B-cells express HLA class II antigens in addition to the class I antigens carried by both B-cells and T-cells, a **positive B- and T-cell crossmatch** implies the presence of anti-class I antibodies (or possibly anti-class I and II antibodies). The presence of a **positive B-cell crossmatch** with a negative T-cell crossmatch implies the presence of anti-class II antibodies (class II HLA antigens are not present on T-cells) and/or the presence of weak anti-class I antibodies (B cells carry HLA class I molecules in greater density than T-cells). A **positive T-cell crossmatch with a negative B-cell crossmatch** usually implies antibodies with non-HLA reactivity (which would not increase the risk of hyperacute rejection). Since class I HLA antigens are present on most nucleated cells of the body, including graft vascular endothelial cells, the presence of a positive T-cell and B-cell crossmatch (indicating the presence of anti-donor class I antibodies) is the strongest predictor of hyperacute rejection. Since class II HLA antigens are normally poorly expressed on vascular endothelium, **a positive B-cell cytotoxic crossmatch with a negative T-cell crossmatch is not predictive of hyperacute rejection.**[15, 51] However, multiple studies have shown that a positive

TABLE 7–6	Interpretation of T-Cell and B-Cell Crossmatches	
T-CELL	B-CELL	ANTIBODY SPECIFICITY
Positive	Positive	HLA class I
Positive	Negative	Non-HLA
Negative	Positive	HLA class II
Negative	Negative	None

B-cell crossmatch is a predictor of increased frequency and severity of rejection in the first 6 months after transplant.[7] The usual interpretation of T- and B-cell crossmatches is summarized in Table 7–6.

FLOW CYTOMETRY CROSSMATCH

Although the CDC crossmatch is the standard crossmatch method, it suffers the disadvantage of its inability to detect non–complement-binding antibodies which may also have anti-HLA activity and precipitate accelerated acute rejection. Furthermore, the standard complement-dependent techniques may not detect weak anti-HLA antibodies or low circulating levels of anti-HLA antibodies.

In recent years, many laboratories have employed flow cytometry for the detection of antibodies that can bind to donor cells. The flow cytometry crossmatch assay was introduced clinically by Garovoy and colleagues in 1983.[46] It is based on immunofluorescence techniques for cell identification which is more sensitive than the standard cytotoxic crossmatch and can be performed on crude cell preparations. Since multiple antibodies can be used, the assay can be extended to multiple cell types.[79] Lymphocytes can be readily distinguished from other cell types in mixed cell preparations. Using monoclonal antibodies against specific cell surface antigens, T-cells can be separated from B-cells (Table 7–7), and IgG antibodies from IgM. The comparative features of flow cytometry and lymphocytotoxicity for crossmatch determination are summarized in Table 7–8.

In a typical flow cytometry crossmatch, the donor cells are treated with patient serum, washed, and treated with two antibodies. One can be an anti-CD3 antibody, which can identify all mature T-cells, and the other can be an anti-human light chain antibody to identify human antibody (such as IgG anti-HLA antibody) that may be bound to the cells. In an analysis such as this one, the anti-CD3 antibody is typically conjugated to a dye called phycoerythrin (PE) that can be excited by laser light at a wavelength of 488 nm, but emits light at 578 nm and fluoresces yellow. Similarly, the anti-light chain antibody is typically conjugated to fluorescein isothiocyanate (FITC), which is also excited by the same wavelength laser, but emits light at a different wavelength than PE and fluoresces green. B-cells can be selectively identified by their binding with a monoclonal antibody against a surface molecule CD19, which is specific for B-cells. The monoclonal antibody is labeled with fluorescence dye molecules such as Peridinin chlorophyll protein (PerCP), which fluoresces red (675 nm) when excited by laser light at 488 nm. When the cell that passes though the flow cell has both antibodies, it emits light that can be detected by two different photomultiplier tubes that are behind the appropriate filters. The signals from the PMTs are sent to a computer, which processes the data for presentation in an understandable form.

Flow cytometry data can be plotted in a number of different ways. One of the simplest and most common ways is in the form of a dot plot, which can show staining by two different antibodies simultaneously. The results of a flow cytometry crossmatch is depicted in Figure 7–10, in which donor cells are treated with anti-CD3 conjugated to phycoerythrin and patient serum plus antihuman antibodies conjugated to fluorescein isothiocyanate. By using different combinations of fluorochromes and antibodies, one can differentiate whether T-cells or B-cells have donor antibodies on the cell surface. Such analyses can be done on any population of cells and with any combination of antibodies, provided that the fluorochrome combination can be unambiguously distinguished. Therefore, on a properly equipped flow cytometer, one can examine a cell population for five to six different parameters simultaneously. In practice, most clinical laboratories use no more than five parameters, three of which are antibodies bearing unique fluorochromes.

The **flow cytometry histogram** typically displays the fluorescence of a group of cells and is represented by a peak that depicts the distribution of cells that fluoresce at a specific intensity on the x-axis and the number of cells on the y-axis. The intensity of fluorescence is a function of the number of fluorescent dye molecules and therefore the antibody concentration on the cell surface. In Figure 7–11 the computer has been set to display data from B-cells (left panel) or T-cells (right panel), a process that is called *gating*, in which certain cell types can be examined (displayed by the computer) and analyzed by excluding or "filtering out" the "unwanted" cells. One may, for example, "gate out" dead cells by eliminating for analysis cells with certain types of scatter. One may gate out B-cells for examination of T-cells only, or vice versa, by displaying cells which fluoresce a given color (as determined by the specific surface molecule and its fluorescent tag). Such displays clearly show the distributions of cells according to the brightness at which they fluoresce with a given fluorochrome. The histograms show that both B-cells and T-

TABLE 7–7	Major T-Cell and B-Cell Antigens
T-CELLS	B-CELLS
CD2	Surface immunoglobulins*
CD3[1]	CD19*
CD4 (subset)*	CD20
CD7 (subset)	CD21 (mature)
CD8 (subset)*	CD25 (activated)
CD25 (activated)	CD39 (mature)
CD28	CD69 (activated)
CD69 (activated)	
T-cell receptor $\alpha, \beta, \gamma, \delta$ chains	

* Antigens most commonly used for identification of lineages and subsets.

TABLE 7-8   Comparison of Flow Cytometric and Lymphocytotoxic Crossmatches

	FLOW CYTOMETRY	LYMPHOCYTOTOXICITY
Sensitivity	50 × more sensitive than standard lymphocytotoxic assays; slightly more sensitive than lymphocytotoxic assays + AHG	Less sensitive
Quantitation	Fluorescence is proportional to the amount of antibody bound; can be performed on multiple dilutions	Tests must be performed on multiple dilutions
Antibodies detected	Complement and noncomplement fixing; can also detect IgM and IgG without additional assays (most commonly used clinically to detect IgG only)	Complement-fixing only; additional assays must be performed to distinguish IgG from IgM
Detection of cell types that bind antibody	Detects anti–T-cell and anti–B-cell antibodies in a single tube	Cell types must be isolated prior to running the test; multiple tests must be performed
Lab-to-lab variability	Higher	Lower

AHG, anti-human globulin.

cells from the potential donor fluoresce brightly when exposed to serum from the potential recipient and goat anti-human immunoglobulin light chain antibody conjugated to fluorescein. The peak, in this case, represents a normal distribution of cells exhibiting a mean fluorescence intensity that corresponds to the middle of the peak. A set of *negative controls* are used to determine the mean fluorescence intensity when no antibody is bound by the cell population. The light intensity generated by the dye bound to the antibodies that nonspecifically stick to the cell surface will establish the light intensity that can be considered negative. This is often established by testing 20–30 sera from unsensitized individuals. A *positive control* includes cells of a specific type (T- or B-cells) which are placed in a tube that contains fluorescent tagged antibodies that are known to react against its HLA surface antigens and therefore will cause the cell to fluoresce brightly. This is typically established by using sera from highly sensitized individuals.

A flow cytometry crossmatch can then be considered positive when the mean fluorescence intensity is 3 SD above the negative control. Depending on how the anal-

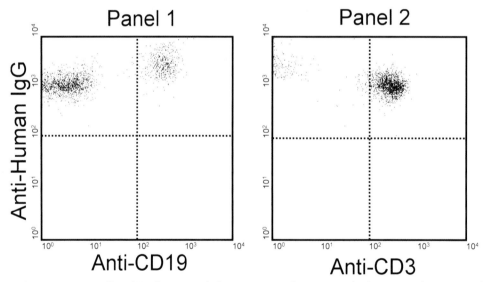

FIGURE **7-10.** A positive B-cell and T-cell crossmatch from a sensitized patient on the heart transplant waiting list. These scatterplots show the brightness of donor peripheral blood mononuclear cells that have been treated with the patient serum, anti-human IgG antibodies conjugated to fluorescein isothiocyanate (to visualize human antibodies that have been bound to the cells), anti-CD19 conjugated to phycoerythrin (to visualize B-cells), and anti-CD3-PerCP (to visualize T-cells). Each of the fluorochromes emit light in a specific wavelength range that is distinct from the other two fluorochromes. Therefore, a computer analysis of the data can distinguish individual cells (each cell is represented by one dot on the scatterplot) bearing zero, one, two, or all three of the antibodies at the same time. *Panel 1,* The two parameter scatterplot shows the brightness of cells bearing either human IgG or CD19. Therefore, since CD19 is a B-cell marker, cells in the upper right hand quadrant are B-cells bearing antibodies specific for human IgG (a positive B-cell crossmatch). A cluster of dots in the lower right hand panel would indicate a negative B-cell crossmatch. A cluster of dots on the left side of the panel represents cells other than B-cells. *Panel 2,* The upper right hand quadrant of the right panel indicates T-cells bearing human IgG antibody (a positive T-cell crossmatch). A cluster of dots in the lower right hand panel would indicate a negative crossmatch. A cluster of dots on the left side of the panel represents cells other than T-cells. Given that both T-cells and B-cells are positive, these results indicate that this patient is highly sensitized for the cells from that donor, and these antibodies are specific for HLA class I.

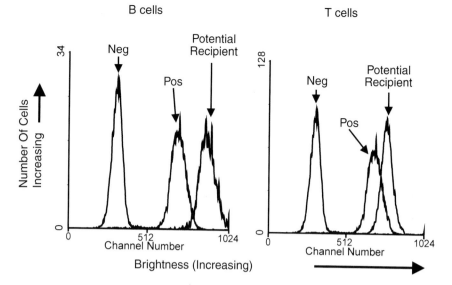

FIGURE **7-11.** Single parameter histograms of the same data used to generate the scatterplots in Figure 7–10. The x-axis shows brightness of fluorescence on a logarithmic scale in "channel units" ranging from 0–1,000 units. The y-axis shows the number of cells exhibiting a given brightness. The negative controls, treated with a known nonreactive isotype matched primary antibody, generate the peak labeled "Neg." Cells treated with positive control sera from highly sensitized patients, are designated "Pos." The test serum from a potential recipient is indicated by "Potential Recip." These B- and T-cell crossmatches are both positive.

ysis is performed, the fluorescence intensity of the cells is depicted on a logarithmic scale, often converted to units called "channels," typically with 1,024 channel units displayed. Therefore, the data may be expressed in units of "channel shift." If the log scale is used, the brightness value may be called the mean or median fluorescence intensity. Based on these determinations, the laboratory will indicate the number of "channel shifts" from the median intensity of a set of negative controls which are required to consider a cell sufficiently coated with tagged antibody to indicate a positive crossmatch. For example, at the University of Alabama at Birmingham (UAB) the channel shift of 40 units from the negative control is the "threshold" for a positive T-cell crossmatch, and a channel shift of 70 units is the "threshold" for a positive B-cell crossmatch. If the typing laboratory has established a protocol for quantitative flow cytometry, the fluorescence can also be expressed as molecule equivalents of soluble fluorochrome (MESF) units. In such a case, the flow cytometer is calibrated using beads on which a known number of fluorochrome molecules have been attached. A standard curve is generated, yielding an equation from which a channel number can be converted to MESF units. The advantage of this scheme is that the fluorescence can be quantitatively compared from one time point to the next. Fluorescence values can also be expressed as a peak displacement in which the values from the normal serum are subtracted, or as a ratio in which the normal values are divided into the patient mean or median intensity.

CONTROVERSIES IN CROSSMATCH INTERPRETATION

IgG CYTOTOXIC T-CELL CROSSMATCH

It is generally accepted that if there are **IgG antibodies** causing a positive cytotoxic crossmatch when recipient

sera is incubated with donor T-cells and B-cells (a positive cytotoxic T-cell and B-cell crossmatch), then cardiac transplantation is contraindicated because of the important probability of hyperacute or severe accelerated acute rejection. However, even with a positive IgG T-cell lymphocytotoxic crossmatch, long-term survival has been reported (57% survival at 2 years) with early posttransplant plasmapheresis.[63] Despite this report, the frequency of serious rejection, with nearly 75% of patients experiencing initial hemodynamically compromising vascular rejection, makes this practice inadvisable. Thus, the presence of a positive cytotoxic T-cell crossmatch should be considered a contraindication to transplantation.

IgM CROSSMATCH

The presence of IgM anti-donor HLA antibody is controversial. The detection of IgM antibodies causing a positive crossmatch usually results from autoantibodies that are not injurious to the graft[88] and can therefore be ignored. The presence of IgM anti-HLA antibodies is rare. Although not proven in cardiac transplantation, studies in renal transplantation suggest that the presence of IgM anti-HLA antibody is not predictive of hyperacute rejection[38, 39, 43, 83, 91] unless the recipient has recently been transfused (with induction of a transient IgM response). Thus, a positive IgM cytotoxic crossmatch in the presence of a negative IgG cytotoxic crossmatch should not be considered a contraindication to cardiac transplantation.

CURRENT VERSUS HISTORIC RECIPIENT SERUM

The standard cytotoxicity crossmatch is usually performed with a current recipient serum sample, although previous (historic) samples may additionally be used when the patient has been sensitized. The presence of a negative crossmatch with current serum but a positive historic serum crossmatch suggests a current low level of circulating anti-donor HLA antibody with the potential risk for an anemnestic response and subsequent accelerated acute rejection. The experiences in renal transplantation in this setting suggest a reduced graft survival in some studies[1] and no change in others.[8, 47] Relevant data have not been reported in cardiac transplantation. If a current cytotoxic T-cell crossmatch is negative and a historic sample ($\geq$ 3 months old) is positive, we recommend proceeding with transplantation with induction therapy; aggressive plasmapheresis; maintenance immunosuppression with prednisone, mycophenolate, and cyclosporine or tacrolimus; and planned photopheresis.

FLOW VERSUS CYTOTOXIC T-CELL CROSSMATCH

The increasing application of flow cytometry crossmatching in solid organ transplantation has introduced new uncertainties in the interpretation of crossmatch data. It is clearly established that flow cytometry is a more sensitive technique than lymphocytotoxicity for the identification of preformed anti-donor HLA antibodies, and in renal transplantation it is likely that a positive flow crossmatch in the presence of a negative cytotoxic crossmatch indicates a greater likelihood of eventual graft loss due to rejection than does a negative flow crossmatch.[13, 56, 82] Ogura and colleagues[56] examined the predictive value of flow cytometry crossmatches in 841 primary cadaver renal transplants. The incidence of early graft failure within 1 month was 20% with a negative CDC T-cell crossmatch and a positive flow cytometry T-cell crossmatch compared to 7% with both negative CDC and flow crossmatches ($p = .001$). The 1-year graft survival was 75% versus 82%, respectively ($p = .01$). No difference in early graft loss or 1-year graft survival was observed between sensitized and nonsensitized patients who had a negative cytotoxic and positive flow crossmatch ($p \geq .2$).

Secure information regarding the relative predictive value of a positive T-cell crossmatch by CDC or flow cytometry in cardiac transplantation is not available. However, several studies suggest that a positive T- and B-cell crossmatch by flow cytometry in the presence of a negative CDC crossmatch may predict a moderate increased incidence of rejection and a mild decrease in survival compared to the combination of a negative T- and B-cell crossmatch by both flow cytometry and CDC.[3, 13] Aziz and colleagues analyzed retrospective flow cytometry crossmatches in 92 patients who underwent cardiac transplantation with a negative cytotoxic anti-human globulin crossmatch, using a protocol of induction therapy with either OKT3 or rabbit anti-human thymocyte globulin and maintenance therapy with cyclosporine, prednisone, and azathioprine.[3] Twenty percent of patients had a positive T- and B-cell flow crossmatch (indicating anti-class I antibodies) in the face of a negative cytotoxic crossmatch. The 6-month mortality in the CDC-negative, flow cytometry T- and B-crossmatch positive patients was only 5%, but the incidence of two or more episodes of cellular rejection was greater in this group than in the flow T-cell and B-cell negative group (45% vs. 11%, $p = .01$). There was no difference between groups in time to first rejection. The experience at both UAB and the Cleveland Clinic indicates that highly sensitized patients can be safely transplanted (although with an increased propensity for early rejection) with a negative T- and B-cell cytotoxic crossmatch in the face of a positive flow cytometry T- and B-cell crossmatch.

The information is critically important in patients who are sensitized from pregnancies or multiple transfusions, especially when confined to an intensive care unit on inotropic support or hospital bound for months on an LVAD with a high PRA and documented anti-HLA antibodies. In such patients, a crossmatch result (e.g., positive flow, negative cytotoxic crossmatch) that gives a low probability of hyperacute rejection and medium risk of aggressive (but potentially treatable) early rejection might be preferable from an overall risk/benefit ratio to the high ongoing risk of death, morbidity, and massive cost of continued hospitalization.

B-CELL CROSSMATCH

The implications of cardiac transplantation in the presence of a positive B-cell, negative T-cell crossmatch remain controversial. In the study by Aziz and colleagues,[3] patients with CDC T- and B-cell negative, flow cytometry T-cell negative and B-cell positive crossmatch had both a higher mortality at 6 months (4 of 12 vs. 2 of 36, $p < .01$) and greater incidence of **vascular rejection** by immunofluorescence studies (5 of 12 vs. 1 of 36, $p < .001$) compared to the T- and B-cell flow cytometry negative crossmatch group, with five of eight episodes of graft dysfunction occurring in the T-cell negative B-cell positive flow cytometry group.

Cook and colleagues[12] reported a 40% incidence of an isolated positive B-cell crossmatch (with negative T-cell crossmatch) by flow cytometry or flow plus CDC. These patients had significantly greater vascular rejection and reduced survival at 3 years compared to patients with cytotoxic and flow B- and T-cell negative crossmatches. Vascular rejection was also more common (one third of patients) when T- and B-cell flow crossmatches were positive and cytotoxic T- and B-cell crossmatches were negative, but survival was unchanged.

RECOMMENDATION

It is appropriate to consider transplantation with either (1) a positive flow IgG T- and B-cell crossmatch when there is a negative AHG or Amos-modified IgG cytotoxic T- and B-cell crossmatch, or (2) an isolated positive B-cell crossmatch by either CDC or flow. However, it should be remembered that, while an isolated positive B-cell crossmatch by flow or CDC and a positive T- and B-cell flow crossmatch (with a negative CDC T- and B-cell crossmatch) do not appear to increase the risk of hyperacute rejection, the incidence of early vascular rejection is significantly increased, and augmented immunosuppression early after transplant is warranted. Our recommendation is to accept donors for transplantation if the Amos-modified or AHG cytotoxic T- and B-cell crossmatch is negative, irrespective of flow T-cell or B-cell crossmatch results. However, we recommend induction therapy in such patients accompanied by close rejection surveillance and aggressive maintenance immunosuppression.

References

1. Alexandre GPJ, Squifflet JP, DeBruyere M, Latinne D, Reding R, Gianello P, Carlier M, Pirson Y: Present experience in a series of 26 ABO-incompatible living donor renal allografts. Transplant Proc 1987;19:4538.
2. Amos DB, Bashir H, Boyle W, MacQueen M, Tiilikaninen A: A simple micro cytotoxicity test. Transplantation 1969;7:220.
3. Aziz S, Hassantash A, Nelson K, Levy W, Kruse A, Reichenbach D, Himes V, Fishbein D, Allen MD: The clinical significance of flow cytometry crossmatching in heart transplantation. J Heart Lung Transplant 1998;17:686.
4. Bodmer JG, Marsh SGE, Albert E, Bodmer WF, Bontrop RE, Charron D, Dupont B, Erlich HA, Fauchet R, Mach B, Mayr WR, Parham P, Sasazuki T, Schreuder GMT, Strominger JL, Svejgaard A, Terasaki PI: 1996 HLA nomenclature report. Hum Immunol 1998;53:98.
5. Breimer ME, Samuelsson BE: The specific distribution of glycolipid-based blood group a antigens in human kidney related to A_1/A_2, Lewis, and secretor status of single individuals. Transplantation 1986;42:88.
6. Brynger H, Rydberg L, Samuelsson B, Blohme I, Lindholm A, Sandberg L: Renal transplantation across a blood group barrier—A_2 kidneys to O recipients. Proc EDTA 1982;19:427.
7. Bunke M, Ganzel B, Klein B, Oldfather J: The effect of a positive B cell crossmatch on early rejection in cardiac transplant recipients. Transplantation 1993;56:758.
8. Cardella CJ, Falk JA, Nicholson MJ, Harding M, Cook GT: Successful renal transplantation in patients with T cell reactivity to donor. Lancet 1982;2:1240.
9. Ceppellini R, Bigliani S, Curtoni ES, Leigheb G: Experimental allotransplantation in man II. The role of A_1, A_2 and B antigens III. Enhancement by circulating antibody. Transplant Proc 1969;1:390.
10. Chien A, Edgar DB, Trela JM: Deoxyribonucleic acid polymerase from the extreme thermophile Thermus aquaticus. J Bacteriol 1976;127:1550.
11. Cicciarelli JC, Helstab K, Mendez R: Flow cytometry PRA, a new test that is highly correlated with graft survival. Clin Transplant 1992;6:159.
12. Cook DJ, Bishay E, Starling RC, Young JB, Smedira N, McCarthy PM: The crossmatch in cardiac transplantation: relative risks [abstract]. J Heart Lung Transplant 2000;19:39.
13. Cook DJ, Terasaki PI, Iwaki Y, Terashita GY, Lau M: An approach to reducing early kidney transplant failure by flow cytometry crossmatching. Clin Transplant 1987;1:253.
14. Cooper DKC: Clinical survey of heart transplantation between ABO blood group-incompatible recipients and donors. J Heart Transplant 1990;9:376.
15. Cross DE, Coxe-Gilliland R, Weaver P: DRW antigen matching and B cell antibody crossmatching: their effect on clinical outcome in renal transplants. Transplant Proc 1978;11:1908.
16. Cummins D, Contreras M, Amin S, Halil O, Downham B, Yacoub MH: Red cell alloantibody development associated with heart and lung transplantation. Transplantation 1995;59:1432.
17. DeMattos AM, Head MA, Everett J, Hosenpud J, Hershberger R, Cobanoglu A, Ott G, Ratkovec R, Norman DJ: HLA-DR mismatching correlates with early cardiac allograft rejection, incidence, and graft survival when high confidence-level serological DR typing is used. Transplantation 1994;57:626.
18. Dowling RD, Jones JW, Carroll MS, Gray LA Jr: Use of intravenous immunoglobulin in sensitized LVAD recipients. Transplant Proc 1998;30:1110.
19. DuToit ED, Oudshoorn M, Smith DC: Pretransplant immunological considerations. In Cooper DKC, Miller LW, Patterson GA (eds): The Transplantation and Replacement of Thoracic Organs. 2nd ed. The Netherlands: Kluwer Academic Publishers, 1996.
20. Everett ET, Kao KJ, Scornik JC: Class I HLA molecules on human erythrocytes: quantitation and transfusion effects. Transplantation 1987;44:123.
21. Farges O, Kalil AN, Samuel D, Saliba F, Arulnaden JL, Debat P, Bismuth A, Castaing D, Bismuth H: The use of ABO-incompatible grafts in liver transplantation: a life-saving procedure in highly selected patients. Transplantation 1995;59:1124.
22. Festenstein H, Banner N, Smith J, Awad J, Burden M, Fitzgerald N, Holmes J, Khaghani A, Smith J, McCloskey D, Yacoub M: The influence of HLA matching lymphocytotoxic status in heart-lung allograft recipients receiving cyclosporin and azathioprine. Transplant Proc 1989;21:797.
23. Fieguth HG, Wahlers T, Schafers HI, Stangel W, Kemnitz J, Haverich A: Impact of HLA-compatibility on rejection sequence and survival rate after orthotopic heart transplantation. Transplant Proc 1991;23:1137.
24. Garcia P, Rodriguez JL, Vinas J: A new rapid and more sensitive microcytotoxicity test. J Immunol Meth 1972;1:303.
25. George JF, Kirklin JK, Shroyer TW, Naftel DC, Bourge RC, McGiffin DC, White-Williams C, Noreuil T: Utility of post-transplantation panel-reactive antibody measurements for the prediction of rejection frequency and survival of heart transplant recipients. J Heart Lung Transplant 1995;14:856.
26. Gibson T, Medawar PB: The fate of skin homografts in man. J Anat 1945;77:299.
27. Gilchrist FC, Bunce M, Lympany PA, Welsh KI, du Bois RM: Comprehensive HLA-DP typing using polymerase chain reaction with sequence-specific primers and 95 sequence-specific primer mixes. Tissue Antigens 1998;51:51.
28. Glotz D, Haymann JP, Sansonetti N, Francois A, Menoyo-Calonge V, Bariety J, Druet P: Suppression of HLA-specific alloantibodies by high-dose intravenous immunoglobulins (IVIg). A potential tool for transplantation of immunized patients. Transplantation 1993;56:335–337.
29. Harmer AW, Heads AJ, Vaughn RW: Detection of HLA class I and class II specific antibodies by flow cytometry and PRA-STAT screening in renal transplant recipients. Transplantation 1997;63:1828.
30. Haymann JP, Glotz D: Intravenous polyclonal immunoglobulin (IVIg): what use in transplantation? Nephrologie 1999;20:139.
31. Hendriks GFJ, Wenting GJ, Mochzar B, Box E, Simoons ML, Balk AHMM, Laird-Meeter K, Essed CE, Weimar W: The influence of ABO blood groups on the incidence of cardiac allograft rejection in males. Transplant Proc 1989;21:803.
32. Jarcho J, Naftel DC, Shroyer TW, Kirklin JK, Bourge RC, Barr ML, Pitts DG, Starling RC, and the Cardiac Transplant Research Database: Influence of HLA mismatch on rejection after heart transplantation; a multi-institutional study. J Heart Lung Transplant 1994;13:583.
33. John R, Lietz K, Burke E, Ankersmit J, Mancini D, Suciu-Foca N, Edwards N, Rose E, Oz M, Itescu S: Intravenous immunoglobulin reduces anti-HLA alloreactivity and shortens waiting time to cardiac transplantation in highly sensitized left ventricular assist device recipients. Circulation 1999;100(suppl):II-229.
34. Johnson AH, Rossen RD, Butler WT: Detection of alloantibodies using a sensitive antiglobulin microcytotoxicity test: identification of low levels of preformed antibodies in accelerated allograft rejection. Tissue Antigens 1972;2:215.
35. Jordan SC, Quartel AW, Czer LS, Admon D, Chen G, Fishbein MC, Schwieger J, Steiner RW, Davis C, Tyan DB: Posttransplant therapy using high-dose human immunoglobulin (intravenous gammaglobulin) to control acute humoral rejection in renal and cardiac allograft recipients and potential mechanism of action. Transplantation 1998;66:800.
36. Kaledin AS, Sliusarenko AG, Gorodetskii SI: Isolation and properties of DNA polymerase from extreme thermophylic bacteria Thermus aquaticus YT-1. [in Russian]. Biokhimiia 1980;45:644.
37. Kerman RH: Clinical immunogenetics: understanding pretransplant crossmatches. In Primer on Transplantation. Thorofare, NJ: American Society of Transplant Physicians, 1998, pp 61–68.

38. Kerman RH, Kimball P, Scheinen S, Radovancevic B, Van Buren CT, Kahan BD, Frazier OH: The relationship among donor-recipient HLA mismatches, rejection and death from coronary artery disease in cardiac transplant recipients. Transplantation 1994;57;884.

39. Kerman RH, Kimball PM, Van Buren CT, Lewis RM, DeVera V, Baghdahsarian V, Heydari A, Kahan BD: AHG and DTE/AHFG procedure identification of crossmatch-appropriate donor-recipient pairings that result in improved graft survival. Transplantation 1991;51:316.

40. Kimball JA, Pescovitz MD, Book BK, Norman DJ: Reduced human IgG anti-ATGAM antibody formation in renal transplant recipients receiving mycophenolate mofetil. Transplantation 1995;60:1379.

41. Kissmeyer-Nielsen F, Olsen S, Peterson VP, Fjeldborg O: Hyperacute rejection of kidney allograft associated with preexisting humoral antibodies against donor cells. Lancet 1966;2:662.

42. Kranetz SA, Pon RT, Dixon GH: Increased efficiency of the Taq polymerase catalyzed polymerase chain reaction. Nucl Acids Res 1989;17:819.

43. Lavee J, Kormos RL, Duquesnoy RJ, Zerbe TR, Armitage JM, Vanek M, Hardesty RL, Griffith BP: Influence of panel reactive antibody and lymphocytotoxic crossmatch on survival after heart transplantation. J Heart Lung Transplant 1991;10:921.

44. Lo C-M, Shaked A, Busuttil RW: Risk factors for liver transplantation across the ABO barrier. Transplantation 1994;58:548.

45. Loh E, Bergin JD, Couper GS, Mudge GH Jr: Role of panel-reactive antibody cross-reactivity in predicting survival after orthotopic heart transplantation. J Heart Lung Transplant 1994;13:194.

46. Lou C, Garovoy MR: Current crossmatch techniques. Scientific and Technical Aspects of the Major Histocompatibility Complex. Arlington, VA: The American Association of Blood Banks, 1989.

47. Matas AJ, Tellis VA, Glicklich D, Soberman R, Veith FJ: Transplantation with a past positive crossmatch and cyclosporine immunosuppression: a 5 year experience. Clin Transplant 1988;2:336.

48. McIntyre JA, Higgins N, Britton R, Faucett S, Johnson S, Beckman D, Hormuth D, Fehrenbacher J, Halbrook H: Utilization of intravenous immunoglobulin to ameliorate alloantibodies in a highly sensitized patient with a cardiac assist device awaiting heart transplantation. Transplantation 1996; 62:691.

49. Medawar PB: The behavior and fate of skin autografts and skin homografts in rabbits. J Anat 1944;78:176.

50. Mittal KK, Mickey MR, Singal DP, Terasaki PI: Serotyping for homotransplantations. Transplantation 1968;6:913.

51. Morris PJ, Ting A, Oliver D: Renal transplantation in the presence of positive crossmatch. Transplant Proc 1978;10:476.

52. Mullis KB, Faloona FA: Specific synthesis of DNA in vitro via a polymerase-catalyzed chain reaction. Meth Enzymol 1987;155:335–350.

53. Mytilineos J: HLA testing: the state of the art of genomic methods in 1996 [editorial; review]. Nephrol Dial Transplant 1996;11:2129.

54. Nelken D, Cohen I, Furcaig I: A method to increase the sensitivity of the lympocyte microcytotoxicity test. Transplantation 1970; 10:346.

55. Norman DJ, Barry JM, Wetzsteon PJ: Successful cadaver kidney transplantation in patients highly sensitized by blood transfusions. Transplantation 1985;39:253.

56. Ogura K, Terasaki PI, Johnson C, Mendez R, Rosenthal JT, Ettenger R, Martin DC, Dainko E, Cohen L, Mackett T, Berne T, Barba L, Lieberman E: The significance of a positive flow cytometry crossmatch test in primary kidney transplantation. Transplantation 1993;56:294.

57. Opelz G: Importance of HLA antigen splits for kidney transplant matching. Lancet 1988;2:61–64.

58. Opelz G: Collaborative Heart Transplant Study. Newsletter 1989.

59. Opelz G, Mytilineos J, Scherer S, Dunckley H, Trejaut J, Chapman J, Fischer G, Fae I, Middleton D, Savage D, Bignon JD, Bensa JC, Noreen H, Albert E, Albrecht G, Schwarz V: Analysis of HLA-DR matching in DNA-typed cadaver kidney transplants. Transplantation 1993;55:782.

60. Opelz G, Terasaki PI: Cadaver kidney transplants in North America: analysis 1978. Dial Transplant 1979;8:167.

61. Opelz G, Wujciak T, Mytilineous J, Scherer S: Revisiting HLA matching for kidney transplantation. Transplant Proc 1993;25:173.

62. Pisani BA, Mullen GM, Malinowska K, Lawless CE, Mendez J, Silver MA, Radvany R, Robinson JA: Plasmapheresis with intravenous immunoglobulin G is effective in patients with elevated panel reactive antibody prior to cardiac transplantation. J Heart Lung Transplant 1999;18:701.

63. Ratkovec RM, Hammond EH, O'Connell JAB, Bristow MR, DeWitt CW, Richenbacher WE, Millar RC, Renlund DG: Outcome of cardiac transplant recipients with a positive donor-specific crossmatch—preliminary results with plasmapheresis. Transplantation 1992;54:651.

64. Renard TH, Andrews WS: An approach to ABO-incompatible liver transplantation in children. Transplantation 1992;53:116.

65. Robinson JA, Radvany RM, Mullen MG, Garrity ER Jr: Plasmapheresis followed by intravenous immunoglobulin in presensitized patients awaiting thoracic organ transplantation. Ther Apheresis 1997;1:147.

66. Rodey GE, Fuller TC: Public epitopes and the antigenic structure of the HLA molecules. Crit Rev Immunol 1987;7:229.

67. Rodey GE, Nylan JF, Whelchel JD, Revels KW, Bray RA: Epitope specificity of HLA Class I alloantibodies. Hum Immunol 1994;39:272.

68. Rozemuller EH, Chadwick B, Charron D, Baxter-Lowe A, Eliaou JF, Johnston-Dow L, Tilanus MGJ: Sequenase sequence profiles used for HLA-DPB1 sequencing-based typing. Tissue Antigens 1996;47:72.

69. Rozemuller EH, Tilanus MG: A computerized method to predict the discriminatory properties for class II sequencing based typing. Hum Immunol 1996;46:27.

70. Sadler AM, Petronzelli F, Krausa P, Marsh SGE, Guttridge MG, Browning MJ, Bodmer JG: Low resolution DNA typing for HLA-B using sequence-specific primers in allele- or group-specific ARMS/PCR. Tissue Antigens 1994;44:148.

71. Saiki RK, Gelfand DH, Stoffel S, Scharf SJ, Highuchi R, Horn GT, Mullis KB, Erllon HA: Primer–directed enzymatic amplification of DNA with a thermostable DNA polymerase. Science 1988; 239:487.

72. Schachter H, Michaels MA, Tilley CA, Crookston MC, Crookston JH: Qualitative differences in the N-acetyl-D-galactosaminyl-transferases produced by human A_1 and A_2 genes. Proc Natl Acad Sci U S A 1973;70:220.

73. Scheltinga SA, Johnson-Dow LA, White CB, Wil van der Zwan A, Bakema JE, Rozemuller EH, van den Tweel JG, Kronick MN, Tilanus MGJ: A generic sequencing based typing approach for the identification of HLA-A diversity. Hum Immunol 1997;57:120.

74. Schmid C, Garritsen HS, Kelsch R, Cassens U, Baba HA, Sibrowski W, Scheld HH: Suppression of panel-reactive antibodies by treatment with mycophenolate mofetil. Thorac Cardiovasc Surg 1998;46:161.

75. Schöne G: Die Heteroplastische und Homöoplastiche Transplantation. Berlini Springer-Verlag, 1912.

76. Scornik JC, Brunson ME, Howard RJ, Pfaff WW: Alloimmunization, Memory, and the interpretation of crossmatch results for renal transplantation. Transplantation 1992;54:389.

77. Scornik JC, Ireland JE, Howard RJ, Pfaff WW: Assessment of the risk for broad sensitization by blood transfusions. Transplantation 1984;37:249.

78. Scornik JC, Ireland JE, Salomon DR, Howard RJ, Fennell RS, Pfaff WW: Pretransplant blood transfusions in patients with previous pregnancies. Transplantation 1987;43:449.

79. Shanahan T: Application of flow cytometry in transplantation medicine [review]. Immunol Invest 1997;26:91.

80. Shroyer TW, Deierhoi MH, Mink CA, Cagle LR, Hudson SL, Rhea SD, Diethelm AG: A rapid flow cytometry assay for HLA antibody detection using a pooled cell panel covering 14 serological cross-reacting groups. Transplantation 1995;59:626.

81. Snell GD: Methods for the study of histocompatibility genes. J Genet 1948;49:87.

82. Stabile C, Bernhardt JP, Colombe BW, et al: Study of pre-sensitization by flow cytometry in cadaveric kidney recipients. Proc Eur Dial Transplant Assoc 1985;22:622.

83. Starzl TE, Marchioro TL, Holmes JH: Renal homografts in patients with major donor-recipient blood group incompatibilities. Surgery 1964;55:195.

84. Tanaka A, Tanaka K, Kitai T, Yanabu M, Tokuka A, Sato B, Mori S, Inomoto T, Shinohara H, Uemoto S, Tokunaga Y, Inomata Y, Yamaoka Y: Living related liver transplantation across ABO blood groups. Transplantation 1994:58:548.

85. Terasaki PI, Marchioro TL, Starzl TED: Sero-typing of human lymphocyte antigens: preliminary trials on long-term kidney homograft survivors. *In* Russell PS, Winn HJ, Amos DB (eds): Histocompatibility Testing 1965. Washington, DC: National Academy of Sciences, 1985, p 83.

86. Terasaki PI, McClelland JD: Microdroplet assay of human serum cytotoxins. Nature 1964;204:998.

87. Thorpe SJ, Hunt B, Yacoub M: Expression of ABH blood group antigents in human heart tissue and its relevance to cardiac transplantation. Transplantation 1991;51:1290.

88. Ting A, Morris PJ: Successful transplantation with a positive T and B cell crossmatch due to autoreactive antibodies. Tissue Antigens 1983;21:219.

89. Voorter CE, Rozemuller EH, de Bruyn-Geraets D, van der Zwan AW, Tilanus MGJ, van den Berg-Loonen EM: Comparison of DRB sequence-based typing using different strategies. Tissue Antigens 1997;49:471.

90. Watkins WM: Genetics and biochemistry of some human blood groups. Proc R Soc Lond Biol 1978;202:31.

91. Zerbe TR, Arena VC, Kormos RL, Griffith BP, Hardesty RL, Duquesnoy RJ: Histocompatibility and other risk factors for histological rejection of human cardiac allografts during the first three months following transplantation. Transplantation 1991:52; 485.

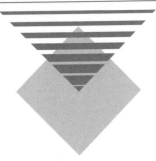

CHAPTER EIGHT

Mechanical Support of the Failing Heart

with the collaboration of
WILLIAM L. HOLMAN, M.D. AND ROBERT L. KORMOS, M.D.

The supply of donor hearts, even with full utilization of the donor pool, will never completely meet the needs of patients awaiting cardiac transplantation.[59] Furthermore, donor heart availability is unpredictable, creating a potentially fatal outcome for the potential recipient who develops acute hemodynamic deterioration. Temporary support of the circulation with mechanical circulatory support systems (MCSS) has allowed patients to survive until a donor heart becomes available. Because of the increasing waiting time required for cardiac transplantation, an increasing number of patients deteriorate prior to transplantation to the point of needing intravenous inotropic support. Without MCSS, 25% or more of such patients die before transplantation can be performed. In 1997, approximately 15% of 2,400 patients undergoing cardiac transplantation in the United States received mechanical circulatory support as a "bridge" to transplantation, and currently at the University of Alabama at Birmingham (UAB), nearly one third of patients are supported by ventricular assist devices prior to transplantation. This chapter describes the general types of MCSS currently available (i.e., ventricular assist devices and total artificial hearts) and their use as a bridge to cardiac transplantation. This chapter will not discuss the use of the intra-aortic balloon pump, since it is a commonly used device in routine cardiac surgery.

DEVELOPMENTAL HISTORY OF MCSS

The possibility of mechanically supporting the circulation for extended periods became feasible after the development of the first blood pumps used in cardiac surgery.[47, 80, 120] Attention was subsequently focused on devices that would provide support for a patient's circulation until recovery of the native heart occurred (bridge to recovery) or until the heart was replaced by a transplanted organ (bridge to transplantation).

Several of the early mechanical assist devices were based on the roller pump.[134, 165, 198] Stucky and Newman[200] reported the concept of limited left ventricular support in cases of acute myocardial infarction, and DeBakey in 1971 reported a left atrial–to–aortic bypass circuit as an assist device for patients who could not be weaned from cardiopulmonary bypass.[48] Although roller pumps were successfully incorporated into extracorporeal membrane oxygenator circuits, they have not proved effective as ventricular assist devices because of limitations imposed by tethering, blood trauma, and difficulties in modulating pump speed according to fluctuations in left atrial or left ventricular pressure.

During the early 1960s, Klaus[121] and others introduced the concept of arterial counterpulsation as a means of providing rapid systolic unloading of the ventricle with diastolic augmentation.[121, 196] This brilliant concept formed the basis for the pioneering work of Moulopoulo and colleagues, who developed the intra-aortic balloon pump for clinical support of the failing heart.[149] Kantrowitz and colleagues first applied counterpulsation with the intra-aortic balloon in 1967 to support patients with cardiogenic shock,[116] and this device is currently the most widely applied mechanical circulatory support device. In 1978, Reemtsma and colleagues reported three patients supported with intra-aortic balloon counterpulsation followed by successful cardiac transplantation.[173] The primary limitation of the intra-aortic balloon pump is that it actually provides little direct flow and cannot adequately support a severely injured left ventricle.

The United States National Institutes of Health (NIH) joined the mechanical circulatory support effort in July 1964, with the establishment of the Artificial Heart Program. The Program's initial plan, presented in 1966, called for the development of emergency support devices, short- and long-term circulatory assist devices, and cardiac replacement pumps.[212]

The primary thrust in early ventricular assist device (VAD) development was to create pneumatically driven pulsatile intra- and paracorporeal pumps. Total artificial heart (TAH) designs for orthotopic cardiac replacement included similar pulsatile pneumatic designs.[94] In 1978, Norman and colleagues[153] reported the employment of an abdominal left ventricular assist device for 5 days while awaiting cardiac transplantation. The patient survived the period of support but died of multiorgan failure following cardiac transplantation. Progress in pump design continued at individual institutions through the 1970s,[153, 154] and in 1980, the Services and Technology Branch, Division of Heart and Vascular Diseases, National Heart, Lung, and Blood Institute, asked for proposals to develop "an implantable, integrated, electrically powered, left heart assist system" that would allow extensive patient mobility.

In September 1984, these extensive research efforts culminated in the first successful cardiac transplant following bridging with a left ventricular assist device, initially by Oyer and colleagues using a Novacor implantable left ventricular assist system[168] and followed by Hill and colleagues using a Pierce-Donachey pneumatic left ventricular assist device.[100] These early successes were the impetus for multi-institutional United States Food and Drug Administration (FDA) sponsored trials of assist devices as bridges to recovery or transplantation.[68, 73, 92, 199] In 1994, the U.S. FDA approved a left ventricular assist device as a bridge to heart trans-

plantation. In the same year, the first wearable left ventricular assist device was used clinically.[81]

Akutsu and Kolff are credited with the first experimental implantation of a TAH in 1958. The dog was supported for 90 minutes,[3] and by 1962 they reported survival in excess of 24 hours.[4]

The TAH was first used as a temporary support device pending transplantation by Cooley in 1969.[35] The circulation of a patient who could not be separated from cardiopulmonary bypass was supported for 64 hours until transplantation could be performed. Although progress with several pneumatic, electric, and even nuclear powered TAH designs continued through the 1980s,[31, 34, 177] it was the Utah group that attracted the attention of the world by performing the first permanent TAH implant (see Box) on December 2, 1982.[54]

The total artificial heart came under early public scrutiny when a clinical trial of the Jarvik-7 total artificial heart was approved by the FDA.[53, 70, 112] This trial demonstrated the shortcomings and strengths of the Jarvik-7 device. Although the Jarvik-7 kept patients who were terminally ill from cardiac disease alive for as long as 620 days, all five of these patients suffered from a variety of adverse events that seriously affected their quality of life while on the pump. All five patients died of complications directly or indirectly associated with the device (i.e., infection, stroke, and hemorrhage). The high incidence of thromboembolic strokes in the patients who survived for greater than 30 days was a major deterrent to its future use.

The initial trial of the Jarvik-7 TAH also generated intense scrutiny from the media. This initial publicity was followed by a period of serious reflection by ethicists, economists, and others concerned with the de-

---

The First Permanent Total Artificial Heart Implant

The heart of Dr. Barney Clark, a 61-year-old retired dentist with end-stage idiopathic dilated cardiomyopathy, was replaced with a Jarvik-7 TAH when the FDA approved a trial of the Jarvik-7 as a permanent replacement device.[53, 70, 112] This experiment lasted 112 days.

Dr. Clark had apparently been denied cardiac transplantation because of "advanced age," and he also suffered from chronic obstructive pulmonary disease. The initial recovery period was marked by numerous complications, including surgical reexploration for subcutaneous emphysema on postoperative day 3, a grand mal seizure associated with elevation of cardiac output to more than 8 L/min on postoperative day 6, and reoperation for acute strut fracture of the total artificial heart mitral prosthesis on day 13. He required tracheostomy because of persistent respiratory insufficiency, and he experienced renal dysfunction related to hemoglobinuria from device-induced hemolysis. Walking with assistance was accomplished only on the 40th postoperative day, but he continued to require ventilatory support intermittently. He eventually succumbed to the complications of aspiration pneumonia, renal failure, and pseudomembranous colitis with septicemia.[26, 53]

ployment of the total artificial heart in clinical practice. Their thoughts and recommendations have helped to establish guidelines for the subsequent use of TAH devices by other investigators.[85, 112, 118]

After completing the initial trial of the Jarvik-7 as a permanent cardiac replacement device, Copeland and colleagues in Arizona subsequently performed the first planned TAH implant as a bridge to transplant in 1985.[38, 132, 133] Multicenter trials of the TAH as a bridge to cardiac transplantation followed.[58, 136, 178] Unresolved problems with the manufacture and investigation of this device under the direction of the Symbion Corporation led to the withdrawal of its FDA Investigational Device Exemption.[70] The CardioWest Corporation, under the leadership of Drs. Jack Copeland and Don Olsen, subsequently revived interest in this model of the total artificial heart, which was modified slightly and renamed the CardioWest C-70. The CardioWest group successfully reinitiated FDA-sponsored trials of the CardioWest C-70 TAH, which is currently used as a bridge to cardiac transplantation. The development of other total artificial heart devices continues under NIH-sponsored and institutionally sponsored programs.[150, 206] The original goal of the NIH initiative was to develop a fully approved total artificial heart by the year 2000.[109] While this has proven to be a somewhat overly optimistic projection, at least one new TAH design is about to enter clinical trials.

DEFINITION AND GENERAL DESCRIPTION

VADs are mechanical pumps that take over the circulatory function for one or both ventricles. VADs are used in a heterotopic position, thus the patient's native heart remains in place and has the potential to support the patient's circulation in the event of total VAD failure. VAD inflow for the pulmonary circulation is usually achieved by right atrial cannulation, although direct right ventricular cannulation is now occasionally employed.[11] VAD inflow for the systemic circulation is usually accomplished with left ventricular apical cannulation, although some devices are designed to accept left atrial cannulas. Ventricular assist pumps have been devised for intracorporeal (within the body) and paracorporeal (outside the body) placement.

VADs have been designed that can support the left (LVAD), right (RVAD), or both ventricles. According to the design of a particular VAD, blood flow is either pulsatile or nonpulsatile. Pulsatile VADs require inflow and outflow valves to maintain unidirectional blood flow. Some pulsatile VADs employ mechanical valves, while others use bioprosthetic valves. Mechanical valves do not require special storage conditions and are more resistant to wear than biologic valves; however, mechanical valves create considerable turbulence in blood and are more thrombogenic than biologic valves. Most VADs and TAHs (and especially those with mechanical valves) require chronic anticoagulation with warfarin. Pulsatile VADs have a higher dp/dt (rate of pressure change

during systole) than the native heart. Bioprosthetic valves and some mechanical valves (e.g., valves with Delrin plastic disks) tolerate this pumping force without perforation or cracking, but more brittle materials such as pyrolytic carbon can shatter.[54]

PUMP BLOOD SURFACE DESIGN

Pumping sacs and diaphragms for pulsatile VADs are fabricated from plastics with high resistance to wear.[113] The most commonly used plastic for pumping surfaces is segmented **polyurethane** (Biomer),[65] and all devices currently in use have linings which are at least in part polyurethane. The relative amounts and chemical composition of the hard and soft segments that are combined in a specific segmented polyurethane determine the plastic's physical properties,[113] and additives that migrate to the surface of a segmented polyurethane can add importantly to the thromboresistance of the plastic.[65]

The linings may be fabricated to have a smooth or rough (e.g., flocked) surface, each of which is intended to minimize thromboembolism. The smooth surface plastics achieve thromboresistance by maintaining high flow over a smooth and relatively nonthrombogenic surface. The goal of flocked surfaces is to promote the rapid development of a protein layer that promotes growth of a pseudoneointima.[175] The specific proteins that cover a blood contacting surface reflect the ionic characteristics of the surface, the surface topography, the relative concentration of proteins in the blood and their avidity for the surface, the duration of surface exposure to the blood, and the effect of flow-induced shear force at the level of the surface.[39, 101, 113]

The deposition of plasma proteins on bioprosthetic surfaces in contact with blood is a dynamic process, and different compositions of this protein layer exist at various times after implantation (shifts in the composition of this protein layer over time is referred to as the Vroman effect). The composition of the protein layer is probably important in determining the interaction of the surface with blood. For instance, a coating film of fibrin tends to activate platelets and clotting factors, while albumin causes less activation of these components. Precoating a blood–biomaterial interface with albumin or gelatin is one method to attenuate blood-biomaterial reactions.[39] Another method is to encourage the rapid deposition of protein by presenting a rough (e.g., flocked polyurethane or sintered titanium) surface to the blood.

Both smooth and rough surfaced devices are in clinical use. The major potential limitation of the surface lining the pump is the development of small thrombi with the potential for embolization. However, secure information about the time-related thromboembolic potential of these surfaces is confounded by the fact that the biomaterial interface is not just the blood sac; it also includes the inflow cannula, the prosthetic inflow valve, the inflow pathway, the outflow valve, and the outflow graft, each of which carries some thromboembolic potential. The measurement of thromboembolic rates is further complicated by the various definitions that are used by different investigators for thromboembolic event and neurologic injury during a VAD support, and by the fact that the end-stage heart is itself an important source of emboli.[40, 77, 84, 174, 187]

In contrast to the smooth polyurethane surface of most chronic pulsatile pumps, the Heartmate TCI VAD has a textured blood contact surface, which has been shown to have low thrombogenicity. Surface imperfections in pumping membranes may predispose to early breakdown due to local failure (tearing) or calcification.[113] Calcification of pumping surfaces has been particularly noticeable in rough-surfaced pumping membranes of mechanical circulatory assist devices that were implanted in calves.[158, 184] This calcification may be related to the adolescent age or species of the host animal, or to the thickness of the protein layer that formed on the experimental rough pumping diaphragm. Calcification has not yet been noted in smooth or rough pumping sacs implanted in humans, although a protein coat and associated cellular deposits have been shown to form on rough pump surfaces in patients.[86, 142, 179] The protein layer over the rough surface of the HeartMate LVAD was found to never exceed 150 μm or contain calcium deposits.[142] Some evidence suggests that cells colonizing the protein layer of a rough surface will express surface molecules similar to those found on endothelial cells, and that these cells will establish themselves over the entire metal and plastic surfaces of the pump. Although the presence of living cells in the protein coat has been demonstrated by several groups, the nature of these cells and their functional properties have not yet been established. As will be discussed later (see later section, Post-VAD Immunologic Sensitization) there are functional properties that may have important immunologic as well as thromboembolic implications.

IMPLANTABLE DEVICES

The VADs that are currently approved by the U.S. FDA are all tethered devices (i.e., they require that the VAD be "continuously connected to external control or energizing systems by wires or tubes leading from the implanted device through the skin to the external component").

Wearable devices (the power supply and controller unit can be carried on a belt, vest, or shoulder harness) currently approved for clinical use have an external power source with a transcutaneous drive line which contains the electrical cable for power and a transcutaneous air vent. A major requirement of electrically powered implantable pumps (VAD or TAH) is the necessity to compensate for changes in air volume within the motor housing; otherwise, negative or positive pressures can develop behind the pumping diaphragm and impede its movement. The two available methods to compensate for changes in air volume are (1) vent the air outside the body through a tube that penetrates the skin, and (2) implant a flexible bag (compliance chamber) in the thorax.

Fully implantable systems are under development which have a self-contained internal power

source[109, 155, 169] and a **compliance chamber** to compensate for air displacement. Refinement of an implantable compliance chamber has been hampered by the tendency for water accumulation in the chamber, escape of gas, and the build-up of fibrous tissue leading to loss of elasticity.[81] Many of the devices covered in this chapter are summarized in Table 8–1.

SHORT-TERM DEVICES ($\leq$ 2 WEEKS)

Short term MCSSs provide circulatory support by means of an external pump and cannulae or drive shafts which penetrate the skin. Patients supported by short-term devices are tethered to the device with little or no mobility. These devices have the advantage of ease of insertion and lower cost compared to chronic devices. The major disadvantage of many short-term devices is the potential for infection (via transcutaneous cannulae in an immobilized patient) and thromboemboli. If cardiac recovery does not occur within a few days to approximately 2 weeks, a decision must be made about the appropriateness of implanting a more chronic device.

NONPULSATILE PUMPS

Roller Pumps

Roller-head pumps are utilized in the majority of cardiopulmonary bypass circuits and act by compressing the flexible tubing circuit, creating a "parasystolic" flow pattern. Continuous anticoagulation with heparin is required. Although historically used for short-term circulatory support in the setting of acute cardiac failure following cardiac surgery, such systems are less suitable for safe bridging to cardiac transplantation due to the high sheer stresses with prolonged use, the constant oversight necessary by perfusionist personnel, and the potential for connection disruption and infection in the circuit.

Centrifugal Pumps

Centrifugal pumps utilize a spinning chamber to generate blood flow, either through rotating cones (Medtronic Bio-Medicus, Inc., Eden Prairie, MN) or by an impeller mechanism (Sarnes/3M Healthcare, Inc., Ann Arbor, MI). Although easily implanted, centrifugal, nonpulsatile pump support through devices such as the Bio-Medicus pump have generally been unsatisfactory for more than 12–24 hours. In our experience, despite heparinization, the incidence of thromboembolic phenomena and hemolysis have been significant after about 24 hours. We no longer employ such devices for isolated ventricular support unless a membrane oxygenator is required in the system.

Extracorporeal Membrane Oxygenation

Extracorporeal membrane oxygenation (ECMO) support combines the use of a centrifugal or roller pump

TABLE 8-1 Summary Features of Devices Described in Text

DEVICE NAME	VENTRICLE(S) SUPPORTED	MECHANISM OF PUMPING	LOCATION OF PUMP	VALVES IN PUMP	CANNULATION SITES FOR INFLOW	PATIENT SIZE	DURATION	POWER SOURCE	ANTI-COAGULATION	PATIENT AMBULATION	PATIENT DISCHARGE	EXPENSE
Biomedicus	Left, right	Centrifugal, nonpulsatile	External	None	Atrium or ventricle	Small to large	Short term	Electric	Yes	No	No	+
ECMO	Cardiopulmonary	Centrifugal, or roller pump, nonpulsatile	External	None	Right atrium	Small to large	Short term	Electric	Yes	No	No	+
Abiomed BVS 500	Left, right	Pneumatic pulsatile	External	Trileaflet polyurethane	Atrium	Small to large	Short term	Pneumatic	Yes	No	No	++
Thoratec	Left, right	Pneumatic, pulsatile	External	Bjork-Shiley	Atrium or ventricle	Medium to large	Intermediate to long	Pneumatic	Yes	Yes	No	+++
HeartMate Pneumatic	Left	Pusher plate	Internal	Porcine bioprosthetic	Left ventricle	Large ($\geq$1.5 m^2)	Longer term	Pneumatic	No	Yes	No	++++
HeartMate Vented Electric	Left	Pusher plate activated by a rotary motor	Internal	Porcine bioprosthetic	Left ventricle	Large ($\geq$1.5 m^2)	Longer term	Electric	No	Yes	Yes	++++
Novacor	Left	Dual pusher plates	Internal	Bovine pericardial bioprosthetic	Left ventricle	Large ($\geq$1.5 m^2)	Longer term	Electric	Yes	Yes	Yes	++++
Nimbus Intra-Corporeal Assist Device	Left	Axial flow	Internal	None	Left ventricle	Medium to large	Longer term	Electric	Yes	Yes	Yes	+++
Jarvik 2000	Left	Axial flow	Internal	None	Left ventricle	Medium to large	Longer term	Electric	Yes	Yes	Yes	+++
DeBakey Micromed	Left	Axial flow	Internal	None	Left ventricle	Medium to large	Longer term	Electric	Yes	Yes	Yes	+++
CardioWest TAH	Left and right	Pneumatic, pulsatile	Internal	Medtronic-Hall	Right & left atria	Large	Longer term	Pneumatic	Yes	Yes	No	+++
Abiomed TAH	Left and right	Centrifugal pump; pulsatile	Internal	Angioflex	Right & left atria	Large	Longer term	Electric	Yes	Yes	Yes	++++
Penn State TAH	Left and right	Push-plate pump; pulsatile	Internal	Bjork-Shiley	Right & left atria	Large	Longer term	Electric	Yes	Yes	Yes	++++

ECMO, extracorporeal membrane oxygenation; TAH, total artificial heart.

and a membrane oxygenator system (usually preferred over a hollow fiber microporous oxygenator) with cannulation in adults either peripherally through the femoral artery and vein or centrally through the ascending aorta and right atrium.

ECMO carries the major advantage of providing an oxygenator in the circuit in the presence of severe pulmonary dysfunction resulting in hypoxemia. In addition, ECMO provides some degree of biventricular support in that the right ventricle is unloaded, greatly decreasing return to the left ventricle. A major disadvantage compared to left atrial to aorta pump support is the inability to effectively decompress the left ventricle when there is essentially no left ventricular output and left ventricular distention results from bronchial collateral flow to the left atrium. When there is essentially no left ventricular contraction, initial decompression of the left atrium is usually necessary through either direct cannulation of the left atrium or a transseptal catheter introduced through the femoral vein and threaded across the atrial septum.

In the adult setting, ECMO has the same anticoagulation requirements as other short-term external pumps, in that continuous heparinization is required, usually aiming for an activated clotting time (ACT) of about 190–220 seconds. The risk of infection is similar to other external roller pumps and is one reason why this support technique should be limited to 5–7 days if possible. Pediatric ECMO support is discussed in the later section on Mechanical Circulatory Support Systems in Children.

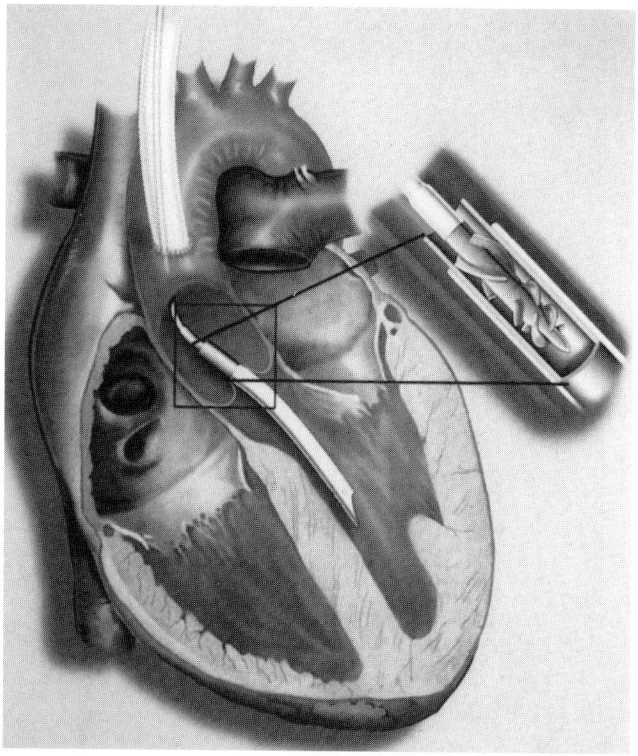

FIGURE **8–1.** Hemopump in position within the heart through a graft anastomosed to the ascending aorta. A cross-section of the pump housing is also shown. See text for further details. (From Lonn U: A Minimally Invasive Axial Blood Flow Pump. Linkoping, Sweden: Linkoping Heart Center, Linkoping University, 1997.)

Axial Flow Pumps

Axial flow pumps use an impeller with turbine blades of highly polished stainless steel to provide continuous blood flow, based on the principle of Archimedes.[21, 215] Axial flow refers to blood movement parallel to the axis defined by the impeller. Since these devices provide continuous forward flow, they do not require valves.[117]

The short-term axial flow pump called the Hemopump was developed by Dr. Richard Wampler in the 1970s.[21, 215] The axial pump (powered by an external motor) lies within a cannula, the tip of which is positioned in the left ventricular cavity through the aortic valve (Fig. 8–1). Blood is then "sucked" out of the left ventricle by the impeller and "expelled" into the ascending aorta,[137] providing circulatory assistance while the heart is in an empty beating mode. The Hemopump system consists of four basic components: a catheter-mounted axial blood flow pump; a small extracorporeal electromagnetic motor; an assembly for purging; and a console which acts as a power source for the pump and the purge set.[137] The Hemopump's impeller and drive shaft are lubricated by a continuous infusion of 40% dextrose and water. The cathetered-mounted Hemopump produces flows of 2.5–4.5 L/min with a blood pump housing about 7 mm in diameter that is mounted on a 9-Fr catheter.[74] This device is no longer manufactured in the United States but is an excellent example of this type of technology.

PULSATILE PUMPS

Abiomed BVS 5000

The Abiomed assist device (BVS 5000) is a pulsatile, asynchronous, right, left, or biventricular support system (Fig. 8–2). It is designed for short-term support for up to 4 weeks. The arterial and atrial cannulae are exteriorized through separate stab wounds, and the cannulae are covered with a Dacron velour sleeve to promote tissue ingrowth and retard ascending bacterial propogation. The atrial cannula is a 46-Fr wire-reinforced cannula which is placed directly into the right or left atrium. The arterial cannula is also 46 Fr, wire reinforced, and attached to a 14-mm preclotted Dacron graft.

The blood pump is filled by passive gravity drainage without vacuum, and consists of two chambers. The upper receiving chamber receives a continuous flow of blood from the patient's atrium. The lower ventricular chamber contains two trileaflet polyurethane valves (Angioflex) as inflow and outflow valves. Since the pump does not employ vacuum for assisted filling, the top of the pump must be maintained below the level of the patient's atria (2–10 inches), and pump filling is dependent upon adequate patient preload. The pump ventricular chamber capacity is 70 mL, and the pump is designed to eject a stroke volume of 70–89 mL. The diastolic time interval and systolic duration are adjusted

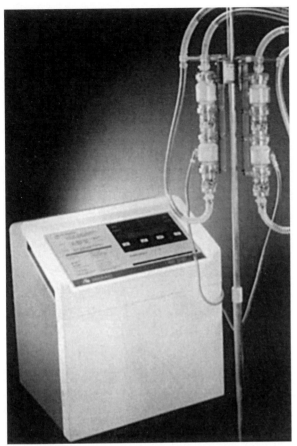

FIGURE **8-2.** Abiomed short-term pulsatile ventricular assist system. (From Abiomed Operations Manual: Abiomed, Inc., Danvers, MA, November 1994, with permission.)

automatically by the console to achieve a consistent stroke volume of 70–80 mL.

The pump is pneumatically driven by compressed room air without the need for gas cylinders. The console is able to provide right or left ventricular support. This extracorporeal pump usually provides 4–5 L/min of pulsatile flow and has the distinctive advantage of simplicity of operation in that the console is highly automated and requires minimal external intervention.

Anticoagulation with heparin is recommended for all patients and is initiated when the postoperative chest tube drainage is minimal, but not more than 24 hours after implant. The recommended ACT during pump utilization is 180–200 seconds. During weaning or in the presence of sustained atrial or ventricular fibrillation, the ACT should be increased to 300 seconds.

The major disadvantage of this system is the lack of patient mobility. Ambulation is not recommended with this system. In addition, the flow rates are frequently less than those achieved with more chronic implantable devices. In general, a decision is made after 5–7 days about the suitability of the patient for transplantation if device weaning has not been possible. If cardiac transplantation is considered to be the appropriate therapy, the Abiomed pump is generally removed and a more chronic bridging device implanted after 5–7 days.

NON–BLOOD CONTACT PUMPS

Other innovative short-term assist device designs have provided direct mechanical support to the ventricles

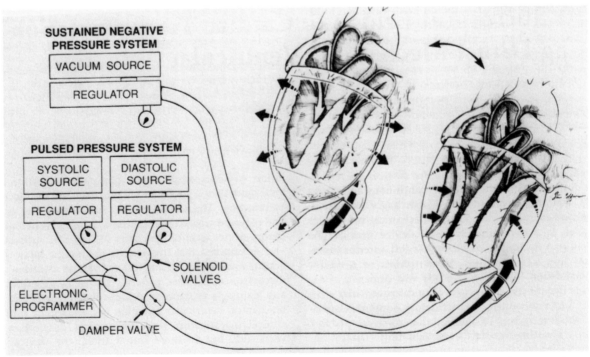

FIGURE **8-3.** Schematic diagram of direct mechanical ventricular actuation drive system and cup. The cup is shown actuating the ventricles into both systolic (right) and diastolic (left) configurations. (From Lowe JE, Anstadt MP, Van Tright P, Smith PK, Hendry PJ, Plunkett MD, Anstadt GL: First successful bridge to cardiac transplantation using direct mechanical ventricular actuation. Ann Thorac Surg 1991;52:1237–1245. Society of Thoracic Surgery, with permission.)

without exposing the blood to artificial surfaces. In the mid 1960s, Anstadt reported successful support of the canine heart with an extracardiac contoured cup which provided pneumatically driven cardiac compression and decompression.[10] The device produced effective cardiac output in a variety of canine experimental models mimmicking left or biventricular failure (or fibrillation).[6–9, 33, 188, 189] This device is unique in its simplicity and lack of blood–foreign surface interface, for which Anstadt coined the term "direct mechanical ventricular actuation."[10] The "Anstadt Cup" is a contoured cup which is placed around both ventricles with firm attachment provided by continuous vacuum at the apex of the cup (Fig. 8–3). The outer cup, the composition of which is either hard (Pyrex) or soft (Dacron-reinforced Silastic), contains an inner flexible diaphragm which is sealed to the myocardial surface by the apical vacuum. This diaphragm "actuates" ventricular compression and decompression by a pneumatic drive system which provides pulsed positive pneumatic pressure for systolic compression and a negative pressure for diastolic filling. A variety of cup sizes have been constructed so that one can be selected which approximates the transverse diameter of the heart.[138] In addition to the advantage of no blood–surface interface, the device is relatively inexpensive and can be rapidly inserted through a left anterior thoracotomy. In 1991, Lowe and colleagues reported two patients who were supported with the Anstadt Cup for up to 56 hours with good hemodynamics, including one patient in continuous ventricular fibrillation for 45 hours with effective biventricular support (after which the device was discontinued due to brain death) and one patient who was successfully transplanted after 56 hours of support.[138] The Anstadt Cup concept has stimulated the development of other more chronic devices such as the Abiomed Heart Booster (see subsequent section).

LONGER TERM DEVICES (> 1 MONTH)

The quest for permanent mechanical circulatory support systems has spawned the development of numerous longer term devices currently in use or under development for bridge-to-transplant support.[114] The general parameters for ideal longer term support systems are listed in Table 8–2, and no device currently available fulfills all these criteria.

PULSATILE EXTRACORPOREAL VENTRICULAR ASSIST DEVICES

Pierce-Donachy Thoratec Ventricular Assist Device

The Thoratec VAD was originally developed by William Pierce and James Donachy at Hershey Medical Center. The pump was first manufactured for clinical investiga-

TABLE 8-2	Important Parameters for an Ideal Longer Term Mechanical Circulatory Support System (Bridge-to-Recovery or Bridge-to-Transplant)

- Effective pressure-flow support of the circulatory system
- Potential for easy removal
  Rapid repair or replacement for pump malfunction
  Ability to explant or shut off and leave in place if heart recovers
  Easy explant during heart transplant
- Small device
  Efficient power source
  Completely implantable
  Quiet
  Little movement that might bother patient
- High reliability
- Long durability
- Low infection risk
- Minimal blood component trauma
- Nonimmunogenic

tion in 1982 and is approved for use in the United States as a bridge to recovery or a bridge to transplantation.

This pneumatically driven extracorporeal system is positioned externally on the abdominal wall and is designed for right ventricular support, left ventricular support, or both (Fig. 8–4). The blood pump contains a smooth seamless polyurethane blood sac enclosed in a rigid polysulfone case.[65, 125] Two Bjork-Shiley mechanical valves with Delrin disks (less potential for breakage than pyrolite carbon) maintain unidirectional flow. Chronic anticoagulation with coumadin (after initial heparin) and antiplatelet agents is necessary for prevention of thromboembolism.

The pump itself consists of two chambers, an air chamber and a blood sac, separated by a polyurethane diaphragm. The surface where the sac and an overlying diaphragm contacts the polysulfone case is lubricated with silicone oil to prevent blood sac friction. The pump case contains a Hall effect sensor which monitors movement of the blood sac. This magnetic switch system allows detection of complete filling of the sac with blood and is the signal that initiates ejection.

Cannulation for right ventricular assistance is through the right atrium or right ventricle with outflow to the pulmonary artery. Cannulation for the left ventricular assist device is through either the left atrium or left ventricular apex. The left atrial cannulation carries the advantage of avoiding damage to the left ventricle in cases where recovery is anticipated. In the "bridge-to-transplant" setting, left ventricular (LV) apical cannulation is preferred because of improved drainage and probably a lesser tendency for systemic embolization (stasis-induced LV thrombus is less likely with apical cannulation). The cannulae are constructed with wire-reinforced polyurethane and covered with an external velour at the exit site to promote tissue ingrowth for the prevention of ascending infection.

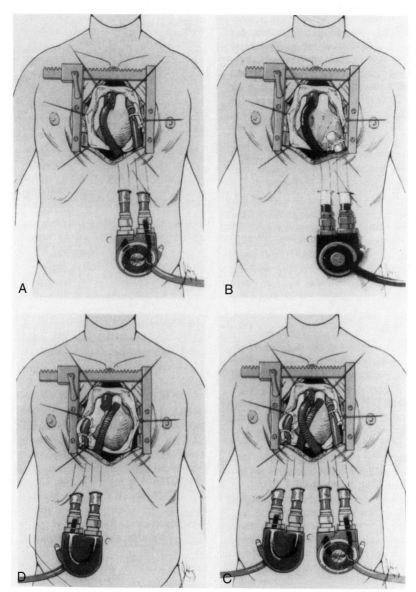

FIGURE **8-4.** Thoratec ventricular assist device in various applications. Clockwise from top left: *A,* Left ventricular assistance with atrial inflow cannulation and blood return to the ascending aorta. *B,* Left ventricular assistance with ventricular inflow cannulation. *C,* Biventricular assistance with left and right atrial cannulation. *D,* Right ventricular assistance with right atrial inflow cannulation and blood return to the pulmonary artery. This pump and a percutaneous wire (left) connects with a portable power supply and control unit. (From Sapirstein JS, Pae WE Jr: Mechanical circulatory support before heart transplantation. *In* Cooper DKC, Miller LW, Patterson GA [eds]: The Transplantation and Replacement of Thoracic Organs. 2nd ed. Boston: Kluwer Academic Publishers, 1996, with permission.)

The Thoratec drive console (see Box) contains two separate pump-control units to provide for biventricular support. The pneumatically driven pumps receive air pressure from the console to produce ejection, while vacuum from the console promotes pump filling. The pump stroke volume is 65 mL, providing outputs up to 7.2 L/min. The Thoratec VAD can be operated in the fixed-rate, volume, or synchronous mode. Volume mode is the preferred mode during support because it maximizes cardiac output. Thoratec drive console adjustments can modulate rate and timing for pump ejection, baseline ejection rate, pump ejection time, ejection drive pressure, and vacuum. The methods of identifying and

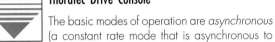

Thoratec Drive Console

The basic modes of operation are *asynchronous* (a constant rate mode that is asynchronous to the heart rate mode) and *volume mode* (a variable rate mode that is asynchronous to the heart and in which the pump empties only when it is completely filled with blood so that the device ejection rate is responsive to preload). When atrial pressure increases, the pump fills more rapidly and the rate and output increase. A third mode is the *external synchronous mode* which is synchronized with the heart rate. This was designed for weaning following native heart recovery, but is rarely used. The volume mode is the recommended mode during standard operation.

Complete filling of the pump bladder is important to maximize VAD output and also to minimize the tendency for blood stasis and thrombus formation. A green "fill light" on the drive console should illuminate with every VAD beat. Failure of illumination indicates incomplete filling. Visual inspection can also identify incomplete pump filling. Inadequate filling of the device from blood in the left (or right) ventricle may result from hypovolemia, right ventricular failure (with decreased left ventricular filling), ventricular recovery (increasing ventricular ejection resulting in lower VAD filling), tamponade, cannula position (resulting in obstruction to filling of the LVAD from left ventricle), cannula pneumatic hose kinking, or vacuum too low. Correction of incomplete VAD filling requires evaluation of possible hemodynamic and pump-related causes and initiation of corrective measures.

Complete VAD ejection (producing a stroke volume of 65 mL) is indicated by visual inspection only. Complete ejection is verified by the "flash test," in which a flashlight will illuminate through the VAD chamber with a complete ejection. Incomplete VAD ejection may be caused by a drive pressure or percent systole setting which is too low, severe systemic (for LVAD) hypertension or pulmonary (RVAD) hypertension, or from kinking of an outflow cannula.

The device contains alarms which sound when the rate is too low in the volume mode ("synch" alarm), drive pressure is too low or too high (pressure alarm), vacuum is too low or too high (vacuum alarm), battery power is low (battery alarm), and when there is loss of a suitable external synchronization signal. In addition, an external alarm can be connected to the hospital remote alarm (nurse call) system which is activated when the console receives no fill signal from the VAD for 8 or more seconds (see Appendix 8–1 for emergency protocol).

correcting ("trouble shooting") device malfunction are summarized in Table 8–3.

In our experience, the Thoratec device carries a somewhat greater potential for thromboembolism than the ThermoCardiosystems LVAD. In addition, the "paracorporeal" position on the abdominal wall and the large console limit patient mobility (although full ambulation within the hospital setting is routine and a smaller drive console has been designed that is currently used in Europe and is under investigation in the United States). This device is particularly useful in the teenage patient or small adult (body surface area less than about 1.5 m²) whose anterior abdominal wall is too small to accommodate an intracorporeal LVAD *or* in circumstances which almost certainly will require biventricular support for more than a few days (incessant ventricular trachcardia or fibrillation, massive right ventricular infarction with biventricular failure, or rarely, severe biventricular failure).

PULSATILE INTRACORPOREAL VADS

Pulsatile intracorporeal pumps are basically designed to be chronic, wearable systems. The ultimate goal has been a totally implantable electric pump, but the development of an effective, implantable compliance chamber has proved difficult. Thus, many intracorporeal pumps have gone through a pneumatic version followed by a vented electric version with external venting and a wearable external power source. Subsequent designs focus on a fully implantable system with an internal compliance chamber and transcutaneous energy transmission system (TETS) coils.

The advantages of implantable VADs are pulsatile flow, high cardiac output capability, good patient mobilization, and the potential for chronic support. Disadvantages include the inability to support right ventricular failure, fit problems in smaller patients (< about 1.5 m²), the requirement for an extensive operation on cardiopulmonary bypass, and the potential for bleeding, infection, and thromboembolism.

HeartMate ThermoCardiosystems Ventricular Assist Device

The HeartMate LVAD (ThermoCardiosystems, Inc., Woburn, MA) is an implantable pulsatile left ventricular support system that is designed to be an easy-to-operate portable "wearable" system for left ventricular support only. Unlike other chronic devices with a smooth polyurethane blood contact surface, the HeartMate LVAD has a textured blood contact surface consisting of a flocked polyurethane pumping diaphragm pushing against a sintered titanium housing, which forms a stable biologic lining that is resistant to thrombus formation[44] (Fig. 8–5). The textured surface of the blood contact surfaces promotes deposition of circulating cells, producing a uniform autologous tissue lining on all of the blood contact surfaces that carries a low tendency for formation of thrombus. Because of the relatively nonthrombogenic surface and unique flow characteris-

TABLE 8-3	**Thoratec Pneumatic LVAD—Problem Analysis**

WARNING SIGNAL	CAUSE	SOLUTION
Alarm plus red **Pressure** light	Drive (eject) pressure <100 mm Hg or >250 mm Hg Possible causes: 1. Pressure change by staff 2. Transducer failure or incorrect calibration 3. Compressor failure or incorrect connection 4. Pneumatic leak	Adjust pressure regulator Check compressors, pneumatic connections, transducer calibration
Alarm plus red Vacuum light	Vacuum less than +4 mm Hg (i.e., +5) or greater than −99 mm Hg (i.e., −100 mm Hg) Possible causes include: Same as above	Same as above
Alarm plus red **Low Battery** light	The module batteries have <30 minutes of power	Plug console into electric outlet to recharge batteries
Failure of green fill light on console to illuminate with every VAD beat and/or visual inspection shows incomplete filling **The external alarm (connected to hospital alarm [nurse call] system); alarm sounds when no fill signals are received from VAD for 8 seconds or longer**	**Incomplete VAD Filling** 1. % systole too high (inadequate time for VAD filling) 2. Set rate too high (inadequate time for VAD filling) if in asynch mode 3. Vacuum too low 4. Cannula or pneumatic hose kinking 5. Poor cannula position 6. Inadequate pharmacologic support (in setting of LVAD with right ventricular failure) 7. Tamponade 8. Ventricular recovery 9. Hypovolemia	1. Decrease % systole (>250 ms to 300 ms) 2. Decrease set rate until fill signal appears or switch to volume mode 3. Increase vacuum (−50 mm Hg) to increase inflow gradient 4. Remove kinks 5. If severe, may need reoperation 6. Adjust support medicines and/or place RVAD 7. Reoperation 8. Administer volume to increase filling and/or wean VAD 9. Administer fluids
Incomplete ejection by flash test (complete ejection indicated by transmission of light from flash light through the VAD chamber) or absence of **eject** light in the manual mode	**Incomplete VAD ejection** 1. Outflow cannula kinked 2. Systolic or pulmonary artery pressure too high 3. Drive pressure too low 4. % systole too low 5. Inadequate ejection time	1. Unkink cannula 2. Lower blood pressure or pulmonary artery pressure if feasible or increase drive pressure to at least 100 mm Hg above systolic pressure 3. Increase drive pressure 4. Increase % systole should be about 25–35% 5. Increase ejection time (should usually be about 300 ms)
-E- in VAD output display window and synch alarm in volume mode	No fill signal received by console (synch alarm will sound in volume mode) Causes include: 1. Fill cable malfunction or disconnection, fill switch failure 2. Incomplete VAD filling (see above for possible causes) 3. Incomplete VAD ejection (see above)	1. Switch to backup console 2. See above 3. See above
Loss of VAD function or unexplained sudden low VAD output	Mechanical failure	1. Glance at patient and assess appearance and tolerance 2. Observe console and identify any alarms 3. Listen to and observe pump 4. If problem not rapidly solved in console, switch to backup console 5. If complete failure, connect drive lines to hand bulbs and squeeze manually at rate of 60 bpm 6. Emergently call appropriate personnel

tics, the device requires only aspirin for antiplatelet action and differs from other available LVADs in that chronic anticoagulation with coumadin is not required.[23, 175] However, if the pump stops operating for more than a few minutes, blood stagnation causes a serious risk of thrombus formation and emboli should the device be restarted.

The inflow and outflow cannulae each contains a 25-mm porcine valve to provide unidirectional flow. Two versions of the HeartMate pump are available, a pneumatic pump and an electric pump. The main difference between the two is the method of actuation of the pusher-plate pump. In both pumps, the inflow cannula is placed in the left ventricular apex and a 20-mm Dacron outflow graft connects to the ascending aorta. The pump is implanted in the left upper quadrant, either in a subrectus position (preferred) or intraperitoneal. The pumps are designed for chronicity and mobility. The

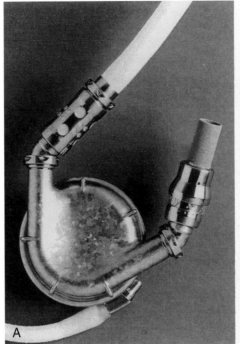
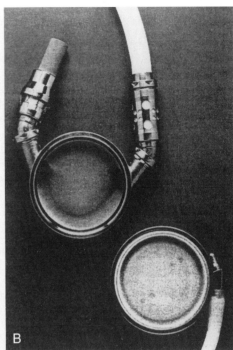

FIGURE **8–5.** *A,* HeartMate vented electric pulsatile left ventricular assist device. *B,* Textured blood contact pump surface of same device. See text for details. (From HeartMate Manual VE Operating Manual: Implantable Vented Electric Left Ventericular Assist System. TCI ThermoCardiosystems, Inc., Woburn, MA, with permission.)

velour covering around the pneumatic drive line at the skin exit site promotes vigorous tissue ingrowth which retards ascending bacterial growth. The devices are capable of delivering blood flows up to 10 L/min. VAD flows are usually adequate even when the left ventricle is asystolic or fibrillating.

The **HeartMate Implantable Pneumatic Left Ventricular Assist Device** (HeartMate 1000 1P) is a pneumatically driven pump with a pusher-plate pump mechanism, an interconnect cable, and an external pneumatic drive console (see Box) that delivers pulses of pressurized air to the pump through a percutaneous drive line.

HeartMate Pneumatic Drive Console

The drive console contains a diaphragm and pusher plate whose displacement compresses a trapped, volume of air within the console diaphragm interconnect cable, and pump air chamber. Over time, the trapped air gradually dissipates due to diffusion through the tubing and diaphragms, which results in gradual reduction in pressure generated to displace the pump diaphragm. In order to restore lost air, the console must be *vented* at least every 8 hours or whenever the console display indicates that the pump is not ejecting completely. The *interconnect cable* also requires maintenance, since water from the blood diffuses through the semipermeable diaphragm. The water vapor which condenses and collects in the interconnect cable (1–2 mL/day) reduces pump efficiency and must be drained at least weekly.

A sensing device within the pump delivers a continuous signal to the console indicating the remaining volume in the blood chamber. The console utilizes this signal to calculate pump stroke volume and flow. The console displays the stroke volume, flow, end diastolic volume, end systolic volume, and pump beat rate.

The drive console has three control modes: *fixed* (pump ejection at a fixed rate of 20–140 bpm, selected by the operator), *automatic* (pump rate is adjusted automatically to maintain a stroke volume of about 78 mL), and *external* (used to synchronize

the LVAD with the heart and will not operate without appropriate external trigger [rarely used]). Other available console adjustments include *ejection duration* (200–450 ms), *rate* (defines the fixed rate or the minimum and maximum rates for automatic and external modes), *synch delay* (during external mode), and *alarm volume.*

A bar graph is displayed on the front panel of the console which provides information about filling and emptying of the pump. The two ends of the graph are labeled E for empty and F for full. The bar graph contains 17 segments, each signifying 5 mL of volume. Dashes at the "empty" end indicate the volume of blood remaining in the pump after ejection (should be only one or two dashes on the E end immediately following systole). Dashes at the "full" end indicate the lack of complete filling (should be no more than two dashes at end of diastole on the F end). The console contains *alarms* which sound when the VAD flow is <1.5 L/min, when battery voltage is low, when the console power is on and there is no pumping function for 2½ minutes, or when neither AC nor battery power is available. A summary of protocols for management of device/console malfunction is contained in Table 8–4. In the event of console failure, there are three back-up systems: a second console, the hand crank, and the hand pump (see Appendix 8–2 for emergency protocol).

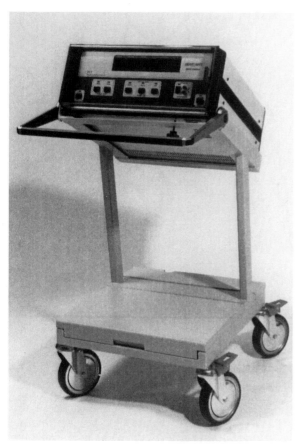

FIGURE **8-6.** Drive console for HeartMate pneumatic left ventricular assist device. (From HeartMate Manual IP LVAS Operating Manual: Drive Console. TCI ThermoCardiosystems, Inc., Woburn, MA, with permission.)

filled chamber and an air-filled chamber (Fig. 8–7). The elastic properties of the diaphragm facilitate diastolic filling of the blood chamber by a restoring force that helps the diaphragm return to its normal position after being deformed during systole. The maximum stroke volume achieved by this system is 83 mL. The methods of identifying and correcting device malfunction are summarized in Table 8–4.

The **ThermoCardiosystems Implantable Vented Electrical Left Ventricular Assist System** (HeartMate VE) is also an intracorporeal, pulsatile pump designed to provide left ventricular circulatory assistance. The HeartMate Vented Electric LVAD and the Novacor LVAD (see next section) are the first **wearable** left ventricular assist devices that allow the patient to reside outside the hospital and resume a semi-independent existence (Fig. 8–8). In the wearable configuration, the pump is powered by two rechargeable batteries that are worn in a belt, vest, or shoulder pack.

The major difference between the pneumatic and electric HeartMate is the pump itself. The vented electric pump has a pusher plate mechanism for blood ejection, activated by a rotary electric motor. The vented electric pump has two compartments: a blood chamber lined with a textured polyurethane/titanium surface (as in the pneumatic device) designed to minimize the development of thrombus and a second portion containing the electrical actuator system. The chambers are separated by a flexible diaphragm. The electric motor positioned below the diaphragm causes a pusher plate to move, which in turn compresses the diaphragm, forcing ejection of blood from the blood pump chamber (Fig. 8–9). This contrasts with the pneumatic devices which use pulses of air to force blood ejection. Unlike the pneumatic device, the vented electric device will completely empty with each ejection and is not sensitive to afterload unless there is severe outlet obstruction of the pump or graft (which increases the pump's electrical current utilization and triggers an alarm).

The low-speed torque electric motor includes a stator (the fixed part which forms the pivot or housing for the rotating motor), an electronic comutator (provides

The console (Fig. 8–6) can be powered by plugging into an AC outlet or battery driven for at least 30 minutes to allow increased mobility. A portable console with battery pack can also be worn by the patient.

The *pumping action* is via a pusher plate that is bonded to a diaphragm which divides the pump into a blood-

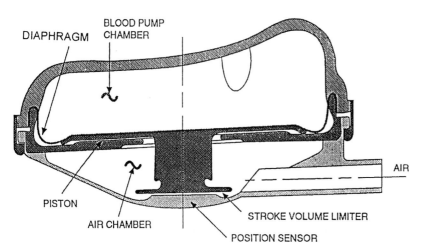

FIGURE **8-7.** Diagram of pusher plate pump mechanism for the pneumatic HeartMate ventricular assist device. (From HeartMate Manual IP LVAS Operating Manual: Drive Console. TCI ThermoCardiosystems, Inc., Woburn, MA, with permission.)

TABLE 8-4	Pneumatic HeartMate LVAD—Problem Analysis	
WARNING SIGNAL	CAUSE	SOLUTION
E----------Stroke---------------F — — — — — ■■■■■■■■ (Inadequate Ejection)	Kinked interconnect cable Eject duration too short Air loss	Straighten interconnect cable; increase **EJECT DURation** 1. Vent 2. If recurs, hand tighten connectors 3. Change console 4. Change cable 5. Examine skin site for air leak 6. Check for fractured drive line (blood in tubing)
	Condensation in interconnect cable Patient arterial pressure is elevated	Drain interconnect cable Adjust patient BP
E----------Stroke---------------F ■■■■■■■■ — — — — — (Inadequate Filling	Rate too fast (fixed rate mode) Hypolemia, right heart failure Kinked inflow tube	Decrease **FIXED RATE** Correct patient condition Change VAD
LOW FLOW ALARM	Flow < 1.5 L/min	Evaluate bar graph for adequate filling and ejection; if persists with stroke volume <30 mL, heparinize and consider pump replacement
LOW BATTERY ALARM	Batteries significantly depleted 10 min battery time left	1. Plug in console 2. Ensure rear AC switch is on
NO OP ALARM	Console in **STOP** mode >2½ minutes	Silence using **ALARM RESET** during implant procedure
NO POWER ALARM	No battery or AC power	1. Plug in console (Turn power off, then on) 2. Press fixed rate 3. If pump doesn't start, turn off console power and use hand crank 4. Replace console
BASAL FIXED RATE ALARM	Microprocessor malfunction	Console defaults to 40 bpm Cannot silence using **ALARM RESET** key Exchange consoles
XX's displayed for volume and stroke	No pump calibration No pump sensor input	**VENT** and cycle console Check connections, **VENT** Exchange console, **VENT** Exchange interconnect cable, **VENT** Exchange pump, **VENT** (if preimplant)
Unexplained internal bleeding beyond peri-implant period *or* red blood from exit site outside tubing	Inflow valve blood leak *or* leak from other components, *or* patient bleed	Operate to fix; note high risk of air embolism if hole in inflow components (use peripheral CPB, then Turn off pump)
CALL SERVICE 01 DISPLAY	Console hardware fault	Console requires service
CALL SERVICE OX (OX=02-06)	Console hardware fault	Console requires service*

*The **CALL SERVICE 02** message may also be displayed if the operator depresses the stop key during a **VENT**. Should the **CALL SERVICE 02** message be displayed, repeat the **VENT** without depressing the **STOP** key. Call service only if the message is repeated after the second **VENT**. See Service Manual for description.

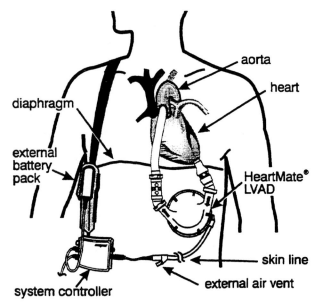

FIGURE **8-8.** Diagram of components of the wearable HeartMate vented electric ventricular assist device. (From HeartMate Manual VE Operating Manual: Implantable Vented Electric Left Ventricular Assist System. TCI ThermoCardiosystems, Inc., Woburn, MA, with permission.)

covered by a polyester velour sheathing to encourage tissue ingrowth and retard ascending infection. The conduit contains two separate lines. The first is an electric cable which connects via an electric lead to the belt mounted TCI vented electric system controller (see Box), which performs control and monitoring functions in the VAD. Controller warning signals and messages describing device or controller malfunction are summarized in Table 8–5. The second line is an external air vent which allows air transfer in and out of the motor chamber to equalize pressure. This vent port can also be used for emergency pneumatic pump activation. The external air vent requires specific management and certain restrictions. The patient must be constantly aware to prevent the vent from being kinked, blocked, or exposed to fluids, which could rapidly decrease or cease LVAD output. Tight clothing that could either bend or kink the tube must be avoided. By placing the external components in a waterproof pouch, the patient is able to shower after the skin exit site is completely healed (and after learning the strict protocol necessary to prevent liquids from contacting the air vent). This device is currently approved and marketed in the United States and many European, Asian, and South American countries.

power to the windings and provides a fixed rate backup of 40 bpm), and a rotator magnet assembly. One motor revolution produces one pump ejection. The actuator converts the rotary motion of the motor to the linear motion of the pusher-plate mechanism. As the cam rotates, the cam/pusher-plate mechanism is forced upward, forcing ejection of blood. The diaphragm is constructed from polyurethane with an integrally textured surface. The blood-contacting metal components are sintered, porous titanium.

The ventricular assist device is implanted in the left upper abdominal region below the diaphgram, usually in a subrectus position. A single drive line conduit exists the abdominal wall on the patient's right side and is

Novacor Left Ventricular Assist Device

The Novacor Left Ventricular Assist Device (Novacor N100, Novacor Division, Baxter Healthcare Corp., Oakland, CA) is an electrically powered device designed for long-term use (Fig. 8–11). Initial experimentation with the Novacor Left Ventricular Assist Device began in 1972 with much of the early experimental work occurring at Stanford University. Early in its development, investigators formulated a vision for a future permanent indwelling circulatory device, focusing on the development of an electrically powered system, miniaturization of parts and electric circuitry, and the development of methodology for monitoring and controlling device function and converting electrical energy to mechanical energy.[192]

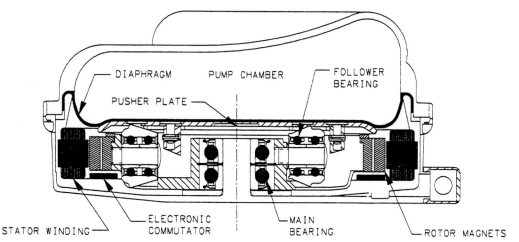

FIGURE **8-9.** Pusher plate pump mechanism for HeartMate vented electric ventricular assist device. (From HeartMate Manual VE Operating Manual: Implantable Vented Electric Left Ventricular Assist System. TCI ThermoCardiosystems, Inc., Woburn, MA, with permission.)

TCI Vented Electric System Controller

The system controller is a complex computerized unit which controls and monitors many details of the pump function. For example, to provide "smooth" pumping action, the controller adjusts the power to the motor unit at the beginning and end of each ejection cycle to "soften" the start and stop of each cycle, a process termed "power conditioning." Other functions include the implementation of rate modes (automatic or fixed) with adjustment of rate according to inflow of blood into the pump, computation of performance data, generation of diagnostic information which is displayed on the system monitor, implementing default operating modes when required, and initiating visual and audible alarm systems. Two operating modes are available: the fixed rate mode (which is preset to 50 bpm, contains a range of 50–120 bpm, and is particularly useful in the operating room) and the auto mode (which is responsive to circulatory demands and maximizes the pumping capacity of the system). The power supply of the vented electric system is provided by two 12-V sealed, lead acid batteries, (which are worn by the patient in "holsters" located under each arm on a waist pack) or by the power base unit (PBU). Each battery is inserted into a battery clip, which in turn receives the cable connected to the controller unit (Fig. 8–10). Each pair of batteries provide about 4–6 hours of operation. Six pairs of batteries last about 1 year. While sleeping and during sedentary periods, the PBU provides power for the device and also acts as a vehicle for charging up to six batteries. The PBU is electrically isolated from the AC electrical ground path to prevent potentially damaging external fault currents gaining access to the controller unit. In the event of an electrical power loss, an emergency power pack and cable kept in the home or near the patient at the hospital provide up to 24 hours of LVAD function. The controller console contains an internal 1-hour backup battery which is automatically activated if wall power fails or if the power switch on the rear panel is turned off while the patient is connected to the power base unit.

A second controller, additional batteries, and a hand pump must always be available as emergency backup components. The controller console contains an internal 1-hour backup battery which is automatically activated if wall power fails or if the power switch on the rear panel is turned off while the patient is connected to the power base unit. The power base unit charges the internal battery whenever it is plugged in and turned on.

The controller contains a switch panel which is comprised of a battery "fuel gauge," two pushbutton switches, and two warning symbols (yellow wrench and a red heart). On the left-hand side of the panel is a pushbutton key marked with an arrow and a spiral, which permits selection of either the fixed rate or auto mode. On the right hand side of the panel, an Alarm Reset button is used to silence the audible alert (for 2 minutes) and to activate the battery "fuel gauge" indicators. In the upper portion of the panel, four green lights indicate the approximate remaining battery capacity (one green light indicates less than 25% full up to four green lights, indicating 75–100% full). Illumination of the right-hand battery symbol with a yellow light indicates less than 15% of battery time remaining, and illumination with a red light

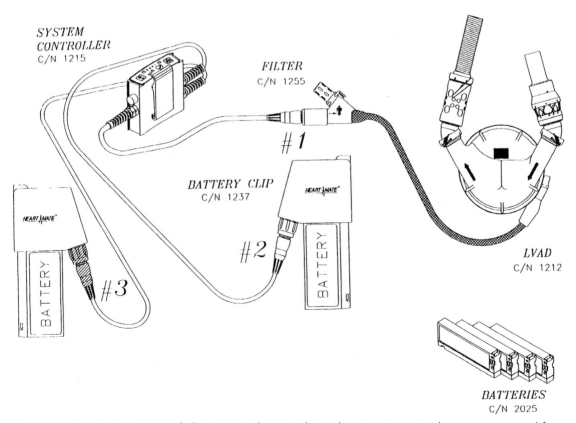

FIGURE **8–10.** HeartMate vented electric ventricular assist device: basic components and connections required for operating the system on rechargeable batteries. (From HeartMate Manual VE Operating Manual: Implantable Vented Electric Left Ventricular Assist System. TCI ThermoCardiosystems, Inc., Woburn, MA, with permission.)

indicates less than 5 minutes remaining. The two alert symbols on the bottom center of the panel provide a number of advisories. The **yellow wrench** indicates malfunctions which have no immediate effect on circulatory support. When the yellow wrench is illuminated, controller connections should be checked and the power base unit and system monitor is utilized to see the message indicating the source of the problem. The yellow wrench provides an alert to power cable disconnection, low stroke volume, low flow, low voltage, controller malfunction, power limit advisory, controller cell low, and rate control fault, among others.

The **red heart** is illuminated when a serious alarm condition is present, indicating that the loss of circulatory support is imminent or present. When the red heart is illuminated, a quick check is made for a blocked vent line and connector and cable integrity. If the connections are intact and there is poor or no VAD function, pneumatic pumping must be immediately initiated while continuing the *problem-solving* algorithm. A summary of *problem analysis and correction* is contained in Table 8–5. Sudden or progressive decrease in VAD output or cessation of pumping are most likely related to loss of battery or external power, broken wires, damage to the controller, or damage to the motor or LVAD parts.

TABLE 8-5	Vented Electric HeartMate LVAD—Problem Analysis		
WARNING SIGNAL	SYSTEM MONITOR MESSAGE	CAUSE	SOLUTION
Red Heart Symbol (with steady tone audio alarm)	Low (or no) Beat Rate (35 bpm) Low stroke volume (25 mL/min) Low flow (<1.5 L/min) Low voltage (below 5 min remaining)	**Potential Causes:** 1. Interruption of power in or to controller 2. Obstruction or kinked vent line 3. ≥ 2 broken power leads in the percutaneous cable 4. Damage to the controller or its connectors 5. Damage to the motor and/or LVAD parts	**Quick check for:** 1. Kinked/blocked vent line 2. All cable connections **If still no VAD function:** 1. Disconnected controller power connection and begin manual hand pumping 2. Switch controller and/or switch to fresh batteries 3. If still no function, switch pneumatic console
Continuous audio alarm without visual symbols and no VAD function	None	All power to controller is lost	1. Plug power source if unplugged 2. If not this, begin manual pumping and check all power sources to controller
Red Battery Symbol with steady audio tone	Low voltage (< 5 min remaining)	Low battery voltage	Change to power base and recharge battery
Yellow battery plus 1 beep per second	Low voltage (< 15 min remaining)	Low battery voltage	Change to power base and recharge battery
Yellow wrench plus 1 beep per second	1. Power cable disconnected from batteries 2. Low stroke volume (<30 mL/min) 3. Low flow (<2 L/min) 4. Controller malfunction 5. Power limit advisory 6. Controller battery cell low 7. Rate control fault	1. Power cable disconnected from batteries 2. Extension cable not properly connected to controller or PBU 3. Broken percutaneous lead 4. Controller malfunction	If VE LVAD is still operating: 1. Check all controller connections 2. Check the vent line for obstruction or kinking 3. Check all connections: Percutaneous electric lead at the "Y" connector, battery or PBU leads 4. If on batteries, change to PowerBase Unit or vice versa; when connection or disconnection the percutaneous cable from the controller to the LVAD, power should be off to minimize risk to the patients 5. Replace controller 6. Replace PBU 20-foot cable 7. Replace PBU 8. Utilize PBU and system monitor to ascertain the source of the problem 9. If yellow alert still persists and the LVAD remains operational, notify perfusionist and call the TCI Heartline for assistance at 800-456-1477

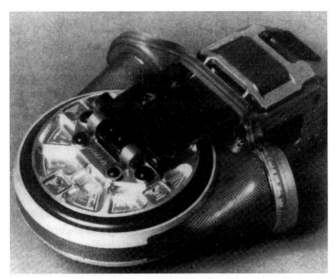

FIGURE **8–11.** Novacor left ventricular assist device. (From Sapirstein JS, Pae WE Jr: Mechanical circulatory support before heart transplantation. *In* Cooper DKC, Miller LW, Patterson GA [eds]: The Transplantation and Replacement of Thoracic Organs. 2nd ed. Boston: Kluwer Academic Publishers, 1996, with permission.)

The device is implanted in the left subrectus position within the abdominal wall. The pump receives blood from the left ventricle through an apical cannula and pumps blood through an outflow conduit to the ascending aorta. A pulsed solenoid (electromagnetic) energy converter is used to activate two opposing pusher plates. The solenoid converts electrical energy to mechanical energy, which is stored in a pair of springs that are attached to two pusher plates (Fig. 8–12). The opposing pusher plates compress the blood sac, producing ejection of blood into the aorta. Electrical input is received via a percutaneous wire. An accompanying percutaneous vent promotes free oscillation of the pusher plates. Unlike the Heartmate VE VAD, the Novacor device does not have a torque vibratory motion within the pocket. Unidirectional flow is maintained by two bovine pericardial bioprosthetic valves.

The external Novacor compact controller (see Box) and power source supply is connected to the pump by a single percutaneous lead brought out through the right abdominal wall, which contains the electrical wires and

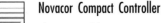

Novacor Compact Controller

The wearable **compact controller** operates and monitors the pump drive unit, and calculates (and displays) pump volume and fill rate in order to coordinate the pump operation with the heart. The controller contains alarms to identify out-of-limit abnormal operation.

Position sensors within pump/drive unit provide continuous pump volume information to the compact controller which can control timing in the Fill Rate Trigger mode (see below), synchronize ejection with the natural heart rhythm (without the need for an electrocardiogram [ECG] signal), and compute values of pump stroke volume and pump output which are displayed on the monitor.

To provide maximal ventricular unloading, the device fills during left ventricular systole and ejects during ventricular diastole, thus operating in synchronous counterpulsation to the natural heart. However, the timing of pump ejection can be altered to provide some ventricular loading if desired during attempts to allow recovery of the natural heart.

The **Fill Rate Trigger** mode is the preferred mode of operation, producing the highest pump output. In this mode, the pump responds to changes in the pump filling rate, and the pump ejection can be triggered to coincide with the end of left ventricular systole (detected by the decrease in fill rate). If there is no left ventricular contraction while in the Fill Rate Trigger mode, the pump will automatically default to the **Fill-to-Empty** mode. If there are conditions of poor pump filling, the pump will default to a minimum pump rate of 60 bpm.

The **Fixed Rate** mode is utilized at the time of implantation in the operating room and rarely thereafter, except possibly during device weaning (anticipating cardiac recovery). The rate settings range from 30–150 bpm. **Status indicators and alarms** are present on the compact controller (Table 8–6), on the left ventricular assist system monitor, and on the personal monitor which advise the patient and physician of abnormal function of some device component.

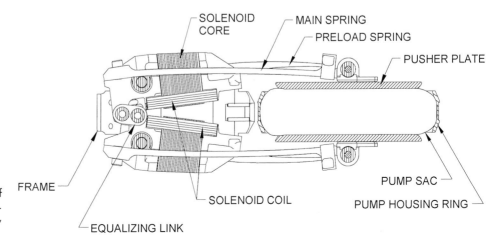

FIGURE **8–12.** Pump mechanism of Novacor ventricular assist device. (From World Heart Corporation, Ottawa, Canada, with permission.)

SOLENOID CORE MAIN SPRING PRELOAD SPRING PUSHER PLATE FRAME SOLENOID COIL EQUALIZING LINK PUMP SAC PUMP HOUSING RING

TABLE 8-6	Novacor LVAD Compact Alarms—Problem Analysis	
WARNING SIGNAL	CAUSE	SOLUTION
"Low Power" red light (with single beep, then continuous beep after 30 seconds)	A viable power source (LVAS monitor, personal monitor, or power pack) is not connected to the port	Reconnect the power source or connect a different power source
"Temp" yellow light (with beep repeated every 15 seconds)	The compact controller internal temperature is too high	Provide good air cooling for the compact controller
"Check" yellow light (with beep repeated every 15 seconds)	1. Low pump output 2. Autostart disabled or the compact controller is not connected	1. Identify/resolve cause of low output 2. Connect to LVAS monitor to get more information on possible fault conditions
"Check" yellow light (with continuous tone)	1. Very low pump output (< 2 L/min) 2. Pump/drive not connected when autostart is enabled	1. Identify and resolve cause of low output 2. Check connection between pump/drive unit and compact controller; replace controller immediately if alarm continues
"Replace" red light and "check" yellow light (with continuous tone)	1. Serious compact controller fault-pump stopped 2. Excessive (dangerous) power being delivered to the pump/drive unit	Replace compact controller immediately

the venting air space. The pump receives blood passively from the left ventricle and delivers a maximum stroke volume of 70 mL, with a sensing mechanism that adjusts beat rate by triggering pump ejection when the rate of filling falls below a threshold level near end diastole. Controller warning signals and alarms are summarized in Table 8–6. The initial anticoagulation consists of low-molecular-weight dextran followed by heparin when surgical bleeding has ceased. Chronic anticoagulation with coumadin and an antiplatelet agent is necessary to prevent thromboembolism.

The device is designed as a portable unit in the outpatient setting. In the wearable configuration, the pump is powered by two rechargeable batteries that provide 4–6 hours of power and are worn in a belt, vest, or shoulder holster. The **wearable (external) power packs** provide power to the compact controller, allowing the patient to have untethered mobility. The primary power pack and a second smaller reserve power pack are rechargeable by a separate power pack charger. A totally implantable electrically powered system with implantable batteries and a volume compensator is under design (Fig. 8–13).

The major weakness of original versions of the Novacor device is stasis at the interface between the inflow valve and the pump, creating a site for possible throm-

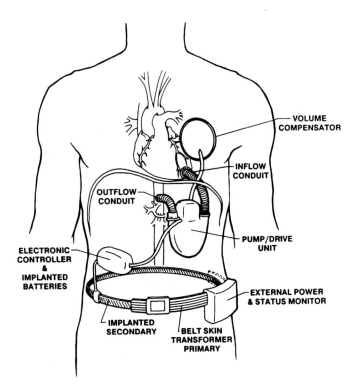

FIGURE **8-13.** The proposed totally implantable Novacor LVAS. (From Smith JA, Oyer PE: Developmetn of the Novacor Left Ventricular Asisst Device. *In* Thoracic Transplantation. Oxford, England: Blackwell Science, 1995, p 134, with permission.)

bus formation. Currently, more than 900 clinical Novacor implants have been performed with an average duration of 4 months and the longest duration exceeding 4 years (Portner, P., personal communication, April 2000).

Other Pulsatile VADs

The **Thoratec Intracorporeal Ventricular Assist Device** contains an implantable blood pump that maintains the same blood flow path, valves, and polyurethane blood pump sac as the paracorporeal Thoratec device. This small, lightweight (about 340 g) pneumatic device can be used for left or biventricular support and is substantially smaller than most other pulsatile VAD systems. It can be implanted in patients ranging in weight from 40–100 kg or more. The small blood pump is implanted in the preperitoneal position, leaving the more complex control unit in an external position where it can be serviced and replaced. A small (9-mm) percutaneous pneumatic drive line for each VAD connects to a portable driver consisting of a small briefcase-sized battery-powered pneumatic control unit.[60, 66, 67]

The **Arrow LionHeart Ventricular Assist Device** is a totally implantable left ventricular device system in which transcutaneous energy is transferred to implanted batteries. A roller screw energy converter causes movement of a pusher plate that compresses a polyurethane blood sac during systole. Unidirectional flow is maintained by tilting disk valves. An intrathoracic compliance chamber maintains near thoracic pressure in the energy converter space. External components consist of the energy transmission source, a power pack, a battery charger, and portable power supplies.

The **WorldHeart HeartSaver Ventricular Assist Device** is also a totally implantable system with an internally implanted and rechargeable battery system. The device is designed for implantation in the left hemithorax adjacent to the natural heart and can be anchored to the rib cage. The device can be implanted without the use of cardiopulmonary bypass. The blood contact surface of the sac is polyurethane and the unidirectional valves are porcine tissue valves.

Several other pulsatile left ventricular assist devices are in various stages of clinical testing in Europe, Japan, the United States, and other countries.[14, 19, 124, 147, 181, 183, 203, 204, 213, 214] In the next few years, these devices will likely become available both as a bridge to transplantation and also potentially as chronic devices intended for long-term treatment of refractory heart failure. In addition to devices mentioned above, the Berlin VAD and TAH from the German Heart Institute; the MEDOS HIA-VAD from Aachen, Germany; the Vienna TAH and VAD from Austria; the Toyobo-National Cardiovascular Center VAD from Osaka, Japan; and the Zeon-Tokyo University VAD from Tokyo, Japan, are pulsatile pneumatic mechanical support systems under investigation or in clinical use. Many other devices not mentioned here are under investigation.

CONTINUOUS FLOW VADS

The unique feature of continuous flow ventricular assist devices is the generation of cardiac output without pulsatility. Since blood flow is continuous (or minimally pulsatile) rather than pulsatile, unidirectional valves are not needed in this system. There are currently two basic types of continuous flow devices: axial flow systems and centrifugal flow systems. These devices have several putative advantages over current pulsatile pumps: (1) they are smaller than most pulsatile pumps and can be used in smaller patients (< 1.5 m^2), even potentially children; (2) they are relatively simple and have fewer moving parts, a potential advantage with respect to mechanical failures; (3) because of the continuous flow characteristics, they do not require a compliance chamber; (4) energy requirements are significantly less than for pulsatile pumps; and (5) with some recovery of heart function, left ventricular ejection of blood through the native aortic valve can provide some pulsatility.

At the current stage of development there are also unresolved potential disadvantages: (1) current axial flow pumps use bearings lubricated by blood and this area of relative stasis is a potential source of thrombus generation; (2) some degree of hemolysis is common, the long-term effects of which are unknown; (3) the long-term effects of nonpulsatile (or essentially nonpulsatile) flow are unknown; (4) current continuous flow devices require chronic anticoagulation; and (5) current devices provide a maximum flow of about 5–6 L/min (moderate flow rates) compared to the 8–11 L/min with chronic pulsatile devices.

Axial Flow Pumps

The axial flow pump motor is small and contains rotor (impeller) blades which spin at 10,000–20,000 rpm. These pumps have an elegant simplicity, in that the pump motor/rotor is the only moving part. A critical feature of the axial flow pump is the requirement for bearings (a device that supports, guides, and reduces friction of motion between fixed and moving parts) which support the rotating impeller. Three basic types of bearings have been employed: blood-immersed bearings, remote-force bearings in which energy is applied across a blood-filled gap, and blood-isolated bearings which require a shaft seal.[113] The design of these bearings appears to be the most critical determinant of the long-term success of these devices.[113] Axial flow pumps are designed to be wearable, easy to manage, and rugged. Several devices are currently undergoing clinical investigation.

The **Nimbus Intracorporeal Ventricular Assist Device (HeartMate II)** is a small (7-cm) axial flow pump that connects to the left ventricle apex for inflow and the ascending aorta for outflow.[22] Blood flow is generated by an electromagnetic power mechanism, in which an internal electric motor provides the torque (developed by an internal magnet in response to an electromagnetic field) required to drive the pump rotor.[208] The pump rotor is supported by two cup-socket ruby bearings, and the outer boundary of the bearing's static and moving surfaces is washed directly by blood flow. A first-generation model has a percutaneous small-diameter electrical cable which passes through the skin and connects to an external electrical controller. Subsequent generations will be totally implantable.

The **Jarvik 2000 Heart** is a similar compact (5.5 cm, 85 g) electrically powered axial flow pump that receives inflow through the left ventricular apex and provides outflow to the descending thoracic aorta.[139] The current version of this device is tethered to its electrical power source by a percutaneous wire.[117] Tiny blood-immersed ceramic bearings which are washed by the rapid flow of blood are used to lubricate the pivot points of the Jarvik 2000 rotor. An implantable microprocessor-based pump speed control system with automatic programmable pump speed adjustment is under development.[110]

The **DeBakey (Micromed) Axial Flow Pump** is an electromagnetically actuated titanium axial flow pump developed in collaboration with engineers from the U.S. National Aeronautics and Space Administration.[46] The pump connects to the left ventricular apex and ascending aorta, and the current design includes a fixed-rpm rate which can be adjusted through an external device. For optimal patient mobilization, power can be supplied by two 12-V DC batteries for several hours. The first clinical implants were performed in Austria.[217]

Centrifugal Flow Pumps

Centrifugal flow pumps are somewhat larger than axial flow pumps and their rotational speeds are slower (about 2,000–4,000 vs. 10,000–20,000 rpm).

The **AB-180 Circulatory Support System** is a small, durable, electromagnetically powered centrifugal pump that receives inflow from the left atrium and empties into the ascending aorta.[29, 88] A solution of distilled water and heparin provides a high local concentration of anticoagulant within the pump. In the event of pump failure, an occluder device prevents retrograde flow form the aorta to the left atrium.

The **HeartMate III** left ventricular assist device is a centrifugal pump powered by magnetic levitation, a process which combines the functions of levitation and rotation. The small pump rotor does not contain bearings and is completely encased in titanium.

TOTAL ARTIFICIAL HEARTS

The total artificial heart is a MCSS that is capable of replacing the function of the entire heart. The patient's native heart is removed when the total artificial heart is implanted, thus there is no fallback mechanism for pumping blood in the event of device failure. Chronic anticoagulation with warfarin is required to prevent thromboembolism.

Compliance chambers pose the same problems for the TAH as they do for VADs, though several TAH designs have eliminated the need for a compliance chamber.[161] Other designs that incorporate an intrathoracic compliance chamber have been used successfully in animals for extended periods. The compliance chamber requires percutaneous recharging of gas, typically with sulfur hexafluoride, about every 2 weeks.[172, 218]

Another factor that must be accounted for by the TAH is the natural **imbalance between the output of the right and left ventricles.** This imbalance is due primarily to the bronchial circulation, with return to the pulmonary veins and left atrium. This effectively produces a left-to-left shunt, increasing the left ventricular output roughly 5–10% above the right ventricular output. Failure to account for this shunt in TAH design would result in left atrial pressure which is unacceptably higher than right atrial pressure.

A variety of methods have been developed to compensate for this difference in native right and left ventricular output, including an interatrial shunt device,[205] a difference in stroke volume reserve between the two prosthetic ventricles, a hydraulic shunt mechanism controlled by left atrial pressure which adjusts the prosthetic right ventricular stroke volume (therefore avoiding shunting of blood within the device),[129, 130] and a pump controller designed to actively balance the output of the right and left ventricles.[194]

The **CardioWest Total Artificial Heart** formerly called the Jarvik or Symbion Total Artificial Heart is a pulsatile biventricular cardiac replacement system that is pneumatically driven (Fig. 8–14). Like many left ventricular assist devices, the blood sac is lined by a smooth polyurethane surface and contains a polyurethane diaphragm that separates the blood chamber from the air chamber (Fig. 8–15). Unidirectional flow is maintained by four Medtronic-Hall mechanical valves. The maximal pump stroke volume is 70 mL with a maximum flow rate of 15 L/min. Initial anticoagulation with heparin followed by chronic anticoagulation with coumadin and antiplatelet agents is necessary to avoid thromboembolism. In its current version, patients can be ambulated,

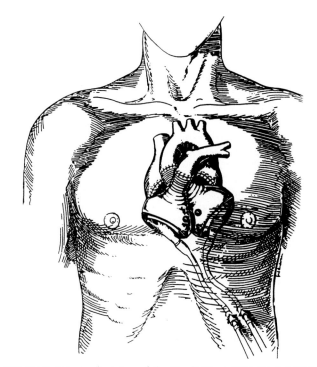

FIGURE 8–14. Implantation of the CardioWest C-70 Total Artificial Heart. (From Sapirstein JS, Pae WE Jr: Mechanical circulatory support before heart transplantation. *In* Copper DKC, Miller LW, Patterson GA [eds]: The Transplantation and Replacement of Thoracic Organs. 2nd ed. Boston: Kluwer Academic Publishers, 1996, with permission.)

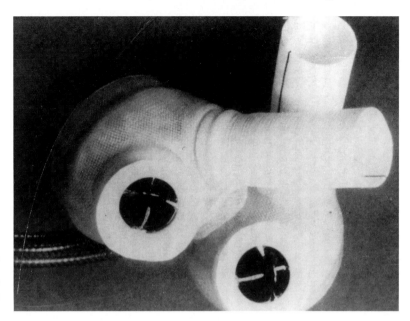

FIGURE **8–15.** Jarvik-7-100 total artificial heart. (From Sapirstein JS, Pae WE Jr: Mechanical circulatory support before heart transplantation. *In* Copper DKC, Miller LW, Patterson GA [eds]: The Transplantation and Replacement of Thoracic Organs. 2nd ed. Boston: Kluwer Academic Publishers, 1996, with permission.)

but their activity is severely restricted by the large drive console.

The **Abiomed Total Artificial Heart** is a totally implantable artificial heart designed for chronic therapy. Blood flow is maintained by a high-efficiency miniature unidirectional centrifugal pump which provides cardiac output in excess of 10 L/min. Unidirectional blood flow is maintained by four trileaflet polyether urethane (Angioflex) valves. The device has a compact electrohydraulically driven energy converter which sits between two blood pumps. A cylindrical rotary valve alternates the direction of hydraulic fluid flow between the left and right pumping chambers.[130] Balance between left and right ventricular blood flow is achieved by a hydraulic fluid balancing chamber which attaches to the left prosthetic ventricle's inflow port. The fluid in this chamber is connected by a shunt to the right prosthetic ventricle's pumping chamber. The shift in hydraulic fluid to and from the right side of the pump adjusts output from the prosthetic right ventricle.[129, 130]

The **Penn State Total Artificial Heart** is a totally implantable device based on dual pusher-plate pumps and a roller screw actuator. Circulatory pusher plates are attached to the two ends of the roller screw shaft, and the motor turns 6.3 revolutions to provide a full 2.6-cm pusher plate stroke. One pump fills while the other empties, and the motor then reverses to eject the opposite pump.[219] A seamless polyurethane blood sac lines each pump, and Bjork-Shiley Convexo-Concave or Delrin monostrut tilting disk valves maintain unidirectional flow in the inlet and outlet ports. Left/right balance is achieved by a controller which adjusts pump output from estimations of end-diastolic volume. The system contains a compliance chamber and transcutaneous energy transmission system.

PUMPS WITHOUT BLOOD CONTACT

An extension of the concepts utilized in the Anstadt Cup (see previous discussion) provided the stimulus

for longer term support devices which augment cardiac output without blood-surface contact. Such devices would combine volume-constraining properties with augmentation of left ventricular stroke volume. By the Laplace relationship, wall stress is a function of intracavitary pressure X radius divided by wall thickness. Thus, larger ventricles with a larger radius develop increased wall stress which increases myocardial oxygen consumption. Devices which limit left ventricular dilatation have been shown to provide a beneficial effect on left ventricular function.[170]

The **Abiomed Heart Booster** adds a contractile component to a volume-constraining device to further augment cardiac output. The contractile element is based on a series of thin-walled tubes which constitute a cone-shaped apparatus that fits over the apex of the heart. Rapid hydraulic actuation of the device inflates the tubes from a flat elliptical shape during diastole to a circular shape in systole, resulting in compression of the ventricle and augmentation of systolic ejection. Rapid deflation of the tubes to the flat elliptical shape occurs during diastole.

MECHANICAL CIRCULATORY SUPPORT SYSTEMS IN CHILDREN

Mechanical circulatory support in infants and children has been much less successful than in adults. Attempts at miniaturization of adult devices has been impeded by the considerable development costs for device companies and the small potential markets. With available devices, thromboembolic episodes, sepsis, and bleeding complications are the major impediments to successful bridging to cardiac transplantation. The shortage of available donors expands the time interval necessary for mechanical support, and transplantation can rarely be accomplished within 1–2 weeks of initiating support.

With most available systems, the child must remain bed-ridden and largely immobile during the support period.

HISTORICAL NOTES

In 1963, Spencer unsuccessfully supported a 6-year-old girl with refractory right ventricular failure and pulmonary hypertension following closure of a ventricular septal defect. The patient died 24 hours following termination of venoarterial bypass.[198] Subsequently, DeBakey reported successful support of a 16-year-old girl with left atrium–to–axillary bypass as therapy for acute cardiac failure following mitral valve replacement.[48] The application of ECMO support for infants and children with cardiac failure followed the development of membrane oxygenators by Clowes[30] and Kolobow.[123] In the early 1970s, Hill[100] and Soeter[195] reported sucessful prolonged ECMO support following repair of tetralogy of Fallot. The success of ECMO for infants with respiratory failure stimulated its subsequent application for infant cardiac failure.

EXTRACORPOREAL MEMBRANE OXYGENATION SUPPORT

A general description of ECMO is found in the section Short Term Devices, above. Use of ECMO as a bridge to cardiac transplantation in infants and children has obvious limitations because of limited patient mobility, requirement for relatively aggressive anticoagulation, short duration of support, and constant need for a trained pump operator to monitor the device at bedside. Nevertheless, ECMO has been used successfully as a bridge to transplantation in a small number of patients.[49]

Much of the information regarding optimal techniques for cannulation, perfusion methods, and expected complications is derived from the application of ECMO after cardiac surgery. Cannulation of the right carotid artery and right internal jugular vein in the neck is the desired route of cannulation in infants whenever possible. Because of the increased incidence of bleeding[42, 216] and mediastinal infection[171, 216, 223] associated with direct cardiac cannulation, patients who are bridged to transplantation following cardiac surgery should be converted to neck cannulation with sternal closure if possible. Bleeding sufficient to require reexploration of the mediastinum is the most frequent complication, occurring in over 40% of patients with mediastinal cannulation.[50, 115, 122, 171, 216] Major bleeding is uncommon with isolated neck cannulation without recent cardiac surgery.

Mediastinal and blood stream infection are also more common with mediastinal than neck cannulation.[25, 171] Fatal mediastinitis with blood stream sepsis occur almost exclusively in patients with mediastinal cannulation.[216, 223]

Acute renal failure requiring dialysis while on ECMO is a strong predictor of subsequent mortality,[171] with fewer than 10% of such patients surviving to hospital discharge.

Neurologic complications are most common in the setting of profound shock with prolonged hypotension prior to initiating ECMO support.[42, 50, 171] Survival is unusual in such patients[40] and survivors frequently have marked developmental abnormalities.[216]

When left ventricular failure is present, left atrial decompression with blade atrial septostomy may be an important adjunct in preventing pulmonary venous hypertension. Maintenance of low left atrial pressure (and therefore low pulmonary artery pressure) during the bridging period is critically important in maintaining normal lung function and minimizing the probability of severe pulmonary hypertension after transplant.

Survival has generally been less good with ECMO for infant cardiac support than for primary respiratory support. Anderson and colleagues reported 47% hospital survival for infants on ECMO for respiratory failure versus 5% with ECMO for cardiac failure[5] during support ranging from 1–25 days.

The likelihood of survival with successful transplantation is variable among institutions,[171] but several centers have reported 40–50% survival in patients supported on ECMO before transplantation, particularly if neck cannulation is utilized.[223]

CENTRIFUGAL PUMP SUPPORT

Centrifugal pumps offer the option of right, left, or biventricular support without the requirement of an oxygenator in the circuit.[210] Thuys and colleagues reported 31% 1-year actuarial survival among 34 infants under 6 kg who required circulatory support with a centrifugal pump after cardiac surgery.[210] However, the potential for thromboembolic and neurologic complications and the necessity for patient immobilization make this an unattractive method for bridging to transplant.

ABIOMED SYSTEM

The Abiomed pulsatile ventricular support system also includes a pediatric device with smaller diameter cannulae which has the same pump design and characteristics as the adult system (see earlier section, Short Term Devices).

MINIATURE AXIAL FLOW PUMPS

Small axial flow pumps for pediatric circulatory support carry the advantage of small size, relative ease of implantation, and less expense than chronic VADS (see earlier section, Continuous Flow VADs). Although the lower size limit has not been determined, these devices would likely be suitable in children of about 1 m² body surface area (BSA).

PARACORPOREAL CHRONIC VAD SUPPORT

Of the chronic VADs available, the intracorporeal Novacor and HeartMate devices are generally not feasible for patients with BSA less than 1.5 m². However, the paracorporeal chronic VADs, with placement of the pump or pumps outside the body cavity, are more readily adaptable to pediatric use. The Thoratec VAD system has been implanted in patients as small as 17 kg and 0.73 m² BSA (age 7 years) as a successful bridge to heart transplantation.[209] As of September 1998, 47 patients with BSA less than 1.5 m² have been supported with the Thoratec device.

A "scaled-down" version of the Pierce-Donachy VAD has been developed for infants as small as 3.0 kg. This pneumatically powered pump contains a polyurethane blood sac which delivers a stroke volume of 11 ml under standard conditions. Unfortunately, the 6-mm inlet and outlet ball valves had an unacceptable thromboembolic rate in animal studies, presumably related to alterations in fluid dynamics in the small system.[41] Further testing was planned with 10-mm bileaflet tilting disk valves.

The Medos HIA-VAD system, developed by the Helmholtz Institute in Aachen, Germany, is a paracorporeal system which has been specifically tailored for pediatric support. In addition to the benefits of a paracorporeal system which allows extubation and mobilization of the patient, this device contains polyurethane valves rather than mechanical valves, which may decrease the incidence of thromboembolism. The pediatric version is available with stroke volumes of 10 or 25 mL.[124] Although only anecdotal case reports have been published,[124, 220] successful bridging to transplant (duration of support, 2 and 7 weeks) has been reported in two infants weighing 3.3 and 3.4 kg. However, despite anticoagulation with heparin, one infant suffered a cerebral thromboembolic event (with resolution), and the polyurethane valves are reliable for only 40 days, requiring multiple pump changes.

A miniaturized version of the pneumatic "Berlin Heart" has also been used for bridging to transplant, but 2 of 11 patients developed thrombus formation in the blood chamber and necessitated multiple pump exchanges in three patients.[108]

Thus, with current support systems available, the adult paracorporeal systems (such as the Pierce-Donachy VAD) are applicable to children over about 15 kg (about 0.7 m²). The development of smaller axial flow devices may provide an alternative for supporting children with an intracorporeal LVAD.[203] For small infants, ECMO support remains the most thoroughly tested system and probably deserves primary consideration. With further testing and refinements, miniature paracorporeal devices will hopefully provide safe support for small infants without the thromboembolic risk of current systems.

INDICATIONS AND TIMING

VADs are used to support the circulation of patients with profound cardiac failure that is refractory to conventional pharmacologic therapy pending cardiac transplantation. Thus, the indications for VAD support describe characteristics of transplant recipients that are markers for severe circulatory failure. It remains controversial whether temporary IABP support should be tried prior to employing LVAD support.

The patient considered for LVAD support should, to the extent that can be ascertained in a critically ill condition, fulfill the general criteria for transplant recipient selection (see Chapter 6). It is clear that patients with irreversible noncardiac pathology (e.g., a fixed neurologic deficit) or other contraindications to transplantation are not candidates for VAD support as a bridge to transplantation. However, it is often difficult to accurately determine the potential for reversing organ dysfunction that results from cardiac failure, and noncardiac subsystem function can clearly improve in patients supported by VADs.[20, 63, 68, 72, 75, 87, 126, 141]

In the absence of severe intrinsic renal disease, renal dysfunction is usually reversible following several weeks of VAD support. Hepatic dysfunction secondary to right ventricular failure and hepatic congestion usually improves after VAD support. Pneumonia in a patient with deteriorating cardiac failure is *not* a contraindication to LVAD support, since improvement in cardiac output and appropriate antibiotics usually provide successful reversal of the process.

The extent of organ damage that can be expected to resolve with successful circulatory support remains poorly defined. Thus, it has been our practice to implant VADs in patients with *potentially* reversible end-organ dysfunction, with the understanding that transplantation will not be offered until the end-organ dysfunction has clearly improved or resolved. The family and patient are told at the time of device implantation that preexisting organ dysfunction may proceed to irreversible organ failure during VAD support. They are further informed that fixed noncardiac organ failure or other complications during VAD support may preclude transplantation and ultimately cause death. Patients who develop irreversible noncardiac organ injury during the period of support (e.g., a debilitating stroke) are given the option of having the VAD removed, recognizing that this may result in the patient's death.

The criteria for profound circulatory failure that is refractory to conventional therapy generally includes a cardiac index less than about 1.8–2.0 L/min/m² or a systemic systolic blood pressure less than 90 mm Hg despite treatment with adequate ventricular preload (e.g., mean atrial pressure of 18–22 mm Hg), intra-aortic balloon counterpulsation, and inotropic therapy. These criteria are only general guidelines, since a more important indicator is the downward trend in hemodynamics or increasing inotropic requirements to maintain hemodynamics. If the patient has a cardiac arrest, there may not be time to gather all the necessary data to assess the hemodynamic criteria for VAD insertion. Persistent hypotension or refractory malignant arrhythmias may demand immediate placement of a VAD if the patient is to survive.

The cardiac index is not an infallible indicator for profound circulatory failure. Some patients with chronic congestive heart failure successfully adapt to a cardiac index that is less than 2.0 L/min/m², while other patients in profound circulatory failure may have a cardiac index greater than or equal to 2.0 L/min/m² by thermodilution. Note that the measurement of cardiac output by thermodilution may be inaccurate in the presence of severe heart failure secondary to tricuspid or pulmonary insufficiency, artificial instability of the baseline blood temperature reading caused by motion (e.g., labored breathing), and low flow rates that allow recirculation before the primary thermodilution curve has been completed.[32] Inspection of the thermodilution curve and a consideration of other findings (e.g., absent distal pulses, oliguria, low mixed venous hemoglobin oxygen saturation, and hypotension) are necessary to appropriately judge the patient's condition.

Disagreement also exists over what types and doses of medication represent optimal therapy for a given patient with acute cardiac failure. This decision is dependent on the knowledge and clinical experience of those caring for the patient. Finally, not every patient requires placement of an intra-aortic balloon pump to demonstrate that counterpulsation cannot reverse severe circulatory failure. In general, patients with ischemic heart disease benefit from counterpulsation, while patients with nonischemic dilated cardiomyopathy and patients with arrhythmias tend to benefit less. A summary of current general criteria for selection of patients with end-stage heart disease who should be considered for LVAD support is presented in Table 8-7.

The experience with the **total artificial heart** as a bridge to cardiac transplantation is small relative to the experience with VADs. Indications for the TAH that overlap with those for biventricular VADs include medically refractory biventricular failure and refractory ventricular arrhythmias. Indications that are unique to the TAH include severe circulatory failure in patients with a prosthetic aortic valve and medically refractory rejection of a transplanted heart.

The replacement of a severely diseased heart in a TAH recipient removes a potential source of morbidity (e.g., morbidity from emboli that originate in the diseased heart or inflammation stimulated by a rejecting heart). However, the native heart that remains in a VAD recipient provides backup pumping in the event of VAD failure. During the earlier experience with the Jarvik-7

TAH, the relatively high incidence of serious mediastinal infection raised the issue of whether or not a large mass of prosthetic material could exist in the mediastinum without infection.[90] While the design of more biocompatible materials will likely decrease the chance of mediastinitis in TAH recipients, the recent results of experienced surgical groups indicate that optimal surgical techniques alone can produce a fairly low incidence of mediastinal infection.[37, 58, 136, 162]

THE CONCEPT OF BRIDGING TO CHRONIC MCS

During the evolution of VAD support as a bridge to transplantation, an important incidence of death between VAD insertion and transplantation was considered an acceptable outcome because of the certainty of death without such support. It is now known that noncardiac organ failure is the major cause of death after implantation. As the field has matured, there is an increasing expectation that patients supported by this very expensive technology should *routinely* survive to transplantation. This changing expectation has given rise to the concept of a "bridge-to-the-bridge."

Patients in profound low cardiac output referred for LVAD bridge undergo rapid assessment of noncardiac organ function, focusing on the severity and immediate sequelae of the acute cardiac failure. Many patients receive IABP support prior to LVAD, but this is frequently insufficient to reverse organ dysfunction. If there are signs of cardiogenic shock or recipient organ failure, the practice of temporary support with a less invasive and expensive device has emerged as a common practice. After 2–7 days, a more accurate assessment can be made of organ function and reversible dysfunction. If dysfunction is deemed irreversible, a decision to terminate support is appropriate before implementing full LVAD support.

An important component of this assessment is neurologic evaluation, since a presenting cardiac arrest or cardiogenic shock may alter mental status and induce obtundation or coma. This period of pre-LVAD support

---

TABLE 8-7 Patient Selection Criteria for VAD Support as a Bridge to Cardiac Transplantation

1. Upper age consistent with successful cardiac transplantation, usually about age 70
2. Lower age limit determined by patient size large enough to accommodate a device
   a. Thoratec VAD: usually ≥ 1.0 m²
   b. HeartMate System: usually ≥ about 1.5 m²
   c. Novacor: usually ≥ about 1.5 m²
   d. Cardiowest total artificial heart: usually ≥ about 1.7 m²
   e. Medos VAD: ≥ about 0.5 m²
3. Suitable candidate for cardiac transplantation
4. Imminent risk of death before donor heart availability; usually with evidence of deterioration on maximal appropriate inotropic support and/or intra-aortic balloon support
5. General hemodynamic guidelines:
   a. Cardiac index < about 1.8 L/min/m²
   b. Systolic arterial blood pressure < about 90 mm Hg
   c. Pulmonary capillary wedge pressure > about 20 mm Hg in spite of appropriate pharmacologic management
6. Adequate psychological criteria and external psychosocial support for transplantation and for potentially prolonged LVAD support
7. Informed consent of patient/family
8. Absence of *fixed* pulmonary hypertension (pulmonary vascular resistance > about 6 WU)
9. Absence of irreversible renal or hepatic failure (LVAD support *not* expected to reverse existing renal or hepatic dysfunction)

allows a more complete evaluation of psychosocial issues, peripheral vascular disease, and other life-limiting conditions which may affect the decision to transplant. If neurologic and other noncardiac function normalizes within the period of preliminary support, full LVAD support can be implemented with a high expectation of successful bridge to transplantation.

DECISIONS REGARDING UNIVENTRICULAR VERSUS BIVENTRICULAR SUPPORT

A key decision during the evaluation of a potential VAD recipient relates to univentricular versus biventricular support[62, 68, 126, 128, 163] (Table 8–8). This decision affects the types of devices that are available for implantation. Furthermore, acute failure of the right ventricle at the initiation of isolated LVAD support remains an important source of VAD-related morbidity and mortality.[72, 190]

Currently, accurate pre-VAD assessment of right ventricular reserves and the ability of the right ventricle to adapt to the volume load delivered by the LVAD remains problematic. To date, no single method for evaluation has been uniformly successful. The simplest technique is measurement of the central venous pressure and evaluation with an echocardiogram to assess right ventricular size, wall motion and ejection fraction prior to surgery. Right ventricular pressure measurements synchronized with transesophageal echocardiographic determinations of ventricular dimensions to derive load-independent measurements of right ventricular function have been used to predict the right ventricular response to LVAD support.[146] A very low right ventricular ejection fraction ($\leq 15\%$) indicates a poor outcome with isolated LVAD support. If central venous pressure remains markedly elevated (> 17 mm Hg) prior to and after LVAD placement, the likelihood of reversal of severe renal or hepatic dysfunction is greater with biventricular than univentricular support.

Malignant ventricular arrhythmias are a relative indication for biventricular support. Medically refractory ventricular arrhythmias that are present prior to VAD implantation often persist despite LVAD support and the return of adequate myocardial perfusion.[64] Biventricular assist or a total artificial heart device provide more secure circulatory support than an isolated LVAD in the setting of sustained ventricular tachycardia or fibrillation.[148] An isolated LVAD can often provide marginally adequate circulatory support in the total absence of native cardiac function if pulmonary vascular resistance is normal,[12, 104, 160] but an LVAD works best with a right ventricle that can respond to demands for increased flow.

An additional important consideration is the potential for improvement in right ventricular function following initiation of left ventricular assistance. In patients with chronic heart failure from ischemic or dilated cardiomyopathy, pulmonary vascular resistance decreases[78] and right ventricular function and myocyte histopathology tend to improve during chronic LVAD support.[131, 182] However, other events may occur that can acutely worsen right ventricular function. For instance, acute ischemia of the right ventricle or ventricular septum has an adverse effect on right ventricular function. Acute increases in pulmonary vascular resistance that may occur in association with cardiopulmonary bypass and blood transfusions may temporarily worsen RV function. Poor right ventricular function will, in turn, impair the delivery of blood to the left VAD.[43, 61] Low (normal) preoperative pulmonary artery pressure may be a risk factor for acute right ventricular failure after-LVAD secondary to inadequate right ventricular adaptation to increased perioperative pulmonary vascular resistance.[76]

Biventricular VADs or a total artificial heart are probably the best options for patients with acute severe biventricular failure (e.g., many of the patients who fail to separate from cardiopulmonary bypass following cardiac operations), patients with chronic severe biventricular failure, and patients with incessant ventricular arrhythmias. For other patients with acute left ventricular failure, isolated LVAD support is nearly always sufficient if the preimplant right atrial pressure is less than about 18 mm Hg.

TIMING OF VAD IMPLANT

Timing the decision to implant a VAD remains imprecise because the exact clinical course of individual patients with severe heart failure is difficult to forsee and donor availability is unpredictable. However, certain general guidelines are appropriate. Once the decision has been made to offer a patient cardiac transplantation and the patient has exhibited signs of severe heart failure with early end-organ injury, there is usually little gained by procrastination about VAD support. If at all possible, education of the patient and family about the potential risks and benefits of VAD support should be well underway before VAD implantation. A minimum 24-hour period of reflection should be provided, unless precluded by the patient's condition. As further experience is gained with VADs, it is likely that results of VAD support will improve. Thus, device placement will be performed somewhat earlier in the patient's course than it is now in order to avoid postimplant complications (e.g., coagulopathic bleeding, infection, and renal dysfunction) and accelerate rehabilitation.

TABLE 8–8	**Typical Settings Necessitating Biventricular Mechanical Circulatory Assistance**

- Bleeding requiring large volumes of transfused blood products
- Failure to separate from cardiopulmonary bypass following cardiac operation (i.e., bridge to recovery patients)
- Signs of overt right ventricular failure in a patient with chronic congestive heart failure
- CVP > 20 mm Hg required for adequate left VAD flow
- Dilated right ventricle with moderate to severe tricuspid regurgitation *prior* to initiation of left VAD pumping
- Recurrent ventricular arrhythmias (sustained ventricular tachycardia or fibrillation)
- Acute myocardial infarction involving the right ventricle or ventricular septum

SURGICAL PLACEMENT OF CHRONIC VENTRICULAR ASSIST DEVICES

The specific technique used for the placement of a VAD is dependent on the device chosen, the condition of the patient, and which ventricles are supported. The following paragraphs describe the general steps involved in placing a chronic left ventricular assist device with either left atrial or left ventricular apical cannulation.[92, 141, 159, 160, 165]

The patient is placed in the standard supine position for a cardiac operation. The groins are left in the operative field in the event that femoral access is needed for cardiopulmonary bypass, and the lateral aspect of the left chest and abdomen are kept within the operative field. The future position of percutaneous drive lines, cannulas, chest tubes, and pressure monitoring lines should be envisioned by the surgeon prior to making the initial skin incision.

Transesophageal echocardiography is routinely employed at many centers to assess specific cardiac abnormalities and assist in de-airing maneuvers following LVAD implantation. Prior to initiating cardiopulmonary bypass, the heart is examined by echocardiography to identify any interatrial communications (which must be surgically closed to prevent desaturation during LVAD support)[18, 185, 193] and to identify aortic regurgitation (which, if more than mild, must be corrected prior to LVAD support).

The heart is exposed using a median sternotomy. If an abdominal incision is necessary for placement of the pump, it is carried in the midline to just above the umbilicus or around the umbilicus and about 2 cm below (depending on the device). Hemostasis is accomplished as completely as possible before heparin is administered. Most pulsatile implantable pumps are placed on the left side of the abdominal wall below both rectus muscles, anterior to the posterior rectus sheath. Complete hemostasis is of critical importance to avoid a pocket hematoma and subsequent infection. Any large arterial or venous perforating vessel should be clipped rather than cauterized. A space is created under both costal margins sufficient for passage of the inlet and outlet portions of the device in a manner which keeps any outflow graft to the ascending aorta away from the sternum. The pocket is filled with surgical lap pads soaked in antibiotic solution. Pneumatic drive lines are often brought out through the left anterior abdominal wall. With electric pumps, the drive line is usually brought out on the patient's right side. Drive lines should exit away from the iliac crest to avoid discomfort from belts and other clothing at waist level.

The pump and its components are prepared on a back table. If bioprosthetic valves are part of the device, they are rinsed in sequential saline solutions. The pump is filled with heparinized saline and the ends of the inlet and outlet ports are covered with a "cap" of latex surgical glove finger. The electrical connections are covered with a threaded component to protect them from blood or other debris prior to the final hookup. If preclotting

of graft components is necessary, cryoprecipitate massaged into the outside surface of the graft followed by topical thrombin spray is highly effective.

LEFT ATRIAL CANNULATION

Before placing the atrial cannula, the aortic graft is preclotted (if necessary) and anastomosed to the ascending aorta. For paracorporeal pumps, the aortic cannula may be passed through the skin before or after the anastomosis is created, depending on the device used. The left atrial cannula can be inserted via the right lateral aspect of the atrium, the roof of the atrium, or the left atrial appendage. We have generally chosen the right lateral aspect of the left atrium, which is exposed by dissecting the inter-atrial groove and freeing the pericardial attachments of the superior vena cava. Two concentric left atrial pursestrings of 3-0 monofilament suture are placed, with felt buttressing of the inner pursestring. The left atrial cannula is passed through the skin prior to inserting it in the atrium.

The use of cardiopulmonary bypass for placement of a left atrial VAD cannula is optional. If the patient is on bypass, blood is diverted to the patient prior to cannula insertion to avoid introduction of air into the left atrium. The wall of the atrium is incised and the cannula is inserted in the direction of the mitral valve. We have found no advantage to placing the tip of the cannula across the mitral valve; rather, we attempt to place the cannula in the midportion of the atrium to prevent the atrial wall from intermittently occluding blood flow to the VAD.

LEFT VENTRICULAR APEX CANNULATION

If left ventricular apical VAD inflow is chosen, cardiopulmonary bypass is mandatory. When the apical cannula is placed, the heart may remain beating, or it can be arrested with continuous warm blood cardioplegia or intermittent cold cardioplegia solution. It is our preference to have the heart beating. The patient is placed in Trendelenburg position and the heart is perfused with oxygenator-derived blood pumped into the cross-clamped aortic root. This maneuver minimizes the chance for coronary or systemic air embolization while maintaining continuous coronary perfusion.

The position of the left ventricular apex relative to the chest wall is assessed and the site for apical cannulation is selected. The inflow portion of the device courses between the costal margin and the diaphragm without entering the peritoneum. A core of the left ventricular apex is removed (and submitted for pathologic examination), and the interior of the left ventricle is inspected for thrombus. The sewing ring of the apical cannula is then anastomosed to the ventricle with individual horizontal pledgeted mattress sutures of 2-0 braided suture material (Fig. 8–16). Large bites of tissue are taken, and the sutures are tied with special care in recently infarcted tissue to avoid tearing. An additional pursestring suture can be placed circumferentially

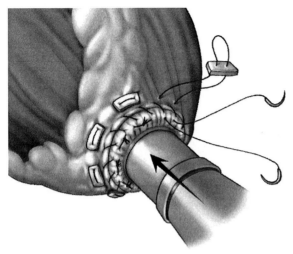

FIGURE **8–16.** Insertion of inflow cannula into left ventricular apex.

through the individual pledgets to provide additional strength at the left ventricular cannulation site.

The anastomosis of the outflow conduit to the ascending aorta is constructed with 4-0 polypropylene (Fig. 8–17) after filling the device and conduit with blood in order to accurately judge its length. Alternatively (UAB), the outflow graft can be anastomosed to the ascending aorta prior to implanting the apical cannula. The completed implantation is shown in Figure 8–18.

DE-AIRING AND INITIATION OF PUMPING

The method for attaching the pump to the inflow and outflow conduits varies with the device. The pump

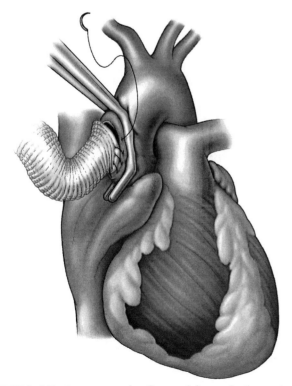

FIGURE **8–17.** Anastomosis of outflow graft from pulsatile ventricular assist device to ascending aorta.

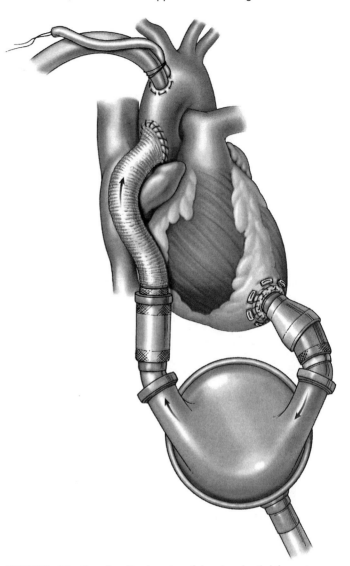

FIGURE **8–18.** Completed implantation of chronic pulsatile left ventricular assist device.

should be filled with saline to minimize air that remains after the pump is connected. If the pump uses a vacuum pressure to enhance filling, the vacuum is *not* activated until the chest is closed. Some devices (e.g., Thermo-Cardiosystems HeartMate) are fabricated with Dacron conduit in the VAD inflow. Air can be sucked through the interstices of the graft by the small negative pressure that is generated by the diaphragm during pump diastole; therefore, it is crucial to keep an adequate preload pressure (by diverting blood from the oxygenator circuit to the patient) in the beating heart to maintain a positive pressure in the inflow cannula.

De-airing is facilitated by venting the aortic root and the Dacron portion of the outflow conduit while running the VAD at a slow rate (e.g., 30–40 bpm) either by hand-pumping the device or utilizing the fixed rate mode. De-airing is monitored by transesophageal echocardiography. A clamp is left on the Dacron outflow conduit during the initial slow pumping of the VAD so that air is expelled through a hole in the graft. The clamp is partially released as the VAD flow is increased when de-airing is nearly complete. The clamp is then removed and the bypass flow rate is reduced to zero as the VAD pumping rate is increased to a level that supports the patient's circulation (left VAD flow index > 2.0 L/min/m²). The VAD flow rate and hemodynamic state are monitored, as is right ventricular function (in isolated LVAD support).

PRESERVATION OF RIGHT VENTRICULAR FUNCTION DURING LVAD IMPLANT

An isolated left ventricular assist device is sufficient to support the failing heart in about 90% of patients who need mechanical circulatory support,[52] even in the presence of significant right ventricular dysfunction, as long as the left ventricle (and therefore left atrium) can be adequately decompressed and pulmonary artery pressure can be normalized. An impaired right ventricle has limited capability to cope with acute increases in pulmonary vascular resistance.

In the absence of severe right-sided failure before implant, it most commonly develops intra- and early postoperatively in the setting of ongoing bleeding and the requirement for multiple blood and platelet transfusions. The associated pulmonary hypertension has been hypothesized to be in part cytokine-mediated, associated with the production of interleukin (IL)-1, IL-6, IL-10, tumor necrosis factor-α (TNF-α), and platelet-activating factor.[24, 105, 106, 157, 186] This problem can be lessened by meticulous hemostasis during implantation and the use of drugs like aprotinin to decrease coagulopathic bleeding. Prostaglandin E₁ has been used as a pulmonary vasodilator, and more recently inhaled nitric oxide has been employed to acutely lower pulmonary vascular resistance and increase right ventricular output in LVAD patients.[79, 143] In institutions where inhaled nitric oxide is available, it is the most effective agent currently available for acute reduction of pulmonary vascular resistance. The weakened right ventricle is also very susceptible to damage from overdistention, ischemic injury, and tamponade, which therefore must be avoided.

COMPLICATIONS OF MECHANICAL CIRCULATORY SUPPORT

The most common complications following VAD or TAH implantation are bleeding requiring reoperation, infection, thromboembolism, renal dysfunction, neurologic dysfunction, and hemolysis.

BLEEDING ASSOCIATED WITH MECHANICAL CIRCULATORY SUPPORT SYSTEMS

Device-related bleeding occasionally occurs during longer term circulatory support, but the most important risk for bleeding occurs at the time of MCSS placement.[127] Patients with end-stage cardiac disease often have liver dysfunction and a coagulopathy related to hepatic con-

gestion. Also, these patients frequently go to the operating room in a state of cardiogenic shock. The usual problems with postcardiopulmonary bypass platelet dysfunction add to this shock-induced coagulopathic state, and persistent bleeding may also occur through nonsealed Dacron surfaces or through nonwatertight connections (e.g., threaded metal connectors).

Aprotinin, a nonspecific serine protease inhibitor, has decreased post-VAD implant blood loss.[83] Aprotinin has an antifibrinolytic effect by blocking plasmin activation, and it blocks contact activation of the kallekrein system during cardiopulmonary bypass. Platelet function is partially preserved by aprotinin's protective effect on platelet surface receptors (e.g., the Gp Ib receptor).[45, 221] No increase in the peri-implant thromboembolic rate has been attributed to the use of aprotinin to date. The risk of an acute allergic reaction to a second dose of aprotinin at the time of transplantation appears to be low.[81] Other drugs, including the less expensive antifibrinolytic drug ε-aminocaproic acid, can used as an alternative medication to diminish fibrinolysis.[27, 95] However, the combined use of aprotinin and ε-aminocaproic acid is *not* recommended because the combination may promote thrombus formation.

In view of the coagulopathic state in many of these seriously ill patients, strict hemostasis in all phases of the operation is the cornerstone for the prevention of both postoperative bleeding and infection. As discussed in the earlier section, Surgical Placement of Chronic Ventricular Assist Devices, the abdominal pocket for the device is a common site of early or delayed bleeding. Application of surgical clips rather than just cautery to any penetrating subcostal or rectus vessels is of particular importance in preventing delayed pocket bleeding, especially with pulsatile devices such as the HeartMate Vented Electric pump which has some vibratory torque which can erode small adjacent vessels.

NEUROLOGIC DYSFUNCTION

Neurologic injury and frank strokes may occur perioperatively or during the weeks/months that follow VAD or TAH implantation. Intraoperative neurologic injury may occur from air embolism at the time of implant. With increasing experience, this complication is now rare with strict attention to filling the device with saline prior to securing connections, filling the left ventricle with blood before allowing device ejection, rigorous de-airing procedures, and intraoperatiave surveillance with transesophageal echocardiography during de-airing and discontinuation of cardiopulmonary bypass. Postoperative neurologic events are most commonly secondary to thromboembolism (see next section) or intracerebral hemorrhage, possibly related to anticoagulation.

THROMBOEMBOLISM ASSOCIATED WITH MCSS

Thromboembolism has been recognized as a problem since the start of MCSS development.[207] Thromboembolic rates for VADs and TAHs have been difficult to quantify precisely because many small emboli are clinically silent,[40, 140] and because enlarged hearts are themselves an important source of emboli.[77, 84, 151, 174] Furthermore, the definition for thromboembolic events used in investigational trials varies from device to device, which makes meaningful comparisons of thromboembolic rates between devices impossible. However, many device designs have components which appear more prone to thrombus formation. For example, the inflow conduit of the Novacor pump has been susceptible to thrombus formation. In axial flow pumps, the bearing sites may be a source of thromboembolism. Centrifugal pumps tend to form thrombus at the cones.[166] Common to all blood–pump contact surfaces is increased thrombogenicity at low-flow states.

All MCSS have some potential for thrombus formation, and all current MCSS are used with some type of anticoagulation regimen. This regimen typically includes heparin immediately after implant with subsequent conversion to coumadin therapy.[202] Of the chronic devices, the Novacor and Thoratec systems require coumadin. The ThermoCardiosystems HeartMate VAD is most often used with only aspirin. As more information is gathered regarding the interaction of specific pump materials and blood, it may be possible to design anticoagulant regimens specific to each pump and to the state of each patient's coagulation system.[15, 16, 39, 55] Other diaphragm/surface modifications like the gelatin-coated surface of the Cleveland Clinic-Nimbus TAH may further reduce blood–surface interactions and the incidence of thromboembolic events.[94, 113]

Patients with indwelling mechanical valve prostheses represent a special problem in VAD support with respect to thromboembolic potential. Although the risk has not been quantified, an indwelling aortic mechanical prosthesis will open only intermittently if at all and represents a definite risk for thromboembolism. In this situation, valve replacement with a bioprosthesis is advisable at the time of VAD implantation.

A mitral mechanical prosthesis is less clearly a risk for thromboembolism (with chronic anticoagulation), since there is normal flow across the mitral valve with left ventricular cannulation.[201] Left atrial cannulation would be contraindicated.

INFECTION

Recipients of mechanical support systems are vulnerable to both device-related and nosocomial infections. The most common site of infection is the drive line, usually confined to the exit site and manageable with local wound care and antibiotics.

Infections in the mediastinum or pump pocket are usually related to a low level of contamination in the operating room (most commonly by skin organisms) in the setting of a large foreign body (the device) in a patient compromised by profound circulatory failure, multiple invasive monitoring devices, nutritional deprivation induced by heart failure, and possible immune derangements. The presence of persistent bleeding or development of hematoma in the device pocket greatly increases the likelihood of infection. Although device-related alterations in the immune system (see subsequent discussion) may play a role in the susceptibility to infection, the overwhelming priority in infection prevention must be strict hemostasis throughout the procedure, rigid adherence to aseptic technique, appropriate prophylactic antibiotics, topical antibiotics directed at skin organisms, and prevention of skin contact with device parts. Additional important maneuvers in infection prevention include minimal pocket dead space, greater drive line tunnel length, and exit of drive line on the patient's right side, away from the device pocket.

In the overall mechanical circulatory support experience, important infections occur in about 25% of patients.[81] Early experience with the TAH suggested that infection would occur in a substantial number of patients supported by these devices,[90, 91] but subsequent experience with the Jarvik-7 and CardioWest-70 devices has shown that the incidence of serious infection in TAH recipients bridged to transplantation is relatively low.[37, 58, 163]

Despite improvements in surgical techniques and antibiotic protocols, device-related infections, usually bacterial, will continue to be a formidable problem because of the compromised state of the patients, the magnitude of the operation, and the presence of a large foreign body. However, despite the presence of extensive drive-line infection, or even gross mediastinal device infection, cardiac transplantation can be safely performed as long as the patient is otherwise in good condition.[13]

Established infection involving the abdominal wall pocket may require open debridement and evacuation of hematoma, occasionally on several occasions. An important advance in the management of established infection on the external (i.e., non–blood contacting) surface of an implanted LVAD is the use of polymethylmethacrylate orthopedic cement to fabricate antibiotic eluting beads which are placed around the pump. This technique, originally described for orthopedic procedures, produces high local antibiotic concentration for weeks with negligible systemic absorption. We have used this technique in a patient who remained free of recurrent device infection for over a year.[101] Rarely, infection on blood-contacting surfaces or device valves may be severe enough to require device replacement. In the future, improved surgical techniques, the development of novel approaches to the control and eradication of biomaterial infections, as well as the discovery of materials that are optimally suited for integration into the environment of the human body will be major steps in solving the problem of device-related infection.

HEMOLYSIS

Hemolysis is an important and sometimes limiting complication of some short-term devices, particularly the centrifugal and axial flow pumps.[152] Important hemolysis is *rare* with the chronic pulsatile devices (Thoratec, HeartMate, and Novacor devices). When clinically important hemolysis occurs, it may be the first sign of cusp rupture of an inflow or outflow bioprosthetic valve (HeartMate or Novacor system). Prompt investigation with transthoracic and/or transesophageal echocardiography is advisable, and device replacement may be necessary if the diagnosis is confirmed.

MECHANICAL CAUSES OF VAD FAILURE

To date, failure of pumping sacs or diaphragms has not been an important problem for VADs that were used for periods of months to a year. However, the development of calcification in the plastic itself or accelerated degradation along microimperfections in plastic pumping surfaces remains a potential problem for VAD implants of several years' duration. In paracorporeal devices such as the Thoratec pump, the polyurethane cannulae can be cut by sharp objects, and the tin alloy solder at the end of the cannula's reinforcement spiraling wire can be degraded by iodine (carried into the polyurethane by the polyethelene glycol of iodine ointments). In one patient at UAB, the wire solder degraded and failed, exposing an end of the reinforcing wire which then cut through the cannula causing a blood leak, necessitating replacement of the VAD. The polysulfone case of the Thoratec VAD can also be severely weakened by exposure to organic solvents (e.g., acetone), leading to extensive cracking of the VAD pumping chamber, which requires pump replacement for correction.[135]

NATIVE VALVE DYSFUNCTION FOLLOWING VAD PLACEMENT

Valvular function changes acutely at the time of VAD placement. Mitral insufficiency typically diminishes following the initiation of left ventricular assistance,[102, 222] particularly if a left ventricular apical cannula is used for left VAD inflow. Upon initiation of isolated left VAD pumping, the dimensions of the right ventricle increase secondary to the volume load imposed on the right ventricle together with a shift in the position of the ventricular septum that occurs with a fall in left ventricular pressure.[102] There may be an increase in tricuspid regurgitation concomitant with the increase in right ventricular dimensions,[102] but this does not produce clinical signs of right ventricular failure.

POST-VAD IMMUNOLOGIC SENSITIZATION

A major current limitation of VAD support prior to transplantation is the formation of anti-HLA antibodies. Although controversy exists regarding the precise stimulus for antibody formation, a major source of sensitization is blood product administration at the time of VAD/TAH implant in an attempt to normalize coagulation. The heavy burden of HLA antigens on leukocytes can be largely (although not completely) eliminated with the routine use of leukocyte filters or leukocyte depletion for red cell and platelet transfusions. Platelet transfusions are a potent source of HLA antigens and have been implicated as a risk factor for sensitization following mechanical circulatory support.[211] The most important preventive measure against sensitization is avoidance of blood product administration, but that is often difficult or impossible in the presence of previous cardiac operations and often reduced hematocrit in a critically ill patient. The incidence of sensitization following VAD placement is 30–70%, and it usually is apparent by panel reactive antibody within 4–6 weeks of implantation.

Recent studies suggest that the VAD **surface** itself may create a milieu that activates the immune system. Spanier and colleagues[197] have hypothesized immunoregulatory dysfunction and compensated coagulaopathy induced by the textured LVAD surface of the TCI HeartMate device. The textured surface selectively absorbs and activates circulating dendritic cells and macrophages, with up-regulation of adhesion molecules such as VCAM and ICAM (see Chapter 2) and increased production of inflammatory cytokines such as TNF-α. A defect in T-cell activation has been identified, with an associated heightened B-cell response which could potentially enhance the production of anti-MHC class I and class II IgG.

Therapeutic strategies to depress the surface-induced inflammatory/immune response are currently directed at blocking NF-κB, a nuclear transcription factor which plays a central role in the activation of endothelial cells and inflammatory leukocytes. Aspirin in animal models inhibits NF-κB gene expression and is recommended at a dose of 325 mg PO/PR qd, beginning within 3 days of VAD implantation. The methods of detecting anti-HLA antibodies (panel reactive antibody) and available pretransplant therapies for sensitization are discussed in Chapter 7.

RESULTS OF BRIDGING TO TRANSPLANT WITH MCSS

PULSATILE VENTRICULAR ASSIST DEVICES

Survival to Transplant

Over the past 10 years, experience with chronically implantable left ventricular assist devices has clearly demonstrated their efficacy in restoring and maintaining excellent hemodynamic function for weeks to months in bridging to heart transplantation. As discussed in earlier sections, the reported successful outcome of transplantation following circulatory support by ventricular assist devices has been consistently superior with chronic devices compared to the short-term devices discussed earlier in this chapter.[126, 128, 141, 169, 175] Nearly a decade ago, the International Society of Heart and Lung Transplantation Registry reported that 67% of LVAD patients went on to transplantation, of which 80% were successfully discharged from the hospital.[144] The success rate in achieving transplantation following bridging with an LVAD is largely dependent upon patient selection criteria for circulatory assistance, but has generally ranged from

60–80%.[141, 144]   In the overall experience of more than 3,000 patients who have received mechanical circulatory support as a bridge to cardiac transplantation, over 60% have actually received a transplant. Over 85% of those transplanted have survived to be discharged from the hospital.[56, 66, 167]

In a controlled study with a chronic implantable pneumatic LVAD in bridge-to-transplant patients, device-supported patients had a major increase in survival to transplantation (71% vs. 36%, $p = .001$) compared to "control" patients (supported with inotropic agents with or without an intra-aortic balloon pump).[73] Among patients receiving "wearable" implantable left ventricular assist devices, greater than 50% are discharged from the hospital while awaiting cardiac transplantation. The major reasons for death prior to transplantation have been early postimplant bleeding, infection, and renal failure.

The superior survival with chronic MCS devices compared to short-term devices relates in part to more effective cardiac output, greater resistance to infection and thromboembolism, increased patient mobility, and greater psychological adjustment provided by chronic support systems. The potential effectiveness of current support systems in terms of survival and rehabilitation potential is exemplified by the superb results after transplantation of patients in New York Heart Association (NYHA) functional Class I (100% survival at 2 years after transplantation) reported by Frazier and colleagues.[71]

Effect of LVAD Support on Right Ventricular Function

In the absence of acute right ventricular injury (such as ischemic injury or air embolism) during LVAD implantation, postimplant right ventricular function is primarily determined by the severity of preexisting right ventricular dysfunction.[61] In the normal right ventricle subjected to left ventricular support, ventricular interactions have relatively little influence on right ventricular performance.[57, 78, 119, 145, 196] Experimental studies of isolated left ventricular support have demonstrated subtle changes in right ventricular function, including a decrease in load-independent contractility secondary to leftward septal shifting, which occurs as a consequence of left ventricular unloading and volume loading of the right ventricle due to increased venous return.[28]

Rehabilitation

The potential for rehabilitation, ambulation, and exercise during chronic mechanical circulatory support is a critical determinant of successful bridge to transplantation as well as definitive therapy for advanced heart failure. The physiology of the VAD-assisted human circulation has been investigated at rest and during exercise in patients with implanted left VADs.[17, 51, 111] At rest and with low levels of exercise, the majority of the systemic circulation is supplied by the VAD. As the patient exercises more strenuously, it appears that the contribution of the native left ventricle to total cardiac output increases. However, the total VAD/native left ventricu-

lar output is limited, and at high levels of exertion, this limitation in VAD/native left ventricular output leads to increasing oxygen extraction to meet the demands of exercise.

TOTAL ARTIFICIAL HEART BRIDGING

The bridge to transplant trial of the Jarvik-7 TAH began in August 1985. A summary of results through 1992 included 175 Jarvik-7 implants in 171 patients.[36] The percentage of implanted patients who survived to undergo cardiac transplantation ranged from 39–89%, with survival at 1 year after transplant ranging from 50–76%. The most prevalent causes of morbidity during the period of support in these patients were infection, renal insufficiency and renal failure, hemorrhage, and thromboembolism. Death most commonly occurred from multiple organ failure and infection. Notably, device failure *per se* has not been an important problem. Pump diaphragm rupture in a right ventricle occurred in one patient. With a mean duration of support approaching 2 months, the reported incidence of thromboembolic events and neurologic injury has been relatively low (< 15%).

In a recent experience at one highly experienced institution, the 2-year posttransplant survival rate of CardioWest patients was 90%, with 62% of implanted patients going to transplantation.[162] Thus, in experienced centers the current results achieved with the CardioWest TAH show that device reliability up to nearly 2 years of use is good, and the effectiveness of bridging to transplant is comparable to VAD support. Device-related infection and thromboembolism are the major current limitations.

FUTURE DIRECTIONS IN MCSS DEVELOPMENT

The long anticipated waiting times for patients supported on mechanical circulatory support systems and the extended hospitalization with the device can be extremely costly. Therefore, the potential for hospital discharge becomes important for the cost of medical care as well as the psychological state of VAD recipients. Only "wearable" left ventricular assist devices or total artificial hearts can be discharged to an outpatient setting as part of the evolution toward chronic mechanical support for some patients with end-stage heart disease. It is anticipated that in the near future most bridge-to-transplant patients will be discharged to an outpatient facility as soon as they are fully ambulatory.

A primary goal of VAD and TAH support is the development of fully implantable systems (i.e., an intracorporeal pump that has no percutaneous connections) that can serve as permanent implants. This requires that energy be transferred to the pump's actuating mechanism without a percutaneous connector, and that a volume reservoir be incorporated in the pump design to compensate for volume changes that occur during cycling of the pump.

Induction coils have been developed that are capable of transferring electrical energy (radiofrequency current) transcutaneously.[2] In addition, storage batteries can be implanted with the VAD, although the battery materials available at present have important limitations. These batteries are designed to provide short periods of support while the patient is disconnected from the transcutaneous power source.

The design of reliable transcutaneous energy transfer systems is a major challenge. The system must be capable of transferring sufficient energy. This requires that the pump motor be energy efficient and that the distance between the transmitting and receiving coils be fairly small. The edges of the implanted portion of the energy transfer coil must be smooth and as compact as possible to minimize the chance of skin erosion over the coil. The transfer of energy must not cause excessive heating of the skin, which will predispose to skin erosion.

The design of compliance chambers for fully implanted devices remains problematic. All plastics and rubber compounds are, to some extent, permeable to gases. Over time, this permeability leads to the loss of volume from the compliance chamber. As gas is lost, the pumping diaphragm begins to work against a vacuum and pumping efficiency is lost. If gas loss from the compliance chamber is severe enough, complete ejection may become impossible. Volume loss is quite slow for some gases; however, even with the use of special gases like sulfur hexafloride, the lost volume must periodically be returned to the compliance chamber. Gas replacement can be accomplished by percutaneous injection of fresh gas into the compliance chamber. Percutaneous vents, like the one currently used in the HeartMate VE left VAD, circumvent this problem altogether.

One example of a material designed to minimize gas loss from the compliance chamber is a composite of polyolefin rubber and butyl rubber co-molded to form a composite that is covered with velour Dacron material. The fusion of these materials combines the fatigue resistance of the polyolefin rubber and the gas diffusion barrier of the butyl rubber in one material. At present, intrathoracic compliance chambers are planned that will attach to the inner chest wall and displace 50–80 mL of lung tissue with each cycle of the pump.

Studies are now underway to evaluate VADs and the TAH as permanent implants.[176] These experiments will provide answers to several important questions. What is the long-term reliability of these devices? Can the modes and timing of device failure be predicted, and can the intracorporeal components of these pumps be replaced with an acceptable morbidity and mortality? What are the mechanisms and limits of cardiac myocyte recovery during protracted periods of mechanical support by a VAD? Is it possible to supplement or augment the repair of the injured heart during support using drugs, myocyte seeding, or genetic manipulations? Is it possible to substantially diminish the chance of infection and thromboembolic injury in a chronically implanted VAD or TAH? Most important, what quality of life can a MCSS provide, and what is the cost?

References

1. Abiomed Operations Manual: Abiomed, Inc, Danvers, MA, November 1994.
2. Ahn JM, Kang DW, Kim HC, Min BG: In vivo performance evaluation of a transcutaneous energy and information transmission system for the total artificial heart. ASAIO J 1993;39:M208–M212.
3. Akutsu T, Kollf WJ: Permanent substitutes for valves and heart. Trans Am Soc Artif Intern Organs 1958;4:230.
4. Akutsu T, Mirkovitch V, Topaz SR: Cylastic type of artifical heart and its use in calves. Trans Am Soc Inern Organs 1963;9:281.
5. Anderson HL III, Attorri RJ, Custer JR, Chapman RA, Bartlett RH: Extracorporeal membrane oxygenation for pediatric cardiopulmonary failure. J Thorac Cardiovasc Surg 1990;99:1011–1021.
6. Anstadt GL, Blakemore, Baue AE: A new instrument for prolonged mechanical massage. Circulation 1965;31 and 32(suppl):II-43–II-44.
7. Anstadt GL, Britz WE Jr: Continued studies in prolonged circulatory support by direct mechanical assistance. Trans Am Soc Artif Intern Organs 1968;14:297–303.
8. Anstadt GL, Camp TF: Acute circulatory suport by mechanical ventricular assistance following myocardial infarction. J Thorac Cardiovasc Surg 1967;54:785–806.
9. Anstadt GL, Rawling CA, Krahwinkel DT, Casey HW, Schiff P: Prolonged circulatory support by direct mechanical ventricular assistance for 2–3 days of ventricular fibrillation. Trans Am Soc Artif Intern Organs 1971;17:174–182.
10. Anstadt MP, Anstadt GL, Lowe JE: Direct mechanical ventricular actuation: a review. Resuscitation 1991;21:7–23.
11. Arabia FA, Paramesh V, Toporoff B, Arzouman DA, Seith GK, Copeland JG: Biventricular cannulation for the Thoratec ventricular assist device. Ann Thorac Surg 1998;66:2119–2120.
12. Arai H, Swartz MT, Pennington DG, Moriyama Y, Miller L, Peigh P, McBride L: Importance of ventricular arrhythmias in bridge patients with ventricular assist devices. ASAIO Trans 1991;37:M427–M428.
13. Argenziano M, Catanese KA, Moazami N, Gardocki MT, Weinberg AD, Clavenna MW, Rose EA, Scully BE, Levin HR, Oz MC: The influence of infection on survival and successful transplantation in patients with left ventricular assist devices. J Heart Lung Transplant 1997;16:822–831.
14. Atsumi K: Research and development of artificial heart in Japan. J Biomater Appl 1990;4:161–224.
15. Bibidakis EJ, Livingston ER, Fisher CA, Todd BA, Furukawa S, Addonizio VP, Jeevanandam V: Inflammatory responses to left ventricular assist device insertion [abstract]. J Heart Lung Transplant 1996;15:S74.
16. Bibidakis EJ, Livingston ER, Pathak AS, Fisher CA, Pendergast TW, Ahmed R, Miraliakbari R, Todd BA, Furukawa S, Addonizio P, Jeevanandam V: The biochemical basis of bleeding during left ventricular assistance [abstract]. J Heart Lung Transplant 1996;15:S66.
17. Branch KR, Dembitsky WP, Peterson KL, Adamson R, Gordon JB, Smith SC, Jaski BE: Physiology of the native heart and Thermo-Cardiosystems left ventricular assist device complex at rest and during exercise: implications for chronic support. J Heart Lung Transplant 1994;13:641–651.
18. Brack M, Olson JD, Pedersen WR, Goldenberg IF, Gobel FL, Pritzker MR, Emery RW, Lange HW: Transesophageal echocardiography in patients with mechanical circulatory assistance. Ann Thorac Surg 1991;52:1306–1309.
19. Bucherl ES: The artificial heart research program in Berlin, Germany. J Heart Transplant 1985;4:510–517.
20. Burnett CM, Duncan JM, Frazier OH, Sweeney MS, Vega JD, Radovancevic B: Improved multiorgan function after prolonged univentricular support. Ann Thorac Surg 1993;55:65–71.
21. Butler KC, Moise JC, Wampler RK: The Hemopump—a new cardiac prothesis device. IEEE Trans Biomed Eng 1990;37:193–196.
22. Butler K, Thomas D, Antaki J, Borovetz H, Griffith B, Kameneva M, Kormos R, Litwak P: Development of the Nimbus/Pittsburgh axial flow left ventricular assist system. Artif Organs 1997;21:602–610.
23. Burton NA, Lefrak EA, Macmanus Q, Hill A, Marino JA, Speir AM, Akl BF, Albus RA, Massimiano PS: A reliable bridge to

cardiac transplantation: the TCI left ventricular assist device. Ann Thorac Surg 1993;55:1425–1431.

24. Camussi G, Bussolino F, Salvidio G, Baglioni C: Tumor necrosis factor/cachectin stimulates peritoneal macrophages, polymorphonuclear neutrophils, and vascular endothelial cells to synthesize and release platelet activating factor. J Exp Med 1987; 166:1390–1404.

25. Cardiac ECMO Registry of the Extracorporeal Life Support Organization (ELSO), Ann Arbor, Michigan, January 1995.

26. Cassell EJ: How is the death of Barney Clark to be understood? *In* Shaw MW (ed): After Barney Clark: Reflections on the Utah Artificial Heart Program. Austin, TX: University of Texas Press, 1984, pp 25–41.

27. Chen RH, Frazier OH, Cooley DA: Antifibrinolytic therapy in cardiac surgery. Tex Heart Inst J 1995;22:211–215.

28. Chow E, Farrar DJ: Right heart function during prosthetic left ventricular assistance in a porcine model of congestive heart failure. J Thorac Cardiovasc Surg 1992;104:569–578.

29. Clark RE, Walters RA, Hughson S, Davis SA Sr, Magovern GJ: Left ventricular support with the implantable AB-180 centrifugal pump in acute myocardial infarction. ASAIO J 1998;44:804–811.

30. Clowes GHA Jr, Hopkins AL, Nevill WE: An artificial lung dependent upon diffusion of oxygen and carbon dioxide through plastic membranes. J Thorac Surg 1956;32:630.

31. Cole DW, Holman WS, Mott WE: Status of the USAEC's nuclear-powered artificial heart. Trans Am Soc Artif Intern Organs 1973;19:537–541.

32. Conway J, Lund-Johansen P: Thermodilution method for measuring cardiac output. *In* Robertson JIS, Birkenhager WH (eds): Cardiac Output Measurement. Philadelphia: WB Saunders, 1991;17:20.

33. Coogan PS, Casey HW, Skinner DB, Anstadt GL: Direct mechanical ventricular assistance: acute and long-term effects in the dog. Arch Pathol 1969;87:423–431.

34. Cooley DA, Akutsu T, Norman JC, Serrato MA, Frazier OH: Total artificial heart in two-staged cardiac transplantation. Tex Heart Inst J 1981;8:305–319.

35. Cooley DA, Liotta D, Hallman GL, Bloodwell RD, Leachman RD, Milam JD: Orthotopic cardiac prosthesis for two-staged cardiac replacement. Am J Cardiol 1969;24:723–730.

36. Copeland JG, Smith RG, Cleavinger MR: Development and current status of the Cardiowest C-70 (Jarvik-7) total artificial heart. *In* Lewis T, Graham TR (eds): Mechanical Circulatory Support. London: Edward Arnold, 1995, pp 186–198.

37. Copeland JG, Smith RG, Icenogle TB, Rhenman B, Williams R, Vasu MA: Early experience with the total artificial heart as a bridge to cardiac transplantation. Surg Clin North Am 1988; 68:621–634.

38. Copeland JG, Smith RG, Icenogle T, Vasu A, Rhenman B, Williams R, Cleavinger M: Orthotopic total artificial heart bridge to transplanation: preliminary results. J Heart Transplant 1989; 8:124–138.

39. Courtney JM, Forbes CD: Thrombosis on foreign surfaces. Br Med Bull 1994;50:966–981.

40. Curtis JJ, Walls JT, Boley TM, Schmaltz RA, Demmy TL: Autopsy findings in patients on postcardiotomy centrifugal ventricular assist. ASAIO J 1992;38:M688–M690.

41. Dailey BB, Pettitt TW, Sutera SP, Pierce WS: Pierce-Donachy pediatric VAD: progress in development. Ann Thorac Surg 1996;61:437–443.

42. Dalton HJ, Siewer RD, Fuhrman BP, del Nido P, Thompson AE, Shaver MD: Extracorporeal membrane oxygenation for cardiac rescue in children with severe myocardial dysfunction. Crit Care Med 1993;21:1020–1028.

43. Daly RC, Chandrasekaran K, Cavarocchhi NC, Tajik AJ, Schaff HV: Ischemia of the ventricular septum: a mechanism of right ventricular failure during mechanical left ventricular assist. J Thorac Cardiovasc Surg 1992;103:1186–1191.

44. Dasse KA, Chipman SD, Sherman CN, Levine AH, Frazier OH: Clinical experience with textured blood-contacting surfaces in ventricular assist devices. ASAIO Trans 1987;33:418.

45. Davis R, Whittington R: Aprotinin. A review of its pharmacology and therapeutic efficacy in reducing blood loss associated with cardiac surgery. Drugs 1995;49:954–983.

46. DeBakey ME: A miniature implantable axial flow ventricular assist device. Ann Thorac Surg 1999;68:637–640.

47. DeBakey ME: A simple continuous flow blood transfusion instrument. New Orleans Med Surg J 1934;87:386–389.

48. DeBakey ME: Left ventricular bypass pump for cardiac assistance. Am J Cardiol 1971;27:3–11.

49. Delius RE: As originally published in 1990: prolonged extracorporeal life support of pediatric and adolescent cardiac transplant patients. Updated in 1998. Ann Thorac Surg 1998;65:877–878.

50. Delius RE, Bove EL, Meliones JN, Custer JR, Moler FW, Crowley D, Amirikia A, Behrendt DM, Bartlett RH: Use of extracorporeal life support in patients with congenital heart disease. Crit Care Med 1992;20:1216–1222.

51. Deng MC: Effects of exercise during long-term support with a left ventricular assist device. Circulation 1998;97:1212–1213.

52. DeRose JJ, Argenziano M, Sun BC, Reemtsma K, Oz MC, Rose EA: Implantable left ventricular assist devices: an evolving long-term cardiac replacement therapy. Ann Surg 1997;226:461–468.

53. DeVries WC: The permanent artificial heart: four case reports. JAMA 1988;259:849–859.

54. DeVries WC, Anderson JL, Joyce LD, Anderson FL, Hammond EH, Jarvik RK, Kolff WJ: Clinical use of the total artificial heart. N Engl J Med 1984;310:273–278.

55. Eidelman BH, Obrist WD, Wagner WR, Kormos RL, Griffith B: Cerebrovascular complications associated with the use of artificial circulatory support services. Neurology Clin 1993; 11:463–474.

56. El-Banayosy A, Deng M, Loisance DY, Gronda E, Loebe M, Vigano M: The European experience of Novacor left ventricular assist (LVAS) therapy as a bridge to transplant: a retrospective multi-center study. Eur J Cardiothorac Surg 1999;15:835–841.

57. Elbeery JR, Owen CH, Savitt MA, Davis JW, Feneley MP, Rankin JS, Van Trigt P: Effects of left ventricular assist device on right ventricular function. J Thorac Cardiovasc Surg 1990;99:809–816.

58. Emery RW, Joyce LD, Prieto M, Johnson K, Goldenberg IF, Pritzker MR: Experience with the Symbion total artificial heart as a bridge to transplantation. Ann Thorac Surg 1992;53:282–288.

59. Evans RW, Orians CE, Ascher NL: The potential supply of organ donors: an assessment of the efficiency of organ procurement efforts in the United States. JAMA 1992;267:239–246.

60. Farrar DJ, Buck KE, Coulter JH, Kupa EJ: Portable pneumatic biventricular driver for the Thoratec ventricular assist device. ASAIO J 1997;43:631–634.

61. Farrar DJ, Chow E, Compton PG, Foppiano L, Woodard J, Hill JD: Effects of acute right ventricular ischemia on ventricular interactions during prosthetic left ventricular support. J Thorac Cardiovasc Surg 1991;102:588–595.

62. Farrar DJ, Hill JD: Univentricular and biventricular Thoratec VAD support as a bridge to transplantation. Ann Thorac Surg 1993;55:276–282.

63. Farrar DJ, Hill JD: Recovery of major organ function in patients awaiting heart transplantation with Thoratec ventricular assist devices. J Heart Lung Transplant 1994;13:1125–1132.

64. Farrar DJ, Hill D, Gray LA Jr, Galbraith TA, Chow E, Hershon JJ: Successful biventricular circulatory support as a bridge to transplantation during prolonged ventricular fibrillation and asystole. Circulation 1989;80:III-147–III-151.

65. Farrar DJ, Hill JD, Gray LA Jr, Pennington G, McBride LR, Pierce WS, Pae WE, Glenville B, Ross D, Galbraith TA, Zumbro GL: Heterotopic prosthetic ventricles as a bridge to cardiac transplantation. N Engl J Med 1988;318:333–340.

66. Farrar DJ, Hill JD, Pennington DG: Preoperative and postoperative comparison of patients with univentricular and biventricular support with the Thoratec ventricular assist device as a bridge to cardiac transplantation. J Thorac Cardiovasc Surg 1997; 113:202–209.

67. Farrar DJ, Korfer R, el-Banayosy A: First clinical use of the Thoratec TLC-II portable VAD driver in ambulatory and patient discharge settings. ASAIO J 1998;44:35A.

68. Farrar DJ, Lawson JH, Litwak P, Cederwall G: Thoratec VAD system as a bridge to heart transplantation. J Heart Transplant 1990;9:415–423.

69. Farrar DJ, Litwak P, Lawson JH, Ward RS, White KA, Robinson AJ, Rodvien R, Hill JD: In vivo evaluations of a new thromboresis-

tant polyurethane for artificial heart blood pumps. J Thorac Cardiovasc Surg 1988;95:191–200.

70. Fox RC, Swazey JP: Desperate appliance: a short history of the Jarvik-7 artificial heart. *In* Fox RC, Swazey JP (eds): Spare Parts: Organ Replacement in American Society. New York: Oxford University Press, 1992, pp 95–153.

71. Frazier OH, Macris MP, Myers TJ, Duncan JM, Radovancevic B, Parnis SM, Cooley DA: Improved survival after extended bridge to cardiac transplantation. Ann Thorac Surg 1994;57:1416–1422.

72. Frazier OH, Rose EA, Macmanus Q, Burton NA, Lefrak EA, Poirier VL, Dasse KA: Multicenter clinical evaluation of the Heart-Mate 1000 IP left ventricular assist device. Ann Thorac Surg 1992;53:1080–1090.

73. Frazier OH, Rose EA, McCarthy PM, Burton NA, Tector A, Levin H, Kayne HL, Poirier VL, Dasse KA: Improved mortality and rehabilitation of transplant candidates treated with a long-term implantable left ventricular assist system. Ann Surg 1995; 222:327–338.

74. Frazier OH, Wampler RK, Duncan JM, Dear WE, Macris MP, Parnis SM, Fuqua JM: First human use of the Hemopump, a catheter-mounted ventricular assist device. Ann Thorac Surg 1990;49:299–304.

75. Friedel N, Viazis P, Schiessler A, Warnecke H, Hennig E, Trittin A, Bottner W, Hetzer R: Recovery of end-organ failure during mechanical circulatory support. Eur J Cardiothorac Surg 1992; 6:519–523.

76. Fukamachi K, McCarthy PM, Smedira NG, Vargo RL, Starling RC, Young JB: Preoperative risk factors for right ventricular failure after implantable left ventricular assist device insertion. Ann Thorac Surg 1999;68:2181–2184.

77. Fuster V, Gersh BJ, Giuliani ER, Tajik AJ, Brandenburg RO, Frye RL: The natural history of idiopathic dilated cardiomyopathy. Am J Cardiol 1981;47:525–531.

78. Gallagher RC, Kormos RL, Gasior T, Murali S, Griffith BP, Hardesty RL: Univentricular support results in reduction of pulmonary resistance and improved right ventricular function. ASAIO Trans 1991;37:M287–M288.

79. George SJ, Black JJM, Boscoe MJ: Nitric oxide: unjustified credit? [letter]. J Thorac Cardiovasc Surg 1996;111:284–285.

80. Gibbon JH Jr: Application of a mechanical heart and lung apparatus to cardiac surgery. Minn Med 1954;37:171–185.

81. Goldstein DJ, Oz MC, Rose EA: Implantable left ventricular assist devices. N Engl J Med 1998;339:1522–1533.

82. Goldstein DJ, Oz MC, Smith CR, Friedlander JP, DeRosa CM, Mongero LB, Delphin E: Safety of repeat aprotinin administration for LVAD recipients undergoing cardiac transplantation. Ann Thorac Surg 1996;61:692–695.

83. Goldstein DJ, Seldomridge JA, Chen JM, Catanese KA, DeRosa CM, Weinberg AD, Smith CR, Rose EA, Levin HR, Oz MC: Use of aprotinin in LVAD recipients reduces blood loss, blood use, and perioperative mortality. Ann Thorac Surg 1995;59:1063–1067.

84. Gottidiener JS, Gay JA, VanVoorhees L, DiBianco R, Fletcher RD: Frequency and embolic potential of left ventricular thrombus in dilated cardiomyopathy: assessment by 2-dimensional echocardiography. Am J Cardiol 1983;52:1281–1285.

85. Grady D: Summary of discussion on ethical perspectives. *In* Shaw MW (ed): After Barney Clark: Reflections on the Utah Artificial Heart Program. Austin, TX: University of Texas Press, 1984, pp 42–52.

86. Graham TR, Dasse K, Coumbe A, Salih V, Marrinan MT, Frazier OH, Lewis CT: Neo-intimal development on textured biomaterial surfaces during clinical use of an implantable left ventricular assist device. Eur J Cardiothorac Surg 1990;4:182–190.

87. Gray LA Jr, Ganzel BL, Mavroudis C, Slater AD: The Pierce-Donachy ventricular assist device as a bridge to cardiac transplantation. Ann Thorac Surg 1989;48:222–227.

88. Griffin WP, Savage EB, Clark RE, Pacella JJ, Johnson GA, Magovern JA, Magovern GJ Sr: AB-180 circulatory support system: summary of development and phase I of trial. ASAIO J 1998; 44:M719–M724.

89. Griffith BP, Kormos RL, Hardesty RL, Armitage JM, Dummer JS: The artificial heart: infection-related morbidity and its effect on transplantation. Ann Thorac Surg 1988;45:409–414.

90. Gristina AG, Dobbins JJ, Giammara B, Lewis JC, DeVries WC: Biomaterial-centered sepsis and the total artificial heart: microbial adhesion vs. tissue integration. JAMA 1988;259:870–874.

91. Gristina AG, Giridhar G, Gabriel BL, Naylor PT, Myrvik QN: Cell biology and molecular mechanisms in artificial device infections. Int J Artif Organs 1993;16:755–764.

92. Guyton RA, Schonberger JPAM, Gray LA Jr, Gielchinsky I, Raess DH, Vlahakes GJ, Woolley SR, Gangahar DM: Postcardiotomy shock: clinical evaluation of the BVS 5000 biventricular support system. Ann Thorac Surg 1993;56:346–356.

93. Hall CP, Liotta D, Henly WS, Crawford ES, DeBakey ME: Development of artificial intrathoracic circulatory pumps. Am J Surg 1964;108:685–692.

94. Harasaki H, Fukamachi K, Massiello A, Chen JF, Himley SC, Fukumura F, Muramoto K, Niu S, Wika K, Davies CR: Progress in Cleveland Clinic-Nimbus total artificial heart development. ASAIO J 1994;40:M494–M498.

95. Hardy JF, Belisle S: Natural and synthetic antifibrinolytics in adult cardiac surgery: efficacy, effectiveness and efficiency. Can J Anaesth 1994;41:1104–1112.

96. HeartMate Manual VE Operating Manual: Implantable Vented Electric Left Ventricular Assist System. TCI ThermoCardiosystems, Inc., Woburn, MA.

97. HeartMate Manual IP LVAS Operating Manual: Drive Console. TCI ThermoCardiosystems, Inc., Woburn, MA.

98. Hennig E: The artificial heart program in Berlin—technical aspects. *In* Unger F (ed): Assisted Circulation 2. Berlin: Springer-Verlag, 1984, pp 229–253.

99. Hill JD, de Leval MR, Fallat RJ, Bramson ML, Eberhart RC, Schulte HD, Osborn JJ, Barber R, Gerbode F: Acute respiratory insufficiency: treatment with prolonged extracorporeal oxygenation. J Thorac Cardiovasc Surg 1972;64:551–562.

100. Hill JD, Farrar DJ, Hershon JJ, Compton PG, Avery GJ, Litwak P, Foan WS, Dunlap TE, Levin BS: Use of a prosthetic ventricle as a bridge to cardiac transplantation for postinfarction cardiogenic shock. N Engl J Med 1986;314:626.

101. Hoffman AS: Modification of material surfaces to affect how they interact with blood. *In* Leonard EF, Turitto VT, Vroman L (eds): Blood in Contact with Natural and Artificial Surfaces. New York: New York Academy of Sciences, 1987, pp 96–101.

102. Holman WL, Bourge RC, Fan P, Kirklin JK, Pacifico AD, Nanda NC: Influence of left ventricular assist on valvular regurgitation. Circulation 1993;88:II-309–II-318.

103. Holman WL, Murrah CP, Ferguson ER, Bourge RC, McGiffin DC, Kirklin JK: Infections during extended circulatory support: University of Alabama at Birmingham experience 1989 to 1994. Ann Thorac Surg 1996;61:366–371.

104. Holman WL, Roye GD, Bourge RC, McGiffin DC, Iyer SS, Kirklin JK: Circulatory support for myocardial infarction with arrhythmias. Ann Thorac Surg 1995;59:1230–1231.

105. Horvath CJ, Ferro TJ, Jesmok G, Malik AB: Recombinant tumor necrosis factor increases pulmonary vascular permeability independent of nutrophils. Proc Natl Acad Sci U S A 1988;85:9219–9223.

106. Horvath CJ, Kaplan JE, Malik AB: Role of platelet-activating factor mediating tumor necrosis factor alpha-induced pulmonary vasoconstriction and plasma-lymph protein transport. Am Rev Respir Dis 1991;144:1337–1341.

107. Hunt SA, Frazier OH, Myers TJ: Mechanical circulatory support and cardiac transplantation. Circulation 1998;97:2079–2090.

108. Inshino K: Circulatory support with paracorporeal pneumatic ventricular assist device (VAD) in infants and children. Eur J Cardiothorac Surg 1997;11:965–972.

109. Institute of Medicine: The Artificial Heart: Prototypes, Policies, and Patients. Washington, DC: National Academy Press, 1991, pp 1–262.

110. Jarvik RK: System considerations favoring rotary artificial hearts with blood-immersed bearings. Artif Organs 1995;19:565–570.

111. Jaski BE: Effects of exercise during long-term support with a left ventricular assist device. Results of the experience with left ventricular assist device with exercise (EVADE) pilot trial. Circulation 1997;95:2401–2406.

112. Jonsen AR: The selection of patients. *In* Shaw MW (ed): After Barney Clark: Reflections on the Utah Artificial Heart Program. Austin, TX: University of Texas Press, 1984, pp 5–10.

113. Kambic HE, Nose Y: Biomaterials for blood pumps. *In* Sharma CP, Szycher M (eds): Blood Compatible Materials and Devices:

Perspectives Towards the 21st Century. Lancaster: Technomic Publishing Co, Inc, 1991, pp 141–151.

114. Kanter KR, McBride LR, Pennington G, Swartz MT, Ruzevich SA, Miller LW, Willman VL: Bridging to cardiac transplantation with pulsatile ventricular assist devices. Ann Thorac Surg 1988;46:134–140.

115. Kanter KR, Pennington DG, Weber TR, Zambie MA, Braun P, Martychenko V: Extracorporeal membrane oxygenation for postoperative cardiac support in children. J Thorac Cardiovasc Surg 1987;93:27–35.

116. Kantrowitz A, Tjonneland S, Freed PS, Phillips SJ, Butner AN, Sherman JL: Initial clinical experience with intraaortic balloon pumping in cardiogenic shock. JAMA 1968;203:135–140.

117. Kaplon RJ, Oz MC, Kwiatkowski PA, Levin HR, Shah AS, Jarvik RK, Rose EA: Miniature axial flow pump for ventricular assistance in children and small adults. J Thorac Cardiovasc Surg 1996;111:13–18.

118. Katz J: Patient autonomy and the process of informed consent. *In* Shaw MW (ed): After Barney Clark: Reflections on the Utah Artificial Heart Program. Austin, TX: University of Texas Press, 1984, pp 11–24.

119. Kinoshita M, Long JW Jr, Pantalos G, Burns GL, Olsen DB: Hemodynamic influence of LVAD on right ventricular failure. ASAIO Trans 1990;36:M538–M541.

120. Kirklin JW, DuShane JW, Patrick RT, Donald DE, Hetzel PS, Harshbarger HG, Wood EH: Intracardiac surgery with the aid of a mechanical pump-oxygenator system (Gibbon type). Report of eight cases. Proc Mayo Clin 1955;30:201–206.

121. Klaus RH, Bitwell WC, Albertal G: Assisted circulation. The arterial counter pulsaor. J Thorac Cardiovasc Surg 1961;41:447.

122. Klein MD, Shaheen KW, Whittlesey GC, Pinsky WW, Arciniegas E: Extracorporeal membrane oxygenation for the circulatory support of children after repair of congenital heart disease. J Thorac Cardiovasc Surg 1990;100:498–505.

123. Kolobar T, Bowman RL: Construction and evaluation of an alveolar membrane artificial heart lung. Trans Am Soc Artif Intern Organs 1963;9:238.

124. Konertz W: Clinical experience with the MEDOS HIA-VAD system in infants and children: a preliminary report. Ann Thorac Surg 1997;63:1138–1144.

125. Korfer R, El-Banayosy A, Arusoglu L, Minami K, Korner MM, Kizner L, Fey O, Schutt U, Morshuis M, Posival H: Single-center experience with the thoratec ventricular assist device. J Thorac Cardiovasc Surg 2000;119:596–600.

126. Kormos RL, Borovetz HS, Armitage JM, Hardesty RL, Marrone GC, Griffith BP: Evolving experience with mechanical circulatory support. Ann Surg 1991;214:471–477.

127. Kormos RL, Borovetz HS, Gasior T, Antaki JF, Armitage JM, Pristas JM, Hardesty RL, Griffith BP: Experience with univentricular support in mortally ill cardiac transplant candidates. Ann Thorac Surg 1990;49:261–272.

128. Kormos RL, Gasior TA, Kawai A, Pham SM, Murali S, Hattler BG, Griffith BP: Transplant candidate's clinical status rather than right ventricular function defines need for univentricular versus biventricular support. J Thorac Cardiovasc Surg 1996;111:773–783.

129. Kung RT, Ochs B, Singh PI: A unique left-right flow imbalance compensation scheme for an implantable total artificial heart. ASAIO Trans 1989;35:468–470.

130. Kung RTV, Yu LS, Ochs S, Parnis S, Frazier OH: An atrial hydraulic shunt in a total artificial heart: a balance mechanism for the bronchial shunt. ASAIO J 1993;39:M213–M217.

131. Levin HR, Oz MC, Chen JM, Packer M, Rose EA, Burkhoff D: Reversal of chronic ventricular dilation in patients with end-stage cardiomyopathy by prolonged mechanical unloading. Circulation 1995;91:2717–2720.

132. Levinson MM, Smith RG, Cork RC, Gallo J, Icenogle T, Emery R, Ott R, Copeland JG: Three recent cases of the total artificial heart before transplantation. J Heart Transplant 1986;5:215–228.

133. Levinson MM, Copeland JG: Technical aspects of the total artificial heart implantation and temporary applications. J Card Surg 1987;2:3–19.

134. Litwak RS, Koffsky RM, Jurado RA, Lukban SB, Ortiz AF, Fischer AP, Sherman JJ, Silvay G, Lajam FA: Use of a left heart assist device after intracardiac surgery: technique and clinical experience. Ann Thorac Surg 1976;21:191–202.

135. Lohmann DP, Pennington DG, McBride LR: Acetone: a hazard to plastic medical products—a case report [letter]. J Thorac Cardiovasc Surg 1991;102:937–938.

136. Lonchyna VA, Pifarre R, Sullivan H, Montoya A, Bakhos M, Grieco J, Foy B, Blakeman B, Altergott R, Calandra D: Successful use of the total artificial heart as a bridge to cardiac transplantation with no mediastinitis. J Heart Lung Transplant 1992;11:803–811.

137. Lonn U: A Minimally Invasive Axial Blood Flow Pump. Linkoping, Sweden: Linkoping Heart Center, Linkoping University, 1997.

138. Lowe JE, Anstadt MP, Van Tright P, Smith PK, Hendry PJ, Plunkett MD, Anstadt GL: First successful bridge to cardiac transplantation using direct mechanical ventricular actuation. Ann Thorac Surg 1991;52:1237–1245.

139. Marlinski E, Jacobs G, Deirmengian C, Jarvik R: Durability testing of components for the Jarvik 2000 completely implantable flow left ventricular assist device. ASAIO J 1998;44:M741–M744.

140. Markus HS, Droste DW, Brown MM: Detection of asymptomatic cerebral embolic signals with Doppler ultrasound. Lancet 1994;343:1011–1012.

141. McCarthy PM, Portner PM, Tobler HG, Starnes VA, Ramasamy N, Oyer PE: Clinical experience with the Novacor ventricular assist system. J Thorac Cardiovasc Surg 1991;102:578–587.

142. Menconi MJ, Pockwinse S, Owen TA, Dasse KA, Stein GS, Lian JB: Properties of blood-contacting surfaces of clinically implanted cardiac assist devices: gene expression, matrix composition, and ultrastructural characterization of cellular linings. J Cell Biochem 1995;57:557–573.

143. Mertes PM, Pinelli G, Hubert T, Carteaux JP, Hottier E, Larcan A, Villemot JP: Impact of nitric oxide inhalation on right ventricular failure after implantation of Novacor left ventricular assist system. J Thorac Cardiovasc Surg 1995;109:1251.

144. Miller CA, Pae WE Jr, Pierce WS: Combined registry for the clinical use of mechanical ventricular assist pumps and the total artificial heart in conjunction with heart transplantation: fourth official report 1989. J Heart Lung Transplant 1990;9:453–458.

145. Morita S, Kormos RL, Eishi K: Left ventricular assistance improves mechanical efficiency of the right ventricle. Surg Forum 1991;42:311–314.

146. Morita S, Kormos RL, Mandarino WA, Eishi K, Kawai A, Gasior TA, Deneault LG, Armitage JM, Hardesty RL, Griffith BP: Right ventricular/arterial coupling in the patient with left ventricular assistance. Circulation 1992;86:II-316–II-325.

147. Moritz A: Mechanical bride to transplantation with the Vienna heart in TAH and LVAD configuration. Int J Artif Organs 1992;15:147–150.

148. Moroney DA, Swartz MT, Reedy JE, Lohmann DP, McBride LR, Pennington DG: Importance of ventricular arrhythmias in recovery patients with ventricular assist devices. ASAIO Trans 1991;37:M516–M517.

149. Moulopoulos SD, Topaz SR, Kolff WJ: Extracorporeal assistance to the circulation and intraaortic balloon pumping. Trans Am Soc Artif Intern Organs 1962;8:85–89.

150. NHLBI Report of the Task Force on Research in Heart Failure: Washington, DC: US Department of Health and Human Services, 1994, pp 1–108.

151. Nakatani T, Noda H, Beppu S, Taenaka Y, Kinoshita M, Tatsumi E, Yutani C, Kumon K, Fujita T, Takano H: Thrombus in a natural left ventricle during left ventricular assist: another thromboembolic risk factor. ASAIO Trans 1990;36:M711–M714.

152. Nakazawa T, Makinouchi K, Takami Y, Glueck J, Takatani S, Nose Y: The effect of the impeller-driver magnetic coupling distance on hemolysis in a compact centrifugal pump. Artif Organs 1996;20:252–257.

153. Norman JC, Cooley DA, Kahan BD, Frazier OH, Keats AS, Hacker J, Massin EK, Duncan JM, Solis RT, Dacso CC, Luper WE, Winston DS, Reul GJ: Total support of the circulation of a patient with post-cardiotomy stone-heart syndrome by a partial artificial heart (ALVAD) for 5 days followed by heart and kidney transplantation. Lancet 1978;1:1125–1127.

154. Norman JC, Duncan JM, Frazier OH, Hallman GL, Ott DA, Reul GJ, Cooley DA: Intracorporeal (abdominal) left ventricular assist devices or partial artificial hearts. Arch Surg 1981;116:1441–1445.

155. Nose Y: Is a totally implantable artificial heart realistic? Artif Organs 1992;16:19–42.

156. Novarcor Operating Manual: Baxter Healthcare Corporation, One Baxter Parkway, Deerfield, IL.

157. Ohar JA, Waller KS, Dahms TE: Platelet-activating factor induces selective pulmonary arterial hyperreactivity in isolate perfused rabbit lungs. Am Rev Respir Dis 1993;148:158–163.

158. Olsen DB, Unger F, Oster H, Lawson J, Kessler T, Kolff J, Kolff WJ: Thrombus generation within the artificial heart. J Thorac Cardiovasc Surg 1975;70:248–255.

159. Oz MC, Goldstein DJ, Rose EA: Preperitoneal placement of ventricular assist devices: an illustrated stepwise approach. J Card Surg 1995;10:288–294.

160. Oz MC, Rose EA, Slater J, Kuiper JJ, Catanese KA, Levin HR: Malignant ventricular arrhythmias are well tolerated in patients receiving long-term left ventricular assist devices. J Am Coll Cardiol 1994;24:1688–1691.

161. Parnis SM, Yu LS, Ochs BD, Macris MP, Frazier OH, Kung RT: Chronic in vivo evaluation of an electrohydraulic total artificial heart. ASAIO J 1994;40:M489–M493.

162. Pavie A, Leger P, Regan M, Nataf P, Bors V, Szefner J, Cabrol C, Gandjbakhch I: Clinical experience with a total artificial heart as a bridge for transplantation: the Pitie experience. J Card Surg 1995;10:552–558.

163. Pennington DG, McBride LR, Swartz MT, Kanter KR, Kaiser GC, Barner HB, Miller LW, Naunheim KS, Fiore AC, Willman VL: Use of the Pierce-Donachy ventricular assist device in patients with cardiogenic shock after cardiac operations. Ann Thorac Surg 1989;47:130–135.

164. Peters JL, McRea JC, Fukumasu H, Mochizuki T, Daitoh N, McGough E, Pearce M, Fee H, Rich G: Recovery of cardiac function with total transapical left ventricular bypass. Trans Am Soc Artif Intern Organs 1980;26:262–267.

165. Phillips WS, Burton NA, Macmanus Q, Lefrak EA: Surgical complications in bridging to transplantation: the ThermoCardiosystems LVAD. Ann Thorac Surg 1992;53:482–486.

166. Pierce WS, Gray LA, McBride LR, Frazier OH: Other postoperative complications: circulatory support—1988. Ann Thorac Surg 1989;47:96–101.

167. Poirier VL: Worldwide experience with the TCI Heart/Mate System: issues and future perspective. Thorac Cardiovasc Surg 1999;47(suppl 2):316–320.

168. Portner PM, Oyer PE, McGregor CGA: First human use of an electrically powered implantable ventricular assist system. Artif Organs 1985;9:36.

169. Portner PM, Oyer PE, Pennington DG, Baumgartner WA, Griffith BP, Frist WR, Magilligan DJ, Noon GP, Ramasamy N, Miller PJ: Implantable electrical left ventricular assist system: bridge to transplantation and the future. Ann Thorac Surg 1989;47:142–150.

170. Power JM, Raman J, Dornom A, Farish SJ, Burrell LM, Tonkin AM, Buxton B, Alferness CA: Passive ventricular constraint amends the course of heart failure: a study in an ovine model of dilated cardiomyopathy. Cardiovasc Res 1999;44:549–555.

171. Raithel SC, Pennington DG, Boegner E, Fiore A, Weber TR: Extracorporeal membrane oxygenation in children after cardiac surgery. Circulation 1992;86(suppl II):II-305–II-310.

172. Reibson JD, Rosenberg G, Snyder AJ, Cleary TJ, Donachy JH, Felder G, Pierce WS: An annular compliance chamber for the Pennsylvania State University electric total artificial heart. ASAIO J 1993;39:M415–M418.

173. Reemtsma K, Krusin R, Edie R, Bergman D, Dobelle W, Hardy M: Cardiac transplantation in patients requiring mechanical circulatory support. N Engl J Med 1978;298:670.

174. Roberts WC, Siegel RJ, McManus BM: Idiopathic dilated cardiomyopathy: analysis of 152 necropsy patients. Am J Cardiol 1987;60:1340–1355.

175. Rose EA, Levin HR, Oz MC, Frazier OH, Macmanus Q, Burton NA, Lefrak EA: Artificial circulatory support with textured interior surfaces: a counter intuitive approach to minimizing thromboembolism. Circulation 1994;90:II-87–II-91.

176. Rose EA, Moskowitz AJ, Packer M: The REMATCH trial: rationale, design and end points. Randomized evaluation of mechanical assistance for the treatment of congestive heart failure. Ann Thorac Surg 1999;67:723–730.

177. Rosenberg G, Pierce WS, Landis DL: Progress in the development of the Pennsylvania State University motor-driven artificial heart. In Unger F (ed): Assisted Circulation 2. Berlin: Springer-Verlag, 1984, pp 270–285.

178. Rowles JR, Mortimer BJ, Olsen DB: Ventricular assist and total artificial heart devices for clinical use in 1993. ASAIO J 1993;39:840–855.

179. Salih V, Graham TR, Berry CL, Coumbe A, Smith SC, Dasse K, Frazier OH: The lining of textured surfaces in implantable left ventricular assist devices. An immunocytochemical and electron-microscopic study. Am J Cardiovasc Pathol 1993;4:317–325.

180. Sapirstein JS, Pae WE Jr: Mechanical circulatory support before heart transplantation. In Cooper DKC, Miller LW, Patterson GA (eds): The Transplantation and Replacement of Thoracic Organs. 2nd ed. Boston: Kluwer Academic Publishers, 1996.

181. Sato N: Multi-institutional evaluation of the Tokyo University Ventricular Assist System. ASAIO Trans 1990;36:M708–M711.

182. Scheinin SA, Capek P, Radovancevic B, Duncan JM, McAllister HA Jr, Frazier OH: The effect of prolonged left ventricular support on myocardial histopathology in patients with end-stage cardiomyopathy. ASAIO J 1992;38:M271–M274.

183. Schiessler A: Clinical use of the Berlin Biventricular Assist Device as a bridge to transplantation. ASAIO Trans 1990;36:M706–M708.

184. Schoen FJ, Harasaki H, Kim KM, Anderson HC, Levy RJ: Biomaterial-associated calcification: pathology, mechanisms, and strategies for prevention. J Biomed Mater Res 1988;22:11–36.

185. Shapiro GC, Leibowitz DW, Oz MC, Weslow RG, Di Tullio MR, Homma S: Diagnosis of patent foramen ovale with transesophageal echocardiography in a patient supported with a left ventricular assist device. J Heart Lung Transplant 1995;14:594–597.

186. Shenkar R, Coulson WF, Abrahm E: Hemorrhage and resuscitation induce alterations in cytokine expression and the development of acute lung injury. Am J Respir Cell Mol Biol 1994;10:290–297.

187. Siostrzonek P, Koppensteiner R, Kreiner G, Madl C, Gossinger HD, Heinz G, Stumpflen A, Wendelin B, Mosslacher H, Ehringer H: Abnormal blood rheology in idiopathic dilated cardiomyopathy. Am J Cardiol 1992;69:1497–1499.

188. Skinner DB, Anstadt GL, Camp TF: Application of mechanical ventricular assistance. Ann Surg 1967;166:500–512.

189. Skinner DB, Anstadt GL, Camp TF Jr: Mechanical ventricular assistance: applications of a method for total cardiac support [review]. Bull Soc Int Chir 1969;3:406–412.

190. Slater JP, Goldstein DJ, Ashton RC Jr, Levin HR, Spotnitz HM, Oz MC: Right-to-left veno-arterial shunting for right-sided circulatory failure. Ann Thorac Surg 1995;60:978–985.

191. Slater JP, Yamada A, Yano OJ, Stennet R, Goldstein DJ, Levin HR, Spotnitz HM, Oz MC: Creation of a controlled venoarterial shunt: a surgical intervention for right-side circulatory failure. Circulation 1995;92:II-467–II-471.

192. Smith JA, Oyer PE: Development of the Novacor Left Ventricular Assist Device. In Thoracic Transplantation. Oxford, England: Blackwell Science, 1995, p 134.

193. Snoddy BD, Nanda NC, Holman WL, Kirklin JK, Chung SM: Usefulness of transesophageal echocardiography in diagnosing and guiding correct placement of a right ventricular assist device malpositioned in the left atrium. Echocardiography 1996;13:159–163.

194. Snyder AJ, Rosenberg G, Weiss WJ, Ford SK, Nazarian RA, Hicks DL, Malotte JA, Kawaguchi O, Prophet GA, Sapirstein JS: In vivo testing of a completely implanted total artificial heart system. ASAIO J 1993;39:M177–M184.

195. Soeter JR, Mamiya RT, Sprague AY, McNamara JJ: Prolonged extracorporeal oxygenation for cardiorespiratory failure after tetralogy correction. J Thorac Cardiovasc Surg 1972;66:551–552.

196. Soreff HS, Levine HJ, Sachs BF: Assisted circulation. Effects of counter pulsation on left ventricular oxygen consumption and hemodynamics. Circulation 1963;27:772.

197. Spanier TB, Oz MC, Levin H, Weinberg A: Activation of coagulation and fibrinolytic pathways in patients with left ventricular assist devices. J Thorac Cardiovasc Surg 1996;112:1090–1097.

198. Spencer FC, Eisman B, Trinkle JK, Rossi NP: Assisted circulation for cardiac failure following intracardiac surgery with cardiopulmonary bypass. J Thorac Cardiovasc Surg 1965;49:56–73.

199. Starnes VA, Oyer PE, Portner PM, Ramasamy N, Miller PJ, Stinson EB, Baldwin JC, Ream AK, Wyner J, Shumway NE: Isolated left ventricular assist as bridge to cardiac transplantation. J Thorac Cardiovasc Surg 1988;96:62–71.

200. Stuckey JH, Newman DC: The use of the heart lung machine in selected cases of acute myocardial infarction. Surg Forum 1957;8:342.

201. Swartz MT, Lowdermilk GA, Moroney DA, McBride LR: Ventricular assist device support in patients with mechanical heart valves. Ann Thorac Surg 1999;68:2248–2251.

202. Szukalski EA, Reedy JE, Pennington DG, Swartz MT, McBride LR, Miller LW: Oral anticoagulation in patients with ventricular assist devices. ASAIO Trans 1990;36:M700–M703.

203. Takano H: Clinical experience with ventricular assist systems in Japan. Ann Thorac Surg 1993;55:250–256.

204. Takano H: Ventricular assist systems: experience in Japan with Toyobo pump and Zeon pump. Ann Thorac Surg 1996; 61:317–322.

205. Tatsumi E, Diegel PD, Holfert JW, Dew PA, Crump KR, Hansen AC, Khanwilkar PS, Rowles JR, Olsen DB: A blood pump with an interatrial shunt for use as an electrohydraulic total artificial heart. ASAIO J 1992;38:M425–M430.

206. Tatsumi E, Khanwilkar PS, Rowles JR, Chiang BY, Burns GL, Long JW, Hansen AC, Holfert JW, Bearnson GB, Crump KR: In vivo long-term evaluation of the Utah electrohydraulic total artificial heart. ASAIO J 1993;39:M373–M380.

207. Termuhlen DF, Swartz MT, Pennington DG: Thromboembolic complications with the Pierce-Donachy ventricular assist device. ASAIO Trans 1989;35:616–618.

208. Thomas DC, Butler KC, Taylor LP, LeBlanc P, Griffith BP, Kormos RL, Borovetz HS, Litwak P, Kameneva MV, Choi S, Burgreen GW, Wagner WR, Wu Z, Antaki JF: Continued development of the Nimbus/University of Pittsburgh (UOP) Axial Flow Left Ventricular Assist System. ASAIO J 1997;43:M564–M566.

209. Thoratec Lab News Letter. March 1998.

210. Thuys CA, Mullaly RJ, Horton SB, O'Connor EB, Cochrane AD, Brizard CPR, Karl TR: Centrifugal ventricular assist in children under 6kg. Eur J Cardiothorac Surg 1998;13:130–134.

211. Tsau PH, Arabia FA, Toporoff B, Paramesh V, Sethi GK, Copeland JG: Positive panel reactive antibody titers in patients bridged to transplantation with a mechanical assist device. ASAIO J 1998; 44:M634–M637.

212. US Department of Health and Human Services: Artificial Heart and Assist Devices: Directions, Needs, Costs, Societal and Ethical Issues. Bethesda, MD: National Institutes of Health, 1985, pp 25–27.

213. Vasku J: Evaluation study of calves with total artificial heart (TAH) surviving for 218-293 days of pumping. Int J Artif Organs 1990;13:830–836.

214. Vasku J: The applicability of experimental experience with the total artificial heart to its clinical use. Int J Artif Organs 1992;15:307–311.

215. Wampler RK, Moise JC, Frazier OH, Olsen DB: In vivo evaluation of a peripheral vascular access axio flow blood pump. ASAIO Trans 1988;34:450–454.

216. Weinhaus L, Canter C, Noetzel M, McAlister W, Spray TL: Extracorporeal membrane oxygenation for circulatory support after repair of congenital heart defects. Ann Thorac Surg 1989; 48:206–212.

217. Wieselthaler GM, Schima H, Hiesmayr M, Pacher R, Laufer G, Noon GP, DeBakey M, Wolner E: First clinical experience with the DeBakey VAD continuous-axial-flow bridge to transplantation. Circulation 2000;101:356–359.

218. Weiss WJ, Rosenberg G, Snyder AJ, Donachy J, Reibson J, Kawaguchi O, Sapirstein JS, Pae WE, Pierce WS: A completely implanted left ventricular assist device. Chronic in vivo testing. ASAIO J 1993;39:M427–M432.

219. Weiss WJ, Rosenberg G, Snyder AJ, Pierce WS, Pae WE, Kuroda H, Rawhuser MA, Felder G, Reibson JD, Cleary TJ, Ford SK, Marlotte JA, Nazarian RA, Hicks DL: Steady state hemodynamic and energetic characterization of the Penn State Health Care Total Artificial Heart. ASAIO J 1999;45:189–193.

220. Weyand M, Kececioglu D, Kehl HG, Schmid C, Lick HM, Vogt J, Scheld HH: Neonatal mechanical bridging to total orthotopic heart transplantation. Ann Thorac Surg 1998;66:519–522.

221. Westaby S: Aprotinin in perspective. Ann Thorac Surg 1993; 55:1033–1041.

222. Ziady GM, Kormos RL, Salerni R, Matesic C, Griffith BP: The effect of mechanical left ventricular assist device on cardiac size and function in end stage heart disease. A Doppler echocardiographic study. Circulation 1991;84:II-490.

223. Ziomek S, Harrell JE, Fasules JW, Faulkner SC, Chipman CW, Moss M, Frazier E, Van Devanter SH: Extracorporeal membrane oxygenation for cardiac failure after congenital heart operation. Ann Thorac Surg 1992;54:861–868.

Appendix

Emergency Protocol For Thoratec Pump Console Failure

1. Remove right and left pneumatic VAD drive line from the nonfunctioning console, attach them to the red hand pumps, and initiate hand pumping at about 60–80 bpm.
2. Be sure that the backup console is plugged in and the POWER button is lit. Now, open the rear door of the backup Thoratec console.
3. Identify the switches for the air compressors, which are located on the floor of the console. These switches are labeled "Top" and "Bottom." Turn both of these switches to the "ON" position. You will hear the compressors working.
4. Activate the upper and lower console panels by pulling the operation-battery charge switches out and then moving them to the "Operation" setting. This is done separately for the upper and lower console panels.
5. Turn the vacuum lever on each console panel to the "ON" position.
6. Close the rear door of the Thoratec console.
7. Set the top console panel to a rate of 60 bpm, 30% systole, positive pressure of 200 mm Hg, negative pressure to –40 mm Hg.
8. Push the "Asynch" button to initiate fixed rate pumping of upper console panel.
9. Attach the left VAD pneumatic drive line to the upper console pneumatic output fitting, which should be emitting pulses of air at 60 bpm.
10. On the lower console, set the rate at 40 bpm, the percent systole at 30%, the positive pressure at 150 mm Hg, and the negative pressure at –40 mm Hg.
11. Push the "Asynch" button and attach the right VAD pneumatic drive line to the lower console pneumatic output fitting, which should be emitting pulses of air at 40 bpm.
12. Connect the electrical cable for the left VAD to the upper console panel "Hall Switch In" connector.
13. Connect the electrical cable for the right VAD to the lower console "Hall Switch In" connector.
14. Press the "Volume" button for the upper and lower console panels to initiate automatic (full-to-empty variable rate) pumping.
15. Page the perfusionist on call and MCSS physician/surgeon to come to the hospital and be certain that the pump is functioning properly and determine that the settings are optimal.
16. Obtain and plug in another Thoratec drive unit as a backup console.

Emergency Protocol for Pneumatic HeartMate Console Failure

- Call MCSS surgery attending and perfusionist
- Perform the following:

  1. Push "Power" on back-out backup console (takes 10 seconds to self-test).
  2. Disconnect the pneumatic and electrical leads and connect them to the backup console.
  3. Push "vent" and wait until the light goes off (6–7 sec).
  4. Push "six" or "auto" (depending on mode of LVAD used). Check to be sure that the options controls on the console are set the same as previously documented.
  5. Assess LVAD ejection and filling.
  6. Assess vital signs and patient's status.

- If backup console fails, use manual crank until console failure is resolved.

  1. Console must be in the **Stop** mode before hand cranking can take place.
  2. Insert the handle mounted on rear panel of console (into the hole in the rear panel of the console) allowing the handle such that you feel the pins engaging in the slots.
  3. Turn handle CLOCKWISE (looking at back panel) to eject blood.
  4. Pause briefly at the end of each rotation to allow the pump to fill.
  5. *Do not* operate console with the crank in place.

- Do not perform chest compression on a patient with implanted LVAD. Defibrillation or cardioversion may be performed.

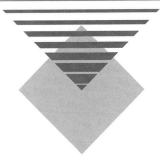

The Transplanted Heart

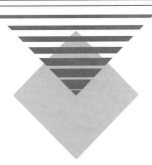

CHAPTER NINE

The Donor Heart

The performance of a cardiac transplantation procedure is a time of elation for the recipient and his or her family, since it brings to an end an often agonizing wait for a donor heart and provides a realistic expectation of a better quality and length of life. However, it is also a time of enormous sadness and tragedy for the donor family. Heart-beating donor organs would not be available but for the humanity of donor families,

a fact that is frequently overshadowed by the more spectacular transplant procedure. Of course, the tragedy of brain death in a usually young and active individual should also be viewed as a societal tragedy because of the epidemic of hand guns, violence, child abuse (as a source of infant donors), and violent death on the roads.

DEFINITION AND DETERMINATION OF BRAIN DEATH

HISTORICAL ASPECTS

For the concept of brain death to be established both in law and medicine, the idea that death occurs when the circulation and respiration ceased had to be replaced by the notion that death occurs when the functions that primarily define a human being as an independent biologic unit (i.e., "as an entity capable of relating to both its external and internal world"[235]) are lost. These functions, consciousness and the capacity to breath spontaneously (and therefore to maintain a heart beat), are in the domain of the brain stem. The relationship between increased intracranial pressure and subsequent death due to cessation of respiration followed by cardiac action can be traced back to the late 1800s in the writings of Horsely[138] and Duckworth.[78] In 1902, Cushing[66] discussed the mode of death due to increased intracranial pressure. The common thread to these writings was the observation that increased intracranial pressure resulted in cessation of respiration followed by the arrest of cardiac action, emphasizing the central nature of brain stem function.

It is interesting to note that before organs for transplantation became a necessity, the Church took a step that opened the way for the development of brain death laws. Pope Pius XII in 1957[250] responded to increasing concern that the lives of patients with irreversible coma were being needlessly prolonged, by declaring that the soul may separate from the body "even when certain organs continue to function." Even though unequivocal principles were not outlined, it was made clear that "the moment of death" in an unconscious patient "was the province of the physician" and "not within the competence of the Church." Furthermore, in the hopelessly unconscious patient the duration of "resuscitation" was covered by his reference to "application of ordinary means of care." The issue of brain death then gained some momentum, probably in part because it was being brought into the consciousness of physicians, perhaps aided by the fact that apparently any potential theological objections regarding the declaration of death in unconscious, apneic, heart-beating patients were dispelled.

The terms *whole brain death* and *brain stem death* gained significance as brain death laws evolved. **Whole brain death** refers to "irreversible cessation of all functions of the entire brain, including the brain stem,"[254] although, from a practical standpoint, it is not possible to determine when all components of the brain have ceased to function. **Brain stem death** is the "physiological cause of brain death,"[235] and hence the central component of the clinical determination of brain death.

The movement towards the eventual development of brain death laws was given considerable impetus by the contributions of French investigators. In 1959, a group of neurophysiologists and neurosurgeons from Lyon, France,[152] described a lesion in patients with traumatic brain injury which had the following features: the injury was complicated by respiratory arrest, and there was persistent apneic coma, absent brain stem and tendon reflexes, and an electrically silent brain. If the patient was disconnected from the ventilator, there was no respiratory response to hypercapnia. These authors attached the term "death of the nervous system" and believed that there was unequivocal evidence of irreversible death of the central nervous system and that continued ventilation was not appropriate. In the same year, two French neurologists (Mollaret and Goulon)[207] described a condition that they called *coma dépassé*, which was essentially the same neurologic condition as described by the Lyon group. The term *coma dépassé* was discontinued in 1988 on the recommendation of the French National Academy of Medicine because of concerns that the term could potentially be construed as describing a situation in which organs were harvested from a comatose patient who was not in fact brain dead.

A number of forums occurred which finally culminated in the acceptance of brain death as equivalent to death of the patient. In 1965, at a Ciba symposium,[350] Alexandra proposed that organs could be available for transplantation from patients who had incontrovertible evidence of brain death and an intact circulation. This visionary view was at a time when a number of senior surgeons had serious reservations about the likelihood

TABLE 9–1   Harvard Criteria of Brain Death
1. No spontaneous respiration
2. No superficial or deep reflexes (pupillary light reflex included)
3. No movements either spontaneous or secondary to painful stimuli
4. Electrocerebral silence (flat) by EEG
5. Apnea (3 minutes off ventilator)
6. All of the above findings unchanged 24 hours later

TABLE 9–2   The "Minnesota Criteria" of Brain Death
1. No spontaneous movement
2. Apnea (for 4 minutes)
3. Absent brain stem reflexes
4. "All findings unchanged for at least 12 hours"
5. The pathologic processes responsible for Numbers 1 through 4 are deemed irreparable

Adapted from Mohandas A, Chou SN: Brain death—a clinical and pathological study. J Neurosurg 1971;35:211–218.

that brain death could ever be equated with death of a patient. There emerged from this meeting the forerunner of the brain death criteria, each criterion being subsequently modified. The criteria upon which there was agreement for diagnosis of brain death of patients with "severe craniocerebral injury" were (1) complete bilateral mydriasis, (2) complete absence of reflexes (including response to profound pain), (3) complete absence of spontaneous respiration 5 minutes after mechanical respiration had been stopped, (4) falling blood pressure necessitating increasing amounts of vasopressive drugs, and (5) a flat electroencephalogram (EEG). Not surprisingly, there was considerable medical, legal, and ethical turmoil which was undoubtedly fueled by the first cardiac transplant, which occurred in December 1967. An historical summary of the development of brain death criteria and the first human heart transplant is found in Chapter 1.

In 1968, the Twenty-second World Medical Assembly which convened in Sydney, Australia,[116] issued a statement on brain death which in essence made the important distinction between death at a cellular level and death of a person, the implications of which are now obvious. In the same year, a *definition of irreversible coma* was proposed that defined irreversible coma as a new criterion for death. The committee determined a number of criteria for the diagnosis of a "permanently nonfunctioning brain" (Table 9–1).[1] The Committee made the very important recommendation that the physician making the decision to declare a patient brain dead should not be involved in any subsequent decision to consider transplantation of the individual's organs or tissues.

The centrality of the brain stem and the distinction between whole brain death and brain stem death were fundamental to the "Minnesota criteria" (Table 9–2).[206] A critical aspect of the Minnesota criteria were that any EEG criteria was considered "extremely questionable," since the emphasis was on brain stem function and not cortical function that was responsible for generation of the EEG. The Minnesota criteria undoubtedly was influential in the genesis of the "UK code" which was published in 1976 and was produced by a conference of the Royal Colleges and faculties of the United Kingdom and had a similar emphasis on the pivitol role of the brain stem in the declaration of brain death.[58]

DIAGNOSIS OF BRAIN DEATH

In 1981, a Presidential Commission for the study of ethical problems in medicine produced a document which contained an appendix entitled "Guidelines for the determination of death," and these criteria have become the basis for the current means of diagnosing brain death.[255]

Criteria for Brain Death

The clinical diagnosis of brain death requires three stages.

1) Preconditions—it is necessary to determine a precise cause of apneic coma and confirm that this cause has resulted in permanent structural damage to the brain. It must also be determined that this structural damage is irreversible, and the irreversibility is determined by a period (usually approximately 12 hours) of observation while resuscitation and measures to correct the underlying cause are instituted. Restoration of normal gas exchange, blood pressure, temperature, and fluid and electrolyte balance is implicit.

2) Exclusions—reversible causes of brain stem dysfunction must be excluded, and these include hypothermia, hypotension, drug intoxication, and a number of metabolic and endocrine disorders.

3) Clinical Testing—the diagnosis of brain stem death relies on the absence of brain stem reflexes (brain stem reflexes are an all or none phenomenon). The brain stem reflexes that are tested are (a) pupillary response to light; (b) corneal reflexes; (c) vestibular ocular reflexes; (d) gag reflex; (e) cough reflex; and (f) apnea. The method of establishing apnea is quite specific and is based on no spontaneous ventilation despite an arterial $Pco_2 > 60$ mm Hg. Hypoxia can be prevented during this test by preoxygenating the patient with 100% oxygen prior to discontinuing ventilation. An EEG, or for that matter any test of brain blood flow, is not required but is at the discretion of the examiners. Brain death should be confirmed by at least two physicians.

Brain Death in Children and the Newborn

Because the Presidential Commission[255] criteria were not extended to children younger than 5 years of age (due to the putative assumption that a younger child's brain is less vulnerable to cerebral injury), it became necessary to formulate guidelines for the determination of brain death in children. In 1987, the Ad Hoc Task Force Committee's guidelines for the determination of brain death in children were introduced (Table 9–3).[262] The committee did not specifically address guidelines for the diagnosis of brain death in preterm and term infants less than 7 days of age. Additional complexities are involved in the determination of brain death in neonates, including the greater resilience of the neonatal central nervous system, the possibility of intrauterine asphyxia and central nervous system malformations which may alter the clinical examination and neurodiagnostic testing,[8] the fact that prior to 34 weeks' reflexes may be incomplete or difficult to test,[9] and the use of anticonvulsants such as phenobarbital for protection in neonates with perinatal

TABLE 9–3	**Guidelines for the Determination of Brain Death in Children**

A. *History*—determination of cause of death and that it is irreversible
B. *Physical examination criteria*
  • Coma and apnea
  • Absence of brain stem function
  • Hypothermia or hypotension for age
  • Flaccid tone and absence of spontaneous or induced movements (excluding those at spinal cord level)
  • Examination consistent with brain death throughout observation period
C. *Laboratory testing*—EEG, if performed, should demonstrate electrocerebral silence

asphyxia. However, there is evidence to suggest that brain death can be readily determined in the newborn, and it has been recommended that[8] the Committee guidelines for determination of brain death can be extended to the preterm infant greater than 32 weeks gestation and the term infant. The diagnosis can be based on clinical assessment without the need for neurodiagnostic studies if the preterm infant is observed for at least 3 days and the term infant observed for 2 days. If neurodiagnostic testing (electrocerebral silence on an EEG and absence of cerebral blood flow) is coupled to clinical examination, then the period of observation can be shortened to 24 hours.[10] Chapter 20 includes further discussion of brain death in infants.

PATHOPHYSIOLOGY OF MYOCARDIAL INJURY ASSOCIATED WITH BRAIN DEATH

The effect of brain death on the myocardium has been of considerable interest in the field of cardiac transplantation for two important reasons: (1) there is a low but not insignificant incidence of primary graft failure following cardiac transplantation (see later section), and (2) many potential donor hearts are not used because of donor heart dysfunction. Successful strategies to improve dysfunctional donor hearts would increase the number of donor hearts available for transplantation.

Contemporary descriptions of the influence of the central nervous system on the heart can be traced back to the work of Byer who, in 1947, described large upright T waves and long Q-T intervals in five patients with severe neurologic injury (four with strokes and one with a hypertensive encephalopathy).[44] Since that time, numerous reports have documented electrocardiographic changes associated with cerebral disease (including subarachnoid hemorrhage,[63, 302] stroke,[92] head injury,[134, 259] and intracranial hemorrhage[64, 306, 332]), which consist of ST-segment elevation, T-wave inversion, and Q waves. While both humoral and neural mechanisms were considered, it was reports of the rapid onset and disappearance of electrocardiographic changes during surgical treatment of cerebral aneurysms that strongly suggested a neural mechanism.[63] A number of these patients had autopsies performed but myocardial injury was not routinely recognized.

Further understanding of myocardial injury due to intracranial disease comes from the production of myocardial injury by catecholamine infusion, the study of stress models, and the study of stimulation of the nervous system. Of particular interest is the effect of catecholamine infusion on the heart. Josué[151] found that infusion with epinephrine could cause cardiac hypertrophy. However, of particular importance was the demonstration that catecholamine infusion produces a characteristic histologic appearance in the myocardium, called **myofibrillar degeneration,** also known as contraction band necrosis or coagulative myocytolysis. This picture is quite distinct from the coagulation necrosis which is the predominant histologic pattern seen in acute myocardial infarction.[19] In coagulation necrosis, myocardial cells die without obvious contraction bands, calcification appears late, and a predominant polymorphonuclear cell response occurs. Coagulation necrosis is not seen histologically for many hours or even days after the onset of the infarction. In contrast, myofibrillar degeneration is histologically detectable early after its onset, and the myofibers die in a hypercontracted state with obvious contraction bands. Furthermore, myofibrillar degeneration elicits a mononuclear cell response and calcification occurs very quickly.[33, 93, 188, 283, 296, 318] The lesion of myofibrillar degeneration can also be seen in humans where the mode of death involves considerable stress, such as physical assault in which death occurred due to the assault but not due to life-threatening injuries, suggesting the association between catecholamine release and myofibrillar degeneration.[48]

Prolonged central nervous system stimulation can also induce myofibrillar degeneration. Bilateral prolonged stimulation of the hypothalamus produces the identical histologic picture to that produced by catecholamine infusions and stress.[196] Myocardial lesions of this type can also be produced by stimulation of the limbic cortex, the mesencephalic reticular formation, and the stellate ganglion. Experimental intracerebral and subarachnoid hemorrhages can also produce these myocardial lesions.[283]

Brain death is frequently accompanied by massive release of endogenous catecholamines.[20, 221, 273] In animal models of acute brain injury, blood epinephrine and norepinephrine levels may increase 100- to 500-fold within 10 seconds of experimental brain injury,[273] with a correlation between severity of injury and magnitude of catecholamine release.[20, 273, 298] In humans, measured catecholamine levels after brain death have been highly variable,[252] likely related to individual variability in neurohumoral response and the mechanism and rapidity of the intracranial catastrophic event. In Novitzky's baboon model, rapid increase in intracranial pressure was accompanied by marked increases in mean arterial, pulmonary wedge, and central venous pressure within 15 minutes (Table 9–4), accompanied by a three- to sevenfold increase in blood norepinephrine and epinephrine levels.[221] A relationship between noradrenaline levels and increases in the plasma level of CK-MB has been demonstrated after acute head injury in man.[64] However,

TABLE 9–4	**Hemodynamic Response to Brain Death in Baboon**		
STAGE	HEMODYNAMICS	ECG	MEAN DURATION
I	Slight fall in: MAP SV CO	Sinus bradycardia AV dissociation Sinus standstill Nodal rhythm	8 min
II	Marked rise in: MAP PCWP PVR CVP Reduction in: SV	Sinus tachycardia	5 min
III	Rise in: MAP PCWP PVR CVP	Ventricular ectopics Ischemic changes	150 min
IV	Fall in: MAP PCWP PVR CVP	Sinus tachycardia Ischemic changes	150 min
V	Low MAP Low PVR Low CVP	Sinus rhythm (rate 50–60 min) Persistent ischemic changes	17 hr

MAP, mean arterial pressure; SV, stroke volume; CO, cardiac output; PCWP, pulmonary capillary wedge pressure; PVR, peripheral vascular resistance; CVP, central venous pressure.
Adapted from Novitzky D, Wicomb WN, Cooper DKC, Rose AG, Fraser RC, Barnard CN: Electrocardiographic, hemodynamic and endocrine changes occurring during experimental brain death in the chacma baboon. Heart Transplant 1984;4:63–69.

patients with acute head injury who received beta blockade did not have a reduction in norepinephrine levels, although the elution of CK-MB was reduced and focal myocardial necrotic lesions were abolished. Novitsky's observation that a total cardiac sympathectomy (but not adrenalectomy) in the baboon prevented myocyte injury after brain death suggests that the **release of catecholamines from postganglionic nerve endings within the myocardium** is more important than circulating catecholamines released from the adrenal glands in producing myocyte injury associated with brain death.[222]

The injury may result from the interplay between coronary vasoconstriction, free radical generation, and reperfusion in association with oxygen-derived free radical generation. Oxidation products of catecholamines, for example, the free radical adrenochrome, may induce myocardial injury,[29] probably resulting from peroxidation of membrane phospholipids. Catecholamine storm may also induce myocardial injury by oxygen-derived free radicals generated by reperfusion of myocardium that has been rendered ischemic by severe coronary vasoconstriction. The physiologic response to the post–brain death "catecholamine storm" in a canine model also demonstrated a reduction in preload independent recruitable stroke work in right and left ventricles.[30] The typical progression of cardiac dysfunction in man due to an expanding supratentorial mass such as incranial bleeding is depicted in Figure 9–1.[106]

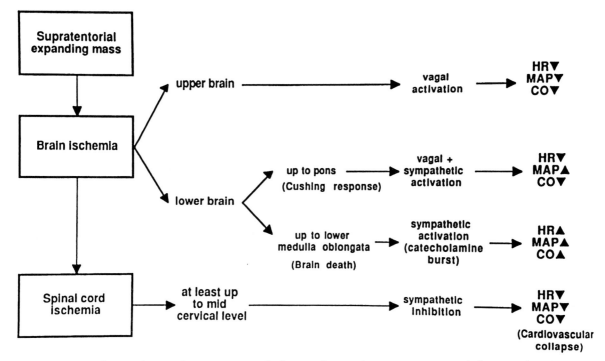

FIGURE **9-1.** Schematic diagram shows progression of ischemia in the central nervous system as a result of an expanding supratentorial mass and summarizes events leading to brain death and eventual collapse. Depending on the anatomical structures involved, there is vagal and/or sympathetic activation and/or inhibition, which in turn causes the hemodynamic changes shown. MAP, mean arterial pressure (mm Hg); HR, heart rate (bpm); CO, cardiac output. (From Freimark D, Czer LSC, Admon D, Aleksic I, Valenza M, Barath P, Harasty D, Queral C, Azen CG, Blanche C, Trento A: Donors with a history of cocaine use: effect on survival and rejection frequency after heart transplanation. J Heart Lung Transplant 1994;13:1138–1144. Copyright 1994, Excerpta Medica Inc., with permission.)

THE PROCESS OF ORGAN DONATION

ORGANIZATION

The process of organ donation in each country involved in organ transplantation includes organization at both a national and local level. In the United States, the pivotal component is the United Network for Organ Sharing (UNOS). The history of UNOS is discussed in Chapter 1, and the organization of UNOS is detailed in Chapter 24.

The event to which the development of a national procurement system can be traced occurred at the Massachusetts General Hospital in 1967.[94] A liver transplant was performed at the Brigham Hospital only because physicians at the Massachusetts General Hospital obtained permission for organ donation from the family of a gunshot victim at the request of a surgeon at the Brigham Hospital who heard about the tragedy on the radio, and the liver was subsequently procured and transplanted at the Brigham Hospital. It then became evident to everybody involved that sharing of organs was crucial, and in 1968 the Massachusetts General Hospital and the Brigham Hospital established the Interhospital Organ Bank Incorporated.

With the demonstration in 1968 and early 1969 that kidneys could be successfully shared over long distance, the Southeastern Regional Organ Procurement Foundation (SEROPF) was established, the ultimate goal being to establish a national renal sharing network. SEROPF, which by 1971 had its own computer system, served 18 trans-plant centers in nine states. With continued addition of transplant centers, SEROPF was in 1975 incorporated into the Southeastern Organ Procurement Foundation (SEOPF), which by 1977 offered an online computer system for matching and sharing kidneys throughout the country. At the same time that this national sharing system was evolving, transplant programs were developing their own organ procurement organizations (OPOs) which early on were hospital based but during the 1980s developed independently of transplant programs and served several transplant centers in a city or state. In 1977,[36] SEOPF developed an online system for matching and sharing kidneys, and this sytem was named UNOS and was based at the UNOS Kidney Center. Since there were no rules for national sharing of organs, a kidney which could not be used locally was placed by accessing either UNOS or a computer generated list at the University of California at Los Angeles. To place nonrenal donor organs, a donor coordinator had to find a potential recipient on the UNOS list or access the Denny-Broznick-Starzl Twenty-Four Hour Alert System, which was based at the University of Pittsburgh Medical Center. Another computer system became available through the North American Transplant Coordinator Organization (NATCO) which was based at the University of Pittsburgh.

Clearly, a national matching and sharing system for all organs was essential, and this came into existence through the establishment of the national Organ Procurement and Transplantation Network (OPTN). OPTN was established in 1984 through the National Organ Transplant Act. In 1986, the administration of OPTN was assigned to UNOS whose central office is based in

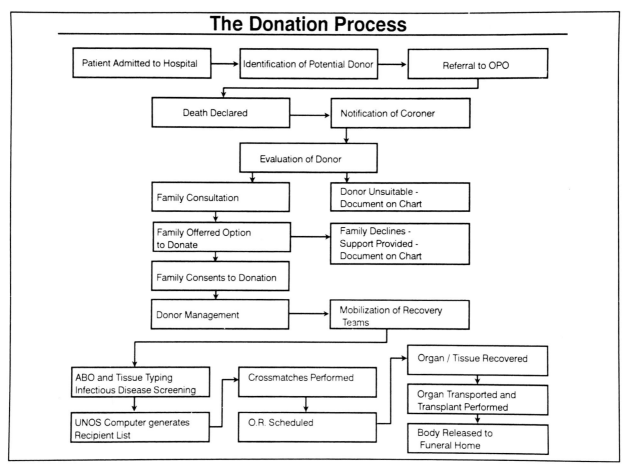

The Donation Process

Patient Admitted to Hospital → Identification of Potential Donor → Referral to OPO

Death Declared → Notification of Coroner

Evaluation of Donor

Family Consultation

Donor Unsuitable - Document on Chart

Family Offered Option to Donate → Family Declines - Support Provided - Document on Chart

Family Consents to Donation

Donor Management → Mobilization of Recovery Teams

ABO and Tissue Typing Infectious Disease Screening → Crossmatches Performed → Organ / Tissue Recovered

UNOS Computer generates Recipient List → O.R. Scheduled → Organ Transported and Transplant Performed

Body Released to Funeral Home

FIGURE **9–2.** The process of organ donation. (From Brennan DC, Lowell JA: Pretransplant preparation of the cadaver donor/ organ procurement. *In* Norman DJ, Suki WN [eds]: Primer on Transplantation. Philadelphia: American Society of Transplant Physicians, 1998.)

Richmond, Virginia. UNOS has a number of important functions (see also Chapter 24), all of which are under the direct oversight of the U. S. Department of Health and Human Services:

1. Provide the infrastructure for coordinating, matching, and sharing of organs throughout the country as well as to improve the effectiveness of this process.
2. Develop and maintain an allocation system which maximizes the access to suitable organs for all potential recipients (with priority to the sickest) and optimizes utilization of appropriate organs.
3. Maintain surveillance over the quality of organ transplantation through:
   a. Specifying the qualifications of transplant surgeons and physicians.
   b. Requiring institutions to have qualified surgeons or physicians, organ procurement agencies, and histocompatibility testing laboratories before listing patients for transplantation.
   c. Collecting information on organ donation and procurement to develop and determine optimal methods and public attitudes for maximal organ donation.
   d. Promoting optimal utilization of organs by monitoring the incidence and reasons for organ usage

and analyzing patient and donor factors which maximize long-term graft function.
4. Provide information to the government, patients, and the transplant community on all aspects of organ donation, procurement and transplantation.
5. Promote exchange of ideas on ethical and moral issues that impact on organ donation.

The UNOS organ center maintains a national computerized list of patients waiting for all transplants in the United States. The organ center adds recipients to the waiting list from each transplant center and deletes recipients or modifies recipient data as required. The national waiting list is accesssible at the Organ Center 24 hours a day by OPOs and a potential recipient list is generated by the UNOS computer for each organ offered for donation. Through an organ-specific algorithm which is determined by the National Organ Allocation Policy, a computer-generated ranked recipient list is immediately available to the OPO offering donor organs. It is then the OPO's responsibility to call recipient transplant centers in order of rank on the list until the organ has been accepted. The UNOS Organ Center will also provide assistance to the OPO for transportation of organs or tissue if required.

The arrangements for donor evaluation and organ procurement, matching, and distribution are the responsibility of the local OPO. Each OPO has its own set of procedures, but these generally follow the sequence outlined in Figure 9–2.[41]

CONSENT

For donation in most countries, including the United States, consent from the next of kin is mandatory. The donor may relieve his family of this decision by previously indicating his or her willingness to donate organs by endorsement of a driver's license or donor card. Obtaining consent from a family requires great sensitivity and compassion. The initial approach to the family regarding organ donation is usually made by the medical and nursing staff caring for the patient. A coordinator from an organ procurement agency is then involved in the process of obtaining consent if the family has not completely dismissed organ donation. The success of organ donation is enhanced by early involvement of organ procurement personnel. The laws which simplified the process of organ donation in the United States are embodied in the Uniform Anatomical Gift Act (UAGA). This law was drafted in 1968 and adopted by all states by 1971. This enactment resulted in the repealing of most of the earlier disconnected legislation relating to authorization of tissue and organ donation.[65] The UAGA contained a number of provisions, including the outlining of donor criteria, prioritizing family members authorized to donate the organs, and allowing an organ donor card or document such as a driver's license to record an individual's willingness to donate organs. To further increase the identification of potential organ donors, a federal "Required Request Law" came into effect in 1987, which mandated that hospitals were required to approach families of brain-dead patients to ask them to consider organ donation. Under this law, hospitals faced the possible loss of Medicare/Medicaid funding if a "Required Request" protocol was not established and used.[230]

In some countries (Denmark, Finland, France, Norway, Austria, Singapore, and others), a law of "presumed consent" is in place allowing the removal of organs unless a prior objection to organ donation has been registered. In the United States and a number of other countries, presumed consent laws have been considered but are not yet enacted because of the potential conflict this could cause between the transplant community and the public. However, in some states presumed consent laws are in place for the removal of corneas.

SPECIAL SITUATIONS

Because there are many more potential recipients than there are donor hearts available, management of potential organ donors to maximize utilization is of paramount importance. So too is the increasing interest in understanding cardiac dysfunction in brain death, optimizing donor heart function, and exploring the probability of using hearts from asystolic donors. One disquieting practice has been the use of organs from executed prisoners (see Box) in China, a practice which has been uniformly rejected in Western countries.

Use of Organs from Executed Prisoners

Based on information obtained by Amnesty International[52, 303] there appears to be use of organs and tissues from executed prisoners in China. Medical and paramedical personnel who have provided information for Amnesty International have indicated that kidneys, hearts, corneas, and skin are used. Amnesty International has documented[52] the process of obtaining organs from executed prisoners. The Deputy Head of the court's executive office is notified by the Head of the Intermediate People's Court of imposed death sentences and this official then informs the government department responsible for health. Members of this department then contact hospitals with transplant programs to inform them of the number of prisoners to be executed, the date of execution, and presumably details such as blood group and serology. It is known that condemned prisoners who have been selected for organ donation have blood samples taken without explanation. As far as Amnesty International is aware, "informed consent" is not usually obtained from the prisoner, although the Chinese Ambassador to the United Kingdom stated in 1994[4] that organs from executed prisoners are used "only if the prisoner has signed his agreement on a voluntary basis or with the consent of the prisoner's family." The prisoner is informed only a few hours before his execution that the death sentence appeal has been unsuccessful. The last night is usually spent shackled to a chair to prevent attempted suicide. On the day of execution the prisoner may be taken to a "mass sentencing rally" where the prisoner's name, crime, and punishment are publicly announced. From there, the prisoner is taken to the place of execution. The method of execution is a single gunshot to the head. Available information suggests that following the execution, the organs are removed from the body in a vehicle at the execution ground.

Amnesty International has also reported a similar practice in Taiwan.[86] In that country, consent for organ donation is obtained from the condemned prisoner.[140] The transplant coordinator is informed 12–24 hours prior to the execution. On the day of execution, an anesthesiologist administers a general anesthetic and intubates the prisoner. A law enforcement officer then delivers a shot through the brain stem, following which the circulation is stabilized and the prisoner ventilated. The pronouncement of brain death is made by an attorney, although other information[237] indicates that this may be made by the anesthesiologist or coroner.[140] The body is then taken to the hospital for organ removal.

Not surprisingly, this practice has received widespread condemnation from the international transplant community and Amnesty International.[237] The procurement of organs from executed prisoners in these countries is embodied in the broader issues of capital punishment, especially for nonviolent crimes and "political crimes," and a judicial system, for example, in China which does not ensure due legal process.

In an address[249] to the Society for Organ Sharing in 1991, Pope John Paul II said "Love, communion, solidarity and absolute respect for the dignity of the human person constitute the only legitimate context of organ transplantation."

DONOR HEART ALLOCATION

CONCEPTS AND CONTROVERSIES IN DONOR ALLOCATION

The stated goals of organ allocation embrace two basic concepts: *fairness* and *utility*. The concept of **fairness** is complex, but basically states that all patients with end-stage heart disease of equivalent severity (time-related probability of death) have an equal chance of obtaining a heart transplant. Unfortunately, quantifying this probability for various patient subsets is currently not possible. Another yardstick of "fairness" has been the duration of **waiting time,** which can readily be compared between patient subsets and institutions. It is, however, generally acknowledged that patients who are critically ill (and therefore more imminently at risk for death) should expect a shorter waiting time for transplantation than those who are less critically ill. The issue is further complicated by the lack of uniform criteria for listing among institutions and even, for that matter, criteria for initiating invasive therapy which justifies a more critical status. There is considerable difference of opinion among transplant experts as to the exact point in the natural progression of heart failure that patients should be listed for transplantation (see Chapter 6). Thus, waiting time as the only or even major criterion is a poor indicator of fairness.

An alternative definition of "fairness" would state that "a fair allocation system would give all patient subsets (from the sickest to the least sick) a similar probability of survival from the time of listing to the period following transplantation." This definition would take into account the chance of the patient dying while awaiting transplantation as well as the risk-adjusted probability of death after transplantation (which would adjust for the fact that some patient subsets will derive less benefit from the transplant procedure if they are too seriously ill before transplantation or have other identifiable risk factors). Thus, if one patient who was waiting at home in stable condition had an 85% chance (from the time of listing) of being alive a year after transplantation if he waited 2 years for a transplant while another critically ill patient had an 80% chance (from the time of listing) of being alive 1 year after transplantation if he only waited 30 days, the allocation of organs between these two patients would be considered "fair." If, however, patient subsets had a widely differing probability of surviving the waiting period and being alive 1 year after their heart transplant procedure (time 0 being the time of listing), then the allocation system would have failed to fulfill the requirements for "fairness."

The concept of **utility** must also be considered in judging any allocation algorithm. This concept embodies the notion that a precious resource like transplant organs should be used to maximally extend life. Inherent is the notion that transplantation should only be offered to patients for whom transplantation would significantly and importantly improve survival over other theraputic options (which would provide a nearly equivalent quality of life). Other therapeutic modalities are discussed in Chapter 5. Thus, if it were ascertained that other medical therapies or surgical therapies (that were not also a limited resource) offered equivalent or nearly equivalent quality and duration of life for an otherwise life-threatening condition, then such patients should not be offered heart transplantation. It must be remembered, however, that there are many conditions for which considerable controversy exists regarding the quality and duration of life which can be expected with transplantation versus alternative therapy. One example is hypoplastic left heart syndrome, in which years of further study and follow-up will be necessary in order to judge whether operations leading to the Fontan pathway can provide equivalent or nearly equivalent quality and duration of life compared to heart transplantation (see also Chapter 20). Other possibly controversial examples would include cardiomyopathy with moderate left ventricular dysfunction and malignant arrhythmias treated with an implantable cardioverter/defibrillater device, and patients with ischemic heart disease, severe left ventricular dysfunction, and marked left ventricular dilation treated with ventricular reduction and remodeling procedures and coronary revascularization (see Chapter 5).

At the other extreme, utility also refers to a level of expected survival following transplantation which would be considered an acceptable use of a scarce resource. Previous risk factor analyses (see Chapter 16) have identified patient subsets with a poor survival following transplantation, usually because of important subsystem dysfunction, disease, or damage. This concept, of course, is the basis behind the identification of relative and absolute contraindications to transplantation. For example, a patient with end-stage heart disease, critically ill in an intensive care unit with cachexia, important renal dysfunction, and the need for ventilator support might have an expected probability of 50% or less of surviving 1 year after cardiac transplantation, even if his or her waiting time was 1 day or 1 week. Allocation of a precious resource to this patient could and would be seriously questioned. These issues impact the decision-making process for recipient selection and are discussed in detail in Chapter 6.

Therefore, it is far too simple (and probably inappropriate) for an allocation system to be driven simply by the concept that "the organs should always go to the sickest patients first," since this would undoubtedly result in poor utilization of this precious resource (which would translate into unacceptably low survival rates following transplantation). Instead, alternative methods of support must be identified to "bridge" these patients to transplantation (e.g., with mechanical assist devices) that would allow for improved expected posttransplant survival. However, even the assessment of "utility" by duration of graft (and patient) survival after transplant is inadequate. It could be argued that allocation of a donor heart to a patient whose 1-year life expectancy was increased from 20% to 70% provided better "utilization" of the organ than allocating the heart to a patient whose 1-year life expectancy was increased from 70%

to 90%. This "increase in survival" provided by cardiac transplantation has been termed the **survival benefit margin.** In this example, the benefit ratio was 50% for the first patient and only 20% for the second patient, although the expected survival of the transplanted heart was 20% lower in the first patient. Although a minimum acceptable graft survival should be expected, the benefit margin to the patient would also be an important determinant of utility. Of course, incorporation of such a concept would require accurate patient specific predictions (see Chapter 3) of survival at a given time in the course of various disease states as well as after transplantation.

Another aspect of "utility" refers to the number of hearts which can and will actually be used for transplantation. Considerable controversy has surrounded the degree to which the local OPO or individual states should have priority for organs procured in that geographical area. On the one hand, "fairness" is potentially violated if a Status II patient (see next section) who has only waited 1 month in that geographical area receives that heart instead of a critically ill Status I patient one or two states away who has also been on the list for 1 month. In terms of "utility," however, there is an unproven but believable assertion that organized, enthusiastic, multidisciplinary, media-supported efforts at the state and local levels aimed at increasing organ donation would be undermined by a single national list or even large regional lists. Furthermore, the proven increased risk of very long ischemic times, which would be necessary for routine long-distance transport of hearts, would be detrimental to patient survival. The total number of hearts utilized would certainly decrease if "extended-criteria" hearts (with suspected increased risk of acute cardiac failure) were either routinely shipped long distance (with poorer outcome) or were utilized locally after great delays caused by multiple attempts to place the heart at distant centers.

These and other complex issues of "fairness" and "utility" underscore the undeniable fact that there is no "perfect" allocation system for a life-saving procedure which is dependent upon the awareness and generosity of donating families, has important constraints of safe ischemic times (the details of which are also dependent upon other variables related to age, cardiac reserves, and damage induced by brain death of the donor), and is applied in the setting of incomplete information about the precise probability of death while waiting of many patient and disease subsets. The most "appropriate," although not perfect, allocation system reflects a balance between these issues to gain the greatest fairness and utility of a precious resource. As new information becomes available in many of these areas, changes in the allocation system are necessary and mandatory in order to maintain the greatest fairness while also maximizing utility.

One area which has long been contested is **identical versus compatible blood group** matching in the allocation algorithm. Until recently, the current UNOS algorithm stated that for Status I patients (see next section), no priority was given for identical over compatible blood group matches. However, multiple analyses have shown that pediatric (see Chaper 20) and adult patients of blood group O have a much longer waiting time than other blood groups, often resulting in higher mortality while waiting, since a blood group O donor heart can go to any recipient but a blood group O recipient can only receive a blood group O heart. A revised UNOS allocation algorithm is described below.

ALLOCATION ALGORITHM

Each country with active transplant programs has evolved an organized system for allocating organs for transplantation. The general mechanism will be illustrated by a detailed discussion of the UNOS allocation system in the United States. The original heart allocation system developed in the 1980s was quite complicated and resulted in confusion and claims of unfairness, principally because of an inability to agree on definitions related to medical urgency.

Over the past 20 years, an evolution of UNOS policies for heart allocation has occurred, always striving for a balance between fairness to patients on the waiting list and maximal utilization of donor organs. The current UNOS allocation algorithm was implemented in January 1999.

1) The definition of a local area has been controversial and the current definition is the OPO unless an alternative local unit has been approved by UNOS. The principles that define an alternative local sharing arrangement are based on a single waiting list with distribution to recipients rather than transplant programs and appropriate monitoring to ensure equitable distribution.
2) Patients awaiting heart transplantation are classified according to medical urgency as determined by the UNOS status codes for medical urgency (see Box). The status codes for pediatric patients are discussed in Chapter 20.
3) The calculation of time that the patient has been waiting for a heart or heart–lung transplant commences with the date and time the patient is added to the UNOS Patient Waiting List with the exception of Status 1 patients, whose waiting time commences only while they are listed as Status 1.
4) Allocation for hearts within the United States follows the algorithm indicated in Tables 9–5 and 9–6.

DONOR HEART SELECTION

Donor selection and management should be considered in the context that most donors will be providing multiple organs for transplantation. There are three levels of screening of a potential donor.[16] Through the system of independent organ procurement agencies, which is operational in most countries of the world, the primary screening is performed by a coordinator at the agency, and the referral is initiated by the medical staff caring for the potential donor. The information required for

UNOS Status Codes for Medical Urgency

Status 1A. A patient listed as Status 1A is admitted to the listing transplant center hospital and has at least one of the following devices or therapies in place:

(a) Mechanical circulatory support for acute hemodynamic decompensation that includes at least one of the following:
  (i) left and/or right ventricular assist device implanted for 30 days or less;
  (ii) total artificial heart;
  (iii) intra-aortic balloon pump; or
  (iv) extracorporeal membrane oxygenator.

(b) Mechanical circulatory support for more than 30 days with objective medical evidence of significant device-related complications such as thromboembolism, device infection, mechanical failure, and/or life-threatening ventricular arrhythmias.

(c) Mechanical ventilation.

(d) Continuous infusion of a single high-dose intravenous inotrope (e.g., dobutamine ≥ 7.5 μg/kg/min, or milrinone ≥ 0.50 μg/kg/min), or multiple intravenous inotropes, in addition to continuous hemodynamic monitoring of left ventricular filling pressures; qualification for Status 1A under this criterion is valid for 7 days with a one-time 7-day renewal for each occurrence of a Status 1A listing for the same patient.

(e) A patient who does not meet the criteria specified in (a), (b), (c), or (d) may be listed as Status 1A if the patient is admitted to the listing transplant center hospital and has a life expectancy without a heart transplant of less than 7 days. Qualification for Status 1A under this criterion is valid for 7 days and must be recertified by an attending physician every 7 days to continue the Status 1A listing. A patient listed as Status 1A under this criterion shall be reviewed by the applicable UNOS Regional Review Board and the UNOS Thoracic Organ Transplantation Committee.

Status 1B. A patient listed as Status 1B has at least one of the following devices or therapies in place:
(a) left and/or right ventricular assist device implanted for more than 30 days; or
(b) continuous infusion of intravenous inotropes.

Status 2. A patient who does not meet the criteria for Status 1A or 1B is listed as Status 2.

Status 7. A patient listed as Status 7 is considered temporarily unsuitable to receive a thoracic organ transplant.

For all adult patients listed as Status 1A, a completed Heart Status 1A Justification Form must be received by the UNOS Organ Center within 24 hours of a patient's listing as Status 1A or continuance as Status 1A in accordance with the criteria in (d) or (e). If a completed Heart Status 1A Justification Form is not received by the UNOS Organ Center within 24 hours of a Status 1A listing, the patient shall be reassigned to his or her previous status.

TABLE 9–5	National Allocation Algorithm (United States)
Local	
1.	Status 1A patients
2.	Status 1B patients
3.	Status 2 patients
Zone A	
4.	Status 1A patients
5.	Status 1B patients
Zone B	
6.	Status 1A patients
7.	Status 1B patients
Zone A	
8.	Status 2 patients
Zone B	
9.	Status 2 patients
Zone C	
10.	Status 1A patients
11.	Status 1B patients
12.	Status 2 patients

Zones are determined by the distance from donor hospital to transplant hospital. Zone A $\leq$ 500 nautical miles, Zone B 500–1000 nautical miles, Zone C > 1000 nautical miles.

this initial screening includes donor age, gender, ABO blood type, confirmation of brain death, consent, donor weight, details of the cause of brain death, the clinical course of the potential donor, and serology for hepatitis B and C and human immunodeficiency virus (HIV). At this stage, the serologic data may not necessarily be available, and acceptance as a potential donor would be contingent upon negative serology (see Chapter 15 for further discussion of hepatitis B and C).

The secondary screening is performed by cardiac transplant cardiologists or surgeons based on information relayed from the organ procurement agency coordinators. The screening information together with an examination of the donor, electrocardiogram, chest x-ray, echocardiogram, and description of the hemodynamic state and inotropic requirements is used to determine the suitability of the heart for transplantation. At this stage, the transplant team may require a coronary arteriogram based on the age of the donor and/or the presence of risk factors for coronary artery disease. In addition, placement of a Swan-Ganz catheter may be

TABLE 9-6	ABO Typing for Heart Allocation (United States)

Within each heart status category, hearts will be allocated to patients according to the following ABO matching requirements:

- Blood type O donor hearts shall only be allocated to blood type O or blood type B patients
- Blood type A donor hearts shall only be allocated to blood type A or blood type AB patients
- Blood type B donor hearts shall only be allocated to blood type B or blood type AB patients
- Blood type AB donor hearts shall only be allocated to blood type AB patients
- If there is no patient available who meets these matching requirements, donor hearts shall be allocated to patients who have a blood type that is compatible with the donor's blood type

required if there are concerns about the performance of the heart.

The tertiary screening process is the inspection of the heart by the procuring cardiac surgeon. Prior to procurement the surgeon must ensure the veracity of the information that has been obtained in the primary and secondary screening levels.

Because of the shortage of donor hearts, transplant centers can no longer afford to adopt rigid exclusion criteria for donor hearts. Instead, it is imperative that a flexible approach be adopted to match donor hearts to recipients. In this matching process, donor variables such as age, presence of donor cardiac dysfunction, and projected ischemic time as well as recipient variables such as age and clinical condition should be considered.

DONOR AGE

For the primary screening process it is necessary for each center to specify an upper age limit for cardiac donors. Most centers have an upper age limit of 55 years although some centers have extended this to 65 years of age. A complete discussion of potentially adverse effects of older donor age on survival and allograft coronary artery disease is found in Chapters 16 and 17.

It is important then that donor age not be viewed in absolute terms, but be considered along with other important variables such as donor cardiac dysfunction, projected ischemic time, and recipient clinical condition. As the donor shortage increases, the need to use older hearts is increasing. From the UNOS scientific registry, 2.1% of heart donors were age 50 or greater in 1982, but by the end of 1994 the percentage had increased to 8.9%.[356] However, currently, older recipients continue to receive younger donor hearts (Fig. 9–3). Since intermediate term survival after adult heart transplantation is also decreased by older donor age, some matching of donor and recipient ages is potentially an important strategy to increase the availability and utilization of donor hearts.

CARDIAC FUNCTION

A donor history of **diabetes mellitus** with microvascular complications or poor diabetic control, longstanding systemic **hypertension,** and a long **smoking history** should alert the transplant team about possible damage to the donor heart. Events during and after brain death may also contribute to graft dysfunction, including prolonged hypotension (systolic blood pressure <60 mm Hg for > about 3 hours), prolonged high-dose inotropic support (dopamine or dobutamine >20 μg/kg/min),[16] or prolonged resuscitation after cardiopulmonary arrest (resuscitation for >30 minutes within 24 hours of cardiac procurement or multiple attempts at cardiopulmonary resuscitation).[16] Other adverse features of the donor heart would include severe left ventricular hypertrophy on either echocardiogram or electrocardiogram and an echocardiogram demonstrating either segmental wall motion abnormalities or global left ventricular dysfunction. The presence of protracted ventricular and supraventricular arrhythmias is also a marker for posttransplant graft dysfunction. Some of these concerns have been handed down from an earlier era in transplantation and have become part of conventional wisdom, but others have been more rigorously tested. It is important to match the donor heart to the clinical situation of the recipient, and for a critically ill recipient, relaxation of these criteria may be appropriate. Donor risk factors which influence posttransplant survival are discussed in Chapter 16.

The electrocardiogram will frequently show nonspecific ST-segment and T-wave changes in the donor, a phenomenon associated with brain death.[59, 92] However,

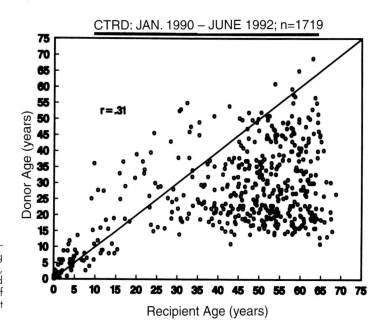

FIGURE **9-3.** Scattergram showing relationship between donor and recipient age at time of transplantation. (From Young JB, Naftel DC, Bourge RC, Kirklin JK, Clemson BS, Porter CB, Rodeheffer RJ, Kenzora JL: Matching the heart donor and heart transplant recipient. Clues for successful expansion of the donor pool: a multivariable multiinstitutional report. J Heart Lung Transplant 1994;13:353.)

these electrocardiographic changes normalize after the donor heart is implanted (Fig. 9–4).

Donor hemodynamic instability is very common and results from complex perturbations of afterload, preload, and myocardial contractility; therefore, proper assessment of cardiac function requires initial optimization of afterload and preload. Determining a rela-

tionship between donor cardiac function and posttransplant graft dysfunction has produced conflicting information. A study by Young and colleagues[356] from the CTRD in adult donors identified diffuse wall motion abnormalities as a risk fctor for death within 30 days of transplantation (see Chapter 16). However, other studies have also emphasized that significant wall motion ab-

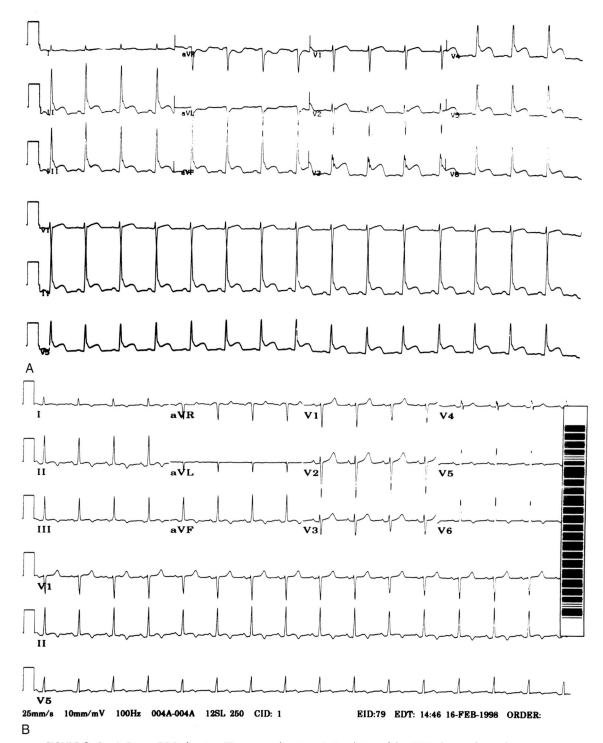

25mm/s   10mm/mV   100Hz   004A-004A   12SL 250   CID: 1   EID:79   EDT: 14:46 16-FEB-1998   ORDER:

B

FIGURE **9–4.** *A,* Donor ECG showing ST-segment elevation. *B,* Resolution of the ECG abnormality in the recipient.

normalities and/or an abnormal ejection fraction does not preclude satisfactory posttransplant graft function.[231]

High-dose inotropic support is often used not to augment myocardial contractility, but to overcome the hemodynamic consequences of a low systemic vascular resistance. It has been recommended[338] that donor hearts not be used if, following optimization of preload and afterload, the inotropic requirements are greater than 20 μg/kg/min of dopamine. The study of Young and colleagues[356] found, by multivariable analysis, that increased inotropic support was a risk factor for death within 30 days of transplantation, but actual differences in survival were small. Likely more important than the independent effect of the level of inotropic support is the interaction of this variable with other factors such as donor age and ischemic time, as discussed in Chapter 16. However, there is not general agreement about the level of inotropic support which indicates structural and functional damage sufficient to compromise posttransplant graft function and increase mortality.

The cornerstone of assessment of donor cardiac function is the transthoracic echocardiogram,[115] although transesophageal echocardiography[307] is also a useful means of screening potential cardiac donors, particularly when transthoracic echocardiography provides inadequate windows, a problem frequently occurring with patients on mechanical ventilation. The insertion of a Swan-Ganz catheter may occasionally be required when there are concerns about the adequacy of fluid resuscitation or there appears to be discordant information between the echocardiogram and clinical assessment. Yokoyama and colleagues[355] have used ventriculoarterial coupling (defined by the ratio of effective arterial elastance and end-systolic elastance), which is derived from a series of pressure–volume loops induced by a decreasing preload and measured by a microtipped manometer and conductance catheter (Millar catheter) inserted into the left ventricle through a pursestring suture in the ascending aorta. This method may be useful in determining contractile function independent of loading conditions, but the logistic difficulties in performing pressure–volume loops in a donor are likely to preclude its use.

The total serum creatine phosphokinase (CPK) and the CPK-MB isoenzyme are routinely measured, but elevations of the total CPK and CKMB in the presence of normal heart function echocardiographically are difficult to interpret and should not preclude use of the heart. Although there is no direct evidence to support this, a markedly elevated CKMB in a potential organ donor likely indicates significant myocardial necrosis, and there usually is other supporting evidence such as cardiac dysfunction on an echocardiogram. Use of such a heart would be inadvisable. Cardiac troponin I is a highly specific marker of myocardial necrosis and may be a useful method of detecting donor myocardial injury.[124] However, it may be overly sensitive, and a high level should not preclude use of the heart if good function is evident echocardiographically.

Perhaps the single most reliable guide to the suitability of a donor heart is the evaluation of an experienced transplant cardiac surgeon procuring the organ (see later section, Techniques of Heart Procurement).

DONOR–RECIPIENT MATCHING

Blood Group Compatibility

ABO blood group compatibility (either ABO-identical or ABO-nonidentical) is a prerequisite because of the substantial risk of hyperacute or accelerated acute rejection in the presence of ABO incompatibility. Rhesus factor blood group incompatibility is inconsequential (see Chapter 7).

Absence of Lymphocytotoxic Antibodies in the Recipient Serum

Absence of lymphocytotoxic antibodies in the recipient serum which react against donor antigens is a prerequisite. Absence of these antibodies can be established either by pretransplant screening against a panel of lymphocytes (panel reactive antibodies) or by a prospective crossmatch (see Chapter 7 for details).

Donor/Recipient Size Matching

A donor–recipient size mismatch in both adult and pediatric transplantation can occur in two directions— oversizing and undersizing. Size mismatch in pediatric patients is considered in Chapter 20. The potential for implanting an importantly oversized heart is greatest when the native heart disease does not result in cardiomegaly, particularly when there has been one or more previous cardiac operations resulting in rigidity of the mediastinum.[232] Severe **oversizing** can produce a serious restrictive physiology (and potentially nonfunction) if the donor heart cannot be accommodated by maneuvers such as incising the pericardium (which allows the donor heart to protrude into the left pleural space), resulting in inability to close the chest without hemodynamically important cardiac compression. Currently, reliable objective guidelines are not available to predict with certainty when the difference in donor-recipient heart size becomes dangerous, but use of a heart from a much larger male donor for a female with a restricted pericardial space secondary to multiple operations or a prior left ventricular assist device may be ill-advised.

Severe **undersizing** is important, not only because of concerns that the donor heart will be unable to support the circulation, but also because of potentially reduced reserves for the load imposed by primary graft dysfunction associated with reperfusion injury or hemodynamically significant rejection. The presence of recipient fixed or reactive pulmonary hypertension has also been regarded as a situation in which an undersized donor heart may be less able to withstand the hemodynamic load; although this remains unproven. Ultimately, there is a limit to how small a donor heart can be used in an individual patient, but defining that limit is not yet possible, partly because it is but one of many factors that determine posttransplant graft function. Determining the size of the donor heart prior to procurement in order to match the heart to an appropriate recipient is highly subjective. Furthermore, it is known from echocardiographic measurements that body weight does not correlate with adult heart size.[50] An athletic young adult male is likely to have a larger heart than an obese female. The chest x-ray of the donor may also prove useful in comparing donor heart size and recipient pericardial cavity size.

Several others have reported their experience with undersized donor hearts. Sethi and colleagues[291] implanted hearts from donors weighing 30–46% of the recipient's weight without adversely affecting survival. A similar finding was made by Costanzo and colleagues[62] using hearts from donors weighing 1–45% less than recipient weight, although it should be noted that the mean difference between donor and recipient weight was only 13.5%. In a study by Blackbourne and colleagues,[31] the survival of recipients receiving undersized donor hearts (donor to recipient body weight ratio of 0.6–0.8) was no different than other donor hearts for nonurgent (UNOS status II) recipients. For UNOS status I recipients, survival was inferior for recipients receiving undersized hearts, which tends to support the notion that undersized hearts have less functional margin than normal or oversized donor hearts when additional hemodynamic load is imposed. The study by Young and colleagues[356] from the CTRD demonstrated that implantation of a smaller female donor heart into a larger male recipient was a risk factor for death within the first 30 days of transplantation (see Chapter 16).

As a general rule, it would appear that using hearts from donors whose body weight is no greater that 30% below that of the intended recipient is safe. In our own experience, a normal heart from a male donor (with a normal physique) weighing 160 pounds or more is considered suitable for any larger recipient, irrespective of weight, without apparent adverse effects. Caution is advised (with a higher inherent risk) when transplanting small female donor hearts into larger male recipients and when using undersized donor hearts if the ischemic time is likely to be prolonged, the recipient is hemodynamically unstable, or the recipient has fixed or reactive pulmonary hypertension.

PROJECTED ISCHEMIC TIME

It remains controversial whether the length of ischemic time (out to at least 4 hours) increases the risk of acute cardiac failure (assuming appropriate methods of myocardial protection). Analyses of longer ischemic time as a risk factor are discussed in Chapter 16 and, for pediatric patients, in Chapter 20. In general, it seems prudent to plan the donor and recipient operations with the goal of keeping the donor ischemic time under 4 hours whenever possible. However, the decision to use a particular donor with a long projected ischemic time may not be an easy one. A long (e.g., >6 hours) ischemic time of a donor heart with excellent pretransplant function on minimal inotropic support is likely to be well tolerated with good graft function. On the other hand, a donor

heart on substantial inotropic support, perhaps with suboptimal function, is highly unlikely to tolerate an ischemic time of greater than 6 hours. Also factored into this decision is the recipient situation. In desperation to save a recipient with substantial hemodynamic instability, a donor receiving significant inotropic support with perhaps suboptimal cardiac function and a long ischemic time may be chosen. On the surface, matching a suboptimal donor to a suboptimal recipient may seem appropriate, but the chances of success are significantly less than if a more robust donor heart was used to provide a greater margin of safety. On the other hand, implanting a suboptimal donor heart with a long projected ischemic time into a perfectly stable recipient who would be more likely to withstand temporary graft dysfunction, may seem appropriate. However, is it fair to expose a stable recipient to anything less than the most optimal graft function? These examples illustrate the medical and philosophical decisions that need to be made by the transplant team, of which projected ischemic time is an integral component.

Although there has been a slight increase in the mean ischemic time over the last few years, most donor ischemic times are still well within the conventional 4 hours. A study by Rodeheffer and colleagues from the CTRD[267] demonstrated that from 1990–1994, the mean donor ischemic time in the participating institutions rose from 150 minutes to 166 minutes, and the proportion of donor hearts with ischemic times greater than 3 hours rose from 30% to 39%.

CONTRAINDICATIONS TO USE OF A DONOR HEART

The following list represents the current contraindications to the use of a donor heart. However, with the inexorable liberalization of donor criteria and changing recipient selection criteria, many contraindications once regarded as absolute are now relative.

1. Positive HIV serology—with the progressive improvement in the outlook of human immunodeficiency virus (HIV) positive individuals, it is conceivable that HIV-positive donors may in the future be implanted into HIV-positive recipients.
2. Positive hepatitis B or C serology—(some centers accept hepatitis C–positive hearts, especially for hepatitis C–positive recipients [see Chapters 6 and 15]). Interpretation of hepatitis B serologies is covered in Chapter 15.
3. Systemic bacterial infection which is not controlled by approprite systemic antibiotics.
4. Malignancies with the exception of primary brain tumors.
5. Cardiac contraindications:
   a. Intractable ventricular arrhythmias.
   b. Recurrent supraventricular arrhythmias.
   c. History of brain death due to cardiac arrest.
   d. The need for excessive inotropic support (the precise definiton of excessive support varies among transplant centers, but generally is more than

about 20 μg/kg/min of dopamine or similar doses of other adrenergic agents despite aggressive optimization of preload and afterload).

e. Cardiac contusion.

f. Severe wall motion abnormalities on echocardiogram and/or persistent severely depressed left ventricular ejection fraction (< about 0.40 despite optimization of preload, afterload, and inotropic support).

g. Preexisting heart disease (see next section).

h. Severe left ventricular hypertrophy on inspection of the heart.

i. Prolonged or repeated episodes of cardiopulmonary resuscitation.

j. Significant congenital cardiac anomalies.

SPECIAL SITUATIONS

Donor Hearts with Identifiable Preexisting Heart Disease

Donor hearts with functionally important anatomic defects are generally rejected for use in transplantation if a significant reduction in myocardial function or reserves has resulted from the defect and/or if prosthetic material or devices would be required for repair. Certain abnormalities (see below), however, may be consistent with successful transplantation.

Coronary Artery Disease

Unrecognized donor obstructive coronary artery disease can potentially result in early posttransplant myocardial ischemia or infarction with resultant hemodynamic instability or acute graft failure. In the long term, the presence of donor coronary artery disease would likely contribute to the early appearance of coronary vasculopathy.[62] The identification of obstructive coronary artery disease becomes increasingly important as transplant programs liberalize donor criteria and accept hearts from older donors. As the donor shortage intensifies, donor hearts with recognizable coronary artery disease may be increasingly utilized for recipients unlikely to survive long enough to receive an "ideal" donor heart or for older recipients. Coronary bypass surgery has been employed prior to implantation on donor hearts with coronary artery disease, either with recipient internal mammary artery[315] or recipient saphenous vein.[167] The use of donors with identifiable coronary artery disease matched to "suboptimal" recipients (patients that would not ordinarily meet criteria for cardiac transplantation or retransplantation) has given rise to the concept of "alternate list" cardiac transplantation.[167]

Coronary angiography is occasionally unobtainable in the donor hospital, and hence there is a need for other techniques to assess donor hearts for the presence and extent of coronary artery disease. Bench coronary angiography has been described and does have potential application. Robicsek and colleagues[266] performed bench angiography on human autopsy hearts by using direct coronary cannulation and cineangiography. Others have demonstrated the feasibility of bench angiography in sheep hearts.[172] The hearts are suspended vertically (if they lay flat the aortic valve became incompetent) and the angiogram is performed by injecting contrast directly into the aortic root and films are taken with a conventional portable x-ray machine. Although these studies produced angiograms of sufficient quality to determine the presence of coronary artery disease, reproducible clinical application in the setting of a donor hospital has not been verified.

Wolff-Parkinson-White Syndrome

The presence of preexcitation on the electrocardiogram of a donor does not necessarily preclude use of the heart. Direct surgical ablation of a left free wall bypass tract after excision of the heart from the donor and prior to implantation in the recipient has been successfully performed,[316] and in the more recent era a left lateral accessory pathway in a heart removed from a donor with recognizable Wolff-Parkinson-White syndrome was successfully ablated by radiofrequency ablation in the postoperative period.[278] Bypass tracts that manifested following cardiac transplantation have undergone successful radiofrequency ablation.[109, 121, 229]

Valvular Heart Disease

A bicuspid aortic valve may be detected on the echocardiogram of the donor heart, and although the natural history of a bicuspid valve in the transplanted heart is unknown, it likely is similar to that of the naturally occurring bicuspid aortic valve. The major concern is the risk of endocarditis; however, given the relatively low risk of endocarditis and the long natural history of progression to hemodynamically significant aortic valve disease, there is no compelling reason to exclude a donor heart with a bicuspid aortic valve. Aortic valve replacement has been successfully performed in a heart transplant recipient for progressive regurgitation of a bicuspid aortic valve.[147]

The same general considerations apply to the echocardiographic findings of mitral valve prolapse. Mitral valve prolapse is common and because of the favorable natural history of this lesion in the absence of important mitral regurgitation, use of such a donor heart should not be contraindicated. If mitral regurgitation is present, consideration can be given to "bench" mitral valve repair. This has been successfully employed in one patient at the University of Alabama at Birmingham (UAB).

Donor Hearts with Potential Toxicity

Cocaine

Recurrent cocaine abuse has important toxic effects on the heart which directly impacts its suitability for transplantation. The effects of cocaine on the heart include (1) cocaine-induced vasoconstriction, (2) coronary endothelial dysfunction, and (3) myocardial toxicity. Cocaine is an alpha$_1$-adrenergic agonist and as such has a potent coronary vasoconstrictor action.[147, 168, 270] The action is both direct and indirect (through release of norepinephrine by the sympathetic nervous system).[81] Cocaine results in deficiency of endothelium-derived relaxation factor (EDRF).[82] The resultant endothelial dysfunction represents an additional mechanism for vasoconstriction which, together with the known increased responsiveness of platelets to thromboxane in the presence of cocaine,[320] produces a substrate for vasoconstriction and thrombosis. Both experimental and clinical studies[21, 34, 103] demonstrate depression of myocardial contractility in response to cocaine.

The two most frequent cardiac abnormalities observed following cocaine abuse are ventricular hypertrophy and a cardiomyopathic process.[82] The ventricular hypertrophy most likely relates to repeated sympathetic stimulation and the cardiomyopathy to recurrent vasoconstriction and ischemia as well as the direct toxic effect of cocaine on the myocardium. Thus, the use of hearts from donors known to be abusing cocaine intravenously is contraindicated. However, the myocardial toxicity of nonintravenous use of cocaine has not been established,[106] and such donors can be considered for transplantation.

The policy at UAB and Cleveland Clinic has been to use hearts from donors with a history of nonintravenous cocaine abuse, provided that at the time of procurement there is normal left ventricular function with no evidence of left ventricular hypertrophy.

Alcohol Abuse

Ethanol has direct toxic effects on the heart. Experimental and clinical evidence suggests that these effects are due to alterations in energy stores, reducing the effectiveness of calcium uptake by the sarcoplasmic reticulum,[280, 284] reducing sodium-potassium adenosine triphosphatase (ATPase) activity,[264] altering ion transport function, and interfering with calcium-troponin binding, all of which attenuates myosin-actin interaction.[257, 280] Myofibril integrity may also be reduced secondary to decreased protein synthesis.[288] An experimental study by Takkenberg[312] showed significantly impaired posttransplant function in a model of hearts from alcohol-fed rats transplanted heterotopically into recipient rats, although this ventricular dysfunction was not evident before the donor heart was transplanted. This suggested that prolonged alcohol exposure produced a subclinical cardiomyopathic process that became evident after transplantation.

Transplantation of a donor heart from an alcoholic may unmask important biochemical abnormalities that manifest as either early graft failure or serious left ventricular dysfunction at the time of acute cardiac rejection. These findings are consistent with the known impairment of left ventricular function characterized by increased wall thickness and abnormal ventricular filling without necessarily a reduction in contractility in asymptomatic alcoholics.[11, 166, 300] The potentially profound biochemical effect of ethanol on the myocardium may importantly reduce posttransplantation cardiac function and recipient survival (Fig. 9–5).[105] At least two clinical studies have identified a history of alcohol abuse as an independent risk factor for death from early graft dysfunction or rejection–related dysfunction.[105, 139] This information suggests that the hearts of organ donors with a history of alcoholism should not be used for

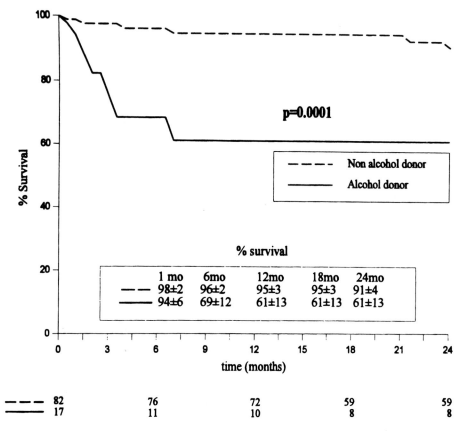

FIGURE **9–5.** Actuarial survival after heart transplantation stratified by donor alcohol usage. Note that most mortalities in the recipients of alcohol-using donors (solid line) occurred within 3 months after transplantation. A statistically significant difference was observed in survival between the two groups ($p = .0001$). All deaths were included in the analysis. Box insert shows the percentage of patients surviving at 1, 6, 12, 18, and 24 months. Numbers below figure indicate patients at risk during follow-up. (From Freimark D, Aleksic I, Trento A, Takkenberg JJ, Valenza M, Admon D, Blanche C, Queral CA, Azen CG, Czer LS: Hearts from donors with chronic alcohol use: a possible risk factor for death after heart transplantation. J Heart Lung Transplant 1996;15:150–159.)

cardiac transplantation. However, a history of intermittent (nonaddictive) alcohol consumption would not be considered a contraindication for donor use.

Carbon Monoxide Poisoning

The hypoxia which occurs from carbon monoxide (CO) poisoning results from a greater affinity (by a factor of 200) of CO compared with oxygen for the hemoglobin molecule, a leftward shift of the oxyhemoglobin dissociation curve resulting in reduced oxygen delivery to the tissues, and an impairment of mitochondrial cellular respiration because of the competition of CO with oxygen for cytochrome a_3.[119] The brain and heart are the organs most susceptible to the hypoxic injury. Myocardial injury due to CO poisoning is variable,[5, 322] but the usual cardiac lesions from acute exposure are focal myocardial necrosis, leukocyte infiltration, and punctate hemorrhages.

Myocardial injury in a potential donor with CO poisoning may be suggested by abnormal findings on the electrocardiogram, cardiac enzymes, and echocardiography. The electrocardiogram may show nonspecific ST-segment changes and T-wave inversion as well as atrial and ventricular premature beats. Elevation of cardiac enzymes suggests myocardial injury but could represent hypoxic injury to other organs.[5, 322] Acute CO exposure can result in echocardiographic findings such as abnormal left ventricular wall motion and papillary muscle dysfunction.[60]

The safety of using hearts from donors dying from CO poisoning has not been fully established, and available publications report variable success.[235] The risk of using such hearts can probably be minimized by restricting the use of hearts from CO poisonings to donors who have (1) normal donor electrocardiogram and echocardiogram, (2) minimal elevation of cardiac enzymes, (3) minimal inotropic requirements, (4) a relatively short ischemic time, (5) favorable donor to recipient weight ratio, and (6) a recipient with normal pulmonary vascular resistance.[297]

Cyanide Poisoning

The probability of a victim of lethal cyanide poisoning becoming an organ donor is extremely remote. Cyanide binds to the iron center of cytochrome oxidase preventing electron transfer from ferric iron to oxygen. The inability to use cellular oxygen results in anaerobic metabolism of glucose producing lactic acidosis. The central nervous system is particularly vulnerable to anoxic injury, and following ingestion of cyanide cerebral edema rapidly ensues.[323] There is a direct toxic effect of cyanide on the myocardium resulting in left ventricular dysfunction and conduction abnormalities. However, the cyanide-cytochrome oxidase complex will dissociate following removal of cyanide with rapid recovery of cellular respiration. Successful transplantation has been reported of a heart from a 19-year-old organ donor who ingested a lethal dose of cyanide.[17] It would appear that in the highly unusual circumstances of a victim of cyanide poisoning surviving to reach medical care and if

brain death ensues, the heart could be considered for transplantation, provided its function is normal.

The Domino Heart

The use of the excised heart from a heart–lung transplant recipient as a donor heart (so-called domino heart) for cardiac transplantation[351, 352] has the special advantage that the right ventricle may have hypertrophied in response to increased pulmonary vascular resistance due to lung disease. Consequently, these domino hearts may possibly better tolerate elevated pulmonary vascular resistance in the cardiac transplant recipient.[224] Most commonly, the diagnosis in the domino heart "donor" has been primary pulmonary hypertension,[224] but could also include Eisenmenger's syndrome secondary to an atrial septal defect or patent ductus arteriosus. Hearts with a ventricular septal defect could theoretically be utilized, but the integrity of the patch utilized for VSD closure could be threatened by future endomyocardial biopsies and it could be a potential site for endocarditis.

The assessment of the "donor" heart should include noninvasive studies of cardiac function and coronary angiography, if feasible, in males over the age of 40 years and females over the age of 45 years as well as donors with a family history of coronary artery disease or diabetes.[224] Hearts should not be used for the domino procedure if the "donor" had a history of recurrent cor pulmonale, the right ventricular cavity is markedly dilated (> about 6 cm by echocardiography), or if there is severe tricuspid or pulmonary incompetence, significant ventricular dysfunction, or coronary artery disease.[224]

The technique of excising a domino heart involves cannulation of the heart–lung transplant recipient close to the diaphragm on the inferior vena cava and cannulation high on the superior vena cava (near its junction with the innominate vein). The domino heart can then be excised with enough superior vena cava to ensure that the sinoatrial node is not injured and allow a bicaval implantation technique. Survival after the domino procedure has been similar to standard orthotopic cadaveric transplantation. The Papworth group reported 53 heart–lung transplant recipients who donated their native hearts in a domino procedure,[224] with domino graft survival equivalent to cadaver heart graft survival. However, since double lung transplantation is assuming a greater role for patients with end-stage lung disease without intrinsic cardiac disease, the technique of domino cardiac transplantation is currently rarely utilized.

Recycled Donor Hearts

A few case reports have documented the reuse of a donor heart in a second recipient following the perioperative or early postoperative development of brain death in the first recipient.[77, 195, 239] Given a shortage of donor hearts, this would seem to be an appropriate use of a donor heart, but it would seem prudent to only use hearts in this exceptional circumstance if the hemodynamics are optimal.

Non–Heart-Beating Donors

There are two situations in which the use of hearts from non–heart-beating donors (see Box) may be considered. First, patients may have a profound and irreversible neurological injury but have residual brain stem function which does not fulfill the legal brain death criteria and hence only become eligible for organ donation following death due to cardiac arrest following withdrawal of ventilatory support. In this setting, the family will have requested that the patient not be maintained on life-support systems if there is no chance for recovery, and they have consented to organ donation. Second, victims of penetrating blunt trauma may either arrive dead in the emergency room or die in the emergency room, at which time consent for organ donation will have been obtained. The usefulness of this source of organs has been demonstrated in renal transplantation

---

Non–Heart-Beating Donors

There is precedence to consider the use of non–heart-beating donors. Until the acceptance of brain death laws, donor death was determined by cessation of cardiac activity. Barnard[18] in his report of the first human-to-human heart transplant, described how the donor was certified dead when there was no electrocardiographic activity for 5 minutes following withdrawal of ventilation. At that time, the donor's chest was opened and the donor was placed on cardiopulmonary bypass and cooled. When 16°C was reached, perfusion was discontinued and the heart was excised and taken to the adjoining operating room for implantation. Contemporary transplant experience adds some credence to the notion of the use of non–heart-beating donors. The experience of Loma Linda with neonatal cardiac transplantation has demonstrated that hearts procured from donors dying of sudden infant death syndrome can have satisfactory function despite documented warm ischemic times of up to 40 minutes before resuscitation was attempted, followed by cardiopulmonary resuscitation of more than an hour before cardiac function was restored.[37] It is on this background that a number of investigators have attempted to resuscitate or "reanimate" animal hearts exposed to warm ischemia by modifying the conditions of reperfusion. Even with quite substantial myocardial insults (such as 60 minutes of warm ischemia following anoxic arrest,[311] or 15 minutes of warm ischemia following exsanguination),[145] return of cardiac function has been demonstrated. A variety of modifications to the reperfusion conditions have been used in these models including controlled reperfusion,[145] Roe's solution,[125] and blood cardioplegia.[145] These experimental data are not, of course, automatically transferable to the human situation, since there are considerable differences in the bioenergetics of the myocardium between humans and the variety of animals used in these experiments. Furthermore, the circumstances, time course, and concomitant injuries associated with the death of human victims of trauma that could result in a situation where they could be potential non–heart-beating donors is usually quite different from the protocols used in these animal experiments.

---

where the long-term outcome of donor kidneys from non–heart-beating donors was similar to that of heart-beating donor kidneys.[47, 79, 287, 345]

Anencephalic Donors

Anencephaly is a condition characterized by the lack of a cranial vault and cerebral hemispheres and usually malformation of the upper brain stem. The majority of anencephalic infants are stillborn, but those that survive do so for a matter of hours to days, although survival can be artificially maintained. Anencephalic donors have been viewed as a source of organs for transplantation,[46, 193, 241, 292, 321] but this issue has been contentious. Those that support the use of anencephalic infants as organ donors argue that from a biological standpoint, anencephaly is incompatible with "life," that without a forebrain there is no possibility of cognition, and the diagnosis using ultrasonography and magnetic resonance is certain.[118] From an ethical standpoint it is argued that an anencephalic infant has no "personhood," since the infant is "cognitively dead." Furthermore, it is argued that parents of anencephalics may derive some emotional benefit from the organs of their infant being used to help others.

On the other hand, there is also considerable argument against the use of anencephalic donors. From an ethical standpoint opponents are concerned that the use of anencephalic infants (who do not satisfy the strict criteria of brain death) as organ donors may be seen as the "slippery slope" toward the use of organs from other neurologically devastated but not brain dead individuals. Furthermore, the organs from anencephalic infants are often not suitable for transplantation. Currently, anencephalic infants are not used as organ donors, and resolution of these important ethical issues is unlikely to occur in the foreseeable future.

DONOR HEART MANAGEMENT

Following the declaration of brain death, the responsibility for donor management is usually transferred from the primary physician to the donor coordinator, although knowledgeable physician input is frequently important. Maintenance of donor stability requires meticulous care to achieve a balance of the somewhat competing therapies to maintain the different organs considered for transplantation. For example, to maintain hemodynamic stability despite adequate fluid resuscitation may require the use of alpha-adrenergic agents which would be discouraged by renal transplant physicians. Maintenance of a good urine output which is an important determinant of renal allograft function may require considerable volume replacement which is potentially deleterious to donor lungs because of the propensity to accumulate interstitial fluid.

Optimal management of the donor includes instrumentation with a urinary catheter, arterial line, and a central line for measuring central venous pressure. Along with continuous monitoring of the donor's hemodynamics, it is essential that the progress of resuscitation and organ viability be assessed by repeated measurements to assess acid base status, gas exchange, electrolytes, and hematocrit.

HEMODYNAMIC INSTABILITY

Profound circulatory changes may occur during the onset of brain death as a result of low systemic vascular resistance (due to loss of vasomotor control), hypovolemia (as a result of the fluid restriction associated with treatment of the brain injury prior to brain death and the presence of diabetes insipidus following brain death), and the direct cardiotoxic effect of the catecholamine storm. Although not always present, a sequence of hemodynamic perturbations is often observed with increasing intracranial pressure leading to brain death (Fig. 9–1). The initial intervention to stabilize the circulation is volume infusion. The usual recommendation is a liter of balance salt solution, the goal being a systolic pressure of no less than 100 mm Hg (mean arterial pressure of 60–80 mm Hg). To maintain stability and ensure urine output of at least 100 mL/hr (which is desired by the renal transplant team), Ringer's lactate (or other balanced salt solution with potassium supplementation) is infused at the rate of 100 mL/hr in addition to the volume of urine from the previous hour. With this volume of urine output it is important to frequently measure serum potassium and replete as necessary. To achieve hemodynamic stability, however, a central venous pressure of between 8 and 12 mm Hg may be required. If the lungs are to be usable for transplantation it is necessary to limit the central venous pressure (and pulmonary wedge pressure) to prevent pulmonary edema. Therefore, under these circumstances, the lowest venous pressure necessary to maintain a systolic blood pressure of 100 mm Hg or greater should be the goal; ideally, this should be 5 mm Hg or less. If after volume replacement the systolic pressure is not greater than 100 mm Hg, then inotropic support should be commenced and dopamine is the drug of first choice. If inotropic support beyond dopamine at about 10–15 μg/kg/min is required to maintain systolic pressure of 100 mm Hg or greater, dobutamine has been recommended,[211, 299] but frequently this drug results in further and unacceptable falls in systemic vascular resistance. The need for adrenergic agents in addition to dopamine including epinephrine and norepinephrine may be required, but this frequently reflects inadequate volume resuscitation or depressed contractility. If on initial evaluation the donor hemodynamics appear unacceptable (central venous pressure >15 mm Hg, inotropic support greater than dopamine 10 μg/kg/min or the equivalent, mean arterial blood pressure <60 mm Hg), insertion of a Swan-Ganz catheter may provide useful information regarding cardiac output and systemic vascular resistance. Occasionally, severe hypertension can develop during the catecholamine storm and this may also require treatment. However, use of blood pressure lowering agents such as nitroprusside or nitroglycerin should be used with extreme caution because of the potential for precipitating hemodynamic instability; therefore, it is usually preferable to tolerate hypertension as long as the systolic pressure is not greater than approximately 160 mm Hg. The infusion of a short-acting beta blocker such as esmolol is usually effective.

Since temperature-regulating ability is lost, it is important to maintain the temperature of the donor by using a warming blanket. If the hematocrit falls below 30%, a blood transfusion is advisable. Leukocyte filters should be used with all red blood cell and platelet transfusions to minimize the introduction of potentially sensitizing HLA antigens and cytomegalovirus (CMV) into the transplanted organs (see also Chapter 12).

PULMONARY DYSFUNCTION

If the lungs are being considered for transplantation, the ventilatory settings are a tidal volume of 10 mL/kg, a positive end-expiratory pressure (PEEP) of 5 cm H_2O to prevent atelectasis, and an FIO_2 to maintain a PO_2 of 90–100 mm Hg. Frequent tracheobronchial suctioning is necessary to keep the airways free of secretions. If the lungs are unsuitable for transplantation, ventilatory settings may need to be altered significantly to maintain oxygenation in the face of deteriorating lung function due, for example, to pulmonary edema.

ENDOCRINE DYSFUNCTION

Diabetes Insipidus

Diabetes insipidus is an almost inevitable consequence of brain death and results in excessive urine output. When the urine output becomes large, maintaining intravascular volume by fluid replacement may exacerbate substantial fluid shifts contributing to interstitial edema, particularly in vulnerable organs like the lungs. The urinary output of diabetes insipidus may be decreased by the use of vasopressin as a continuous low-dose infusion (20 units of aqueous vasopressin in 500 mL of 5% dextrose) at an initial starting dose of 0.8–1 units/hr and titrated to maintain a urine output of approximately 1–2 mL/kg/hr. Alternatively, desmopressin (desamino-cys-D-arginine-vasopressin) may be used, since it does not have the vasoconstrictor properties of aqueous vasopressin, and this is given in a dose of 0.5–2.0 μg intravenously every 8–12 hours. (For other uses of vasopressin, please see Chapter 12.)

Triiodothyronine (T_3)

The incidence and degree of T_3 insufficiency in brain dead organ donors remains controversial. Both tetraiodothyronine (T_4) and T_3 are synthesized in the thyroid gland by iodination of tyrosine. The formation of T_3, which contains three atoms of iodine, occurs largely peripherally through the deiodination of T_4. T_4 binds to serum proteins more tightly than does T_3, and it must be converted to T_3 in order to exert its biologic effects. T_3 readily enters peripheral tissues such as the myocardium, where it increases the synthesis and utilization of high-energy phosphates by stimulation of mitochondrial aerobic activity, thereby enhancing myosin ATPase activity. Alteration of peripheral thyroid hormone metabolism has been demonstrated in a variety of stress states including patients undergoing cardiopulmonary bypass.[40, 54, 137, 220, 238, 282] The mechanism may relate to a high endogenous catecholamine release which results in preferential conversion of thyroxine (T_4) to reverse triiodothyronine (rT_3), which is a nonactive metabolite of T_3 occurring through an alternative deiodination pathway.[35, 181] In this situation, T_4 levels are either low or normal and thyroid-stimulating hormone (TSH) levels are normal, a condition that has been termed the "sick euthyroid syndrome."[132] A similar reduction of free T_3 has been observed in brain death both experimentally[221] and in up to 85% of brain dead organ donors,[114, 185, 218, 251, 313] although this has not been a universal finding. Furthermore, this reduction in free T_3 is not necessarily associated with donor cardiac dysfunction.

In an experimental isolated porcine model, Walker and colleagues demonstrated that T_3 improves myocardial contractility by increasing intracellular calcium, a phenomenon potentiated by adrenergic stimulation.[328, 329] T_3 has been shown to significantly improve postischemic left ventricular function in an ischemic rabbit Langendorff preparation,[80] and following clinical cardiac surgery.[220] This notion is supported by a randomized trial of T_3 administration after reperfusion in patients undergoing coronary artery bypass surgery. Utilizing an initial T_3 bolus of 0.8 μg/kg following removal of aortic crossclamp, followed by a continuous infusion of 0.1 μg/kg/hr for 6 hours, the authors noted improvement in cardiac index, lower inotropic requirement, fewer ischemic events, and improved survival among patients receiving intravenous T_3.

Brain death is associated with profound changes in metabolic processes characterized by tissue hypoxia despite normal oxygen delivery systems likely resulting from impaired oxygen extraction[72] and impaired mitochondrial oxidative phosphorylation.[217, 219] Several experimental models have demonstrated improvement in myocardial function with the administration of T_3 following brain death,[223] but other studies have failed to corroborate these findings.[204] Although administration of T_3 to organ donors is often associated with improvement in cardiac function,[150] this has not been a universal finding.[260] Currently, we believe there is insufficient information to recommend its routine use, although T_3 administration may have a role in improving the function of donor hearts with initially depressed contractile function.[205]

COAGULOPATHY

There is frequently a prominent coagulopathy which may have an association with the amount of brain injury,[205] and this may be exacerbated by hypothermia. Administration of fresh frozen plasma and platelets, maintenance of normal body temperature, and maintaining the hematocrit at approximately 30% are the usual measures taken.

OTHER MEASURES

It is important to obtain regular (every 2–4 hours unless otherwise indicated) measurement of serum electrolytes including sodium, potassium, magnesium, calcium, and phosphate. Use of 0.9% saline for urinary replacement fluid should ensure a normal sodium. There may be significant urinary loss of potassium, which can be repleted by adding 20 mEq of potassium chloride to each liter of intravenous fluid administered. If further supplementation is required, an additional 20 mEq of potassium chloride can be given over 20 minutes in 100 mL of intravenous fluid. Magnesium depletion associated with a large urine output does not usually require correction in the organ donor, but if ventricular arrhythmias were to occur magnesium can be repleted by administering 1–2 g (8–16 mEq) of magnesium sulfate intravenously over 5 minutes as tolerated by the blood pressure. This bolus may then need to be followed by an ongoing infusion of 2 g of magnesium sulfate every hour for the next few hours, carefully monitoring serum magnesium levels to avoid hypermagnesemia. Hypocalcemia in the organ donor may need to be corrected as part of the process of improving a dysfunctional donor heart by administering 100 mg of elemental calcium over 10 minutes followed by a maintenance infusion of 0.3–2 mg/kg/hr. Calcium may be administered as calcium chloride (13.6 mEq [272 mg] elemental Calcium per 10-mL amp = 1 g $CaCl^2$), calcium gluconate (4.5 mEq [90 mg] elemental Calcium per 10-mL amp = 1 g $CaCl^2$), or calcium gluceptate (4.5 mEq [90 mg] elemental Calcium per 5-mL amp = 1 g $CaCl^2$).

Hypophosphatemia, which may be a contributing factor to impaired cardiac function, can be corrected by intravenous administration of 30 mmol of potassium phosphate per liter of 0.45% normal saline.[299]

An antibiotic is usually administered prior to procurement. The protocol used at UAB calls for cefazolin 1 g administered 4 hours prior to procurement. Additional antibiotic coverage may be dictated based on other cultural information, such as the sputum from potential lung donors.

DONOR HEART PRESERVATION

CARDIAC ENERGETICS

Energy Supply for Myocyte Function

In order to discuss the concepts and components of reproducible myocardial protection during the prolonged ischemia frequently necessary for cardiac transplantation, it is useful to review the biochemical basis of myocardial energetics. Myocardial energetics as related to heart failure is discussed in Chapter 4. Glucose, free fatty acids, triglyceride, glycogen, and certain amino

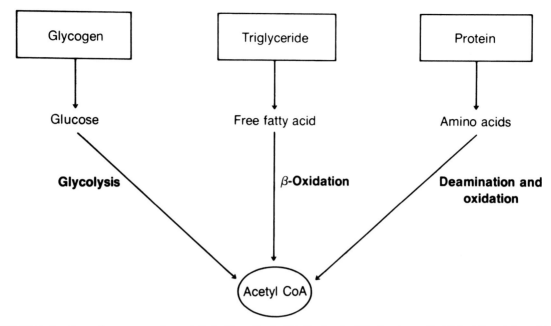

FIGURE **9–6.** General precursors of acetyl CoA. (From Devlin TM: Textbook of Biochemistry with Clinical Correlations. New York: John Wiley & Sons, 1982.)

acids can provide the metabolic fuel for ATP generation in the heart under various conditions. It has been estimated that over 50% of the heart's total oxidative metabolism is supplied by oxidation of fatty acids.[73] However, during anoxia, glucose and glycogen are the only available energy sources.

During **aerobic** glycolysis, the major energy-producing pathways converge at the generation of acetyl-CoA (Fig. 9–6).[73] In the metabolism of carbohydrates, glucose penetrates the plasma membrane by facilitated diffusion and is converted to pyruvate in the cytoplasm via the Embden-Meyerhof glycolytic pathway. Pyruvate is converted to the 2-carbon unit acetyl-CoA by the pyruvate dehydrogenase enzyme complex located exclusively in the mitochondria. The highly aerobic cardiac cells contain a high concentration of mitochondria in the cytoplasm, accounting for nearly half the cytoplasmic volume.[73] The rate-limiting enzyme in the glycolytic pathway is phosphofructokinase, which is stimulated by ATP in low concentrations and inhibited by high ATP concentrations, with further modification by citrate and adenosine monophosphate (AMP) (Fig. 9–7).[73] Hydrogen ions (low pH) also inhibit phosphofructokinase.

With the availability of oxygen, the primary fate of acetyl-CoA in cardiac cells is its complete oxidation in the tricarboxylic acid (or Krebs) cycle (Fig. 9–8),[73] the enzymes of which are primarily located in the mitochondria (Fig. 9–9).[73] The products of one cycle are two CO_2 plus one high-energy phosphate bond and four reducing equivalents per unit of acetyl-CoA (Fig. 9–10). The complete oxidation in the Krebs cycle of 1 mole of acetyl-CoA yields 11 moles of ATP. The net energy yield per mole of glucose metabolized aerobically via the Embden-Meyerhof pathway and the Krebs cycle is 38

moles of ATP (Fig. 9–11), which is the major energy currency of the body and of cardiac contraction. When hydrolyzed to adenosine diphosphate (ADP), it liberates energy directly to processes necessary to maintain cellular integrity and initiate cardiac contraction and relaxation. The Krebs cycle is critically dependent on a continuous supply of oxygen, ADP, and inorganic phosphorus (Pi), which, through oxidative phosphorylation and the election transport system, provide a continuous source of the oxidized form of nicotinamide adenine dinucleotide (NAD^+) and flavin adenine dinucleotide (FAD^+) to fuel the primary dehydrogenase reactions of the Krebs cycle.

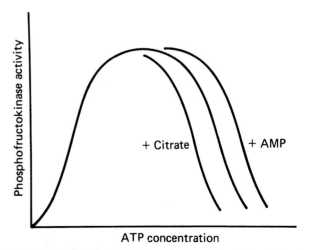

FIGURE **9–7.** Effect of ATP, citrate, and AMP on the activity of phosphofructokinase. (From Devlin TM: Textbook of Biochemistry with Clinical Correlations. New York: John Wiley & Sons, 1982.)

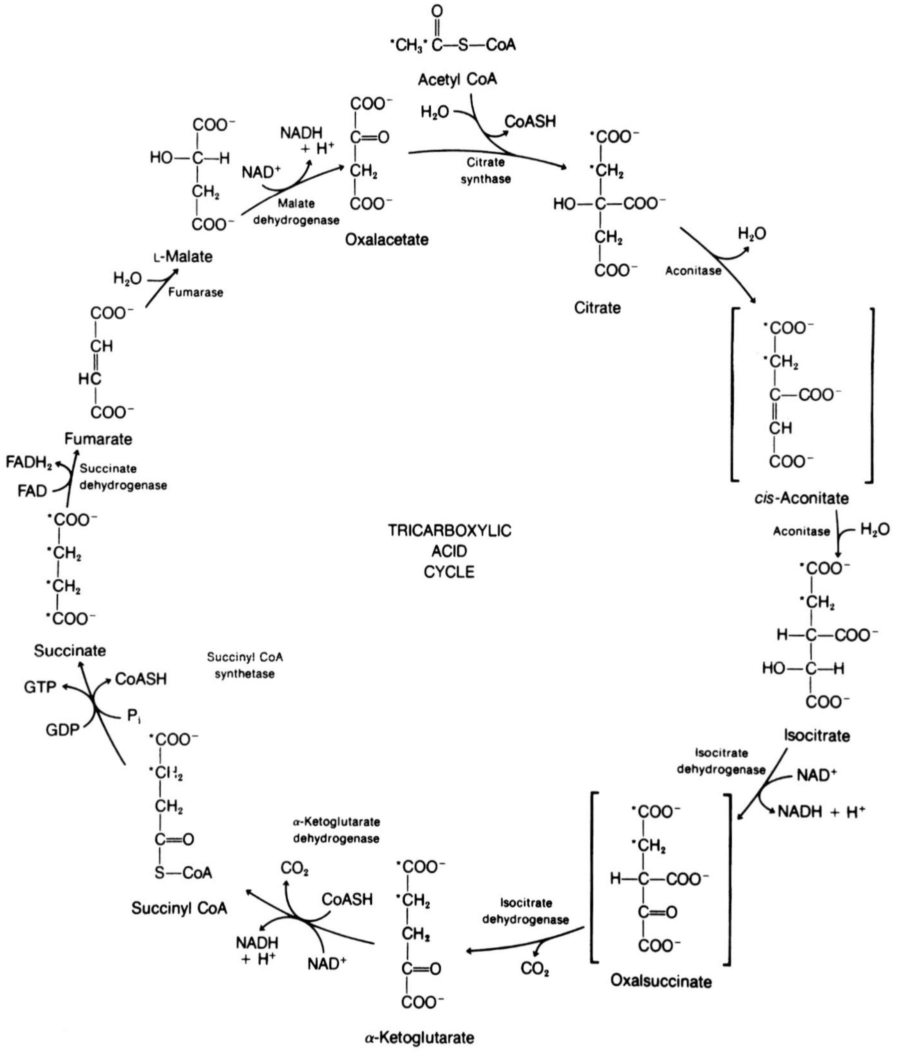

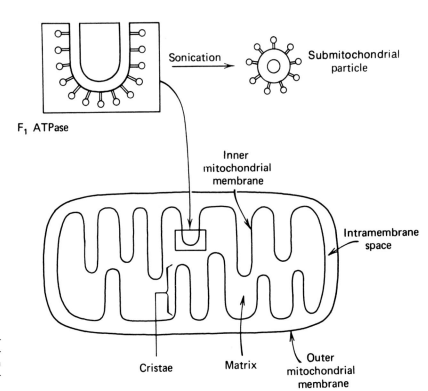

FIGURE **9-8.** The tricarboxylic acid cycle. (From Devlin TM: Textbook of Biochemistry with Clinical Correlations. New York: John Wiley & Sons, 1982.)

FIGURE **9-9.** Diagram of the various submitochondrial compartments. (From Devlin TM: Textbook of Biochemistry with Clinical Correlations. New York: John Wiley & Sons. © John Wiley & Sons, 1982, with permission.)

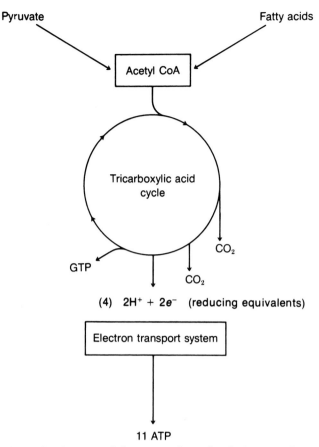

Pyruvate → Acetyl CoA ← Fatty acids

Tricarboxylic acid cycle

GTP

CO_2

CO_2

(4) $2H^+ + 2e^-$ (reducing equivalents)

Electron transport system

11 ATP

FIGURE **9-10.** General description of mitochondrial ATP synthesis. (From Devlin TM: Textbook of Biochemistry with Clinical Correlations. New York: John Wiley & Sons. © John Wiley & Sons, 1982, with permission.)

The rapid formation of the high-energy ATP molecules during oxidative phosphorylation is the main source of cellular energy and is tightly coupled with the mitochondrial electron transport system, a sequence of linked oxidation-reduction reactions in which electrons are transferred from a suitable electron donor (reductant) to a suitable electron acceptor (oxidant) (Fig. 9–12).[110] The major enzymes involved in the transfer of electrons in this system are associated with the inner mitochondrial membrane and convert reducing equivalents plus ADP and inorganic phosphorus to ATP in the presence of oxygen. These enzymes include NAD-linked dehydrogenases, flavin-linked dehydrogenases, iron-sulfur proteins, and cytochromes. The terminal electron acceptor in the sequence is oxygen ($1/2 O_2$) which receives two hydrogen ions and two electrons to form H_2O.

Maintenance of Cellular Integrity

As in all mammals, the integrity of the cardiac myocyte depends on a variety of transport systems which require active energy in order to maintain the intracellular ionic environment against a concentration gradient. A key active transport system is the Na-K pump, which utilizes the enzyme ATPase in the plasma membrane to catalyze the hydrolysis of ATP to ADP and inorganic phosphate (Fig. 9–13). In this process, three molecules of Na^+ are moved out of the cell and two molecules of K^+ moved in

for each molecule of ATP hydrolyzed. Conformational changes in the ATPase enzyme likely produce changes in the affinity constants for Na^+ and K^+. Maintenance of cellular integrity through the Na^+-K^+-ATPase pump utilizes a major (perhaps 50% or more) portion of the ATP synthesized by the cell.[73]

Anatomy of the Cardiac Cell

Each ventricular myocardial cell (myocyte) contains a complex array of organelles which facilitate the energy-driven contractile process. A detailed description of the contractile apparatus within the myocyte is found in Chapter 4. Mitochondria which provide ATP for contraction are densely positioned between myofibrils and occupy about 33% of the cell volume.[67] The sarcoplasmic reticulum (SR) takes up and releases calcium during the contraction process. It occupies about 2% of the cell volume. This contrasts with the neonate, in which the mitochondria occupy only about 16% of the cell volume and sarcoplasmic reticulum about 33%.[67]

The sarcolemma (outer cell membrane) is composed of a bimolecular phospholipid layer called the plas-

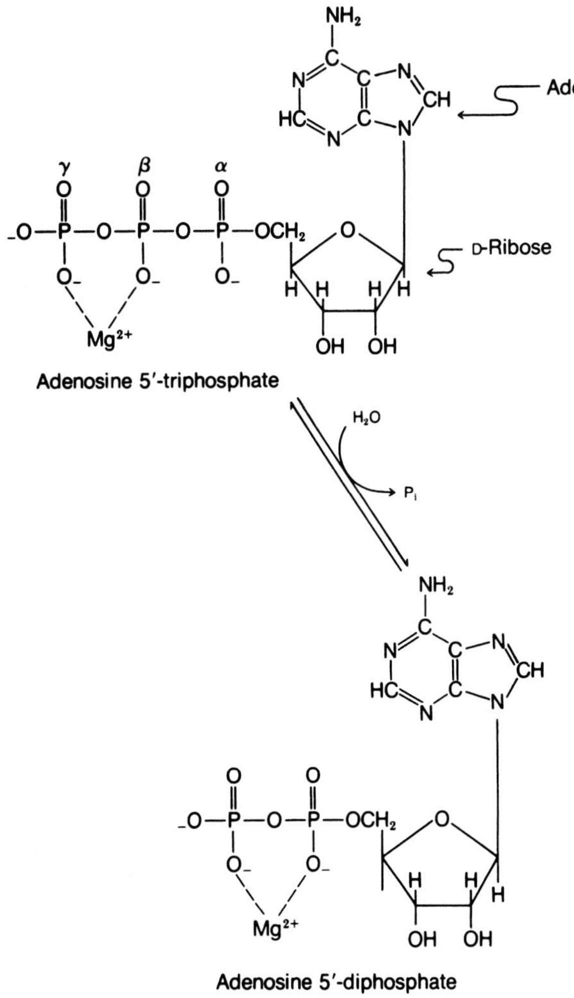

Adenine

D-Ribose

Adenosine 5'-triphosphate

H_2O

P_i

Adenosine 5'-diphosphate

FIGURE **9-11.** Structure of ATP and ADP. (From Devlin TM: Textbook of Biochemistry with Clinical Correlations. New York: John Wiley & Sons, 1982.)

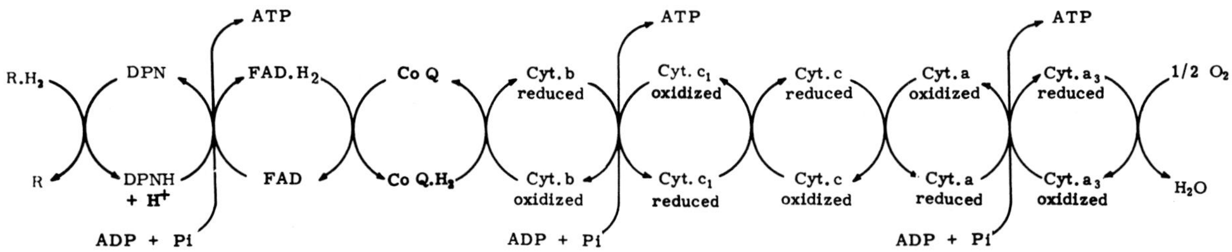

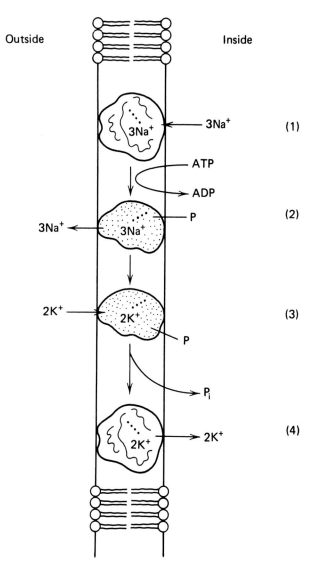

FIGURE **9–12.** Outline of respiratory chain oxidation. Pi, inorganic phosphate; FAD, flavoprotein; Co Q, coenzyme Q; R, proton donor. (From Ganong WF: Review of Medical Physiology. Los Altos, CA: Lange Medical Publishers, 1969, p 225.)

FIGURE **9–13.** A hypothetical model for the translocation of Na^+ and K^+ across the plasma membrane by the Na^+-K^+-ATPase. (1) Transporter in conformation 1 picks up Na^+. (2) Transporter in conformation 2 translocates and releases Na^+. (3) Transporter in conformation 2 picks up K^+. (4) Transporter in conformation 1 translocates and releases K^+. (From Devlin TM: Textbook of Biochemistry with Clinical Correlations. New York: John Wiley & Sons. © John Wiley & Sons, 1982, with permission.)

malemma, which contains the Na-K-ATPase pump and other passive and energy-dependent ion channels for maintenance of cell integrity and development of action potentials. The electrical signals are transmitted to the interior of the cell through the transverse tubules (T-tubules), which are contiguous with the sarcoplasmic reticulum. The sarcoplasm is the cytoplasm of the myocyte and provides a specialized milieu for changing the concentration of ionized calcium necessary for myofibril contraction.

The intracellular myofibrils account for about 50% of the cell volume and are composed of serially connected sarcomeres (Fig. 9–14).[26] Sarcomeres contain the contractile apparatus, made up of thicker filaments containing myosin molecules and thinner filaments of actin molecules. The regulatory proteins troponin and tropomyosin are linked to the thin filaments.

The Role of Calcium in Cardiac Contraction

In the absence of Ca^{2+} activation, tropomyosin and troponin I inhibit the actin-myosin interaction and prevent contraction. The onset of cardiac contraction depends on the presence of calcium, which enters the cell and is bound to the SR, T-system, mitochondria, sarcolemma, and nucleus.[87, 90] Depolarization of the cell membrane causes release of Ca^{2+} from the cisternae of the SR[87, 90, 310] into the cytoplasm. The Ca^{2+} binds to troponin C which inhibits troponin I and produces a conformational change in tropomyosin that allows the interaction between actin and myosin to initiate contraction (see Chapter 4 for further details). Relaxation is induced by the active uptake of Ca^{2+} into the SR, which, in the presence of ATP (an energy-requiring process) reaccumulates Ca^{2+} against a concentration gradient and the low calcium concentration results in its detachment from troponin, producing inhibition of actin-myosin interaction, and thus initiating relaxation.

A number of cellular mechanisms have been described which contribute to maintenance of the appropriate intramyocyte calcium concentration, as described in Chapter 4. The control of calcium concentration within the myocardium is of importance not only to cardiac contraction and relaxation, but also to events during and following ischemia, in which injury to energy-requiring control processes may lead to uncontrolled entry of calcium into the cell with resultant contracture and cell death.

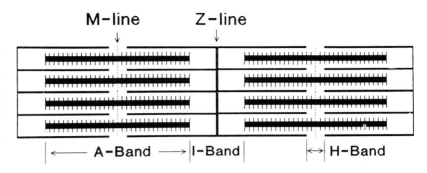

FIGURE **9-14.** The organization of the sarcomere. The thin filaments meet at the Z-lines and the center of the thick filaments is known as the M-line. The I-band (or isotropic band) is the area where there are only thin filaments and the A-band (or anisotropic band) is the length of the thick filaments. The region of the thick filament where there is no overlap with thin filaments is known as the H-band (or H-zone). (From Bers DM: Excitation-Contraction Coupling and Cardiac Contractile Force. Boston: Kluwer Academic Publishers, 1991, with permission.)

CONSEQUENCES OF ISCHEMIA

When the blood supply to the donor heart (or any other organ) is interrupted, intracellular biochemical changes rapidly occur in the cytosol and in the mitochondria which, if persistent, lead to cell injury or death.

Anaerobic Energy Production in the Heart

When the supply of oxygen is critically reduced at the cellular level, the mitochondrial electron transport–oxidative phosphorylation process is inhibited, resulting in rapidly declining levels of ATP and creatine phosphate. In the absence of sufficient cellular oxygen supply, anaerobic glycolysis is rapidly initiated. In this setting, pyruvate undergoes reduction and NADH is oxidized to form lactate and NAD^+ (1) instead of undergoing oxidative decarboxylation by the pyruvate dehydrogenase–multienzymes complex to form acetyl-CoA (2).

(1) Pyruvate + NADH

$$+ H^+ \xrightarrow{\text{lactate dehydrogenase}} \text{L-lactate} + NAD^+$$

(2) Pyruvate + NAD^+ + CoASH $\xrightarrow{\text{lactate dehydrogenase}}$ acetyl-CoA

$$+ CO_2 + NADH + H^+$$

The lactate which is produced by the cell is transported out of the cell in exchange for hydroxide ion (Fig. 9–15).[73] When localized tissues become ischemic and generate large amounts of lactate through anaerobic glycolysis, it is pumped out of the cells and produces lactic acidosis in the blood stream. The energy production is drastically reduced under these conditions, with the net production of only 2 moles of ATP for each mole of glucose (compared to 38 moles of ATP during complete oxidation of glucose). In the heart, this very limited production of ATP under normothermic ischemic conditions is not sufficient to meet the metabolic demands of the myocyte to maintain cellular integrity.

The Effect of Acidosis

In the presence of acute cardiac ischemia with cessation of blood flow, the extracellular lactate accumulates and impedes the extrusion of lactate and accompanying hydrogen ions from the cell. Lactate itself does not inhibit glycolysis. It is the build-up of intracellular hydrogen

ions (intracellular acidosis) which is directly toxic to the cell, inhibiting phosphofructokinase, the rate-limiting step of glycolysis. Although generation of lactate has traditionally been linked to the progressive intracellular acidosis of ischemia, the sources of proton (H^+) formation during ischemia are likely multifactorial and complex.[71] With reduction of ATP generation to critically low levels, the membrane transport pumps (which maintain the normal intracellular ion concentrations) are paralyzed. Na^+ and H_2O enter the cell along concentration and osmotic gradients and cellular swelling occurs, particularly in endothelial cells. The translocation of H_2O from the intravascular space into the endothelial cells increases the viscosity of the intravascular space. The resultant changes in blood properties combined with the decreased lumen diameter secondary to endothelial cell swelling may produce capillary lumen obstruction and decreased flow during reperfusion. In its severe form, extensive capillary occlusion may produce the **"no reflow phenomenon,"** with inability to reper-

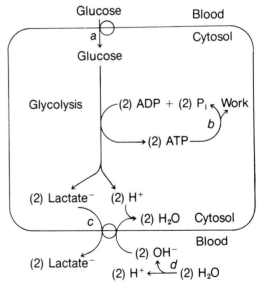

FIGURE **9-15.** Fate of lactate formed by glycolysis. Unless lactate is released from the cell, the intracellular pH is decreased as a consequence of the accumulation of intracellular lactic acid. The low pH decreases phosphofructokinase activity so that further lactic acid production by glycolysis is shut off. a, Glucose transport into the cell. b, All work peformances which convert ATP back to ADP and P_i. c, Lactate-hydroxide ion antiport. d, Ionization of water in the blood to give hydroxide ions for exchange with lactate. (From Devlin TM: Textbook of Biochemistry with Clinical Correlations. New York: John Wiley & Sons, 1982.)

fuse areas of ischemic myocardium. Mitochondria also begin to swell and accumulate calcium, which impairs mitochondrial function. As intracellular acidosis progresses, lysomal membranes are damaged, with release of hydrolytic proteases. Intracellular acidosis inhibits the binding of transitional metals such as iron to their carrier proteins (transferrin and ferritin) and increases free intracellular iron, an important catalyst for production of free radicals. Lipases, phosphatases, and glucosidase are released, and the end result of these processes, if uncontrolled, is autolysis of cell components and cell death.

Summary of Potential Damage Prior to Reperfusion of the Heart at Transplantation

The hostile environment of the donor contributes to the myocyte damage which can occur during initial harvesting, transport of the heart, and implantation unless special interventions occur which retard progressive tissue acidosis, critical depletion of ATP, membrane damage, and release of hydrolytic enzymes. This has all occurred before the massive release of free radicals and the inflammatory response which can occur during early reperfusion. Thus, ischemic injury may induce irreversible damage to the myocyte as well as reversible injury which renders the myocyte susceptible to the additional damaging effects of reperfusion.

REPERFUSION INJURY

The reintroduction of blood flow after the period of prolonged ischemia during transport and implantation provides oxygen and substrate necessary for the return of oxidative metabolism, and rewarming increases the metabolic rate toward normal. However, these life-sustaining components also have the potential to induce further damage to cells which were reversibly injured during the ischemic period. Ischemic injury followed by reperfusion is a potent stimulus for a localized inflammatory response, the basic components of which are discussed below.

Free Radical Injury

During the initial phase of myocardial reperfusion with oxygenated blood after the period of prolonged ischemia, potentially toxic oxygen species called **oxygen-derived free radicals** are generated which can induce direct myocardial injury. Free radicals are neutral molecular species which contain one or more unpaired electrons. They are unstable, exist mainly as short-lived intermediates, and are particularly reactive against electron-rich double bonds. There are numerous sources of intracellular free radicals, including endoplasmic reticulum, nuclear membrane and mitochondrial electron transport systems, plasma membranes, and soluble enzymes.[55] The knowledge base about these extremely labile molecules has been enhanced by the technology of electron spin resonance spectroscopy.[15, 111, 164, 357, 358]

Under physiologic conditions, about 5% of available oxygen is diverted toward a "univalent reduction pathway,"[200] in which oxygen gains electrons in a sequential fashion, leading to the formation of free radicals. The acceptance of the first electron generates the **superoxide anion** ($O_2^{\cdot-}$):

$$O_2 \xrightarrow{e^-} O_2^{\cdot-}$$

The gain of a second electron generates hydrogen peroxide (H_2O_2).

$$O_2^{\cdot-} \xrightarrow{e^- + 2H^+} H_2O_2$$

The gain of a third electron generates the **hydroxyl radical** ($^{\cdot}OH$)

The hydroxyl radical ($^{\cdot}OH$) can be generated by the reaction of superoxide anion ($O_2^{\cdot-}$) and hydrogen peroxide (H_2O_2): $O_2^{\cdot-} + H_2O_2 \xrightarrow{Fe} O_2 + {^{\cdot}OH} + {^{\cdot}OH}$. This reaction is known as the Haber-Weiss reaction and requires a *transitional metal* catalyst, usually iron.[112, 126] This reaction may play an important role in reperfusion injury with increased availability of free iron.[143] Transitional metals also catalyze the breakdown of lipid peroxides into unstable and damaging intermediates.[200]

These free radicals are generated in limited amounts under normal aerobic conditions and their potentially toxic effects are rapidly neutralized by intracellular enzymatic free radical scavengers which act as the natural antioxidant defense (see Box). Under conditions of isch-

Natural Antioxidant Defense

Under normal physiologic conditions, free radicals generated during cell metabolism are rapidly scavenged by the natural free radical defense system, which acts against the toxic intermediates formed by the univalent reduction of oxygen molecules.[107] The first line of defense is *cytochrome oxidase*, which reduces molecular oxygen to water without producing reactive oxygen radicals. The second line of defense is *superoxide dismutases*, which catalyze the formation of hydrogen peroxide from superoxide anions.[107] The third line of antioxidant defense includes *catalase* and *glutathione peroxidase*, which eliminate hydrogen peroxide. Catalase catalyzes the conversion of H_2O_2 to oxygen and water, but catalase concentration in the myocardium is much lower than gluthathione peroxidase,[96, 153] which catalyzes the reduction of H_2O_2 to water by oxidizing glutathione to glutathione disulfide dinucleotide phosphate.[55] *Reduced glutathione* (GSH) is thus a critical part of the native defense against oxidant injury, acting as a substrate for glutathione peroxidase, which reduces H_2O_2 to water (and avoids formation of OH radicals). GSH also is a direct scavenger of free radicals through trapping of unpaired electrons. GSH stores are also important in maintaining protein sulfhydryl groups in a reduced state.[95, 277] Ischemia leads to a critical reduction in GSH stores, which in turn limits the activity of glutathione peroxidase, and the depleted sulfhydryl groups of certain proteins makes them more susceptible to enzymatic hydrolysis and loss of function.[144, 154] A fourth layer of defense is biological antioxidants such as vitamins E and C, which function to maintain tocopherol in a reduced active form for neutralization of free radicals.[104, 107]

emia/reperfusion, however, their quantities may increase in the presence of reduced availability of natural scavengers, setting the stage for free radical injury.

These inadequately controlled free radicals are typically cytotoxic by attacking the bilipid layer of cell membranes (Fig. 9–16) through reactions with unsaturated fatty acid side chains to form lipid peroxides, which can decompose in the presence of transition metals such as iron to form unstable (and toxic) peroxy radicals. **Malondialdehyde**, a by-product of lipid peroxidation, can initiate damaging cross-linking reactions in plasma membrane proteins. Free radicals also react with and damage membrane proteins by oxidation of amino acids, oxidation of sulfhydryl groups, and polypeptide chain scission.[317] Amino acids which have sulfhydryl groups such as tryptophan, tyrosine, phenylalanine, histidine, methionine, and cystine are particularly susceptible to free radical damage.[104]

The hydroxyl radical is particularly reactive and destructive, promoting marked cellular swelling, mitochondrial disruption, breaks within the sarcolemmal membrane,[43, 256, 340] and damage to membrane transport systems, cytochrome enzymes, and nucleic acids. The hydroxyl radical is especially dangerous if produced in excessive quantities, since there is no effective natural scavenging system for this radical.

The role of the **xanthine oxidase** system in human myocardial reperfusion injury is controversial, since studies have not identified appreciable quantities of the enzyme in human myocardium.[212] In the presence of O_2, xanthine oxidase catalyzes the conversion of hypoxanthine (a breakdown product of ATP during ischemia) to xanthine, which is then converted to superoxide anions + uric acid.

Although free radicals are generated during ischemia (particularly through the mitochondrial electron transport system and the arachidonic acid pathway),[127, 258] their production is especially pronounced during reperfusion, with the respiratory burst initiated by the sudden increase in oxygen tension[112] and by free radical genera-

tion and release by activated neutrophils (see below). The potential for cellular damage is increased by the relative mismatch between free radical generation and availability of natural scavengers such as reduced glutathione, superoxide dismutase, catalase, and peroxidase, which are depleted during ischemia.[95, 131, 153, 194, 277]

Quantitative assessment of the role of oxygen radicals in ischemic/reperfusion injury is confounded by the inability to directly measure free radical injury. Since the major site of free radical injury is the lipid component of cell membranes, the measurement of lipid peroxidation products is often used to approximate free radical injury. **Malondialdehyde** (an end product of the cyclooxygenase pathway of arachidonic acid metabolism) is often used as an index of lipid peroxidation, but it may lack specificity.[104, 154, 336] The measurement of **conjugated dienes** (a stabilized form of lipid radicals which have undergone molecular rearrangement) is probably more reliable,[268] but the assay is complex.

Calcium Overload

During the initial myocardial reperfusion with blood following a period of prolonged ischemia, damaged myocytes have reduced energy stores available for maintaining membrane integrity and proper function of the sarcoplasmic reticulum. The mechanisms necessary for maintaining appropriate intracellular calcium concentrations (Fig. 9–17) may be inactivated as a consequence.[26] Calcium in the reperfusion blood may rapidly enter the cell across "injured" membranes and activate the contractile apparatus. If the injured sarcoplasmic reticulum is unable to properly sequester the cytosolic calcium, potentially fatal myocyte contracture may occur.

Complement Activation

Complement plays a central role in the inflammatory response to infection and injury through a series of reac-

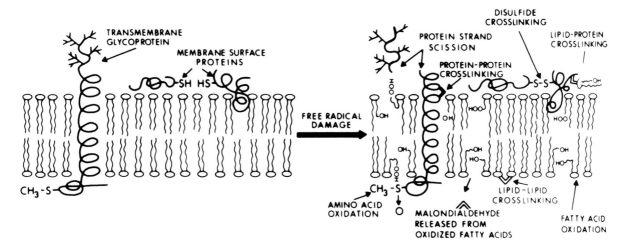

FIGURE **9–16.** Potential sites of free radical damage to plasma membranes. Free radicals can initiate lipid peroxidation, which produces short chain fatty acyl derivatives and the by-product malondialdehyde. Reactions with malondialdehyde can mediate a variety of cross-linking reactions. Free radicals can also catalyze amino acid oxidation, protein-protein cross-linking, and protein strand scission. (From Freeman BA, Crapo JD: Biology of disease: free radicals and tissue injury. Lab Invest 1982;47:412–426, with permission.)

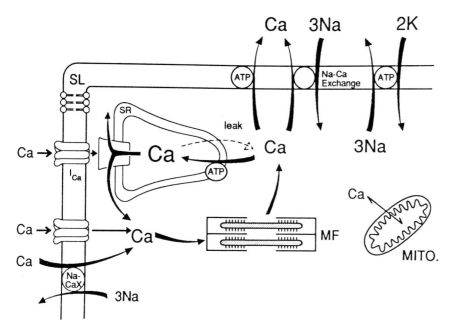

FIGURE **9–17.** General scheme of calcium (Ca) cycle in a cardiac myocyte. Ca can enter via Ca channels and Na/Ca exchange. Ca current may also control the sarcoplasmic reticulum (SR) Ca release. Ca is removed from the myofilaments (MF) and cytoplasm by the SR Ca-ATPase pump and the sarcolemmal Ca-ATPase pump and Na/Ca exchange. SL, sarcolemma; Mito, mitochondria. (From Bers DM: Excitation-Contraction Coupling and Cardiac Contractile Force. Boston: Kluwer Academic Publishers, 1991, with permission.)

tions called the **humoral amplification system** consisting of the coagulation, fibrinolytic, bradykinin-kallikrein, and complement cascades. The complement system consists of a group of circulating glycoproteins whose immunologic function is described in Chapter 2. Activation of the complement cascade results in the elaboration of the potent anaphylatoxins C3a and C5a,[142] which act as inflammatory mediators by increasing vascular permeability, inducing vascular smooth muscle contraction, mediating leukocyte chemotaxis, and promoting leukocyte adhesion and activation.[120, 122] Complement is activated through either the classical or the alternative pathways (see also description in Chapter 2). The alternative pathway of complement is also activated by cardiopulmonary bypass (Fig. 9–18) with resultant activation of the anaphylatoxins C3a and C5a.[51] C5a is a potent neutrophil chemoattractant and elaboration of C3bi from the damaged endothelial cell surface produces CD11b/CD18-dependent neutrophil adhesion.[186] Neutrophils further activate complement through the action of protease[242] and oxygen free radicals[294] released from activated neutrophils. Complement is also activated by myocardial protease elaborated from disrupted myocytes[136, 148] and by the interaction between C1 and damaged mitochondrial membranes.[275] Complement-derived products may also induce left ventricular dysfunction by mechanisms independent of neutrophil activation.[69]

Neutrophil Activation

Neutrophils entering the vasculature of the heart during reperfusion are a critical component of the reperfusion injury. Leukocyte chemotaxis following myocardial ischemia is facilitated by at least two mediators: complement activation and products of the arachidonic acid cascade.[317]

The initial "rolling" of neutrophils along the endothelium is mediated by the **selectin** adhesion molecules,

including E-selectin, L-selectin, and P-selectin.[27, 129] A detailed discussion of selectins as they relate to the immunology of allograft rejection is found in Chapter 2. E-selectin is expressed on endothelial cells following stimulation by inflammatory cytokines such as tumor necrosis factor (TNF).[28] L-selectin is a leukocyte surface molecule which is rapidly shed after neutrophil activation.[163] P-selectin is stored in platelets and also expressed on endothelial cell surfaces after exposure to various inflammatory mediators.[177, 240] P-selectin may be particularly important during reperfusion because it may be the most rapidly available adhesion molecule, in that it is stored in cytoplasmic vacuoles (Weibel-Palade bodies)

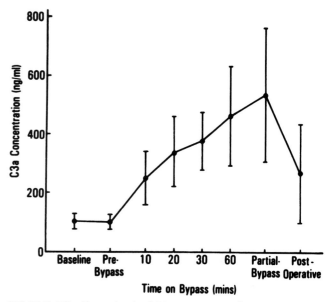

FIGURE **9–18.** Plasma levels of C3a in patients undergoing cardiopulmonary bypass. (From Chenoweth DE, Cooper SW, Hugli TE, Stewart RW, Blackstone EH, Kirklin JW: Complement activation during cardiopulmonary bypass. Evidence for generation of C3a and C5a anaphylatoxins. N Engl J Med 1981;304:497–503.)

and can rapidly reach the luminal surface for activation by exocytosis.[326] **C5a** is a potent agonist for P-selectin endothelial surface expression and may play a pivotal role in rapid neutrophil recruitment. Neutrophils express beta-2 **integrins,** which are surface glycoproteins which contain a common beta-2 chain and one of three separate alpha chains (CD11a, CD11b, or CD11c)[7] (see also Chapter 2 for further discussion of integrins). Neutrophil activation produces transient up-regulation of CD11b/CD18 on the neutrophil surface. Integrins bind to the endothelial intracellular adhesion molecule-1 (ICAM-1), which is the principal ligand for neutrophil CD11b/CD18. This binding process between neutrophil and endothelial cell is necessary for neutrophil attachment to the endothelium and subsequent diapedesis (Fig. 9–19).[2, 3, 85, 191, 301] Neutrophil accumulation along the endothelial surfaces may also plug small capillaries and contribute to the no-reflow phenomenon.[83, 84]

As activated neutrophils undergo rolling, adhesion, and diapedesis in the coronary microvasculature, a variety of mechanisms normally employed by the neutrophil in host defense can potentiate cardiac damage (Fig. 9–20). The burst of respiratory activity following activation and diapedesis stimulates the surface-bound NADPH-ase system, which stimulates the production of free radical superoxide anions with subsequent production of H_2O_2 and hydroxyl radicals,[14, 334] which themselves further activate complement and promote leukocyte chemotaxis in addition to their direct cellular toxic effects.[330] The exocytosed granules release proteolytic enzymes into the extracellular space (Fig. 9–21).[14, 129, 133] Elastase is a particularly potent protease which can hydrolyze numerous extracellular proteins.[148, 183] Myeloperoxidase released from the azurophil granules catalyzes the formation of hypochlorous acid from hydrogen peroxide and chloride. Hypochlorous acid's reactivity with primary amines and ammonia produces the major neutrophil oxygen free radical (OFR)-induced toxcity.[14, 334] Activated neutrophils also release lactoferrin (a protein which stores iron) making "free" ion (through a reaction with superoxide anion)[91] available to catalyze the formation of hydroxyl radicals. Neutrophil-induced OFRs also induce vascular contraction and coronary endothelial dysfunction by inactivation of endothelial nitric oxide.[123, 279]

Activated neutrophils also release inflammatory mediators via the **arachidonic acid** pathways. Neutrophil activation results in stimulation of phospholipase A_2, which promotes the generation of lipoxygenase products such as leukotriene B_4 and platelet-activating factor (PAF), which in turn stimulate neutrophil chemotaxis, adhesion to endothelial cells and disruption of endothelial integrity, all of which promotes leakage of macromolecules and interstitial edema.[128, 289, 331] Thus, it appears likely that a major mechanism of neutrophil-mediated local tissue injury and inflammatory amplification results from the generation of oxygen free radicals.

Cytokine System

The cytokine system also contributes to the local inflammatory response (see also Chapter 2). TNF and interleukin (IL)-1 are activated by tissue breakdown and stimulate IL-8 synthesis by endothelial cells. IL-8 is a potent chemoattractant[308] which can induce transendothelial neutrophil migration.[141, 276] These and other mediators promote amplification of the inflammatory re-

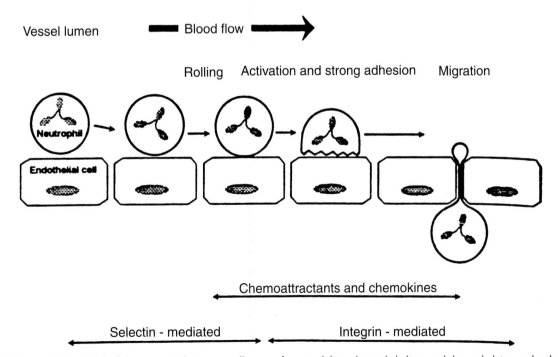

FIGURE **9–19.** Model of the sequential steps in adhesion of neutrophils to the endothelium and the underlying molecular mechanisms. (From Hansen PR: Role of neutrophils in myocardial ischemia and reperfusion. Circulation 1995;91:1872–1885, with permission.)

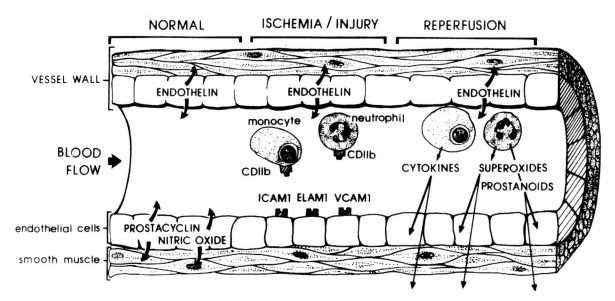

FIGURE **9–20.** Endothelial cells produce and secrete several factors under normal circumstances to maintain the vessel integrity. During ischemia or injury, there is a decrese in the production of nitric oxide and prostacyclin and an increase in the production of endothelin. There is also an activation of leukocytes and an increase in the presence of endothelial adhesion molecules. In reperfusion injury, there is leukocyte adherence, movement through vascular intima, capillary leakage, and production of cytokines, prostanoids, and superoxides that cause further cellular damage, edema, and fluid sequestration. (From McMillen MA, Huribal M, Sumpio B: Common pathway of endothelial-leukocyte interaction in shock ischemia, and reperfusion. Am J Surg 1993;166:557–562, with permission.)

sponse. Other cytokine-endothelial interactions are discussed in the next section.

Endothelial Response to Ischemia/ Reperfusion Injury

Endothelial cells, which cover the luminal surface of the vascular bed, are activated by ischemia/reperfusion injury to produce a variety of inflammatory mediators. Oxygen free radical generation promotes activation of plasma membrane phospholipase A_2, which catalyzes synthesis of PAF from membrane phospholipids. PAF likely participates in ischemic/reperfusion injury by increasing vascular permeability, promoting leukocyte adherence to endothelium,[49] and facilitating leukocyte chemotaxis.

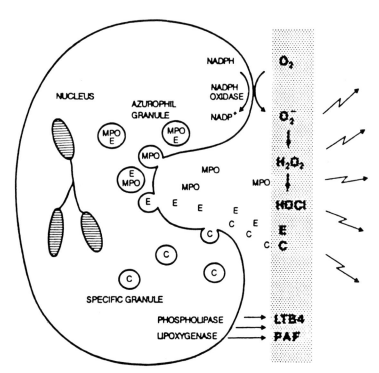

FIGURE **9–21.** Schematic representation of important inflammatory mediators with cardiotoxic potential released from activated neutrophils. O_2^-, superoxide anion; HCl, hypochlorous acid; H_2O_2, hydrogen peroxide; MPO, myeloperoxidase; E, elastase; C, collagenase; LTB4, leukotriene B_4; PAF, plateletactivating factor. (From Hansen PR: Role of neutrophils in myocardial ischemia and reperfusion. Circulation 1995;91:1872–1885, with permission.)

Cytokines are released from injured tissue as discussed above, but they are also specifically produced by the activated endothelium, particularly IL-1, IL-6, IL-8, and TNF.[214] IL-1 and TNF promote expression of endothelial adhesion molecules.[173] Leukotriene B$_4$ and thromboxane A$_2$ are also produced by activated endothelial cells and participate in the inflammatory response as noted in the section Neutrophil Activation.

Endothelial cells also play a pivotal role in reperfusion injury through regulation of vasomotor tone and expression of adhesion molecules. Normally, endothelial cells synthesize several important vaodilators: prostacyclin (a direct smooth muscle relaxant which is a product of arachadonic acid metabolism and is also produced by platelets and monocytes), and nitric oxide (EDRF).[175]

Nitric Oxide (NO) is synthesized from L-arginine by the enzyme nitric oxide synthase (NOS). The clinical use of nitric oxide is discussed in Chapters 6, 12, and 20. The two major subtypes of NOS are the calcium/calmodulin-dependent constitutive enzymes (cNOS) and inducible forms (iNOS). The endothelial cNOS is expressed in arteriolar endothelial cells, where the production of NO induces marked vasodilation and inhibits neutrophil adherence and chemotaxis.[75, 346] NO is generally believed to play a protective role during reperfusion, on the basis of its vasodilator and neutrophil inhibition properties. Experimentally, addition of L-arginine has enhanced postreperfusion recovery and blockade of NOS has increased injury.[74, 157, 244] However, certain of its actions may be detrimental in that NO also reacts with the superoxide radical to form peroxynitrite, which induces mitochondrial damage.[228, 236, 346]

Endothelial cells are also a potent source of **adenosine,** which promotes vasorelaxation. The vasoconstriction function of endothelial cells may play an important role in reperfusion injury. **Endothelin** is a potent endothelial derived vasoconstriction factor which is released following ischemia/reperfusion.[295, 353] Endothelin, a 21-amino-acid peptide, has four known isoforms, the first two (ET-1 and ET-2) of which are mainly in peripheral, coronary, and renal vessels.[290] Endothelial cells also produce thromboxane A$_2$ and angiotensin II, also potent vasoconstrictors.[178]

The specific alterations in vasomotor tone and permeability with ischemia/reperfusion injury result from a complex interplay between these and other regulatory substances. In general, ischemia or injury results in a decrease in nitric oxide and prostacyclin production and an increase in endothelin production. This enhances neutrophil activity, since nitric oxide and prostacyclin inhibit neutrophil adherence and activation.[38, 102, 175] The interaction between endothelium and neutrophils is critical to the body's defense against invasion by foreign organisms, but unfortunately many of the same mechanisms (as discussed earlier in the section Neutrophil Activation) act to perpetuate and augment tissue damage during ischemia/reperfusion injury. Endothelial cells which are injured, ischemic, or exposed to inflammatory cytokines such as TNF or IL-1 greatly increase their surface expression of adhesion molecules. Endothelial leukocyte adhesion molecule (ELAM-1) is expressed on endothelial cells within 2 hours after exposure to TNF or IL-1 and binds to neutrophils even before they are activated.[192, 247] Intercellular adhesion molecule (ICAM-1) undergoes up-regulation with exposure to TNF, IL-1, or interferon-γ and binds with the CDIIa/CD18 beta$_2$ integrin on lymphocytes and the CDIIb/CD18 beta$_2$ integrin or neutrophils and monocytes. Vascular cell adhesion molecule (VCAM-1) shows increased expression after exposure to TNF, IL-1, or IL-4 and binds only to activated T-lymphocytes and monocytes (not neutrophils).[263]

As ischemia/reperfusion injury progresses, the competing forces promoting vasodilation (with greater local blood flow but also greater damaging neutrophil accumulation) versus vasoconstriction (with decreased local blood flow) yield an unpredictable outcome in the stages when injury is still potentially reversible. **Local vasodilation** is promoted by production of carbon dioxide, lactate, hydrogen ions, histamine, and adenosine in ischemic tissues; loss of sympathetic neuronal control; and systemic infusion of platelet-derived serotonin, histamine released from mast cells, kinins released from plasma proteins, and prostaglandins produced by cell membrane phospholipids.[192] **Local vasoconstriction** is promoted by the increased endothelial production of endothelin; impaired nitric oxide and prostacyclin production; impaired nitric oxide-induced vasorelaxation by oxygen free radicals,[279] systemic catecholamines, and angiotensin; decreased lumen size secondary to endothelial cell swelling; and "no-reflow" lesions induced by capillary plugging. The damage is amplified by neutrophil adherence and chemotaxis followed by additional neutrophil migration into the ischemic zone.[175]

The complex process of endothelial cell activation may involve a single signal transduction pathway utilizing the transcription factor **NF-κB** which appears to play a key role in the regulation of genes that respond to various external stimuli (Fig. 9–22).[39, 155, 182, 314] Normally, NF-κB is bound to a cytosolic inhibitor protein called IκB which keeps NF-κB inactive.[57] When the NF-κB – IκB complex is activated by various cytokines and other products of ischemia/repefusion, the complex dissociates and free IκB is rapidly degraded. This allows NF-κB to accumulate and translocate to the nucleus, where it binds to specific DNA sequences resulting in transcription of various activation genes, a process which takes about 4 hours and peaks within 24 hours.[28, 208] This basic mechanism may underline the expression of E-selectin, ICAM, IL-8, and other tissue factors.[39]

In experimental models, very high potassium concentration (> about 100 mEq/L) in cardioplegia solutions has been implicated in endothelial damage, inducing vasospasm and increased capillary permeability.[13] High potassium concentrations promote calcium influx into myocardial cells during ischemia and reperfusion, potentially promoting increased resting wall tension and possibly subsequent diastolic dysfunction. Endothelial dysfunction may also be exacerbated by high initial reperfusion pressure (> about 60 mm Hg)[286] and very cold cardioplegia temperatue (<4°C).[6]

The events of ischemia and reperfusion which may produce acute allograft injury and potentiate chronic endothelial injury are summarized in Figure 9–23. The

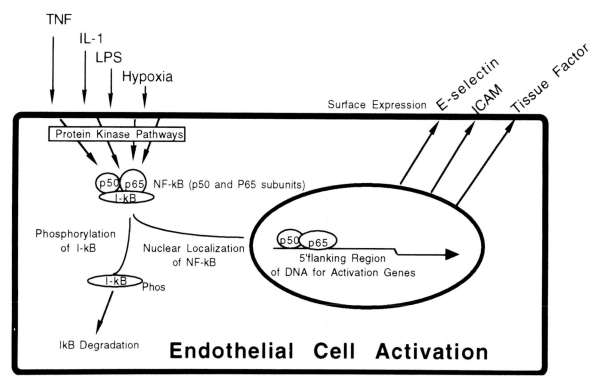

FIGURE **9–22.** Signal transduction through NF-κB. P$_{50}$ and P$_{65}$ are subunits of NF-κB. (From Boyle EM Jr, Pohlman TH, Johnson MC, Verrier ED: The systemic inflammatory response. Ann Thorac Surg 1997;64:S31–S37. Reprinted with permission from the Society of Thoracic Surgeons.)

relationship between endothelial cell injury at the time of implantation and subsequent chronic endothelial injury manifesting as allograft vasculopathy remains speculative, as indicated by the "?" in the lower right box in Figure 9–23. However, considerable evidence suggests that such a relationship may exist (see also Chapter 17).

The term "**endothelial cell activation**" has been used to describe the endothelial response to injury or ischemia which includes the release of endothelial factors which promote leukocyte adhesion and diapedesis, procoagulant effects, vasoconstriction, and smooth muscle cell proliferation. Endothelial cells act as a source of platelet-

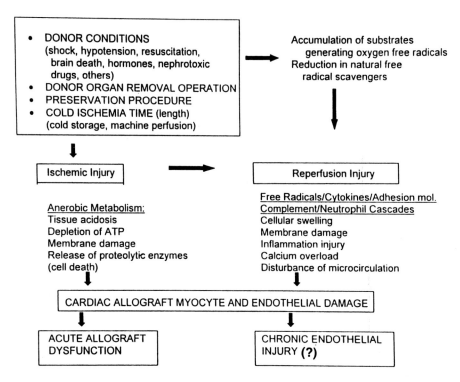

FIGURE **9–23.** Mechanisms of donor heart ischemic and reperfusion injury.

derived growth factor and basic fibroblast growth factor, which stimulate smooth muscle proliferation in the media, detectable within 24 hours of endothelial injury.[56, 274] Smooth muscle cell proliferation is known to be an important component of allograft vasculopathy and atherosclerosis.

PRINCIPLES OF EXTENDED MYOCARDIAL PRESERVATION

The basic goal of myocardial preservation for heart transplantation is to preserve the microvascular, cellular, and functional integrity of the heart during the transplant process. Cellular and microvascular damage should be minimal and reversible such that systolic and diastolic function are either normal or reversibly and mildly abnormal following the period of reperfusion and cessation of cardiopulmonary bypass.

Initial Flushing Solution

The basic aims of the initial flush solution for organs preserved for transplantation, as articulated by Belzer,[22] include prevention of cellular swelling, prevention of intracellular acidosis, and maintenance of intracellular ATP levels sufficient to preserve membrane function.

Hypothermia

The most important (and simplest) maneuver in donor heart preservation is the induction of hypothermia, which decreases (but does not eliminate) cellular metabolic activity. Most mammalian enzyme systems show a 1.5- to 2.5-fold increase in reaction rate for every 10°C increase in temperature. This has been numerically expressed as van't Hoff's law, which relates the logarithm of a chemical reaction rate to temperature. The term Q_{10} refers to the increase in the reaction rate for every 10°C increase in temperature.[108] If we assume a heart temperature of 3° to 5°C during storage, the metabolic rate would be about 1/10 that at 37°C. From many studies it is clear that profound hypothermia to near freezing drastically reduces metabolic activity, but does not eliminate it. Some ongoing energy requirement exists for maintaining the Na-K-ATPase pump and other active membrane transport systems which maintain the intracellular ionic milieu and thereby prevent cellular swelling.

Though profound hypothermia is clearly advisable, controversy exists about the safety of maintaining the heart temperature near 0°C and therefore potentially inducing freezing and crystalization. Until further information is available regarding its safety, we recommend maintaining the myocardial temperature not less than 3°C.

Controversy exists regarding the temperature at which initial induction of a diastolic arrest should be accomplished. The introduction of a profoundly cool solution to the normothermic, beating heart may theoretically increase cytosolic free calcium, which is known to accelerate the depletion of ATP and predispose to contracture under ischemic conditions.[156, 215, 248, 304] Furthermore, Rosenkrantz, Buckberg, and colleagues have shown experimentally that warm blood induction of cardioplegia after initially placing the aortic cross-clamp improves recovery following an ischemic period.[71, 97] However, induction of diastolic arrest with an initial warm solution is currently impractical in the donor setting, so design of the arrest solution to contain low calcium concentration and induce rapid diastolic arrest is probably the best compromise.

Prevention of Cellular Swelling

The sodium and potassium concentration of the preservation solution may affect cellular swelling by altering the ionic concentration gradient. Theoretically, an intracellular-based solution (low sodium, high potassium concentration) would minimize the tendency for intracellular accumulation of Na^+ (and therefore H_2O). However, high-molecular-weight impermeants such as lactobionate and raffinose, and to a lesser extent pentastarch, hydroxyethyl starch, and mannitol may be more important additives in the prevention of intracellular edema.[22, 203, 227, 319]

Intracellular Versus Extracellular Solutions

"Extracellular" solutions refer to those which mimic the ionic concentration of the extracellular milieu. Practically speaking, cardioplegic solutions are so labeled when the Na^+ concentration exceeds about 100 mEq/L. Such solutions generally have potassium concentration of less than about 40 mEq/L. "Intracellular" solutions mimmick the intracellular ionic milieu, which is high in potassium and low in sodium. Such solutions generally have potassium concentration which exceeds 100 mEq/L. Historically, cardioplegic solutions for cardiac surgery have been extracellular solutions, partly related to adverse effects reported by solutions with very high potassium concentration (>100 mEq/L). However, intracellular solutions have gained prominence as the standard solution for preservation of most solid organs and also provide excellent myocardial protection (see below).

Prevention of Calcium Overload

Maintenance of cell membrane integrity and prevention of cellular swelling coupled with a low ionized calcium concentration in the initial flush solution and reperfusion solution offers the best protection against calcium overload. Additional conditions which retard calcium influx include a high magnesium concentration,[243] slightly acidic pH,[25] and the presence of calcium chelators (possibly lactobionate).[199]

Free Radical Scavengers

The importance of free radical injury and free radical scavengers has been previously discussed. Increasingly, initial flush solutions have been designed to include antioxidants for the inactivation of free radicals generated during ischemia and for the provision of free radical scavengers to the intravascular and possibly interstitial compartments that will be available during initial reperfusion.

GSH, as discussed earlier, is one of the most effective naturally occurring scavengers.[159, 202, 343] GSH is a low-molecular-weight antioxidant shown to improve recovery when administered as part of the cardioplegia solution[198, 200] or in the reperfusate.[32] The thiol residue on the reduced form of the molecule is extremely effective in trapping unpaired electrons: GSH is the cofactor for glutathione peroxidase, an enzyme which inactivates H_2O_2 and prevents formation of toxic hydroxyl radicals. GSH is depleted during ischemia,[95] and exogenously supplied GSH in preservation solutions partly compensates for this loss.[253] However, oxidized glutathione (GSSG) increases in concentration as the solution ages by the process of auto-oxidation, and GSSG is potentially damaging to the myocardial collagen network.[349]

Mannitol, in addition to an osmotic agent, has antioxidant properties, particularly against hydroxyl radicals.[233] Enzymatic scavengers such as **superoxide dismutase,**[107] **catalase,**[96, 153] and **peroxidases**[135, 198] have been added to experimental cardioplegic solutions with improved myocardial recovery after ischemia.

Additional antioxidants which have shown promise as additives in experimental solutions include N-acetylcysteine, a low-molecular-weight thiol group donor which can penetrate cells and replenish intracellular stores of GSH,[197] and iron chelating agents such as deferoxamine, which likely act by inhibition of the Haber-Weiss reaction through chelation of transitional metal catalysts such as Fe that are needed for generation of hydroxyl radicals.[210]

Allopurinol has improved myocardial recovery in some experimental preparations, but the antioxidant effects of allopurinol in the human heart may relate to its ability to scavenge hydroxyl radicals rather than through the inhibition of xanthine oxidase, which has a very low concentration in human cardiac muscle.[23, 209, 212, 213]

Preservation of Energy Substrate

Preservation of ATP levels during ischemia likely translates into greater preservation of membrane integrity. Enhancement of flush solutions with Krebs cycle intermediates such as glutamate has improved ATP preservation in experimental studies[246, 272, 335] and is a standard part of the current Buckberg cardioplegia solution.[25]

Available Flush Solutions in Clinical Transplantation

The ideal solution for clinical cardiac transplantation has not yet been established, and several solutions are used clinically. A major distinguishing feature relates to the ionic composition of Na^+ and K^+ and whether the solution should mimic the extracellular or intracellular milieu. The transmembrane sodium-potassium adenosine triphosphatase is inactivated by profound hypothermia,[22] resulting in movement of potassium out of the cell and Na, Cl, and water into the cell. The ionic gradient and probably the net effect is reduced by a high potassium concentration. In addition, the specific combination of protective additives varies greatly.[344]

Two clinical solutions are discussed in detail below which contain an attractive combination of protectants and have been extensively clinically studied.

UW Solution is a flush and storage solution developed by Wahlberg, Southard, and Belzer at the University of Wisconsin for pancreatic transplantation,[22, 327] and successfully extended to liver, kidney, heart, and lung preservation. UW solution is an intracellular based (low sodium, high potassium) solution ([Na] ~20 mEq/L) which contains the impermeable molecules lactobionate (molecular weight, 358), raffinose (molecular weight, 594), and pentastarch to prevent cellular swelling, adenosine as a precursor for ATP generation during reperfusion, magnesium sulfate to retard calcium influx and promote membrane stabilization, glutathione as an antioxidant, and allopurinol to potentially reduce free radical generation (Table 9–7). Experimental[309, 354] and clinical studies[149, 305] have demonstrated excellent myocardial preservation with UW solution out to about 6 hours and possibly beyond. There currently is an extensive clinical experience with UW solution in heart transplantation for neonates, children, and adults. The experimental data and clinical experience support the safety of the UW intracellular formulation.

Despite these excellent results, there continues to be concern about the potentially deleterious effects of high concentrations of potassium. Previous experimental studies indicated that very hyperkalemic solutions (> about 100 mEq/L) may damage the coronary endothelium.[158, 184, 281] One study suggested that standard UW solution (K^+ ~120 mEq/L) impairs endothelial-dependent vasodilator responses and nitric oxide release following reperfusion and that this response is preserved by reducing the potassium concentration of UW solution to about 24 mEq/L.[174] Temperature of the solution is also important, in that endothelial dysfunction after standard UW solution is minimized with temperatures of 4° to 10°C.[184]

Given the potentially deleterious effects of high potassium concentration coupled with the evidence that impermeants such as lactobionate and raffinose may be more important in retarding cellular edema than ionic composition, recent experimental and clinical studies have focused on an "extracellular" composition **(Cel-**

TABLE 9–7	UW Solution
Pentafraction	50 g
Lactobionic acid	100 mmol
Phosphate	25 mmol
Magnesium sulfate	5 mmol
Raffinose	30 mmol
Adenosine	5 mmol
Allopurinol	1 mmol
Gluthathione reduced	3 mmol
Insulin	40 units
Dexamethasone	16 mg
Potassium	120 mEq
Sodium	30 mEq
Total osmolarity	323
pH	7.4

1 liter solution

TABLE 9-8	Celsior Solution
Mannitol	60 mmol
Lactobionate	80 mmol
Glutamate	20 mmol
Histidine	30 mmol
Calcium chloride	0.25 mmol
Potassium chloride	15 mmol
Magnesium chloride	113 mmol
Sodium hydroxide	100 mmol
Reduced gluthione	3 mmol
pH	7.30

1 liter solution

sior) (Table 9–8) with similar additives as UW solution. In addition to lactobionate and mannnitol as impermeants, this solution contains glutamate as substrate for energy production and as a possible antioxidant. Glutamate may decrease the formation of damaging superoxide anions from oxygen, a reaction which is promoted by the buildup of cytoplasmic NADH. With provision of excess glutamate, the malate-aspartate shunt is activated and facilitates transport of cytoplasmic NADH into the mitochondria for oxidation.[24, 68] Other antioxidants in the solution include reduced glutathione, histidine, and mannitol. Calcium overload is limited by a high magnesium content, a low ionized calcium content, and maintenance of very slight acidosis (pH, 7.3) by histidine buffer. The Na^+ concentration is approximately 100 mEq/L and $[K^+]$ about 15 mEq/L. Experimental studies[199, 245, 261] suggest that this extracellular formulation is similar to UW solution in its effectiveness.

Storage

The primary goal of effective storage is maintenance of profound hypothermia during transport in order to minimize cellular energy requirements. Although unproven, a storage temperature near 4°C seems desirable, usually attained by placing the donor heart in a plastic bag submerged in a cold storage solution with crushed ice in contact with the outside of the bag. Temperatures near or at 0°C may be damaging to intracellular structures such as sarcoplasmic reticulum,[146] and ice in prolonged direct contact with the heart may cause thermal injury.[265] Other methods of maintaining hypothermia with inflatable devices have also been proposed.[339]

Reperfusion

Pressure

Initial reperfusion pressure after a period of global cardiac ischemia is known to affect functional recovery, and pressures exceeding about 70–80 mm Hg have been shown to increase myocardial edema,[226, 286] decrease ventricular compliance,[159, 234, 324] and impair endothelium-dependent vasodilation.[159]

Excessively low perfusion pressure (<30 mm Hg) during initial and subsequent reperfusion may risk inadequate perfusion of areas of myocardium with increased microvascular resistance secondary to reversibly injured

(and therefore activated) endothelium. An effective method of removing the influence of low systemic resistance (which is common during cardiopulmonary bypass and heart transplantation) is "controlled aortic root reperfusion,"[161] in which normokalemic blood or other reperfusion solutions[53, 113, 169, 170, 271] can be infused at a desired pressure.

Prevention of Neutrophil-Induced Reperfusion Injury

The modalities for neutrophil depletion or neutralization of neutrophil-induced toxicity are not yet a routine part of clinical extended myocardial preservation for cardiac transplantation, and their discussion is currently largely experimental and theoretical (Table 9–9). However, several lines of investigation suggest that preventing neutrophil adhesion and diapedesis would provide a major increment in recovery following reperfusion. Filtering of leukocytes (three parallel pall filters) during a 10-minute period of reperfusion in a neonatal piglet heart model[305] provided a further increment in myocardial recovery. Others have also demonstrated benefit with neutrophil filtering during reperfusion.[347, 348]

Effective reduction in neutrophil-endothelial adhesion in experimental models has been reported by inhibition of neutrophil CD11b/CD18 up-regulation by monoclonal antibodies against CD18,[76] pharmacologic blockade of the CDIIb/CD18,[117] and administration of acadesine or adenosine.[190] Reduction in postischemic reperfusion injury has also been demonstrated experimentally with monoclonal antibodies against L-selectin,[179] P-selectin,[337] and ICAM-1.[179] Perfluorocarbons have been shown to inhibit neutrophil adherence to endothelial cells during postischemic reperfusion.[13, 100, 101] Inhibition of complement activation with synthetic soluble complement receptors has been demonstrated in rodent models to decrease neutrophil accumulation in postischemic myocardium.[136, 187, 333] Inhibition of neutrophil inflammatory mediators by inhibitors of elastase,[216] lipoxygenase,[285] cyclooxygenase,[269] and PAF[179, 189] have all shown promise in experimental preparation for the blunting of neutrophil-induced postischemic injury.

Heart Preservation By Perfusion

Charles Lindbergh has been credited with the first successful perfusion of organs.[176] From the earliest days of cardiac transplantation, perfusion methods have been available to core cool the donor. This was initially necessary because brain death laws had not been enacted and immediate cooling of the heart was required on

TABLE 9-9	Proposed Methods of Decreasing Neutrophil-Induced Reperfusion Injury

- Neutrophil depletion
- Inhibition of complement activation
- Inhibition of neutrophil adhesion
- Inhibition of neutrophil inflammatory mediators

cessation of the circulation. This methodology became unnecessary with brain death laws and the simplicity and efficacy of single flush and hypothermic storage methods, although some centers still pursued donor core cooling with a portable pump oxygenator for heart–lung block preservation.

The first use of **autoperfusion** of a heart–lung preparation can be traced to Demikhov[70] for short-term preservation of an experimental donor heart. Robicsek in 1959[265] also demonstrated that autoperfusion was feasible for experimental transplantation of the heart. Autoperfusion has been used for clinical heart and heart–lung transplantation,[130] but the system was too cumbersome for widespread applicability.

From a technical and biological standpoint, **hypothermic perfusion** offers the possibility of longer term donor heart preservation than is currently available from simple flush and hypothermic storage. A number of reports have documented preservation out to 12 hours with a continuous hypothermic perfusion system[293] or a combination of coronary perfusion and cold storage[225] in experimental models. Calhoon and colleagues[45] described a portable continuous hypothermic preservation system in which 12 hours of canine heart preservation and subsequent transplantation was possible using oxygenated UW solution. Wicomb[341] achieved 24 hours of preservation and subsequent transplantation by continuous hypothermic perfusion in baboon hearts with an oxygenated hyperosmolor solution. A similar system was used[342] in clinical heterotopic cardiac transplantation but delayed donor function was common, with the circulation being temporarily supported by the recipient's own heart.

Currently, the technical and biological problems associated with normothermic or hypothermic perfusion preclude its routine use in clinical transplantation. However, it could play a future role in cardiac transplantation if ischemia times exceeding about 5 hours (after which the risk of donor heart dysfunction increases with current flush and storage techniques) become routine. Such longer ischemic times might occur with longer distance procurement if, for example, closer donor-recipient matching (HLA matching or donor alteration via gene therapy) improves survival.

STRATEGY OF DONOR HEART MYOCARDIAL PROTECTION

At UAB we have employed standard UW solution (Via Span by DuPont) (Table 9–6) for over 10 years. With current methods of preparation, oxidation of reduced glutathione can be detected by the presence of a cloudiness of the solution. In an adult, 1 L of UW solution is infused by gravity at a temperature of 4°–6°C. Infusion of UW or any other cardioplegic solution through a pressurized bag carries a potential danger of high-pressure infusion injury and, in our opinion, should always be avoided. In pediatric patients, the dose utilized is 25 mL/kg of body weight. Profound hypothermia is further maintained during the infusion by topical 4°C saline slush. After removal of the heart, it is placed

in UW solution for storage during transport. The solution is maintained at about 4°–6°C by packing the plastic bag in ice, which does not come in direct contact with the heart.

During implantation, we do not infuse additional cardioplegic solutions. Moderate hypothermic systemic perfusion and profound topical cooling with cold saline is maintained during implantation to minimize myocardial warming.

We have employed hyperkalemic blood cardioplegia solution as described by Buckberg[42, 98, 99] during initial reperfusion with good results.[162] However, because of occasional prolonged asystole, we currently initiate reperfusion with normokalemic blood from the oxygenator (simple removal of cross-clamp). If systemic perfusion pressure is less than about 50 mm Hg and cardiac contraction remains weak after 10–15 minutes of reperfusion, controlled aortic root perfusion[160] is established with normokalemic blood infused through the cardioplegic needle into the aortic root (with crossclamp in place) to maintain a perfusion pressure of 50–70 mm Hg. This is considered preferable to initiating high-dose vasoconstrictive agents such as phenylephrine or norepinephrine, which can importantly increase pulmonary vascular resistance. If the heart becomes vigorous enough to produce pulsatile flow in the aortic root during controlled reperfusion, both the systolic and diastolic aortic root pressures should be monitored. If the systolic pressure exceeds about 80 mm Hg, the crossclamp is partially or completely removed to avoid high-pressure infusion into the coronary arteries.

During initial reperfusion, the left ventricle is intermittently gently palpated for signs of firmness. Usually during this time, the ventricular myocardium continues to be soft until effective contraction is established. If an area of firmness is palpable, we believe this represents a clinical sequela of ischemic/reperfusion injury, in which endothelial cell swelling and localized myocardial edema have likely occurred with marked increase in microvascular resistance and therefore a decreased ability to provide sufficient substrate to that area for recovery and membrane stabilization. We have occasionally encountered this phenomenon if ventricular fibrillation occurs following reperfusion and prompt electrical cardioversion is not initiated. Another sign of increased microvascular resistance, probably at the subendocardial level, is prolonged quiesence (asystole) during reperfusion. We hypothesize that the Purkinje system is inadequately perfused if quiesence persists, which suggests inadequate subendocardial perfusion.

If, during reperfusion following transplantation, prolonged cardiac quiescence, ventricular myocardial firmness, or frequent ventricular arrhythmias are observed, we intervene by infusion of 2–5 mL of dilute nitroglycerin (50 mg nitroglycerin diluted with 25 mL of normal saline solution) injected into the aortic root. If this is not effective, an injection of 2–3 mg of dilute adenosine (diluted with 10 mL of normal saline) is often effective in restoring sinus rhythm (likely resulting from marked coronary vasodilation and improved subendocardial perfusion). If such a situation occurs during reperfusion, it is important to **avoid** infusion of calcium or inotropic agents (which increase myocardial oxygen consumption and adversely affect the balance between oxygen supply and demand) until the heart has fully recovered. Such a situation is rare, in that over 90% of transplanted hearts regain a regular rhythm within about 1–2 minutes of initiating reperfusion.

We do not currently employ techniques of leukocyte depletion, but available experimental evidence suggests that a technique of leukocyte depletion or blockade of neutrophil adhesion should be employed when a simple and effective method is clinically available.

TECHNIQUES OF HEART PROCUREMENT

Once the decision has been made to utilize a donor heart, considerable coordination and communication is required. Invariably, multiorgan donation will occur and frequently with more than one organ procurement team. It is the responsibility of the organ procurement organization managing the donor to communicate with each of the procurement teams to establish a time to take the donor to the operating room, and it is the responsibility of each team to arrange transportation to arrive at the donor hospital in a timely manner and communicate any delays. The heart procurement team establishes communication with the recipient hospital for later decisions regarding suitability of the donor heart and to coordinate arrival of the donor heart with preparation of the recipient. When a long ischemic time is anticipated, precise coordination is especially important.

The donor should be managed throughout the procurement by an anesthesiologist or nurse anesthetist. A central venous pressure line and an arterial line are useful for the management of donors during the procurement, particularly when there may be hemodynamic instability. The donor is placed supine on the operating table on a heating blanket and the arms placed by the sides. A muscle relaxant should be administered to prevent limb or abdominal wall movement due to spinal reflexes, which can be distressing to personnel unfamiliar with the procedure. The procurement coordinators with each team are responsible for the smooth organization of the procurement, assistance at the operating table, packaging of the organs, and most importantly, treating the operating room staff with an attitude of professionalism, cordiality, and gratitude for their role in the transplant process.

The donor is prepped from neck to midthigh and widely draped. Two electrocautery units and two suction units should be provided, one each for the surgeons working in the abdominal cavity and the surgeon working in the thoracic cavity. A midline incision is made from the sternal notch to the pubis. The abdominal procurement surgeons proceed with mobilization of the abdominal organs. A median sternotomy is performed with a sternal saw or, on occasions when that is not available, a Lebsche knife. Bone wax and liberal cautery is required because of the coagulopathic state. The pericardium is opened and pericardial sutures are placed. The right pleural space is widely opened and the pericardium at the diaphragm is incised down toward the inferior vena cava (IVC) to allow blood and hepatic preservation solutions to drain into the right pleural space after the IVC has been partially divided. The heart is inspected for overall size, evidence of contusion, and any wall motion abnormalities of right or left ventricle. The course of the coronary arteries is palpated for evidence of wall disease. The heart is palpated for evidence of valvular heart disease, although this is unlikely to be discovered in the face of a normal echocardiogram. When the procurement surgeon is satisfied that the heart is suitable, this is communicated to the recipient hospital.

For the **bicaval insertion technique,** a length of superior vena cava is required. The superior vena cava is freed from its pericardial reflection up to the innominate vein. The ascending aorta is then dissected from the main pulmonary artery. A pursestring suture of 4.0 polypropylene is placed in the ascending aorta.

If there is hemodynamic instability during the dissection process, ligation of the abdominal aorta at the bifurcation is usually effective in improving the blood pressure. When mobilization of the abdominal organs is complete and blood is collected for crossmatching purposes, heparin at a dose of 300 units/kg of body weight is administered. A cardioplegic needle is inserted in the ascending aorta and connected to the cardiac preservation solution and at the same time the flush lines for the abdominal organs are placed. After at least 2 minutes of heparin circulation, the procurement can proceed.

The superior vena cava is cross-clamped and the inferior vena cava is nearly completely divided at the right atrial-inferior vena caval junction to allow sufficient inferior vena caval tissue for the liver transplant surgeon. The heart should be allowed to continue beating to partially exsanguinate the donor (into the right pleural space) through this inferior vena caval incision. When the heart is empty (and this may be after 5–10 beats) the ascending aorta is cross-clamped and the preservation solution is commenced by gravity infusion (a pressurized bag should never be used because of the potential for high-pressure infusion injury) (Fig. 9–24). To prevent any left ventricular distention, the right pulmonary veins are divided (Fig. 9–25). If a heart–lung block is being procured, the left atrial appendage is amputated. If the lungs are being procured for lung transplantation, then the interatrial groove is partially dissected and the pulmonary venous circuit can be decompressed by incising the left atrium so as to commence the left atrial cuff of the left lung. The heart is topically cooled with saline slush. When the preservation solution infusion is complete, the heart is excised by completing the transection of the inferior vena cava transecting the superior vena cava as cephalad as possible (for bicaval implantation) and all pulmonary veins (Fig. 9–26). The left and right pulmonary arteries are divided (main pulmonary artery is divided if the lungs are being procured for lung transplantation) and the ascending aorta is divided, usually distal to the innominate artery (Figs. 9–27 and 9–28). There are occasions when the recipient may require

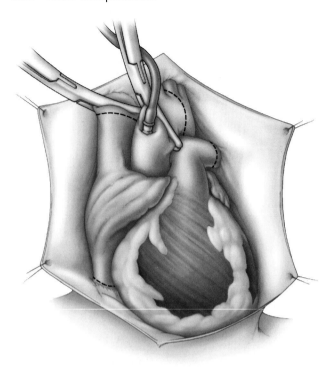

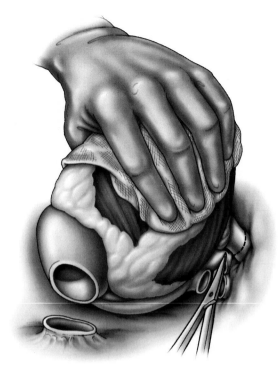

FIGURE **9–24.** Diagram of the donor heart immediately prior to harvesting. The aorta and SVC are clamped and a cardioplegia catheter has been inserted into the ascending aorta. The dashed lines indicate the places where the SVC, IVC, ascending aorta, and left pulmonary artery will be divided. SVC, superior vena cava; IVC, inferior vena cava.

FIGURE **9–26.** Division of the left pulmonary veins during cardiac procurement. The inferior vena cava, superior vena cava, and right pulmonary veins have already been divided. The dashed line indicates the point of transection of the left pulmonary artery.

more donor ascending aorta than usual (previous aortic root surgery, left ventricular assist device implantation, some forms of congenital heart disease) and under those circumstances the donor aorta should be divided at the distal aortic arch. A complete description of procure-

ment for neonates and infants with congenital heart disease is found in Chapter 20. The pericardial attachments are then divided. The heart should be taken to the back table and inspected for a patent foramen ovale (which should be closed), the atrioventricular valves should be inspected, and the normal drainage of the coronary sinus to the right atrium should be confirmed. The heart is

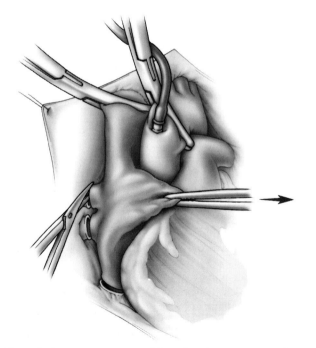

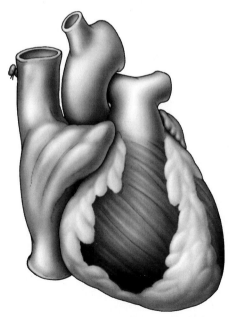

FIGURE **9–25.** Decompression of the right pulmonary veins to decompress the left ventricle during cardioplegia infusion. The inferior vena cava has already been nearly transected.

FIGURE **9–27.** Completed excision of donor heart. Additional length of superior vena cava has been obtained in preparation for a bicaval implantation.

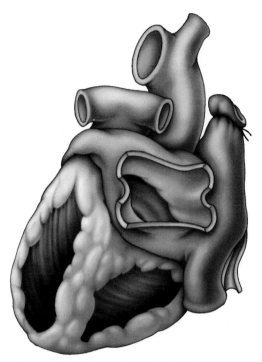

FIGURE **9–28.** Posterior view of excised donor heart. Incisions have been made through the orifices of the pulmonary veins to prepare the left atrium. The superior vena cava has been ligated and an incision has been made through the inferior vena caval opening onto the body of the right atrium, in preparation for a standard orthotopic implantation.

then packed in cold UW solution, double bagged, and placed in a hard plastic container with cold saline. The plastic container is enclosed by an outer bag. The heart is then placed in a transport cooler surrounded by ice. Several lymph nodes are placed in the container with transport medium to be taken to the recipient hospital for a prospective crossmatch.

References

1. Ad Hoc Committee of the Harvard Medical School: Definition of irreversible coma. JAMA 1968;205:85–88.
2. Adams DH, Shaw S: Leukocyte-endothelial interactions and regulation of leukocyte migration. Lancet 1994;343:831–836.
3. Adams DH, Wang LF, Neuberger JM, Elias E: Inhibition of leukocyte chemotaxis by immunosuppressive agents. Specific inhibition of lymphocyte chemotaxis by cyclosporine. Transplantation 1990;50:845–850.
4. Ambassador of the People's Republic of China. Transplants in China, Times (London), December 5, 1994.
5. Anderson RF, Allensworth DC, deGroot WJ: Myocardial toxicity from carbon monoxide poisoning. Ann Intern Med 1967;67:1172–1182.
6. Aoki M, Kawata H, Mayer JE Jr: Coronary endothelial injury by cold crystalloid cardioplegic. Circulation 1992;86(suppl II):346–351.
7. Aranaout MA: Structure and function of the leukocyte adhesion molecules CD11/CD18. Blood 1990;75:1037–1050.
8. Ashwal S: Brain death in the newborn. Clin Perinatol 1989;16:501–518.
9. Ashwal S, Schneider S: Pediatric brain death: current perspectives. Adv Pediatr 1991;38:181–202.
10. Ashwal S, Schneider S: Brain death in the newborn (articles continued). Pediatrics 1989;84:429–437.
11. Askanas A, Udoshi M, Sadjadi SA: The heart in chronic alcoholism: a noninvasive study. Am Heart J 1980;99:9–16.
12. Aust SD, Morehouse LA, Thomas CE: Role of metals in oxygen radical reactions. J Free Radic Biol Med 1985;1:3–25.
13. Babbitt DG, Forman MB, Jones R, Bajaj AK, Hoover RL: Prevention of neutrophil-mediated injury to endothelial cells by perfluorochemical. Am J Pathol 1990;136:451–459.
14. Badwey JA, Karnovsky ML: Active oxygen species and the functions of phagocytic leukocytes. Annu Rev Biochem 1980;49:695–726.
15. Baker JE, Felix CC, Olinger GN, Kalyanaraman B: Myocardial ischemia and reperfusion: direct evidence for free radical generation by electron spin resonance spectroscopy. Proc Natl Acad Sci U S A 1988;85:2786–2789.
16. Baldwin JC, Anderson JL, Boucek MM, Bristow MR, Jennings B, Ritsch ME, Silverman NA: Task Force 2: Donor Guidelines. J Am Coll Cardiol 1993;22:1–64.
17. Barkoukis TJ, Sarbak CA, Lewis D: Multiorgan procurement from a victim of cyanide poisoning. Transplantation 1992;55:1434.
18. Barnard CN: The operation: a human cardiac transplant: an interim report of a successful operation performed at Grrote Schuur Hospital, Cape Town. S Afr Med J 1967;41:1271–1274.
19. Baroldi G: Different morphological types of myocardial cell death in man. In Fleckenstein A, Rona G (eds): Recent Advances in Studies of Cardiac Structure and Metabolism. Vol 6. Pathophysiology and Morphology of Myocardial Cell Alteration. Baltimore: University Park Press, 1975, pp 385–397.
20. Beckman DL, Iams SG: Circulating catecholamines in cats before and after lethal head injury. Proc Soc Exp Biol Med 1979;160:200–202.
21. Bedotto JB, Lee RW, Lancaster LD, Olajos M, Goldman S: Cocaine and cardiovascular function in dogs: effects on heart and peripheral circulation. J Am Coll Cardiol 1988;11:1337–1342.
22. Belzer FO, Southard JH: Principles of solid-organ preservation by cold storage. Transplantation 1988;45:673–676.
23. Bergsland J, Lobalsamo L, Lajos P, Feldman MJ, Mookerjee B: Allopurinol in prevention of reperfusion injury of hypoxically stored rat hearts. J Heart Transplant 1987;6:137–140.
24. Berkowitz S, Perille T, Leach M: Anaerobic amino acid metabolism as a potential energy source in mammalian hearts. Clin Res 1978;26:219A.
25. Bernard M, Menasche P, Canioni P, Fontanarava E, Grousset C, Piwnica A, Cozzone P: Influence of the pH of cardioplegic solution on intracellular pH, high-energy phosphates, and postarrest performance. J Thorac Cardiovasc Surg 1985;90:235–242.
26. Bers DM: Excitation-Contraction Coupling and Cardiac Contractile Force. Boston: Kluwer Academic Publishers, 1991.
27. Bevilacqua MP, Nelson RM: Selectins. J Clin Invest 1993;91:379–387.
28. Bevilacqua MP, Pober JS, Mendrick DL, Cotran RS, Gimbrone MA Jr: Identification of an inducible endothelial-leukocyte adhesion molecule. Proc Natl Acad Sci U S A 1987;84:9238–9242.
29. Bittner HB, Kendall SWH, Chen EP, Davis RD, van Trigt P: Myocardial performance after graft preservation and subsequent cardiac transplantation from brain-dead donors. Ann Thorac Surg 1995;60:47–54.
30. Bittner HB, Kendall WH, Campbell KA, Montine TJ, van Trigt P: A valid experimental brain death organ donor model. J Heart Lung Transplant 1995;14:308–317.
31. Blackbourne LH, Tribble CG, Langenburg SE, Sinclair KN, Rucker GB, Chan BBK, Spotnitz WD, Bergin JD, Kron IL: Successful use of undersized donors for orthotopic heart transplantation—with a caveat. Ann Thorac Surg 1994;57:1472.
32. Blaustein AS, Deneke SM, Fanburg BL: Glutathione enriched reperfusate improves recovery of myocardial function following ischemia [abstract]. Circulation 1987;76(suppl 4):197.
33. Bloom S, David D: Isoproterenol myocytolysis and myocardial calcium. Recent Adv Stud Card Struct Metab 1974;4:581.
34. Boehrer JD, Moliterno DJ, Willard JE, Snyder RW, Horton RP, Glamann DB, Lange RA, Hillis LD: Hemodynamic effects of intranasal cocaine in humans. J Am Coll Cardiol 1992;10:90.
35. Boles JG, Garre M: Thyroid function in non-thyroidal illness: "the euthyroid sick syndrome." In Vincent JL (ed): Update in Intensive Care and Emergency Medicine. New York: Springer, 1986, p 239.
36. Bollinger RR: The role of UNOS in thoracic organ transplantation. In Shumway SJ, Shumway NE (eds): Thoracic Transplantation. Boston: Blackwell Science, 1995, pp 141–148.

37. Boucek MM, Mathis CM, McCormack J, Gundry SR, Bailey LL: Sudden infant death syndrome (SIDS) and heart transplant donors: evidence against an intrinsic cardiac abnormality. Circulation 1990;82(suppl 3):352.

38. Boxer LA, Allen JM, Schmidt M, Yoder M, Baehner RL: Inhibition of polymorphonuclear leukocyte adherence by prostacyclin. J Lab Clin Med 1980;95:672–678.

39. Boyle EM Jr, Pohlman TH, Johnson MC, Verrier ED: The systemic inflammatory response. Ann Thorac Surg 1997;64:S31–S37.

40. Bremner WF, Taylor KM, Baird S, Thomas JE, Thomson JA, Ratcliffe JG, Lawrie TDV, Bain WH: Hypothalamopituitary-thyroid axis function during cardiopulmonary bypass. J Thorac Cardiovasc Surg 1978;75:392.

41. Brennan DC, Lowell JA: Pretransplant preparation of the cadaver donor/organ procurement. In Norman DJ, Suki WN (eds): Primer on Transplantation. Philadelphia: American Society of Transplant Physicians, 1998.

42. Buckberg GD: Oxygenated cardioplegia: blood is a many splendored thing. Ann Thorac Surg 1990;50:175.

43. Burton KP: Evidence of direct toxic effects of free radicals on the myocardium. Free Radic Biol Med 1988;4:15–24.

44. Byer E, Ashman R, Toth LA: Electrocardiogram with large upright T wave and long Q-T intervals. Am Heart J 1947;33:796–801.

45. Calhoon JH, Bunegin L, Gelineau JF, Felger MC, Naples JJ, Miller OL, Sako EY: Twelve-hour canine heart preservation with a simple, portable hypothermic organ perfusion device. Ann Thorac Surg 1996;62:91–93.

46. Cabasson J, Blanc WA, Joos HA: The anencephalic infant as a possible donor for cardiac transplantation. Clin Pediatr 1969; 8:86–89.

47. Cassavilla A, Ramirez C, Shapiro R, Nghiem D, Miraclee K, Fung JJ, Starzl TE: Experience with liver and kidney allografts from non-heart-beating donors. Transplant Proc 1995;27:2898.

48. Cebelin J, Hirsch SC: Human stress cardiomyopathy. Hum Pathol 1980;2:123–132.

49. Cecka JM, Terasaki PI: Optimal use for older donor kidneys: older recipients. Transplant Proc 1995;27:801.

50. Chan BBK, Fleischer KJ, Bergin JD, Peyton VC, Flanagan TL, Kern JA, Tribble CG, Gibson RS, Kron IL: Weight is not an accurate criterion for adult cardiac transplant size matching. Ann Thorac Surg 1991;52:1230.

51. Chenoweth DE, Cooper SW, Hugli TE, Stewart RW, Blackstone EH, Kirklin JW: Complement activation during cardiopulmonary bypass. Evidence for generation of C3a and C5a anaphylatoxins. N Engl J Med 1981;304:497–503.

52. China: The use of organs from executed prisoners. AI Index: ASA 17/01/95: March 1995.

53. Choong YS, Gavin JB: L-aspartate improves the functional recovery of explanted hearts stored in St. Thomas' Hospital cardioplegic solutions at 4°C. J Thorac Cardiovasc Surg 1990;99:510.

54. Chu SH, Huang TS, Hsu RB, Wang SS, Wang CJ: Thyroid hormone changes after cardiovascular surgery and clinical implications. Ann Thorac Surg 1991;52:791.

55. Clark JM: Oxygen toxicity. In Bennett P, Elliott D (eds): The Physiology and Medicine of Diving. Philadelphia: WB Saunders 1993.

56. Clowes AW: Prevention and management of current disease after arterial reconstruction: new prospects of pharmacologic control. Thromb Haemost 1991;66:2–66.

57. Collins T, Read MA, Neish AS, Whitley MZ, Thanos D, Maniatis T: Transcriptional regulation of endothelial cell adhesion molecules: NFkB and cytokine-inducible enhancers. FASEB J 1995; 9:899–909.

58. Conference of the Royal Colleges and Faculties of the United Kingdom: Diagnosis of brain death. Lancet 1976;2:1069–1070.

59. Cooper DKC: The donor heart; the present position with regard to resuscitation, storage, and assessment of viability. J Surg Res 1976;21:363.

60. Corya BC, Black MJ, McHenry PL: Echocardiographic findings after acute carbon monoxide poisoning. Br Heart J 1976; 38:712–717.

61. Costanzo M, Naftel DC, Pritzker MR, Heilman JK III, Boehmer JP, Brozena SC, Dec GW, Ventura HO, Kirklin JK, Bourge RC, Miller LW, and the Cardiac Transplant Research Database: Heart transplant coronary artery disease detected by coronary angiography: a multiinstitutional study of preoperative donor and recipient risk factors. J Heart Lung Transplant 1998;17:744–753.

62. Costanzo-Nordin MR, Liao Y, Grusk BB, O'Sullivan EJ, Cooper RS, Johnson MR, Siebold KM, Sullivan HJ, Heroux AH, Robinson JA, Pifarre R: Oversizing of donor hearts: beneficial or detrimental? J Heart Lung Transplant 1991;10:717.

63. Cropp GJ, Manning GW: Electrocardiographic changes simulating myocardial ischemia and interactions associated with spontaneous intracranial hemorrhage. Circulation 1960;22:25–38.

64. Cruickshank JM, Neil-Dwyer G, Scott A: The possible role of catecholamines, corticosteroids, and potassium in the production of ECG changes with subarachnoid hemorrhage. Br Heart J 1974;36:697–706.

65. Cullpepper MI Jr: Legal aspects of organ and tissue procurement and transplantation. In Phillips MG (ed): UNOS Organ Procurement, Preservation and Distribution in Transplantation. 2nd ed. Richmond, VA: UNOS, 1996.

66. Cushing H: Some experimental and clinical observations concerning states of increased intracranial tension. Am J Med Sci 1902;124:375–400.

67. David M, Meyer R, Marx I, Guski H, Wenzelides K: Morphometric characterization of left ventricular myocardial cells of male rats during postnatal development. J Mol Cell Cardiol 1979;11:63.

68. Davis EJ, Bremmer J: Studies with isolated surviving rat hearts. Interdependence of free amino acids and citric acid-cycle intermediate. Eur J Biochem 1973;38:86.

69. Del Balzo UH, Levi R, Polley MJ: Cardiac dysfunction caused by purified human C3a anaphylatoxin. Proc Natl Acad Sci U S A 1985;82:886–890.

70. Demikhov VP: Experimental Transplantation of Vital Organs. Authorized transplantation from the Russian by Haigh B. New York: Consultants Bureaus, 1962.

71. Dennis SC, Gevers W, Opie LH: Protons in ischemia: where do they come from; where do they go to? J Mol Cell Cardiol 1991;23:1077–1086.

72. Depret J, Teboul JL, Benoit G, Mercat A, Richard C: Global energetic failure in brain-dead patients. Transplantation 1995;60:966.

73. Devlin TM: Textbook of Biochemistry with Clinical Correlations. New York: John Wiley & Sons, 1982.

74. Diamond JR, Karnovsky MJ: Focal and segmental glomerulosclerosis: analogies to atherosclerosis. Kidney Int 1988;33:917.

75. Donadio JV Jr, Torres VE, Velosa JA, Wagoner RD, Holley KE, Okamura M, Ilstrup DM, Chu CP: Idiopathic membranous nephropathy: the natural history of untreated patients. Kidney Int 1988;33:708.

76. Dreyer WJ, Michael LH, Millman EE, Berens KL: Neutrophil sequestration and pulmonary dysfunction in a canine model of open heart surgery with cardiopulmonary bypass. Evidence for a CD18-dependent mechanism. Circulation 1995;92:2276–2283.

77. Drinkwater D: Personal communication. In Meiser BM, Uberfuhr P, Reichenspurner H, Stang A, Kreuzer E, Reichart B (eds): One heart transplanted successfully twice. J Heart Lung Transplant 1994;13:339.

78. Duckworth D: Some cases of cerebral disease in which the function of respiration entirely ceases for some hours before that of the circulation. Edinb Med J 1898;3:145–152.

79. Dunlop P, Varty K, Veitch PS, Nicholson ML, Bell PRF: Non-heart-beating donors: the Leicester experience. Transplant Proc 1995;27:2940.

80. Dyke CM, Yeh T, Lehman JD, Abd-Elfattah A, Ding M, Wechsler AD, Salter DR: Triiodothyronine-enhanced left ventricular function after ischemic injury. Ann Thorac Surg 1991;52:14.

81. Eichhorn EJ, Grayburn PA: Substance abuse and the heart. In Willerson JT, Cohn JN (eds): Cardiovascular Medicine. New York: Churchill Livingstone, 1995, pp 1687–1701.

82. Eichhorn EJ, Peacock E, Grayburn PA, Bedotto JB, Willard JE, Willerson JT, Demian SE: Chronic cocaine abuse is associated with accelerated atherosclerosis in human coronary arteries [abstract]. J Am Coll Cardiol 1992;19:105A.

83. Engler RL, Dahlgren MD, Peterson MA, Dobbs A, Schmid-Schonbein GW: Accumulation of polymorphonuclear leukocytes during 3-h experimental myocardial ischemia. Am J Physiol 1986;2251:H93–H100.

84. Engler RL, Schmid-Schonbein GW, Pavelec RS: Leukocyte capillary plugging in myocardial ischemia and reperfusion in the dog. Am J Pathol 1983;111:98–111.

85. Entman ML, Michael L, Rossen RD, Dreyer WJ, Anderson DC, Taylor AA, Smith CW: Inflammation in the course of early myocardial ischemia. FASEB J 1991;5:2529–2537.

86. Executions and Organ Transplantation: Taiwan. AI Index: ASA 38/04/92: March 1992.

87. Fabiato A: Calcium-induced release of calcium from the cardiac sarcoplasmic reticulum. Am J Physiol 1993;2245:C1.

88. Fabiato A: Simulated calcium current can both cause calcium loading in and trigger calcium release from the sarcoplasmic reticulum of a skinned canine cardiac Purkinje cell. J Gen Physiol 1985;85:291.

89. Fabiato A, Baumgarten CM: Methods for detecting calcium release from the sarcoplasmic reticulum of skinned cardiac cells and the relationships between calculated transsarcolemmal calcium movements and calcium release. *In* Sperelakis N (ed): The Physiology and Pathophysiology of the Heart. Boston: Martinus Nijhoff, 1984, p 215.

90. Fabiato A, Fabiato F: Calcium and cardiac excitation muscle. Mayo Clin Proc 1982;57(suppl):6.

91. Fantone JC, Ward PA: Role of oxygen-derived free radicals and metabolites in leukocyte-dependent inflammatory reactions. Am J Pathol 1982;107:397–418.

92. Fentz V, Gormson J: Electrocardiographic patterns in patients with cerebrovascular accidents. Circulation 1962;25:22–28.

93. Ferrans FJ, Hobbs RG, Black WC, Weilbaecher DG: Isoproterenol-induced myocardial necrosis. A histo-chemical and electron microscopic study. Am Heart J 1964;68:71.

94. Ferree DM, Stearns JM, Stockdreher DD: Organ sharing: UNOS organ center. *In* Phillips MG (ed): UNOS Organ Procurement, Preservation and Distribution in Transplantation. 2nd ed. Richmond, VA: UNOS, 1996.

95. Ferrari R, Ceconi C, Curello S, Guarnieri C, Caldarera CM, Albertini A, Visioli O: Oxygen-mediated myocardial damage during ischaemia and reperfusion: role of the cellular defences against oxygen toxicity. J Mol Cell Cardiol 1985;17:937–945.

96. Flohe L: Glutathione peroxidase brought into focus. *In* Pryor WA (ed): Free Radical in Biology. New York: Academic Press, 1982, 223–254.

97. Follette DM, Fey K, Buckberg GD, Helly JJ Jr, Steed DL, Foglia RP, Maloney JV Jr: Reducing postischemic damage by temporary modification of reperfusate calcium, potassium, pH, and osmolarity. J Thorac Cardiovasc Surg 1981;81:493.

98. Follette DM, Fey K, Mulder DG, Maloney JV Jr, Buckberg GD: Prolonged safe aortic clamping by combining membrane stabilization, multidose cardioplegia and appropriate pH reperfusion. J Thorac Cardiovasc Surg 1977;74:682.

99. Follette DM, Mulder DG, Maloney JV Jr, Buckberg GD: Advantages of blood cardioplegia over continuous coronary perfusion or intermittent ischemia: experimental and clinical study. J Thorac Cardiovasc Surg 1978;76:604.

100. Forman KE, Ingram D, Murray JJ: Role of perfluorochemical emulsions in the treatment of myocardial reperfusion injury. Am Heart J 1992;124:1347–1357.

101. Forman MB, Puett DW, Bingham SE, Virmani R, Tantangco MV, Light RT, Bajaj A, Price R, Friesinger G: Preservation of endothelial cell structure and function by intracoronary perfluorochemical in a canine preparation of reperfusion. Circulation 1987;76:469–479.

102. Fostermann U, Mugge A, Alheid U, Bode SM, Frolich JC: Endothelium-derived relaxing factor (EDRF): a defense mechanism against platelet aggregation and vasospasm in human coronary arteries. Eur Heart J 1989;10:36–43.

103. Fraker TD Jr, Temesy-Armos PN, Brewster PS, Wilkerson RD: Mechanism of cocaine-induced myocardial depression in dogs. Circulation 1990;81:1012–1016.

104. Freeman BA, Crapo JD: Biology of disease: free radicals and tissue injury. Lab Invest 1982;47:412–426.

105. Freimark D, Aleksic I, Trento A, Takkenberg JJ, Valenza M, Admon D, Blanche C, Queral CA, Azen CG, Czer LS: Hearts from donors with chronic alcohol use: a possible risk factor for death after heart transplantation. J Heart Lung Transplant 1996;15:150–159.

106. Freimark D, Czer LSC, Admon D, Aleksic I, Valenza M, Barath P, Harasty D, Queral C, Azen CG, Blanche C, Trento A: Donors with a history of cocaine use: effect on survival and rejection

107. Fridovich I, Freeman B: Antioxidant defenses in the lung. Ann Rev Physiol 1986;48:693–702.

108. Fuhrman GJ, Fuhrman FA: Oxygen consumption of animals and tissues as a function of temperature. J Gen Physiol 1959;42:715.

109. Gallay P, Albat B, Thevenet A, Grolleau R: Direct current catheter ablation of an accessory pathway in a recipient with refractory reciprocal tachycardia. J Heart Lung Transplant 1992;11:442–445.

110. Ganong WF: Review of Medical Physiology. Los Altos, CA: Lange Medical Publishers, 1969, p 225.

111. Garlick PP, Davies MJ, Hearse DJ, Slater TF: Direct detection of free radicals in the reperfused rat heart using electron spin resonance spectroscopy. Circ Res 1987;61:757–760.

112. Gauduel Y, Duvelleroy MA: Role of oxygen radicals in cardiac injury due to reoxygenation. J Mol Cell Cardiol 1984;16:459–470.

113. Gharagozloo F, Melendez FJ, Hein RA, Laurence RG, Shemin RJ, DiSesa VJ, Cohn LH: The effect of amino acid L-glutamate on the extended preservation ex vivo of the heart for transplantation. Circulation 1987;76(suppl V):V65.

114. Gifford RR, Weaver AS, Burg JE, Romano PJ, Demers LM, Pennock JL: Thyroid hormone levels in heart and kidney cadaver donors. J Heart Transplant 1986;5:249–253.

115. Gilbert EM, Krueger SK, Murray JL, Renlund DG, O'Connell JB, Gay WA, Bristow MR: Echocardiographic evaluation of potential cardiac transplant donors. J Thorac Cardiovasc Surg 1988;95:1003.

116. Gilder SSB: Twenty-second World Medical Assembly. BMJ 1968;3:493–494.

117. Gillinov AM, Redmond JM, Zehr KJ, Wilson IC, Curtis WE, Bator JM, Burch RM, Reitz BA, Baumgartner WA, Herskowitz A, Cameron DE: Inhibition of neutrophil adhesion during cardiopulmonary bypass. Ann Thorac Surg 1994;57:126–133.

118. Girvin J: The use of anencephalic infants for organ procurement. J Heart Lung Transplant 1993;12:S369–S378.

119. Goldbaum LR, Orellano T, Dergel E: Mechanism of the toxic action of carbon monoxide. Am Clin Lab Sci 1976;6:372–376.

120. Goldstein IM, Brai M, Osler AG, Weissmann G: Lysosomal enzyme release from human leukocytes: mediation by the alternative pathway of complement activation. J Immunol 1973;III:33.

121. Goy JJ, Kappenberger TM: Wolff-Parkinson-White syndrome after transplantation of the heart. Br Heart J 1989;61:368–371.

122. Grant JA, Dupree E, Goldman AS, Schultz OR, Jackson AL: Complement-mediated release of histamine from human leukocytes. J Immunol 1975;114:1101.

123. Gryglewski RJ, Palmer RMJ, Moncada S: Superoxide anion is involved in the breakdown of endothelium-derived vascular relaxing factor. Nature 1986;320:454–456.

124. Guest TM, Ramanathan AV, Tuteur PG, Schechtman KB, Ladenson JH, Jaffe AS: Myocardial injury in critically ill patients. A frequently unrecognized complication. JAMA 1995;273:1945.

125. Gundry SR, de Begona JA, Kawauchi M, Bailey LL: Successful transplantation of hearts harvested 30 minutes after death from exsanguination. Ann Thorac Surg 1992;53:772.

126. Gutteridge JMC, Richmond R, Halliwell B: Inhibition of the iron-catalysed formation of hydroxyl radicals from superoxide and of lipid peroxidation by desferrioxamine. Biochem J 1979;184:469–472.

127. Hammond B, Hess ML: The oxygen free radical system: potential mediator of myocardial injury. J Am Coll Cardiol 1985;6:215–220.

128. Hanahan DJ: Platelet-activating factor: a biologically active phosphoglyceride. Annu Rev Biochem 1986;55:483–509.

129. Hansen PR: Role of neutrophils in myocardial ischemia and reperfusion. Circulation 1995;91:1872–1885.

130. Hardesty RL, Griffith BP: Autoperfusion of the heart and lungs for preservation during distant procurement. J Thorac Cardiovasc Surg 1987;93:11.

131. Harlan JM, Callahan KS: Role of hydrogen peroxide in the neutrophil-mediated release of prostacyclin from cultured endothelial cells. J Clin Invest 1984;74:442–448.

132. Hays JH: Thyroid disease. *In* Zaloga G (ed): Problems in Critical Care, Endocrine Emergencies. Vol 4. Philadelphia: JB Lippincott, 1990, p 325.

133. Henson PM, Johnston RB: Tissue injury in inflammation. J Clin Invest 1987;79:669–674.

134. Hersch C: Electrocardiographic changes in head injury. Circulation 1961;23:853–866.
135. Hess ML, Manson NH: Molecular oxygen: friend and foe. The role of the oxygen free radical system in the calcium paradox, the oxygen paradox and ischemia reperfusion injury. J Mol Cell Cardiol 1984;16:969–985.
136. Hill JH, Ward PA: The phlogistic role of C3 leukotactic fragments in myocardial infarcts of rats. J Exp Med 1971;133:885–900.
137. Holland FW II, Brown PS Jr, Weintraub BD, Clark RE: Cardiopulmonary bypass and thyroid function: a "euthyroid sick syndrome." Ann Thorac Surg 1991;52:791.
138. Horsley V: On the mode of death in cerebral compression and its prevention. Q Med J 1894;2:305–309.
139. Houyel L, Petit J, Nottin R, Duffet JP, Macé L, Neveux JY: Adult heart transplantation: adverse role of chronic alcoholism in donors on early graft function. J Heart Lung Transplant 1992;11:1184–1187.
140. Hsieh H, Yu TJ, Yang WC, Chu SS, Lai MK: The gift of life from prisoners sentenced to death: preliminary report. Transplant Proc 1992;24:1335–1336.
141. Huber AR, Kunkel SL, Todd RF III, Weiss SJ: Regulation of transendothelial neutrophil migration by endogenous interleukin-8. Science 1991;250:99–102.
142. Hugli T: Chemical aspects of the serum anaphylatoxins. Contempo Top Mol Immunol 1978;7:181.
143. Hunt LP, Short CD, Mallick NP: Prognostic indicators in patients presenting with the nephrotic syndrome. Kidney Int 1988;34:382.
144. Hyslop PA, Hinshaw DB, Halsey WA, Schraufstatter IU, Sauerheber RD, Spragg RG, Jackson JH, Cochrane CG: Mechanisms of oxidant-mediated cell injury: the glycolytic and mitochondrial pathways of ADP phosphorylation are major intracellular targets inactivated by hydrogen peroxide. J Biol Chem 1988;263:1665–1675.
145. Illes RW, Asimakis GK, Inners-McBride K, Buckingham ED: Donor management and organ distribution: recovery of nonbeating donor hearts. J Heart Lung Transplant 1995;14:553.
146. Inesi G, Millman M, Eletr S: Temperature-induced transitions of function and structure in sarcoplasmic reticulum membranes. J Mol Biol 1973;81:483–504.
147. Isner JM, Chokshi SK: Cardiovascular complications of cocaine. Curr Probl Cardiol 1991;16:89.
148. Janoff A: Elastase in tissue injury. Annu Rev Med 1985;36:207–216.
149. Jeevanandam V, Barr ML, Auteri JS, Sanchez JA, Fong J, Schenkel FA, Marboe CC, Michler RE, Smith CR, Rose EA: University of Wisconsin solution versus crystalloid cardioplegia for human donor heart preservation. J Thorac Cardiovasc Surg 1992;103:194–199.
150. Jeevanandam V, Todd B, Regillo T, Hellman S, Eldridge C, McClurken J: Reversal of donor myocardial dysfunction by triiodothyronine replacement therapy. J Heart Lung Transplant 1994;13:681.
151. Josué O: Hypertrophie cardiaque causee par l'adrenaline et la toxine typhique. C R Soc Biol (Paris) 1807;63:285–287.
152. Jouvett M: Diganostic électro-sousscorticographique de la mort du système nerveux central au cours de certains comas. Electroencephalogr Clin Neurophysiol 1959;II:805–808.
153. Julicher RHM, Tijburg LBM, Sterrenberg L, Bast A, Koomen JM, Noordhoek J: Decreased defence against free radicals in rat heart during normal reperfusion after hypoxic, ischemic and calcium-free perfusion. Life Sci 1984;35:1281–1288.
154. Kako KJ: Free radical effects on membrane protein in myocardial ischemia/reperfusion injury. J Mol Cell Cardiol 1987;19:209–211.
155. Karin M: Signal transduction from cell surface to nucleus in development and disease. FASEB J 1992;8:2581–2590.
156. Katz AM, Reuter H: Cellular calcium and cardiac cell death. Am J Cardiol 1979;44:188–190.
157. Keane WF, Kasiske BL, O'Donnell MP, Kim Y: The role of altered lipid metabolism in the progression of renal disease: experimental evidence. Am J Kidney Dis 1991;17(suppl 1):38.
158. Kempsford RD, Hearse DJ: Protection of the immature myocardum during global ischemia: a comparison of four clinical cardioplegic solutions in the rabbit heart. J Thorac Cardiovasc Surg 1989;97:856–863.
159. Kevelaitis E, Mouas C, Menasche P: Poststorage diastolic abnormalities of heart transplants: is vascular dysfunction or myocardial contracture the culprit? J Heart Lung Transplant 1996;15:461–469.
160. Kirklin JK, Neves J, Naftel DC, Digerness SB, Kirklin JW, Blackstone EH: Controlled initial hyperkalemic reperfusion after cardiac transplantation: coronary vascular resistance and blood flow. Ann Thorac Surg 1990;49:625–631.
161. Kirklin JW, Barratt-Boyes BG: Cardiac Surgery. 2nd ed. New York: Churchill Livingstone, 1993.
162. Kirklin JW, Digerness SB, Fontan FM, Kirklin JK: Controlled aortic root reperfusion in cardiac surgery. Semin Thorac Cardiovasc Surg 1993;5:134–140.
163. Kishiamako TK, Jutila MA, Berg EL, Butcher EC: Neutrophil Mac-1 and MEL-14 adhesion proteins inversely regulated by chemotactic factors. Science 1989;245:1238–1241.
164. Kramer JH, Arroyo CM, Dickens BF, Weglicki WB: Spin-trapping evidence that graded myocardial ischemia alters post-ischemic superoxide production. Free Radic Biol Med 1987;3:153–159.
165. Kuo P, Monaco AP: Chronic rejection and suboptimal immunosuppression. Transplant Poc 1993;25:2082.
166. Kupari M, Koskinen P, Suokas A, Ventila M: Left ventricular filling impairment in asymptomatic chronic alcoholics. Am J Cardiol 1990;66:1473–1477.
167. Laks H, Scholl FG, Drinkwater DC, Blitz A, Hamilton M, Moriguchi J, Fonarrow G, Kobashigawa J: The alternate recipient list for heart transplantation: does it work? J Heart Lung Transplant 1997;16:735–742.
168. Lange RA, Cogarroa RG, Yancy CW, Willard JE, Popma JJ, Sills MN, McBride W, Kim AS, Hillis LD: Cocaine-induced coronary artery vasoconstriction. N Engl J Med 1989;321:1557–1562.
169. Lazar HL, Buckberg GD, Manganaro AM, Becker H: Myocardial energy replenishment of secondary blood cardioplegic with amino acids during reperfusion. J Thorac Crdiovasc Surg 1980;80:350.
170. Lazar HL, Buckberg GD, Manganaro AM, Becker H, Maloney JV Jr: Reversal of ischemic damage with amino acid substrate enhancement during reperfusion. Surgery 1980;80:702.
171. Lazar HL, Buckberg GD, Manganaro A, Becker H, Mulder DG, Maloney JV Jr: Limitation imposed by hypothermia during recovery from ischemia. Surg Forum 1980;31:312.
172. Lee CC, Aruny JE, Laurence RG, Appleyard RF, Couper GS, Cohn LH: Bench coronary angiography: a potentially useful method to assess coronary artery disease in the older donor heart without catheterization laboratory angiography. J Heart Lung Transplant 1992;11:693–697.
173. Lee LK, Meyer TW, Pollock AS, Lovett DH: Endothelial cell injury initiates glomerula sclerosis in the rat remnant kidney. J Clin Invest 1995;96:953.
174. Lee J, Drinkwater DC Jr, Laks H, Chong A, Blitz A, Chen MA, Ignarro LJ, Chang P: Preservation of endothelium-dependent vasodilation with low-potassium University of Wisconsin solution. J Thorac Cardiovasc Surg 1996;112:103–110.
175. Lefer AM, Tsao PS, Lefer DJ, Ma XL: Role of endothelial dysfunction in the pathogenesis of reperfusion injury after myocardial ischemia. FASEB J 1991;5:2029–2034.
176. Lindbergh CA: An apparatus for the culture of whole organs. J Exp Med 1935;62:409.
177. Lorant DE, Patel KD, McIntyre TM, McEver RP, Prewscott SM, Zimmerman GA: Coexpression of GMP-140 and PAF by endothelium stimulated by histamine or thrombin: a juxtacrine system for adhesion and activation of neutrophils. J Cell Biol 1991;115:223–234.
178. Luscher TF: Vascular biology of coronary artery bypass grafts. J Coronary Artery Dis 1992;3:157–165.
179. Ma X, Weyrich AS, Lefer DJ, Lefer AM: Diminished basal nitric oxide release after myocardial ischemia and reperfusion promotes neutrophil adherence to coronary endothelium. Circ Res 1993;72:403–412.
180. Macoviak JA, McDougall IR, Bayer MF, Brown M, Tazelaar H, Stinson EB: Significance of thyroid dysfunction in human cardiac allograft procurement. Transplantation 1987;43:824.
181. Madsden M: The low T3 state, an experimental study. Medical dissertations. No. 229, Linkoping University, Sweden, 1986; cited in Novitzky D: Heart transplantation, euthyroid sick syndrome,

and triiodothyronine replacement. J Heart Lung Transplant 1992;11:S196.

182. Magnuson DK, Maier RV, Pohlman TH: Proetein kinase C: a potential pathway of endothelial cell activation by endotoxin, tumor necrosis factor, and interleukin-1. Surgery 1989;106:216–223.

183. Mainardi CL, Hasty DL, Seyer JM, Kang AH: Specific cleavage of human type III collagen by human polymorphonuclear leukocyte elastase. J Biol Chem 1980;255:12006–12010.

184. Mankad PS, Chester AH, Yacoub MH: Role of potassium concentration in cardioplegic solutions in mediating endothelial damage. Ann Thorac Surg 1991;51:89–93.

185. Mariot J, Jacob F, Voltz C, Perrioer JF, Strub P: Hormonal therapy in human brain-dead potential organ donors: comparative study. Anesthesiology 1990;73:A246.

186. Marks RM, Todd RF III, Ward PA: Rapid induction of neutrophil-endothelial adhesion by complement fixation. Nature 1989;339:314–317.

187. Maroko PR, Carpenter CB, Chiariello M, Fishbein MC, Radvany P, Knostman JD, Hale SL: Reduction by cobra venom factor of myocardial necrosis after coronary artery occlusion. J Clin Invest 1978;61:661–670.

188. Maruffo CA: Fine structural study of myocardial changes induced by isoproterenol in rhesus monkeys (Macaca mulatta). Am J Pathol 1967;50:27.

189. Maruyama M, Farber NE, Vercellotti GM, Jacob HS, Gross GJ: Evidence for a role of platelet activating factor in the pathogenesis of irreversible but not reversible myocardial injury after reperfusion in dogs. Am Heart J 1990;120:510–520.

190. Mathew JP, Rinder CS, Tracey JB, Auszura LA, O'Connor T, David E, Smith BR: Acadesine inhibits neutrophil CD11B upregulation in vitro and during in vivo cardiopulmonary bypass. J Thorac Cardiovasc Surg 1995;109:448–456.

191. McEver RP: Leukocyte-endothelial cell interactions. Curr Opin Cell Biol 1992;4:840–849.

192. McMillen MA, Huribal M, Sumpio B: Common pathway of endothelial–leukocyte interaction in shock, ischemia, and reperfusion. Am J Surg 1993;166:557–562.

193. Medearis DN, Holmes LB: On the use of anencephalic infants as organ donors. N Engl J Med 1989;321:391–393.

194. Meerson FZ, Kagan VE, Kozlov YP, Belkina LM, Arkhipenko YV: The role of lipid peroxidation in pathogenesis of ischemic damage and the antioxidant protection of the heart. Basic Res Cardiol 1982;77:465–485.

195. Meiser BM, Uberfuhr P, Reichenspurner H, Stang A, Kreuzer E, Reichart B: One heart transplanted successfully twice. J Heart Lung Transplant 1994;13:339.

196. Melville KI, Blum B, Shister HE, Silver MD: Cardiac ischemic changes and arrhythmias induced by hypothalamic stimulation. Am J Cardiol 1963;12:781–791.

197. Menasche P, Grousset C, Gauduel Y, Mouas C, Piwnica A: Maintenance of the myocardial thiol pool by N-acetylcysteine. J Thorac Cardiovasc Surg 1992;103:936–944.

198. Menasche P, Grousset C, Gauduel Y, Piwnica A: A comparative study of free radical scavengers in cardioplegic solution. J Thorac Cardiovasc Surg 1986;92:264–271.

199. Menasche P, Hricak B, Pradier F, Cheav SL, Grousset C, Mouas C, Alberici G, Bloch G, Piwnica A: Efficacy of lactobionate-enriched cardioplegic solution in preserving compliance of cold-stored heart transplants. J Heart Lung Transplant 1993;10:53–61.

200. Menasche P, Piwnica A: Free radicals and myocardial protection: a surgical viewpoint. Ann Thorac Surg 1989;47:939–945.

201. Menasche P, Pradier F, Grousset C, Peynet J, Mouas C, Bloch G, Piwnica A: Improved recovery of heart transplants with a specific kit of preservation solutions. J Thorac Cardiovasc Surg 1993;105:353–363.

202. Menasche P, Pradier F, Peynet J, Grousset C, Mouas C, Bloch G, Piwnica A: Limitation of free radical injury by reduced glutathione: an effective means of improving the recovery of heart transplants. Transplant Proc 1991;23:2440–2442.

203. Menasche P, Termignon JL, Pradier F, Grousset C, Mouas C, Alberici G, Weiss M, Piwnica A, Bloch G: Experimental evaluation of Celsior®, a new heart preservation solution. Eur J Cardiothorac Surg 1994;8:207–213.

204. Meyers CH, D'Amico TA, Peterseim DS, Jayawant AM, Steenbergen C, Sabiston DC, Van Trigt P: Effects of triiodothyronine and vasopressin on cardiac function and myocardial blood flow after brain death. J Heart Lung Transplant 1991;12:68.

205. Minek ME, Kaufman HH, Graham SH, Haar FB: Disseminated intravascular coagulation fibrinolytic syndrome following head injury in children: frequency and prognostic implications. J Pediatr 1982;100:687.

206. Mohandas A, Chou SN: Brain death—a clinical and pathological study. J Neurosurg 1971;35:211–218.

207. Mollaret P, Goulon M: Le coma dépassé (mémoire préliminaire). Rev Neurol 1959;101:3–15.

208. Montgomery KF, Osborn L, Hession C, Tizard R, Goff D, Vassallo C, Tarr PI, Bomsztyk K, Lobb R, Harlan JM, Pohlman TH: Activation of endothelial-leukocyte adhesion molecule 1 (ELAM-1) gene transcription. Proc Natl Acad Sci U S A 1991;88:6523–6527.

209. Moorhouse PC, Grootveld M, Halliwell B, Quinlan JG, Gutteridge JMC: Allopurinol and oxypurinol are hydroxyl radical scavengers. FEBS Lett 1987;213:23.

210. Morita K, Ihnken K, Buckberg GD, Sherman MP, Young HH: Studies of hypoxemic/reoxygenation injury: without aortic clamping. J Thorac Cardiovasc Surg 1995;110:1190–1199.

211. Muhlbert J, Wagner W, Rohling R, Link J, Neumayer HH: Hemodynamic and metabolic problems in the preparation for organ donation. Transplant Proc 1987;18:391.

212. Muxfeldt M, Schaper W: The activity of xanthine oxidase in heart and liver of rats, guinea pigs, pigs, rabbit, and human beings [abstract]. Circulation 1987;76(suppl 4):198.

213. Meyers CH, D'Amico TA, Peterseim DS, Jayawant AM, Steenbergen C, Sabiston DC, Van Trigt P: Effects of triiodothyronine and vasopressin on cardiac function and myocardial blood flow after brain death. J Heart Lung Transplant 1993;12:68.

214. Najarian JS, Gillingham KJ, Sutherland DE, Reinsmoen NL, Payne WD, Matas AJ: The impact of the quality of initial graft function on cadaver kidney transplants. Transplantation 1994;57:812.

215. Nayler WG: The role of calcium in the ischemic myocardium. Am J Pathol 1981;102:262–270.

216. Nicolini FA, Mehta JL, Nichols WW, Donnelly WH, Luostarinen R, Saldeen TGP: Leukocyte elastase inhibition and t-PA-induced coronary artery thrombosis in dogs: beneficial effects on myocardial histology. Am Heart J 1991;122:1245–1251.

217. Novitzky D: Change from aerobic anaerobic metabolism after brain death, and reversal following triiodothyronine therapy. Transplantation 1988;45:32.

218. Novitzky D, Cooper DKC, Morrell D, Isaacs S: Brain death, triiodothyronine depletion, inhibition of oxidative phosphorylation; relevance to management of organ donors. Transplant Proc 1987;19:4110.

219. Novitzky D, Cooper DKC, Reichart B: Hemodynamic and metabolic responses to hormonal therapy in brain-dead potential organ donors. Transplantation 1987;43:852.

220. Novitzky D, Cooper DKC, Swanepoel A: Inotropic effect of triiodothyronine (T3) in low cardiac output following cardioplegic arrest and cardiopulmonary bypass: an initial experience in patients undergoing open heart surgery. Eur J Cardiothorac Surg 1989;3:140.

221. Novitzky D, Wicomb WN, Cooper DKC, Rose AG, Fraser RC, Barnard CN: Electrocardiographic, hemodynamic & endocrine changes occurring during experimental brain death in the chacma baboon. Heart Transplant 1984;4:63–69.

222. Novitzky D, Wicomb WN, Cooper DKC, Rose AG, Reichart B: Prevention of myocardial injury during brain death by total cardiac sympathectomy in the chacma baboon. Ann Thorac Surg 1986;41:520–524.

223. Novitzky D, Wicomb WN, Cooper DKC, Tjaalgard MA: Improved cardiac function following hormonal therapy in brain dead pigs: relevance to organ donation. Cryobiology 1987;24:1–10.

224. Oaks TE, Aravot D, Dennis C, Wells FC, Large SR, Wallwork J: Domino heart transplantation: the Papworth experience. J Heart Lung Transplant 1994;13:433–437.

225. Ohtaki A, Ogiwara H, Sakata K, Takahashi T, Morishita Y: Long-term heart preservation by the combined method of simple immersion and coronary perfusion. J Heart Lung Transplant 1996;15:269–274.

226. Okamoto F, Allen BS, Buckberg GD, Bugi H, Leaf J: Studies of controlled reperfusion after ischemia. XIV. Reperfusion conditions: importance of ensuring gentle versus sudden reperfusion during relief of coronary occlusion. J Thorac Cardiovasc Surg 1986;92:613.

227. Okouchi Y, Shimizu K, Yamaguchi A, Kamada N: Effectiveness of modified University of Wisconsin solution for heart preservation as assessed in heterotopic rat heart transplant model. J Thorac Cardiovasc Surg 1990;99:1104–1108.

228. Olbricht CJ, Cannon JK, Garg LC, Tisher CC: Activities of cathepsins B and L in isolated nephron segments from proteinuric and nonproteinuric rats. Am J Physiol 1986;250:F1055.

229. Ollitrault J, Daubert JC, Ramee MP, Ritter P, Mabo P, Leguerrier A, Rioux C, Logeais Y: Wolff-Parkinson-White syndrome in a case of acute rejection of cardiac transplantation. Arch Mal Coeur 1990;83:1603–1606.

230. Omnibus Budget Reconciliation Act of 1986, P.L. No. 99-509, Sec 9318, 100 stat 2009, (42 U.S.C. sec. 1320 6-8, 1986) contained the "Required Request" provision, which made Medicare/Medicaid funds contingent upon the hospital establishing a required request protocol.

231. Ott GY, Herschberger RE, Ratkovek RR, Norman D, Hosenpud JD, Cobanoglu A: Cardiac allografts from high-risk donors: excellent clinical results. Ann Thorac Surg 1994;57:76.

232. Ott GY, Norman DJ, Hosenpud JD, Hershberger RE, Ratkovec RM, Cobanoglu A: Heart transplantation in patients with previous cardiac operations. Excellent clinical results. J Thor Cardiovasc Surg 1994;107:203–209.

233. Ouriel K, Ginsburg ME, Patti CS, Pearce FJ, Hicks GL: Preservation of myocardial function with mannitol reperfusate. Circulation 1985;72(suppl 2):254–258.

234. Ouyang P, Becker LCJ, Effron MB, Herskowitz A, Weisfeldt ML: Hemodynamic vascular forces contribute to impaired endothelium-dependent vasodilation in reperfused canine epicardial coronary arteries. J Am Coll Cardiol 1994;23:1216–1223.

235. Pallis C: Brainstem death: the evolution of a concept. In Morris PJ (ed): Kidney Transplantation. London: Grune & Stratton, 1984.

236. Park CH, Maack T: Albumin absorption and catabolism by isolated perfused proximal convoluted tubules of the rabbit. J Clin Invest 1984;73:767.

237. Parry J: Organ donation after execution in Taiwan. BMJ 1991; 303:1420.

238. Paschen U, Muller MJ, Darup J, Kalmer P, Seitz JH: Alteration in the thyroid hormone concentration during and after coronary bypass operation. Ann Endocrinol (Paris) 1983;44:239.

239. Pasic M, Gallino A, Carrel T, Maggiorini M, Laske A, von Segesser L, Turina M: Brief report: reuse of a transplanted heart. N Engl J Med 1993;328:319.

240. Patel KD, Zimmerman GA, Prescott SM, McEver RP, McIntyre TM: Oxygen radicals induce human endothelial cells to express GMP-140 and bind neutrophils. J Cell Biol 1991:112:749–759.

241. Peabody JL, Emery JR, Ashwal S: Experience with anencephalic infants as prospective organ donors. N Engl J Med 1989;321: 344–350.

242. Perez HD, Ohtani O, Banda D, Ong R, Fukuyama K, Goldstein IM: Generation of biologically active complement-(C5) derived peptides by cathepsin H1. J Immunol 1983;131:397–402.

243. Pernot AN, Ingwall JS, Menasche P, Grousset C, Bercot M, Mollet M, Piwnica A, Fossel ET: Limitations of potassium cardioplegia during cardiac ischemic arrest: a phosphorus 31 nuclear magnetic resonance study. Ann Thorac Surg 1981;32:536–545.

244. Peterson JC, Adler S, Burkart JM, Green T, Hebert LA, Hunsicker LG, King AJ, Klahr S, Massry SH, Seifter JL: Blood pressure control, proteinuria, and the progression of renal disease: the modification of diet in renal disease study. Ann Intern Med 1995;123:754.

245. Pietri S, Culcash M, Albat B, Alberii G, Menasche P: Direct assessment of the antioxidant effects of a new heart preservation Solution, Celsior. Transplantation 1994;6:739–742.

246. Pisarenko OI, Portnoy VF, Studneva IM, Arapov AD, Korostylev AN: Glutamate-blood cardioplegia improves ATP preservation in human myocardium. Biomed Biochim Acta 1987;46:499–504.

247. Pober JS, Bevilacqua MP, Mendrick DL, Lapierre LA, Fiers W, Gimbrone MA: Two distinct monokines, interleukin-1 and tumor necrosis factor, each independently induce biosynthesis and tran-

248. Pool Wilson PA, Harding DP, Bourdillon PDV, Tones MA: Calcium out of control. J Mol Cell Cardiol 1984;16:175–187.

249. Pope John Paul II: Address of The Holy Father to the Participants of The Society for Organ Sharing. Transplant Proc 1991;23: xvii-xviii.

250. Pope Pius XII: Replies to some important questions concerning reanimation. In Wolstenhome GEW, O'Connor M (eds): Ethics in Medical Progress: With Special Reference to Transplantation. London: J & A Churchill, 1966.

251. Powner DJ, Hendrich A, Lagler RG, Ng RH, Madden RL: Hormonal changes in brain dead patients. Crit Care Med 1990;18:702.

252. Powner DJ, Hendrich A, Nyhuis A, Strate R: Changes in serum catecholamine levels in patients who are brain dead. J Heart Lung Transplant 1992;11:1046–1053.

253. Prescott LF, Illingworth RN, Critchley JAJH, Stewart MJ, Adam RD, Proudfoot AD: Intravenous N-acetylcysteine, the treatment of choice for paracetamol poisoning. BMJ 1979;2:1097–1100.

254. President's Commission for the Study of Ethical Problems in Medicine and Biomedical and Behavioral Research. Defining Death: A Report on the Medical, Legal, and Ethical Issues in the Determination of Death. Washington, DC: US Government Printing Office, 1981, pp 1–66.

255. President's Commission for the Study of Ethical Problems in Medicine and Biomedical and Behavioral Research: Guidelines for the Determination of Death. Special Communication. JAMA 1981;246:2184–2186.

256. Przyklenk K, Whittaker P, Kloner RA: Direct evidence that oxygen free radicals cause contractile dysfunction in vivo. Circulation 1988;78(suppl II):II-264.

257. Puszkin S, Rubin E: Adenosine diphosphate effect on contractility of human muscle actomyosin: inhibition by ethanol and acetaldehyde. Science 1975;188:1319–1320.

258. Rao PS: Production of free radicals and lipid peroxides in early experimental myocardial ischemia. J Mol Cell Cardiol 1983;10: 713–716.

259. Rajs J, Jakofsson S: Severe trauma and subsequent cardiac lesion causing heart failure and death. Forensic Sci 1976;8:13–21.

260. Randell TT, Hockerstedt KAV: Triiodothyronine treatment is not indicated in brain-dead multiorgan donors; a controlled study. Transplant Proc 1993;25:1552.

261. Reigner J, Mazmanian M, Chapelier A, Alberici G, Menasche P, Weiss M, Herve P, and the Paris-Sud University Lung Transplantation Group: Evaluation of a new preservation solution: Celsior in the isolated rat lung. J Heart Lung Transplant 1995;14: 601–604.

262. Report of Special Task Force: Guidelines for the determination of brain death in children. Pediatrics 1987;80:298–300.

263. Rice CE, Munro JM, Corless C, Bevilacqua MP: Vascular and nonvascular expression of INCAM-110: a target for mononuclear leukocyte adhesion in normal and inflamed human tissue. Am J Pathol 1991;138:385–393.

264. Roach MK: Changes in the activity of Na+K+ -ATPase during acute and chronic administration of ethanol. In Majchrowicz E, Noble EP (eds): Biochemistry and Pharmacology of Ethanol. Vol 2. New York, Plenum Press, 1979, pp 67–80.

265. Robicsek F, Masters TN, Duncan GD, Denyer MH, Rise HE, Etchison M: An autoperfused heart lung preparation: metabolism and function. J Heart Transplant 1985;4:333.

266. Robiscek F, Masters TN, Thomley AM, Rice HE, Morales-Reyna J: Bench coronary cineangiography: a possible way to increase the number of hearts available for transplantation. J Thorac Cardiovasc Surg 1992;103:490–495.

267. Rodeheffer FJ, Naftel DC, Stevenson LW, Porter CB, Young JB, Miller LW, Kenzora JL, Haas GJ, Kirklin JK, Bourge RC: Secular trends in cardiac transplant recipient and donor management in the United States, 1990 to 1994: a multiinstitutional study. Circulation 1996;94:2883.

268. Romaschin AD, Rebeyka I, Wilson GJ, Mickle DAG: Conjugated dienes in ischemic and reperfused myocardium: an in vivo chemical signature of oxygen free radical mediated injury. J Mol Cell Cardiol 1987;19:289–302.

269. Romson JL, Hook BG, Kunkel SL, Abrams GD, Schork MA, Lucchesi BR: Reduction of the extent of ischaemic myocardial injury

by neutrophil depletion in the dog. Circulation 1983;67:1016–1023.

270. Rongione AJ, Steg PG, Gal D, Isner JM: Cocaine causes endothelium-independent vasoconstriction of vascular smooth muscle [abstract]. Circulation 1988;78:II-436.

271. Rosenkranz ER, Okamoto F, Buckberg GD, Vinten-Johansen J, Edwards H, Bugyi H: Advantages of glutamate-enriched cold blood cardioplegia in energy-depleted hearts. Circulation 1982;66(suppl II):11–151.

272. Rosenkranz ER, Okamoto F, Buckberg GD, Vinten-Johansen J, Robertson JM, Bugyi H: Safety of prolonged aortic clamping with blood cardioplegia. II. Glutamate enrichment in energy-depleted hearts. J Thorac Cardiovasc Surg 1984;88:402.

273. Rosner MJ, Newsome HH, Becker DP: Mechanical brain injury: the sympathoadrenal response. J Neurosurg 1984;61:76–86.

274. Ross R, Glomset JA: Atherosclerosis and arterial smooth muscle cell science. Science 1973;180:1332–1339.

275. Rossen RD, Michael LH, Kagiyama A, Savage HE, Hanson G, Reisberg MA, Moake JN, Kim SH, Self D, Weakley S, Giannini E, Entman ML: Mechanism of complement activation after coronary artery occlusion: evidence that myocardial ischemia in dogs causes release of constituents of myocardial subcellular origin that complex with human C1q in vivo. Circ Res 1988;62:572–584.

276. Rot A: Endothelial cell binding of NAP-1/IL-8:role in neutrophil emigration. Immunol Today 1992;13:291–294.

277. Roth E, Torok B, Zsoldos T, Matkowics B: Lipid peroxidation and scavenger mechanism in experimentally induced heart infarcts. Basic Res Cardiol 1985;80:530–536.

278. Rothman SA, Hsia HH, Bove AA, Jeevanandam V, Miller JM: Radiofrequency ablation of Wolff-Parkinson-White syndrome in a donor heart after orthotopic heart transplantation. J Heart Lung Transplant 1994;13:905–909.

279. Rubanyi GM, Vanhoutte PM: Superoxide anions and hyperoxia inactivate endothelium-derived relaxing factor. Am J Physiol 1986;2250:H822–H827.

280. Rubin E: Alcoholic myopathy in heart and skeletal muscle. N Engl J Med 1979;301:28–33.

281. Saldanha C, Hearse DJ: Coronary vascular responsiveness to 5-hydroxytryptamine before and after infusion of hyperkalemic crystalloid cardioplegic solution in the rat heart: possible evidence of endothelial damage. J Thorac Cardiovasc Surg 1998;98:783–787.

282. Salter DR, Dyke CM, Wechsler AS: Triiodothyronine (T3) and cardiovascular therapeutics: a review. J Cardiol Surg 1992;7:363.

283. Samuels MA: Neurogenic heart disease: a unifying hypothesis. Am J Cardiol 1987;60:15J–19J.

284. Sarma JS, Ikeda S, Fischer R, Maruyama Y, Weishaar R, Bing RJ: Biochemical and contractile properties of heart muscle after prolonged alcohol administration. J Mol Cell Cardiol 1976;8:951–972.

285. Sasaki K, Ueno A, Katori M, Kikawada R: Detection of leukotriene B4 in cardiac tissue and its role in infarct extension through leukocyte migration. Cardiovasc Res 1988;22:142–148.

286. Sawatari K, Kadoba K, Bergner KA, Mayer JE Jr: Influence of initial reperfusion pressure after hypothermic cardioplegic ischemia on endothelial modulation of coronary tone in neonatal lambs: impaired coronary vasodilator response to acetylcholine. J Thorac Cardiovasc Surg 1991;101:777.

287. Schlumpf R, Weber M, Weinreich T, Klotz H, Zollinger A, Candinas D: Transplantation of kidneys from non-heart-beating donors: an update. Transplant Proc 1995;27:2942.

288. Schreiber SS, Reff F, Evans CD, Rothschild MA, Oratz M: Prolonged feeding of ethanol to the young growing guinea pig. III. Effect on the synthesis of the myocardial contractile proteins. Alcoholism 1986;10:531–534.

289. Serhan CN, Radin A, Smolen E: Leukotriene B4 is a complete secretagogue in human neutrophils: a kinetic analysis. Biochem Biophys Res Commun 1982;107:1006–1012.

290. Sessa WC, Kaw S, Hecker M, Vane JR: The biosynthesis of endothelin-1 by human polymorphonuclear leukocytes. Biochem Biophys Res Commun 1991;174:613–618.

291. Sethi GK, Lanauze P, Rosado LJ, Huston C, McCarthy MS, Butman S, Copeland JG: Clinical significance of weight difference between donor and recipient in heart transplantation. J Thorac Cardiovasc Surg 1993;106:444.

292. Shewmon DA, Capron AM, Peacock WJ, Schulman BL: The use of anencephalic infants as organ sources. JAMA 1989;261:1773–1781.

293. Shimada Y, Yamamoto F, Yamamoto H, Oka T, Kawashima Y: Temperature-dependent cardioprotection of exogenous substrates in long-term heart preservation with continuous perfusion: twenty four hour preservation of isolated rat heart with St. Thomas' Hospital solution containing glucose, insulin, and aspartate. J Heart Lung Transplant 1996;15:485–495.

294. Shingu M, Nobunaga M: Chemotactic activity generated in human serum from the fifth component on hydrogen peroxide. Am J Pathol 1984;117:201–206.

295. Simonson MS, Dunn MJ: Cellular signaling by peptides of the endothelin gene family. FASEB J 1990;4:2989–3000.

296. Singal PK, Dhillon KS, Beamish RK, Napur N, Dhalla NS: Myocardial cell damage and cardiovascular changes due to IV infusion of adrenochrome in rats. Br J Exp Pathol 1982;63:167–176.

297. Smith JA, Bergin PJ, Williams TJ, Esmore DS: Successful heart transplantation with cardiac allografts exposed to carbon monoxide poisoning. J Heart Lung Transplant 1992;11:698–700.

298. Soblosky JS, Rogers NL, Adams JA, Farrell JB, Davidson JF, Carey ME: Central and peripheral biogenic amine effects of brain missile wounding and increased intracranial pressure. J Neurosurg 1992;76:119–126.

299. Soifer BE, Gelb AW: The multiple organ donor: identification and management. Ann Intern Med 1989;110:814.

300. Spodick DH, Pigott VM, Chirife R: Preclinical cardiac malfunction in chronic alcoholism. N Engl J Med 1972;287:677–680.

301. Springer TA: Traffic signals for lymphocyte recirculation and leukocyte emigration: the multistep paradigm. Cell 1994;76:301–314.

302. Srivastava SC, Robson AO: Electrocardiographic abnormalities associated with subarachnoid hemorrhage. Lancet 1964;2:431–433.

303. Statement of Amnesty International USA: On the Harvesting of Organs from Executed Prisoners in The People's Republic of China. May 1995.

304. Steenbergen C, Murphy E, Watts JA, London RE: Correlation between cytosolic free calcium, contracture, ATP, and irreversible ischemic injury in perfused rat heart. Circ Res 1990;66:1135–1146.

305. Stein DG, Drinkwater DC, Laks H, Permut LC, Sangwan S, Chait HI, Child JS, Bhuta S: Cardiac preservation in patients undergoing transplantation. J Thorac Cardiovasc Surg 1991;102:657–665.

306. Stern S, Lavy S, Carmon A, Herishianu Y: Electrocardiographic changes in hemorrhagic stroke. J Neurol Sci 1968;8:61–67.

307. Stoddard MF, Longaker RA: The role of transesophageal echocardiography in cardiac donor screening. Am Heart J 1993;125:1676.

308. Strieter RM, Kunkel SL, Showell HJ, Remick DG, Phan SH, Ward PA, Marks RM: Endothelial cell gene expression of a neutrophil chemotactic factor by TNF, LPS, and IL-1. Science 1989;243:1467–1469.

309. Swanson DK, Pasaoglu I, Berkoff HA, Southard JA, Hegge JO: Improved heart preservation with UW preservation solution. J Heart Lung Transplant 1988;7:456–467.

310. Tada M, Shigekawa M, Nimura Y: Uptake of calcium by the sarcoplasmic reticulum and its regulation and functional consequences. *In* Speerelakis N (ed): Physiology and Pathophysiology of the Heart. Boston: Kluwer Publishers, 1984, pp 255–277.

311. Takagaki M, Hisamochi K, Morimoto T, Bando K, Sano S, Shimizu N: Successful transplantation of cadaver hearts harvested one hour after hypoxic cardiac arrest. J Heart Lung Transplant 1996;15:527.

312. Takkenberg JJM, Wang HM, Trento A, Popov A, Freimark D, Eghbali K, Wang CHK, Blanche C, Czer LSC: The effect of chronic alcohol use on the heart before and after transplantation in an experimental model in the rat. J Heart Lung Transplant 1997;16:939–945.

313. Taniguchi S, Kitamura S, Kawachi K, Dou Y, Aoyama N: Effects of hormonal supplements on the maintenance of cardiac function in potential donor patients after cerebral death. Eur J Cardiothorac Surg 1992;6:96.

314. Thanos D, Maniatis T: NF-kB; a lesson in family values. Cell 1995;80:529–532.

315. Thomason DJ, Kostuk W, Pflugfelder P, Menkis A, McKenzie FN: De novo coronary artery grafting in a heart transplant recipient. J Heart Lung Transplant 1988:7:468–470.

316. Thompson E, Steinhaus D, Long N, Borkon AM: Preexcitation syndrome in a donor heart. J Heart Transplant 1989;8:177–180.

317. Thompson JA, Hess ML: The oxygen free radical system: a fundamental mechanism in the production of myocardial necrosis. Prog Cardiovasc Dis 1986;6:449–462.

318. Todd GL, Baroldi G, Pieper GM, Clayton FC, Eliot RS: Experimental catecholamine-induced myocardial necrosis I. Morphology, quantification and regional distribution of acute contraction band lesions. J Mol Cell Cardiol 1985;17:317–338.

319. Tokunaga Y, Wicomb WN, Concepcion W, Nakazato P, Collins GM, Esquivel CO: Successful 20-hour rat liver preservation with chlorpromazine in sodium lactobionate sucrose solution. Surgery 1991;110:80–86.

320. Togna G, Tempesta E, Togna AR, Dolci N, Cebo B, Caprino L: Platelet responsiveness and biosynthesis of thromboxane and prostacyclin in response to in vitro cocaine treatment. Hemostasis 1985;15:100.

321. Truog RD, Fletcher JC: Anencephalic newborns. Can organs be transplanted before brain death? N Engl J Med 1989;321:388–391.

322. Turino GM: Effect of carbon monoxide on the cardiorespiratory system. Carbon monoxide toxicity: physiology and biochemistry. Circulation 1981;63:253-259A.

323. Varnell RM, Stimac GK, Fligner CL: CT diagnosis of toxic brain injury in cyanide poisoning: considerations for forensic medicine. Am J Neuroradiol 1987;8:1063.

324. Vogel WM, Briggs LL, Apstein CS: Separation of inherent diastolic myocardial fiber tension and coronary vascular erectile contributions to wall stiffness of rabbit hearts damaged by ischemia, hypoxia, calcium paradox and reperfusion. J Mol Cell Cardiol 1985;17:57–70.

325. Votapka TV, Canvasser DA, Pennington DG, Koga M, Swartz MT: Effect of triiodothyronine on graft function in a model of heart transplantation. Ann Thorac Surg 1996;62:78.

326. Wagner DD: The Weibel Palade body: the storage granule for von Willebrand factor and P-selectin. J Thromb Haemost 1993;70:105–110.

327. Wahlberg JA, Southard JH, Belzer FO: Development of a cold storage solution for pancreas preservation. Cryobiology 1986;23:466–482.

328. Walker JD, Crawford FA, Mukhejee R, Spinale FG: The direct effects of 3,5,3′-triiodo-L-thyronine (T3) on myocyte contractile processes: insights into mechanisms of action. J Thorac Cardiovasc Surg 1995;110:1369.

329. Walker JD, Crawford FA, Spinale FG: Pretreatment with 3.5.3′ triiodo-L-thyronine (T3): effects on myocyte contractile function after hypothermic cardioplegic arrest and rewarming. J Thorac Cardiovasc Surg 1995;110:315.

330. Ward PA, Till GO, Kunkel R, Beauchamp C: Evidence for role of hydroxyl radical in complement and neutrophil dependent tissue injury. J Clin Invest 1983;72:789–801.

331. Wedmore CV, Williams TJ: Control of vascular permeability by polymorphonuclear leukocytes in inflammation. Nature 1981;289:646–650.

332. Weidler DJ: Myocardial damage and cardiac arrhythmias after intracranial hemorrhage. Stroke 1974;5:759–764.

333. Weisman HF, Bartow T, Leppo MK, Marsh HC Jr, Carson GR, Concino MF, Boyle MP, Roux KH, Weisfeld ML, Fearon DT: Soluble human complement receptor type 1: in vivo inhibitor of complement suppressing post-ischemic myocardial inflammation and necrosis. Science 1990;249:146–151.

334. Weiss SJ: Tissue destruction by neutrophils. N Engl J Med 1989;320:365–376.

335. Weldner PW, Myers JL, Miller CA, Arenas JD, Waldhausen JA: Improved recovery of immature myocardium with L-glutamate blood cardioplegia. Ann Thorac Surg 1993;55:102–105.

336. Werns SW, Shea MJ, Lucchesi BR: Free radicals and myocardial injury: pharmacologic implications. J Am Coll Cardiol 1986;74:1–5.

337. Weyrich AS, Ma X-L, Lefer DJ, Albertine KH, Lefer AM: In vivo neutralization of P-selectin protects feline heart and endothelium

338. Wheeldon DR, Potter CDO, Jonas M, Wallwork J, Large SR: Transplantation of ''unsuitable'' organs? Transplant Proc 1993;25:3104.

339. Wheeldon DR, Potter CDO, Oduro A, Wallwork J, Large SR: Donor management and organ distribution: transforming the ''unacceptable'' donor: outcomes from the adoption of a standardized donor management technique. J Heart Lung Transplant 1995;14:734.

340. Whittaker P, Kloner RA, Przyklenk K: In vivo damage by exogenous oxygen radicals mimics ischemia/reperfusion injury. Circulation 1988;78(suppl II):II-30.

341. Wicomb WN, Cooper DKC, Hassoulas J, Rose AG, Barnard CN: Orthotopic transplantation of the baboon heart after 20 to 24 hours preservation by continuous hypothermic perfusion with an oxygenated hyperosmolor solution. J Thorac Cardiovasc Surg 1982;83:133.

342. Wicomb WN, Cooper DKC, Novizky D, Barnard CN: Cardiac transplantation following storage of the donor heart by a portable hypothermic perfusion system. Ann Thorac Surg 1984;37:143.

343. Wicomb WN, Perey R, Portnoy V, Collins GM: The role of reduced glutathione in heart preservation using a polyethylene glycol solution, Cardiosol. Transplantation 1992;54:1181–1182.

344. Wicomb WN, Portnoy VF, Collins GM: In Cooper DKC, Miller LW, Patterson GA (eds): The Transplantation and Replacement of Thoracic Organs. 2nd ed. Boston: Kluwer Publishers, 1996, pp 675–687.

345. Wijnen RMH, Booster MH, Stubenitsky BM, deBoer J, Heineman E, Kootstra G: Outcome of transplantation of non-heart-beating donor kidneys. Lancet 1995;345:1067.

346. Williams JD, Czop JK, Abrahamson DR, Davies M, Austen KF: Activation of the alternative complement pathway by isolated human glomerular basement membrane. J Immunol 1984;133:394.

347. Wilson IC: Leukocyte depletion in a neonatal model of cardiac surgery. Ann Thorac Surg 1993;55:12–19.

348. Wilson IC, Gardner TJ, DiNatale JM, Gillinov AM, Curtis WE, Cameron DE: Temporary leukocyte depletion reduces ventricular dysfunction during prolonged postischemic reperfusion. J Thor Cardiovasc Surg 1993;106:805–810.

349. Wolkowicz PE, Caulfield JB: Cardioplegia with aged UW solution induces loss of cardiac collagen. Transplantation 1991;51:898–901.

350. Wolstenholme GEW, O'Connor M: Ethics in Medical Progress. Ciba Foundation Symposium. London: J & A Churchill, 1966.

351. Yacoub MH, Banner NR, Khaghani A, Fizgerald M, Madden B, Tsang V, Radley-Smith R, Hodson M: Heart-lung transplantation for cystic fibrosis and subsequent domino heart transplantation. J Heart Transplant 1990;9:459–467.

352. Yacoub M, Khaghani A, Aravot D: Cardiac transplantation from live donors [abstract]. Am Coll Cardiol 1988;11:102.

353. Yanagisawa M, Kurihara H, Kimura S, Tomobe Y, Kobayashi M, Mitsui Y, Yazaki Y, Goto K, Masaki T: A novel potent vasoconstrictor peptide produced by vascular endothelial cells. Nature 1988;332:411–415.

354. Yeh T Jr, Hanan SA, Johnson DE, Rebeyka IM, Abd-Elfattah AS, Lee KF, Wechsler AS: Superior myocardial preservation with modified UW solution after prolonged ischemia in the rat heart. Ann Thorac Surg 1990;49:932–939.

355. Yokoyama MD, Cooper DKC, Sasaki H, Snow TR, Akutsu T, Zuhdi N: Donor-heart evaluation by monitoring the left ventricular pressure-volume relationship. Clinical observations. J Heart Lung Transplant 1992;11:685.

356. Young JB, Naftel DC, Bourge RC, Kirklin JK, Clemson BS, Porter CB, Rodeheffer RJ, Kenzora JL: Matching the heart donor and heart transplant recipient. Clues for successful expansion of the donor pool: a multivariable multiinstitutional report. J Heart Lung Transplant 1994;13:353.

357. Zweier JL: Measurement of superoxide-derived free radicals in the reperfused heart: evidence for a free radical mechanism of reperfusion injury. J Biol Chem 1988;263:1353–1357.

358. Zweier JL, Rayburn BR, Flaherty JT, Weisfeldt ML: Recombinant superoxide dismutase reduces oxygen free radical concentration in reperfused myocardium. J Clin Invest 1987;80:1728–1734.

in myocardial ischemia and reperfusion injury. J Clin Invest 1993;91:2620–2629.

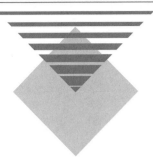

The Heart Transplant Operation

This chapter will describe the surgical details of the cardiac transplant operation. However, some of the operative procedures are discussed in other chapters to facilitate the reader's convenience. The **donor operation** for adult cardiac transplantation is covered in Chapter 9. **Pediatric cardiac transplantation,** including both donor and recipient operations, is discussed in Chapter 20. Both donor and recipient aspects of **combined heart and lung transplantation** are covered in Chapter 21. Implantation of **ventricular assist devices** is considered in Chapter 8.

STANDARD ORTHOTOPIC CARDIAC TRANSPLANTATION

The standard technique of orthotopic cardiac transplantation was developed by Lower and Shumway in their early experimental studies (see Chapter 1).[33,60] Since the original human-to-human heart transplant by Christiaan Barnard in 1967, this technique has remained the primary method of heart transplantation for nearly 30 years.

OPERATIVE TECHNIQUE

In addition to the usual preparations for cardiac operations, a large-gauge triple-lumen catheter is placed through the left internal jugular vein after induction of anesthesia. The right internal jugular vein is left undisturbed if possible to preserve it as access for future endomyocardial biopsies. After endotracheal intubation, a transesophageal echo probe is passed into the esophagus for later monitoring during de-airing maneuvers and assessment of ventricular function. The heart is exposed through a median sternotomy. In the presence of previous cardiac operations, a femoral artery catheter is inserted percutaneously in case acute cardiac decompensation requires insertion of an intra-aortic balloon pump or emergent institution of cardiopulmonary bypass.

When arrival of the donor heart is imminent, cardiopulmonary bypass is established with separate caval cannulation. Additional time is allotted if extensive dissection is necessary. The aorta is cross-clamped and a standard cardiectomy is performed, leaving a cuff of left and right atrium and dividing the great vessels proximally (Fig. 10–1). The great vessels are accurately dissected free one from the other to facilitate the great vessel anastomoses.

The donor heart is removed from its cannister and the fluid from the inner bag is cultured. The roof of the left atrium is dissected free from the posterior aspect of the right and left pulmonary artery segments. The aorta is dissected from the pulmonary artery, which is then divided just proximal to the bifurcation unless additional pulmonary artery is necessary for reconstruction. A cuff of left atrium is created by incising through the pulmonary vein orifices (Fig. 10–2). The right atrium is prepared by incising through the inferior vena caval orifice and extending the incision toward the base of the right atrial appendage approximately equidistant from the sulcus terminalis and the atrioventricular groove (Fig. 10–3).

During implantation, the perfusate temperature is generally 28°C with intermittent topical cooling using 4°C saline. No additional cardioplegic solution is infused. The left atrial anastomosis is constructed first using continuous 3.0 polypropylene (Fig. 10–4). When constructing the left atrial anastomosis, the first few stitches are placed "at a distance" before lowering the

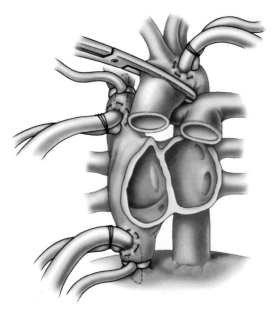

FIGURE **10–1.** Completed recipient cardiectomy in preparation for standard orthotopic transplantation.

donor heart into the pericardial space. The remainder of the entire left atrial anastomosis is constructed in an everting fashion to provide endothelium–to–endothelium apposition, thereby reducing the chance of thrombus formation along the suture line. Construction of the far leftward portion of the anastomosis (along the left pulmonary veins) is often facilitated by retracting the donor ascending aorta inferiorly with a traction suture. The right atrial anastomosis is also constructed with continuous 3.0 polypropylene. In the area over the interatrial septum, the suture lines are partially overlap-

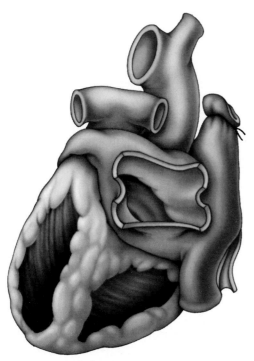

FIGURE **10–2.** Creation of the donor heart left atrial cuff by incising through the pulmonary vein orifices.

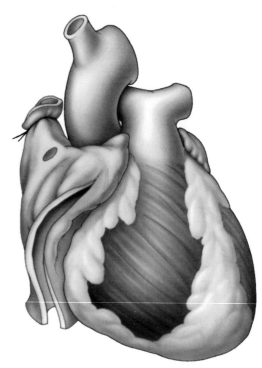

FIGURE **10–3.** Creation of the donor heart right atrial cuff. The incision begins at the orifice of the inferior vena cava and extends toward the right atrial appendage approximately halfway between the sulcus terminalis and the atrioventricular groove.

ping (Fig. 10–5). Each chamber is filled with cold saline before securing the suture lines.

The aortic anastomosis is constructed with continuous 4.0 polypropylene after the donor and native aorta are cut to an appropriate length. A cardioplegia catheter to be used as a "needle vent" for aspirating air is placed in the donor ascending aorta. Air is evacuated from the heart through the aortic suture line and the suture line is secured. The aortic cross-clamp is removed with strong suction on the needle vent. This is a critical period during the operation, since the donor heart is being reperfused after a prolonged period of global ischemia. A detailed discussion of the pathophysiology of reperfusion injury and the management of this stage of reperfusion is found in Chapter 9. In most instances, the donor heart will begin rhythmic contractions within 1–3 minutes of cross-clamp removal. If ventricular fibrillation or tachycardia occurs the heart should be promptly defibrillated. In addition to the maneuvers discussed in Chapter 9 for signs of early reperfusion injury, an esmolol infusion is initiated temporarily if marked sinus tachycardia or frequent ventricular arrhythmias occur during early reperfusion. We believe esmolol is particularly useful in this setting, since it reduces myocardial oxygen consumption when the heart is recovering from the period of ischemia, and its duration of action is very short (and therefore its effects will have dissipated before discontinuation of cardiopulmonary bypass).

When a gentle sinus rhythm is established, preparations are made for the pulmonary artery anastomosis. (Some surgeons prefer to complete this anastomosis before removing the cross-clamp.) The pulmonary artery

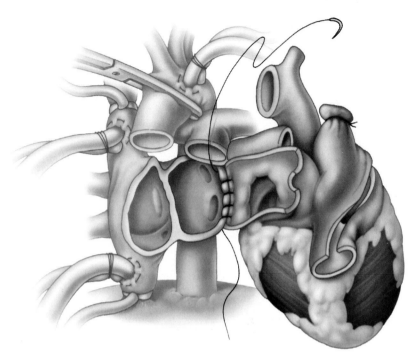

FIGURE **10–4.** Commencement of the left atrial anastomosis.

segments are cut to an appropriate length and the anastomosis is constructed, usually with 5.0 polypropylene (Fig. 10–6).

The remainder of the operation is conducted as usual during rewarming, and cardiopulmonary bypass (CPB) is gradually discontinued after thoroughly debubbling the heart through the aortic needle vent while examining the heart for residual air with transesophageal echocardiography (TEE). Immediately before and after discontinuation of CPB, the function of each ventricle is assessed with TEE and appropriate interventions are made, if necessary, to improve function.

SPECIAL CONSIDERATIONS

In patients with a **previous sternotomy,** particularly with previous bypass surgery, the likelihood of acute, severe, cardiac decompensation is greatly increased if there is inadvertent injury to a patient's saphenous or internal mammary graft. In this situation, routine insertion of a percutaneous femoral artery catheter for arterial pressure monitoring is advantageous. Should decompensation occur, a guidewire for insertion of an intra-aortic balloon pump can be rapidly accomplished or CPB established with a percutaneously inserted arterial

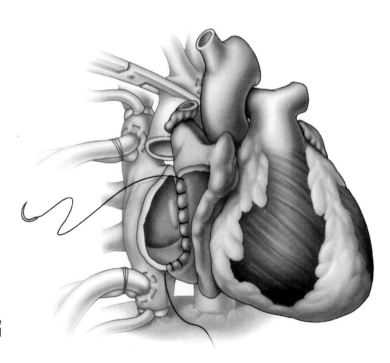

FIGURE **10–5.** Right atrial anastomosis is commenced on the interatrial septum, this suture line overlapping with the atrial septal portion of the left atrial anastomosis.

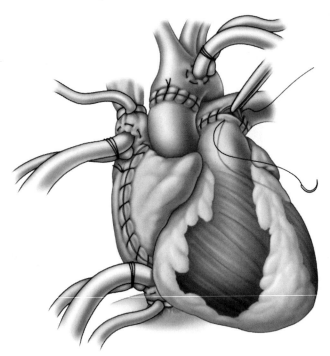

FIGURE **10–6.** Completion of the aortic and pulmonary artery anastomoses.

cannula. In situations in which sternotomy is considered very high risk, a guidewire can also be placed in the femoral vein for percutaneous venous cannulation, if necessary.

In the preparation of every donor heart prior to implantation, the area of the fossa ovalis should be specifically examined. If a **patent foramen ovale** is identified, it must be surgically closed. Failure to do so has resulted in severe hypoxemia and right-to-left shunting early after cardiac transplantation in a situation of right ventricular dysfunction, particularly in the presence of elevated pulmonary artery pressure.[59]

Tricuspid insufficiency detected by Doppler echocardiography is common after standard orthotopic cardiac transplantation. This may relate to the geometry of the newly constructed right atrium, and an association has been suggested between a larger relative size of the donor right atrium and the likelihood of tricuspid insufficiency.[53] Thus, consideration should be given to excising excess right atrial tissue, particularly on the lower side of the anastomosis (without jeopardizing the sinoatrial node). Tricuspid insufficiency as a late complication is discussed in Chapter 18. Less commonly, mitral valve regurgitation has been observed after standard orthotopic transplantation, associated with the "snowman" configuration formed by the donor–recipient left atrial anastomosis.[61]

During construction of the left atrial suture line, the **orifice of the left pulmonary vein** should be observed. Excessive protrusion of tissue in the suture line with an inverting technique can potentially obstruct pulmonary venous inflow (and may also be thrombogenic). In extreme cases, surgically induced cor triatriatum secondary to anastomotic obstruction of pulmonary venous inlet has been reported.[11]

Sinus node dysfunction occasionally occurs after standard orthotopic cardiac transplantation (see Chapter 12). Therefore, specific attention to avoiding damage to the sinoatrial node is important during harvesting and implantation. The ligature on the superior vena cava should be placed 1–2 cm above the superior vena cava–right atrial junction. The incision in the donor right atrium should be kept well above the sulcus terminalis to avoid damage to the sinoatrial node during construction of the lower right atrial suture line.

Kinking of the **main pulmonary artery** may occur if the length of the newly constructed pulmonary artery is redundant.[66] Therefore, care must be taken to trim sufficient donor and recipient main pulmonary artery to avoid redundancy after construction of the anastomosis. The newly constructed main pulmonary artery is particularly vulnerable with an oversized heart relative to the size of the recipient pericardial space. Redundancy which results in kinking of the main pulmonary artery can produce an important gradient across the pulmonary artery anastomosis with resultant severe right ventricular hypertension.

Adverse **neurological events** after orthotopic cardiac transplants are uncommon,[25] but may be affected by the technique of implantation. Mural thrombus may be potentiated by an excessively inverting suture line, particularly in the left atrium. Effective and complete de-airing of the heart is extremely important in order to minimize the risk of cerebral air embolism. When systemic vascular resistance is very low following implantation of the heart, flow rates during cardiopulmonary bypass must be adequate. Although the precise level of perfusion pressure and flow rate which contribute to neurologic events has not been clearly defined, we attempt to maintain a systemic mean perfusion pressure of 40 mm Hg or greater during rewarming with perfusion flow rates of 2.5 L/min/m^2 in pediatric patients and 4.2–4.5 L/min in adult patients.

In the presence of important **right ventricular dysfunction** during rewarming, a second left atrial catheter is placed for infusion of inotropic agents,[7] and prostaglandin E_1 and other vasodilator agents can be infused into the central venous line. If this is not successful and pulmonary hypertension is present, nitric oxide[7, 29, 65] can be employed as an inhalational agent. A detailed discussion of inotropic and vasodilator agents for the management of early right and left ventricular dysfunction is found in Chapter 12.

ORTHOTOPIC CARDIAC TRANSPLANTATION WITH BICAVAL TECHNIQUE

Although used experimentally in the early era of experimental cardiac transplantation, the bicaval anastomotic technique was not described clinically until 1991 with the report of Dreyfus and colleagues.[20] Subsequently, several studies have identified abnormal atrial contribution to ventricular filling,[62] tricuspid insufficiency,[28] and mitral insufficiency with the standard orthotopic technique, which may be reduced with the bicaval method.[12, 13, 22, 54] At the University of Alabama at Birmingham (UAB), the bicaval technique is currently the method of choice except in small infants and children.

After initiating cardiopulmonary bypass, the aorta is cross-clamped as usual. The pericardial reflection between the inferior vena cava and inferior right pulmonary vein is extensively opened. The superior vena cava is dissected circumferentially at its junction with the right atrium, taking care to avoid injury to the adjacent phrenic nerve. The left atrium is entered anterior to the pulmonary veins as in the standard approach for mitral valve surgery. The incision is carried superiorly under the superior vena cava and inferiorly under the inferior vena cava (Fig. 10–7). The right atrium is divided approximately 1–2 cm on the atrial side of the junction of the superior vena cava with the right atrium. This leaves a generous cuff of right atrial wall which can, if necessary, be utilized in the anastomosis. The superior vena cava and remnant of right atrium are dissected free from the right pulmonary artery below. Near the inferior vena cava, the right atrium is divided 2–3 cm above the entrance of the inferior vena cava (Fig. 10–8). It is important to leave a large cuff of right atrium to facilitate anastomosis with the donor heart. Particularly in the era of nearly routine harvesting of multiple organs, a generous segment of donor inferior vena cava is not available if the liver is also harvested. If the donor heart is considerably smaller than the recipient heart, there

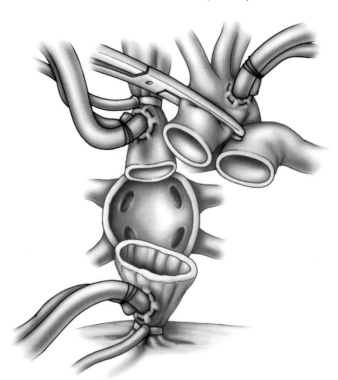

FIGURE **10–8.** Division of the right atrium to create superior and inferior vena caval cuffs for bicaval technique. The great vessels are divided as in the standard orthotopic method.

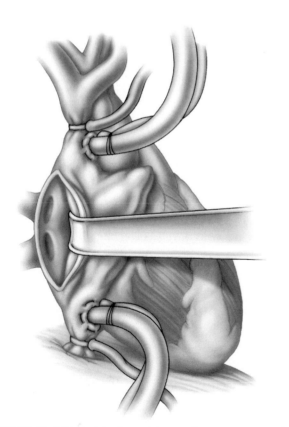

FIGURE **10–7.** Initial incision for recipient cardiectomy in preparation for bicaval technique. The left atrium is entered anterior to the right pulmonary veins and the incision carried beneath the superior and inferior vena cavae.

must be enough recipient right atrium around the inferior vena cava entrance to allow a tension-free anastomosis to the donor right atrium. The great vessels are divided as in the standard recipient cardiectomy.

The donor left atrium is prepared as usual. No incisions are made in the right atrium. The atrial septum is examined through the inferior vena caval orifice for a possible patent foramen ovale. A generous length of the superior vena cava has generally been harvested to facilitate the bicaval anastomosis. The aorta and pulmonary artery are prepared as for the standard orthotopic technique.

The left atrial anastomosis is constructed in the same fashion as for standard orthotopic transplantation (Fig. 10–9). It is noteworthy that the orifice for the left atrium is larger with the bicaval technique than when a remnant of septum is left as in the standard orthotopic technique. Particularly when a smaller donor is utilized and two lungs are also harvested, the circumference of the left atrial opening in the donor heart may be considerably smaller than in the recipient. Therefore, it may be necessary to extend the incision into the left atrial appendage to make up for this discrepancy.

The inferior vena cava (IVC) anastomosis is generally constructed after the left atrial anastomosis. An oblique anastomosis is constructed with continuous 4.0 polypropylene (Fig. 10–10). Commonly, the anterior aspect of the donor IVC opening must be incised slightly to enlarge the anastomotic opening.

The superior vena cava (SVC) anastomosis is usually constructed during the rewarming phase (prior to the pulmonary artery anastomosis) with a beating, reper-

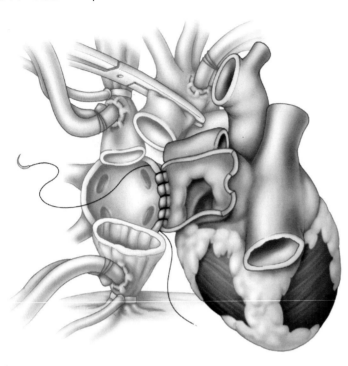

FIGURE **10-9.** Commencement of left atrial anastomosis in the bicaval technique (same as for standard orthotopic cardiac transplantation).

fused heart. The donor and recipient SVC must be trimmed to avoid redundancy, which may cause angulation of the new SVC and create a pressure gradient or increase the difficulty of passing a bioptome during performance of endomyocardial biopsies. The anastomosis is constructed with continuous 5-0 polypropylene. Other aspects of the operation are performed in the same manner as described for standard orthotopic transplantation (Fig. 10–11).

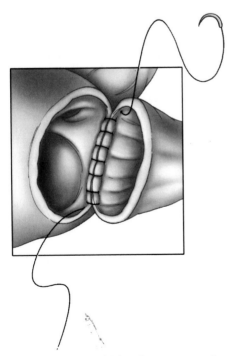

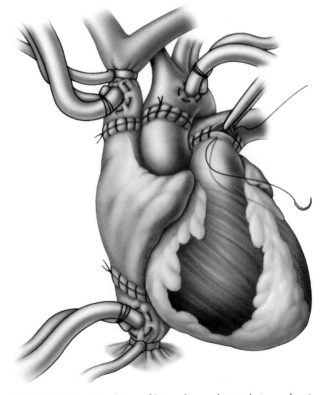

FIGURE **10-10.** Construction of the inferior vena caval anastomosis.

FIGURE **10-11.** Completion of bicaval transplant technique, showing the inferior vena caval, superior vena caval, aortic, and pulmonary artery anastomoses.

HETEROTOPIC HEART TRANSPLANTATION

The term "heterotopic cardiac transplantation" is used to describe the placement of the heart in an abnormal anatomical position (as opposed to the orthotopic or normal anatomical position). Although this term, when used in the clinical setting, has become synonymous with intrathoracic placement of the donor heart in parallel with the native heart,[50] the terms "auxiliary" and "parallel" were used in the original publications of this technique. Heterotopic transplantation of the heart as an auxiliary pump was first described in the early 1960s.[35, 49] Since that time, heterotopic transplantation has found divergent roles as an experimental model and in clinical practice. In view of the current rarity of this procedure, a complete discussion of the procedure, results, indications, and special features will be included in this section.

Since the first description of heterotopically transplanted hearts into the abdominal cavity in rats by Abbott in 1964,[1] multiple variations have been reported in several experimental models in differing positions.[21] Working left heart models have been described in the intrathoracic[64] as well as abdominal position.[44] Heterotopic transplantation has been used to study such diverse areas as the electrophysiology of denervation,[4, 45] noninvasive diagnosis of acute allograft rejection,[58] kinetics of acute cardiac rejection,[57] cardiac allograft function after ischemia and reperfusion,[5] and myocardial preservation.[67]

Heterotopic cardiac transplantation was first performed clinically in 1974 in South Africa,[10] and this procedure was used exclusively in Cape Town for many years.[23] A number of putative advantages of heterotopic transplantation over orthotopic transplantation were felt to justify this procedure, including (1) support of a dysfunctional donor heart (due to an excessively long ischemic time) by the residual native heart until donor heart recovery occurs,[23] (2) management of elevated pulmonary vascular resistance with a heterotopic heart so that the native right ventricle can continue to support the right side of the circulation after transplantation,[9] (3) the use of a small donor heart for a larger recipient, (4) the potential to function as a "a built-in assist device" at the time of hemodynamically significant acute cardiac rejection,[32] (5) support of the native heart with the development of coronary vasculopathy, as protection against sudden cardiac death until retransplantation can be undertaken,[8] and (6) rare circumstances when native cardiac failure may result from a process such as acute myocarditis where there is the potential for recovery and subsequent removal of the heterotopic transplant.

The initial clinical experience of heterotopic cardiac transplantation in Cape Town included the use of the donor heart purely for left ventricular assist,[10] with the donor pulmonary artery being anastomosed to the recipient right atrium for donor coronary sinus venous return. The technique of heterotopic transplantation was subsequently altered in favor of biventricular support.[40]

In 1983, Cooper and colleagues reported two patients who underwent heterotopic heart transplantation with donor heart ischemic times of 8 hours and nearly 13 hours, respectively, preserved with a portable hypothermic perfusion apparatus. Initial donor heart function was poor for approximately 20 hours, the circulation being supported by the recipient's own heart until the donor heart recovered.[16]

A number of novel variations of heterotopic transplantation have been proposed, investigated experimentally, and in some cases used clinically. In one model,[55] implantation of the donor heart was performed through a left thoracotomy without cardiopulmonary bypass. The technique involved creation of a large atrial septal defect in the donor heart, closing the inferior vena cava, defunctioning the donor right ventricle by excision of the tricuspid valve, oversewing the pulmonary artery and pulmonary veins, and implanting the donor heart by anastomosing the donor superior vena cava to the recipient left inferior pulmonary vein or left atrium and anastomosing the donor aorta to the recipient descending thoracic aorta (Fig. 10–12).

Heterotopic transplantation has been used clinically for purely left ventricular support[51] and has also been performed in patients with end-stage ischemic heart disease in association with other procedures such as left ventricular aneurysmectomy and coronary bypass surgery.[51]

Right ventricular assistance has been used experimentally in a model of right ventricular failure, using the right ventricle of the heterotopically placed donor heart for recipient right ventricular assist.[27] The use of the donor left ventricle for right ventricular support has been investigated experimentally and involved anastomosis of the donor left atrium to the recipient right atrium, connection of a left ventricular apical valved conduit from the donor left ventricle to the recipient pulmonary artery, and anastomosis of the donor ascending aorta to the recipient ascending aorta (to provide coronary circulation). The donor pulmonary artery is anastomosed to the donor left atrial appendage to drain coronary sinus return (Fig. 10–13).[17] A variation of the use of the donor left ventricle to support the pulmonary circulation was proposed by Novitzky,[39] and involved anastomosing the donor left atrium to the right atrium of the recipient and ascending aorta of the donor left ventricle to the pulmonary artery of the recipient, coronary blood flow being provided by saphenous vein grafts from the ascending aorta of the recipient aorta directly to the coronary arteries. Heterotopic heart and single lung transplantation has been performed (unsuccessfully) for a patient with end stage cardiopulmonary disease due to pulmonary hypertension secondary to a patent ductus arteriosus where entry into the left pleural space was deemed inadvisable because of previous surgery.[15]

Biological bridging to recovery of patients with native heart disease using heterotopic transplantation, although conceptually possible, would be a highly unusual strategy given the availability of extracorporeal membrane oxygenation and ventricular assist devices. However, a case has been reported[56] of repair of anoma-

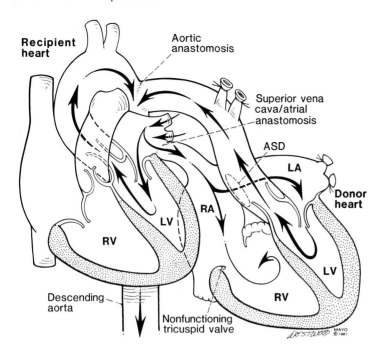

FIGURE **10–12.** Experimental heterotopic heart transplant for left ventricular assist, implanted in the left thorax. Blood in the high-pressure left atrium of the failing recipient heart passes through superior vena cava into right atrium of recipient heart; there blood crosses atrial septal defect into left atrium and is ejected into the aorta. The right ventricle is defunctionalized by excision of the tricuspid valve, and the pulmonary artery and inferior vena cava are oversewn. RV, right ventricle; LV, left ventricle; RA, right atrium; LA, left atrium; ASD, atrial septal defect. (From Schaff HV, Tago M, Gersh BJ, Pluth JR, Fetter J, Kaye MP: Simplified method of heterotopic cardiac transplantation of left ventricular assist. J Thorac Cardiovasc Surg 1983;85:434, with permission.)

lous origin of the coronary artery from the pulmonary artery associated with concomitant heterotopic transplantation using the left ventricular only assist configuration with subsequent removal of the donor heart 4 years following recovery of recipient native cardiac function.

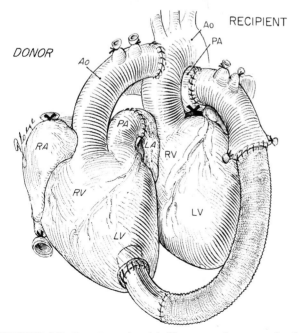

FIGURE **10–13.** Experimental model of heterotopic heart transplant for right ventricular assist. See text for anatomic details. Ao, aorta; LA, left atrium; LV, left ventricle; PA, pulmonary artery; RA, right atrium; RV, right ventricle. (From Corno AF, Laks H, Davtyan H, Flynn WM, Chang P, Drinkwater DC: The heterotopic right heart assist transplantation. J Heart Transplant 1988;7:183. Copyright 1988, Excerpta Medica Inc., with permission.)

CURRENT INDICATIONS FOR HETEROTOPIC TRANSPLANTATION

Although the use of heterotopic transplantation for right ventricular assist (particularly for patients with a univentricular heart for which the Fontan operation is contraindicated) seems attractive, this must currently be regarded as experimental.

In the current era, there are two basic indications for hetertopic transplantation. First, this procedure should be considered when there is marked elevation of pulmonary vascular resistance in the recipient, with systolic pressure greater than about 60 mm Hg and little or no pulmonary reactivity despite pharmacologic intervention (see Chapter 6). The situation is particularly dangerous for orthotopic transplantation if the pulmonary artery systolic pressure remains above 55 mm Hg when the pulmonary capillary wedge pressure is below about 20 mm Hg. Second, heterotopic transplantation may be considered when the donor heart is from a considerably smaller donor than the recipient (in body surface area). The limits of safe orthotopic cardiac transplantation from a smaller donor into a larger recipient are not well established, but the risk is known to be increased when a smaller female heart is transplanted into a considerably larger male recipient[68] and probably from a smaller sized young teenage donor into a larger adult male recipient. It should be emphasized that every effort should be made to find a suitable teenage recipient for a teenage donor before resorting to this extreme procedure in an adult recipient.

OPERATIVE TECHNIQUE

Preparation of the Donor Heart

The donor heart is procured in the standard way except that the entire ascending aorta and aortic arch are harvested. The orifices of the right pulmonary veins are oversewn with continuous 5.0 polypropylene. The inferior vena caval orifice is also oversewn, taking care to avoid impingement upon the coronary sinus. The partition between the left superior and inferior pulmonary veins is excised and the incision extended slightly into the base of the left atrial appendage, as necessary to create an opening as large as the mitral valve orifice. A marking suture is placed on the posteriormost aspect of this opening, opposite the left atrial appendage. In addition, the entire superior vena cava and proximal innominate vein is harvested.

Preparation of the Recipient

A standard median sternotomy is made. The right pleural space is widely opened to accommodate the donor heart. The pericardium is opened in the midline, and a pericardial flap for support of the transplanted heart is fashioned by making two perpendicular incisions on the right side which stop approximately 2 cm from the phrenic nerve. Careful hemostasis of this flap is important because it will not be accessible after the heart is implanted. Great care must be taken to avoid any coagulation near the phrenic nerve. Small bleeding points at the extent of these pericardial incisions should be controlled with fine polypropylene sutures.

Construction of the Heterotopic Transplant

Cardiopulmonary bypass is established with separate caval cannulation and moderate hypothermic perfusion at 25°–28°C. Myocardial preservation of the native heart is extremely important, since most of the pulmonary ventricular function will arise from the native right ventricle, and the native left ventricle may be required to contribute to systemic support early after the transplant. The aorta is cross-clamped and multidose cardioplegic techniques are employed for the native heart as in stan-

dard cardiac operations. Intermittent topical cooling with cold saline is employed. A left atriotomy is made in the inter-atrial groove as for standard mitral valve surgery except that the incision does not extend under the superior or inferior vena cava. The opening in the donor left atrium is anastomosed to the corresponding opening in the native left atrium using continuous 3.0 polypropylene. The anastomosis is oriented such that the midportion of the posterior lip of the incision on the native heart corresponds with the marking suture placed on the donor left atrial opening (Fig. 10–14).

The donor superior vena cava is then anastomosed end to side to the anterolateral aspect of the recipient superior vena cava near the junction of the native right subclavian and innominate veins. This anastomosis is constructed with continuous 5.0 polypropylene, and the opening should be as large as the circumference of the donor superior vena cava (Fig. 10–15). This will provide access for endomyocardial biopsies of the donor right ventricle. The donor aorta is then anastomosed end to side to the anterolateral aspect of the native aorta with continuous 4.0 polypropylene (Fig. 10–16). Air is thoroughly evacuated from both hearts and the aortic cross-clamp is removed with the same attention to the details of reperfusion as in orthotopic cardiac transplantation (see preceding sections and Chapter 9). While rewarming, the donor pulmonary artery is lengthened with an appropriate sized woven graft (Hemishield), which is then anastomosed end to side to the anterior aspect of the native pulmonary artery (Fig. 10–17). The remainder of the operation is completed as usual, taking care to leave atrial and ventricular pacing wires on both the native and the transplanted heart for use if necessary during the postoperative period.

The use of the direct superior vena caval connection simplifies the passage of an endomyocardial biopsy forceps into the donor right ventricle.[6, 51] Infection of the pulmonary artery conduit is a potential risk of hetero-

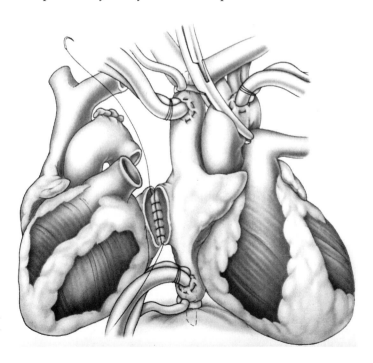

FIGURE **10–14.** Heterotopic transplantation. Donor and recipient hearts, showing the beginning of the posterior suture line of the left atrial anastomosis.

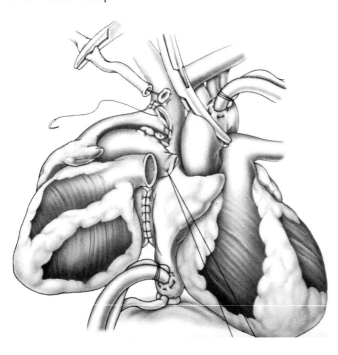

FIGURE **10–15.** Heterotopic transplantation. The donor superior vena cava is anastomosed end to side to the recipient superior vena cava. Construction of the anastomosis may be facilitated by transient removal of the superior vena caval cannula.

topic transplantation using this method, and this complication has previously been described,[48] requiring removal of the conduit and replacement with an aortic allograft. A technique has been described[18] that avoids the use of a pulmonary artery conduit by anastomosing the donor pulmonary artery directly to the recipient right pulmonary artery which was facilitated by an anastomosis between the recipient superior vena cava and donor superior vena cava as well as another right atrial connection towards the recipient inferior vena cava.

Permanent anticoagulation is required after heterotopic cardiac transplantation, since the native heart is a source of thrombus formation which may be ejected through the native aortic valve. Despite adequate anticoagulation, systemic emboli can still occur.[9, 37] The presence of a mechanical valve in the native heart increases the risk of thrombosis and is regarded as a contraindication to heterotopic heart transplantation.

The management of patients after heterotopic transplantation, including immunosuppression and surveillance for and treatment of acute cardiac rejection, is the same as that for patients after orthotopic transplantation. Endomyocardial biopsy is accomplished via the right internal jugular approach when a superior vena caval anastomosis has been performed,[6] but other approaches have been used, including the right femoral vein.[14, 34]

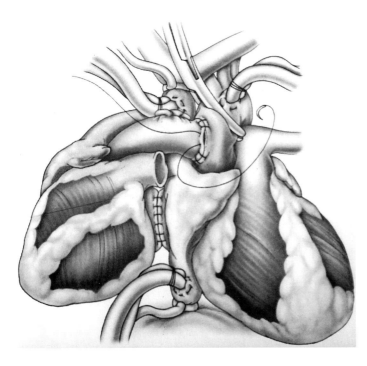

FIGURE **10–16.** Heterotopic transplantation, completion of the aortic anastomosis.

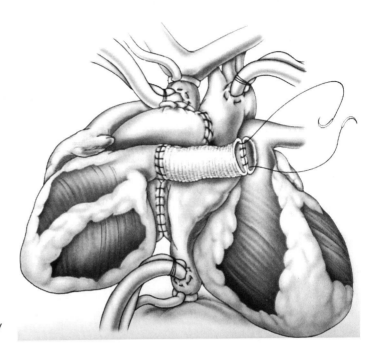

FIGURE **10–17.** Heterotopic transplantation. The pulmonary artery connection requires interposition of a Dacron graft.

The femoral approach allows more directional control over the tip of the biopsy forceps given the course that the biopsy forceps may have to take when a side-to-side right atrial anastomosis has been performed. Surgical clips can be placed around this anastomosis to visually facilitate passage of the endomyocardial biopsy forceps from the recipient to the donor right atrium.[2]

The usual practice in clinical heterotopic heart transplantation has been to allow donor and recipient hearts to beat asynchronously, the differential flow to donor or recipient heart being determined by such factors as ventricular contractility and compliance. However, an experimental study by Raza and colleagues[47] demonstrated that sequential pacing (depolarization of either atrium was sensed resulting in pacing of the other ventricle at the end of a programmed delay) as opposed to synchronous pacing (depolarization of either ventricle resulted in immediate stimulation of the opposite ventricle) resulted in a marginally greater cardiac index. Of potentially more relevance was a study by Morris-Thurgood and colleagues[36] which demonstrated in patients who had undergone heterotopic cardiac transplantation that paced linkage (recipient heart systole occurred during donor heart diastole by sensing the donor atrium and pacing the recipient atrium) improved systolic ventricular performance of the recipient heart as a result of a reduction in recipient heart afterload. This is in contrast to the usual unpaced situation in heterotopic heart transplantation where the recipient heart may not make any contribution to cardiac output and the aortic valve may open very infrequently. In asynchronously beating hearts, some patients with very poor recipient heart function will have almost continuous aortic and mitral regurgitation resulting in retrograde flow.[3]

Following heterotopic transplantation in patients with pulmonary hypertension there is good evidence that the pulmonary hypertension frequently regresses[37, 52] (Fig.

10–18), making it possible for the donor right ventricle to take over the right side of the circulation. The relative contribution of each ventricle of each heart is highly dependant on a number of factors including native left and right ventricular systolic function, native left and right ventricular compliance, and pulmonary vascular resistance; but it appears that in patients with the severest preoperative left ventricular dysfunction, the heterotopic heart assumes almost total biventricular assist, whereas in patients with less severe preoperative left ventricular dysfunction the heterotopic heart provides partial assist.[52]

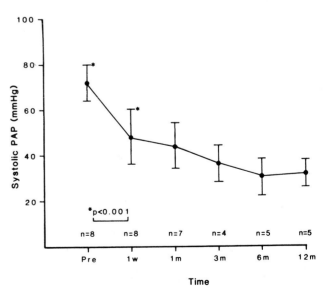

FIGURE **10–18.** Progressive fall in pulmonary artery pressure in patients undergoing heterotopic cardiac transplantation because of pulmonary hypertension. (From Nakatani T, Frazier OH, Lammermeier DE, Macris MP, Radovancevic B: Heterotopic heart transplantation: a reliable option for a select group of high-risk patients. J Heart Transplant 1989;8:40.)

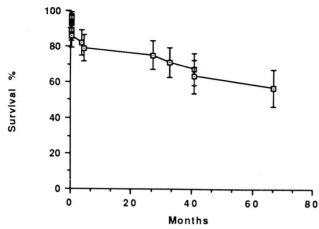

FIGURE 10-19. Actuarial survival of patients undergoing heterotopic heart transplantation together with concomitant procedures on the native heart of patients with ischemic heart disease. (From Ridley PD, Khaghani A, Musumeci F, Favaloro R, Akl ES, Banner NR, Mitchell AG, Yacoub MH: Heterotopic heart transplantation and recipient heart operation in ischemic heart disease. Ann Thorac Surg 1992;54:333.)

RESULTS OF HETEROTOPIC TRANSPLANTATION

In an earlier era, survival after heterotopic and orthotopic heart transplantation were similar.[37] However, the results of heterotopic cardiac transplantation are generally inferior to that of orthotopic cardiac transplantation,[26] and the procedure currently is rarely used. Nevertheless, satisfactory results have been reported with heterotopic transplantation and concomitant procedures (coronary artery bypass surgery with and without aneurysmectomy) for ischemic heart disease in a group of patients that were judged unable to undergo conventional procedures for ischemic heart disease without associated heterotopic transplantation (Fig. 10–19).[51] The survival of pediatric patients undergoing heterotopic transplantation for dilated or restrictive cardiomyopathy (the indication for heterotopic transplantation being either an undersized donor or significant pulmonary hypertension)[30] is generally less good than for orthotopic transplantation (Fig. 10–20).

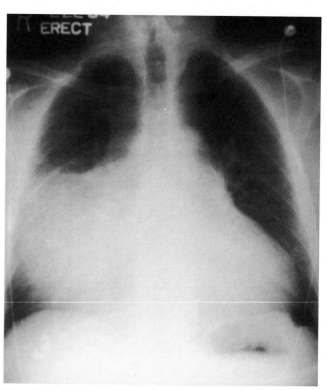

FIGURE 10-21. Chest x-ray in the posteroanterior projection of a patient with heterotopic transplantation with placement of the donor heart in the right pleural cavity.

There are a number of disadvantages and complications associated with heterotopic heart transplantation. The placement of the donor heart in the right pleural space can potentially cause obstructive collapse of the right middle and lower lobes resulting in an increased risk of pulmonary infection[37] (Fig. 10–21). In patients undergoing heterotopic transplantation for ischemic heart disease, angina from the native heart may recur.[51] One of the long-term concerns after heterotopic heart transplantation is the development of mitral and tricuspid regurgitation in the native heart,[19, 24] as well as significant mitral regurgitation in the donor heart.[24] The potential for the native heart to develop malignant ventricular arrhythmias has posed a concern for heterotopic

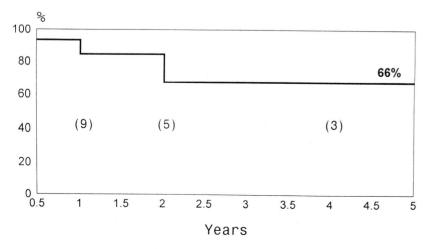

FIGURE 10-20. Actuarial survival curve of pediatric heterotopic transplant recipients. One- and 5-year actuarial survivals were 83% and 66%, respectively. Number of patients at risk at each time point are shown in parentheses. (From Khaghani A, Santini F, Dyke CM, Onuzu O, Radley-Smith R, Yacoub MH: Heterotopic cardiac transplantation in infants and children. J Thorac Cardiovasc Surg 1997;113:1042.)

transplantation, but there are reports of patients who developed native heart ventricular tachycardia being able to maintain satisfactory hemodynamics because of the presence of the donor heart.[31, 38] Definitive localization of a wide complex rhythm to the donor or recipient heart may require examining the precordial ECG leads from both the right and left chest.[38, 63]

Rarely, additional cardiac procedures have been performed following heterotopic heart transplantation. These include excision of the native heart (for severe regurgitation of the native aortic and mitral valves),[46] replacement of the heterotopic heart (for irreversible acute rejection or coronary vasculopathy),[43] excision of the donor and recipient hearts followed by orthotopic cardiac transplantation, and excision of the native heart and performance of orthotopic cardiac transplantation without removal of the heterotopic heart (patient has two donor hearts).[41, 42]

The potential role of heterotopic heart transplantation has diminished in recent years. The recognition that orthotopic cardiac transplantation can be performed with quite significant donor–recipient weight discrepancy, the availability of extracorporeal membrane oxygenation and left ventricular assist devices that render obsolete the use of small donor hearts as an auxiliary pump in a rapidly deteriorating patient, and the numerous pharmacological manipulations that are available for pulmonary hypertension limit the applicability of heterotopic cardiac transplantation. However, the one absolute indication for heterotopic cardiac transplantation is fixed high pulmonary vascular resistance, although the use of small donor hearts as an auxiliary pump is still worthy of consideration, particularly when there remains such a differential between donor hearts available and hearts required for transplantation.

References

1. Abbott CP, Lindsey ES, Creach O Jr, DeWitt CW: A technique for heart transplantation in the rat. Arch Surg 1964;98:645.
2. Adey C, Nath PH, Soto B, Shin MS, Schwartz M, Epstein AE, Kirklin JK: Heterotopic heart transplantation: a radiographic review. Radiographics 1987;7:151.
3. Akasaka T, Lythall D, Cheng A, Yoshida K, Yoshikawa J, Mitchell A, Yacoub MH: Continuous aortic regurgitation in several dysfunctional native hearts after heterotopic cardiac transplantation. Am J Cardiol 1989;63:1483.
4. Alvarez L, Escudero C, Alzueta J, Marquez-Montes J, Castillo-Olivares JL: Electrophysiology of heterotopic heart transplant: experimental study in dogs. Eur Heart J 1990;11:517.
5. Alyono D, Crumbley AJ, Schneider JR: Early mechanical function in the heterotopic heart transplant. J Surg Res 1984;37:55.
6. Arzouman DA, Arabia FA, Sethi GK, Copeland JG: Endomyocardial biopsy in the heterotopic heart transplant patient. Ann Thorac Surg 1998;65:857.
7. Baldwin JC: Heart and lung transplantation. New Dev Transplant Med 1995;2:8–9.
8. Barnard CN, Barnard MS, Curchio CA, Hassoulas J, Novitsky D, Wolpowitz A: The present status of heterotopic cardiac transplantation. J Thorac Cardiovasc Surg 1981;81:433–439.
9. Barnard CN, Cooper DKC: Clinical transplantation of the heart: a review of 13 years' personal experience. J R Soc Med 1981;74:670.
10. Barnard CN, Losman JG: Left ventricular bypass. S Afr Med J 1975;49:303.
11. Bjerke RJ, Zoiady GM, Matesic C, Marrone G: Early diagnosis and followup by echocardiography of acquired cor triatriatum after orthotopic heart transplantation. J Heart Lung Transplant 1992;11:1073-1077.
12. Blanche C, Czer LSC, Valenza M, Trento A: Alternative technique for orthotopic heart transplantation. Ann Thorac Surg 1994; 57:765–767.
13. Blanche C, Valenza M, Czer LSC, Barath P, Admon D, Harasty D, Utley C, Freimark D, Aleksic I, Matloff J, Trento A: Orthotopic heart transplantation with bicaval and pulmonary venous anastomoses. Ann Thorac Surg 1994;58:1505–1509.
14. Boffa GM, Grassi G, Cocco P, Razzolini R, Isabella GB, Livi U, Thiene G, Chioin R: Endomyocardial biopsy in heterotopic heart transplant recipients via the femoral vein. Cathet Cardiovasc Diagn 1993;28:18.
15. Cooley DA, Frazier OH, Macris MP, Duncan JM: Heterotopic heart-single lung transplantation: report of a new technique: J Heart Transplant 1987;6:112.
16. Cooper DKC, Novitzky D, Hassoulas J, Barnard CN: Heart transplantation: the South African experience. Heart Transplant 1982;2:151.
17. Corno AF, Laks H, Davtyan H, Flynn WM, Chang P, Drinkwater DC: The heterotopic right heart assist transplantation. J Heart Transplant 1988;7:183.
18. Da Silva JP, Cascudo MM, Baumgratz JF, Vila JHA, Filho MW, Neto DOB, Fonseca LD: Heterotopic heart transplantation: a direct pulmonary artery anastomosis technique. J Thorac Cardiovasc Surg 1994;108:795.
19. Desruennes M, Muneretto C, Gandjbakhch I: Heterotopic heart transplantation: current status in 1988. J Heart Transplant 1989;8:479.
20. Dreyfus G, Jebara V, Mihaileanu S, Carpentier AF: Total orthotopic heart transplantation: an alternative to the standard technique. Ann Thorac Surg 1991;52:1181–1184.
21. Dworkin GH, Eich DM, Allen C, Wechsler AS: Revised technique of heterotopic heart transplantation in rabbits. J Heart Transplant 1991;10:591.
22. Freimark D, Silverman JM, Aleksic I, Crues JV, Blanche C, Trento A, Admon D, Queral CA, Harasty DA, Czer LSC: Atrial emptying with orthotopic heart transplantation using bicaval and pulmonary venous anastomoses: a magnetic resonance imaging study. J Am Coll Cardiol 1995;25:932–936.
23. Hassoulas J, Barnard CN: Heterotopic cardiac transplantation: a 7-year experience at Groote Schuur Hospital, Cape Town. S Afr Med J 1984;65:675.
24. Hildebrandt A, Reichenspurner H, Gordon GD, Horak AR, Odell JA, Reichart B: Heterotopic heart transplantation: mid-term hemodynamic and echocardiographic analysis—the concern of arteriovenous-valve incompetence. J Heart Transplant 1990;9:675.
25. Jessen ME, Meyer DM, Moncrief CL, Wait MA, Melamed NB, Ring WS: Reducing neurological complications after cardiac transplantation: technical considerations. J Card Surg 1993;8:546–553.
26. Kawaguchi A, Gandjbakhch I, Pavie A, Muneretto C, Bors V, Leger P, Cabrol A, Desruennes M, Cabrol C: Factors affecting survival after heterotopic heart transplantation. J Thorac Cardiovasc Surg 1989;98:928.
27. Kazakov EN, Ryklin VA, Kriuchkov AI, Ustinov DV, Kobakhidze EA: Experimental model of right ventricular failure with heterotopic heart transplantation for assisted circulation. Cor Vasa 1985;27:374.
28. Kendall SWH, Ciulli F, Mullins PA, Biocina B, Dunning JJ, Large SR: Total orthotopic heart transplantation: an alternative to the standard technique. Ann Thorac Surg 1992;54:187–192.
29. Kieler-Jensen N, Lundin S, Ricksten SE: Vasodilator therapy after heart transplantation: effects of inhaled nitric oxide and intravenous prostacyclin, prostaglandin E1, and sodium nitroprusside. J Heart Lung Transplant 1995;14:436–443.
30. Khaghani A, Santini F, Dyke CM, Onuzu O, Radley-Smith R, Yacoub MH: Heterotopic cardiac transplantation in infants and children. J Thorac Cardiovasc Surg 1997;113:1042.
31. Kotliar C, Smart FW, Sekela ME: Heterotopic heart transplantation and native heart ventricular arrhythmias. Ann Thorac Surg 1991; 51:987.
32. Losman JG, Levine H, Campbell CD, Replogle RL, Hassoulas J, Novitsky D, Cooper DKC, Barnard CN: Changes in indications for heart transplantation. J Thorac Cardiovasc Surg 1982;84:716–726.

33. Lower RR, Shumway NE: Studies of the orthotopic homotransplantation of the canine heart. Surg Forum 1960;11:18–23.

34. Lowry RW, Bitar JN, Grinstead WC, Young JB, Noon GP, Vardan S, Cocanougher B, Kleiman NS: Heterotopic heart transplantation: catheterization, endomyocardial biopsy, and coronary angiography of the donor heart. Cathet Cardiovasc Diagn 1994;32:18.

35. McGough EC, Brewer PL, Reemtsma K: The parallel heart: studies of intrathoracic auxiliary cardiac transplants. Surgery 1966;60:153.

36. Morris-Thurgood J, Cowell R, Paul V, Kalsi K, Seymour AM, Ilsley C, Mitchell A, Khaghani A, Yacoub M: Hemodynamic and metabolic effects of paced linkage following heterotopic cardiac transplantation. Circulation 1994;90:2342.

37. Nakatani T, Frazier OH, Lammermeier DE, Macris MP, Radovancevic B: Heterotopic heart transplantation: a reliable option for a select group of high-risk patients. J Heart Transplant 1989;8:40.

38. Neerukonda SK, Schoonmaker FW, Nampalli VK, Narod JA: Ventricular dysrhythmia and heterotopic heart transplantation. J Heart Lung Transplant 1992;11:793.

39. Novitzky D, Cooper DKC: Letter to the Editor: right ventricular assist by a heterotopic left ventricle. J Heart Transplant 1989;8:345.

40. Novitzky D, Cooper DKC, Barnard CN: The surgical technique of heterotopic heart transplantation. Ann Thorac Surg 1983; 36:476–482.

41. Novitzky D, Cooper DKC: Surgical techniques of orthotopic and heterotopic heart transplantation. In Cooper DKC, Lanza RD (eds): Heart Transplantation: The Presentation Status of Orthotopic and Heterotopic Heart Transplantation. Lancaster, England: MTP Press Limited, 1984.

42. Novitzky D, Cooper DKC, Brink JG, Reichart BA: Sequential—second and third—transplants in patients with heterotopic heart allografts. Clin Transplant 1987;1:57.

43. Novitzky D, Cooper DKC, Lanza RP, Barnard CN: Further cardiac transplant procedures in patients with heterotopic heart transplants. Ann Thorac Surg 1985;39:149.

44. Ohmi M, Yokoyama H, Nakame T, Murata S, Akimoto H, Tabayashi K, Mohri H: Hemodynamic performance in a heterotopically transplanted dog heart: proposal of techniques for working left heart model of heterotopic (abdominal) heart transplantation. J Heart Lung Transplant 1992;11:1147.

45. Osorio ML, Stefano FJE, Langer SZ: Heterotopic heart transplant in the cat: an experimental model for the study of the development of sympathetic denervation and of allograft rejection. Pharmacology 1974;283:389.

46. Pham SM, Kormos RL, Griffith BP: Native cardiectomy in a heterotopic heart transplant recipient. J Thorac Cardiovasc Surg 1996;112:1109.

47. Raza ST, Tam SKC, Sun SC, Laurance R, Berkovitz B, Shemin R, Cohn LH: Sequentially paced heterotopic heart transplant in the left chest provides improved circulatory support for the failed left ventricle: a potential biologic bridge to orthotopic transplantation. J Thorac Cardiovasc Surg 1989;98:266.

48. Reddy SC, Katz WE, Medich GE, Gasior TA, Quinlan JJ, Pham SM, Ziady GM, Kormos RL: Infective endocarditis of the pulmonary artery conduit in a recipient with a heterotopic heart transplant: diagnosis by transesophageal echocardiography. J Heart Lung Transplant 1994;13:139.

49. Reemtsma K: The heart as a test organ in transplantation studies. Ann N Y Acad Sci 1964;120:778.

50. Reemtsma K: Cardiac and pulmonary replacement: editorial: cardiac transplantation for auxiliary circulatory support. J Thorac Cardiovasc Surg 1997;113:1041.

51. Ridley PD, Khaghani A, Musumeci F, Favaloro R, Akl ES, Banner NR, Mitchell AG, Yacoub MH: Heterotopic heart transplantation and recipient heart operation in ischemic heart disease. Ann Thorac Surg 1992;54:333.

52. Rigaud M, Bourdarias JP, Khoury EE, Beauchet A, Labedan F, Bardet J, Gandjbakhch I, Cabrol C: Hemodynamic evaluation of heterotopic heart transplantation. J Thorac Cardiovasc Surg 1992;104:248.

53. Sack FU, Lange R, DeSimone R, Mehmanesh H, Hagi S: Influence of atrial geometry on tricuspid valve insufficiency after orthotopic heart transplantation: intraoperative echocardiography [abstract]. J Heart Lung Transplant 1993;12:S102.

54. Sarsam MAI, Campbell CS, Yonan NA, Deiraniya AK, Rahman AN: An alternative surgical technique in orthotopic cardiac transplantation. J Card Surg 1993;8:344–349.

55. Schaff HV, Tago M, Gersh BJ, Pluth JR, Fetter J, Kaye MP: Simplified method of heterotopic cardiac transplantation for left ventricular assist. J Thorac Cardiovasc Surg 1983;85:434.

56. Schmid C, Kececioglu D, Konertz W, Möllhoff T, Scheld HH: Biological bridging after repair of an anomalous origin of a left coronary artery. Ann Thorac Surg 1996;62:1839.

57. Schüetz A, Kemkes BM, Breuer M, Brandl U, Engelhardt M, Kugler C, Manz C, Hatz R, Gokel JM, Hammer C: Kinetics and dynamics of acute rejection after heterotopic heart transplantation. J Heart Lung Transplant 1992;11:289.

58. Scott GE, Nath RL, Friedlich JA, Fallon JT, Erdmann AJ: Usefulness of myocardial edema to assess heterotopic allograft rejection in dogs. Heart Transplant 1983;II:232.

59. Shulman LL, Smith CR, Drusin R, Rose EA, Enson Y, Reemtsma K: Patent foramen ovale complicating heart transplantation. Chest 1987;92:569–572.

60. Shumway NE, Lower RR, Stouffer RC: Transplantation of the heart. Adv Surg 1966;2:265–284.

61. Stevenson LW, Dadourian BJ, Kobashigawa J, Child JS, Clark SH, Laks H: Mitral regurgitation after cardiac transplantation. Am J Cardiol 1987;60:119–122.

62. Valantine HA, Appleton CP, Hatle LK, Hunt SA, Stinson EB, Popp RL: Influence of recipient atrial contraction on left ventricular filling dynamics of the transplanted heart assessed by Doppler echocardiography. Am J Cardiol 1987;59:1159–1163.

63. Vanderheyden M, de Sutter J, Goethals M: ECG diagnosis of native heart ventricular tachycardia in a heterotopic heart transplant recipient. Heart 1999;81:323.

64. Verrier ED, Crombleholme TM, Sauer L, Longaker M, Langer JC, Flake AW, Dae M, Brem H, Harrison MR: Neonatal model of heterotopic heart transplantation in pigs. J Thorac Cardiovasc Surg 1989;98:127.

65. Williams TJ, Salamonsen RF, Snell G, Kaye D, Esmore DS: Clinical heart transplantation. Preliminary experience with inhaled nitric oxide for acute pulmonary hypertension after heart transplantation. J Heart Lung Transplant 1995;14:419–423.

66. Wolfsohn AL, Walley VM, Masters RG, Davies RA, Boone SA, Keon WJ: The surgical anastomoses after orthotopic heart transplantation: clinical complications and morphologic observations. J Heart Lung Transplant 1994;13:455–465.

67. Yeh T, Rebeyka IM, Jakoi ER, Johnson DE, Dignan RJ, Dyke CM, Wechsler AS: Orotic acid improves left ventricular recovery four days after heterotopic transplantation. Ann Thorac Surg 1994; 58:409.

68. Young JB, Naftel DC, Bourge RC, Kirklin JK, Clemson BS, Porter CB, Rodeheffer RJ, Kenzora JL: Matching the heart donor and heart transplant recipient. Clues for successful expansion of the donor pool: a multivariable, multiinstitutional report. J Heart Lung Transplant 1994;13:353–365.

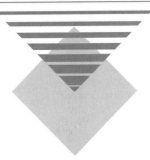

CHAPTER ELEVEN

Physiology of the Transplanted Heart

Few things in medicine are more dramatic than observing the functional improvement that occurs when patients with advanced heart failure or cardiogenic shock undergo successful heart transplantation.[108] It is clear that the cardiac allograft affords profound circulatory rehabilitation to patients with advanced heart failure. In the severely symptomatic end-stage heart failure patient, cardiac transplantation is superior to any other therapy available and generally immediately improves functional capacity while extending life. Functional limitations that are clearly related to hemodynamic abnormalities will improve substantially, and, when a heart transplant is completely successful, often resolve totally. The fact, however, that outcomes sometimes are relative and related to the severity of heart failure at the time of transplantation implies that residual dysfunction of the cardiac allograft can be problematic.[149]

The function of the transplanted heart is a complex interplay between intrinsic myocardial contractility, ventricular loading conditions, catecholamine levels, donor–recipient size relations, pulmonary vascular resistance, and the state of denervation. Though cardiac transplantation provides remarkable rehabilitation to profoundly disturbed heart failure physiology, it is extraordinarily important to remember that **cardiac allografts do not function normally.** In the absence of substantive rejection, significant allograft vasculopathy, or hypertension, the transplanted heart performs **at rest** in a similar but not identical fashion to a healthy, age- and sex-matched normal heart. However, exercise tolerance in transplant recipients can be much less than in normal individuals.

A key to understanding subtleties in dysfunction of the transplanted denervated heart is understanding allograft responses to brain death (Chapter 9), harvesting injury (Chapter 9), allograft rejection (acute and chronic inflammation) (Chapter 14), ischemic injury from allograft arteriopathy (Chapter 17), and hypertension related to immunosuppressive agents (Chapter 16). Preexisting donor cardiac pathology can also contribute to pump dysfunction, particularly in the setting of rejection or allograft vasculopathy. All of these factors can contribute to the physiologic environment that characterizes

353

TABLE 11–1	Factors Which Alter Function of the Transplanted Heart

Hemodynamic Issues
  Donor–recipient atrial asynchrony
  Early postoperative restrictive physiology
  Late occult restrictive physiology
  Tricuspid insufficiency
Allograft Denervation
  Afferent denervation
    Altered reflex control of peripheral vasoconstriction/vasodilation
    Altered Na$^+$/H$_2$O regulation via central nervous system–dependent vasopressin,
      renin, angiotensin, aldosterone secretion
    Absence of anginal syndrome during ischemia
  Efferent denervation
    Absent vagal nerve control
    Rapid heart rate at rest
    Attenuated heart rate response to exercise
  Hypersensitivity to circulating catecholamines
  Exaggerated response to acetylcholine
Altered Hormonal Milieu
  ANP secretion enhanced
  Elevated exercise circulating catecholamines
  Increased circulating paracrine peptides (endothelin)

Myocardial Injury/Maladaptation
  Organ preservation and recovery injury
  Rejection
  Ventricular hypertrophy
  Hypertension (increased ventricular wall stress)

Donor-Related Issues
  Effect of brain death
  Donor–recipient size mismatch
  Age-related diastolic dysfunction
  Preexisting hypertrophy
  Preexisting myopathy
  Preexisting structural heart disease

Allograft Arteriopathy (ischemia)

cardiac allograft physiology and pathophysiology in the months and years after transplantation (Table 11–1) and help explain the deterioration in function over time observed in some transplanted hearts.

HISTORICAL PERSPECTIVE

Early heart transplant animal models gave insight into the potential for adequate function of cardiac allografts. Mann et al. in 1933[74] suggested that circulatory physiology after cardiac transplantation would be "excellent" if the "biologic factors" that caused organ failure (now understood as "rejection") during experimental transplantation could be identified and controlled. Obviously, this related to long-term cardiac allograft performance, but function of transplanted hearts in that era was impaired immediately after implantation of the organ. Without immunosuppression, these early experiments were quickly doomed by cellular and humoral rejection which caused substantive systolic and diastolic ventricular dysfunction and rapid demise of the organ.

Autotransplantation models demonstrated longer durability but still suggested that cardiac performance was not normal.[28, 139] Indeed, some of these early experiments with heart excision and subsequent reimplantation demonstrated that cardioplegia, duration of ischemia, and denervation altered performance characteristics. Most of these studies were done to clarify the effects of cardiac innervation by creating the scenario of denervation.[139] Autotransplant experiments demonstrated that right and left heart filling pressures were elevated, which generally returned to more normal levels over time. Also, exercise tolerance in canine models of autotransplantation seemed similar to control animals.[36, 37]

Autotransplantation experiments also demonstrated that total blood volume increased substantially. Blunted diuretic and natriuretic response to volume expansion was also shown in a denervated canine autotransplant preparation.[47, 86, 140] Interruption of afferent neurocardiac innervation systems seemed to affect circulatory system volume homeostasis. Early observations suggested that the circulatory milieu of a cardiac transplant recipient was one of a volume-expanded state.

The observation that the denervated heart is associated with rapid and profound reduction of myocardial catecholamine levels that leads to a loss of feedback inhibition of circulatory catecholamine increase had great implications regarding posttransplant hypertension, which is seen so often today.[28, 78, 95] Nonetheless, in animal models, giving us our initial insight into physiology of transplanted hearts, auto- and allotransplant canine experiments generally demonstrated substantial capability for exercise despite physiologic abnormalities.[37]

DENERVATION

THE ANATOMY OF CARDIAC INNERVATION

Afferent and Efferent Fibers

The heart is supplied by **sympathetic** and **parasympathetic** nerves, most of which arise in the neck. Embryologic development of the heart begins in the neck, followed later by migration of the heart and its accompanying nerve supply to the thorax. Cardiac sympathetic and parasympathetic nerves carry both afferent and efferent fibers. **Afferent** fibers (nerve fibers which convey sensory impulses from the periphery, in this case the heart, to the central nervous system) transmit impulses to the central nervous system from cardiac receptors located predominantly in the endocardium around the orifices of the caval and pulmonary veins, over the interatrial septum, and in the atrioventricular valves.[82] **Efferent** fibers (nerve fibers which carry impulses from the central nervous system to the periphery) to the heart are controlled by the brain stem, hypothalamus, and higher brain centers; and they are modified reflexly by cardiac, aortic, and pulmonary artery afferent impulses. Afferent fibers from the heart and great vessels largely travel to the spinal cord via the sympathetic cardiac nerves, and to the medulla oblongata of the brain stem via the vagus nerves. Efferent fibers follow similar routes. The cell bodies of the afferent fibers lie in dorsal root ganglia of the upper four or five thoracic spinal nerves and in the inferior vagal ganglia. These relationships are depicted in Figure 11–1. All of the parasympathetic (vagal) and sympathetic cardiac nerves converge to form the **cardiac plexus,** which lies between the posterior aspect of the concavity of the distal ascending aorta/proximal aortic arch and the tracheal bifurcation. Fibers

from the left and right side surround and accompany the coronary arteries and their branches.

Sympathetic Cardiac Nerves

Cervical and upper thoracic sympathetic trunk ganglia give off cardiac branches, all of which pass through the cardiac plexus. Three pairs of sympathetic cardiac nerves arise from cervical ganglia of the sympathetic trunks, and others originate from the upper thoracic ganglia. The **superior cervical sympathetic cardiac nerve** arises from the superior cervical sympathetic ganglion, and it often unites with the superior cervical vagal cardiac nerves and descends posterior to the carotid sheath on each side. The **middle cervical sympathetic cardiac nerve** receives filaments from the middle and

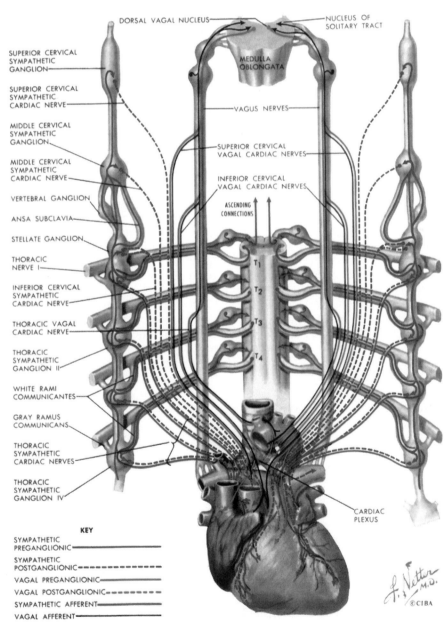

FIGURE **11–1.** Sympathetic and parasympathetic (vagal) innervation of the heart. See text for discussion. (From Netter FH: The Ciba Collection of Medical Illustrations Summit, NJ: Ciba, 1969, with permission.)

vertebral ganglia of the sympathetic trunk and is often the largest cervical cardiac nerve. The **inferior cervical sympathetic cardiac nerve** receives filaments from the stellate ganglion and the ansa subclavia and courses toward the cardiac plexus. The **thoracic sympathetic cardiac nerves** consist of four or five small branches which originate from the corresponding upper thoracic sympathetic trunk ganglia and course forward and medially to the cardiac plexus.

The **preganglionic sympathetic fibers** are the axons of cells in the lateral gray columns of the upper four or five thoracic spinal segments. These fibers enter the corresponding spinal nerves and exit them in white rami communicantes which travel to adjacent ganglia in the sympathetic trunks.[82] Some of these fibers relay in these ganglia, and their axons (postganglionic fibers) course to the heart in the thoracic sympathetic cardiac nerves (see again Fig. 11–1). Thus, the **sympathetic ganglia are located at some distance from the heart. Cardiac pain fibers** arising from the heart pass through the cardiac plexus, then course in the thoracic, inferior cervical, and middle cervical sympathetic nerves.

Parasympathetic Cardiac Nerves

The vagal (parasympathetic) branches are grouped as the superior and inferior cervical and thoracic vagal cardiac nerves. The **superior cervical vagal cardiac nerve** is formed by several filaments which leave the vagus in the upper neck and travel with the corresponding sympathetic cardiac nerve to the cardiac plexus. The **inferior cervical vagal cardiac nerve** arises in the lower third of the neck and often joins with branches from the middle cervical, vertebral, and/or stellate sympathetic ganglia in their course toward the cardiac plexus. The **thoracic vagal cardiac nerve** arises from the vagus nerves at the thoracic inlet and the recurrent laryngeal nerves and travels to the cardic plexus. In contrast to the sympathetic nerves, the **parasympathetic relays occur in ganglia near or in the heart,** thereby making the postganglionic parasympathetic fibers relatively short.

EFFECTS OF CARDIAC DENERVATION

Donor heart cardiectomy severs both afferent and efferent nervous system connections, and these are not restored during subsequent heart implantation. This creates a state of complete cardiac denervation. Interruption of afferent and efferent innervation affects different aspects of cardiovascular homeostasis.

Afferent Denervation

Afferent neurocardiac innervation systems seem to mediate, at least in part, **circulatory system volume homeostasis.** In the innervated heart, sensory receptors in the cardiopulmonary region of the ventricles served by vagal fibers provide the afferent limb (traveling away from the heart) which exerts a tonic restraining influence on sympathetic outflow to the heart and peripheral circulation.[1, 2, 72] A decrease in cardiac filling pressures and volume normally results in decreased activity of these

sensory receptors and therefore decreases tonic vagal inhibition of sympathetic outflow. The abrupt loss of vagal tone causes marked reflex activation of the sympathetic nervous system. These receptors may reside predominantly in the ventricles and, to a lesser degree, in the atria and lungs.[72, 80] In the transplanted heart, the absence of these afferent fibers produces a **reduced augmentation of peripheral vascular resistance and blunted plasma norepinephrine response to an abrupt decrease in central venous pressure.**[80, 125]

Interruption of the afferent nervous pathways impairs normal **renin-angiotensin-aldosterone regulation** (see Chapter 4). Normally, in response to various metabolic stimuli, renin is released into the blood from the kidney and catalyzes cleavage of angiotensinogen to generate angiotensin I. Angiotensin-converting enzyme catalyzes the conversion of angiotensin I to the active form, angiotensin II, in the lungs, blood vessel walls, and other sites. Angiotensin II has a potent vasoconstrictor effect and stimulates aldosterone secretion by the adrenal cortex, which promotes retention of sodium and water and increases circulating plasma volume. Afferent stretch receptors in the heart normally provide a feedback mechanism which acts to decrease renin and antidiuretic hormone secretion when the blood volume is increased, thus returning plasma volume to normal levels.[44–47, 121, 132, 140] By interrupting the afferent neural fibers from the heart, this feedback mechanism (which normally counterbalances sympathetic renal stimulation) is lost, resulting in chronically increased sympathetic stimulation of the renin-angiotensin-aldosterone axis. This engenders fluid retention with altered cardiac loading conditions because of a new volume steady state. Thus the general circulatory milieu of a cardiac transplant recipient is one of **a volume-expanded state** with increased total blood volume. **Blunted diuretic and natriuretic responses to volume expansion** have also been shown in denervated canine autotransplant preparations.[47, 86, 140]

The general decrease in vagal inhibitory effect of sympathetic output may also aggravate the **hypertensive tendency** after transplant. Scherrer and colleagues[103] noted that cyclosporine directly increases sympathetic activation (as measured by the rate of sympathetic nerve firing), which is accentuated in heart transplant patients. The degree of sympathetic overactivity does not appear to decrease with time after transplant (at least out to 18 months) and may account in part for the persistent hypertension associated with cyclosporine.

Loss of afferent nervous signaling is likely also responsible for **the absence of angina pectoris** being sensed when patients after heart transplant are experiencing cardiac ischemia or having an actual myocardial infarction.[112]

Efferent Denervation

Efferent cardiac innervation mediates sympathetic and parasympathetic nervous system effects on the heart and, thus, denervation will cause the **resting heart rate to be higher** by eliminating vagal-mediated parasympathetic influences. Largely because of the higher resting heart rate, 24-hour variations in heart rate are less in the transplanted heart than in the normal heart.[4] The

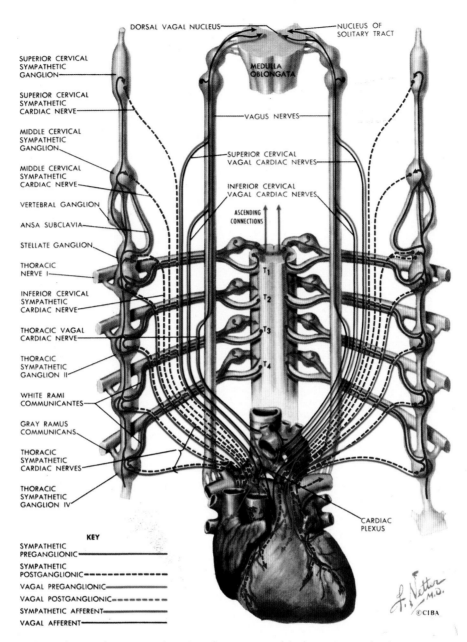

DORSAL VAGAL NUCLEUS

NUCLEUS OF
SOLITARY TRACT

MEDULLA
OBLONGATA

SUPERIOR CERVICAL
SYMPATHETIC
GANGLION

SUPERIOR CERVICAL
SYMPATHETIC
CARDIAC NERVE

MIDDLE CERVICAL
SYMPATHETIC
GANGLION

MIDDLE CERVICAL
SYMPATHETIC
CARDIAC NERVE

VERTEBRAL GANGLION

ANSA SUBCLAVIA

STELLATE GANGLION

THORACIC
NERVE I

INFERIOR CERVICAL
SYMPATHETIC
CARDIAC NERVE

THORACIC VAGAL
CARDIAC NERVE

THORACIC
SYMPATHETIC
GANGLION II

WHITE RAMI
COMMUNICANTES

GRAY RAMUS
COMMUNICANS

THORACIC
SYMPATHETIC
CARDIAC NERVES

THORACIC
SYMPATHETIC
GANGLION IV

VAGUS NERVES

SUPERIOR CERVICAL
VAGAL CARDIAC NERVES

INFERIOR CERVICAL
VAGAL CARDIAC NERVES

ASCENDING
CONNECTIONS

T₁

T₂

T₃

T₄

CARDIAC
PLEXUS

KEY

SYMPATHETIC
PREGANGLIONIC

SYMPATHETIC
POSTGANGLIONIC

VAGAL PREGANGLIONIC

VAGAL POSTGANGLIONIC

SYMPATHETIC AFFERENT

VAGAL AFFERENT

FIGURE 11–1. Sympathetic and parasympathetic (vagal) innervation of the heart. See text for discussion. (From Netter FH: The Ciba Collection of Medical Illustrations Summit, NJ: Ciba, 1969, with permission.)

largest variation from normal occurs during sleep, when the denervated heart shows minimal slowing.

Also absent will be the influence on the heart of vaso-signaling from the central nervous system. This loss of autonomic signaling attenuates the usual rapid changes in heart rate and contractility normally noted during exercise. **Hypovolemia** or **vasodilation** also reflexly activates autonomic adrenergic signaling mechanisms, and these central reactions to peripheral events will not be sensed by the denervated heart (see below).

Effect of Denervation on Other Stresses

Cardiac denervation after heart transplantation also creates altered responses to other forms of physiologic stress. In general, the denervated heart appears to respond adequately to increased stresses **except in situations which require an abrupt major increase in heart rate** to maintain or increase cardiac output. Based on experimental studies,[125] acute hypertension is generally well tolerated with only a slight decrease in cardiac output and small increase in left ventricular end-diastolic pressure, but **acute hypotension** is far less well tolerated because a prompt circulatory response requires intact afferent and efferent cardiac pathways (see above sections). Baroreflex-induced volume regulation after heart transplantation is impaired, resulting in minimal reflex increase in cardiac output because of little, and late occurring, heart rate responsiveness.[80] For example, by placing the lower body of a transplant patient in a negative pressure chamber to mimic central venous volume reduction, Mohanty and colleagues noted that the reflex increase in vascular resistance (measured in the forearm) was smaller in transplant patients than in normal subjects.[80]

The complex interaction between the denervated left ventricle and the peripheral vasculature has been characterized by Borow and colleagues[17] as having an exaggerated myocardial beta$_1$- or beta$_2$-mediated positive chronotropic effect and a reduced sensitivity to alpha$_1$ receptor peripheral stimulation. It has also been suggested that the inability to autoregulate blood flow by reflex sympathetic nervous system mediated vasoconstriction to nonworking muscles plays a role in limiting the maximal exercise capacity of heart transplant recipients[128] (see later section, Cardiac Allograft Response to Exercise).

REINNERVATION

A variety of studies indicate that some heart transplant patients reinnervate their cardiac allograft. **Immunohistochemical staining** of transplanted hearts indicates that viable intrinsic nerve fibers are present despite the extrinsic denervation.[138] Perhaps the best evidence indicating reconnection of these intrinsic nerve fibers to the extrinsic nervous system is the fact that some patients late after transplantation begin to sense **angina pectoris** that is quite classic during bouts of cardiac ischemia.[112] This suggests that at least some heart transplant recipients can reestablish at least partial afferent reinnervation.

During donor cardiectomy the **sympathetic nerves** are severed from the nerve cell bodies located in the thoracic and cervical ganglia. Subsequently, norepinephrine stores in the cardiac sympathetic nerve terminals are rapidly depleted[87] because the enzymes and vesicles necessary for the synthesis of norepinephrine must be transported from the cell body in the ganglion to the nerve terminal via an intact axon.[64] This fact provides the basis for an important test to examine reinnervation following cardiac transplantation. The substance **tyramine,** when infused intravenously in the vicinity of sympathetic nerve terminals, causes neuronal release of norepinephprine.[122] The displaced norepinephprine can be detected by measuring the cardiac norepinephprine gradient (the concentration of plasma norepinephrine in the coronary sinus minus the plasma concentration of norepinephrine in the aortic root entering the coronary arteries) before and after the administration of tyramine.[42, 112] A significant increase in the norepinephrine gradient [Δ(NE)CS–Ao] in the transplanted heart implies significant release of norepinephprine from sympathetic nerve terminals, which indirectly implies reestablishment of postganglionic nerve connections, thus indicating **sympathetic reinnervation** (Fig. 11–2).

Stark et al.[112] showed that in two patients with angina pectoris and allograft vasculopathy, a tyramine-induced increase in cardiac release of norepinephrine was present, indicating reinnervation. Using this methodology, Wilson et al.[144] found that approximately 70% of patients have evidence of reinnervation after 1 year and about 80% after 5 years. The extent of reinnervation as judged by tyramine infusion is very heterogenous by regions of the heart,[142] and studies by DiCarli et al. indicate that (based on a small number of patients) recipients 5 or more years after transplant show greater reinnervation of the left anterior descending region than either the circumflex or right coronary regions.[33] The overall mean norepinephrine release increases with time after transplantation[144] (Fig. 11–3), suggesting a greater degree of reinnervation. Using both tyramine infusion and sustained hand grip exercise (a reflex sympathetic stimulus), Wilson and colleagues found no evidence of reinnervation within the first 5 months and limited sympathetic reinnervation in most patients after 1 year.[144]

Other end points have also been examined following intracoronary tyramine administration to infer reinnervation. Release of norepinephprine from the intact sympathetic nerve terminals within the ventricular myocardium produces an increase in left ventricular contractility (measured as dp/dt). A change in dp/dt before and after tyramine infusion into the left coronary artery provides evidence of reinnervation.[20] In addition, coronary blood flow can be assessed by an intracoronary Doppler catheter. With intact sympathetic innervation, intracoronary injection of tyramine results in release of norepinephprine from sympathetic terminals and a brief microvascular constriction response (usually in vessels < 400 μm in diameter).[134] This results in a demonstrable decrease in coronary blood flow. In the denervated state, no change in coronary blood flow would be observed. Burke and colleagues[20] found that by stimulation of reinnervating sympathetic neurons with tyramine, a sig-

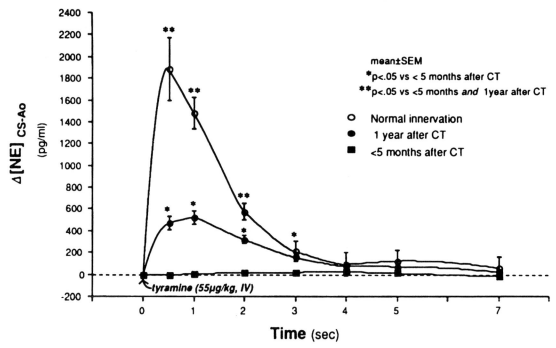

FIGURE **11–2.** Plot of time course of norepinephrine release as $\Delta[NE]_{CS-Ao}$ after tyramine administration. Patients studied early after cardiac transplantation (CT) had no significant change in $\Delta[NE]_{CS-Ao}$. Patients studied 1 year or more after cardiac transplantation had a significant increase in $\Delta[NE]_{CS-Ao}$, but less than that seen in normally innervated controls. In both groups, the peak norepinephrine release occurred 30 seconds to 1 minute after intravenous tyramine injection. $\Delta[NE]_{CS-Ao}$, difference in plasma norepinephrine concentration between the coronary sinus and aorta. (From Wilson RF, McGinn AL, Johnson TH, Christensen BV, Laxson DD: Sympathetic reinnervation after heart transplantation in human beings. J Heart Transplant 1992;11:S88–S89.)

nificant but subnormal increase in dp/dt and a transient decrease in coronary blood flow occurred which suggested that reinnervating sympathetic neurons were seemingly associated with meaningful physiologic changes in ventricular function and coronary artery tone. Sympathetic reinnervation of the heart after cardiac transplantation has also been demonstrated by **catecholamine uptake in the myocardial nerve ending**[31, 106] and by **carotid baroreflex modulation of the electrocardiographic RR interval.**[10]

Sinus node sympathetic reinnervation can also be inferred by an increase in heart rate with injection of

tyramine into the sinus node artery (Fig. 11–4). Wilson and colleagues[142, 143] demonstrated sinus node reinnervation and/or regional left ventricular reinnervation (norepinephrine response after selective injection of tyramine into the left anterior descending or circumflex arteries) in a majority of cardiac transplant recipients more than 1 year after transplantation. However, there was often disparity between sinus node and left ventricular reinnervation, in that about 50% of patients demonstrated reinnervation of both the left ventricle and sinus node, whereas about 20% had only left ventricular reinnervation and 20% only sinus node reinnervation.[142] As

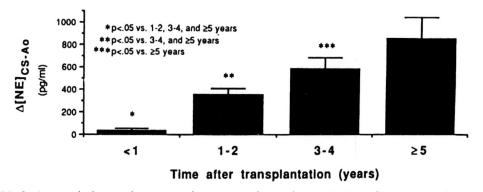

FIGURE **11–3.** Bar graph showing the mean cardiac norepinephrine release $\Delta[NE]_{CS-Ao}$ after tyramine administration with respect to time after cardiac transplantation. (From Wilson RF, McGinn AL, Johnson TH, Christensen BV, Laxson DD: Sympathetic reinnervation after heart transplantation in human beings. J Heart Transplant 1992;11:S88–S89.)

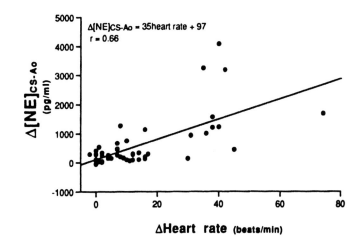

FIGURE **11-4.** Scatterplot of peak cardiac release of norepinephrine $\Delta[NE]_{CS-Ao}$ in response to injection of tyramine into the left main coronary artery (Y-axis) compared with change in heart rate after tyramine injection into the sinus node artery (X-axis). (From Wilson RF, Christensen BV, Olivari MT, Simon A, White CW, Laxson DD: Evidence for structural sympathetic reinnervation after orthotopic cardiac transplantation in humans. Circulation 1991;83:1210–1220.)

with ventricular reinnervation, the degree of sinus node reinnervation appears to increase with time after transplant (Fig. 11–5). Those patients with evidence of sinus node reinnervation demonstrated a higher peak exercise heart rate and greater maximal oxygen consumption (200 ± 2.3 vs. 17.6 ± 2.7 mL/kg/min) than those without sinus node reinnervation. Also, patients with left ventricular reinnervation demonstrated a normal coronary small vessel constrictive response to sympathetic stimulation, which was not seen in patients without evidence of left ventricular reinnervation.[143]

Vagal (parasympathetic) reinnervation is still a matter of conjecture. In a study by Uberfuhr[127] of heart transplant recipients, sympathetic innervation was demonstrated, and in a small proportion of these patients there

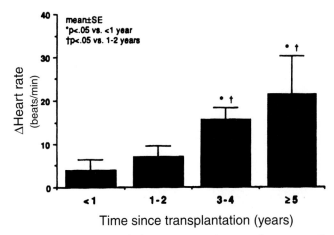

FIGURE **11-5.** Bar graph shows average change in heart rate with respect to time in transplant recipients after injection of tyramine into the artery perfusing the sinus node. Heart rate response increased significantly with the time interval between transplantation and study. (From Wilson RF, Christensen BV, Olivari MT, Simon A, White CW, Laxson DD: Evidence for structural sympathetic reinnervation after orthotopic cardiac transplantation in humans. Circulation 1991;83:1210–1220.)

was evidence of vagal reinnervation inferred from the abolition by atropine of a baroreflex-induced variability in the RR interval of the surface electrocardiogram. It is important to note that the proportion of patients demonstrating vagal reinnervtion was considerably less than those demonstrating sympathetic innervtion.

ELECTROPHYSIOLOGY

ELECTROCARDIOGRAPHIC PATTERNS

It has been known for some time that electrocardiographic changes can be seen after transplantation. The earliest method of monitoring for heart transplant rejection, indeed, quantified changes in electrocardiographic QRS voltage patterns. Reduction in quantitative voltage suggested cell-mediated allograft rejection.[7, 116] Though this finding is now believed to be insensitive and indiscriminate, the observation undoubtedly reflected attenuation of electrical signals during inflammation. Certainly, electrocardiographic abnormalities in the most general sense are frequently noted after heart transplantation. Leonelli et al.[69] suggested that almost 75% of first postoperative electrocardiograms demonstrated changes that would not be expected in normal patients. There was no difference with respect to patient age, donor age, ischemic time, and prior drug therapy between patients with normal and those with abnormal electrocardiograms. Clearly, there are evolutionary changes taking place during the initial post–heart transplant period. Patients having progressive deterioration of the conduction system manifested by widening QRS complexes or worsening preexisting conduction defects irrespective of other aspects of their clinical course seemingly have a higher early postoperative mortality. These changes can also become an important prognostic finding for subsequent left ventricular dysfunction and mortality.[68] Sudden death in such patients in some cases relates to complete heart block, which potentially could be prevented with a pacemaker system.

SINUS NODE DYSFUNCTION

Normal sinus node function is dependent on a complex interplay between intrinsic electrophysiologic properties of the sinus node, sinoatrial conduction properties, and extrinsic factors such as the autonomic nervous system.[34, 59] Sinus node dysfunction in the transplanted heart may be caused by injury during graft harvesting, ischemic injury during the transplant procedure, distortion of the atria during implantation, acute cell-mediated rejection, or, during longer term follow-up, ischemia caused by allograft vasculopathy. Approximately 20% of heart transplant patients during the early postoperative period demonstrate sinus node dysfunction with slow or no spontaneous depolarization.[71, 93] Most often noted is simply a sinus rhythm with a lower resting heart rate (< 70 bpm). Fortunately, sinus node dysfunction is usually transient, with corrected sinus node recovery time (the interval before resuming sinus rhythm following a 15- to 60-second period of overdrive suppression by rapid atrial pacing) reported to be longest about 2 weeks after transplant.[55] When this is associated with sinus bradycardia (rather than junctional escape rhythms), the likelihood of subsequent normal sinus node function is high.[54] However, a resting heart rate persistently less than 70 bpm, even though in sinus rhythm, or a junctional rhythm at the time of hospital discharge is predictive of long-term sinus node dysfunction. One note of interest relates to the frequent use of amiodarone before transplantation (see Chapters 5 and 12). In addition to other deleterious effects, this drug may induce a sinus bradycardia after transplantation which may persist for weeks (until the drug is mostly excreted) but eventually is totally reversible.[22]

Some studies suggest that the escape mechanism of "lower pacemakers" in the denervated heart is less reliable, which may increase the risk of an adverse event in the presence of sinus node dysfunction.[12] The rare posttransplant patient who dies in sudden and unexpected fashion early, as well as late, after heart transplantation[51] may have sinus node dysfunction. Thus, the presence of persistent relative bradycardia after cardiac transplantation suggests sinus node dysfunction, and resultant bradyarrhythmic events might be more significant than ventricular tachyarrhythmias. Indeed, some patients receive permanent pacemaker implantation for persistent sinus node dysfunction.[32, 93] Some transplant physicians recommend placement of permanent pacemakers after heart transplantation in patients with unexplained recurrent syncope or near syncope, particularly in the setting of allograft vasculopathy, where sinus node dysfunction may be intermittent and difficult to document.[51] The treatment of early and late sinus node dysfunction is discussed in Chapters 12 and 18.

ATRIOVENTRICULAR CONDUCTION

Electrophysiologic studies performed after cardiac transplantation demonstrate that atrioventricular node conduction times are similar to those of normal subjects both at rest and during pacing.[13, 126] Atrial-His and His-ventricular intervals are also normal. The atrioventricular node is known to alter conductivity in relation to the rate of stimulation, but this response requires more time to occur in the transplanted heart.[15] In normal hearts these changes occur almost instantaneously, but in the denervated heart several seconds are required. These observations reemphasize the fact that atrioventricular node impulse transmission is controlled intrinsically with autonomic innervation not being essential for underlying function. Autonomic innervation, however, likely enhances this activity.

VENTRICULAR ARRHYTHMIAS

Ventricular arrhythmias in the heart transplant patient, in contradistinction to bradyarrhythmias, are uncommon. Animal models have suggested that cardiac denervation is an antiarrhythmic maneuver, particularly in terms of ischemia-related ventricular arrhythmias.[104] Because ventricular tachycardia is uncommon in long-term survivors of orthotopic heart transplantation, when serious ventricular arrhythmias do occur, they seem mostly associated with development of allograft vasculopathy and myocardial ischemia.[3, 41, 75] This is not to discount the fact that when seen early, ventricular arrhythmias can signal acute inflammation associated with cell-mediated rejection. Again, the relationship of ischemic disease in the transplanted heart to bradyarrhythmias may be more important and ominous. These findings could herald problems and be sensed as nonspecific "spells" or near-syncopal episodes that may be difficult to characterize. Interestingly, heart transplant patients do not seem to sense their arrhythmias with the same frequency or intensity as nontransplant patients, and one wonders about the relationship of cardiac denervation to this observation.

HEMODYNAMIC FUNCTION

Hemodynamic derangements, often quite subtle, are usually apparent in the cardiac allograft. Nonetheless, despite sometimes significant hemodynamic perturbation, these hearts are, for the most part, functioning far better than the organs they replaced. Indeed, the initial reports of human heart transplantation gave insight into this fact, though rejection was likely much more profound in those experiences.[118]

HEART RATE

As discussed earlier, one important characteristic of the transplanted heart without vagal innervation is a higher resting heart rate (90–115 bpm) compared to normal hearts of similar age (60–90 bpm). As is discussed in the later section Cardiac Allograft Response to Exercise, the heart rate response is also blunted during exercise, which adversely affects exercise performance. Increases in heart rate in response to stress or exercise appear to be mediated mainly by circulating catecholamines. Following denervation, beta-receptor density in the myocardium increases, as does myocyte chronotropic sensitivity to circulating catecholamines.[150] It is of interest that chronic vigorous exercise training in heart transplant patients is associated with a decrease in resting heart rate.[63] The heart rate does not respond to carotid sinus massage or to innervation-dependent drugs such as atropine.

SYSTOLIC FUNCTION

Following the denervation which accompanies cardiac transplantation, myocardial catecholamine stores are completely depleted within days. However, intrinsic myocardial contractility remains unaffected by this change. Experimental studies in denervated heart preparations indicate that isolated papillary muscle length–tension relationship[27] and ventricular function curves[30] remain normal. When the cardiac allograft is not rejecting and in the absence of allograft vasculopathy, left ventricular systolic function is usually normal during long-term follow-up. In an elegant study utilizing fluoroscopic analysis of radiopaque myocardial markers implanted surgically at the time of transplantation, shortening fractions were within normal baseline ranges (compared to nontransplant controls) and an appropriate increase in cardiac output occurred during low-intensity exercise resulting from augmentation in end-diastolic volume and a subsequent increase in left ventricular stroke volume.[58] Verani et al.[135] demonstrated that systolic ventricular performance of the transplanted heart (both right and left ventricular ejection fraction) was comparable to that of controls when radionuclide angiography was used. With this technique, resting peak diastolic filling rates and time to peak diastolic filling rate were also normal.

ATRIAL DYNAMICS

In the traditional orthotopic transplant, atrial dynamics are abnormal because of the midatrial anastomosis required to effect allograft implantation.[130] Varying-sized portions of donor and recipient atria will be present with the native atria not necessarily contracting synchronously with the allograft atria. The left atrium (with its combined donor and recipient components) is generally larger with depressed emptying fraction compared to normal controls.[29] Normally, 15–20% of net stroke volume is contributed by atrial systole, and this is not the

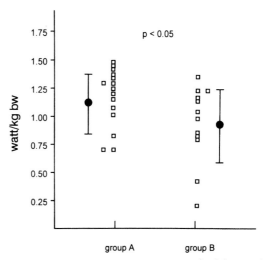

FIGURE **11–7.** Exercise capacity (mean $\pm$ 1 standard deviation) of 27 patients after orthotopic heart transplantation. Exercise capacity was significantly greater in the bicaval transplantation group (group A, $n = 15$) (1.17 ± 0.25 watt/kg body weight) compared with the standard transplantation group (group B, $n = 12$) (0.93 ± 0.34 watt/kg body weight). (From Leyh RG, Jahnke AW, Kraatz EG, Sievers HH: Cardiovascular dynamics and dimensions after bicaval and standard cardiac transplantation. Ann Thorac Surg 1995;59:1495–1500.)

case in cardiac allografts. Since native sinus node electrical activity is not transmitted across the atrial suture line, the normal atrial contribution to net stroke volume is generally less in heart transplant patients than in normal subjects.[29, 124]

More recent reports suggest that improved atrial transport function can be achieved following the **bicaval** anastomotic technique (see Chapter 10) compared to the more traditional "biatrial" anastomosis.[43, 70] Freimark et al.[43] reported more normal atrial transport function and greater atrial ejection force with the bicaval technique. Leyh and colleagues noted more synchronous right atrial contraction, smaller right ventricular end-diastolic diameter, and smaller right ventricular end-diastolic area (Fig. 11–6) in hearts implanted with the bicaval compared to the biatrial technique.[70] During exercise, bicaval hearts had a lower incidence and lesser severity of tricuspid regurgitation, and exercise capacity was better in the bicaval group (Fig. 11–7). The bicaval technique is increasingly utilized by transplant surgeons, and, if properly performed, it does not increase ischemic time (see Chapter 10). It does, however, carry the potential for subsequent superior vena caval stenosis, particularly in infants and children. This complication is rare in adults.

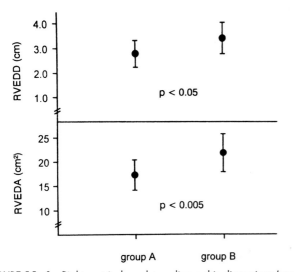

FIGURE **11–6.** Right ventricular echocardiographic dimensions (mean $\pm$ 1 standard deviation) in 27 patients after orthotopic heart transplantation. Right ventricular end-diastolic dimension (RVEDD) and right ventricular end-diastolic area (RVEDA) were significantly greater in the group having standard transplantation (group B, $n = 12$) compared with the group having bicaval transplantation (group A, $n = 15$). (From Leyh RG, Jahnke AW, Kraatz EG, Sievers HH: Cardiovascular dynamics and dimensions after bicaval and standard cardiac transplantation. Ann Thorac Surg 1995;59:1495–1500.)

DIASTOLIC FUNCTION

Right and left atrial pressures are often somewhat elevated during the first few days or weeks following cardiac transplantation, reflecting **decreased diastolic compliance.**[147] Similar findings have been noted in experimental studies.[115] When these diastolic abnormalities occur, they likely relate to reversible (although rarely it is irreversible and persistent) dysfunction secondary to ischemia/reperfusion injury, a smaller donor heart in a larger recipient, elevation of pulmonary vascular resistance, or a larger donor heart implanted into a restricted pericardial space secondary to multiple prior operations.

St Goar and colleagues[111] utilized Doppler echocardiographic techniques early after transplantation to assess left ventricular diastolic function serially and noted that isovolumic relaxation time and time to peak ventricular filling were suggestive of restrictive myocardial physiology. The restrictive hemodynamic patterns noted early after transplantation seemed to normalize within days or weeks, and the findings did not correlate well with preoperative pulmonary artery pressure or pulmonary vascular resistance. Also, there did not appear to be a correlation between observed restrictive myocardial changes and donor age or ischemic times.

Although obvious restrictive myocardial contractile patterns usually disappear early after transplantation, a subclinical, **occult, restrictive hemodynamic state** may persist that can be uncovered with an acute volume challenge or other preload/afterload modulation techniques. This subtle abnormality is present in most heart transplant recipients, but its significance is uncertain. Nonetheless, this finding likely impacts cardiac performance and may also contribute to molecular biodynamic and physical remodeling of the heart (see Chapter 4). Sometimes, more profound diastolic dysfunction can be noted, and it has been suggested by Doppler echocardiographic studies that impaired ventricular filling is significant and overt in 10–15% of patients long-term after heart transplantation. This abnormality is most often noted when significant cellular allograft rejection is apparent.[48, 131]

DONOR–RECIPIENT SIZE MATCH

There continues to be controversy over the relationship between donor–recipient size mismatch and hemodynamic performance after cardiac transplantation. Although the traditional recommendation is to accept donor hearts within 20% of the recipient weight, it has become common (University of Alabama at Birmingham experience) to allocate hearts from male donors who are 70 kg or greater to essentially any sized recipient (up to 110–120 kg). Hosenpud et al. examined the impact of size mismatch on several hemodynamic indices and found that smaller hearts into larger recipients achieved normal cardiac outputs at increased heart rates and higher filling pressures (right atrial and pulmonary capillary wedge pressures).[57] However, it is important to note that there was considerable scatter in the data, and none of the resting right atrial pressures exceeded 12 mm Hg (very mild elevation). Thus, secure information about the influence of and adaptation to considerable donor–recipient size mismatch is still lacking. However, we must underscore the potential dangers of transplanting smaller female donor hearts into larger male recipients[148] (see Chapter 16).

LEFT VENTRICULAR MASS/VOLUME

Left ventricular mass is known to increase in patients who suffer recurrent rejection after cardiac transplantation.[123] In the absence of recurrent rejection, however, left ventricular mass generally remains within the normal range.[123] Of note, Tischler et al. reported small but significant increases in left ventricular end-systolic volume during the first 4 years after transplantation, despite normal ejection fraction and ventricular mass.[19, 123] The resultant decrease in mass/volume ratio and increase in end-systolic wall stress suggest that the transplanted heart may respond to chronic pressure overload (e.g., with cyclosporine-induced hypertension) with ventricular dilatation more than hypertrophy. The explanation for this response in the denervated heart is unclear.

PREEXISTING CARDIAC DISEASE

Preexisting disease in a donor heart may also account for physiologic abnormalities after implantation. Older donor hearts may have occult but significant coronary artery disease, which will further contribute to diastolic dysfunction. Mitral valve prolapse may predispose to subsequent mitral regurgitation. Hypertension in the donor may lead to increased ventricular mass, left ventricular hypertrophy, and diastolic dysfunction. Clearly, whenever one is evaluating function of a transplanted heart, the patient status with respect to these confounding variables must be considered.

CARDIAC ALLOGRAFT RESPONSE TO EXERCISE

In the absence of rejection, allograft vasculopathy, or severe forms of diastolic dysfunction, transplant patients can engage in moderate exercise, and with proper conditioning, even high levels of exercise; this clearly offers great improvement over their prior state of heart failure (see Chapter 4). Although some studies suggest normal exercise capacity in heart transplant patients,[78, 92, 152] it appears that transplant recipients have, for the most part, diminished maximal exercise tolerance when compared with that of age- and sex-matched normal controls.[60, 61, 90, 100, 101, 114] The subnormal exercise tolerance is largely related to a **limitation of maximal cardiac output during exercise**. The hemodynamic alterations which contribute to this limitation are listed in Table 11–2.

TABLE 11–2	Factors Contributing to Reduction in Peak Cardiac Output of Heart Allografts During Exercise

- Delayed and blunted increase in heart rate
- Mismatch of heart rate and venous return
- Exaggerated increase in intracardiac filling pressures during early exercise (diastolic dysfunction)
- Reduced systolic reserves
- Decreased coronary flow reserves

HEART RATE RESPONSE DURING EXERCISE

Animal and human transplant studies have documented a distinct pattern of chronotropic response to exercise. The major impediment to high levels of exercise is the **limited ability to rapidly augment heart rate** with exertion. Cannon[24] and Donald[36] first demonstrated that the denervated heart increases heart rate in response to exercise, but the response is delayed and, in experimental models, the peak heart rate response is considerably less than in normal controls (Fig. 11–8).[36] When a human heart transplant recipient initiates exercise, the initial (resting) heart rate is higher than normal controls. However, within moments, the normal control subject demonstrates a prompt acceleration of heart rate, driven by central sympathetic nerve activity, and the heart rate quickly (within several minutes) surpasses the transplanted heart rate. This blunting of chronotropic response during early exercise results from the lack of sympathetic innervation. As documented in animal studies (see again Fig. 11–8), the tranplant heart rate has a delayed but steady rise during increasing exercise which generally is less than in control subjects at similar levels of exercise.[128] Typically, peak transplant heart rate may not be achieved until about 15 minutes into exercise. Eventually, if exercise is continued to near exhaustion the heart rate approaches that of normal subjects.[107] Thus, exercise after heart transplantation eventually induces tachycardia and an increased contractile state, but this takes time to develop and is seemingly related to the effects of increased circulating catecholamine levels.[105] The dynamics of this exercise response may account for the fact that maximal stress cardiac output after heart transplantation is usually lower than that seen in normal subjects.[9, 23, 26, 90, 92, 118, 151]

SYSTOLIC RESPONSE TO EXERCISE

The transplant left ventricular **ejection fraction** shows significant increase during exercise,[135] typically from about 0.60 at rest to 0.70 or more during exercise,[77] likely due to increased circulating catecholamines. However, studies by Verani and colleagues[135] concluded that peak right and left ventricular ejection fractions were significantly less than normal, suggesting mild impairment of systolic reserves.

DIASTOLIC FUNCTION DURING EXERCISE

As noted in the earlier section, Diastolic Function, most transplanted hearts show evidence of subtle diastolic dysfunction. Intracardiac filling pressures elevate quickly during exercise, with the left ventricle operating at normal or reduced left ventricular volumes on a pressure–volume curve that is steeper and shifted to the left (Fig. 11–9), indicative of a stiff (less compliant) ventricle with diastolic dysfunction.[8, 50, 107, 117, 123, 147] In many patients this abnormality may be quite subtle, as noted by a nearly normal increase in peak diastolic filling rate during exercise.[135] The impact of diastolic function on supine versus upright exercise is discussed in a subsequent section.

MECHANISMS FOR INCREASING CARDIAC OUTPUT DURING EXERCISE

The earliest and probably most important mechanism for increasing cardiac output is **increased venous return** during initial exercise, producing an increase in ventric-

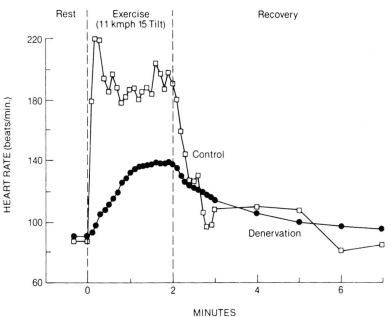

FIGURE **11–8.** The heart rate increase with exercise in a dog before and after cardiac denervation is shown. Cardiac denervation produces a slower rise in heart rate with exercise and a slower decline in heart rate after exercise. (From Donald DE, Shephard JT: Response to exercise in dogs with cardiac denervation. Am J Physiol 1963; 205:494–500.)

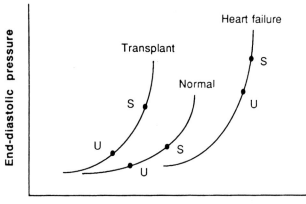

FIGURE **11–9.** Theoretical end-diastolic pressure–volume relations in normal, failing, and transplanted hearts based on current and reported exercise hemodynamic data. S, supine exercise; U, upright exercise. (From Rudas L, Pflugfelder PW, McKenzie FN, Menkis ANRJ, Kostuk WJ: Normalization of upright exercise hemodynamics and improved exercise capacity one year after orthotopic cardiac transplantation. Am J Cardiol 1992;69:1336–1339.)

ular end-diastolic volume and pressure which results in increased stroke volume (Starling mechanism) (Table 11–3). As exercise progresses, adrenal output of **endogenous catecholamines** increases, which **accelerates heart rate** and **increases contractility.** Indeed, the ultimate increase in heart rate and cardiac output has been shown in experimental and clinical studies[35, 92] to parallel the increase in circulating adrenal catecholamines.

Observations in canine studies following cardiac autotransplantation (producing a denervated heart) indicate an excellent exercise capacity which is largely dependent on circulating catecholamines during peak exercise, as evidenced by greyhounds running at competitive levels.[36] Cardiac output increases in proportion to minute volume of oxygen consumption in a similar ratio as before denervation, accomplished by a greater increase in stroke volume early in exercise to compensate for the blunted heart rate response.[36]

It is of interest that despite the strong dependence on circulating catecholamines, the reported rise in plasma norepinephrine levels during exercise is similar to levels in normal subjects,[99] suggesting that any enhanced effect on the denervated heart relates to increased myocardial sensitivity to beta-adrenergic compounds. Other mechanisms are undoubtedly also involved, since animals can exercise after autotransplantation and bilateral adrena-

TABLE 11–3	**Mechanisms for Increasing Cardiac Output in the Transplanted Heart**

- Increased venous return during initial exercise is accompanied by increased ventricular end-diastolic pressure–volume and stroke volume (Starling mechanism)
- Increased circulating adrenal catecholamines produce increased heart rate and contractility
- Increased heart rate contributes to increased cardiac output
- Increased heart rate leads to increased contractility (Bowditch effect)
- Release of atrial natriuretic peptide promotes arteriolar vasodilation (decreased systemic vascular resistance)

lectomy,[36] and transplant recipients can perform some exercise after acute beta blockade.[14, 35, 107, 152]

The accelerated heart rate is itself a stimulus for increased contractility, referred to as the **Bowditch** or treppe (staircase) **effect.**[145] The effect is small compared to that of circulating catecholamines, but it may be clinically significant.

Atrial natriuretic peptide (see later section, Endocrine Abnormalities) may also have a beneficial effect on cardiac output during exercise. As atrial and ventricular stretch receptors rapidly stimulate increased cardiac secretion of this cardiac hormone, arterial vasodilation is enhanced and afterload is reduced.

EARLY STAGES OF EXERCISE

During the early stages of exercise, the increase in allograft cardiac output results primarily from an increase in stroke volume secondary to an **increase in end-diastolic volume** and pressure, with little change in end-systolic volume. Pflugfelder and colleagues compared exercise responses in a group of transplant patients 1 month to 2 years after transplant who exercised regularly with those of an age- and sex-matched normal control group.[90] The transplant group had a 30% higher heart rate at rest. During initial stages of exercise, the transplant group increased their heart rate by only 3% (compared to 37% in the normal group). The increase in cardiac output in transplant patients resulted from a 20% increase in stroke volume (3% increase in controls), accompanied by a 14% increase in end-diastolic volume index (unchanged in controls) and a 6% increase in end-systolic volume index (decreased in controls). Thus, the abnormal response of the transplant heart to early stages of exercise is majorly influenced by the **blunted chronotropic response,** which contrasts with normal subjects, in whom heart rate increases by 30% or more quickly after initiating exercise[90, 91] and prompt cardiac sympathetic stimulation also increases both inotropy and lusitropy.[81, 97] In the denervated heart, the prompt increase in venous return with initiation of exercise is not accompanied by a prompt chronotropic response, resulting in the recognized abnormal elevation of end-diastolic volume to augment cardiac output. Thus, a hallmark of the initial response to exercise in the transplanted heart is a **mismatch of heart rate and venous return.**[100] This and other factors contributing to increased ventricular filling pressures during exercise are summarized in Figure 11–10.[100]

EFFECT OF POSTURAL CHANGES

Additional insight is gained from studies on the impact of posture on cardiac function. Cardiac allograft performance is quite dependent on loading conditions, which can be significantly influenced by postural changes that alter intracardiac volume.[101] During **supine exercise,** augmented venous return with leg raising contributes to significant increase in end-diastolic volume.[92] As expected, heart rate increases slowly and subnormally[102]

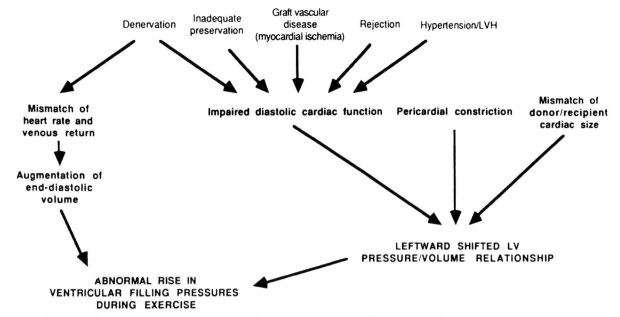

FIGURE **11–10.** Postulated mechanisms responsible for elevated ventricular filling pressures during exercise in cardiac transplant recipients. LV, left ventricular; LVH, left ventricular hypertrophy. (From Rudas L, Pflugfelder PW, McKenzie FN, Menkis ANRJ, Kostuk WJ: Normalization of upright exercise hemodynamics and improved exercise capacity one year after orthotopic cardiac transplantation. Am J Cardiol 1992;69:1336–1339.)

during exercise, very different from the innervated heart. The importance of heart rate in maintaining cardiac output is evident in the transition from supine to upright position in healthy untrained subjects, in whom a 15–20% increase in heart rate[11, 120, 137] accompanies the decrease in ventricular filling pressures and stroke volume secondary to venous pooling and decrease in venous return. In posttransplant patients, ventricular filling pressures are generally significantly lower during upright than supine exercise,[100] and abnormally high pulmonary wedge (>20 mm Hg) and right atrial (10–15 mm Hg) pressures have been documented during supine exercise.[100] Heart rate increases slowly in both forms of exercise, and peak heart rates are similar in both positions. Similarly, peak stroke index and cardiac index are similar in both situations.

CHANGE IN EXERCISE PERFORMANCE OVER TIME

In many patients, the hemodynamic derangement appears to improve somewhat during the first year after transplantation, characterized by an increased heart rate responsiveness from lying to sitting, higher peak heart rate, higher peak cardiac index, and lower mean pulmonary capillary wedge and right atrial pressures during exercise at 12 months compared to 3 months after transplant.[101] A number of factors may contribute to this improvement, including greater recovery from the pretransplant heart failure state (see Chapter 4), partial cardiac reinnervation, and other unidentified factors. In addition, less hemodynamic perturbation seems apparent in patients who have optimized their body weight and trained regularly in aerobic fashion.

ROLE OF PULMONARY DYSFUNCTION IN REDUCED EXERCISE CAPACITY

Other systems may participate in the exercise limitations of some transplant patients. Reports of exercise-induced hypoxemia in some heart transplant recipients indicate that not all of the exercise and resting hemodynamic impairment noted in cardiac allografts is due entirely to changes within the heart. Braith et al.[18] studied whether heart transplantation was associated with **abnormal pulmonary diffusion capacity** and attempted to clarify potentially deleterious effects of impaired pulmonary diffusion on arterial blood-gas dynamics during exercise. Preexisting conditions known to affect diffusion adversely include congestive heart failure, presence of comorbid primary lung disease, pulmonary infection in an immunocompromised host, and prior drug administration causing pulmonary toxicity such as seen with amiodarone. In this evaluation, patients underwent pulmonary function testing with bicycle ergometric exercise 13 months before and 18 months after cardiac transplantation. Despite improvements in pulmonary function, post–heart transplant vital capacity, forced expiratory volume, and diffusion capacity were lower than in matched control subjects. Changes in arterial blood-gas findings were similar between groups at 40% of peak exercise, but at 70% of peak exercise arterial blood gases and blood pH were significantly different in allograft patients having low diffusion capacity than in patients with normal diffusion or in control subjects. Cardiac index did not differ between the transplant patients with normal or low diffusion at rest or during exercise and, therefore, it appears that exercise-induced relative hypoxemia secondary to pulmonary dysfunction can limit exercise capacity after cardiac transplantation[85] (see Pulmonary Function section in Chapter 6).[39, 52]

SKELETAL MUSCLE PERFORMANCE AFTER TRANSPLANTATION

It is also important to relate post–heart transplant exercise performance to other determinants of peak exercise function such as peripheral muscle performance.[38, 73] Patients with advanced heart failure often have **skeletal muscle atrophy** and **metabolic abnormalities** which contribute to exercise intolerance above and beyond that to be expected from altered cardiac output and abnormal pulmonary filling pressures. Wilson et al.[141] performed hemodynamic monitoring during maximal treadmill exercise testing, demonstrating that the level of exercise intolerance perceived by patients with heart failure had little or no relation to objective measures of circulatory, ventilatory, or metabolic dysfunction produced during aerobic stress. Therefore, simply altering blood flow and pressure to more normal levels after heart transplantation may not entirely improve exercise intolerance, since intrinsic muscle oxidative problems could persist after heart transplantation and, in fact, be exacerbated by immunotherapeutic drug administration. Peak oxygen utilization and time taken to reach anaerobic threshold may be impaired after transplantation[60, 114] because of residual peripheral skeletal muscle abnormalities (such as depressed skeletal muscle oxidative metabolism and subnormal rate of mitochondrial adenosine triphosphate [ATP] synthesis)[119] originally precipitated by the heart failure syndrome. Indeed, peak exertional oxygen utilization after cardiac transplantation is often surprisingly low, and sometimes, despite time, does not improve dramatically. At any level of oxygen consumption during exercise, cardiac output is generally lower in transplant recipients than in normal controls.[26] Savin et al.[102] demonstrated that patients after heart transplantation have higher peak lactate levels but lower peak oxygen uptake and lower peak work rates than those of normal age- and sex-matched controls. Nonetheless, as has been previously emphasized, allograft recipients are still capable of participating in most desired physical activities and, in comparison to their pretransplant morbid states, are usually dramatically improved.

EXERCISE RESPONSE DURING BETA BLOCKADE

Under conditions of high levels of exercise, the increased sensitivity of myocardial beta receptors to circulating catecholamines seems to compensate for the absence of sympathetic nerve stimulation, such that, as noted previously, the heart rate of the transplanted heart responds to exercise demands, although more slowly than normally innervated hearts. Because of this reliance on myocardial beta-adrenergic receptors, the administration of beta-adrenergic blocking agents may have deleterious effects during situations of increased circulatory stress. During acute beta blockade, Yusuf and colleagues[152] noted a blunting of exercise-induced tachycardia and a reduction in peak exercise capacity by about 15%.

ENDOCRINE ABNORMALITIES

NATRIURETIC PEPTIDE

The heart is also an endocrine gland, in that **atrial natriuretic peptide** (ANP) is normally synthesized, stored, and released from the right atrium in response to atrial stretch.[5, 66, 89, 146] Brain natriuretic peptide (BNP) is stored mainly in the ventricles and may respond similarly to ventricular stretch, which reflects increased ventricular pressure and volume.[79] Many studies have documented that the autonomic nervous system is not necessary for the release of ANP and BNP. These hormones play a role in sodium and water homeostasis, acting to enhance sodium and water excretion in states of cardiac and/or circulatory volume overload, apparently through inhibition of aldosterone and vasopressin secretion. They also promote arterial vasodilation.[16, 98, 154]

In heart transplant patients, **plasma ANP levels are generally elevated** (Fig. 11–11) and further increases occur in response to volume loading.[109, 125] Available evidence suggests that ANP levels are higher than would be expected by atrial and ventricular stretch alone.[6] The role of partial reinnervation or inflammation (secondary to rejection) on ANP secretion after transplantation remains to be clarified.

Graded exercise significantly increases ANP levels in both the right atrium and the main pulmonary artery, thus indicating that heart transplant recipients still retain the ability to increase ANP synthesis and release in response to exercise.[88] Bussieres-Chafe et al.[21] further studied ANP dynamics by attempting to clarify the relationship of plasma levels of ANP to body position and central hemodynamics. Hemodynamics, mixed expiratory gas exchange analysis, ventilatory measurements, and venous blood levels of ANP were determined at

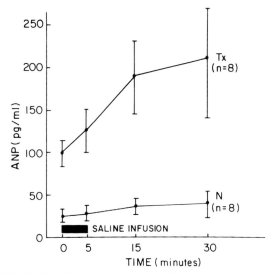

FIGURE **11–11.** The response to a rapid (6-minute) infusion of a liter of normal saline solution to a group of transplant patients (n = 8) and normal subjects (n = 8). Note the higher baseline level of ANP in transplant patients and the increase in ANP with volume loading. (From Uretsky BF: Physiology of the transplanted heart. Cardiovasc Clin 1990;20:23–56.)

rest and during graded bicycle ergometric study. These investigators noted a change in exercise ANP levels from rest, and the degree of change correlated with increases in pulmonary capillary wedge pressure, systolic pulmonary artery pressure, and right atrial pressure. No correlation existed between changes in ANP level and peak oxygen consumption, heart rate, or mean arterial blood pressure. Clearly, exercise in the heart transplant recipient is a stimulus for ANP secretion with augmentation of plasma ANP levels during exercise modulated by changes in central hemodynamics.

ENDOTHELIN

Paracrine system perturbations are also apparent in heart transplant patients. Cyclosporine-treated individuals exhibit a high index of systemic hypertension as already alluded to, and endothelin, a potent vasoconstrictor peptide of endothelial origin, may contribute to this complication. Haas and colleagues[53] detected increased endothelin-1 levels in heart transplant patients, and the increase persisted during short-term follow-up, but did not correlate with hemodynamic variables, serum creatinine, or cyclosporine levels. The observation of increased endothelin in these patients raises some concern because of the rather substantial hemodynamic effects of this peptide which functions in a paracrine fashion.

CORONARY CIRCULATION

In the denervated transplanted heart, resting coronary blood flow (in the absence of rejection or allograft vasculopathy) is similar to or slightly higher[83] than in normal hearts.[33] Despite documented differences in regional myocardial reinnervation, basal coronary blood flow remains similar in all major coronary territories, which suggests that resting coronary flow is not substantially influenced by neural adrenergic influences.[25, 33, 56] Furthermore, in the absence of allograft vasculopathy, coronary flow reserve, as assessed by intracoronary papaverine or adenosine, is similar to that observed in normal (innervated) hearts. Importantly, however, cardiac efferent adrenergic signals play a prominent role in augmenting coronary blood flow during periods of stress such as with exercise or exposure to cold, in which the sympathetic nervous system is activated. Denervated transplant hearts (or denervated areas of transplant myocardium) have a limited ability to augment coronary blood flow in such situations, which may contribute to subnormal cardiac performance during exercise.[33]

PHARMACOLOGIC RESPONSES OF THE CARDIAC ALLOGRAFT

Numerous cardiovascular drugs affect physiologic responses through autonomic nervous system activation or blockade and therefore will be different, with respect to response, when given to transplant rather than nontransplant patients.

PARASYMPATHETIC BLOCKING AGENTS

The effects of atropine are mediated by a parasympatholytic mechanism. Therefore, given the generally denervated state of the transplanted heart, atropine does not increase the allograft ventricular rate when bradycardia is present.[67] **Atropine** is, therefore, a useless drug in heart transplant patients when bradycardia, sudden heart block, or asystole develops. In a similar vein, edrophonium, a cholinesterase-inhibiting compound, has no effect on heart rate in the transplanted patient.[113]

BETA-ADRENERGIC DRUGS

Sympathetic agents which have a direct effect on myocardial beta-adrenergic receptors appear to have exaggerated effects on heart rate and cardiac contractility after heart transplantation.[153] The human transplanted, denervated heart demonstrates increased sensitivity to the chronotropic effects of catecholamines such as isoproterenol[153] and dobutamine.[17] Experimental[134] and clinical studies[153] suggest that the increased sensitivity is secondary to an increase in beta-receptor density. Direct-acting beta-adrenergic stimulating drugs, such as isoproterenol or epinephrine, are effective agents to treat sinus bradycardia.[67, 113, 153]

ADENOSINE

Exaggerated sensitivity to acetylcholine in denervated cardiac animal models has been documented.[62] Acetylcholine and the endogenous nucleoside adenosine have similar electrophysiologic effects.[40] The denervated donor sinus node has greater sensitivity to exogenous adenosine than does the normal innervated sinus node.[40] The fact that a denervated sinus node drives intrinsic heart rate after heart transplant mandates that care should be taken to prevent bradycardia when adenosine is used during diagnostic scintigraphic studies or to attempt cardioversion in patients having paroxysmal supraventricular arrhythmias (which can be seen in the setting of acute cellular rejection). Perhaps it is best to avoid adenosine administration entirely after cardiac transplantation because of these altered pharmacologic properties.

BETA-ADRENERGIC BLOCKING AGENTS

Beta-adrenergic blocking agents are sometimes used for control of difficult chronic hypertension after transplantation. However, these agents may have deleterious effects on the denervated heart, which relies extensively on circulating catecholamine stimulation of myocardial beta-adrenergic receptors for enhancement of ventricular performance. Verani et al.[136] studied beta-adrenergic blockade in heart transplant patients using propranolol administration. Acutely, this agent produced a decrease in ventricular performance at rest that was characterized by a lower stroke volume index, lower cardiac index, and lower ejection fraction in both heart transplant patients and control subjects with the ejection fraction significantly lower in the heart transplant recipients. As the ejection fraction decreased, end-systolic volume increased substantially. In normal subjects there was a reduction in heart rate, but there was only a minimal reduction in ejection fraction and no change in end-systolic volume. Circulating neurohormones appear crucial in heart transplant patients to enable reasonable exercise performance which, as detailed previously, is not normal. Therefore, caution is advised with the use of beta blockers in this setting.[152] Despite these general limitations, beta blocking agents used chronically are usually tolerated reasonably well in transplant patients with difficult hypertension.[50]

DIGOXIN

The electrophysiologic effects of digoxin are primarily on sympathetic and parasympathetic mediated sinoatrial and atrioventricular node function; therefore, this agent has little electrophysiologic activity in the transplanted heart.[49] The inotropic effect of digoxin, which is not mediated by the autonomic nervous system, remains intact but is minimal. Digoxin is therefore likely not to be effective when given to induce atrioventricular block in patients with atrial fibrillation or supraventricular tachycardia after transplant.

OTHER ANTIARRHYTHMIC AGENTS

Certain antiarrhythmic agents, such as Vaughn Williams Class IA agents quinidine and disopyramide, have vagolytic effects that increase resting heart rate in nontransplant patients.[13, 76] These changes are not seen in the denervated cardiac allograft and, instead, the direct effects of decreased sinus rate and increased atrioventricular conduction times can be noted.[13, 76]

CALCIUM CHANNEL BLOCKING AGENTS

Calcium channel blockers demonstrate an attenuated response with respect to electrophysiologic and electrocardiographic changes in heart transplant patients. **Diltiazem,** a calcium channel blocker frequently used to control post–heart transplant hypertension and allograft vasculopathy, does not seem to cause substantial decline in resting heart rate.[12, 94] **Verapamil** produces a slight increase in atrial-His interval.[12] The dihydropyridine calcium channel blocker **nifedipine** produces a minimal reflex increase in heart rate that is coincident with decrement in blood pressure and has been shown to produce a slight decrease in atrial-His interval.[12]

PHYSIOLOGY OF HETEROTOPIC HEART TRANSPLANTS

Though the so-called "piggyback" or heterotopic cardiac transplant is rarely performed today, the procedure may still serve a specific purpose and play a role in managing selected patients.[57, 65, 96] Utilizing a heterotopic heart is, in effect, using the allograft as a "biologic" ventricular assist device.[65, 96, 133] Because heterotopic heart transplantation historically had been performed in the setting of a very elevated pulmonary artery pressure or when donor size seemed inadequate in relation to needs dictated by the potential recipient's size, central hemodynamics after heterotopic transplantation have been somewhat difficult to interpret. Furthermore, central circulatory hemodynamics are often difficult to assess, since the heterotopic implant is placed in parallel to the existing native circulation. Hemodynamic function of the heterotopic heart is dependent, therefore, on additional physiologic variables such as the contribution to overall native cardiac output by the native heart, patency of venous anastomoses, presence of pulmonary hypertension, and the ability or inability to fill the heterotopic right heart system. Heterotopic implants have been demonstrated capable of completely supporting a patient's circulation when the native heart becomes asystolic or develops ventricular fibrillation.[65] Furthermore, over time, reduction in pulmonary hypertension has been noted after heterotopic transplantation with right heart hemodynamics in the native heart becoming similar to those noted in an orthotopic heart transplant recipient.[133] Heterotopic cardiac transplantation can provide hemodynamic support sufficient enough to ameliorate many of the abnormalities and limitations caused by advanced left ventricular dysfunction and congestive heart failure, but little data is available that suggests substantial increase in exercise tolerance develops. For further discussion of heterotopic transplants, see Chapter 10.

CONFOUNDING ISSUES

Many additional factors can contribute to functional alteration in the transplanted heart. Obviously, cell-mediated or humoral rejection with its subsequent myocarditis adversely affects cardiac pump performance. During acute rejection, whether it be humoral or cellular mediated, coronary vascular reserve is compromised with varying degrees of systolic and diastolic ventricular dysfunction (see Chapter 14). Profound reduction in cardiac output and ejection fraction with concomitant acute rise in ventricular filling pressures are often noted when rejection develops rapidly and is fulminant. Indeed, a sudden drop in blood pressure and cardiogenic shock early after transplant suggests profound rejection. Treatment of rejection often reverses these abnormalities, resulting in improved graft function.[84, 110] Nonetheless, permanent biventricular diastolic dysfunction and, sometimes, concomitant systolic dysfunction may result from frequent and severe episodes of histologic documented rejection. As alluded to previously, it has been suggested that the restrictive hemodynamic pattern noted after cardiac transplantation may result from inflammation that is chronic with acute intervals of worsening inflammatory activity.

With the use of cyclosporine-based immunosuppression, **hypertension** is very frequent after cardiac transplantation, with all of its subsequent effects on left ventricular afterload. In general, hypertension is well tolerated, but cardiac hypertrophy likely develops in response to hypertension and contributes to a detrimental remodeling process with all of its associated long-term functional alterations. Though hypertrophy seems intimately related to hypertension and afterload increases, one must remember that hypertrophy is also a response to inflammation and, therefore, the immunologic milieu of the transplant patient also contributes to this difficulty.

Chronic rejection or allograft vasculopathy also causes functional graft impairment (see Chapter 17). Left ventricular systolic dysfunction can occur in the setting of ischemic heart disease and, particularly, when coronary angiography defines high-risk groups such as those having myocardial infarction and heart failure.[129] Also important is the fact that the physiologic changes associated with allograft arteriopathy might precipitate sudden cardiac death from bradyarrhythmic events. Generally, as allograft arteriopathy progresses, slow deterioration in systolic and diastolic function is apparent with profound congestive heart failure often developing in a setting of low ejection fraction, small left ventricular chamber, and increased stiffness of the heart.

References

1. Abboud FM, Heistad DD, Mark AL, Schmid PG: Reflex control of the peripheral circulation. Prog Cardiovasc Dis 1976;18:371.
2. Abboud FM, Thames MD: Interaction of cardiovascular reflexes in circulation control. In Shepherd JT, Abboud FM (eds): Handbook of Physiology: The Cardiovascular System. Baltimore: Williams & Wilkins, 1983, p 675.
3. Alexopoulos D, Yusuf S: Ventricular arrhythmias in long term survivors of orthotopic and heterotopic heart transplantation. Br Heart J 1988;59:648–652.
4. Alexopoulos D, Yusuf S, Johnston JA, Bostock J, Sleight P, Yacoub MH: The 24-hour heart rate behavior in long term survivors of cardiac transplantation. Am J Cardiol 1988;61:880–884.
5. Anderson JV, Millar ND, O'Hare JP, Mackenzie JC: CRBS. Atrial natriuretic peptide: physiologic release associated with natriuresis during water immersion in man. Clin Sci 1986;71:319.
6. Ationu A, Burch M, Singer D, Littleton P, Carter N: Cardiac transplantation affects ventricular expression of brain natriuretic peptide. Cardiovasc Res 1993;27:188–191.
7. Barnard CA: Human heart transplantation: the diagnosis of rejection. Am J Cardiol 1968;22:811–819.
8. Barrow KM, Neumann A, Arensman FW, Yacoub MH: Left ventricular contractility and contractile reserve in humans after cardiac transplantation. Circulation 1985;71:866–872.
9. Beck W, Barnard CN, Schrire V: Heart rate after heart transplantation. Circulation 1969;40:437.
10. Bernardi L, Bianchini B, Spadacini G, Leuzzi S, Valle F, Marachesi E, Passino C, Calciati A, Vigano M, Rinaldi M, Martinelli L, Finardi G, Sleight P: Demonstrable cardiac reinnervation after human heart transplantation by carotid baroreflex modulation of RR interval. Circulation 1995;92:2895–2903.
11. Bevegard S, Homgren A, Jonsson B: The effect of body position on the circulation at rest and during exercise, with special reference to the influence on the stroke volume. Acta Physiol Scand 1960;49:279–298.
12. Bexton RS, Cory-Pearce R, Spurrell FAJ, Nathan AW, English TAH, Camm AJ: Electrophysiological effects of nifedipine and verapamil in the transplanted human heart. J Heart Transplant 1984;3:97–104.
13. Bexton RS, Hellerstrand KJ, Cory-Pearce R, Spurrell RA, English TA, Camm AJ: The direct electrophysiologic effects of disopyramide phosphate in the transplanted human heart. Circulation 1983;67:38–45.
14. Bexton RS, Milne JR, Cory-Pearce R: Effect of beta blockade on exercise response after cardiac transplantation. Br Heart J 1983;49:584.
15. Bexton RS, Nathan AW, Hellerstrand KJ, Cory-Pearce R, Spurrell FAJ, English TA, Camm AJ: Electrophysiologic abnormalities in the transplanted human heart. Br Heart J 1983;50:555–563.
16. Biollaz J, Nussberger J, Porchet M, Brunner-Feber F, Otterbein ES, Gomez H, Waeber B, Brunner HR: Four hour infusion of synthetic atrial natriuretic peptide in normal volunteers. Hypertension 1986;8(suppl):96.
17. Borow KM, Neumann A, Arensman FW, Yacoub MH: Cardiac and peripheral vascular responses to adrenoceptor stimulation and blockade after cardiac transplantation. J Am Coll Cardiol 1989;14:1229–1238.
18. Braith RW, Limacher MC, Mills RM Jr, Leggett SH, Pollack ML, Staples ED: Exercise-induced hypoxemia in heart transplant recipients. J Am Coll Cardiol 1993;22:768–776.
19. Brockway BA: Echocardiography and cardiac transplantation: a literature review on practical approach. J Am Soc Echocardiogr 1989;2:72–78.
20. Burke MN, McGinn AL, Homan DC, Christensen BV, Kubo SH, Wilson RF: Evidence for functional sympathetic reinnervation of left ventricle and coronary arteries after orthotopic cardiac transplantation in humans. Circulation 1995;91:72–78.
21. Bussieres-Chafe LM, Pflugfelder PW, Henderson AR, MacKinnon D, Taylor AW, Kostuk WJ: Effect of cardiac filling pressures on the release of atrial natriuretic peptide during exercise in heart transplant recipients. Can J Cardiol 1994;10:245–250.
22. Cameron DE, Augustine SM, Gardner TJ, Baumgartner WA, Reitz BA: Preoperative amiodarone therapy causes graft bradycardia following orthotopic heart transplantation. J Heart Transplant 1988;7:67.
23. Campeau L, Pospisil L, Grondin P, Dyrda I, Lepage G: Cardiac catheterization findings at rest and after exercise in patients following cardiac transplantation. Am J Cardiol 1970;25:523.
24. Cannon WB, Lewis JT, Britton SW: A lasting preparaton of the denervated heart for detecting internal secretion, with evidence from accessory accelerator fibers from the thoracic sympathetic chain. Am J Physiol 1926;77:326.
25. Chilian WM, Boatwright RB, Shoji T, Griggs DM: Evidence against significant resting sympathetic coronary vasoconstrictor tone in the conscious dog. Circ Res 1981;49:866–876.
26. Clark DA, Schroeder JS, Griepp RB, Stinson EB, Dong E, Shumway NE, Harrison DC: Cardiac transplantation in man: review of first three years' experience. Am J Med 1973;54:563.
27. Coleman HN, Dempsey RJ, Cooper T: Myocardial oxygen consumption following chronic cardiac denervation. Am J Physiol 1970;218:475.
28. Cooper T, Willman VL, Jellinek M, Hanlon CR: Heart transplantation: effect on myocardial catecholamine and histamine. Science 1962;138:40–41.
29. Cresci S, Goldstein JA, Hiram C, Waggoner AD, Perez JE: Impaired left atrial function after heart transplantation: disparate contribution of donor and recipient atrial components studied on-line with quantitative echocardiography. J Heart Transplant 1995;14:647–653.
30. Daggett W, William VL, Cooper T: Work capacity and efficiency of the autotransplanted heart. Circulation 1967;35(suppl):96–104.
31. DeMarco T, Dae M, Yuen-Green MSF, Kumar S, Sudhir K, Keith F, Amidon TM, Rifkin C, Klinski C, Lau D, Botvinick EH, Chatterjee K: Iodine-123-metaiodobenzylguanidine scintigraphic assessment of the transplanted human heart. Evidence of late reinnervation. J Am Coll Cardiol 1995;25:927–931.

32. DiBiase A, Tse TM, Schnittger I, Wexler L, Stinson EB, Valantine HA: Frequency and mechanism of bradycardia in cardiac transplant recipients and need for pacemakers. Am J Cardiol 1991; 67:1385–1389.

33. DiCarli MF, Tobes MC, Mangner TL, Levine AB, Muzik O, Chakroborty P, Levine TB: Effects of cardiac sympathetic innervation on coronary blood flow. N Engl J Med 1997;336:1208–1215.

34. Dighton DH: Autonomic influences and clinical assessment. Br Heart J 1974;36:791–797.

35. Donald DE, Ferguson DA, Milburn SE: Effect of beta adrenergic receptor blockade on racing performance of greyhounds with normal and denervated hearts. Circ Res 1968;22:127.

36. Donald DE, Shephard JT: Response to exercise in dogs with cardiac denervation. Am J Physiol 1963;205:494–500.

37. Dong E Jr, Hurley EJ: Performance of the heart two years after autotransplantation. Surgery 1964;56:270–240.

38. Drexler H: Skeletal muscle failure in heart failure. Circulation 1992;85:1621–1622.

39. Egan JJ, Kalra S, Yonan N, Hasleton PS, Brooks N, Woodcock AA: Pulmonary diffusion abnormalities in heart transplant recipients. Chest 1993;104:1085–1089.

40. Ellenbogen KA, Stamble BS, Wood MA, Mohanty PK: Electrophysiological effects of adenosine in the transplanted human heart. Evidence of supersensitivity. Circulation 1990;81:821–828.

41. Ellenbogen KA, Stamble BS, Wood MA, Mohanty PK: Division of mechanoelectrical feedback in the transplanted human heart. Am J Cardiol 1995;76:51–55.

42. Forman MB, Robertson D, Goldberg M, Bostick D, Uderman H, Perry JM, Robertson RM: Effect of tyramine on myocardial catecholamine release in coronary heart disease. Am J Cardiol 1984;53:80.

43. Freimark D, Czer LS, Aleksic I, Barthold C, Admon D, Trento A, Blanche C, Valenza M, Siegel RJ: Improved left atrial transport and function with orthotopic heart transplantation by bicaval and pulmonary venous anastomoses. Am Heart J 1995;130:121–126.

44. Gauer OH: Osmocontrol versus volume control. Fed Proc 1968;27:1134–1135.

45. Gauer OH, Henry JP: Circulatory basis of fluid volume control. Physiol Rev 1963;43:423–481.

46. Gauer OH, Henry JP, Behn C: The regulation of extracellular fluid volume. Ann Rev Physiol 1970;32:547–595.

47. Gilmore JP, Daggett W: Response of the chronic cardiac denervated dog to acute volume expansion. Am J Physiol 1966;210:509–512.

48. Glazier JJ, Mullen GM, Johnson MR, Lung CT, Heroux AL, Kao WG, Koch D, Khatib Y, Fisher SG, Costanzo MR: Factors associated with the development of persistently depressed cardiac output during the first year after cardiac transplantation. Clin Cardiol 1994;17:489–494.

49. Goodman DJ, Rossen RM, Cannom DS, Rider AK, Harrison DC: Effect of digoxin on atrioventricular conduction: studies in patients with and without cardiac autonomic innervation. Circulation 1975;51:251–256.

50. Greenberg MD, Uretsky BF, Reddy S, Bernstein RL, Griffith BP, Hardesty RL, Thompson ME, Bahnson HT: Long term hemodynamic followup of cardiac transplant patients treated with cyclosporine and prednisone. Circulation 1985;71:487–494.

51. Grinstead WC, Smart FW, Pratt CM, Weilbaecher DG, Sekela ME, Noon GP, Young JB: Sudden death caused by bradycardia and asystole in a heart transplant patient with coronary arteriopathy. J Heart Transplant 1991;10:931–936.

52. Groen HJ, Bogaard JM, Balk AH, Kho SG, Hop WC, Hilvering C: Diffusion capacity in heart transplant recipients. Chest 1992;102:456–460.

53. Haas GH, Wooding-Scott M, Binkley PF, Myerowitz PD, Kelley R, Cody RJ: Effects of successful cardiac transplantation on plasma endothelin. Am J Cardiol 1993;71:237–240.

54. Heinz G, Hirschl M, Buxbaum P, Laufer G, Gasic S, Laczkovics A: Sinus node dysfunction after orthotopic cardiac transplantation: postoperative incidence and long term implications. PACE 1992;15:731–737.

55. Heinz G, Ohner T, Laufer G, Gasic S, Laczkovics A: Clinical and electrophysiologic correlates of sinus node dysfunction after orthotopic heart transplantation. Chest 1990;4:890–895.

56. Hodgson JMB, Cohen MD, Szentpetery S, Thames MD: Effects of regional (alpha)- and (abeta) - blockade on resting and hyperemic coronary blood flow in conscious, unstressed humans. Circulation 1989;79:797–809.

57. Hosenpud JD, Pantely GA, Morton MJ, Norman DJ, Cobanoglu AM, Starr A: Relationship between recipient, donor body size matching, and hemodynamics three months following cardiac transplantation. J Heart Transplant 1989;8:241–243.

58. Ingels NB Jr, Hansen DE, Daughters GT, Stinson EB, Alderman EL, Miller DC: Relation between longitudinal, circumferential, and oblique shortening and torsional deformation in the left ventricle of the transplanted human heart. Circ Res 1989; 64:915–927.

59. James TN: The sinus node as a servomechanism. Circ Res 1973; 32:307–313.

60. Kao A, VanTrigt P, Shaffer-McCall G, Shaw JP, Kuzil BB, Page RD, Higginbotham MB: Allograft diastolic dysfunction and chronotropic incompetence limit cardiac output response to exercise two to six years after heart transplantation. J Heart Transplant 1995;14:11–22.

61. Kao AC, Trigt PV, Shaeffer-McCall GS, Shaw JP, Kuzil BB, Page RD, Higginbotham MB: Central and peripheral limitations to upright exercise in untrained cardiac transplant recipients. Circulation 1994;89:2605–2615.

62. Kaseda S, Zipes DP: Super-sensitivity to acetylcholine of canine sinus and atrial ventricular nodes after parasympathetic denervation. Am J Physiol 1988;225:H534–H539.

63. Kavanaugh T, Yacoub MH, Mertens D, Kennedy J, Campbell RB, Sawyer P: Cardiorespiratory responses to exercise training after orthotopic cardiac transplantation. Circulation 1988;77:162.

64. Klein RL, Lagercrantz H, Zimmerman H: Chemical Neurotransmission—An Introduction. New York: Academic Press, 1982.

65. Kotliar CD, Smart FM, Sekela ME, Pacifico A, Pratt CM, Noon GP, DeBakey ME, Young JB: Heterotopic heart transplantation and native heart ventricular arrhythmias. Ann Thorac Surg 1991;51:987–991.

66. Lang RE, Tholken H, Ganten D, Luft FC, Ruskoaho H, Unger T: Atrial natriuretic factor—a circulating hormone stimulated by volume loading. Nature 1985;314:264.

67. Leachman RD, Kokkinos DV, Cabrera R, Leatherman LL, Rochelle DG: Response of the transplanted,denervated human heart to cardiovascular drugs. Am J Cardiol 1977;27:272–276.

68. Leonelli FM, Dunn JK, Young JB, Pacifico A: Natural history, determinants, and clinical relevance of conduction abnormalities following orthotopic heart transplantation. Am J Cardiol 1996; 77:47–51.

69. Leonelli FM, Pacifico A, Young JB: Frequency and significance of conduction defects early after orthotopic heart transplantation. Am J Cardiol 1994;73:175–179.

70. Leyh RG, Jahnke AW, Kraatz EG, Sievers HH: Cardiovascular dynamics and dimensions after bicaval and standard cardiac transplantation. Ann Thorac Surg 1995;59:1495–1500.

71. Mackintosh AF, Carmichael DZJ, Wren C, Cory-Pearace R, English TA: Sinus node function in the first three weeks after cardiac transplantation. Br Heart J 1982;48:584–588.

72. Mancia G, Donald DE: Demonstrations that atria, ventricles and lungs each are responsible for a tonic inhibition of the vasomotor center in the dog. Circ Res 1975;36:310.

73. Mancini DM, Walter G, Reichek N, Lenkinski R, McCully KK, Mullen JL, Wilson JR: Contribution of skeletal muscle atrophy to exercise intolerance and altered metabolism in heart failure. Circulation 1992;85:1364–1373.

74. Mann RC, Priestley JT, Markowitz J, Yater WM: Transplantation and the intact mammalian heart. Arch Surg 1933;26:219–224.

75. Mason JW, Stinson EB, Harrison DC: Autonomic nervous system and arrhythmias: studies in the transplanted denervated human heart. Cardiology 1967;61:75–87.

76. Mason JW, Winkle RA, Rider AK, Stinson EB, Harrison DC: The electrophysiologic effects of quinidine in the transplanted human heart. J Clin Invest 1977;59:481–489.

77. McGiffin DC, Karp RB, Logic JR, Tauxe WN, Ceballos R: Results of radionuclide assessment of cardiac function following transplantation of the heart. Ann Thorac Surg 1984;37:382–386.

78. McLaughlin PR, Kleiman JH, Martin RP: The effects of exercise and atrial pacing on left ventricular volume and contractility in

patients with innervated and denervated hearts. Circulation 1980;61:897.

79. Moe GW, Grima EA, Wong NL, Howard RJ, Armstrong PW: Dual natriuretic peptide system in experimental heart failure. J Am Coll Cardiol 1993;22:891.

80. Mohanty PK, Thomas MD, Arrowood JA, Sowers JR, McNamara C, Szentpetery S: Impairment of cardiopulmonary baroreflex after cardiac transplantation in humans. Circulation 1987;75:21.

81. Morad M, Rolett EL: Relaxing effects of catecholamines on mammalian heart. J Physiol (Lond) 1972;224:537–558.

82. Netter FH: The Ciba Collection of Medical Illustrations. Summit, NJ: Ciba, 1969.

83. Nitenberg A, Tavolaro O, Loisance D, Foult JM, Cachera JP: Dynamic evaluation of the coronary circulation in human orthotopic heart transplants. Transplant Proc 1987;19:3772.

84. Nitenberg A, Tavollaro O, Benvenuti C, Loisance D, Foult JM, Hittinger L, Castaigne A, Cachera JP, Vernant P: Recovery of a normal vascular reserve after rejection therapy in acute human cardiac allograft rejection. Circulation 1990;81:1312–1318.

85. Ohar J, Osterloh J, Ahmed N, Miller L: Diffusing capacity decreases after heart transplantation. Chest 1993;103:857–861.

86. Parent R, Stanley P, Chartrand C: Long-term daily study of blood volume in cardiac autotransplanted dogs. Eur Surg Res 1987; 19:193–199.

87. Peiss CN, Cooper T, William VL, Randall WC: Circulatory responses to electrical and reflex activation of the nervous system after cardiac denervation. Circ Res 1966;19:153–166.

88. Pepke-Zaba J, Higenbottam TW, Morice A, Dinh-Xuan AT, Raine AE, Wallwork J: Exercise increases the release of atrial natriuretic peptide in heart transplant recipients. Eur J Clin Pharmacol 1992;42:21–24.

89. Petterson A, Hedner J, Rieksten SE, Towle AC, Hedner T: Acute volume expansion as a physiologic stimulus for the release of atrial natriuretic peptides in the rat. Life Sci 1986;38:1127.

90. Pflugfelder PW, Purves PD, McKenzie FN, Kostuk WJ: Cardiac dynamics during supine exercise in cyclosporine treated orthotopic heart transplant recipients. Assessment by radionuclide angiography. J Am Coll Cardiol 1987;10:336–341.

91. Pflugfelder PW, Purves PD, Menkis AH, McKenzie FN, Kostuk WJ: Rest and exercise left ventricular ejection and filling characteristics following orthotopic cardiac transplantation. Can J Cardiol 1989;5:161–167.

92. Pope SE, Stinson EB, Daughters GT, Schroeder JS, Ingels NB, Alderman E: Exercise response of the denervated heart in long-term cardiac transplant recipients. Am J Cardiol 1980;46:213–218.

93. Raghavan C, Malone JD, Nitta J, Lowry RW, Saliba WI, Cocanougher B, Zhu WX, Young JB: Long-term followup of heart transplant recipients requiring permanent pacemakers. Transplantation 1995;14:1081–1089.

94. Ray LF, East DS, Browning FM, Shaw D, Ogilvie RI, Cardella C, Leenen FH: Short term effects of calcium antagonists on hemodynamics and cyclosporine pharmacokinetics in heart transplant and kidney transplant patients. Clin Pharmacol Ther 1989;36: 657–667.

95. Regitz V, Bossaller C, Strasser R, Schuler S, Hetzer R, Fleck E: Myocardial catecholamine content after heart transplantation. Circulation 1990;82:620–623.

96. Reichenspurner H, Hildebrandt A, Boehm D, Kaulbach HG, Willems S, Odell JA, Horak A, Reichart B: Heterotopic heart transplantation in 1988. Recent selective indications and outcome. J Heart Transplant 1989;8:381–386.

97. Ricci DR, Orblick AE, Alderman EL, Ingels NB, Daughters GT, Kusnick CA, Reitz BA, Stinson EB: Role of tachycardia as an inotropic stimulus in man. J Clin Invest 1979;63:695–703.

98. Richards AM, Ikram H, Yandle TG, Espiner EA: Renal, hemodynamic, and hormonal effects of human alpha atrial natriuretic peptide in healthy volunteers. Lancet 1985;1:545.

99. Robertson D, Johnson GA, Robertson RM, Nies AS, Shand DG, Oates JA: Comparative assessment of stimuli that release neuronal and adrenomedullary catecholamines in man. Circulation 1979;59:637.

100. Rudas L, Pflugfelder PW, Kostuk WJ: Comparison of hemodynamic responses during dynamic exercise in the upright and supine postures after orthotopic cardiac transplantation. J Am Coll Cardiol 1990;16:1367–1373.

101. Rudas L, Pflugfelder PW, McKenzie FN, Menkis FN, Novick RJ, Kostuk WJ: Normalization of upright exercise hemodynamics and improved exercise capacity one year after orthotopic cardiac transplantation. Am J Cardiol 1992;69:1336–1339.

102. Savin WM, Haskell WL, Schroeder JS, Stinson EB: Cardiorespiratory responses of cardiac transplant patients to graded, symptom limited exercise. Circulation 1980;62:55–60.

103. Scherrer U, Vissing SF, Morgan BJ, Rollins JA, Tindall RS, Ring S, Hanson P, Mohanty PK, Victor RG: Cyclosporine induced sympathetic activation and hypertension after heart transplantation. N Engl J Med 1990;323:693–699.

104. Schoal SF, Wallace AG, Sealy WC: Protective influence of cardiac denervation against arrhythmias of myocardial infarction. Cardiovasc Res 1969;3:241–244.

105. Schuler S, Thomas D, Thebken M, Frei U, Wagner T, Warnecke H, Hetzer R: Endocrine response to exercise in cardiac transplant patients. Transplant Proc 1987;19:2506–2509.

106. Schwaiger M, Hutchins GD, Kalff V, Rosenspire K, Haka MS, Mallette S, Deeb GM, Abrams GD, Wieland D: Evidence for regional catecholamine uptake and storage sites in the transplanted human heart by positron emission tomography. J Clin Invest 1991;87:1681–1690.

107. Shaver S, Leon EF, Gray S, Leonard JJ, Bahnson HT: Hemodynamic observations after cardiac transplantation. N Engl J Med 1969;281:822–824.

108. Shumway NE: Cardiac transplantation. J Am Coll Cardiol 1993;22:66–68.

109. Singer DRJ, Buckley MG, MacGregor CA, Khaghani A, Banner NR, Yacoub MH: Increased concentration of plasma atrial natriuretic peptides in cardiac transplant recipients. BMJ 1986;293: 1391–1392.

110. Skowronski EW, Epstein M, Ota D, Hoagland PM, Gordon JB, Adamson RM, McDaniel M, Peterson KL, Smith SC, Jaski BE: Right and left ventricular function after cardiac transplantation. Changes during and after rejection. Circulation 1981;84:2409–2417.

111. St Goar FG, Gibbons R, Schnittger I, Valantine HA, Popp RL: Left ventricular diastolic function. Doppler echocardiographic changes soon after cardiac transplantation. Circulation 1990;82: 872–878.

112. Stark RP, McGinn AL, Wilson RF: Chest pain in cardiac transplant recipients. Evidence of sensory reinnervation after cardiac transplantation. N Engl J Med 1991;324:1791–1794.

113. Stemple DR, Hall RJC, Mason JW, Harrison DC: Electrophysiological effects of edrophonium in the innervated and the transplanted denervated human heart. Br Heart J 1978;40:644–649.

114. Stevenson LW, Sietsema K, Tillisch JH, Lem V, Walden J, Kobashigawa JA, Moriguchi J: Exercise capacity for survivors of cardiac transplantation or sustained medical therapy for heart failure. Circulation 1990;81:78–85.

115. Stinson EB, Caves PK, Griepp RB: Hemodynamic observation in the early period after human heart transplantation. J Thorac Cardiovasc Surg 1975;69:264.

116. Stinson EB, Dong E Jr, Bieber CP, Schroeder JS, Shumway NE: Cardiac transplantation in man: early rejection. JAMA 1969;207: 2233–2242.

117. Stinson EB, Dong E Jr, Schroeder JS, Harrison DC, Shumway NE: Initial clinical experience with heart transplantation. Am J Cardiol 1972;22:791–803.

118. Stinson EB, Friepp RB, Schroeder JS, Dong E Jr, Shumway NE: Hemodynamic observations one and two years after cardiac transplantation in man. Circulation 1972;45:1183–1193.

119. Stratton JR, Kemp GJ, Daly RC, Yacoub SM, Rajagopalan B: Effects of cardiac transplantation on bioenergetic abnormalities of skeletal muscle in congestive heart failure. Circulation 1994;89:1624–1631.

120. Thadani U, Parker JO: Hemodynamics at rest and during supine and sitting bicycle exercise in normal subjects. Am J Cardiol 1978;41:52–59.

121. Thames MD, Hassan ZU, Brackett NC, Lower RR, Kontos HA: Plasma renin responses to hemorrhage after cardiac transplantation. Am J Physiol 1971;221:1115–1119.

122. Thureson-Klein A: Fine Structure of the Isolated Noradrenergic Vesicles. New York: Academic Press, 1982.

123. Tischler MD, Lee RT, Plappert T, Mudge GH, St John SM, Parker JD: Serial assessment of left ventricular function and mass after orthotopic heart transplantation: a four year longitudinal study. J Am Coll Cardiol 1992;6:60–66.

124. Triposkiadis F, Starling RC, Haas GJ, Sparks E, Myerowitz PD, Boudoulas H: Timing of recipient atrial contraction: a major determinant of transmitral diastolic flow in orthotopic cardiac transplantation. Am Heart J 1993;126:1175–1181.

125. Tsakiris AG, Donald DE, Rutishaver WJ, Banchero N, Wood EH: Cardiovascular responses to hypertension and hypotension in dogs with denervated hearts. J Appl Physiol 1969;27:817–821.

126. Tuna I, Barragry T, Walker M, Lillehei T, Blatachford JW, Gornick C, Ring WS, Bolman RM, Benditt DG: Effects of transplantation on atrial ventricular nodal accommodation and hysteresis. Am J Physiol 1987;253:H1514–H1522.

127. Uberfuhr P, Frey AW, Reichart B: Vagal reinnervation in the long term after orthotopic heart transplantation. J Heart Lung Transplant 2000;19:946–950.

128. Uretsky BF: Physiology of the transplanted heart. Cardiovasc Clin 1990;20:23–56.

129. Uretsky BF, Kormos RL, Zerbe TR, Lee A, Tokaraczyk TR, Murali S, Reddy PS, Denys BG, Griffith BP, Hardesty RL, Armitage JM, Arena VC: Cardiac events after heart transplantation: increase and predictive value of coronary angiography. J Heart Transplant 1992;11:S44–S51.

130. Valantine HA, Appleton CP, Hatle LV, Hunt SA, Stinson EB, Popp RL: Influence of recipient atrial contraction on left ventricular filling dynamics of the transplanted heart assessed by Doppler echocardiography. Am J Cardiol 1987;59:1159–1163.

131. Valantine HA, Fowler MB, Hunt SA, Naasz C, Hatle LK, Billingham ME, Stinson EB, Popp RL: Changes in Doppler echocardiographic indices of left ventricular function as potential markers of acute cardiac rejection. Circulation 1987;76(suppl):V-82–V-92.

132. Vander AJ: Control of renin release. Physiol Rev 1967;47:359–382.

133. Vardan S, Bitar JN, Lowry RW: The evolution of hemodynamic parameters following heterotopic cardiac transplantation. Proc Am Soc Transplant Physicians 1993;60: 19th Scientific Session.

134. Vatner DE, Lavallee M, Amano J, Finizola A, Homcy CJ, Vatner SF: Mechanisms of supersensitivity to sympathomimetic amines in the chronically denervated heart of the conscious dog. Circ Res 1985;57:55–64.

135. Verani MS, Geroge SE, Leon CA, Whisenand HH, Noon GP, Short HD, DeBakey ME, Young JB: Systolic and diastolic ventricular performance at rest and during exercise in heart transplant recipients. J Heart Transplant 1988;7:145–151.

136. Verani MS, Nishimura S, Mahmarian JJ, Hays JT, Young JB: Cardiac function after orthotopic heart transplantation: response to postural changes, exercise, and beta-adrenergic blockade. J Heart Transplant 1994;13:181–193.

137. Ward RJ, Danziger F, Bonica JJ, Allen GD, Tolas AG: Cardiovascular effects of change of posture. Aerosp Med 1966;37:257–259.

138. Wharton J, Polak JM, Gordon L, Banner NR, Springall DR, Rose M, Khagani A, Wallwork J, Yacoub MH: Immunohistochemical demonstration of human cardiac innervation before and after transplantation. N Engl J Med 1990;323:693–699.

139. Willman VL, Cooper T, Cian LG, Hanlon CR: Neural responses following autotransplantation of the canine heart. Circulation 1963;27:713–716.

140. Willman VL, Jerjovy JP, Pennell R, Hanlon CR: Response of the autotransplanted heart to blood volume expansion. Ann Surg 1967;166:513–517.

141. Wilson JR, Rayos G, Yeoh TK, Gothard P, Bak K: Dissociation between exertional symptoms and circulatory function in patients with heart failure. Circulation 1995;92:47–53.

142. Wilson RF, Christensen BV, Olivari MT, Simon A, White CW, Laxson DD: Evidence for structural sympathetic reinnervation after orthotopic cardiac transplantation in humans. Circulation 1991;83:1210–1220.

143. Wilson RF, Laxon DD, Christensen BV, McGinn AL, Kubo SH: Regional differences in sympathetic reinnervation after human orthotopic cardiac transplantation. Circulation 1993;88:165–171.

144. Wilson RF, McGinn AL, Johnson TH, Christensen BV, Laxson DD: Sympathetic reinnervation after heart transplantation in human beings. J Heart Transplant 1992;11:S88–S89.

145. Woodworth RS: Maximal contraction, "staircase" contraction, refractory period, and compensatory pause of the heart. Am J Physiol 1902;8:213.

146. Yamaji T, Ishibashi M, Takaku F: Atrial natriuretic factor in human blood. J Clin Invest 1985;76:1705.

147. Young JB, Leon CA, Short HD, Noon GP, Lawrence EC, Whisennand HH, Pratt CM, Goodman DA, Weilbaecher D, Quinones MA, DeBakey ME: Evolution of hemodynamics after orthotopic heart and heart/lung transplantation: early restrictive patterns persisting in occult fashion. J Heart Transplant 1987;6:34–43.

148. Young JB, Naftel DC, Bourge RC, Kirklin JK, Clemson BS, Porter CB, Rodeheffer RJ, Kenzora JL: Matching the heart donor and heart transplant recipient. Clues for successful expansion of the donor pool: a multi-variable, multi-institutional report. J Heart Transplant 1994;13:353–365.

149. Young JB, Winters WL, Bourge RC, Uretsky BF: 24th Bethesda conference: cardiac transplantation. Task Force 4: function of the heart transplant recipient. J Am Coll Cardiol 1993;22:45.

150. Younis L, Melin J, Schoevaerdts J, Van Dyck M, Detry JM, Robert A, Chalant C, Goenen M: Left ventricular systolic function and diastolic filling at rest and during upright exercise after orthotopic heart transplantation: comparison with young and aged normal subjects. J Heart Transplant 1990;9:683–692.

151. Yusuf S, Mitchell A, Yacoub MH: Interrelation between donor and recipient heart rates during exercise after heterotopic cardiac transplantation. Br Heart J 1985;54:173.

152. Yusuf S, Theodoropoulos S, Dhalia N, Mathias C, Yacoub M: Effect of beta blockade on dynamic exercise in human heart transplant recipients. Heart Transplant 1985;4:312.

153. Yusuf S, Theodoropoulos S, Mathias CJ, Dhalla N, Wittes J, Mitchell A, Yacoub M: Increased sensitivity of the denervated transplanted human heart to isoprenaline both before and after beta adrenergic blockade. Circulation 1987;75:696–704.

154. Zimmerman RS, Schirger JA, Edwarads BS, Schwab TR, Heublein DM, Burnett JC: Cardiac-renal endocrine dynamics during stepwise infusion of physiologic and pharmacologic concentrations of atrial natriuretic factor in the dog. Circ Res 1987;60:63.

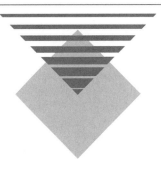

Management of the Transplant Patient

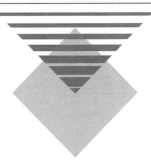

Management of the Recipient During the Transplant Hospitalization

The ultimate goal of cardiac transplantation is to provide high-quality, long-term survival for patients with end-stage heart disease. The probability of such an outcome is determined in a major way during the hospitalizationfor the transplant procedure. This chapter discusses the major areas of recipient management during the posttransplant hospitalization. The accomplishment of the therapeutic goals set forth in Table 12–1 requires a wide range of physician and nonphysician medical expertise in the hospital setting. Although a variety of hospital organizational plans have provided outstanding results in cardiac transplantation, we believe a dedicated unit for the care of patients with advanced heart failure and patients undergoing cardiac transplantation facilitates the concentration of necessary expertise and services to optimize their care.

PREPARATION OF THE PATIENT FOR CARDIAC TRANSPLANTATION

Whether the patient is already hospitalized or admitted from an outpatient status at the time of transplantation, a brief reevaluation of the potential recipient is made to ensure that the goals listed in Table 12–1 are not seriously compromised by the patient's pretransplant condition. The blood type of the donor and proposed recipient are rechecked to verify the recipient–donor compatibility. The donor and recipient weight are verified to ensure appropriate recipient–donor size match (see also Chapters 6 and 16). The recipient clinical summaries dictated by the transplant surgeon and cardiologist at the time of evaluation are reviewed for additional medical conditions which will require specialized care during and after cardiac transplantation.

In patients with a history of **reactive pulmonary vascular resistance** and prior pulmonary hypertension, placement of a pulmonary artery catheter may be advisable prior to transplantation. If pulmonary artery systolic pressure is markedly elevated (> about 55 mm Hg), the pulmonary artery pressure is again adjusted pharmacologically to demonstrate reactivity immediately prior to transplantation. This information may be particularly important in the final decision regarding the suitability of a heart from a smaller donor, particularly when transplanting from a smaller female donor into a

TABLE 12-1	Goals of Early Management of the Heart Transplant Recipient

- Maintenance of graft function
- Recovery (maintenance) of organ subsytem function
- Establishment of the immunologic environment for graft acceptance
- Prevention and treatment of early infectious complications
- Promotion of a psychological and education milieu for long-term rehabilitation and compliance

larger male recipient (see Chapter 9). The history of pulmonary hypertension may alert the operative team to the possible need for prostaglandin infusion or inhaled nitric oxide[53] during the process of weaning from cardiopulmonary bypass.[5]

If **serum creatinine** and blood urea nitrogen levels are abnormal, adjustments are necessary in the perioperative administration of cyclosporine or tacrolimus with their known nephrotoxicity. If the preoperative serum creatinine exceeds about 1.5 mg/dL, renal dose dopamine is initiated with the induction of anesthesia for the transplant operation and continued for at least 24–48 hours thereafter.

The potentially deleterious effects of **amiodarone** on pulmonary function after transplantation are discussed in detail later in this chapter. All patients receiving amiodarone have a special sign attached to the medical record indicating the presence of amiodarone therapy, and this is communicated to the anesthesia staff prior to transplantation so that every effort can be made to maintain the lowest safe concentration of inspired oxygen during the procedure and in the intensive care unit.

Preoperative steroids have been a standard part of perioperative immunosuppressive protocols, but they may also play a role in ameliorating the damaging effects of cardiopulmonary bypass. Experimental and clinical studies have suggested that the effectiveness of steroids in this regard is enhanced if they are administered 4–6 hours prior to cardiopulmonary bypass. We recommend whenever possible intravenous administration of methylprednisolone at a dose of 500 mg (15 mg/kg in infants and children) 4 hours prior to transplantation and 250 mg (10 mg/kg in infants and children) intravenously 1 hour before transplant.

Preoperative **immunosuppressive protocols** are highly variable among institutions, but generally include the administration of steroids as discussed above, azathioprine or mycophenolate mofetil, and usually a preoperative dose of cyclosporine or tacrolimus. The selection and administration of immunosuppressive agents before and early after transplantation is discussed later in this chapter and in Chapter 13.

Preoperative antibiotic prophylaxis includes coverage for gram-positive organisms (including coagulase-negative staphylococcus) and gram-negative organisms. The dosing regimen is discussed later in this chapter and in Chapter 15.

Patients with **previous mediastinal operations,** long-standing right-sided congestive heart failure, and those

Aprotinin

Aprotinin, a bovine serine protease inhibitor, is known to attenuate the systemic inflammatory response associated with cardiopulmonary bypass. Aprotinin has been long recognized as an inhibitor of plasmin and kallikrien, thus producing an antifibrinolytic effect and attenuating the inflammatory response to cardiopulmonary bypass.[35, 38] Furthermore, aprotinin has been shown to inhibit proinflammatory cytokine release and prevents the expression of proinflammatory adhesive glycoproteins such as CD11B in granulocytes. Although the mechanism remains speculative, the aprotinin likely inhibits the turnover of coagulation factors and maintains platelet adhesiveness, making them less susceptible to the damaging effects of cardiopulmonary bypass.[12, 34, 77, 96] Several studies have demonstrated reduced bleeding with aprotinin following implantation of left ventricular assist devices as a bridge to cardiac transplantation.[38, 77, 78] Other studies indicate that aprotinin reduces the need for blood transfusions after primary[12, 23, 24, 41, 42, 97] and reoperative[3, 86] cardiac surgery.

Hypersensitivity reactions have been reported following aprotinin administration, including histamine-mediated cardiovascular collapse,[80] potentiation of muscle relaxants, prolongation of the activating clotting time, nephrotoxicity, and potentially a hypercoagulable state.[10, 16, 20, 31, 48, 68, 78, 80] However, the experience in cardiac surgery and in cardiac transplantation suggests that these adverse events occur rarely. Particularly with prior cardiac operations, the use of aprotinin in cardiac transplantation, with the likely reduction in blood transfusion requirements, appears justified.

on chronic coumadin therapy are anticipated to have an increased bleeding diathesis. Such patients routinely receive vitamin K 10 mg subcutaneously (1 mg in infants and small children) prior to operation. Platelets and fresh frozen plasma are ordered as desired by the surgical team. In addition, consideration should be given to the use of aprotinin[3, 10, 20, 23, 24, 31, 34, 35] (see Box), particularly in patients with previous cardiac operations (Table 12–2). The effects of aprotinin are also discussed in Chapter 8.

TABLE 12-2	Aprotinin Protocol During Cardiac Transplantation

Test dose for hypersensitivity: 1 mL* IV
Initial loading dose: 100 mL over 30 minutes
Maintenance dose: 50 mL/hr for duration of procedure (initiated prior to CPB)
Dose added to CPB circuit: 200 mL

IV, intravenous; CPB, cardiopulmonary bypass.
*Each mL contains 10,000 kallikrein inhibitor units.

TABLE 12–3	Major Adrenergic Receptors	
RECEPTOR	LOCATION	EFFECT
Beta₁	Myocardium	Increase atrial and ventricular contractility
	Sinoatrial node	Increase heart rate
	Atrioventricular conduction system	Enhance atrioventricular conduction
Beta₂	Arterioles	Vasodilation
	Lungs	Bronchodilation
Alpha	Arterioles	Vasoconstriction

TABLE 12–5	Standard Inotropic Doses	
DRUG	STARTING DOSE	DOSING RANGE
Dopamine	2.5 μg/kg/min	2.5–20 μg/kg/min
Dobutamine	2.5 μg/kg/min	2.5–20 μg/kg/min
Milrinone	0.2–0.3 μg/kg/min	0.2–1.0 μg/kg/min
Epinephrine	0.025 μg/kg/min	0.025–0.1 μg/kg/min
Norepinephrine	0.025 μg/kg/min	0.025–0.1 μg/kg/min
Isoproterenol	0.025 μg/kg/min	0.025–0.1 μg/kg/min

MAINTENANCE OF GRAFT FUNCTION (CARDIAC PERFORMANCE)

The ability of the transplanted heart to generate adequate cardiac output in the early hours and days following cardiac transplantation is perhaps the primary determinant of posttransplant survival. The donor heart can sustain injury during trauma leading to death (myocardial contusion), in the process of brain death, and during implantation and subsequent reperfusion (see Chapter 9), all of which may contribute to initial systolic and/or diastolic dysfunction.[76, 84, 95] Some degree of initial donor heart dysfunction occurs in 30–50% of transplanted hearts, but fortunately with current methods of preservation, less than 2% of patients die from early graft failure.[67] Most forms of early graft dysfunction are reversible, resulting in normal donor heart function if the heart is properly supported during its recovery phase.

HEMODYNAMIC MONITORING

The assessment and management of cardiac function in the transplanted heart begins in the operating room during the final phases and discontinuation of cardiopulmonary bypass. Systolic function may be directly assessed with transesophageal echocardiography, which is also useful to ensure effective de-airing of the heart. Left atrial pressure is directly measured and monitored for 12–24 hours following transplantation. Central venous pressure is monitored and the relationship between right and left atrial pressure is observed for signs

of isolated right or left ventricular dysfunction. If depressed cardiac performance is detected, a pulmonary artery catheter with continuous cardiac output and mixed venous oxygen saturation monitoring can be placed in the intensive care unit and provides excellent continuous assessment of cardiac performance and evaluation of the response to pharmacologic interventions.

INOTROPIC AGENTS USEFUL EARLY AFTER CARDIAC TRANSPLANTATION

Dopamine is an endogenous catecholamine which is the biosynthetic precursor of norepinephrine and directly stimulates myocardial beta₁-adrenergic receptors (Table 12–3). It also stimulates release of norepinephrine from sympathetic nerve terminals. At low doses ($\leq$2.5 μg/kg/min), dopamine causes relatively selective vasodilation of the renal and splanchnic arterial beds. Specific dopamine presynaptic as well as postsynaptic receptors have been identified in the peripheral arterioles and on the luminal membranes of renal tubular cells, particularly in the proximal tubules.[60] Although the effectiveness of low-dose dopamine in specifically increasing renal blood flow remains controversial,[7, 27, 32] dopamine remains the most commonly utilized inotropic agent after cardiac transplantation.

Doses between 5 and 20 μg/kg/min cause progressive peripheral vasoconstriction secondary to alpha-adrenergic receptor stimulation, making high-dose dopamine undesirable except in the presence of low systemic vascular resistance. In addition, higher dose dopamine is often accompanied by tachycardia (see Tables 12–4 and 12–5). Large doses of dopamine may also increase coronary vascular resistance by direct cardiac alpha₁-adrenergic stimulation.

Dobutamine is a sympathomimetic agent which stimulates beta₁-, beta₂- and alpha-adrenergic receptors, but

TABLE 12–4	Adrenergic Receptor Activity and Other Properties of Sympathomimetic Amines Following Cardiac Surgery				
	ALPHA (PERIPHERAL VASOCONSTRICTION)	BETA₁ (CARDIAC CONTRACTILITY)	BETA₂ (PERIPHERAL VASODILATION)	CHRONOTROPIC EFFECT	ARRHYTHMIA RISK
Norepinephrine	++++	+++	0	+	+
Epinephrine	+++	++++	+	++	+++
Dopamine*	++	+++	+	+	+
Dobutamine	0	+++	++	+	+
Isoproterenol	0	++++	+++	++++	++++
Phenylephrine	++++	0	0	0	0

*Causes renal arteriolar dilatation at low doses by stimulating dopaminergic receptors, moderate diuretic effect.

unlike dopamine, it does not release norepinephrine from adrenergic nerve endings. Its positive inotropic effects are less than isoproterenol or epinephrine (Table 12–4). Dobutamine usually reduces pulmonary vascular resistance, and systemic vascular resistance usually decreases secondary to an increase in cardiac output and the predominance of beta$_2$ activity over peripheral alpha-adrenergic activity. Tachycardia is usually less pronounced with dobutamine than dopamine. When moderate increases in inotropic support are required after cardiac transplantation, the combination of dopamine and dobutamine at doses of 2.5–7 μg/kg/min are usually effective.

Norepinephrine is a potent endogenous catecholamine with pronounced beta$_1$-adrenergic and peripheral alpha-adrenergic effects (Table 12–4). Unless profound low cardiac output is present, norepinephrine should be reserved for the situations in which marked peripheral vasodilation (decreased peripheral vascular resistance) is severe enough to compromise arterial perfusion pressure. In severe low cardiac output states, the marked vasoconstrictive effects of norepinephrine usually further compromise organ perfusion and increase cardiac afterload.

Epinephrine is an endogenous sympathomimetic agent with marked positive inotropic action and predominance of peripheral alpha-adrenergic over beta$_2$-adrenergic effects. In the setting of severe donor heart dysfunction and peripheral hypotension, epinephrine combined with dopamine and dobutamine often further increases cardiac contractility. If the systemic blood pressure increases after initiating epinephrine, its vasoconstrictive effects can be ameliorated with additional agents such as milrinone (see below) or nitroprusside.

Isoproterenol is a potent beta$_1$- beta$_2$- adrenergic receptor agonist that does not cause vasoconstriction and, in fact, is associated with a fall in mean blood pressure despite generally increasing the systolic pressure. It may have some beneficial effects with respect to lowering pulmonary artery pressures. Isoproterenol's use is somewhat limited by the tachycardia (and other arrhythmias) it can produce, but the chronotropic effects of this agent are sometimes advantageous. Indeed, in the denervated posttransplant heart struggling to regain sinus node function, this agent can be effective in keeping the heart rate up and maintaining a sinus mechanism. There is some argument about whether or not it is better to accomplish this with atrial pacing, but the advantage of using isoproterenol may also be its beta$_1$ effects which can help to improve cardiac contractility in the stunned postoperative heart. Some caution should be used when starting this agent, as the arrhythmias can be problematic and hypotension may occur.

Milrinone is the preferred intravenous inotropic agent in the class of phosphodiesterase inhibitors. Milrinone exerts its inotropic and vasodilator effects through inhibition of the enzyme phosphodiesterase F-3, a membrane-bound enzyme responsible for the breakdown of cyclic adenosine monophosphate (cAMP). The increase in intracellular cAMP concentrations causes an increase in calcium influx through slow calcium channels, which augments contractility.[18] Phosphodiesterase inhibitors do not act through direct stimulation of adrenergic receptors. Milrinone is particularly useful after cardiac transplantation in the setting of elevated systemic or pulmonary vascular resistance and is the preferred agent over amrinone, in that it is approximately 10 times more potent, has a shorter half-life, and is not associated with thrombocytopenia, which frequently occurs with amrinone.

LEFT VENTRICULAR SYSTOLIC DYSFUNCTION

When catecholamine support is required early after cardiac transplantation, dopamine, dobutamine, amrinone, and milrinone are effective in augmenting cardiac output without the deleterious severe peripheral vasoconstrictive effects of epinephrine and norepinephrine. Isoproterenol was often used in the past for its chronotropic effects, but currently it is rarely needed with the availability of temporary postoperative atrial pacing. When more than moderate doses of combined inotropic agents (such as dopamine, dobutamine, and milrinone) are required, circulatory assistance with an intra-aortic balloon pump (IABP) is recommended.[29, 81] Under rare circumstances, the depression of left ventricular function may be so profound that mechanical circulatory support is necessary as a life-sustaining maneuver (see Chapter 8).

Rarely, extremely low systemic vascular resistance will occur during and following cardiopulmonary bypass in patients undergoing cardiac transplantation. The mechanism of this phenomenon is unclear, but it has been variously attributed to chronic administration of angiotensin-converting enzyme inhibitors in the treatment of heart failure, circulatory hypoperfusion states followed by exposure to the inflammatory effects of cardiopulmonary bypass, and/or a deficiency of circulating vasopressin.[15, 56] When systemic vascular resistance is unresponsive to moderate doses of the alpha-adrenergic agent phenylephrine or norepinephrine, an intra-aortic balloon pump is often effective in establishing sufficient pulsatility to improve coronary perfusion and cardiac performance prior to discontinuation of cardiopulmonary bypass. With reestablishment of pulsatile flow, peripheral vascular resistance often progressively improves. In the rare situation in which very low systemic vascular resistance persists despite these interventions, infusion of arginine vasopressin (0.04–0.1 units/min) is sometimes effective in reversing catecholamine-resistant low systemic resistance.[4, 15, 56] If cardiac function is otherwise good, the systemic resistance usually normalizes within 6–12 hours, and these agents can be gradually discontinued.

LEFT VENTRICULAR DIASTOLIC DYSFUNCTION

The hallmark of isolated left ventricular diastolic dysfunction is an elevated left atrial (and left ventricular end-diastolic) pressure required to produce effective cardiac output in the presence of normal or near normal systolic function. Chronic diastolic dysfunction after cardiac transplantation is discussed in Chapter 11. Temporary diastolic dysfunction of either the right or left ventricle occurs commonly after cardiac transplantation,[103] usually secondary to reversible myocardial injury associated with ischemia/reperfusion. Resolution usually occurs within a few days. The relationship of this phenomenon to later (>3 months) restrictive physiology patterns which occasionally occur remains speculative, but it seems likely that severe subendocardial ischemic injury with subsequent fibrosis may contribute to the rare development of permanent diastolic derangement. Acquired diastolic dysfunction may also result from an "oversized" heart placed in a smaller pericardial space (usually after previous cardiac operations) or accumulation of blood in the mediastinum after transplant with resultant tamponade.

Treatment of diastolic dysfunction in the operating room usually begins with intravenous nitroglycerin, usually at a dose of 0.5–2 μg/kg/min. Attention must be paid to the total volume infused with a nitroglycerin drip, since the standard concentration often requires 30 or more mL/hour of fluid administration. Further concentration of the nitroglycerin preparation may be advisable when urine output is not robust. Diuretic therapy and intravenous fluid restriction may also be useful. When calculated systemic vascular resistance is increased, further afterload reduction with nitroprusside in the first 24–48 hours and subsequent oral afterload-reducing agents is indicated. Inotropic agents such as milrinone may also favorably impact peripheral vascular resistance while increasing cardiac output.

The sudden appearance of apparent right or left ventricular dysfunction during the first several postoperative days may indicate cardiac tamponade from blood accumulation in the mediastinum. A transthoracic echocardiogram may indicate retained blood, which, if accompanied by altered hemodynamics, should prompt surgical evacuation of retained hematoma. In any case, an echocardiogram should be routinely obtained prior to hospital dismissal to evaluate heart function and identify any pericardial effusion, which, if large, should be surgically drained.

RIGHT VENTRICULAR DYSFUNCTION

The thin-walled right ventricle is particularly susceptible to injury during the period of ischemia and reperfusion, and also compensates poorly for any increase in afterload (pulmonary vascular resistance) which is typically elevated to some degree due to longstanding elevation of left atrial pressure in patients with heart failure.[9, 54] Although pulmonary vascular resistance generally falls rapidly following cardiac transplantation, it frequently takes 1–2 two weeks for near normalization to occur[54] (Fig. 12–1). The likelihood and degree of right ventricular dysfunction is highly correlated with the level of pulmonary vascular resistance immediately following transplantation. When additional functional disadvantage of the right ventricle is induced by inadequate right ventricular preservation or possibly a considerably smaller donor heart transplanted into a larger recipient, the deleterious effects of increased right

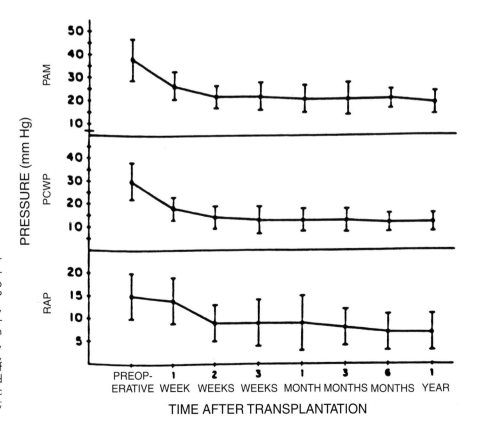

FIGURE **12–1.** Serial hemodynamics after cardiac transplantation compared with pre-operative measurements. Depicted are group means ± 1 SD for RAP, PAM, and PCWP (in mm Hg). RAP, right atrial pressure; PAM, pulmonary artery mean pressure; PCWP, pulmonary capillary wedge pressure. (From Bhatia SJS, Kirshenbaum JM, Shemin RJ, Cohn LH, Collins JJ, DiSesa VJ, Young PJ, Mudge GH Jr, Sutton MGS: Time course of resolution of pulmonary hypertension and right ventricular remodeling after orthotopic cardiac transplantation. Circulation 1987; 76:819–826.)

PRESSURE (mm Hg)

PREOPERATIVE   1 WEEK   2 WEEKS   3 WEEKS   1 MONTH   3 MONTHS   6 MONTHS   1 YEAR

TIME AFTER TRANSPLANTATION

TABLE 12-6	Management of Right Ventricular (RV) Dysfunction

- Evaluate pulmonary artery (PA) anastomosis for possible obstruction (measure RV and PA pressures); surgical revision if systolic gradient ≥10 mm Hg
- If PA pressure normal or near normal, add inotropic support for RV contractility and adjust RV preload
- If PA pressure and transpulmonary gradient are elevated, add vasodilator agents (via central venous pressure line) and alpha-adrenergic agents (via left atrial catheter) as necessary to support systemic perfusion pressure ± intra-aortic balloon pump
- If PA systolic pressure elevation persists (≥45 mm Hg) with important RV dysfunction, initiate inhaled nitric oxide
- RV assist device if above measures fail

ventricular afterload are especially important. The management of right ventricular dysfunction is summarized in Table 12–6.

A rare but treatable cause of right ventricular dysfunction is obstruction at the pulmonary artery anastomosis secondary to torsion or redundancy of the donor or recipient pulmonary artery.[62] A large "athletic" donor heart transplanted into a restricted pericardial space secondary to previous surgery may increase the likelihood of obstruction adjacent to the anastomosis by partial compression of the proximal left pulmonary artery by the donor heart. Right ventricular pressure and pulmonary artery pressure should always be measured in the operating room when any signs of right ventricular dysfunction occur; an important systolic gradient (≥10 mm Hg) indicates the need for surgical revision.

Mild right ventricular dysfunction generally responds well to a vasodilating agent such as nitroglycerin and inotropic support with dobutamine or milrinone. If vasodilatory therapy results in systemic arterial hypotension, a second left atrial catheter can be placed so that inotropic agents with alpha-adrenergic effects such as phenylephrine, higher dose dopamine, or norepinephrine can be infused through the left atrial catheter to maintain systemic perfusion pressure while infusing vasodilator agents through the central venous catheter (Table 12–7). Infusion of alpha-adrenergic agents through a left atrial catheter induces less pulmonary hypertension than does infusion directly into the central venous catheter.[66] If more than moderate alpha-adrenergic support is required to offset the vasodilator effects of nitroglycerin and milrinone on systemic perfusion pressure, an intra-aortic balloon pump is a useful intervention to maintain

coronary perfusion pressure while treating right ventricular dysfunction with higher dose vasodilator agents.

When right ventricular dysfunction is accompanied by marked pulmonary hypertension, (pulmonary artery systolic pressure exceeding about 50 mm Hg), primary attention must focus on reducing the pulmonary vascular resistance. Although intravenous infusions of isoproterenol, nitroprusside, aminophylline, and nitroglycerin are useful in reducing moderate elevations of pulmonary artery pressure, intravenous prostaglandin E_1 (0.01–0.1 μg/kg/min)[5] and prostacyclin are more effective. Inhaled nitric oxide is the agent with the most specific and pronounced effect on lowering pulmonary vascular resistance without affecting systemic resistance.[53, 89] The dose is usually 20–60 parts per million, with monitoring of methemoglobin levels, reducing the dose if levels exceed about 4 mg/dL. The pharmacology and administration of nitric oxide are discussed in Chapter 20.

DISTURBANCES OF CARDIAC RATE AND RHYTHM

SINUS NODE DYSFUNCTION/BRADYCARDIA

The majority of transplanted hearts exhibit normal sinus rhythm in the operating room soon after reperfusing the transplanted heart, and clinically important arrhythmias are uncommon in the weeks following transplantation. However, electrophysiologic studies have established that 25–50% of heart transplant patients have sinus node dysfunction including prolonged sinus node recovery time (>1,400 ms),[49] prolonged corrected sinus node recovery time (>520 ms),[45] and abnormal sinoatrial conduction time.[8] The cause of sinus node dysfunction following cardiac transplantation is incompletely understood but may relate to surgical trauma, imperfect myocardial preservation, cardiac denervation, or underlying sinus node dysfunction in the donor. Although controversial, at least one study has suggested that the bicaval technique (see Chapter 10) is associated with a lower incidence of sinus node dysfunction (and presumably damage) compared to the standard orthotopic technique.[11] The reported incidence of pacemaker implantation during the transplant admission varies from about 2–10%,[14, 22, 47, 69, 72, 79] but the incidence of early pacemaker implantation in the current era is likely considerably

TABLE 12-7	Properties of Vasodilator Agents			
	SYSTEMIC ARTERIAL VASODILATION	PULMONARY ARTERIAL VASODILATION	POSITIVE INOTROPIC EFFECT	INCREASE IN SYSTEMIC VENOUS CAPACITANCE
Isoproterenol	++	+++	++++	0
Milrinone	+++	+++	+++	0
Nitroprusside	++++	+++	0	0
Nitroglycerin	++	++	0	+++
Prostaglandin E_1	+++	+++	0	0
Prostacyclin	++	+++	0	0
Nitric oxide	0	++++	0	0

lower. In our experience, less than 2% of patients require early pacemaker implantation. This likely reflects a better understanding of the favorable natural history of early bradycardia and possibly improvement in myocardial preservation and avoidance of surgical trauma to the sinoatrial (SA) node. Miyamoto and colleagues noted a correlation between the incidence of sinus node dysfunction and longer donor ischemic times.[72] Sinus node dysfunction may manifest as junctional bradycardia, sinus bradycardia (<70 bpm), or dysfunction detectable only on electrophysiologic studies. Rarely, sinus arrest or atrioventricular (AV) block may occur.[69] The natural history of this sinus dysfunction is normalization in approximately 50–75% of cases within 3 months following transplantation and 90% of patients within 1 year.[43, 72, 88] Despite this favorable natural history, several studies have raised cautionary notes because of occasional sudden deaths following hospital discharge in patients with bradycardia and sinus node dysfunction.[14, 61] However, a more recent study by Heinz and colleagues demonstrated that sinus node dysfunction early after cardiac transplantation is not predictive of an adverse outcome.[45]

When sinus node dysfunction is manifested as important sinus bradycardia (< about 80 bpm), atrial pacing can be initiated through the temporary atrial wires which are placed at time of transplantation. Isoproterenol is usually unnecessary unless the atrial wires are nonfunctional. If important bradycardia persists after 4 or 5 days, methylxanthines such as intravenous aminophylline or oral theophylline may be effective at augmenting heart rate.[19, 44] It has been hypothesized that early sinus node dysfunction may be in part related to the effects of adenosine release from ischemic myocardium.[33, 46, 49, 72, 104] Methylxanthines antagonize the effects of adenosine,[100] and intravenous aminophylline has been shown to normalize sinus node dysfunction occurring early after transplantation.[44] The standard oral dose of theophylline is 100–200 mg twice daily.

The indications for early pacemaker implantation remain controversial, particularly in view of the favorable natural history of early sinus node dysfunction. However, pacemaker implantation is probably advisable for patients with persistent symptomatic bradycardia associated with depressed cardiac output or symptoms despite theophylline therapy, and probably those with persistent junctional escape rhythms or persistent sinus bradycardia of less than 70 bpm more than 2 weeks after transplantation.[87] If a pacing device is required, dual chamber pacing is recommended, utilizing atrial pacing whenever possible to preserve the atrial contribution to cardiac output in the transplanted heart.

ATRIAL ARRHYTHMIAS

Asymptomatic, transient atrial arrhythmias are common following cardiac transplantation, occurring in about one fourth of patients during the transplant hospitalization.[59] Little and colleagues identified premature atrial complexes as the most common *atrial arrhythmia* (24% of patients) during the transplant hospitalization, with atrial flutter, atrial tachycardia, and atrial fibrillation occurring rarely. Although atrial fibrillation and flutter have been associated with acute rejection, these arrhythmias are clearly not specific for rejection and occur less commonly with rejection in the cyclosporine era than in the azathioprine/prednisone era.[59] There is no difference in the incidence of atrial arrhythmias between patients who experience rejection during initial hospitalization and those who do not.[59]

When atrial fibrillation and atrial flutter do occur in the setting of rejection, they may be responsive to antirejection therapy. Conversion to sinus rhythm with intravenous methylprednisolone provides presumptive evidence for acute rejection. Atrial flutter can be managed with rapid atrial pacing if the temporary atrial pacing wires are in place. In the absence of rejection, atrial fibrillation or flutter with a rapid ventricular response rate can be managed with intravenous diltiazem or a short-acting beta blocking agent such as esmolol if the hemodynamics are good. Otherwise, cardioversion should be considered. Digoxin is relatively ineffective in reducing the rate of ventricular response in atrial fibrillation following heart transplantation because of the limited action of digoxin in the denervated heart.[30, 58, 65, 83]

VENTRICULAR ARRHYTHMIAS

Ventricular arrhythmias are more common than atrial arrhythmias early following transplantation, occurring in up to 65% of patients during the transplant admission.[59] In a telemetry study by Little et al.,[59] the most common ventricular arrhythmia was premature ventricular complexes (65% of patients), followed by nonsustained ventricular tachycardia (47%) and accelerated idioventricular rhythms (12%). Ventricular arrhythmias may result from ischemic/reperfusion injury such as with prolonged ischemic time[59] or metabolic disturbances such as hypokalemia or hypomagnesemia. Intravenous lidocaine is usually effective, along with correction of associated electrolyte abnormalities. Unless severe myocardial dysfunction is present, malignant ventricular arrhythmias are extremely rare.[59] Ventricular arrhythmias have not been identified as a marker for rejection.

MAINTENANCE OF RENAL FUNCTION

Renal reserves may be impaired prior to transplantation secondary to prolonged low cardiac output and chronic high-dose diuretic therapy. In such a state, kidney function is particularly vulnerable following transplantation due to the combination of abnormal renal perfusion during cardiopulmonary bypass, the potential for early graft dysfunction and associated low cardiac output, and the deleterious effects of cyclosporine on renal function.

The primary determinant of effective renal function early after transplant is robust cardiac performance. Appropriate support of the cardiovascular subsystem will minimize the probability of important renal dysfunction. In the presence of oliguria or rising creatinine (particularly if > about 1.7 mg/dL), initiation of cyclosporine therapy should be delayed until renal function normalizes. If more than 48 hours elapse after transplant before cyclosporine therapy can be initiated, it is advisable to begin cytolytic therapy with OKT3 or ATG. If early renal dysfunction is reversed, there is generally no deleterious effect on long-term posttransplant renal function.

Dopamine may be routinely employed after cardiac transplantation in a "renal dose" of 2.5 μg/kg/min in order to maximize renal blood flow. The use of diuretic therapy in the first few days after cardiac transplantation is controversial. There is a known tendency for patients receiving high-dose diuretics prior to transplantation to exhibit relative oliguria if diuretic therapy is suddenly stopped. Therefore, diuretic therapy may require reinitiation in order to maintain adequate urine output in such patients. When oliguria (urine output < about 50 mL/hr) is present early after transplantation, preload is augmented with volume administration to increase the central venous pressure or left atrial pressure to 12–13 mm Hg. Cardiac output should be measured and optimized as discussed in the preceding section. If a cyclosporine infusion has been initiated, it should be stopped. If urine output remains low, furosemide may be administered at an initial dose of 20–40 mg (or 1 mg/kg in pediatric patients). If blood urea nitrogen (BUN) and creatinine are elevated (BUN > about 40 mg/dL and/or creatinine >1.6 mg/dL), special care is required to maintain intravascular volume while administering diuretics. If a brisk diuresis occurs after diuretic administration, it may be useful to perform "urine output replacement" in which hourly urine output is matched with an infusion of normal or half normal saline up to a maximum left atrial or central venous pressure of 13 or 14 mm Hg. If renal dysfunction is severe and refractory to other measures, the rarely needed temporary options of dialysis and continuous hemofiltration are usually well tolerated if the cardiac performance is robust.

PULMONARY MANAGEMENT

Ventilator management, weaning, and extubation criteria following cardiac transplantation follow the same general protocols utilized for cardiac operations employing cardiopulmonary bypass, with the exception that 8–12 hours are usually necessary to assess adequacy of graft function prior to extubation. Management of **persistent pulmonary hypertension** should include (in addition to the pharmacologic interventions discussed above) mechanical hyperventilation with P_{CO_2} maintained at 25–35 mm Hg and oxygen saturation in excess of 95% if possible, to minimize the tendency for pulmonary vasoconstriction. When prolonged mechanical ventilation is required (>4 or 5 days), early consideration

for tracheostomy facilitates patient mobilization, comfort, and gradual weaning.

Special considerations in pulmonary management are necessary for patients receiving chronic administration of **amiodarone** therapy before transplant for life-threatening ventricular arrhythmias. Although it remains controversial whether amiodarone use is a risk factor for early mortality following cardiac transplantation, patients on chronic amiodarone are at increased risk for serious and potentially fatal postoperative pulmonary dysfunction.[75] The mechanism of postoperative acute amiodarone lung injury (see Box) is unknown, but may relate to the generation of oxygen free radicals, which could be potentiated by high inspired oxygen concentration during the transplant procedure.[28, 64] The clinical manifestation is the acute onset of dyspnea, often requiring reintubation 2–5 days following cardiac transplantation. There is radiographic evidence of acute pulmonary edema in the absence of left atrial hypertension. Such patients are likely prone to superimposed pulmonary infection. The only recognized (though not proven) preventive measures against amiodarone-induced pulmonary toxicity following cardiac transplantation are (1) maintenance of the lowest possible amiodarone dose which prevents ventricular tachycardia prior to transplantation (about 200 mg daily if possible) and (2) **strict avoidance of high inspired oxygen fraction during and after the transplant procedure**. Whenever possible, the inspired oxygen fraction should be maintained at 0.40 or lower.

ESTABLISHMENT OF THE IMMUNOLOGIC ENVIRONMENT FOR GRAFT ACCEPTANCE

Although a variety of protocols exist for the induction of allograft acceptance with immunosuppressive therapy, most include preoperative methylprednisolone, azathioprine or mycophenolate mofetil, and cyclosporine (or tacrolimus) combined with maintenance therapy using cyclosporine (or tacrolimus), azathioprine (or mycophenolate mofetil), with or without prednisone. The protocol at the University of Alabama at Birmingham (UAB) for early administration of immunosuppression includes preoperative administration of methylprednisolone (see earlier section, Preparation of the Patient for Cardiac Transplantation), azathioprine 4 mg/kg orally (PO) (or mycophenolate 10 mg/kg in pediatric patients and 500 mg in adults) and cyclosporine 0–3 mg/kg PO (Table 12–8). Methylprednisolone is administered intravenously (IV) at the end of cardiopulmonary bypass at a dose of 500 mg (10 mg/kg in infants and children), and three subsequent doses of 150 mg IV (3 mg/kg in infants and children) are given at 8-hour intervals. Prednisone at 1 mg/kg/day PO is initiated on the first postoperative day and continued for 3 weeks, after which the dose is gradually tapered to 0–10 mg (0–0.2 mg/kg in pediatric patients) daily, depending on rejection frequency.

Acute Amiodarone Lung Injury

Since the first reported observation in 1980,[85] lung injury has been recognized in approximately 5–7% of patients receiving chronic amiodarone therapy.[28, 63, 64, 91] Clinical manifestations include the insidious onset of cough and dyspnea, often associated with roentgenographic evidence of diffuse pulmonary infiltrates. Characteristic pathologic findings include alveolar deposition of foamy macrophages, thickening of the interalveolar septae, and progressive interstitial and alveolar fibrosis.[51, 74]

With the increasing experience of cardiac surgical and other procedures performed in patients receiving chronic amiodarone therapy, the syndrome of *acute* amiodarone-associated lung injury has been recognized,[40, 51, 75, 85] with an incidence of 12% or more[51] in an era before the practice of focused efforts to avoid high intraoperative oxygen concentrations. The efficacy of preventive measures is of particular significance in cardiac transplantation, where a major proportion of listed patients are maintained on chronic amiodarone therapy for treatment of recurrent ventricular arrhythmias.

The precise pathogenesis of the acute lung injury with acute pulmonary decompensation which occasionally occurs within 3–5 days following transplantation in patients on amiodarone remains elusive, but several lines of investigation implicate oxygen free radical species as a critical catalyst in the environment of high inspired concentrations of oxygen during and after the transplant operation.[52] Amiodarone may react with the oxygen in high concentrations, generating reactive oxygen intermediates. Amiodarone is an iodinated benzofuran derivative which participates readily in redox reactions (Fig. 12–2). Benzofurans are effective scavengers of singlet oxygen molecules[90] in which the reduction of amiodarone is accompanied by the simultaneous generation of a highly reactive aryl radical. Chemiluminescence studies in rats demonstrate that amiodarone produces such free radicals,[55, 99] which play a role in the pathologic development of thickening of interalveolar septae, accumulation of foamy macrophages, and variable degrees of interstitial fibrosis observed after 3 days of amiodarone therapy. Mice treated with amiodarone have exacerbation of alveolar edema within 3 days after exposure to 6 hours of 100% oxygen.[26]

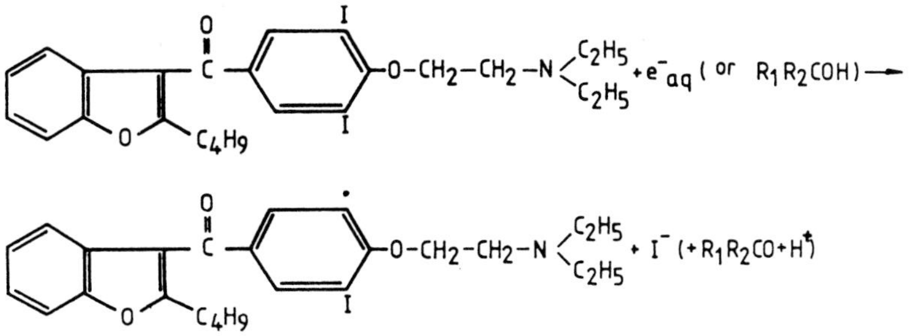

FIGURE 12–2. The formation of aryl radical from amoidarone in a reducing environment, with the simultaneous release of an iodine (I⁻) molecule. e⁻aq, hydrated electron; $R_1 R_2 COH$, α-hydroxy radical situated on an organic molecule; $R_1 R_2 CO$, carbonyl group situated on an organic molecule; H⁺, hydrogen ion. (From Vereckei A, Blazovics A, Gyorgy I, Feher E, Toth M, Szenasi G, Zsinka A, Foldiak G, Feher J: The role of free radicals in the pathogenesis of amiodarone toxicity. J Cardiovasc Electrophysiol 1993;4:161–177.)

Cyclosporine is generally withheld for the first 12 hours after transplant and then initiated at 1 mg/hr by continuous infusion (0.02 mg/kg/hr in infants and children) if urine output and cardiac performance are good. If urine output decreases, the infusion is temporarily discontinued. Oral cyclosporine is initiated following extubation when renal function is normalized and is gradually increased to achieve target levels of 300–400 ng/mL while in hospital. Postoperative azathioprine is dosed at 1–3 mg/kg/day to keep the white cell count about 3,000–5,000/mL. If mycophenolate is

selected instead of azathioprine, the initial dose is 500 mg PO or IV twice daily (10 mg/kg in pediatric patients) and rapidly increased over 3–4 days to a target dose of 1,750 mg PO bid in adults (22 mg/kg bid in infants and children). If gastrointestinal symptoms persist or leukopenia develops, the dose is reduced.

Induction therapy with OKT3 (7–10 days) is currently recommended for patients with depressed renal function (serum creatinine >1.7 mg/dL) for more than 2 days after transplant, thus limiting the usual progressive increase in cyclosporine dosage, and in patients at risk for accelerated acute rejection, highly sensitized patients, and those with positive B-cell crossmatch (by either flow cytometry or cytotoxic method). The usual dose is 5 mg day IV (0.1–0.2 mg/kg/day in infants and children) with the first daily dose divided into three smaller doses (1 mg, 1 mg, 2.5 mg) administered 3–4 hours apart to possibly decrease the initial dose "cytokine effect" (see Chapter 13).

With the availability of "humanized" monoclonal antibodies against interleukin-2 receptors, many cardiac

TABLE 12–8	**Protocol for Pretransplant Cyclosporine Administration**
SERUM CREATININE (mg/dL)	ORAL DOSE
<1	3 mg/kg
1.0–1.5	2 mg/kg
1.5–2.0	1 mg/kg
>2	None

transplant programs are developing protocols for their use as induction therapy. A more complete discussion of induction and maintenance immunosuppression strategies is found in Chapter 13.

PREVENTION OF EARLY INFECTION

Infection remains a major cause of morbidity and mortality early after cardiac transplantation, with approximately 25% of patients experiencing one or more major infections within the first 2 months.[70] Bacterial infections predominate during the initial transplant hospitalization, with a peak risk during the first posttransplant week. Successful prevention of infection contributes immensely to the reduction of long-term morbidity and increased patient survival. Strict surgical aseptic technique and proper care of indwelling lines and devices postoperatively is of obvious importance. Strict handwashing before and after examining the postoperative transplant patient is routinely recommended. Protective isolation has not proved beneficial in reducing infection incidence or mortality,[36, 102] and is not currently recommended unless severe bone marrow suppression is present. A detailed discussion of prevention and treatment of posttransplant infection is found in Chapter 15.

PROPHYLACTIC ANTIMICROBIAL THERAPY

Perioperative prophylactic antibiotics (vancomycin and ceftazidime at UAB) are routinely employed. In order to provide effective circulating levels prior to skin incision, the preoperative IV dose of each antibiotic (15 mg/kg) is administered 1 hour before operation. Vancomycin (10 mg/kg) is readministered at the conclusion of cardiopulmonary bypass (CPB) to overcome the dilutional effects of CPB. Vancomycin (10 mg/kg IV q 8 hr initially and then adjusted for renal function) and Ceftazidine (1 gm IV q 8 hr) are routinely administered for 4 days. A detailed listing of infection prophylaxis after cardiac transplantation is found in Table 15–9.

MANAGEMENT OF THE SURGICAL WOUND

The same surgical concepts of strict asepsis, hemostasis, and secure wound closure are applied during closure of the sternum and superficial incisions after cardiac transplantation as for routine cardiac surgery. Irrigation of the mediastinum and superficial wounds with dilute vancomycin is employed by some groups to decrease colony counts of gram-positive skin organisms. The surgical dressing is left in place for 48 hours to allow sealing of the skin edges unless bleeding under the dressing necessitates earlier wound examination. The wound is painted with an iodine-containing solution such as Betadine once or twice daily for several days until the wound is well sealed.

Because the pericardial space is frequently large in the transplant recipient with previous heart failure and marked cardiomegaly, there is frequently excess "dead space" following implantation of the donor heart. In addition to standard angled and straight Argyle chest tubes, a useful maneuver to decrease the incidence of postoperative pericardial effusions is placement of a soft surgical drainage catheter (Blake) in the posterior pericardial space connected to a drainage bulb which can be compressed to induce negative pressure drainage. Such drains can be left in place for 3–4 days (following removal of standard chest tubes) to allow evacuation of fluid collecting in the posterior mediastinal space. They are generally removed when the total drainage is less than about 40 mL in a 24-hour period.

DIAGNOSIS AND MANAGEMENT OF NEUROLOGIC DYSFUNCTION AFTER HEART TRANSPLANTATION

Multiple mechanisms may predispose to neurologic dysfunction following cardiac transplantation, including low cardiac output with hypotension and watershed infarction, cerebral emboli from a dilated left ventricle with thrombus, and side effects of medications. The neurological manifestations of low cardiac output are dependent on both the rate at which low cardiac output develops as well as its severity.[37, 82] Chronic low cardiac output may produce fatigue, headache, and tremor, and chronic cerebral hypoperfusion may result in a vascular dementia.[94] Acute and subacute hypotensive neurologic injury produces the pathological changes of diffuse neuronal loss in the cerebral cortex, Purkinje cells, thalamus, and striatum.[2] A number of medications used in the pre- and posttransplant period may contribute to neurological symptoms, including beta blockers (depression and confusion), calcium channel blockers (vertigo, headache, tremor, confusion), amiodarone (tremor, ataxia, neuropathy), and digoxin (visual disturbances, seizures, and syncope).[57] The neurological side effects of these medications may be more pronounced with the presence of impaired renal and hepatic function, and may produce residual neurologic sequalae in the posttransplant period. Central nervous system infection should be considered in all patients presenting with cerebral dysfunction (see Chapter 15), but is unlikely in the early posttransplant period.

Neurological complications in the early postoperative period can be grouped into one of three broad categories—encephalopathy, focal cerebral abnormalities, and seizures.

ENCEPHALOPATHY

An encephalopathic picture may range from mild confusion to obtundation and coma. If the symptoms develop within the first 48 hours of transplantation, the most likely causes are an operative or postoperative global hypoxic-ischemic insult and metabolic abnormalities. A rare but important cause of postoperative encephalopathy is cyclosporine-induced headache, depression, obtundation, cortical blindness, visual hallucinations, and seizures.[101] This picture is usually seen in patients with an elevated cyclosporine level, but may be exacerbated by hypomagnesemia, high-dose steroids, hypertension, and uremia. A similar picture may be seen with tacrolimus. The magnetic resonance imaging (MRI) scan is usually normal. OKT3 may produce aseptic meningitis manifested by fever, photophobia, and headache, as well as a milder encephalopathic picture with altered mentation.[1] High-dose steroids may produce psychosis.

FOCAL CEREBRAL ABNORMALITIES

In the early postoperative period, focal neurological disorders after cardiac transplantation are usually due to embolic events. However, focal neurologic disorders that are associated with dysarthria or mental state change can be misinterpreted as an encephalopathy. Within the first 24–48 hours, the computed tomographic (CT) scan may appear normal with small ischemic strokes.

SEIZURES

In the early posttransplant period, seizures occasionally occur, the most likely cause being a drug toxicity, especially due to cyclosporine, tacrolimus, and OKT3. Other causes include metabolic abnormalities and hypoxic-ischemic injury. Imaging with MRI is important to exclude a structural abnormality such as an infarct, hemorrhage, or abscess,[57] and an electroencephalogram is useful to confirm the diagnosis and aid in therapy selection. Anticonvulsants, such as phenytoin, phenobarbital, carbamazepine (because of their metabolism by the hepatic cytochrome P-450 system) may accelerate the metabolism of cyclosporine and tacrolimus, resulting in lowering of the drug levels. Other anticonvulsants that may be effective but do not interfere with the metabolism of cyclosporine or tacrolimus are valproic acid and gabapentin.

DIAGNOSIS AND MANAGEMENT OF GASTROINTESTINAL DYSFUNCTION AFTER TRANSPLANTATION

Intra-abdominal complications are recognized as potential risks following cardiac transplantation in the setting of a nutritionally compromised patient with advanced heart failure who undergoes the stress of cardiac surgery with initial high-dose immunosuppression. All of these elements are known to potentiate the development of intra-abdominal complications.

PANCREATITIS

Pancreatitis has been recognized after transplantation since Starzl's initial report in 1962.[92] Although this complication generally occurs later after transplantation (see Chapter 18), it may be rarely observed during the transplant admission. No specific risk factors have been identified for its early occurrence, and diagnosis is often delayed because of the nonspecific nature of the initial symptoms, which may include anorexia, vague abdominal discomfort, intense nausea, or nonspecific crampy abdominal pain during the first week following transplantation. The diagnostic process is complicated by the similarity of symptoms to nonspecific postoperative ileus or the gastrointestinal side effects of medications such as mycophenolate mofetil. The diagnosis of pancreatitis should be suspected whenever such gastrointestinal symptoms persist for more than about 24 hours. Serum amylase and lipase levels should be obtained and if markedly elevated strongly suggest the diagnosis of pancreatitis.[71] A CT scan should be obtained to evaluate the pancreas for signs of edema and inflammation. The gallbladder is examined for evidence of stones and the bile ducts are assessed for signs of dilation indicating obstruction.

Pancreatitis induced by gallstones is an indication for prompt surgical intervention. More commonly, no specific etiology is identified for the pancreatitis. The mortality of early pancreatitis is considerably less than pancreatitis occurring after the first 3 months.[6, 17, 25, 93] Pancreatitis without evidence of inflammation or edema by CT scan generally has a benign course and usually responds to nasogastric suction and avoidance of oral feedings, particularly if an ileus is present. When there is evidence of extensive peripancreatic inflammation, extravasation of fluid, or circulatory instability, severe pancreatitis should be suspected and, in the absence of rapid signs of improvement (within 24–48 hours), surgical exploration should be considered.

BILIARY COMPLICATIONS

The most common biliary complication early after cardiac transplantation is acute cholecystitis. The usual manifestation is abdominal pain or discomfort associated with right upper quadrant tenderness, rarely with a palpable distended gallbladder. The diagnosis is supported by the finding of gallstones with inflammation of the gallbladder wall on CT scan and/or a poorly functioning gallbladder on HIDA (dimethyl iminodiacetic acid) scan. Unless there is prompt resolution of symptoms with conservative therapy, including antibiotics, early surgical intervention is necessary. If the cardiac performance is good after cardiac transplantation, the mortality is generally low.

OTHER GASTROINTESTINAL COMPLICATIONS

Histamine receptor-blocking antacids are generally administered following transplantation to decrease gastric secretions and reduce the propensity for gastric and duodenal ulcer formation. Persistent midepigastric discomfort or dysphagia should prompt endoscopic evaluation of the esophagus and stomach for signs of gastric stress ulcers, cytomegalovirus (CMV)-induced gastritis and gastric ulcerations, and *Candida* esophagitis. Treatment of *Candida* esophagitis and cytomegalovirus infections are covered in Chapter 15. In the presence of gastric or duodenal ulcer disease, it may be advisable to taper steroid dosage more rapidly than usual. Repeat endoscopic evaluation is advisable within 2 weeks to ascertain healing of the gastric mucosa. Rarely, gastric or duodenal perforation may occur early after transplantation and require prompt surgical therapy. Transplant physicians and surgeons must be cognizant of the potential for steroids to mask traditional signs of abdominal viscus perforation.

ADDITIONAL POSTOPERATIVE CONSIDERATIONS

FLUID MANAGEMENT

Because of the tendency for extravascular fluid accumulation during cardiopulmonary bypass and the obligatory associated weight gain, maintenance intravenous fluid administration (in addition to the fluid requirements for monitoring devices and intravenous medications) is unnecessary for the first 24–48 hours. Colloid and packed red blood cells for maintenance of a desired hemoglobulin level are administered as needed to maintain the desired level of cardiac preload indicated by left and right atrial pressures.

TRANSFUSIONS

Although undesirable because of the potential for sensitization and transmission of transfusion-related infections, transfusion of packed red cells,[73] platelets, and fresh frozen plasma may be necessary to correct clotting abnormalities following cardiopulmonary bypass and to maintain the desired level of hemoglobin/hematocrit. Because of the known risk of transmitting cytomegalovirus in transfused red blood cells and platelets, all platelet transfusions should be administered through a leukocyte filter and packed red cells should be leukoreduced when possible or infused through a leukocyte filter, since the CMV virus is carried within leukocytes which accompany red cells and platelets in standard transfusions.[98] Numerous other viruses, including Epstein-Barr virus and human T-cell lymphotropic virus, are associated exclusively with leukocytes. The use of leukocyte-depleted transfusions of platelets and red cells rather than standard transfusion without leukocyte depletion is supported by several clinical studies suggesting a reduction in postsurgical morbidity and/or infection with the use of leukoreduced red cells and platelets rather than standard transfusions without leukocyte depletion.[13, 50]

PAIN RELIEF AND SEDATION

The standard agent for pain relief after cardiac surgery and cardiac transplantation is morphine sulfate in IV doses of 1–3 mg (0.05 mg/kg in pediatric patients). Additional sedation with diazepam in 1–2 mg IV doses (0.05 mg/kg in pediatric patients) or midazolam hydrochloride at doses of 1–1.5 mg as needed every 2–3 hours is useful while the patient is intubated. A continuous fentanil or propofol infusion provides effective analgesia and sedation in patients who are hemodynamically unstable or unusually agitated.

OTHER ROUTINE MEDICATIONS

Table 12–9 contains a list of other medications which are commonly initiated during the transplant admission. These and other drugs are aimed at reducing late complications as discussed in Chapters 17 and 18.

PHYSICAL ACTIVITY

Early ambulation and physical therapy are of great importance following extubation. As soon as the patient is physically able, convalescence is expedited by a program of progressive ambulation and physical therapy. More intensive physical therapy programs are necessary for patients who are severely physically deconditioned or who have been largely bedridden from severe heart failure requiring inotropic support.

PROMOTION OF A PSYCHOLOGICAL AND EDUCATIONAL MILIEU FOR LONG-TERM REHABILITATION AND COMPLIANCE

Most heart transplant programs have organized protocols for in-hospital education of transplant recipients

TABLE 12–9	**Additional Routine Medications Initiated During Transplant Hospitalization**		
MEDICATION	INDICATION	DOSE	DURATION
Calcium carbonate	Calcium supplement	10 ml PO tid	1 year
Acetylsalicylic acid (aspirin)	Antiplatelet action	81 mg PO qd	Chronic
Diltiazem	Reduction in cyclosporine dose, retardant of allograft vasculopathy	90 mg SR PO bid, then 180 mg CD qd	Chronic
Pravastatin	Lipid reduction	10 mg PO qd (increased as outpatient to target dose of 40 mg qd if liver function remains normal)	Chronic

TABLE 12–10	**Risk Factors for Noncompliance**
AREA OF NONCOMPLIANCE	PSYCHOSOCIAL RISK FACTORS
• Failure to take medications (≥1 time/month)	High anger-hostility level
• Failure to keep 1 or more clinic appointments or failure to have blood work done	High anxiety level
• Resumption of smoking	High anxiety level Poor relationship with caregivers Use of avoidance strategies for coping
• Failure to follow diet	High anxiety level Use of avoidance strategies for coping
• Failure to follow exercise regimen	High anxiety level

Adapted from Dew MA, Roth LH, Thompson ME, Kormos RL, Griffith BP: Medical compliance and its predictors in the first year after heart transplantation. J Heart Lung Transplant 1996;15:631–645.

and their families by transplant coordinators, a pharmacist, and transplant physicians. Such education typically includes intensive instruction about medications, including the timing of administration and dosage as well as potential side effects. The patients should learn about the clinical symptoms of rejection and infection so they understand when to call the transplant team. Clinical appointments and outpatient blood work schedules are reviewed with the patient and their family.

Long-term outcome and rehabilitative potential after cardiac transplantation are affected in a major way by patient compliance[21] (Table 12–10). Neurocognitive function is often abnormal early following transplantation[55] and can affect the ability of patients to comprehend and follow the complex medical regimen. Specific attempts to identify such deficits are important, since they are often not discovered with routine physician–patient interaction.

References

1. Adair JC, Woodley SL, O'Connell JB, Call GK, Baringer JR: Aseptic meningitis following cardiac transplantation: clinical characteristics relationship to immunosuppressive regimen. Neurology 1991;41:249–252.
2. Adams J, Brierly J, Connor R: The effects of systemic hypotension upon the human brain: clinical and neuropathological observations in eleven cases. Brain 1966;89:235.
3. Alajmo F, Calamai G, Perna A, Melissano G, Pretelli P, Palmarini MF, Carbonetto F, Noferi D, Boddi V, Palminiello A, Vaccari M: High-dose aprotinin: hemostatic effects in open heart operations. Ann Thorac Surg 1989;48:536–539.
4. Argenziano M, Choudhri AF, Oz MC, Rose EA, Smith CR, Landry DW: A prospective randomized trial of arginine vasopressin in the treatment of vasodilatory shock after left ventricular assist device placement. Circulation 1997;96(suppl II):II-286–II-290.
5. Armitage JM, Hardesty RL, Griffith BP: Prostaglandin E₁: an effective treatment of right heart failure after orthotopic heart transplantation. J Heart Transplant 1987;6:348–351.
6. Aziz S, Bergdahl L, Baldwin JC, Weiss LM, Jamieson SW, Oyer PE, Stinson EB, Shumway NE: Pancreatitis after cardiac and cardiopulmonary transplantation. Surgery 1985;97:653–661.
7. Baldwin L, Henderson A, Hickman P: Effect of postoperative low-dose dopamine on renal function after elective major vascular surgery. Ann Intern Med 1994;120:744.
8. Bexton RS, Nathan AW, Hellestrand KJ, Cory-Pearce R, Spurrell RAJ, English TAH, Camm AJ: Sinoatrial function after cardiac transplantation. J Am Coll Cardiol 1984;3:712–723.
9. Bhatia SJS, Kirshenbaum JM, Shemin RJ, Cohn LH, Collins JJ, DiSesa VJ, Young PJ, Mudge GH Jr, Sutton MGS: Time course

10. of resolution of pulmonary hypertension and right ventricular remodeling after orthotopic cardiac transplantation. Circulation 1987;76:819–826.
10. Bidstrup BP, Royston D, Sapsford RN, Taylor KM: Reduction in blood loss and blood use after cardiopulmonary bypass with high dose aprotinin (Trasylol). J Cardiovasc Surg 1989;97:364–372.
11. Blanche C, Nessim S, Quartel A: Heart transplantation with bicaval and pulmonary venous anastomoses. A hemodynamic analysis of the first 117 patients. J Cardiovasc Surg (Torino) 1997;38:561–566.
12. Blauhut B, Gross C, Necek S, Doran JE, Spath P, Lundsgaard-Hansen P: Effects of high-dose aprotinin on blood loss, platelet function, fibrinolysis, complement, and renal function after cardiopulmonary bypass. J Thorac Cardiovasc Surg 1991;101:958–967.
13. Blumberg N, Triuizi DJ, Heal JM: Transfusion-induced immunomodulation and its clinical consequences. Transfus Med Rev 1990;4(suppl):24–35.
14. Buja G, Miorelli M, Livi U: Complete atrioventricular block after orthotopic heart transplantation: incidence, electrocardiographic-electrophysiological evolution and clinical importance. Eur J Card Pacing Electrophysiol 1992;3:173–179.
15. Carp H, Vadhera R, Jayaram A, Garvey D: Endogenous vasopressin and renin-angiotensin systems support blood pressure after epidural block in humans. Anesthesiology 1994;80:1000–1007.
16. Chasapakis G, Dimas C: Possible interaction between muscle relaxants and the kallikrein-trypsin inactivator "Trasylol". Br J Anaesth 1966;38:838–839.
17. Colon R, Frazier OH, Kahan BD, Radovancevic B, Duncan JM, Lorber MI, VanBuren CT: Complications in cardiac transplant patients requiring general surgery. Surgery 1988;103:32–38.
18. Colucci WS, Wright RF, Braunwald E: New positive inotropic agents in the treatment of congestive heart failure. N Engl J Med 314:292, 1986.
19. Cook LS, Will KR, Moran J: Treatment of junctional rhythm after heart transplantation with terbutaline. J Heart Transplant 1989;8:342–344.
20. Cosgrove DM, Heric B, Lytle BW, Taylor PC, Novoa R, Golding AR, Stewart RW, McCarthy PM, Loop FD: Aprotinin therapy for preoperative myocardial revascularization: a placebo-controlled study. Ann Thorac Surg 1992;54:1031–1038.
21. Dew MA, Roth LH, Thompson ME, Kormos RL, Griffith BP: Medical compliance and its predictors in the first year after heart transplantation. J Heart Lung Transplant 1996;15:631–645.
22. DiBiase A, Tse TM, Schnittger I, Wexler L, Stinson EB, Valantine HA: Frequency and mechanism of bradycardia in cardiac transplant recipients and need for pacemakers. Am J Cardiol 1991;67:1385–1389.
23. Dietrich W, Barankay A, Dilthey G, Henze R, Niekau E, Sebening F, Richter JA: Reduction of homologous blood requirement in cardiac surgery by intra-operative aprotinin application: clinical experience in 152 cardiac surgical patients. Thorac Cardiovasc Surg 1989;37:92–98.

24. Dietrich W, Spannagl M, Jochum M, Wendt P, Schramm W, Barankay A, Sebening F: Influence of high-dose aprotinin treatment on blood loss and coagulation patterns in patients undergoing myocardial revascularization. Anesthesiology 1990;73:1119–1126.

25. DiSesa VJ, Kirkman RL, Tilney NL, Mudge GH, Collins JJ Jr, Cohn LH: Management of general surgical complications following cardiac transplantation. Arch Surg 1989;124:539–541.

26. Donica SK, Paulson AW, Simpson BR, Ramsay MAE, Saunders CT, Swygert TH, Tappe J: Danger of amiodarone therapy and elevated inspired oxygen concentrations in mice. Am J Cardiol 1996;77:109–110.

27. Duke GJ, Briedis JH, Weaver RA: Renal support in critically ill patients: low-dose dopamine or low-dose dobutamine? Crit Care Med 22:1919, 1994.

28. Dusman RE, Stanton MS, Miles WM, Klein LS, Zipes DP, Fineberg NS, Heger JJ: Clinical features of amiodarone-induced pulmonary toxicity. Circulation 1990;82:51–59.

29. Emery RW, Eales F, Joyce LD, Von Rueden TJ, King RM, Jorgensen CR, Pritzker MR, Johnson KE, Lake KD, Arom KV: Mechanical circulatory assistance after heart transplantation. Ann Thorac Surg 1991;51:43–47.

30. Farrell TG, Camm AJ: Action of drugs in the denervated heart. Semin Thorac Cardiovasc Surg 1990;2:279–289.

31. Fischer JH: Effects of Trasylol on the kidneys: dependence on temperature and dose. In Dudziak R, Reuter HD, Kirchhoff PG, Schumann F (eds): Proteolysis and Proteinase Inhibition in Cardiac Vascular Surgery. Stuttgart: Schattauer Verlag, 1985, pp 127–135.

32. Flancbaum L, Choban PS, Dasta JF: Quantitative effects of low-dose dopamine on urine output in oliguric surgical intensive care unit patients. Crit Care Med 1994;22:61.

33. Fox AC, Reed GE, Glassman E, Kaltman AJ, Silk BB: Release of adenosine from human hearts during angina induced by rapid atrial pacing. J Clin Invest 1974;53:1447–1457.

34. Fritz H, Wunderer G: Biochemistry and applications of aprotinin, the kallikrein inhibitor from bovine organs. Arzneimittelforsch 1983;33:479–494.

35. Fuhrer F, Gallimore MJ, Heller W, Hoffmeister HE: Aprotinin in cardiopulmonary bypass: effects on the Hageman factor (FXII)-kallikrein system and blood loss. Blood Coagul Fibrinolysis 1992;3:99–104.

36. Gamberg P, Miller JL, Lough ME: Impact of protection isolation on the incidence of infection after heart transplantation. J Heart Transplant 1987;6:147–149.

37. Ginsberg M, Hedley-White T, Richardson E: Hypoxic ischemic leukoencephalopathy in man. Arch Neurol 1976;33:5.

38. Goldstein DJ, Seldomridge JA, Chen JM, Catanese KA, DeRosa CM, Weinberg AD, Rose EA, Levin HR, Oz MC: Use of aprotinin in LVAD recipients reduces blood loss, blood use, and perioperative mortality. Ann Thorac Surg 1995;59:1063–1068.

39. Gott JP, Cooper WA, Schmidt FE Jr, Brown WM, Wright CE, Merlino JD, Fortenberry JD, Guyton RA: Modifying risk for extracorporeal circulation: trial of four anti-inflammatory strategies. Ann Thorac Surg 1998;66:747–754.

40. Greenspon AJ, Kidwell GA, Hurley W, Mannion J: Amiodarone-related postoperative adult respiratory distress syndrome. Circulation 1991;84(suppl III):III-407–III-415.

41. Harder MP, Eijsman L, Roozendaal KJ, van Oeveren W, Wildevuur CRH: Aprotinin reduces intraoperative and postoperative blood loss in membrane oxygenator cardiopulmonary bypass. Ann Thorac Surg 1991;51:936–941.

42. Havel M, Teufelsbauer H, Knobl P, Dalmatiner R, Jaksch P, Zwolfer W, Muller M, Vukov T: Effect of intraoperative aprotinin administration on postoperative bleeding in patients undergoing cardiopulmonary bypass operation. J Thorac Cardiovasc Surg 1991;101:968–972.

43. Heinz G, Hirschl M, Buxbaum P, Laufer G, Gasic S, Laczkovic S: Sinus node dysfunction after orthotopic cardiac transplantation: postoperative incidence and long-term implications. PACE 1992;15:731–737.

44. Heinz G, Kratochwill C, Buxbaum P, Laufer G, Kreiner G, Siostrzonek P, Gasic S, Derfler K, Gossinger H: Immediate normalization of profound sinus node dysfunction by aminophylline after cardiac transplantation. Am J Cardiol 1993;71:346–349.

45. Heinz G, Kratochwill C, Koller-Strametz J, Kreiner G, Grimm M, Grabenwoger M, Laufer G, Gossinger H: Benign prognosis of early sinus node dysfunction after orthotopic cardiac transplantation. PACE 1998;21:422–429.

46. Heinz G, Ohner T, Laufer G, Gossinger H, Gasic S, Laczkovics A: Demographic and perioperative factors associated with initial and prolonged sinus node dysfunction after orthotopic heart transplantation: the impact of ischemic time. Transplantation 1991;51;1217–1232.

47. Holt ND, McComb JM: Late atrioventricular (AV) block and permanent pacemaker implantation after orthotopic cardiac transplantation [letter]. PACE 1996;19:1272.

48. Horl WH: Effect of aprotinin on renal function. In Dudziak R, Reuter HD, Kirchhoff PG, Schumann F (eds): Proteolysis and Proteinase Inhibition in Cardiac and Vascular Surgery. Stuttgart: Schattauer Verlag, 1985, pp 137–142.

49. Jacquet L, Ziady G, Stein K, Griffith B, Armitae J, Hardesty R, Kormos R: Cardiac rhythm disturbances early after orthotopic heart transplantation: prevalence and clinical importance of the observed Abnormalities. J Am Coll Cardiol 1990;16:832–837.

50. Jensen LS, Kissmeyer-Nielsen P, Wolfe B, Ovist N: Randomized comparison of leucocyte-depleted versus buffy-coat poor blood transfusion and complications after colorectal surgery. Lancet 1996;348:841–845.

51. Kay GN, Epstein AE, Kirklin JK, Diethelm AG, Graybar G, Plumb VJ: Fatal postoperative amiodarone pulmonary toxicity. Am J Cardiol 1988;62:490–492.

52. Kennedy TP, Gordon GB, Paky A, McShane A, Adkinson NF, Peters SP, Friday K, Jackman W, Sciuto AM, Gurtner GH: Amiodarone causes acute oxidant lung injury in ventilated and perfused rabbit lungs. J Cardiovasc Pharmacol 1988;12:23–36.

53. Kieler-Jenson N, Lundin S, Ricksten SE: Vasodilator therapy after heart transplantation: effects of inhaled nitric oxide and intravenous prostacyclin, prostaglandin E1, and sodium nitroprusside. J Heart Lung Transplant 1995;14:436–443.

54. Kirklin JK, Naftel DC, Kirklin JW, Blackstone EH, White-Williams C, Bourge RC: Pulmonary vascular resistance and the risk of heart transplantation. J Heart Transplant 1988;7:331–336.

55. LaMarche J, Naftel D, Smith R, Kirklin J, Bourge R, McGiffin D, Weiss T: Neurocognitive impairment as a factor in cardiac transplant candidate selection [abstract]. Program Issue–J Heart Lung Transplant 1995;14:S36.

56. Landry DW, Levin HR, Gallant EM, Ashton RC Jr, Seo S, D'Alessandro A, Oz MC, Oliver JA: Vasopressin deficiency contributes to the vasodilation of septic shock. Circulation 1997;95:1122–1125.

57. Lee JM, Raps EC: Neurologic complications of transplantation. Neurol Clin North Am 1998;16:21–33.

58. Liem LB, DiBiase A, Schroeder JS: Arrhythmias and clinical electrophysiology of the transplanted human heart. Semin Thorac Cardiovasc Surg 1990;2:271–278.

59. Little RE, Kay GN, Epstein AE, Plumb VJ, Bourge RC, Neves J, Kirklin JK: Arrhythmias after orthotopic cardiac transplantation. Circulation 1989;80(suppl III):III-140–III-146.

60. Lokhandwala MF, Amenta F: Anatomical distribution and function of dopamine receptors in the kidney. FASEB J 1991;5:3023.

61. Mackintosh AF, Carmichael DJ, Wren C, Cory-Pearce R, English TA: Sinus node function in first three weeks after cardiac transplantation. Br Heart J 1982;48:584–588.

62. Marchena ED, Futterman L, Wozniak P, Madrid W, Mitrani A, Myerburg RJ, Bolooki H: Pulmonary artery torsion: a potentially lethal complication after orthotopic heart transplantation. J Heart Transplant 1989;8:499–502.

63. Marchlinski FE, Gansler TS, Waxman HL, Josephson ME: Amiodarone pulmonary toxicity. Ann Intern Med 1982;97:839–845.

64. Martin WJ, Rosenow EC: Amiodarone pulmonary toxicity: recognition and pathogenesis. Chest 1988;93(pt 1):1067–1074.

65. Mason JW, Harrison DC: Electrophysiology and electropharmacology of the transplanted human heart. In Narula OS (ed): Cardiac Arrhythmias: Electrophysiology Diagnosis and Management. Baltimore: Williams & Wilkins, 1979, pp 69–81.

66. McEnany MT, Morgan RJ, Mundth ED, Austen WG: Circumvention of detrimental pulmonary vasoactivity of exogenous catecholamines in cardiac resuscitation. Surg Forum 1975;26:98.

67. McGiffin DC, Kirklin JK, Naftel DC, Bourge RC: Competing outcomes after heart transplantation: a comparison of eras and outcomes. J Heart Lung Transplant 1997;16:190–198.

68. McMahon MJ, Axon ATR: Anaphylactic reaction to aprotinin [letter]. BMJ 1984;289:1696.

69. Melton IC, Gilligan DM, Wood MA, Ellenbogen KA: Optimal cardiac pacing after heart transplantation. PACE 1999;22:1510–1527.

70. Miller LW, Naftel DC, Bourge RC, Kirklin JK, Brozena SC, Jarcho J, Hobbs RE, Mills RM, and the Cardiac Transplant Research Database Group: Infection after heart transplantation: a multiinstitutional study. J Heart Lung Transplant 1994;13:381–393.

71. Missavage A, Weaver D, Bouwman D, Parnell V, Wilson R: Hyperamylasemia after cardiopulmonary bypass. Am Surg 1984;50:297–300.

72. Miyamoto Y, Curtiss E, Kormos RL, Armitage JM, Hardesty RL, Griffith BP: Bradyarrhythmia after heart transplantation: incidence, time course and outcome. Circulation 1990;82(suppl IV):313–317.

73. Murphy PJ, Connery C, Hicks GI Jr, Blumberg N: Homologous blood transfusion as a risk factor for postoperative infection after coronary artery bypass graft operations. J Thorac Cardiovasc Surg 1992;104:1092–1099.

74. Myers JL, Kennedy JI, Plumb VJ: Amiodarone lung: pathologic findings in clinically toxic patients. Hum Pathol 1987;18:349–354.

75. Nalos PC, Kass RM, Gang ES, Fishbein MC, Mandel WJ, Peter T: Life-threatening postoperative pulmonary complications in patients with previous amiodarone pulmonary toxicity undergoing cardiothoracic operations. J Thorac Cardiovasc Surg 1987;93:904–912.

76. Okereke OUJ, Frazier OH, Reece IJ, Painvin GA, Radovancevic B, Cooley DA: Experimental heart and heart/lung transplantation. Transplant Proc 1987;XIX:1034–1035.

77. Pae WE: Ventricular assist devices and total artificial hearts: a combined registry experience. Ann Thorac Surg 1993;55:295–298.

78. Pae WE Jr, Aufiero TX, Weldner PW, Miller CA, Pierce WS: Aprotinin therapy for insertion of ventricular assist devices for staged heart transplantation. J Heart Lung Transplant 1994;13:811–816.

79. Pavri BB, O'Nunain SS, Newell JB, Ruskin JN, William G: Prevalence and prognostic significance of atrial arrhythmias after orthotopic cardiac transplantation. J Am Coll Cardiol 1995;25:1673–1680.

80. Proud G, Chamberlain J: Anaphylactic reaction to aprotinin. Lancet 1976;2:48–49.

81. Radovancevic B, Nakatani T, Frazier OH, Moncrief C, Vega J, Haupt H, Duncan JM: Mechanical circulatory support for perioperative donor heart failure. ASAIO Trans 1989;35:539–541.

82. Read W, Anderson R: Effects of rapid blood pressure reduction on cerebral blood flow. Am Heart J 1986;111:226.

83. Ricci DR, Orlick AE, Reitz BA, Mason JW, Stinson EB, Harrison DC: Depressant effect of digoxin on atrioventricular conduction in man. Circulation 1978;57:898–905.

84. Rosner MJ, Newsome HH, Becker DP: Mechanical brain injury: the sympathoadrenal response. J Neurosurg 1984;61:76–86.

85. Rotmensch HH, Liron M, Tupilski M, Laniado S: Possible association of pneumonitis with amiodarone therapy. Am Heart J 1980;100:412–413.

86. Royston D, Bidstrup BP, Taylor KM, Sapsford RN: Effect of aprotinin on need for blood transfusion after repeat open-heart surgery. Lancet 1987;2:1289–1291.

87. Scott CD, Dark JH, McComb JM: Sinus node function after cardiac transplantation. J Am Coll Cardiol 1994;24:1334–1341.

88. Scott CD, McComb JM, Dark JH, Bexton RD: Permanent pacing after cardiac transplantation. Br Heart J 1993;59:399–403.

89. Semigran MJ, Cockrill BA, Kacmarek R: Nitric oxide is an effective pulmonary vasodilator in cardiac transplant candidates with pulmonary hypertension [abstract]. J Heart Lung Transplant 1993;12:S67.

90. Singh A: Chemical and biochemical aspects of super-oxide radicals and related species of activated oxygen. Can J Physiol Pharmacol 1982;60:1330–1345.

91. Sobol SM, Rakita L: Pneumonitis and pulmonary fibrosis associated with amiodarone treatment: possible complication of a new antiarrhythmic drug. Circulation 1982;65:819–824.

92. Starzl TE: Experience in Renal Transplantation. Philadelphia: WB Saunders Company, 1962.

93. Steed DL, Brown B, Reilly JJ, Peitzman AB, Griffith BP, Hardesty RL, Webster MW: General surgical complications in heart and heart-lung transplantation. Surgery 1985;98:739–745.

94. Sulkawa R, Erkinjuntii T: Vascular dementia and systemic hypotension. Acta Neurol Scand 1987;76:123.

95. Todd GL, Baroldi G, Pieper GM, Clayton FC, Eliot RS: Experimental catecholamine-induced myocardial necrosis I. Morphology, quantification and regional distribution of acute contraction band lesions. J Mol Cell Cardiol 1985;17:317–338.

96. Van Oeveren W, Harder MP, Roozendaal KJ, Eijsman L, Wildevuur CR: Aprotinin protects platelets against the initial effect of cardiopulmonary bypass. J Thorac Cardiovasc Surg 1990;99:788–797.

97. Van Oeveren W, Jansen NJG, Bidstrup BP, Royston D, Westaby S, Neuhof H, Wildevuur CR: Effects of aprotinin on hemostatic mechanisms during cardiopulmonary bypass. Ann Thorac Surg 1987;44:640–645.

98. VanProoijen HC, Visser JJ, vanOostendorp WR, deGast GC, Verdonck LF: Prevention of primary transfusion-associated cytomegalovirus infection in bone marrow transplant recipients by the removal of white cells from blood components with high-affinity filters. Br J Haematol 1994;87:144–147.

99. Vereckei A, Blazovics A, Gyorgy I, Feher E, Toth M, Szenasi G, Zsinka A, Foldiak G, Feher J: The role of free radicals in the pathogenesis of amiodarone toxicity. J Cardiovasc Electrophysiol 1993;4:161–177.

100. Vestal RE, Eiriksson CE, Musser B, Ozaki LK, Halter JB: Effect of intravenous aminophylline on plasma levels of catecholamines and related cardiovascular and metabolic responses in man. Circulation 1983;67:162–171.

101. Walker R, Brochstein J: Neurologic complications of immunosuppression agents. Neurol Clin 1988;6:261.

102. Walsh TR, Gutendorf J, Dummer S, Hardesty RL, Armitage JM, Kormos RL, Griffith BP: The value of protective isolation procedures in cardiac allograft recipients. Ann Thorac Surg 1989;47:539–545.

103. Young JB, Leon CA, Short HD, Noon GP, Lawrence EC, Whisennand HH, Pratt CM, Goodman DA, Weilbaecher D, Quinones MA, DeBakey ME: Evolution of Hemodynamics after orthotopic heart and heart-lung transplantation: early restrictive patterns persisting in occult fashion. J Heart Transplant 1987;6:34–43.

104. Zmyslinski RW, Warner MG, Dietrich EB: Symptomatic sinus node dysfunction after heart transplantation. PACE 1988;11:445–448.

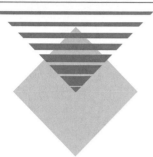

CHAPTER THIRTEEN

Immunosuppressive Modalities

with the collaboration of
JAMES F. GEORGE, PH.D.

TABLE 13–1 Evolution of Immunosuppression in Organ Transplantation

YEAR	APPROACHES
1959	Total body irradiation
1960–1962	6-Mercaptopurine and azathioprine
1960–1965	Additional myelotoxic agents
1962–1963	Steroids used systematically
1966	Lymphocytotoxic sera/antibodies
1978	Cyclosporine
1989	Tacrolimus
1997	Mycophenolate mofetil
1998	Sirolimus

Immunotherapeutic modalities in transplantation are designed to reduce the intensity of the immune response to a degree that allows acceptance of the allograft and provide sufficiently low toxicity to allow prolonged survival of the organism. The historical evolution of immunosuppressive modalities applied to organ transplantation is reviewed in Table 13–1. Pharmacologic agents have evolved from general suppression of the host immunologic defenses to selective blockade of intracellular immune events that maximize graft acceptance while minimizing toxicity. In the case of patients following organ transplantation, there are three basic situations which require specific combinations of immunosuppressive therapies: (1) high-dose initial immunosuppression to facilitate graft acceptance, minimize the chance of early rejection, and potentially favor induction of tolerance; (2) maintenance therapy for chronic acceptance of the allograft; and (3) augmented immunosuppression to reverse episodes of acute rejection. In cardiac transplantation, there is also increasing interest in specific immunotherapeutic modalities to prevent or reverse chronic rejection in the form of allograft vasculopathy.

The immune response to transplantation is highly dependent on T-cell activation and proliferation. The cellular events of T-cell activation are of great importance because many of the current immunosuppressive drugs target specific intracellular pathways of T-cell activation. These events are detailed in Chapter 2. A recapitulation of the three "signals" of T-cell activation is presented in Table 13–2.

TABLE 13–2 T-Cell Response to Transplantation

Signal 1:	Antigenic peptide engages and triggers the T-cell receptor (TCR) in the context of self MHC class II molecule, which requires the presence of CD3 and CD4 molecules. This interaction activates transduction pathways in the cytosol such as the calcineurin pathway which are necessary for transcription of cytokine genes and subsequent cytokine production.
Signal 2:	Costimulation of CD28 and other receptors on the T-cell by ligands on the antigen-presenting cell such as B7-1 or B7-2. Signals 1 and 2 act synergistically to induce cytokine production.
Signal 3:	Cytokines produced by the activated T-cells engage cytokine receptors on the cell surface which initiate cell division and proliferation.

TABLE 13-3   Actions of Immunosuppressive Modalities

	Corticosteroids	Cyclosporine	Tacrolimus	Azathioprine	Mycophenolate Mofetil	Cyclophosphamide	Methotrexate	Actinomycin D	Sirolimus	Mizoribine	Brequinar Sodium	Leflunomide	Gusperimus	ATG	OKT3	Basiliximab, Daclizumab	OKT4	Plasmapheresis	Photopheresis	TLI
Inhibition of T-cell Activation Decreased APC effectiveness	X												X							
Inhibition of TCR/antigen binding	X													X	X					
Inhibition of accessory molecules	X													X	X		X			
Inhibition of IL-2 production	X	X	X																	
Inhibition of T-cell proliferation Inhibition of IL-2/IL-2R interaction																X				
Inhibition of proliferative response to cytokine	X								X			X								
Inhibition of DNA synthesis				X	X	X	X	X		X	X	X								X
T-cell depletion														X	X		X			X
Inhibition of B-cell proliferation	X	X	X	X	X	X	X	X	X	X	X	X	X	X	X	X	X			X
B-cell/antibody depletion														X					X	X
Inhibition of smooth muscle proliferation (? Allograft vasculopathy)					X				X			X	X							
Promotion of suppressor cells																			X	X

A general classification of immunosuppressive modalities discussed in this chapter, categorized by their primary mechanism of action, is presented in Table 13-3 and Figure 13-1 which is adapted from Figure 2-19. As future knowledge refines our understanding of the immune system and the basic mechanisms underlying allograft rejection, more selective and less toxic immunotherapeutic modalities will target specific T-cell subsets, cytokines, and adhesion molecules which participate in the rejection process.

CORTICOSTEROIDS

HISTORICAL NOTE

The immunosuppressive effects of steroids on the immune system have been known for over 50 years. The effectiveness of corticosteroids in suppressing rejection of rabbit skin homografts was demonstrated by Billingham and colleagues in 1951.[50] Steroids were first employed in clinical transplantation in 1960, when cortisone was used to reverse an acute rejection episode after renal transplantation at the Peter Bent Brigham Hospital. By 1962, steroids were a standard part of maintenance immunosuppression.

CHEMICAL STRUCTURE

Prednisone, prednisolone, and methylprednisolone are synthetic corticosteroids. The chemical structure of prednisone is illustrated in Figure 13-2.

MECHANISM OF IMMUNOSUPPRESSION

The importance of steroids in transplantation relates both to their immunosuppressive action and to their anti-inflammatory properties. The anti-inflammatory effects result in part, from inhibition of inflammatory mediators such as leukotrienes and prostaglandins. Steroids induce the release of lipocortin, a regulatory protein that inhibits phosphodiesterase A2. These actions undoubtedly play an important role in the reversal of symptoms of clinical rejection, in that a beneficial effect of high-dose methylprednisolone on symptomatic rejection may be apparent within 1-2 hours (even occasionally in the presence of hemodynamic compromise), which is too fast to be explained by purely immunosuppressive effects.

The immunosuppressive actions of steroids are complex, but a principal effect on T-lymphocytes is the impairment of the rate of transcription of specific genes which encode important regulatory cytokines involved in the immune response (Fig. 13-1). After entering a target cell, corticosteroids bind to their intracytoplasmic receptors, and the steroid-receptor complex migrates into the nucleus, where it retards gene transcription through its interaction with certain gene promoters and inhibition of nuclear factor of activated T-cells (NFAT). The result is inhibition of expression of interleukin-2 (IL-2) and other cytokines, including IL-1, IL-3, IL-6, tumor necrosis factor-α (TNF-α), and interferon-γ (IFN-γ).[226] Other corticosteroid actions include suppression of macrophage function, reduction in adhesion molecule expression, inhibition of leukocyte transmigration through blood vessels, induction of lymphocyte

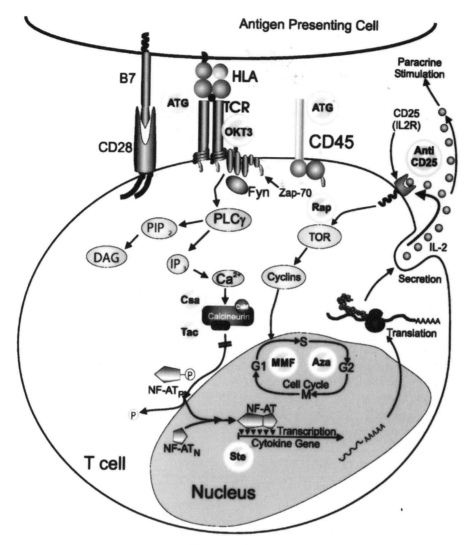

FIGURE 13-1. Immunosuppressants are directed against multiple targets in the cellular activation pathway. Refer to discussion of individual agents for further details. Antithymocyte globulins (ATG) and OKT3 target the T-cell receptor and cause it to be removed from the cell surface, or they cause destruction of the entire cell through multiple mechanisms. ATG also contains antibodies that bind to CD45 and interfere with T-cell activation via an unknown mechanism. Cyclosporine (CsA) and tacrolimus (Tac) interfere with calcium-mediated signaling via calcineurin. Steroids (Ste) have multiple actions, including inhibition of transcription of multiple cytokines. Mycophenolate mofetil (MMF) and azathioprine (Aza) target cellular replication, and rapamycin (Rap) binds to a protein involved in IL-2 receptor signaling called the target of rapamycin (TOR), therefore indirectly inhibiting cellular replication. Finally, anti-CD25 blocks ligation of the IL-2 receptor by IL-2.

apoptosis, and reduction of major histocompatibility complex expression.[137, 208]

PHARMACOKINETICS

Prednisone and prednisolone are rapidly absorbed from the upper gastrointestinal tract, yielding peak plasma concentrations within 1–3 hours.[119] Prednisone undergoes hepatic conversion to prednisolone, which is the biologically active form. The average bioavailability is about 80% of an oral dose of prednisolone.[423] Corticosteroids exist in plasma in two forms: protein-bound and free. Normally, 90% or more of prednisolone is bound

in plasma by cortisone-binding globulin or albumin, but only the free steroid is available to react with cytosol receptors. Cortisone-binding globulin has low total binding capacity, but high affinity; whereas albumin has high total binding capacity but low affinity. Thus, changes in the state of circulating albumin have the greatest impact on available free prednisolone. Conditions in which plasma-binding capacity is increased (such as pregnancy) will decrease the bioavailability of steroids, whereas conditions that decrease plasma-binding capacity (such as hypoalbuminemia) will increase steroid bioavailability and therefore side effects.[316]

The half-life of prednisolone is about 3 hours.[37] Steroids are inactivated almost exclusively in the liver; thus,

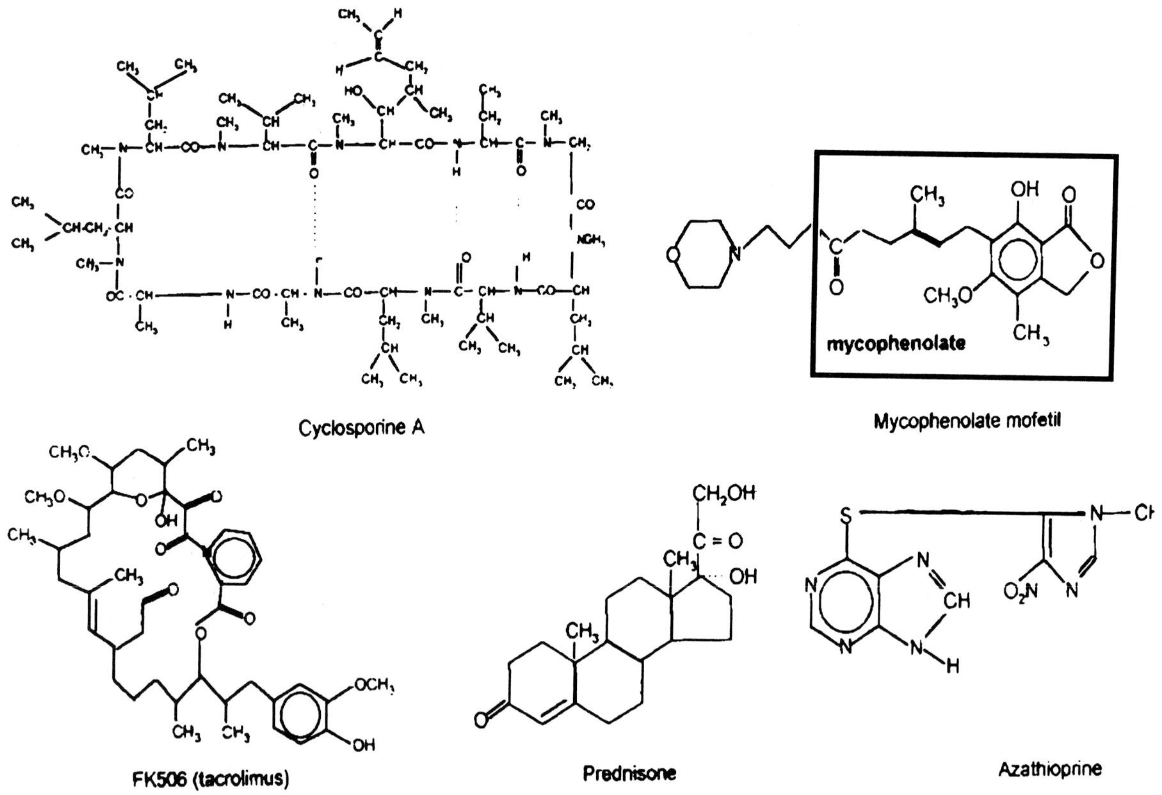

FIGURE **13-2.** Structural formulas of azathioprine, corticosteroids, cyclosporine, tacrolimus (FK-506), and mycophenolate mofetil. (From Halloran PF, Lui SL: Approved immunosuppressants. *In* Norman DJ, Suki WN [eds]: Primer on Transplantation. Thorofare, NJ: American Society of Transplant Physicians, 1998.)

depressed hepatic function increases the half-life of steroids, while some drugs such as phenytoin, barbituates, and rifampin, which induce hepatic enzyme systems, will shorten the half-life.[119]

DOSING

Many different dosing regimens for corticosteroids have been employed after cardiac transplantation. There are no specific measurable parameters which indicate therapeutic efficacy (such as cyclosporine blood levels) or toxicity (such as leukocyte count in azathioprine therapy). The immunosuppressive strength of prednisone, prednisolone, and methylprednisolone are similar on a per-milligram basis, so the same dose is usually maintained when converting from oral prednisone or prednisolone to intravenous methylprednisolone.

Considerable variability exists in the dosing schedules of steroids used in cardiac transplantation (Table 13–4). In general, high-dose methylprednisolone is administered prior to transplant at a dose of 250–500 mg (or 5–10 mg/kg) and a similar dose immediately after transplantation. A smaller dose is usually administered at 8 hourly intervals for 24–48 hours. Steroids are usually part of induction therapy, in which 0.5–1 mg/kg/day of prednisone is administered for 1–3 weeks, after which it is tapered to either low-dose daily steroids (10 mg/day in an adult or 0.1 mg/kg/day in an infant), alternate-day steroids, or no steroids (see also Chapter 14 for specific

TABLE 13-4	**Corticosteroids**

Clinical Use
- Maintenance immunosuppression.
- Pulse therapy for acute rejection.

Mechanism
- Anti-inflammatory action.
- Inhibition of IL-2 production by impairment of gene transcription.
- Suppression of antigen-presenting cell function, reduction in adhesion molecule expression, inhibition of leukocyte transmigration, inhibition of lymphocyte proliferation.

Dose

Maintenance immunosuppression
- Individual protocols are highly variable. A standard regimen is an initial prednisone dose of 1 mg/kg tapered to an every-other-day dose of approximately 0.1–0.2 mg/kg or no steroids by 6 months. Some programs use no maintenance corticosteroids. Daily steroids (approximately 0.2 mg/kg/day) are maintained in the setting of recurrent rejection.

Treatment of acute rejection
- Adults: 500–1,000 mg methylprednisolone IV daily for 3 days or prednisone 2–3 mg/kg PO for 3 days with or without a rapid taper thereafter.
- Pediatric: For neonates and small infants (<7 kg), generally 100 mg methylprednisolone IV daily for 3 days. For older infants and children, methylprednisolone 15 mg/kg IV daily × 3 or prednisolone 2–4 mg/kg PO daily × 3 with or without a subsequent taper.

Target levels
- None available.

Adverse effects
- Diabetes, bone disorders, obesity, cushingoid changes, decreased wound healing, cataracts, peptic ulcer disease, hypertension, psychiatric disorders.

protocols). In the presence of recurrent rejection, chronic prednisone or prednisolone therapy is maintained at about 0.2 mg/kg/day.

TOXICITY

Of all the drugs used in maintenance immunosuppression, corticosteroids are responsible for the greatest number of important side effects. The chronic adverse effects of steroids are also discussed in Chapter 18.

Diabetes

Approximately 5–10% of transplant patients on chronic steroids require diabetic therapy, usually with oral hypoglycemic agents. Patients with pre-existing diabetes usually experience worsening of hyperglycemia with daily prednisone. Steroid-induced diabetes is frequently improved on an every-other-day prednisone regimen.

Obesity

Steroid therapy markedly increases appetite, often in a dose-related manner. For patients with a natural tendency to gain weight, daily prednisone therapy may induce marked obesity.

Cushingoid Features

In patients with higher dose chronic steroids ($\geq$15 mg/day), the development of the characteristic moon face, altered hair distribution, and truncal obesity with thin extremeties is common. The myopathy associated with Cushing's syndrome is particularly severe during the first few months after transplant.

Wound Healing

Chronic steroid administration decreases collagen content of the dermis, resulting in thin and easily damaged skin and retarded wound healing. Although unproven, these features are thought to improve with alternate-day steroids.

Bone Disorders

Chronic steroid therapy predisposes to the development of osteoporosis and avascular necrosis. Avascular necrosis of the femoral head occurs in 2–15% of transplant patients with osteoporosis and is related to chronic steroid administration. The hips are the most frequently involved joints, frequently with bilateral disease. Less commonly, shoulders, wrists, elbows, and knees are involved.

Cataracts

Approximately 5–10% of transplant patients on chronic steroids develop posterior lenticular cataracts. In less than 5% of cases, the cataracts are severe enough to require removal of the lens. At least one study suggests that the inciting events for cataracts occur during the peritransplant period of high-dose steroids.[475]

Peptic Ulcer Disease

Although it is controversial whether acute and chronic steroid therapy actually causes peptic ulcer disease, steroid therapy increases the likelihood of complications of peptic ulcers. Prophylactic H_2 antagonists are recommended during the period of high-dose steroid therapy.

Colonic Perforation

Chronic steroid therapy may increase the likelihood of perforation in the presence of diverticulosis or cytomegalovirus (CMV) colitis. Once a perforation occurs, chronic steroids may mask the symptoms of perforation, increasing the dangers of unrecognized peritonitis.

Pancreatitis

In the absence of identifiable etiologies such as gallstones, alcohol, preexisting pancreatic disease, or viral etiologies, steroids have been implicated in idiopathic pancreatitis after transplantation. An etiologic role of steroids, however, is unproven.

Psychiatric Disorders

High-dose steroids (1 mg/kg) during the first several weeks post transplant may induce euphoria, insomina, and/or confusion. Rarely, psychosis may occur if there is an underlying psychiatric disorder. Reduction of steroid dose usually relieves the symptoms.

Hypertension

Steroids contribute to posttransplant hypertension through retention of salt and water. In the absence of cyclosporine, prednisone-induced hypertension is rare.

CLINICAL USE

Corticosteroids are an integral part of initial and early maintenance immunosuppression after cardiac transplantation. Because of the considerable morbidity associated with chronic steroid administration, most heart transplant programs attempt weaning of prednisone or prednisolone to every-other-day low-dose ($\leq$0.1 mg/kg) or no steroids by 3–6 months following transplantation. However, many patients develop recurrent or even severe rejection off steroids and require chronic steroid administration. Intravenous methylprednisolone or oral prednisone (or prednisolone) are the standard initial therapy for acute allograft rejection.[380] Further details about steroid administration after cardiac transplantation and the use of steroids in the treatment of acute rejection are discussed in Chapters 12 and 14. The long-term complications of steroid use are discussed in Chapter 18.

CYCLOSPORINE

HISTORICAL NOTE

The critical experiments by Borel and colleagues between 1972 and 1976 led to the discovery of cyclosporine's immunosuppressive powers (see Box). These studies brought attention to the unique immunosuppressive effects and low toxicity of cyclosporine A[285] (CyA), paving the way for clinical trials in transplantation. The first clinical use of CyA in human transplantation was reported in 1979.[71]

CHEMICAL STRUCTURE

CsA is a metabolic product of two strains of fungi imperfecti: *Cylindrocarpon lucidum Booth* and *Tolypocladium inflatum Gams*. CsA is a neutral hydrophobic cyclic polypeptide composed of 11 amino acid residues (Fig. 13–2). The empirical formula is $C_{62}H_{111}N_{11}O_{12}$. The three-dimensional structure has been determined by nuclear magnetic resonance and x-ray crystallography (Fig. 13–3).

The relationship between the structure of the CsA molecule and its immunosuppressive properties is not completely understood, but it is known that the immunosuppressive effect is importantly related to the 9-carbon unsaturated amino acid in position 1 as well as amino acids 2, 3, and 11, and its overall conformational shape (Fig. 13–4).

MECHANISM OF IMMUNOSUPPRESSION

In normal T-cell activation, Signal 1 (the HLA antigen in the presence of a self-MHC class II molecule) engages and triggers the T-cell receptor to activate the calcineurin pathway within the cytoplasm. Calcineurin is a calcium calmodulin-dependent phosphatase which plays an integral part in the calcium-dependent signal which is generated after recognition of antigen by the T-cell receptor.[403] This signal transduction pathway activates the binding of a number of DNA-binding proteins (such as NFAT) to the enhancer region of the IL-2 gene, which results in IL-2 gene transcription.[477] Calcineurin also stimulates synthesis of other cytokines, particularly IL-3, IL-4, TNF-α, and IFN-γ.[581] Cyclosporine is a **prodrug,** in that its immunosuppressive properties depend on the formation of a complex with cellular proteins called **immunophilins,** which include two basic families: the cyclophilins (which bind to CsA) and the FK-binding proteins (which bind to tacrolimus and rapamycin). The CsA-cyclophilin complex binds to calcineurin,[248] thus inhibiting calcineurin phosphatase activity.[364] There are at least five cyclophilins of which all have peptidyl-prolyl *cis/trans* isomerase activity that appears to take part in protein traffic, stability, and folding.[161] Cyclosporine's basic mechanism is **blockade of**

The Discovery of Cyclosporine's Immunosuppressive Powers

The discovery and subsequent development of cyclosporine into an immunosuppressive agent was the product of both an organized scientific program and serendipity. In the 1950s Sandoz laboratories in Basel, Switzerland, made a critical decision to investigate active fungal metabolic compounds for effects other than antimicrobial activity. Sandoz investigators became interested in the P-815 mouse mastocytoma-tumor strain because it was known to produce histamine and serotonin.[487] To their good fortune, Sandoz used P-815 mouse mastocytoma cells in their drug screening program, and this proved critical to the subsequent discovery of cyclosporine. A fungal metabolite ovalicin was noted to strongly inhibit proliferation of mouse mastocytoma cells, but no other cell lines that were examined. Although ovalicin never proved useful clinically, interest in this compound stimulated Sandoz researchers to maintain tests assaying the immune system as part of their screening program, eventually resulting in the discovery of cyclosporine.

In 1971, Haerri and Ruegger isolated a metabolite mixture with the code 24-556 as a product of the soil fungus *Tolypocladium inflatum Gams*. The main component of 24-556 was later identified as cyclosporine A. The initial interest in metabolite 24-556 stemmed from its antifungal activity against *Aspergillus niger* and *Neurosporg crassa* with an unusually low level of toxicity. In January of 1972, Jean F. Borel discovered the marked immunosuppressive properties of 24-556. Of critical importance was the observation that the suppression of humoral and cellular immunity was accomplished without general cytostatic effects and without demonstrable circulatory or central nervous system toxicity.

Further experimentation with cyclosporine was facilitated by the purification of cyclosporine A by Ruegger in 1973[56] and elucidation of the structure of CyA by Petcher, Ruegger, and colleagues in 1975, using chemical degradation and x-ray analysis.[420] The complete synthesis of CyA was accomplished by Wenger in 1980.[565]

In the Proceedings of an International Conference on Cyclosporine A in 1981, Borel summarized the experimental data which he first presented to the British Society of Immunology in 1976: "(1) CyA shows selectivity for lymphocytes; mainly for T helper cells; sometimes for T-effector cells, depending on the test model used. It is clearly not myelotoxic in immunosuppressive doses. (2) It exerts an immunosuppressive action on humoral and cell-mediated immunity and in chronic but not in acute inflammatory reactions. (3) CyA inhibits the induction phase of lymphoid cell proliferation. It affects the early mitogenic triggering, but not mitosis. (4) It is not lymphocytotoxic, because the reversibility of the effect can be demonstrated. (5) CyA is effective in all species tested, i.e. in the mouse, rat, guinea pig, rabbit and monkey."

Soon other groups reported experimental transplantation models, such as work from Cambridge, England, in heterotopic heart allografts in rats.[285] These observations were quickly followed by other impressive experimental reports from multiple investigators.[70, 136, 570]

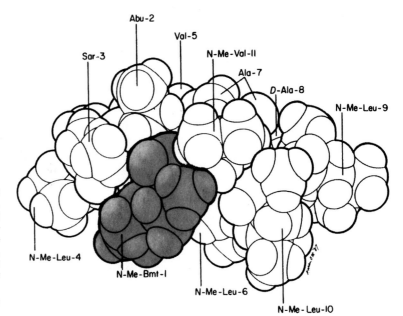

FIGURE **13–3.** A space-filling model of cyclosporine. Each amino acid residue and its sequence number are indicated. N-Me-Bm, is (4R)-4-[(E)-2-butenyl]-4, N-di-methyl-ʟ-threonine; Abu, α-aminobutyric acid; Sar, sarcosine; Me-Leu, N-methyl-ʟ-leucine; Val, ʟ-valine; Ala, ʟ-alanine; D-Ala, ᴅ-alanine; Me-Val, N-methyl-ʟ-valine. (From Tax WJ, van de Heijden HM, Willems HW, Hoitsma AJ, Berden JH, Capel PJ, Koene RA: Immunosuppression with monoclonal anti-T3 antibody [WT32] in renal transplantation. Transplant Proc 1987;19[1 pt 3]:1905–1907. Copyright 1987, Elsevier Science, with permission.)

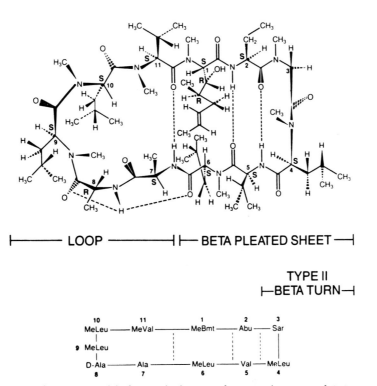

FIGURE **13–4.** Conformational structure model of CsA. The basic conformational structure of CsA consists of an open loop (amino acid position 7–11) and a beta pleated sheet (amino acid positions 1–6) with a type 2 beta turn (amino acid positions 3–4). The biological activity of CsA resides in a major portion of the CsA molecule including amino acids 1, 2, 3, and 11 as well as its conformational structure. (From Hess A: Cyclosporine in Clinical Use. World Medical Press, 1988.)

TABLE 13-5	Cyclosporine

Clinical use
- Chronic maintenance immunosuppression, usually combined with azathioprine or mycophenolate mofitel, with or without corticosteroids.

Mechanism
- Calcineurin blockade, inhibition of IL-2 production, inhibition of T-cell proliferation.

Dose
  Adults:
  - Initial posttransplant infusion of 0.5–1 mg/hr continuous infusion.
  - Initial oral dose of 25–50 mg bid and, if renal function remains normal, rapidly increase over 3–4 days to achieve whole blood trough level of 300–400 ng/mL.

  Pediatric:
  - Initial infusion of 0.25–0.5 mg/kg/day as continuous infusion while observing urine output and renal function. If renal function stable, begin PO dose at 1 mg/kg/day in three divided doses. If renal function remains normal, rapidly increase over 3–4 days to achieve target trough levels.

Target levels
- See Table 13–8 for target levels.

Toxicity
- Nephrotoxicity, neurotoxicity, hypertension, hypercholesterolemia, hepatotoxicity, hyperkalemia, renal tubular acidosis, hypermagnesemia, hyperuricemia, hypertrichosis, gingival hyperplasia.

Drug Interactions
- See Tables 13–9 to 13–13.

the calcineurin pathway (Table 13–5), thereby inhibiting production of IL-2 and other cytokines (Fig. 13–5).

CsA blocks the T-cell cycle (see Box) at the G_0–G_1 phase and limits the activation of cytotoxic T-lymphocytes, but it does not impair the ability of an activated cytotoxic T-cell to kill its target cells. CsA **inhibits the gene expression for interleukin-2** and other lymphokines such as IL-4, and IFN-γ, which are critical for the differentiation and proliferation of cytotoxic T-cells (Fig. 13–6). CsA also inhibits IL-2 receptor formation (further impairing the cytotoxic T-cell responsiveness to IL-2) and[294] impairs responsiveness to and production of

T-Cell Cycle

The cell cycle is the collection of events involved in cell division and is the fundamental basis of reproduction in all living things. The cell cycle of eukaryotic cells is divided into four successive phases called G_1, S, G_2, and M. Some cell types, such as lymphocytes, can exist in a specialized resting state within G_1, sometimes called G_o, in which there is a pause that can sometimes last for years. The G_1 phase encompasses the entire period between the last cell division cycle (the M, or mitosis phase) and the beginning of the S (synthesis) phase in which a doubling of DNA content occurs. The G_2 phase follows the S phase. Both G_1 and G_2 are periods that allow for cell growth before division, which is usually inhibited until a doubling in cell volume is achieved. The completion of the M (mitosis) phase, which follows G_2, results in cellular division. These events are called the cell cycle because they are repeated in sequence each time the cell divides.

IL-1, a cytokine which promotes production of IL-2. The specific actions of CsA are dose-dependent *in vivo* with inhibition of IL-2 production occurring at low CsA concentrations. However, CsA does not completely block IL-2 production, since a second signaling pathway mediated by CD28 through protein kinase C also stimulates IL-2 production, and this pathway is resistant to CsA.[217]

The immunologic activity of CsA appears restricted to its effects on **cytotoxic T-cells** and **T-helper cells,** with little or no effect on suppressor T-cells.[216] Through its inhibitory effect on T-cell activation, CsA inhibits primary B-cell (humoral) responses that are T-cell dependent, but not secondary T-cell independent B-cell responses. CsA appears to have little effect on granulocyte or macrophage migration or phagocytosis activity and does not induce bone marrow suppression.

The effect of cyclosporine on atherogenesis and allograft vasculopathy is controversial. *In vitro* studies of human umbilical vein endothelial cells indicate that cyclosporine may impair atherogenesis by inhibiting endothelial cell apoptosis induced by oxidatively modified low-density lipoprotein, an early event in atherogenesis.[28, 240, 494, 558] On the other hand, other studies indicate that cyclosporine may promote allograft vasculopathy by up-regulation of vascular growth factors.

PHARMACOKINETICS

Standard CsA is a highly lipophilic compound which, after oral ingestion, is absorbed through the upper gastrointestinal tract where it enters the portal circulatory system. This accounts for approximately 99% of a dose, and the other 1% passes directly into intestinal lymphatics.[196] Cycosporine is transported across the intestinal epithelium by P-glycoprotein, a countertransport protein in the brush border membrane of intestinal epithelial cells. After a single oral dose, peak serum concentrations (designated C_{max} to indicate the highest blood level achieved) are reached within 3–4 hours (average, 3.5 hours).[46] This time required to reach C_{max} is termed T_{max}. Ingestion of a fatty meal significantly delays absorption of the standard formulation (but not the microemulsion).

The **bioavailability** of oral CsA is the pharmacokinetic parameter which shows the greatest variability among transplant patients.[318] Bioavailability is the actual percent of administered drug that is absorbed and is calculated as the ratio of the area under the concentration-versus-time curve (AUC) after an oral and an intravenous dose ($AUC_{oral}/AUC_{iv} \times 100$). The area under the AUC is calculated from the point of initial dosing to the subsequent dose and represents the total blood exposure of the drug between doses (Fig. 13–7).[72] The bioavailability of an oral dose of the original soft gelatin capsule (Sandimmune) is approximately 30% of an intravenous dose, with considerable intra- and interindividual variability in absorption. The original oil-based formulation of CsA is pH neutral and has low aqueous solubility. The lipophilic makeup (low aqueous solubility), the high molecular weight (1,203 daltons), and the restriction of absorption to

Text continues on page 402

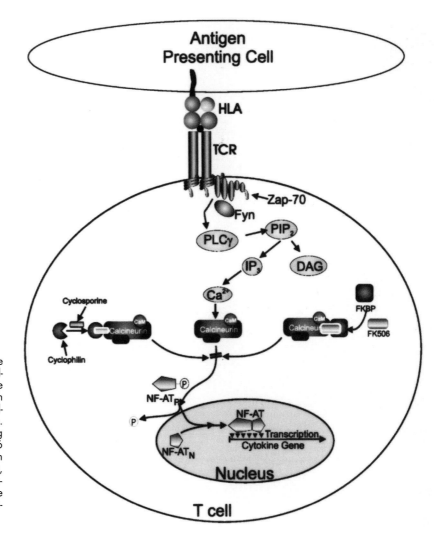

FIGURE **13–5.** Differing effects of cyclosporine and tacrolimus on calcineurin. The initial steps leading to calcineurin activation are as depicted in Figure 13–1. Cyclosporine and tacrolimus (FK506) both interfere with calcium-mediated signaling via calcineurin, but through different mechanisms. Cyclosporine binds a cyclophilin and the resulting complex causes the inhibition of calcineurin. FK506 binds to FK506-binding protein (FKBP), which then causes the inhibition of calcineurin. In either case, calcineurin cannot dephosphorylate NF-AT$_P$. Therefore, NF-AT$_P$ does not bind to NF-AT$_N$ and mediate transcription of cytokines through promotors that contain NF-AT binding sites.

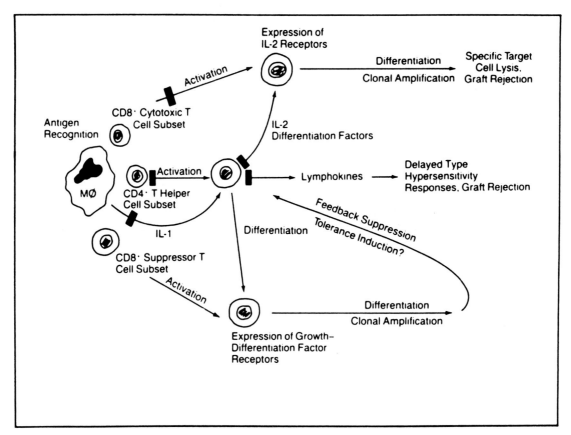

FIGURE **13-6.** Schematic representation of an allograft response and the primary effect of cyclosporine. (From Hess A: Cyclosporine in Clinical Use. World Medical Press, 1988.)

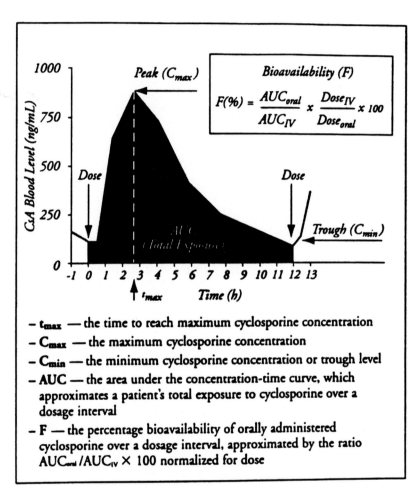

FIGURE **13–7.** Area under the curve monitoring of cyclosporine therapy. (Adapted from Canafax DM: Immunosuppressant Pharmacokinetics and Product Performance. Current Trends: Setting Performance Standards for Immunosuppressive Drugs. Booklet sponsored by University of Minnesota [office of Continuing Medical Education], 1996.)

TABLE 13-6	Physiologic Factors Affecting Bioavailability of Cyclosporine		
GI FACTORS INFLUENCING ABSORPTION	PHYSIOCHEMICAL FACTORS	PATIENT FACTORS	DRUG FACTORS
Gastric mixing and gastric emptying	pH (drug and intestinal)	Volume of distribution	Gut transport and metabolism
Absorptive surface	Polarity	Age	Hepatic metabolism
Splanchnic flow	Particle size	Cholesterol	Renal clearance
Bile flow	Dosing frequency	Albumin	
	Dosage	RBC mass	

GI, gastrointestinal.

the upper small intestine all contribute to the marked variability of absorption.[541] The oil-in-water mixture within the gastrointestinal (GI) tract must undergo emulsion of the oily droplets by bile salts, then digestion by pancreatic enzymes.[541] Effective gastrointestinal motility and sufficient pancreatic, biliary, and small bowel secretions are necessary for the absorption process. The amount of lipophilic cyclosporine absorbed in the GI tract is importantly reduced with a reduction in available bile acids and with reduced GI motility.[344, 387] The effect of simultaneously administered food on absorption of cyclosporine is variable, but a high-fat meal with cyclosporine increases its absorption.[203, 309] The physiologic factors which influence bioavailability of cyclosporine are summarized in Table 13-6.

Cyclosporine is distributed extensively outside the blood stream, with highest levels detected in liver, pancreas, and fat (Fig. 13-8).[247] Lowest levels are detected in spinal cord and brain. Within blood, 33–47% of CsA is in plasma, of which 90% of drug is bound to proteins, particularly lipoproteins[216] (Table 13-7). In the one half to two thirds of blood cyclosporine which is localized in blood cell elements, 40–60% is found in erythrocytes (lower temperatures increase erythrocyte-CsA binding), 5–12% in granulocytes, and 4–9% in lymphocytes.

Cyclosporine is **metabolized** by the enzyme CYP 3A4, a member of the cytochrome P-450 enzyme system (see Box) which is present in hepatocytes within the liver.[115, 389] This enzyme is also present in enterocytes that line the intestine, which with the involvement of P-glycoprotein, may play an important role in CsA metabolism and exert an effect on bioavailability.[281] Expression of cytochrome P-450 3A4 and intestinal P-glycoprotein may differ up to 10- to 20-fold between individual patients and within the same patient as influenced by other drugs which may induce or inhibit this enzyme system, accounting for a major part of the inter- and intrapatient variability in CsA blood levels with the same CsA dose.

The half-life of CsA is about 19 hours. Metabolism occurs by hydroxylation, demethylation, carboxylation, and/or saturation of the double bond. The major metabolites of CsA retain the cyclic oligopeptide structure of the parent compound (Fig. 13-9).[338] Metabolites 1, 17,

and 21 have immunosuppressive effects *in vitro*. The major metabolites in urine and bile are 1, 17, and 21.[450] Approximately 90% of drug is excreted in the feces and about 10% in urine.

MICROEMULSION FORMULATION

The microemulsion formation of CsA (CsA-ME) (Neoral) is an oral formulation that immediately forms a microemulsion in an aqueous milieu. It was developed to reduce the variability in absorption (bioavailability) of standard CsA. The active form of the drug is unaltered, but absorption is more rapid and less dependent on bile flow than standard CsA, which is mainly distributed in lipid droplets. The time to peak blood

Cytochrome P-450 Enzymes System

Cytochrome P-450 is the name of a superfamily of enzymes that are bound hemethiolate proteins which are critical for oxidative, peroxidative, and reductive metabolism of a large number of compounds. They catalyze reactions of the overall stoichiometry $NAD(P)H + H^+ O_2 + R \rightarrow NAD(P)^+ + H_2O + RO$, where R is an organic substrate.[202] There are 36 gene families that code for these proteins, and it is believed that they arose from a single ancestral gene approximately 3.6×10^9 years ago. It is estimated that there are at least 60 cytochrome P-450 genes in humans. The cytochrome P-450 enzymes are designated by the letters "CYP" followed by a number, a letter, and a number (e.g., CYP2D6).[115, 389] The members of the CYP3A family are the most abundant cytochromes in humans. They account for 30% of the cytochrome P-450 enzymes in the liver and are also expressed in the intestines.[115]

Many of these enzymes play a major role in drug metabolism. As discussed elsewhere in this chapter, the major pathway of cyclosporine, tacrolimus, and rapamycin metabolism is via CYP3A4. Therefore, drugs such as rifampicin and erythromycin, which affect the activity of CYPA4 enzymes, can drastically affect levels of these agents.

CYCLOSPORINE TISSUE LEVELS

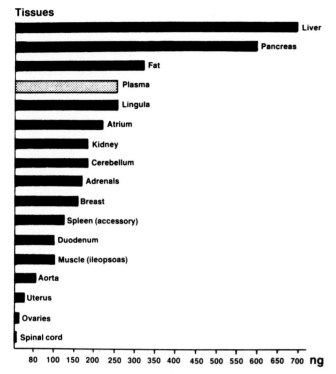

FIGURE 13-8. Cyclosporine tissue levels expressed as nanograms per gram of tissue wet weight. (From Kahan BD, Reid M, Newburger J: Pharmacokinetics of cyclosporine in human renal transplantation. Transplant Proc 1983;15:446–453.)

cyclosporine concentration (T_{max}) following oral administration of CsA-ME is approximately 1.5–2.0 hours (vs. about 2.5 hours for CsA). Compared to CsA, the AUC with CsA-ME is increased about 30%.[551] The CsA AUC and C_{max} are decreased if Neoral is administered with food. Compared to standard CsA, Neoral provides less inter- and intrapatient variability in blood levels,[221, 287, 551] as measured by AUC and C_{max}.[31, 157, 355]

Conversion from standard CsA to the microemulsion formulation is generally recommended with a 1:1 conversion followed by blood level monitoring every 4–7 days for several weeks with appropriate dose adjustment until preconversion target levels are reached. In patients who require greater than 10 mg/kg/day of standard CsA (indicating reduced absorption), important reduction of dosage with Neoral should be anticipated (with appropriate blood level monitoring).

DOSING

Standard cyclosporine (Sandimmune) is supplied orally as soft gelatin capsules in 25-mg, 50-mg, and 100-mg strengths. Each capsule contains the designated weight of cyclosporine plus alcohol, maximum volume of 12.7%. Oral solution is also available in 50-mL bottles, each milliliter containing 100 mg of cyclosporine. Cyclosporine for intravenous administration is dis-

pensed in 5-mL vials, each of which contains 50 mg cyclosporine per milliliter. Prior to administration, the cyclosporine is further diluted with 0.9% sodium chloride or 5% dextrose.

The microemulsion form of cyclosporine (Neoral) is available in oral soft gel capsules (25-mg and 100-mg strengths) and an oral solution (100 mg cyclosporine/mL).

Recently, the U.S. Food and Drug Administration (FDA) has approved two generic AB-rated equivalents to Neoral capsules, Abbott's Gengraf and EON's Cyclosporin Capsules, USP [Modified], and withdrew approval of SangStat's generic SangCya because of concern over impaired absorption when taken with apple juice. There will likely be great interest in using generic formulations of microemulsion cyclosporine because of the cost of this drug. The generics may be less expensive, but concern has been voiced about the true equivalence of these preparations to Novartis' Neoral. A report by the United States National Kidney Foundation[454] recommended that therapeutic substitution of generic cyclosporine formulations should not be done without the specific approval of the prescribing physician. As discussed in this chapter, cyclosporine administration, whatever the formulation, must be guided by appropriate surveillance drug level monitoring. When switching from one preparation to another, frequent drug level monitoring is mandatory. Though subtle, the different absorption characteristics of these preparations could, theoretically, produce clinically important changes in immunosuppressive efficacy that the physician should be aware of.[213, 249, 319, 374]

PLASMA/BLOOD LEVEL MONITORING

The importance of blood level monitoring stems from two basic factors: (1) the therapeutic window between inadequate immunosuppression and toxicity is very narrow and (2) there is large inter- and intrapatient variability in drug bioavailability. Currently, the immunosuppressive and toxic effects of cyclosporine are most accurately predicted by blood levels.[243, 244, 247, 511]

The two most widely used cyclosporine assays are based on monoclonal antibodies or high-pressure liquid

TABLE 13-7	**Characteristics and Distribution of Cyclosporine in Whole Blood**
CHARACTERISTICS	PROPORTION OF DISTRIBUTION
Liquid element	33–47%
Plasma	Most lipoprotein bound
Cellular elements	
Lymphocytes	4–9%
Granulocytes	5–12%
Erythrocytes	41–58%
Other features	
Binding to erythrocytes	Increased binding at lower temperatures

chromatography (see Box). High-pressure liquid chromatography (HPLC) has the advantage of being specific for not only parent compound, but also metabolites such as 17 and 18. However, HPLC is complex and labor intensive. It currently is rarely used in clinical transplantation.

Cyclosporine levels are generally measured in either whole blood or plasma. The temperature of blood samples collected and transported to the laboratory for cyclosporine level determination may have an important effect on levels. When a blood sample is collected and plasma is separated from red cells at room temperature, plasma concentration of CsA decreases by 20–50% due to the increased binding to erythrocytes at lower temperatures.[310] Furthermore, even if samples are separated at 37°C, there is variability in the whole blood/plasma ratio, partly related to variations in hematocrit

---

High-Performance Liquid Chromatography (HPLC)

Chromatography is used for the separation of macromolecules and other compounds for analysis or preparative purposes. Simple liquid chromatography is performed using a cylindrical column containing a packed matrix of porous beads in liquid. The material to be separated is placed at the top of the matrix and passed into the column by the application of liquid to the top of the column (assuming that one end of the column faces upward). As the material passes through the matrix, the movement of the molecules through the column bed is dependent on the flow of the liquid (liquid phase) and on Brownian motion of the solute molecules into the porous bead matrix (stationary phase). Larger molecules cannot enter the stationary phase because they are unable to enter the pores of the matrix. Smaller molecules, which can enter the pores of the stationary phase, move through the column more slowly, since they spend more time in the stationary phase. Therefore, the molecules emerge from the other end of the column in order of decreasing molecular size. By using different matrices in the column, one can adjust the size range of molecules that are separated by this method. There is a nearly infinite array of matrices that can be used to separate molecules based on size, as discussed above, or on other principles.

Column liquid chromatography was the first chromatographic method to be developed for the separation of compounds in liquid, and is often used as a method to prepare large quantities of a purified material. The use of chromatography as an analytical method was not as useful until there were improvements in instrumentation and matrices that were used for packing the columns. Earlier chromatography columns were packed with particles of 100–200 μm in diameter, and the liquid phase was controlled by gravity feed. HPLC is an improved form of liquid chromatography in which particles of much smaller diameters ($\sim$ 5 μm), higher solvent velocities (typically at pressures $>7 \times 10^6$ N/m^2 or 1,000 psi), and much narrower column bores (2–3 mm) are used. Thus, the capability of the columns to resolve different molecules is enhanced by several orders of magnitude.

---

and lipoprotein concentration. In contrast, cyclosporine in whole blood samples remains stable at temperatures up to 40°C for a week. This provides a major advantage over plasma levels, since no special handling is required for whole blood samples, either within the hospital or when mailing samples. Thus, most centers currently base therapeutic decisions on whole blood rather than plasma cyclosporine levels.

Assays have been developed to measure cyclosporine alone (parent compound) or cyclosporine and various metabolites. Controversy exists regarding the methodology which most closely reflects immunologic activity. There is a rational basis for including metabolites in the assay, since certain metabolites such as numbers 1, 17, and 21 possess some immunosuppressive properties.[450, 471, 472, 559, 564] However, since different assays measure different metabolites, caution is advised when comparing one assay to another, especially monoclonal specific (parent compound alone), and monoclonal-nonspecific (parent compound plus metabolites).[58] If a transplant program switches from one assay to another, it is advisable to make duplicate assays on all patient samples for some period so that the correlation between assays can be determined (Fig. 13–10). Currently, most clinical programs utilize commercial monoclonal assays for parent compound only.

The current standard for immunosuppressive monitoring is a trough level drawn just before the morning dose administration. In practice, any time within an hour of dosing is adequate for dosing decisions. Calculation of AUC provides the best estimate of total drug exposure, but it is too time consuming and expensive for routine clinical use.[197] The use of peak blood levels and peak/trough ratios is not reproducible because of the variability in the time to achieve peak levels, although they may provide useful information in selected patients suspected of having malabsorption or hepatic dysfunction.

There is general agreement that higher blood levels of cyclosporine are necessary during the first 3–6 months for prevention of acute allograft rejection, after which the target level can be safely reduced. The general guidelines for target levels are presented in Table 13–8. However, the correlation between specific CsA levels and either toxicity or freedom from rejection is weak,[568] and these target levels must be adjusted according to individual patient responses. Lower cyclosporine trough levels (<200 ng/mL) during the first year are probably advisable in the setting of chronic renal dysfunction (serum creatinine ≥ 2 mg/dL), recurrent infection, or malignancy as long as serial surveillance endomyocardial biopsies are performed to monitor allograft rejection.

TOXICITY

Nephrotoxicity

Nephrotoxicity is the most important complication limiting the chronic use of CsA immunosuppression. The

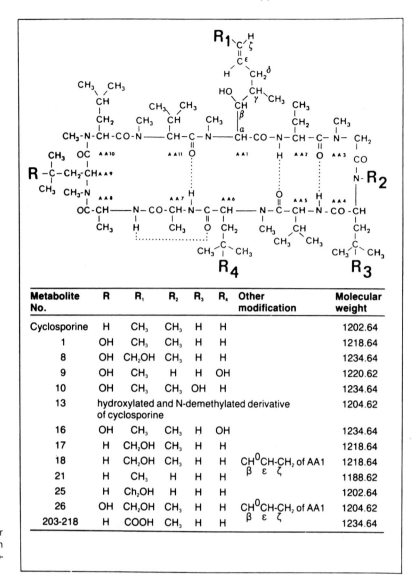

Metabolite No.	R	R_1	R_2	R_3	R_4	Other modification	Molecular weight
Cyclosporine	H	CH_3	CH_3	H	H		1202.64
1	OH	CH_3	CH_3	H	H		1218.64
8	OH	CH_2OH	CH_3	H	H		1234.64
9	OH	CH_3	H	H	OH		1220.62
10	OH	CH_3	CH_3	OH	H		1234.64
13	hydroxylated and N-demethylated derivative of cyclosporine						1204.62
16	OH	CH_3	CH_3	H	OH		1234.64
17	H	CH_2OH	CH_3	H	H		1218.64
18	H	CH_2OH	CH_3	H	H	$CH^O_\beta CH_\varepsilon\text{-}CH_{2\zeta}$ of AA1	1218.64
21	H	CH_3	H	H	H		1188.62
25	H	Ch_2OH	H	H	H		1202.64
26	OH	CH_2OH	CH_3	H	H	$CH^O_\beta CH_\varepsilon\text{-}CH_{2\zeta}$ of AA1	1204.62
203-218	H	COOH	CH_3	H	H		1234.64

FIGURE 13-9. Structure of cyclosporine and its major metabolites. (From Maurer G, Lemair M: Biotransformation and distribution in blood of cyclosporine and its metabolism. Transplant Proc 1986;18[suppl 5]:25–35.)

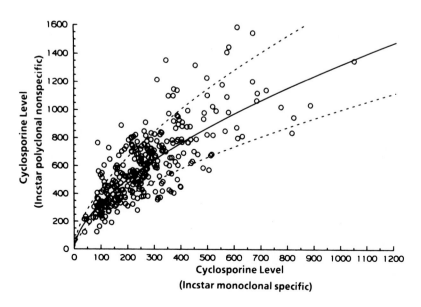

FIGURE 13-10. Comparison of cyclosporine levels using a monoclonal specific versus a monoclonal nonspecific assay (UAB; n = 247). The basic regression line (before multivariate analysis) and the 70% confidence limits (± 1 SD) are depicted. Cyclosporine units are nanograms per milliliter of whole blood. (From Bourge RC, Kirklin JK, Ketchum C, Naftel DC, Mason DA, Siegel AL, Scott JW, White-Williams C: Cyclosporine blood monitoring after heart transplantation: a prospective comparison of monoclonal and polyclonal radioimmunoassays. J Heart Lung Transplant 1992;11:522–529.)

TABLE 13-8	Recommended Cyclosporine Levels*
MONTHS POSTTRANSPLANT	TARGET LEVEL (ng/mL)†
0–3	350–450
3–6	250–350
6–12	200–300
>12	100–200

*Whole blood, parent compound trough levels.
†Higher levels (up to 400) may be advisable with recurrent rejection; lower levels may be desirable with renal dysfunction, recurrent infection, or malignancy.

acute phase of cyclosporine-induced nephrotoxicity typically occurs with the initial dose or doses of cyclosporine and is manifested by acute oliguria and rise in blood urea nitrogen and serum creatinine. These effects are largely initiated by **renal arteriolar vasoconstriction,** which occurs mainly at the level of the preglomerular arterioles (Fig. 13–11).[146, 396]

Intravenous and oral administration of CsA are known to induce an initial dose-dependent increase in renal vascular resistance which produces a reduction in renal blood flow.[377] This cyclosporine-induced vasoconstriction may result in part from an **imbalance between vasodilator and vasoconstrictor prostaglandins.**[97] Available evidence suggests a generalized defect in phospholipase activity,[97] though the precise alterations in the synthesis of each prostanoid with cyclosporine administration remains to be established (Fig. 13–12). Cyclosporine mediates inhibition of local prostacyclin (PGI₂) synthesis with its known vasodilator effect and inhibition of platelet aggregation.[543] CsA increases thromboxane A₂ production (a cyclooxygenase metabolite of arachidonic acid), which increases renal arteriolar resistance and mesangial cell contraction.[349, 417]

Endothelium-derived vasoconstrictor, **endothelin,** may also play an important role in cyclosporine-mediated vasoconstriction. In experimental studies, endothelin-1 is released into the renal vein following

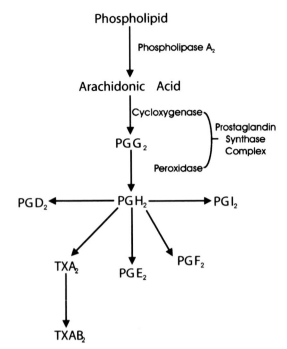

FIGURE **13-12.** Synthetic pathway for prostaglandin and thromboxane. PG, prostaglandin; Tx, thromboxane.

renal artery injection of cyclosporine,[77] and renal tubular cells and endothelial cells *in vitro* increase secretion of endothelin in response to cyclosporine stimulation.[64, 386] The role of endothelin is further supported by the experimental finding that anti-endothelin antibodies injected into the renal arteries protect against CsA-induced acute vasoconstriction.[102, 164, 282]

The **intrarenal renin angiotensin system** may contribute to both the nephrotoxic and hypertensive effects of CsA. CsA stimulates renin synthesis and release from isolated renal juxtaglomerular cells and the afferent arteriolar vessel wall.[298] It remains unclear, however,

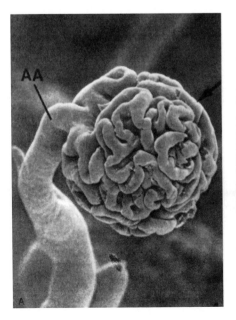

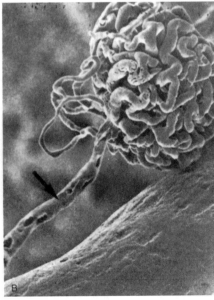

FIGURE **13-11.** Cast of rat vasculature with CSA. *A,* Control kidney. AA, afferent arteriole; arrow, efferent arteriole. *B,* Afferent arteriole (arrow) after CSA 50 mg/kg/day × 14 days. (From English J, Evan A, Houghton DC, Bennett WM: Cyclosporine-induced acute renal dysfunction in the rat. Evidence of arteriovasoconstriction with preservation of tubular fuction. Transplantation 1987;44:135–141.)

whether the increase in angiotensin II mediates or is induced by the renal arteriolar vasoconstriction. The partially protective effects of captopril and verapamil suggest a role of the renin-angiotensin system and cellular calcium channel entry (necessary for vessel wall contraction) on the decrease in renal plasma flow.[33, 76, 493]

Nitric oxide inhibition by CsA may also increase renal arteriolar vascular resistance. Experimentally, cyclosporine inhibits endothelium-dependent vasodilation.[442] Furthermore, endothelin-mediated vasoconstriction is inhanced by inhibition of nitric oxide.[312] CsA-induced generation of oxygen free radicals has been demonstrated *in vitro*,[557] and free radicals may react with nitric oxide, inhibiting the normal vasorelaxation response.

The hallmark of **subacute cyclosporine nephrotoxicity** is reduction in renal blood flow. This renal dysfunction typically manifests within the first few weeks after transplantation as a gradual increase in serum creatinine and reduction in glomerular filtration rate. The mechanisms are likely the same as in the acute phase. Thromboxane A_2 synthesis is increased, but it is unknown whether this is a causal or secondary phenomenon. In a rat cyclosporine model, administration of CsA produces infiltration of renal interstitium by macrophages that synthesize increased amounts of thromboxane B_2 with decreased production of PGE_2.[443] This phase of renal dysfunction is usually responsive to a reduction in CsA dosage.

Chronic cyclosporine nephrotoxicity after prolonged cyclosporine therapy is characterized by patchy glomerular sclerosis, with interstitial fibrosis (in striped or patchy distribution corresponding to the vascular lesions)[354, 470] and thickening of capillary basement membranes. The pathophysiology of these lesions is not yet clear, but a proposed mechanism is presented in (Fig. 13–13).[41] In a study of liver transplant recipients on cyclosporine 1.5–4.5 years after transplant, about 25% of glomeruli examined in a biopsy study showed extensive sclerosis,[132] which was the most common pathologic finding. Transforming growth factor-β1 (TGF-β1), which promotes fibrogenesis, may play a role in the changes in extracellular matrix observed in chronic CsA nephrotoxicity. CsA stimulates expression of TGF-β1 which directly stimulates collagen production in human renal fibroblasts and tubular cells.[181] In a rat model, vacuolization of the proximal tubule and loss of brush border membranes are noted after CsA therapy with focal interstitial fibrosis prominent after 3 months.

Two risk factors which are known to predispose to chronic cyclosporine-induced nephrotoxicity are the presence of underlying renal disease and the maintenance of chronically high cyclosporine blood levels. In addition, older age, high initial dosages, high maintenance doses, and large AUC may increase the likelihood of chronic renal dysfunction.[155] Once chronic renal damage has occurred, it is usually not responsive to decrease in CsA dosage or drug withdrawal.

Cyclosporine-Induced Hypertension

Most patients (>80%) that receive maintenance cyclosporine therapy will develop hypertension.[42, 85] Al-

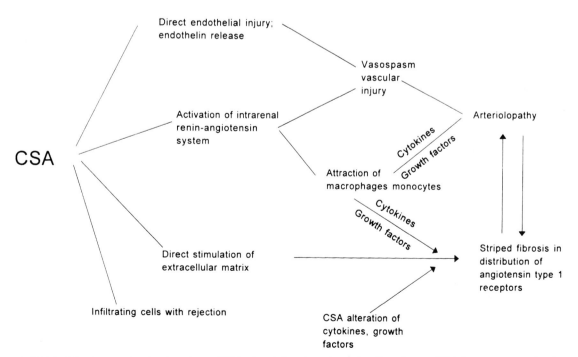

FIGURE **13–13.** Proposed pathophysiology of CSA-related chronic nephropathy. (From Bennett WM: Immunosuppressive drug nephrotoxicity. *In* Tilne NL, Strom TB, Paul LC [eds]: Transplantation Biology—Cellular and Molecular Aspects. Philadelphia: Lippincott-Raven, 1996.)

though not completely understood, the mechanism likely relates to a combination of intrarenal and systemic vasoconstriction[117] and increased sodium and water retention by the kidney. Cyclosporine promotes vasoconstriction by stimulating endothelin and thromboxane production[184, 229, 282, 321, 323] and by promoting influx of extravascular calcium.[64] The cyclosporine-induced sodium retention is most likely a consequence of preglomerular arteriolar vasoconstriction which results in decreased renal plasma flow and the renal perception of decreased effective arterial blood volume. This in turn activates the renin-angiotensin-aldosterone system, promoting increased tubular reabsorption of sodium.[372] Although unproven, cyclosporine may also have a direct antinatriuretic effect independent of vasoconstriction. The role of the sympathetic nervous system has been controversial, with some studies supporting[324, 325, 334, 377] the concept of increased sympathetic activity with cyclosporine. Urinary catecholamine levels usually remain normal.[523]

Hepatotoxicity

Hepatotoxicity is an uncommon and reversible effect of cyclosporine that is generally dose-related rather than idiosyncratic. Alterations in hepatic function are common at CsA doses exceeding 25 mg/kg/day. The usual enzyme changes are an increase in serum glutamate-pyruvate transaminase (SGPT), serum glutamic oxaloacetic transaminase (SGOT), and bilirubin.[339] The major histologic change is centrilobular fatty changes. The hepatic enzyme abnormalities are usually readily reversible with CsA dose reduction and rarely require drug discontinuation.[242, 274]

Biliary stones (usually gallstones) are observed with increased frequency in patients on chronic CsA. The high concentration of CsA metabolites in bile presumably promotes gallstone formation.

Hyperkalemia

Mild hyperkalemia is common in patients on chronic CsA, usually in the presence of normal or low aldosterone levels and low or normal plasma renin levels.[7, 385] Cyclosporine inhibits the Na^+/K^+-ATPase activity in the distal tubule which may decrease potassium excretion.[36] Although unproven, there appears to be a distal tubule resistance to aldosterone which impairs the ability to excrete potassium or a primary suppression of the adrenal aldosterone response to angiotensin II.[497]

Acidosis

Pediatric patients on CsA are prone to the development of metabolic acidosis which mimics renal tubular acidosis and is responsive to oral bicarbonate administration.

Hypomagnesemia

Low magnesium levels (≤ 1 mEq/L) are common if supplemental magnesium is not provided. Urinary magnesium excretion is increased, suggesting distal tubule wasting of magnesium.[35]

Hyperuricemia

Elevated serum uric acid levels are observed in some patients on chronic CsA. There may be a defect in renal tubular secretion of uric acid,[98] but alterations in clearance of uric acid may also result from CsA-induced depression of GFR.

Neurologic Sequelae

Hand tremors are common in CsA-treated patients but usually subside with gradual dose reduction, especially at doses below 5 mg/kg/day.[242] Paresthesias of distal extremeties are less common, and seizures are rare. Seizures may be either petit mal or grand mal, and may be potentiated by hypomagnesemia. Rarely, neurologic syndromes associated with white matter degeneration have been attributed to cyclosporine.

Hypertrichosis

Excessive hair growth is common and may be an important cosmetic problem in pediatric and female patients. Hair removal creams are usually effective therapy.

Gingival Hyperplasia

Gingival hyperplasia is common after several months of CsA therapy and may be pronounced in patients with poor dental hygiene. Concomitant use of diphenylhydantoin may aggravate this complication. Rarely, gingivectomy may be necessary.

Hyperlipidemia

Cyclosporine increases total cholesterol, low-density lipoprotein, and apolipoprotein B.[27]

Cardiac Toxicity

It remains controversial whether cyclosporine itself may induce chronic myocardial damage in some patients. Diffuse fine interstitial fibrosis has been reported in cardiac transplant patients on chronic cyclosporine,[49] unlike patients receiving azathioprine and steroids only.[254, 426, 498]

TABLE 13-9	Drugs that *Increase* Cyclosporine Blood Concentration
MECHANISM	DRUG
Decreased metabolism (competition for cytochrome P-450 system)	Erythromycin Ketoconazole* Itraconazole Diltiazem* Verapamil Nicardipine Cimetidine Methylprednisolone
Increased bioavailability (increased GI absorption)	Metoclopramide

GI, gastrointestinal.
*↑ Cyclosporine blood levels by 2–10 times.

TABLE 13-10	Drugs that *Decrease* Cyclosporine Blood Levels by Induction of Cytochrome P-450 System

Rifampin
Isoniazid
Phenobarbital
Phenytoin
Carbamazepine

In an isolated rodent heart model, cyclosporine-induced increases in myocyte cytoplasmic free calcium concentration, vacuolization and focal necrosis of myocytes, and focal areas of fibrosis have been demonstrated.[409, 430, 523] The effect, if any, of these findings on long-term cardiac allograft function remains to be elucidated.

DRUG INTERACTIONS WITH CSA

Other drugs taken concurrently with CsA may increase or decrease CsA blood levels or increase CsA toxicity. Tables 13–9 through 13–12[260, 430] summarize the important drug interactions affecting cyclosporine, and Table 13–13 summarizes important effects that cyclosporine may have on other drugs used in transplant recipients.[233] Some special features of these drug interactions are discussed below.

Anticonvulsants

Medications administered for seizure control in transplant recipients may importantly complicate cyclosporine management. Phenobarbital and phenytoin profoundly increase cyclosporine metabolism (and lower cyclosporine blood levels by induction of the hepatic cytochrome P-450 enzyme system) (Table 13–10). To a lesser degree, carbamazepine also lowers cyclosporine

TABLE 13-11	Drugs which Increase Nephrotoxicity of Cyclosporine*	
MECHANISM		**DRUGS**
• Renal vasoconstriction and/or renal tubular injury		Amphotericin Aminoglycosides
• Inhibition of cyclooxygenase, resulting in decreased renal prostaglandin synthesis and decrease in renal vasodilation with potentation of CsA decrease in renal blood flow		Nonsteroidal anti-inflammatory agents
• Inhibition of creatinine secretion by the renal tubules (potentiates similar action of CsA)		Trimethoprim sulfamethoxazole
• Other mechanisms		Radiocontrast agents Melphalan Sirolimus

*Drugs that act by increasing CsA blood levels are not included in this table.

TABLE 13-12	Other Drugs Which Alter Cyclosporine Effects
DRUG	**EFFECT**
Bromocriptine	May ↑ immunosuppressive effect of CsA by inhibition of prolactin
Dopamine	May decrease CsA nephrotoxicity
Minoxidil	↑ hirsutism
Nifedipine	↑ gingival hyperplasia
Ranitidine	Additive hepatotoxicity

levels. Valproic acid has little effect on cyclosporine metabolism and is often used as the drug of first choice in the posttransplant setting.

Gastrointestinal Agents

H_2 blocker drugs, particularly cimetidine, famotidine, and omeprazole, have opposing effects on cyclosporine levels. When cyclosporine is administered orally, these agents decrease its absorption because gastric acid (which is reduced by H_2 blocker agents) is an important factor necessary for absorption of hydrophobic substances in the small bowel. The result of this interaction would be a reduction in the cyclosporine level for a given dose.[438] However, the ultimate effect of these agents is to *increase* cyclosporine levels, likely through inhibition of the hepatic cytochrome P-450 enzyme system.[25, 202, 438] Metoclopramide, a drug which enhances gastric emptying, increases cyclosporine bioavailability and therefore blood levels by increasing absorption in the small intestine.[545]

Calcium Channel Blockers

Certain calcium channel blocking agents, particularly **diltiazem** and verapamil, are known to interact with cyclosporine in a manner that increases circulating cyclosporine levels for a given cyclosporine dose (Table 13–9). This action results from interference with the metabolism of cyclosporine A in the cytochrome P-450 hepatic enzyme system. The interaction between diltiazem and cyclosporine not only increases the trough of cyclosporine level but also the total amount of drug exposure as determined by the AUC for cyclosporine.[548] However, the magnitude of diltiazem effect on reduction of cyclosporine dose is not as great as ketoconazole (see next section). Currently, a diltiazem dose of 90 mg SR bid or 180 mg CD once a day is a standard dose with

TABLE 13-13	Effect of CsA on Other Drug Toxicity
DRUG	**EFFECT**
Digoxin	↑ serum digoxin levels
Lovastatin	↑ lovastatin levels, possible rhabdomyolysis, myalgia, muscle weakness
Pancuronium	Potentiation of neuromuscular blockade
Prednisolone	↑ prednisolone levels due to ↓ hepatic metabolizing activity
Vaccines	↓ efficacy of vaccine prophylaxis

cyclosporine. It is noteworthy that other calcium channel blockers, such as the dihydropyridine derivatives nifedipine and isradipine, do not significantly alter cyclosporine levels.[61, 148, 547] In a randomized trial of cyclosporine with or without diltiazem, Valentine and colleagues noted a 40% reduction in immunosuppression costs during the first 2 years with diltiazem plus cyclosporine.[532] However, the combination of cyclosporine and diltiazem is associated with higher serum creatinine levels,[532] so close surveillance of renal function is important during combined therapy. Because of this property of diltiazem and verapamil, many transplant centers routinely employ diltiazem or verapamil following transplantation in order to maintain therapeutic levels of cyclosporine at lower doses. This has the advantage of decreasing costs of immunosuppressive medications.[58, 532] However, there is not uniform agreement with this policy, since patients are at risk for acute allograft rejection initiated by a fall in cyclosporine levels should the calcium channel blocker require discontinuation or be stopped inadvertently by the patient.

Calcium channel blocking agents are generally considered a first line of therapy for cyclosporine-induced hypertension. They have been shown to facilitate sodium and water excretion, likely by a direct effect on renal tubules.[328, 394, 444] In addition, renal plasma flow and glomerular filtration rate may be enhanced through afferent arteriolar dilatation.[444] *In vitro* studies indicate that calcium channel blocking agents antagonize the vasoconstriction effects of neurohormonal factors such as angiotensin II, norepinephrine, thromboxane, and endothelin.[184, 229, 321, 323]

Controversy exists about the role of calcium channel blockers in attenuating cyclosporine-induced nephrotoxicity.[144, 322] Clinical and experimental studies have demonstrated a reduction in cyclosporine-mediated intrarenal vasoconstriction with diltiazem and other calcium channel blockers.[33, 55, 76, 229, 321-323] Wagner and colleagues reported a decreased incidence of delayed graft function after renal transplantation with pre- and post-transplant diltiazem therapy.[546] The exact mechanism is unknown, but it does not appear to act by prevention of endothelin release.[76] Other studies have demonstrated improved glomerular filtration rate with verapamil[65] and nifedipine[262] during cyclosporine therapy. Pretreatment with verapamil in a mouse model improved subcapsular renal microcirculation during cyclosporine infusion.[449] In clinical studies, verapamil has been shown to improve parenchymal diastolic blood flow following cyclosporine administration.[120] However, long-term studies of renal function after heart transplantation failed to demonstrate a beneficial effect of diltiazem on renal function during cyclosporine therapy 12 or more months after transplant.[390]

Calcium channel blocking agents may have a role in attenuating allograft vasculopathy. Schroeder and colleagues[461] have demonstrated that diltiazem attenuates progressive coronary artery narrowing following heart transplantation.[461] Further studies are necessary to clarify this possible beneficial effect (see also Chapter 17).

Antifungal Agents

Imidazole antimycotic agents such as **ketoconazole** markedly increase cyclosporine levels by inhibition of cytochrome P-450 enzymes responsible for cyclosporine metabolism.[569] The known interaction between ketoconazole and cyclosporine has been used to reduce the dose of cyclosporine needed to maintain therapeutic levels. Ketoconazole is a synthetic imidazole agent with antifungal action but also with broad-spectrum antimicrobial activity against *Staphylococcus epidermidis*, nocardia, candida, herpes simplex, and microsporum. Ketoconazole also reduces the metabolism of corticosteroids, effectively increasing levels of steroids administered as immunosuppression. However, the overall effect on steroid immunosuppression is uncertain, since ketoconazole may also act as a glucocorticoid antagonist by binding with glucocorticoid receptors.[259] Side effects of ketoconazole include nausea, vomiting, diarrhea, gynecomastia, pruritus, and hepatic toxicity.

In a randomized clinical trial, heart transplant recipients who received ketoconazole 200 mg/day had a significant reduction in cyclosporine dosage necessary to achieve therapeutic levels (60% reduction at 1 week and 80% reduction at 1 year).[259] This resulted in a cost saving of over $5,000 (U.S.) per patient in the first year after transplantation with reduction in rates of rejection and infection.

Compared to diltiazem, ketoconazole produces a more rapid increase in cyclosporine levels (1–2 days vs. 4–7 days), and the magnitude of reduction in cyclosporine dose is more sustained with ketoconazole.[413] Ketoconazole has the additional advantage of reducing the level of low-density lipoprotein cholesterol. It is currently recommended that cyclosporine cost savings should be achieved with either diltiazem or ketoconazole.

Miconazole has a similar effect but of lesser magnitude than ketoconazole.[222] **Intraconazole** has also been reported to modestly increase cyclosporine levels.[288] Conflicting information has been reported about the interaction between **fluconazole** and cyclosporine,[99, 103, 140, 191, 295, 502] but there appears to be little effect except at high doses of fluconazole.

Cilastatin

Cilastatin, an inhibitor of the brush border enzyme dehydropeptidase I, rapidly hydrolyzes the beta-lactam ring and is a component of the beta-lactam antibiotic imipenem. It also inhibits uptake of organic substances by renal tubular cells and may reduce cyclosporine uptake. A nephroprotective effect of cilastatin early after cardiac transplantation with cyclosporine has been reported,[335] but the initial doses of cyclosporine in that study were much higher than would be currently recommended.

Miscellaneous Drug Interactions

Troglitazone, an oral hypoglycemic agent, decreases cyclosporine levels,[252] although the mechanism and magnitude of the effect have not been established. Nafcillin has also been reported to decrease cyclosporine blood levels.[537]

CLINICAL USE

Since the early 1980s, cyclosporine has been the critical component of most immunosuppressive protocols, usually in combination with prednisone and either azathioprine or, more recently, mycophenolate mofetil. The recommended target levels are listed in Table 13–8. Currently, tacrolimus (see next section) may be used instead of cyclosporine in the immunosuppressive protocol. In the presence of chronic, progressive renal dysfunction, cyclosporine is generally discontinued in favor of prednisone and mycophenolate mofetil (or azathioprine) or continued at very low doses (whole blood CsA levels ≤70 ng/mL). Details of cyclosporine use are discussed further in Chapter 14.

CYCLOSPORINE ANALOGS

Norvaline–cyclosporine G was examined as a possible immunosuppressive agent because of potentially less nephrotoxicity than cyclosporine A (standard cyclosporine).[66, 228, 514] Isolated from the same fungus that produces cyclosporine A (*Tolypocladium inflatum Gams*), it differs from cyclosporine A only by the presence of a methylene group at amino acid number 2. The mechanism of immunosuppressive action appears to be similar to cyclosporine A, with blockade of calcineurin inhibiting cytokine gene activation.[81, 342] Animal studies suggested similar levels of immunosuppression with cyclosporine A and G.[72, 152, 524] The pharmacokinetic profile shows rapid absorption following an oral dose, though bioavailability decreases with higher dosages, like cyclosporine A. Peak serum concentration occurs 2–3 hours after an oral dose.[332] Distribution in blood has a plasma/blood ratio of 0.8, with most of the drug in plasma bound to high-density lipoproteins. Excretion is predominantly fecal, with only 3% of an oral dose excreted in the urine (compared to 6% for cyclosporine A).[332] Clinical trials with Norvaline–cyclosporine G suggested similar efficacy as cyclosporine A against rejection in renal transplantation, except in lower dosing ranges, where Norvaline–cyclosporine G was inferior. Transient elevation of liver enzymes has been observed in 30–40% of patients receiving Norvaline–cyclosporine G. Renal toxicity appears to be less with Norvaline-cyclosporine G during the first 3–4 months, but longer term reduction in nephrotoxicity compared to cyclosporine A has been inconsistent.[580] Cyclosporine G is currently not clinically available.

TACROLIMUS

HISTORICAL NOTE

Tacrolimus (initially called FK506) was first isolated in 1984 from the bacteria *Streptomyces tsukubaensis*.[264] It was first used clinically in 1989 as replacement therapy for cyclosporine in liver transplantation patients with intractable rejection.[174]

CHEMICAL STRUCTURE

Tacrolimus is a macrolide compound with the empirical formula $C_{44} H_{69} NO_{12} \cdot H_2O$. The chemical structure (Fig. 13–14) is unrelated to cyclosporine, and the binding sites are different; however, their immunosuppressive effects are similar. Tacrolimus is essentially insoluble in water and freely soluble in ethanol.

MECHANISM OF IMMUNOSUPPRESSION

Like cyclosporine, tacrolimus is a **prodrug,** in that the complex of the drug and its immunophilin (rather than either the drug or the immunophilin alone) binds with calcineurin[121, 459] (Fig. 13–5). Through its blockade of calcineurin, tacrolimus inhibits the calcium-dependent transcription of other early activation genes. However, the specific immunophilin for tacrolimus is different from cyclophilin, the immunophilin for cyclosporine. The specific immunophilin which binds with tacrolimus is a binding protein within the cytoplasm called FK binding protein (FKBP)-12, which is one of a family of four FKBP's. Like cyclophilin, FKBP-12 is a peptidyl-prolyl isomerase, which catalyzes the *cis-trans* isomerization of peptidyl-prolyl bonds in peptides and proteins, an action which is inhibited by tacrolimus. Tacrolimus gains its **immunosuppressive** effect by binding to FKBP-12 and producing the FKBP-12–tacrolimus complex, whose target is calcineurin.

On a milligram-per-miligram basis, tacrolimus is about 100 times more potent[234] and also more toxic than cyclosporine. The increased potency of tacrolimus may relate to its binding affinity to FKBP, which is much

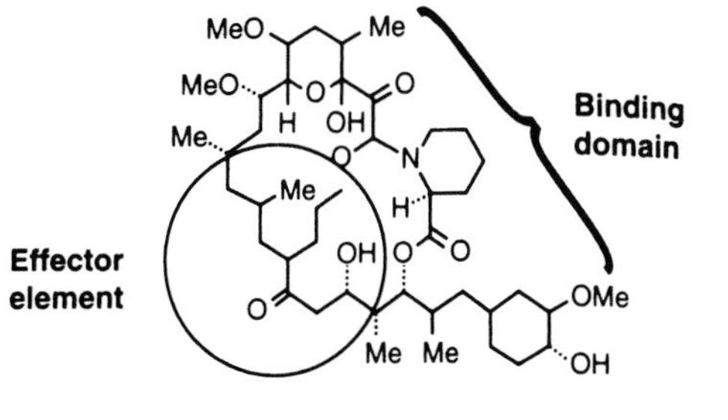

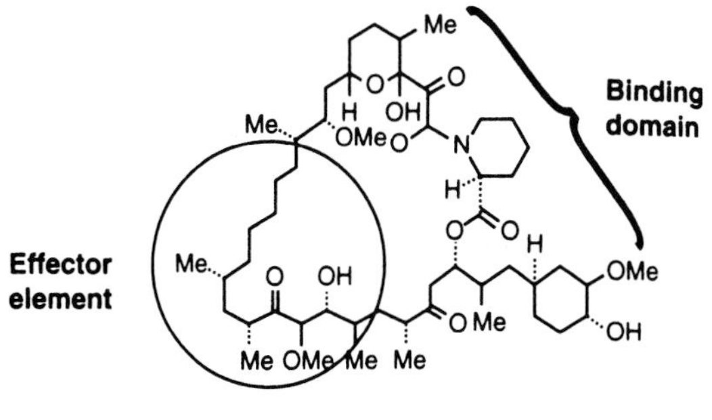

FIGURE **13–14.** Molecular structure of tacrolimus (FK506) and sirolimus (rapamycin). (From Morris PJ: New immunosuppressive agents. *In* Kidney Transplantation 4th ed. Philadelphia: WB Saunders Company, 1994, pp 233–243.)

greater than the binding affinity of cyclosporine to cyclophilin, and its ability to turn off the synthesis of cytokines by graft infiltrating T-cells.[366] This ability to reverse ongoing rejection in patients receiving cyclosporine clearly differentiates tacrolimus from cyclosporine.

The prevention of T-cell activation by tacrolimus is not complete, since it only blocks calcium-dependent pathways. Full activation mediated by CD28 or protein kinase C is unaffected.[48, 84, 256] Tacrolimus inhibits the production of a number of cytokines by activated T-cells, including IL-2, IL-3, IL-4, and IL-5, and TNF.[264] Tacrolimus does not inhibit cytotoxicity mediated by natural killer cells or antibody-dependent cell-mediated cytotoxicity.[560] Tacrolimus also appears to inhibit primary lymphokine-driven B-cell proliferation, but not T-cell independent secondary B-cell responses.[362] Cyclosporine and tacrolimus appear to have similar effects on the allograft lymphocytic infiltrate.[526]

PHARMACOKINETICS

Tacrolimus is highly lipophilic, and the bioavailability is quite variable after oral administration. Tacrolimus is absorbed through the small intestinal mucosa, with about 25% of the dose absorbed, independent of bile formation.[231] Maximal blood levels are generally achieved within 2–3 hours of ingestion. Like cyclosporine, tacrolimus is heavily absorbed by erythrocytes, and whole blood levels are 10–30 times higher than plasma levels. Metabolism is predominately in the liver via the cytochrome P-450 enzyme system and the metabolites are excreted via bile and stool, with less than 1% of parent compound excreted in the urine. The terminal half-life for elimination ranges from 11–21 hours.[201] Table 13–14 compares the pharmacokinetic profiles of cyclosporine and tacrolimus.

The precise metabolic pathway *in vivo* has not been determined, but demethylation and hydroxylation reactions have been identified *in vitro*. Ten metabolites have been identified in human plasma, the major metabolite identified as 13-demethyl tacrolimus. Low levels of T-cell suppression (<10% of parent compound potency) have been found in two metabolites.

DOSING

Tacrolimus is supplied as 1- and 5-mg capsules for oral administration. The intravenous preparation is supplied in 1-mL ampules, each containing 5 mg of tacrolimus.

Initial recommended oral dose of tacrolimus is 1–2 mg bid in an adult early after transplantation with normal renal function (Table 13–14). The dose is progressively increased thereafter to achieve target levels of 10–20 ng/mL. With initial intravenous administration, a starting dose of 0.01–0.02 mg/kg/day as a continuous infusion is recommended. Sublingual tacrolimus has been suggested (same dose as oral administration) as a useful method in the early postoperative period or in the presence of ileus (the capsules are opened and the powder is placed sublingually).[178] In pediatric patients, the initial oral dose is 0.05–0.15 mg/kg/day in two oral doses followed by gradual increases to achieve targeted blood levels as indicated above.

When converting patients from cyclosporine to tacrolimus in the presence of normal renal function, cyclosporine can be discontinued in the evening and tacrolimus initiated the following day at 5 mg bid (0.1 mg/kg bid in pediatric patients) and gradually increased to achieve target levels while monitoring renal function. When renal function is impaired (creatinine > about 1.5 mg/dL), the initial tacrolimus dose should be reduced to about 1–2 mg orally (PO) bid with close

TABLE 13–14	**Comparison of Pharmacokinetics of Cyclosporine and Tacrolimus**	
PARAMETER	CYCLOSPORINE (ORIGINAL FORMULATION)	TACROLIMUS
Chemical structure	Cyclic polypeptide	Macrolide
Solubility (aqueous)	Very low, < 7 mg/L	Very low, <1 mg/L
Absorption		
Rate	Variable	Variable
Bioavailability	Low (30%)	Low (25%)
T_{max} (mean)	3.5 h	2 h
Distribution		
Blood:plasma ratio	2:1	15:1
Major binding plasma proteins	Lipoproteins	α_2-acid glycoprotein
Metabolism		
Enzyme pathways	Highly metabolized by cytochrome P-450 hydroxylation, demethylation, conjugation	Highly metabolized by cytochrome P-450 hydroxylation, demethylation, minimal conjugation
Elimination		
Parent drug	Very low in urine	Very low in urine
Metablites	Excreted primarily in bile	Excreted primarily in bile
Terminal disposition half-life (h)	19	12–14 (range)
Therapeutic range		
Blood	100–400 ng/mL	5–20 ng/mL
Plasma	50–200 ng/mL	—

surveillance of renal function. If serum creatinine increases, dose reduction of tacrolimus usually results in prompt fall in creatinine.

BLOOD LEVELS

Currently recommended target trough whole blood levels are 10–20 ng/mL measured by enzyme-linked immunosorbent assay (ELISA). Although incomplete data are available, levels at the higher range are probably advisable during the first 6 months and somewhat lower levels thereafter, as with cyclosporine (Table 13–15). Pharmacokinetic studies in children suggest that, like cyclosporine, higher doses (per kilogram body weight) are needed than in adults to achieve similar trough blood levels.

TOXICITY

The major side effects of tacrolimus are nephrotoxicity, glucose intolerance, hyperkalemia, and neurotoxicity. Unlike cyclosporine, tacrolimus does not cause gingival hyperplasia or hirsutism, and hypertension is less common.

Nephrotoxicity

The dose-related effects on renal function are similar to those seen with cyclosporine, although several clinical

---

TABLE 13–15 Tacrolimus

Clinical use
- Chronic maintenance immunosuppression (alternative to cyclosporine), either as primary choice or conversion from cyclosporine due to recurrent or hemodynamically compromising rejection.

Mechanism
- Calcineurin blockade, inhibition of IL-2 production, inhibition of T-cell proliferation.

Dose
  Adults:
  - Initial intravenous dose of 0.01–0.05 mg/kg/day as a continuous infusion to gradually achieve whole blood trough levels of 10–20 ng/mL. The initial oral dose early posttransplant is 1–2 mg q 12 h. Close monitoring of renal function is necessary while doses are progressively increased to achieve target blood levels.
  - When converting from cyclosporine to tacrolimus with normal renal function, discontinue cyclosporine and begin tacrolimus at approximately 5 mg PO bid (adults) and adjust dosage according to trough levels.
  - In the presence of renal dysfunction (creatinine ≥ 1.7), begin with very-low-dose tacrolimus both early after transplant and when converting from cyclosporine (1–2 mg bid in adults).
  Pediatric:
  - 0.05–0.15 mg/kg/day PO in 2 divided doses. Once stable, renal function is verified after initial 1–2 days of therapy, dosage can be rapidly increased to attain target level (with continued surveillance of renal function).

Target levels

Days posttransplant	Whole blood trough levels (ng/mL)
0–31	17–23
31–90	15–20
>90	10–15

Common adverse effects
- Nephrotoxicity, neurotoxicity, glucose intolerance, hyperkalemia.

---

studies have reported greater nephrotoxicity with tacrolimus.[151, 531] The mechanism of nephrotoxicity is incompletely understood, but tacrolimus appears to induce less increase in renovascular resistance,[40, 486] does not stimulate thromboxane release from glomerular mesangial cells in culture,[432] and does not induce secretion of endothelin-1 from endothelial cells at clinical dosing levels.[432] Animal studies suggest that the intrarenal renin-angiotensin system plays a role in tacrolimus nephrotoxicity, since renal damage is reduced with angiotensin-blocking drugs.[43] The chronic lesions of interstitial fibrosis seen with tacrolimus are similar to the chronic changes observed with cyclosporine nephrotoxicity.

Neurologic Effects

A variety of effects have been observed, including tremor, headache, insomnia, nightmares, and rarely, aphasia,[441] confusion, psychosis, seizures, encephalopathy, and coma. In general, these side effects are dose related and more frequent than with cyclosporine, with an overall reported incidence of 8–20%.[9, 130, 141, 441]

Glucose Intolerance

This complication also appears to be dose-related, and approximately 10–30% of patients require temporary insulin therapy. Dose reduction leads to resolution of insulin requirement in up to half of those affected.[9] At 1 year, less than 10% of patients on tacrolimus require diabetic therapy. Diabetes requiring insulin is uncommon in children receiving maintenance tacrolimus.[78]

Hyperkalemia

Hyperkalemia is common and usually responds to dose reduction. Potassium-sparing diuretics should not be used with tacrolimus.

Posttransplant Lymphoproliferative Disorder

The risk of posttransplant lymphoproliferative disorder (PTLD) during tacrolimus therapy is probably similar to that with cyclosporine, with reported overall incidence of less than 2%.[441] However, a somewhat higher risk compared to cyclosporine in pediatric patients has been suggested,[113] which may in part relate to additional immunotherapy, such as induction with OKT3 or ATG.

Other Side Effects

Hyperuricemia and hypomagnesemia occur occasionally and are dose-related. Anemia and chronic diarrhea have been reported in pediatric patients.[21] Hypercholesterolemia and hypertension[421] are less common than with cyclosporine. A rare observation of hypertrophic cardiomyopathy associated with tacrolimus was reported in five pediatric patients following small bowel and/or liver transplantation, with regression after discontinuation of tacrolimus.[22] Rare allergic reactions, including anaphylaxis, have been reported primarily with intravenous injection.

Drug Interactions

Since tacrolimus, like cyclosporine, undergoes metabolic degradation primarily through the hepatic cytochrome P-450 enzyme system, drugs that affect cyclosporine levels will also likely affect tacrolimus levels (see Tables 13–9 through 13–12). Coadministration of tacrolimus with other nephrotoxic drugs, such as cyclosporine, amphotericin, and aminoglycosides may cause additive nephrotoxicity.

CLINICAL USE

Tacrolimus is employed as an alternative to cyclosporine in current immunosuppressive regimens. In contrast to cyclosporine, the increased potency of tacrolimus allows it to be used frequently as a sole immunosuppressive agent. Because of the additive renal toxicity with cyclosporine, tacrolimus and cyclosporine should not be used concurrently. Among patients receiving initial cyclosporine-based immunosuppression, tacrolimus has proven to be a highly effective "rescue" therapy for patients with persistent rejection after renal, lung, and cardiac transplantation.[238] In general, patients receiving triple-drug immunosuppression with cyclosporine, prednisone, and azathioprine usually first undergo conversion from azathioprine to mycophenolate in the setting of recurrent allograft rejection. If frequent rejection persists, cyclosporine is then converted to tacrolimus. Among centers that preferentially employ tacrolimus instead of cyclosporine, tacrolimus is generally employed in a two-drug protocol with prednisone or as monotherapy. Among pediatric heart transplant recipients, the University of Pittsburgh has reported excellent long-term results with initial maintenance using prednisone and tacrolimus, weaning off prednisone by about 6 months. Over half the patients received tacrolimus as sole maintenance immunosuppression after the first year.[21]

AZATHIOPRINE

HISTORICAL NOTE

The synthesis of 6-mercaptopurine (6-MP) and other purine analogues in 1952 resulted from experimental work by Hitchings and colleagues.[142] In the late 1950s, Schwartz and Damashek showed that 6-MP had important immunosuppressive properties. Azathioprine was first synthesized by Elion and colleagues in 1961, and later that year was first used clinically in renal transplantation.[378]

CHEMICAL STRUCTURE

Azathioprine belongs to the class of drugs called thiopurines. It is the nitroimidazole derivative of 6-MP (Fig. 13–2) which is a sulfite derivative of hypoxanthine.

MECHANISM OF IMMUNOSUPPRESSION

Azathioprine is a purine analog which impairs DNA synthesis and acts as an antiproliferative agent (Table 13–16). Azathioprine is a prodrug that is metabolized in the liver to 6-MP, which is converted to the active metabolite, thio-inosine-monophosphate (TIMP). TIMP interferes with the synthesis of adenylic and guanylic acid from inosinic acid by inhibiting the enzymes adenylsuccinate synthetase, adenylsuccinate lyase, and inosine monophosphate dehydrogenase. TIMP is converted to thioguanylic acid, a precursor for thiodeoxyguanosine which is incorporated into DNA and impairs its synthesis. The initial steps of the *de novo* purine synthesis pathway are impaired by the thiopurine ribonucleotides through a feedback inhibition of the enzyme glutamine phosphoribosyl pyrophosphate amidotransferase. By inhibiting DNA and RNA synthesis, azathioprine suppresses both T- and B-lymphocyte proliferation, although antibody production is thought to be less affected than T-cell activity. Incorporation of TIMP into nucleic acids can result in chromosome breakage,[26] which may predispose to malignancies. An important part of the immunologic effect of azathioprine and 6-MP is blockade of IL-2 production in mixed lymphocyte culture, but by a different mechanism than cyclosporine or tacrolimus.

PHARMACOKINETICS

Azathioprine is well-absorbed from the upper gastrointestinal tract after oral administration. Peak immunosuppressive activity in blood occurs within 1–2 hours and declines over 12–24 hours. The effects likely persist considerably longer in tissues, since only a once daily dose is necessary for immunosuppression. Azathioprine is metabolized in the liver to the active metabolite 6-thioinosinic acid via 6-MP and probably other pathways.

TABLE 13-16	**Azathioprine**

Clinical use
- Maintenance immunosuppression usually combined with either cyclosporine or tacrolimus, with or without steroids.

Mechanism
- Impairment of lymphocyte proliferation by inhibition of purine synthesis.

Dose
- When used with cyclosporine or tacrolimus, maximum dose of 2–2.5 mg/kg/day. Dose reduced as necessary to maintain white blood cell count ≥ 3,000/mL.

Target levels
- Blood levels not monitored.

Adverse effects
- Myelosuppression (leukopenia most common, rarely accompanied by thrombocytopenia and/or anemia). Bone marrow suppression effects may be additive with other myelosuppressive drugs.
- Hepatic toxicity, pancreatitis, alopecia (uncommon).
- Malignancies, especially cutaneous, may be more common with chronic azathioprine therapy.
- Concomitant use of allopurinol, an inhibitor of xanthine oxidase, may increase myelosuppression. When using allopurinol, azathioprine dose should be reduced to 25–33% of preallopurinol dose.

Catabolism occurs by direct oxidation via xanthine oxidase and by methylation of the sulfur group in the thiopurine methyltransferase (see Box) pathway. The final inactive metabolites are excreted in the urine.

The role of xanthine oxidase in the metabolism of azathioprine is of great clinical importance, since the concomitant administration of a drug such as allopurinol, which blocks the xanthine oxidase pathway, results in an approximately fourfold increase in immunosuppression and a two- to fourfold increase in myelosuppression for the same azathioprine dose.[143]

DOSING

In the precyclosporine era, the recommended dose of azathioprine was generally 2–4 mg/kg/day intrave-

nously (IV) or PO to maintain the total leukocyte count between 3,000 and 5,000/mL. In the current era, however, lower doses of 1–2 mg/kg/day are recommended in combination with cyclosporine or tacrolimus. The dose is reduced as needed to keep the leukocyte count above about 3,000/mL, platelet count above about 100,000, and hematocrit about 27% or higher.

TOXICITY

The major toxicity of azathioprine is myelosuppression, which is usually dose dependent and delayed in onset. Leukopenia is most common, but thrombocytopenia and anemia may also occur. Dose reduction or drug discontinuation usually results in reversal of the myelo-

 ### Thiopurine Methyltransferase

A small subpopulation of patients experience severe myelosuppression when they receive azathioprine. This problem is directly related to the intracellular accumulation of 6-thioguanine nucleotides, which are the major toxic species of 6-thiopurine derivatives such as azathioprine, and these toxic species are catabolized by xanthine oxidase and thiopurine methyl transferase (TPMT) into 6-methyl-thiuric acid. The xanthine oxidase gene is not polymorphic, but there are several codominant polymorphisms of the thiopurine methyl transferase gene that result in the reduction or complete abrogation of enzyme activity. Approximately 10% of Caucasian patients have intermediate TPMT activity because they are heterozygous for one of

the TPMT polymorphisms (Fig. 13–15). Since they only have one working copy of the gene instead of two, the enzyme activity is only 40–60% of that found in cells from individuals who are homozygous for the functional TPMT alleles. Clinical studies have found an inverse correlation between TPMT activity and the accumulation of thioguanine metabolites. Approximately 1 in 300 individuals are homozygous for nonfunctional variants of the gene and are therefore at risk for severe hematopoietic toxicity unless dose is reduced to a fraction of normal (8- to 15-fold lower).[578] In the clinical setting, TPMT polymorphisms are detected by measuring the levels of 6-thioguanine metabolites in erythrocytes.

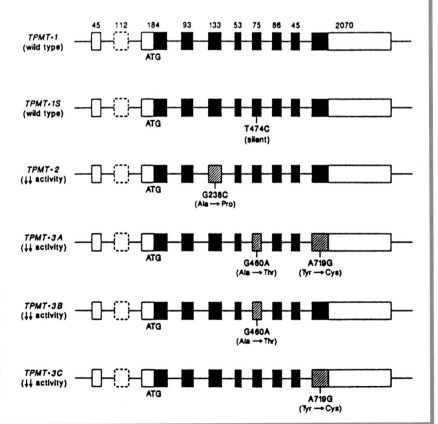

FIGURE **13–15.** Allelic variants at the human thiopurine S-methyltransferase (TPMT) locus. White boxes are untranslated regions, black boxes represent portions of the gene that are transcribed and translated into proteins, and the hatched boxes represent the areas of the gene that result in an altered amino acid sequence due to a mutation. (From Yates CR, Krynetski EY, Loennechen T, Fessing MY, Tai HL, Pui CH, Relling MV, Evans WE: Molecular diagnosis of thiopurine S-methyltransferase deficiency: genetic basis for azathioprine and mercaptopurine intolerance. Ann Intern Med 1997;126:608–614.)

suppression within 7–10 days unless other causes of bone marrow suppression are present (CMV infection, other myelosuppressive drugs, or previous myelosuppression).

Hepatotoxicity (transaminase elevation or rarely hyperbilirubinemia[418]) and pancreatitis are uncommon complications. Alopecia is usually reversible. Megaloblastic anemia occurs rarely.

Malignancies, especially cutaneous, may be more common with chronic azathioprine therapy, possibly secondary to chromosomal breakage. Genetic predisposition and exposure to sunlight are the two greatest risk factors for cutaneous squamous cell carcinoma. Ultraviolet light from sun exposure induces DNA damage, which plays a direct etiologic role in squamous cell carcinoma.[258] Azathioprine and other antimetabolites which impair DNA synthesis and induce chromosomal breakage likely impair DNA repair mechanisms[567] and increase susceptibility to malignant transformation.

DRUG INTERACTIONS

Caution is advised when azathioprine is administered with other drugs with potential for bone marrow suppression. The most important single drug interaction is with allopurinol, a xanthine oxidase inhibitor that interferes with the breakdown of azathioprine and its metabolites. Azathioprine dose should be reduced to 25–30% of usual. Failure to appropriately reduce the azathioprine dose may lead to accumulation of metabolites and prolonged leukopenia.

CLINICAL USE

Although initially used in a two-drug maintenance regimen with prednisone, azathioprine is currently most commonly employed as part of a three-drug immunosuppression regimen of either cyclosporine, azathioprine, and prednisone, or less commonly, tacrolimus, azathioprine, and prednisone. In steroid-free protocols, azathioprine is used with either cyclosporine or tacrolimus. In the presence of malignancies, recurrent viral infections or prolonged bone marrow suppression, azathioprine is usually discontinued or converted to mycophenolate (if recurrent rejection is an issue).

MYCOPHENOLATE MOFETIL

HISTORICAL NOTE

Mycophenolic acid, the immunologically active metabolite of mycophenolate mofetil, was first isolated by Gosio in 1898 from a *Penicillium* culture.[185] Alsberg and Black provided the name "mycophenolic acid" in 1913 after isolating it from *Penicillium stoloniferum*,[15] and the chemical structure was later elucidated by Birkinshaw and colleagues.[51] Initial clinical interest focused on the treatment of psoriasis.[235, 333] In the mid 1970s, Allison and colleagues demonstrated that children with the Lesch-Nyhan syndrome had essentially normal T- and B-lymphocyte function.[11] This was a critical observation, since the Lesch-Nyhan syndrome is characterized by a deficiency in hypoxanthine-guanine phosphoribosyl transferase, a key enzyme in the salvage pathway for purine synthesis. Allison and colleagues subsequently proved that lymphocytes, in contrast to other cell lines, depend primarily on the *de novo* pathway for purine synthesis.[11, 12, 150] Mycophenolic acid was known to be a potent inhibitor of guanine synthesis, a critical step in *de novo* synthesis.[13] Thus, mycophenolic acid was a potentially important lymphocyte-specific immunosuppressive agent. Syntex Corporation initiated a research program to develop a form of mycophenolic acid with greater bioavailability.[308] The result of this effort was the synthesis of mycophenolate mofetil by Dr. Peter Nelson and colleagues at Syntex laboratories,[308] which has about twice the bioavailability of mycophenolic acid.[308]

CHEMICAL STRUCTURE

Mycophenolate mofetil is the morpholinoethyl ester of mycophenolic acid (Fig. 13–2), which is a fungal metabolite. The empirical formula is $C_{23}H_{31}NO_7$.

MECHANISM OF IMMUNOSUPPRESSION

Mycophenolate mofetil (MM) is a prodrug that is rapidly hydrolyzed to form mycophenolic acid (MPA), which blocks the *de novo* pathway for purine synthesis by producing reversible noncompetitive inhibition of the enzyme inosine monophosphate dehydrogenase (IMPDH), which converts inosine monophosphate to xanthine monophosphate, which is in turn converted to guanine monophosphate[504] (Fig. 13–16). Most human cells can synthesize purines for DNA through either the *de novo* purine pathway or the salvage purine pathway. Human lymphocytes are unique in that they are *only* able to synthesize purines for DNA synthesis through the *de novo* pathway, making them susceptible to the action of MPA. There are two isoforms of IMPDH, types I and II. MPA has greater activity against the type II isoform, which is also the most prevalant type in proliferating T- and B-lymphocytes.[383, 388] Thus, MPA acts to selectively inhibit proliferation of lymphocytes (Fig. 13–1), and inhibits mixed lymphocyte responses when added as late as 3 days following initial stimulation.[68, 150] MPA primarily affects this later stage of lymphocyte response because, unlike cyclosporine and tacrolimus, it does not inhibit IL-2 production.[150, 371]

In vitro and *in vivo* studies indicate its ability to inhibit both T- and B-cell proliferation in response to antigen stimulation.[10, 150, 369, 584] MPA is also a potent inhibitor of B-cell lines transformed by Epstein-Barr virus.[150, 584] Other studies also suggest that MPA may retard adhesion of lymphocytes to endothelial surfaces.[10, 13] Of particular interest is the unique ability of MPA to prevent proliferation of smooth muscle cells *in vitro*[10] and *in vivo* in a rat aortic allograft model,[492] a rat heterotopic cardiac allograft model, and in a baboon heterotopic cardiac allograft model.[343] Although unproven in human cardiac

Pathways of Purine Biosynthesis

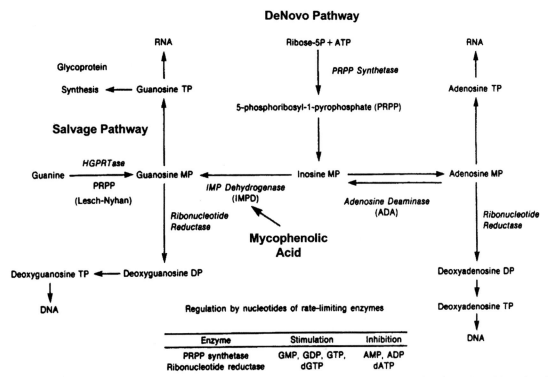

FIGURE **13–16.** Pathways of purine biosynthesis, showing the central position of inosine monophosphate (IMP). Mycophenolic acid inhibits IMP dehydrogenase thereby depleting GMP, GTP, and dGTP. (From Allison AC, Eugui EM, Sollinger HW: Mycophenolate mofetil [RS-61443]: mechanisms of action and effects in transplantation. Transplant Rev 1993;7:129.)

transplantation, long-term clinical studies are in progress to examine the potential beneficial effect of mycophenolate on the development of allograft vasculopathy, as suggested by primate xenotransplantation studies.[400]

PHARMACOKINETICS

MM is rapidly absorbed across the gastrointestinal tract and converted to the active form MPA by the action of gastric and hepatic hydrolysis (Fig. 13–17). The bioavailability of an ingested dose of MM is greater than 90%. Peak blood levels of MPA are reached within 1–2 hours of oral administration, with a secondary peak 6–8 hours later caused by the enterohepatic circulation.[308, 504] The half-life for drug elimination is approximately 11–17 hours. MPA is conjugated with glucuronic acid by glucuronyl transferase in the liver to form an inactive metabolite mycophenolic acid glucuronide (MPAG), which is then excreted in the bile where it enters the enterohepatic circulation.[504] About 90% of ingested drug is excreted within 24 hours in the urine and feces as MPAG.[504] Renal function does not affect circulating levels. The major determinant of MPA levels appears to be changes in absorption from the gastrointestinal tract.

DOSING

Mycophenolate mofetil is supplied in 250-mg capsules and 500-mg tablets. An intravenous preparation is also available and is equivalent to the oral dose. In *adult* patients, oral or intravenous dosing is generally initiated at 250–500 mg bid, with daily dose increments of 250–500 mg unless gastrointestinal symptoms develop (Table 13–17). The usual target dose is 1,500–1,750 mg PO bid. In *pediatric* patients, the usual starting dose is approximately 5 mg/kg PO or IV bid, with 2.5- to 5-mg/kg increments, to a target dose of 20–22 mg/kg bid in the absence of gastrointestinal symptoms. If patients are unable to take oral medications, the intravenous preparation can be administered in the same doses.

BLOOD LEVEL MONITORING

Until recently, blood level determinations of MPA have not been generally available in clinical transplantation. Recent studies suggest that trough whole blood levels of 2.5–5 μg/mL are desirable for immunosuppression effect, although the experience with blood levels is limited.[348]

TOXICITY

The major side effects of MM are gastrointestinal symptoms, most commonly nausea, vomiting, and/or diarrhea,[122, 148, 149, 236, 273, 425] which are experienced in over one-third of patients and are generally responsive to temporary dose reduction. Rarely, severe diarrhea may be related to villous atrophy, which is reversible following

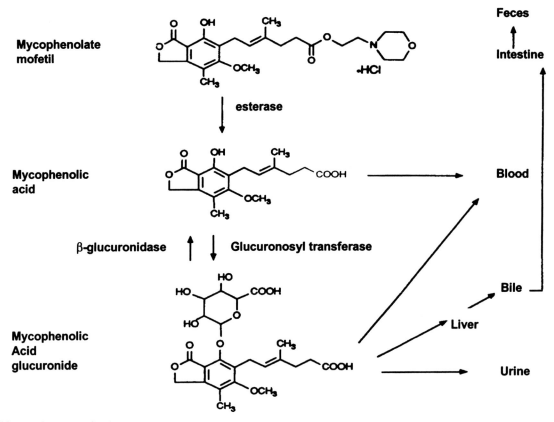

Mycophenolate mofetil

esterase

Mycophenolic acid

β-glucuronidase   Glucuronosyl transferase

Mycophenolic Acid glucuronide

Feces
Intestine
Blood
Bile
Liver
Urine

FIGURE **13–17.** Molecular structure of the morpholinoethyl ester of mycophenolic acid (mycophenolate mofetil) and its glucuronide, and sites of their interconversion and excretion. (From Allison AC, Eugui EM, Sollinger HW: Mycophenolate mofetil [RS-61443]: mechanisms of action and effects of transplantation. Transplant Rev 1993;7:129.)

TABLE 13–17	**Mycophenolate Mofetil**

Clinical use
- Chronic maintenance immunosuppression with cyclosporine or tacrolimus, with or without corticosteroids. Replaces azathioprine in chronic immunosuppression regimen.

Mechanism
- Hydrolyzed to mycophenolic acid, the active immunosuppressive component, which inhibits inosine monophosphate dehydrogenase, thereby inhibiting *de novo* purine synthesis. Selective inhibitory effects on T- and B-cell proliferation.

Dose
- Adults: Begin at 500 mg bid and progressively increase to a target dose of 1,500–1,750 mg bid, if tolerated (GI symptoms).
- Pediatric: Begin at 5 mg/kg PO bid and progressively increase to a target dose of 20–23 mg/kg bid if tolerated (GI symptoms).
- When administered intravenously, the dose is equivalent to the oral dose.

Target levels
- Limited experience with blood level monitoring, but current recommendations include a target level of 2–5 ng/mL.

Adverse effects
- Gastrointestinal: nausea, vomiting, abdominal pain, diarrhea, loss of appetite; rarely, gastric ulceration, gastritis, GI bleeding, jaundice, pancreatitis.
- Leukopenia (uncommon), effects may be additive with other myelosuppressive agents.

GI, gastrointestinal.

MM withdrawal.[133] Less common symptoms include gastritis, urinary urgency or dysuria (10–20%), and cholestasis.[149, 236]

Initial studies in clinical cardiac transplantation indicated that MM had minimal myelosuppressive effects.[148, 265] However, a multicenter randomized trial found that the incidence of leukopenia was similar in the mycophenolate and azathioprine groups.[277] As clinical experience has increased, it clearly has been established that occasional patients will have marked leukopenia requiring dose reduction or drug discontinuation (more common at doses exceeding 2 g/day of MM). Mycophenolate mofetil does not cause renal toxicity.

DRUG INTERACTIONS

The absorption of MM is decreased in the presence of antacids containing magnesium and aluminum hydroxides. Peak concentration may be reduced as much as 33%. Therefore, patients receiving antacids should not have them administered simultaneously with MM. Drugs which interfere with enterohepatic recirculation (such as cholestyramine) may reduce the MPA AUC by as much as 40% and therefore should not be administered in patients taking MM. Drugs which alter intestinal flora may also interfere with MM absorption by disrupting enterohepatic recirculation. MM should be administered on an empty stomach, since coadministration of food may importantly reduce absorption. Since clearance of MPAG occurs by renal tubular secretion as well as glomerular filtration, drugs such as probenecid (which inhibit tubular secretion) may greatly increase MPA AUC concentrations. No important interaction has been detected between MM and cyclosporine, acyclovir, ganciclovir, or trimethoprim/sulfamethoxazole.

CLINICAL USE

The first clinical trial of mycophenolate in human transplantation was reported by Sollinger in 1992.[485] In that phase I clinical trial in renal transplant patients, the frequency of rejection decreased with increasing doses of mycophenolate (substituted for azathioprine) up to a dose of 3,500 mg/day.[484] A subsequent multi-institutional study indicated that 69% of patients with refractory renal allograft rejection had "successful long-term rescue" with conversion from azathioprine to MMF.[485] Similar findings were noted in liver transplantation.[167, 273] Early clinical studies in cardiac transplantation showed that MM was safe in doses up to 3,000 mg/day.[148] Subsequent studies have shown that MM is frequently an effective therapy for recurrent cardiac allograft rejection.[265, 278, 513] When used to treat recurrent rejection, the reduction in rejection frequency is similar to that achieved with methotrexate and total lymphoid irradiation.[268]

In current immunosuppressive strategies with triple-drug immunosuppression, MMF is frequently substituted for azathioprine and used with either cyclosporine or tacrolimus, usually in combination with low-dose steroids. Although there is clinical evidence and experience to support conversion from azathioprine to MM with recurrent or persistent rejection, the advisability of *routine* use of MM instead of azathioprine remains contentious. MM has certain advantages over azathioprine: (1) the lymphocyte-specific effect of MM versus the generalized myelosuppressive effects of azathioprine, resulting in a lesser potential for anemia, neutropenia, thrombocytopenia, and stomatitis; (2) the favorable effect of MM on recurrent rejection; (3) a possibly lower potential for induction of malignancies (especially combined with cyclosporine and tacrolimus) with MM than with azathioprine (which is more likely to cause chromosomal abnormalities)[17, 225, 535]; and (4) experimental evidence suggesting the potential for MM to impede the development of allograft vasculopathy.

In a randomized, multicenter trial comparing MM with azathioprine in combination with cyclosporine and prednisone in cardiac transplantation, patients treated with MM had a lower mortality at 1 year (6.2% vs. 11.4%, $p = .03$), a reduction in the requirement for rejection treatment ($p = .03$), and fewer patients with grade $\geq$3A rejection ($p = .055$).[277] Despite these many advantages, MM has the distinct disadvantage of cost, which is many fold higher than an equivalent dose of azathioprine. Future studies will delineate the overall cost/benefit comparison of these two drugs in terms of actual drug costs/charges versus the potential cost-saving of

MM in treatment and rehospitalization for recurrent rejection.

One option is to initially use azathioprine (because of lower cost) in patients at low risk for rejection, selecting MM for patients with any risk factors for early or recurrent rejection (see Chapter 14). MM can be substituted for azathioprine in patients with recurrent rejection or rejection with hemodynamic compromise.

CYCLOPHOSPHAMIDE (CYTOXAN)

HISTORICAL NOTE

The discovery of cyclophosphamide by Arnold and Bourseaux[20] resulted from attempts to chemically alter mechlorethamine to achieve greater selectivity for neoplasms.

CHEMICAL STRUCTURE

Cyclophosphamide is an alkylating agent that is a derivative of nitrogen mustard. The empirical formula is $C_7H_{15}C_{12}N_2O_2 P \cdot H_2O$.

MECHANISM OF IMMUNOSUPPRESSION

Cyclophosphamide interferes with DNA replication by alkylating and crosslinking DNA strands (Table 13-18). Thus, its action is primarily on actively dividing cells. Both B-cells and T-cells are affected by cyclophosphamide, but the toxicity is greater in B-cells, since their recovery is slower. Some experimental studies suggest that cyclophosphamide has greater specificity for B-cells than azathioprine.[116, 330, 463, 528, 588] In a guinea pig model, Turk and colleagues showed that the B-cell response (but not T-cell response) to soluble antigen was completely blocked by cyclophosphamide.[528]

TABLE 13-18 Cyclophosphamide

Clinical use
- Maintenance immunosuppressive agent; may be substituted for azathioprine if antibody-mediated rejection suspected.

Mechanism
- Inhibition of lymphocyte proliferation by interference with DNA replication.
- Inhibition of B-cell response.

Dose
- When used with cyclosporine or tacrolimus, maximum dose generally 1–1.5 mg/kg/day. Dose is reduced as necessary to maintain white blood cell count $\geq$3,000/mL.

Target levels
- Blood levels not monitored.

Adverse effects
- Myelosuppression with maximal effect at approximately 7–10 days. Bone marrow suppression effects may be additive with other myelosuppressive drugs.
- Hemorrhagic cystitis, alopecia, gastrointestinal distress, interstitial pneumonitis (rare).

PHARMACOKINETICS

Cyclophosphamide is well absorbed from the upper gastrointestinal tract after oral administration, with extensive distribution throughout the body. It is metabolized by the hepatic cytochrome P-450 enzyme system, and about 15% is excreted in the urine.

DOSING

Cyclophosphamide is supplied in 25-mg and 50-mg tablets and as an intravenous preparation. The usual starting dose is 0.5 mg/kg/day. Dosage can be slowly titrated to maximum of 1 to 1.5 mg/kg/day with triple-drug immunosuppression while monitoring the peripheral leukocyte count (Table 13–18). When converting patients from azathioprine to cytoxan, the usual conversion dose is one half the azathioprine dose because of the greater bone marrow toxicity of cyclophosphamide. Some studies have suggested that a somewhat lower dose of cyclophosphamide (25–35% of azathioprine dose in milligrams) would produce a similar target white blood cell (WBC) count.[549, 550, 576] When given intravenously, the dose is the same as the oral dose.

An alternative dosing regimen has been utilized at Columbia Presbyterian Hospital (Itescu 1999, personal communication), in which cytoxan is administered intravenously every 3 weeks at a dose of 0.5–1 g/m^2, adjusted according to the nadir WBC count achieved.

TOXICITY

The major side effect is myelosuppression. All cell lines are affected and the bone marrow suppressive effect is generally slightly longer than with azathioprine. With normal hepatic function the nadir of leukopenia is generally about 7 days after the last dose of azathioprine, versus about 7–10 days with cyclophosphamide. Hemorrhagic cystitis may occur due to direct irritation of the bladder wall by the drug. This side effect is minimized by routinely administering the drug in the morning so that urine containing drug metabolites is not sitting in the bladder for a prolonged period. Other side effects include alopecia (at higher doses), gastrointestinal distress, and interstitial pneumonitis. All of these are rare at low doses of about 0.5–1.5 mg/kg/day.[576] Potential long-term effects include malignancy, decreased reproductive potential, cardiomyopathy, and teratogenesis.

DRUG INTERACTIONS

Caution is advised when using cyclophosphamide together with other drugs with the potential for myelosuppression, since the bone marrow effects may be additive.

CLINICAL USE

Cyclophosphamide is likely as effective as azathioprine in preventing allograft rejection early after cardiac trans-

plantation in a cyclosporine-based regimen. It may be useful in preventing antimurine antibody formation following OKT3 administration. Based on experimental studies suggesting its superior action (compared to azathioprine) against humoral immunity,[528] cyclophosphamide is often substituted for azathioprine in the setting of suspected humoral mediated rejection. However, this has not been proven in clinical studies.

METHOTREXATE

HISTORICAL NOTE

Methotrexate is primarily an antineoplastic agent which produced the first remissions in leukemia. During the last 30 years it has also proven beneficial in the treatment of psoriasis and adult rheumatoid arthritis.

CHEMICAL STRUCTURE

Methotrexate is the 4-amino, N^{10}-methyl analog of folic acid.

MECHANISM OF IMMUNOSUPPRESSION

Methotrexate, a folic acid antagonist, binds competitively to the enzyme dehydrofolate reductase, which catalyzes the conversion of folic acid to tetrahydrofolic acid. It thereby acts to inhibit both purine synthesis and the interconversion of amino acids such as glycine to serine and homocysteine to methionine. This antiproliferative effect inhibits proliferation of lymphocytes as well as other rapidly dividing cell lineages, and has important inhibitory effects on both humoral and cellular immunity.[196, 249, 320] The ability of methotrexate to inhibit IL-1 and IL-6 production may contribute to its immunosuppressive effect.[450, 472] It has been used in lower doses to successfully treat psoriasis and rheumatoid arthritis and in higher doses in the treatment of certain malignancies.

PHARMACOKINETICS

Methotrexate is rapidly absorbed following oral administration, with peak levels in 1/2 to 2 hours. The half-life is 8–12 hours with high doses and 3–10 hours with low doses. The half-life may be significantly increased with renal dysfunction, hepatic dysfunction, ascites, or pleural effusions. There is limited biliary excretion, but the primary route of excretion is via the kidney, with approximately 90% of drug excreted unchanged in the urine.

DOSING

Methotrexate may be administered orally or intravenously, but in cardiac transplantation it is generally administered orally. The standard adult dose is 1–5 mg every 8–12 hours for three doses per week, generally administered for 3–12 weeks as adjunctive therapy for recurrent or recalcitrant rejection. When administered, other myelosuppressive agents such as azathioprine are either reduced or discontinued. For pediatric patients, the standard dose is 5–10 mg/m^2/pr wk in 3 q-12-h doses. A pediatric intravenous dose of 150–300 μg/kg daily for 7–14 days has also been recommended,[57] but the incidence of severe bone marrow suppression is greater with intravenous administration. When administering methotrexate, close surveillance of leukocyte count, platelet count, hematocrit, and renal function are necessary to prevent toxic bone marrow suppression and subsequent serious infections.

TOXICITY

The major toxicity is bone marrow suppression, resulting in leukopenia, anemia, and thrombocytopenia. Fatal infection associated with profound bone marrow suppression has occurred in cardiac transplant recipients, possibly related to interactions with other drugs. Therefore, it is advisable to start therapy with very low doses while closely monitoring leukocyte counts. Other uncommon side effects of low-dose therapy include stomatitis, alopecia, GI distress, hepatotoxicity (including cirrhosis), dizziness, nephrotoxicity (in higher doses) and, rarely, hypersensitivity pneumonitis or severe dermatologic reactions.

DRUG INTERACTIONS

Salicylates, nonsteroidal anti-inflammatory drugs, and penicillins decrease tubular secretion of methotrexate and can increase methotrexate levels. Salicylates, phenytoin, and sulfonamides can displace protein-bound methotrexate and increase its toxicity. Trimethoprim plus sulfamethoxazole (Bactrim, Septra) and pyrimethamine may increase its bone marrow suppression. Leucovorin (folinic acid) can overcome the methotrexate-induced inhibition of dihydrofolate reductase and is useful in the treatment of inadvertant overdose. However, it must be administered before the onset of irreversible cell damage, usually within about 4 hours.

CLINICAL USE

Methotrexate is an effective adjunct to standard immunosuppression for recurrent or persistent acute rejection[108, 223] and may allow reduction in maintenance steroids during therapy.[405] Methotrexate has been successfully employed as an immunosuppressive adjunct in pediatric heart transplantation for persistent or recurrent rejection despite steroids and antilymphocyte serum.[57, 467]

ACTINOMYCIN D

BACKGROUND

Actinomycin D (ACD) is an effective chemotherapeutic agent that has been employed in the treatment of Ewing's sarcoma, Wilms' tumor, Kaposi's sarcoma, rhabdomyosarcoma, advanced cases of choriocarcinoma, and testicular carcinoma.[424] In low doses, actinomycin D has been an effective adjunct in the treatment of recurrent renal allograft rejection.[131]

CHEMICAL STRUCTURE

Actinomycin D, an antibiotic derived from streptomyces yeast, is a crystalline chromopeptide with both a phenoxazone ring and a polypeptide chain.[556]

MECHANISM OF IMMUNOSUPPRESSION

Actinomycin D requires the presence of guanine for its action. The phenoxazone ring intercalates between adjacent guanine-cytosine base pairs in DNA, resulting in inhibition of DNA transcription by RNA polymerase and the induction of single-strand DNA breakage.

PHARMACOKINETICS

The drug is most effective if administered intravenously. Approximately 50% of the drug is excreted unchanged in the bile and about 10% in urine.

DOSING

As an immunosuppressive agent for heart transplantation, ACD has been administered at an initial dose of 5 μg/kg by slow intravenous infusion over 5 minutes once every 6 weeks. A complete blood count is obtained before each dose, and the dose is reduced if there is evidence of myelosuppression.

TOXICITY

With higher dose ACD, frequent side effects include bone marrow suppression, stomatitis, gastrointestinal toxicity, and dermatologic reactions. In a small clinical experience, these side effects were not observed with this dose schedule in the presence of three-drug maintenance immunosuppression.[131]

DRUG INTERACTIONS

As with cyclophosphamide, the administration of ACD with other myelosuppressive agents may increase bone marrow suppression.

CLINICAL USE

DiSalvo and colleagues reported the use of ACD in the treatment of recurrent allograft rejection in a small number of patients after cardiac transplantation. Each patient received an intravenous ACD dose of 5 μg/kg every 6 weeks. Minimal toxicity was observed and an important reduction in rejection frequency was noted during the 6 months after initiating ACD therapy. The daily corticosteroid dose was also significantly reduced following actinomycin D therapy.[131] Thus, although uncommonly employed, actinomycin D may be an effective adjunct (similar to methotrexate but with perhaps less toxicity) in the treatment of recurrent allograft rejection.

SIROLIMUS (RAPAMYCIN)

HISTORICAL NOTE

Sirolimus is a natural product of the actinomycete (not a fungus) *Streptomyces hygroscopicus*, first isolated from Rapa-Nui, the Easter Islands, in the early 1970s.[465, 538] Sirolimus was the by-product of an antifungal drug discovery program at Ayerst Research Laboratory in Montreal, Canada. The potential of sirolimus as an immunosuppressive agent for transplantation was discovered by Morris at Stanford University working with Schgal at Wyeth-Ayerst Research and by Calne at Cambridge University, England, in 1988.[368]

In 1999, the U.S. FDA granted approval for the use of sirolimus as prophylaxis against organ rejection following renal transplantation.

CHEMICAL STRUCTURE

Sirolimus is a macrolide antibiotic with a structure similar to tacrolimus (Fig. 13–14). Rapamycin has a ring structure of 31 members compared to 23 in tacrolimus. It is highly lipophilic and therefore passes through cell membranes readily. Because of its insolubility in aqueous physiologic buffers, it is poorly absorbed after oral ingestion.

MECHANISM OF IMMUNOSUPPRESSION

Sirolimus belongs to a new class of immunosuppressive agents called **inhibitors of** TOR (see Box) (Table 13–19). TOR refers to the target of rapamycin, a cytoplasmic enzyme that plays a critical role in connecting signals from the T-cell surface to the cell nucleus for the stimulation of growth and proliferation of lymphocytes[2, 215] (Fig. 13–1). Once activated, TOR transduces signals to a series of inducible pathways which result in T-cell proliferation and differentiation and B-cell activation, proliferation, and antibody production. Thus, TOR appears to play an important role in cellular and humoral "effector" functions.[1, 460]

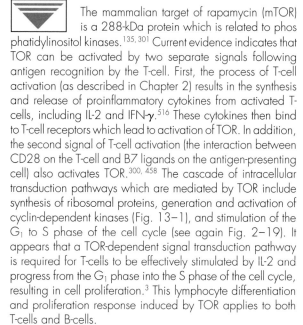

TOR

The mammalian target of rapamycin (mTOR) is a 288-kDa protein which is related to phosphatidylinositol kinases.[135, 301] Current evidence indicates that TOR can be activated by two separate signals following antigen recognition by the T-cell. First, the process of T-cell activation (as described in Chapter 2) results in the synthesis and release of proinflammatory cytokines from activated T-cells, including IL-2 and IFN-γ.[516] These cytokines then bind to T-cell receptors which lead to activation of TOR. In addition, the second signal of T-cell activation (the interaction between CD28 on the T-cell and B7 ligands on the antigen-presenting cell) also activates TOR.[300, 458] The cascade of intracellular transduction pathways which are mediated by TOR include synthesis of ribosomal proteins, generation and activation of cyclin-dependent kinases (Fig. 13–1), and stimulation of the G_1 to S phase of the cell cycle (see again Fig. 2–19). It appears that a TOR-dependent signal transduction pathway is required for T-cells to be effectively stimulated by IL-2 and progress from the G_1 phase into the S phase of the cell cycle, resulting in cell proliferation.[3] This lymphocyte differentiation and proliferation response induced by TOR applies to both T-cells and B-cells.

TOR also has another important role which may have implications in the development of allograft vasculopathy. The activation of TOR triggers the proliferation of endothelial and smooth muscle cells and release of growth factors in vessel walls and in the airways. Via this mechanism, intimal proliferation may result after vessel wall trauma, ischemia, or immune-mediated inflammation.[163] The release of growth factors (such as platelet-derived growth factor, fibroblast growth factor, endothelial growth factor, and transforming growth factor-β) from proliferating T-cells can also induce activation of TOR within mesenchymal cells, promoting proliferation of vascular smooth muscle cells, endothelial cells, and fibroblasts.[317, 460]

Finally, the TOR mechanism may have relevance in the induction of tolerance, since TOR may play a role in the delivery of signals which prevent apoptosis within cells.[2] It is speculated that apoptosis of activated T-cells may facilitate the induction of tolerance, and thus inhibitors of TOR could potentially be useful in a regimen of tolerance induction.

Like cyclosporine and tacrolimus, sirolimus is a prodrug which must bind to an immunophilin in order to exert its immunologic effects. In the cytoplasm, sirolimus binds to the same immunophilin as does tacrolimus, namely, FKBP12. However, important differences occur in the details after binding with FKBP12. Whereas the FKBP12-tacrolimus complex binds to calcineurin, the FKBP12-rapamicin complex (which exerts the immunosuppressive activity of sirolimus) targets TOR. Thus, the immunosuppressive effects of sirolimus can be predicted by the result of blockade of TOR (Table 13–2).

Sirolimus (via its binding and inhibition of mTOR) acts at the G_1–S phase of the cell cycle, later than cyclosporine or tacrolimus (which block the T-cell cycle at the G_0–G_1 stage)[411] (Fig. 13–18). Cyclosporine and tacrolimus inhibit gene expression for IL-2, IL-4, IFN-γ,

TABLE 13–19	TOR Inhibitors

Clinical use
- Approved for maintenance immunosuppression following renal transplantation combined with a calcineurin inhibitor and prednisone or azathioprine and prednisone. The use of this agent and RAD in heart and heart–lung transplantation will likely be similar.

Mechanism: Inhibition of TOR
- Inhibition of T-cell differentiation and proliferation.
- Inhibition of B-cell activation and proliferation.
- Inhibition of mesenchymal cell proliferation.
- Preservation of T-cell apoptosis.

Dose
- Sirolimus: 2–5 mg/day PO.
- RAD: dose not established.

Target levels
- Preliminary and clinical studies suggest a whole blood trough level of 5–20 ng/mL.

Adverse effects
- Hypercholesteremia.
- Elevated triglyceride.
- Thrombocytopenia (dose related).

and IL-2 receptor. Sirolimus inhibits neither calcineurin phosphatase nor the production of T-cell cytokines. In contrast to cyclosporine and tacrolimus, sirolimus **inhibits cell proliferation stimulated by growth factors.** Sirolimus inhibits lymphocyte proliferative responses to cytokines such as IL-2, IL-4, and IL-6[363] after the cytokine is bound to its receptor, and inhibits gene expression of IL-10, whose regulation is not dependent on calcium or protein kinase C.[587] The net effect is **selective blockade of cytokine signal-mediated cell division and proliferation with arrest of the cell cycle in the G_1 phase.** Since the action is distinct from calcineurin inhibitors, these two classes when combined have **synergistic effects.** Sirolimus inhibits T-cell activation initiated by the same calcium-dependent reactions that are sensitive to inhibition by cyclosporine and tacrolimus, but in addition sirolimus inhibits the calcium-independent signaling pathways for both T- and B-cell activation, which are not affected by tacrolimus and cyclosporine.[134, 257, 352, 365]

In contrast to cyclosporine and tacrolimus, whose antiproliferative effects are primarily restricted to T- and B-cells, sirolimus also has important effects outside the immune system, particularly in relationship to growth factors. A potentially important effect in relationship to heart and lung transplantation is the observation that sirolimus inhibits arterial smooth muscle cell and endothelial cell proliferation induced by platelet-derived growth factor and basic fibroblast growth factor,[357] which does not occur with cyclosporine or tacrolimus except at very high concentrations.[162] Although unproven in humans, it has been shown to prevent arterial disease in rat cardiac allografts.[345] Like mycophenolate, sirolimus appears to inhibit arterial intimal thickening caused by both an alloimmune and a mechanical injury both *in vivo* and *in vitro*.[193, 195] Extrapolating from its anti-TOR effects, TOR inhibitors such as sirolimus may also inhibit the proliferative response of mesenchymal cells (including fibroblasts) within the bronchioles of pulmonary allografts. These properties make TOR inhibitors appealing as immunosuppressive agents which could potentially attenuate allograft vasculopathy in heart

transplantation and obliterative bronchiolitis in lung transplantation. In contrast to TOR inhibitors, calcineurin blockers may actually promote chronic rejection by the enhancement of mesenchymal proliferation due to up-regulation of growth factors.[126]

Sirolimus and **cyclosporine** appear to have **synergistic** effects. Sirolimus appears to be 10- to 100-fold more potent than cyclosporine,[145, 496] and equivalent immunosuppression is produced with much lower doses of cyclosporine and sirolimus than with either alone.[365] Sirolimus potentiates the inhibitory effect of cyclosporine on cytotoxic T-cell generation and proliferation, while cyclosporine potentiates the inhibitory effect of sirolimus on lymphokine signal transduction.[365] A possible mechanism is that cyclosporine blocks T-cell induced cytokine synthesis, while sirolimus blocks the responsiveness of receptor-positive lymphocytes to the cytokine that is produced. There is evidence that the combination of a calcineurin inhibitor and a TOR inhibitor will have a synergistic effect in blocking G_1 phase T-cell proliferation.[263] Although **sirolimus and tacrolimus** are potentially antagonistic for many of their actions because of competition for the same binding protein (FKBP),[365] in clinical doses the synergism between sirolimus and tacrolimus appears similar to that between sirolimus and cyclosporine.

Sirolimus prevents acute rejection in rodent models of heart, renal, and small bowel transplantation.[496] In addition, its application in rodent models has promoted the induction of alloantigen-specific tolerance. Thus, substantial animal data indicate that sirolimus can prevent and reverse acute cellular rejection, suppress primary and secondary antibody production, and inhibit allograft vasculopathy.

PHARMACOKINETICS

The oral administration of sirolimus has a long terminal half-life of approximately 60 hours, indicating that a once-daily administration will sustain steady-state concentrations, which are reached within 7–14 days. After a single dose, 90% of sirolimus is recovered from feces, with only about 2% excreted in urine.[166] After a single

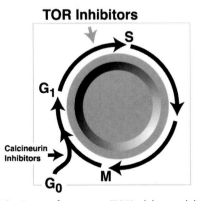

FIGURE 13–18. Target of rapamycin (TOR) inhibitors inhibit the molecular reactions during the G_1 phase of T-cell proliferation. In contrast, calcineurin inhibitors suppress interleukin-2 synthesis during the G_0 phase of T-cell activation.

oral dose, 70% of patients achieve maximal concentration within 1 hour and 100% within 3 hours.[589] As in calcineurin inhibitors, sirolimus (and RAD) is transported back into the intestinal lumen by P-glycoprotein countertransport carriers.[114] The distribution of drug among cellular components is 95% red blood cells (RBC), 3% plasma, 1% lymphs, and 1% granulocytes.[579]

Since cyclosporine microemulsion and sirolimus both involve P-glycoprotein carrier systems, it has been observed that simultaneous administration of sirolimus and cyclosporine results in high peak and trough sirolimus concentration and significantly shorter time to maximum concentration during simultaneous administration.[252] This may in part relate to inhibition of CYPA4 metabolism and/or decreased P-glycoprotein countertransport of sirolimus in the intestine.

DOSING

Based on renal transplant studies, the recommended loading dose of 6–15 mg PO should be administered as soon as possible after transplantation. The daily maintenance dose is 2–5 mg/day PO, with dose reduction for adverse events such as severe thrombocytopenia, hypertriglyceridemia, and hypercholesteremia.

BLOOD LEVEL MONITORING

Based on the available studies in renal transplantation, whole blood monitoring of sirolimus is advisable (sirolimus is highly sequestered in erythrocytes). The steady-state trough levels correlate well with the area under the curve in renal transplant patients, and therapeutic trough levels are considered to be 5–20 ng/mL. No commercial sirolimus immunoassays are currently available, and HPLC has been utilized.

TOXICITY

Toxicity of sirolimus differs markedly from cyclosporine and tacrolimus, perhaps because inhibition of the calcineurin activity in nonimmune cells (not affected by sirolimus) may account for many of the toxic effects of cyclosporine and tacrolimus. Sirolimus has minimal nephrotoxic effects but is associated with elevation of triglycerides or cholesterol and occasional thrombocytopenia or mild leukopenia.[368] Weight loss, testicular atrophy, and lethargy have rarely been observed.

In a phase III multicenter study in renal transplantation,[166] the major hematologic effect of sirolimus over a 12-month trial was a dose-related, reversible mild decrease in platelet counts. Severe thrombocytopenia (platelet count <20,000/mL) was rare (0.2%). The decrease in platelet count was greater with the 5-mg/day dose of sirolimus than the 2-mg dose, and the overall level of platelet counts was similar to those seen with azathioprine. Clinically important thrombocytopenia usually responded to dose reduction. No patient in this study demonstrated absolute neutropenia. Mild de-

crease in mean hemoglobin level was observed in the 5-mg/day sirolimus group, but remained greater than 13 g/dL.

Sirolimus has minimal effects on renal function in most trials. However, a dose related increase in serum creatinine may occur when sirolimus is combined with cyclosporine, likely reflecting cyclosporine-associated renal effects.[165] Sirolimus used in psoriasis patients as monotherapy had no effect on renal function compared to placebo, and when combined with corticosteroids and mycophenolate and compared to a regimen of cyclosporine, corticosteroids, and mycophenolate, serum creatinine in the sirolimus group was significantly lower at 12 months compared to the cyclosporine cohort ($p = .007$).[199, 289] In addition, sirolimus does not produce the hypertensive effects associated with cyclosporine therapy.

The magnitude of hypercholesterolemia and hypertriglyceridemia has been examined in a phase III multicenter trial in renal transplantation. In the global study, the incidence of hypercholesterolemia (cholesterol level ≥ 240 mg/dL) was 46% in the sirolimus 5-mg/day group, 43% in the 2-mg/day group, and 23% in the placebo group.[525] Similarly, approximately 50% of patients in the sirolimus group experienced hypertriglyceridemia (triglyceride level ≥ 400 mg/dL), about twice that observed in the placebo group. At the end of the first year of the phase III study, the mean cholesterol levels of the sirolimus groups averaged approximately 20 mg/dL greater than the mean levels in the nonsirolimus groups. Elevations of cholesterol and triglyceride levels are at least partially responsive to medical intervention with HMG-CoA reductase inhibitors and fibrates. The long-term effects of these lipid abnormalities and the potential for control with drug therapy and/or sirolimus dose reduction remains to be established.

ANIMAL AND CLINICAL STUDIES

Sirolimus has been most extensively studied in renal transplantation.[244, 376] In a multicenter phase III United States and international randomized trial in renal transplantation, sirolimus in two doses (2 mg/day and 5 mg/day) was combined with cyclosporine microemulsion and corticosteroids and compared with azathioprine or placebo as part of a triple-drug regimen. This study, involving over 1,200 renal allograft recipients, provided useful insight into the potential role of sirolimus.[166] The mean incidence of acute rejection during the first 6 months was significantly lower in both sirolimus groups (2 and 5 mg/day) compared to either azathioprine or placebo groups ($p < .002$). Severe histologic damage associated with the first rejection episode (biopsy proven) was the lowest in the 5-mg sirolimus group (4.4%), 9.2% in a 2-mg sirolimus group, and 17.4% in the azathioprine group ($p < .01$). An analysis by MacDonald and colleagues[326] revealed that the combination of sirolimus and cyclosporine provided the same protection against early acute rejection *irrespective* of the cyclosporine trough level (range, 100–500 ng/mL) as long as the sirolimus concentration was at least 10 ng/

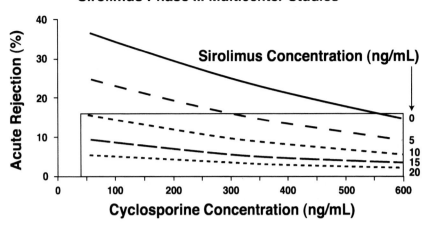

Sirolimus Phase III Multicenter Studies*

FIGURE **13–19.** The almost flat pharmacodynamic–efficacy response curve (day 0 to day 75) for cyclosporine (CsA) suggests that it is not necessary to keep CsA levels high for the combined therapy to be effective. As indicated in the figure, the combined therapy is effective at a wide range of CsA trough levels as long as the sirolimus trough concentration is maintained at approximately 10 ng/mL, which was approximately the median value for the study population treated with sirolimus in the phase III studies. (From TOR Inhibition—a new therapeutic pathway to immunosuppression. Sponsored by the AST and funded through an unrestricted educational grant from Wyeth-Ayerst Laboratories. April 2000.)

*U.S./Global clinical study data combined.
Adapted from MacDonald et al.[326]

mL. The lowest incidence of rejection was in the sirolimus group, with a target level of 20 ng/mL[326, 525] (Fig. 13–19). This important information suggests that, at least in renal transplantation, the combination of sirolimus and cyclosporine may allow important reduction in the cyclosporine levels early after transplantation with no increase in the likelihood of allograft rejection.[246, 249]

In a European randomized trial in renal transplantation, sirolimus was as effective as cyclosporine when combined with azathioprine and prednisolone in preventing acute rejection and graft loss.[199] Another randomized trial in renal transplantation also found equivalent efficacy between sirolimus and cyclosporine when combined with mycophenolate mofetil and prednisone.[289] In both trials, renal function at 1 year was significantly better with sirolimus than with cyclosporine.

POTENTIAL CLINICAL ROLE

Sirolimus holds promise as a maintenance immunosuppressive agent which can be combined with cyclosporine (or tacrolimus) in place of azathioprine or mycophenolate, or combined with mycophenolate and prednisone in place of cyclosporine (particularly useful in the presence of renal dysfunction). Further studies in heart and lung transplantation will be necessary to elucidate a possibly beneficial role in the prevention of allograft coronary artery disease or obliterative bronchiolitis.

RAD

The poor oral bioavailability of sirolimus has been an impediment to the exploration of this drug as a clinical immunosuppressive agent. RAD001 is the product of efforts to develop a TOR inhibitor with greater absorption after oral administration than sirolimus.

CHEMICAL STRUCTURE

RAD is the O-alkylated analogue of sirolimus; their structures are identical except that RAD contains a hydroxyethyl group at position 40 (Fig. 13–20)[464] conferring increased polarity and rendering greater solubility in ethereal solvents.

MECHANISM OF IMMUNOSUPPRESSION

From available studies, the immunosuppressive action and effects are identical to sirolimus (see previous section).

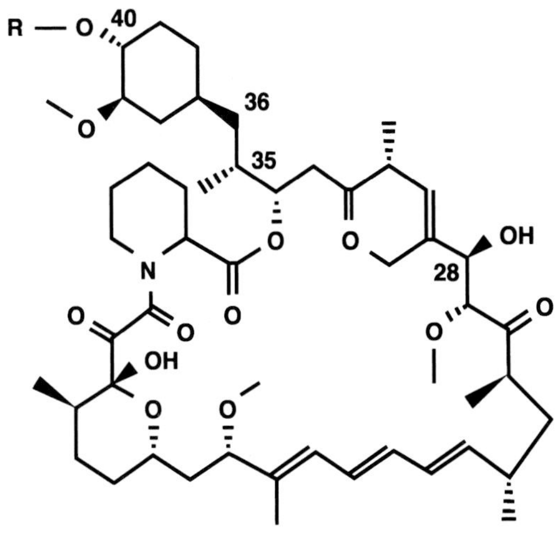

1. Sirolimus   R = H
2. SDZ RAD   R = HO(CH₂)₂-

FIGURE **13–20.** Structural differences between target of rapamycin (TOR) inhibitors sirolimus and RAD (SDZ RAD). The structures are identical except at position 40, where RAD contains a hydroxyethyl group. (From Sedrani R, Cottens J, Kallen J, Schuler W: Chemical modification of rapamycin: the discovery of SDZ RAD. Transplant Proc 1998;30: 2192–2194.)

PHARMACOKINETICS

The half-life of RAD001 is approximately 30 hours, which is considerably shorter than an oral preparation of sirolimus. In animals, RAD001 is cleared metabolically, and there is no significant concentration in the urine or bile.

DOSING

The recommended dose of RAD001 is yet to be determined. At a total dose of 10 mg/day, RAD001 does not appear to be well tolerated, and current phase III trials are using RAD001 doses of 5 mg/day or less.

TOXICITY

The toxicity associated with RAD001 appears to be the same as that of sirolimus and includes principally thrombocytopenia, leukopenia, and increased cholesterol and triglyceride levels.[245, 376]

HUMAN STUDIES

RAD is currently an investigational agent. A number of studies have either been completed or are currently underway in renal, liver, heart, heart–lung, and lung transplant recipients to determine the safety and efficacy of RAD001.

MIZORIBINE

HISTORICAL NOTE

Mizoribine, also known as bredinin, was first isolated in 1974 by Mizuno in Japan as a product of the soil fungus *Eupnicillium brefeldianum*.[358] In 1975, it was discovered to have important immunosuppressive qualities as an inhibitor of the enzyme inosine monophosphate dehydrogenase, which was the first evidence of the critical role of the *de novo* purine biosynthesis pathway during lymphocyte activation. This line of investigation revealed that inhibitors of inosine monophosphate dehydrogenase produce relatively selective inhibition of lymphocyte proliferation, indicating that the *de novo* pathway for purine synthesis is more important for lymphocytes than for other rapidly dividing cells. It was approved for use in transplantation in Japan in 1984.

CHEMISTRY

Mizoribine is an imidazole nucleoside antibiotic (Fig. 13–21). Mizoribine itself is a prodrug, requiring phosphorylation by adenosine kinase to form mizoribine 5′-monophosphate, which competitively inhibits inosine monophosphate dehydrogenase.

MECHANISM OF IMMUNOSUPPRESSION

Mizoribine has the same basic mechanism of action as mycophenolate mofetil, in that it inhibits inosine monophosphate dehydrogenase of the *de novo* pathway for purine biosynthesis. Like mycophenolate, mizoribine suppresses the primary antibody response and production of memory B-cells and T-helper cells. It does not reduce IL-2 synthesis or expression and does not block the cytotoxic effects of effector T-cells.

PHARMACOKINETICS

Rodent and canine studies indicate that mizoribine is rapidly absorbed from the gastrointestinal tract with peak serum levels achieved within 1.5 hours. Greater than 80% of drug is excreted unchanged in the urine by

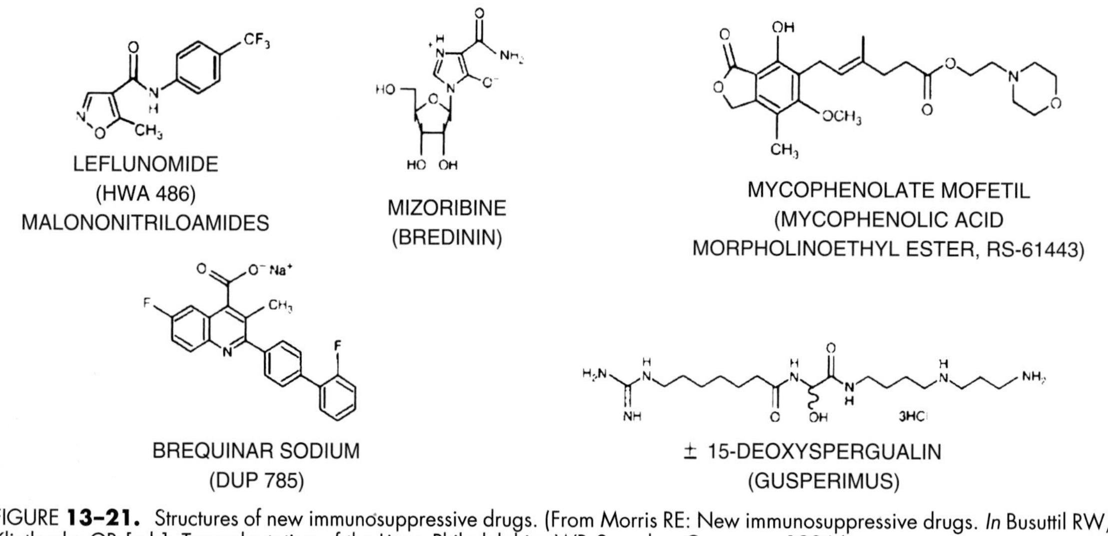

LEFLUNOMIDE
(HWA 486)
MALONONITRILOAMIDES

MIZORIBINE
(BREDININ)

MYCOPHENOLATE MOFETIL
(MYCOPHENOLIC ACID
MORPHOLINOETHYL ESTER, RS-61443)

BREQUINAR SODIUM
(DUP 785)

± 15-DEOXYSPERGUALIN
(GUSPERIMUS)

FIGURE **13–21.** Structures of new immunosuppressive drugs. (From Morris RE: New immunosuppressive drugs. *In* Busuttil RW, Klintlmalm GB [eds]: Transplantation of the Liver. Philadelphia: WB Saunders Company, 1996.)

24 hours.[200] The half-life of mizoribine is approximately 3 hours in the presence of normal renal function.

TOXICITY

Mizoribine has considerably less myelotoxicity and hepatotoxicity than azathioprine. In canine models, mizoribine has produced hemorrhagic enteritis and erosive intestinal mucosal changes, particularly in the presence of high serum drug levels.[368] Because of its renal clearance, toxic effects are especially likely in the presence of renal dysfunction.

CLINICAL USE

Mizoribine has been approved in Japan for clinical transplantation, where it has generally replaced azathioprine in the immunosuppressive regimen for renal transplantation. European trials[307] also suggest efficacy in renal transplantation, but caution is advised in the presence of renal dysfunction. When combined with cyclosporine, it has produced impressive survival in experimental studies on heart transplantation, liver transplantation, and pancreas transplantation.

BREQUINAR SODIUM

HISTORICAL NOTE

Brequinar was synthesized at Dupont Merck in the United States in a program targeting new anticancer agents. It was subsequently found to have better immunosuppressive effects than antitumor activity, and Murphy and Morris at Stanford demonstrated its ability to suppress transplant rejection in 1991.[368, 577]

CHEMICAL STRUCTURE

Brequinar sodium is a quinoline carboxylic acid analogue produced by organic synthesis (Fig. 13–21).

MECHANISM OF IMMUNOSUPPRESSION

Brequinar is a reversible, noncompetitive inhibitor of dihydroorotate dehydrogenase, the fourth enzyme in the *de novo* pathway of pyrimidine synthesis. Its actions are relatively selective for inhibition of T- and B-cell proliferation, presumably because of the high level of RNA and DNA synthesis in activated immune cells which requires pyrimidine production via *de novo* as well as the salvage pathways. Brequinar suppresses antibody production response to both T-dependent and T-independent antigens and suppresses the induction of ICAM-1 and LFA-2 on activated lymphocytes.[356, 363] In mouse cardiac allografts, brequinar is as effective as sirolimus for reversing ongoing rejection in sensitized

recipients. However, the immunosuppressive efficacy is somewhat less in large animals. Of note, brequinar seems to be uniquely effective in suppressing the production of antidonor antibodies, and it has been shown to prolong allograft survival in presensitized rodents and to prolong concordant xenograft survival in rodents.[368] The effect of brequinar is potentiated by cyclosporine.

PHARMACOKINETICS

Brequinar is water soluble and has greater than 90% bioavailability after oral administration. It is metabolized primarily in the liver (66%) by the cytochrome P-450 enzyme system and by the kidney (23%).

DOSING

Appropriate dosing has not been established.

TOXICITY

Primary toxic effects in animals are leukopenia, thrombocytopenia, and diarrhea. This suggests that proliferation of bone marrow and epithelial cells depend more on the *de novo* pathway for pyrimidine synthesis than on the *de novo* pathway for purine synthesis. The toxic effects have not yet been well studied in man and the therapeutic window may be narrow.

LEFLUNOMIDE AND MALONONITRILAMIDE ANALOGS

HISTORICAL NOTE

Leflunomide, formerly called HWA-486, was derived from a group of compounds that were targeted as agricultural herbicides.

STRUCTURE

Leflunomide is a synthetic organic isoxazole derivative (Fig. 13–21). It is a prodrug with the active metabolite A77 1726, which is classified as a malononitrilamide.

MECHANISM OF IMMUNOSUPPRESSION

Leflunomide is unique from other immunosuppressive agents in that it provides effective suppression of both cellular and humoral immunity in many animal transplant models.[363] The active component inhibits proliferation of B-cells more strongly than T-cells and antagonizes cytokine effects on immune cells. Although the precise mechanisms of action are unknown, inhibition of *de novo* pyrimidine biosynthesis and inhibition of

IL-2 receptor-associated tyrosine kinases are likely mechanisms.[74]

In animal models, leflunomide successfully prevents and reverses acute allograft rejection in rats and potentiates the effects of low-dose cyclosporine.[366] This drug may have unique qualities in inhibiting the proliferation of smooth muscle cells and airway fibroblasts in a rat model of lung transplantation, suggesting a potential beneficial effect in experimental obliterative bronchiolitis.[368] Leflunomide inhibits antidonor antibody synthesis in rat heart transplant models and suppresses coronary artery narrowing.[327, 370]

PHARMACOKINETICS

Leflunomide is metabolized to its active form, A77 1726, which is water-soluble and comprises 90% of its metabolites.

DOSING

Clinical dosing in organ transplantation has not been established.

TOXICITY

No major toxicity has yet been identified with the clinical use of leflunomide in rheumatoid arthritis.[34] Anemia and loss of appetite have been identified in animal studies,[370] but further studies are needed to evaluate its toxicology in transplant patients.

CLINICAL EXPERIENCE

Leflunomide has been used in clinical trials of rheumatoid arthritis with minimal side effects.[95, 379] Although its future role in clinical cardiac transplantation is unknown, it is particularly attractive, since it appears to exhibit little myelotoxicity or nephrotoxicity compared to other clinical immunosuppressive agents.[34, 95, 296, 366, 367]

GUSPERIMUS (DEOXYSPERGUALIN)

HISTORICAL NOTE

Spergualin, the parent compound of gusperimus, was first isolated by Takeuchi in Tokyo from the microorganism *Bacillus laterosporus*.[507, 530]

CHEMICAL STRUCTURE

Gusperimus is a guanidino analog of the common polyamine spermidine (Fig. 13–21). The formula is $C_{17}H_{37}N_7O_3HCl$.

MECHANISM OF IMMUNOSUPPRESSION

The mechanism of action is unclear, but gusperimus binds to a cytosolic protein called heat shock cognate 70 (Hsc70) which is a member of the heat shock protein family.[382] Heat shock proteins may be involved in lymphocyte activation and they affect the folding and unfolding of proteins as well as the processing of class II MHC antigens.[534] Gusperimus is a potent inhibitor of the humoral response to B-cells.[172, 313, 508, 515, 530] In several animal systems, gusperimus produces donor-specific tolerance. It is also an effective agent for control of rejection, perhaps related to inhibition of macrophage proliferation. Based on rodent studies, gusperimus appears superior to cyclosporine in preventing allograft vasculopathy after cardiac transplantation, perhaps related to suppression of macrophage function and antibody production.[129, 172] However, its effect on preventing intimal proliferation is less than observed with mycophenolate mofetil or sirolimus.[194] Gusperimus is active against gram-positive and gram-negative bacteria and inhibits growth of some tumors. Unlike cyclosporine and tacrolimus, gusperimus does not inhibit IL-2 production.[129, 172]

Some experimental evidence points to blockade of NF-κB as an important immunosuppressive effect of gusperimus. NF-κB is a critical transcription factor for endothelial activation (gene up-regulation) in response to ischemia, atherosclerosis, and probably rejection.[154] It may be important in the induction of endogenous genes which are up-regulated during cytokine-induced endothelial activation. NF-κB is also required for expression of E-selection and ICAM-1.[566]

BIOAVAILABILITY

The oral availability of gusperimus is extremely low and it must therefore be administered intravenously.

TOXICITY

Reported side effects include leukopenia, thrombocytopenia, anemia, hepatotoxicity, facial numbness, and gastrointestinal disturbance.[16]

CLINICAL USE

Gusperimus has been approved for renal transplantation in Japan since 1994, but its potential role in cardiac transplantation remains to be clarified.[402]

POLYCLONAL ANTIBODIES

HISTORICAL NOTE

Polyclonal antilymphocyte preparations were the first lymphocyte-specific agents to be used in clinical transplantation. The first reports in the literature regarding the use of antilymphocyte sera as immunosuppressive agents appeared in the early 1960s.[192, 314, 359, 360, 574] These antisera were produced in rabbits by immunizing them with thoracic duct lymphocytes or thymocytes and then collecting the serum after a sufficient period for antilymphocyte antibodies to appear as assayed by the ability of the serum to deplete circulating lymphocytes.[574] Later, the antisera were assayed for their ability to inhibit graft rejection. These early papers showed the validity of the concept that depletion of lymphocytes or inhibition of their activity could prolong allograft survival. Initially employed as prophylaxis against rejection, these preparations were subsequently demonstrated to be highly effective against steroid-resistant rejection.[105, 491] The preparations have included a variety of immunogenic lymphoid cells, producing antilymphocyte serum (ALS), antilymphoblast globulin (ALG), and antithymocyte globulin (ATG).

MECHANISM OF IMMUNOSUPPRESSION

Polyclonal ATG preparations contain variable amounts of specific antibodies directed against T-cell molecules such as CD2, CD3, CD4, and CD8, and against B-cell molecules such as CD19, CD20, and CD21. Antibodies with preparations directed against HLA class I and class II antigens and adhesion molecules (CD 11a/CD18) have been identified[52] (Table 13–20). Several studies suggest that anti-CD45 antibodies in RATG (see Box) could play an important role in reversing rejection[52-54, 436] (Fig. 13–6).

Effective ATG preparations induce lymphocyte depletion which persists during and beyond the period of treatment. Proposed mechanisms for lymphocyte depletion include complement-dependent cytolysis[88] and induction of apoptosis through a Fas/Fas ligand activation.[63, 128, 239] Other possible mechanisms without supporting data include opsonization, homocytolysis, and margination (see section Anti-CD3 [OKT3, Muromonab, Orthoclone]). It has been postulated that the

Anti-CD45 Antibodies in RATG

A comprehensive study of the specificities within clinical ATG shows that the antibodies that persist the longest in vivo are specific for CD3, CD4, CD8, CD11a, CD40, CD45, and CD54. Of these, the CD45 antigen is interesting because the expression of different isoforms of CD45 has been associated with particular populations of T-cells. The higher molecular weight isoform, called CD45α (formely called CD45RA), has been used as a marker for unprimed, naive T-cells. The smaller isoform, CD45O (formerly called CD45RO) is associated with memory T-cells. CD45 is a protein tyrosine phosphorylase that plays a role in T-cell activation by regulating inducible tyrosine phosphorylation in cells of the hematopietic lineage. Perturbation of this molecule with antibodies can affect T-cell activation.[241] Monoclonal antibodies specific for CD45 have been shown to induce tolerance or reverse allograft rejection in animal models.[24, 303, 304, 586] Therefore, the ability of RATG to reverse allograft rejection is multifactorial, but the specificities directed against CD45 could play a significant role.

initial immunosuppressive effect is related to elimination of circulating T-cells and that the subsequent more prolonged effect may be in part due to suppressor cells.[331]

The ATG response is not limited to T-cells and B-cells, since it may also contain antibodies which react against monocytes, macrophages, neutrophils, platelets, and endothelial cells.[52, 54]

PREPARATION

In clinical transplantation, the animal source of antibody has typically been rabbit, horse, or goat. The immunogenic cells have been thymocytes from human thymus, thoracic duct lymphocytes, or lymphoblast (B-cells). Following administration of the selected immunogen, the animal is allowed to produce antibody after which serum is extracted and the IgG fraction is isolated.

METHOD OF ADMINISTRATION

Various preparations have been administered subcutaneously, intramuscularly, or intravenously; however, intravenous administration seems most desirable, since local tissue necrosis and painful sterile abscesses have occurred following subcutaneous or intramuscular injection. **Antithymocyte globulin (Atgam)** is a commercial preparation of purified equine immunoglobulin generated by immunization with human thymic lymphocytes. It must be administered through a central vein over 6–8 hours, at a dose of 15 mg/kg. The dose must occasionally be reduced or discontinued due to thrombocytopenia. The half-life of the immunoglobulins is approximately 3–10 days.

Another commercially available ATG preparation is a rabbit antithymocyte globulin **(Thymoglobulin)**. The

TABLE 13–20	Antithymocyte Globulin

Clinical use
- Antirejection prophylaxis (induction therapy), steroid-resistant or recurrent rejection, rejection with hemodynamic compromise.

Mechanism
- Polyclonal anti–T-cell antibody preparation that blocks surface receptors (inhibition of TCR/antigenic peptide interaction), impairs effectiveness of antigen-presenting cells, destroys T-lymphocytes.
- B-cell/antibody depletion.

Dose
- Specifics regarding dosage, premedications, and hypersensitivity testing vary according to specific antithymocyte preparation.

Monitoring parameters
- T-cell counts below 10% of pretreatment levels, but not routinely measured in many transplant centers.

Adverse effects
- Thrombocytopenia, arthralgias, edema, hives, fever, chills; vary according to preparation.
- Rarely major systemic reactions including hypotension, anaphylaxis, respiratory distress, serum sickness.

TCR, T-cell receptor.

reconstituted preparation contains 5 mg Thymoglobulin of which greater than 90% is rabbit gamma immune globulin. The standard dose of 1.5 mg/kg/day is infused through a central venous catheter over 4–6 hours, and administered for 7–14 days.[75]

MONITORING DURING ALS THERAPY

A major disadvantage of antilymphocyte preparation is the variability in potency of various batches due to the variable immune response of different animals. Furthermore, differing preparations vary greatly in their potency. Therefore, monitoring of T-cell numbers in peripheral blood with the use of T-cell-specific monoclonal antibodies is helpful in determining effect. T-cell markers should be obtained during the first 5 days of therapy. In general, depression of CD3+ cells to less than 10% of pretreatment values has correlated with efficacy. CD2 and CD3 T-cells are typically depressed to levels of 25 cells/mL within 48 hours of ATG administration. In pediatric patients, similar suppression of CD2+ and CD3+ cells has been documented.[306]

TOXICITY

Following a course of polyclonal antilymphocyte therapy, the development of serum antibodies to the antilymphocyte preparation is common.[393] If present in sufficient quantities, such antibodies could neutralize the effect of subsequent administration of the preparation. Although serum sickness is a potential complication of these preparations, it fortunately is rarely observed.[510] Patients are routinely tested with small epidermal injections of the polyclonal antibody preparation prior to receiving the first dose in order to minimize the possibility of anaphylactic reactions. Other side effects include chills and febrile reactions in 70–80% of patients with initial infusion, but in only 5–10% with subsequent infusions. These polyclonal preparations include significant quantities of extraneous antibodies that are reactive against antigens which may have wide tissue and cell distribution (e.g., on erythrocytes and platelets). Thrombocytopenia is particularly common with the commercial preparations of equine antithymocyte globulin (Atgam). Uncommonly, erythema and local phlebitis are observed.

Polyclonal antilymphocyte preparations share with monoclonal preparations such as OKT3 the propensity for subsequent viral infections[219] and viral driven malignancies. This is discussed in detail under OKT3 toxicity.

Two commercial preparations, Thymoglobulin and Atgam, share the same toxicity profile. In a multicenter, double-blind, randomized clinical trial comparing Thymoglobulin and Atgam in renal transplant recipients, the reported adverse effects were similar, and included fever and chills in over 50% of patients, and headache, abdominal pain, diarrhea, hypertension, and/or nausea in about one third of patients.[175] Malaise and/or dizziness occured in 5–25% of patients. The most important side effects during drug administration are leukopenia and thrombocytopenia, which are generally dose re-

lated. In a multicenter trial,[175] leukopenia was more common with Thymoglobulin than Atgam (57% vs. 30% p <.001), and the incidence of thrombocytopenia was similar between the two agents (36–44%). CMV and posttransplant lymphoproliferative disease (PTLD) are more common following cytolytic therapy with antilymphocyte preparations.

About two thirds of recipients receiving Thymoglobulin will develop anti-rabbit antibodies, and about three fourths of patients receiving Atgam develop anti-horse antibodies. Patients with an allergy to rabbits should not receive Thymoglobulin and those with horse allergies should not receive Atgam.

CLINICAL USE

Some antilymphocyte preparations have been extremely effective as induction therapy and as therapy for steroid-resistant rejection (Table 13–20). They are currently most commonly used in place of OKT3, either as induction therapy or when the patient has already received a course of OKT3 (see section on clinical use of OKT3). Several studies have found increased freedom from rejection and rejection mortality with RATG compared to OKT3 prophylaxis.[302] Rabbit antithymocyte globulin has been successfully applied as prophylacic "induction" therapy in pediatric heart transplantation.[306] The major disadvantage of such sera is the marked differences in potency of different preparations, as noted above. The equine antithymocyte globulin Atgam has been generally disappointing because of great variability in observed potency and the frequency (>30%) of thrombocytopenia with its use. The rabbit antithymocyte globulin (Thymoglobulin) has undergone extensive clinical trials as an antirejection therapy in renal transplantation.[175, 205] Compared to an equine antithymocyte globulin (Atgam), Thymoglobulin was more successful in reversing acute renal allograft rejection (78% vs. 67.5%) in a 7- to 14-day course of therapy.

Thymoglobulin is currently our polyclonal preparation of choice, administered for either prophylactic induction therapy or steroid-resistant recurrent rejection (see Chapter 14). Because of the potential for CMV, patients undergoing ATG should receive intravenous ganciclovir while receiving ATG and oral ganciclivir for 6 weeks following treatment (see Table 15–9). Because of the risk of overimmunosuppression and possible posttransplant lymphoproliferative disease, the duration of therapy should be limited to 14 days or less unless life-threatening rejection is persisting.

MONOCLONAL ANTIBODIES

Monoclonal antibodies provide an attractive method for immunosuppression therapy because their specificity provides a means by which specific cell surface molecules can be targeted. The specificity and uniformity of monoclonal antibodies offers a potential advantage over the variability and lack of specificity of polyclonal preparations. They can be used as a blockade of specific receptor-ligand interactions, or they can be used to deplete cells bearing a particular cell surface molecule. Therefore, the mechanism by which immunosuppression occurs and the side effects associated with that activity depends on the target of the antibody and the isotype and species used to generate the antibody. Monoclonal antibodies are usually derived from mice or rats and can also be composed of a number of different isotypes that can strongly affect the *in vivo* effector activity. These same variables also affect the probability that a human transplant recipient treated with the monoclonal antibody will produce antibodies specific for the portions of the monoclonal antibody that are antigenic to humans. In some cases such as the current anti–IL-2 receptor drugs, the antibodies have been "humanized." This means that the portions of the genes that do not code for the antigen-binding regions of the mouse monoclonal antibody have been removed and replaced with genes that code for the nonantigen-binding portions of a human antibody molecule. The end result is a human antibody with the specificity of the mouse monoclonal antibody. Since most of the resulting molecule is from a human, the probability that an individual who received the monoclonal antibody would produce antibodies specific for the parts of the molecule other than the variable region are greatly reduced.

The ultimate goal of monoclonal antibody antirejection therapy is the induction of short-term, highly selective inhibition of the immune system to induce donor-specific unresponsiveness, possibly with a combination of antibodies. A large number of monoclonal antibodies have been tested in clinical and experimental transplantation, but currently only OKT3, basiliximab, and daclizumab are approved by the FDA for clinical use in solid organ transplantation in the United States (Table 13–21).

ANTI-CD3 (OKT3, MUROMONAB, ORTHOCLONE)

Historical Note

The development of monoclonal antibodies was dependent on the observations that each B-lymphocyte of an

TABLE 13–21	Monoclonal Antibodies Used in Clinical Organ Transplantation			
ANTIBODY NAME	TARGET ANTIGEN	ANTIGEN FUNCTION	ANTIGEN DISTRIBUTION	EVIDENCE OF EFFICACY (Y/N)
BTI-332	CD2	Adhesion/activation		N
BMA031	T-cell receptor heterodimer	Antigen/MHC receptor	All T-cells	?
T10B9.1A-31				Y
OKT3	CD3			Y
WT-32				Y
OKT4	CD4	Accessory molecule	T-cell subpopulations	Y
Cdr4a				Y
BL4				N
B-F5				N
MAX. 16H5				Y
MT151				N
Anti-T12	CD6(T12)	Signal transduction?	Peripheral blood T-cells, thymocytes	Y
SDZCHH380	CD7	Unknown	Hematopoietic cells, mostly of T-cell lineage	N
Leu-2A	CD8	Accessory molecule	T-cell subpopulation	N
Basiliximab (Simulect)	CD25	IL-2 receptor	Activated T-cells	Y
Daclizumab (Zenopax)				Y
AntiCD45	CD45	Phosphotyrosine phosphatase	All hematopoietic derived cells except erythrocytes, including APCs	Y
Campath 1	CD52	Unknown	Thymocytes, T-cells, B-cells	Y
25-3	CD11a/CD18 (LFA-1)	Adhesion	Lymphocytes, monocytes, granulocytes, macrophages	N
BIRRI	CD54(ICAM-1)	Adhesion	Activated T-cells and B-cells, monocytes	Y

APCs, antigen-presenting cells.

immunized animal produces a single specific antibody and that malignant myeloma cells can be grown permanently in culture and produce antibodies with no predefined specificity. The critical breakthrough in monoclonal technology occurred in 1975 when Kohler and Milstein succeeded in fusing both cell types. This produced a hybridoma cell line with permanent growth and the production of a monoclonal antibody with known specificity and a useless myeloma protein.[280] The significance of the production of monoclonal antibodies with antilymphocyte activity[297, 439] was soon appreciated, and clinical trials of the use of such antibodies as immunosuppressants were initiated in 1980,[124] beginning with a trial in renal transplantation reported by Cosimi and colleagues.[105]

Preparation

Monoclonal antibodies differ from other antilymphocyte preparations by their purity. Each molecule of the specific monoclonal product is identical to other molecules in both the constant and variable regions of the immunoglobulin, since each molecule is produced by a single clone of immunized lymphocytes which are fused with myeloma cells and maintained in tissue culture. The use of humanized antibodies also allows the initiation of antibody-mediated effector responses in contrast to murine antibodies that are unable to mediate functions such as antibody-dependent cytotoxicity.

To prepare murine monoclonal antibodies, mice are injected with a "priming" dose of the specific T-cell component as antigen, followed by a subsequent booster dose. In 4–6 weeks, spleen cells are extracted from the immunized mice, isolated, and fused with mouse myeloma cells (Fig. 13–22).[428]

Chemistry/Mechanism of Immunosuppression

The CD3 antigen is present on essentially all mature T-lymphocytes and is closely linked to the antigen recognition site of the T-cell receptor. Following engagement of the T-cell receptor to antigen outside the cell, the CD3 complex transmits an intracellular signal which initiates T-cell activation.[392, 563]

OKT3 is a murine monoclonal antibody of the IgG2a isotype that is specific for the 20-kDa ε-chain of the CD3 complex, which constitutes the part of the T-cell receptor that is involved in transmembrane signaling following the binding of an antigen–MHC complex (Fig. 13–1). Since CD3 is expressed only on T-cells, administration of OKT3 results in depletion of CD3 cells from the peripheral blood in 30–60 minutes[90, 91, 517] as indicated by a lack of staining for CD3+ cells and a similar lack of cells staining for CD4 or CD8.[100] After 3–5 days, CD3- lymphocytes expressing CD4 or CD8 can be found in the circulation, indicating the presence of T-cells in which modulation of the T-cell receptor (see Box) has occurred[90, 91] by either endocytosis or shedding of the CD3 antigen.[93, 428] These T-cells are unresponsive to mitogens and to alloantigens in vitro,[90, 91] a state that correlates with the lack of responsiveness to alloantigens in vivo.

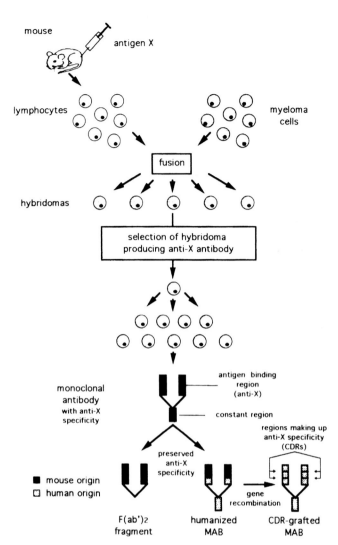

FIGURE **13–22.** Fusion of a myeloma cell with a lymphocyte produces an immortal cell line that secretes a specific monoclonal antibody (MAB). This murine MAB can then be humanized with recombinant DNA technology. (From Powelson JA, Knowles RW, Delmonico FL, Kawai T, Mourad G, Preffer FI, Colvin RB, Cosimi B: CDR-grafted OKT4A monoclonal antibody in cynomolgus renal allograft recipients. Transplantation 1994;57:788–793, with permission.)

The number of T-cells increases more rapidly after cessation of treatment than with ATG, and often reaches pretreatment levels within days.

Several mechanisms have been invoked to explain the rapid depletion of T-cells following OKT3 administration, including opsonization and phagocytosis with subsequent removal by the reticuloendothelial system, lysis of bystander T-cells (homocytolysis),[573] margination of the cells after up-regulation of adhesion molecules,[69] induction of apoptosis,[232] and complement activation (Fig. 13–24). Homocytolysis may be mediated by bivalent anti-CD3 antibodies crosslinking CD3 molecules on different T-cells, therefore causing them to contact each other, activate, and lyse the other T-cell. Induction of apoptosis following cell activation is an important means by which the immune system maintains homeostasis, particularly as a means of limiting the clonal expansion of T-cells. Therefore, continued stimulation

Modulation of the T-cell Receptor

The term "modulation" in this context refers to the disappearance of an antigen from the cell surface following exposure to monoclonal or polyclonal antibodies specific for that surface antigen. One of the earliest observations of this phenomenon was made when B-cells were studied by immunofluorescence microscopy using antibodies specific for surface immunoglobulins. When B-cells are stained using such antibodies (e.g., fluoresceinated anti-IgG), the entire cell surface is stained diffusely. After several minutes, the staining begins to coalesce into patches and then aggregates into a single area of the cell such that the staining is highly polarized. This polarized staining, called "capping," lasts from minutes to hours depending on the cell type. The caps are eventually internalized and degraded, or are shed. The aggregation of molecules on the cell surface following exposure to antibody is a function of crosslinking molecules with two or more antigenic epitopes on the cell surface by divalent antibodies. The process of forming patches of fluorescence is apparently passive, but the forma-

tion of caps requires an active metabolic process and membrane movement.

The process of capping, when it culminates in the disappearance of an antigen from the cell surface, is called *modulation* (Fig. 13–23). Cells that modulate surface antigens will usually reexpress them in a matter of hours. OKT3 causes capping of CD3 molecules on the surface of T-lymphocytes *in vitro* within 30 minutes[91] and modulation in a few hours.[329] This same process also occurs *in vivo* when transplant recipients are treated with OKT3. Administration of OKT3 results in a rapid decline (within 1 hour) in the proportion of CD3+, CD4+, and CD8+ lymphocytes,[90, 91] indicating that T-cells have been removed from the circulation. By days 2–5, the proportion of CD3+ cells is nearly 0%,[90, 91, 180, 329] although approximately 30–40% of the lymphoid cells that remain express CD4 and CD8, indicating that there is a subpopulation of T-cells in which the CD3 complex is masked, modulated, or shed.[90, 91, 180, 329] This process appears to require the continuous presence of OKT3, since incubation of the cells *in vitro* results in the reexpression of the CD3 complex within 24 hours.[90, 91, 180, 329]

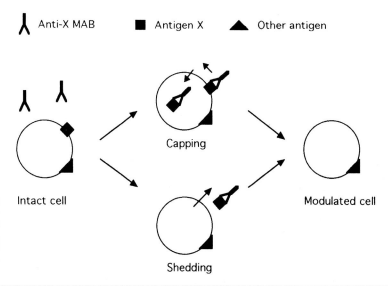

FIGURE **13–23.** Antigenic modulation. Some MABs modify the antigenic characteristics of target cells without changing their number. (From Powelson JA, Knowles RW, Delmonico FL, Kawai T, Mourad G, Preffer FI, Colvin RB, Cosimi B: CDR-grafted OKT4A monoclonal antibody in cynomolgus renal allograft recipients. Transplantation 1994;57:788–793, with permission.)

of the T-cells via the antigen receptor following activation in the absence of a costimulatory signal could result in the induction of apoptosis.[101, 353, 433, 434] Furthermore, OKT3 induces the expression of Fas, a cell surface molecule that induces apoptosis following its ligation with Fas-ligand.

When OKT3 is discontinued or the serum level of OKT3 falls below therapeutic levels, the CD3 molecules are reexpressed on the TCR complex within a few hours.[90, 91] The rapidity of return of CD3+ T-cells to the circulation is probably a function of the relative number of T-cells that are destroyed during the OKT3 therapy versus circulating or demarginated cells that are intact but modulated.

This phenomenon of rapid reappearance of CD3+ cells soon after discontinuation of therapy (which does not occur after treatment with polyclonal ATG), coupled with clinical observations of occasional acute rejection

episodes within a week of ending OKT3 therapy, have prompted some transplant programs to routinely augment steroid doses for several days after completing OKT3.

There is a theoretical basis for an additional effect of cytolytic therapy on antibody production. Except for a special class of antigens called T-independent antigens, the **generation of an antibody response requires the participation of T-cells** in the form of contact between T-cells and B-cells and through the secretion of cytokines by T-cells. The central point of interaction between T-cells and B-cells is through the antigen/MHC receptor on T-cells and antigen presented in the context of MHC class II on the surface of B-cells. A number of other molecules also participate in this interaction, including leukocyte function associated molecule (LFA)-3 with CD2, intercellular adhesion molecule (ICAM)-1 or ICAM-3 with LFA-1, B7-1 or B7-2 with CD28, and CD40

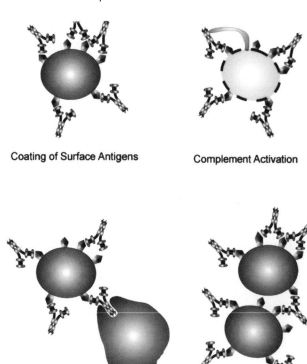

Coating of Surface Antigens

Complement Activation

Fc Receptor Mediated
Conjugation & Cytolysis

Crosslinking

FIGURE **13–24.** Antibodies can interfere with immune responses by a variety of mechanisms. The antibody binds to a surface molecule and, if situated in the appropriate place, can hinder the function of a molecule by binding directly to an active site, or by steric hindrance because of proximity to the active site. If the antibody is of the appropriate isotype, it can activate complement, resulting in the lysis of the target cell. The Fc region of antibody molecules can also serve as a ligand for Fc receptors of inflammatory cells, which can then mediate the destruction of a cell by secretion of lethal soluble factors. Crosslinking of molecules on the cell surface can interfere with the membrane mobility of surface molecules and can also cause aggregation of cells, therefore interfering with mobility and homing.

with CD40-ligand. The latter interaction is particularly important in the activation of B-cells. The interaction of CD40 with CD40-ligand on T-cells delivers a potent activating signal in B-cells that results in the entry of B-cells into the cell cycle. This is an important component in the formation of germinal centers in lymph nodes. This signal via CD40 is apparently required for isotype switching by B-cells. Patients that have the immune deficiency disease, hyper-IgM syndrome, have a mutation in the gene that codes for CD40-ligand. These patients can produce low-affinity IgM antibodies, but cannot switch to the production of high-affinity antibodies of the IgG and IgA isotypes because contact between CD40-ligand on T-cells with CD40 on B-cells is required for isotype switching. T-cells also produce a number of cytokines that act on B-cells. IL-2 is a growth factor for both T-cells and B-cells. IL-4 has effects on B-cell differentiation and proliferation, as does IL-6, IFN-γ, IL-11, and IL-13. Therefore, a reduction of the mass of T-cells in the lymph nodes could have the effect of inhibiting B-cell activation and isotype switching. Modulation of the T-cell receptor from the surface of T-cells will

also interfere with this process. Further discussion of B-cell activation is found in Chapter 2.

Dosing and Duration of Therapy

OKT3 is usually administered in a dose of 5 mg (one vial contains 5 mL with 1 mg/mL) daily for 7–14 days (Table 13–22). In most adults, 2.5 mg/day is also effective in depleting CD3$^+$ cells,[14] but its effectiveness should be ascertained by monitoring with lymphocyte phenotyping (T-cell markers). If sufficient T-cell suppression is not achieved with 5-mg doses, then 7.5- or, rarely, 10-mg doses may be effective. In pediatric patients, a dose of 0.1–0.2 mg/kg/dose is usually effective, but monitoring of T-cell markers is necessary to ensure effective T-cell depletion.

The recommended duration of OKT3 therapy is highly variable and without clear data to support a given protocol. Most centers currently employ a 5- to 10-day course of OKT3 for induction therapy (prophylaxis), aiming for therapeutic cyclosporine levels (300–400 ng/mL) by the completion of OKT3. When used for rejection therapy, 7–10 days are recommended, with augmentation of prednisone doses (for several days to a week) following completion of OKT3 because of the subsequent rapid reappearance of CD3$^+$ lymphocytes.

Monitoring of Blood Levels/T-Cell Markers

In patients treated with 5 mg/day for 14 days, mean serum trough levels steadily rise to approximately 900 ng/mL and remain there for the succeeding 11 days. Effective and continuous depletion of T-cells requires serum levels higher than 800 ng/mL.[462] However, in clinical practice OKT3 levels are rarely employed. Quantitative lymphocyte phenotyping (T-cell markers) is often performed, especially when doses less than 5 mg/day are utilized in adults, in children, or when OKT3 has been previously administered. The target is nearly complete suppression of CD3$^+$ peripheral blood lym-

TABLE 13-22	OKT3

Clinical use
- Antirejection prophylaxis (induction therapy), steroid-resistant or recurrent rejection, rejection with hemodynamic compromise.

Mechanism
- Monoclonal anti-CD3 antibody that blocks alloantigen recognition by modulation or depletion of CD3 molecules from T-cell surface.
- T-cell depletion.

Dose
- 2.5–5 mg IV daily usually for 7–14 days. In pediatric patients, 0.1–0.2 mg/kg/dose with dose adjustment by T-cell markers.

Monitoring parameters
- Measurement of T-cell markers, with a target suppression of CD3$^+$ cells to an absolute cell count of < 10 cells/mL and less than 5% of total lymphocytes.

Adverse effects
- Cytokine release syndrome: fever, chills, headache, nausea, myalgias, mild hypertension. Rarely, bronchospasm, and profound hypotension.
- Production of antimurine antibodies.
- Increased susceptibility to CMV infection and posttransplant lymphoproliferative disorder, particularly with repeat or prolonged administration.

phocytes (<10% of total lymphocytes and absolute count <20/mL).

Sensitization

Since OKT3 is a murine antibody, human anti-mouse antibodies may form following initial administration or during prolonged administration (> about 14 days).[399] Using the ELISA method, O'Connell and colleagues reported a 14% incidence of human anti-mouse antibody formation following a 14-day induction protocol. Others have reported greater than 50% incidence,[218] particularly with more prolonged administration.[399]

Thus, it is advisable to measure for the production of human anti-mouse antibodies when a second course of OKT3 is administered or if CD3+ lymphocytes cannot be suppressed. This is typically done using an ELISA to measure human anti-mouse antibodies in serial dilutions of the patient serum. If antibodies develop, they are generally present in titers >1:1,000 3–4 weeks after completing OKT3 therapy. When sensitization is identified, OKT3 is unlikely to be effective and should be discontinued in favor of other immunosuppressive modalities.

Adverse Reactions/Toxicity

A number of adverse reactions can occur following the administration of OKT3. The most common is chills and fever approximately 30–60 minutes after injection, a phenomenon that has been termed "cytokine release syndrome." It is characterized by fever, chills, generalized weakness, myalgias, and mild hypotension. Less commonly, the patient experiences nausea, vomiting, diarrhea, and rarely bronchospasm or severe hypotension. When the OKT3 antibody molecules coat T-cells and then bind to Fc receptors on monocytes, the T-cells are transiently activated, resulting in the production of a number of cytokines, including IL-2, IL-6, IFN-γ, and TNF.[87, 88, 92, 186, 391] Treatment of patients with agents that reduce the release of cytokines or that effectively remove some cytokines from the circulation tend to reduce the severity of the symptoms.[86, 88, 89, 337, 401] Initially, this phenomenon was called a "first dose reaction" by some groups, but further evidence suggests that these effects may recur (usually to a lesser degree) after subsequent doses.[536] Occasional patients develop a flu-like syndrome for 3–5 days following the first dose. Treatment of these side effects has included administration of corticosteroids before and following administration of OKT3,[159] antihistamines, and antipyretics.[160] A variety of treatment protocols have been used, and a typical protocol is presented in Table 13–23. Although unproven, our own experience suggests that the first dose cytokine syndrome may be ameliorated by administering the first day's dose in three separate doses of 1, 1, and 2.5 mg about 4 hours apart. Alternatively, prevention of the cytokine syndrome has been reported by infusing the first dose of 5 mg over 2 hours instead of as a bolus.

Rarely, aseptic meningitis or encephalopathy have been associated with OKT3 administration.[52, 198]

Anti–T-cell preparations like OKT3 and polyclonal antilymphocyte preparations suppress cell-mediated

TABLE 13–23	Protocol for Reduction of Adverse Reactions During OKT3 Administration

Adult patients
- Administer methylprednisolone 1 g IV 1 h prior to first 3 OKT3 doses
- Benadryl 50 mg IV prior to first OKT3 doses, then 25 mg IV prior to subsequent doses
- Tylenol 650 mg PO or PR prior to each OKT3 dose
- Pepcid 20 mg IV prior to and bid for first 3 OKT3 doses, then bid for remaining doses
- If symptoms of fever, chills, nausea continue, increase Benadryl to bid or tid and Tylenol to every 6–12 h

Pediatric patients
- Methylprednisolone 15–20 mg/kg IV 1 h prior to first 3 OKT3 doses
- Benadryl 1 mg/kg IV prior to first 3 doses
- Tylenol 10 mg/kg PO/PV prior to each dose
- Pepcid 0.5 mg/kg IV prior to and bid first 3 doses and bid thereafter
- If symptoms of fever or chills persist, continue Tylenol and Benedryl bid or tid throughout OKT3 course

immunity against viruses.[94] Herpes simplex stomatitis and CMV infections have been reported with greater frequency after antilymphocyte cytolytic therapy.[452] The risk of CMV infection following ATG or OKT3 induction therapy is greatest in the setting of a recipient with negative CMV serology who receives a heart from a donor with positive CMV serology.[216, 268] Although unproven, extensive clinical experience suggests that ganciclovir prophylaxis during and following OKT3 or ATG decreases the likelihood of subsequent CMV infection (see Chapter 15).

Latent Epstein-Barr virus (EBV) may also be reactivated following OKT3 or ATG therapy, potentially inducing transformation of an EBV-dependent polyclonal B-cell population to a malignant monoclonal B-cell lymphoma.[414] An increased incidence of PTLD has been noted among heart transplant patients treated with OKT3, particularly with a cumulative dose of 75 mg or more in adults.[505] Lymphomas have included B-cell, T-cell, large cell, Burkitt's, and other cell types (see Chapter 18 for further discussions).

Drug Interactions

Drug interactions are uncommon. Encephalopathy has been reported in association with the use of indomethicin at the time of OKT3 administration.[83]

Clinical Use

Early studies in renal transplantation demonstrated that OKT3 was highly effective in reversing acute allograft rejection.[512] Subsequent studies in liver transplantation and heart transplantation (both in pediatric and adult)[214, 467] have confirmed this finding. In cardiac transplantation, OKT3 with continued maintenance immunosuppression plus augmented steroids reverses over 90% of acute rejection episodes which do not respond to pulse steroid therapy.[214]

OKT3 has also been widely employed as **"induction" therapy** at the time of transplantation for the first 7–14 days.[168, 467] Although renal allograft survival was clearly increased when OKT3 induction was used with azathioprine and steroids, its benefit with cyclosporine-based immunosuppression has been controversial. In heart transplantation, numerous studies have reported similar rejection frequency and survival with and without OKT3 induction. Multiple studies comparing polyclonal (ATG) preparations versus OKT3 as induction therapy have failed to show clear superiority of either approach.[5, 111, 112, 266, 284, 293, 299, 350, 351, 375, 440, 488, 572] In a single institutional study, OKT3 and equine anti-human thymocyte globulin as prophylactic therapy produced similar survival and freedom from rejection. Using multivariable analyses of multi-institutional data, OKT3 prophylaxis does not appear to improve survival. It does delay the onset of initial rejection, but the frequency of rejection during the first year is unchanged.[279] Similar findings have been noted in pediatric cardiac transplantation.[467]

The major **current indication for OKT3** is recurrent or persistent rejection despite pulse therapy with intravenous methylprednisolone. A standard protocol would utilize OKT3 for the second of two rejection episodes occurring within a 1-month period during the first 3–6 months following transplantation. In the presence of hemodynamic compromise, OKT3 should be considered as part of an initial antirejection strategy (if it has not previously been utilized) (see also Chapter 14 for further discussion of rejection therapy).

Prophylactic use of OKT3 as induction therapy is probably not advisable on a routine basis. However, it is particularly useful in two general situations: (1) patients at higher risk for early rejection, including patients with prior sensitization (elevated pretransplant panel reactive antibody screen) and patients with a positive B-cell crossmatch at the time of transplant (see Chapter 7), and (2) patients with renal dysfunction in whom cyclosporine target blood levels will be delayed.

ANTI-CD25 (BASILIXIMAB, DACLIZUMAB)

The ideal immunosuppressive agent would have the ability to suppress or neutralize only those T-cell subsets which were destined to attack the allograft, while leaving other immunity intact. The properties of anti-CD25 monoclonal antibodies are a step in that direction.

Background

The first anti–IL-2 receptor (anti-CD25) monoclonal antibody was produced by immunizing mice with a peripheral blood T-cell line that had been actively proliferating.[188] One hybridoma that was produced by fusion of B-cells from these mice reacted to T-cells stimulated by mitogens or alloantigens, but not with freshly isolated resting T-cells. More complete characterization of the antibody showed that it bound to a surface antigen (Tac) primarily found on activated T-cells.[529] From the perspective of immunosuppression, more interesting properties of anti-Tac soon emerged. It was found to inhibit the appearance of the Tac antigen and also to inhibit the appearance of MHC class II antigens on T-

cells.[527] We now know that both of the surface antigens are markers of T-cell activation; therefore, it is apparent that the anti-Tac antibody suppressed T-cell activation. This important property was quickly appreciated when the Tac antigen was identified as a receptor for IL-2, and the antibody could abrogate IL-2 dependent proliferation of cultured T-cells and also suppress IL-2–induced RNA synthesis. Furthermore, it was found that the addition of IL-2 could reverse the anti-Tac inhibition.[127] Molecular cloning of the human IL-2 receptor showed that the Tac surface antigen and the IL-2 receptor are, in fact, identical.[311, 395] The possibility that anti–IL-2 receptor antibodies could be used for immunosuppression was demonstrated in rodents in which the anti–IL-2 receptor antibodies inhibited allograft rejection[270, 320, 509] and reduced cellular infiltration in cyclosporine-treated animals.[320] A preliminary trial in monkeys showed a modest but significant prolongation of renal allograft survival.[437] In humans, the same monoclonal antibodies were shown to reduce the number of rejection episodes during the first 10 days after transplantation, provided that they were administered with cyclosporine.[272] Since these initial observations, a number of clinical studies have been performed.

Chemistry/Mechanism of Immunosuppression

Since the first anti-Tac antibody was produced, a number of monoclonal antibodies have been generated. One of the primary disadvantages of the use of murine and rat monoclonal antibodies as immunosuppressive agents is that they are xenogeneic proteins and therefore are highly immunogenic. This can result in a poor antibody persistence. To counteract this problem, two approved antibodies are "humanized," meaning that most of the variable region, which determines the specificity of binding, is derived from the original hybridoma (except for the framework regions), but the constant regions are human. The rationale is that the humanized antibody will be less antigenic and therefore not elicit as much antibody production. There is evidence that the response to isotypic (i.e., constant region) determinants is reduced.[206]

Two of the currently approved antibodies, **basiliximab** (Simulect) and **daclizumab** (Zenopax), are humanized IgG1 monoclonal antibodies that bind specifically to the α-chain (Tac subunit) of the high-affinity IL-2 receptor on activated T-lymphocytes (Fig. 13–1). They are composed of approximately 90% human and 10% murine antibody sequences. However, they are distinctly different antibodies with different pharmacokinetics. These antibodies compete with the cytokine IL-2 for occupancy of the IL-2 receptor. A necessary step in T-cell activation is the secretion of IL-2 by a T-cell, which itself is stimulated by IL-2 in an autocrine fashion, and also serves to recruit other T-cells by stimulation in a paracrine fashion, all via the IL-2 receptor. This interaction between IL-2 and its receptor is necessary for clonal expansion. The IL-2 receptor is composed of three transmembrane proteins: a 55-kDa α-chain (CD25, also called Tac antigen) and 70-kDa β- (CD122) and γ-

(CD132) chains. The IL-2 receptors are present on the T-cell surface as high-, intermediate- and low-affinity binding sites. The high-affinity site is a complex of CD25 (Tac antigen) and the β-chain. The isolated β-chain has an intermediate affinity and the isolated CD25 site is a low-affinity site. The β- and γ-chains transduce a signal that results in differentiation and entry into the cell cycle. The IL-2 and IL-15 receptors share the β-chain, and the β-chain is also shared by other cytokine receptors, including the IL-7 receptor.[29, 283, 397] The specificity of the inhibition of alloreactive T-cell proliferation by anti–IL-2R antibodies arises from the fact that resting T-cells do not express appreciable quantities of CD25. Following antigenic stimulation and T-cell activation, CD25 is up-regulated and therefore susceptible to anti-Tac antibodies. Thus, resting T-cells reactive with other antigens (e.g., CMV) are relatively unaffected.

Basiliximab is a chimeric antibody, retaining the murine elements of the variable portion of the immunoglobulin chain. Daclizumab is more completely humanized, retaining a smaller region of the murine antibody. Daclizumab requires a higher concentration (about 10-fold) than basiliximab for effective binding to IL-2 receptors, though daclizumab may have less immunogenicity. However, the incidence of human anti-mouse antibodies has been low (<1%) with either agent.[431, 540]

These anti–IL-2 receptor monoclonal antibodies are designed to be used with a calcineurin blocking agent (cyclosporine or tacrolimus) to decrease the amount of IL-2 which would be available for any unblocked IL-2 receptors. Controversey exits regarding how soon cyclosporine or tacrolimus should be administered after transplant in order to get the maximal synergistic effect, but cyclosporine should probably be started within 2–4 days after transplantation.

Pharmacokinetics

Basiliximab has a terminal half-life of about 7 days in adults and 11–12 days in children. Saturation of IL-2 receptors is obtained *in vivo* as long as serum levels are greater than 0.2 μg/mL. At the recommended dosing schedules, the average time that IL-2 receptor saturation is maintained is 36 days.

Daclizumab using the recommended dosing schedule yields a peak serum concentration after the first dose of about 21 μg/mL and 32 μg/mL after the fifth dose. Mean trough level after the fifth dose is about 7.5 μg/mL. The terminal half-life for elimination is about 20 days.

Dosing

Basiliximab is supplied as a buffered saline solution containing 20 mg antibody. The recommended administration is in 50 mL normal saline via a peripheral (not central) line over 20–30 minutes. Adults should be given two doses of 20 mg each, with the first dose administered within 2 hours prior to transplantation. The second dose should be administered 4 days later. Children and adolescents (2–15 years of age) should be given 12-mg doses using the same schedule as adults.

Daclizumab is supplied in 5 mL buffered saline at 5 mg/mL. The recommended dose is 1 mg/kg. The calculated dose should be diluted in 50 mL normal saline and administered intravenously over 15 minutes. Each patient is given five doses, with the first dose given no more than 24 hours prior to transplantation. The next four doses are administered every 14 days.

These dosing schedules were determined in renal transplant patients. Given the importance of achieving suitable blood levels for effective IL-2 receptor blockade, the dilutional effect of cardiopulmonary bypass (CPB) and the potential for antibody loss in the perfusion circuit must be considered when establishing dosing protocols in heart transplantation. It has not been established whether it is most efficacious to give the initial dose prior to CPB (as the standard dose or a higher dose), immediately following CPB, or when the patient arrives in the intensive care unit.

Plasma/Blood Monitoring

Blood levels can be determined using ELISA, but are generally not used clinically.

Toxicity

No overdoses have been reported, and the maximum tolerated dose has not been determined. No serious adverse reactions have been reported in patients given 60 mg of basiliximab in a single dose or 1.5 mg/kg of daclizumab. The cytokine "first-dose" effect seen with OKT3 does not occur with anti-Tac preparations. Insufficient clinical experience exists to make definitive statements about late complications.

Drug Interactions

No significant interactions are known. Both agents have been administered with azathioprine, cyclosporine, tacrolimus, ATG, OKT3, mycophenolate mofetil, and steroids without apparent adverse effects. It should be noted that OKT3 has been administered following both agents, without an apparent increase in the incidence of anti-mouse human antibodies.

Clinical Use

Studies in renal transplantation suggest that prophylactic use of anti–IL-2 receptor monoclonal antibodies delays the onset of rejection.[73] A multi-institutional study in renal transplantation compared daclizumab to placebo in a dose of 1 mg/kg IV before transplant and every other week after transplant for a total of five doses.[539] Fewer patients had rejection with daclizumab than with placebo (22% vs. 35%, $p = .03$) at 12 months. No differences were observed in the incidence of infection or lymphoma. In another study, an anti-Tac monoclonal antibody significantly delayed the time to first rejection after renal transplantation without a clear benefit in patient or graft survival.[271] Anti–IL-2 receptor antibodies were not effective in reversing acute ongoing allograft rejection.

The exact role of monoclonal antibodies against IL-2R in cardiac transplantation remains to be determined. In one randomized trial comparing OKT3 with anti–IL-2R monoclonal antibodies, the incidence of early rejection was 50% with IL-2R therapy versus 9% with OKT3.[181] Furthermore, although the anti–IL-2R treatment eliminated CD25+ cells from peripheral blood, CD25+ cells were found in 80% of endomyocardial specimens from rejecting hearts. It is also noteworthy that the anti–IL-2R antibodies were started after the patient returned from the transplant procedure rather than preoperatively. The authors hypothesized that the synergistic effect of cyclosporine with anti–IL-2R therapy may require early initiation of cyclosporine (within the first 1–2 days after transplant).

In another study of 34 primary heart transplant recipients randomized to daclizumab plus triple-drug immunosuppression (cyclosporine, prednisone, and mycophenolate) versus triple drug alone, daclizumab was administered at a dose of 1 mg/kg IV prior to transplant and every 2 weeks for a total of five doses. Patients who received daclizumab experienced fewer rejection episodes and a longer interval to the first rejection episode.[39]

Future Role of Anti-CD25 Blockade

If studies in heart transplant recipients are as promising with as few side effects as those in renal transplantation, anti-CD25 therapy will likely become a routine component of initial "induction" immunosuppression in heart transplantation. Protocols will need to be evaluated which specify the optimal timing of administration with respect to cardiopulmonary bypass and the number of days that cyclosporine can be held (in the presence of renal dysfunction) and the anti-CD25 blockade still be effective.

MONOCLONAL ANTIBODIES AGAINST CO-STIMULATORY MOLECULES

Anti-CD4 Monoclonal Antibodies

Background and Mechanism of Action

CD4+ cells are important in the early phases of responses to alloantigens. The CD4 molecule functions as an accessory molecule during interactions between helper-inducer T-cells and antigen-presenting cells bearing MHC class II gene products by binding to a monomorphic domain of the MHC molecule. It increases the affinity of binding between T-cells and the antigen-presenting cells,[291] and is also associated with the p56 lck tyrosine kinase that mediates a signal into the interior of the T-cell (see also Chapter 2). Thus, the CD4 molecule plays an important role in T-cell activation, particularly during the early phases when antigen presentation takes place. By functionally inactivating CD4+ T-cells, anti-CD4 monoclonal antibodies inhibit cell-mediated alloimmunity and prevent the participation of CD4+ T-cells in antibody responses. Although CD4+ cells are typically removed from the circulation by these antibodies, some antibodies extend graft survival without removing CD4+ cells from the circulation. The reasons for this variability are unclear, but they relate to the fact that each of these monoclonal antibodies binds to different epitopes of the CD4 molecule. Possible explanations for the mechanism of CD4 suppression could be: (1) blocking of the CD4/MHC class II interaction resulting in a failure to activate T-cells; (2) blocking as above, but resulting in a single signal to graft MHC-specific T-cells (cells that receive signals via the T-cell receptor but do not receive a signal via the CD4 accessory molecule can be anergized, i.e., they will not respond to further stimulation); and (3) the anti-CD4 antibody could stimulate active suppression directly.

Experimental Results

Experimental models have been used to show that treatment with anti-CD4 can extend graft survival. In rodents, a number of different anti-CD4 monoclonal antibodies have been tested, and the degree to which they can extend graft survival is highly variable.[455] However, some reports indicate induction of allograft unresponsiveness for 90 days or more using OKT4 as monotherapy.[474] Trials in monkeys with OKT4A, a murine IgG2a monoclonal antibody, showed extension of renal allograft survival from a mean survival time of 8–39 days with a single 10-mg/kg dose on the day of transplantation.[125] This antibody does not cause depletion of circulating CD4+ cells; therefore, removal of CD4+ cells was not the mechanism of suppression. Most animals in this trial and others like it developed anti-mouse immunoglobulin antibodies that limited the pharmacological half-life of the antibody in the circulation. "Humanization" of the antibody in which the antigen-binding region of the antibody was grafted to human IgG resulted in extension of primate graft survival to as long as 8 weeks[125, 427] and the only antibodies to the injected antibody were directed to the idiotypic determinants (from the mouse). Other anti-CD4 antibodies have been tested in animal models with similar results.[237]

Clinical Results

Several clinical studies in renal transplantation have evaluated anti-CD4 monoclonal antibodies.[398, 501] Induction therapy with OKT4A plus triple-drug immunosuppression had modest success, with greater than 80% of patients developing anti-murine antibodies and over one third of patients developing rejection within 3 months. CD4+ cells were not depleted. An IgG4 humanized monoclonal antibody against CD4, called OKTcdr4a, with only 8% of the murine OKT4A sequence, was more successful in preventing, but not eliminating, early renal rejection, and no antibody response to OKTcdr4a was detected.[123]

Few clinical trials have examined the safety and efficacy of anti-CD4 antibodies in cardiac transplantation. The use of a chimeric murine/human, monoclonal CD4 antibody has been studied in heart transplant patients as adjunctive therapy to conventional immunotherapy. After 1 year, the anti-CD4 group had fewer rejection episodes, delayed time to first rejection, and improved survival compared to ATG prophylaxis.[398]

Anti–Adhesion Molecule Antibodies

Anti-LFA-1

LFA-1, also called CD11a/CD18, is a member of the beta$_2$-integrin family, and consists of a beta$_2$ (CD18) and a beta$_1$ (CD11a) chain. It mediates cell-to-cell and cell-to-matrix adhesion via ICAM-1 and it is important in the binding of T-cells to endothelium and a number of other targets. Monoclonal antibodies against LFA-1 and those against ICAM-1 have drawn particular attention because of their ability to induce tolerance in rodent models. In those experiments, prolongation of graft survival was achieved with either antibody, but the best results were obtained when both were used in combination. A multicenter randomized trial in France tested the 25-3 anti-LFA monoclonal antibody in a quadruple immunosuppression protocol and compared it to rabbit antithymocyte globulin (RATG). They found that short-term rejection rates were the same in patients that received anti-LFA in comparison to RATG.[224] This raises the possibility that the anti-LFA antibody could be useful as an adjunct immunosuppressant.

Anti–ICAM-1

ICAM-1, also called CD54, serves as a ligand for LFA-1 and is present on the vascular endothelium and about 20% of peripheral blood mononuclear cells. This molecule is expressed at low levels on most peripheral blood mononuclear cells and is also present on follicular dendritic cells and the vascular endothelium. This molecule can be important in T-cell activation and migration because it is present at high levels on vascular endothelium and T-cell–dependent areas of the lymph nodes. Thus, this and other adhesion molecules may play an important role in the rejection process.

Trials of the anti–ICAM-1 monoclonal antibody, BIRR1, as a sole immunosuppressant in a monkey renal allograft model showed prolonged allograft survival at 24.2 days versus 9.2 days for the controls.[107] Further testing of the antibody in 18 highly sensitized renal allograft recipients showed that an adequate BIRRI serum level was associated with less delayed graft function, suggesting that the antibody could ameliorate damage due to ischemia/reperfusion injury and reduce rejection.[212] Although the combination of anti–LFA-1 and anti–ICAM-1 antibodies can produce indefinite survival in murine cardiac transplant models with MHC-incompatible strains,[230] no clinical trials have yet been published in which both anti–LFA-1 and anti–ICAM-1 antibodies have been used in concert.

ANTI-CD45 MONOCLONAL ANTIBODIES

CD45 (leukocyte common antigen) interacts with antigen-presenting cells via phosphotyrosine phosphatase. Anti-CD45 monoclonal antibodies can reduce renal allograft rejection when used to flush the renal allograft prior to its implantation.[60, 182, 183, 585]

MONOCLONAL ANTIBODIES AGAINST THE TCR/CD3 COMPLEX

The TCR/CD3 complex on the T-cell surface is essential for antigen recognition and T-cell activation (Fig. 13–1). Murine monoclonal antibodies against the TCR/CD3 complex, such as T10B9-31,[552, 555] have successfully reversed renal allograft rejection. A randomized trial showed it to be as effective as OKT3 without the cytokine release symptoms.[553] Since this IgM antibody does not bind the Fc receptor of monocytes (a binding process required for T-cell activation and the cytokine release induced by anti-CD3 IgG antibodies), the cytokine release syndrome is avoided with T10B9-31. In vitro studies indicate failure of T10B9-31 to induce release of IFN-γ, TNF-α, IL-6, or IL-2.[62] In a small group (phase I study) of patients undergoing cardiac transplantation, T10B9-31 was similar to OKT3 in preventing acute rejection as induction therapy. T10B9-31 successfully reversed rejection in a patient who rejected while receiving OKT3.[554]

OTHER MONOCLONAL ANTIBODIES

Other monoclonal antibodies[106, 373] tested for anti-rejection therapy in solid organ transplantation are listed in Table 13–21. These include BTI-332, an anti-CD2 monoclonal antibody[4, 45]; BMAO31, an anti-T-cell receptor heterodimer monoclonal antibody[38]; WT-32, an anti-CD3 monoclonal antibody[168, 512]; Max 16 H5, an anti-CD4 monoclonal antibody[123]; BL4, an anti-CD4 monoclonal antibody[361]; an anti-CD4 monoclonal antibody[118]; anti-T12, an anti-CD6 monoclonal antibody[124, 269]; SDZCHH 380, an anti-CD7 monoclonal antibody[305, 469]; anti-Leu2a, an anti-CD8 monoclonal antibody[561]; and Compath 1, an anti-CD52 monoclonal antibody.[169, 170, 207, 542]

APHERESIS PROCEDURES

Apheresis refers to the use of extracorporal fluid and cell separation technology. The use of apheresis techniques for treatment of rejection is relatively recent and is primarily reserved for the treatment of rejection episodes that are refractory to the usual armamentarium of immunosuppressive drugs.

PLASMAPHERESIS

Background

Plasmapheresis, also known as plasma exchange, involves the removal of blood from the patient, separation of plasma by centrifugation or membrane filtration, and reconstitution of the remaining blood to the original volume with fresh plasma or 5% albumin. The removal of plasma results in depletion of substances contained within the plasma that are capable of passing through the plasma separator. As a result, this technique has been used for many years as a means to remove undesirable soluble mediators such as immune complexes from the blood. Plasmapheresis is a standard therapy for a number of autoimmune diseases, including idiopathic thrombocytopenic purpura, hemolytic uremic syndrome, Goodpasture's syndrome, Guillain-Barré syndrome, and myasthenia gravis.

Mechanism of Immunosuppression

Virtually any molecule in the plasma small enough to pass through the filtration membrane is removed from the vascular compartment. This has been the basis for the use of plasmapheresis in the removal of drugs resulting from overdose.[251] Given that large macromolecules can be removed from the blood, a natural extension of this technique has been the **removal of antibodies** from transplant patients who are believed to be experiencing antibody-mediated rejection. Thus, one possibility is that the favorable effect of plasmapheresis on rejection with hemodynamic compromise results from the removal of antibody.[79] The effectiveness of removal of antibodies by plasmapheresis is dependent on the immunoglobulin class and whether the antibody is bound to tissues or immune complexes. IgG is distributed in both the intravascular and extracellular spaces. Therefore, only approximately 40% of IgG is accessible to removal from the blood. Of that, approximately 50% can be removed by a single treatment of plasmapheresis. This would explain why multiple treatments are often necessary before a significant effect on rejection is observed. Approximately 90% of IgM antibodies are in the vascular compartment and therefore would be removed with greater efficiency. One should be cautioned, however, that the causal relationship between this type of rejection and the appearance of serum antibodies has not been established. In addition, plasmapheresis results in a decrease in **soluble mediators** potentially released during acute rejection, including IL-1,[406] IL-6, TNF-α,[23, 177] and the anaphylatoxin C3a.[407] Some of these mediators, such as TNF-α and IL-1, have been shown to have a direct depressant effect on myocyte contractility,[156, 562] so the effect of plasmapheresis on cardiac performance could potentially be quite direct.

Technique of Administration

The technique of plasmapheresis generally requires a large-bore indwelling catheter inserted into the internal jugular, subclavian, or femoral vein. The apparatus and circuitry are diagrammed in Fig. 13–25.

Adverse Effects

Complications include infections because of the removal of antibodies, bleeding disorders, and citrate-induced disorders resulting from the anticoagulation. Transient reduction in white blood cell count and platelet count, depletion of fibrinogen, and activation of the classical

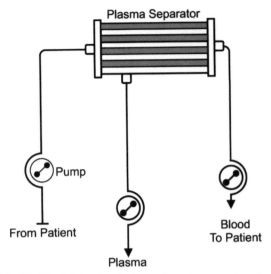

FIGURE **13–25.** Schematic of plasmapheresis apparatus. See text for description.

pathway for complement (elevation of C4 levels) are observed following plasmapheresis.[406, 408] Compared to the effect of other augmented immunosuppressive agents, the potential for infection after plasmapheresis seems relatively low. The potential for bleeding complications after plasmapheresis appears to be low as long as the fibrinogen level is maintained above 100 mg/dL.

Clinical Use

In 1992, two reports of the use of plasmapheresis as a rescue therapy for rejection after cardiac transplantation were published. The first report described a cohort of 11 patients who had an IgG-positive crossmatch. The authors noted that 73% of these patients experienced rejection episodes with hemodynamic compromise. Eight of these patients were treated with plasmapheresis daily for 3 days in addition to augmentation of immunosuppression. Survival among those patients was 75%.[435] Other anecdotal reports have also suggested successful reversal of hemodynamically compromising rejection with plasmapheresis treatment for 3–4 days.[44, 82]

Our experience with plasmapheresis at the University of Alabama at Birmingham (UAB) includes a cohort of patients treated for rejection with hemodynamic compromise. Although unproven, our anecdotal experience strongly suggests that plasmapheresis is a powerful adjunct in the treatment of left ventricular dysfunction associated with acute rejection. When left ventricular function as assessed by transthoracic echocardiogram is profoundly depressed, plasmapheresis is usually combined with methylprednisolone, cytolytic therapy, inotropic support, and heparin. Rarely observed in the absence of plasmapheresis, it is common for ejection fraction (even with initial ejection fraction as low as 0.15–0.20) to promptly improve after the first plasmapheresis treatment, with normalization or near normalization of ejection fraction after the first two treatments. The response appears to be similar whether or not there is evidence of acute cellular rejection on biopsy. Daily plasmapheresis is typically continued for 3 consecutive days. Therapy is temporarily interrupted if the fibrinogen level falls below about 100 mg/dL.

The role of plasmapheresis in the treatment of cardiac rejection is not yet certain, since clear elucidation of its mechanism and controlled studies of its benefit are lacking. However, the many reported experiences of successful reversal of difficult rejection with plasmapheresis strongly support its efficacy. The most common indications for the use of plasmapheresis have been rejection that was unresponsive to augmentation of immunosuppression or cytolytic therapy, rejection with the appearance of donor-specific panel reactive antibodies, a positive crossmatch, rejection with vasculitis or other evidence of humoral rejection,[189] and rejection with hemodynamic compromise (see also Chapter 14).

IMMUNOADSORPTION

Background

Plasmapheresis is a passive process in which immunoglobulins pass through the filtration membranes with the removed plasma. If one subscribes to the hypothesis that the primary pathogenic components in the circulation are antibodies, then the removal of other elements in the plasma is potentially detrimental, and it would be desirable to remove the antibodies in a specific fashion. To address this issue, some centers have used columns containing immunoadsorbents that specifically bind to immunoglobulins. These immunoadsorbents are typically utilized in the form of columns filled with a porous bead matrix covalently coupled to polyclonal anti-human IgG antibodies or to protein A, a natural cell wall constituent of Staphylococcus aureus which has the unique property of binding to circulating immune complex and immunoglobulin G with high avidity. Plasma is removed at about 20–30 mL/min, passed through the column, and returned to the patient. Protein A specifically binds to IgG1, IgG2, and IgG4, but does not bind well to IgG3, IgM, or IgA. Each column can typically bind 1–2 g of antibody and can be regenerated when the binding capacity is reached. Like other extracorporeal treatments, immunoadsorption is most effective when performed repeatedly because these techniques can only remove antibodies in the peripheral circulation and do not directly affect tissue-bound antibodies.

Mechanism of Immunosuppression

The most direct proposed mechanism of action is removal of circulating IgG antibodies, some of which may be anti-HLA class I antibodies. Some have speculated that immunoadsorption can also stimulate the production of anti-idiotypic antibodies, which are believed to regulate antibody production and B-cell differentiation.[483]

Adverse Effects

Side effects are usually mild and include occasional nausea, vomiting, headache, fever, and rarely cutaneous rash and hypotension.

Clinical Use

Favorable results of immunoadsorption therapy have been reported in the treatment of idiopathic thrombocytopenic purpura when caused by a 7S gamma globulin antibody directed at the platelet membrane.[209, 255]

Treatments using this procedure have been associated with a drop in the concentration of anti-HLA antibodies and in the concentration of IgG present in the peripheral circulation.[8, 220, 292, 404, 410, 453] Anecdotal cases of successful treatment of acute vascular rejection with improvement in ejection fraction and decrease in panel reactive antibodies have been reported.[404] At present, there are no published reports of randomized studies to compare the efficacy of immunoadsorption with plasmapheresis.

PHOTOPHERESIS

Historical Note

The medical use of psoralens can be traced back to the observations by Egyptian physicians, who noted that individuals who ingested the leaves of a plant (Ammi majus) found by the Nile River were particularly prone to sunburn.[179] Psoralens, the active ingredient in these plants, are a class of compounds that include 8-methoxypsoralen (8-MOP), the drug which makes photopheresis possible. In 1903, Niels Finsen received the Nobel Prize in Medicine for his pioneering efforts in the application of artificial light to the treatment of cutaneous disorders.[179]

Formal studies of psoralens as a therapeutic agent in the modern era began at the University of Cairo in the 1940s, in which Elmofty and colleagues noted that ingestion of extracts from the Ammi plant combined with exposure to sunlight were effective therapy for vitiligo.[138] Lerner and Fitzpatrick studied purified 8-MOP in the 1950s, and the drug was utilized in the treatment of psoriasis in the 1970s. The application of 8-MOP in the treatment of the skin lesions of cutaneous T-cell lymphoma (CTCL) was initiated by Gilchrest and colleagues at Harvard Medical School. Edelson and colleagues at Yale University reported the first application of photopheresis in the treatment of CTCL.[139]

Background

Extracorporeal photopheresis is a relatively new therapy for modulation of immune responses in autoimmune diseases, transplantation, and the treatment of cutaneous T-cell lymphoma. Photopheresis, also called extracorporeal photochemotherapy, involves the extracorporeal administration of ultraviolet light to leukocytes treated with 8-MOP. This modality has induced prolonged remissions in about 75% of treated patients with cutaneous T-cell lymphoma, a malignancy of T-helper cells. Even the advanced form of the disease, called Sézary syndrome, has responded to a combination of extracorporeal photochemotherapy and low-dose interferon.[447] Favorable clinical responses have also been observed in autoimmune disorders such as rheumatoid arthritis, pemphigus vulgaris, and systemic sclerosis.[445]

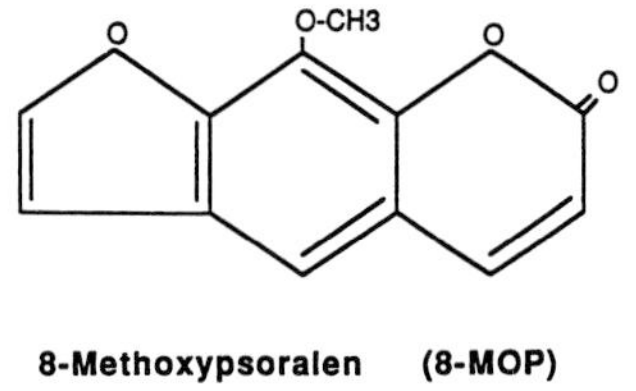

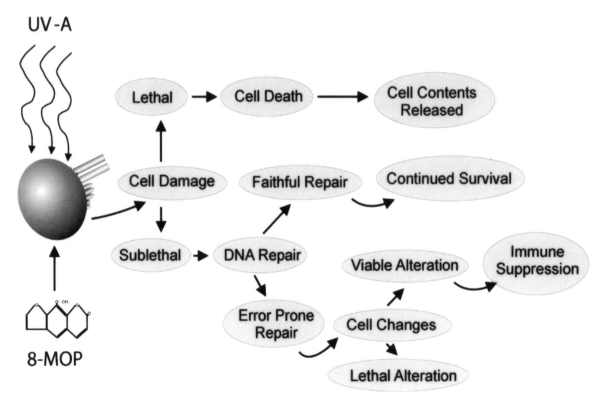

8-Methoxypsoralen   (8-MOP)

FIGURE **13-26.** The chemical strucure of 8-methoxypsoralen (8-MOP).

Photopheresis utilizes a photoactivatable compound, 8-MOP, which is administered to the patient orally, reaching peak levels in blood within 2 hours and excreted almost completely within 24 hours. After 2 hours, blood is withdrawn via a peripheral intravenous line, heparinized, and collected into a cell separator in which leukocyte-depleted blood is returned to the patient and a leukocyte-enriched fraction is sent to a thin transparent disposable chamber. The chamber is surrounded by a light source emitting ultraviolet A (UVA) light at a range of 320–400 nm. Since UVA is a weak form of ultraviolet radiation, the layer of exposed blood must be very thin to allow penetration of the lymphocytes. The exposed cells are then sent back to the patient.

Mechanism of Immunosuppression

8-MOP is a tricyclic aromatic photoactivatable compound (Fig. 13–26). The unique property of 8-MOP and other psoralens is their capacity to absorb ultraviolet light of specific wavelengths and undergo activation. The wavelengths included in UVA light induce activation of 8-MOP. UVA readily penetrates glass and certain plastics, unlike ultraviolet B, which causes sunburn. In the absence of UVA, psoralens are very safe, but once activated they induce severe DNA damage. Furthermore, the activation is extremely brief, lasting only several millionths of a second following UVA exposure. Therefore, when the source of UV irradiation is turned off, the drug promptly reverts to its inactive form.[138] In its active form, the aromatic rings of 8-MOP confer a highly planar structure that allows the molecule to intercalate into DNA strands. Following exposure to ultraviolet light at an optimal wavelength, 8-MOP crosslinks with pyrimidines in cellular DNA[179] in such a way that strands of the DNA helix are unable to separate, thus inhibiting DNA replication. 8-MOP also binds to cell membrane proteins and fatty acids, suggesting that other mechanisms may be involved in the effect of 8-MOP on cells.

The exact mechanism of immunosuppression with photopheresis is unknown, but several studies suggest the induction of a **suppressor T-cell response.** Treatment of lymphocytes by photopheresis results in cell damage followed by death (Fig. 13–27). Increased levels of CD95 (Fas) and increased rates of apoptosis have been observed in these populations after photopheresis, suggesting that these cells are induced to undergo apoptosis.[18, 147, 582] The simplest mechanism that could be invoked to explain the effect of photopheresis is that activated cells are likely targets for damage. However, photopheresis directly affects only a small number of leukocytes relative to the total pool of cells that reside in different cellular compartments of the body. Photopheresis performed for 2 consecutive days every 4 weeks alters approximately 2–5% of the total T-cell pool.[571]

FIGURE **13-27.** Schematic depiction of the fate of cells exposed to photoactivated 8-methoxypsoralen.

More illuminating has been the finding that photopheresis appears to induce specific suppression of immunity. In T-cell lymphoma, Perez and Khavari have demonstrated that photopheresis induces a clone-specific T-cell response that suppresses proliferation of the pathogenic T-cells.[261, 416] This has led to the concept of "T-cell vaccination" in which it is believed that treatment of leukocytes in the peripheral blood with photopheresis leads to suppression of untreated T-cell clones. Similar results have been generated in a mouse system of skin allograft immunity in which immunity to specific skin allografts could be adoptively transferred from an immunized recipient to a naive individual. But, pretreatment of the naive recipient with cells treated with 8-MOP and UV irradiation conferred resistance to the adoptively transferred immunity, implying an antigen-specific suppressor T-cell response. Such **anti-idiotypic responses** (T-cell response against T-cell receptor portions of the same organism) are hypothesized as the primary mechanism for the efficacy of photopheresis as an antirejection therapy. **Theoretically, T-cells activated by the allograft are damaged by the 8-MOP/UVA treatment and when returned to the body act as a stimulus for an anti-idiotypic, suppressor T-cell response.**

Clinical studies in autoimmune disorders such as pemphigus vulgaris suggest that patients who receive photopheresis show a correlation between clinical improvement and an increase in the number of peripheral lymphocytes that have phenotypic features of suppressor T-cells.[446] Photopheresis may also induce morphologic and functional alterations in antigen-presenting cells such as B-cells and macrophages[190, 204, 419] and induces production of TNF-α by monocytes.[544]

Method of Administration

8-MOP is administered orally in a dose (0.6 mg/kg) sufficient to achieve a blood level of 50 ng/mL. Since venous flow rates of 25–50 mL/min are necessary for the initial leukopheresis phase, a noncollapsing large-bore (16-gauge) peripheral intravenous catheter or central venous catheter is necessary. After 90–120 minutes (time to peak 8-MOP blood levels), an enriched lymphocyte solution from the patient is passed through the photopheresis system (UVAR, Therakos, Inc.) (Fig. 13–28).[138] Blood is first withdrawn, heparinized, and collected in the photopheresis unit. The blood is centrifuged to separate the blood into a leukocyte-rich buffy coat fraction, red blood cells, and plasma. The enriched lymphocyte solution is generated by removing 240 mL of buffy coat and 300 mL of plasma, diluted with 200 mL of saline plus 10,000 units of heparin. The solution contains about 30–50% of the patient's circulating lymphocytes and is passed through a six-chambered photoactivation unit as a 1-mm film to expose it to ultraviolet light delivered by a fluorescent source. Following exposure, the entire solution is returned to the patient.

Psoralen levels within the photopheresis buffy-coat bag should be greater than 50 ng/mL. A liquid form of psoralen that can be mixed directly with the lymphocytes within the photopheresis devices[276] may allow more precise regulation of psoralen levels and eliminate the need for oral administration of 8-MOP.

Adverse Effects

Photopheresis is generally well tolerated. Generalized depletion of leukocytes does not occur with photopheresis. Occasional psoralen-induced nausea may occur, but it typically only lasts for 30–60 minutes. Nervousness, vertigo, headache, and mental depression have been observed with psoralen therapy. Inadvertent overdosage of methoxy-psoralen or overexposure to UV light during psoralen administration may cause severe burning of skin and retinal injury. The patient is instructed to avoid direct sunlight and wear UV-light-blocking dark glasses during and for 24 hours following photopheresis treatment. Rarely, transient hypotension may occur during the leukopheresis phase which is responsive to volume administration. Low-grade fever may occur 4–12 hours after reinfusion of treated cells, likely related to cytokine release.[571]

Studies in T-cell lymphoma and systemic sclerosis suggest that delayed-type hypersensitivity[544] and general cell-mediated immunity are unaffected by a 6-month course of photopheresis therapy.[571]

Drug Interactions

Concomitant administration of other photosensitizing agents while undergoing phototherapy may increase the photosensitizing effects of psoralen.

Clinical Use

A number of single-center experiences with the use of photopheresis for the treatment of cardiac allograft rejection have been published since 1992. Early reports described the use of photopheresis as a rescue therapy for acute rejection episodes[109, 110] or as chronic therapy resulting in a decrease in the frequency of rejection episodes over time, particularly in patients with posttransplant anti-HLA antibodies.[8, 451] Other studies have also suggested a protective effect against recurrent rejection.[32, 346–448] Barr and colleagues noted less coronary intimal thickening after 1 year when photopheresis was added to standard immunosuppression.[32] Between 1991 and November 1995, 27 patients at UAB received photophesis therapy for recurrent rejection, recurrent rejection with hemodynamic compromise, or a positive cross-match. Among the 17 patients who completed 6 months of photopheresis, the rejection rates decreased significantly ($p < .001$) following treatment. Infection rates were also noted to be lower following photopheresis ($p = .01$).

Although photopheresis is still undergoing active evaluation as an antirejection modality, there clearly remains an important subset of patients who continue to experience recurrent rejection despite OKT3 (and/or ATG), multiple courses of methylprednisolone, conversion from azathioprine to mycophenolate, and conversion from cyclosporine to tacrolimus. Preliminary data, as noted above, and our clinical experience suggest that

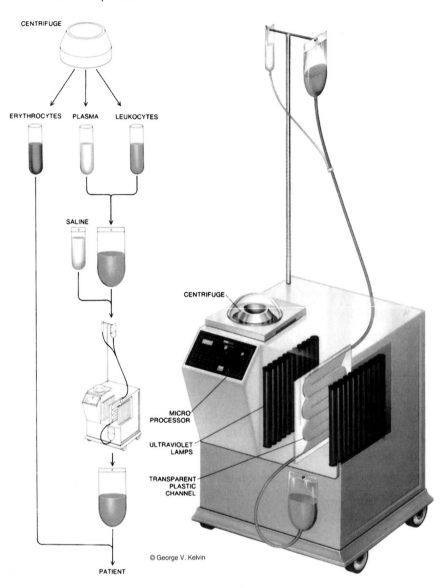

FIGURE **13–28.** Diagram of photopheresis machine (Therakos) and procedure. See text for description. (From Edelson R: Light-activated drugs. Scientific American 1988;259:68–75, with permission.)

in this subset a 6 to 12-month course of photopheresis therapy is the most effective treatment currently available for recurrent allograft rejection. When recurrent rejection is complicated by hemodynamic compromise, photopheresis is combined with initial plasmapheresis. There is currently insufficient information to indicate whether photopheresis (combined with initial plasmapheresis) would be equally as effective against humoral rejection.

TOTAL LYMPHOID IRRADIATION

BACKGROUND

The use of irradiation in clinical transplantation was contemplated 30 years ago, but it was found that whole body irradiation was too toxic, resulting in bone marrow suppression and gastrointestinal symptoms. Work with radiation treatments for Hodgkin's disease had shown that using a more restrictive field of irradiation (i.e., to

the lymphoid tissues only) was more easily tolerated, and was not associated with an increase in the incidence of cancer. It was also noted that patients treated with total lymphoid irradiation (TLI) for Hodgkin's disease also sustained a significant and long-lasting impairment of cell-mediated immune responses.

TLI is a low-dose radiotherapy that targets lymphoid tissues, including the cervical, axillary, mediastinal, periaortic, and iliofemoral lymph nodes, the thymus, and the spleen. Nonlymphoid tissue is shielded during treatment. Experimental evidence using animal models has shown that TLI can prolong allograft survival in hamsters,[495] rats,[293, 495] mice, and nonhuman primates.[518] Administration of bone marrow intravenously 1 week after TLI in mice can induce a state of permanent chimerism in which the recipient is specifically tolerant to the bone marrow donor and will reject third-party grafts.[478–480] The extent and type of antigens to which the recipient is tolerant is partially dependent on the dose of radiation, the proximity of the antigen exposure to the time of TLI administration, and the type of antigen. The "window of tolerance" induced by TLI is very short for allogeneic cells such as bone marrow, but soluble proteins such as bovine serum albumin can abrogate or reduce immune responses approximately 100 days after TLI.[583] Subsequent challenge with that same antigen plus an adjuvant (a coinjected substance used to intensify antibody production) results in 10-fold less antibody production compared to that generated by animals not treated with TLI.[583]

Large animal studies have consistently shown prolongation of graft survival with TLI, but only with concomitant immunosuppression with ATG, azathioprine, and/or cyclosporine.[47, 415] However, some primate studies in renal transplantation showed worse results when TLI was combined with cyclosporine.[381] When cumulative dose has exceeded 2,000 rad, radiation-related deaths were more common.

MECHANISM OF IMMUNOSUPPRESSION

The precise molecular/cellular mechanisms by which TLI reduces the immune response are unclear, but effects of radiation at the molecular level are likely of central importance. Radiation induces ionization of atoms and initiates physiochemical reactions that result in formation and breakage of new chemical bonds. Cell death results from alterations in the configuration of DNA, producing structural damage such as chromosomal breakage, translocations, and bridges associated with breaks or damage to purine and pyrimidine base pairs.[253] Double-strand breakage is usually lethal to the cell, whereas single-strand breaks are usually amenable to enzymatic repair. However, the resultant chromosomal damage may potentially set the stage for increased damage by other antiproliferative agents in the future.

Both T-cells and B-cells are susceptible to radiation injury. Sublethal irradiation to the thymus and peripheral lymphoid tissue in mice results in loss of normal thymic cytoarchitecture, with transient depletion of the medulla and long-term effects on the stromal tissue, including a loss of macrophages. Normal cytoarchitecture returns after 1–2 months.[6] Treatment alone, or in combination with immunosuppressive drugs, also results in an initial depression in lymphocyte counts that recover after 3–4 months. However, the distribution of T-cell subpopulations and their expression of surface antigens also show long-term changes. It has been noted that the immune systems of TLI-treated mice exhibit characteristics normally found in neonates, particularly if one examines the time course of immunofluorescent staining for cell surface markers following treatment.

Some have hypothesized that TLI induces a population of cells called "natural suppressor cells" that have similarities to natural killer (NK) cells.[482] These cells, which have nonspecific suppressor activity, were originally isolated from neonatal spleen cells by negative selection (i.e., they were the cells left behind after an extensive sorting using a number of surface markers), and were therefore called "null cells" because of their lack of known lineage markers (see also Chapter 2). Null cells were shown to nonspecifically inhibit mixed

lymphocyte cultures and graft-versus-host disease *in vivo*. More recent evidence suggests that "null cells" are, in fact, CD34+ stem cells, suggesting that TLI may reduce or eliminate rejection by facilitating the establishment of microchimerism, which has been postulated to be a necessary step for the induction of donor-specific unresponsiveness.[67, 489, 490, 499, 506]

TLI DOSING PROTOCOLS

Three separate fields are used to provide radiation exposure to all major lymphoid bearing areas. A supradiaphragmatic mantle allows treatment of the base of the skull to the T8 and T9 areas with lateral extensions to treat the axillary lymph nodes. This area has been called the mantle[227] (Fig. 13–29). The rest of the field, consisting of an "inverted Y," encompasses a periaortic and splenic field extending to the L4 and L5 levels and a field that includes the pelvic and inguinal lymph nodes. These areas are treated with a total target dose of 800 cGy using twice-weekly doses of 80 cGy each. Azathioprine is discontinued just before intiation of TLI to reduce the suppression of bone marrow associated with the irradiation. The treatment schedule for TLI may be adjusted depending on the white blood cell counts, which must be monitored during therapy. TLI is generally

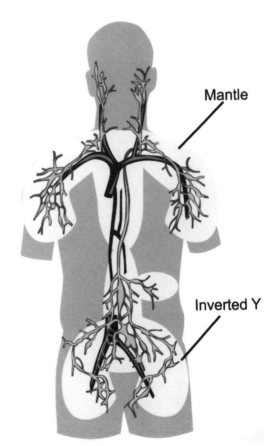

FIGURE **13–29.** Fields of irradiation used for clinical total lymphoid irradiation. (From Hunt SA, Strober S, Hoppe RT, Stinson EB: Total lymphoid irradiation for treatment of intractable cardiac allograft rejection. J Heart Transplant 1991;10:211–216. Copyright 1991, Elsevier Science, with permission.)

withheld when the leukocyte count drops below 2,700/mL, granulocytes are less than 1,500/mL, or the platelet count is less than 125,000/mL (or falling rapidly). Individual doses can be reduced or given at increased intervals. Treatment should be discontinued if leukopenia is sustained.

CLINICAL USE

Studies of renal allograft patients given pretransplant TLI showed that maintenance immunosuppression could be reduced.[457] Donor-specific unresponsiveness to donor antigens (usually with cryopreserved donor spleen cells) in mixed leukocyte reactions (MLR) has been demonstrated 18–30 months following renal transplantation with pretransplant TLI and RATG and prednisone after transplant.[96, 500] Pretransplant TLI and donor bone marrow at the time of heart transplant has also been reported to induce donor-specific unresponsiveness.[250]

A number of case reports describe the use of posttransplant TLI as a treatment for intractable or recurrent rejection episodes.[227, 315] Subsequent extensive experiences have provided strong clinical support to the efficacy of TLI as highly effective therapy for persistent or recurrent rejection.

The UAB experience with TLI in the therapy of recurrent or severe rejection was initially reported in 1992[456] and updated in 1998.[59] Among 91 patients receiving 40–840 cGy of TLI, the rejection frequency fell from 1.0 ± 0.07 rejection episodes per month before TLI to 0.08 ± 0.02 episodes after TLI, with no further increases in rejection frequency out to 5 years or more. Similar favorable results have been reported with the use of TLI in children.[267]

TOXICITY

The most common early complications of TLI are leukopenia and thrombocytopenia, which, as noted above, may necessitate interruption or discontinuation of therapy. A major concern with TLI in transplantation is possible mutagenesis. The anticipated relative safety of TLI has been largely based on the absence of an increased incidence of subsequent leukemia or lymphoma in patients with Hodgkin's disease who receive up to 4,500 rad of TLI. However, the addition of other immunosuppressive agents in the transplant patient may induce an unquantified increased risk of malignancy, even with low-dose TLI. Lymphoma following TLI in clinical renal transplantation has been reported,[384] and metastatic lymphoma was observed following primate cardiac transplantation plus TLI.[415]

A disturbing incidence of late leukemia has been noted after TLI in heart transplantation. In 1994, Frist reported a case of chronic myelogenous leukemia 5 years after receiving TLI for recurrent rejection.[171] In the UAB experience with TLI between 1986 and 1996, 91 patients received TLI therapy (40–800 cGy over a planned 5-week period) for recurrent or severe rejection. Four pa-

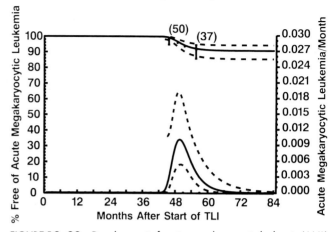

Total Lymphoid Irradiation
UAB Heart Transplantation; n = 89

FIGURE **13–30.** Development of acute megakaryocytic leukemia (AML) following total lymphoid irradiation (TLI) at UAB (n = 89). The upper curve is the actuarial freedom from AML with the 70% confidence limits (dashed lines). The numbers in parentheses indicate the number of patients at risk at the designated time of follow-up. The lower curve (and 70% CL) is the associated hazard function (instantaneous risk) for AML. Note that the greatest risk for AML occurs about 4–5 years following TLI.

tients developed fatal **acute megakaryocytic leukemia** between 4 and 5 years following TLI. No patient developed this malignancy who did not receive TLI. The actuarial likelihood of acute megakaryocytic leukemia was 9% at 5 years after TLI (Fig. 13–30). This rare leukemia was heralded by the onset of progressive thrombocytopenia (platelet count <70,000/mL) with death within 3 months of diagnosis.

CLINICAL INDICATIONS

It has been clearly established that TLI is an effective adjunctive therapy for the treatment of recurrent or severe rejection after cardiac transplantation. TLI is not effective, however, in reversing an ongoing episode of acute rejection, as 5 or more weeks are likely required for it to be effective. Other therapies (such as methylprednisolone and/or cytolytic therapy) are necessary for reversal of the acute episode.

Unfortunately, its effectiveness as an immunotherapeutic modality is clouded by the possible predisposition to late leukemia. Until further clarification of this fatal complication is available, we believe TLI should not be used after cardiac transplantation unless no other effective anti-rejection modalities are available.

BONE MARROW INFUSION

BACKGROUND/MECHANISMS OF IMMUNOSUPPRESSION

Early studies by Medawar had shown that administration of donor lymphoid cells or bone marrow during fetal life resulted in the establishment of tolerance in neonates or adults. They later showed that ablation of circulating lymphocytes followed by administration of bone marrow cells resulted in the induction of tolerance in adult animals as well. This concept has been extended into a number of different experimental systems in which the recipient is preconditioned by treatment with antilymphocyte globulins, or is subjected to radiation-induced ablation. Many of these protocols have been devised and studied in rodent experimental systems, but have been difficult to translate into outbred large animal systems. In addition, protocols that involve preconditioning of more than 3–4 hours prior to transplantation are poorly suited for heart transplantation. Therefore, from the perspective of heart transplantation, the most interesting protocols are those that involve perioperative treatment of the recipient.

Conceptually, the practice of donor bone marrow administration can be observed from two perspectives. The first is that the administration of donor cells results in the establishment of an anergic state that is dependent on the presence of donor antigen, but does not require an active role by the infused donor cells beyond the requirement to replicate in order to provide a continuously renewing source of antigen. The second perspective is that infused donor cells actively suppress or delete recipient T-cells that can react with donor HLA antigens. In either case, animal experiments have unambiguously shown that administration of viable bone marrow cells can result in the extension of graft survival or the induction of tolerance (Fig. 13–31).[187, 210, 211, 466, 482, 519, 520]

EXPERIMENTAL RESULTS

Clinical application of this technique was first discussed in a case report in which a 38-year-old kidney recipient

immunosuppressed with azathioprine, prednisolone, and antilymphocyte serum (for 14 days after transplant) was infused with 11×10^9 cryopreserved bone marrow cells on posttransplant day 25. The patient died with a functioning allograft from peritonitis secondary to perforated sigmoid diverticulitis at 8 months. There were no rejection episodes, and since the resident immune system was left largely intact, there was no evidence of graft-versus-host disease.[358]

This report was followed by a large series of experiments in rhesus monkeys by Judy Thomas and colleagues in which kidney transplant recipients were treated with RATG and donor bone marrow. They showed that antigen-specific tolerance could be induced in rhesus monkeys, particularly when $CD3^-$, $CD16^+$, $CD2^+$, $CD8^+$ bone marrow subpopulations were used in recipients that were also treated with total lymphoid irradiation. This treatment resulted in greater than 50% permanent graft survival among recipients that shared one HLA-DR antigen and did not develop anti-donor IgG antibodies.[80, 518, 522]

CLINICAL TRIALS

These encouraging results have led to cautious clinical trials of bone marrow administration in conventionally immunosuppressed patients. The first large-scale trial was conducted at UAB in a group of 57 renal allograft patients that received immunosuppression with cyclosporine, azathioprine, prednisone, and a 10- to 14-day course of Minnesota antilymphocyte globulin (MALG). Seven days following the last MALG dose, patients were infused with $2–3 \times 10^8$ cryopreserved donor bone marrow cells. At a median follow-up of 16 months, 85% graft survival was observed in the group that received donor bone marrow versus 67% in the control group. There was no difference in the number of rejection episodes experienced by each group.[30] It is interesting to note that this group of patients showed no evidence of induction of tolerance or unresponsiveness as observed in the primate model investigated by Thomas. It is likely that this differential response is due to the differences in immunosuppression. It is not clear whether drugs that inhibit T-cell activation, such as cyclosporine or tacrolimus, facilitate or hinder the development of tolerance in this system. Cyclosporine has been shown to interfere with thymic deletion during T-cell development.[173, 286, 473]

Some studies have been based on the simple concept that **chimerism** is necessary for the long-term establishment of unresponsiveness; therefore, augmentation of chimerism by administration of bone marrow can be beneficial. In these studies, the recipient is not treated with drugs that deplete circulating T-cells, but is treated with tacrolimus and given a dose of $3–5 \times 10^8$ fresh bone marrow cells at the time of transplantation. In renal allograft recipients, this resulted in 97% 1-year and 87% 3-year actuarial graft survival compared to 92% and 82%, but this was not found to be statistically significant. Another center used a similar protocol in which patients received OKT3 induction therapy (postoperative days

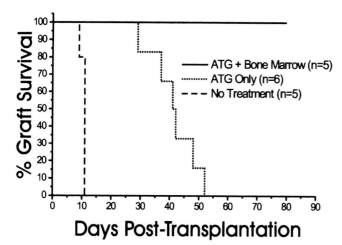

FIGURE **13–31.** Induction of tolerance by administration of donor bone marrow. C57BL/6 strain mice were treated with 400 mg/kg rabbit antithymocyte globulin on days −1 and +2 relative to the application of a skin graft from a mouse of the B10.D2(R107) strain. On day +7, the mice received 2.5×10^7 bone marrow cells from a C57BL/6 mouse. Mice treated in this manner did not reject their skin grafts within 90 days after transplantation (solid line). Mice treated only with rabbit antithymocyte globulin rejected their grafts within 55 days (dotted line). The dashed line represents animals that received no treatment. (Courtesy of J. George, unpublished data.)

1–10), tacrolimus, and methylprednisolone with cryo-preserved bone marrow infusions at days 1 and 4 after transplantation.[468] These patients were extensively studied to determine levels of chimerism in various cellular compartments. Compared to 100 concurrent kidney transplant recipients that did not receive bone marrow, they found a 10-fold higher level of chimerism in recipient iliac crest bone marrow, and significantly lower levels of chimerism in patients that experienced rejection episodes. However, the actuarial patient and graft survival was lower in patients that received donor bone marrow, apparently due to increased susceptibility of these patients to viral infections.[176] There is one randomized clinical trial underway in which cardiac transplant recipients are being treated with donor bone marrow.[341] The treatment has been found to be safe, but no other outcome data are currently available.

All but one trial suggests that treatment with donor bone marrow is, at worst, benign, and at best, offers a clear survival advantage over conventional treatment. It is also clear that the mechanisms by which bone marrow would confer graft unresponsiveness is poorly understood, which increases the risk that small changes in the protocols could have unforseen consequences. Animal models have clearly shown that the effect of donor bone marrow administration is considerably enhanced as the resident immune system of the host is ablated. However, increasing recipient T-cell ablation increases the risk that the recipient will experience graft-versus-host disease. Situations in which the ablation of the resident T-cell population is nearly complete have resulted in the development of graft-versus-host disease symptoms in rhesus monkeys when bone marrow cells are administered even in very small quantities (J. M. Thomas, personal communication).

IMMUNOTOXINS

Antibodies, by virtue of their ability to bind specifically to an antigen, can serve as a tool for the specific identification and targeting of cells and tissues. In general, monoclonal and polyclonal antibody therapies target lymphocytes and rely on the native effector mechanisms of the body for the removal of the target cell population, or they modulate or interfere with function by blocking or perturbing a molecule. However, given that antibodies are highly specific, it is possible that they could also be used as delivery systems in which a particular drug or toxin could be transported to a specific cell population. Immunotoxins are such reagents, and in the context of transplantation, have been envisioned as a means to deplete T-cells or subpopulations of T-cells. One of the most recent examples of this therapeutic modality is the use of an anti-CD3 monoclonal antibody coupled to a genetically engineered form of diphtheria toxin. The enzymatically active domain of diphtheria toxin is an ADP-ribosyl transferase that targets elongation factor-2, which is an essential component of the process of translation during protein synthesis. When the translocation domain of diphtheria toxin is inactivated or re-moved, the systemic toxicity of the toxin is drastically reduced. When coupled to an antibody against the CD3 complex, it serves as an effective means by which noncycling memory T-cells as well as activated T-cells can be depleted.[19, 275, 521] This type of immunotoxin can target T-cells in a highly specific fashion and can effect depletion following intracellular uptake without the intervention and limitations of native effector mechanisms.

In nonhuman primates, pretreatment of recipients with anti-CD3 immunotoxin results in significant *in vivo* suppression and extension of graft survival in a group of rhesus monkey renal allograft recipients.[153] More importantly, this immunotoxin has been successfully used to induce stable renal graft tolerance in rhesus monkeys treated on the day of transplantation. In that study, four of five recipients that received fully histoincompatible renal allografts exhibited survival times of 120 days to >1.5 years with no further immunosuppression.[521] Examination of the peripheral lymphoid organs shows that immunotoxin administration results in extensive depletion of peripheral T-cells in the circulation and in the peripheral lymphoid organs, which has not been reported for any other cytolytic agent used in a large animal model. The depletion of circulating CD3+ cells is transient, recovering to pretreatment levels in 30–40 days.[521] Further examination has shown that the coadministration of 15-deoxyspergualin and methylprednisolone results in rejection-free kidney allograft acceptance in 75% of recipients for up to 550 days.[104]

Other immunotoxins have been devised using antibodies specific for a variety of surface antigens on different cell types, such as MHC class II antigens on antigen-presenting cells, CD5, which is present on both T-cells and B-cells,[336, 422, 429, 476, 481, 533] and CD25 (IL-2 receptor).[290, 340, 412, 533] All of these have been tested as a means of inhibiting or preventing graft-versus-host disease in bone marrow transplant recipients. Anti-CD25 coupled to yttrium has been tested in a cynomolgus monkey cardiac transplant model, but there was severe bone marrow depression unless granulocyte colony-stimulating factor was also used.

Immunotoxins are subject to some of the same limitations as other monoclonal antibody based therapies in which the recipients can develop antibodies against the xenogeneic antibodies. In the case of the anti-monkey CD3-diphtheria conjugate in which only a short course of the antibody appears to be necessary, this is not a limitation, provided that there are no preexisting antibodies against mouse proteins or the diphtheria organism.

References

1. Aagaard-Tillery KM, Jelinek DF: Inhibition of human B lymphocyte cell cycle progression and differentiation by rapamycin. Cell Immunol 1994;152:493–507.
2. Abraham RT: Mammalian target of rapamycin: immunosuppressive drugs uncover a novel pathway of cytokine receptor signaling. Curr Opin Immunol 1998;10:330–336.
3. Abraham RT, Wiederrecht GJ: Immunopharmacology of rapamycin. Annu Rev Immunol 1996;14:483–510.
4. Abramowicz D, Schandene L, Goldman M, Crusiaux A, Vereerstraeten P, DePauw L, Wybran J, Kinnaert P, Dupont E, Toussaint C: Release of tumor necrosis factor, interleukin-2 and gamma-

interferon in rejection of OKT2 monoclonal antibody in kidney transplant recipients. Transplantation 1989;47:606–608.

5. Adamson RM, Demritsky WP, Wormsley SB. OKT3 vs ATG: is there really a difference in immunosuppressive potency? Evaluation of rejection and effect on peripheral blood lymphocytes in heart transplantation recipients. J Heart Transplant 1989;8:74.

6. Adkins B, Gandour D, Strober S, Weissman I: Total lymphoid irradiation leads to transient depletion of the mouse thymic medulla and persistant abnormalities among medullary stromal cells. J Immunol 1988;140:3373–3379.

7. Adu D, Michael J, Turney J, McMaster P: Hyperkalemia in cyclosporine-treated renal allograft recipients. Lancet 1983;2: 370–372.

8. Alarabi AA, Wikstrom B, Backman U, Danielson BG, Tufvesson G, Sjoberg O: Pretransplantation immunoadsorption therapy in patients immunized with human lymphocyte antigen: effect of treatment and three years' clinical follow-up of grafts. Artifi Organs 1993;17:702–707.

9. Alessiani M, Cillo U, Fung JJ, Irish W, Abu-Elmagd K, Jain A, Takaya S, Van Thiel D, Starzl TE: Adverse effects of FK506 overdosage after liver transplantation. Transplant Proc 1993;25:628.

10. Allison AC, Eugui EM, Sollinger HW: Mycophenolate mofetil (RS-61443): mechanisms of action and effects in transplantation. Transplant Rev 1993;7:129.

11. Allison AC, Hovi T, Watts RWE, Webster ADB: Immunological observations on patients with Lesch-Nyhan syndrome, and on the role of *de novo* purine synthesis in lymphocyte transformation. Lancet 1975;2:1179–1183.

12. Allison AC, Hovi T, Watts RWE, Webster ADB: The role of *de novo* purine synthesis in lymphocyte transformation. Ciba Found Symp 1977;48:207–224.

13. Allison AC, Kowalski WJ, Muller CJ, Waters RV, Eugui EM: Mycophenolic acid and brequinar, inhibitors of purine and pyrimidine synthesis, block the glycosylation of adhesion molecules. Transplant Proc 1993;25(suppl 2):67.

14. Alonso-Pulpon L, Serano-Fiz S, Rubio JA, Cavero MA, Silva L, Sanchez-Vegazo I, Burgos R, Montero CG, Maicas C, Kreisler M, Crespo ML, Tellez G, Ugarte J: Efficacy of low-dose OKT3 as cytolytic induction therapy in heart transplantation. J Heart Lung Transplant 1995;14:136–142.

15. Alsberg CL, Black OF: Contribution to the study of maize deterioration: biochemical and toxicological investigations of *Penicillium puberulum* and *Penicillium stoloniferum*. US Dept Agr Plant Ind Bull 1912;270:7–48.

16. Amemiya H, Suzuki S, Ota K, Takahashi K, Sonoda T, Ishibashi M, Omoto R, Koyama I, Dohi K, Fukuda Y, Fukao K: A novel for rescue drug, 15-deoxyspergualin: first clinical trials for recurrent graft rejection in renal recipients. Transplantation 1990;49: 337–343.

17. Apelt F, Kolin-Gerresheim J, Bauchinger M: Azathioprine, a clastogen in human somatic cells? Analysis of chromosome damage and SCE in lymphocytes after exposure in vivo and in vitro. Mutat Res 1981;88:61–72.

18. Aringer M, Graninger WB, Smolen JS, Kiener HP, Steiner CW, Trautinger F, Knobler R: Photopheresis treatment enhances CD95 (fas) expression in circulating lymphocytes of patients with systemic sclerosis and induces apoptosis. Br J Rheumatol 1997; 36:1276–1282.

19. Armstrong N, Buckley P, Oberley T, Fechner J Jr, Dong Y, Hong X, Kirk A, Neville D, Knechtl S: Analysis of primate renal allografts after T-cell depletion with anti-CD3-CRM9. Transplantation 1998;66:5–13.

20. Arnold H, Bourseaux F: Synthese and Abbau cytostatisch wirksamer cyclischer N-Phosphamidester des Bis (-Chloraethyl)-amins. Angew Chem 1958;70:539–544.

21. Asante-Korang A, Boyle GJ, Webber SA, Miller SA, Fricker FJ: Experience of FK506 immune suppression in paediatric heart transplantation of long-term adverse effects. J Heart Lung Transplant 1996;15:415–422.

22. Atkison P, Joubert G, Barron A, Grant D, Paradis K, Seidman E, Wall W, Rosenberg H, Howard J, Williams S, Stiller C: Hypertrophic cardiomyopathy associated with tacrolimus in paediatric transplant patients. Lancet 1995;345:894–896.

23. Atsumi T, Kato K, Kurosawa S, Abe M, Fujisaku A: A case of Crow-Fukase syndrome with elevated soluble interleukin-6 receptor in cerebrospinal fluid. Response to double-filtration plasmapheresis and corticosteroids. Acta Haematol 1995;94:90–94.

24. Auersvald LA, Rothstein DM, Oliveira SC, Khuong CQ, Onodera H, Lazarovits AI, Basadonna GP: Indefinite islet allograft survival in mice after a short course of treatment with anti-CD45 monoclonal antibodies. Transplantation 1997;63:1355–1358.

25. Babany G, Morris R, Babaney I, Shepherd S, Kates RE: In vivo evaluation of the effects of altered cyclosporine metabolism on its immunosuppressive potency. J Pharmacol Exp Ther 1988; 248:893–899.

26. Bach JF: The Mode of Action of Immunosuppressive Agents. Oxford: North Holland Publishing Company, 1975.

27. Ballantyne CM, Podet EJ, Patsch WP, Harati Y, Appel V, Gotto AM Jr, Young JB: Effects of cyclosporine therapy on plasma lipoprotein levels. JAMA 1989;262:53–56.

28. Ballantyne CM, Radovancevic B, Farmer JA, Frazier OH, Chandler L, Payton-Ross C, Cocanougher B, Jones PH, Young JB, Gotto AM: Hyperlipidemia after heart transplantation: report of a 6-year experience with treatment recommendations. J Am Coll Cardiol 1992;19:1315–1321.

29. Bamford RN, Grant AJ, Burton JD, Peters C, Kurys G, Goldman CK, Brennan J, Roessler E, Waldmann TA: The interleukin (IL) 2 receptor beta chain is shared by IL-2 and a cytokine, provisionally designated IL-T, that stimulates T-cell proliferation and the induction of lymphokine-activated killer cells. Proc Natl Acad Sci U S A 1994;91:4940–4944.

30. Barber WH, Mankin JA, Laskow DA, Deierhoi MH, Julian BA, Curtis JJ, Diethelm AG: Long term results of a controlled prospective study with transfusion of donor-specific bone marrow in 57 cadaveric renal allograft recipients. Transplantation 1991;51: 70–75.

31. Barone G, Chang CT, Choc MG Jr, Klein JB, Marsh CL, Meligeni JA, Min DI, Pescovitz MD, Pollak R, Pruett TL, Stinson JB, Thompson JS, Vasquez E, Waid T, Wombolt DG, Wong RL: The pharmacokinetics of a microemulsion formulation of cyclosporine in primary renal allograft recipients. Transplantation 1996;61: 875–880.

32. Barr ML, Berger CL, Wiedermann JG, Murphy MP, Jorgensen BA, McLauglin SN, Schenkel FA, Pepino P, He X, Marobe CC, Rose EA: Photochemotherapy for the prevention of graft atherosclerosis in cardiac transplantation. J Heart Lung Transplant 1993;12:S85.

33. Barros EJG, Boim MA, Ajzen H, Ramos OL, Schor N: Glomerular hemodynamics and hormonal participation on cyclosporine nephrotoxicity. Kidney Int 1987;32:19–25.

34. Bartlett PR, Dimitrijevic M, Mattar T: Leflunomide (HWA 486), a novel immunomodulating compound for the treatment of autoimmune disorders and reactions leading to transplantation rejection. Agents Actions 1991;32:10–21.

35. Barton CH, Vaziri ND, Martin DC, Choi S, Alikhani S: Hypomagnesemia and renal magnesium wasting in renal transplant recipients receiving cyclosporine. Am J Med 1987;83:693–699.

36. Battle DC, Gutterman C, Tarka J, Prasad R: Effect of short-term of cyclosporine A administration on urinary acidification. Clin Nephrol 1986;25:S62.

37. Baxter JD, Forsham PH: Tissue effects of glucocorticoids. Am J Med 1972;53, 573.

38. Beelen DW, Graeven U, Schulz G, Grosse-Wilde H, Doxiadis I, Schaefer UW, Quabeck K, Sayer H, Schmidt CG: Treatment of acute graft-versus-host disease after HLA-partially matched marrow transplantation with a monoclonal antibody (BMA031) against the T cell receptor. First results of a phase I/II trial. Onkologie 1988;11:56–58.

39. Beniaminovitz A, Donovan M, Itescu S, Burke E, Edwards N, Oz M, Mancini D: Use of daclizumab decreases the frequency of early allograft in *de novo* heart transplant recipients [abstract]. JACC Program, February 1999.

40. Benigni A, Morigi M, Perico N, Zoja C, Amuchastegui CS, Piccinelli A, Donadelli R, Remuzzi G: The acute effect of FK 506 and cyclosporine on endothelial cell function and renal vascular resistance. Transplantation 1992;54:775–780.

41. Bennett WM: Immunosuppressive drug nephrotoxicity. *In* Tilne NL, Strom TB, Paul LC (eds): Transplantation Biology—Cellular and Molecular Aspects. Philadelphia: Lippincott-Raven, 1996.

42. Bennett WM, Porter JA: Cyclosporine-associated hypertension. Am J Med 1988;85:131–133.

43. Bennett WM, Walker RG, Kincaid-Smith P: Renal cortical interstitial volume in mesangial IgA nephropathy: dissociation from creatinine clearance in serially biopsied patients. Lab Invest 1982;47:330–335.

44. Berglin E, Kjellstrom C, Mantovani V, Stelin G, Svalander C, Wiklund L: Plasmapheresis as a rescue therapy to resolve cardiac rejection with vasculitis and severe heart failure. A report of five cases. Transplant Int 1995;8:382–387.

45. Besse T, Malaise J, Mourad M, Pirson Y, Hope J, Awwad M, White-Scharf M, Squifflet JP: Prevention of rejection with BTI-322 after renal transplantation (results at 9 months). Transplant Proc 1997;29:L2425–L2426.

46. Beveridge T, Gratwohl A, Michot F, Niederberger W, Nuesch E, Nussbaumer K, Schaub P, Speck B: Cyclosporin A: pharmacokinetics after a single dose in man and serum levels after multiple dosing in recipients of allogenic bone marrow grafts. Curr Ther Res 1981;30:5–17.

47. Bieber CP, Jamieson S, Raney A, Burton N, Bogarty S, Hoppe R, Kaplan HS, Strober S, Stinson EB: Cardiac allograft survival in rhesus primates treated with combined total lymphoid irradiation and rabbit antithymocyte globulin. Transplantation 1979;28:347–350.

48. Bierer B, Schreiber SL, Burakoff SJ: The effect of the immunosuppressant FK506 on alternate pathways of T cell activation. Eur J Immunol 1991;21:439.

49. Billingham ME: Diagnosis of cardiac rejection by endomyocardial biopsy. Heart Transplant 1981;1:25–30.

50. Billingham RE, Krohn PL, Medawar PB: Effect of cortisone on survival of skin homografts in rabbits. BMJ 1951;1:4716.

51. Birkinshaw JH, Raistrick H, Ross DJ: Studies in the biochemistry of micro-organisms. Biochem J 1952;50:630–634.

52. Bonnefoy-Berard N, Flacher M, Revillard JP: Antiproliferative effect of antilymphocyte globulins on B cells and B-cell lines. Blood 1992;79:2164–2170.

53. Bonnefoy-Berard N, Revillard JP: Mechanisms of immunosuppression induced by antithymocyte globulins and OKT3. J Heart Lung Transplant 1996;15:435–442.

54. Bonnefoy-Berard N, Vincent C, Revillard JP: Antibodies against functional leukocyte surface molecules in polyclonal antilymphocyte and antithymocyte globulins. Transplantation 1991;51:669–673.

55. Bonventre JV, Skorecki KL, Kreisberg JI, Cheung JY: Vasopressin increases cytosolic free calcium concentration in glomerular mesangial cells. Am J Physiol 1986;251:F94–F102.

56. Borel JF: The history of cyclosporin A and its significance. In White DJG (ed): Cyclosporin A; Proceedings of an International Conference on Cyclosporin A. London: Elsevier Biomedical Press, 1982.

57. Bouchart F, Gundry SR, Schaack-Gonzales, Razzouk AJ, Marsa RJ, Kawauchi M, deBegona JA, Bailey LL: Methotrexate as rescue/adjunctive immunotherapy in infant and adult heart transplantation. J Heart Lung Transplant 1993;12:427–433.

58. Bourge RC, Kirklin JK, Ketchum C, Naftel DC, Mason DA, Siegel AL, Scott JW, White-Williams C: Cyclosporine blood monitoring after heart transplantation: a prospective comparison of monoclonal and polyclonal radioimmunoassays. J Heart Lung Transplant 1992;11:522–529.

59. Bourge RC, Kirklin JK, McGiffin DC, Naftel DC, White-Williams C, Bhatnagar RM, Benza RL, Rayburn BK, Foley B: Total lymphoid irradiation after cardiac transplantation: is there a risk of late leukemia? [abstract]. J Heart Lung Transpl Program Issue, 1998.

60. Brewer Y, Palmer A, Taube D, Welsh K, Bewick M, Bindon C, Hale G, Waldmann H, Dische F, Parsons V: Effect of graft perfusion with two CD45 monoclonal antibodies on incidence of kidney allograft rejection. Lancet 1989;3:935–937.

61. Brockmoller J, Neumayer HH, Wagner K, Weber W, Heinemer G, Kewitz H, Roots I: Pharmacokinetic interaction between cyclosporin and diltiazem. Eur J Clin Pharmacol 1990;38:237–242.

62. Brown SA, Lucas BA, Waid TH, McKeown JW, Barve S, Jackson LR, Thompson JS: T10B9(MEDI-500) mediated immunosuppression: studies on the mechanism of action. Clin Transplant 1996;10(6 pt 2):607–613.

63. Brunner T, Mogil RJ, LaFace D, Yoo N, Mahboubl A, Echeverrl F, Martin SJ, Force WR, Lynch DH, Ware CF, Green DR: Cell-autonomous Fas (CD95)/Fas-ligand interaction mediates activation-induced apoptosis in T-cell hybridomas. Nature 1995;373:441–444.

64. Bunchman TE, Brookshire CA: Cyclosporine-induced synthesis of endothelin by cultured human endothelial cells. J Clin Invest 1991;88:310–314.

65. Bunke M, Wilder L: Effect of verapamil on glomerular filtration rate and glomerular prostaglandin production during cyclosporine administration. Transplantation 1988;46:433–437.

66. Burdman EA, Rosen S, Lindsley J, Elzinga L, Andoh T, Bennett WM: Production of less chronic nephrotoxicity by cyclosporine G than cyclosporine A in a low-salt rat model. Transplantation 1993;55:963.

67. Burlingham WJ: Chimerism after organ transplantation: is there any clinical significance? [review]. Clin Transplant 1996;10:110–117.

68. Burlingham WJ, Grailer AP, Hullett DA, Sollinger HW: Inhibition of both MLC and in vitro IgG memory response to tetanus toxoid by RS-61443. Transplantation 1991;51:545–547.

69. Buysmann S, Bemelman FJ, Schellekens PT, van Kooyk Y, Figdor CG, ten Berge IJM. Activation and increased expression of adhesion molecules on peripheral blood lymphocytes is a mechanism for the immediate lymphocytopenia after administration of OKT3. Blood 1996;87:404–411.

70. Calne RY, White DJG: Cyclosporin A—a powerful immunosuppressant in dogs with renal allografts. IRCS Med Sci 1977;5:595.

71. Calne RY, White DJG, Thir S, Evans DB, McMaster P, Dunn DC, Craddock GN, Henderson RG, Azia S, Lewis P: Cyclosporin A initially as the only immunosuppressant in 36 recipients of cadaveric organs: 32 kidney, 2 pancreas and 2 livers. Lancet 1979;2:1033.

72. Canafax DM: Immunosuppressant Pharmacokinetics and Product Performance. Current Trends: Setting Performance Standards for Immunosuppressive Drugs. Booklet sponsored by University of Minnesota (office of Continuing Medical Education), 1996.

73. Cantarovich D, Le Mauff B, Hourmant M, Peyronnet P, Jacques Y, Boeffard F, Hirn M, Soulillou JP: Prophylactic use of a monoclonal antibody (33B3.1) directed against interleukin 2 receptor following human renal transplantation. Am J Kidney Dis 1988;20:101–106.

74. Cao WW, Kao PN, Chao AC, Gardner P, Ng J, Morris RE: Mechanism of the antiproliferative action of leflunomide. J Heart Lung Transplant 1995;14:1016–1030.

75. Carrier M, White M, Perrault LP, Pelletier GB, Pellerin M, Robitaille D, Pelletier LC: A 10-year experience with intravenous thymoglobuline in induction of immunosuppression following heart transplantation. J Heart Lung Transplant 1999;18:1218–1223.

76. Carrier M, Trone F, Stewart D, Nattel S, Pelletier LC: Blockade of cyclosporine-induced vasoconstriction by the calcium channel blocker diltiazem in dogs. J Thorac Cardiovasc Surg 1993;106:487–490.

77. Carrier M, Tronc F, Stewart D, Pelletier LC: Dose-dependent effect of cyclosporine on renal arterial resistance in dogs. Am J Physiol 1991;261:H1791–H1796.

78. Carroll PB, Rilo H, Reyes J, Alejandro R, Zeng Y, Ricordi C, Tzakis A, Shapiro R, Starzl TED: FK506 associated diabetes mellitus in the pediatric transplant population is a rare complication. Transplant Proc 1991;26:3171.

79. Caruana RJ, Zumbro GL, Hoff RG, Rao RN, Daspit SA: Successful cardiac transplantation across an ABO blood group barrier. Transplantation 1988;46:472–474.

80. Carver M, Alqaisi M, Cunningham P, Gross U, Thomas F, Thomas JM: Posttransplant TLI is effective in nonhuman primates if combined with rabbit ATG. Transplant Proc 1991;23:480–482.

81. Caspi RR, McAllister CG, Gery I, Nussenblatt RB: Differential effects of cyclosporins A and G on functional activation of T-helper lymphocyte line mediating experimental autoimmune uveoretinitis. Cell Immunol 1988;113:350–360.

82. Catalan M, Llorens R, Legarra JJ, Segura I, Sarralde A, Rabago G: Plasmapheresis as therapy to resolve vascular rejection in heart transplantation with severe heart failure: "a report of one case" [review]. Transplant Proc 1998;30:176–179.

83. Chan GL, Weinstein SS, Wright CE, Bowers VD, Alveranga DY, Shires DL, Ackermann JR, LeFor WW, Kahana L: Encephalopathy associated with OKT3 administration. Possible interaction with indomethacin. Transplantation 1991;52:148–150.

84. Chang JY, Sehgal SN, Bansbach CC: FK506 and rapamycin: novel pharmacological probes of the immune response. Trends Pharmacol Sci 1991;12:218.

85. Chapman JR, Marcen R, Arias M, Raine AEG, Dunnill MS, Morris PJ: Hypertension after renal transplantation. Transplantation 1987;43:860–864.

86. Charpentier B, Hiesse C, Ferran C: Acute clinical syndrome associated with OKT3 administration. Prevention by single injection of an anti-human TNF monoclonal antibody [in French]. Presse Med 1991;20:2009–2011.

87. Charpentier B, Hiesse C, Lantz O, Ferran C, Stephens S, O'Shaugnessy D, Bodmer M, Benoit G, Bach JF, Chatenoud L: Evidence that antihuman tumor necrosis factor monoclonal antibody prevents OKT3-induced acute syndrome. Transplantation 1992;54:997–1002.

88. Chatenoud L: OKT3-induced cytokine-release syndrome: prevention effect of anti-tumor necrosis factor monoclonal antibody [review]. Transplant Proc 1993;25:47–51.

89. Chatenoud L, Bach JF: T lymphocyte activation induced by monoclonal anti-CD3 antibodies: physiopathology of cytokine release. [in French]. C R Seances Soc Biol Fil 1991;185:268–277.

90. Chatenoud L, Baudrihaye M, Schindler J, Kreis H, Goldstein G, Bach JF: In vivo induction of antigenic modulation in man by an anti-T cell monoclonal antibody (author's transl). [in French]. C R Seances Acad Sci III 1982;294:805–807.

91. Chatenoud L, Baudrihaye MF, Kreis H, Goldstein G, Schindler J, Bach JF: Human in vivo antigenic modulation induced by the anti-T cell OKT3 monoclonal antibody. Eur J Immunol 1982;12:979–982.

92. Chatenoud L, Ferran C, Bach JF: The anti-CD3-induced syndrome: a consequence of massive in vivo cell activation [review]. Curr Top Microbiol Immunol 1991;174:121–134.

93. Chatenoud L, Ferran C, Legendre C: In vivo cell activation following OKT3 administration. Systemic cytokine release and modulation by corticosteroids. Transplantation 1990;49:697–702.

94. Chatenoud L, Ferran C, Reuter A, Legendre C, Gevaert Y, Kreis H, Franchimont P, Bach JF: Systemic reaction to the monoclonal antibody OKT3 in relation to serum levels of tumor necrosis factor and interferon. N Engl J Med 1989;320:1420–1421.

95. Chong ASF, Finnegan A, Jiang X, Gebel H, Sankary HN, Foster P, Williams JW: Leflunomide, a novel immunosuppressive agent. Transplantation 1993;55:1361–1366.

96. Chow D, Saper V, Strober S: Renal transplant patients treated with total lymphoid irradiation show specific unresponsiveness to donor antigens in the mixed leukocyte reaction (MLR). J Immunol 1987;138:3746–3750.

97. Coffman TM, Carr DR, Yarger WE, Klotman PE: Evidence that renal prostaglandin and thromboxane production is stimulate in chronic cyclosporine nephrotoxicity. Transplantation 1987;43:282–285.

98. Cohen SL, Boner G, Rosenfeld JB, Shmueli D, Sperling O, Yusim A, Todd-Pokropek A, Shapira Z: The mechanisms of hyperuricaemia in cyclosporine-treated renal transplant recipients. Transplant Proc 1987;19:1829–1830.

99. Collignon P, Hurley B, Mitchell D: Interaction of fluconazole with cyclosporin. Lancet 1989;333:1262.

100. Colvin RB, Preffer FI: Laboratory monitoring of therapy with OKT3 and other murine monoclonal antibodies [review]. Clin Lab Med 1991;11:693–714.

101. Combadiere B, Sousa CR, Germain RN, Lenardo MJ: Selective induction of apoptosis in mature T lymphocytes by variant T cell receptor ligands. J Exp Med 1998;187:349–355.

102. Conger JD, Kim GE, Robinette JB: Effects of ANG II ET$_2$ and TXA$_2$ receptor antagonists on cyclosporin A renal vasoconstriction. Am Physiol Soc 1994;267:F443–F449.

103. Conti DJ, Tolkoff-Rubin NE, Baker GP, Doran M, Cosimi AB, Delmonico F, Auchincloss H, Russell PS, Rubin RH: Successful treatment of invasive fungal infection with fluconazole in organ transplant recipients. Transplantation 1989;48:692–695.

104. Contreras JL, Wang PX, Eckhoff DE, Lobashevsky AL, Asiedu C, Frenette L, Robbin ML, Hubbard WJ, Cartner S, Nadler S, Cook WJ, Sharff J, Shiloach J, Thomas FT, Neville DM, Thomas JM: Peritransplant tolerance induction with anti-CD3-immunotoxin: a matter of proinflammatory cytokine control. Transplantation 1998;65:1159–1169.

105. Cosimi AB: The clinical value of antilymphocyte antibodies. N Engl J Med 1981;305:308–314.

106. Cosimi AB, Conti D, Delmonico FL, Preffer FI, Wee SL, Rothlein R, Faanes R, Colvin RB: In vivo effects of monoclonal antibody to ICA1 (CD54) in nonhuman primates with renal allografts. J Immunol 1990;144:4604–4612.

107. Cosimi AB, Conti D, Delmonico FL, Preffer FI, Wee SL, Rothlein R, Faanes R, Colvin RB: In vivo effects of monoclonal antibody to ICAM-1(CD54) in nonhuman primates with renal allografts. J Immunol 1990;144:4604–4612.

108. Costanzo-Nordin MR, Grusk BB, Silver MA: Reversal of recalcitrant cardiac allograft rejection with methotrexate. Circulation 1988;78(suppl III):III-47–III-57.

109. Costanzo-Nordin MR, Hubbell EA, O'Sullivan EJ, Johnson MR, Mullen GM, Heroux AL, Kao WG, McManus BM, Pifarre R, Robinson JA: Photopheresis versus corticosteroids in the therapy of heart transplant rejection. Preliminary clinical report. Circulation 1992;86:II-242–II-250.

110. Costanzo-Nordin MR, McManus BM, Wilson JE, O'Sullivan EJ, Hubbell EA, Robinson JA: Efficacy of photopheresis in the rescue therapy of acute cellular rejection in human heart allografts: a preliminary clinical and immunopathologic report. Transplant Proc 1993;25:881–883.

111. Costanzo-Nordin MR, O'Sullivan EJ, Hubbel EA, Zucker MJ, Pifarre R, McManus BM, Winters GL, Scanlon PJ, Robinson JA: Long-term follow-up of heart transplant recipients treated with murine anti-human mature T cell monoclonal antibody (OKT3): the Loyola experience. J Heart Transplant 1989;8:288–295.

112. Costanzo-Nordin MR, O'Sullivan EJ, Johnson MR, Winters GL, Pifarre R, Radvany R, Zucker MJ, Scanlon PJ, Robinson JA: Prospective randomized trial of OKT3 versus horse antithymocyte globulin-based immunosuppressive prophylaxis in heart transplantation. J Heart Lung Transplant 1990;9(3 pt 2):306–315.

113. Cox KL, Lawrence-Miyasaki LS, Garacia-Kennedy R, Lennette ET, Martinez OM, Krams SM, Berquist WE, So SKS, Esquivel CO: An increased incidence of Epstein-Barr virus infection and lymphoproliferative disorder in young children on FK506 after liver transplantation. Transplantation 1995;59:524–539.

114. Crow A, Lemaire M: In vitro and in situ absorption of SDZ RAD using a human intestinal cell line (Caco-2) and a single-pass perfusion model in rats. Pharm Res 1998;15:1666–1672.

115. Cupp MJ, Tracy TS: Cytochrome P450: New nomenclature and clinical implications. Am Fami Physician 1998;57:107–116.

116. Cupps TR, Edgar LC, Fauci AS: Suppression of human B lymphocyte function by cyclophosphamide. J Immunol 1982;128:2453.

117. Curtis JJ, Luke RG, Jones P, Diethelm AG: Hypertension in cyclosporine treated renal transplant recipients is sodium dependent. Am J Med 1988;85:134–138.

118. Dantal J, Ninin E, Hourmant M, Boeffard R, Cantarovich D, Giral M, Wijdenes J, Soulillou JP, LeMauff B: Anti-CD4 MoAb therapy in kidney transplantation—a pilot study in early prophylaxis of rejection. Transplantation 1996;162:1502–1506.

119. Davis M, Williams R, Chakraborty J, English J, Marks V, Ideo G, Tempini S: Prednisone or prednisolone for the treatment of chronic active hepatitis? A comparison of plasma availability. Br J Clin Pharmacol 1978;5:501–505.

120. Dawidson I, Rooth P, Dulzo AT, Palmer B, Peters LP, Sagalowsky A, Sandor Z: Verapamil prevents posttransplant delayed function and cyclosporine A nephrotoxicity. Transplant Proc 1990;22:1379–1380.

121. DeFranco AL: Immunosuppressants at work. Nature 1991;352:754–755.

122. Deierhoi MH, Sollinger HW, Diethelm AG, Belzer FO, Kauffman RS: One year followup results of a phase I trial of mycophenolate mofetil (RS 61443) in cadaveric renal transplantation. Transplant Proc 1993;25:693–694.

123. Delmonico FL, Cosimi AB: Anti-CD4 monoclonal antibody therapy. Clin Transplant 1996;10:397–403.

124. Delmonico FL, Cosimi AB: Monoclonal antibody treatment of human allograft recipients. Surg Gynecol Obstet 1988;166:89–98.

125. Delmonico FL, Cosimi AB, Kawai T, Cavender D, Lee W, Jolliffe LK, Knowles RW: Nonhuman primate responses to murine and humanized OKT4A. Transplantation 1993;55:722–728.

126. Denton MD, Magee CC, Sayegh MH: Immunosuppressive strategies in transplantation. Lancet 1999;353:1083–1091.

127. Depper JM, Leonard WJ, Robb RJ, Waldmann TA, Greene WC: Blockade of the interleukin-2 receptor by anti-Tac antibody: inhibition of human lymphocyte activation. J Immunol 1983;131:690–696.

128. Dhein J, Walczak H, Baumier C, Debatin KM, Krammer PH: Autocrine T cell suicide mediated by APO-1/(FAS/CD95). Nature 1995;373:438–441.

129. Dickneite G, Schorlemmer HU, Sedlacek HH, Falk W, Ulrichs K, Muller-Ruchholtz WM: Suppression of macrophage function and prolongation of graft survival by the new guanidinic-like structure, 15-deoxyspergualin. Transplant Proc 1987;19:1301–1304.

130. DiMartini A, Pajer K, Trzepacz P: Psychiatric morbidity in liver transplant patients. Transplant Proc 1991;23:3179–3180.

131. DiSalvo TG, Narula J, Cosimi AB, Keck S, Dec GW, Semigran MJ: Actinomycin D is an effective adjunctive immunosuppressive agent in recurrent cardiac allograft rejection. J Heart Lung Transplant 1995;14:955–962.

132. Dische FE, Neuberger J, Keating J, Parsons V, Calne RY, Williams R: Kidney pathology in liver allograft recipients after long-term treatment with cyclosporin A. Lab Invest 1988;58:395–401.

133. Ducloux D, Ottignon Y, Semhoun-Ducloux S, Labbe S, Saint-Hillier Y, Miguet JP, Carayon P, Chalopin JM: Mycophenolate mofetil-induced villous atrophy. Transplantation 1998;66:1115–1116.

134. Dumont FJ, Melino MR, Staruch MJ, Koprak SL, Fischer PA, Sigal NH: The immunosuppressive macrolides FK 506 and rapamycin act as reciprocal antagonists in murine T cells. J Immunol 1990;144:1418.

135. Dumont FJ, Su Q: Mechanism of action of the immunosuppressant rapamycin. Life Sci 1996;58:373–395.

136. Dunn DC, White DJG, Wade J: Survival of first and second kidney allografts after withdrawal of cyclosporin A therapy. IRCS Med Sci 1978;6:464.

137. Dupont E, Schandene L, Denys C, Wybran J: Differential in-vitro actions of cyclosporin, methylprednisolone, and 6-metacaptopurine; implications for drugs' influence on lymphocyte activation mechanisms. Clin Immunol Immunopathol 1986;40:422–428.

138. Edelson R: Light-activated drugs. Sci Am 1988;259:68–75.

139. Edelson R, Berger C, Gasparro F, Jegasothy B, Heald P, Wintroub B, Vonderheid E, Knobler R, Wolfe K, Plewig G, McKiernan G, Christiansen I, Oster M, Honigsmann H, Wilford H, Kokoschka E, Rehle T, Perez M, Stingl G, Laroche L: Treatment of cutaneous T-cell lymphoma by extracorporeal photochemotherapy. Preliminary results. N Engl J Med 1987;316:297–303.

140. Ehninger G, Jaschonek K, Schuler U, Kruger HU: Interaction of luconazole with cyclosporin. Lancet 1989;334:104–105.

141. Eidelman BH, Abu-Elmagd K, Wilson J, Fung JJ, Alessiani M, Jain A, Takaya S, Todo SN, Tzakis A, Van Thiel D: Neurologic complications of FK506. Transplant Proc 1991;23:3175.

142. Elion GB, Burgi E, Hitchings GH: Studies on condensed pyrimidine systems. IX. Synthesis of some six substituted purines. J Am Chem Soc 1952;74:411.

143. Elion GB, Callahan S, Nathan H, Beiber S: Potentiation by inhibition of drug degradation: 6-substituted purines and xanthine oxidase. Biochem Pharmacol 1963;12:85.

144. Endresen E, Bergan S, Holdaas H, Pran T, Sinding-Larsen B, Berg KJ: Lack of effect of the calcium antagonist isradipine on cyclosporine pharmacokinetics in renal transplant patients. Ther Drug Monit 1991;13:490–495.

145. Eng CP, Gullo-Brow J, Chang JY, Sehgal SN: Inhibition of skin graft rejection in mice by rapamycin: a novel immunosuppressive macrolide. Transplant Proc 1991;23:868–869.

146. English J, Evan A, Houghton DC, Bennett WM: Cyclosporine-induced acute renal dysfunction in the rat. Evidence of arteriovasoconstriction with preservation of tubular function. Transplantation 1987;44:135–141.

147. Enomoto DN, Schellekens PT, Yong SL, Ten B, Mekkes JR, Bos JD: Extracorporeal photochemotherapy (photopheresis) induces apoptosis in lymphocytes: a possible mechanism of action of PUVA therapy. Photochemi Photobiol 1997;65:177–180.

148. Ensley RD, Bristow MR, Olsen SL, Taylor DO, Hammond E, O'Connell JB, Dunn D, Osburn L, Jones KW, Kauffman RS, Gay WA, Renlund DG: The use of mycophenolate mofetil (RS-61443) in human heart transplant recipients. Transplantation 1993;56:75–82.

149. Epinette WW, Parker CM, Jones EL, Greist MC: Mycophenolic acid for psoriasis: a review of pharmacology, long-term efficacy and safety. J Am Acad Dermatol 1987;17:962–971.

150. Eugui EM, Almquist SJ, Muller CD, Allison AC: Lymphocyte-selective cytostatic and immunosuppressive effects of mycophenolic acid in vitro: role of deoxyguanosine nucleotide depletion. Scand J Immunol 1991;33:175–183.

151. European FK506 Multicentre Liver Study Group: Randomized trial comparing tacrolimus (FK506) and cyclosporine in prevention of liver allograft rejection. Lancet 1994;344:423–428.

152. Faraci M, Vigeant C, Yale JF: Pharmacokinetic profile of cyclosporine A and G and their effects on cellular immunity and glucose tolerance in male and female Wistar rats. Transplantation 1988;45:617.

153. Fechner JHJ, Vargo DJ, Geissler EK, Graeb C, Wang J, Hanaway MJ, Watkins DI, Piekarczyk M, Neville DM, Knechtle SJ: Split tolerance induced by immunotoxin in a rhesus kidney allograft model. Transplantation 1997;63:1339–1345.

154. Ferran C, Millan MT, Csizmadia V, Cooper JT, Brostjan C, Bach FH, Winkler H: Inhibition of NF-κB by pyrrolidine dithiocarbamate blocks endothelial cell activation. Biochem Biophys Res Commun 1995;214:212–223.

155. Feutren G, Mihatsch MJ: Risk factors for a cyclosporine-induced nephropathy in patients with autoimmune disease. International kidney biopsy registry of cyclosporine in autoimmune diseases. N Engl J Med 1992;326:1654–1660.

156. Finkel MS, Oddis CV, Jacob TD, Watkins SC, Hattler BG, Simmons RL: Negative inotropic effects of cytokines on the heart mediated by nitric oxide. Science 1992;257:387–389.

157. Fiocchi R, Mamprin F, Gamba A, Glauber M, Catania S, Cattaneo G, Torre L, Bertocchi C, Ruhrmann R, Colombo D, Binetti G, Ferrazzi P: Pharmacokinetics profile of cyclosporine in long-term heart transplanted patients treated with a new oral formulation. Transplant Proc 1994;26:2994–2995.

158. Firpo EJ, Koff A, Solomon MJ, Roberts JM: Inactivation of a Cdk2 inhibitor during interleukin 2-induced proliferation of human T lymphocytes. Mol Cell Biol 1994;14:4889–4901.

159. First MR, Schroeder TJ, Hariharan S, Alexander JW, Weiskittel P: The effect of indomethacin on the febrile response following OKT3 therapy. Transplantation 1992;53:91–94.

160. First MR, Schroeder TJ, Hariharan S, Weiskittel P: Reduction of the initial febrile response to OKT3 with indomethacin. Transplant Proc 1993;25:52–54.

161. Fischer G, Schmid FX: The mechanism of protein folding. Implications of in vitro refolding to de novo protein folding and translocation in the cell. Biochemistry 1990;29:2205.

162. Floyd KC, Hricik DE, Simonson MS: Cyclosporine but not rapamycin stimulates endothelin-1 secretion by endothelial cells: potential significance in transplant vasculopathy. American Society of Transplantation. Accessed November 14, 1999.

163. Foegh ML, Virmani R: Molecular biology intimal proliferation. Curr Opin Cardiol 1993;8:938–950.

164. Fogo A, Hellings SE, Inagami T, Kon V: Endothelin receptor antagonism is protective in in vivo acute cyclosporine toxicity. Kidney Int 1992;42:770–774.

165. Food and Drug Administration (FDA): Center for Drug Evaluation and Research (CDER). NDA 21-083. Rapamune (sirolimus) oral solution: medical officer's review and clinical pharmacology and biopharmaceutics review(s). Accessed January 2000.

166. Food and Drug Administration (FDA): NDA 21-083 Sirolimus Rapamune. 11/29/99.

167. Freise CE, Hebert M, Osorio RW, Nikolai B, Lake JR, Kauffman RS, Ascher NL, Roberts JP: Maintenance immunosuppression with prednisone and RS-61443 alone following liver transplantation. Transplant Proc 1993;25:1758–1759.

168. Frenken LA, Hoitsma AJ, Tax WJ, Koene RA: Prophylactic use of anti-CD3 monoclonal antibody WT32 in kidney transplantation. Transplant Proc 1991;23:1072.

169. Friend PJ, Rebello P, Oliveira D, Manna V, Cobbold SP, Hale G, Jamieson NV, Jamieson I, Calne RY, Harris DT: Successful

treatment of renal allograft rejection with a humanized antilymphocyte monoclonal antibody. Transplant Proc 1995;27:869–870.

170. Friend PJ, Waldmann H, Hale G, Cobbold S, Rebella P, Thiru S, Jamieson NV, Johnston PS, Calne RY: Reversal of allograft rejection using the monoclonal antibody, Campath-1G. Transplant Proc 1991;23:2253–2254.

171. Frist WH, Biggs VJ: Chronic myelogenous leukemia after lymphoid irradiation and heart transplantation. Ann Thorac Surg 1994;57:214–216.

172. Fujii JJ, Takada T, Nemoto K, Yamashita Y, Abe F, Fujii A, Takeuchi T: Deoxyspergualin directly suppresses antibody formation *in vivo* and *in vitro*. J Antibiot (Tokyo)1990;43:213–219.

173. Fukuzawa M, Sharrow SO, Shearer GM: Effect of cyclosporin A on T cell immunity. II. Defective thymic education of CD4 T helper cell function in cyclosporin A-treated mice. Eur J Immunol 1989;19:1147–1152.

174. Fung JJ, Eliasziw M, Todo S, Jain A, Demetris AJ, McMichael JP, Starzl TE, Meier P, Donner A: The Pittsburgh randomized trial of tacrolimus compared to cyclosporine for hepatic transplantation. J Am Coll Surg 1996;183:117–125.

175. Gaber AO: Results of the double-blind, randomized, multicenter, phase III clinical trial of Thymoglobulin versus Atgam in the treatment of acute graft rejection episodes after renal transplantation. Transplantation 1998;66:29–37.

176. Garcia-Morales R, Carreno M, Mathew J, Zucker K, Cirocco R, Ciancio G, Burke G, Roth D, Temple D, Rosen A, Fuller L, Esquenazi V, Karatzas T, Ricordi C, Tzakis A, Miller J: The effects of chimeric cells following donor bone marrow infusions as detected by PCR-flow assays in kidney transplant recipients [published erratum appears in J Clin Invest 1997 May;99(9):2295]. J Clin Invest 1997;99:1118–1129.

177. Gardlund B, Sjolin J, Nilsson A, Roll M, Wickerts CJ, Wretlind B: Plasma levels of cytokines in primary septic shock in humans: correlation with disease severity. J Infect Dis 1995;172:296–301.

178. Garrity ER Jr, Hertz M, Trulock EP, Keenan R, Love R: Suggested guidelines for the use of tacrolimus in lung-transplant recipients. J Heart Lung Transplant 1999;18:175–176.

179. Gasparro FP, Chan G, Edelson RL: Phototherapy and photopharmacology. Yale J Biol Med 1985;58:519–534.

180. Gebel HM, Lebeck LK, Jensik SC, Webster K, Bray RA: T cells from patients successfully treated with OKT3 do not react with the T-cell receptor antibody. Hum Immunol 1989;26:123–129.

181. van Gelder T, Mulder AH, Balk AHMM, Mochtar B, Hesse CJ, Baan CC, Vaessen LMB, Weimar W: Intragraft monitoring of rejection after prophylactic treatment with monoclonal anti-interleukin-2 receptor antibody (BT563) in heart transplant recipients. J Heart Lung Transplant 1995;14:346–350.

182. Goldberg LC, Bradley JA, Connolly J, Friend PJ, Oliveira DB, Parrott NR, Rodger RS, Taube D, Thick MG: Anti-CD45 monoclonal antibody perfusion of human renal allografts prior to transplantation. A safety and immunohistological study. CD45 Study Group. Transplantation 1995;59:1285–1293.

183. Goldberg LC, Cook T, Taube D: Pretreatment of renal transplants with anti-CD45 antibodies: optimization of perfusion technique. Transplant Immunol 1994;2:27–34.

184. Goldberg JP, Schrier RW: Effect of calcium membrane blockers on in vivo vasoconstrictor properties norepinephrine, angiotensin II and vasopressin. Miner Electrolyte Metab 1984;10:178–183.

185. Gosio B: Ricerche bacteriologiche e chimiche sulle alter-azioni del mais. Riv Igiene Sanita Pubblica 1899;7:825–868.

186. Goumy L, Ferran C, Merite S, Bach JF, Chatenoud L: In vivo anti-CD3-driven cell activation. Cellular source of induced tumor necrosis factor, interleukin-1 beta, and interleukin-6. Transplantation 1996;61:83–87.

187. Gozzo JJ, Wood ML, Monaco AP: Use of allogenic, homozygous bone marrow cells for the induction of specific immunologic tolerance in mice treated with antilymphocyte serum. Surg Forum 1970;21:281–284.

188. Grabstein KH, Eisenman J, Shanebeck K, Rauch C, Srinivasan S, Fung V, Beers C, Richardson J, Schoenborn MA, Ahdieh M, Johnson L, Alderson MR, Watson JD, Anderson DM, Giri JG: Cloning of a T cell growth factor that interacts with the beta chain of the interleukin-2 receptor. Science 1994;264:965–968.

189. Grandtnerova B, Javorsky P, Kolacny J, Hovoricova B, Dedic P, Laca L: Treatment of acute humoral rejection in kidney trans-

plantation with plasmapheresis. Transplant Proc 1995;27:934–935.

190. Granstein RD, Tominaga A, Mizel SB: Molecular signals in antigen presentation. J Immunol 1984;132:2210.

191. Graves NM, Matas AJ, Hilligoss DM, Canafax DM: Fluconazole/cyclosporine interaction [abstract]. Clin Pharmacol Ther 1990;47:208.

192. Gray JG, Monaco AP, Wood ML, Russell PS: Studies on heterologous antilymphocyte serum in mice. I. In vitro and in vivo properties. J Immunol 1966;96:217–228.

193. Gregory CR, Huang X, Pratt RE, Dzau VJ, Shorthouse R, Billingham ME, Morris RE: Treatment with rapamycin and mycophenolic acid reduces arterial intimal thickening produced by mechanical injury and allows endothelial replacement. Transplantation 1995;59:655–661.

194. Gregory CR, Huie P, Billingham ME, Morris RE: Rapamycin inhibits arterial intimal thickening caused by both alloimmune and mechanical injury. Transplantation 1993;55:1409–1418.

195. Gregory CR, Pratt RE, Shorthouse HR, Dzau VJ, Billingham ME, Morris RE: Effects of treatment with cyclosporine, FK506, rapamycin, mycophenolic acid, or deoxyspergualin on vascular muscle proliferation in vitro and in vivo. Transplant Proc 1993;25:770–771.

196. Grevel J: Cyclosporine pharmacokinetics. Transplant Proc 1988;20 (suppl 2):428–434.

197. Grevel J, Kahan BD: Area under the curve monitoring of cyclosporine therapy: the early posttransplant period. Ther Drug Monit 1991;13:89–95.

198. Griffith BP, Kormos RI, Armitage JM, Dummer JS, Hardesty RL: Comparative trial of immunoprophylaxis with RATG versus OKT3. J Heart Transplant 1990;9:301.

199. Groth CG, Backman L, Morals JM, Calne R, Kreis H, Lang P, Touraine JL, Claesson K, Campistol JM, Durand D, Wramner L, Brattstrom C, Charpentier B: Sirolimus (rapamycin)-based therapy in human renal transplantation. Transplantation 1999;67:1036–1042.

200. Gruber S, Erdman GR, Burke BA: Mizoribine pharmacokinetics and pharmacodynamics in a canine renal allograft model of local immunosuppression. Transplantation 1992;53:12–19.

201. Gruber SA, Hewitt JM, Sorenson AL, Barber D, Bowers L, Rynders G, Arrazola L, Matas AJ, Rosenberg ME, Canafax DM: Pharmacokinetics of FK506 after intravenous and oral administration in patients awaiting renal transplantation. J Clin Pharmacol 1994;34:859–864.

202. Guengerich FP: Role of cytochrome P450 enzymes in drug-interactions. Adv Pharmacol 1997;43:7–35.

203. Gupta SK, Manfro RC, Tomlanovich SJ, Gambertoglio JG, Garovoy MR, Benet LZ: Effect of food on the pharmacokinetics of cyclosporine in health subjects following oral and intravenous administration. J Clin Pharmacol 1990;30:643–653.

204. Gurish MF, Lynch DG, Daynes RA: Changes in antigen-presenting cell function in the spleen and lymph nodes of ultraviolet-irradiated mice. Transplantation 1982;33:280–284.

205. Guttmann RD: Pharmacokinetics, foreign protein immune response, cytokine release, and lymphocyte subsets in patients receiving Thymoglobulin and immunosuppression. Transplant Proc 1997;29(suppl A):24S–26S.

206. Hakimi J, Chizzonite R, Luke DR, Familletti PC, Bailon P, Kondas JA, Pilson RS, Lin P, Weber DV, Spence C, Mondini LJ, Tsien WH, Levin JL, Gallati VH, Korn L, Waldmann TA, Queen C, Baenjamin WR: Reduced immunogenicity and improved pharmacokinetics of humanized anti-Tac in cynomolgus monkeys. J Immunol 1991;147:1352–1359.

207. Hale G, Waldmann H, Friend P, Calne R: Pilot study of CAMPATH-1, a rat monoclonal antibody that fixes human complement, as an immunosuppressant in organ transplantation. Transplantation 1986;42:308–311.

208. Halloran PF, Lui SL: Approved immunosuppressants. In Norman DJ, Suki WN (eds): Primer on Transplantation. Thorofare, NJ: American Society of Transplant Physicians, 1998.

209. Harrington WJ, Minnieh V, Hollingsworth WJ: Demonstration of a thrombocytopenia factor in the blood of patients with thrombocytopenia purpura. J Clin Lab Med 1951;38:1–11.

210. Hartner WC, De Fazio SR, Maki T, Markees TG, Monaco AP, Gozzo JJ: Prolongation of renal allograft survival in antilympho-

cyte-serum-treated dogs by postoperative injection of density-gradient-fractionated donor bone marrow. Transplantation 1986; 42:593–597.

211. Hartner WC, De Fazio SR, Markees TG, Maki T, Monaco AP, Gozzo JJ: Specific tolerance to canine renal allografts following treatment with fractionated bone marrow and antilymphocyte serum. Transplant Proc 1987;19:476–477.

212. Haug CE, Colvin RB, Delmonico FL, Auchincloss H, Tolkoff-Rubin N, Preffer FI, Rothlein R, Norris S, Scharschmidt L, Cosimi AB: A phase I trial of immunosuppression with anti-ICAM-1 (CD54) mAb in renal allograft recipients. Transplantation 1993;55: 766–773.

213. Haug M III, Wimberley SL: Problems with the automatic switching of generic cyclosporine oral solution for the innovator product. Am J Health Syst Pharm 2000;57:1349–1353.

214. Haverty TP, Sanders M, Sheahan M: OKT3 treatment of cardiac allograft rejection. J Heart Lung Transplant 1993;12:591–598.

215. Heitman J, Movva NR, Hall MN: Targets for cell cycle arrest by the immunosuppressant rapamycin in yeast. Science 1991;253: 905–909.

216. Hess A: Cyclosporine in Clinical Use. New York: World Medical Press, 1988.

217. Hess AD, Bright EC: Cyclosporin inhibits T-cell activation at two distinct levels: role of the CD28 activation pathway. Transplant Proc 1991;23:961.

218. Hesse CJ, Heyse P, Stolk BJM, Hendriks GFJ, Weimar W, Balk AHMM, Mochtar B, Jutte NHPM: Differences in antibody formation to OKT3 between kidney and heart transplant recipients. Transplant Proc 1989;21:979–980.

219. Hibberd PL, Tolkoff-Rubin NE, Cosimi AB, Schooley RT, Isaacson D, Doran M, Delvecchio A, Delmonico FL, Auchincloss H, Rubin RH: Symptomatic cytomegalovirus disease in the cytomegalovirus antibody seropositive renal transplant recipient treated with OKT3. Transplantation 1992;53:68–72.

220. Hiesse C, Kriaa F, Rousseau P, Farahmand H, Bismuth A, Fries D, Charpentier B: Immunoadsorption of anti-HLA antibodies for highly sensitized patients awaiting renal transplantation. Nephrol Dial Transplant 1992;7:944–951.

221. Holt DW, Mueller EA, Kovarik JM, van Bree JB, Kutz K: The pharmacokinetics of Sandimmune Neoral: a new formulation of cyclosporine. Transplant Proc 1993;26:2935–2939.

222. Horton CM, Freeman CD, Nolan PE, Copeland JG: Cyclosporine Interactions with miconazole and other azole-antimycotics: a case report and review of the literature. J Heart Lung Transplant 1992;11:1127–1132.

223. Hosenpud J, Hershberger R, Ratkovec R, Hovaguimian H, Ott G, Cobanoglu A, Norman D: Methotrexate for the treatment of patients with multiple episodes of acute cardiac allograft rejection. J Heart Lung Transplant 1992;11:739–745.

224. Hourmant M, Bedrossian J, Durand D, Lebranchu Y, Renoult E, Caudrelier P, Buffet R, Soulillou JP: A randomized multi-center trial comparing leukocyte function associated antigen-1 monoclonal antibody with rabbit antithymocyte globulin as induction treatment in first kidney transplantations. Transplantation 1996; 62:1565–1570.

225. Hrelia P, Murelli L, Scotti M, Paolini M, Cantelli-Forti G: Organo-specific activation of azathioprine in mice: role of liver metabolism in mutation induction. Carcinogenesis 1988;9:1011–1015.

226. Hricik DE, Almawi WY, Stromm TB: Trends in the use of glucocorticoids in renal transplantation. Transplantation 1994;57:979.

227. Hunt SA, Strober S, Hoppe RT, Stinson EB: Total lymphoid irradiation for treatment of intractable cardiac allograft rejection. J Heart Transplant 1991;10:211–216.

228. Huser B, Thiel O, Oberholzer M, Beveridge T, Bianchi L, Mihatsch MJ, Landmann J: The efficacy and tolerability of cyclosporin G in human kidney transplant recipients. Transplantation 1992; 54:65–69.

229. Ichikawa I, Miele JF, Brenner BM: Reversal of renal cortical actions of angiotensin II by verapamil and manganese. Kidney Inte 1979;16:137–147.

230. Isobe M, Yagita H, Okumura K, Ihara A: Specific acceptance of cardiac allograft after treatment with antibodies to ICAM-1 and LFA-1. Science 1992;255:1125–1127.

231. Jain AB, Venkataramanan R, Cadoff E, Fung JJ, Todo S, Krajack A, Starzl TE: Effect of hepatic dysfunction and T tube clamping on FK 506 pharmacokinetics and trough concentrations. Transplant Proc 1990;22(suppl 1):57–59.

232. Janssen O, Wesselborg S, Kabelitz D: Immunosuppression by OKT3—induction of programmed cell death (apoptosis) mechanism of action. Transplantation 1992;53:233–234.

233. Jensen CWB, Flechner SM, Van Buren CT, Frazier OH, Cooley DA, Lorber MI, Kahan BD: Exacerbation of cyclosporine toxicity by concomitant administration of erythromycin. Transplantation 1987;43:263–270.

234. Jiang H, Suguo H, Takahara S, Takano Y, Li D, Kameoka H, Moutabarrik A: Combined immunosuppressive effect of FK506 and other immunosuppressive agents on PhA- and CD3-stimulated human lymphocyte proliferation in vitro. Transplant Proc 1991;23:2933–2936.

235. Jones EL, Epinette WW, Hackney VC, Menendez L, Frost P: Treatment of psoriasis with oral mycophenolic acid. J Invest Dermatol 1975;65:537–542.

236. Jones EL, Frost P, Epinette WW, Gomez E: Mycophenolic acid: an evaluation of long-term safety. In Faraber EM, Cox AJ, Jacobs PH, Nall ML (eds): Psoriasis: Proceedings of the Second International Symposium. New York: Yorke, 1977, pp 442–443.

237. Jonker M, Malissen B, Mawas C: The effect of in vivo application of monoclonal antibodies specific for human cytotoxic T cells in rhesus monkeys. Transplantation 1983;35:374.

238. Jordan ML, Shapiro R, Vivas CA, Scantlebury VP, Rhandhawa P, Carrieri G, McCauley J: FK506 "rescue" for resistant rejection of renal allografts under primary cyclosporine immunosuppression. Transplantation 1994;57:860–865.

239. Ju ST, Panka DJ, Cui H, Ettinger R, El-Khatib M, Sherr DH, Stanger BZ, Marshak-Rothstein A: Fas (CD95)/FasL interactions required for programmed cell death after T-cell activation. Nature 1995;373:444–448.

240. Juckett MB, Balla J, Balla G, Jessurun J, Jacob HS, Vercellotti GM: Ferritin protects endothelial cells from oxidized low density lipoprotein in vitro. J Pathol 1995;1147:782–789.

241. Justement LB: The role of CD45 in signal transduction. Adv Immunol 1997;66:1–65.

242. Kahan BD: Cyclosporine. N Engl J Med 1989;321:1725–1738.

243. Kahan BD, Dunn J, Fitts C, Van Buren D, Wombolt D, Pollak R, Carson R, Alexandewr JW, Choc M, Wong R, Hwang DS: Reduced inter- and intrasubject variability in cyclosporine pharmacokinetics in renal transplant formulation in conjunction with fasting, low-fat meals, or high-fat meals. Transplantation 1995;59:505–511.

244. Kahan BD, Flechner SM, Lorber MI, Jensen C, Golden D, Van Buren CT: Complications of cyclosporine therapy. World J Surg 1986;10:348–360.

245. Kahan BD, Gibbons S, Chou TC: Synergistic interactions of cyclosporine and rapamycin to inhibit immune performances of normal human peripheral blood lymphocytes in vitro. Transplantation 1991;51:232–239.

246. Kahan BD, Julian BA, Pescovitz MD, Vanrenterghem Y, Neylan J: Sirolimus reduces the incidence of acute rejection episodes despite lower cyclosporine doses in Caucasian recipients of mismatched primary renal allografts: a phase II trial. Transplantation 1999;68:1526–1532.

247. Kahan BD, Reid M, Newburger J: Pharmacokinetics of cyclosporine in human renal transplantation. Transplant Proc 1983;15:446–453.

248. Kahan BD, Welsh M, Rutzky LP: Challenges in cyclosporine therapy: the role of therapeutic monitoring by area under the curve monitoring. Ther Drug Monit 1995;17:621–624.

249. Kahan BD, Wong RL, Carter C, Katz SH, Fellenberg JV, Van Buren CT, Appel-Dingemanse S: A phase I study of a 4-week course of SDZ-RAD (RAD) in quiescent cyclosporine-prednisone-treated renal transplant recipients. Transplantation 1999;68:1100–1106.

250. Kahn DR, Hong R, Greenberg AJ, Gilbert EF, Dacumos GC, Dufek JH: Total lymphatic irradiation and bone marrow in human heart transplantation. Ann Thorac Surg 1984;38:169–171.

251. Kale-Pradhan P, Woo MH: A review of the effects of plasmapheresis on drug clearance. Pharmacotherapy 1997;17:684–695.

252. Kaplan B, Meier-Kriesch HU, Napoli KL, Kahan BD: The effects of relative timing of sirolimus and cyclosporine microemulsion

formulation coadministration on the pharmacokinetics of each agent. Clin Pharmacol Ther 1998;63:48–53.

253. Kaplan HS: Selective effects of total lymphoid irradiation (TLI) on the immune response. Transplant Proc 1981;13:425–428.

254. Karch SB, Billingham ME: Cyclosporine induced myocardial fibrosis: a unique controlled case report. J Heart Tranplant 1985;4: 210–212.

255. Karpatkin S, Strick N, Karpatkin MN, Siskind GW: Cumulative experience on the detection of anti-platelet antibodies in 234 patients with idiopathic thrombocytopenic purpura, systemic lupus erythematosus, and other clinical disorders. Am J Med 1972;52:776–785.

256. Kay JE, Benzie CR: T lymphocyte activation through the CD28 pathway is insensitive to inhibition by the immunosuppressive drug FK506. Immunol Lett 1989;23:155.

257. Kay JE, Kromwel L, Does SE: Inhibition of T and B lymphocyte proliferation by rapamycin. Immunology 1991;72:544–549.

258. Kelly GE, Mahony JF, Sheil AGR, Meikle WD, Tiller DJ, Horvath J: Risk factors for skin carcinogenesis in immunosuppressed kidney transplant recipients. Clin Transplant 1987;271:1987.

259. Keogh A, Spratt P, McCosker C, Macdonald P, Mundy J, Kaan A: Ketoconazole to reduce the need for cyclosporine after cardiac transplantation. N Engl J Med 1995;333:628–633.

260. Kennedy MS, Deeg HJ, Siegel M, Crowley JJ, Storb R, Thomas ED: Acute renal toxicity with combined use of amphotericin B and cyclosporine after marrow transplantation. Transplantation 1983;35:211–215.

261. Khavari PA, Edelson R, Lider O, Gasparro FP, Weiner HL, Cohen IR: Specific vaccination against photoinactivated cloned T cells [abstract]. Clin Res 1988;36;662A.

262. Kiberd BA: Cyclosporine-induced renal dysfunction in human renal allograft recipients. Transplantation 1989;48:965–969.

263. Kimball PM, Kerman RH, Kahan BD: Production of synergistic but nonidentical mechanisms of immunosuppression by CsA and RAPA. Transplantation 1991;51:486.

264. Kino T, Hatanaka H, Miyata S, Inamura N, Nishiyama M, Yajima T, Goto T, Okuhara M, Kohsaka M, Aoki H, Ochiai T: FK50–6 a novel immunosuppressant isolated from a Streptomyces. II. Immunosuppressive effect of FK506 in vitro. J Antibiot 1987; 40:1256.

265. Kirklin JK, Bourge RC, Naftel DC, Morrow WR, Deierhoi MH, Kauffman RS, White-Williams C, Nomberg RI, Holman WL, Smith DC Jr: Treatment of recurrent heart rejection with mycophenolate mofetil (RS-61443): initial clinical experience. J Heart Lung Transplant 1994;13:444–450.

266. Kirklin JK, Bourge RC, White-Williams C, Naftel DC, Thomas FT, Thomas JM, Phillips MG: Prophylactic therapy for rejection after cardiac transplantation; a comparison of rabbit antithymocyte globulin and OKT3. J Thorac Cardiovasc Surg 1990;99: 716–724.

267. Kirklin JK, George JF, McGiffin DC, Naftel DC, Salter MM, Bourge RB: Total lymphoid irradiation: is there a role in pediatric heart transplantation? J Heart Lung Transplant 1993;12:S293–S300.

268. Kirklin JK, Naftel DC, Levine TB, Bourge RC, Pelletier GB, O'Donnell J, Miller LW, Pritzker MR, and the Transplant Cardiologist Research Database (TCRD) Group: Cytomegalovirus after heart transplantation: risk factors for infection and mortality: a multi-institutional study. J Heart Lung Transplant 1994:13:394–404.

269. Kirkman RL, Araujo JL, Busch GJ, Carpenter CB, Milford EL, Reinherz EL, Schlossman SF, Strom TB, Tilney NL: Treatment of acute renal allograft rejection with monoclonal anti-T12 antibody. Transplantation 1983;36:620–626.

270. Kirkman RL, Barrett LV, Gaulton GN: Administration of an anti-interleukin 2 receptor monoclonal antibody prolongs cardiac allograft survival in mice. J Exp Med 1985;162:358–362.

271. Kirkman RL, Shapiro ME, Carpenter CB, McKay DB, Milford EL, Ramos EL, Tilney NL, Waldmann TA, Zimmerman CE, Strom TB: A randomized prospective trial of anti-Tac monoclonal antibody in human renal transplantation. Transplantation 1991;51: 107–113.

272. Kirkman RL, Shapiro ME, Carpenter CB, Milford EL, Ramos EL, Tilney NL, Waldmann TA, Zimmerman CE, Strom TB: Early experience with anti-Tac in clinical renal transplantation. Transplant Proc 1989;21:1766–1768.

273. Klintmalm GB, Ascher NL, Busuttil RW, Deierhoi M, Gonwa TA, Kauffman R, McDiarmid S, Poplawski S, Sollinger H, Roberts J: RS-61443 for treatment-resistant human liver rejection. Transplant Proc 1993;25:697.

274. Klintmalm GBG, Iwatsuki S, Starzl TE: Cyclosporine A hepatotoxicity in 66 renal allograft recipients. Transplantation 1981;32: 488–489.

275. Knechtle SJ, Fechner JHJ, Dong Y, Stavrou S, Neville DM, Oberley T, Buckley P, Armstrong N: Primate renal transplants using immunotoxin. Surgery 1998;124:438–446.

276. Knobler R, Trautinger F, Graninger W, Macheiner W, Gruenwald C, Neumann R, Ramer W: Parenteral administration of 8-methoxypsoralen in photopheresis. J Am Acad Dermatol 1993;28: 580–584.

277. Kobashigawa J, Miller L, Renlund D, Mentzer R, Alderman E, Bourge R, Costanzo M, Eisen H, Dureau G, Ratkovec R, Hummel M, Johnson J, Ipe D, Keogh A, Mamelok R, Mancini D, Smart F, Valantine H, for the Mycophenolate Mofetil Investigators: A randomized active-controlled trial of mycophenolate mofetil in heart transplant recipients. Transplantation 1998;66:507–515.

278. Kobashigawa JA, Renlund DG, Olsen SL, Stevenson LW, McDiarmid SV, Swanson S, Albanese E, Taylor DO, Dunn D, Brown E, Kauffman RS, Laks H: Initial results of RS-61443 for refractory cardiac rejection [abstract]. J Am Coll Cardiol 1992;19:203A.

279. Kobashigawa JA, Stevenson LW, Brownfield E, Moriguchi JD, Kawata N, Hamilton M, Minkely R, Drinkwater D, Laks H: Does short-course induction with OKT3 improve outcome after heart transplantation? A randomized trial. J Heart Lung Transplant 1993;12:250–258.

280. Kohler G, Milstein C: Continuous cultures of fused cells secreting antibody of predefined specificity. Nature 1975;256:495–497.

281. Kolars JC, Awni WM, Merion RM, Watkins PB: First-pass metabolism of cyclosporine by the gut. Lancet 1991;338:1488–1490.

282. Kon V, Sugiura M, Inagami T, Harvie BR, Ichikawa I, Hoover RL: Role of Endothelin in cyclosporine-induced glomerular dysfunction. Kidney Int 1990;37:1487–1491.

283. Kondo M, Takeshita S, Ishii N, Nakamura M, Watanabe S, Arai K, Sugamura K: Sharing of the interleukin-2 (IL-2) receptor gamma chain between receptors for IL-2 and IL-4. Science 1993;262:1874–1877.

284. Kormos RL, Herlan DB, Armitage JM, Stein K, Kaufman C, Zeevi A, Duquesnoy R, Hardesty RL, Griffith BP: Monoclonal versus polyclonal antibody therapy for prophylaxis against rejection after heart transplantation. J Heart Lung Transplant 1990;9:1–9.

285. Kostakis AJ, White DJG, Calne RY: Prolongation of the heart allograft survival by cyclosporin A. IRCS Med Sci 1977;5:280.

286. Kosugi A, Zuniga-Pflucker JC, Sharrow SO, Kruisbeek AM, Shearer GM: Effect of cyclosporin A on lymphopoiesis. II. Developmental defects of immature and mature thymocytes in fetal thymus organ cultures treated with cyclosporin A. J Immunol 1989;143:3134–3140.

287. Kovarik JM, Mueller EA, van Bree JB, Fluckiger SS, Lange H, Schmidt B, Boesken WH, Lison AE, Kutz K: Cyclosporine pharmacokinetics and variability from a microemulsion formulation multicenter investigation in kidney transplant patients. Transplantation 1994;58:658–663.

288. Kramer MR, Marshall SE, Denning DW, Keogh AM, Tucker RM, Galgiani JN, Lewiston NJ, Stevens DA, Theodore J: Cyclosporine and itraconazole interaction in heart and lung transplant patients. Ann Intern Med 1990;113:327–329.

289. Kreis H, Durand D, Land W, for the Sirolimus European Renal Transplant Study Group: Sirolimus in association with mycophenolate mofetil induction for the prevention of acute graft rejection in renal allograft recipients. Transplantation (in press).

290. Kreitman RJ, Chang CN, Hudson DV, Queen C, Bailon P, Pastan I: Anti-Tac(Fab)-PE40, a recombinant double-chain immunotoxin which kills interleukin-2-receptor-bearing cells and induces complete remission in an in vivo tumor model. Int J Cancer 1994; 57:856–864.

291. Krenski AM, Weiss A, Crabtree G, David MM, Poorham P: T-lymphocyte-antigen interaction in transplant rejection. N Engl J Med 1990;322:510–517.

292. Kriaa F, Rousseau P, Hiesse C, Farahmand H, Brocard JF, Rieu P, Lantz O, Farquet C, Bismuth A, Benoit G, Charpentier B: Anti-HLA antibodies depletion on protein A-sepharose columns in

hyperimmunized patients awaiting renal transplantation. Ann Med Interne 1992;143(suppl 1):39–42.

293. Krieger NR, Quezada VR, Huie P, Holm B, Sibley RK, Dafoe DC, Alfrey EJ: Cardiac allograft unresponsiveness using a posttransplant strategy: characterization of the graft infiltrate. J Surg Res 1996;63:86–92.

294. Kroczek RA, Black CDV, Barbet J, Shevach EM: Mechanism of action of cyclosporine A in vivo. I. Cyclosporine A fails to inhibit T lymphocyte activation in response to allo-antigens. J Immunol 1987;139:3597–3603.

295. Kruger HU, Schuler U, Zimmerman R, Ehninger G: Absence of significant interaction of fluconazole with cyclosporin. J Antimicrob Chemother 1989;24:781–786.

296. Kuchle CCA, Thoenes GH, Langer KH, Schorlemmer HU, Bartlett RR, Schleyerbach R: Prevention of kidney and skin allograft rejection in rats by leflunomide, a new immunomodulating agent. Transplant Proc 1991;23:1083–1086.

297. Kung PC, Goldstein G, Reinherz EL, Schlossman SF: Monoclonal antibodies defining distinctive human T cell surface antigens. Science 1979;206:347–349.

298. Kurtz A, Bruna RD, Kuhn K: Cyclosporine A enhances renin secretion and production in isolated juxtaglomerular cells. Kidney Int 1998;33:947–953.

299. Ladowski JS, Dillon T, Schatzlein MH, Peterson AC, Deschner WP, Beatty L, Sullivan M, Scheeringa RH, Clark WR: Prophylaxis of heart transplant rejection with either antithymocyte globulin-, Minnesota antilymphocyte globulin-, or an OKT2-based protocol. J Cardiovasc Surg 1993;34:135–140.

300. Lai J-H, Tan TH: CD28 signaling causes a sustained downregulation of IκBα which can be prevented by the immunosuppressant rapamycin. J Biol Chem 1994;269:30077–30080.

301. Lam E, Martin MM, Timermans AP, Sabers C, Fleischers S, Lukas T, Abraham RT, O'Keefe SJ, O'Neill EA, Wiederrecht GJ: A novel FK506 binding protein can mediate the immunosuppressive effects of FK506 and is associated with the cardiac ryanodine receptor. J Biol Chem 1995;270:26511–26522.

302. Laske A, Gallino A, Schneider J, Bauer EP, Carrel T, Pasic M, von Segesser LK, Turina MI: Prophylactic cytolytic therapy in heart transplantation: monoclonal versus polyclonal antibody therapy. J Heart Lung Transplant 1992;11:557–563.

303. Lazarovits AI, Poppema S, Zhang Z, Khandaker M, LeFeuvre CE, Singhal SK, Garcia BM, Ogasa N, Jevnikar AM, White MJ, Singh G, Stiller CR, Zhong RZ: Prevention and reversal of renal allograft rejection by antibody against CD45RB. Nature 1996; 380:717–720.

304. Lazarovits AI, Poppema S, Zhang Z, Khandaker M, LeFeuvre CE, Singhal SK, Garcia BM, Ogasa N, Jevnikar AM, White MJ, Singh G, Stiller CR, Zhong RZ: Therapy for mouse renal allograft rejection by monoclonal antibody to CD45RB. Transplant Proc 1996;28:3208–3209.

305. Lazarovits AI, Rochon J, Banks L, Hollomby DJ, Muirhead N, Jevnikar AM, White MJ, Amlot PL, Beauregard-Zollinger L, Stiller CR: Human mouse chimeric CD7 monoclonal antibody (SDZCHH380) for the prophylaxis of kidney transplant rejection. J Immunol 1993;150:5163–5174.

306. Lebeck LK, Chang L, Lopez-McCormack C, Chinnock R, Boucek M: Polyclonal antithymocyte serum: immune prophylaxis and rejection therapy in pediatric heart transplantation patients. J Heart Lung Transplant 1993;12:S286-S92.

307. Lee H, Slapak M, Venkatraman G, Mason J, Digard N, Wise M: Mizoribine as an alternative to azathioprine in triple-therapy immunosuppressant regimens in cadaveric renal transplantation. Transplant Proc 1994;25:2699–2700.

308. Lee WA, Gu L, Miksztal AR, Chu M, Leung K, Nelson PH: Bioavailability improvement of mycophenolic acid through amino ester derivation. Pharm Res 1990;7:161–166.

309. Lemaire M, Maurer G, Wood AJ: Cyclosporin. Pharmacokinetics and metabolism. Prog Allerg 1986;38:93–107.

310. Lensmeyer GL, Wiebe DA, Carlson IH: Distribution of cyclosporin-A metabolites among plasma and cells in whole blood: effect of temperature, hematocrit, and metabolite concentration. Clin Chem 1989;35:56–63.

311. Leonard WJ, Depper JM, Crabtree GR, Rudikoff S, Pumphre J, Robb RJ, Ronke M, Vetlik PB, Peffer NJ, Idmann TA, Eene WC:

312. Lerman A, Sandok EK, Hildebrand FL Jr, Burnett JC Jr: Inhibition of endothelium-derived relaxing factor enhances endothelin-mediated vasoconstriction. Circulation 1992;85:1894–1898.

313. Leventhal JR, Flores HC, Gruber SA, Figueroa J, Platt JL, Manivel JC, Bach FH, Matas AJ, Bolman RM: Evidence that 15-deoxyspergualin inhibits natural antibody production but fails to prevent hyperacute rejection in a discordant xenograft model. Transplantation 1992;54:26–31.

314. Levey RH, Medawar PB: Nature and mode of action of antilymphocytic serum. Proc Natl Acad Sci USA 1966;56:1130–1137.

315. Levin B, Bohannan L, Warvariv V, Bry W, Collins G: Total lymphoid irradiation (TLI) in the cyclosporine era—use of TLI in resistant cardiac allograft rejection. Transplant Proc 1989;21: 1793–1795.

316. Lewis GP, Jusko WJ, Burke CW, Graves L: Prednisone side-effects and serum-protein levels. A collaborative study. Lancet 1971;2: 778–778.

317. Li Y, Li XC, Zheng XX, Wells AD, Tuka LA, Strom TB: Blocking both signal 1 and signal 2 of T-cell activation prevents apoptosis of alloreactive T cells and induction of peripheral allograft tolerance. Nat Med 1999;5:1298–1302.

318. Lindholm A, Kahan BD: Influence of cyclosporine pharmacokinetics, trough concentrations, and AUC monitoring on outcome after kidney transplantation. Clin Pharmacol Ther 1993;54: 205–218.

319. Lokiec F, Fischer A, Gluckman E: A safer approach to the clinical use of cyclosporine: the predose calculation. Transplant Proc 1986;18(suppl 5):194–199.

320. Lord RH, Hancock WW, Colby AJ, Padberg W, Diamanstein T, Kupiec-Weglinski JW, Tilney NL: Effects of anti-IL 2 receptor monoclonal antibody and cyclosporine on IL 2 receptor-positive cells infiltrating cardiac allografts in the rat. Transplant Proc 1987;19:354–355.

321. Loutzenhiser R, Epstein M. The renal hemodynamic effects of calcium antagonists. In Epstein M, Loutzenhiser R (eds): Calcium Antagonists and the Kidney. Philadelphia: Hanley & Belfus, 1990, p 33.

322. Loutzenhiser R, Epstein M: Effects of calcium antagonists on renal hemodynamics. Am J Physiol 1985;249:F619-F629.

323. Loutzenhiser R, Epstein M, Horton C, Sonke P: Reversal of renal and smooth muscle actions of the thromboxane mimetic U-44069 by diltiazem. Am J Physiol 1986;250:F619-F626.

324. Lucini D, Milani RV, Ventura HO, Mehra MR, Messerli FH, Murgo JP, Regenstein F, Copley B, Malliani A, Pagani M: Cyclosporine-induced hypertension: evidence for maintained baroreflex circulatory control. J Heart Lung Transplant 1997;16: 615–620.

325. Lyson T, McMullan DM, Ermel LD, Morgan BJ, Victor RG: Mechanisms of cyclosporine-induced sympathetic activation and acute hypertension in rats. Hypertension 1994;23:667–675.

326. MacDonald A, Scarola J, Burke JT: Clinical pharmacokinetics and therapeutic drug monitoring of sirolimus. Clin Ther (in press).

327. MacDonald AS, Sabr K, MacAuley MA, McAlister VC, Bitter-Suermann H, Lee T: Effects of leflunomide and cyclosporine on aortic allograft chronic rejection in the rat. Transplant Proc 1994;26:3244–3245.

328. MacGregor GA, Capuccio FP, Markandu ND: Sodium intake, high blood pressure, and calcium channel blockers. Am J Med 1987;82(suppl 3B):16–22.

329. Magnussen K, Klug B, Moller B: CD3 antigen modulation in T-lymphocytes during OKT3 treatment. Transplant Proc 1994;26: 1731.

330. Maguire HC, Maibach HI: Specific immmune tolerance to anaphylactic sensitization (egg albumin) induced in the guinea pig by cyclophosphamide (Cytoxan). J Allergy 1961;32:406.

331. Maik T, Simpson M, Monaco AP: Development of suppressor T-cells by antilymphocyte serum treatment in mice. Transplantation 1982;34:376–381.

332. Mangold JB, Schran HF, Yatscoff RW: Biotransformation of cyclosporin G in comparison to cyclosporin A. Transplant Proc 1994;26:3013–3015.

333. Marinari R, Fleischmajor R, Schragger AH, Rosenthal AL: Mycophenolic acid in the treatment of psoriasis. Arch Dermatol 1977;113:930–932.

Molecular cloning and expression of cDNAa for the human interleukin-2 receptor. Nature 1984;311:626–631.

334. Mark AL: Cyclosporine, sympathetic activity and hypertension. N Engl J Med 1990;323:748–750.
335. Marketwitz A, Hammer C, Pfeiffer M, Zahn S, Drechsel J, Reichenspurner H, Reichart B: Reduction of cyclosporine-induced nephrotoxicity by cilastatin following clinical heart transplantation. Transplantation 1994;57:865–870.
336. Martin PJ, Nelson BJ, Appelbaum FR, Anasetti C, Deeg HJ, Hansen JA, McDonald GB, Nash RA, Sullivan KM, Witherspoon RP, Scannon PJ, Friedmann N, Storb R: Evaluation of a CD5-specific immunotoxin for treatment of acute graft-versus-host disease after allogeneic marrow transplantation. Blood 1996;88:824–830.
337. Matthys P, Dillen C, Proost P, Heremans H, Van Damme J, Billiau A: Modification of the anti-CD3-induced cytokine release syndrome by anti-interferon-gamma or anti-interleukin-6 antibody treatment: protective effects and biphasic changes in blood cytokine levels. Eur J Immunol 1993;23:2209–2216.
338. Maurer G, Lemaire M: Biotransformation and distribution in blood of cyclosporine and its metabolism. Transplant Proc 1986; 18(suppl 5):25–34.
339. Mauer G, Loosli HR, Schrier E, Keller B: Disposition of cyclosporine in several animal species and man. Structural elucidation of its metabolites. Drug Metab Dispos 1984;12:120–126.
340. Mavroudis DA, Jiang YZ, Hensel N, Lewalle P, Couriel D, Kreitman RJ, Pastan I, Barrett AJ: Specific depletion of alloreactivity against haplotype mismatched related individuals by a recombinant immunotoxin: a new approach to graft-versus-host disease prophylaxis in haploidentical bone marrow transplantation. Bone Marrow Transplant 1996;17:793–799.
341. McGurl PA, Platsoucas CD, Ricordi C, Slachta CA, Goldman BI, Fedalen P, Gaughman JP, Xu B, Eisen HJ, Furukawa S, Jeevanandam V: Efficacy of donor specific bone marrow in reducing frequency of rejection following heart transplantation [abstract]. J Heart Lung Transplant 1999;18:93.
342. McKenna RM, Szturm K, Jeffrey JR, Rush DN: Inhibition of cytokine production by cyclosporin A and G. Transplantation 1989; 47:343–348.
343. McManus RP, O'Hair DP, Hunter JB, Komorowski R: Spectrum of vascular changes in primate cardiac xenografts. Transplant Proc 1992;24:619–624.
344. Mehta MU, Venkataramanan R, Burkart GJ: Effect of bile on cyclosporine absorption in liver transplant patients. Br J Clin Pharmacol 1988;25:579–584.
345. Meiser BM, Billingham ME, Morris RE: Graft vessel disease: the role of rejection and the effect of cyclosporine, FK506, and rapamycin. Lancet 1991;338:1297–1298.
346. Meiser BM, Kur F, Reichenspurner H, Wagner F, Boos KS, Vielhauer S, Weiss M, Rohrbach H, Kreuzer E, Uberfuhr P, Reichart B: Reduction of the incidence of rejection by adjunct immunosuppression with photochemotherapy after heart transplantation. Transplantation 1994;57:563–568.
347. Meiser BM, Kur F, Uberfuhr P, Reichenspurner H, Kreuzer E, Reichart B: Modern application for an old compound: 8-methoxypsoralen for photochemotherapy after heart transplantation. Transplant Proc 1993;25:3307–3308.
348. Meiser BM, Pfeiffer M, Schmidt D, Reichenspurner H, Ueberfuhr P, Paulus D, von Scheidt W, Kreuzer E, Seidel D, Reichart B: Combination therapy with tacrolimus and mycophenolate mofetil following cardiac transplantation: importance of mycophenolic acid therapeutic drug monitoring. J Heart Lung Transplant 1999;18:143–149.
349. Mene P, Dunn MJ: Contractile effects of TxA$_2$ and endoperoxide analogues on cultured rat glomerular mesangial cells. Am J Physiol 1986;251:F1029–F1035.
350. Menkis AH, Powell AM, Novick RJ, McKenzie FN, Kostuk WJ, Pflugfelder PW, Brown J, Rochon J, Chan L, Stiller C: Prospective randomized trial of short-term immunosuppressive prophylaxis using OKAT3 or Minnesota equine ALG. J Heart Transplant 1991;10:163.
351. Menkis AH, Powell AM, Novick RJ, McKenzie FN, Kostuk WJ, Pflugfelder PW, Brown JE, Rochon J, Chow LH, Stiller C: A prospective randomized controlled trial of initial immunosuppression with ALG versus OKT3 in recipients of cardiac allografts. J Heart Lung Transplant 1992;11:569–576.
352. Metcalfe SM, Richards FM: Cyclosporine, FK 506 and rapamycin: some effects on early activation events in serum-free, mitogen-stimulated mouse spleen cells. Transplantation 1990;49:798–802.
353. Miethke T, Vabulas R, Bittlingmaier R, Heeg K, Wagner H: Mechanisms of peripheral T cell deletion: anergized T cells are Fas resistant but undergo proliferation-associated apoptosis. Eur J Immunol 1996;26:1459–1467.
354. Mihatsch MJ, Antonovych T, Bohman SO, Habib R, Helmchen U, Noel LH, Olsen S, Sibley RK, Kemeny E, Feutren G: Cyclosporin A nephropathy: standardization of the evaluation of kidney biopsy. Clin Nephrol 1994;41:23–32.
355. Mikhail G, Eadon H, Leaver N, Yacoub M: Use of Neoral in heart transplant recipients. Transplant Proc 1994;26:2985–2987.
356. Mizuno K, Tsujino M, Takada M, Hayashi M, Atsumi K, Asano K, Matsuda T: Studies on Bredinin. I. Isolation, characterization and biological properties. J Antibiot 1974;27:775–782.
357. Mohacsi PJ, Tuller D, Hulliger B, Wijngaard PLJ: Different inhibitory effects of immunosuppressive drugs on human and rat aortic smooth muscle and endothelial cell proliferation stimulated by platelet-derived growth factor or endothelial cell growth factor. J Heart Lung Transplant 1997;16:484–492.
358. Monaco AP, Clark AW, Wood ML, Sahyoun AI, Codish SD, Brown RW: Possible active enhancement of a human cadaver renal allograft with antilymphocyte serum (ALS) and donor bone marrow: case report of an initial attempt. Surgery 1976;79: 384–392.
359. Monaco AP, Wood ML, Russell PS: Effect of adult thymectomy on the recovery from immunologic depression induced by heterologous antilymphocyte serum. Science 1965;149:423.
360. Monaco AP, Wood ML, Russell PS: Effect of adult thymectomy on the recovery from immunological depression induced by antilymphocyte serum. Surg Forum 1965;16:209–211.
361. Morel P, Vincent C, Cordier G, Panaye G, Carosella E: Anti-CD4 monoclonal antibody administration in renal transplanted patients. Clin Immunol Immunopathol 1990;56:311–322.
362. Morikawa K, Oseko F, Morikawa S: The distinct effects of FK506 on the activation proliferation, and differentiation of human B lymphocytes. Transplantation 1992;54:1025–1030.
363. Morris PJ: New immunosuppressive agents. In Kidney Transplantation. 4th ed. Philadelphia: WB Saunders Company 1994, pp 233–243.
364. Morris R: Modes of action of FK 506, cyclosporine A, and rapamycin. Transplant Proc 1994;26:3272–3275.
365. Morris RE: 15-Rapamycin: antifungal, antitumor, antiproliferative and immunosuppressive macrolides. Transplant Rev 1992; 6:39.
366. Morris RE: New small molecule immunosuppressants for transplantation: review of essential concepts. J Heart Lung Transplant 1993;12:S275-S286.
367. Morris RE: New immunosuppressive drugs. In Busuttil RW, Klintmalm GB (eds): Transplantation of the Liver. Philadelphia: WB Saunders Company, 1996.
368. Morris RE: Investigational immunosuppressants: nonbiologics. In Norman DJ, Suki WN (eds): Primer on Transplantation. Thorofare, NJ: American Society of Transplant Physicians 1998, pp 103–112.
369. Morris RE, Hot EG, Murphy MP, Eugui EM, Allison AC: Mycophenolic acid morpholinoethylester (RS 61443) is a new immunosuppressant that prevents and halts heart allograft rejection by selective inhibition of T- and B-cell purine synthesis. Transplant Proc 1990;22:1659–1662.
370. Morris RE, Huang X, Cao W, Zheng B, Shorthouse RA: Leflunomide and its analog suppress T and B cell proliferation in vitro, acute rejection, ongoing rejection and anti-donor antibody synthesis in mouse, rat, and Cynomolgus monkey transplant recipients as well as arterial intimal thickening after balloon catheter injury. Transplant Proc 1995;27:445–447.
371. Morris RE, Wang J, Blum JR, Flavin T, Murphy MP, Almquist SJ, Chu N, Tam YL, Kaloostian M, Allison AC: Immunosuppressive effects of the morpholinoethyl ester of mycophenolic acid (RS 61443) in rat and nonhuman primate recipients of heart allografts. Transplant Proc 1991;23(suppl 2):19–25.
372. Moss NG, Powell SL, Falk RJ: Intravenous cyclosporine activates afferent renal nerves and causes sodium retention in innervated kidneys in rats. Proc Natl Acad Sci U S A 1985;82:8222–8226.
373. Mourad M, Besse T, Malaise J, Baldi A, Latinne D, Bazin H, Pirson Y, Hope J, Squifflet JP: BTI-322 for acute rejection after renal transplantation. Transplant Proc 1997;29:2353.

374. Mueller EA, Kovarik JM, van Bree JB, Grevel J, Lucker PW, Kutz K: Influence of a fat-free meal on the pharmacokinetics of a new oral formulation of cyclosporine in a crossover comparison with the market formulation. Pharm Res 1994;11:151–155.

375. Mundy J, Chang J, Keogh A: Prophylactic OKT3 versus equine antithymocyte globulin after heart transplantation: increased morbidity with OKT3 [abstract]. J Heart Transplant 1991;10:163.

376. Murgia MG, Jordan S, Kahan BD: The side effect profile of sirolimus: a phase I study in quiescent cyclosporine-prednisone-treated renal transplant patients. Kidney Int 1996;49:209–216.

377. Murray BM, Paller MS, Ferris TF: Effect of cyclosporine administration on renal hemodynamics in conscious rats. Kidney Int 1985;28:767–774.

378. Murray JE, Merrill JP, Harrison JH, Wilson RE, Dammin G: Prolonged survival of human-kidney homograft by immunosuppressive drug therapy. N Engl J Med 1963;268:1315.

379. Musikic P, Logar D, Mladenovic V, Rozman B, Domljan Z, Jajic I: Efficacy of leflunomide in patients with rheumatoid arthritis. Rheumatology 1992;51(suppl):58–59.

380. Mussche MM, Ringoir SGM, Lamiere NN: High intravenous doses of methylprednisolone for acute cadaveric renal allograft rejection. Nephron 1976;16:289.

381. Myburgh JA, Smit JA, Browde S, Stark JH: Current status of total lymphoid irradiation. Transplant Proc 1983;15:659–667.

382. Nadler SG, Tepper MA, Schacter B, Mazzucco CE: Interaction of the immunosuppressant deoxyspergualin with a member of the Hsp70 family of heat shock proteins. Science 1992;258:484–486.

383. Nagai M, Natsumeda Y, Webster G: Proliferation-linked regulation of the type II IMP dehydrogenase gene in human normal lymphocytes and HL-60 leukemic cells. Cancer Res 1992;52:258.

384. Najarian JS, Ferguson RM, Sutherland DER, Slavin S, Kim T, Kersey J, Simmons RL: Fractionated total lymphoid irradiation as preparative immunosuppression in high risk renal transplantation. Ann Surg 1982;196:442–452.

385. Najarian JS, Strand M, Fryd DS: Comparison of cyclosporine versus azathioprine-antilymphocyte globulin in renal transplantation. Transplant Proc 1983;15:438–441.

386. Nakahama H: Stimulatory effect of cyclosporin A on endothelin secretion by a cultured renal epithelial cell line. LLC-PK1 cells. Eur J Pharmacol 1990;180:191–192.

387. Naoumov NV, Tredger J, Steward CM, O'Grady O, Grevel J, Niven A, Whiting B, Williams R: Cyclosporin A pharmacokinetics in liver transplant recipients in relation to biliary T tube clamping and liver dysfunction. Gut 1989;30:391–396.

388. Natsumeda Y, Ohno S, Kawasaki H, Konno Y, Weber G, Suzuki K: Two distinct cDNAs for human IMP dehydrogenase. J Biol Chem 1990;265:5292.

389. Nelson DR, Kamataki T, Waxman DJ, Guengerick FP, Estabrook RW, Feyereisen R: The P450 superfamily: update on new sequences, gene mapping, accession numbers, early trivial names of enzymes, and nomenclature. DNA Cell Biol 1993;12:1–51.

390. Neumayer HH, Schreiber M, Wagner K: Prevention of delayed graft function in cadaveric kidney transplants by the antagonist diltiazem and the prostacyclin-analogue iloprost—outcome of a prospective randomized clinical trial. Prog Clin Biol Res 1989; 301:289–295.

391. Neumann MC, Muller TF, Sprenger H, Gemsa D, Lange H: The influence of the immunosuppressants OKT3 and ATG on immunological parameters. Clin Nephrol 1996;45:345–348.

392. Neville DM Jr, Scharff J, Hu HZ, Rigaut K, Shiloach J, Slingerland W, Jonker M: A new reagent for the induction of T-cell depletion, anti-CD3-CRM9. J Immunother Emphasis Tumor Immunol 1996;19:85–92.

393. Niblack G, Johnson K, Williams T, Green W, Richie R, MacDonell R: Antibody formulation following administration of antilymphocyte serum. Transplant Proc 1987;19:1896–1897.

394. Nicholson JP, Resnick LM, Laragh JH: The antihypertensive effect of verapamil at extremes of dietary sodium intake. Ann Intern Med 1987;107:329–334.

395. Nikaido A, Shimizu N, Sabe H, Teshigawara K, Maeda M, Uchiyama T, Yodoi J, Honjo T: Molecular cloning of cDNA encoding human interleukin-2 receptor. Nature 1984;311:631–635.

396. Nizze H, Mihatsch MJ, Zollinger HU, Brocheriou C, Gokel JM, Henry K, Sloane JP, Stovin PG: Cyclosporine-associated nephropathy in patients with heart and bone marrow transplants. Clin Nephrol 1988;30:248–260.

397. Noguchi M, Nakamura Y, Russell SM, Ziegler SF, Tsang M, Cao X, Leonard WJ: Interleukin-2 receptor gamma chain: a functional component of the interleukin-7 receptor. Science 1993;262:1877–1880.

398. Norman DJ, Bennett WM, Cobanoglu A, Hershberger R, Hosenpud JD, Meyer MM, Misiti J, Ott G, Ratkovec R, Shihab F, Vitow C, Barry JM: Use of OKT4 (a murine monoclonal anti-CD4 antibody) in human organ transplantation: initial clinical experience. Transplant Proc 1993;25(1 pt 1):802–803.

399. O'Connell JB, Renlund DG, Hammond EH, Wittwer CT, Yowell RL, DeWitt CW, Jones KW, Gay WA Jr, Menlove RL, Bristow MR: Sensitization to OKT3 monoclonal antibody in heart transplantation: correlation with early allograft loss. J Heart Lung Transplant 1991;10:217–222.

400. O'Hair DP, McManus RP, Komorowski R: Inhibition of chronic vascular rejection in primate cardiac xenografts using mycophenolate mofetil. Ann Thorac Surg 1994;58:1311–1315.

401. Oettinger CW, D'Souza M, Milton GV: In vitro comparison of cytokine release from antithymocyte serum and OKT3. Inhibition with soluble and microencapsulated neutralizing antibodies. Transplantation 1996;62:1690–1693.

402. Ohlman S, Gannedahl G, Tyden G, Tufveson G, Groth CG: Treatment of renal transplant rejection with 15-deoxyspergualin—a dose finding study in man. Transplant Proc 1992;24:318–320.

403. Olbrich HG, Donck LV, Geerts H, Mutschler E, Kober G, Kaltenbach M: Cyclosporine increases the intracellular free calcium concentration in electric passed isolated rat cardiomyocytes. J Heart Lung Transplant 1993;12:652–658.

404. Olivari MT, May CB, Johnson NA, Ring WS, Stephens MK: Treatment of acute vascular rejection with immunoadsorption. Circulation 1994;90(p 2):II-70–II-73.

405. Olsen SL, O'Connel JB, Bristow MR, Renlund DG: Methotrexate as an adjunct in the treatment of persistent mild cardiac allograft rejection. Transplantation 1990;50:773–775.

406. Omokawa S, Malchesky PS, Sakamoto H, Flynn A, Loftus MA, Nose Y: Changes in interleukin-1 during membrane plasmapheresis. ASAIO Trans 1986;32:392–396.

407. Omokawa S, Malchesky PS, Yamashita M, Goldcamp JB, Nose Y: Anticoagulant and membrane effects on humoral and cellular changes during plasmapheresis. ASAIO Trans 1988;34:404–409.

408. Omokawa S, Suzuki T, Dustoor MM, Uchida N, Malchesky PS, Nose Y: Humoral, cellular, and hemodynamic changes induced by blood-material interaction in membrane plasmapheresis. Trans Am Soc Artif Intern Organs 1987;33:112–117.

409. Owunwanne A, Shihab-Eldeen A, Sadek S, Junaid T, Yacoub T, Abdel-Dayem HM: Is cyclosporine toxic to the heart? J Heart Lung Transplant 1993;12:199–204.

410. Palmer A, Taube D, Welsh K, Bewick M, Gjorstrup P, Thick M: Removal of anti-HLA antibodies by extracorporeal immunoadsorption to enable renal transplantation. Lancet 1989;1:10–12.

411. Pardee AB: G$_1$ events and regulation of cell proliferation. Science 1989;246:603–608.

412. Parenteau GL, Dirbas FM, Garmestani K, Brechbiel MW, Bukowski MA, Goldman CK, Clark R, Gansow OA, Waldmann TA: Prolongation of graft survival in primate allograft transplantation by yttrium-90-labeled anti-tac in conjunction with granulocyte colony-stimulating factor. Transplantation 1992;54:963–968.

413. Patton PR, Brunson ME, Pfaff WW, Howard RJ, Peterson JC, Ramos EL, Karlix JL: A preliminary report of diltiazem and ketoconazole. Transplantation 1994;57:889–892.

414. Penn I: Lymphomas complicating organ transplantation. Transplant Proc 1983;15:2790.

415. Pennock JL, Reitz BA, Bieber CP, Aziz S, Oyer PE, Strober S, Hoppe R, Kaplan HS, Stinson EB, Shumway NE: Survival of primates following orthotopic cardiac transplantation treated with total lymphoid irradiation and chemical immunosuppression. Transplantation 1981;32:467–473.

416. Perez M, Edelson R, LaRoche L, Berger C: Inhibition of antiskin allograft immunity by infusions with syngeneic photoinactivated effector lymphocytes. J Invest Dermatol 1989;92:669–676.

417. Perico N, Zoja C, Benigni A, Ghilardi F, Gualandris L, Remuzzi G: Effect of short-term cyclosporine administration in rats on renin-angiotensin and thromboxane A$_2$: possible relevance to the

reduction in glomerular filtration rate. J Pharmacol Exp Ther 1986;239:229–235.

418. Perini GP, Bonadiman C, Fraccaroli GP, Vantini I: Azathioprine-related cholestatic jaundice in heart transplant patients. J Heart Transplant 1990;9:577–578.

419. Perry LL, Green MI: Antigen presentation by epidermal Langerhans cells: loss of function following ultraviolet (UV) irradiation in vivo. Clin Immunol Immunopathol 1982;24:204–219.

420. Petcher TJ, Weber HP, Ruegger A: Crystal and molecular structure of an iododerivative of the cyclic undecapeptide cyclosporin A. Helv Chim Acta 1976;59:1480–1489.

421. Pham SM, Kormos RL, Hattler BG, Kawai A, Tsamandas AC, Demetris AJ, Murali S, Fricker FJ, Chang HC, Jain AB, Starzl TE, Hardesty RL, Griffith BP: Cardiac pulmonary replacement—a prospective trial of tacrolimus (FK506) in clinical heart transplantation: intermediate term results. J Thorac Cardiovasc Surg 1996;111:764–772.

422. Phillips GL, Nevill TJ, Spinelli JJ, Nantel SH, Klingemann HG, Barnett MJ, Shepherd JD, Chan KW, Meharchand JM, Sutherland HJ: Prophylaxis for acute graft-versus-host disease following unrelated donor bone marrow transplantation. Bone Marrow Transplant 1995;15:213–219.

423. Pickup ME: Clinical pharmacokinetics of prednisone and prednisolone. Clin Pharmacokinet 1979;4:111–128.

424. Pinkel D, Howarth C: Pediatriac neoplasms: In Sartorelli AC, Johns DG (eds): Antineoplastic and Immunosuppressive Agents. Part II. New York: Macmillan, 1985, pp 1226–1258.

425. Platz KP, Sollinger HW, Hullett DA, Eckhoff DE, Eugui EM, Allison AC: RS-61443, a new, potent immunosuppressive agent. Transplantation 1991;51:27–31.

426. Pomerance A, Stovin PGI: Heart transplant pathology: the British experience. J Clin Pathol 1985;38:146–159.

427. Powelson JA, Cosimi AB: Antilymphocyte globulin and monoclonal antibodies. In Morris RE (ed): Kidney Transplantation. Philadelphia: WB Saunders Company, 1993.

428. Powelson JA, Knowles RW, Delmonico FL, Kawai T, Mourad G, Preffer FI, Colvin RB, Cosimi B: CDR-grafted OKT4A monoclonal antibody in cynomolgus renal allograft recipients. Transplantation 1994;57:788–793.

429. Przepiorka D, Chan KW, Champlin RE, Culbert SJ, Petropoulos D, Ippoliti C, Khouri I, Huh YO, Vreisendorp H, Deisseroth AB: Prevention of graft-versus-host disease with anti-CD5 ricin A chain immunotoxin after CD3-depleted HLA-nonidentical marrow transplantation in pediatric leukemia patients. Bone Marrow Transplant 1995;16:737–741.

430. Ptachcinski RJ, Venkataramanan R, Burckart GJ: Clinical pharmacokinetics of cyclosporin. Clin Pharmacokinet 1986;11:107–132.

431. Queen C: A humanized antibody that binds to the interleukin 2 receptor. Proc Natl Acad Sci U S A 1989;86:10029–10033.

432. Radeke HH, Kuster S, Kaever V, Resch K: Effects of cyclosporine and FK-506 on glomerular mesangial cells: evidence for direct inhibition of thromboxane synthase by low cyclosporine concentrations. Eur J Clin Pharmacol 1993;44(suppl 1):S11–S16.

433. Radvanyi LG, Mills GB, Miller RG: Religation of the T cell receptor after primary activation of mature T cells inhibits proliferation and induces apoptotic cell death. J Immunol 1993;150:5704–5715.

434. Radvanyi LG, Shi Y, Mills GB, Miller RG: Cell cycle progression out of G1 sensitizes primary-cultured nontransformed T cells to TCR-mediated apoptosis. Cell Immunol 1996;170:260–273.

435. Ratkovec RM, Hammond EH, O'Connell JB, Bristow MR, DeWitt CW, Richenbacher WE, Millar RC, Renlund DG: Outcome of cardiac transplant recipients with a positive donor-specific crossmatch—preliminary results with plasmapheresis. Transplantation 1992;54:651–655.

436. Rebellato LM, Gross U, Verbanac KM, Thomas JM: A comprehensive definition of the major antibody specificities in polyclonal rabbit antithymocyte globulin. Transplantation 1994;57:685–694.

437. Reed MH, Shapiro ME, Strom TB, Milford EL, Carpenter CB, Letvin NL, Waldmann TA, Kirkman RL: Prolongation of primate renal allografts with anti-Tac monoclonal antibody. Curr Surg 1988;45:28–30.

438. Reichenspurner H, Meiser BM, Muschiol F, Nollert G, Uberfuhr P, Markewitz A, Wagner F, Pfeiffer M, Reichart B: The influence of gastrointestinal agents on resorption and metabolism of cyclosporine after heart transplantation: experimental and clinical results. J Heart Lung Transplant 1993;12:987–992.

439. Reinherz EL, Kung PC, Goldstein G, Schlossman SF: A monoclonal antibody with selective reactivity with functionally mature human thymocytes and all peripheral human T cells. J Immunol 1979;123:1312–1317.

440. Renlund DG, O'Connell JB, Gilbert EM, Hammond ME, Burton NA, Jones KW, Karwande SV, Doty DB, Menlove RL, Herrick CM: A prospective comparison of murine monoclonal CD-3 (OKT3) antibody-based and equine antithymocyte globulin-based rejection prophylaxis in cardiac transplantation. Transplantation 1989;47:599–605.

441. Reyes J, Gayowski T, Fung J, Todo S, Alessiani M, Starzl TE: Expressive dysphasia possibly related to FK506 in two liver transplant recipients. Transplantation 1990;50:1043.

442. Richards NT, Poston L, Hilston PJ: Cyclosporin A inhibits endothelium-dependent, prostanoid-induced relaxation in human subcutaneous resistance vessels. J Hypertens 1990;8:159–163.

443. Rogers TS, Elzinga L, Bennett WM, Kelley VE: Selective enhancement of thromboxane in macrophages and kidneys in cyclosporine-induced nephrotoxicity. Dietary protection by fish oil. Transplantation 1988;45:153–156.

444. Romero JC, Raij L, Granger JP, Ruilope LM, Rodicio JL: Multiple effects of calcium entry blockers on renal function in hypertension. Hypertension 1987;10:140–151.

445. Rook AH, Freundlich B, Jegasothy BV, Perez MI, Barr WG, Jimenezz GA, Rietschel RL, Wintroub B, Kahaleh B, Varga J, Heald W, Steen V, Massa MC, Murphy GF, Perniciaro C, Istfan M, Ballas SK, Edelson RL: Treatment of systemic sclerosis with extracorporeal photochemotherapy. Arch Dermatol 1992;128:337–346.

446. Rook AH, Heald PW, Nahass GT, Macey W, Witmer WK, Lazarus GS, Jegasothy BV: Treatment of autoimmune disease with extracorporeal photochemotherapy: pemphigus vulgaris: preliminary report. Yale J Biol Med 1989;62:647–652.

447. Rook AH, Prystowsky MB, Cassin M, Boufal M, Lessin SR: Combined therapy for Sezary syndrome with extracorporeal photochemotherapy and low-dose interferon alfa therapy. Arch Dermatol 1991;127:1535–1540.

448. Rook AH, Wolfe JT: Role of extracorporeal photopheresis in the treatment of cutaneous T-cell lymphoma, autoimmune disease, and allograft rejection. J Clin Apheresis 1994;9:28–30.

449. Rooth P, Dawidson I, Diller K, Taljedal IB: Protection against cyclosporine-induced impairment of renal microcirculation by verapamil in mice. Transplantation 1988;45:433–437.

450. Rosano TG, Fred BM, Pell MA, Lempert N: Cyclosporine metabolites in human blood and renal tissue. Transplant Proc 1986;18 (suppl 5):35–40.

451. Rose EA, Barr ML, Xu H, Pepino P, Murphy MP, McGovern MA, Ratner AJ, Watkins JF, Marboe CC, Berger CL: Photochemotherapy in human heart transplant recipients at high risk for fatal rejection. J Heart Lung Transplant 1992;11:746–750.

452. Rubin RH, Tolkoff-Rubin NE: The impact of infection on the outcome of transplantation. Transplant Proc 1991;23:2068–2074.

453. Ruiz JC, de Francisco AL, Vazquez de Prada JA, Ruano J, Pastor JM, Alcalde G, Arias M: Successful heart transplantation after anti-HLA antibody removal with protein-A immunoadsorption in a hyperimmunized patient [letter]. J Thorac Cardiovasc Surg 1994;107:1366–1367.

454. Sabatini S, Ferguson RM, Helderman JH, Hull AR, Kirkpatrick BS, Barr WH: Drug substitution in transplantation: a National Kidney Foundation White Paper. Am J Kidney Dis 1999;33:389–397.

455. Sablinski T, Hancock WW, Tilney NL: CD4 monoclonal antibodies in organ transplantation—a review of the progress. Transplantation 1991;52:579–589.

456. Salter MM, Kirklin JK, Bourge RC, Naftel DC, White-Williams C, Tarkka M, Waits E, Bucy RP: Total lymphoid irradiation in the treatment of early or recurrent heart rejection. J Heart Lung Transplant 1992;11:902–912.

457. Saper V, Chow D, Engleman E, Hoppe RT, Levin B, Collins G, Strober S: Clinical and immunologic studies of cadaveric renal transplant recipients given total lymphoid irradiation and maintained on low dose prednisone. Transplantation 1988;45:540–546.

458. Sayegh MH, Turka LA: The role of T-cell costimulatory activation pathways in transplant rejection. N Engl J Med 1998;338:1813–1821.

459. Schreiber SL: Chemistry and biology of the immunophilins and their immunosuppressive ligands. Science 1991;251:283.

460. Schmidbauer G, Hancock WW, Wasowska B, Badger AM, Kupiec-Weglinski JW: Abrogation by rapamycin of accelerated rejection in sensitized rats by inhibition of alloantibody responses and selective suppression of intragraft mononuclear and endothelial cell activation, cytokine production, and cell adhesion. Transplantation 1994;57:933–941.

461. Schroeder JS, Gao SZ, Alderman EL, Hunt SA, Johnstone I, Boothroyd DB, Wiederhold V, Stinson EB: A preliminary study of diltiazem in the prevention of coronary artery disease in heart transplant recipients. N Engl J Med 1993;328:164–170.

462. Schroeder TJ, First MR, Hurtubise PE, Marmer DJ, Martin DM, Mansour ME, Melvin DB: Immunologic monitoring with orthoclone OKT3 therapy. J Heart Transplant 1989;8:371–380.

463. Schulak JA, McBride JL: Cyclophosphamide inhibition of anamnestic humoral immunity. Transplant Proc 1989;21:1147–1149.

464. Sedrani R, Cottens J, Kallen J, Schuler W: Chemical modification of rapamycin: the discovery of SDZ RAD. Transplant Proc 1998;30:2192–2194.

465. Sehgal SW, Baker H, Vezina C: Rapamycin (AY-22,989), a new antifungal antibiotic. II. Fermentation, isolation and characterisation. J Antibiot 1975;28:727–732.

466. Seledtsov VI, Avdeev IV, Morenkov AV, Seledtsova GV, Kozlov VA: Antiproliferative effect of bone marrow cells on leukemic cells. Immunobiology 1995;192:205–217.

467. Shaddy RE, Bullock EA, Morwessel NJ, Hannon DW, Renlund DG, Karwande SV, McGough EC, Hawkins JA: Murine monoclonal CD3 antibody (OKT3)-based early rejection prophylaxis in pediatric heart transplantation. J Heart Lung Transplant 1993;12:434–439.

468. Shapiro R, Starzl TE: Bone marrow augmentation in renal transplant recipients. Transplant Proc 1998;30:1371–1374.

469. Sharma LC, Muirhead N, Lazarovits AI: Human mouse chimeric CD7 monoclonal antibody (SDZCHH380) for the prophylaxis of kidney transplant rejection: analysis beyond 4 years. Transplant Proc 1997;29(1–2):323–324.

470. Sharma VK, Bologa RM, Xu GP, Li B, Mouradian J, Wang J, Serur D, Rao V, Suthanthiran M: Intragraft TGF-beta 1 mRNA: a correlate of interstitial fibrosis and chronic allograft nephropathy. Kidney Int 1996;49:1297–1303.

471. Shaw LM: Critical issues in cyclosporine monitoring: report of the task force on cyclosporine monitoring. Clin Chem 1987;33:1269–1288.

472. Shaw LM: Cyclosporine monitoring. Clin Chem 1989;35:5–6.

473. Shi Y, Sahai BM, Green DR: Cyclosporin A inhibits activation induced cell death in T-cell hybridomas and thymocytes. Nature 1989;339:625–626.

474. Shizuru JA, Seydel KB, Flavin TF, Wu AP, Kong CC, Hoyt EG, Fujimoto N, Billingham ME, Starnes VA, Fathman CG: Induction of donor-specific unresponsiveness to cardiac allografts in rats by pretransplant antiCD4 monoclonal antibody therapy. Transplantation 1990;50:366–373.

475. Shun-Shin GA, Ratacliffe P, Bron AJ, Brown NP, Sparrow JM: The lens after renal transplantation. Br J Ophthalmol 1990;74:261.

476. Siena S, Villa S, Bonadonna G, Bregni M, Gianni AM: Specific ex-vivo depletion of human bone marrow T lymphocytes by an anti-pan-T cell (CD5) ricin A-chain immunotoxin. Transplantation 1987;43:421–426.

477. Sigal NH, Dumont FK: Cyclosporin A, FK506 and rapamycin: pharmacologic probes of lymphocyte signal transduction. Am Rev Immunol 1992;10:519.

478. Slavin S, Fuks Z, Kaplan HS, Strober S: Transplantation of allogeneic bone marrow without graft-versus-host disease using total lymphoid irradiation. J Exp Med 1978;147:963–972.

479. Slavin S, Strober S, Fuks Z, Kaplan HS: Induction of specific tissue transplantation tolerance using fractionated total lymphoid irradiation in adult mice: long-term survival of allogeneic bone marrow and skin grafts. J Exp Med 1977;146:34–48.

480. Slavin S, Strober S, Fuks Z, Kaplan HS: Use of total lymphoid irradiation in tissue transplantation in mice. Transplant Proc 1977;9:1001–1004.

481. Smith GJ, Ingham-Clark C, Crane P, Lear P, Wood RF, Fabre JW: Ex vivo perfusion of intestinal allografts with anti-T cell monoclonal antibody/ricin A chain conjugates for the suppression of graft-versus-host disease. Transplantation 1992;53:717–722.

482. Snyder DS, Lu CY, Unanue ER: Control of macrophage Ia expression in neonatal mice–role of a splenic suppressor cell. J Immunol 1982;128:1458–1465.

483. Snyder HW, Bertram JH, Channel ME: Reduction in platelet-binding immunoglobulins and improvement in platelet counts in patients with HIV-associated idiopathic thrombocytopenic purpura (ITP) following extracorporeal immunoadsorption of plasma over staphylococcal protein A-silica (PROSORBA Columns). Arti Organs 1999;13:71–77.

484. Sollinger HW, Belzer FO, Deierhoi MH, Belzer FO, Diethelm AG, Kauffman RS: RS-61443: a phase I clinical trial and pilot rescue study. Transplantation 1992;53:428–432.

485. Sollinger HW, Belzer FO, Deierhoi MH, Gonwa TA, Kauffman RS, Klintmalm GB, McDiarmid SV, Roberts J, Rosenthal JT: RS-611443 (mycophenolate mofetil): a multicenter study for refractory kidney transplant rejection. Ann Surg 1992;216:513–519.

486. Souza ERM, Boim MA, Bergamaschi C, Versolato C, Pestana JOM, Schor N: Acute effects of FK 506 on glomerular hemodynamics. Transplant Proc 1992;24:3082.

487. Stahelin H: Historical Background. Prog Allerg 1986;38:19–27.

488. Starnes JA, Oyer PE, Stinson EP, Dein JR, Shumway NE: Prophylactic OKT3 used as induction therapy for heart transplantation. Circulation 1989;80(suppl III):III-9.

489. Starzl TE, Demetris AJ, Trucco M, Murase N, Ricordi C, Ildstad S, Ramos H, Todo S, Tzakis A, Fung JJ: Cell migration and chimerism after whole-organ transplantation: the basis of graft acceptance [review]. Hepatology 1993b;17:1127–1152.

490. Starzl TE, Demetris AJ, Trucco M, Zeevi A, Ramos H, Terasaki P, Rudert WA, Kocova M, Ricordi C, Ildstad S: Chimerism and donor-specific nonreactivity 27 to 29 years after kidney allotransplantation. Transplantation 1993;55:1272–1277.

491. Starzl TE, Porter KA, Iwaski Y: The use of heterologous antilymphocyte globulins in human homotransplantations. In Wolstenholme GEW, O'Connor M (eds): Antilymphocyte Serum. Boston: Little, Brown, 1967, p 1.

492. Steele DM, Hullett DA, Bechstein WO, Kowalski J, Smith LS, Kennedy E, Allison AC, Sollinger HW: Effects of immunosuppressive therapy on the rat aortic allograft model. Transplant Proc 1993;25:754–755.

493. Stein CM, He H, Pincus T, Wood AJJ: Cyclosporine impairs vasodilation without increased sympathetic activity in humans. Hypertension 1995;26:705–710.

494. Steinberg D, Parthasarathy S, Carew TE, Khoo JC, Witztum JL: Beyond cholesterol: modifications of low-denisty lipoprotein that increase its atherogenicity. N Engl J Med 1989;320:915–924.

495. Steinbruchel DA, Madsen HH, Nielsen B, Kemp E, Larsen S, Koch C: Graft survival in a hamster-to-rat heart transplantation model after treatment with total lymphoid irradiation, cyclosporine A, and a monoclonal anti-T-cell antibody. Transplant Proc 1990;22:1088–1088.

496. Stepkowski SM, Chen H, Daloze P, Kahan BD: Rapamycin, a potent immunosuppressive drug for vascularized heart, kidney, and small bowel transplantation in the rat. Transplantation 1991;51:22–26.

497. Stern N, Lustig S, Petrasek D, Jensen G, Eggena P, Lee DBN, Tuck ML: Cyclosporin A-induced hyperreninemic hypoaldosteronism. Hypertension 1987;9(suppl 3):III-31–III-35.

498. Stovin PGI, English TAH: Effects of cyclosporine on the transplanted human heart. J Heart Transplant 1987;6:180–185.

499. Strober S: Natural suppressor (NS) cells, neonatal tolerance, and total lymphoid irradiation: exploring obscure relationships. Ann Rev Immunol 1984;2:219–237.

500. Strober S, Dhillon M, Schubert M, Holm B, Engleman E, Benike C, Hoppe R, Sibley R, Myburgh JA, Collins G: Acquired immune tolerance to cadaveric renal allografts: a study of three patients treated with total lymphoid irradiation. N Engl J Med 1989;321:28–33.

501. Strom TB, Ettenger RB: Investigational immunosuppressants: Biologics. In Norman DJ, Suki WN (eds): Primer on Transplantation. Thorofare, NJ: American Society of Transplant Physicians, 1998.

502. Sugar AM, Saunders C, Idelson BA, Bernard DB: Interaction of fluconazole and cyclosporine [letter]. Ann Intern Med 1989;110:844.

503. Sugiura K, Pahwa S, Yamamoto Y, Borisov K, Pahwa R, Nelson RP, Ishikawa J, Iguchi T, Oyaizu N, Good RA, Idehara S: Characterization of natural suppressor cells in human bone marrow. Stem Cells 1998;16:99–106.

504. Sweeney MJ, Hoffman DH, Esterman MA: Metabolism and biochemistry of mycophenolic acid. Cancer Res 1972;2232:1803–1809.

505. Swinnen LJ, Costanzo-Nordin MR, Fisher SG, O'Sullivan EJ, Johnson MR, Heroux AL, Dizikes GJ, Pifarre R, Fisher RI: Increased incidence of lymphoproliferative disorder after immunosuppression with the monoclonal antibody OKT3 in cardiac transplant recipients. N Engl J Med 1990;323:1723–1728.

506. Sykes M, Sachs DH: Mixed allogeneic chimerism as an approach to transplantation tolerance [published erratum appears in Immunol Today 1988 May;9:131]. [review]. Immunol Today 1988;9:23–27.

507. Takahashi K, Ota K, Tanabe K, Oba S, Teraoka S, Toma H, Agishi T, Kawaaguchi H, Ito K: Effect of a novel immunosuppressive agent, deoxyspergualin, on rejection in kidney transplant recipients. Transplant Proc 1990;22:1606–1612.

508. Takeuchi T, Iinuma H, Kunimoto S, Masuda T, Ishizuka M, Takeuchi M, Hamada M, Naganawa H, Kondo S, Umezawa H: A new antitumor antibiotic, spergualin: isolation and antitumor activity. J Antibiot 1981;27:1619–1621.

509. Taniguchi N, Miyawaki T, Yachie A: A monoclonal anti-tac antibody may interfere with receptor binding of interleukin 2. Lymphokine Res 1982;1:107–112.

510. Tatum AH, Bollinger RR, Sanfilippo F: Rapid serologic diagnosis of serum sickness from antilymphocyte globulin therapy using enzyme immunoassay. Transplantation 1984;38:582–586.

511. Task Force Members: Critical issues in cyclosporine monitoring: report of the task force on cyclosporine. Clin Chem 1987;33:1269–1288.

512. Tax WJ, van de Heijden HM, Willems HW, Hoitsma AJ, Berden JH, Capel PJ, Koene RA: Immunosuppression with monoclonal anti-T3 antibody (WT32) in renal transplantation. Transplant Proc 1987;19(1 pt 3):1905–1907.

513. Taylor DO, Ensley RD, Olsen SL, Dunn D, Renlund DG: Mycophenolate mofetil (RS-61443): preclinical, clinical and three-year experience in heart transplantation. J Heart Lung Transplant 1994;113:571–582.

514. Tejani A, Lancman I, Pomrantz A, Khawar M, Chen C: Nephrotoxicity of cyclosporine A and cyclosporine G in rat model. Transplantation 1988;45:184.

515. Tepper MA, Petty B, Bursuker I, Pasternak RD, Cleaveland J, Spitalny GL, Schacter B: Inhibition of antibody production by the immunosuppressive agent 15-deoxyspergualin. Transplant Proc 1991;23:328–331.

516. Terada N, Lucas JJ, Szepesi A, Franklin RA, Domenico J, Gelfand EW: Rapamycin blocks cell cycle progression of activated T cells prior to event characteristic of the middle to late G_1 phase of the cycle. J Cell Physiol 1993;154:7–15.

517. Thistlethwaite JRJ, Cosimi AB, Delmonico FL, Rubin RH, Talkoff-Rubin N, Nelson PW, Fang L, Russell PS: Evolving use of OKT3 monoclonal antibody for treatment of renal allograft rejection. Transplantation 1984;38:695–701.

518. Thomas JM, Alqaisi M, Cunningham P, Carver M, Rebellato L, Gross U, Patselas T, Araneda D, Thomas F: The development of a posttransplant TLI treatment strategy that promotes organ allograft acceptance without chronic immunosuppression. Transplantation 1992;53:247–258.

519. Thomas JM, Carver FM, Burnett CM, Thomas FT: Enhanced allograft survival in rhesus monkeys treated with anti-human thymocyte globulin and donor lymphoid cells. Transplant Proc 1981;13:599–602.

520. Thomas JM, Carver FM, Foil MB, Hall WR, Adams C, Fahrenbruch GBTFT: Renal allograft tolerance induced with ATG and donor bone marrow in outbred rhesus monkeys. Transplantation 1983;36:104–106.

521. Thomas JM, Neville DM, Contreras JL, Eckhoff DE, Meng G, Lobashevsky AL, Wang PX, Huang ZQ, Verbanac KM, Haisch CE, Thomas FT: Preclinical studies of allograft tolerance in rhesus monkeys: a novel anti-CD3-immunotoxin given peritransplant with donor bone marrow induces operational tolerance to kidney allografts. Transplantation 1997;64:124–135.

522. Thomas JM, Verbanac KM, Carver FM, Kasten-Jolly J, Haisch CE, Gross U, Smith JP: Veto cells in transplantation tolerance [review]. Clin Transplant 1994;8:195–203.

523. Thompson ME, Shapiro AP, Johnson AM, Reeves R, Itzkoff J, Ginchereau E, Hardesty RL, Griffith BL, Bahnson HT, McDonald R Jr: New onset of hypertension following cardiac transplantation: a preliminary report and analysis. Transplant Proc 1983;15:2573–2577.

524. Todo S, Porter KA, Kam I, Lynch S, Venkataramanan R, DeWolf A, Starzl TE: Canine liver transplantation under Nva²-cyclosporine versus cyclosporine. Transplantation 1986;41:296.

525. TOR Inhibition—a new therapeutic pathway to immunosuppression. Sponsored by the AST and funded through an unrestricted educational grant from Wyeth-Ayerst Laboratories. April 2000.

526. Tsamandas AC, Pham SM, Seaberg EC, Pappo O, Kormos RL, Kawai A, Griffith BP, Zeevi A, Duquesnoy R, Fung JJ, Starzl TE, Demetris AJ: Adult heart transplantation under tacrolimus (FK506) immunosuppression: histopathologic observations and comparison to a cyclosporine based regimen with lymphocytic (ATG) induction. J Heart Lung Transplant 1997;16:723–734.

527. Tsudo M, Uchiyama T, Takatsuki K, Uchino H, Yodoi J: Modulation of Tac antigen on activated human T cells by anti-Tac monoclonal antibody. J Immunol 1982;129:592–595.

528. Turk JL, Parker D, Poulter LW: Functional aspects of the selective depletion of lymphoid tissue by cyclophosphamide. Immunology 1972;23:493–501.

529. Uchiyama T, Nelson DL, Fleisher TA, Waldmann TA: A monoclonal antibody (anti-Tac) reactive with activated and functionally mature human T cells. II. Expression of Tac antigen on activated cytotoxic killer T cells, suppressor cells, and on one of two types of helper T cells. J Immunol 1981;126:1398–1403.

530. Umezawa H, Kondo S, Inuma H, Kunimoto S, Ikeda D, Takeuchi T: Structure of an antitumor antibiotic spergualin. J Antibiot 1981;34:1622–1624.

531. U.S. Multicenter FK506 Liver Study Group: A comparison of tacrolimus (FK506) and cyclosporine for immunosuppression in liver transplantation. N Engl J Med 1994;331:1110–1115.

532. Valantine H, Keogh A, McIntosh N, Hunt S, Oyer P, Schroeder J: Cost containment: coadministration of diltiazem with cyclosporine after heart transplantation. J Heart Lung Transplant 1992;11:1–8.

533. Vallera DA, Carroll SF, Snover DC, Carlson GJ, Blazar BR: Toxicity and efficacy of anti-T-cell ricin toxin a chain immunotoxins in a murine model of established graft-versus-host disease induced across the major histocompatibility barrier. Blood 1991;77:182–194.

534. Van Buskirk AM, DeNagel DC, Guagliardi LE, Brodsky FM, Pierce SK: Cellular and subcellular distribution of PBP72/74, a peptide-binding protein that plays a role in antigen processing. J Immunol 1991;146:500–506.

535. Van Went GF: Investigation into mutagenic activity of azathioprine (Imuran) in different test systems. Mutat Res 1979;68:153–160.

536. Vasquez EM, Fabrega AJ, Pollak R: OKT3-induced cytokine-release syndrome: occurrence beyond the second dose and association with rejection severity. Transplant Proc 1995;27:873–874.

537. Veremus SA: Subtherapeutic cyclosporine concentrations during nafcillin therapy. Transplantation 1987;43:913–915.

538. Vezina C, Kudelski A, Sehgal SN: Rapamycin (AY-22, 989) a new antifungal antibiotic. I. Taxonomy of the producing streptomycete and isolation of the active principle. J Antibiot 1975;23:2736.

539. Vincenti F, Kirkman R, Light S, Bumgardner G, Pescovitz M, Halloran P, Neylan J, Wilkinson A, Ekberg H, Gaston R, Backman L, Burdick J: Interleukin-2 receptor blockade with daclizumab to prevent acute rejection renal transplantation. N Engl J Med 1998;338:161–165.

540. Vincenti F, Nashan B, Light S: Daclizumab: outcome of phase III trials and mechanism of action. Double blind and the triple therapy study groups. Transplant Proc 1998;30:2155–2158.

541. Vonderscher J, Meinzer A: Rationale for the development of Sandimmune Neoral. Transplant Proc 1994;26:2925–2927.

542. Voraberger G, Schafer R, Stratowa C: Cloning of the human gene for intercellular adhesion molecule 1 and analysis of its 5'-regulatory region. J Immunol 1991;147:2777–2786.

543. Voss BL, Hamilton KK, Samara ENS, McKee PA: Cyclosporine suppression of endothelial prostacyclin generation. Transplantation 1988;45:799–796.

544. Vowels BR, Cassin M, Boufal MH, Walsh LJ, Rook AH: Extracorporeal photochemotherapy induces the production of tumor necrosis factor-alpha by monocytes: implications for treatment of cutaneous T cell lymphoma and systemic sclerosis. J Invest Dermatol 1992;98:686–692.

545. Wadhwa NK, Schroeder TJ, O'Flaherty E, Pesce AJ, Myre SA, First MR: The effect of oral metoclopramide on the absorption of cyclosporine. Transplantation 1987;43:211–213.

546. Wagner K, Albrecht S, Neumayer HH: Prevention of delayed graft function by a calcium antagonist—a randomized trial in renal graft recipients on cyclosporine A. Transplant Proc 1986;18:1269–1271.

547. Wagner K, Henkel M, Heinemeyer G, Neumayer HH: Interaction of calcium blockers and cyclosporine. Transplant Proc 1988;2 (suppl 2):561–568.

548. Wagner K, Neumayer HH: Influence of the calcium antagonist diltiazem on delayed graft function in cadaveric kidney transplantation: results of a 6-month follow-up. Transplant Proc 1987;1:1353–1357.

549. Wagoner LE, Olsen SL, Bristow MR, O'Connell JB, Taylor DO, Lappe DL, Renlund DG: Cyclophosphamide as an alternative to azathioprine in cardiac transplant recipients with suspected azathioprine-induced hepatotoxicity. Transplantation 1993;56:1415–1418.

550. Wagoner LE, Olsen SL, Taylor DO, Rasmussen LG, Ensley RD, Renlund DG: Cyclophosphamide as an alternative immunosuppressive agent in cardiac transplant recipients with recurrent rejection. J Heart Lung Transplant 1992;11(pt II):199.

551. Wahlberg J, Wilczek HE, Fauchald P, Nordal KP, Heaf JG, Olgaard K, Hansen JM, Lokkegaard H, Mueller EA, Kovarik JM: Consistent absorption of cyclosporine from a microemulsion formulation assessed in stable recipients over a one-year study period. Transplantation 1995;60:648–652.

552. Waid TH, Lucas BA, Thompson JS, Brown SA, Munch L, Prebeck RJ, Jezek D: Treatment of acute cellular rejection with T10B9.1A-31 or OKT3 in renal allograft recipients. Transplantation 1992;53:80–86.

553. Waid TH, Lucas BA, Thompson JS, McKeown JW, Brown S, Kryscio R, Skeeters LJ: Treatment of renal allograft rejection with T10B9.1A31 or OKT: final analysis of a phase II clinical trial. Transplantation 1997;64:274–281.

554. Waid TH, Thompson JS, McKeown JW, Brown SA, Sekela ME: Induction immunotherapy in heart transplantation with T10B9.1A-31: a phase I study. J Heart Lung Transplant 1997;16:913–916.

555. Waid TH, Lucas BA, Thompson JS, Munch LC, Brown S, Kryscio R, Prebec R, VanHoy MA, Jezek D: Treatment of acute rejection with anti-T-cell antigen receptor complex alpha beta (T10B9.1A-31) or anti-CD3 (OKT3) monoclonal antibody: results of a prospective randomized double-blind trial. Transplant Proc 1991;23(1 pt 2):1062–1065.

556. Waksman S, Woodruff H: Bacteriostatic and bactericidal substances produced by a soil actinomyces. Proc Soc Exp Biol Med 1940;45:609–614.

557. Walker PD, Lazzaro VA, Duggin GG, Horvat JS, Tiller DJ: Evidence that alteration in renal metabolism and lipid peroxidation may contribute to nephrotoxicity. Transplantation 1990;50:487–492.

558. Walter DH, Haendeler J, Galle J, Zeiher AM, Dimmeler S: Cyclosporin A inhibits apoptosis of human endothelial cells by preventing release of cytochrome C from mitochondria. Circulation 1998;98:1153–1157.

559. Wang CP, Burckart GJ, Ptachcinski RJ, Venkataramanan R, Schwinghammer T, Hakala T, Griffith B, Hardesty R, Shadduck R, Knapp J, Van Thiel DH, Makowa L, Starzl TE: Cyclosporine metabolite concentrations in the blood of liver, heart, kidney, and bone marrow transplant patients. Transplant Proc 1988;20 (suppl 2):591–596.

560. Wasik M, Gorski A, Stepien-Sopniewska B: Effect of FK506 versus cyclosporine on human natural and antibody dependent acytoxicity reactions in vitro. Transplantation 1991;51:268.

561. Wee SL, Colvin RB, Phelan JM, Preffer FI, Reichert TA, Berd D, Cosimi AB: Fc-receptor for mouse IgG1 (Fc gamma RII) and antibody-mediated cell clearance in patients treated with Leu2a antibody. Transplantation 1989;48:1012–1017.

562. Weisensee D, Bereiter-Hahn J, Schoeppe W, Low-Friedrich I: Effects of cytokines on the contractility of cultured cardiac myocytes. Int J Immunopharmacol 1993;15:581–587.

563. Weiss A: T lymphocyte activation. In Paul WE (ed): Fundamental Immunology. New York: Raven Press, 1989, p 359.

564. Wenger R: Cyclosporine and analogues: structural requirements for immunosuppressive activity. Transplant Proc 1986;18(suppl 5):213–218.

565. Wenger RM: In White DJG (ed): Cyclosporin A. Amsterdam: Elsevier Biomedical, 1982.

566. Whalen J, Ghersa P, Hooft van Huijsduijnen R, Gray G, Chandra F, Talabot F, DeLamarter JF: An NF kappa B-like factor is essential but not sufficient for cytokine induction of endothelial leukocyte adhesion molecule 1 (ELAM-1) gene transcription. Nucl Acids Res 1991;19:2645–2653.

567. Wheeler GP, Bowdon BJ, Adamson DJ: Comparison of the effects of several inhibitors of the synthesis of nucleic acids upon the viability and progression through the cell cycle of cultures. H. Ep. No. 2 cells. Cancer Res 1972;32:2661–2669.

568. White D, Rose M, Wright L: Failure of whole blood cyclosporine levels to provide a reliable measure of immunosuppression in clinical heart and heart/lung transplantation. Transplant Proc 1988;20(suppl 2):422–425.

569. White DJG, Blatchford NR, Cauwenbergh G: Cyclosporine and ketoconazole. Transplantation 1984;37:214–215.

570. White DJG, Plumb AM, Pawelec G, Brons G: Cyclosporin A: an immunosuppressive agent preferentially active against proliferating T cells. Transplantation 1979;27:55–58.

571. Wolfe JT, Lessin SR, Singh AH, Rook AH: Review of immunomodulation by photopheresis: treatment of cutaneous T-cell lymphoma, autoimmune disease, and allograft rejection. Artif Organs 1994;18:888–897.

572. Wollenek G, Laufer G, Laczkovics A, Buxbaum P, Kober I: Comparison of a monoclonal anti-T cell antibody versus ATG as prophylaxis after heart transplantation. Transplant Proc 1989;21:2499–2501.

573. Wong JT, Eylath AA, Ghobrial I, Colvin RB: The mechanism of anti-CD3 monoclonal antibodies. Transplantation 1990;50:683–689.

574. Woodruff MFA, Anderson NF: Effect of lymphocyte depletion by thoracic duct fistula and administration of anti-lymphocytic serum on the survival of skin homografts in rats. Nature 1963;200:702.

575. Wrighton CJ, Hofer-Warbinek R, Moll T, Eytner R, Bach FH, deMartin R: Inhibition of endothelial cell activation by adenovirus-mediated expression of IκBα, an inhibitor of the transcription factor NF-κB. J Exp Med 1996;183:1013–1022.

576. Yadav RV, Indudhara R, Kumar P, Ghugh KS, Gupta KL: Cyclophosphamide in renal transplantation. Transplantation 1988;45:421–424.

577. Yasunaga C, Cramer DV, Chapman FA, Wang HK, Barnett M, Wu GD, Makowka L: The prevention of accelerated cardiac allograft rejection in sensitized recipients after treatment with brequinar sodium. Transplantation 1993;56:898–904.

578. Yates CR, Krynetski EY, Loennechen T, Fessing MY, Tai HL, Pui CH, Relling MV, Evans WE: Molecular diagnosis of thiopurine S-methyltransferase deficiency: genetic basis for azathioprine and mercaptopurine intolerance. Ann Intern Med 1997;126:608–614.

579. Yatscoff RW, LeGatt DF, Kneteman NM: Therapeutic monitoring of rapamycin: a new immunosuppressive drug. Ther Drug Monit 1993;15:478–482.

580. Yatscoff RW, Rosano TG, Bowers LD: The clinical significance of cyclosporin metabolites. Clin Biochem 1991;24:23–35.

581. Yokum DE: Cyclosporine, FK506, rapamycin, and other immunomodulators. Rheum Dis Clin North Am 1996;22:133–154.

582. Yoo EK, Rook AH, Elenitsas R, Gasparro FP, Vowels BR: Apoptosis induction of ultraviolet light A and photochemotherapy in cutaneous T-cell lymphoma: relevance to mechanism of therapeutic action. J Invest Dermatol 1996;107:235–242.

583. Zan-Bar I, Slavin S, Strober S: Induction and mechanism of tolerance to bovine serum albumin in mice given total lymphoid irradiation (TLI). J Immunol 1978;121:1400–1404.

584. Zeevi A, Woan M, Yao GZ, Venkataramanan S, Todo S, Starz TE, Duquesnoy RJ: Comparative *in vitro* studies on the immunosuppressive activities of mycophenolic acid, bredinin, FK506, cyclosporine, and rapamycin. Transplant Proc 1991;23:2928–2930.
585. Zhang Z, Lazarovits A, Grant D, Garcia B, Stiller C, Zhong R: CD45RB monoclonal antibody induces tolerance in the mouse kidney graft, but fails to prevent small bowel graft rejection. Transplant Proc 1996;28:2514.
586. Zhang Z, Zhong R, Grant D, Garcia B, White M, Stiller C, Lazarovits A: Prevention and reversal of renal allograft rejection by monoclonal antibody to CD45RB in the mouse model. Transplant Proc 1995;27:389.
587. Zheng XX, Strom TB, Steele AW: Quantitative comparison of rapamycin and cyclosporine effects on cytokine gene expression studied by reverse transcriptase-competitive polymerase chain reaction. Transplantation 1994;59:87–92.
588. Zhu LP, Cupps TR, Whalen G, Fauci AS: Selective effects of cyclophosphamide therapy on activation, proliferation, and differentiation of human B cells. J Clin Invest 1987;79:1082–1090.
589. Zimmerman JJ, Kahan BD: Pharmacokinetics of sirolimus in stable renal transplant patients after multiple oral dose administration. J Clin Pharmacol 1997;37:405–415.

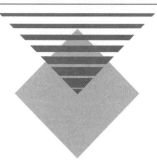

CHAPTER FOURTEEN

Cardiac Allograft Rejection

with the collaboration of
ROBERT C. BOURGE, M.D., E. RENE RODRIGUEZ, M.D.,
AND CARMELA D. TAN, M.D.

The immunologic response to transplantation is discussed in detail in Chapter 2. **Cardiac allograft rejection** represents the histologic result of this immunologic process within the cardiac allograft. The potential target cells within the heart include, among others, the myocyte and endothelial cells of the coronary vasculature which provide the interface between recipient immune cells and donor allograft. The recipient alloimmune response includes presentation of donor peptide antigens by donor antigen-presenting cells (donor vascular endothelial cells and so-called "passenger leukocytes") and recipient antigen-presenting cells. The immune system, and specifically the alloimmune response (against the transplanted organ) is composed of multiple redundant pathways for activation and attack of the foreign organ. The presentation or exposure of donor antigens by antigen-presenting cells to the appropriate recipient T-cells leads to T-cell activation and clonal proliferation in the presence of the appropriate costimulatory molecules. The endothelial lining of the vasculature of the cardiac allograft plays a critical role in the rejection process. Although the primary function of the vascular endothelium is maintenance of an anticoagulated milieu to prevent intravascular thrombosis, it participates directly in the rejection process by recruiting immune cells to the allograft. Up-regulation of endothelial adhesion molecules causes circulating activated lymphocytes to stick to the endothelial surface and extravasate into the interstitium of the allograft. The production and release of cytokines from activated T-cells and the up-regulation of their surface receptors leads to a proliferation of immune cells and recruitment of macrophages. If unabated by immunosuppressive agents, the result of these events is the release of powerful biologic effectors of myocyte injury and necrosis, which can be recognized by histologic examination. The evidence of cellular injury in the presence of immunologic effector cells (T-lymphocytes, macrophages, neutrophils) can be detected and graded by histologic examination of myocardial tissue obtained by endomyocardial biopsy. Thus, this technique forms the cornerstone of rejection identification and surveillance in heart transplant patients.

The success of organ transplantation is based on the premise that immunosuppressive modalities can effectively suppress those aspects of the immune system which, when stimulated by donor HLA antigens, ultimately lead to destruction of the transplanted organ. The process of controlling and/or preventing allograft rejection in order to promote long-term graft (and patient) survival with nearly normal graft function involves a strategy of initial immunosuppressive therapy, a program of chronic maintenance immunosuppression, methods of monitoring the graft for early detection of rejection, and specific strategies for treating rejection. As the science and practice of organ transplantation has evolved, multiple drugs and therapies have been developed which interfere with or block certain aspects of the alloimmune response. These modalities and their mechanism of action are discussed in Chapter 13.

With the use of one or more antirejection drugs or modalities, ideally rejection could be completely prevented through the inability of the immune system to mount an effective attack of the transplanted organ; or in the "perfect" situation, the immune system could be prevented from recognizing the transplanted organ as "foreign" (induction of tolerance), and therefore the immune system would not be stimulated to attack the transplanted organ.

Over the nearly 40 years of clinical organ transplantation (and over 30 years of cardiac transplantation) no immunosuppressive regimen has been identified which uniformly prevents rejection without unacceptable toxicity. To date, no modalities have been identified which specifically block rejection of the transplanted heart while leaving intact the remainder of the immune system to combat infection and malignancy. Thus, the problem of rejection prevention is further complicated by the additional effects of immunosuppressive drugs and other modalities on the overall immune system. If the dose of one or multiple immunosuppressive agents becomes high enough, interference with the immune system will create a situation where the risk of fatal or serious infection or malignancy exceeds the risk of fatal rejection.

Therefore, current strategies of immunosuppression focus on controlling or preventing rejection that is severe enough to destroy or cripple the cardiac allograft while at the same time maintaining immunosuppression at a level low enough to prevent fatal infection and malignancy. The difficulty of this task is confounded by the great variability among patients with respect to the vigor of their immune response (attack) against the allograft as well as the variable degree of immunosuppression achieved with a given dose of one or more immunosuppressive agents.

Another perplexing aspect of the immune response to transplantation is the observation of long periods of apparent quiescence (absence of rejection) of immune activity against the allograft only to be suddenly interrupted (without apparent reason) by a vigorous immunologic attack of the allograft. Our understanding of the reasons for these apparently sudden increases in the intensity of the immune response to the allograft is incomplete, but extensive clinical experience supported by surveillance endomyocardial biopsies indicates that the rejection process occurs in "waves" of heightened immunologic activity within the allograft. The precise factors which may stimulate the immune response and initiate active rejection (as evidenced by myocyte and/or endothelial injury in the presence of immune cells) are incompletely understood, but include reduction of immunosuppression, stimulation of the immune system by infectious illness (particularly viral), and possibly stress. In most instances, however, an inciting stimulus is not identified.

With current maintenance immunosuppressive therapy, the frequency and severity of rejection episodes tends to decrease over time, presumably related to adaptation of the host immune system to the allograft and its histocompatibility antigens. A state of partial unresponsiveness can be detected in many patients after transplantation, in which donor antigens will illicit a much weaker immune response from the host than cells from a third party. The possible reasons for this are discussed in Chapter 2.

PATHOLOGY OF ALLOGRAFT REJECTION

The following discussion will focus on the histologic examination of the transplanted heart based on **tissue obtained by endomyocardial biopsy.** The same general principles apply to the histologic examination of explanted heart or transplanted hearts at autopsy. The description of hyperacute rejection later in this section is based on autopsy and experimental observations, since hyperacute rejection is nearly uniformly fatal and not amenable to endomyocardial biopsy.

The histologic examination of endomyocardial tissue obtained by biopsy of the allograft has, since 1972, provided the basis ("gold standard") for diagnosing rejection. The techniques of endomyocardial biopsy are discussed later in this chapter. A histologic grading system for rejection was developed by Billingham and colleagues at Stanford University.[13] Over the ensuing years, numerous pathologic classifications of rejection have been developed. Unfortunately, the lack of standardization hampered the understanding of the rejection process, indications for therapy, and outcome. In 1990, the concerted efforts of many pathologists and other heart transplant professionals resulted in the publication of the **Working Formulation of the International Society of Heart and Lung Transplantation (ISHLT),** which established the standard methodology and criteria for the histopathologic diagnosis of rejection[15] (Table 14–1).

PROCESSING AND FIXATION OF BIOPSY SPECIMENS

An analysis of biopsy specimens indicated that 95% of inflammatory infiltrates can be detected with three pieces, and up to 98% of infiltrates will be detected with four pieces.[212] The Working Formulation for allograft monitoring recommends the examination of at least four pieces of tissue,[14] usually 3–4 mm in diameter (Fig. 14–1). All pieces obtained should be submitted, since they may yield valuable information with microscopic examination. Pieces that look white, suggesting that they are made up of thick endocardium, may actually be curled up and conceal some myocardium that is visible on

TABLE 14–1	**ISHLT Standardized Endomyocardial Biopsy Grading Scheme**	
GRADE*	DESCRIPTION	NOMENCLATURE
0	No lymphocytic infiltrate	No rejection
1A	Focal (perivascular or interstitial) lymphocytic infiltrate without myocyte necrosis	Focal mild acute rejection
1B	Diffuse but sparse lymphocytic infiltrate without myocyte necrosis	Diffuse mild acute rejection
2	One focus only with "aggressive" lymphocytic infiltrate and/or focal myocyte injury	Focal moderate rejection
3A	Multifocal aggressive lymphocytic infiltrates and/or myocyte necrosis	Multifocal moderate acute rejection
3B	Diffuse, inflammatory process with myocyte necrosis	Diffuse borderline severe acute rejection
4	Diffuse, aggressive, polymorphous infiltrate with necrosis (± edema; ± hemorrhage; ± vasculitis)	Severe acute rejection

* Biopsy graded by worst infiltrate noted on at least 3 to 5 specimens reviewed.

Additional Information Which Should Be Reported
- Biopsy less than 4 pieces
- Resolving rejection—denoted by a lesser grade than prior biopsy.
- Humoral rejection (positive immunofluorescence, vasculitis, or severe edema in absence of cellular infiltrate)
- "Quilty" effect
  - A = No myocyte encroachment
  - B = With myocyte encroachment
- Ischemia
  - A = Up to 3 weeks after transplant
  - B = Late ischemia
- Infection present
- Lymphoproliferative disorder
- Other

From Billingham ME, Cary NRB, Hammond ME, Kemnitz J, Marboe C, McCallister HA, Snovar DC, Winters GL, Zerbe A: A working formulation for the standardization of nomenclature in the diagnosis of heart and lung rejection. J Heart Lung Transplant 1990;9:587–593.

histologic sections. Likewise, pieces that look like blood clot may harbor a piece of myocardium in their core.

The tissue should be fixed immediately in the desired fixative that has been allowed to reach room temperature. The tissue should not be allowed to sit on filter paper, gauze, or any other surface impregnated with saline. Saline is a very poor solution to preserve the morphology of myocardium and creates artifacts readily.

The standard fixative for **routine light microscopic examination** is 10% phosphate-buffered formalin. At least three biopsy specimens should be handled in this way. If **electron microscopic studies** are desired for certain research protocols, one piece may be preserved in 2.5% buffered glutaraldehyde. If **immunofluorescence or immunohistochemical** studies are requested, one or more biopsy pieces are frozen. A specific freezing protocol is important in order to achieve the best preservation of morphology possible. The Working Formulation recommends freezing the tissue in OCT compound (Miles Inc., Diagnostics Division, Elkhart, IN).[15] Another effective protocol utilizes isopentane to freeze the tissue. The isopentane should be chilled to –20°C in a small 1.8-mL cryogenic vial. The biopsy tissue is immersed in this prechilled isopentane cryovial, the cap is tightened, and the container is immersed in liquid nitrogen. At this point the tissue can be processed for immunofluorescence or stored at –80°C for future study.

It should be noted that the Working Formulation does not require routine submission of tissue from cardiac allograft biopsies for electron microscopy.[14] This is due to the delay and expense of processing the tissue and the fact that there is relatively low clinical relevance of the pathologic findings seen on ultrastructural examination.[14] However, this procedure has value in some research protocols.[126] Immunofluorescence studies are also not routinely employed for the diagnosis of rejection.

In the pathology laboratory, the **gross description** should include the demographic data of the patient, the number of tissue pieces, the average size, and color. Careful gross examination provides in most instances important information regarding the presence of myocardium, thickened endocardium, adipose tissue, chordae tendineae,[235] blood clot, or small endocardial thrombi. The number of pieces submitted should be stated in the requisition form, verified on gross examination, and always correlated with the number of pieces present in the paraffin block and in the hematoxylin and eosin–stained slides. This is important because the Working Formulation calls for the examination of at least four pieces of myocardium, 50% of which must contain myocardium and not previous biopsy site or scar.[14] Specimens that do not meet these criteria should be diagnosed as "inadequate biopsy."[14]

Whenever possible, the tissue should not be handled with forceps during gross exam in the pathology lab-

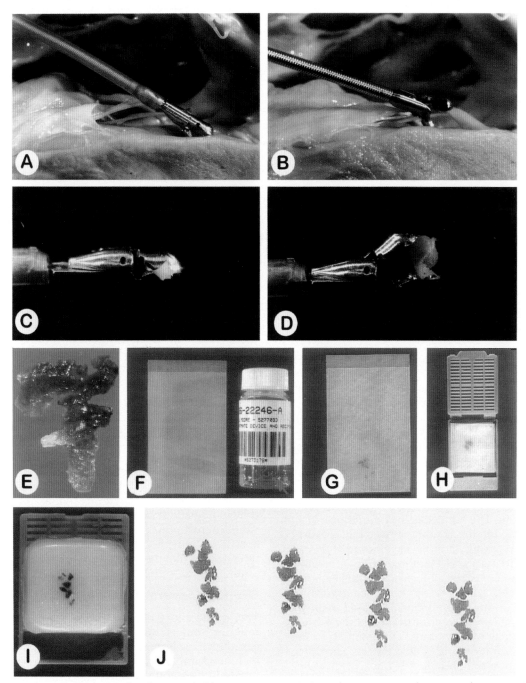

FIGURE **14-1.** Procurement of endomyocardial biopsy specimen. *A,* Caves bioptome opened against right interventricular endocardium. The cutting mechanism has one rigid and one mobile ''jaw.'' The tricuspid valve is seen to the left of the bioptome. The tip of the bioptome measures 3.0 mm in diameter. *B,* Cordis bioptome showing that the cutting mechanism has two flexible, but slightly smaller ''jaws.'' The tip of the bioptome measures 2.5 mm in diameter. *C,* Caves bioptome showing the biopsy sample as it is retrieved. Most of the tissue is inside the cutting ''jaws''; however, some tissue is noticeable outside of cutter. This represents torn tissue rather than cut tissue. *D,* Same as *C* but with the cutter opened, revealing the size of the biopsy tissue (usually 2 × 2 × 2 mm). *E,* Fresh pieces of myocardium before being placed in fixative. *F,* Specimen mesh-bag and container with the fixed specimen in it (arrow). *G,* Specimen is transferred to the mesh bag. *H,* Specimen bag is folded into processing tissue cassette. *I,* Paraffin-embedded tissue. *J,* Ribbon of paraffin sections stained with hematoxylin and eosin.

oratory. It can be safely transferred into a specimen-mesh-bag securely folded into the processing cassette. The small size of the biopsy pieces allows any pathology laboratory to process the specimen in about 4 hours without compromising the quality of the final slides.

Following fixation, the biopsy is generally processed in paraffin. The Working Formulation recommends a minimum of three step levels through the paraffin block with at least three sections of each level. If possible, the sections should be cut at a thickness of 4 μm. Slides should be stained routinely with **hematoxylin and eosin,** and one additional slide should be stained with a connective tissue stain such as **Masson's trichrome,** which is useful for identifying myocyte damage, indicating whether a cellular infiltrate is contained within scar tissue, and to delineate the endocardium in a "Quilty" lesion (see later section). Any unstained slides are archived for later study, if necessary. The method of tissue processing and histologic examination should allow reporting of about 90% of all heart biopsies within 8 hours, greater than 97% within 24 hours, and only about 3% later than 24 hours after they are received in the pathology laboratory.

ACUTE CELLULAR REJECTION

Morphologically, acute cellular rejection is a mononuclear inflammatory response, predominantly lymphocytic,[26] directed against the cardiac allograft. Autopsy studies have demonstrated that both ventricles are equally involved in the rejection process; thus, sampling of the right ventricular septum is usually indicative of histologic changes in the left ventricle.[190] The key histologic feature which identifies rejection of a sufficient degree ("moderate") to warrant immunosuppressive intervention is the presence of **myocyte damage.** In severe cases, there is also participation of granulocytes in the rejection process. The subtleties and variations of this response are used in the grading of rejection. It must be noted that the Working Formulation grading of rejection was designed to assess rejection in endomyocardial biopsies and cannot be applied to whole grafts examined at autopsy or following explantation. The grades proposed in the Working Formulation are based mainly on the amount of **inflammatory infiltrate** and the presence of **myocyte damage;** the pattern of inflammatory infiltration plays a minor role (Table 14–1). The ISHLT grades of rejection are presented below.

Grade 0 (No Acute Rejection)

A lymphocytic infiltrate is absent. There is no evidence of acute rejection or myocyte damage on the biopsy specimens. The findings are consistent with normal myocardium.

Grade 1A (Focal Mild Acute Rejection)

Focal, perivascular, or interstitial infiltrates of large lymphocytes are present that cause no myocyte damage.

One or more pieces of the biopsy tissue may be involved (Fig. 14–2).

Grade 1B (Diffuse Mild Acute Rejection)

A more diffuse, perivascular, or interstitial (or both) infiltrate of large lymphocytes with no myocyte damage is present. Although described as a "diffuse" infiltrate, the infiltrate is locally diffuse, not present throughout the biopsy piece. One or more pieces of biopsy tissue may be involved (Fig. 14–3).

Grade 2 (Focal Moderate Acute Rejection)

This grade indicates only one focus of inflammatory infiltrate (large aggressive lymphocytes with or without eosinophils), which is sharply circumscribed. Architectural distortion with myocyte damage should be present within the solitary focus (Fig. 14–4).

Grade 3A (Multifocal Moderate Acute Rejection)

Multifocal inflammatory infiltrates are present, consisting of large lymphocytes with or without eosinophils and possibly neutrophils. There should be evidence of myocyte damage in some areas of infiltrate. These infiltrates may involve one or more pieces of biopsy tissue (Fig. 14–5). Nearly all transplant centers agree that grade 3A rejection or higher warrants specific immunosuppressive treatment.

Grade 3B (Diffuse Borderline Severe Acute Rejection)

This represents a diffuse inflammatory process within several of the pieces of biopsy tissue. Myocyte damage is present, as well as an aggressive inflammatory infiltrate of large lymphocytes and eosinophils with an occasional neutrophil. The multifocal infiltrates are more confluent than in grade 3A. Focal hemorrhage in the interstitium may be seen in this grade (Fig. 14–5).

Grade 4 (Severe Acute Rejection)

This grade represents the most severe form of acute rejection and is rarely observed clinically. A diffuse aggressive, polymorphous inflammatory infiltrate that includes lymphocytes, eosinophils, and neutrophils is invariably present. Myocyte necrosis and damage is always seen. Edema, interstitial hemorrhage, and vasculitis are usually present. In some cases in which the patient has been treated aggressively with immunosuppression for some time, edema and hemorrhage may be more prominent than the cellular infiltrate (Fig. 14–5). Graft loss should be considered imminent without aggressive immunosuppressive therapy (see later sections).

Resolving Rejection

Biopsies taken to evaluate the results of therapy after an episode of moderate rejection are graded in the same

Text continues on page 472

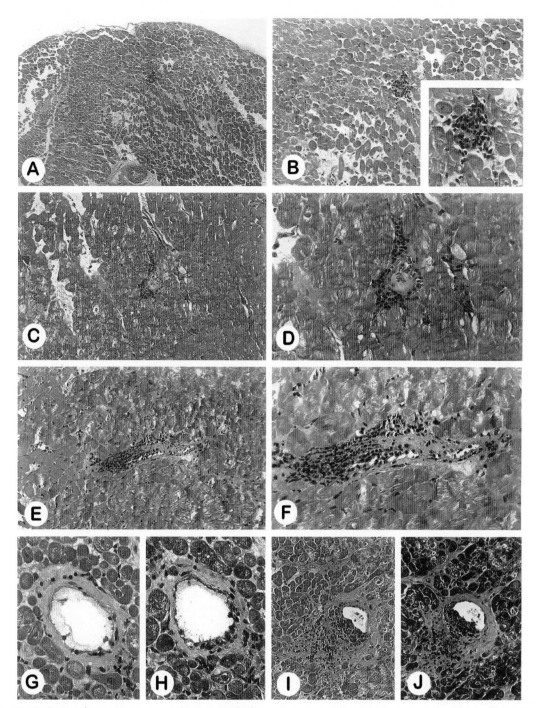

FIGURE **14–2.** Grade 1A rejection. *A,* Light micrograph of an endomyocardial biopsy showing a focus of lymphocytic infiltrate evident at low magnification. The endocardium is thin and myocytes sectioned in an oblique to transverse plane are of normal size. Note a small artery present in the bottom part (middle) of the biopsy without any inflammatory infiltrate (hematoxylin and eosin stain [H&E], 10 ×). *B,* The same biopsy at higher magnification shows a few red blood cells in the center of the infiltrate which represents a perivascular cuff of mononuclear cells. The infiltrate is beginning to extend into the interstitial space between the myocytes (inset). There is no evidence of myocyte damage (H&E, 16 ×; Inset, 40 ×). *C,* Another perivascular infiltrate around a venule with open lumen and intravascular red cells. There is very early expansion of the interstitial space without evidence of myocyte damage. Note the presence of contraction band artifact in the myocytes (H&E, 16 ×). *D,* Higher magnification of the same field as *C* (H&E, 40 ×). *E,* A small vessel longitudinally cut is shown with a cuff of mononuclear cells. The inflammatory infiltrate is asymmetrically distributed giving an impression of widening of the interstitial space at the left end of the vessel (H&E, 16 ×). *F,* Higher magnification of the same vessel showing rows of lymphocytes parallel to the axis of the arteriole (H&E, 40 ×). *G,* If a cross-section is made through the right end of the arteriole in *E,* the infiltrate would look similar to this small dilated postcapillary venule (note the large diameter but the absence of media). The sparse infiltrate consists of a few lymphocytes subjacent to the endothelial cell layer and lymphocytes that have crossed this layer into the collagenous adventitia (H&E, 40 ×). *H,* An adjacent section of the same field as *G* demonstrating more subendothelial lymphocytes. Note the collagen-stained blue in the adventitia and the small foci of lymphocytes that have reached the interstitial space between the myocytes (Masson's trichrome, 40 ×). *I,* Another example of venular infiltration with extension into and expansion of the perivascular and interstitial space (H&E, 16 ×). *J,* A section adjacent to the field shown in *I* reveals perivascular scar around the venule and a slight increase in collagen (Masson's trichrome, 16 ×).

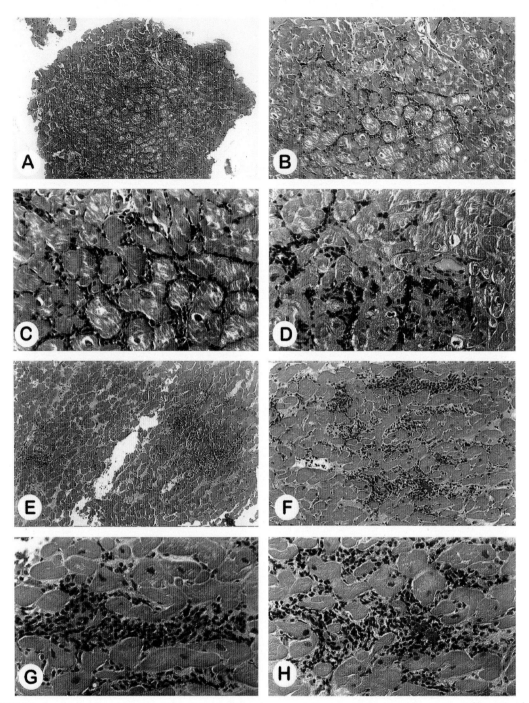

FIGURE **14–3.** Grade 1B rejection. *A*, Light micrograph showing a conspicuous mononuclear inflammatory infiltrate that forms a network-like pattern of interstitial dark blue cells surrounding individual myocytes. (H&E, 10 ×). *B*, Higher magnification of the biopsy shown in *A*, lymphocytes form one to three rows of "Indian files" in between myocytes. There is no myocyte damage; however, there is contraction band artifact. When examined in cross-sections or oblique sections, contraction band artifact shows a pattern of hypereosinophilic cytoplasm alternating with areas that are somewhat emptier. Therefore, the "bands" are not as readily apparent (H&E, 20 ×). *C*, Higher magnification of the same focus as in *B* (H&E, 40 ×). *D*, This micrograph shows another example of grade 1B rejection. The infiltrate is less evenly distributed with areas that are more basophilic, but an overall diffuse pattern is readily discernible. There is no evidence of myocyte damage (H&E, 40 ×). *E*, Low magnification of another example of grade 1B with more conspicuous inflammatory infiltrates than in *A*. There are two distinct areas of involvement (H&E, 16 ×). *F*, At the same magnification as *B* these foci even show greater widening of the interstitial space due to the inflammatory infiltrate (H&E, 20 ×). *G*, At higher magnification, it is obvious that some of the increase in interstitial space is because the inflammatory infiltrates are also surrounding small arterioles, which in turn gives the appearance of a wider interstitial space. (Note the red blood cells in the lumen of the arteriole.) The myocyte hypertrophy is more evident. If one considers that the average lymphocyte nucleus with condensed chromatin measures 10 μm, then the average myocyte in this field measures about 50 μm. (The average myocyte diameter in adults is ~ 20 μm.) This field is a higher magnification of the upper portion of *F*. There is no evidence of myocyte damage or dropout (H&E, 40 ×). *H*, Higher magnification of the lower portion of *F*. Once again, it shows how the inflammatory infiltrate surrounds an arteriole, and even individual myocytes. There is no evidence of myocyte damage or dropout. These widened spaces are no wider than the average diameter of two adjacent myocytes seen in this field (H&E, 40×).

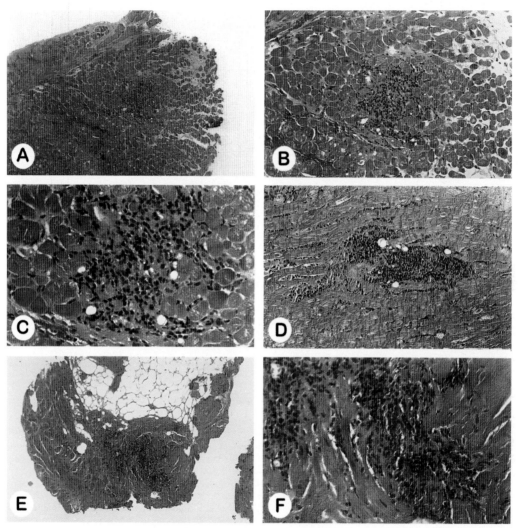

FIGURE **14–4.** Grade 2 rejection. Several examples illustrating the spectrum of lesions seen in this grade are shown. *A,* Light micrograph of a biopsy showing a single focus of mononuclear inflammatory infiltrate which clearly expands the interstitial space. The visible endocardium is thin. There are some areas of "pseudohemorrhage" (see text) (H&E, 10 ×). *B,* Higher magnification shows some vacuolar spaces near the focus of inflammation. The interstitial red blood cells are not associated with myocyte damage (H&E, 20 ×). *C,* Higher magnification shows that the inflammatory infiltrate consists mostly of lymphocytes and some macrophages. There is no clear evidence of myocyte damage or necrosis. However, the infiltrate covers an area of about 300 × 500 μm, thus representing a large area of myocyte dropout. Vacuoles are present, some are clearly within myocytes, but others are difficult to assign to a specific cell type as no visible rim of cytoplasm remains (H&E, 40 ×). *D,* A section from a different biopsy shows a somewhat elongated focus of inflammatory infiltrate. It follows the course of a small arteriole (seen to the left of the infiltrate). Compared with the focus of rejection seen in *F,* this infiltrate again covers a much greater area similar to that seen in *A–C.* There is myocyte dropout and some extension of the inflammatory infiltrate into the perimyocytic spaces adjacent to the main focus of rejection. There are also a few vacuoles present. Note the absence of clear-cut necrosis of myocytes (H&E, 20 ×) *E,* This biopsy piece shows about 40% adipose tissue. There is a large mononuclear infiltrate in the center of the piece (H&E, 4 ×). *F,* Higher magnification of the focus seen in *E* shows a dense mononuclear infiltrate, myocyte dropout, and absence of clear-cut necrosis and vacuoles. There are some hypereosinophilic myocytes present near the focus of rejection (H&E, 40 ×).

Illustration continued on following page

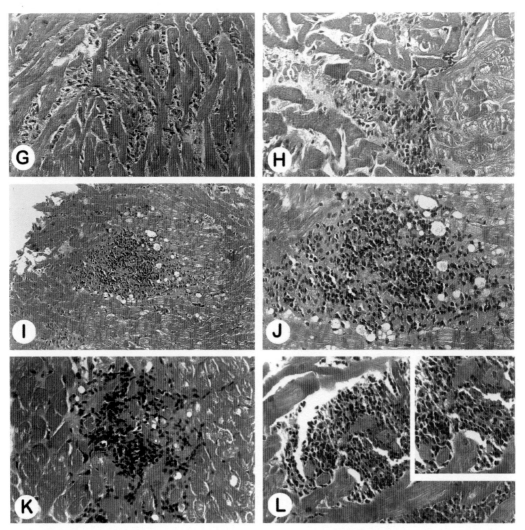

FIGURE **14–4.** *Continued. G,* This focus of rejection shows an inflammatory infiltrate that clearly is less dense than those seen in *A–F.* However, there is myocyte damage present as seen in the center of the micrograph. They are much thinner, have irregular borders and fragmented sarcoplasm (H&E, 40 ×). *H,* Another focus of rejection that shows myocyte damage and less inflammatory infiltrate than in *A–F.* Some of the damaged myocytes are thinner and disrupted. Others are hypereosinophilic (H&E, 40 ×). *I,* Large focus of mononuclear inflammatory infiltrate that replaces the myocardium. Numerous vacuolated structures are present. There is also abundant contraction band artifact (H&E, 20 ×). *J,* Higher magnification of the focus seen in *I.* The vacuolated cells seem to be macrophages. There are no visible myocytes with damage or necrosis. Contraction band artifact is abundant (H&E, 40 ×). *K,* This example shows a small focus of dense inflammatory infiltrate. There are the remnants of several hypereosinophilic myocytes intermingled with some red blood cells entrapped within capillaries and the inflammatory infiltrate (H&E, 40 ×). *L,* This focus shows a large lesion consisting of lymphocytes and macrophages which has disrupted the architecture and is associated with some necrotic myocytes. There are occasional extravasated red blood cells. This infiltrate was the only one seen and was present in only one of the biopsy pieces in 30 slides representing all levels of sections through the biopsy. Therefore, the diagnosis of a more severe grade of rejection was not made. The inset shows the area of myocyte damage (H&E, 40 ×; Inset, 60 ×).

manner as any other allograft monitoring biopsy. The Working Formulation allows the terms "resolving" or "resolved" to be added to the report in parenthesis after the grade (Fig. 14–6).

Sampling Error

The occasional clinical experience of clear clinical rejection, occasionally with hemodynamic compromise, which improves with augmented "bolus" immunosuppression despite an initial biopsy of grade 0, 1A, 1B, or 2 raises the possibility of "sampling error" in the biopsy. This notion is reinforced by the occasional observation

of a subsequent biopsy about 3 days later which reveals clear 3A rejection or an autopsy which demonstrates severe acute rejection several days after a biopsy revealed no or low-grade rejection. Such "sampling errors," in which 3A or greater rejection is present but not identified in the biopsy sample, are estimated to occur in about 2–15% of actual rejection episodes.[236]

PITFALLS AND OTHER FINDINGS IN THE ENDOMYOCARDIAL BIOPSY

The common pitfalls in the interpretation of endomyocardial biopsies and important observations that gener-

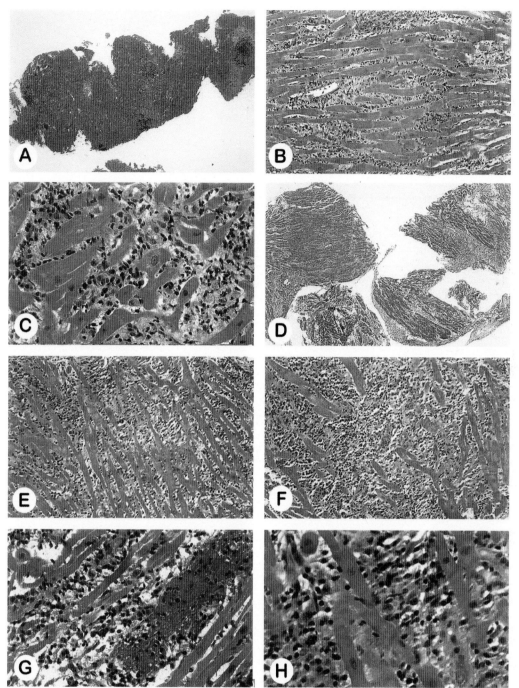

FIGURE **14–5.** Grade 3A, 3B, and 4 rejection. *A,* Low-power view of a biopsy piece showing grade 3A rejection. Several foci of mononuclear inflammatory infiltrate are present. Each focus measures > 300 μm. Vacuoles are noted in the focus located in the upper center region of the biopsy. The focus to the far right also shows scarring around it. Each focus in this piece individually fulfills the requirements of a grade 2 lesion, thus making it a grade 3A lesion (H&E, 4 ×). *B,* An example of diffuse extensive infiltrate of the myocardium in grade 3B rejection. Instead of making small nests of lymphocytes, the inflammatory infiltrate extends through the interstitial space, separating the myocytes and in some areas destroying the myocytes (H&E, 20 ×). *C,* Higher magnification of a similar focus showing myocyte damage and dropout. Notice the presence of an occasional polymorphonuclear leukocyte and some myocyte debris among the inflammatory cells (H&E, 40 ×). *D,* Low-power view of a biopsy sample showing that four out of four pieces have abundant inflammatory infiltration which markedly expands the interstitial space. If all the pieces look like the piece on the upper left side of the micrograph, it may be easy to make the diagnosis of grade 3B. However, the large infiltrate seen in the piece at the right upper corner of the field should prompt for further examination at higher magnification to rule out diagnostic features of grade 4 rejection (H&E, 4 ×). *E,* At higher magnification, there is no evidence of abundant neutrophils, eosinophils, hemorrhage, and/or vasculitis. Therefore, this particular field has only diagnostic features of grade 3B if seen as an extensive infiltrate in several pieces (H&E, 20 ×). *F,* Another example of grade 3B rejection, this field shows more extensive infiltrate with myocyte debris, some neutrophils but no hemorrhage present (H&E, 20 ×). *G,* Grade 4 rejection shows more abundant myocyte necrosis, pyknosis, a mixed infiltrate showing lymphocytes, macrophages, some neutrophils, and an area of interstitial hemorrhage (H&E, 40 ×). *H,* Another field of the same biopsy piece shows myocyte necrosis, and abundant mixed inflammatory infiltrate. Although no hemorrhage is present, some eosinophils are seen in this field (H&E, 40 ×).

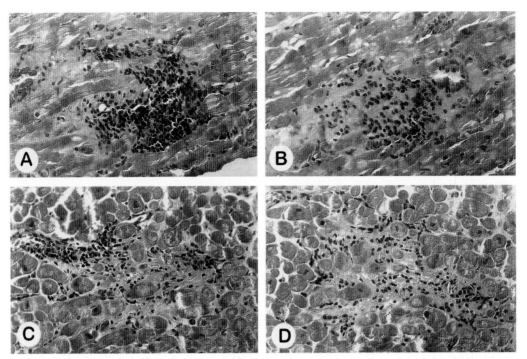

FIGURE **14-6.** Follow-up biopsies after a grade 3A rejection. *A,* This is a biopsy from a patient who had grade 3A rejection 1 week before this specimen was obtained. After therapy, the new biopsy shows one focus of grade 2 rejection in this field (H&E, 40 ×). *B,* The same focus was followed through serial sections and now illustrates an involuting focus of rejection. Although the mononuclear inflammatory cells are abundant, there is clear evidence of collagen deposition in the area of myocyte loss. (H&E, 40 ×). *C,* This field shows an area that at first glance suggests grade 1A rejection. However, note the slight disproportion between the widened interstitial space and the scant amount of inflammatory infiltrate. This is a clue that in fact there may have been a more abundant inflammatory infiltrate in this place before therapy. Note that the interstitial space between the myocytes in areas peripheral to the inflammatory focus is normal. This indicates that there is no edema in this biopsy to account for the widening of the interstitium (H&E, 40 ×). *D,* In subsequent sections, the same focus shows an area of myocyte dropout that is now replaced by loose connective tissue. Persistent lymphocytic infiltrate is out of proportion to the expanded interstitial space. Again, notice the absence of edema (H&E, 40 ×).

ally do not relate to allograft rejection are summarized in Table 14–2.

Procedural Artifacts

Artifacts produced by the sampling process can obscure the interpretation of the endomyocardial biopsy (Fig.

TABLE 14-2	Pitfalls and Other Findings in the Endomyocardial Biopsies

Procedural artifacts
 Contraction bands
 Bioptome distortion
 Pseudohemorrhage
 Telescoping
Sampling issues
 Previous biopsy site
 Adipose tissue
 Extracardiac tissue/perforation
 Valvular apparatus
 Inadequate tissue
Transplant-related conditions
 Ischemic injury
 Myocyte damage
 Quilty effect
 Opportunistic infections
 PTLD
 Dystrophic calcification
 Transmitted conditions

PTLD, posttransplant lymphoproliferative disease.

14–7). **Contraction bands** are a common artifact seen in transplant and nontransplant heart biopsies. This artifact may result from trauma to the myocardium induced when the bioptome cuts the tissue. It may also be induced by poor osmolarity of the medium in which the biopsy is placed before and during fixation, as well as the cool temperature of the medium (i.e., 4°C vs. 22°C). Because they are a common artifact, contraction bands should never be the only criterion used to make a diagnosis of myocyte necrosis or ischemic damage. **Bioptome distortion** represents mechanical distortion of the tissue due to manipulation. The bioptome itself can induce this artifact, especially if its cutters are not very sharp (in the case of reusable bioptomes). It can also be induced during processing of the tissue in the pathology laboratory. **Pseudohemorrhage** represents red blood cells that are embedded into the tissue by the pressure of the bioptome on the myocardium being sampled. This produces artifactual pools that mimic hemorrhage. They are usually not accompanied by inflammatory cells or pathologic changes in the myocytes, thus making the distinction between artifact and rejection fairly easy. **"Telescoping" or intussusception of small arteries** may occur when a small muscular artery is sampled by the bioptome. Just before the bioptome cutters actually cut the tissue, the small artery is stretched, and as soon as it is cut, it recoils into its own lumen. This can give the appearance of an occluded vessel or a small artery

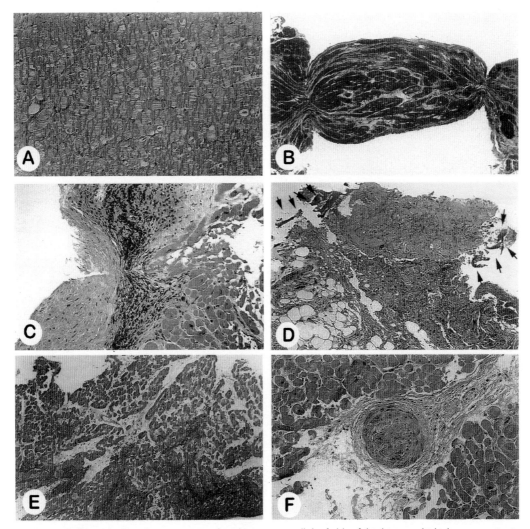

FIGURE **14–7.** Artifacts. *A,* Abundant contraction bands present in all the fields of this biopsy which shows no rejection. The myocyte nuclei show no evidence of pyknotic changes (H&E, 16 ×). *B,* This symmetric area of pinching artifact is probably due to a bioptome that ripped rather than cut the biopsy piece. Compare with the gross photograph in Figure 14–1*C.* A similar artifact can be induced by careless use of forceps while handling the biopsy in the pathology laboratory, but is usually not symmetric (Masson's trichrome, 20 ×). *C,* A crush artifact renders an inflammatory infiltrate uninterpretable (H&E, 20 ×). *D,* An area of perforation showing epicardial "gel foam" material (arrows) embedded in a mesh of organizing pericarditis (H&E, 20 ×). *E,* Pseudohemorrhage and artifactual separation of the myocyte fascicles that mimics edema are seen in this biopsy. Note the absence of rejection, neutrophilic infiltrates, or myocyte necrosis (H&E, 20 ×). *F,* Intussusception of a small artery. Note the slightly wavy birefringent internal elastic lamina separating the media from the intussuscepted and distorted arterial wall filling the lumen (H&E, 40 ×).

with vasculopathy. However, the elastic lamina is usually determinant in showing that in fact there is an intussusception of the artery.

Sampling Issues

Previous Biopsy Site

The average heart transplant recipient undergoes 15–20 cardiac biopsies during the first posttransplant year, of which up to 50%[59] or more[205] show evidence of a previous biopsy site. This high frequency is due to the tendency for the bioptome to follow the same path through the right ventricle. During the biopsy procedure using the jugular approach, the ridges of the atrial anastomotic site, the right ventricular trabeculations, and the moderator band all contribute to guide the tip of the bioptome

towards the same site in the interventricular septum. Gross examination at autopsy may show a patch of thickened endocardium measuring 1–2 cm in diameter in the mid-third of the right ventricular septum in patients who survived several months to years after the transplant. On light microscopy, the findings of this repetitive sampling of a small area of the septum vary with the interval between biopsies. These changes are illustrated in Figure 14–8 and may include hemorrhage in a recent biopsy site, granulation tissue with mononuclear inflammatory cells and myocyte disarray, and fibrous tissue.

Adipose Tissue: Perforation Versus Infiltration

Adipocytes are normal cellular components of the heart, mostly present in the epicardium. Microscopic foci of

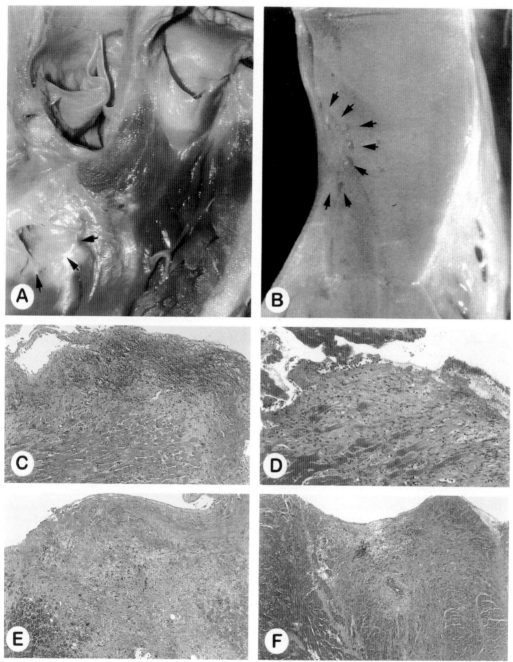

FIGURE **14–8.** Previous biopsy site. *A,* Outflow tract of the right ventricle. A focus of endocardial thickening (arrows) is present below the tricuspid valve. This is an area where many previous biopsies have led to scarring of the endocardium. The yellow discoloration is due to abundant hemosiderin-laden macrophages. *B,* Coronal view of the interventricular septum. There is a depression of the endocardial contour in the right ventricular side of the septum. The endocardium lining this area of depression is thickened and somewhat opalescent. The arrows show that the scar replaces several millimeters of myocardium representing scars from repeated biopsies. *C,* Light micrograph of an area of previous biopsy site. There is hemorrhage and fibrin deposition on the endocardial side of this specimen (top) (H&E, 16 ×). *D,* This previous biopsy site is composed mostly of granulation tissue, with the remnants of some necrotic myocytes indicating that it has had some time to begin healing (about 7 days). However, the surface of this biopsy (top of the picture) shows fibrin deposition and with entrapment of platelets and red blood cells. This indicates a very recent event. What in fact this biopsy represents is sampling of an area of a previous biopsy site. The fresh fibrin microthrombus indicates that this particular biopsy piece was not the first to be obtained in the current procedure. Very likely another piece(s) was (were) obtained a few minutes earlier, thus, the bioptome eroded the endocardium and triggered the formation of this microthrombus (H&E, 20 ×). *E,* This micrograph illustrates that in later stages granulation tissue appears with variable amounts of mononuclear inflammatory infiltrate and abundant hemosiderin-laden macrophages. This gives the yellow discoloration of the scar on gross examination such as the one shown in *A* (H&E, 10 ×). *F,* Further organization shows less inflammatory infiltrate and a different stage of maturation of the collagen deposition which is still somewhat loose and spongy in appearance (H&E, 10 ×).

Illustration continued on opposite page

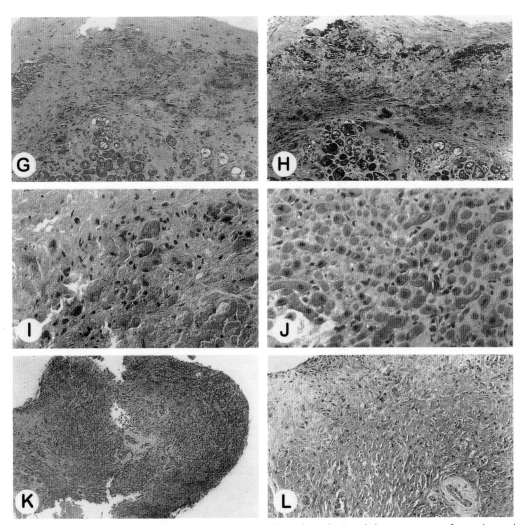

FIGURE **14–8.** *Continued. G,* Organizing scar which thickens the endocardium and shows presence of smooth muscle cells within the endocardium. Vacuolated cardiac myocytes as seen in the lower part of the picture are usually present beneath thick endocardial scars (H&E, 40 ×). *H,* This section shows the dense collagenous thickening of the endocardium seen in G. It confirms the presence of many spindly-looking smooth muscle cells within the thickened endocardium (red spindly cells) (Masson's trichrome, 40×). *I,* A tangential section of an area of previous biopsy site shows numerous enlarged myocytes and some endothelial cells with enlarged, hyperchromatic, bizarre-shaped nuclei. These nuclear changes in the myocytes and endothelial cells are reactive. The changes are common in areas of healing previous biopsy site scar and should not be confused with viral inclusions (H&E, 40 ×). *J,* Another artifact seen in areas of previous biopsy site is the entrapment of myocytes within the scar. When these myocytes do not undergo lethal injury, they survive and become embedded within the scar. This pattern of eosinophilic fibrous tissue surrounding individual myocytes can be readily differentiated from other types of connective tissue infiltrates such as amyloid (H&E, 40 ×). *K,* Low magnification of an area of previous biopsy site with heavy infiltration of lymphocyte forming a nest of Quilty-like effect. The myocytes subjacent to the scar show disarray (H&E, 10 ×). *L,* Higher magnification of such an area confirms the artifactual disarray of the myocytes. This is another relatively common artifact in areas of previous biopsy site. Note the normal arteriole in the bottom right part of the figure (H&E, 20 ×).

adipose tissue are usually present in the subendocardium and within the myocardium. These foci can be seen in all chambers but are more commonly found in the right ventricular wall (Fig. 14–9). Small foci of adipose tissue are more common in obese patients and patients taking steroid hormones. Thus, finding adipose tissue per se is not pathologic. An attempt should be made to define whether the adipose tissue seen in an endomyocardial biopsy is part of the ventricular wall, since it may also come from the epicardium. The pathologist must remember that although the aim of a right ventricular biopsy procedure is to obtain samples from the right side of the interventricular septum, the bioptome may actually sample the right ventricular free wall.

Therefore, when a focus of adipose tissue is found in an endomyocardial biopsy, the pathologist should make an effort to determine if it is subendocardial or subepicardial adipose tissue. This can sometimes be easily determined by looking for the presence of mesothelial cell lining, which indicates that the surface is actually epicardium. The presence of ganglion cells or nerves is suggestive of epicardial location (and therefore possible right ventricular perforation). The presence of adipose tissue in endomyocardial biopsies has been reported[33] and classified[17] in non-transplant patients. In transplant biopsies, there is also some tendency to see fat deposits in areas of previous biopsy or perhaps foci of healing ischemic damage. Whether the use of steroids for the treatment

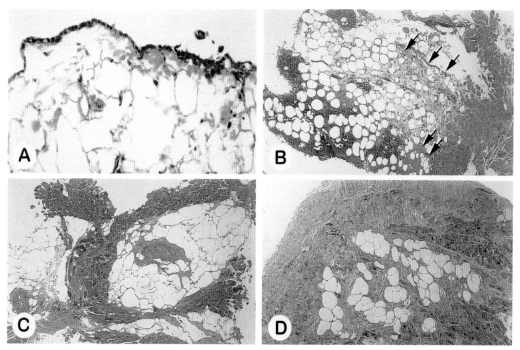

FIGURE **14–9.** Adipose tissue. *A,* Light micrograph of epicardial adipose tissue covered by a single layer of mesothelial cells from a nontransplant patient with dilated cardiomyopathy. The presence of mesothelium clearly indicates perforation of the right ventricular free wall (H&E, 40 ×). *B,* Adipose tissue with focal necrosis and pseudohemorrhage seen in an early posttransplant biopsy. Tamponade as a result of perforation is rare in posttransplant hearts because of the adhesive pericarditis that develops after surgery (H&E, 16 ×). *C,* Abundant adipose tissue infiltration of the myocardium without clear evidence of perforation (H&E, 16 ×). *D,* This biopsy shows adipose tissue subjacent to the endocardium which is thickened as a result of a previous biopsy (H&E, 16 ×).

of rejection increases the amount of adipose tissue in the endocardium is not known.

Valvular Apparatus

Fragments of **chordae tendineae and valvular tissue** are occasionally seen as part of the biopsy specimen. They should be described and processed along with the biopsy. The clinical significance with regard to tricuspid dysfunction secondary to chordal rupture is varied.[213, 235]

Inadequate Tissue

Appropriate histologic examination of four pieces obtained from endomyocardial biopsy yields a sensitivity as high as 95–98% for the diagnosis of acute rejection.[212] The sensitivity decreases greatly with three or fewer pieces to examine. Some cardiac pathologists have recommended that the term "inadequate biopsy" should be used when the specimen consists of less than four pieces[14] or when the number of pieces examined under the microscope is four, but the myocardium present in one or more of these pieces is less than 50% of the piece. The inadequate pieces usually consist of mostly or only endocardium, thrombus, or granulation tissue from a previous biopsy site. It should be recognized, however, that in some instances valuable information (such as rejection) is present in the other (adequate) biopsy pieces, and although a histologic diagnosis of rejection cannot be rendered, the findings should be documented in the report as part of the histologic description.

Transplant-Related Conditions

A number of specific histologic findings are unique to heart transplant patients and must be distinguished from (or correlated with) acute rejection (Table 14–3).

Ischemic Injury

Particularly early after transplantation, areas of acute ischemic damage can be identified by subendocardial foci of myocytes showing myocytolysis or coagulation necrosis with variable amounts of polymorphonuclear inflammatory infiltrates (Fig. 14–10). These areas are usually conspicuous, especially when stained with Masson's trichrome. The finding of such foci may persist for several weeks in a given patient. It has been postulated that this persistence is due to a delayed inflammatory response secondary to immunosuppression.[61] In the healing stages, these ischemic foci usually show a few lymphocytes, hemosiderin-laden macrophages, a somewhat loose connective tissue scar, and scant granulation

TABLE 14-3	Entities that May Mimic the Histologic Features of Rejection

- Ischemic injury
- Quilty effect
- Infection
- Posttransplant lymphoproliferative disorder
- Previous biopsy site

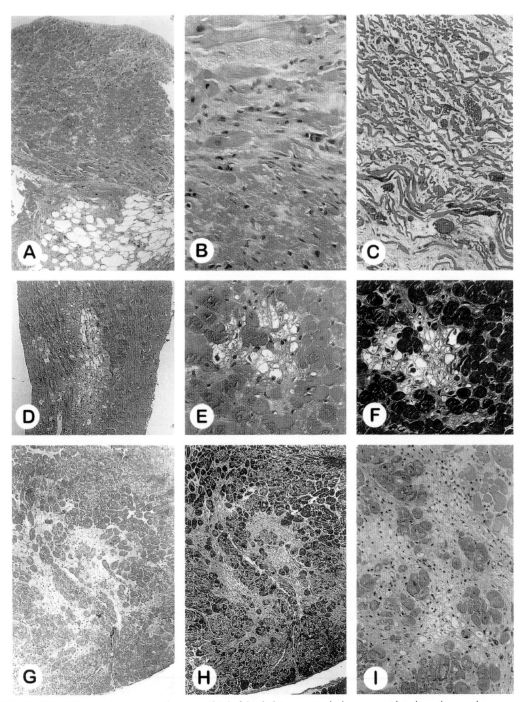

FIGURE **14-10.** Ischemic changes. *A,* The upper third of this light micrograph shows normal endocardium and myocytes. The middle third shows myocytes with coagulation necrosis evidenced by hypereosinophilia and loss of nuclei. The bottom third shows an area of adipose tissue infiltration (H&E, 10 ×). *B,* Higher magnification of an area similar to *A* shows normal myocytes with striations and normal nuclei in the upper half of the biopsy. The bottom half shows myocytes that are hypereosinophilic and fragmented, with loss of striations and nuclei. The only nuclei seen are those of interstitial cells (i.e., capillary endothelial cells, pericytes, and fibroblasts) (H&E, 40 ×). *C,* Focus of coagulation necrosis. The myocytes show hypereosinophilia, loss of striations, and loss of nuclei. There is interstitial edema which exaggerates the thin appearance of the myocytes. Some myocytes show calcification of the mitochondria which shows as dark blue granular material that fills the myocyte sarcoplasm (one in the center of field, several others towards the lower third). Note the absence of inflammatory infiltrate (H&E, 40 ×). *D,* Low magnification of an ischemic focus. The area of myocyte dropout does not show any type of inflammatory response. The neutrophils have disappeared and there is the beginning of deposition of new collagen (H&E, 10 ×). *E,* A similar focus as seen in *E* shows myocyte dropout with early loose collagen deposition. There are no inflammatory cells (H&E, 40 ×). *F,* The trichrome stain of an adjacent section confirms the presence of a delicate collagen network (blue material) in the area of myocyte dropout (Masson's trichrome, 40 ×). *G,* A larger area of ischemic damage showing a further stage of healing with an increase in the density of the collagen network. There are no inflammatory cells except for hemosiderin-laden macrophages and fibroblasts (H&E, 16 ×). *H,* The trichrome stain confirms the extent of the scar being formed (Masson's trichrome, 16 ×). *I,* At higher magnification it is evident that there are many hemosiderin-laden macrophages and fibroblasts within the organizing scar. Some myocytes show vacuolation. Note the absence of neutrophils or lymphocytes (H&E, 40 ×).

tissue. Early perioperative necrosis may be due to events that affect the donor such as catecholamine discharge, pressor therapy given during acute care, severe donor trauma, reimplantation (reperfusion) damage, or early postoperative damage.[61]

During allograft monitoring, the Working Formulation makes a distinction between ischemic changes commonly seen up to the third week after transplant representing perioperative injury and late ischemic changes that occur after 3 or more months. Morphologically, there is clear evidence of myocyte necrosis, usually coagulative type, with hypereosinophilic myocytes and pyknotic nuclei. In hearts receiving high-dose catecholamines, there may be multiple focal lesions with damaged myocytes surrounded by inflammatory cells, including neutrophils. Myocyte necrosis is usually out of proportion to the inflammatory infiltrate, in contrast to acute rejection, in which the cellular infiltrate predominates.

Healing may be delayed due to immunosuppression.[61] Although this type of necrosis can be clinically silent, these changes, if severe, can compromise graft function. Another possible implication in hearts that had damage during the peritransplant period is the development of interstitial fibrosis.[172]

Myocyte Damage

The single most difficult issue in the interpretation of endomyocardial biopsies from human allografts has been the inability to obtain consensus among experienced cardiovascular pathologists about the definition of myocyte damage. The morphologic spectrum of myocyte damage that can be seen in the myocardium on light microscopic examination varies from vacuolization, hydropic change, or perinuclear halos[104, 105] at the somewhat milder side of the spectrum to coagulation

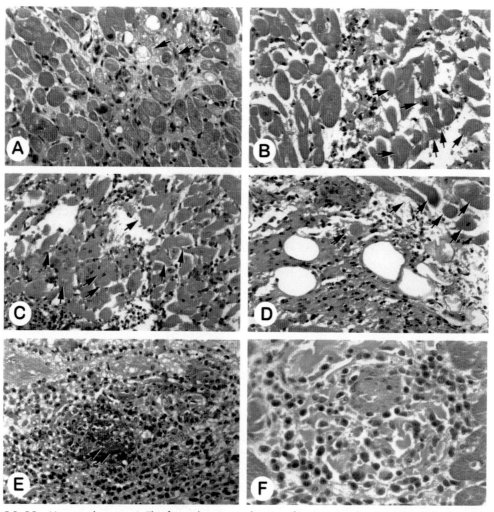

FIGURE **14-11.** Myocyte damage. *A,* This focus shows vacuolization of myocytes with perinuclear halos (arrows). There is no evidence of frank necrosis or pyknotic changes (H&E, 40 ×). *B,* This focus shows several necrotic (hypereosinophilic) myocytes (arrows). Some of them have lost their nuclei and show only lipofuscin pigment in the area of the sarcoplasm where the nucleus used to be (H&E, 40 ×). *C,* Another focus of myocyte necrosis showing multiple necrotic myocytes without nuclei (arrows) and fragment of myocytes scattered between the inflammatory infiltrate (H&E, 40 ×). *D,* This focus shows myocyte necrosis (arrows) as well as infiltration of the adipose tissue by inflammatory cells (H&E, 40 ×). *E,* Severe necrosis, with myocyte and inflammatory cell debris constitute most of the cells in the center of this field. The myocyte debris are marked by the arrows. There are also some eosinophils seen within the inflammatory infiltrate (H&E, 40 ×). *F,* This focus shows an inflammatory infiltrate composed of lymphocytes and abundant eosinophils. There are some amorphous eosinophilic structures in the center of the field which represent dense bundles of collagen. A focus like this should not be confused with myocyte damage (H&E, 40 ×).

necrosis, myocytolysis, and nuclear pyknosis at the worst end of the spectrum (Fig. 14–11). Thus, the term "damage" is rather ambiguous. Unless there is clear coagulative necrosis or fragmentation of the sarcoplasm or typical nuclear changes such as pyknosis in the myocytes, the identification of "damaged" cells in hematoxylin and eosin–stained paraffin sections is a subjective matter. By light microscopy, some of the myocyte changes that represent sublethal (and reversible) damage are indistinguishable from actual early necrosis.[148, 160] Ultrastructural studies can clearly distinguish myocyte degeneration from necrosis.[160] Damage to endothelial cells, basal lamina, or other components is also easily recognized.[81] Myocyte necrosis as defined by ultrastructural criteria is common in humoral rejection, whereas myocyte degeneration (with the potential for recovery) is more common in cellular rejection.[91]

Quilty Effect or Endocardial Lymphocytic Infiltrates

Endocardial lymphocytic infiltrates[216] also known as "Quilty effect"[101] or "lymphoma-like lesions,"[105] are collections of T- and B-cells with histiocytes[125, 145] seen in the endocardium of transplanted hearts (Fig. 14–12). Controversy exists whether these lymphocytic infiltrates are benign or actually predict subsequent rejection. Plasma cells are present in about half of these infiltrates. Occasional eosinophils and neutrophils may be seen.[145] Capillaries with red blood cells and sometimes prominent endothelial cells may be seen within the infiltrate. They vary in size from 0.01–1.9 mm².[125] Several hypotheses have been proposed to explain the pathogenesis of these infiltrates, including an effect of cyclosporine,[60, 125, 216] a concomitant infection with

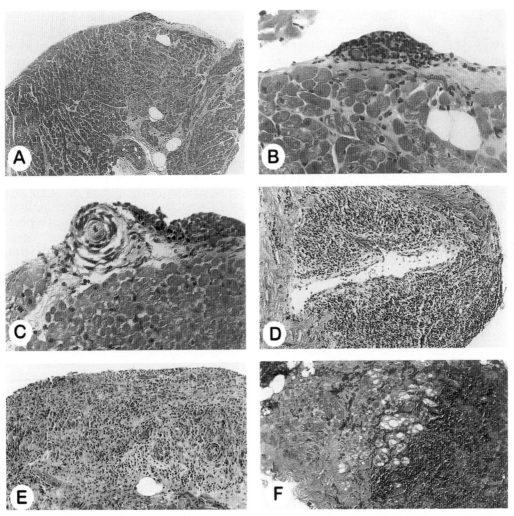

FIGURE **14–12.** Endocardial lymphocytic infiltrates (ELI) (Quilty effect). *A,* Light micrograph of a biopsy piece showing an endocardial lymphocytic infiltrate. Note the absence of rejection infiltrates in the myocardium (H&E, 10 ×). *B,* A close up of the ELI shown in *A* reveals layers of lymphocytes within the endocardium proper. There is no extension into the subjacent myocardium. There is a small vessel filled with red blood cells noted to the left of the ELI. Small networks of open capillaries are a common feature in larger ELI's (H&E, 40 ×). *C,* A focus of ELI shows layering within the endocardium. There is a brisk stop at the myocardial border (H&E, 40 ×). *D,* Exuberant ELI producing marked thickening of the endocardium, but no infiltration into the myocardium (Quilty type A) (H&E, 20 ×). *E,* Another focus of ELI producing marked thickening of the endocardium. There are numerous vessels (capillaries and dilated venules) present within the infiltrate. The ELI does not infiltrate the myocardium (H&E, 20 ×). *F,* Invasive ELI (Quilty type B) shows that the lymphocytic infiltrate extends into the myocardium (H&E, 20 ×).

Epstein-Barr virus (EBV),[161] and early rejection. However, one striking observation is that Quilty effect does not occur in the hearts of patients who are taking cyclosporin A for noncardiac organ transplantation (i.e., liver, kidney)[9]; it seems to be a phenomenon that only occurs in the endocardium of cardiac allografts.

The size of these infiltrates varies greatly. Two morphologic patterns are recognized, type A and type B. Type A infiltrates are confined to the endocardium. The term type B, also known as "invasive Quilty," is used if the Quilty effect encroaches into the myocardium from the endocardium.[14] The myocardial interstitium can appear "expanded" or in other instances individual myocytes are surrounded by the infiltrate. It has been suggested that the number of Quilty effect infiltrates is somewhat higher in patients treated with OKT3 antibody prophylaxis.[105] The ultrastructure of Quilty type infiltrates has been described.[125, 126]

The relationship, if any, between Quilty infiltrates and **acute allograft rejection** remains controversial. Several studies have found no correlation between Quilty effects and the presence of rejection on endomyocardial biopsy.[216] However, Costanzo and colleagues studied the presence of Quilty effect in over 5,000 endomyocardial biopsies and found that histologic evidence of rejection was more common in biopsies with Quilty effect than in those without (44% vs. 24%, $p < .001$). Furthermore, rejection on the subsequent biopsy was more common when a biopsy contained Quilty lesions than when none were present (37% vs. 24%, $p < .01$).[41]

The possibility also exists that Quilty type B infiltrates may be confused histologically with grade 2 (focal moderate) rejection[46] (Fig. 14–13). This indeed is a problem for pathologists because of the obvious implications for therapy. Quilty type B infiltrates can extend deep into the subjacent myocardium. The **hallmark** of the Quilty type B infiltrate is **continuity** of the lymphocytic infiltrate within the endocardium and underlying myocardium, in contrast to a grade 2 infiltrate within the myocardium (which may be easily confused with a Quilty B infiltrate).[55] One may imagine how a tangential section through the deeper (myocardial) end of a biopsy may show inflammatory infiltrates that look like rejection if only a few levels of section are examined. However, if deeper sections are made or, better yet, if all the biopsy tissue is examined, it would soon become evident that in fact the inflammatory infiltrate in the myocardium is connected to a Quilty type lesion in the endocardium, thus representing a Quilty type B infiltrate.

Differentiation between these two infiltrates is facilitated by examining all the tissues available. A possible focus of grade 2 rejection can easily be tracked down through all the subsequent levels of section of that particular biopsy piece to determine whether a focus of mononuclear inflammation in question is part of an endocardial Quilty type B infiltrate that has penetrated deep into the myocardium or is indeed a focus of grade 2 rejection. Areas of the endocardium that contain dilated capillaries may be a site for "homing" of lymphocytes before they actually infiltrate the endocardium.

In a recent report including 217 adults and 22 children studied during a period of 10 years, 49% of adults and 68% of children demonstrated these infiltrates.[101] The authors found no correlation between the endocardial infiltrates and (1) grade of rejection, (2) subsequent development of vasculopathy (vascular chronic rejection), (3) development of lymphoma, or (4) viral infections (cytomegalovirus [CMV] or EBV). There was no difference whether the infiltrate was type A or type B.[101]

Opportunistic Infections

It is a well known fact that the chronic therapy with immunosuppressive drugs to control rejection predisposes these patients to a large number of opportunistic infections including viruses, bacteria, fungi, and protozoa. Most of these infectious processes are systemic, and some may infect the heart (Fig. 14–14). Some of the organisms identified in heart allografts include **viruses** (CMV, enteroviruses, EBV), **bacteria** (including norcardia and mycobacteria),[136, 169, 170] **fungi** (aspergillus,[95] candida, mucor,[215] pneumocystis,[35] and others), and **protozoa**[42, 90, 228] (toxoplasmosis, leishmania,[68] and reactivation of Chagas' disease).[137] In the pediatric population, the pathogens reported include viruses (CMV, herpes simplex, varicella-zoster, respiratory viruses, and EBV), bacteria (mycobacteria, gram-positive and gram-negative), toxoplasmosis, and pneumocystis.[23, 44] Although the above infections have been reported, the **most commonly recognized infections on endomyocardial biopsy are CMV and *Toxoplasma gondii*.**

It should be noted that the identification of microorganisms in an endomyocardial biopsy is difficult and should never be the only method to identify infection. When examining a biopsy, always look for hints of infection such as unusual inflammatory infiltrates, with granulocytes, plasma cells, and/or macrophages in a focus of inflammation without overt myocyte necrosis or dropout. Areas like these may harbor intracellular parasites (such as *Toxoplasma*) or fungal organisms which can be elusive on hematoxylin and eosin stain. Special stains for microorganisms should then be performed. One should also look for viral inclusions in the nuclei of endothelial cells, smooth muscle cells, or miscellaneous perivascular cells. Inclusions seen by light microscopy within the cardiac myocytes are rare.

Posttransplant Lymphoproliferative Disorder

Rarely, a lymphoproliferative infiltrate may be identified as posttransplant lymphoproliferative disorder (PTLD) on endomyocardial biopsy. The distinction between this infiltrate and the lymphocytic infiltrate of acute rejection may be subtle. The presence of PTLD is suggested by the presence of atypical lymphocytes, frequent mitoses, and lymphoplasmacytoid mononuclear infiltrates.

Dystrophic Calcification

There have been reports of various forms of calcification in the heart after transplantation. In some patients, radiographic evidence of dystrophic calcification has been shown in the native atria and rarely in biopsy tissue[34]

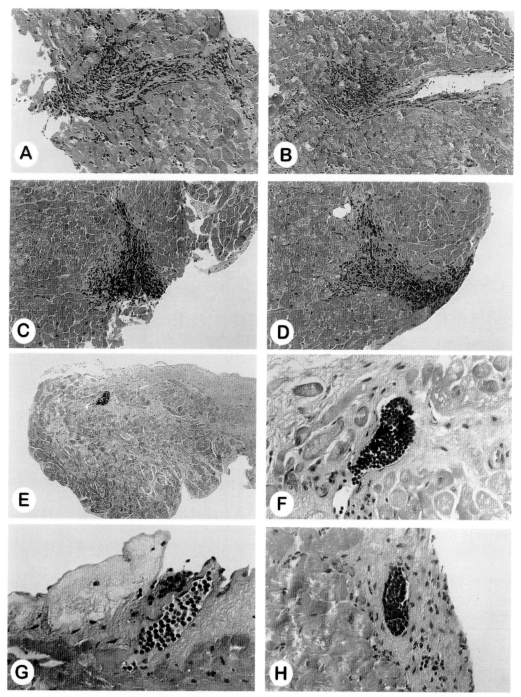

FIGURE **14-13.** Grade 2 vs. Quilty effect. *A,* This section shows a large perivascular mononuclear inflammatory infiltrate which expands the interstitial space (upper portion of the field). If evaluated in this section only, this focus of inflammation could be called a grade 2 lesion (H&E, 20 ×). *B,* When serial sections at many levels are examined this focus is shown to surround a small venule that opens into the ventricular cavity (H&E, 20 ×). *C,* Further sections show this focus of inflammation becoming more dense (H&E, 20 ×). *D,* Clear association with an area of ELI is shown in this micrograph (H&E, 20 ×). *E,* Light micrograph of a focus mononuclear cell near the endocardium (H&E, 10 ×). *F,* Higher magnification shows that these lymphocytes are all contained within the lumen of a venule. This may represent homing of the lymphocytes before they actually penetrate the endocardial connective tissue (H&E, 40 ×). *G,* Another example from a different patient showing a similar event (H&E, 40 ×). *H,* In this micrograph there is a cluster of lymphocytes within the venule, whereas other lymphocytes have already migrated into the endocardial stroma (H&E, 40 ×).

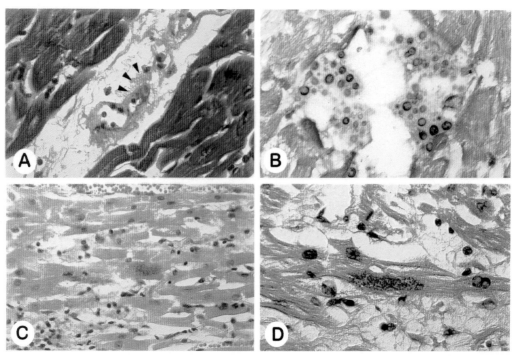

FIGURE **14–14.** Opportunistic infections. *A*, Light micrograph showing a cytomegalovirus-induced nuclear inclusion in an endothelial cell (arrows) (H&E, 40 ×). *B*, Collection of *Cryptococcus* species organisms are seen in the myocardium (mucicarmine stain, 40 ×). *C, Toxoplasma* trophozoites are seen within a cardiac myocyte (H&E, 40 ×). *D*, Higher magnification of another myocyte parasitized by *Toxoplasma* (H&E, 40 ×).

(Fig. 14–15). On light microscopy, dystrophic calcification of the mitochondria is easily recognized as dark blue granular material within the myocytes. These granules are 1–2.5 μm in diameter. The granules may be seen in perinuclear location and also following the pattern of the sarcomeres. When abundant, they follow the contour of the whole myocyte. In some cases, a relationship between calcification of the mitochondria and cyclosporine therapy has been suggested.[214] Some conditions that have been associated are sepsis, temporary uremia, hypomagnesemia, steroid therapy, and alcoholism.[34]

Transmitted Conditions

Several conditions which may be present in the recipient at the time of transplantation can be transmitted to the donor heart. Amyloidosis, sarcoidosis, and giant-cell myocarditis may be mistaken for idiopathic cardiomyopathy and can be transmitted to the transplanted heart.

Immunofluorescence

If immunofluorescence is performed, the results should be included in the biopsy report. The Working Formulation even suggests that when available, immunofluorescence should be done on every biopsy for the first 6 weeks after the transplant.[14] In most institutions, however, immunofluorescence is performed only when the clinical suspicion of humoral rejection is high and the biopsy result shows grade 0 or 1A rejection that is unchanged when compared to the previous biopsy. The panel of antibodies typically detects fibrinogen, IgG, IgM, IgA, Clq, and C3. Other antibodies for surface mol-

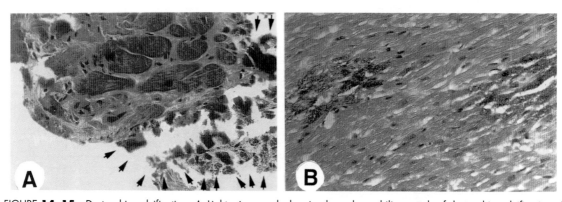

FIGURE **14–15.** Dystrophic calcification. *A*, Light micrograph showing large basophilic crystals of dystrophic calcification of the endocardium (arrows) (H&E, 40 ×). *B*, Small basophilic intracellular granules corresponding to calcified mitochondria are seen in two separate groups of myocytes (H&E, 20 ×).

ecules have been reported but are not widely recommended. Immunofluorescence studies are described in more detail in the section Microvascular ("Humoral") Rejection, below.

Lymphocyte Subtypes and Other Immunohistochemical Markers

It remains contentious whether detection of specific **lymphocyte subtypes** (CD4, CD8) in cardiac biopsy tissue correlates with the grade of rejection.[89] The discrepancy in these studies may relate to the fact that the immune response to the allograft is a continuous process in flux that is usually dissected in small "time lapsed" views for pathologic study. Some support to this notion is provided by the fact that if phenotypes of lymphocytes are further subclassified on the basis of the presence of naive cells (CD45RA) and memory cells (CD45RO), naive cells are more abundant in biopsy tissue during mild as opposed to moderate rejection.[97] B-cells are also found in allografts and do not correlate with the degree of rejection.[200] Other immunohistochemical markers (see Box) have been examined, but they have not been predictive enough to guide therapy.

MICROVASCULAR ("HUMORAL") REJECTION

Basic Description

Humoral rejection in cardiac transplantation refers to a rejection process resulting from immunoglobulin (antibody) directed against donor antigens located on the endothelial surface of the allograft coronary microvasculature.[22,222] Immunoglobin and complement are localized in the microvasculature of the transplanted heart, involving arterioles, capillaries, and venules. The resulting inflammatory process invades the vessel wall with neutrophils and macrophages, producing arteritis and venulitis which may be seen on endomyocardial biopsy. Complement and other inflammatory mediators induce endothelial cell swelling and interstitial edema. Antithrombin III (ATT), a marker of the natural anticoagulant pathway, is reduced or absent in the presence of microvascular damage.[51] Tissue plasminogen activator (t-PA) (a stimulus for the fibrinolytic pathway and normally present in smooth muscle cells of myocardial arterioles) is also lost in allograft microvascular injury. Plasminogen activator inhibitor-1 (PAI-1) has been identified in complexes with t-PA within the microvasculature of allografts.[51,52,130] Interstitial fibrin deposition and microvascular thrombosis occur when the process is advanced. Macrophages are likely a critical component of this process, with their known ability to alter the normal fibrinolytic process. Macrophages from atherosclerotic lesions are able to make PAI-1 and stimulate endothelial cells to generate PAI-1, possibly mediated through the secretion of IL-1 and tumor necrosis factor-α (TNF-α).[220]

Thus, the hallmarks of microvascular rejection are **endothelial cell activation, increased vascular permeability,** and in severe forms **microvascular thrombosis** and subsequent myocardial cell degeneration. The evidence

Other Immunohistochemical Markers

Many molecules have been detected by immunohistochemistry in human endomyocardial biopsy tissue. HLA class I and II antigens have been studied in the heart and are found to be expressed readily in any inflammatory condition ranging from myocarditis to rejection. Unlike the good correlation found between serologic HLA mismatches between donor and recipient and the subsequent development of rejection,[210] detection of these molecules in tissue sections does not have a predictive value. Detection of interleukin (IL)-2 expression in cardiac tissue has been reported in cases of severe rejection.[194] Endothelial antigens such as vascular endothelial growth factor (VEGF) are expressed in the microcirculation of the graft, and are confined to areas where there is fibrin deposition, macrophages, and neutrophils.[221] VEGF may act to modulate the phenotype of microvascular endothelial cells during episodes of thrombosis and endothelial damage that accompany rejection.[221] The localization of several cytokines in heart biopsies has been examined during rejection.[226] Expression of cytokines IL-2, IL-3, and IL-10 can be detected in biopsies with high-grade rejection, whereas few cells express IL-6, IL-8, and interferon (IFN)-γ. In biopsies with lower grades of rejection, a weaker expression of these cytokines can be observed. Expression of IL-12 is detectable in most biopsies, and IL-4 is rarely detected. IL-3, IL-6, IL-10, and IL-12 can be detected both in lymphocytes and macrophages. Among the adhesion molecules, expression of intracellular adhesion molecule-1 (ICAM-1)[46,177,194,221,226] and E-selectin[25,53,218] seems to correlate with up-coming rejection, whereas VCAM-1[7,163] seems to be a somewhat better marker to evaluate the effect of therapy of an acute episode of rejection.[25] It is speculated that alloantibodies may enhance cellular rejection by promoting the interaction between alloreactive T-cells and the allograft endothelium.[93]

implicating antigen-antibody complexes as the definite cause of this type of rejection is lacking, but the pathogenic vascular inflammatory processes associated with microvascular rejection, including complement activation, cytokine release, chemotaxis and activation of neutrophils and macrophages, and microvascular thrombosis are very similar to the morphologic changes observed with humorally mediated rejection documented by immunofluorescence studies.[1,32,167,173]

There is undoubtedly a spectrum of acute cellular rejection (see previous section) and microvascular (humoral) rejection as described here. The endothelium plays a critical role in both processes, since expression of adhesion molecules, certain cytokines, ATT, and PAI-1 is limited to microvascular endothelium. Endothelial cells stimulated by IFN-γ can induce T-lymphocyte proliferation without macrophages.[93] In the presence of vascular rejection with vasculitis, there is also up-regulation (increased expression) of endothelial MHC class II antigens.[28,80] The mixture of cellular and vascular (humoral) rejection occurring simultaneously after cardiac transplantation has been well documented by Hammond[79] and others.[80, 82, 83]

The reported frequency of humoral rejection has been reported as high as 40% or more in some institutions,[18, 82, 140] but most institutions rarely report evidence of humoral rejection on biopsy.

Although more common early after transplantation, particularly in the presence of a positive donor-specific crossmatch or a sensitized recipient with preformed anti-HLA antibodies, humoral rejection can also occur later after transplantation. Its presence is suspected when rejection with hemodynamic compromise occurs in the setting of a low endomyocardial biopsy score (0–2). Although the exact mechanisms of graft dysfunction during humoral rejection remain speculative, antibody-mediated arteritis may induce vasospasm and possibly microvasular thrombosis. The term "humoral rejection" should not be confused with the term "chronic rejection," which refers to allograft vasculopathy (see Chapter 17).

Pathology

Humoral rejection affects most notably the components of the capillary network of the heart[82] and includes the pathological findings of prominent endothelial cell swelling and/or vasculitis on light microscopy (Table 14–4) and the identification of immunoglobulin (IgM or IgG) and complement deposition by immunofluorescence.[82, 106] A recent clinicopathologic study expands the definition of humoral rejection by adding hemorrhage and neutrophilic infiltrates to the spectrum.[140] The **minimal criteria** to diagnose humoral rejection include capillary endothelial cell swelling and any immunoglobulin and complement staining in the capillaries. However, a surprising and important finding is that most swollen cells in capillaries are macrophages when stained with appropriate cell markers. On light microscopic exam, the capillary endothelial cells are thicker and plumper than usual and their nuclei may be hyperchromatic. Sometimes, damage to the endothelium of small arterioles can also be documented. Other morphologic findings are inconsistent and nonspecific. Interstitial edema has been described, but the assessment of edema in endomyocardial biopsy specimens can be inaccurate, since slight variability in handling, processing, and fixation conditions may result in prominent changes that mimic edema. Furthermore, the assessment of humoral rejection usually includes immunofluorescence, which in turn requires frozen tissue. Even under the best circumstances, freezing can create artifacts that mimic edema, making accurate interpretation difficult. Thus,

TABLE 14-4	Signs of Microvascular (Humoral) Rejection on Endomyocardial Biopsy

- Endothelial cell swelling
- Endothelial cell necrosis
- Inflammatory infiltrates in the walls of microvessels (vasculitis)
- Microvascular thrombosis
- Interstitial edema
- Interstitial hemorrhage

TABLE 14-5	Humoral Rejection

GRADE	HISTOLOGIC CRITERIA
Mild vascular rejection	LM: Endothelial cell activation, edema, hemorrhage
	IMF: Immunoglobulin, complement deposition within vessels ± interstitial fibrin
Moderate vascular rejection	LM: Endothelial cell activation, edema, hemorrhage ± vasculitis
	IMF: Immunoglobulin, complement deposition within vessels, abundant interstitial fibrin
Severe vascular rejection	LM: Extensive infiltrates of lymphocytes, plasma cells, neutrophils with myocyte necrosis, edema, hemorrhage
	IMF: Immunoglobulin, complement deposition within vessels; interstitial leakage of immunoglobulin, complement, and fibrin

LM, light microscopy; IMF, immunofluorescence.
Adapted from Olsen SL, Yowell RL, Ensley D, Bristow MR, OConnell JB, Renlund DG: Vascular rejection in heart transplantation: clinical correlation treatment options, and future considerations. J Heart Lung Transplant 1993;12:S135–S142.

evaluation of edema in small biopsy pieces is unreliable and should be avoided in frozen tissue.

The Working Formulation makes brief mention that an entry should be made to indicate if there is humoral rejection, and on this category the following items should be recorded; "positive immunofluorescence, vasculitis or severe edema in the absence of cellular infiltrate."[14] However, it does not indicate how many pieces of endomyocardium should be examined in this manner, or whether both the light microscopic and immunofluorescence findings must be present. A grading system for humoral rejection has been suggested by Olsen and colleagues (Table 14–5).[166]

Immunofluorescence Studies

Perhaps the most common way to evaluate humoral rejection is the use of immunofluorescence to identify fibrinogen, IgG, IgM, and complement components C1q and C3 in frozen sections.[82] Deposits of IgM, IgG, or complement deposition in the microvasculature[140] and/or myocytes[146, 200] is indicative of humoral rejection (Fig. 14–16). In the pediatric population, the findings of humoral rejection have been documented to occur concomitantly with cellular rejection and persist after treatment.[242] It should be noted that while immunofluorescence may be clinically useful, immunohistochemistry in paraffin-embedded tissue for the detection of humoral rejection markers (e.g., IgG, IgM) is not reliable, since the fixation process may absorb many serum proteins into the tissue and give a high false-positive rate.[143]

The value of immunofluorescence remains controversial. First, interpretation of positive results varies among different observers.[18, 82, 140] Second, some reports show a greater incidence of positive immunofluorescence in controls (63%) than in transplanted patients.[18] Third, the interpretation and methods of examination in studies of humoral rejection have not been standardized. For

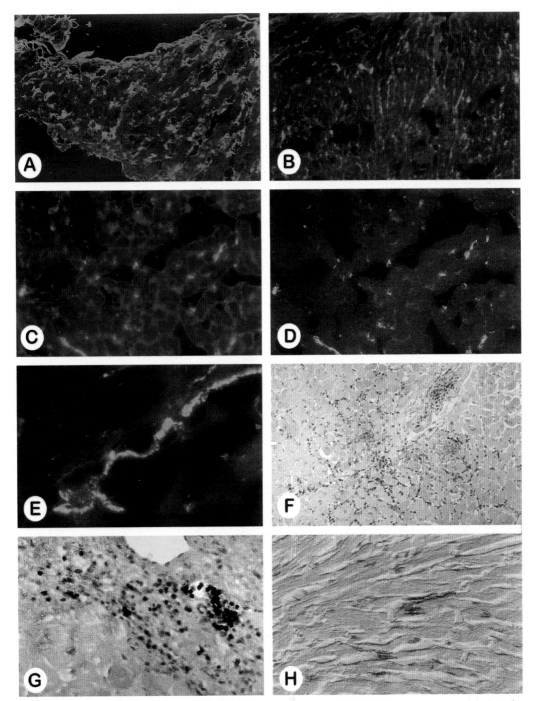

FIGURE **14–16.** Immunohistochemical staining of endomyocardial biopsies. *A,* Indirect immunofluorescence labeling of myocardium with antifibrinogen antibodies. There is deposition of fibrinogen around the myocytes (green fluorescence) and in the endocardium. These deposits are seen in every biopsy and serve as positive internal control. Secondary antibody is labeled with fluorescein isothiocyanate (FITC, 61 ×). *B,* Indirect immunofluorescence of myocardium labeled with anti-IgG antibodies. Note the linear pattern of deposits around the contours of the myocytes but not in the lumina of venules and endocardial spaces (black spaces). Secondary antibody is labeled with FITC (10 ×). *C,* Indirect immunofluorescence of a myocardial biopsy labeled with anti-C1q antibody. The individual capillaries are labeled but not the myocytes. Secondary antibody is labeled with FITC (40 ×). *D,* Same field as *C* analyzed after staining with Evans blue. This technique provides better contrast than FITC-labeled secondary antibody alone by staining the myocyte sarcoplasm which then fluoresces in red (40 ×). *E,* Indirect immunofluorescence staining of a small venule with anti-factor VIII antibody. Note the strong stain of the venule and the small capillaries present in this section parallel to the long axis of a fascicle of myocytes (60 ×). *F,* Immunoperoxidase stain of T-lymphocytes in an endomyocardial biopsy with grade 1B rejection (16 ×). *G,* Immunoperoxidase stain of B-lymphocytes in a focus of Quilty effect inflammatory infiltrate (40 ×). *H,* Immunoperoxidase stain of dendritic cells in the myocardium. Note the long processes extending in between the myocytes (40 ×).

example, the Working Formulation does not specify how many of the biopsy pieces should be examined in this manner, and it does not clearly define the methods and the interpretation criteria in the way it does for light microscopic histologic examination.

Clinical Correlates with Humoral Rejection

In some studies, humoral rejection correlates well with the presence of anti-HLA antibodies in serum,[31, 186] perhaps indicating that a more reliable way to diagnose humoral rejection could be the combined use of immunofluorescence and serologic measurement of anti-HLA antibodies, and that one test alone may not be sufficient to make this diagnosis. In one study, serum specimens were obtained an average of 1.8 days before or after the cardiac biopsy and analyzed for anti-HLA antibodies.[31] Done in this manner, there was good correlation between the presence of these antibodies and the finding of linear deposits of immunoglobulins or complement components in biopsies.

Humoral rejection is usually suspected clinically when there is evidence of suboptimal graft function and the endomyocardial biopsy shows either no evidence of cellular rejection (i.e., grade 0) or mild rejection (grade 1 or 2) (see later section). This combination of findings may prompt the transplant physicians to request the performance of immunofluorescence in a given specimen.

HYPERACUTE REJECTION

Hyperacute rejection consists of a violent lethal immune attack on the graft which is triggered by preformed antibodies and occurs very quickly after graft implantation, usually within minutes to hours. The preformed antibodies are usually directed against epitopes of the HLA system of the donor heart which usually can be detected by a prospective cytotoxic crossmatch (see Chapter 7) or the ABO system (in the event of inadvertent transplantation across a major blood group incompatibility). Rarely, hyperacute rejection may result from anti-endothelial antibodies.[11] The result is essentially always loss of the graft. An essential feature is rapid activation of the complement cascade producing severe damage to the endothelial cells, platelet activation, initiation of the clotting cascade, and widespread microvascular thrombosis. The morphologic findings include swelling of the endothelial cells, microthrombosis, extravasation of red blood cells, massive interstitial hemorrhage, interstitial edema, and subsequently polymorphonuclear inflammatory infiltrates followed by tissue necrosis. These changes occur focally but rapidly spread through the organ. On gross exam, the changes may be inconspicuous or may show hemorrhages or the combination of pallor and hemorrhages. Immunohistochemical studies may show deposits of IgM, IgG, and complement in the vessel walls as well as interstitial fibrin.[189] Unfortunately, the pathologic examination of this type of rejection is done during the autopsy.

DIAGNOSIS OF ACUTE CARDIAC REJECTION

Although the current gold standard for diagnosis of acute cardiac allograft rejection is the endomyocardial biopsy, the histologic findings of rejection are not uniformly present throughout the myocardium. Autopsy studies have documented extensive acute rejection which was not demonstrated by endomyocardial biopsy of the right ventricular septum several days prior to death. Because of this discrepancy, acute rejection has become a "clinical" diagnosis which usually, but not always, is supported by histologic findings on endomyocardial biopsy. Thus, many studies of acute rejection after clinical cardiac transplantation have defined rejection as a "clinical event in which temporary augmentation of immunosuppression is initiated to treat presumed acute rejection."[113, 116] It is therefore of particular importance to review the means by which the "clinical" diagnosis of rejection is made.

CLINICAL MANIFESTATIONS

Most episodes of cardiac rejection are asymptomatic, detected only on endomyocardial biopsy. Thus, with current methods of immunosuppression, no clinical signs or symptoms are specific for rejection. However, when symptoms occur, they fall into three major categories: nonspecific constitutional symptoms, signs of cardiac irritation, and signs/symptoms of cardiac dysfunction and low cardiac output. **Constitutional symptoms** include fever, malaise, myalgias, joint discomfort, and flu-like symptoms. Signs of **cardiac irritation,** which may occur without evidence of depressed cardiac function, include sinus tachycardia (heart rate > 120 bpm); pericardial friction rub; new onset of frequent atrial premature contractions, atrial fibrillation, or atrial flutter[201]; and new or enlarging pericardial effusion by echocardiogram. Arrhythmias early after cardiac transplantation are also discussed in Chapter 12. Patients who develop new-onset atrial fibrillation or flutter after cardiac transplantation should be evaluated for possible rejection with endomyocardial biopsy. In general, these first two categories of suggestive signs and symptoms should prompt an **echocardiogram** (to assess right and left ventricular function) and an **endomyocardial biopsy** (to look for histological evidence of rejection).

If there are no clinical signs of low cardiac output, **if** the echocardiogram shows normal right and left ventricular function, and **if** the endomyocardial biopsy is grade 0 or 1A, then **rejection** is considered **absent,** and antirejection therapy is not initiated. However, there are exceptions to this general statement, since each physician caring for the transplant patient must evaluate the clinical and laboratory information, the patient's recent and remote rejection history, the current status of immunosuppressive therapy (are the cyclosporine or tacrolimus levels therapeutic, is the patient undergoing a steroid taper?), and the interval since transplant. A decision to initiate temporary augmentation of immunosuppression indicates that the physician has called this an "acute rejection episode."

The third category of clinical manifestations, **signs and symptoms of cardiac dysfunction and low cardiac output,** is much more serious because of the possibility of **rejection with hemodynamic compromise,** which has an important associated early and intermediate mortality (see later section). Symptoms which suggest important dysfunction of the cardiac allograft include a history of severe fatigue, loss of energy, or listlessness; sudden onset of progressive dyspnea at low levels of activity; syncope or presyncope; and orthopnea and paroxysmal nocturnal dyspnea. Physical findings which suggest a state of congestive heart failure and/or low cardiac output include rales on chest auscultation, jugular venous distention, S_3 or S_4 gallop rhythm, a prominent P_2 suggesting pulmonary hypertension, hepatomegaly, peripheral edema, diminished peripheral pulses (in the absence of peripheral vascular disease), and hypotension (or normalization of blood pressure in the presence of prior hypertension). When the constellation of signs and symptoms suggests the new onset of congestive heart failure or low cardiac output, urgent (or emergent) further evaluation of allograft function is mandatory. In the current era, an **echocardiogram** is usually the most expeditious method to evaluate cardiac systolic function. If systolic function is normal and the primary hemodynamic alteration appears to be diastolic dysfunction, direct measurement of central venous pressure, pulmonary artery systolic and diastolic pressure, pulmonary capillary wedge pressure, and cardiac output at the time of endomyocardial biopsy is warranted in order to focus hemodynamic therapy as well as immunologic treatment (see later sections). In the presence of new onset hemodynamic compromise, especially in the presence of new depressed ejection fraction without another established etiology, severe rejection should be suspected and therapy initiated, regardless of the histology on endomyocardial biopsy.

ENDOMYOCARDIAL BIOPSY

As previously discussed, the endomyocardial biopsy and its histologic evaluation remains the standard method for detection of rejection following cardiac transplantation. Unfortunately, the invasive nature of this procedure creates a potentially unpleasant experience for the patient, and along with its cost, limits the frequency with which the myocardium can be "examined." A more desirable diagnostic method would be one that provides nearly continuous information about rejection phenomena. However, until other noninvasive techniques of rejection detection prove reliable, the endomyocardial biopsy will remain the cornerstone of rejection surveillance. Although it will never be a pleasant experience, the skilled and careful operator can ensure that "the biopsy" is not something for the patient to fear.

Historical Note

The routine histologic examination of tissue from the allograft was dependent on the development of a technique for safe, intermittent access. In 1962, Sakakibara and Konno provided the major breakthrough in the technique of transvenous endomyocardial biopsy.[124,196] They developed a bioptome with two large, mobile cutting cusps capable of venous insertion for multiple biopsy specimens via the internal jugular vein. However, the bioptome was stiff, difficult to maneuver, and because of the large outer jaws it required a venous cutdown for insertion. In 1972, Caves, while working at Stanford, modified the Konno bioptome into what is now known as the Stanford or Caves-Schultz bioptome that was optimized for the transvenous approach via the right internal jugular vein.[30] Scholten at Stanford developed the Scholten bioptome for the internal jugular approach. Improvements in these bioptomes included an adjustable cutting force via a spring mechanism and an adjustable bend to facilitate proper positioning against the interventricular septum. This type of bioptome, or one of the newer disposable modified models, is probably the most widely used type in the United States. In 1974, Richardson introduced the King's bioptome (from King's College Hospital in London), a modified bronchoscope biopsy forceps. This device has a thin shaft coated with Teflon, and is therefore easier to insert through a small sheath. It is very "flexible" and may be less prone to myocardial perforation, but it requires a guiding sheath and the bioptome procures a relatively small biopsy specimen.[3]

Biopsy Techniques

The technique of endomyocardial biopsy is currently extremely safe and easy to perform. Catheter manufacturing companies have improved on the designs of bioptomes, having introduced disposable bioptomes with different types of cutting jaws, which are smaller and easier to bend. These disposable products offer the advantage of alleviating the need to clean, sterilize, and resharpen the nondisposable devices such as the Caves-Schultz bioptome. Bioptomes are available in different sizes; therefore the sizes of the pieces of tissue retrieved are slightly different. The common sizes used are 9 Fr (French) and 7 Fr in adults and 3 Fr, 5 Fr, and 7 Fr in pediatric patients.[8] A 7- or 9-Fr bioptome generally provides a specimen size of 3–4 mm in diameter, and the 3–5 Fr bioptomes yield specimens of 1–2 mm.

Venous Access

The bioptome may be inserted through the internal jugular, subclavian, or femoral vein. At most cardiac transplant programs, endomyocardial biopsies are performed via the **right internal jugular vein** using the "middle" approach (Fig. 14–17). Cannulation of the internal jugular vein in the middle third of the neck avoids the right apical pleural reflection (decreasing the risk of pneumothorax). This point of access also allows effective arterial and/or venous compression if necessary. The right internal jugular vein is the closest large easily accessible vein to the right ventricle. One is therefore able to use a relatively short bioptome (50 cm in the adult) with nearly a "straight shot" to the right heart. Physi-

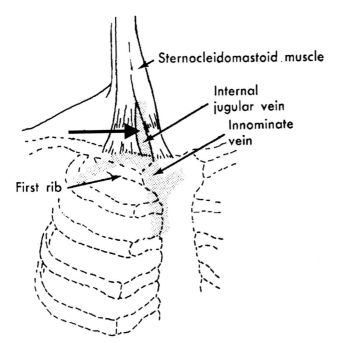

FIGURE **14-17.** Diagrammatic representation of the relationship between the right internal jugular vein and the sternal and clavicular bellies of the sternocleidomastoid muscle. The optimum guide needle insertion site is noted by the large arrow.

cians involved in the performance of endomyocardial biopsies should be proficient in the performance of endomyocardial biopsies from other venous approaches, including the femoral vein (see below) and subclavian vein.

To allow **cannulation of the right internal jugular vein** (RIJ), the patient is placed in a prone position with the head turned slightly to the left. The sternal (medial) and clavicular (lateral) bellies of the sternocleidomastoid are identified (Fig. 14–17). If needed, the sternocleidomastoid muscle bellies may be made more evident by having the patient tense these muscles by lifting up the head or by having the patient press the right cheek against resistance. The RIJ is usually found running between and deeper than these muscles.

The right neck area is cleansed, prepped, and draped (just as for a nonbiopsy cardiac catheterization). A small amount of local anesthetic (1 mL) is slowly introduced into the subcutaneous tissue at the superior angle of the triangle formed by the clavicle and the two bellies of the sternocleidomastoid muscle using a 25-gauge needle. After skin anesthesia, a 21-gauge 2-inch-long needle is used to anesthetize the deeper tissues. Aspiration of the syringe prior to anesthetic injection is important to avoid direct intravenous injection. This "finder needle" is directed at an angle 60 degrees posterior to the horizontal and 30 degrees laterally toward the right nipple. The finder needle is often used to locate the vein, which usually lies 1–3 cm below the skin. To enlarge the jugular vein and allow easier cannulation, the patient's feet are elevated (or the patient is placed in the Trendelenburg position) to increase venous return, and/or the patient is asked to create a slight Valsalva, decreasing venous flow into the right heart and distending the upper body venous system.

After the vein is located with the finder needle, the angle and location is noted and the needle is removed prior to introduction of a larger, 18-gauge needle via the same route. Some operators prefer to introduce the larger needle before withdrawal of the finder needle (which acts as a guide). After venous cannulation with the 18-gauge needle, a 0.035-inch flexible tipped guidewire is introduced, the position of the wire is verified under fluoroscopy, and the 18-gauge needle is removed. A 3-mm incision in the skin is made at the site of the guidewire penetration to allow insertion of the venous sheath. An incision is made at the guidewire site, incising first in a lateral direction and then in a medial direction. One should *not* "jab" the blade into the skin to a depth sufficient to create a wide enough incision, as overly deep penetration of the blade into the skin may lead to persistent bleeding.

After wiping off the guidewire with a normal saline-soaked sponge to remove any particles of clotted blood, a sheath large enough to allow passage of the bioptome with a central dilator is introduced over the wire (8- or 9-Fr sheath). The dilator and guidewire are then removed and discarded. The sheath should have both a side port to allow flushing and a rubber or latex diaphragm to prevent blood back-flow and also prevent air emboli. A slow continuous infusion of intravenous fluids is attached to the side port via a sterile tubing extension to prevent clots from forming in the sheath and obviate the need to intermittently flush the sheath.

Prior to the performance of the biopsy, many programs utilize the opportunity gained by obtaining central venous access to perform a right heart catheterization. A Swan-Ganz balloon-tipped flow-directed catheter can be inserted through the venous sheath to assess volume status (right atrial and pulmonary capillary wedge pressure), cardiac function (cardiac index), and systemic vascular resistance. This assessment of cardiac function may reveal diastolic dysfunction or depressed cardiac output suggesting rejection, sometimes hours before the biopsy is processed and interpreted. Any unsuspected deterioration of cardiac function should be reported to the transplant physician primarily responsible for the patient's care, as the flow-directed catheter may be left in place to guide therapy.

Internal jugular access, even under unusual circumstances such as volume depletion, small vein size, and unusual location of the vein, can usually be accomplished by experienced operators. However, under adverse conditions, the procedure may become time consuming and may result in inadvertent entry into the carotid artery. These more difficult procedures extend the need for local anesthesia; cause local trauma, edema, and hematoma formation; and increase scar tissue of the skin and subcutaneous tissues. Due to these problems, **ultrasound instruments** with small, high-frequency, two-dimensional ultrasound probes have been designed to aide in obtaining venous access (SiteRite Scanner, Dymax Corporation, Philadelphia, PA). These devices allow the assessment of vein position, size, and patency.[47] Such devices may be used in several ways to facilitate rapid venous access. These include (1) a preprocedure ultrasound scan of the neck prior to patient prep to identify the internal jugular vein location, vein size and response to slight Valsalva, the location and relationship of the carotid artery to the jugular vein, and the relationship of these structures to external landmarks; (2) a preprocedure ultrasound scan after patient preparation utilizing a sterile probe cover to obtain similar information as noted in number 1 above; and (3) an intraprocedure ultrasound scan to allow direct visualization of needle penetration of the vein using either a hand-held syringe and needle or applying a sterile needle guide attached to the ultrasound probe.

Biopsy Procurement Under Fluoroscopic Guidance

From the right internal jugular approach, the bioptome is inserted through the sheath. The tip of the bioptome has an adjustable bend which is in the direction of the handle of the bioptome. The tip of the bioptome therefore turns in the direction of the handle (or a notation on the handle on some disposable instruments). The bioptome is passed through the diaphragm of the sheath and into the lower third of the right atrium with the tip pointed to the right lateral side of the patient (Fig. 14–18 see position 1).

Any resistance to passage of the bioptome is transmitted well via the relatively stiff shaft. Occasionally, the tip of the bioptome "hangs up" at the recipient–donor right atrial anastomotic site, and passage is facilitated by gentle counterclockwise torque on the bioptome. **The bioptome should never be introduced forcibly against resistance!** At the level of the mid to lower third of the

right atrium, the handle of the bioptome is rotated 135 degrees counterclockwise (to approximately the 10:30 position if looking toward the patient's feet from the head) and is usually advanced easily through the tricuspid valve (see position 2 in Fig. 14–18). One should not turn the bioptome in the clockwise direction in the right atrium, as it may enter the coronary sinus.

Once in the right ventricle, the bioptome is rotated another 80–90 degrees counterclockwise to point directly toward the interventricular septum. The catheter is then advanced until it "touches" the septal wall (Fig. 14–18 see position 3). One can usually detect the transmitted septal motion on the tip of the bioptome and premature ventricular contractions (PVCs) often occur. Correct catheter position is verified by the bioptome tip pointed to the right of the screen (to the left of the patient) on the anteroposterior fluoroscopy image, and toward the spine in the left anterior oblique and lateral fluoroscopy images (Figs. 14–19 and 14–20).

After confirmation of bioptome position, it is withdrawn approximately 1.5 cm, and the jaws are opened. The bioptome is then advanced until it again touches the septum, the jaws are closed, and the bioptome is slowly withdrawn. Some slight resistance is often encountered during withdrawal. If marked resistance is encountered, the jaws should be opened and another attempt at obtaining a specimen should be made.

After withdrawal of the bioptome, the operator opens the jaws over a sterile field (catheterization table) and an assistant carefully removes the specimen from the bioptome jaws, taking care not to crush the specimen.

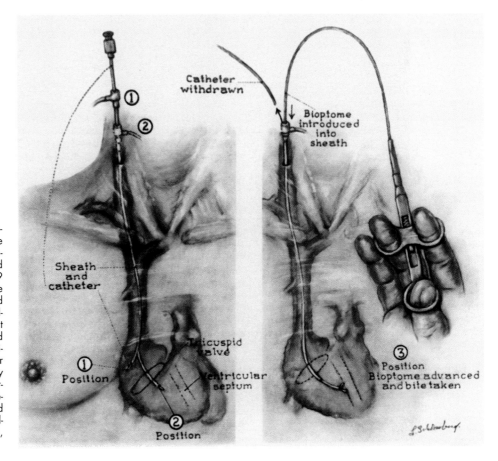

FIGURE **14–18.** Technique of endomyocardial biopsy using a disposable system. 1, The disposable system, consisting of a 7-Fr long biopsy sheath and catheter, is inserted through a No. 9 self-sealing sheath and directed into the right atrium. 2, The bioptome is inserted and then rotated anteriorly and advanced under fluoroscopy into the right ventricle. 3, The bioptome is directed to the ventricular septum, where a biopsy is obtained. See text for further details. (From Baughman KL: History and current techniques of endomyocardial biopsy. In Baumgartener WA, Reitz BA, Achuff SC [eds]: Heart and Heart Lung Transplantation. Philadelphia: WB Saunders Company, 1990, pp 165–182.)

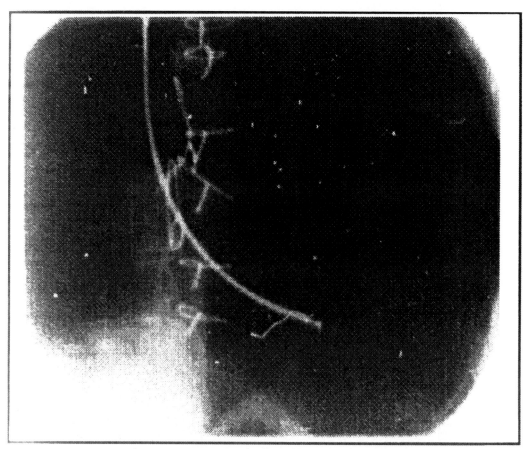

FIGURE **14–19.** Anteroposterior fluoroscopy image of a bioptome in the right ventricle with the tip pointed posterolateral toward the ventricular septum. In this view, the tip points to the right of the screen (the left of the patient).

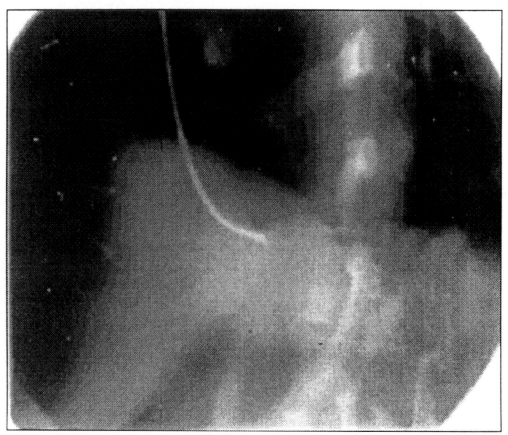

FIGURE **14–20.** Left anterior oblique fluoroscopy image of a bioptome in the right ventricle with the tip pointed posterolateral toward the ventricular septum. In this view, the tip again points to the right of the screen (the posterior-left of the patient).

492

An 18-gauge needle is often used (in order to avoid crush artifact) to gently remove the specimen and transfer it to an appropriate specimen container. The needle should be discarded after each use to prevent unforeseen contamination of the bioptome. The tissue should not be handled with forceps or divided with a scalpel. Squeezing the tissue can produce artifacts that upon microscopic exam will render it uninterpretable. Approximately four to five specimens are obtained in the same manner to ensure adequate sample size. The bend on the end of the bioptome should be varied to prevent the procurement of multiple specimens from the same area of the ventricular septum. The size and gross characteristics of the obtained specimens should be studied prior to ending the procedure. "Good" specimens are usually pink to red, are of adequate size (3–4 mm), and usually sink when placed into formalin. Specimens containing "scar" from previous biopsy sites are often white or gray-white and occasionally float on formalin. Utilizing these techniques, adequate specimens can be obtained over 98% of the time.

When neck access is not available, the **femoral vein approach** is most often utilized. The femoral vein approach requires a longer bioptome (100 cm in the adult) which is curved at a 135-degree angle to allow access to the right ventricular septum through the tricuspid valve from an inferior approach (Fig. 14–21).

Echocardiography-Guided Endomyocardial Biopsy

Most endomyocardial biopsies are performed using fluoroscopic guidance because such invasive procedures have traditionally been performed in cardiac catheterization laboratories or operating suites. Fluoroscopy exposes the patient and the operator to cumulative doses of radiation, and the equipment needed is expensive, bulky, and limits biopsies to specifically designated areas. Endomyocardial biopsy under echocardiographic guidance[154] eliminates radiation exposure and allows the operator to absolutely confirm the correct position of the bioptome against the myocardium prior to the bi-

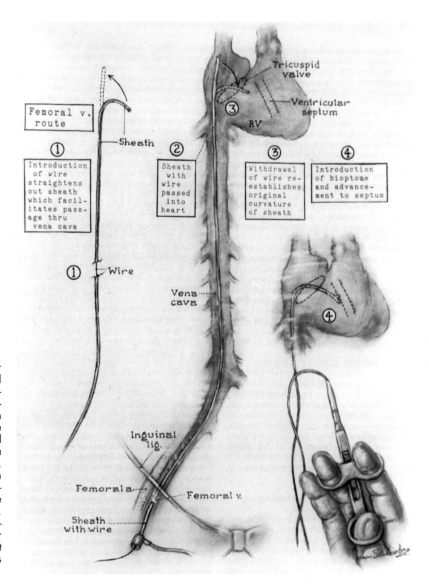

FIGURE **14–21.** Femoral venous approach for endomyocardial biopsy. 1, The 98-cm femoral venous bioptome sheath is curved at a 135-degree angle to allow positioning in the right ventricle. A guidewire is inserted through the sheath to straighten this angulation to facilitate passage through the inferior vena cava. 2, The sheath and guidewire are inserted into the right atrium via the femoral vein using a Seldinger technique. 3, The guidewire is withdrawn, allowing restoration of the sheath angle. 4, The bioptome is then inserted through the sheath and is directed to the ventricular septum, where a biopsy is obtained. (From Baughman KL: History and current techniques endomyocardial biopsy. In Baumgartener WA, Reitz BA, Achuff SC [eds]: Heart and Heart Lung Transplantation. Philadelphia: WB Saunders Company, 1990, pp 165–182.)

opsy. The echocardiogram also allows assessment of cardiac function and detection of right ventricular perforation. The relative advantages of fluoroscopy- versus echocardiography-guided myocardial biopsies are noted in Table 14–6. As with fluoroscopic guidance, cardiac biopsy under echocardiographic guidance is associated with a very low incidence of myocardial perforation and other complications.[154, 179]

Complications

The major disadvantage of the endomyocaradial biopsy is its invasive nature. In experienced hands, the performance of endomyocardial biopsies in the post–cardiac transplant population is extremely safe. The safety of endomyocardial biopsy is documented in the Stanford experience of over 25,000 biopsies performed on over 740 human heart transplant recipients since 1972 without biopsy-related mortality in adult patients.[15] Miller and colleagues reported 2 complications (one apparent myocardial perforation and one chordal injury) during the acquisition of over 4,700 biopsy specimens under echocardiographic guidance over a 4.5-year period, and neither episode resulted in significant sequelae.[154] Similarly, at the University of Alabama at Birmingham (UAB) there have been no fatal complications (but one hemodynamically significant episode of tamponade, treated with urgent pericardiocentesis) in over 5,000 biopsies since 1981. However, rare complications do occur, reported in 0.3–13% of biopsies.

Right Ventricular Perforation and Pericardial Tamponade

As noted above, this is fortunately a rare complication in the cardiac transplant patient, in part related to (1) obliteration of the pericardial space in most posttransplant patients, (2) the "normal" myocardium that is being biopsied (compared to the diseased and thin myocardium of the cardiomyopathy patient), and (3) the frequent development of ventricular hypertrophy following transplantation. Patients are observed carefully with frequent vital signs for 2 hours after an endomyocardial biopsy. Any patient complaining of sharp chest pain during the procedure should be monitored

closely and have an echocardiogram performed. Acute tamponade is usually treated with emergency pericardiocentesis, and if blood reaccumulates, it is treated by insertion of a drain and/or pericardial exploration and repair. A pericardiocentesis needle and accompanying equipment should be available in the area that endomyocardial biopsies are performed.

Pneumothorax

This complication is related to venous access and is more common when the subclavian route is utilized or if a long (>2 inch) needle is utilized via the middle internal jugular approach. A right pneumothorax generally results from needle puncture of the right apical pleura. Occurrence may be lessened by approaching the internal jugular in the middle third of the neck. Patient complaints of right pleuritic chest pain or sudden dyspnea should prompt careful ascultation of the lungs and chest radiograph for evalution of possible pneumothorax. A pneumothorax of about 15% or more should usually be treated with catheter aspiration or chest tube evacuation.

Nerve Paresis

The use of local anesthesia, especially if infused excessively into the deep tissues or the carotid sheath, may result in a Horner's syndrome, vocal cord paralysis, or rarely, diaphragmatic paralysis. The problem usually resolves in 1–2 hours unless direct nerve damage occurred due to the needle or the sheath insertion.

Venous Hematoma

A hematoma at the primary biopsy site may be painful and temporarily limit further access to the vein for the performance of needed biopsies. Excess sheath manipulation, prolonged and repeated passes with the "finder" needle or the 18-gauge insertion needle, inadequate pressure at the venous entry site after the procedure, and high venous pressures (chronic, or due to coughing, straining, etc.), are associated with this complication. A significant hematoma may lead to internal jugular vein thrombosis subsequently precluding further use of this important venous access site.

Carotid Artery Puncture

Utilizing proper technique and a "finder needle," significant laceration is rare. If the artery is punctured by the "finder needle," then direct pressure for 5 minutes usually prevents any complication. This probably occurs more frequently in the patient with a small internal jugular vein or a carotid artery which lies just posterior to the internal jugular. The use of an ultrasound scanner virtually eliminates this problem.

Tricuspid Valve Injury

Repeated biopsies may inadvertently trap and damage or sever parts of the chordal apparatus of the tricuspid valve. If recurrent damage occurs, severe tricuspid insuf-

TABLE 14–6	Myocardial Biopsy: Comparison of Guidance by Fluoroscopy Versus Echocardiography	
	TECHNIQUE	
PARAMETER	Fluoroscopy	Echocardiography
Radiation dose	++	0
Portability	0/+	++++
Accessible sampling area	+	++++
Assessment of cardiac function	0*	++++
Cost	++	+

*Cardiac hemodynamics may be assessed using Swan-Ganz catheterization with either technique.
Adapted from Miller LW, Labovitz AJ, McBride LA, Pennington DG, Kanter K: Echocardiography-guided endomyocardial biopsy: a 5-year experience. Circulation 1988;78S:99–102.

ficiency may occur.[214] Rarely, the chronic sequelae of tricuspid insufficiency may require surgical intervention with tricuspid valve repair or replacement (see Chapter 18).

Malignant Ventricular Arrhythmia

The presence of PVCs during the biopsy procedure confirms the location of the bioptome in the right ventricle. Short runs (2–10 beats) of nonsustained ventricular tachycardia may occur during sampling but almost universally end with removal of the bioptome. In our experience with biopsies in cardiac transplant patients, we have never noted sustained ventricular tachycardia or ventricular fibrillation associated with an endomyocardial biopsy. The nontransplant patient, especially with a history of ventricular ectopy, is at higher risk for this complication.

Transient Complete Heart Block

This complication occurs rarely in the posttransplant population, primarily in patients with preexisting left bundle branch block who experience pressure against the right bundle. It is usually transient and responds to removal of the bioptome (and/or the venous sheath) but occasionally requires temporary transvenous pacing. A temporary transvenous pacing wire, a pacemaker, and all associated connecting cables should be readily available in the biopsy area. Patients with preexisting left bundle branch block are coached extensively to cough on command. We have documented systemic blood pressures of 100–110 mm Hg for up to 3 minutes during "cough" cardiopulmonary resuscitation in nontransplant patients with left bundle branch block that developed complete heart block during endomyocardial biopsy procedures.

Supraventricular Tachycardia

Atrial flutter may be induced by the occurrence of premature atrial contractions during the passage of the sheath or the bioptome into the right atrium. The arrhythmia is usually terminated by removal of the bioptome and/or the sheath. Occasionally, especially early following transplantation, patients will require rapid atrial pacing to terminate atrial flutter (easy to perform via the venous sheath), or direct current cardioversion.

ECHOCARDIOGRAPHY

Two-dimensional echocardiography with Doppler has been extensively studied as a tool for detecting rejection after cardiac transplantation. Since many of the histologic changes observed with acute rejection may alter diastolic function, the evaluation of diastolic function by echocardiography has been correlated with acute rejection. Worsening rejection has been associated with progressive shortening of isovolumic relaxation time, increases in peak early initial valve flow velocity,[223] and increased pressure half-time (a parameter determined

by the analysis of the Doppler mitral flow velocity curve). Another echocardiographic indicator of rejection is new or progressive mitral insufficiency identified by echo Doppler.[50] New-onset or increasing pericardial effusion has also been correlated with acute rejection.[224] While these findings raise the index of suspicion for acute rejection (and the need for endomyocardial biopsy), none of these findings, either individually or collectively, has proven sensitive or specific enough to routinely initiate antirejection therapy without confirmation by endomyocardial biopsy. These echocardiographic findings, although not specific for rejection, suggest the need for endomyocardial biopsy.

Perhaps the most important application of echocardiography to transplantation in children and adults is the identification of **systolic dysfunction.** It is well established that the histologic findings on endomyocardial biopsy are not predictive of hemodynamics obtained at right heart catheterization or left ventricular function assessed by echocardiography. Left ventricular ejection fraction remains within normal limits in 95% of rejection episodes.[157] However, with the exception of the usually transient systolic dysfunction occasionally observed in the first several days after-transplant secondary to donor heart dysfunction or inadequate myocardial preservation, acute rejection is overwhelmingly the most common cause of acute depression of systolic function. Other causes include advanced allograft vasculopathy (which may cause segmental wall dysfunction), nonspecific unexplained graft failure without acute rejection or vasculopathy, and, rarely, infection. However, unless another cause has been clearly identified, acute depression of systolic function (ejection fraction <50%) more than several days after transplant should be assumed secondary to acute cellular or humoral rejection and treated as such, with or without confirmation by endomyocardial biopsy. The serious prognosis of hemodynamically compromising rejection and its treatment is discussed in detail later in this chapter.

A special situation exists with the **neonate and infant** following cardiac transplantation, in whom repeated surveillance cardiac biopsies may not be feasible. In this age group, echocardiographic parameters have been identified which are predictive of acute rejection. These are discussed in Chapter 20.

OTHER NONINVASIVE METHODS

Electrocardiographic Analysis

The **electrocardiogram (ECG)** is primarily useful to establish the new onset of atrial fibrillation and atrial flutter. In patients receiving cyclosporine immunosuppression, new onset of frequent atrial premature contractions, atrial fibrillation, and atrial flutter has been correlated with acute rejection.[138, 201] However, these findings are not specific enough to justify antirejection therapy without biopsy. Ventricular arrhythmias are not predictive of acute rejection[98, 138] (see further discussion in Chapter 12).

In the precyclosporine era, a greater than 20% reduction in the summed QRS complex voltage in leads I, II,

III, V_1, and V_6 in serial ECGs was considered a marker of acute rejection and indicated the need for prompt endomyocardial biopsy.[63] In the current era of cyclosporine- and tacrolimus-based immunosuppression, the summed ORS complex voltage has *not* proved helpful in the diagnosis of acute rejection, presumably in part because of less myocardial tissue edema with current antirejection therapies.

Electrocardiographic signal averaging, a technique that averages together multiple samples of repeating complexes and enhances the signal-to-noise ratio by electronic filtering, increases the sensitivity of the ECG in predicting rejection,[109] but it has not proved useful enough to be routinely employed.[85, 103, 122, 131]

Another electrocardiographic technique which has been evaluated for the detection of rejection is the frequency analysis of the electrocardiogram by **fast-Fourier transformation,**[74] a technique which analyzes frequencies not detected on the surface ECG and is independent of signal amplitude. Analysis of the QRS complex and ST segments with this technique has been reported to identify rejection with a sensitivity of 90% but a specificity of only 40%.[74, 122] In its current form, the technique is not reproducible or predictive enough to gain widespread application in clinical cardiac transplantation.[122]

Beat-to-beat fluctuations in heart rate reflect modulations in sinus node activity and can be quantified by the techniques of **power spectrum analysis.** Cardiac transplantation and the resultant cardiac denervation results in a reduction of heart rate variability, whereas acute rejection tends to increase heart rate variability.[198] However, this like most other electrocardiographic techniques, has not demonstrated the specificity or sensitivity to replace the cardiac biopsy.

Electrocardiographic changes during high-dose **dipyridamole infusion** indicate reduction of coronary reserves in the presence of normal epicardial vessels. Acute allograft rejection has been shown to induce ST-segment depression during dipyridamole infusion, but the sensitivity is too low to be useful in the diagnosis of acute rejection.[171]

One of the more promising techniques for daily long-distance rejection surveillance is the intramyocardial ECG utilizing **intramyocaradial electrograms (IMEG).**[123, 193, 231] The technique requires an implantable pacemaker and an epicardial lead system, usually placed at the time of transplantation, for telemetric monitoring of myocardial voltage amplitudes. Rejection is known to decrease the myocardial voltage amplitude, and a 15% decrease in QRS voltage compared to control has been reported to indicate rejection. In some studies, the sensitivity of this technique in predicting acute rejection approaches 100%.[230] The specificity is considerably less, since infection and ventricular dysrhythmias can also decrease voltage amplitude. However, several centers with an extensive experience using IMEG report that clinical rejection is extremely rare in the presence of a normal IMEG and a normal echocardiogram, thus avoiding the need for endomyocardial biopsy.[230] Currently, the major limitations to widespread acceptance of this method have been (1) the need for pacemaker and epicardial lead implantation, (2) variations in the IMEG patterns, and (3) insufficient documentation of its long-term usefulness.

Cytoimmunologic Monitoring

Methods of detecting T-lymphocyte activation in the peripheral blood as a reflection of T-cell activity in the allograft form the basis for techniques of cytoimmunologic monitoring.[78] Although activated lymphocytes comprising greater than 5% of the lymphocyte population has been correlated with acute rejection, similar results have been found with acute infections, particularly viral.[48, 54, 181] Similarly, circulating CD4/CD8 lymphocyte ratios (CD4/CD8 ratio >1.0 correlated with rejection)[102, 114, 234] have not provided the necessary sensitivity and specificity to replace cardiac biopsies. A number of immunologic and biochemical markers of T-cell activation have shown some correlation with acute rejection, including IL-2 receptors on lymphocytes,[45, 94, 158, 188] soluble IL-2 receptors,[133, 134, 195] plasma TNF-α, thromboxane B_2 in urine,[56, 57] urine and serum neopterin levels,[84, 147] transferrin receptors,[95] prolactin levels,[29, 37] serum β_2-microglobulins,[67] plasma P-selectin levels, plasma prothrombin fragment levels,[58, 202, 239] and expression of adhesion molecules (VCAM-1, E-selectin, ICAM-1) in the allograft.[25, 218] Although in individual studies these and other cytoimmunologic markers have shown a significant correlation with rejection in a group of patients, none have demonstrated the sensitivity or specificity in multiple clinical studies to replace the more invasive endomyocardial biopsy. To date, techniques which identify lymphocyte activation in the peripheral blood do not accurately reflect immunologic activity in the allograft.

Nuclear Magnetic Resonance Imaging

Nuclear magnetic resonance (NMR) imaging for the detection of acute rejection is based on the premise that cellular infiltrates, myocardial edema, myocyte damage, and interstitial hemorrhage may alter proton relaxation times (so called T^1, the spin-lattice relaxation time, and T^2, the spin-spin relaxation time), proton concentration, and flow/diffusion characteristics.[129, 144] Prolonged T^1 and T^2 can result from myocardial edema and have been correlated with acute rejection,[2, 27, 129, 185, 237] as has left ventricular wall thickness by magnetic resonance imaging.[31] P NMR spectroscopy has demonstrated decreases in phosphate metabolites during acute rejection, presumably from alterations in high-energy phosphate metabolism,[77] with a decrease in phosphocreatine/inorganic phosphate ratio and a decrease in the phosphocreatine/adenosine triphosphate ratio.[27] Unfortunately, the current indicies identified by NMR are poorly predictive of rejection during the first few weeks after transplantation and later are only indicative of more advanced degrees of rejection.[208, 237]

Radionuclide Methods

A variety of radionuclide techniques have been evaluated for the identification of acute rejection. Radionuclide imaging techniques such as ^{99}TcPP or ^{201}Th are not sensitive or specific enough to detect rejection unless it is very advanced. [111]Indium-radiolabeled Fab fragments of monoclonal antibodies against myosin can detect histologic myocyte necrosis. A comparison can be made between lung and heart antibody uptake with a heart/lung ratio exceeding 1.5 being highly predictive of rejection. The method is somewhat limited by its detection of myocyte necrosis from any cause, not just rejection. Although promising, clinical experience and controlled studies with this and other radionuclide techniques are currently too limited to warrant omission of the endomyocardial biopsy.

TIME-RELATED NATURE AND RISK FACTORS FOR REJECTION AFTER CARDIAC TRANSPLANTATION

Although allograft rejection is one of the critical biologic phenomena which limits the long-term outcome after cardiac transplantation, the difficulty of precise definition and identification of allograft rejection has impaired our ability to fully understand this phenomenon and its risk factors. In cardiac transplantation the endomyocardial biopsy has been the standard method of identifying the rejection process, but controversy exists regarding the precise correlation between histopathologic changes and the rejection process. For purposes of clinical investigations, any analysis of clinical rejection phenomena must account for differences among institutions in the threshold for "treatment of rejection" based on histopathologic criteria and the frequency of surveillance sampling by endomyocardial biopsy during the first 6–12 months following cardiac transplantation. Realizing the imperfections and limitations of any clinical diagnosis of "rejection," the multi-institutional Cardiac Transplant Research Database (CTRD) has adopted a definition of rejection which acknowledges subtle differences among transplant physicians and institutions and their criteria for treatment of a rejection episode. For purposes of analysis, they define a **rejection episode** as "a clinical event, usually but not always accompanied by an abnormal myocardial biopsy, which results in acute and temporary augmentation of a patient's immunosuppression."[116] In a CTRD study by Kobashawaga and colleagues, 70% of rejection episodes were associated with an endomyocardial biopsy grade 3A or higher.[116]

TIME-RELATED NATURE OF REJECTION

The frequency of rejection episodes tends to decrease with increasing interval since transplantation, related to the acquired state of partial unresponsiveness achieved with current maintenance immunosuppression. This fact must be considered in evaluating the effect of therapeutic interventions aimed at reducing rejection frequency.

The time-related depictions of rejection generally include a description of the time until initial rejection,

cumulative rejection over a defined period, and the tendency (risk) for recurrent rejection. Actuarial and parametric depictions are used to describe time to first rejection and time to a subsequent rejection (recurrent rejection). Cumulative rejection is described by the frequency distribution curve (see Chapter 3).

Time to First Rejection

The simplest and most common depiction of rejection is "freedom from any rejection" or "time to first rejection." Such a depiction from the CTRD is depicted in Figure 14–22. Nearly 40% of adult transplant patients have one or more rejection episodes within the first month, and over 60% experience one or more rejections within 6 months. By 1 year after-transplant only about one third of patients remain free of rejection. The hazard function (instantaneous risk) for initial rejection (Fig. 14–23) peaks at 1–2 months, then rapidly decreases thereafter, merging with a low constant risk of rejection after about 1 year.

Although this depiction of rejection is convenient for actuarial and parametric illustrations and risk factor analysis, it does not fully describe the patient's tendency for rejection phenomena. The initial rejection episode, unless severe, is usually easily treated and would be a minor problem if it were the only rejection experienced by the patient.

Of much greater concern is those patients who suffer recurring (repeated) rejection, with the need for repeated augmentation of immunosuppression, the possibility of hemodynamic compromise (graft dysfunction), the increased risk of infection, and the potential contribution of recurrent rejection to allograft vasculopathy.

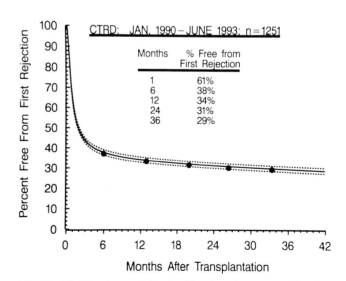

FIGURE **14–22.** Actuarial (Kaplan-Meier) and parametric freedom from initial rejection after heart transplantation. The dotted lines indicate the enclosed 70% confidence limits. Closed circles represent the Kaplan-Meier survival estimates at approximately 6-month intervals. CTRD, Cardiac Transplant Research Database. (From Kubo SH, Naftel DC, Mills RM Jr, O'Donnell J, Rodeheffer RJ, Cintron GB, Kenzora JL, Bourge RC, Kirklin JK, and The Transplant Research Database: Risk factors for late recurrent rejection after heart transplantation: a multi-institutional, multivariable analysis. J Heart Lung Transplant 1995;14:409–418.)

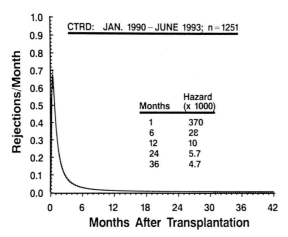

FIGURE 14-23. Hazard function for initial rejection episode after heart transplantation. Dashed lines indicate the enclosed 70% confidence limits. CTRD, Cardiac Transplant Research Database. (From Kubo SH, Naftel DC, Mills RM Jr, O'Donnell J, Rodeheffer RJ, Cintron GB, Kenzora JL, Bourge RC, Kirklin JK, and The Transplant Research Database: Risk factors for late recurrent rejection after heart transplantation: a multi-institutional, multivariable analysis. J Heart Lung Transplant 1995;14:409–418.)

Although unproven, the overwhelming opinion among transplant physicians is that repeated evidence of acute cellular rejection (grade 3A or higher) on endomyocardial biopsy indicates a higher risk of irreversible graft damage or graft loss.

Cumulative Rejection

A convenient way to display the frequency of rejection for a group of patients is the cumulative frequency distribution of the mean rejection episodes per patient over time (Fig. 14–24). Risk factors for a greater cumulative

number of rejection episodes in a given time period can be identified by multiple regression analysis (see Chapter 3). In the interpretation of data such as this, it must be remembered that any calculation of frequency of rejection is heavily dependent on the frequency of rejection surveillance with endomyocardial biopsies, which varies considerably among institutions. This also is a description of the "average" patient and provides no information about the extremes of rejection tendency.

Recurrent Rejection

Another useful method of examining repeated or recurrent rejection depicts the time-related probability of rejection after a prior rejection episode. This type of analysis is considerably more complex than the first two depictions, in that "time O" changes for each new rejection episode. Thus, time "O" is the time of transplantation for the first rejection, and for each subsequent episode, time O is the time of the prior rejection episode. Such a depiction for recurrent rejection is displayed in Figure 14–25. In this depiction, recurrent rejection is examined during the first year. Thus, during the first posttransplant year, approximately 25% of patients will experience another rejection episode within 1 month of the previous one. The risk, or hazard function, for the next rejection episode peaks at about 2 weeks after the previous episode and rapidly declines thereafter, merging with a low constant risk of subsequent rejection about 4–6 months later. Thus, during the first posttransplant year, patients are most vulnerable to a recurrent rejection episode within the first month following treated rejection. Although this probably reflects the biologic nature of allograft rejection, there is a certain artificiality in this concept, since all analyses are totally dependent upon the timing of follow-up surveillance

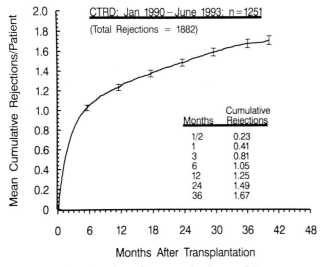

FIGURE 14-24. Cumulative frequency distribution of the mean rejection episodes per patient after heart transplantation. Vertical bars represent the 70% confidence limits. CTRD, Cardiac Transplant Research Database. (From Kubo SH, Naftel DC, Mills RM Jr, O'Donnell J, Rodeheffer RJ, Cintron GB, Kenzora JL, Bourge RC, Kirklin JK, and The Transplant Research Database: Risk factors for late recurrent rejection after heart transplantation: a multi-institutional, multivariable analysis. J Heart Lung Transplant 1995;14:409–418.)

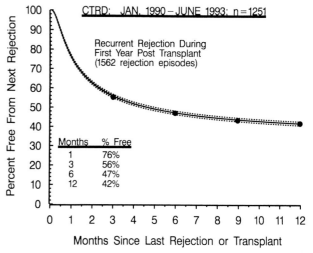

FIGURE 14-25. Actuarial and parametric freedom from the next rejection episode after either heart transplantation or any rejection episode during the first year after heart transplantation. The depiction is as in Figure 14–22. CTRD, Cardiac Transplant Research Database. (From Kubo SH, Naftel DC, Mills RM Jr, O'Donnell J, Rodeheffer RJ, Cintron GB, Kenzora JL, Bourge RC, Kirklin JK, and The Transplant Research Database: Risk factors for late recurrent rejection after heart transplantation: a multi-institutional, multivariable analysis. J Heart Lung Transplant 1995;14:409–418.)

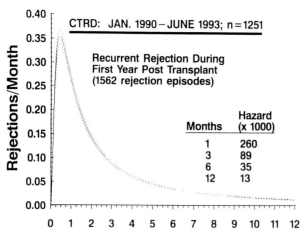

FIGURE 14–26. Hazard function for subsequent rejection after either heart transplantation or any rejection episode during the first year after heart transplantation. The depiction is as in Figure 14–23. CTRD, Cardiac Transplant Research Database. (From Kubo SH, Naftel DC, Mills RM Jr, O'Donnell J, Rodeheffer RJ, Cintron GB, Kenzora JL, Bourge RC, Kirklin JK, and The Transplant Research Database: Risk factors for late recurrent rejection after heart transplantation: a multi-institutional, multivariable analysis. J Heart Lung Transplant 1995;14:409–418.)

biopsies (unless the patient exhibits clinical symptoms of recurrent rejection). However, whatever the method of surveillance, multiple studies have shown that the tendency for recurrent rejection progressively decreases with time after about the first month (Fig. 14–26). The further decrease in the tendency for recurrent rejection after the first posttransplant year is reflected in the much lower hazard function for subsequent rejection (Fig. 14–27).

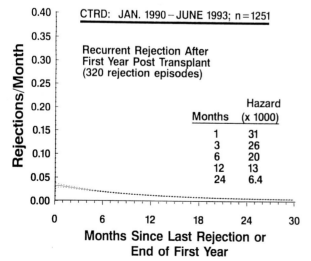

FIGURE 14–27. Hazard function for subsequent rejection after either 1 year or any rejection episode thereafter. (From Kubo SH, Naftel DC, Mills RM Jr, O'Donnell J, Rodeheffer RJ, Cintron GB, Kenzora JL, Bourge RC, Kirklin, and The Transplant Research Database: Risk factors for late recurrent rejection after heart transplantation: a multi-institutional, multivariable analysis. J Heart Lung Transplant 1995;14:409–418.)

TABLE 14-7	Risk Factors for Earlier Initial Rejection after Cardiac Transplantation (CTRD 1990-1992, n = 1,719)

RISK FACTOR	p VALUE
Early phase	
• Younger age (among adult recipients)	<.0001
• Female gender (donor and recipient)	.0006
• If white recipient: higher number of HLA mismatches	.01
Constant phase	
• Black recipient race	.004

Adapted from Jarcho J, Naftel DC, Shroyer TW, Kirklin JK, Bourge RC, Barr ML, Pitts DG, Starling RC: Influence of HLA mismatch on rejection after heart transplantation: a multi-institutional study. The Cardiac Transplant Research Database Group. J Heart Lung Transplant 1994;13:583–596.

RISK FACTORS FOR INITIAL OR RECURRENT REJECTION

Using techniques of multivariable analysis, a number of risk factors have been identified for earlier onset of **initial** rejection following transplantation (Table 14–7). Similar risk factors have been identified for **cumulative** rejection during the first year (Table 14–8).[99]

The presence of preformed anti-HLA antibodies against the allograft, particularly if directed against class I HLA antigens (**positive T-cell** crossmatch), is perhaps the most powerful predictor of hyperacute or aggressive potentially fatal acute rejection. The importance of minimizing this possibility by appropriate pretransplant immunologic evaluation is emphasized in Chapter 7. It is predictable that this overwhelming risk factor would not be identified by multivariable analysis, since donor hearts with a positive T-cell and B-cell crossmatch are rarely selected for cardiac transplantation.

There is less certainty about the implications of an isolated positive B-cell crossmatch (anti-HLA class II antibodies) at transplant. However, as discussed in Chapter 7, there are several studies suggesting that a positive B-cell crossmatch predicts a greater chance of rejection-induced graft dysfunction.

Perhaps the most useful type of analysis examines risk factors which include not only patient variables identified before the transplant but also events following transplantation which are associated with a greater tendency for repeated rejection episodes. Such an analysis of risk factors for **recurrent rejection** during the first year in a large multi-institutional study is depicted in

TABLE 14-8	Risk Factors for Increased Cumulative Rejection Episodes During First Year After Transplantation (CTRD, 1990-1992, n = 1,719)

RISK FACTOR	p VALUE
• Younger age of recipient	.02
• Female gender (donor and recipient)	<.0001
• HLA-DR mismatches	.04
• Induction therapy	<.0001

Adapted from Jarcho J, Naftel DC, Shroyer TW, Kirklin JK, Bourge RC, Barr ML, Pitts DG, Starling RC: Influence of HLA mismatch on rejection after heart transplantation: a multi-institutional study. The Cardiac Transplant Research Database Group. J Heart Lung Transplant 1994;13:583–596.

TABLE 14-9	Risk Factors for Recurrent Rejection During the First Year After Transplantation (CTRD, 1990–1993, n = 1,251)

RISK FACTOR	p VALUE
Demographic (recipient)	
Female	.03
Younger age (except infants)	<.0001
Clinical	
Positive CMV serology (before transplant)	.005
Donor	
Female	.03
Induction therapy	
Use of OKT3	<.0001
Time-related factors	
Fewer months since transplantation	<.0001
Fewer months since last rejection	<.0004
Greater number of previous infections	.05

Adapted from Kubo SH, Naftel DC, Mills RM Jr, O'Donnell J, Rodeheffer RJ, Cintron GB, Kenzora JL, Bourge RC, Kirklin JK, and The Transplant Research Database: Risk factors for late recurrent rejection after heart transplantation: a multi-institutional, multivariable analysis. J Heart Lung Transplant 1995;14: 409–418.

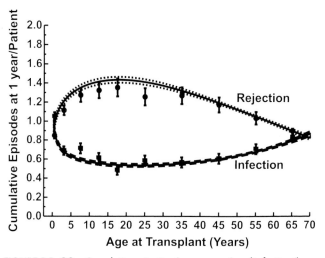

FIGURE **14-28.** Cumulative rejection (upper curve) and infection (lower curve) episodes at 1 year plotted against age at transplant, including both pediatric patients (from the Pediatric Heart Transplant Study, n = 961) and adult patients (from the Cardiac Transplant Research Database, n = 7,283) between 1990 and 1999. The dashed lines indicate the 70% confidence intervals around the parametric estimate, and the error bars represent the 70% confidence intervals around the point estimates. (Unpublished data, 2000.)

Table 14–9.[128] This study, however, did not analyze HLA data. A similar type of analysis can be employed to identify risk factors for later recurrent rejection, for example after the first post transplant year (Table 14–10). A number of single and multi-institutional clinical studies have examined the impact of these risk factors.

Younger recipient age at transplant among adults is known to increase the tendency for rejection.[99, 113, 120, 128, 183] Among younger children, especially in small infants and neonates, there may be a slightly lower tendency for rejection (Fig. 14–28) (see Chapter 20). Although the exact mechanism is unknown, the immune system likely becomes generally less responsive with advancing age and very young age. This notion is also supported by the slightly increased frequency of infection at the extremes of age after transplantation shown in Figure 14–28.

Numerous studies have examined the relationship between **gender** and rejection tendency, and female gender is frequently identified as a risk factor for earlier rejection.[43, 49, 108, 113, 116] The probable explanation for gender

TABLE 14-10	Risk Factors for Recurrent Rejection After First Posttransplant Year (CTRD, 1990–1993, n = 1,251)

RISK FACTOR	p VALUE
Demographic (recipient)	
Female	.01
Black race	.0009
Induction therapy	
Use of OKT3	.003
Events during first year	
Greater number of rejections	<.0001
Prior CMV infections	.003

Adapted from Kubo SH, Naftel DC, Mills RM Jr, O'Donnell J, Rodeheffer RJ, Cintron GB, Kenzora JL, Bourge RC, Kirklin JK, and The Transplant Research Database: Risk factors for late recurrent rejection after heart transplantation: a multi-institutional, multivariable analysis. J Heart Lung Transplant 1995;14:409–418.

differences relates to sensitization to HLA antigens at the time of pregnancy. Johnson and colleagues demonstrated in a multi-institutional study that the "gender effect" in rejection was entirely related to the earlier onset and increased frequency of rejection in *parous females*,[100] and increasing number of prior pregnancies did not further increase the rejection risk. Nulliparous females have the same rejection tendency as male recipients.[100]

Donor female gender appears in several studies to be an additional independent risk factor for rejection,[99, 108, 116] but the mechanism is unknown.

Studies in cadaveric renal transplantation have identified a clear relationship between increasing levels of HLA matching and increased graft survival.[244] Several studies in cardiac transplantation have identified a relationship between an increasing number of **HLA mismatches** and rejection propensity. In a multi-institutional CTRD study, Jarcho and colleagues[99] identified three or more HLA mismatches to be a predictor of earlier rejection (Fig. 14–29). The DR locus exerted a beneficial effect on time to first rejection only if there were no DR mismatches (Fig. 14–30), but there was a progressive effect of increasing number of DR mismatches on cumulative rejection during the first year[99] (Table 14–8; Fig. 14–31). Smith and colleagues from Harefield noted a correlation between increasing HLA - DR mismatching and both a shorter time to first rejection and a greater number of rejection episodes in the first 3 months following cardiac transplantation.[209] Others have noted similar findings.[204] A relationship has also been noted between class I HLA mismatch and rejection.[99, 243] These studies support the immunologic concepts that disparity between donor and recipient class I as well as class II HLA antigens play a role in graft recognition and rejection by the immune system (see

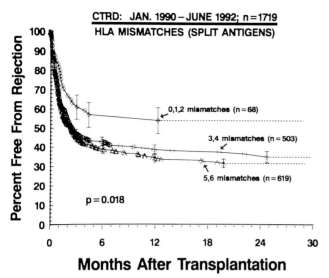

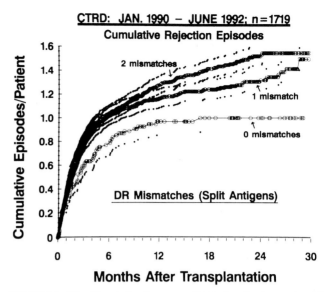

FIGURE **14–29.** Actuarial (Kaplan-Meier) freedom from initial rejection, stratified according to the number of HLA mismatches calculated with split antigens. The p value refers to overall differences between any of the actuarial curves presented. CTRD, Cardiac Transplant Research Database. (From Jarcho J, Naftel DC, Shroyer TW, Kirklin JK, Bourge RC, Barr ML, Pitts DG, Starling RC: Influence of HLA mismatch on rejection after heart transplantation: a multi-institutional study. The cardiac Transplant Research Database Group. J Heart Lung Transplant 1994;13:583–596.)

FIGURE **14–31.** Cumulative frequency distribution for the number of rejection episodes during the first year, stratified according to HLA-DR mismatches. Dotted lines indicate the 70% confidence limits around the cumulative distribution curve. (From Jarcho J, Naftel DC, Shroyer TW, Kirklin JK, Bourge RC, Barr ML, Pitts DG, Starling RC: Influence of HLA mismatch on rejection after heart transplantation: a multi-institutional study. The cardiac Transplant Research Database Group. J Heart Lung Transplant 1994;13:583–596.)

Chapter 2). The relationship between HLA mismatch and rejection tendency is less clear among recipients of Black race compared to Caucasians, partly because of the greater genetic HLA heterogeneity among Blacks with more poorly defined HLA antigens.[135]

The increased tendency for rejection among recipients with **previous serious infection** has been noted after renal transplantation[142, 206] and after cardiac transplanta-

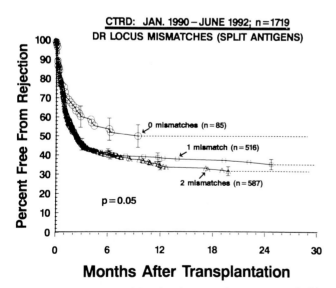

FIGURE **14–30.** Actuarial freedom from initial rejection stratified by the number of HLA mismatches (split antigens) for DR locus. (From Jarcho J, Naftel DC, Shroyer TW, Kirklin JK, Bourge RC, Barr ML, Pitts DG, Starling RC: Influence of HLA mismatch on rejection after heart transplantation: a multi-institutional study. The cardiac Transplant Research Database Group. J Heart Lung Transplant 1994;13:583–596.)

tion (Table 14–9 and Fig. 14–32).[113, 128] Recent evidence suggests that **cytomegalovirus** could promote or augment acute rejection by directly or indirectly enhancing the expression of HLA antigens and adhesion molecules on the graft endothelium.[225, 227] Human endothelial cells infected with cytomegalovirus can activate T-lymphocytes *in vitro*, and these activated lymphocytes may mediate allograft rejection.[64, 229] In a large multi-institutional study, recurrent rejection after the first year was related to the presence of prior CMV infections (Table 14–10, and Figs. 14–33 and 14–34).[128] The association between cytomegalovirus infection and allograft rejection was also noted in an earlier study from Stanford.[69]

Recipients of Black race are known to have a higher tendency for rejection, both early and late after cardiac transplantation[113, 128] and are at greater risk for rejection episodes severe enough to cause death or the need for retransplantation.[99] This may in part relate to the greater heterogeneity of the HLA system among Blacks, with the resultant potential for greater HLA disparity between donor and recipient.

Induction therapy (particularly with the monoclonal antibody OKT3 or polyclonal antithymocyte globulin) has been employed as a means to prevent or retard early rejection (see Chapter 13). A study at UAB examined rejection and survival in 32 consecutive patients who received either OKT3 or RATG as induction therapy. Although the survival was excellent (100% survival at 2 years), the tendency for early rejection remained high, with only about 30% of patients in each group free from rejection at 1 month and about 10% at 6 months.[111] Although OKT3 generally delays the time to first rejection (see Chapter 13), multicenter studies indicated that the prophylactic use of OKT3 was actually associated

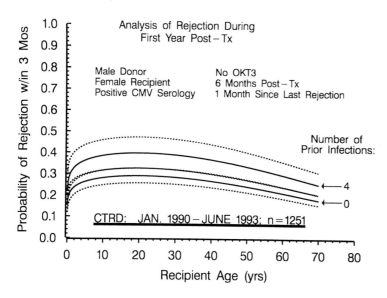

FIGURE **14–32.** A nomogram from the solution of the multivariable equation for recurrent rejection during the first posttransplantation year. The nomogram is stratified according to number of prior infection episodes. Dashed lines represent the 70% confidence limits. CTRD, Cardiac Transplant Research Database; Post Tx, posttransplantation. (From Kubo SH, Naftel DC, Mills RM Jr, O'Donnell J, Rodenheffer RJ, Cintron GB, Kenzora JL, Bourge RC, Kirklin JK, and The Transplant Research Database: Risk factors for late recurrent rejection after heart transplantation: a multi-institutional, multivariable analysis. J Heart Lung Transplant 1995;14:409–418.)

with greater cumulative rejection frequency (Table 14–8).[99, 113, 128] The explanation for this observation remains obscure, but it seems apparent that OKT3 does not favorably affect cumulative rejection tendency when used as prophylaxis.

The relationship between **ischemic damage** at the time of transplant and the tendency for early rejection is controversial, but ischemic injury may lead to greater indirect antigen presentation (see Chapter 2) secondary to the associated inflammatory response in the graft.

This concept is indirectly supported by the identification of longer ischemic time as a risk factor for recurrent rejection in an era before the availability of current preservation.[113]

Despite the numerous risk factors which are predictive of future rejection events, the complex interaction between the immunologic milieu of donor and recipient is altered by immunosuppressive therapy in a way which currently is incompletely understood. Thus, it is not surprising that a patient's prior tendency for rejection, as measured by his or her **prior rejection history** (rather than other specified risk factors), has the greatest

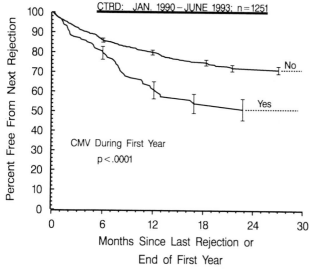

FIGURE **14–33.** Stratified actuarial for freedom from subsequent rejection after the first year or after any rejection episode after 1 year, stratified according to the presence or absence of cytomegalovirus (CMV) infection during the first year. Vertical bars represent 70% confidence limits. CTRD, Cardiac Transplant Research Database. (From Kubo SH, Naftel DC, Mills RM Jr, O'Donnell J, Rodeheffer RJ, Cintron GB, Kenzora JL, Bourge RC, Kirklin JK, and The Transplant Research Database: Risk factors for late recurrent rejection after heart transplantation: a multi-institutional, multivariable analysis. J Heart Lung Transplant 1995;14:409–418.)

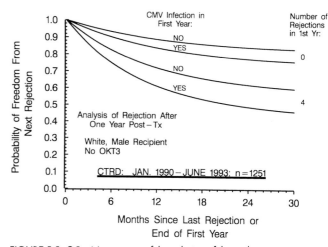

FIGURE **14–34.** Nomogram of the solution of the multivariate equation for subsequent rejection after the first year, stratified according to number of rejections during the first year and cytomegalovirus (CMV) infection. CTRD, Cardiac Transplant Research Database; Post-Tx, posttransplantation. (From Kubo SH, Naftel DC, Mills RM Jr, O'Donnell J, Rodeheffer RJ, Cintron GB, Kenzora JL, Bourge RC, Kirklin JK, and The Transplant Research Database: Risk factors for late recurrent rejection after heart transplantation: a multi-institutional, multivariable analysis. J Heart Lung Transplant 1995;14:409–418.)

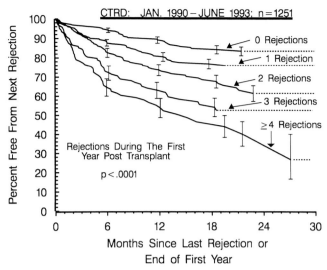

FIGURE **14-35.** Stratified actuarial for freedom from subsequent rejection after 1 year or any rejection episode later than 1 year, stratified according to the number of rejection episodes during the first year after transplantation. Vertical bars represent 70% confidence limits. CTRD, Cardiac Transplant Research Database. (From Kubo SH, Naftel DC, Mills RM Jr, O'Donnell J, Rodeheffer RJ, Cintron GB, Kenzora JL, Bourge RC, Kirklin JK, and The Transplant Research Database: Risk factors for late recurrent rejection after heart transplantation: a multi-institutional, multivariable analysis. J Heart Lung Transplant 1995;14:409–418.)

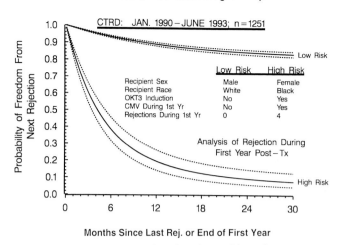

FIGURE **14-37.** Nomograms from the solution of the multivariate equation for subsequent rejection later than 1 year, showing high-risk and low-risk patient for the subsequent rejection. Dashed lines represent 70% confidence limits. CTRD, Cardiac Transplant Research Database; CMV, cytomegalovirus; Post-Tx, posttransplantation. (From Kubo SH, Naftel DC, Mills RM Jr, O'Donnell J, Rodeheffer RJ, Cintron GB, Kenzora JL, Bourge RC, Kirklin JK, and The Transplant Research Database: Risk factors for late recurrent rejection after heart transplantation: a multi-institutional, multivariable analysis. J Heart Lung Transplant 1995;14:409–418.)

predictive impact on the likelihood of future rejection (Fig. 14–35).[128]

An important future goal of such analyses is the "tailoring" of individual patient immunotherapy programs to maintain sufficient immunosuppression to prevent recurrent rejection while keeping the global immunosuppressive level low enough to minimize the complications of "overimmunosuppression," such as infection and malignancies (see Chapter 18). Using the techniques of multivariable analysis discussed in Chapter 3, nomograms can be generated which illustrate interactions between risk factors. Identification of patients (before transplantation or 6–12 months after transplant) with low-risk and high-risk "rejection profiles" (Figs. 14–36 and 14–37)[128] would contribute greatly to this tailoring process.

HIGH-RISK FORMS OF REJECTION

The highest risk form of rejection is **hyperacute rejection,** which is secondary to preformed antibodies directed against HLA antigens on the donor heart or against an inadvertent mismatch of blood groups (see Chapter 7). This form of rejection is currently extremely rare but is almost uniformly fatal. Other high-risk forms of acute rejection (associated with an increased chance of graft loss and death) are of three basic types (which are not mutually exclusive): (1) biopsy grades 3B and higher, (2) evidence of vasculitis or humoral rejection on biopsy, (3) rejection (with any biopsy score) accompanied by hemodynamic compromise, and (4) acute rejection in the presence of circulating antidonor antibodies.

GRADE 3B OR 4 REJECTION ON BIOPSY

These very aggressive histologic grades of rejection are, fortunately, rarely observed clinically, even in patients

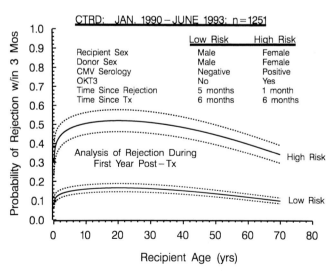

FIGURE **14-36.** Nomogram from the solution of the multivariable equation for recurrent rejection within the first year. A high-risk and low-risk patient are shown. Dashed line represents 70% confidence limits. CTRD, Cardiac Transplant Research Database; Post-Tx, posttransplantation; CMV, cytomegalovirus. (From Kubo SH, Naftel DC, Mills RM Jr, O'Donnell J, Rodeheffer RJ, Cintron GB, Kenzora JL, Bourge RC, Kirklin JK, and The Transplant Research Database: Risk factors for late recurrent rejection after heart transplantation: a multi-institutional, multivariable analysis. J Heart Lung Transplant 1995;14:409–418.)

with hemodynamic compromise. Despite the lack of clinical outcome studies with these advanced histologic grades of rejection, the prognosis is likely poor without prompt reversal of this process.

VASCULITIS AND EVIDENCE OF HUMORAL REJECTION ON BIOPSY

As discussed earlier in this chapter, microvascular rejection typically includes the finding of vasculitis on endomyocardial biopsy. This finding suggests the possibility of an active humoral component to the rejection process, which often also shows elements of cellular rejection.[82, 140, 242] Vasculitis (with transmural arterial wall infiltration of lymphocytes and monocytes, with or without neutrophils) has been associated with a high incidence of fatal rejection or graft loss within 6–12 months.[211] Similarly, evidence of humoral rejection (see section Microvascular [Humoral] Rejection, above) by immunofluoresence studies suggests a more ominous prognosis. Hammond and colleagues reported a 40% mortality at 1 year in patients who suffered early humoral rejection,[82] and Lones et al. noted a 32% incidence of hemodynamic compromise when humoral rejection was identified on biopsy.[140]

REJECTION WITH HEMODYNAMIC COMPROMISE

In about 5% of rejection episodes, hemodynamic compromise accompanies the episode, as evidenced by clinical signs of low cardiac output, decreased ejection fraction by echo, and/or decreased cardiac index, prompting the use of inotropic agents to support the circulation. This serious complication can be rapidly fatal if not promptly reversed. The mechanism of depressed systolic function is unclear, but experimental studies indicate that IL-1, IL-2, and TNF may participate in the production of graft dysfunction during rejection.[73, 92, 241]

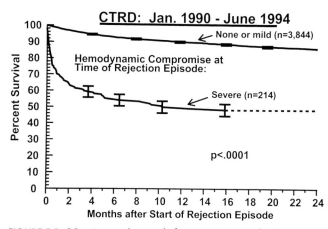

FIGURE 14–38. Actuarial survival after rejection episode. Upper curve indicates rejection with no or mild hemodynamic compromise, and lower curve rejection with severe hemodynamic compromise. Error bars enclose 70% confidence limits. (From Mills RM Jr, Naftel DC, Kirklin JK, VanBakel AB, Jaski B, Massin EK, Eisen HJ, Eisen HJ, Lee FA, Fishbein D, Bourge RC, and The Transplant Research Database: Heart transplant rejection with hemodynamic compromise: a multi-institutional study of the role of endomyocardial cellular infiltrate. J Heart Lung Transplant 1997;16: 813–821.)

Mills and colleagues examined the outcome of patients experiencing rejection with hemodynamic compromise in a multi-institutional database (CTRD).[157] A similar analysis in pediatric patients is discussed in Chapter 20. Approximately 5% of all rejection episodes have hemodynamic compromise at the onset of rejection, and that percentage remains relatively constant over time; that is, irrespective of the time after transplantation, there is less than 5% chance of any given rejection episode having evidence of hemodynamic compromise. By multivariable analysis, female gender, Black race, recipient diabetes, older age donor, donor Black race, and donor diabetes have been identified as risk factors for rejection with hemodynamic compromise.[157]

The serious consequences of rejection with hemodynamic compromise are apparent in Figure 14–38.[157] The

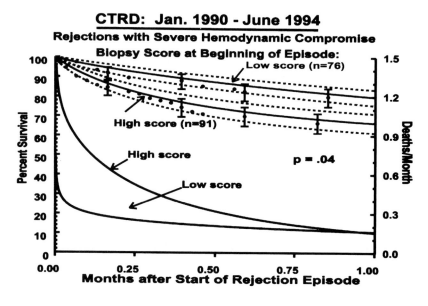

FIGURE 14–39. Survival after rejection with hemodynamic compromise. Upper curves represent actuarial survival rates after rejection associated with severe hemodynamic compromise, stratified according to biopsy score at beginning of rejection. "Low score" includes biopsy scores of 2 or less. "High score" includes biopsy scores of 3A or higher. Lower curves represent hazard function for death after onset of rejection, stratified by biopsy score. Dashed lines enclose 70% confidence limits. (From Mills RM Jr, Naftel DC, Kirklin JK, VanBakel AB, Jaski B, Massin EK, Eisen HJ, Eisen HJ, Lee FA, Fishbein D, Bourge RC, and The Transplant Research Database: Heart transplant rejection with hemodynamic compromise: a multi-institutional study of the role of endomyocardial cellular infiltrate. J Heart Lung Transplant 1997;16:813–821.)

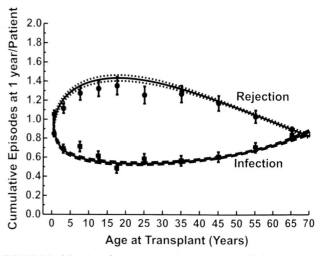

FIGURE **14-28.** Cumulative rejection (upper curve) and infection (lower curve) episodes at 1 year plotted against age at transplant, including both pediatric patients (from the Pediatric Heart Transplant Study, n = 961) and adult patients (from the Cardiac Transplant Research Database, n = 7,283) between 1990 and 1999. The dashed lines indicate the 70% confidence intervals around the parametric estimate, and the error bars represent the 70% confidence intervals around the point estimates. (Unpublished data, 2000.)

roids undoubtedly relate to the underlying rejection tendency and the other elements of the immunosuppressive program. Although definitive studies are not available, single-institution studies have identified several factors which likely influence the success of steroid withdrawal. **Women** are known to have a lower success rate in steroid withdrawal (by 15–20%)[115] than men, likely related to the effect of prior pregnancy on rejection tendencies.[100, 232] The **prior rejection history** is a strong predictor of subsequent rejection.[110, 127] Among patients with no prior rejection while taking corticosteroids, the chances of successful steroid withdrawal are about twice as high as among patients with prior rejection on steroids.[156] Although controversial, at least one HLA-DR match between recipient and donor is predictive of successful steroid withdrawal.[119]

Method of Steroid Withdrawal

There are four general philosophies regarding steroid withdrawal: no maintenance steroids from the time of transplant, early steroid withdrawal during the first month, steroid withdrawal after the first 3–6 months, and late steroid withdrawal (after the first year). There is no clear evidence to suggest superiority of one method over another, but our recommended protocol in adults is routine steroid taper beginning about 3 weeks after transplantation with steroid discontinuation between 3 and 6 months (Table 14–13). The steroid withdrawal is *not* completed if (1) two rejection episodes occur during the tapering process, (2) there is any rejection with hemodynamic compromise, or (3) any endomyocardial biopsy shows vasculitis, grade 3B, or grade 4 rejection.

In planning long-term immunosuppressive management, it is important to remember that there may be an

TABLE 14-13	Prednisone Taper Protocol and Exceptions

Early prednisone taper protocol (patient weight ≥50 kg)*
- Begin prednisone taper on POD 21 (or 14 days after discontinuing OKT3)
- Decrease prednisone 5 mg qod until 10 mg qd, then decrease the alternate-day dose by 2.5 mg every other day until this dose is 0 mg
- Continue routine biopsy schedule (see Table 14–19)
- When 10 mg alternating with 0 mg is reached, maintain that dose for 1 mo
- If no rejection occurs, then taper steroids off as follows:
    7.5 mg/0 mg for 1 mo with echo at 1 mo
    5 mg/0 mg for 1 mo with biopsy at 1 mo
    2.5 mg/0 mg for 1 mo with echo at 1 mo
    0 mg prednisone with biopsy at 1 mo

Protocol exceptions
- If 2 or more biopsies are grade 1B or more, or if hemodynamic compromise occurs, hold steroids at 10 mg qd
- If no further rejection (≥1B) occurs for 3 mo, attempt steroid taper again:
    10 mg/7.5 mg for 1 mo with echo at 4 wk
    10 mg/5.0 mg for 2 mo with biopsy at 1 mo
    10 mg/2.5 mg for 1 mo with echo at 1 mo
    10 mg/0 mg with biopsy at 1 mo
- If there is any rejection (≥1B) during this taper, remain at 10 mg qd

POD, postoperative day.
*UAB protocol.

TABLE 14-14	Late Prednisone Taper and Protocol Exceptions

Late Prednisone Taper (> 1 year after transplantation)*
- Decrease from 15 mg qd to 12.5 mg for 4 wk (biopsy at 4 wk)
- 10 mg qd × 4 wk (echo at 4 wk)
- 10 mg/7.5 mg × 4 wk (biopsy at 4 wk)
- 10 mg/5.0 mg × 4 wk (echo at 4 wk)
- 10 mg/2.5 mg × 4 wk (biopsy at 4 wk)
- 10 mg/0 mg with biopsy at 4 wk, then 2 mo, 3 mo

Protocol Exceptions
1. If patient has steroid complications, continue taper down to 5 mg alternating with 0 mg
2. If obtain biopsy of grade 2 or more during taper, resume prerejection dose and hold there
3. If rejection with hemodynamic compromise, abandon steroid taper and resume pretaper dose indefinitely

*UAB protocol.

increased risk of rejection and graft loss in the months following steroid withdrawal. Therefore, patients who are on maintenance corticosteroids after the first year should be removed from corticosteroids with caution. In view of this potential, we have avoided late (> 2 years after transplant) steroid withdrawal unless important complications of steroids are present. Instead, late steroid tapering (in the absence of important steroid complications) aims for a goal of 5–10 mg prednisone every other day (Table 14–14).

ROLE OF INHIBITORS OF TOR

There are currently no published clinical studies on the use of TOR (target of rapamycin) inhibitors in cardiac transplantation. However, the data reviewed in Chapter 13 in renal transplantation suggests that inhibitors of TOR (such as sirolimus and/or RAD) may have an important role as a maintenance immunosuppressive agent. As discussed in Chapter 13, the primary action of TOR inhibitors is the blockade of the transduction of cell surface cytokine signals to the nucleus which stimulate growth and proliferation of lymphocytes. Thus, sirolimus is an antiproliferative agent with no direct anticalcineurin effect. It is synergistic with both cyclosporine and tacrolimus.

In cyclosporine-based immunosuppression, sirolimus may be an excellent agent in combination with cyclosporine, potentially providing effective protection against rejection with lower doses (and levels) of cyclosporine. Thus, early and late after cardiac transplantation, sirolimus may have a "cyclosporine-sparing" effect which could be particularly useful in the presence of renal dysfunction.

In tacrolimus-based immunosuppression, sirolimus may also have a role.[207] Although both agents bind the immunophilin FK-binding protein, the sirolimus–FK binding protein complex inhibits TOR (rather than calcineurin), and the synergism between sirolimus and tacrolimus appears similar to that between sirolimus and cyclosporine.

As shown in renal transplantation trials, sirolimus also appears to be effective when combined with mycophenolate (without a calcineurin-blocking drug). Even though both mycophenolate and sirolimus are primarily antiproliferataive agents, sirolimus (in contrast to mycophenolate) does not directly block nucleotide synthesis. Thus, sirolimus combined with mycophenolate (with or without prednisone) could possibly provide an option for patients with prolonged or chronic posttransplant renal dysfunction.

TREATMENT OF ACUTE REJECTION

The standard primary treatment for cardiac allograft rejection (usually indicated by a grade 3A biopsy) is **intravenous or oral steroid** therapy, which usually is successful in reversing the rejection process. When such therapy does not lead to resolution of the histologic signs of rejection (persistent rejection) or is followed by recurrent rejection after a short time interval, steroid therapy alone may be ineffective at clearing the rejection process. The diversity of therapies for recurrent or persistent allograft rejection reflects the lack of secure information about basic issues such as (1) the precise definition of cardiac allograft rejection, (2) the prognostic implications of persisting or recurring cellular infiltrates on endomyocardial biopsy with regard to subsequent rejection or graft loss, (3) the effectiveness of various immunosuppressive interventions at eliminating such infiltrates, and (4) the long-term risks of such interventions. Some have questioned the necessity of treating moderate (3A) rejection in the absence of symptoms or hemodynamic compromise.[96] Despite these important uncertainties, the bulk of indirect evidence suggests that persisting or recurrent cellular infiltrates of ISHLT grade 3A or higher adversely affect long-term graft function and may contribute to the development of allograft vasculopathy.[4, 119] Strategies to reduce or eliminate such a pattern of histologic rejection are therefore justified.

For purposes of this discussion, **persistent steroid-resistant rejection** is rejection in which a biopsy grade of 3A or greater is present on two or more successive biopsies 7–10 days apart, each treated with augmented intravenous or oral steroid therapy. **Recurrent steroid-resistant rejection** is defined as three or more rejection episodes treated with augmented immunosuppression occurring within a 2-month period.

INITIAL THERAPY FOR ACUTE CELLULAR REJECTION GRADE 3A

Approximately 95% of rejection episodes occur in the setting of normal hemodynamics.[157] The standard initial therapy for an isolated grade 3A biopsy (moderate rejection) without hemodynamic compromise is intravenous or oral corticosteroids (Table 14–15). In most transplant programs, rejection within the first 2 months after transplantation is treated with a "pulse" of intravenous methylprednisolone at a dose of 1 g/day for 3 days with continuation of maintenance doses of prednisone. Although rare hemodynamic side effects of intravenous methylprednisolone have been reported,[211] this therapy is usually well tolerated. For patients less than about 60 kg, our standard dose of methylprednisolone is 15 mg/kg intravenously. Typically, in the absence of hemodynamic derangement, the methylprednisolone is administered on an outpatient basis. Although this is our recommended protocol, other protocols have proven equally as effective. In a randomized trial, a dose of 500 mg methylprednisolone for 3 days has been compared to the standard dose of 1 g, with no difference in effectiveness of reversing acute rejection.[88]

For isolated uncomplicated moderate rejection more than 2 months after transplant, steroids are generally administered as oral prednisone in a dose of 2–3 mg/kg/day for 3 days followed by either a gradual taper of prednisone or abrupt continuation of the prior maintenance dose of prednisone. The oral administration of 100 mg of prednisone (followed by a taper over 2 weeks) in one study was as effective as a 1-g dose of methylprednisolone for 3 days in providing prompt resolution of a grade 3A biopsy with no difference in the incidence of subsequent infection or rejection.[120]

The necessity for gradually tapering prednisone after a 3-day oral bolus is also controversial. From available studies, there does not appear to be a clear advantage of a slow taper compared to returning directly to the prebolus prednisone dose.[141] Our practice is to omit a "taper" unless there is a pattern of recurrent rejection.

The response rate (resolution of rejection on follow-up biopsy 7–14 days later) following treatment with intravenous or oral corticosteroids is greater than 80% for an isolated grade 3A biopsy in the asymptomatic patient without hemodynamic compromise.[116, 153] If rejection is persistent on the follow-up biopsy (without he-

TABLE 14–15	Treatment of Isolated Acute Cellular Rejection Without Hemodynamic Compromise	
BIOPSY GRADE	THERAPY	FOLLOW-UP
1A	None	Routine follow-up
1B	Prednisone (3 mg/kg PO) × 3 days ± taper*	Re-biopsy in 2–4 wk
2	Prednisone (3 mg/kg PO) × 3 days ± taper*	Same as above
3A	Methylprednisolone (IV) or prednisone (same dose as above)	Re-biopsy in 1–2 wk
3B	Same protocol as for recurrent or persistent rejection†	Re-biopsy in 1 wk
4	Same protocol as for rejection with hemodynamic compromise†	Re-biopsy in 1 wk

PO, oral; IV, intravenous.
*Treatment recommended during first 3–6 mo after transplant. Isolated grade 1B or 2 after 6 mo usually receives no therapy, with follow-up biopsy in 2–4 wk.
†See text for further details.

modynamic compromise) or recurrent within 2 months, the standard therapy is a repeat 3-day course of corticosteroids, usually with intravenous methylprednisolone, again with about an 80% chance of resolution.[153]

Although corticosteroid therapy is the mainstay of therapy for isolated, uncomplicated rejection, several studies indicate that augmentation of cyclosporine is also usually effective, either by high-dose oral (14 mg/kg/day) plus intravenous (1–3 mg/kg/day) cyclosporine[178] or, for lower grades of rejection, increasing the cyclosporine level by 50%.[121]

TREATMENT OF ACUTE REJECTION WITH LOW BIOPSY SCORE

Controversy exists regarding the implications of biopsy scores of grades 1B and 2[14] in asymptomatic patients. The decision to treat a biopsy with a low grade of rejection is influenced by several factors, including the time after-transplant, the grade of recent biopsies, the level of maintenance immunosuppression, and clinical signs or symptoms. The likelihood that a biopsy score of 1B or 2 will progress to moderate or greater rejection (≥3A) on the subsequent biopsy is highly dependent on the elapsed time since transplant. During the first 6 months after-transplant, greater than 25% of untreated grade 1B or 2 biopsies will progress to grade 3A on the subsequent biopsy,[187] with an even higher likelihood in the presence of multiple prior rejection episodes.[139] In contrast, after the first year, the likelihood of progression falls to about 7% or less. Thus, we currently recommend treatment of low grades of rejection (grade 1B and 2) as isolated findings during the first 4–6 months and, if recurrent, during the first year following transplantation. Therapy generally includes pulse steroid therapy (intravenous or oral) and/or augmentation of maintenance immunosuppression. After the first year, isolated grade 1B or 2 biopsy scores are poorly predictive of future rejection and probably do not warrant therapy.[236] A follow-up surveillance biopsy is recommended within 3–4 weeks. Repetitive episodes of grade 1B or 2 rejection have been associated with long-term graft damage.[4] Therefore, if a cluster of late (>1 year) grade 1B or 2 biopsies occurs, augmentation or alteration of baseline immunosuppression is probably advisable.

THERAPEUTIC OPTIONS FOR RECURRENT/ PERSISTENT REJECTION

In an immunosuppressive program based on cyclosporine, azathioprine, and prednisone, the second line of therapy after corticosteroids for persistent or recurrent rejection is usually either OKT3 or a polyclonal antilymphocyte (or antithymocyte) preparation (if these modalities have not been employed as initial "induction" therapy), with an expected response rate of about 80%.[66] OKT3 should be administered for 7–14 days, with frequent monitoring of circulating T-cell markers to document effective T-cell suppression (see Chapter 13). Since IgM and/or IgG anti-OKT3 antibodies may de-

velop 2–3 weeks after initiating OKT3 therapy, it is advisable to limit the duration of therapy to 14 days or less. More prolonged therapy may increase the likelihood of microvascular rejection presumably secondary to deposition of anti-OKT3 antibodies along the coronary endothelium.[79] After these have been administered once, the probability of CMV infections and lymphoproliferative disease (see Chapter 13) may increase with additional administrations. Thus, multiple "courses" of such therapy are generally avoided except in the circumstance of life-threatening rejection with severe hemodynamic compromise.

The remainder of this discussion, then, will focus on the therapeutic options for recurrent or persistent allograft rejection *after* administration of OKT3 and/or an antilymphocyte preparation. The most common options for subsequent treatment are listed in Table 14–16. Information is not yet available which indicates the most efficacious (and least toxic) treatment, so we will review the merits of each and offer our own recommendations. When applying the therapies listed below, episodes of acute rejection should also receive pulse therapy with methylprednisolone.

Conversion from Azathioprine to Mycophenolate Mofetil

Mycophenolate has a potential role in recurrent rejection of either cellular or humoral type, since it provides suppression of T-cell and B-cell activity.[159] As noted in Chapter 13, available data from a randomized multicenter trial indicates its superiority over azathioprine in freedom from rejection. Other studies suggest a reduction in rejection frequency and depression of antibody production.[191] Thus, during initial therapy of the acute rejection episode, intravenous methylprednisolone is administered and mycophenolate is generally substituted for azathioprine.

Conversion from Azathioprine to Methotrexate

As discussed in Chapter 13, methotrexate is a potent antiproliferatiave agent. Conversion from azathioprine to methotrexate (with or without azathioprine) has proven beneficial in controlling recurrent acute allograft

TABLE 14-16	**Strategies for Treatment of Recurrent or Persistent Rejection Without Hemodynamic Compromise**

- Initial treatment with intravenous methylprednisolone ± cytolytic therapy (Thymoglobulin or OKT3)
- Consider 1 or more of the following:
  1. Convert from azathioprine to mycophenolate or cyclophosphamide (if evidence of humoral rejection)
  2. Convert from cyclosporine to tacrolimus
  3. Raise maintenance prednisone to 0.2 mg/kg/day
  4. Initiate photopheresis
  5. Add methotrexate (rarely needed)
  6. TLI (only as last resort because of potential for late megakaryocytic leukemia)

TLI, total lymphoid irradiation.

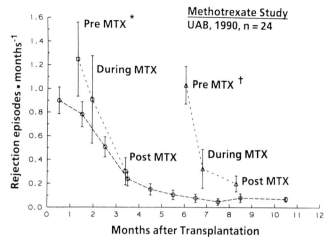

FIGURE **14–42.** Rejection rates during methotrexate (Mtx) therapy. The squares represent the mean rejection incidences and mean times since transplantation for the group of patients who started methotrexate therapy (n = 9) less than 2 months after transplantation; the triangles represent those patients who started methotrexate therapy more than 2 months after transplantation. Pre-Mtx includes the period after transplantation within 3 months of methotrexate therapy. Post-Mtx includes the 3 months immediately after methotrexate therapy. The circles represent the time-related rejection rates for all other patients (who were not treated with methotrexate therapy; n = 73) undergoing heart transplantation between January 1, 1987, and January 1, 1990. *p = .11, compared with all other patients at same interval after transplantation (circles). †p = .0001, compared with all other patients at same interval after transplantation (circles).

rejection (Fig. 14–42),[20, 21, 38, 165, 203] usually in a dose of 2.5–5 mg orally every 12 hours for three doses at weekly intervals for 6–8 weeks in adults.[203] Azathioprine dosage is reduced during methotrexate therapy and may need temporary discontinuation.

Conversion from Azathioprine to Cyclophosphamide

Because of more pronounced anti–B-cell activity (see Chapter 13), cyclophosphamide is often selected to replace azathioprine as part of a three-drug regimen in the suspected presence of humoral-mediated rejection.[70] The usual dose is one-half the azathioprine dose (milli-

grams). There are no clinical studies which have compared the effectiveness of cyclophosphamide to mycophenolate in the treatment of recurrent humoral-mediated rejection.

Conversion from Cyclosporine to Tacrolimus

Tacrolimus, like cyclosporine, inhibits the activity of calcineurin and may be more immunosuppressive than cyclosporine at clinical doses. Several studies suggest that conversion from cyclosporine to tacrolimus provides highly effective therapy for recurrent or persistent allograft rejection.[75, 86, 149–151]

When conversion from cyclosporine to tacrolimus is undertaken in the setting of persisting and/or hemodynamically compromising rejection, it is important to avoid a prolonged period without effective calcineurin blockade (low levels of both cyclosporine and tacrolimus). However, the nephrotoxic effects may be additive, so the two drugs should not be administered concurrently. In general, cyclosporine should be discontinued and tacrolimus started 12–24 hours after the last cyclosporine dose at an oral dose of 0.05–0.15 mg/kg/day. If renal function remains stable, dosing should be rapidly increased to achieve a therapeutic level >10 ng/mL within about 3 days. The recommended doses and levels of tacrolimus are discussed in Chapter 13. In the presence of severe rejection, intravenous tacrolimus (0.01–0.02 mg/kg/24 h) usually provides therapeutic levels within 1–2 days.[149]

Total Lymphoid Irradiation

The application of radiation to lymphoid tissue using an inverted Y-mantle field induces delayed immunosuppression that is highly effective in the treatment of recurrent rejection.[112] Patients with increased rejection tendency usually experience a reduction in the frequency of rejection episodes to that of standard patients within 2 months of completing total lymphoid irradiation (TLI) (Fig. 14–43).[112, 197] The mechanisms of immunosuppression, dosing schedule, and toxicity are discussed in Chapter 13. It is important to note that TLI, while effec-

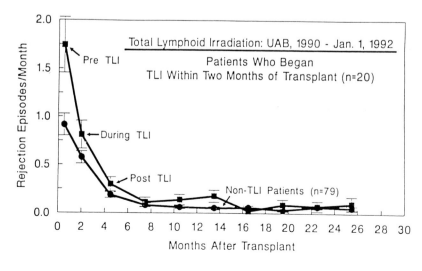

FIGURE **14–43.** Rejection rates during and after total lymphoid radiation. The solid line depicts patients (adult plus pediatric, n = 20) who underwent heart transplantation between January 1, 1990, and January 1, 1992, and received TLI within 2 months of transplantation. The dotted line depicts all patients (adult plus pediatric, n = 79) who underwent heart transplantation between January 1, 1987, and January 1, 1992, who did not receive TLI but received a uniform protocol of triple-drug immunosuppression plus OKT3 or rabbit antithymocyte globulin induction. The enclosed bars represent ± 1 standard error.

TABLE 14–17	Photopheresis Protocol*

Photopheresis on 2 consecutive days:
- 3-wk intervals × 6 sessions, then
- 4-wk intervals × 3 sessions, then
- 5-wk intervals × 3 sessions, then
- 6-wk intervals × 3 sessions

Contraindications
- Absolute lymphocyte count <500/mL
- Contraindication to heparin use
- Hematocrit <20%
- Extracorporeal volume of device >15% total blood volume; lower limit of patient size is about 15 kg

*UAB protocol.

tive against recurrent rejection, is not effective against ongoing acute rejection, and its utility depends on reversing acute rejection with other modalities. However, as discussed in Chapter 13, the occasional development of fatal megakaryocytic leukemia about 5 years after TLI has severely dampened our enthusiasm for TLI, and we currently believe its use is rarely indicated because of the availability of other safer alternatives.

Photopheresis

Clinical studies have demonstrated the effectiveness of photopheresis in treating recurrent acute allograft rejection.[39] We have used photopheresis following plasmapheresis for the treatment of recurrent or persistent allograft rejection, particularly early after transplantation and when the rejection is associated with hemodynamic compromise. Rejection frequency has been reduced significantly during photopheresis, and posttransplant panel reactive antibody levels have declined following photopheresis therapy. Although photopheresis is theoretically effective against B-cell as well as T-cell populations via development of anti-idiotypic antibodies, there as yet are no clinical data to substantiate its effectiveness against humoral rejection. The frequency of photopheresis treatments is outlined in Table 14–17.

Considerations in Selection of Therapy

In selecting a specific regimen for the treatment of recurrent or persistent allograft rejection, one should consider several general factors. Infants and children receiving cyclosporine immunosuppression should probably undergo conversion to tacrolimus in the presence of persistent or recurrent rejection, since the excellent results with tacrolimus are well established. The presence of hemodynamic compromise or evidence of humoral rejection are important and may affect the specific recommendations (see next section). The patient travel distance from the medical center may affect the feasibility of using TLI, which requires twice-weekly therapies for 5 weeks, or photopheresis, which requires treatments every 3–4 weeks for up to 12–15 months. There are also important cost differentials between various therapeutic options. Methotrexate and cyclophosphamide are about equal in cost to azathioprine, but mycophenolate is many times more expensive than an equivalent dose of azathioprine. Tacrolimus is slightly more expensive than

cyclosporine. The cost of TLI is typically about one tenth the cost of a 1-year course of photopheresis.

THERAPY FOR HIGH-RISK FORMS OF REJECTION

General Considerations

In each of these settings, treatment should **not** be limited to corticosteroids, but should also include cytolytic therapy (unless multiple courses of OKT3 or ATG have previously been administered). If humoral rejection is suspected or identified, mycophenolate or cyclophosphamide is advisable as an antiproliferative agent, and plasmapheresis should be routinely employed during the rejection episode. Additional therapeutic considerations are discussed below. Biopsy grades 3B and 4 are rare, but indicate advanced forms of rejection which (even if asymptomatic) should receive treatment as discussed in the next section, with additional consideration of therapeutic options for recurrent/persistent rejection (see above).

Rejection with Hemodynamic Compromise

As noted previously in this chapter, the presence of hemodynamic compromise (with clinical signs of low cardiac output and/or important reduction of ejection fraction by echocardiogram) indicates a major risk of subsequent death from rejection. Therefore, hospitalization with prompt aggressive therapy is mandatory to prevent fatality. The primary (simultaneous) goals of therapy are (1) initiation of strong anti–T-cell therapy, (2) prompt reversal of left (and right) ventricular dysfunction, (3) depletion of circulating antigraft antibodies (and possibly circulating cytokines), and (4) suppression of antibody formulation (Table 14–18). Initial therapy of rejection with hemodynamic compromise should include intravenous methylprednisolone, inotropic support, prompt plasmapheresis, and cytolytic therapy with either OKT3 or antithymocyte globulin.

TABLE 14–18	Therapeutic Strategy for Rejection with Hemodynamic Compromise

- Always consider this a life-threatening event
- Methylprednisolone 1 g IV and daily for 3 days
- Prompt inotropic support (preferably with dopamine, milrinone, or dobutamine, depending on blood pressure and heart rate)* to maintain effective cardiac output
- If cardiac output is clinically depressed and/or there is more than mild decrease in ejection fraction (≤ .35), place Swan-Ganz catheter for hemodynamic monitoring
- Prompt plasmapheresis (patients ≥ 15 kg) and daily for 3 days
- Cytolytic therapy with thymoglobulin or OKT3
- Heparinize
- Continue maintenance immunosuppression†
- Schedule photopheresis‡

IV, intravenous.
*Dopamine is preferable if blood pressure is low; milrinone is preferable if blood pressure is normal and tachycardia is present (see also Chapter 12).
†Reduce or hold cyclosporine and tacrolimus if renal function depressed. Switch to mycophenolate if on azathioprine. Begin daily steroids if off prednisone.
‡First treatment usually during the hospitalization for rejection.

If the ejection fraction by echocardiography shows new-onset depression to about 0.35 or less, if a measured cardiac index at time of endomyocardial biopsy is acutely depressed (<2.0 l/min/m^2 by thermodilution in the absence of severe tricuspid regurgitation), and/or if clinical signs of low cardiac output are present, the patient should be considered in danger of fatal decompensation. Prompt monitoring with an indwelling pulmonary artery catheter with continuous cardiac output and mixed venous oxygen saturation is advisable. After a bolus of methylprednisolone, initial inotropic support with dopamine, dobutamine, and/or milrinone is indicated. If the systolic blood pressure is depressed, dopamine is the first-line inotrope. However, marked sinus tachycardia (130–150 bpm) often accompanies severe rejection with depressed hemodynamics, and this tachycardia may be worsened with dopamine or dobutamine. In that circumstance, milrinone is preferred if the systolic blood pressure is adequate (>95 mm Hg).

Because of the potential for alteration in local plasminogen activators, endothelial inflammation, and microvascular thrombosis in the presence of humoral rejection, full heparinization is advisable. Azathioprine is converted to mycophenolate, and if recurrent rejection persists, cyclosporine is switched to tacrolimus.

Multiple studies in renal[19] as well as cardiac transplantation have demonstrated the efficacy of **plasmapheresis** (see Chapter 13) in the treatment of humoral rejection by reducing circulating titers of anti-HLA antibodies.[71, 168] Plasmapheresis generally requires about 3 hours to perform and rarely results in hemodynamic compromise. It is a critically important component of early treatment for rejection with hemodynamic compromise. In fact, it is common to see prompt improvement, or normalization, of left ventricular ejection fraction by echocardiogram immediately following the first session of plasmapheresis.

Although plasmapheresis likely reduces the circulating titer of anti-HLA antibodies, the rapidity of its effect on improving left ventricular function suggests additional mechanisms such as removal of cytokines and other inflammatory mediators which may directly depress left ventricular function. For that reason, plasmapheresis should be promptly instituted for hemodynamically compromising rejection, irrespective of biopsy score (i.e., whether the basic process is thought to be cellular or humoral). Plasmapheresis should be repeated daily for 3 days (occasionally 4 days if left ventricular function has not normalized). Occasionally, it is necessary to skip a day because of low fibrinogin levels (<100 mg/dL). Because of the ongoing risk of subsequent graft dysfunction, photopheresis is recommended after control of the rejection episode (see Chapter 13). Photopheresis is usually initiated during the hospitalization for acute rejection and continued for 12–15 months on an outpatient basis (Table 14–17).

LONG TERM REJECTION SURVEILLANCE

With current methods of immunotherapy, the risk of rejection continues throughout the life of the recipient,

TABLE 14–19	Schedule for Surveillance Endomyocardial Biopsies*

TIME AFTER TRANSPLANT	BIOPSY FREQUENCY
Wk 1–6	Weekly
Wk 7–6 mo	Gradual increase in interval between biopsies from 2 wk to 1 mo, 2 mo, then 3 mo
7 mo–2 yr	Every 3 mo
Yr 2–3	Biopsy during yearly catheterization for coronary angiography

*This UAB protocol applies only to surveillance biopsies for asymptomatic patients. Additional biopsies are performed as dictated by rejection history and symptoms or signs of rejection. An echocardiogram is usually also performed when a biopsy is obtained. If there is a favorable rejection history, discontinuation of annual surveillance biopsies is considered after 2–3 yr.

although it becomes quite low after the first year, with a low constant hazard for many years after cardiac transplantation. To date, there are no noninvasive tests which have demonstrated sufficient sensitivity among multiple centers to warrant complete reliance on such methods. Since most episodes of rejection are asymptomatic, most programs have established protocols for routine, gradually decreasing rejection surveillance by endomyocardial biopsy for at least several years following transplantation. One such protocol is presented in Table 14–19. The concept of examining the endomyocardium for signs of asymptomatic rejection once or twice a year is contentious and probably is not cost-effective after the first several years.

The most effective surveillance for rejection lies in appropriate education of the patient and his or her family or support members about the signs and symptoms of possible rejection, including signs of congestion (elevated atrial pressures) and low cardiac output. Despite the rarity of this event, late rejection with hemodynamic compromise remains an important cause of late mortality. Thus, patient and family must understand the critical importance of contacting the transplant center and/or transplant physician early in the course of such symptoms so that prompt evaluation may be undertaken, usually including an echocardiogram and, if indicated, an endomyocardial biopsy. The best chance for a successful outcome is early recognition of subtle signs of congestion and low cardiac output, followed by prompt investigation and aggressive treatment. In the presence of rejection with hemodynamic compromise, prolonged delays (days or weeks) between onset of symptoms and initiation of therapy carries a high mortality, but therapeutic intervention **early in the process** (with the methods discussed in this chapter) is highly successful.

References

1. Abramowicz D, Schandene L, Goldman M, Crusiaux A, Vereerstraeten P, DePau WL, Wybran J, Kinnaert P, Dupont E, Toussaint C: Release of tumor necrosis factor, interleukin-2, and gamma-interferon in serum after injection of OKT3 monoclonal antibody in kidney transplant recipients. Transplantation 1989;47:606.
2. Aherne T, Tscholakoff D, Finkbeiner W, Sechtem U, Derugin N, Yee E, Higgins CB: Magnetic resonance imaging of cardiac transplants: the evolution of rejection of cardiac allografts with and without immunosuppression. Circulation 1986;74:1145–1156.

3. Anderson JL, Marshall HAW, Allison SIB: The femoral venous approach to endomyocardial biopsy: comparison with internal jugular and transarterial approaches. Am J Cardiol 1984;53:833–837.

4. Anguita M, Lopez-Rubio F, Arizon JM, Latre JM, Casares J, Lopez-Granados A, Mesa D, Gimenez D, Torres F, Concha M, Valles F: Repetitive nontreated episodes of grade 1B or 1 acute rejection impair long-term graft function. J Heart Lung Transplant 1995;14:452–460.

5. Armitage JM, Fricker FJ, del Nido P, Cipriani L, Starzl TE: The clinical trial of FK506 as primary and rescue immunosuppression in pediatric cardiac transplantation. Transplant Proc 1991;23:3058–3060.

6. Armitage JM, Kormos RL, Morita S, Fung J, Marrone GC, Hardesty RL, Griffith BP, Starzl TE: Clinical trial of FK506 immunosuppression in adult cardiac transplantation. Ann Thorac Surg 1992;54:205–210.

7. Baan CC, Vaessen LM, Loonen EH, Balk AH, Jutte NH, Claas FH, Weimar W: The effect of antithymocyte globulin therapy on frequency and avidity of allospecific ommitted CTL in clinical heart transplants. Transplant Proc 1995;27:482–484.

8. Balzer D, Moorhead S, Saffitz JE, Skarski DR, Canter CE: Pediatric endomyocardial biopsy performed solely with echocardiographic guidance. J Am Soc Echocardiogr 1993;6:510–515.

9. Barone JH, Fishbein MC, Czer LSC, Blanche C, Trento A, Luthringer DJ: Absence of endocardial lymphoid infiltrates (quilty lesions) in the non-cardiac transplant patients treated with cyclosporin. J Heart Lung Transplant 1997;16:600–603.

10. Barr ML, Sanchez JA, Seche LA, Schulman LL, Smith CR, Rose EA: Anti-CD3 monoclonal antibody induction therapy. Immunological equivalency with triple drug therapy in heart transplantation. Circulation 1990;82(suppl):291.

11. Basile L, Zerbe T, Rabin B, Clarke J, Abrams A, Cerilli J: Identification of the antibody to vascular endothelial cells in patients undergoing cardiac transplantation. Transplantation 1985;40:670–674.

12. Baughman KL: History and current techniques of endomyocardial biopsy. In Baumgartener WA, Reitz BA, Achuff, SC (eds): Heart and Heart Lung Transplantation. Philadelphia: WB Saunders Company, 1990, pp 165–182.

13. Billingham ME: Diagnosis of cardiac rejection by endomyocardial biopsy. Heart Transplant 1982;1:25–30.

14. Billingham ME: Dilemma of variety of histopathologic grading systems for acute cardiac allograft rejection by endomyocardial biopsy. J Heart Lung Transplant 1990;9:272–276.

15. Billingham ME, Cary NRB, Hammond ME, Kemnitz J, Marboe C, McCallister HA, Snovar DC, Winters GL, Zerbe A: A working formulation for the standardization of nomenclature in the diagnosis of heart and lung rejection. J Heart Lung Transplant 1990;9:587–593.

16. Bolman RM, Elick B, Olivari MT, Ring WS, Arentzen CE: Improved immunosuppression for heart transplantation. Heart Transplant 1985;4:315–318.

17. Bonacina E, Recalcati F, Mangiavacchi M, Gronda E: Interstitital myocardial lipomatosis: morphological study on endomyocardial biopsies and diseased hearts surgically removed for heart transplantation. Eur Heart J 1989;10(suppl):100–102.

18. Bonnaud E, Lewis NP, Masek MA, Billingham ME: Reliability and usefulness of immunofluorescence in heart transplantation. J Heart Lung Transplant 1995;14:163–171.

19. Bonomini V: Value of plasma exchange in renal transplant rejection induced by specific anti-HLA antibodies. Trans Am Soc Artif Intern Organs 1982;28:599–603.

20. Bouchart F, Gundry SR, VanSchaack-Gonzales J, Razzouk AJ, Marsa RJ, Kawauchi M, AlonsodeBegona J, Bailey LL: Methotrexate as rescue/adjunctive immunotherapy in infant and adult heart transplantation. J Heart Lung Transplant 1993;12:427–433.

21. Bourge RC, Kirklin JK, Naftel DC, White-Williams CW, George JF, Morrow R, Tarkka M, Welborn JM: Methotrexate pulse therapy in the treatment of recurrent acute heart rejection. J Heart Lung Transplant 1992;11:1116–1124.

22. Brasile L, Zerbe T, Rabin B, Clarke J, Abrams A, Cerilli J: Identification of the antibody to vascular endothelial cells in patients undergoing cardiac transplantation. Transplantation 1985;40:672.

23. Braunlin EA, Canter CE, Olivari MT, Ring WS, Spray TL, Bolman RM: Rejection and infection after pediatric cardiac transplantation. Ann Thorac Surg 1990;49:385–390.

24. Breisblatt WM, Schulman DS, Stein K, Wolfe CJ, Whiteside T, Kormos R, Hardesty RL: Hemodynamic response to OKT3 in orthotopic heart transplant recipients: evidence of reversible myocardial dysfunction. J Heart Lung Transplant 1991;10:359.

25. Briscoe DM, Yeung AC, Schoen FJ, Allred EM, Stavrakis G, Ganz P, Cotran RS, Pober JS, Schoen EL: Predictive value of inducible endothelial cell adhesion molecule expression for acute rejection of human cardiac allografts [published erratum appears in Transplantation 1995 Mar 27,59(6):928]. Transplantation 1995;59:204–211.

26. Briscoe DM, Alexander SI, Lichtman AH: Interactions between T lymphocytes and endothelial cells in allograft rejection. Curr Opin Immunol 1998;10:525–531.

27. Canby RC, Evanochko WT, Barrett LV, Kirklin JK, McGiffin DC, Sakai TT, Brown ME, Foster RE, Reeves RC, Pohost GM: Monitoring the bioenergetics of cardiac allograft rejection using in vivo P-331 nuclear magnetic resonance spectroscopy. J Am Coll Cardiol 1987;9:1067–1074.

28. Carlquist JF, Hammond EH, Yowell RL, O'Connell JB, Anderson JL: Correlation between class II antigen (DR) expression and interleukin 2 induced lymphocyte proliferation during acute cardiac allograft rejection. Transplantation 1990;50:582.

29. Carrier M, Russel DH, Wild JC, Emery RW, Copeland JG: Prolactin as a marker of rejection in human heart transplantation. J Heart Lung Transplant 1987;6:290–292.

30. Caves PK, Stinson EB, Billingham ME: Serial transvenous biopsy of the transplanted human heart. Lancet 1974;2:821–826.

31. Cherry R, Nielsen H, Reed E, Reemtsma K, Suciu-Foca N, Marboe CC: Vascular (humoral) rejection in human cardiac allograft biopsies: relation to circulating anti-HLA antibodies. J Heart Lung Transplant 1992;11:24–29.

32. Cines DB, Lyss AP, Bina M: Fc and C3 receptors induced by herpes simplex virus on cultured human endothelial cells. J Clin Invest 1982;69:123.

33. Cladellas M, Abadal ML, Ballester M, Obrador D, Crexells C, Matias-Guiu X, Bordes R, Bonnin O: Endomyocardial diagnosis of cardiac lipomatosis. Cathet Cardiovasc Diagn 1988;13:2269–2270.

34. Cohnert TR, Kemnitz J, Haverich A, Dralle H: Myocardial calcification after orthotopic heart transplantation. J Heart Lung Transplant 1988;7:304–308.

35. Conrad SA, Chhabra A, Vay D: Long-term followup and complications after cardiac transplantation. J La State Med Soc 1993;145:217–210.

36. Copeland JG, Icenogl TB, Williams RJ, Rosado LJ, Butman SM, Vasu MA, Sethi GK, McDonald AN, Klees E, Rhenman MJ, Copeland JA, Wild JC, McCarthy M, Martinez JD, Christensen R: Rabbit antithymocyte globulin. A 10-year experience in cardiac transplantation. J Thorac Cardiovasc Surg 1990;99:852.

37. Cosson C, Myara I, Guillemain R, Amrein C, Dreyfus G, Moatti N: Serum prolactin as a rejection marker in heart transplantation. Clin Chem 1989;35:492–493.

38. Costanzo-Nordin MR, Grusk BB, Silver MA, Sobotka PA, Winters GL, OConnell JB, Pifarre R, Robinson JA: Reversal of recalcitrant cardiac allograft rejection with methotrexate. Circulation 1988;78(suppl):47–57.

39. Costanzo-Nordin MR, McManus BM, Wilson JE, OSullivan JE, Hubbell EA, Robinson JA: Efficacy of photopheresis in the rescue therapy of acute cellular rejection in human heart allografts: a preliminary clinical and immunopathologic report. Transplant Proc 1993;25:881–883.

40. Costanzo-Nordin MR, O'Sullivan JE, Johnson MR, Winters GL, Pifarre R, Radvany R, Zucker MJ, Scanlon PJ, Robinson JA: Prospective randomized trial of OKT3 versus horse antithymocyte globulin-based immunosuppressive prophylaxis in heart transplantation. J Heart Lung Transplant 1990;9:306.

41. Costanzo-Nordin MR, Winters GL, Fisher SG, O'Sullivan J, Heroux AL, Kao W, Mullen GM, Johnson MR: Endocardial infiltrates in the transplanted heart: clinical significance emerging from the analysis of 5026 endomyocaradial biopsy specimens. J Heart Lung Transplant 1994;13:733–734.

42. Couvreur J, Tournier G, Sardet-Frismand A, Fauroux B: Heart or heart-lung transplantation and toxoplasmosis. Presse Med 1992;21:1569–1574.

43. Crandall BG, Renlund DG, O'Connell JB, Burton NA, Jones KW, Gay WA, Doty DB, Karwande SV, Lee HW, Holland C, Menlove RL, Hammond E, Bristow MR: Increased cardiac allograft in female heart transplant recipients. J Heart Lung Transplant 1988;7:419–423.

44. Deen JL, Blumberg DA: Infectious disease considerations in pediatric organ transplantation. Semin Pediatr Surg 1993;2:218–234.

45. DeMaria R, Zuccelli QC, Masini S, Caroli A, Brando B, Gronda E, Donato L: Nonspecific increase of interleukin 2 receptor serum levels during immune events in heart transplantation. Transplant Proc 1989;21:440–441.

46. Deng MC, Bell S, Huie P, Pinto F, Hunt SA, Stinson EB, Sibley R, Hall BM: Cardiac allograft vascular disease. Relationship to microvascular cell surface markers and inflammatory cell phenotypes on endomyocardial biopsy. Circulation 1995;91:1647–1654.

47. Denys BG, Uretsky BF: Anatomical variations of internal jugular vein location: impact on central venous access. Crit Care Med 1991;19:1516–1519.

48. Ertel W, Reichenspurner H, Hammer C, Plahl M, Lehmann M, Kemkes BM, Osterholzer G, Reble B, Reichart B: Cytoimmunologic monitoring: a method to reduce biopsy frequency after cardiac transplantation. Transplant Proc 1985;17:204–206.

49. Esmore D, Keogh A, Spratt P, Jones B, Chang V: Heart transplantation in females. J Heart Lung Transplant 1991;10:335–341.

50. Fan PH, Kirklin JK, Naftel DC, Bourge RC, Nanda NC, White-Williams CW, Smith S: Application of echo color flow Doppler mitral regurgitation to the diagnosis of acute cardiac transplant rejection. Echocardiography 1992;8:169–174.

51. Faulk WP, Laberrere CA: Antithrombin-III in normal and transplanted human hearts: indications of vascular disease. Semin Hematol 1994;31:1.

52. Faulk WP, Laberrere CA, Pitts D, Halbrook H: Laboratory clinical correlates of time-associated lesions in the vascular immunopathology of human cardiac allografts. J Heart Lung Transplant 1993;12(suppl):125.

53. Ferran C, Peuchmaur M, Desruennes M, Ghoussoub JJ, Cabrol A, Brousse N, Cabrol C, Bach JF, Chatenoud L: Implications of de novo ELAM-1 and VCAM-1 expression in human cardiac allograft rejection. Transplantation 1993;55:605–609.

54. Fieguth HG, Haverich A, Schaefers JH: Cytoimmunologic monitoring for the invasive diagnosis of cardiac rejection. Transplant Proc 1987;19:2541–2542.

55. Fishbein MC, Bell G, Lones MA, Czer LSC, Miller JM, Harasty D, Trento A: Grade 2 cellular heart rejection: does it exist? J Heart Lung Transplant 1994;13:1051–1057.

56. Foegh ML: Eicosanoids and platelet activating factor mechanisms in organ rejection. Transplantation Proc 1988;20:1260–1263.

57. Foegh ML, Alijani MR, Helfrich GB, Khirabadi BS, Goldman MH, Lower RR, Ramwell PW: Thromboxane and leukotrienes in clinical and experimental transplant rejection. Adv Prostaglandin Thromboxane Leukot Res 1985;13:209–217.

58. Foegh ML, Khirabadi BS, Shapiro R: Monitoring of rat heart allograft rejection by urinary thromboxane. Transplant Proc 1984;16:1606–1608.

59. Foerster A, Simonsen S, Froysaker T: Morphological monitoring of cardiac allograft rejection. A 3-year followup. APMIS 1988;96:14–24.

60. Freimark D, Czer LSC, Aleksic I, Ruan XM, Admon D, Blanche C, Trento A, Fishbien MC: Pathogenesis of quilty lesion in cardiac allografts: relationship to reduced endocardial cyclosporine A. J Heart Lung Transplant 1995;14:1197–1203.

61. Fyfe B, Loh E, Wingers GL, Couper GS, Kartashov A, Schoen FJ: Heart transplantation-associated perioperative ischemic myocardial injury. Morphological features and clinical significance. Circulation 1996;93:1133–1140.

62. Gammie JS, Pham SM: Tacrolimus (FK506) in thoracic organ transplantation. In Cooper DKC, Miller LW, Patterson GA (eds): The Transplantation and Replacement of Thoracic Organs. Boston: Kluwer Publisher, 1996.

63. Gao SZ, Hunt SA, Wiederhold MA, Schroeder JS: Characteristiacs of serial electrocardiograms in heart transplant recipients. Am Heart J 1991;122:771–774.

64. Gaston JSH, Waer M: Virus-specific MHC restricted T-lymphocytes may initiate allograft rejection. Immunol Today 1985;6:237–241.

65. George JF, Kirklin JK, Shroyer TW, Naftel DC, Bourge RC, McGiffin DC, White-Williams CW, Noreuil T: Utility of posttransplantation panel-reactive antibody measurements for the prediction of rejection frequency and survival of heart transplant recipients. J Heart Lung Transplant 1995;14:856–864.

66. Gilbert E, DeWitt C, Eiswirth C, Renlund DG, Menlove RL, Freedman LA, Herrick CM, Gay WA, Bristow MR: Treatment of refractory cardiac allograft rejection with OKT3 monoclonal antibody. Am J Med 1987;1987:202.

67. Goldman MH, Lippman R, Landwehr D, Szentpetery S, Wolfgang T, Lee HM, Hess M, Mendez-Picon G, Hastillo A, Lower RR: Beta 2 microglobulin and the diagnosis of cardiac transplant rejection. Transplantation 1983;36:209–211.

68. Golino A, Duncan JM, Zeluff B, DePriest J, McAllister HA, Radovancevic B, Frazier OH: Leishmaniasis in a heart transplant patient. J Heart Lung Transplant 1992;11:820–823.

69. Grattan MT, Moreno-Cabral CE, Starnes VA, Oyer PE, Stinson EB, Shumway NE: Cytomegalovirus infection is associated with cardiac allograft rejection and atherosclerosis. JAMA 1989;261:3561–3566.

70. Grauhan O, Muller J, Warnecke H, Baeter HV, Cohnert T, Mansfeld H, Volk D, Fietze E, Gossel H, Hetzer R: Impact of apheresis and cyclophosphamide in the treatment of vascular rejection following heart transplantation. J Heart Lung Transplant 1994;13S:74.

71. Grauhan O, Knosalla C, Ewert R, Hummel M, Loebe M, Weng YG, Hetzer R: Plasmapheresis and cyclophosphamide in the treatment of humoral rejection after heart transplantation. J Heart Lung Transplant 2001;20:316–321.

72. Griffith BP, Kormos RL, Armitage JM, Dummer JS, Hardesty RL: Comparative trial of immunoprophylaxis with RATG versus OKT3. J Heart Lung Transplant 1990;13S:74.

73. Gulick T, Chung MK, Pieper SJ, Lange LG, Schreiner GF: Interleukin-1 and tumor necrosis factor inhibit cardiac myocyte beta-adrenergic responsiveness. Proc Natl Acad Sci U S A 1989;86:6753–6757.

74. Haberl R, Weber M, Reichenspurner H, Kemkes BM, Osterholzer G, Anthuber M, Steinbeck G: Frequency analysis of the surface electrogram for recognition of acute rejection after orthotopic cardiac transplantation in man. Circulation 1987;76:108.

75. Hachida M, Hoshi H, Maeda T, Koyanagi H, Takahashi K, Yoyama N: The rescue effect of FK506 in refractory rejection after cardiac transplantation. J Jpn Assoc Thorac Surg 1994;42:1972–1976.

76. Hagan ME, Holland CS, Herrick CM, and Utah Cardiac Transplant Program: Amelioration of weight gain after heart transplantation by corticosteroid-free maintenance immunosuppression. J Heart Lung Transplant 1990;9:382.

77. Hall TS, Baumgartener WA, Borkon AM, LaFrance ND, Traill TA, Norris S, Hutachins GM, Brawn J, Reitz BA: Diagnosis of acute cardiac rejection with antimyosin monoclonal antibody, phosphorus nuclear magnetic resonance imaging, two-dimensional echocardiography and endocardial biopsy. J Heart Lung Transplant 1986;5:4119–4424.

78. Hammer C, Reichenspurner H, Ertel W, Lersch C, Plahl M, Brendel W, Reichart B, Uberfuhr P, Welz A, Kemkes BM, Reble B, Funccius W, Gokel M: Cytological and immunological monitoring of cyclosporine treated human heart recipients. J Heart Lung Transplant 1984;3:4430–4443.

79. Hammond EH: Paathology of cardiac allograft rejection. In Cooper DKC, Miller LW, Patterson GA (eds): The Transplantation and Replacement of Thoracic Organs. Boston: Kluwer, 1996, pp 239–252.

80. Hammond EH, Hansen J, Spencer LS, Jensen A, Riddell D, Craven CM, Yowell RL: Vascular rejection in cardiac transplantation: histologic, immunopathologic, and ultrastructural features. Cardiovasc Pathol 1993;2:21.

81. Hammond EH, Yowell RL: Ultrastructural findings in cardiac transplant recipients. Ultrastruct Pathol 1994;18:213–220.

82. Hammond EH, Yowell RL, Nunoda S, Menlove RL, Renlund DG, Bristow MR, Gay WA, Jones KW, OConnell JB: Vascular (humoral) rejection in heart transplantation: pathologic observations and clinical implications. J Heart Lung Transplant 1989;8:4430–4443.

83. Hammond EH, Yowell RL, Price GD, Menlove RL, Olsen SL, O'Connell JB, Bristow MR, Doty DB, Millar RC, Karwande SV, Jones KW, Gay WA, Renlund DG: Vascular rejection and its relationshiip to allograft coronary artery disease. J Heart Lung Transplant 1992;11:111.

84. Havel M, Laczkovics A, Teufelsbauer H, Muller MM, Wolner E: Neopterine as a new marker to detect acute rejection after heart transplantation. J Heart Lung Transplant 1989;8:167–170.

85. Hayry P, Renkonen R, Leszenznski D, Mattila P, Tiisala S, Halttunen J, Turunen JP, Partanen T: Local events in graft rejection. Transplant Proc 1989;21:3716.

86. Herget S, Heemann U, Friedrich J, Kribben A, Wagner K, Philipp T: Initial experience with tacrolimus rescue therapy in OKT3 resistant rejection. Clin Nephrol 1996;1996:352–354.

87. Herskowitz A, Soule LM, Ueda K, Tamura F, Baumgartener WA, Borkon AM: Arteriolar vasculitis on endomyocardial biopsy: a histologic predictor of poor outcome in cyclosporine-treated heart transplant recipients. J Heart Lung Transplant 1987;6:127–136.

88. Heublein B, Wahler T, Haverich A: Pulsed steroids for treatment of cardiac rejection after transplantation. Circulation 1989;80 (suppl):97–99.

89. Higuchi ML, deAssis RV, Sambiase NV, Reis MM, Kalil J, Bocchi E, Fiorelli A, Stolf N, Bellotti G, Pileggi F: Usefulness of T-cell phenotype characterization in endomyocardial biopsy fragments from human cardiac allografts. J Heart Lung Transplant 1991;10:235–242.

90. Holliman R, Johnson J, Savva D, Cary N, Wreghitt T: Diagnosis of toxoplasma infection in cardiac transplant recipients using the polymerase chain reaction. J Clin Pathol 1992;11:820–3.

91. Hook S, Caple JF, McMahon JT, Myles JL, Ratliff NB: Comparison of myocardial cell injury in acute cellular rejection versus acute vascular rejection in cyclosporine-treated heart transplant. J Heart Lung Transplant 1995;14:351–358.

92. Hosenpud JD, Campbell SM, Mendelson DJ: Interleukin-1 induced myocardial depression in an isolated heart preparation. J Heart Lung Transplant 1989;8:460–464.

93. Hosenpud JD, Shipley GD, Morris TE, Hefeider SH, Wagner CR: The modulation of human aortic endothelial cell ICAM-1 (CD54) expression by serum containing high titers of anti-HLA antibodies. Transplantation 1993;55:405–411.

94. Hoshinaga K, Mohanakumar K, Pascoe EA, Szentpetery S, Lee HM, Lower RR: Expression of transferrin receptors on lymphocytes: its correlation with T helper/T suppressor cytoxic ratio and rejection in heart transplant recipients. J Heart Lung Transplant 1988;7:198–204.

95. Hoshinaga K, Mohanakumar T, Pascoe EA, Szentpetery S, Lower RR: Increase in trans-Ferring receptors as a marker for rejection and infection in human cardiac transplantation. J Heart Transplant 1988;7:198–204.

96. Hutter JA, Wallwork J, English TAH: Management of rejection in heart transplant recipients: does moderate rejection always require treatment? J Heart Lung Transplant 1990;9:87–91.

97. Ibrahim S, Dawson DV, VanTrigt P, Sanfilipp F: Differential infiltration by CD45RO and CD45RA subsets of T cells associated with human heart allograft rejection. Am J Pathol 1993;1142:1794–1837.

98. Jacquet L, Ziady G, Stein K, Griffith B, Armitage JM, Hardesty R, Kormos R: Cardiac rhythm disturbances early after orthotopic heart transplantation: prevalence and clinical importance of the observed abnormalities. J Am Coll Cardiol 1990;16:832–837.

99. Jarcho J, Naftel DC, Shroyer TW, Kirklin JK, Bourge RC, Barr ML, Pitts DG, Starling RC: Influence of HLA mismatch on rejection after heart transplantation: a multi-institutional study. The Cardiac Transplant Research Database Group. J Heart Lung Transplant 1994;13:583–596.

100. Johnson MR, Naftel DC, Hobbs RE, Kobashigawa JA, Pitts D, Levine TB, Tolman D, Bhat G, Kirklin JK, Bourge RC, and The Transplant Research Database: The incremental risk of female gender in cardiac transplanation: a multi-institutional study of peripartum cardiomyopathy and pregnancy. J Heart Lung Transplant 1997;16:801–812.

101. Joshi A, Masek MA, Brown BW, Weiss LM, Billingham ME: "Quilty" revisited: a 10 year perspective. Hum Pathol 1995;26:547–557.

102. Jutte NH, Daane R, Bemd JMG, Hop WCJ, Essed CE, Simoons ML, Bos E, Weimar W: Cytoimmunologic monitoring to detect rejection after heart transplantation. Transplant Proc 1989;21:2519–2520.

103. Kemkes BM, Schutz A, Englehardt M, Brandl U, Breuer M: Noninvasive methods of rejection diagnosis after heart transplantation. J Heart Lung Transplant 1992;11S:221–231.

104. Kemnitz J, Cohnert T, Schaefers JH, Helmke M, Wahler T, Herrmann G, Schmidt RM, Haverich A: A classification of cardiac allograft rejection. A modification of the classification by Billingham. Am J Surg Pathol 1987;11:503–515.

105. Kemnitz J, Cremer J, Gebel M, Uysal A, Haverich A, Uysal A, Heublein B, Wirth S: Some aspects of changed histopathologic appearance of acute rejection in cardiac allografts after prophylactic application of OKT3. J Heart Lung Transplant 1991;10:366–372.

106. Kemnitz J, Restrepot-Specht I, Haverich A, Cremer J: Acute humoral rejection: a new entity in the histopathology of heart transplantation. J Heart Lung Transplant 1990;9:447–449.

107. Keogh A, Macdonald P, Harvison A, Richens D, Mundy J, Spratt P: Initial steroid-free vs steroid-based maintenance therapy and steroid withdrawal after heart transplantation. J Heart Lung Transplant 1992;11:421.

108. Keogh A, Valentine HA, Humst SA, Schroeder JS, Oyer PE: Increased rejection in gender-mismatched grafts: amelioration by triple therapy. J Heart Lung Transplant 1991;10:375–341.

109. Keren A, Gillis AM, Freeddman RA: Heart transplantation rejection monitored by signal averaged electrocardiography in patients receiving cyclosporine. Circulation 1984;70S:123–129.

110. Kirklin JK, Bourge RC, Naftel DC, Morrow R, Deierhoi MH, Kauffman RS, White-Williams CW, Nomberg RI, Holman WL, Smith DC: Treatment of recurrent heart rejection with mycophenolate mofetil (RS-61443): initial clinical experience. J Heart Lung Transplant 1994;13:444–450.

111. Kirklin JK, Bourge RC, White-Williams CW, Naftel DC, Thomas F, Thomas JM: Prophylactic therapy for rejection following cardiac transplantation. A comparison of RATG and OKT3. J Thorac Cardiovasc Surg 1990;99:716–724.

112. Kirklin JK, George JF, McGiffin DC, Naftel DC, Salter MM, Bourge RC: Total lymphoid irradiation: is there a role in pediatric heart transplantation? J Heart Lung Transplant 1993;13:293–300.

113. Kirklin JK, Naftel DC, Bourge RC, White-Williams CW, Caulfield JB, Tarkka MR, Holman WL, Zorn GL Jr: Rejection after cardiac transplantation. Circulation 1992;86S:236–241.

114. Klanke D, Hammer C, Schulman DS: Reproducibility and reliability of cytoimmunologic monitoring of heart transplanted patients. Transplant Proc 1989;21:2512–2513.

115. Kobashigawa JA: Trends in immunosuppressive therapy with regard to cytolytic induction therapy and corticosteroid withdrawal. In Cooper DKC, Miller JM, Patterson GA (eds): The Transplantation and Replacment of Thoracic Organs. Boston: Kluwer, 1996.

116. Kobashigawa JA, Kirklin JK, Naftel DC, Bourge RC, Ventura HO, Mohanty PK, Cintron GB, Bhat G, and The Transplant Research Database: Pretransplantation risk factors for acute rejection after heart transplantation: a multiinstitutional study. J Heart Lung Transplant 1993;12:355–366.

117. Kobashigawa JA, Miller L, Renlund DG, Mentzer R, Alderman E, Bourge RC, Costanzo-Nordin MR: A randomized active controlled trial of mycophenolate mofetil in heart transplant recipients. Transplantation 1998;66:507–515.

118. Kobashigawa JA, Stevenson L, Brownfield ED, Gleeson M, Moriguchi JD, Kawata N, Minkley R, Drinkwater DC, Laks H: Corticosteroid weaning late after heart transplantation: relation to HLA-DAR mismatching and long-term metabolic benefits. J Heart Lung Transplant 1995;14:963.

119. Kobashigawa JA, Stevenson L, Brownfield ED, Moriguchi JD, Kawata N, Fandrich R, Drinkwater D, Laks H: Initial success of steroid weaning late after heart transplantation. J Heart Lung Transplant 1992;11:428.

120. Kobashigawa JA, Stevenson L, Moriguchi J: Is intravenous glucocorticoid therapy better than an oral regimen for asymptomatic cardiac rejection a randomized trial. J Am Coll Cardiol 1993;21:1142.

121. Kobashigawa JA, Stevenson L, Moriguchi J, Westlake C, Wilmarth J, Kawata N, Chuck C, Lewis W, Drinkwater D, Laks H:

Randomized study of high-dose oral cyclosporine therapy for mild acute cardiac rejection. J Heart Lung Transplant 1989;8:53.

122. Kobashigawa JA, Warner-Stevenson L: Noninvasive detection of acute cardiac allograft rejection. *In* Kapoor AS, Laks H, Schroeder JS, Yacoub MH (eds): Cardiomyopathies and Heart-Lung Transplantation. New York: McGraw-Hill, 1991, pp 293–303.

123. Koike K, Hesslein PS, Dasmahaptra HK, Wilson GJ, Finlay CD, David SL, Kielmanowicz S, Coles JG: Telemetric detection of cardiac allograft rejection. Circulation 1988;78S:106–112.

124. Konno S, Sekiguchi M, Sakakibara S: Catheter biopsy of the heart. Radiol Clin North Am 1971;9:491–510.

125. Kottke-Marchant K, Ratliff NB: Endomyocardial lymphocytic infiltrates in cardiac transplant recipients. Incidence and characterization [published erratum appears in Arch Pathol Lab Med 1989 Dec;113(12):1348]. Arch Pathol Lab Med 1989;113:690–698.

126. Kottke-Marchant K, Ratliff NB: Endomyocardial biopsy. Pathologic findings in cardiac transplant recipients. Pathol Annu 1990;225:211–244.

127. Kubo SH, Naftel DC, Mills RM, O'Donnell J, Rodeheffer RJ, Vijay RR, Kenzora JL, Bourge RC, Kirklin JK, and The Transplant Research Database: Who is at risk for late recurrent rejection after cardiac transplantation? J Heart Lung Transplant 1994;13:S71.

128. Kubo SH, Naftel DC, Mills RM Jr, O'Donnell J, Rodeheffer RJ, Cintron GB, Kenzora JL, Bourge RC, Kirklin JK, and The Transplant Research Database: Risk factors for late recurrent rejection after heart transplantation: a multi-institutional, multivariable analysis. J Heart Lung Transplant 1995;14:409–418.

129. Kurland RJ, West J, Kelley S, Shoop JD, Harris R, Carr EA, Bergsland J, Wright J, Carroll M: Magnetic resonance imaging to detect heart transplant rejection; sensitivity and specificity. Transplant Proc 1989;221:2537–2543.

130. Labarrere CA, Pitts D, Halbrook HFWP: Tissue plasminogen activator, plasminogen activator inhibitor-1, and fibrin as indexes of clinical course in cardiac allograft recipients: an immunocytochemical study. Circulation 1994;89:1599.

131. Lacroix D, Kacet S, Savard P, Molin F, Dagano J, Pol A, Lekieffre J: Signal-averaged electrocardiography and detection of heart transplant rejection: comparison of time and frequency domain analyzes. J Am Coll Cardiol 1992;19:553.

132. Ladowski JS, Dillon T, Schatzlein MH, Peterson AC, Deschner WP, Beatty L, Sullivan M, Scheeringa RH, Clark WR: Prophylaxis of heart transplant rejection with either antithymocyte globulin, Minnesota antilymphocyte globulin, or an OKT3 based protocol. J Cardiovasc Surg 1993;34:135.

133. Lawrence EC: Diagnosis and management of lung allograft rejection. *In* Grossman RF, Maurer JR (eds): Pulmonary Considerations in Transplantation. Clinics in Chest Medicine. Philadelphia: WB Saunders Company, 1990, pp 369–378.

134. Lawrence EC, Holland VA, Young JB, Windsor NT, Brousseau KP, Noon GP, Whisennand HH, Debakey ME, Nelson DL: Dynamic changes in soluble interleukin-2 receptor levels following lung or heart-lung transplantation. Am Rev Respir Dis 1989; 140:7879–7896.

135. Lazda VA: The impact of HLA frequency differences in races on the access to optimally HLA-matched cadaver renal transplants. Transplantation 1992;53:352–357.

136. LeMense GP, VanBakel AB, Crumbley AJ, Judson MA: Mycobacterium scrofulaceum infection presenting as lung nodules in a heart transplant recipient. Chest 1994;106:1918–1920.

137. Libow LF, Beltrani VP, Silvers DN, Grossman ME: Post-cardiac transplant reactivation of Chagas' disese diagnosed by skin biopsy. Curtis 1991;48:37–40.

138. Little RE, Kay N, Epstein AE, Plumb VJ, Bourge RC, Neves J, Kirklin JK: Arrhythmias after orthotopic cardiac transplantation. Circulation 1989;80:140–146.

139. Lloveras JJ, Escourrou G, Delisle MB, Fournial G, Cerene A, Bassanetti I, Durand D: Evolution of untreated mild rejection in heart transplant recipients. J Heart Lung Transplant 1992;11:757–756.

140. Lones MA, Czer LS, Trento A, Harasty D, Miller JM, Fishbein MC: Clinical-pathologic features of humoral rejection in cardiac allografts; a study in 81 consecutive patients. J Heart Lung Transplant 1995;14:151–162.

141. Lonquist J, Radovancevic B, Vega J, Burnett CM, Birovljev S, Saade NG, Duncan JM, Frazier OH: Reevaluation of steroid taper-

ing after steroid pulse therapy for heart rejection. J Heart Lung Transplant 1992;11:913.

142. Lopez C, Simmons RL, Mauer SM, Najarian JS, Good RA: Association of renal allograft rejection with virus infections. Am J Med 1974;56:280–289.

143. Loy TS, Bulatao IS, Darkow GV, Demmy TL, Reddy HK, Curtis J, Bickel JT: Immunostaining of cardiac biopsy specimens in the diagnosis of acute vascular (humoral) rejection: a control study. J Heart Lung Transplant 1993;12:736–740.

144. Lund G, Letourneau JG, Day DL, Crass JR: MRI in organ transplantation. Radiol Clin North Am 1987;25:281–288.

145. Luthringer DJ, Yamashita JT, Czer LS, Trento A, Fishbein MC: Nature and significance of epicardial lymphoid infiltrates in cardiac allografts. J Heart Lung Transplant 1995;14:537–543.

146. Malafa M, Mancini MC, Myles JL, Gohara A, Dickinson JM, Walsh TE: Successful treatment of acute humoral rejection in a heart transplant patient. J Heart Lung Transplant 1992;11:486–491.

147. Maragreiter R, Fuchs D, Hausen A, Huber C, Reibnegger G, Spielberger M, Wachter H: Neopterine as a new biochemical marker for diagnosis of allograft rejection. Transplantation 1983;36:650–653.

148. McMahon JT, Ratliff NB: Regeneration of adult human myocardium after acute heart transplant rejection. J Heart Lung Transplant 1990;9:554–567.

149. Meiser BM, Uberfuhr P, Fuchs A: Single-center randomized trial comparing tacrolimus (FK506) and cyclosporine in the prevention of acute myocardial rejection. J Heart Lung Transplant 1998;17:782–788.

150. Meiser BM, Uberfuhr P, Fuchs D: Tacrolimus: a superior agent to OKT3 for treating cases of persistent rejection after intrathoracic transplantation. J Heart Lung Transplant 1997;17:795–800.

151. Mentzer R, Jahania MS, Lasley RD: Tacrolimus as a rescue immunosuppressant after heart and lung transplantation. Transplantation 1998;65:109–113.

152. Merrell SW, Ames SA, Nelson EW, Renlund DG, Karwande SV, Burton NA, Sullivan JJ, Jones KW, Gay WA: Major abdominal complications following cardiac transplantation. Arch Surg 1989;124:88–89.

153. Miller LW: Treatment of cardiac allograft rejection with intravenous corticosteroids. J Heart Lung Transplant 1990;9:2283.

154. Miller LW, Labovitz AJ, McBride LA, Pennington DG, Kanter K: Echocardiography-guided endomyocardial biopsy: a 5-year experience. Circulation 1988;78S:99–102.

155. Miller LW, Schlant RC, Kobashigawa JA, Kubo SH, Renlund DG: 24th Bethesda Conference: Cardiac Transplantation (Task Force 5: Complications). J Am Coll Cardiol 1993;22:41.

156. Miller LW, Wolford T, McBride LA, Peigh P, Pennington DG: Successful withdrawal of corticosteroids in heart transplant. J Heart Lung Transplant 1992;11:431.

157. Mills RM Jr, Naftel DC, Kirklin JK, VanBakel AB, Jaski B, Massin EK, Eisen HJ, Lee FA, Fishbein D, Bourge RC, and The Transplant Research Database: Heart transplant rejection with hemodynamic compromise: a multi-institutional study of the role of endomyocardial cellular infiltrate. J Heart Lung Transplant 1997;16:813–821.

158. Mohanakumar T, Hoshinaga K, Wood NL, Szentpetery S, Lower RR: Enumeration of transferrin-receptor-expressing lymphocytes as a potential marker for rejection in human cardiac transplant recipients. Transplantation 1986;42:691–694.

159. Morris RE, Hoyt EG, Murphy MP, Eugui EM, Allison AC: Mycophenolic acid morpholinoethylester (RS 61443) is a new immunosuppressant that prevents and halts heart allograft rejection by selective inhibition of T and B cell purine synthesis. Transplant Proc 1990;22:1659–1662.

160. Myles JL, Ratliff NB, McMahon JT, Golding LR, Hobbs RE, Rincon G, Sterba RW, Stewart R: Reversibility of myocyte injury in moderate and severe acute rejection in cyclosporine-treated cardiac transplant patients. Arch Pathol Lab Med 1987;111:947–952.

161. Nakhleh RE, Copenhaver CM, Werdin K, McDonald K, Kubo SH, Strickler JG: Lack of evidence for involvement of Epstein-Barr virus in the development of the "Quilty" lesion of transplanted hearts: an in situ hybridization study. J Heart Lung Transplant 1991;10:504–507.

162. OHair DP, McManus RP, Komorowski R: Inhibition of chronic vascular rejection in primate cardiac xenografts using mycophenolate mofetil. Ann Thorac Surg 1994;58:1311–1315.

163. Ohtani H, Strauss HW, Southern JF, Tamatani T, Miyasaka M, Sekiguchi M, Isobe M: Intercellular adhesion molecule-1 induction: a sensitive and quantitative marker for cardiac allograft rejection. J Am Coll Cardiol 1995;26:793–799.

164. Olivari MT, Kubo SH, Braunlin EA, Bolman RM, Ring WS: Five year experience with triple-drug immunosuppressive therapy in cardiac transplantation. Circulation 1990;82S:276.

165. Olsen SL, OConnell JB, Bristow MR, Renlund DG: Methotrexate as an adjunct in the treatment of persistent mild cardiac allograft rejection. Transplantation 1990;50:773–775.

166. Olsen SL, Yowell RL, Ensley D, Bristow MR, OConnell JB, Renlund DG: Vascular rejection in heart transplantation: clinical correlation treatment options, and future considerations. J Heart Lung Transplant 1993;12:S135–S142.

167. Oluwole SF, Tezuka K, Wasfie T, Stegall MD, Reemtsma K, Hardy MA: Humoral immunity in allograft rejection. Transplantation 1989;48:751–755.

168. Partanen J, Nieminen MS, Krogerus L, Harjula ALJ, Mattila S: Heart transplant rejection treated with plasmapheresis. J Heart Lung Transplant 1992;11:301–305.

169. Patel R, Roberts GD, Keating MR, Paya CV: Infections due to nontuberculous mycobacteria in kidney, heart, and lung transplant recipients. Clin Infect Dis 1994;106:1918–1920.

170. Peters M, Schurmann D, Mayr AC, Heterzer R, Pohle HD, Ruf B: Immunosuppression and mycobacteria other than Mycobacterium tuberculosis: results from patients with and without HIV infection. Epidemiol Infect 1989;103:293–300.

171. Picano E, DePieri G, Salerno JA, Arbustini E, Distante A, Martinelli L, Pucci A, Montemartini C, Vigano M, Donato L: Electrocardiographic changes suggestive of myocardial ischemia elicited by dipyridamole infusion in acute rejection early after heart transplantation. Circulation 1990;81:72–77.

172. Pickering JG, Bourhner DR: Fibrosis in the transplanted heart and its relation to donor ischemic time. Assessment with polarized light microscopy and digital image analysis. Circulation 1990;81:309–313.

173. Platt JL, Fischel RJ, Matas AJ, Reif SA, Bolman RM, Bach FH: Immunopathology of hyperacute xenograft rejection in a swine-to-primate model. Transplantation 1991;52:214.

174. Price GD, Olsen SL, Taylor DO, O'Connell JB, Bristow MR, Renlund DG: Corticosteroid-free maintenance immunosuppression after heart transplantation; feasibility and beneficial effect. J Heart Lung Transplant 1992;11:403.

175. Prieto M, Lake KD, Pritzker MR, Jorgensen CR, Arom KV, Love KR, Emery RW: OKT3 induction and steroid-free maintenance immunosuppression for treatment of high-risk heart transplant recipients. J Heart Lung Transplant 1991;10:901.

176. Pritzker MR, Lake KD, Reutzel T: Minneapolis Heart Institute Experience. J Heart Lung Transplant 1992;11:415.

177. Qiao JH, Ruan XM, Trento A, Czer LS, Blanche C, Fishbein MS: Expression of cell adhesion molecules in human cardiac allograft rejection. J Heart Lung Transplant 1992;5:307.

178. Radovancevic B, Frazier OH: Treatment of moderate heart allograft rejection with cyclosporine. J Heart Lung Transplant 1986;5:307.

179. Ragni T, Martinelli L, Goggi C, Speziali G, Rinaldi M, Roda G, Pederzolli C, Intili PA, Raisaro A, Vigano M: Echo-controlled endomyocardial biopsy. J Heart Lung Transplant 1990;9:538–542.

180. Reichart BR, Meiser BM, Vigano M: European multicenter tacrolimus (FK506) heart pilot study: one-year results—European Tacrolimus Multicenter Heart Study Group. J Heart Lung Transplant 1998;17:775–781.

181. Reichenspurner H, Kemkes BM, Osterholzer G, Reble B, Ertel W, Reichart B, Lersch C, Hammer C, Haberl R, Steinbeck G, Gokel J: Special control of infection and rejection episodes. Tex Heart Inst J 1986;13:5–12.

182. Renlund DG, Bristow MR, Crandall BG, Burton NA, Doty DB, Karwande SV, Gay WA, Jones KW, Hegewald MG, Hagan ME: Hypercholesterolemia after heart transplantation; amelioration by corticosteroid-free maintenance immunosuppression. J Heart Lung Transplant 1989;8:214.

183. Renlund DG, Gilbert E, O'Connell JB, Gay WA, Jones KW, Burton NA, Doty DB, Karwande SV, DeWitt C, Menlove RL, Herrick CM, Bristow MR: Age-associated decline in cardiac allograft rejection. Am J Med 1987;83:391–398.

184. Renlund DG, O'Connell JB, Gilbert E, Hammond ME, Burton NA, Jones KW, Karwande SV, Doty DB, Menlove RI, Herrick CM: A prospective comparison of murine monoclonal CD-3 (OKT3) antibody and equine antithymocyte globulin-based rejection prophylaxis in cardiac transplantation. Transplantation 1989;47:599.

185. Revel D, Chapeon C, Malhieu D, Cochet P, Ninet J, Chuzel M, Champsaur G, Dureau G, Amiel A, Helenon O, Vasile N, Cachera JP, Loisance D: Magnetic resonance imaging of human orthotopic heart transplantation: correlation with endomyocardial biopsy. J Heart Lung Transplant 1989;8:139–146.

186. Rhynes VK, McDonald JC, Gelder FB, Aultman DF, Hayes JM, McMillan RW, Mancini MC: Soluble HLA class I in the serum of transplant recipients. Am Surg 1993;217:485–489.

187. Rizeq MN, Masek MA, Billingham ME: Acute rejection: significance of elapsed time after transplantation. J Heart Lung Transplant 1994;13:862–868.

188. Roodman ST, Miller LW, Tsai CC: Role of interleukin 2 receptors in immunologic monitoring following cardiac transplantation. Transplantation 1988;45:1050–1056.

189. Rose AG, Cooper DKC, Human PA, Reichenspurner H, Reichart B: Histopathology of hyperacute rejection of the heart: experimental and clinical observations in allografts and xenografts. J Heart Lung Transplant 1991;10:223–234.

190. Rose AG, Uys CJ, Losman JG, Barnard CN: Evaluation of endomyocardial biopsy in the diagnosis of cardiac rejection. A study using bioptome samples of formalin-fixed tissue. Transplantation 1978;26:10.

191. Rose ML, Danskine AJ, Smith JD, Keogh A, Dureau G, Kobashigawa JA, Dunn MJ: Mycophenolate mofetil (MMF) depresses antibody production after cardiac transplantation [abstract]. Circulation 2000;102:II-490.

192. Rosenberg PB, Drazner MH, Dimaio JM, Kaiser PA, Meyer DM, Ring WS, Yancy CW: Induction with basiliximab preserves renal function following cardiac transplantation [abstract]. Circulation 2000;102:II-738.

193. Rosenbloom M, Laschinger JC, Saffitz JE, Cox JL, Bolman RM, Branham BH: Noninvasive detection of cardiac allograft rejection by analysis of the unipolar peak-to-peak amplitude of intramyocardial electrograms. Ann Thorac Surg 1989;47:407–411.

194. Ruan XM, Qiao JH, Trento A, Czer LS, Blanche C, Fishbein MC: Cytokine expression and endothelial cell and lymphocyte activation in human cardiac allograft rejection: an immunohistochemical study of endomyocardial biopsy samples. J Heart Lung Transplant 1992;11:1110–1115.

195. Rubin XM, Kurman CC, Fritz ME, Biddison WE, Boutin B, Yarchoan R, Nelson DL: Soluble interleukin-2 receptors are released from activated human lymphoid cells in vitro. J Immunol 1985;135:3172–3177.

196. Sakakibara S, Konno S: Endomyocardial biopsy. Jpn Heart J 1962;3:537–543.

197. Salter MM, Kirklin JK, Bourge RC, Naftel DC, White-Williams CW, Tarkka M, Waits E, Bucy RP: Total lymphoid irradiation in the treatment of early or recurrent heart rejection. J Heart Lung Transplant 1992;11:902–912.

198. Sands KEF, Appel ML, Lilly LS, Schoen FJ, Mudge GH, Cohen RJ: Power spectrum analysis of heart rate variability in human cardiac transplant recipients. Circulation 1989;79:76–82.

199. Sangrigoli RD, Eisen HJ: Recovery of left ventricular function is more delayed in non-cellular than cellular rejection [abstract]. Circulation 2000;102:II-817.

200. Schuurman HJ, Meyling FH, Wijngaard PL, vanderMeulen A, Slootweg PJ, Jambroes G: Endomyocardial biopsies after heart transplantation. The presence of immunoglobulin/immune complex deposits. Transplantation 1989;48:435–438.

201. Scott CD, Dark JH, McComb JM: Arrhythmias after cardiac transplantation. Am J Cardiol 1992;70:1061–1063.

202. Segal JB, Kasper EK, Rohde C, Bray PF, Baldwin WM, Resar JR, Hruban RH, Kickler TS: Coagulation markers predicting cardiac transplant rejection [abstract]. Circulation 2000;102:II-763.

203. Shaddy RE, Bulock EA, Tani LY, Orsmond GS, Olsen SL, Taylor DO, McGough EC, Hawkins JA, Renlund DG: Methotrexate therapy in pediatric heart transplantation as treatment of recurrent mild to moderate acute cellular rejection. J Heart Lung Transplant 1994;13:1009–1013.

204. Sheldon ST, Hasleton PS, Yonan NA, Rhaman AN, Deiraniya AK, Campbell CS, Brooks NH, Dyer PA: Rejection in heart transplantation strongly correlates with HLA-DR antigen mismatch. Transplantation 1994;58:719–722.

205. Sibley RK, Olivari MT, Ring WS, Bolman RM: Endomyocardial biopsy in the cardiac allograft recipient. A review of 570 biopsies. Ann Surg 1986;203:177–187.

206. Simmons RL, Well R, Tallent MB, Kjellstrand CM, Najarian JS: Do mild infections trigger the rejection of renal allografts? Transplant Proc 1970;2:419–423.

207. Simmons RL, Wang SC: New horizons in immunosuppression. Transplant Proc 1991;23:2152–2156.

208. Smart FW, Young JB, Weilbaecher D: Magnetic resonance imaging for assessment of tissue rejection after heterotopic heart transplantation. J Heart Lung Transplant 1993;12:403–410.

209. Smith JD, Danskine AJ, Pomerance A, Rose ML, Yacoub MH: The beneficial effect of HLA-DR matching on rejection episodes following cardiac transplantation. J Heart Lung Transplant 1993; (Abstract)12:76S.

210. Smith JD, Rose ML, Pomerance A, Burke M, Yacoub MH: The beneficial effect of HLA-DR matching on rejection episodes following cardiac transplantation. Lancet 1995;346:1318–1322.

211. Smith SH, Kirklin JK, Geer JC, Abadal ML, Caulfield JB, McGiffin DC: Arteritis in cardiac rejection after transplantatiaon. Am J Cardiol 1987;59:1171–1173.

212. Spiegelhalter DJ, Stovin PG: An analysis of repeated biopsies following cardiac transplantation. Stat Med 1983;2:33–40.

213. Stahl RD, Karwande SV, Olsen SL, Taylor DO, Hawkins JA, Renlund DG: Tricuspid valve dysfunction in the transplanted heart. Ann Thorac Surg 1995;59:477–480.

214. Stahl RD, Karwande SV, Olsen SL, Taylor DO, Hawkins JA, Renlund DG: Tricuspid valve dysfunction in the transplanted heart. Ann Thorac Surg 1995;59:477–480.

215. Studemeister AE, Kozak K, Garrity E, Venezio FR: Survival of a heart transplant recipient after pulmonary cavitary mucormycosis. J Heart Lung Transplant 1988;7:159–161.

216. Suit PF, Kottke-Marchant K, Ratliff NB, Pippenger CE, Easley K: Comparison of whole-blood cyclosporine levels and the frequency of endomyocardial lymphocytic infiltrates (the Quilty lesion) in cardiac transplantation. Transplantation 1989;48:618–621.

217. Swinnen LJ, Costanzo-Nordin MR, Fisher SG, O'Sullivan JE, Johnson MR, Heroux AL, Dizikes GJ, Pifarre R, Fisher RI: Increased incidence of lymphoproliferative disorder after immunosuppression with the monoclonal antibody OKT3. N Engl J Med 1990;323:1723.

218. Tanio JW, Basu CB, Albelda SM, Eisen HJ: Differential expression of the cell adhesion molecules ICAM-1, VCAM-1, and E-selectin in normal and posttransplantation myocardium. Cell adhesion molecule expression in human cardiac allografts. Circulation 1994;89:1760–1768.

219. Taylor DO, Barr ML, Radovancevic B: Randomized, multicenter comparison of tacrolimus and cyclosporine immunosuppressive regimens in cardiac transplantation: decreased hyperlipidemia and hypertension with tacrolimus. J Heart Lung Transplant 1999;18:336–345.

220. Tipping PG, Davenport P, Gallicchio M: Atheromatous plaque macrophages produce plasminogen activator inhibitor type-1 and stimulate its production by endothelial cells and vascular smooth muscle cells. Am J Pathol 1993;143:875.

221. Torry RJ, Labarrere CA, Torry DS, Holt VJ, Faulk WP: Vascular endothelial growth factor expression in transplanted human hearts. Transplantation 1995;60:1451–1457.

222. Trento A, Hardesty RL, Griffith BP: Role of the antibody to vascular endothelial cells in hyperacute rejection in patients undergoing cardiac transplantation. J Thorac Cardiovasc Surg 1988;95:37.

223. Valantine HA, Fowler M, Hatle L: Doppler echocardiographic indices of diastolic function as markers of acute cardiac rejection. Transplant Proc 1987;19:2556–2559.

224. Valantine HA, Hunt SA, Gibbons R, Billingham ME, Stinson EB, Popp RL: Increasing pericardial effusion in cardiac transplant recipients. Circulation 1989;79:603–609.

225. VanDorp WT, vanWieringen PAM, Marselis-Jonges E: Cytomegalovirus directly enhances MHC class I and intercellular adhesion molecule I expression on cultured proximal tubular epithelial cells. Transplantation 1993;55:1367–1371.

226. VanHoffen E, vanWichen D, Stuij I, deJonge N, Klopping C, Lahpor J, vandenTweel J, Gmelig-Meyling F, DeWeger R: In situ expression of cytokines in human heart allografts. Am J Pathol 1996;1149:1991–2003.

227. VonWilleban E, Petterson E, Ahonen J, Hayry P: CMV infection, class II antigen expression, and human kidney allograft rejection. Transplantation 1986;42:364–367.

228. Wagner FM, Reichenspurner H, Uberfuhr P, Weiss M, Fingerle V, Reichart B: Toxoplasmosis after heart transplantation: diagnosis by endomyocardial biopsy. J Heart Lung Transplant 1994;13:916–918.

229. Waldman WJ, Adams PW, Orosz CG, Sedmak DD: T-lymphocyte activation by cytomegalovirus-infected, allogeneic cultured human endothelial cells. Transplantation 1992;54:887–896.

230. Warnecke H, Muller J, Cohnert T, Hummel M, Spiegelsberger S, Siniawski HK, Lieback E, Hetzer R: Clinical heart transplantation without routine endomyocardial biopsy. J Heart Lung Transplant 1992;11:1093–1102.

231. Warnecke H, Schuler S, Goetze HJ, Matheis G, Suthoff U, Muller J, Tietze U, Hetzer R: Noninvasive monitoring of cardiac allograft rejection by intramyocardial electrogram recordings. Circulation 1986;74S:72–76.

232. Wechsler ME, Giardina EG, Sciacca RR, Rose EA, Barr ML: Increased early mortality in women undergoing cardiac transplantation. Circulation 1995;91:1029.

233. Weimar W, Essed CE, Balk ML, Simoons ML, Hendriks GF, Wenting GJ, Mochtar B, Bos E: OKT3 delays rejection crisis after heart transplantation. Transplant Proc 1989;21:2497–2498.

234. Wijngaard PL, Muelen A, Schuurman HJ, Gmelig-Meyling F, Heyn A, Borleffs JC, Jambroes G: Cytoimmunologic monitoring for the diagnosis of acute rejection after heart transplantation. Tranplant Proc 1989;21:25211–2522.

235. Wiklund L, Suurkula MB, Kjellstrom C, Berglin E: Chordal tissue in endomyocardial biopsies. Scand J Thorac Cardiovasc Surg 1994;28:13–18.

236. Winters GL: The pathology of heart allograft rejection. Arch Pathol Lab Med 1991;115:266–272.

237. Wisenberg G, Pflugfelder PW, Kostuck WJ, McKenzie FN, Prato FS: Diagnostic applicability of magnetic resonance imaging in assessing human cardiac allograft rejection. Am J Cardiol 1987;60:1130–1136.

238. Wollnek G, Laufer G, Laczkovis A, Buxbaum P, Kober I: Comparison of monoclonal anti-T-cell antibody vs ATG as prophylaxis after heart transplantation. Tranplant Proc 1989;21:2499.

239. Womble JR, Larson DF, Copeland JG, Russel DH: Urinary polyamine levels are markers of altered T lymphocyte proliferation/loss and rejection in heart transplant recipients. Tranplant Proc 1984;16:1573–1575.

240. Yacoub MH, Aalivizatos P, Khaghani A, Mitchell A: The use of cyclosporin, azathioprine, and antithymocyte globulin with or without low-dose steroids for immunosuppression of cardiac transplant patients. Tranplant Proc 1985;17:221.

241. Yeoh TK, Frist WHY, Eastburn TE, Atkinson J: Clinical significance of mild rejection of the cardiac allograft. Circulation 1992;86:2267–2271.

242. Zales VR, Crawford S, Backer CL, Lynch P, Benson DW, Mavroudis C: Spectrum of humoral rejection after pediatric heart transplantation. J Heart Lung Transplant 1993;12:563–571.

243. Zerbe TR, Arena VC, Kormos RL, Griffith BP, Hardesty RL, Duquesnoy RJ: Histocompatibility and other risk factors for histological rejection of human cardiac allografts during the first three months following transplantation. Transplantation 1991;52:485–490.

244. Zhou YC, Cecka CM: Effect of HLA matching on renal transplant survival. In Terasaki PI (ed): Clinical Transplants. Los Angeles: UCLA Tissue Typing Laboratory, 1993, p 499.

245. Zucker K, Rosen A, Tsaroucha A: Unexpected augmentation of mycophenolic acid pharmacokinetics in renal transplant patients receiving tacrolimus and mycophenolate mofetil in combination therapy, and analogous in vitro finding. Transplant Immunol 1997;5:225–232.

246. Zucker K, Tsaroucha A, Olson L, Esquenazi V, Tzakis A, Miller J: Evidence that tacrolimus augments the bioavailability of mycophenolate mofetil through the inhibition of mycophenolic acid glucuronidation. Ther Drug Monit 1999;21:35–43.

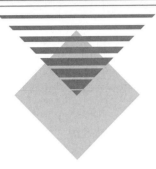

CHAPTER FIFTEEN

Infections After Heart (and Heart/Lung) Transplantation

with the collaboration of
ROBIN K. AVERY, M.D. AND PETER G. PAPPAS, M.D.

Infections after organ transplantation result in so much of the work load of transplantation, both in terms of the incidence of infectious complications and diagnostic and therapeutic complexity, that a solid understanding of infection should be an important component of the knowledge base of all transplant physicians and surgeons. Infectious complications pervade

transplantation for a number of reasons[375]: (1) a broad range of organisms may be involved in infectious disease, including the usual pathogenic organisms, organisms that are not usually pathogenic except in immunocompromised hosts, endogenous organisms, and donor-transmitted infectious disease; (2) the presentation of infectious disease in immunocompromised patients may be atypical because of blunted signs and symptoms due to the effect of immunosuppression on the inflammatory response resulting in a delay in diagnosis and institution of therapy; consequently, a diagnostically and therapeutically aggressive policy is required for the diagnosis of infectious disease in immunocompromised patients; (3) infections are not only important because of the syndromes that they cause but also indirectly through modulation of the immune response, injury to the transplanted organs, and malignant transformation; and (4) infection and rejection are not mutually exclusive conditions, since treatment of rejection may precipitate infectious complications, and certain infections, especially immunomodulating viruses such as cytomegalovirus may precipitate the rejection process.

The **immunocompromised host** is a term that refers to patients whose natural and/or specific immunity to infection is impaired[483] and in the context of transplantation refers to impaired host defenses due to iatrogenic immunosuppression. These patients are susceptible to three major groups of infection[483]: (1) infection due to **true pathogens,** which are organisms with sufficient virulence to overwhelm the natural defense mechanism of a nonimmunocompromised host; (2) organisms that may colonize the mucocutaneous surfaces of the body, called **sometime pathogens,** which may cause infection when there is a breach in a mucocutaneous surface; and (3) organisms that do not present a risk to the normal host, called **nonpathogens,** due to the susceptibility of these organisms to nonspecific host defenses, but may cause infectious disease in immunocompromised patients.

Opportunistic infection is a term that refers to infectious processes in immunocompromised patients, not

521

only as a result of invasive infection due to nonpathogens, but also infections with sometime pathogens or true pathogens which may produce an illness that is different from that typically produced in a host with normal defense mechanisms.[483]

NORMAL HOST DEFENSE MECHANISMS

Maintaining freedom from infectious diseases is an enormous physiological challenge. Host defense mechanisms (Table 15–1) against microorganisms are a complex interplay between three major lines of defense.

EPITHELIAL AND MUCOSAL BARRIER

Epithelial and mucosal surfaces which are exposed to the external environment require mechanisms to defend against microbiological penetration. Skin defense mechanisms include exfoliation of the epidermis and the chemical milieu of the skin that is produced by the sebaceous glands and lactic acid in sweat which either inhibit growth of bacteria or promote colonization resistance (see Box).

The **lung** (which is an important site of infection after heart and heart/lung transplantation) has an elaborate system that maintains sterility in the airways. The mucociliary transport system, which is characterized by cilia that beat in a coordinated fashion within a layer of periciliary fluid, transports mucus. Particles that enter the alveoli are phagocytosed by alveolar macrophages and subsequently removed by mucociliary transport. Secretory immunoglobulin A (IgA) is also an important barrier to epithelial microbiological penetration by the prevention of bacterial adhesion to mucosal cells. Coughing and forced expiration is a means of mucus clearance

and is a secondary system to mucociliary transport for mucus mobilization. Even in immunosuppressed patients, the airways are quite resistant to colonization.

The **gastrointestinal tract** has luminal mechanisms that are a barrier to microorganisms, including gastric acid secretion, intestinal motility, and unconjugated bile acid, all acting to inhibit bacterial overgrowth. Urinary tract colonization is inhibited by the simple method of frequent voiding. Saliva and tears have lysozyme and lactoferrin, which have antibacterial properties.

After heart and heart/lung transplantation, there are many opportunities for these primary defense mechanisms to be breached, and epithelial and mucosal surface penetration by microorganisms are an important portal for microorganism entry and invasion.

IMMUNOLOGICAL DEFENSE

Immunological defense mechanisms are the second line of defense,[446] with a variety of humoral and cellular

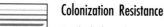

Colonization Resistance

Epithelial and mucosal surfaces are normally colonized by large populations of microorganisms, with each area having a distinct flora, determined by the specificity of organism adhesion to epithelial cells.[1, 39] The existing stable flora of a specific epithelial or mucosal area forms a barrier against entry of other microorganisms, a phenomenon known as colonization resistance,[447] which occurs because of the production of bacteriocins[386] and competition for nutrients.[195] The pattern of microbiological colonization is influenced by a multitude of factors such as diet,[272] diabetes,[272] cancer,[241] renal failure,[93] alcohol abuse,[272] pregnancy,[429] race,[9, 314] and the use of antibiotics.

TABLE 15–1	Host-Defense Mechanisms	
LINE OF DEFENSE	NONSPECIFIC	SPECIFIC
Surface defense (skin, mucous membranes)	Mechanical barrier Secretory barrier Ciliary motion Movement (ventilation, intestinal motility)	Immunoglobulins
Humoral defense	Complement system	Immunoglobulins
Cellular defense	Natural killer cells Interferons	Cell-mediated immunity (T-lymphocytes and macrophages)
Phagocytic defense	Neutrophilic granulocytes Eosinophilic granulocytes Mononuclear phagocytes Fibronectin Lysozyme and lactoferrin	

Modified from van der Meer JWM: Defects in host defense mechanisms. *In* Rubin R, Young L (eds): Clinical Approach to Infection in the Compromised Host. 3rd ed. New York: Plenum Medical Book Company, 1994.

components. With any infectious invasion, multiple components of the immune system may be rapidly activated. The components of the immune system are discussed in detail in Chapter 2 and are briefly summarized here.

Humoral Defense

Immunoglobulins have been discussed in detail in Chapter 2. In the context of infection, immunoglobulins interact with microorganisms through a number of processes including neutralization, agglutination of the antigen, complement activation and binding, opsonization, and prevention of epithelial and mucosal attachment of the antigen.[446] The extent to which each class of immunoglobulin performs these functions varies and can be demonstrated by the effect of immunoglobulin deficiency disorders. For example, deficiency of IgG (hypogammaglobulinemia) predisposes to infection with encapsulated bacteria (*Streptococcus pneumoniae*, *Haemophilus influenzae*, and *Neisseria meningitidis*[209, 397, 446]) enteric pathogens such as *Salmonella* and *Campylobacter*,[371] protozoal infections such as *Giardia lamblia*[319] and certain viral infections including poliovirus, echovirus, and rotavirus.[385, 482] Patients with IgA deficiency are at risk of recurrent respiratory infections.

In the context of defense against microorganisms, the **complement cascade** is activated by the alternative pathway prior to the development of a specific immune response, while the presence of a specific antibody response initiates the classical complement pathway.[446] Complement deficiency can be associated with an increased susceptibility to bacterial infection. For example, deficiency of terminal complement (C^6, C^7, C^8) has been associated with recurrent infection due to *Neisseria* species.

Cellular Defense

Effector T-cells are capable of killing virus-infected cells[446] and also participate in microbiological cellular defense by activating macrophages. Macrophages are generally unable to kill microorganisms until they are activated by cytokines released by the immune response cascade[304] (see Chapter 2).

Natural killer (NK) cells have the ability to kill certain virus-infected cells[202] without a requirement for antibody, complement, or the presence of major histocompatability antigens (see Chapter 2). Cell lysis occurs via a system that is similar to the membrane-attack complex of the complement cascade.[248]

The **interferons** are glycoproteins which consist of three main classes—α-interferon, β-interferon and γ-interferon.[446] α-Interferon and β-interferon are principally antiviral agents, whereas the role of γ-interferon is primarily immune modulation. The antiviral effects, which are not virus specific, are mediated by a number of actions which occur principally at the site of infection (Fig. 15–1).[446] The effect of the interferon appears to be locally at the site of infection.[446]

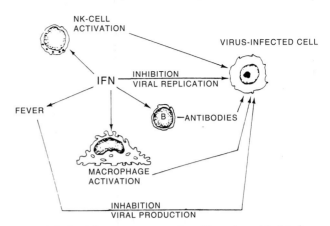

FIGURE 15–1. Schematic representation of the actions of the interferons (IFNs) (modified after a model proposed by Dr. H. Schellekens). No attempt has been made to separate the functions of the various types of interferons. (From van der Meer JWM: Defects in host defense mechanisms. *In* Rubin R, Young L (eds): Clinical Approach to infection in Compromised Host. 3rd ed. New York: Plenum Medical Book Company, 1994, with permission.)

Phagocytic Defense

The phagocytic cells are comprised of the neutrophil granulocytes, eosinophilic granulocytes, and the mononuclear phagocytes. **Neutrophils** arise from a bone marrow stem cell, and their differentiation and proliferation result from the interaction of a number of hematopoietic growth factors.[446] Once released into the circulation they exist as either circulating neutrophils or are attached to the vascular endothelium as a marginating pool of cells.[446] Endothelial adhesion molecules (Chapter 2) control the adhesion of neutrophils to endothelial cells, and the dynamics of the circulating versus marginated pool of neutrophils as well as neutrophil function is modulated by many factors associated with heart and heart/lung transplantation including the whole body inflammatory response to cardiopulmonary bypass, ischemia/reperfusion injury of the donor organs, and immunosuppressive agents (most notably glucocorticoids). **Eosinophils,** also derived from a bone marrow stem cell, are under the control of a number of hematopoietic factors, and they also have a role in cellular defense due to their participation in the inflammatory response.

Mononuclear phagocytes originate in the bone marrow and enter the circulation as monocytes, from which they subsequently differentiate into many different types of macrophages, depending on the tissue of residence (pulmonary macrophages, Kupffer cells in the liver, pleural macrophages, and histiocytes).[446] An intact monocyte-macrophage system is particularly important for cellular immunity against intracellular pathogens such as *Legionella, Salmonella, Listeria* and *Mycobacterium.*

Fibronectin is a globulin produced by hepatocytes[425, 446] and secreted on mucosal surfaces. It's major function in the context of infection is adherence of microorganisms to cells, promoting endocytosis (see Chapter 2).

Lysozyme (an enzyme found in polymorphonuclear phagocytes as well as other body fluids) interferes with cell wall synthesis, particularly that occurring in Gram-positive bacteria. Lactoferrin is a protein which inhibits the growth of Gram-negative and Gram-positive bacteria and also *Candida* by chelating iron.[446]

INFLAMMATORY RESPONSES TO INFECTION

There are a limited number of inflammatory responses to microbiological infection, and the pattern that occurs in an individual patient is a product of the interaction between the microorganism and the host defenses, which may be substantially modified by immunosuppression. These responses may be grouped into five major patterns, with considerable overlap.[382]

Suppurative (Polymorphonuclear) Inflammation

The hallmark of this inflammatory response is accumulation of neutrophils at the site of infection in response to chemoattractants released from pyrogenic bacteria. Depending on the virulence of the organism and the host response, there may be extensive tissue destruction and abscess formation.

Mononuclear and Granulomatous Inflammation

This pattern is characterized by a mostly mononuclear interstitial infiltrate as a response to infection by viruses, intracellular bacteria, spirochetes, intracellular parasites, and helminths. Accumulation of lymphocytes occurs in response to cell-mediated immunity against the organism or the organism-infected cell. Macrophages aggregate around a central necrotic focus and sometimes fuse to form giant cells, resulting in granulomatous inflammation, a response characteristic of slowly dividing infectious organisms.

Cytopathic-Cytoproliferative Inflammation

Certain viruses may damage cells without an accompanying inflammatory response. Viruses such as cytomegalovirus (CMV) or adenovirus may replicate within cells resulting in aggregates of viral material that form inclusion bodies. Measles virus and some herpes viruses may induce cells to fuse and form polykaryons, resulting in epithelial injury and blister formation. Papilloma virus and pox virus may cause epithelial cells to proliferate and produce lesions such as venereal warts or the papules of molluscum contagiosum.

Necrotizing Inflammation

Because of the release of powerful toxins from organisms such as *Clostridium perfringens,* severe tissue injury may occur which resembles ischemic necrosis. Viruses such as hepatitis B virus (HBV) may induce an immune-mediated response which causes necrotizing inflammation with widespread host cell damage.

Chronic Inflammation and Scarring

Chronic inflammation may be the end result of any form of inflammatory response, and the clinical consequence depends on the site and extensiveness of the fibrotic process.

HOST SUSCEPTIBILITY TO INFECTION

The susceptibility of a patient after heart or heart/lung transplantation to infection is a combination of a number of interacting factors which contribute to the "net state of immunosuppression,"[374] including immunosuppressive agents, age, comorbid disease (such as diabetes, malnutrition, hepatic dysfunction, renal dysfunction), integrity of the skin surfaces, and the presence of immunomodulating infections such as CMV and Epstein-Barr virus (EBV).

Immunosuppressive agents make the major contribution to the predisposition to infection after transplantation. The immunosuppressive properties of these agents are detailed in Chapter 13, and this section addresses their impact on infection.

Glucocorticoids have long been linked to an increased predilection for infection. Both the immunosuppressive effects and the anti-inflammatory effects of glucocorticoids increases susceptibility to infection as well as impairment of wound healing. Glucocorticoids reduce the accumulation of neutrophils at the site of inflammation due to reduced chemotactic activity.[475] The mononuclear phagocytic system is impaired by glucocorticoids because of reduced monocyte chemotaxis[368] and because of a reduction in the production of macrophages.[243] The T-cell activation cascade is blunted, leading to an impaired cellular response and also impaired antibody production. The lung is a major site of infection after transplantation, and glucocorticoids may contribute to this by inhibiting the function of alveolar macrophages.[146] In renal transplantation, a low-dose steroid regimen is associated with less infection than a high-dose steroid regimen.[457]

Cytolytic therapy with antilymphocyte serum and polyclonal or monoclonal antibodies can profoundly deplete circulating lymphocytes (see Chapter 13). This depression of cell mediated immunity has been associated with an increased incidence of CMV infection in heart[236] as well as other solid organ transplants.[205, 376]

There is considerable evidence linking the development of posttransplant lymphoproliferative disorder with EBV infection. The use of OKT3 has been associated with an increased incidence of posttransplant lymphoproliferative disorder,[423] which may be the result of primary or reactivated EBV infection.

Azathioprine, because of its inhibitory effect on purine nucleotide synthesis, impairs lymphocyte proliferation and results in decreased antibody production by B-cells, decreased cytotoxic T-cell proliferation, and impaired NK cell activity.[479] Azathioprine also causes leukopenia, further impairing cellular defenses.

Cyclosporine has powerful immunosuppressive effects which are mediated through its blocking action on antigen-induced T-cell expression, although cytotoxic T-cell function, NK cell function, and macrophage function is retained. Cyclosporine does not appear to result in significant infection complications when used in non-transplant patients, such as in the treatment of patients with ocular inflammatory disorders,[328] myasthenia gravis,[432] and diabetes.[27] When used as an immunosuppressive agent for organ transplantation, the use of cyclosporine does not appear to increase the risk of infection as much as azathioprine/prednisone with or without cytolytic therapy.[147] There is even some evidence that the incidence and severity of infection with cyclosporine-based immunosuppression (with lower doses of azathioprine and prednisone) is less than that with azathioprine/prednisone therapy.[35, 70, 71, 152, 291, 309]

Although infection is relatively common during methotrexate therapy, no doubt due in part to concomitant immunosuppressive therapy, the incidence of infection is not importantly increased following a course of methotrexate therapy.[51]

Although some controversy exists, an immunosuppressive protocol which includes mycophenolate mofetil does not appear to increase the risk of CMV over other agents (particularly azathioprine).[235, 244] However, a multicenter trial[244] did report an increased likelihood of viral opportunistic infections (herpes simplex and herpes zoster) in the mycophenolate mofetil group compared to azathioprine.

Use of plasmapheresis and photopheresis does not appear to increase the risk of infection. However, the possibility that plasmapheresis may reduce overall IgG levels and contribute to hypogammaglobulinemia should be considered.

GENERAL ASPECTS OF INFECTION IN THE TRANSPLANT PATIENT

TIME-RELATED NATURE OF INFECTION

Infection is an important cause of mortality and morbidity after heart and heart/lung transplantation, as it is with any patient receiving immunosuppression after

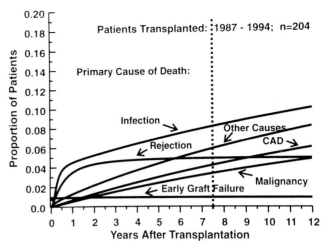

FIGURE **15–3.** Competing risk depiction of proportion of patients dying from each of a number of causes during time frame 1987 through June 1994. Dotted vertical line indicates that there is no follow-up beyond this time. CAD, coronary artery disease. (From McGiffin DC, Kirklin JK, Naftel DC, Bourge RC: Competing outcomes after heart transplantation: a comparison of eras and outcomes. J Heart Lung Transplant 1997; 16:190–198.)

solid organ transplantation.[216, 262, 297] A number of studies[17, 131, 186] have demonstrated a reduction in the incidence of infection in the current compared to earlier eras of transplantation. However, using a competing outcomes analysis (see Chapter 3) in a single institutional study, the proportion of patients dying of infection after cardiac transplantation in the 1981–1986 (Fig. 15–2) era was essentially the same as that in the 1987–1994 era[287] (Fig. 15–3).

Approximately 40% of patients suffer one or more infections during the first year following cardiac transplanation (Fig. 15–4).[297] Fortunately, most infections in

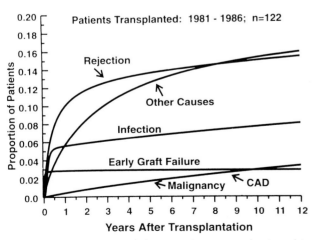

FIGURE **15–2.** Competing risk depiction of proportion of patients dying from each of a number of causes during time frame 1981 through 1986. CAD, coronary artery disease. (From McGiffin DC, Kirklin JK, Naftel DC, Bourge RC: Competing outcomes after heart transplantation: a comparison of eras and outcomes. J Heart Lung Transplant 1997;16:190–198.)

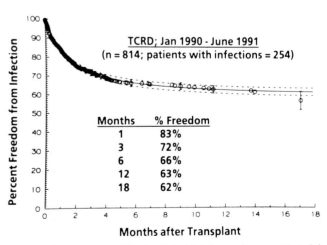

FIGURE **15–4.** Actuarial (Kaplan-Meier) (circles) and parametric (solid lines) depiction of freedom from first infection. Error bars indicate ± 1 standard error. Dashed lines enclose the 70% confidence limits around the parametric curve. TCRD, Transplant Cardiologist Research Database. (From Miller LW, Naftel DC, Bourge RC, Kirklin JK, Brozena SC, Jaracho J, Hobbs RE, Mills RM, and the Cardiac Transplant Research Database Group: Infection after heart transplantation: a multiinstitutional study, J Heart Lung Transplant 1994;13:381–393.)

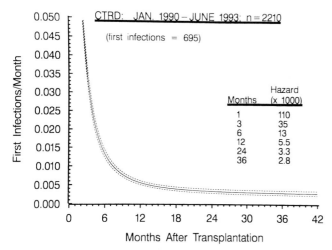

FIGURE **15–5.** Hazard function for initial infection. Dashed lines represent the 70% confidence limits. CTRD, Cardiac Transplant Researach Database. (From Smart FW, Naftel DC, Costanzo MR, Levine TB, Pelletier GB, Yancy CW, Hobbs RE, Kirklin JK, Bourge RC: Risk factors for early, cumulative, and fatal infections after heart transplantation: a multiinstitutional study. J Heart Lung Transplant 1996;15:329–341.)

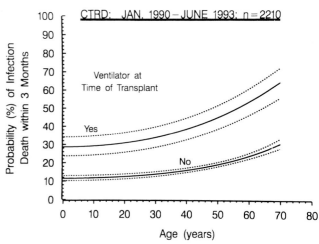

FIGURE **15–6.** Nomogram from the solution of the multivariate equation for time to first infection (see Table 15–2). Dashed lines represent the 70% confidence limits. "Yes" indicates patients receiving ventilator support at time of transplantation, "No" indicates no ventilator support. The variables in the equation are set such that ventricular assist device at transplantation = no; induction therapy = no; donor cytomegalovirus = negative. (From Smart FW, Naftel DC, Costanzo MR, Levine TB, Pelletier GB, Yancy CW, Hobbs RE, Kirklin JK, Bourge RC: Risk factors for early, cumulative, and fatal infections after heart transplantation: a multiinstitutional study. J Heart Lung Transplant 1996;15:329–341.)

the current era are successfully treated, as evidenced by only a 4% actuarial probability of death from infection at 6 and 12 months. Most infection episodes associated with heart and heart/lung transplantation are likely related to intensity of immunosuppression, and there is evidence[17, 363] that less intense immunosuppression is associated with less infectious complications. In a study by Smart and colleagues,[405] the risk for a first infection was highest during the first month after transplantation and then declined rapidly to merge with a constant risk of initial infection at approximately 10 months (Fig. 15–5). Risk factors identified for infection early after transplantation were older recipient age, ventilator support at the time of transplantation, ventricular assist support at the time of transplantation, the use of OKT3

induction therapy, and a positive donor CMV serology (Table 15–2).[405] The interaction between increasing recipient age and ventilator support at the time of transplantation is depicted in Figure 15–6. The greatest risk of death due to infection is approximately 2 months after transplantation, and this risk falls to a constant level at approximately 6 months (Fig. 15–7). Not surprisingly, many of the same risk factors identified for infec-

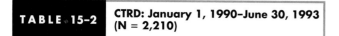

TABLE 15–2	CTRD: January 1, 1990–June 30, 1993 (N = 2,210)

	p VALUE	
RISK FACTORS FOR FIRST INFECTION	Early Phase	Constant Phase
Demographic		
Age (older)	<.0001	—
Clinical		
Ventilator at transplantation	<.0001	—
VAD at transplantation	.02	—
Induction therapy: OKT3	<.0001	—
Donor		
CMV (positive)	.0007	—
Black race	—	.0007

VAD, ventricular assist device; CMV, cytomegalovirus.
From Smart FW, Naftel DC, Costanzo MR, Levine TB, Pelletier GB, Yancy CW, Hobbs RE, Kirklin JK, Bourge RC: Risk factors for early, cumulative, and fatal infections after heart transplantation: a multiinstitutional study. J Heart Lung Transplant 1996;15:329–341.

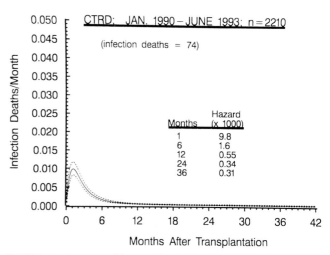

FIGURE **15–7.** Hazard function for infection as the primary cause of death. Dashed lines represent the 70% confidence limits. (From Smart FW, Naftel DC, Costanzo MR, Levine TB, Pelletier GB, Yancy CW, Hobbs RE, Kirklin JK, Bourge RC: Risk factors for early, cumulative, and fatal infections after heart transplantation: a multiinstitutional study. J Heart Lung Transplant 1996;15:329–341.)

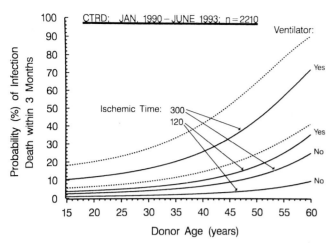

FIGURE **15-8.** Nomogram of the solution for the multivariate equation for death caused by infection. The variables in the equation are set such that recipient is a 55-year-old man and donor ischemic time of 120 and 300 minutes are displayed. The 70% confidence limits are shown only for the patient with ventilator support with 300 minutes of donor ischemic time (upper curve). (From Smart FW, Naftel DC, Costanzo MR, Levine TB, Pelletier GB, Yancy CW, Hobbs RE, Kirklin JK, Bourge RC: Risk factors for early, cumulative, and fatal infections after heart transplantation: a multiinstitutional study. J Heart Lung Transplant 1996;15:329–341.)

tion occurrence also predict early fatal infection; namely, older donor and recipient age, ventilator support at transplant, and longer donor ischemic time (Fig. 15–8). These analyses underscore the poorer tolerance of older patients for the ravages of prolonged cardiac dysfunction after transplant (more likely with longer ischemic times), with the associated periods of instrumentation in an intensive care unit and increased chance of invasive infection. The decreased ability of the older patients to withstand pneumonia (undoubtedly associated with prolonged intubation) is supported by the nomogram in Figure 15–6.

Following cardiac transplantation, bacterial infection is the most common type of infection (50%), followed by viral infection (40%), fungal infection (5%), and protozoal infection (5%).[297] Of the bacterial infections, approximately equal numbers are caused by Gram-positive organisms (50%) (75% due to staphylococci) and Gram-negative rods (40%).[297] In a multi-institutional study, the most common **sites of infection** during the first 18 months after cardiac transplantation were the lung (28% of all infections), blood stream (26%), gastrointestinal tract (17%), urinary tract (12%), skin (8%), and wound (7%).[297] Approximately 50% of pulmonary infections were bacterial in origin.

There is a quite distinct time course for the different infectious agents after cardiac transplantation (Fig. 15–9).[297] Bacterial infection is mostly likely to occur within the first month, typical of nosocomial infection in postoperative surgical patients. The peak incidence of viral infection at 2 months after transplantation reflects the time course of CMV and other herpes virus infections after transplantation. The peak incidence of fungal infection is within the first month after trans-

plantation, and the peak incidence of the very uncommon protozoal infection is delayed to 3–5 months. Despite all the changes in many facets of cardiac transplantation including immunosuppression and prophylaxis against infectious disease, the classic representation of the time course of infections after solid organ transplantation by Rubin[374] is still relevant (Fig. 15–10).

SCREENING OF POTENTIAL ORGAN DONORS FOR TRANSMISSIBLE INFECTIOUS DISEASE

Organ donors represent an important potential source of disease transmission to the recipient. Serologic testing of the donor is intended to minimize exposure of the recipient to potentially life-threatening donor infection without limiting the number of organ donors. Infectious disease screening encompasses not only the serological tests that are routinely performed (Table 15–3) on organ donors,[324] but also screening for possible transmission of bacterial infection.

Bacterial or Fungal Transmission

Transmission of bacterial infection to a recipient may occur through the contamination of the heart or heart/lung block during the procurement process, during transport, or as a result of donor bacterial infection. Contamination of the graft should be a very low probability event, but there are rare circumstances where this is more likely, such as inadvertent spillage of intraperitoneal infection into the pericardial cavity during procurement. The more likely source is a donor bacterial infection with blood stream involvement, such as pneumonia, cellulitis surrounding a traumatic injury, intra-abdominal sepsis from traumatic bowel injury, and

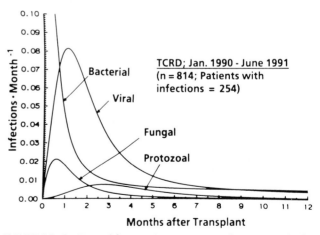

FIGURE **15-9.** Hazard function (instantaneous risk over time) for first infection of each major category of infectious agent. TCRD, Transplant Cardiologist Research Database. (From Miller LW, Naftel DC, Bouge RC, Kirklin JK, Brozena SC, Jaracho J, Hobbs RE, Mills RM, and the Cardiac Transplant Reaserch Database Group: Infection after heat transplantation: a multiinstitutional study. J Heart Lung Transplant 1993; 13:381–393.)

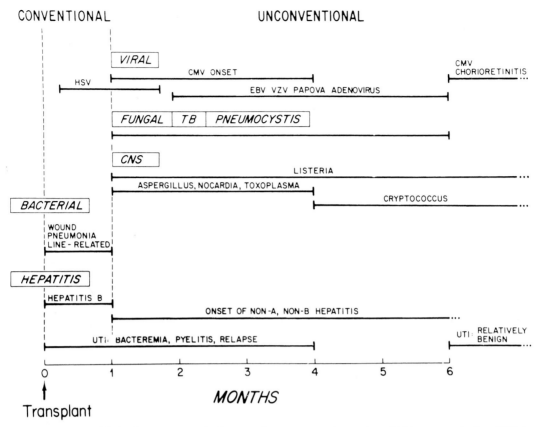

FIGURE **15-10.** Timetable for the occurrence of infection in the organ transplant patient. CMV, cytomegalovirus; HSV, herpes simplex virus; EBV, Epstein-Barr virus; VZV, varicella-zoster virus; CNS, central nervous system; UTI, urinary tract infection; Papova, papillomavirus; TB, tuberculous. (From Rubin RH: Infection in the organ transplant recipient. *In* Rubin R, Young L (eds): Clinical Approach to infection in the Compromised Host. 3rd ed. New York: Plenum Medical Book Company, 1994, pp 629–705.)

line sepsis. As part of the evaluation of a potential organ donor, blood cultures are routinely performed. Transmission of bacteria from donor to recipient with serious infective complications (especially invasive arterial infection) has been described: *Staphylococcus aureus* (renal transplant—arterial anastomotic rupture),[127] *Bacteroides* species (renal transplant—arterial anastomotic rupture), *Klebsiella* and *Enterobacter* species (renal transplant—rupture of the arterial anastomosis requiring nephrectomy),[463] *Pseudomonas aeruginosa* (renal transplant—arterial anastomotic infection requiring nephrectomy),[312]

TABLE 15-3	Routine Serology Screening of the Organ Donor

HIV antibody
HTLV-I antibody
Hepatitis B virus surface antigen (HBsAg)
Hepatitis B virus surface antibody (anti-HBs)
Hepatitis B virus core antibody (anti-HBc)
Hepatitis C virus antibody (HCV)
Cytomegalovirus antibody (CMV)
Treponemal antigen (syphilis)
Toxoplasma antibody
Epstein-Barr antibody

and *Escherichia coli* (renal transplant—fatal rupture of arterial anastomosis).[463] Transmission of fungi from donor to recipient has also been reported, including *Candida albicans* (pancreatic transplant—recipient intra—abdominal fungal infection,[40] and renal transplant—arterial anastomotic rupture requiring nephrectomy),[409] *Cryptococcus neoformans* (renal transplant—recipient urinary infection),[322] and *Histoplasma capsulatum* (renal transplant—fatal disseminated histoplasmosis).[273]

Despite these troubling reports, there are published reports of patients receiving contaminated kidneys (based on positive bacterial cultures from blood, urine, wound, or flush solution) with little or no evidence of posttransplant infection with the donor organism.[15, 45, 320] Several studies have demonstrated the safety of using organs from donors with positive blood cultures with no evidence of bacterial transmission and no difference in 30-day graft and patient survival compared with recipients receiving organs from nonbacteremic donors.[161, 257] It appears that the use of hearts or heart/lungs from donors with systemic infection appears relatively safe, but the risk can be minimized by administering a pathogen-specific antibiotic (or if the organism is unknown, broad-spectrum antibiotic coverage) for as long as is practicable in the donor and continuing that antibiotic (or antibiotics) for at least 10 days in the recipient.

The use of hearts or heart/lungs from donors who are brain dead due to bacterial meningitis can be a vexing question. The organisms most likely to be involved are *Haemophilus influenzae* (although becoming uncommon due to *Haemophilus influenzae* type B vaccine), *Streptococcus pneumoniae*, or *Neisseria meningitidis*.[356] Procurement after administration of a broad-spectrum cephalosporin (although *S. pneumoniae* resistance must be considered) is likely safe.

Heart/lung transplantation is a special situation where transmission of contaminated airways could result in recipient infection, but even in this seemingly high-risk situation, donor transmitted bacterial infection seems to be quite uncommon.[94] A related question is the significance of perioperative cultures from the donor heart and donor heart transport solution. A study by Mossad and colleagues[302] studied donor left atrial and transport fluid cultures and found no evidence that positive cultures increased the risk of recipient infection. The authors did, however, suggest that the growth of indolent organisms (coagulase-negative staphylococci, diphtheroids) can be discounted, but the growth of more virulent organisms should prompt a short course of specific antibacterial therapy, which seems prudent advice.

The finding of positive serology for **syphilis** in a donor does not contraindicate the use of the heart or lungs. There have been no cases reported in which syphilis has been transmitted from donor to recipient. There was one case reported where two kidneys were taken from a donor with syphilis and subsequently transplanted, but neither recipient developed syphilis following a course of penicillin.[175] The recipient should receive a posttransplant course of either benzathine penicillin 2.4 million units intramuscularly once weekly for 3 weeks or ceftriaxone 2 g daily for 14 days (based on the strategy for patients with late latent syphillis).

The heart or lungs from a donor with known *Mycobacterium tuberculosis* infection should **not** be used for transplantation. Disseminated tuberculosis from a donor source has occurred after renal transplantation[342] and unequivocal transmission of donor *M. tuberculosis* (confirmed by DNA fingerprinting) from donor to recipient has occurred following single-lung transplantation.[367]

Viral Transmission

Hepatitis B Virus Infection

The long-term consequences of renal transplantation in patients who are chronic carriers of hepatitis B surface antigen (HBsAg) is still a matter of controversy. There is evidence[330] that the risk of developing chronic liver disease in these patients is prohibitively high, and this contributed to the belief that HBsAg positivity is a contraindication to renal transplantation. However, other studies found no increase in the probability of liver disease[162] or only a very small difference in patient and graft survival in HBsAg-positive renal transplant recipients.[344] The study by Fornairon and colleagues[159] demonstrated that although there was no difference in survival between HBsAg-positive and HBsAg-negative renal recipients, there was a high rate of persistent viral replication (50%) and reactivation (30%), and a high frequency of histological deterioration (85%) accompanied by cirrhosis in 28% and by hepatocellular carcinoma in 23% of patients with cirrhosis. In a study by Kliem,[239] survival to 10 years was no different between HBsAg-positive and HBsAg-negative renal recipients, but after 10 years, survival was inferior in the HBsAg-positive patients, death most frequently occurring as the result of complications of hepatitis B. In renal transplant patients with allografts functioning for more than 20 years who were chronically infected with hepatotropic viruses (HBV and HCV), survival was inferior to that of uninfected patients, but long-term survival is still possible.[485] The increased mortality from liver disease in HBsAg-positive renal transplant recipients is most likely to occur in patients with persistent active viral replication (HBeAg and/or HBV DNA).

In a small series of HBV-infected heart transplant recipients,[66] all patients developed persistently abnormal liver function tests when followed up for 5 years. In another study of heart transplant recipients who acquired HBsAg positivity after transplantation, 56% of patients developed severe fibrosis/cirrhosis within a mean of 7.4 years after infection and 18% of deaths in HBsAg-positive patients were due to HBV-related liver failure. However, the impact on survival of patients with HBsAg positivity after heart transplantation is not apparent until beyond 10 years after transplantation (Fig. 15–11).[464] Although these studies do not deal with transmission of HBV infection from donor to recipient, the impact is almost certainly identical.

The serological tests for HBV infection in donors reflect the three antigen-antibody systems that are associated with the virus. Hepatitis B virus is a DNA virus of the hepadnavirus family. HBsAg is a protein associated with the surface coat of the virus. Hepatitis core antigen (HBcAg) is a protein in the inner core of the virus. HBe antigen (HBeAg) is a protein also associated with the inner core and is only found in patients that are HBsAg positive. The serologic assays for hepatitis B infections are sensitive and specific and are important clues to the stage of the disease (acute resolving infection, acute disease proceeding to chronic infection) (Fig. 15–12).[214] HBsAg indicates acute infection, and persistence for greater than 6 months usually indicates a chronic hepatitis B carrier state. **HBsAb indicates immunity to hepatitis B (vaccination produces HBsAb and not HBcAb positivity).** HBcAg cannot be detected in blood. A high titer of IgM HBcAb indicates acute hepatitis B, whereas a low titer implies ongoing hepatitis B–related chronic disease, usually chronic active hepatitis. IgG HBcAb with negative HBsAg indicates a past exposure to hepatitis B, whereas if it is associated with positive HBsAg, it indicates chronic hepatitis B. HBeAg indicates acute hepatitis B and, if it persists, indicates chronic infection. HBeAb is an indication of low infectivity. HBV DNA, which is a highly sensitive index of viral replication, indicates an ongoing infectious state.

Because of the important incidence of liver disease in heart transplant recipients with chronic hepatitis B

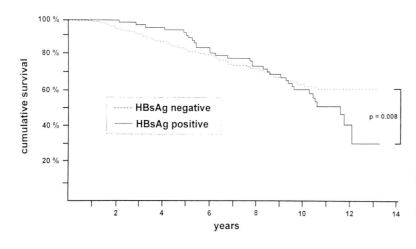

FIGURE **15–11.** Cumulative survival of heart transplant recipients with (n = 74) and without (n = 271) hepatitis B infection. Operation mortality was excluded, as only patients with at least 1 year of survival were included. Cumulative survival was significantly reduced after more than 10 years of follow-up. (From Wedemeyer H, Pethig K, Wagner D, Flemming P, Oppelt P, Petzold DR, Haverich A, Manns MP, Boeker KHW: Long-term outcome of chronic hepatitis B in heart transplant recipients. Transplantation 1998;66:1347–1353.)

infection, the **conservative approach is to avoid the use of organs from donors with evidence of hepatitis B infection, the only exception being donors who are HBsAb positive with a clear history of hepatitis B vaccination.** However, there are geographic areas such as Hong Kong and Saudi Arabia where the HBsAg carrier rate is very high and naturally occurring immunity to hepatitis B infection is as high as 40–50%. Living-related renal transplantation has been performed using HBsAg-positive HBeAg-negative donors into HBsAg-negative recipients without evidence of subsequent seroconversion or manifestation of liver dysfunction, although all recipients were given hyperimmune gammaglobulin at the time of transplantation.[86,89] Madayag[274] has demonstrated the safety of renal transplantation from IgG HBcAb–positive, IgM HBcAb–negative, HBsAg–negative donors into recipients with either a history of previous vaccination or hepatitis B virus infection, and this policy did not result in clinically detectable antigenemia or hepatitis B viral disease, although there was a significant incidence of hepatitis B seroconversion. A similar study reported[452] the outcome of the use of IgG

HBcAb-positive, IgM HBcAb-negative, HBsAg-negative donors in recipients of heart, liver, or kidney transplants (the majority being HBsAb- and HBcAb-negative). None of the HBsAb-negative, HBcAb-negative heart transplant recipients seroconverted, an identical finding to that in 12 heart transplant recipients in a similar study by Kadian.[229] However, although the use of IgG HBcAb-positive, IgM HBcAb-negative, HBsAg-negative donors for heart transplantation appears safe, it should be tempered by the finding[452] that three of six liver transplant recipients of similar donors became HBsAg-positive after transplantation. Furthermore, HBV-DNA has been demonstrated[129] in the serum and liver biopsies of IgG HBcAb-positive, HBsAg-negative donors, where HBV infection was transmitted to the liver recipient. The use of IgG HBcAb-positive, IgM HBcAb-negative, HBsAg-negative donors for heart transplantation should probably still be regarded as carrying a likely low but as yet uncertain risk of HBV transmission.

The use of a **HBsAg-positive donor for heart transplantation must be currently regarded as a procedure carrying a significant risk for HBV transmission.** How-

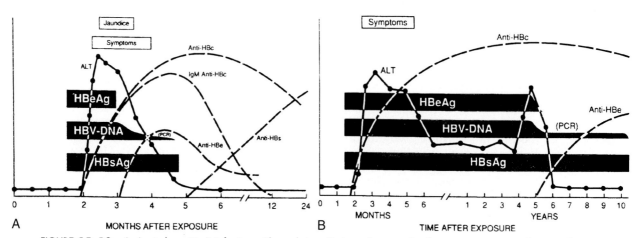

FIGURE **15–12.** *A,* Acute hepatitis B infection with resolution. *B,* Acute hepatitis B infection converting to chronic infection. (From Hoofnagle JH, Di Bisceglie AM: Serologic diagnosis of acute and chronic viral hepatitis. Semin Liver Dis 1991;11:73–83.)

ever, there are reports[257, 437] of HBsAg-positive donor hearts transplanted to serologically negative recipients using pre- and postoperative hepatitis B vaccine and hepatitis B immune globulin without subsequent HBV infection. This strategy must currently be regarded as experimental.

Hepatitis C Virus

After acute HCV infection, 75–80% of normal hosts develop chronic HCV infection with the development of active liver disease in 60–70% of these chronically infected patients, and 10–20% of these patients will develop cirrhosis over a period of 20–30 years. Hepatitis C infection after renal transplantation generally has a benign course,[416] but there are reports[87] of renal transplant recipients developing severe liver disease. The expected outcome of heart transplant recipients who contract HCV is uncertain. The study by Lake and colleagues[256] found no difference in survival between heart transplant recipients that were HCV positive compared with survival of a United Network of Organ Sharing (UNOS) control group. However, there was a 50% incidence of liver dysfunction, and a greater proportion of the deaths were due to liver disease in the HCV-positive group. There are anecdotal reports of cholestatic liver disease in heart transplant recipients leading to liver failure,[487] although it would appear that a relatively small percentage of HCV-negative recipients of HCV-positive hearts will develop progressive HCV liver disease.[339]

Ong and colleagues[321] reviewed the results of HCV antibody-negative cardiac transplant recipients receiving HCV antibody-positive donor hearts. Twenty-three of 28 patients developed detectable viremia, of whom 7 developed HCV-related liver disease. Four of the seven patients developed severe acute cholestatic hepatitis which contributed to a significantly poorer survival compared with those patients receiving hearts from HCV antibody negative donors.

Unfortunately, the diagnostic tests for HCV infection (see Box) have not always been sufficiently sensitive and specific. Using second-generation enzyme-linked immunoassay (EIA) tests to detect HCV exposure in organ donors, HCV transmission from donor to recipient should be rare. In Pereira's study,[340] the second-generation EIA assay was highly specific (98.1%). There is enough information for us to recommend that **transplantation of HCV-positive donor hearts to HCV-negative recipients should be avoided** unless it is the rare circumstance of a critically ill patient where bridging with a ventricular assist device is not possible,[82, 339] and with full disclosure to the recipient of the potential risks. It has also been suggested[346] that anti–HCV-positive donors be reserved for anti–HCV-positive recipients, a strategy that has not been fully evaluated.

Cytomegalovirus

The donor heart and heart/lung block is an important source of CMV infection in the recipient. The prevalence of CMV positivity in organ donors is between 40 and 80% depending on age, socioeconomic status, and geographic distribution.[113] All organ donors must have CMV serological status determined, as donor and recipient serological status defines risk groups for which prophylaxis and monitoring are indicated, with the highest risk group being those at risk for primary infection (CMV-positive donor to CMV-negative recipient). Because of the success of CMV prophylaxis and treatment, donor CMV-positive to recipient CMV-negative heart and heart/lung transplantation is not contraindicated. Ideally, organ donors should have blood drawn for CMV serology before blood or blood products are transfused, but this may not always be possible. The risk of an organ donor acquiring CMV from blood product transfusion is less than 1%.[113] If the organ donor blood is tested after donor transfusion, there is the possibility of a false-positive result because of passively transmitted anti-CMV antibody in the blood products.[113] CMV IgG antibody is the assay usually performed to screen for CMV in the organ donor, but CMV IgM antibody assay may be requested. Current evidence suggests that adding IgM assay to an IgG assay is unnecessary, since IgM anti-CMV will not be present if IgG antibody is absent.[116, 410]

Human Immunodeficiency Virus

Testing of donors for the human immunodeficiency virus (HIV) is mandatory, since transmission of HIV from donor to recipient has occurred after solid organ transplantation[134, 144, 399] most of these occurring prior to routine HIV-1 antibody screening in 1985. HIV transmission to a heart transplant recipient has also been reported[18] following transfusion of contaminated blood products during the procedure. A negative enzyme-linked immunosorbent assay (ELISA) for HIV in the donor is not a complete guarantee that HIV infection will not be transmitted to a recipient. If the testing is performed in the "window period" which lasts from several weeks to several months from the time of contraction of the infection to development of detectable HIV-1 antibody, the ELISA will be negative. Transmission of HIV infection

---

Diagnostic Tests for HCV

There are two means of detecting HCV infection—detection of antibodies to HCV by a serological assay, and tests detecting the presence of HCV RNA using a virological assay. The serological tests (anti-HCV) detect antibodies to HCV-specific proteins and include the EIA and the recombinant immunoblot assay (RIBA). The sensitivity and specificity of the serologic tests have improved with each generation (currently three generations). The virological tests include a polymerase chain reaction (PCR) assay to detect HCV RNA and the branched-chain DNA assay (b-DNA) in which the probe as opposed to the viral RNA is amplified to detect viral RNA. The major role of these virological assays is to confirm active viral replication and assess the therapeutic response.

from an organ donor with a negative HIV-1 antibody assay at the time of procurement to four solid organ recipients and 52 tissue recipients has been reported.[399] All solid organ recipients including the heart recipient became HIV-1 antibody positive. Donor frozen spleen cells were available for retrospective testing and HIV-1 was cultured and HIV-1 RNA was identified by PCR. Therefore, it is important that organ procurement coordinators obtain a detailed social history on the potential donor, and if a social risk factor for HIV is uncovered based on the Centers for Disease Control (CDC) criteria (Table 15–4)[80] in the face of a negative HIV-1 antibody assay, the heart or heart/lung block should not be transplanted unless the risk in a life-threatening situation on balance is in favor of transplantation. The recipient, however, must be informed by the transplant center of the possible risk of HIV infection with a negative HIV-1 antibody assay, but a positive social history.[83] Another possible way in which HIV can be transmitted from donor to recipient with a negative HIV-1 antibody assay is if the donor has received massive transfusion leading to a false-negative result, a situation that has been reported.[52] In the future, the use of the HIV p24 antigen (the core structural protein of the HIV virus) test for screening of organ donors will allow detection of HIV antigen within 30 days of exposure to the virus,[77, 122] prior to the development of an antibody response. The development of rapid testing for HIV viral load (HIV-RNA) will be even more sensitive than the p24 test.

Human T-cell Lymphotropic Virus Type I

Human T-cell lymphtropic virus type I (HTLV-I) infection may result in the subsequent development of adult T-cell leukemia and tropical spastic paraparesis. The latter condition has been linked to transmission of this virus by transfusion,[126] and therefore, UNOS policy is to not use organ donors who are HTLV-I positive. Interestingly, a survey[128] of Organ Procurement Organization practices found that, in fact, some would accept donors with positive HTLV-I antibody, presumably because although transmission of HTLV has been demonstrated with blood transfusion[422] it has not been clearly demonstrated with organ donation. In a life-threatening situation, a heart from a HTLV-I–positive donor could possibly be used. HTLV-II has also been associated with T-cell malignancies, but clinical studies of this infection have been hampered by the fact the HTLV-I and HTLV-II cross-react in standard serological assays.

Creutzfeldt-Jakob Disease

Creutzfeldt-Jakob disease (CJD) is an encephalopathy with a clinical picture of dementia, and the disease is progressive and ultimately fatal. It is caused by a prion and may have a long incubation period. The prion has been isolated from liver, kidney, and lung of humans.[26, 164] CJD has been transmitted through cadaveric-harvested growth hormone therapy[64] and cadaveric dura mater grafts.[76] A case was described[132] of a corneal graft being removed from a cadaver with CJD being confirmed at autopsy and was transplanted into a patient who died 18 months later of CJD. Mink encephalopathy (an animal model for CJD) has been demonstrated experimentally to be transmissible through corneal tissue.[276] Consequently, use of hearts and heart/lung blocks for transplantation from patients who have died from CJD is contraindicated. It is also important to consider the possibility of CJD in potential donors who have died with dementia or other neurological disorders of unknown etiology.

Rabies

Although rabies in humans is a rare disease, it should nevertheless be considered, given the circumstances of an animal bite and a neurologic death. Rare cases have been reported of transmission of rabies to recipients of corneal grafts[74, 75, 217] and therefore, donors with rabies should not be considered for organ donation.

Protozoan Transmission

Transmission of the protozoan *Toxoplasma gondii* from donor to recipient after cardiac transplantation is an important consideration, particularly since this parasite preferentially resides in muscle tissue. The demonstration of seropositivity for this organism in a donor does not contraindicate the use of heart or lungs, but can be used as a means of identifying recipients who have a toxoplasma mismatch and require prophylactic therapy after transplantation.

Malaria has been transmitted from donor to recipient,[438] and a history of malaria in a donor should generally contraindicate organ donation.

TABLE 15-4	**Social Risk Factors for HIV Infection* (Centers for Disease Control Guidelines)**

A. In the preceding 5 years:
   Men who have had sex with another man.
   Persons who report nonmedical intravenous, intramuscular, or subcutaneous injection of drugs.
   Men and women who have engaged in sex in exchange for money or drugs.
B. Persons with hemophilia or related clotting disorders who have received human-derived clotting factor concentrates.
C. In the preceding 12 months:
   Persons who have had sex with any person described in items A and B above or with a person known or suspected to have HIV infection.
   Persons who have been exposed to known or suspected HIV-infected blood through percutaneous inoculation or through contact with an open wound, nonintact skin, or mucous membrane.
D. Current inmates of correctional systems.

*Centers for Disease Control Guidelines. This social history presents an increased risk of HIV transmission despite negative serology screening of a potential organ donor.

POSTTRANSPLANT INFECTIOUS AGENTS

BACTERIAL INFECTIONS

Bacteria are the most common cause of infectious morbidity in cardiac transplant patients, particularly in the early posttransplantation period (i.e., the first 30 days). Wound infection, pneumonia, urinary tract, infection, and intravenous catheter-associated sepsis are most commonly secondary to bacterial agents during this early period. Overall, bacterial infections occur in over 40% of cardiac transplant recipients.[62, 135, 156, 211, 249, 297, 301, 343, 418]

Gram-Positive Organisms

Staphylococci

Staphylococcus species (Gram-positive cocci) including *S. aureus* (coagulase positive) and coagulase-negative staphylococci are the most common Gram-positive bacterial organisms causing disease in cardiac transplant patients.[301] *S. aureus* which is acquired in the community is usually methicillin-sensitive, although methicillin-resistant *S. aureus* (MRSA) can occur in this setting. Nosocomially acquired *S. aureus* infection may be due to MRSA, which appears to be an increasing problem. In a study of liver transplant recipients,[401] the incidence of MRSA infections has progressively increased and, when it is the cause of deep-seated bacteremic infections, there is a high associated mortality (86% in this study). There appears to be a greater risk of developing MRSA infections in CMV-seronegative recipients, and in those developing primary CMV infection. *S. aureus* infections early after heart or heart/lung transplantation usually manifest as wound infections (such as mediastinitis),[32] bacteremia from line sepsis, pneumonia, and urinary tract infection.[171] The presence of resistant *S. aureus* in the lungs of patients with cystic fibrosis who are undergoing heart/lung transplantation importantly increases the risk of posttransplant pulmonary infection.

The treatment of choice for methicillin-sensitive *S. aureus* is a semi-synthetic penicillin such as oxacillin or nafcillin. Alternatives include vancomycin or a first-generation cephalosporin such as cefazolin. For methicillin-resistant *S. aureus*, vancomycin (a tricyclic glycopeptide) is the first-line drug (Table 15–5). In the case of severe *S. aureus* infections, rifampin or gentamicin may be added. For wound infections, surgical debridement is usually required in addition to antimicrobial therapy. The doses of a variety of antimicrobial agents are listed in Table 15–6.

The incidence of *S. aureus* infections can be reduced by appropriate perioperative prophylactic antibiotics, strict attention to sterile technique in the operating room and during postoperative procedures, and prevention of line-related bacteremia by following published guidelines.[84]

Coagulase-negative staphylococcal infections after heart and heart/lung transplantation are similar to those caused by *S. aureus*. *S. epidermidis* (comprising 65–90% of all coagulase-negative staphylococcal species), is the most prevalent bacterial species on human skin and mucous membranes. Nearly all coagulase-negative staphylococcal infections are hospital acquired. Coagulase-negative staphylococci may cause wound infections and are particularly associated with line infections, likely due to the ability of these organisms to adhere to the surface of catheters. Nosocomially acquired coagulase-negative staphylococcal infections are usually resistant to methicillin and β-lactam antibiotics (see Box). Infections due to resistant coagulase-negative staphylococci tend to occur later in the hospitalization course than infections due to methicillin-sensitive coagulase-negative staphylococci.[142]

The treatment of choice for methicillin-sensitive coagulase-negative staphylococcal infection is oxacillin, nafcillin, or first-generation cephalosporins; and vancomycin should be used for methicillin-resistant coagulase-negative staphylococci. Patients with line-related sepsis due to coagulase-negative staphylococci can often be treated without catheter removal except in cases of tunnel infection, in which case removal is required to clear the infection. For patients with line related sepsis where the organism has not been identified, removal is recommended. Empiric therapy in these cases should include vancomycin because of possible coagulase-negative staphylococcal involvement. The in-

β-Lactam Antibiotics

β-Lactam antibiotics inhibit the synthesis of bacterial peptidoglycan, a critical component of the bacterial cell wall. Multiple side chains can be added to the basic β-lactam ring to produce different antibiotics. β-lactam antibiotics include the penicillins, cephalosporins, and carbapenems (including imipenem).

Resistance to β-lactam antibiotics stems from several mechanisms. Many bacteria produce enzymes called β-lactamases, which are capable of inactivating certain β-lactam antibiotics. The narrow specificity of these β-lactamases typically restricts their activity to certain penicillins or cephalosporins. Some bacteria are resistant to β-lactams because of the inability of the drug to penetrate to its intracellular site of action. The protein targets for the action of these antibiotics are called penicillin-binding proteins, of which there are a large variety. Some bacteria develop altered penicillin-binding proteins which have a lower affinity for the antibiotic.

The activity of some β-lactam antibiotics has been increased by combining them with β-lactamase inhibitors, which bind irreversibly to β-lactamases produced by gram-positive and Gram-negative bacteria. One such agent is clavulinic acid, which has been combined with amoxicillin as an oral agent (Augmentin) and with ticarcillin to produce Timentin. Others include sulbactam and tazobactam.

TABLE 15–5   Therapeutic Choices for Selected Infections in Cardiac Transplant Recipients

ORGANISM	FIRST CHOICE	ALTERNATIVE
Gram-Positive Bacteria		
Staphylococcus species		
Methicillin-susceptible	Nafcillin or oxacillin	Cefazolin
Methicillin-resistant	Vancomycin	Synercid or linezolid
Streptococcus species (e.g., beta-hemolytics streptococci and viridans streptococci)	Penicillin or ampicillin or clindamycin	Cefazolin or erythromycin
Streptococcus pneumoniae		
Penicillin-susceptible	Penicillin	Erythromycin or azithromycin or ceftriaxone
Pencillin-resistant	Vancomycin or ceftriaxone	Levofloxacin
Enterococcus species		
Vancomycin-sensitive	Ampicillin plus gentamicin	Vancomycin plus gentamicin
Vancomycin-resistant	Quinupristin/dalfopristin or linezolid	Ampicillin or gentamicin plus chloramphenicol
Listeria monocytogenes	Ampicillin usually with gentamicin	Trimethoprim/sulfamethoxazole
Nocardia species	Sulfisoxazole or trimethoprim/ sulfamethoxazole	Imipenem/cilastatin or cefotaxime
Gram-Negative Bacteria		
Initial therapy for gram-negative organisms (prior to identification)	Empiric therapy with an aminoglycoside and/or third-generation cephalosporin or higher level pencillin (ticarcillin, piperacillin) (specific therapy is based on susceptibility data)	Imipenem/cilastatin or quinolone
Legionella species	Erythromycin (with rifampin or levofloxacin or ciprofloxacin)	Azithromycin or clarithromycin
Mycobacteria		
M. tuberculosis	Isoniazid, rifampin, ethambutol and pyrazinamide (multi-drug regimens based on susceptibility data)	—
M. kansasii	Isoniazid, rifampin and ethambutol	—
M. avium-intracellulare	Ethambutol and clarithromycin	—
M. chelonae/fortuitum	Clarithromycin or ciprofloxacin	—
Viruses		
Cytomegalovirus	Ganciclovir*	Foscarnet
Herpes simplex virus		
Severe disease	Acyclovir and valacyclovir	Foscarnet
Mild-moderate mucosal disease	Acyclovir or valacyclovir	Famciclovir
Varicella zoster	Acyclovir	Valacyclovir or famciclovir
Human herpes virus-6	Ganciclovir	Foscarnet
Hepatitis B	Lamivudine (with or without IFN)	—
Hepatitis C	IFN alfa and ribavirin	—
Fungi		
Aspergillus sp.	Amphotericin B or lipid amphotericin	Itraconazole or caspofungin
Blastomyces dermatitidis	Amphotericin B	Itraconazole
Candida species		
Mucosal (oral or esophageal)	Fluconazole	Amphotericin B
Candidemia (uncomplicated)	Fluconazole	Amphotericin B
Candidemia with organ involvement	Amphotericin B plus flucytosine	Fluconazole
Pneumocystis carinii	Trimethoprim/sulfamethoxazole	Pentamidine, dapsone/trimethaprim, atovaquone or clindamycin/primaquine
Cryptococcus neoformans		
Complicated pulmonary and extrapulmonary	Amphotericin B ± flucytosine	Fluconazole
Uncomplicated pulmonary	Fluconazole	Amphotericin ± flucytosine
Coccidioides immitis		
Pulmonary	Fluconazole or itraconazole	Amphotericin B
Non-CNS extrapulmonary	Fluconazole or itraconazole	Amphotericin B
CNS	Amphotericin B	Fluconazole
Histoplasma capsulatum		
Pulmonary	Itraconazole	Amphotericin B
Disseminated (non-CNS)	Amphotericin B	Itraconazole
CNS	Amphotericin B	Fluconazole
Zygomycosis	Amphotericin B or lipid amphotericin	—
Parasites		
Toxoplasma gondii	Pyrimethamine and sulfadiazine plus leucovorin	Primaquine and clindamycin
Strongyloides stercoralis	Ivermectin or albendazole	Thiabendazole

IFN, interferon.

* May substitute valganciclovir (oral administration) for intravenous ganciclovir.

TABLE 15-6	Doses for Common Drugs Used to Treat Posttransplant Infections

DRUG*	DOSE Adult	DOSE Pediatric
Bacterial		
Ampicillin	1–2 g q 4–6 h IV	100–200 mg/kg/day IV in 4 divided doses
Azithromycin	500 mg PO qd	5–20 mg/kg/day PO or IV
Cefazolin	1 g IV q 8 h	50–100 mg/kg/day IV in 3 divided doses
Ceftriaxone	1–2 g IV q 12 h	50–75 mg/kg/day IV in 2 divided doses
Chloramphenicol	1 g IV q 6 h	50–75 mg/kg/day IV in 4 divided doses
Ciprofloxacin	500–750 mg PO (or 400 mg IV) q 12 h	—
Clarithromycin	0.5–1.0 g PO q 12 h	—
Clindamycin	600 mg IV q 8 h	25–40 mg/kg/day IV in 4 divided doses
Erythromycin	500–1,000 mg IV q 6 h	15–50 mg/kg/day IV in 4 divided doses
Gentamicin	1 mg/kg IV q 8 h (adjusted for renal function and blood levels)	Same
Imipenem/cilastatin	500 mg IV q 6 h	60–100 mg/kg/day IV in 4 divided doses
Levofloxacin	500 mg IV qd	—
Linezolid	600 mg IV q 12 h	—
Nafcillin	1–2 g IV q 4–6 h	100 mg/kg/day IV in 4 divided doses
Oxacillin	1–2 g IV q 4–6 h	100–150 mg/kg/day IV in 4 divided doses
Penicillin	2–4 million units IV q 4 h for most serious infections (1 million units q 4 h for mild infections)	100,000–200,000 units/kg/day IV in 4 divided doses
Quinupristin/dalfopristin	7.5 mg/kg IV q 8 h	Same
Sulfisoxazole	2 g PO qid	—
Vancomycin	15 mg/kg IV q 12 h (adjust for renal function and blood levels)	Same
Ethambutol	15–25 mg/kg/day PO	Same
Isoniazid	10–20 mg/kg/day PO (max dose 300 mg/day)	—
Pyrazinamide	15–30 mg/kg/day PO (max dose 2,000 mg/day)	Same
Rifampin	10–20 mg/kg/day PO (max dose 600 mg)	Same
Viral		
Acyclovir	5–10 mg/kg IV q 8 h for severe disease; dose for moderate disease depends on disease being treated	Same
Famciclovir	500 mg PO q 8 h	—
Foscarnet	60 mg/kg IV q 8 h	Same
Ganciclovir	See Table 15–8	Same
Interferon	Dose depends on disease	—
Lamivudine	100–300 mg PO qd	—
Valaciclovir	See Table 15–10	—
Fungal		
Amphotericin B	1.0–1.5 mg/kg/day IV	Same
Amphotericin B (lipid)	3.0–5.0 mg/kg/day PO (see Table 15–11)	Same
Fluconazole	200–400 mg/day PO or IV	6–12 mg/kg/day PO or IV
Flucytosine	100 mg/kg/day PO in 4 divided doses	Same
Itraconazole	100–200 mg PO bid	—
Pentamidine	4 mg/kg/day IV	Same
Parasitic		
Albendazole	400 mg PO qd × 3 days	—
Ivermectin	200 microgrms/kg/day PO × 2 days	Same
Leucovorin	10 mg/day PO	—
Pyrimethamine	50–100 mg PO bid on 1st day then 50–75 mg PO qd	2 mg/kg/day PO in 2 doses for 3 days then 1 mg/kg/day in 2 doses
Sulfadiazine	4–6 mg PO qd in 4 doses	—
Thiabendazole	20 mg/kg PO bid × 2 days	Same

*Drugs are listed alphabetically under each major category of infection. Doses may need adjustment with altered renal function.

cidence of nosocomial acquired staphylococcal infections can be reduced by proper infection control measures including strict hand washing (see later section, Infection Control) and contact isolation for patients with MRSA.

Enterococci

Enterococci (*Enterococcus faecalis, E. faecium, E. durans*) are Gram-positive facultative anaerobes that are impor-

tant pathogens in many immunocompromised patients, including those receiving heart and heart/lung transplants. Enterococci are constituents of the normal flora of the gastrointestinal tract, and infection in transplant recipients may be acquired either from their own flora or transmission from hospital staff or other sources within the hospital environment. Whereas infections in the general population are much more likely to be due to *E. faecalis,* in transplant recipients, particularly liver transplant recipients, *E. faecium* may be more common.[453]

Enterococcal infections occur most frequently in the first few weeks after cardiac transplantation and are most likely to manifest as wound infections, intravascular line infections, and urinary tract infections.[171, 211] Enterococci have the propensity for synergistic relationships with other organisms and hence are likely to be involved in polymicrobial infections, contributing to the significant morbidity and mortality associated with enterococcal infections. Of particular concern is the recent emergence of vancomycin-resistant enterococci (VRE) (usually *E. faecium*), which have become an important source of infection in many solid organ and bone marrow transplant recipients. In a study of enterococcal infections in organ transplant recipients (which included patients undergoing heart and lung as well as other solid organ transplants), enterococcal infections were associated with a 25% mortality, of which 50% were due to VRE infections.[384] Vancomycin-resistant enterococcal infections are particularly likely to occur in patients who have a complicated and prolonged postoperative course and particularly those patients who have invasive devices, have been treated for rejection, and have received antibiotics, especially vancomycin.[384] Vancomycin-resistant enterococci can be isolated in up to 75% of patients within 6 months of solid organ transplantation.[384]

Treatment of enterococcal infections may be particularly difficult because of frequent involvement in polymicrobial infections, antibiotic resistance (in particular vancomycin), and the difficulty in demonstrating antibiotic sensitivity.[143] For infections due to sensitive enterococci, the first-line antibiotic is ampicillin. For patients who are allergic to penicillin, vancomycin may be used (Tables 15–5 and 15–6). For intravascular infections, gentamicin should be added. The current recommendation for infections due to vancomycin-resistant enterococci is Synercid (quinupristin/dalfopristin), but these infections are notoriously difficult to treat and antimicrobial therapy may be ineffective. The recently approved anti–Gram-positive drug linezolid appears to have excellent activity against vancomycin-resistant enterococci. Alternative choices include ampicillin or gentamicin plus chloramphenicol. Removal of foreign material such as intravascular lines is critical.

Prevention of enterococcal infections, particularly glycopeptide-resistant enterococcal infections, requires scrupulous hand-washing procedures, thorough cleaning of patient rooms, and reverse barrier nursing of patients with enterococcal infections. The widespread use of prophylactic antibiotics in organ transplantation and empiric antibiotic therapy for infections is no doubt a contributing factor for the emergence of glycopeptide-resistant enterococci. An important preventative measure is limiting the use of antibiotics for both prophylaxis and empiric therapy.

Viridans Streptococci

Viridans streptococci (Gram-positive cocci) are a normal constituent of the flora in the oral cavity and in the upper respiratory tract and gastrointestinal tract. These sites may be the portal of entry into the circulation. Since viridans streptococcal bacteremia is most likely to occur during neutropenia, this infection is of particular importance in bone marrow transplant recipients and does not appear to be an important problem in solid organ transplant recipients.[143] The treatment of choice for viridans streptococci is penicillin (Tables 15–5 and 15–6), and vancomycin is the antibiotic of choice for penicillin-resistant strains.

Streptococcus pneumoniae

Bone marrow transplant recipients are at much greater risk of pneumococcal infection than solid organ transplant recipients, who are at increased risk of pneumococcal infection over the normal population. The most common manifesting syndromes are bacteremia, meningitis and pulmonary infection (including sinus infection and middle ear infection).[10, 263] Pneumococcal endocarditis has been described in a heart transplant recipient.[10] Pneumococcal infection is more likely to present as a community-acquired infection late after transplantation rather than during the transplant hospitalization. While most *S. pneumoniae* (a Gram-positive diplococcus) remain susceptible to penicillin, penicillin resistance occurs in up to 40% of strains, and these can usually be effectively treated with ceftriaxone (Tables 15–5 and 15–6). Cephalosporin-resistant *S. pneumoniae* have also emerged (15–20% in some areas), and for these infections vancomycin is the drug of choice.[306] The mortality associated with pneumococcal infection in solid organ transplant recipients is generally low, but the presence of blood stream invasion increases the risk. When sepsis due to penicillin-resistant pneumococci is a possibility, vancomycin should be included in the initial empiric regimen.

Listeria monocytogenes

Listeria monocytogenes (a Gram-positive bacillus) is a well-recognized pathogen in immunocompromised patients. It is a leading cause of bacterial meningitis in solid organ transplant recipients,[59, 198, 211, 412, 488] but appears to be most prevalent after renal transplantation. *L. monocytogenes* also causes other types of central nervous system (CNS) infection including cerebritis, encephalitis, and brain abscess.[413] Less common sites of primary involvement are blood and lungs. Most infections occur early after transplantation or during treatment for rejection. Stamm and co-workers,[411] in a review of 102 cases of listeriosis among renal transplant recipients, found that two thirds of patients presented with meningitis and/or parenchymal CNS disease and one third presented with primary bacteremia. Patients with listerial meningitis commonly present with fever, headache, meningismus, altered mental status, and, uncommonly, frank coma. Sixty percent of transplant patients with listerial meningitis have associated bacteremia. Parenchymal CNS disease may occur with or without associated meningitis. The most common presenting symptoms are a febrile illness and/or headache, with variable progression to altered mental state, coma, seizures, cranial nerve palsies, and hemiparesis or hemiplegia. Bacteremia occurs in 90% of cases. Seizure activity or focal neurologic findings necessitate computerized tomographic (CT) scanning or magnetic resonance imaging (MRI) to exclude an intracerebral abscess or other focal lesion. In patients with listeria meningitis, the cerebrospinal fluid (CSF) usually demonstrates a mixture of neutrophils and lymphocytes with an absolute white cell count of less than 1,000, an elevated CSF protein, and often decreased CSF glucose. *L. monocytogenes* will infrequently be seen on Gram stain of the CSF. The overall mortality for listeriosis in transplant patients is about 30%, with mortality approaching 50% in patients with parenchymal CNS disease.

The antimicrobial regimen of choice for listeriosis in the transplant patient is ampicillin (often in combination with an aminoglycoside) for at least 3 weeks to reduce the risk of relapsing disease (Table 15–5). In the penicillin-allergic patient, trimethoprim/sulfamethoxazole or imipenem are acceptable alternatives.

Listeriosis is often a food-borne illness associated with soft cheeses, certain dairy products, deli foods, and hot dogs. Listeria may survive in a cold environment such as a refrigerator, and thus it is important in educational programs to emphasize food preparation precautions, such as ensuring that leftovers are reheated to steaming hot and, if possible, avoiding foods such as soft cheeses, unpasteurized dairy foods, and deli foods.[424]

Nocardia

Nocardia species are aerobic Gram-positive rods with filamentous branching chains (actinomycetes). Infectious complications due to *Nocardia* species are relatively common among transplant patients, particularly cardiac and renal transplant recipients,[23, 261] although the incidence in heart transplant recipients appears to have fallen with cyclosporine-based immunosuppression.[211] Disease caused by *Nocardia* species may occur in a localized or disseminated form, the lungs being the most common site of localized disease, followed by skin, CNS, bone, joint, eye, and kidney.[398, 400, 478] Disseminated nocardiosis may rarely present as a subcutaneous or a primary soft tissue mass.[362] Overall, about 70% of patients have disease localized to one organ system (lung, skin, CNS, or bone and joint). Nocardiosis may occur at any time following transplantation, but most commonly occurs between the first and fourth months after transplantation. A prior CMV infection appears to increase the risk of developing nocardiosis.[91]

The clinical presentation is usually that of a subacute pneumonia, often with symptoms for 1 or more weeks. Symptoms include cough with thick, purulent sputum, pleuritic chest pain, shortness of breath, anorexia, weight loss, and hemoptysis. If CNS disease is present, the symptoms and signs are those typical of a brain abscess, with headache, nausea, vomiting, and changes in mental state. Soft tissue infection due to *Nocardia* may present as cellulitis, a lymphocutaneous form (cutaneous ulcer with nodular lesions along the course of lymphatics), or a mycetoma (nodular lesion with a draining fistula).[154] Nonfluctuant nodules are most commonly seen.

Radiographically, pulmonary infections usually manifest as solitary or multiple pulmonary nodules (often with cavitation), while lobar and segmental infiltrates occur less commonly. Central nervous system disease is usually manifest as a solitary intracerebral abscess, though multiple abscesses may occur (Fig. 15–13). However, even in the absence of neurological signs and symptoms, CNS imaging studies should be performed, since brain abscesses may be clinically silent.[413]

The histologic diagnosis depends on the finding of Gram-positive, branching filamentous organisms obtained either from culture or biopsy specimens.

Survival is the rule among transplant patients infected with *Nocardia* sp., provided the diagnosis is made early, but survival is less likely in patients with CNS disease. In a series of cardiac transplant patients[400] with nocardiosis, none died as a direct result of their infection. Importantly, none of the patients had developed clinically apparent CNS nocardiosis.

Treatment of *Nocardia* infections includes trimethoprim/sulfamethoxazole or a sulfonamide (see Box) alone. Alternative drugs include cefotaxime or imipenem/cilastatin. Duration of therapy should be prolonged, often 6 months or longer, depending on clinical response to therapy.

Clostridium difficile

Antibiotic-associated colitis secondary to *C. difficile* (a Gram-positive bacillus) has been reported after solid organ transplantation (including heart transplanta-

Sulfonamides

Sulfonamides bind the bacterial enzyme dihydropteroate synthetase by competing with *para*-aminobenzoic acid, resulting in prevention of folic acid synthesis and inhibition of nucleic acid formation. The term sulfonamides is a generic term which applies to any antibiotic which is derived from *para*-aminobenzene sulfonamide.

Bacterial resistance to sulfonamides has diminished the effectiveness of these agents in recent years. The potency of sulfonamides in the immunosuppressed patient is also diminished because these agents generally exert only a bacteriostatic effect, requiring cellular and humoral defense mechanisms for final eradication of the infection process. Bacterial resistance appears to originate largely from random mutations in the enzymatic makeup of the bacterial cell which alters the utilization of *para*-aminobenzoic acid.

The combination of **trimethoprim** and **sulfamethoxazole** provides an important added effectiveness because the two drugs act on sequential steps in the synthetic pathway for tetrahydrofolic acid. There appears to be an optimal ratio of the concentration of the two agents for maximal synergism, and the ratio of 20 parts of sulfamethoxazole to one part of trimethoprim appears optimal for the greatest number of microorganisms.

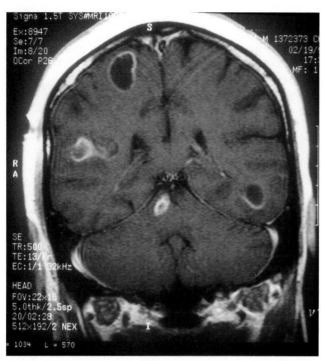

FIGURE **15–13.** MRI of the brain in a cardiac transplant recipient with CNS nocardiosis with typical multifocal abscesses involving both hemispheres and the cerebellum.

tion).[237] The source of *C. difficile* may be endogenous (part of the normal intestinal flora) or it may be transmitted nosocomially, due in part to selection of this organism by multiple antibiotics. The usual presentation is watery diarrhea and abdominal pain in a patient who is receiving a course of antibiotics. The diagnosis is made by the detection of *C. difficile* cytotoxin in the stool. If the diagnosis is uncertain, sigmoidoscopy may be helpful in demonstrating the typical mucosal changes with ulceration and pseudomembranes. Culture of the organism is less useful and more difficult than detection of the toxin. The treatment is withdrawal of the antibiotic and treatment with oral metronidazole 250–500 mg three times a day for 10 days. Oral vancomycin should be reserved for failure of metronidazole therapy.

Rhodococcus equi

R. equi is an aerobic Gram-positive coccobacillus whose natural habitat is soil and typically causes disease in horses, swine, and cows. Human infection with this organism usually involves the lungs, resulting in a febrile illness, cough, shortness of breath, and pleuritic chest pain. Chest x-ray typically reveals nodular opacities which may cavitate. This infection has been described in renal transplant patients[448] and has been reported in a cardiac transplant recipient[392] who was successfully treated by a course of intravenous vancomycin and ciprofloxacin followed by oral ciprofloxacin and amoxicillin-clavulanate.

Gram-Negative Bacilli

Aerobic Gram-negative bacilli are particularly important organisms in the immunosuppressed patient and are agents of pneumonia, wound infection, urinary tract infection, intra-abdominal sepsis, and primary bacteremia. The most common sources of Gram-negative pathogens in heart and heart/lung transplant recipients are the upper respiratory tract (*Haemophilus influenzae*) and gut (Enterobacteriaceae).[456] Another common source is colonization of the recipient prior to transplantation such as in colonization of the airways in patients with cystic fibrosis by Gram-negative bacilli including *Pseudomonas aeruginosa*, *Burkholderia cepacia*, and *Stenotrophomonas maltophilia*,[415] which may be multidrug resistant. Following heart/lung transplantation, pulmonary grafts may become contaminated by colonization of the trachea and paranasal sinuses. Prolonged ventilation and an indwelling urinary tract catheter are common sources of colonization–induced infection.

Infections with Gram-negative organisms are most likely to occur in the first 1–2 months after transplantation, at a time when immunosuppression is augmented (and hence neutrophil function, which is the primary defense against enteric Gram-negative bacilli, may be impaired) and when epithelial and mucosal barriers are most likely to have been breached. Likely infection syndromes include pneumonia, wound infection, urinary tract infection, and mediastinitis. Rarely, Gram-negative endocarditis or infection of the aortic suture line may involve the transplanted heart. The enteric Gram negative bacilli that are most frequently seen in heart transplant recipients are *Escherichia coli*, *Pseudomonas* spp., *Enterobacter* spp., *Serratia* spp., *Klebsiella* spp., *Proteus* spp., and *Citrobacter* spp.[297]

The treatment of infections due to Gram-negative bacilli can be based on susceptibility data, but empiric therapy should include an aminoglycoside (see Box) and/or an extended-spectrum penicillin with or without

Aminoglycosides

This group of antibiotics includes gentamicin, tobramycin, amikacin, kanamycin, streptomycin, and neomycin. The primary mechanism of action is inhibition of microbial protein synthesis. In contrast to most drugs which act by blocking protein synthesis (and are bacteriostatic), aminoglycosides are rapidly bactericidal. These agents are employed primarily to treat aerobic gram-negative bacteria. Mechanisms of bacterial resistance include mutations affecting proteins in the bacterial ribosome (the target for drug action), bacterial acquisition of plasmids that contain genes which code for enzymes that degrade aminoglycosides, and loss of ability to effectively transport the drug into the bacterial cell. All aminoglycosides possess the important potential for nephrotoxicity and ototoxicity (which can affect both the auditory and vestibular functions of the eighth cranial nerve).

a β-lactamase inhibitor. An alternative strategy is to primarily use an extended-spectrum penicillin with or without a β-lactamase inhibitor, a higher generation cephalosporin, a quinolone, a carbapenem, or a combination of the above and reserve aminoglycosides for use in synergistic combination for septic patients with *Pseudomonas*, for severely ill patients with suspected Gram-negative sepsis, resistant organisms, or severely β-lactam–allergic patients. Empiric antimicrobial therapy of nosocomial Gram-negative infections should be based on institution-specific susceptibility patterns.

Stenotrophomonas maltophilia

S. maltophilia is an uncommon but potentially serious cause of pneumonia and bacteremia associated with indwelling lines. The reported mortality with infection due to this organism is approximately 20%.[456] Therapy consists of trimethoprim/sulfamethoxazole alone or in combination with either minocycline or ticarcillin, since this organism is usually resistant to cephalosporins and aminoglycosides.[456] This organism also colonizes the airway of intubated patients and may colonize surgical wounds. Although the source of invasive infection with *S. maltophilia* is colonization, treatment of colonization with *S. maltophilia* is not advisable, since this organism is difficult to eradicate, resistance may increase, and prolonged antibiotics may precipitate a fungal infection.

Salmonella

Salmonellosis is a rare complication in solid organ transplant recipients, although their risk for developing *Salmonella* infection is much greater than the normal population. Whereas salmonellosis in the normal population presents as an intestinal infection, transplant recipients are more likely to have a secondary bacteremia, setting the stage for unusual presentations such as pneumonia, septic thrombophlebitis, osteomyelitis, and mycotic aneurysms.[456] Salmonellal empyema (successfully treated by decortication and ampicillin therapy)[44] and salmonellal arthritis[278] have been described in heart transplant recipients. It is important to note that salmonellosis is usually a food-borne illness, and food precautions should be emphasized to transplant patients (see later section, Prevention of Infection).[78] The antibiotic of choice for the treatment of salmonellosis is a quinolone, such as ciprofloxacin. Quinolones have broad antimicrobial activity, and development of resistance, although uncommon in the past, is on the rise. These agents act by inhibiting a bacterial enzyme called DNA gyrase, which mediates DNA supercoiling, a process required for bacterial growth.

Vibrio vulnificus

Vibrio vulnificus (part of the normal marine flora in estuaries around the United States Gulf, Atlantic, and Pacific coasts) is known to be pathogenic in patients with underlying chronic disease, particularly cirrhosis of the liver. It may cause primary sepsis from ingestion of contaminated seafood, soft tissue infection by direct inoculation, and gastroenteritis. A heart transplant recipient developed rapidly progressive cellulitis from this organism after a crab scratch, which required an amputation to control the infection.[8]

Legionella Species

Though potentially any *Legionella* species may cause pneumonia, *L. pneumophila* and *L. micdadei* have a particular proclivity for renal and cardiac transplant recipients.[160, 163, 215, 476] The source of *Legionella* is commonly a contaminated water source within the hospital. *Legionella* contamination of cold water intakes may set the stage for dispersion to hot water heaters and then through the plumbing system.[454] The clinical features of legionellosis are nonspecific, consisting of fever, myalgias and malaise, followed by dyspnea, cough, and pleuritic chest pain.[413] Watery diarrhea occurs in at least 50% of patients, and headache and confusion are common.[413] The physical signs are those associated with the pneumonic process. Chest x-ray findings are usually not distinctive and may consist of segmental, diffuse alveolar or nodular parenchymal lesions. Unilateral or bilateral involvement may occur, and cavitation can be seen in more advanced cases.

Definitive diagnosis of *Legionella* pneumonia is based on isolation of the pathogen from sputum or bronchial washings. It is noteworthy that *Legionella* is usually not visualized on a Gram stain. If a "conventional" sputum Gram stain and culture is ordered, the diagnosis will likely be missed. This fastidious pathogen requires special media (charcoal-yeast extract) for culture and is typically slow growing, usually taking 72 hours to grow. For this reason, a fluorescent antibody technique is often used on sputum or bronchial washings for rapid identification of *Legionella* antigen in these specimens. The recently licensed *Legionella* urine antigen assay is both sensitive and specific and has become the diagnostic assay of choice among patients with suspected acute disease with *Legionella pneumophila*. Serologic tests for *Legionella* sp. are available, but because of the typically slow response (weeks) in developing specific antibody and the need to obtain acute and convalescent sera, the diagnostic usefulness of these assays in acutely ill patients is limited.

Erythromycin (a macrolide) is the drug of choice for *Legionella* sp. infections (Table 15–5). Before erythromycin therapy, 80% of renal transplant patients with *L. pneumophila* died.[277] Even with effective therapy, mortality is significant and in part is dependent on the virulence of the individual *Legionella* sp. and the degree of host immunocompromise.[378]

In patients seriously ill at time of diagnosis or who fail to respond to erythromycin, rifampin may be added. However, the concomitant use of cyclosporine and rifampin greatly complicates management of cyclosporine due to significant lowering of cyclosporine levels (see Chapter 13). Likewise, cyclosporine levels must be carefully followed in patients receiving erythromycin due to altered cyclosporine clearance. Newer macrolides

Macrolides

Macrolide antibiotics are bacteriostatic drugs that are named for the presence of a many-membered lactone ring to which are attached one or more deoxysugars. The major macrolide antibiotics are erythromycin, clarithromycin, and azithromycin, all of which inhibit bacterial protein synthesis by binding reversibly to the 50S ribosomal subunits of susceptible microorganisms. Mutational changes in this ribosomal subunit promote drug resistance.

(see Box) such as clarithromycin and azithromycin, as well as quinolones such as ciprofloxacin, levofloxacin, and trovafloxacin, also have excellent *in vitro* activity against *Legionella* sp., but clinical data in transplant recipients are limited.[137, 138]

Bartonella

Although the natural reservoir for *Bartonella henselae* is controversial, infection due to this organism is strongly related to domestic cat and/or cat flea exposure. In normal hosts, *Bartonella* is responsible for a number of illnesses, most notably cat scratch disease. *Bartonella* infection has been described in renal,[47] liver,[20] and heart[231] transplant recipients, and may be responsible for a variety of presentations including cat scratch disease (lymph nodes which have the histological appearance of necrotizing granulomas with microabscesses[413]) and systemic lymphadenopathy associated with multiple nodules throughout the liver and spleen (epitheloid hemangiomatous lesions). The mechanism of transmission of the disease is uncertain but is associated with recent contact with young cats, usually with a scratch or bite.[37] The diagnosis involves staining tissue (Warthin-Starry stain), since the organism is not usually obtained from the blood stream except by special isolator cultures.[413] Information on the effectiveness of antibiotics in this disease is limited, since cat scratch disease in normal hosts is a self-limiting disease.[413] Antibiotics that appear effective include erythromycin, doxycycline, clarithromycin, and azithromycin.

MYCOBACTERIAL INFECTIONS

The occurrence of mycobacterial disease in transplant patients is relatively uncommon in the United States, although the incidence clearly exceeds that in the general population.[303, 310, 332] In areas of the world where tuberculosis is endemic, this infection accounts for important morbidity and mortality in organ transplant recipients. All potential heart and heart/lung transplant recipients should have purified protein derivative (PPD) and anergy skin testing performed prior to transplantation, particularly in countries where tuberculosis is endemic. Of particular importance is *M. tuberculosis*, which may

cause localized pulmonary as well as disseminated disease. If diagnosis is not delayed, an excellent response to antituberculosis therapy is expected. Recommendations for specific antituberculous therapy in the transplant population do not differ from those in the normal host (Table 15–5).

Infections due to nontuberculous mycobacteria, although less common than *M. tuberculosis* infections, have received increased attention in recent years.[332] Localized and disseminated infections due to *M. kansasii*, *M. chelonae*, and *M. fortuitum* are the most commonly encountered nontuberculous isolates in transplant patients. Cutaneous and/or pulmonary disease is the most common presentation of nontuberculous mycobacterial infections. Skin infections (*M. chelonae*, *M. fortuitum*) manifest as localized skin nodules or abscesses occurring on the extremities. Isolates of nontuberculous mycobacteria from respiratory secretions have been reported in cardiac transplant recipients; most of these individuals have localized parenchymal disease.[332] Specific therapy for common nontuberculous mycobacteria is outlined in Table 15–5. Nontuberculous mycobacterial infections in cardiac transplant recipients generally present with either pulmonary or subcutaneous manifestations, and the response to therapy is generally good.[317]

MYCOPLASMA INFECTIONS

Mycoplasma (organisms that differ from bacteria in that a cell wall is absent) is a common cause of infection in the normal population, generally causing a relatively mild respiratory illness (*Mycoplasma pneumoniae*), and is known to cause infection in transplant recipients. *Mycoplasma pneumoniae* respiratory infections do not pose an inordinate risk for transplant patients, but *M. hominis* has been responsible for superficial and deep sternal wound infections after heart and heart/lung transplantation.[219, 414] Characteristically, the presentation is of a pyogenic infection, but no organisms are seen on Gram stain and cultures fail to grow an organism. Cell wall active agents such as β-lactams, and also many other antibiotics such as aminoglycosides, sulfonamides, and erythromycin, are ineffective against *M. hominis*. *M. hominis* is sensitive to tetracycline, clindamycin, rifampin, and fluoroquinolones.

VIRAL INFECTIONS

Viruses are minute infectious agents (usually not visible under light microscopy) which contain either DNA or RNA and a protein shell, lack the capability of independent metabolism, and require entry into a living host cell for replication. Viral infections, particularly those in the herpesvirus family, are common complications in heart transplant recipients and are second only to bacterial infections in overall frequency. The definitive diagnosis of most viral infections requires isolation of the organism in cell culture or the demonstration of the organism in pathologic specimens using special stains or PCR technology. In the herpesvirus family, serodiagnostic assays are most useful in documenting seroconversion, but are less specific in demonstrating reactivation or reinfection. For other viral infections, especially the hepatitis viruses and HIV, serodiagnosis is central to the detection of infection. Serologic assays are widely available, but viral isolation requires cell culture and is not generally available outside of research medical centers.

The human herpesvirus family is an important cause of severe and sometimes life threatening disease in transplant recipients and accounts for the majority of viral infections. Members of the human herpesvirus family that cause infection following transplantation include cytomegalovirus, herpes simplex, varicella-zoster, human herpesvirus-6, herpesvirus-8, and EBV. Herpesviruses produce illness that has a greater incidence, is more severe and more prolonged than that seen in immunocompetent individuals. An important feature in all herpesviruses is latency (after a primary infection the viral genome establishes residency in specific tissues but does not complete replication and produce infectious progeny virus). If the latent virus completes a replication cycle (e.g., in association with augmentation of immunosuppression), symptomatic recurrent herpesvirus infection will result.[180]

Cytomegalovirus

Cytomegaloviruses (members of the herpesvirus family) are ubiquitous agents that commonly infect humans. Man is the only reservoir for human CMV, and transmission occurs through direct or indirect person-to-person contact. Natural infection is often a function of socioeconomic status, with early infection being more prevalent in lower socioeconomic groups and in populations from developing countries. In many parts of the world, as many as 90% of adults have been infected with CMV.[250]

Cytomegalovirus is a double-stranded DNA virus that has a capsid, a matrix, and an envelope. Receptors on the viral envelope facilitate entry into the host cell and incorporate the viral DNA into the nucleus, following which the host machinery produces viral DNA and viral proteins which are assembled and released as new viral particles. In the normal host, primary CMV infection stimulates the development of long-term cellular and humoral immunity, thus controlling viral persistence. However, in the immunocompromised patient, latent CMV can become reactivated (characteristic of the herpesvirus family). The sites at which the latent CMV lodges remain uncertain, but may be endothelial cells,[190] lymphocytes,[390] neutrophils,[174] and macrophages.[408]

Types of CMV Infection

The term **CMV syndrome** refers to the flu-like illness manifested by fever, chills, malaise, and often leukopenia and thrombocytopenia, accompanied by CMV viremia. The term **CMV disease** refers to symptomatic CMV syndrome as well as tissue invasive disease. **CMV infection** includes asymptomatic viremia, CMV syndrome, and CMV disease.[28]

Primary CMV infection occurs because a CMV-seronegative recipient receives a CMV-positive donor organ or a CMV-seronegative recipient receives blood or blood products from CMV-positive donors that have not been depleted of leukocytes (the site of CMV virus among blood elements). **Secondary infection,** or reactivation infection, is the result of reactivation of a latent virus in a CMV-seropositive recipient following transplantation. **Superinfection**[331] or reinfection occurs when a seropositive recipient receives a seropositive donor organ with CMV of a different strain than the recipient's latent CMV.[92]

Time-Related and Organ-Specific Occurrence of CMV Infections

Following cardiac transplantation, approximately 20% of recipients will have experienced one or more CMV infections by 2 years (Fig. 15–14),[238] the peak incidence occurring between the first and second posttransplant months (Fig. 15–15).[238] The peak incidence of CMV infection after heart/lung transplantation appears to be the same as that after heart transplantation. In a multiinstitutional study in cardiac transplantation from the Cardiac Transplant Research Database (CTRD), CMV was the single most common infectious agent producing serious infection after cardiac transplantation.[297]

A number of **risk factors** have been identified for CMV infection early after cardiac transplantation. The pretransplant CMV serologic status of donor and recipient appears to be the most important risk factor, a CMV-positive donor into a CMV-negative recipient resulting in the highest risk (Fig. 15–16).[238] The use of induction therapy with antilymphocyte preparations (OKT3 or antilymphocyte globulin) enhances the susceptibility to CMV infection, especially in CMV-seropositive pa-

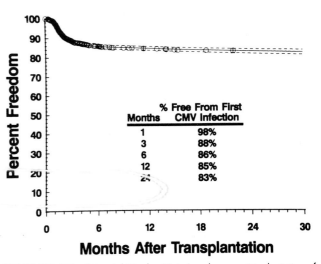

FIGURE 15–14. Actuarial (Kaplan-Meier) and parametric depiction of freedom from initial cytomegalovirus (CMV) infection. Circles represent individual cytomegalovirus infection episodes. Dashed lines surrounding solid parametric line indicate 70% confidence limits. (From Kirklin JK, Naftel DC, Levine TB, Bourge RC, Pelletier GB, O'Donnell J, Miller LW, Pritzker MR, and the Cardiac Transplant Research Database Group: Cytomegalovirus after heart transplantation. Risk factor for infection and death: a multiinstitutional study. J Heart Lung Treansplant 1994;13:394–404.)

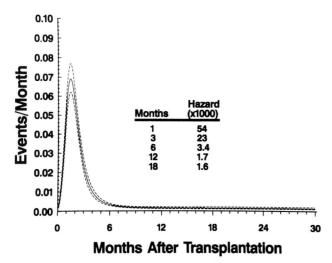

FIGURE **15-15.** Hazard function for initial CMV infection. Dashed lines indicate 70% confidence limits. (From Kirklin JK, Naftel DC, Levine TB, Bourge RC, Pelletier GB, O'Donnell J, Miller LW, Pritzker MR, and the Cardiac Transplant Research Database Group: Cytomegalovirus after heart transplantation. Risk factors for infection and death: a multiinstitutional study. J Heart Lung Transplant 1994;13:394–404.)

tients.[206,235,353] Others[102] have demonstrated an association between the use of increasing doses of OKT3 (for either treatment of rejection or induction therapy) and the subsequent development of CMV infection, although this is not a uniform finding.[255] The mechanism of enhanced reactivation of latent CMV infection with antilymphocyte agents has not been established, but may involve induction of cytokines such as tumor necrosis factor.[153] The incidence of CMV disease in heart/lung transplant recipients may be higher than that in heart transplant recipients because of the larger amount of endothelial and lymphoid tissue with the possibility of a greater viral load.

Clinical manifestations of CMV infections range from mild flu-like symptoms to life-threatening visceral organ dysfunction, and the likelihood of clinical symptomatology is a direct function of type of infection (primary versus reactivation) and the degree of immunosuppression. For instance, patients experiencing primary CMV infection are at least twice as likely to have symptomatic infection and greater severity of symptoms. Moreover, the greater the net state of immunosuppression, the more likely that symptomatic CMV infections will occur in seropositive individuals. Tacrolimus has anecdotally been associated with a slightly higher incidence of CMV infection consistent with its more potent immunosuppression, but this has not been universally observed.

Blood stream CMV infection without invasive organ disease is often associated with fever, myalgia, and other constitutional symptoms as well as leukopenia and thrombocytopenia (CMV syndrome). Identification of CMV in only the blood stream is the most common form of CMV infection (43% of CMV infections).[238] Any visceral organ may be involved, but the lungs, gastrointestinal tract, liver, and CNS are most common.[178] For some types of transplantation, the organ system most commonly involved reflects the organ transplanted; for example, CMV pneumonitis most frequently occurs in lung and heart/lung transplant recipients, and CMV hepatitis occurs most frequently in liver transplant recipients. However, direct cardiac involvement which is clinically apparent is rare, even among heart transplant recipients (see below).

CMV pneumonitis is the most serious form of CMV disease and is the second most common form of the disease (after isolated blood stream involvement),[235] accounting for about 30% of CMV infection. In patients with symptomatic disease, CMV pneumonia is associated with nonproductive cough, dyspnea, hypoxia, and chest roentgenographic abnormalities. Diffuse interstitial infiltrates are most common, but lobar infiltrates, focal opacities, and pleural effusion may be seen. CMV pneumonitis in heart or heart/lung transplant recipients has the poorest outcome, with a reported mortality of nearly 15%, even in the era of ganciclovir.[235] CMV pneumonitis is more frequent after heart/lung or isolated lung transplantation (compared to heart transplantation) and accounts for about half of all CMV infections.[109,223,406]

CMV gastrointestinal involvement may occur in up to 8% of heart transplant recipients[21] and usually manifests as gastritis, duodenitis, or hemorrhagic colitis; although any portion of the gastrointestinal tract from esophagus to large bowel may be involved. Upper gastrointestinal symptoms include dysphagia, odynophagia, nausea, vomiting and delayed gastric emptying, and abdominal pain.[331] Focal or multiple ulcerations[21,403] of the gastrointestinal tract may occur anywhere from the esophagus to the rectum and can lead to perforation and hemorrhage. On endoscopy, the findings of ulceration,

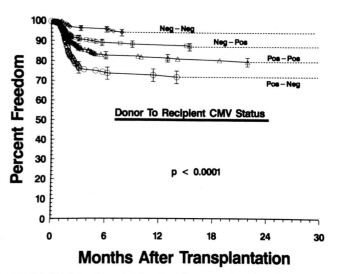

FIGURE **15-16.** Actuarial freedom from initial CMV infection according to CMV serologic status of donor and recipient before transplantation. Dashed lines indicate duration of follow-up. Error bars indicate ± 1 standard error. (From Kirklin JK, Naftel DC, Levine TB, Bourge RC, Pelletier GB, O'Donnell J, Miller LW, Pritzker MR, and the Cardiac Transplant Research Database Group: Cytomegalovirus after heart transplantation. Risk factor for infection and death: a multiinstitutional study. J Heart Lung Transplant 1994;13:394–404.)

erosions, and erythema are nonspecific; therefore, biopsy is required to confirm the diagnosis.[331] The **histological picture** demonstrates mucosal ulceration with a vasculitis picture and giant cells with characteristic CMV intranuclear and intracytoplasmic inclusions. Fatal hemorrhage from CMV duodenitis after heart transplantation has been described.[57] Colonic involvement with CMV in heart transplant recipients has been responsible for diarrhea, massive lower gastrointestinal bleeding,[145] colonic perforation,[169] and stricture formation mimicking a colonic carcinoma.[105, 123]

Severe **CMV hepatitis** is rare in cardiac transplant recipients (being much more common in liver transplant recipients), but may present with fever, nonspecific constitutional symptoms, and elevation of transminase and alkaline phosphatase levels. The distinction between CMV hepatitis and other forms of viral and chemical hepatitis may require liver biopsy.

Central nervous system involvement with CMV is uncommon, but mild encephalopathy to severe progressive meningoencephalitis may be seen and must be distinguished from other causes of encephalitis, including herpes simplex virus and toxoplasmosis.

Myocardial CMV invasive infection is rare, even among heart transplant recipients. Necrotizing myocarditis (with myocyte intranuclear inclusions typical of CMV)[194] and coronary arterial thrombosis (with coronary endothelial cell intranuclear inclusions) have been reported.[298] In heart transplant recipients with CMV antigenemia, endomyocardial biopsies have demonstrated subendothelial lymphocyte accumulation and endothelial cell proliferation in arterioles, resulting in luminal narrowing.[246] CMV DNA has been detected by PCR from endomyocardial biopsies in patients with CMV infections. This must be interpreted with some caution, since the highly sensitive technique of PCR may have detected CMV genome in a leukocyte in the biopsy rather than necessarily in a myocyte.[22, 355]

CMV retinitis, though uncommon, usually occurs greater than 6 months after transplantation and can be devastating. The process results in full-thickness retinal necrosis with a sharp border between necrotic and normal appearing retina. The histologic feature of CMV retinitis is intracytoplasmic and intranuclear ("owl's eye") inclusions.[338] There may be a sparse lymphocytic infiltrate in the retina or no inflammatory infiltrate, which is in contradistinction to acquired immunodeficiency syndrome (AIDS) patients with CMV retinitis who usually have a neutrophilic infiltrate. CMV antigens can be found in all layers of the retina[338] and may also be found in the choroid and the optic nerve. CMV retinitis involving the periphery of the retina may present as blind spots or floaters, but when the posterior pole of the retina is involved, the patient experiences blurred vision and visual field loss. When the process causes an optic neuritis and papillitis, there may be sudden loss of vision.[338] Because of the perivascular distribution of CMV retinitis, in the early stages the lesions resemble granular foci of infection. Because of cell-to-cell spread of the infection over a period of weeks to months, these lesions tend to grow, producing an irregular granular border.[338] If the process is not arrested, blindness may result.

In the differential diagnosis of posttransplant retinitis, other causes of chorioretinitis including toxoplasma, herpes simplex virus, varicella-zoster virus, *Candida* spp., and *C. neoformans*[338] should be considered. CMV retinitis may coexist with other retinal infections.

CMV infection has been implicated in a number of other complications in heart and heart/lung transplant recipients. Based partly on the demonstration experimentally[436, 441] that CMV induces expression of class II and class I MHC antigens, CMV has been hypothesized to play a role in precipitating acute cardiac rejection and the development of coronary vasculopathy (see Chapter 17). CMV infection may also initiate or accelerate the development of obliterative bronchiolitis in heart/lung transplant recipients (see Chapter 22). CMV infections may also increase susceptibility to other infections.[97, 172, 185] In liver transplantation, CMV has been identified as a risk factor for developing EBV-related posttransplant lymphoproliferative disease.[275] CMV immunoglobulin prophylaxis in renal transplant recipients was associated with a reduced incidence of fungal infections and *Pneumocystis carinii* pneumonia.[407] A relationship between CMV and other types of infections has not been clearly established in heart and heart/lung transplant recipients, but it seems likely given the evidence in other solid organ transplants.

Diagnosis

In view of the nonspecific signs and symptoms of CMV infection, CMV diagnostic studies (see Box) play a pivotal role in establishing the clinical diagnosis. The diagnosis of CMV infection is supported by the isolation of the organism from peripheral white blood cells and/or involved tissue together with demonstration of the characteristic histopathologic findings in tissue specimens, which include viral inclusions (Fig. 15–17) and positive immunoperoxidase staining (Fig. 15–18). Isolation of CMV from bronchoalveolar lavage or bronchial washings without histologic confirmation provides only presumptive evidence of disease. Rapid culture techniques such as the shell vial assay have replaced preexisting standard cultures, which often require up to 28 days for viral isolation. **Serologic assays** for CMV are valuable only for purposes of documenting seroconversion in previously seronegative patients and are not generally useful in following seropositive individuals. The **CMV antigenemia** assay is currently the standard method in many centers for detection of CMV in peripheral blood, and **quantitative PCR** or hybrid capture assay for CMV DNA provide the most sensitive technology available for detection of CMV in virtually any tissue or fluid sample. The prognostic value of various methods for CMV detection in blood are listed in Table 15–7.

Treatment of CMV Disease

Despite the lack of randomized controlled trials for the treatment of CMV disease with ganciclovir, numerous nonrandomized studies support the use of ganciclovir

CMV Diagnostic Studies

Serology

The presence of IgG antibodies against CMV is clear evidence of past infection, but the measurement of these antibodies has a limited role in the diagnosis of acute CMV disease in the solid organ recipient. Many assays are described for detection of IgG and IgM antibodies against CMV, including neutralization, complement fixation, indirect hemagglutinin, indirect immunofluorescence, latex agglutination, radioimmunoassay, and enzyme immunoassays. The usefulness of CMV antibody detection is generally limited to epidemiological studies and pretransplant screening. Among patients who were seronegative before transplant, measurement of IgG and IgM antibodies against CMV in the posttransplant period can confirm seroconversion.

Cell Culture

Human fibroblasts are the only cells fully permissive to CMV infection in vitro, and the technique is time consuming and cumbersome. The cells must be fresh, and after inoculation with the specimen for 1 hour at 37°C, the cells are washed and cell culture media is added to sustain cell growth. The cell culture should be observed every other day for typical cytopathic effect (CPE) produced by CMV, though the CPE develops slowly and cultures must be maintained for at least 21 days. Traditional cell culture is rarely used in the management of transplant recipients due to lengthy delays in obtaining results and because of the availability of more rapid and sensitive assays. However, cell culture still retains importance for CMV susceptibility testing in the setting of antiviral agent resistance.

Rapid Detection of CMV Gene Products

The **detection of early antigen fluorescent foci (DEAFF) test** retains the sensitivity and specificity of cell culture, but through the detection of early or intermediate-early gene products of CMV replication, the need to wait for full viral replication (often up to 21 days) is eliminated. Clinical specimens are inoculated onto cell cultures in the traditional manner. After 18–24 hours of incubation, the cells are fixed and stained with monoclonal antibodies directed against early and intermediate CMV gene products that are present within the cell nuclei. Cells are stained with a fluorescent antibody, and a positive result reveals fluorescent nuclei when viewed under an ultraviolet microscope.

The **shell vial** assay also allows the early detection of gene products of CMV replication. Fibroblasts are grown on round coverslips which are placed at the bottom of shell vials. After inoculation with clinical specimens, they are centrifuged for 1 hour at $700 \times g$. The cultures are incubated 18–24 hours and the coverslips processed and interpreted in the same manner as for the DEAFF test. The centrifugation step is felt to enhance the sensitivity of the test. The CMV **antigenemia test** and other new tests have largely replaced traditional CMV culture, shell vial assay, and DEAFF for the detection of CMV in peripheral blood. For the antigenemia assay, polymorphonuclear leukocytes (PMNLs) from peripheral blood are separated and stained with monoclonal antibodies directed against pp65, an early matrix protein of CMV, followed by immunoperoxidase staining. This process detects pp65 in the PMNLs, and the number of positive PMNLs provides a semiquantitative estimate of viral load. The method is rapid and reproducible, but optimal accuracy is dependent on a fresh whole blood sample. The assay is most useful in the management of solid-organ transplant recipients in guiding therapy, and the test is of limited use among neutropenic patients. There is disagreement as to what represents "significant" antigenemia.

The **hybrid capture CMV DNA assay** (Version 2.0) involves unlabeled RNA probes which hybridize with CMV DNA. Antibodies to the RNA-DNA hybrids are used to amplify this signal and the detection system involves a chemiluminescent system. The hybrid capture is more sensitive than standard culture shell vial assays for the detection of CMV viremia.[283] The sensitivity and specificity is equivalent to the pp65 antigenemia assay. The advantage of the hybrid capture technique is that it can be performed on blood that has been stored up to 48 hours and detects CMV DNA in leukocytes, which may more closely parallel clinical symptoms and the response to CMV therapy.[173]

PCR represents the most sensitive method of detecting CMV antigen. The methodology involves amplification of various target epitopes in the CMV DNA sequence that are highly specific for CMV. The **advantage of PCR** is the ability to test virtually any tissue or fluid sample; its primary disadvantages are the relative difficulty in quantitation, poor standardization between laboratories, and the difficulty in performing the assays in comparison with the pp65 CMV antigenemia assay. A related technology referred to as the **branched-chain DNA assay** (B-DNA), another unlicensed test, is a chemiluminescence assay that has excellent promise as a semiquantitative CMV assay.

CMV antigenemia assay, hybrid capture, and CMV-PCR have proven to be highly sensitive for the detection of active CMV infection and CMV disease[148, 426, 430, 445] following renal transplantation. CMV antigenemia turns positive a median of 7 days before the onset of CMV disease and PCR turns positive a median of 11 days before the onset of CMV disease. However, given the fact that the antigenemia assay requires several hours as opposed to the PCR assay, which requires several days, these tests are equivalent for the early diagnosis of CMV disease. CMV antigenemia appears to reflect the clinical course when it is used for surveillance for CMV infection early after transplantation better than the CMV-PCR assay, serology, or shell vial assay.[426]

for the treatment of CMV disease. Prior to the availability of ganciclovir, the mortality associated with CMV pneumonitis after heart and heart/lung transplantation was 75% in one study,[136] which is substantially greater than the mortality (<15%) associated with CMV pneumonitis in the current ganciclovir era. Ganciclovir (see Box) (a synthetic purine nucleoside analogue of guanine) is active against all members of the herpesvirus family.

The usual dose of ganciclovir is 5 mg/kg every 12 hours by intravenous infusion over 1 hour. In patients with renal dysfunction the dose of ganciclovir must be modified based on the estimated creatinine clearance

Ganciclovir

Ganciclovir is an acyclic guanine nucleoside analog which is similar in structure to acyclovir except that it has an additional hydroxymethyl group on the acyclic side chain. All herpesviruses are susceptible to the inhibitory efforts of ganciclovir, but it is especially effective against CMV, where its inhibitory concentrations are 10– to 100–fold lower than acyclovir.[348] Ganciclovir competitively inhibits viral DNA polymerase and is incorporated into viral DNA as a false nucleotide which terminates DNA synthesis. Although it is incorporated into both viral and cellular DNA, it preferentially inhibits viral rather than host cellular DNA polymerases. Ganciclovir is virostatic and *in vitro* viral DNA synthesis may resume after ganciclovir inhibition is removed. When CMV resistance to ganciclovir occurs, the two major mechanisms are viral point mutations, which reduce intracellular ganciclovir phosphorylation, and mutations in viral DNA polymerase, which prevent inhibition of viral replication.

The major dose-limiting toxicity of ganciclovir is myelosuppression, neutropenia occurring in about 15–40% of patients, and thrombocytopenia in 5–20%.[149] Central nervous system effects are reported in 5–15% of patients, manifesting most commonly as headaches or behavioral changes, but rarely producing convulsions and coma.

(Table 15–8).[4] The duration of therapy has not been clearly established, but traditionally 2–3 weeks is recommended. Many clinicians feel that tissue-invasive disease should be treated for longer periods of time (up to 6 weeks). With the current availability of quantitative measures of CMV viral load, it may be advisable to continue treatment until at least one viral load measure is zero, with all symptoms having resolved. In patients with severe CMV disease, particularly CMV pneumonitis, CMV hyperimmune globulin may be used in combination with ganciclovir, although this combination has not been clearly substantiated outside of bone marrow transplant recipients. The CMV infection relapse rate can be as high as 20% in seropositive individuals and even higher among patients with primary infection.[377] Despite such reports, the observed recurrence of CMV infection among heart transplant patients in a multiinstitutional study has been low (12%) in the current era with ganciclovir therapy.[238] In patients with a recurrence of CMV disease, several months of oral ganciclovir following intravenous therapy is advisable to suppress recurrences.

There are a number of important side effects associated with the use of ganciclovir. The hematologic side effects include neutropenia and thrombocytopenia due to a direct myelotoxic effect of the drug.[4] One study indicated that 15–20% of patients who are receiving ganciclovir for the treatment of cytomegalovirus infection experience a decline in the absolute neutrophil count to less than 500/mL.[4] A decrease in the dose or

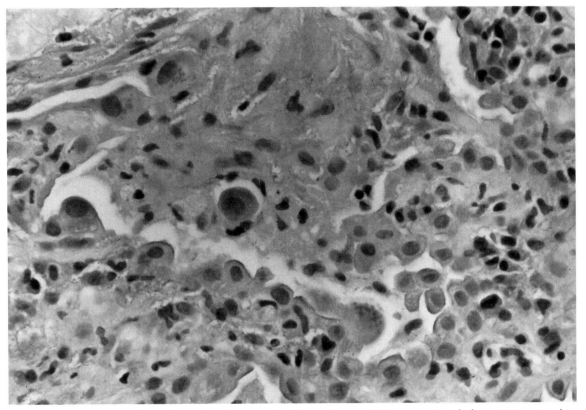

FIGURE 15–17. Hematoxylin and eosin stain of an open lung biopsy showing CMV pneumonitis with characteristic cytopathic changes (intranuclear and intracytoplasmic inclusion bodies).

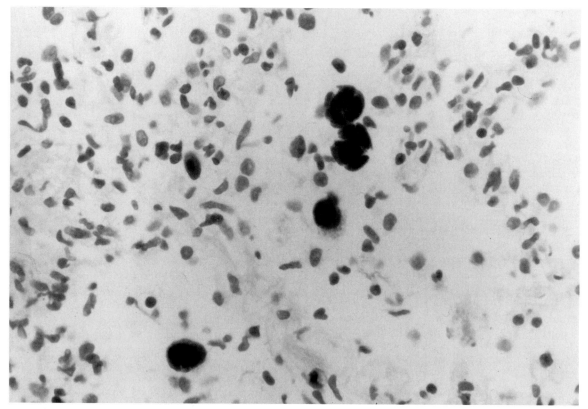

FIGURE **15–18.** Open lung biopsy in a patient with CMV pneumonitis confirmed by a positive immunoperoxidase stain.

temporary discontinuation of ganciclovir will usually result in an increase in the neutrophil count within 3–7 days. However, an important question arises when the clinician observes progressive leukopenia at the beginning of ganciclovir therapy: is the leukopenia resulting from the CMV infection (indicting the need for continued high-dose ganciclovir) or the ganciclovir therapy (indicating the need for ganciclovir dose reduction or discontinuation)? In our experience, leukopenia early in the course of ganciclovir therapy is more likely caused by the CMV infection, and ganciclovir therapy is contin-

ued. However, if the leukopenia persists, the likelihood increases that ganciclovir is the cause.

In patients with severe neutropenia that is not recovering by ganciclovir dose reduction or interruption, granulocyte colony-stimulating factor (G-CSF) or granulocyte-macrophage colony-stimulating factor (GM-CSF)

TABLE 15-7	Prognostic Values of Methods for CMV Detection in Blood*	
METHOD	SENSITIVITY (%)	SPECIFICITY (%)
Shell vial assay[345]	63	88
Polymerase chain reaction		
Serum[333]	83	57
Peripheral blood mononuclear cells[112]	57	35
Antigenemia[246]	83	71
Digene hybrid capture CMV DNA assay[283]	95	95
Quantitative PCR[220] in serum (2,000–5,000 copies/ mL)	86	87

*Sensitivity and specificity were used as markers of future CMV disease.
Adapted from Patel R, Snydman DR, Rubin RH, Ho M, Pescovitz M, Martin M, Paya CV: Cytomegalovirus prophylaxis in solid organ transplant recipients. Transplantation 1996;61:1279–1289.

TABLE 15-8	Intravenous Ganciclovir: Adjustment for Renal Function	
CREATININE CLEARANCE (mL/min)	DOSE (mg/kg)	INTERVAL (hr)
Treatment doses		
>70	5	12
50–69	2.5	12
25–49	2.5	24
10–24	1.25	24
<10	1.25	3 times/wk (following hemodialysis)
Prophylaxis doses		
>70	5	24
50–69	2.5	24
25–49	1.25	24
10–24	0.625	24
<10	0.625	3 times/wk (following hemodialysis)

Estimate of creatinine clearance (Ccr)[4]

$$Ccr\ (male) = \frac{(140 - age) \times weight}{72 \times serum\ creatinine}$$

Ccr (female) = 0.85 × Ccr (male)

where age is in years, weight is in kg, and serum creatinine is in mg/dL.

can be used, and this therapy has had success in the treatment of AIDS patients, including continuation of ganciclovir therapy in combination with GM-CSF. Thrombocytopenia may also occur in patients receiving ganciclovir, but a decrease to less than 25,000/mm³ occurs in only 3% of heart transplant recipients.[4] As with neutropenia, a platelet count of less than 25,000/mm³ should prompt discontinuation of ganciclovir until bone marrow recovery is evident.

Transient impairment of renal function may occur with ganciclovir therapy, but this may represent an interaction with other nephrotoxic drugs such as cyclosporine or tacrolimus. Central nervous system side effects have been reported in a small proportion of patients receiving ganciclovir, and these include headache, confusion and, rarely, seizures.[4]

One of the most important recent developments in the treatment of CMV is the measurement of viral load by quantitative methods to direct and monitor therapy. In a series of liver transplant patients,[220] the plasma viral load by quantitative PCR predicted the development of CMV disease (similar results from the antigenemia assay), suggesting its usefulness for the initiation of preemptive therapy. In another series of liver transplant patients,[293] quantification of the viral load (quantitative PCR) proved useful for the diagnosis of established CMV disease. CMV viral load also predicts the likelihood of relapsing CMV infection in a number of solid organ transplant recipients (including heart transplant recipients).[396] Therefore, quantification of viral load in CMV infection or disease may be useful for initiating preemptive therapy, monitoring the success of therapy, and may have a role in determining the duration of therapy based on the probability of recurrent disease.

Most of the experience in treating **CMV retinitis** stems from AIDS patients, but CMV retinitis occasionally occurs after heart and heart/lung transplantation. Repeated episodes of CMV retinitis are a significant risk and are probably due to the emergence of antiviral resistance secondary to chronic subtherapeutic intraocular levels in patients receiving systemic therapy.[253] Persistent or relapsing CMV retinitis may require the combination of systemic therapy and local therapy by either intraocular injection of ganciclovir or foscarnet or the use of a sustained-release ganciclovir implant. The device is implanted in the pars plana and delivers a sustained amount of ganciclovir for approximately 8 months. In AIDS patients, the use of ganciclovir implants appears to be effective, but systemic therapy is probably also required.[201, 305, 351]

Ganciclovir-resistant CMV strains are well known in AIDS patients but are uncommon in solid organ transplant recipients, although they have been identified following heart,[31] lung,[6, 252, 269] and liver transplantation.[372] It has been speculated that oral ganciclovir may contribute to selection of resistant strains.[31] Of interest is the case of a renal transplant patient[294] who had undergone prolonged ganciclovir therapy for CMV disease without resolution. A codon deletion in CMV DNA was found after prolonged therapy with ganciclovir, this deletion not being present before the commencement of therapy. The clinical CMV disease resolved when ganciclovir was switched to foscarnet therapy. Identification of these deletion mutations associated with ganciclovir resistance may find a role in treating patients with CMV disease that is unresponsive to ganciclovir.

Trisodium phosphonoformate (foscarnet) is an organic analogue of inorganic pyrophosphate which inhibits viral DNA polymerase, and it is structurally dissimilar to all other current antiviral drugs. Foscarnet has a high toxicity profile, particularly because of its nephrotoxicity and other toxic effects including headache and seizures (which may include grand mal seizures) and electrolyte disturbances including hypocalcemia, hypophosphatemia, hyperphosphatemia, hypomagnesemia, and hypokalemia. Foscarnet has considerable use in AIDS patients, particularly for CMV retinitis, but has had only limited use in heart and heart/lung transplant recipients because of its toxicity. In heart and heart/lung transplantation, foscarnet should currently be reserved for recipients with ganciclovir-resistant CMV disease. The dose of the drug must be adjusted for renal impairment and the usual recommended intravenous dose is 60 mg/kg every 8 hours for 14–21 days, although higher doses may be used in patients with CMV disease progression.

Cidofovir, a purine nucleotide analogue of cytosine, has shown antiviral effects in patients with ganciclovir-resistant strains of CMV. Cidofovir has been used in the treatment of CMV retinitis in patients with AIDS, but there is currently insufficient information on the use of this drug in transplant recipients to assess its role. Like foscarnet, it is potentially nephrotoxic.

CMV Prophylaxis

A number of strategies have been recommended for the prevention of CMV disease in heart and heart/lung transplant recipients.[28]

1) *Donor and recipient CMV serology matching.* Although prevention of serious CMV disease by avoiding the situation likely to produce the highest risk of CMV disease (CMV-positive donor to CMV-negative recipient) seems logical, the use of this strategy, given the shortage of donor organs, is impractical.

2) *CMV seronegative or filtered blood products.* Use of CMV-seronegative blood products is an effective means of reducing the incidence of CMV transmission,[387] but because of the high prevelance of seropositivity in the community, CMV-seronegative blood products may not necessarily be available. In the absence of CMV seronegative blood products, all blood products should be either passed through a high-efficiency leukocyte filter or leukocyte-poor blood should be used, both of which are associated with removal of greater than 99% of leukocytes and a very low risk of CMV transmission.[387]

3) *Vaccination.* Pretransplant vaccination against CMV disease in seronegative potential heart and heart/lung transplant recipients seems attractive. However, producing a reliable vaccine has proven

difficult. A live attenuated CMV Towne strain vaccine has been tested in renal transplant recipients[33, 349] and successfully decreased the severity of symptoms in the CMV-positive donor to CMV-negative recipient patients, but it did not reduce the overall incidence of CMV disease. Work on other CMV vaccines that are not derived from live viral strains is in progress. Complete protection seems unlikely, but partial protection is probable with future preparations.

4) *Passive immunoprophylaxis.* Hyperimmune CMV immunoglobulin (obtained from CMV-positive donors and standardized to ensure a high titer of anti-CMV antibodies) and unselected immune globulin preparations to confer passive immunization have been tested in solid organ transplant recipients. A number of randomized trials have been performed using hyperimmune CMV globulin and unselected immune globulin preparations in solid organ transplant recipients, and the results have been variable, possibly related to the variation in the doses and duration of therapy and the use of both unscreened and hyperimmune globulin.[331] A study of the use of unscreened immunoglobulin together with acyclovir in donor CMV-seropositive to CMV-seronegative recipients after heart and heart/lung transplantation did not show a benefit,[29] whereas other studies in liver and renal transplant recipients did demonstrate a benefit. Several studies in thoracic transplantation indicate a favorable effect of ganciclovir plus CMV hyperimmune globulin as prophylaxis against CMV infection, particularly when a CMV-negative recipient receives a CMV-positive organ.[442–444] When all of the studies are examined, CMV hyperimmune globulin appears effective in providing additional protection against CMV disease, and potentially some benefit against allograft coronary artery disease and obliterative bronchiolitis (OB) (in heart/lung transplant recipients).[331, 442] The main disadvantage is cost, with the greatest net savings likely to be on hospitalizations for CMV pneumonia (and possibly OB) in heart/lung recipients.

5) *Antiviral drug therapy.* The use of antiviral agents is now considered an essential strategy in the prevention of CMV infection and CMV disease after heart and heart/lung transplantation. There are a number of randomized trials that demonstrate some protection against CMV disease and infection after solid organ transplantation but with varying degrees of success, reflecting the heterogeneity of the antiviral drug protocols, the definition of CMV disease, and different immunosuppressive protocols.[334] In heart transplantation, there is compelling evidence of the effectiveness of ganciclovir prophylaxis in reducing the incidence of cytomegalovirus disease in CMV-positive recipients (Fig. 15–19).[295] Macdonald and colleagues[271] demonstrated a reduced incidence of CMV disease in CMV-mismatched patients and reduction in the morbidity of CMV disease in CMV-positive recipients.[271] In a meta-analysis,[103] patients of solid organ transplantation, including heart transplant recipients, did demonstrate a significant benefit of antiviral agents as prophylaxis against CMV infection and CMV disease. Ganciclovir is currently the antiviral agent of choice for prophylaxis. Many different dosing regimens have been investigated, and currently there is no consensus. Oral ganciclovir is generally effective as a prophylactic agent against CMV,[168] but ganciclovir levels following oral ingestion are highly variable, and it is not a reliable form of therapy when treating active disease. The CMV prophylaxis regimen used at the University of Alabama at Birmingham (UAB) is outlined in Table 15–9. Although acyclovir has been thought to reduce the incidence of CMV disease,[140] its effectiveness as an anti-CMV drug is suboptimal, with little demonstrative *in vitro* activity against CMV. Valacyclovir is a valine ester of acyclovir and has demonstrated some effectiveness in preventing CMV disease in both CMV-positive recipients and CMV-negative renal transplant recipients receiving CMV-positive kidneys.[267] This drug, like ganciclovir, is effective in reducing the risk of herpes simplex virus infection. Valganciclovir, an oral

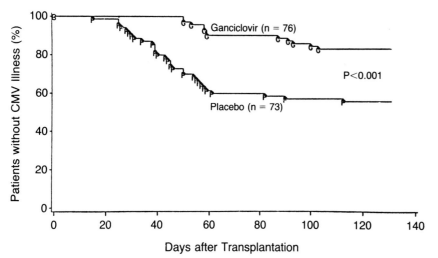

FIGURE **15–19.** Incidence of CMV illness in pretransplant CMV-positive recipients and pretransplant seronegative recipients receiving seropositive donor hearts stratified by randomization to either intravenous ganciclovir or placebo (although the beneficial effect was only seen in CMV positive recipients). (From Merigan TC, Renlund DG, Keay S, Bristlow MR, Starnes V, O'Connell JB, Resta S, Dunn D, Gamberg P, Ratkovec RM, Richenbacher WE, Millar RC, DuMond C, DeAmond B, Sullivan V, Cheney T, Buhles W, Stinson EB: A controlled trial of ganciclovir to prevent cytomegalovirus disease after heart transplantation. N Engl J Med 1992;326:1182.)

TABLE 15-9	Infection Prophylaxis After Heart And Heart/Lung Transplantation (UAB)

INFECTIOUS COMPLICATION	PROPHYLAXIS
Perioperative wound and line sepsis	Vancomycin 15 mg/kg preop, then 10 mg/kg q 8 h × 4 days Ceftazidime 15 mg/kg preop, then 1 g q 8 h × 4 days
Pneumocystis carinii	Trimethoprim/sulfamethoxazole 1 qd (1 yr); for patients allergic to sulfonamides, dapsone 50 mg qd (1 yr) or pentamidine 300 mg via nebulizer every month (1 yr)
Mucocutaneous candidiasis	Topical, nonabsorbable antifungal (nystatin) 500,000 units tid (6 mo)
Toxoplasmosis	
Recipient negative, donor positive	Pyrimethamine 25 mg qd and leucovorin 10 mg qd (6 mo) serology is checked at 3 mo, 6 mo and 1 yr
Cytomegalovirus*	
Recipient negative, donor positive	Ganciclovir† IV (6 wk) then ganciclovir 1 g tid PO (6 wk) Cytogam 150 mg/kg IV within 72 hr after transplant then every 2 wk × 4 doses; then 100 mg/kg IV every 4 wk × 2 doses (round dose to nearest 2,500)
Recipient positive or any course of OKT3 or antithymocyte globulin	Ganciclovir† IV during hospitalization then ganciclovir 1 g tid PO (6 wk) then acyclovir 200 mg PO tid for 6 mo
Recipient negative, donor negative	Acyclovir 200 mg tid PO (6 mo)
Epstein-Barr virus	
Recipient negative, donor positive	EBV IgM IgG serologies are checked at 6 wk, 3 mo and every 3 mo for the first year and then every 6 mo until seroconversion; at seroconversion patient is treated with ganciclovir IV (6 wk) then ganciclovir PO 1 g tid for 6 mo then acyclovir 200 mg PO tid for 6 mo†
Herpes simplex 1 and 2	Acyclovir 200 mg tid PO (6 mo)§

*CMV antigenemia test obtained monthly for the first 5 months after transplant.
†See Table 15–8 for doses.
‡The dose is adjusted according to renal function.
§Acyclovir is held during administration of ganciclovir.

agent which results in levels similar to intravenous ganciclovir, is currently under study.

6) *Preemptive therapy.* Preemptive therapy refers to the administration of antiviral agents to patients who have laboratory markers and clinical features that indicate high risk of CMV disease prior to the appearance of the disease. A number of laboratory markers indicating the likely onset of CMV infection have been investigated (Table 15–7). The use of CMV antigenemia[247] and quantitative PCR[220] appear to be effective means of predicting the subsequent development of symptomatic CMV infection, and the effectiveness of antigenemia-directed preemptive antiviral therapy after heart transplantation has been demonstrated.[224] Antigenemia was shown in one study to have an 83% sensitivity as a marker for future CMV disease, preceding the onset of infection by a mean of 5 days.[246] Preemp-

tive therapy for CMV disease has been found effective in liver transplant recipients, therapy being prompted by viral shedding determined by surveillance cultures (buffy coat and urine) and in renal transplant recipients who had positive serology for CMV and who were receiving antilymphocyte antibody therapy.[206] Preemptive therapy for CMV infection in heart and lung transplant recipients has been reported,[139] but requires further investigation, especially using markers such as antigenemia and CMV DNA by PCR.

We conclude that surveillance by antigenemia testing should focus on the first 3–5 months after transplant (the period of greatest risk), obtaining blood samples for testing every 2–4 weeks, depending on patient risk factors, including patient–donor CMV serology mismatch, CMV-positive recipients, and recipients who receive antilymphocyte therapy (OKT3, ATG). Although the benefit of preemptive therapy is unproven in heart and heart/lung transplantation, we believe it is advisable and recommend the same course of ganciclovir as in established disease.

CMV Mortality

In the current era, the probability of death due to or associated with CMV infection is low with the availability of ganciclovir therapy. In a multi-institutional study, the actuarial freedom from fatal CMV infection at 2 years after cardiac transplantation was 98.6%[238] (Fig. 15–20), the peak hazard for CMV mortality occurring between 2 and 3 months after transplantation (Fig. 15–21).[238] The overall current mortality for an episode of CMV infection is 7% (70% confidence limits 5–9%) based on multi-institutional data.[238] The highest mortality is in CMV

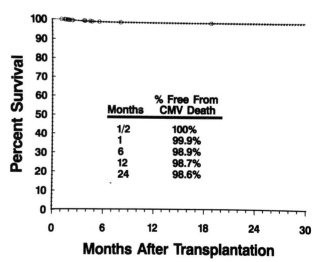

FIGURE **15–20.** Actuarial and parametric freedom from death associated with CMV infection. Dashed lines indicate 70% confidence limits around the parametric curve, and circles indicate individual cytomegalovirus-related deaths in actuarial depiction. (From Kirklin JK, Naftel DC, Levine TB, Bourge RC, Pelletier GB, O'Donnell J, Miller LW, Pritzker MR, and the Cardiac Transplant Research Database Group: Cytomegalovirus after heart transplantation. Risk factors for infection and death: a multiinstitutional study. J Heart Lung Transplant 1994;13:394–404.)

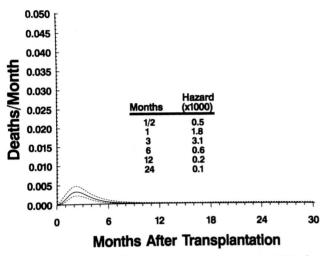

FIGURE **15-21.** Hazard function for death associated with CMV infection after heart transplantation. Dashed lines indicate 70% confidence limits. (From Kirklin JK, Naftel DC, Levine TB, Bourge RC, Pelletier GB, O'Donnell J, Miller LW, Pritzker MR, and the Cardiac Transplant Research Database Group: Cytomegalovirus after heart transplantation. Risk factors for infection and death: a multiinstitutional study. J Heart Lung Transplant 1994;13:394–404.)

lung infections (13%), followed by gastrointestinal tract (6%) and blood (4%).[238] The only risk factor that was identified for death with CMV infection was a higher number of infections of any type during the first month after transplantation. Interestingly, the donor–recipient CMV serologic status at transplantation was not a risk factor for death, suggesting that even in the most unfavorable setting of CMV-positive donor to CMV-negative recipient, prophylaxis and therapy for CMV disease is effective in preventing mortality. Also, there was no difference in mortality between initial and subsequent CMV infections.

Herpes Simplex Virus

Herpes simplex virus (HSV) (of the herpesvirus family) infections are worldwide in distribution. HSV-1 usually infects children between ages 2 and 10, although primary infection may be delayed until adolescence or early adulthood. Primary infection usually occurs through direct contact with oral secretions. HSV-2 primary infection usually occurs in sexually active adolescents and adults and is spread through sexual contact. It has been associated with penile vesicular lesions, cervicovaginitis, proctitis, and disseminated infection in the neonate. Most reactivation disease involving the mouth, lips, and face is due to HSV-1, whereas recurrent disease in the anogenital region is typically due to HSV-2.

Latency with HSV is established by transport of the virus following replication on the mucocutaneous surface along cutaneous neurons to cell bodies in ganglia. When reactivation occurs, the virus travels back to the mucocutaneous surface along peripheral sensory nerves followed by replication in the dermal and epidermal layers, resulting in painful vesicles.[100]

Among solid organ transplant recipients, HSV is second only to CMV as a cause of proven viral infection.

Unlike CMV, primary infection is rarely transmitted from the donor organ,[133, 245] and most cases are due to reactivation in previously infected patients. Peak incidence of HSV reactivation occurs at approximately 1 month after transplant during the period of maximum immunosuppression. Reactivation infection due to HSV-1 or HSV-2 typically presents as vesicular or ulcerative lesions of the mouth, lips, nose, face, or anogenital region. Any cutaneous site may be involved, however, and lesions tend to be more severe and protracted than in normal patients. Chronic, large ulcerated areas may persist for weeks or months in the most severe cases. As in other immunocompromised patients, esophagitis may occur and is characterized by odynophagia and multiple, confluent, shallow ulcerations throughout the esophagus. Tracheobronchitis can be seen in patients with long-term endotracheal intubation. Disseminated disease may be associated with diffuse pneumonitis, fulminant hepatitis, encephalitis, and disseminated intravascular coagulation. Mortality associated with disseminated disease approaches 100%.[208]

The clinical diagnosis of HSV mucocutaneous infection is not difficult and is suspected based on the appearance of typical vesiculoulcerative lesions. Visceral involvement with HSV may present difficult diagnostic problems. In either event, confirmation of the diagnosis is based on isolation of the organism in cell culture from clinical specimens. Histologic confirmation is usually based on the presence of multinucleated giant cells and a positive immunofluorescent stain specific for HSV. Serologic assays for HSV-1 and HSV-2 are available but of limited value under ordinary circumstances except to define susceptibility or to document seroconversion. The ELISA assay is not able to reliably distinguish antibodies against HSV-1 or HSV-2. However, PCR is becoming increasingly employed and is now the standard diagnostic technique for CNS infection due to suspected HSV.

The drug of choice for prophylaxis against HSV-1 and HSV-2 infection is acyclovir (Table 15–9). It is important to emphasize that in patients who are receiving ganciclovir prophylaxis or therapy, simultaneous acyclovir for HSV prevention is not required.

Acyclovir remains the treatment of choice for HSV infections in most patients. Serious life-threatening infections are treated with intravenous acyclovir (15–30 mg/kg/day), and less severe mucocutaneous disease is adequately treated with oral acyclovir (1–2 g/day) (Tables 15–5 and 15–6). Length of therapy is dependent on clinical and virologic responses, and may range between 2 weeks and several months. Newer agents including valacyclovir and famciclovir offer improved pharmacokinetics and less frequent dosing, but must be given orally and are probably not superior to acyclovir. Acyclovir-resistant HSV strains have been identified among immunocompromised patients,[90] and therapy with foscarnet is probably warranted in these cases. Cidofovir, although investigational, may be useful in this setting. However, the widespread use of prophylactic oral acyclovir in patients for the first 3–12 months after transplant has led to a dramatic decrease in the incidence of clinically apparent HSV infections, and to date, significant acyclovir resistance has not developed in this population.

Varicella-Zoster Virus

Varicella–zoster virus (VZV) (a member of the herpesvirus family) is responsible for two distinct clinical syndromes, primary infection (chickenpox) and its recurrent form (herpes zoster or shingles). Humans are the only known reservoir of VZV. Chickenpox is highly contagious, with an attack rate of at least 90% (via airborne transmission) among susceptible seronegative individuals. The virus is endemic in the population at large, but may become epidemic seasonally, especially late winter and early spring in temperate zones. The virus enters through the mucosal surfaces of the respiratory tract, produces a primary viremia with widespread dissemination of the virus to the reticuloendothelial system. Seven days later, a second viremic phase occurs at which time the symptoms and cutaneous manifestations of chickenpox develop.[192] Children less than 3 years of age account for about 90% of cases of chickenpox, most other cases occurring between the ages of 4 and 10 years. Over the ages of 15 years, between 10 and 25% of the population is susceptible to infection. Thus, for organ transplant recipients, the majority of adults are at risk only for recurrent infection. However, chickenpox does occur in previously seronegative transplant recipients, and can be a devastating infection in bone marrow[265] and solid organ transplant recipients.[270] The incubation period ranges between 10 and 21 days, and patients are infectious for approximately 48 hours prior to the onset of rash and until complete scabbing of all lesions. Latency is established by the transport of viruses during the chickenpox illness along sensory nerves to the corresponding dorsal root ganglia.

In contrast to chickenpox, herpes zoster is a sporadic disease which is a consequence of reactivation of latent virus from the dorsal root ganglia. It occurs in all ages, but primarily in the elderly, with peak incidence between the sixth and eighth decades of life. Impairment of cell-mediated immunity associated with immunosuppression in solid organ transplant recipients renders these patients at especially high risk of herpes zoster.[357] Unlike HSV infection, which usually occurs early after transplantation, zoster generally occurs after the first 3 posttransplant months.

Herpes zoster typically occurs in a dermatomal distribution with a vesicular rash. Pain may precede the rash by 48 hours. Lesions evolve within the dermatome in a manner similar to chickenpox with complete healing occurring in 14–21 days, although the disease may be protracted in immunocompromised hosts with prolonged vesicle formation and delayed healing. Cutaneous dissemination occurs in up to 25% of patients depending on the degree of immunosuppression, and visceral dissemination can also occur.

In contrast to the normal host, primary VZV infection in transplant recipients is often protracted with delayed healing of vesicles, and hemorrhagic lesions are much more common. There is a propensity to develop visceral complications with primary VZV infection, and this can

occur in 25–50% of individuals (bone marrow transplantation).[265] Visceral involvement may also occur in reactivation VZV (disseminated zoster), although less likely than with primary VZV. Pneumonia, encephalitis, hepatitis, bleeding diatheses, and pancreatitis are the most common visceral complications, and overall mortality in the compromised host with primary VZV without therapy is as high as 20% (children with malignancy).[151] A similar picture of widely disseminated disease has also been described in pediatric solid organ transplant recipients following renal transplantation[150, 270] and liver transplantation.[289] Residual complications of varicella infection include blindness from retinal necrosis, cutaneous scarring, and postherpetic neuralgia.

The diagnosis of chickenpox and herpes zoster can usually be made on clinical grounds with characteristic history and presentation. Distinguishing between VZV infection and HSV infection when the disease is on the face or genital region can be difficult, and laboratory confirmation may be required.[180] VZV is not shed in asymptomatic patients (unlike HSV or CMV), and therefore the finding of VZV antigens or virus particles indicates active infection.[180] Serological tests for VZV are not useful for diagnosing acute infection. A number of laboratory tests are available to confirm the diagnosis based on vesicular fluid or tissue biopsies. These include tissue culture looking for characteristic cytopathic effects, direct immunofluorescent staining using a VZV-specific monoclonal antibody staining of a VZV glycoprotein antigen, direct fluorescent antigen (DFA) assay, and PCR for detecting VZV DNA.

Treatment of primary or recurrent VZV infection in transplant recipients should involve the use of acyclovir or one of its derivatives, valacyclovir or famciclovir. Treatment with one of these agents is effective in shortening the duration of illness, limiting viral shedding, speeding healing, and is associated with decreased morbidity and mortality probably through reducing the risk of cutaneous and visceral dissemination.[394] Acyclovir is available parenterally and is the agent of choice in severely ill patients and is given at a dose of 30 mg/kg/day in three divided doses for 10–14 days. The treatment of cutaneous zoster with an outpatient regimen of oral acyclovir (Table 15–10) appears safe[264] but close follow-up is essential, and the patient must be instructed to

TABLE 15-10	Herpes-Zoster Treatment Protocol (Oral Therapy) (UAB)
Acyclovir 800 mg 5 times a day × 14 days, then	Valacyclovir 1,000 mg tid × 14 days
Acyclovir 800 mg tid × 7 days, then	Valacyclovir 1,000 mg bid × 7 days
Acyclovir 400 mg tid × 14 days, then OR	Valacyclovir 500 mg bid × 14 days
Acyclovir 200 mg tid × 6 mo	Valacyclovir 500 mg qd × 6 mo

1. Renal profiles should be checked weekly × 2 for elevations in creatinine and BUN.
2. Follow-up at 2 wk. Lesions should become crusted during the initial 2 wk of therapy.
3. Dose adjustment required for renal insufficiency.

report any new symptoms or spread of the lesions beyond the initial dermatome. Renal function must be closely monitored, and dose reduction is necessary with depressed renal function. Patients with dermatomal zoster involving the head and neck should probably not be treated with outpatient therapy because of the increased likelihood of complications. This outpatient treatment strategy does result in a significant incidence of nausea and vomiting due to the high doses of antiviral drugs.

Patients evaluated for cardiac transplantation who are seronegative for VZV should receive vaccination with the recently licensed live varicella vaccine prior to transplantation. While there is limited data suggesting acceptable safety and efficacy in severely immunocompromised patients, vaccination among VZV seronegative patients who have already received transplantation cannot be endorsed until further data are available. For nonvaccinated, seronegative patients with significant exposure to chickenpox, immune prophylaxis with varicella-zoster immune globulin (VZIG) is recommended, although protection against primary varicella will not occur in all cases.[270] Administration should occur within 96 hours of exposure. An alternative strategy for postexposure prophylaxis is high-dose oral acyclovir, although effectiveness has not been confirmed.

Human Herpes Virus-6

Human herpes virus-6 (HHV-6) (a member of the herpesvirus family) is a recently discovered virus (1986) that is the etiologic agent of the childhood exanthem roseola (exanthem subitum) and has been associated with acute and reactivation disease. Among herpesviruses, HHV-6 is most closely related to CMV. Approximately 80% of the adult population is seropositive for HHV-6. It has been primarily recognized as a cause of undifferentiated fever, bone marrow suppression, and interstitial pneumonitis in allogeneic bone marrow transplant recipients.[72, 98] Among solid organ transplant patients, kidney and liver recipients have been most carefully studied, and it remains unclear whether significant disease is caused by this organism in the absence of CMV co-infection. In a study of liver transplant patients, HHV-6 appeared to be a more frequent cause of fever than CMV.[89] There are reports that HHV-6 and CMV act as co-pathogens causing pneumonitis as well as other diseases in solid organ transplant recipients.[225, 242, 360] HHV-6 could be considered as another "immunomodulatory virus," since it is closely associated with CMV infection after renal transplantation[121] and after liver transplantation[125] and also appears to be associated with an increased risk of fungal infection in liver transplant recipients (pretransplant HHV-6 seronegativity being a marker for primary HHV-6 infection after transplantation).[124, 125] HHV-6 has not been well studied in cardiac transplant patients. A diagnosis of acute or reactivation HHV-6 is based on demonstration of viremia (using the shell vial assay), seroconversion, or a significant rise in specific HHV-6 antibody titer, although the latter is very nonspecific. Demonstration of HHV-6 in tissue using immunohistochemical stains may also be useful. Treatment for acute or presumed reactiva-

tion HHV-6 requires ganciclovir or foscarnet as the organism is resistant to acyclovir. Randomized, controlled studies of HHV-6 therapy have not been conducted, thus optimal dose and duration of therapy is unclear.[323]

Human Herpes Virus-8

There is good evidence from patients with AIDS, bone marrow transplantation, and solid organ transplantation that HHV-8 (a member of the herpesvirus family) infection is associated with Kaposi's sarcoma. The incidence of Kaposi's sarcoma in solid organ transplant recipients is approximately 0.5%[393] and has been reported after heart transplantation.[3] There is no information currently available on the role of antiviral drugs as prophylaxis against HHV-8 infection, although prophylaxis may possibly have a role in AIDS patients.

Epstein-Barr Virus

Like other herpesviruses, EBV has the ability to establish latency and to recur. Unlike other herpesviruses, it does not lead to cytopathic effect, although its lymphotropic nature can result in transformation of cell lines leading to immortalization of lymphocytes. Among transplant recipients, EBV causes two well-recognized disorders. The first is acute mononucleosis associated with fever, lymphadenopathy, pharyngitis, tonsillitis, hepatosplenomegaly, and lymphocytosis seen in otherwise normal adolescents and young adults. This disorder has also been described in solid organ transplant recipients, but it is relatively uncommon. The second disorder related to EBV is the posttransplantation lymphoproliferative disorder (PTLD), a malignant disorder associated with EBV-induced B-cell proliferation.[36, 199, 337] PTLD occurs almost exclusively in EBV seropositive patients and is strongly associated with net state of immunosuppression and recent EBV seroconversion. A detailed discussion of PTLD is found in Chapter 16.

In Western society, at least 90% of the population has immunity to EBV by the age of 40 years, with infection occuring as a subclinical infection or a mononucleosis syndrome which is a self-limited lymphoproliferative process.[354] Latency of EBV infection is established in resting nonproliferative B-cells in the peripheral blood,[300] lymphoid tissues, and in the oropharynx. In heart and heart/lung transplant recipients who are EBV seronegative, transplantation from an EBV-seropositive donor is almost certain to cause a primary EBV infection. In a study by Gray and colleagues,[187] 23% of patients after heart and heart/lung transplantation had serological evidence of EBV infection after transplantation, of which 6% had primary EBV infection (EBV-positive donor to EBV-negative recipient) and 17% had reactivation of past infection. Of the patients who had posttransplant EBV infection, 11% of the heart/lung transplant recipients and 10% of the heart transplant recipients developed lymphoproliferative disorder or lymphoma. The strong association between posttransplant primary EBV infection and PTLD has also been demonstrated in pediatric heart transplant patients[486] (see Chapter 20).

Both acyclovir and ganciclovir have shown some benefit as prophylactic agents in the prevention of PTLD.[108,

[110, 111] Consequently, EBV serology after transplantation, particularly in those patients who are at high risk of primary EBV infection (EBV-positive donor to EBV-negative recipient) should be monitored and the use of acyclovir may be advisable (see Table 15–9). A promising strategy that appears to decrease the incidence of PTLD in pediatric liver transplant patients[285] involves EBV-PCR (semiquantitative viral load) to detect an increase in viral copies. Immunosuppression is reduced together with increasing the intravenous ganciclovir dose or reinstitution of intravenous ganciclovir until viral copies fall to a low level. In another study,[188] pediatric liver transplant patients with PTLD had EBV viral load monitoring during treatment, and clearance of the EBV virus appeared to be associated with regression of the PTLD. Using preemptive therapy for EBV based on EBV viral load may be a useful component of prevention and treatment of EBV-associated PTLD.

There is no reliable antiviral therapy for acute EBV-associated mononucleosis and no vaccination (passive or active) is available for EBV prevention.

Human Immunodeficiency Virus

As mentioned in an earlier section (Screening of Potential Organ Donors for Transmissible Infectious Disease), HIV may be transmitted to a solid organ transplant recipient. Over 80 cases of HIV infection in solid organ recipients have been documented,[144] including five cases in cardiac transplant recipients. Seventy-five percent of the cases were seronegative prior to transplant, the remainder being HIV-positive at the time of transplant. Almost 30% developed AIDS in less than 3 years, and among those who developed AIDS, 80% died of AIDS-related complications. In the highly unlikely event of posttransplant development of HIV infection and AIDS in a heart or heart/lung transplant recipient, treatment should be similar to that of a nontransplant patient, but the protease inhibitors used in most regimens have many drug interactions which must be considered.

Hepatitis B

Transmission of HBV infection following cardiac transplantation may occur through the usual modes of transmission (blood, blood products, or sexual contact), but transmission has also been described in cardiac transplant recipients as a direct result of endomyocardial biopsy.[114, 326] As indicated previously (in the section Screening of Potential Organ Donors for Transmissible Infectious Disease), HBV infection in heart transplant recipients has a likelihood of progressing to chronic liver disease. Currently, there is little information regarding the treatment of heart or heart/lung transplant recipients with hepatitis B infection, but ganciclovir has been shown to suppress HBV DNA in HBV infected liver transplant recipients.[177] Famciclovir[49] and lamivudine,[439] which also suppress HBV DNA, may also be useful. Lamivudine appears to be emerging as the drug of choice for the treatment of HBV after transplantation and for posttransplant prophylaxis (together with HBIg in liver transplant recipients at risk for HBV recurrence).

However, the usefulness of this drug may be limited by the development of HBV resistance, so that combination antiviral therapy may be preferable. There is a report of the use of ganciclovir to treat a heart transplant recipient with active hepatitis B virus infection and hepatic decompensation.[14] Following treatment, the patient became asymptomatic, liver function tests normalized, and serum HBV DNA became undetectable. The use of interferon in HBV infected liver transplant recipients[428] has had some limited success in eliminating HBV DNA, and this therapy may be considered in the HBV-infected heart or heart/lung transplant recipient. With the availability of more effective antiviral agents against HBV such as lamivudine, famciclovir, and adefovir, there may be a shift in the risk/benefit ratio in favor of cardiac transplantation for potential recipients who are HBsAg positive. A patient at the Cleveland Clinic who was HBsAg positive underwent cardiac transplantation and was treated initially with ganciclovir followed by famciclovir and then lamivudine and is free of evident liver disease 3.5 years after transplantation.

Hepatitis C

As previously mentioned (Screening of Potential Organ Donors for Transmissible Infectious Disease), this virus has been transmitted from donor to recipient after heart transplantation. There are at least six recognized genotypes of hepatitis C virus: 1a, 1b, 2, 3a, 4, and 5. There is currently no secure information regarding the treatment of heart transplant recipients with HCV infection. Because of the relatively benign course of this disease in many patients over many years, treatment may not be advisable, although recent reports of rapidly progressive liver disease early after heart transplantation[321] may change that recommendation. There is evidence that the combination of ribavirin with interferon (Tables 15–5 and 15–6), which has been tested in liver transplant recipients,[46] can produce normalization of liver function tests, improve the histological picture of the infection, and suppress serum levels of HCV RNA. Identification of the genotype is advisable, since there are differences in response to therapy among genotypes. In the United States, about 70% of infected persons are genotype 1a or 1b. Rates of response (clearing of virus by quantitative PCR) to interferon alfa-2b and ribavirin therapy are substantially less for genotype 1b and mixed 1a/1b compared to other genotypes.[85] Substantial clearing of virus from the blood stream after 6 months of interferon/ribavirin therapy is more likely in the presence of low viral load (<2 million copies/mL), genotype 2 or 3, absence of cirrhosis on liver biopsy, and negative serum hepatitis C viral RNA test at 4 weeks (i.e., a prompt response to therapy).[213] Thus, although no controlled studies are available in solid organ transplantation, infected heart transplant patients should be evaluated for possible treatment.

The major side effects of the combination of interferon alfa-2b/ribavirin therapy are chronic weakness, irritability, abdominal pain, diarrhea, flu-like syndrome, and ribavirin-induced (dose-related) anemia, leukopenia, and occasional thrombocytopenia. Interferon therapy has been associated with an increase in rejection propensity, so increased rejection surveillance is warranted during therapy. Although it remains speculative whether certain immunosuppressive agents may potentiate progression of HCV infection, one study in renal transplant recipients concluded that mycophenolate may promote HCV viral replication and should be used with caution in HCV-infected transplant patients.[373] Hepatitis C in potential transplant recipients is also discussed in Chapter 6.

Parvovirus B19

Parvovirus is a member of the family Parvoviridae, and its genome is a small single-stranded DNA molecule. The blood group P antigen has been demonstrated as the cellular receptor for parvovirus B19,[63] and this antigen has also been found on endothelial cells[391] and fetal myocardial cells.[308, 352] The finding of this distribution of receptors in part explains the increasing array of diseases due to parvovirus B19 in immunocompetent and immunocompromised humans. Serologic evidence of previous parvovirus B19 infection increases with age, approximately 50% of the population having IgG antibodies by age 15 and 90% in the elderly.[96] In the normal population, infection may be asymptomatic or result in erythema infectiosum or "fifth disease."[434] Suppression of erythrocyte production may occur but is usually not clinically apparent, although in patients with diseases such as sickle cell anemia or thalassemia where red blood cell life is shortened, aplastic crises may occur.[336] Other illnesses caused by parvovirus B19 in immunocompetent patients include polyarthropathy syndrome,[308] fetal hydrops,[50] and myocarditis.[141, 388]

Reports have appeared of a severe erythroblastopenic anemia associated with active parvovirus B19 infection in renal,[43, 101, 311, 421, 440] liver,[88] lung,[474] and heart[12, 41, 474] transplant recipients. In a review of parvovirus B19-induced erythroblastopenic anemia in 14 solid organ transplant recipients[474] (of which two were heart/lung transplant recipients), the mean time from transplantation to development of anemia was 11.5 months (range, 0.5–34 months). Additional presentations occurred in half of the patients and included pancytopenia, leukopenia, flu-like syndrome with myalgia, and in one child erythema infectiosum. The mean value of hemoglobin at presentation was 6.0 g/dL (4.6–8.6 g/dL). In the immunocompetent patients with parvovirus B19, a rise of IgM with parvovirus is invariably present, but the antibody response may not occur in immunocompromised patients. In 2 of the 14 patients, there was no detectable level of IgM antibody, and in other patients the immune response was substantially delayed. Therefore, in immunocompromised patients, parvovirus B19 infection should be determined by either detection of parvovirus B19 DNA in the serum or bone marrow, or the presence of specific morphologic features in bone marrow specimens. A number of methods have been used to detect viral genome including PCR, Southern-blot analysis, and dot-blot analysis, but the most sensitive is PCR.[73] The specific morphologic features seen in the bone marrow include giant proerythroblasts, vacuolization of the cytoplasm, and intranuclear inclusions which are limited to erythroid cells. In the review by Wicki,[474] all patients who underwent a bone marrow examination had at least one of the morphologic patterns. A severe pneumonia due to parvovirus B19 has been reported[227] in a pediatric heart transplant recipient.

Although parvovirus B19-induced anemia in solid organ transplant patients has been reported to spontaneously recover,[88, 311, 315] the current therapy is a course of intravenous immunoglobulin (IVIG) which, because of the prevalence of this infection in the community, is a good source of anti–parvovirus B19 antibodies. No firm recommendations can be made currently regarding the dosage and duration of IVIG; however, protocols have ranged between 0.4 and 1 g/kg/day for between 3 and 10 days.[41, 227, 315, 474] Because of potential recurrent viremia and reticulocytopenia after cessation of IVIG treatment, repeated doses may be required.[88, 358] Use of recombinant human erythropoietin (r-HuE) in the belief that it will stimulate proliferation and maturation of erythroid precursors is controversial, but has been used in conjunction with IVIG.[474] Normalization of the hemoglobin level and an increase in the reticulocyte count can be expected within 2 to 4 weeks after commencement of treatment.[474]

There is evidence[292] that the method for inactivation of parvovirus B19 in donated blood (dry heat treatment at 80°C for 72 hours) may not completely eliminate parvovirus B19 infectivity, and this does raise the issue of the advisability of screening blood donors for this virus, since blood may potentially be a source of parvovirus B19 infection after heart transplantation.

Papillomavirus

Human papillomavirus (HPV) is a double-stranded DNA virus which is responsible for a number of conditions in transplant patients including cutaneous warts, urogenital and anal warts, and malignant transformation resulting in squamous cell carcinoma and urogenital cancer.

The markedly increased prevalence of HPV-associated cutaneous warts with increasing duration of immunosuppression has been demonstrated after renal transplantation.[170, 379] Risk factors for HPV-associated cutaneous warts include not only increased duration of immunosuppression, but also sun exposure[54] and possibly azathioprine- and prednisone-based immunosuppression as opposed to cyclosporine-based immunosuppression.[290]

Treatment is the same as in nonimmunosuppressed patients and may include topical salicylic acid (common warts), tretinoin cream (flat warts), 5-fluorouracil cream (flat warts), podophyllin, cryotherapy, and electrocautery. HPV-associated cutaneous warts in immunosuppressed patients tend to be disseminated, are often resistant to treatment, and may recur after treatment. The urogenital and anal warts associated with HPV infection appear identical to condylomata acuminata and, as with HPV-associated cutaneous warts, may be resistant to therapy.

The findings of HPV DNA in squamous cell carcinoma, transitional cell carcinoma, and cervical cancers suggest that this virus may be responsible for malignant transformation. This is supported by evidence that immunosuppressed patients are at increased risk of squamous cell carcinoma.[218, 259] Squamous cell carcinomas may arise in HPV-associated cutaneous warts and a number of specific types of HPV (HPV 16 and 18) are more likely to be associated with malignant transformation. Urogenital cancers, as with squamous cell carcinomas, occur with increased frequency in immunosuppressed patients who have HPV infection. Avoidance of sun exposure in immunosuppressed patients, particularly those with cutaneous warts, is a particularly important preventative measure. The management of patients with HPV-associated cancer is similar to that in nonimmunosuppressed patients and includes surgical resection, radiation therapy, chemotherapy, and reduction in immunosuppression.

Adenovirus

In the normal population, adenoviral infection is a self-limited illness occurring in children between the ages of 6 months and 5 years, and is spread by person-to-person contact. There is evidence[389] that adenovirus infection may cause a myocardial inflammatory process in pediatric cardiac transplant recipients. These patients were described as presenting with a history of an upper respiratory infection and subsequent development of cardiogenic shock with histological features of severe rejection on endomyocardial biopsy, and adenoviral genome was found by PCR in the endomyocardial biopsy specimens. Adenoviral infection has also been implicated in acute pulmonary failure in pediatric lung and heart/lung transplant recipients[58] (see Chapter 21).

Respiratory Syncytial Virus

In normal infants, respiratory syncytial virus (RSV) causes bronchiolitis and tracheobronchitis which can progress to a pneumonic illness. RSV infection can also occur in adults and older children, usually resulting in upper respiratory infections and tracheobronchitis. Although not extensively studied, RSV infection in solid organ transplant recipients results in illnesses manifesting as upper respiratory infections, bronchiolitis, and rarely life-threatening pneumonic illness. Respiratory tract RSV infection has been reported[465] in lung transplant recipients, and this infection was associated with a low mortality, most patients being treated with aerosolized ribavirin.

Influenza Virus

There is little information on influenza in solid organ transplant recipients, but influenza is known to cause severe illness in pediatric solid organ transplant recipients,[282] resulting in potentially fatal respiratory failure. Because of the high attack rate of the influenza virus in the general community, heart and heart/lung transplant recipients are at risk of developing influenza infection. Prophylactic measures should include annual vaccination of the patient and their families and strict avoidance

of contact with individuals with influenza. In the general community, because of the antigenic variation of the influenza virus, the severity of the illness will vary from year to year. Rimantadine or amantidine may be used for postexposure prophylaxis and both also have been used for therapy of established disease. The treatment of severe influenza illness in solid organ transplant recipients has not been established, but a number of drugs are under investigation, including ribavirin (intravenous or aerosolized) and neuraminidase inhibitors.

Parainfluenza Virus

Parainfluenza viruses 1, 2, 3, 4a, and 4b cause a wide range of respiratory infection in infants and children including croup, bronchiolitis, and viral pneumonia. Types 1 and 2 usually cause epidemic disease in the fall and type 3 produces perennial disease.[189, 203] A typical feature of parainfluenza virus infection is reinfection within 3 months of primary infection.[179] Parainfluenza virus infection in immunocompromised patients where the infection involves the lower respiratory tract has a high mortality (32% in bone marrow transplant recipients).[466] Parainfluenza virus infection has been described in pediatric patients undergoing organ transplantation,[19] particularly after lung transplantation,[465] and parainfluenza virus pneumonia has been described in a heart transplant recipient, resolution occurring with aerosolized ribavirin therapy.[95] Even in immunosuppressed patients, the disease is usually self-limited, resolution occurring even without antiviral therapy.[473]

Rhinovirus and Coronavirus

These viruses typically cause a coryzal syndrome that is similar to the self-limited course seen in the normal population except that it may be a little more severe and prolonged. Heart and heart/lung transplant recipients should use the same infection control measures for avoidance of these infections as they would for any community respiratory virus infections.

Polyoma Viruses (BK Virus and JC Virus)

The JC and related BK viruses, although infecting most normal children, rarely cause disease. However, the JC virus results in progressive multifocal leukoencephalopathy, which is a demyelinating disease of the central nervous system and has been described after cardiac transplantation[157, 197] (see section Central Nervous System Infection in the section Approach to Infection Syndromes and Specific Infections). The BK virus is known to occur in renal transplant patients, can mimic acute rejection, and is associated with urethral stricture.[115] It is not known whether this virus causes disease in heart transplant recipients.

FUNGAL INFECTIONS

Invasive fungi (nucleated parasitic organisms with a polysaccharide cell wall) represent a serious threat to the cardiac transplant patient, and may occur at any time following transplantation, although there is an early increased peak of risk (Fig. 15–9). Locally invasive disease or widespread dissemination may occur with almost any of the mycoses, and if unrecognized and untreated, these infections result in serious sequelae, including death.

The development of fungal disease in a heart or heart/lung transplant recipient usually results from the breakdown of specific and nonspecific host defenses, such as breaching of skin and mucosal barriers (intravenous lines, urinary catheterization, arterial line, intubation), immunosuppression with impairment of nonspecific defenses (phagocytic cells) and specific defense mechanisms (humoral and cellular immunity), the effect of broad-spectrum antibiotic administration, and immunomodulation with viral infection such as CMV and EBV. The most frequently occuring fungal infections in heart transplant recipients are[297] Candida spp., Aspergillus spp., Pneumocystis carinii, and Cryptococcus neoformans.

Candida spp.

Invasive candidiasis is the commonest invasive fungal infection in cardiac transplant recipients and occurs almost exclusively as a nosocomial infection, usually within the first 30 days following transplantation. Candida infection usually originates from endogenous flora but can also be transmitted from the hospital environment. There are a large number of Candida spp. that are pathogenic to man, but it is C. albicans and C. tropicalis that are most likely to cause candidiasis after heart and heart/lung transplantation. The types of infections caused by the Candida include mucosal colonization or infection, candidemia (blood stream Candida without obvious visceral disease), and disseminated candidiasis (blood stream and visceral involvement by invasive candidiasis).

Colonization and infection may be seen in a number of mucosal surfaces including the mouth (most common), vagina, and esophagus, producing typical candidal lesions which may coalesce if untreated. In heart and heart/lung transplantation, locally invasive candidiasis has been described causing constrictive pericarditis,[69] mycotic aneurysms of the aortic anastomosis (see later section, Donor Heart Infection), tracheal anastomotic infection and dehiscence (see Chapter 21), and candidal sternal wound infection. Asymptomatic candiduria due to bladder colonization can also be seen.

Disseminated candidiasis may involve most organ systems. The principal symptom is fever, and other signs and symptoms may be either nonspecific or referrable to the involved organ. With the possible exception of endophthalmitis (classic white retinal lesion with vitreal extension which is seen relatively infrequently[61]), there are no reliable physical findings that support this diagnosis. Nodular cutaneous lesions may be seen in disseminated candidiasis, but these usually only occur in neutropenic patients. Leukocytosis is usually present but is nonspecific. Blood cultures are the only reliable diagnostic tool, but have relatively limited sensitivity. The sensitivity of blood culture appears increased somewhat by use of such newer techniques as lysis-centrifugation, BAC-TEC high-blood volume fungal media (HBV-FM) system, and the BAC-TEC system,[176, 477] but probably remains less than 60%. Unfortunately, proven serodiagnostic tests are not yet available,[119, 281] and the diagnosis often depends on maintaining a high index of suspicion for this infection. This requires recognition of the important risk factors (prolonged stay in an intensive care unit, prolonged use of antimicrobial agents, use of central venous catheters, and colonization with Candida spp.). Of these factors, colonization at one or more sites (e.g., sputum, urine, wound, stool) seems very powerful,[347] and its absence makes invasive candidiasis less likely.

Treatment of invasive candidiasis requires systemic therapy with either fluconazole or amphotericin B (see Box) (Tables 15–5 and 15–6). These drugs appear to be equally effective for uncomplicated candidemia. There are fewer data supporting the use of fluconazole in visceral invasive disease, and most experts prefer amphotericin B as "induction therapy" in these cases followed by "consolidation therapy" with fluconazole. The current Food and Drug Administration (FDA)-approved indications for lipid formulations of amphotericin B are outlined in Table 15–11.

Mucocutaneous candidiasis is treated topically with nonabsorbable antifungal agents such as nystatin or clotrimazole. Systemic therapy with fluconazole or low-dose amphotericin B may be required if topical therapy is unsuccessful. Candiduria is treated with oral fluconazole.

The emergence of azole-resistant yeasts such as C. glabrata and C. krusei may be related to extensive use of azoles in many centers. For this reason, patients with suspected severe disseminated candidal infection should be treated at least initially with amphotericin.

Aspergillus spp.

Invasive aspergillosis may be caused by any of several Aspergillus species, most importantly A. fumigatus, A.

Amphotericin B

Amphotericin B (AmB) is a successful antifungal agent for treating severe systemic mycotic infections, but its use is limited by adverse reactions including nephrotoxicity and infusion-related events. The toxicity of amphotericin B is related to its propensity to bind cholesterol. In order to improve the therapeutic index of amphotericin B, delivery systems have been developed which reduce the exposure of amphotericin to host cells while still achieving a therapeutic level at the site of infection. These lipid-based amphotericin B preparations include amphotericin B lipid complex (ABLC), amphotericin B cholesteryl sulfate complex (also called amphotericin B colloidal dispersion) (ABCD), and liposomal amphotericin B (L-AmB). Each lipid formulation has its distinct pharmacological properties, but they have in common less nephrotoxicity than the conventional formulation of amphotericin B. However, superior efficacy of these lipid preparations has not been established, and they cost significantly more than conventional AmB.

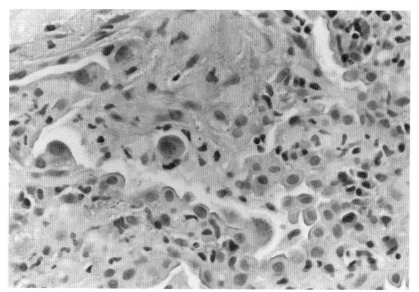

FIGURE **15–17.** Hematoxylin and eosin stain of an open lung biopsy showing CMV pneumonitis with characteristic cytopathic changes (intranuclear and intracytoplasmic inclusion bodies).

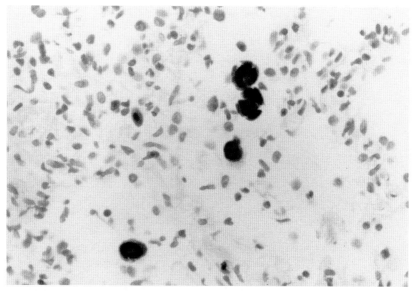

FIGURE **15–18.** Open lung biopsy in a patient with CMV pneumonitis confirmed by a positive immunoperoxidase stain.

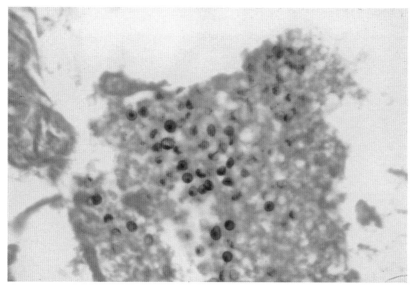

FIGURE **15-23.** Transbronchial lung biopsy demonstrating multiple organisms consistent with *Pneumocystis carinii* (Gomori's methenamine silver stain).

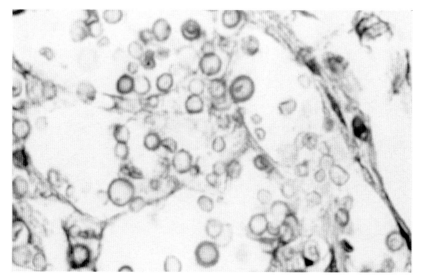

FIGURE **15-24.** Periodic acid–Schiff stain from lung tissue demonstrating multiple encapsulated yeast consistent with *Cryptococcus neoformans.*

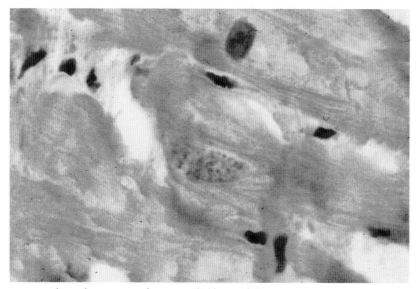

FIGURE **15-26.** Hematoxylin and eosin stain of a myocardial biopsy following recent cardiac transplantation demonstrating the tachyzoite of a *Toxoplasma gondii.*

TABLE 15–11 FDA-Approved Indications for Lipid Formulations of Amphotericin B

FDA-APPROVED INDICATION	ABLC	ABCD	L-AmB
1. Treatment of the following conditions in patients who are refractory to AmBD or in whom renal impairment or unacceptable toxicity precludes use of AmBD:			
• Invasive fungal infection	✔[1]		
• *Aspergillus* species		✔[2]	✔[3]
• *Candida* species			✔[3]
• *Cryptococcus* species			✔[3]
2. Empiric therapy for presumed fungal infection in febrile, neutropenic patients			✔[4]

AmBD, amphotericin B desoxycholate; ABLC, amphotericin B lipid complex; ABCD, amphotericin B colloidal dispersion; L-AmB, liposomal amphotericin B. Recommended dosing: [1]ABLC 5 mg/kg/day; [2]ABCD 3–4 mg/kg/day; [3]L-AmB 3–5 mg/kg/day; [4]L-AmB 3 mg/kg/day (immunocompromised patients will require higher and more frequent dosing).
Adapted from Hoesley CJ, Dismukes WE: New antifungal agents: emphasis on lipid formulations of amphotericin B. Clin Updates Fungal Infect 1999;2:1–5.

flavus, A. niger, and *A. terreus.*[365] *Aspergillus* species are ubiquitous soil-dwelling molds. Exposure almost always occurs via the respiratory route, making pulmonary and sinus presentations the most common form of the disease.[279] *Aspergillus* spp. infections are often acquired from within the hospital, and there have been reports of outbreaks of *Aspergillus* infection associated with construction work (the density of airborne spores is known to be increased at construction sites[370, 383]) and contaminated air-conditioning systems.[24, 260] Once the conidia germinate, there is endobronchial proliferation of hyphae into the pulmonary arterioles. This blood vessel invasion results in thrombosis, ischemic necrosis of lung parenchyma, hemorrhage, and hematogenous dissemination to distant organs.[280] The central nervous system is the most commonly recognized extrapulmonary site among patients with disseminated disease, although any organ may be involved.[460] A case of vetebral osteomyelitis and diskitis (successfully treated by surgical resection and antifungal agents) after heart transplantation has been described.[221] The pathology of CNS aspergillosis is single or multiple abscesses associated with hemorrhagic infarction and is usually found in the cortex. Patients may present with a clinical picture similar to that of a stroke or altered mental status. In disseminated aspergillosis, there may be widespread involvement of other organs such as kidney, liver, and spleen with necrosis and abscess formation. In lung transplant recipients, CMV infection was found to be a risk factor for invasive aspergillosis.[222]

The diagnosis of aspergillosis is suspected on the basis of clinical and radiographic findings in patients at risk for invasive disease. Blood cultures are rarely positive. The characteristic appearance on chest x-ray is one of nodules with associated infiltrates. Cavitation may be present and sometimes diffuse pulmonary infiltrates may occur (Fig. 15–22). A negative computerized tomographic study of the chest strongly reduces the likelihood of invasive aspergillosis.[67, 68, 451] Serologic assays are available but are rarely helpful in the diagnosis of invasive aspergillosis among severely immunocompromised patients. Thus, the diagnosis of invasive aspergillosis is confirmed based on histological evidence of tissue invasion by characteristic appearing organisms and isolation of *Aspergillus* spp. from involved tissue.[117] Isolation of *Aspergillus* spp. from biologic specimens in an immunosuppressed patient indicates the presence of actual or imminent invasive infection.[484] The treatment of invasive aspergillosis at present requires amphotericin B (preferably a lipid AMB formulation) (Table 15–11) given at doses of 1.0-1.5 mg/kg/day (or 3–5 mg/kg/day for lipid AMB) (Table 15–6) until all evidence of disease is resolved. Among patients with focal pulmonary involvement, surgical excision may be curative. Untreated invasive aspergillosis in the cardiac transplant patient is uniformly fatal. Even with aggressive therapy, success rates exceeding 50% are uncommon.

Pneumocystis Carinii

Pneumocystis carinii is an organism of low virulence found in the lungs of humans and a variety of animals. The taxonomy of *P. carinii* has long been a matter of controversy, with the weight of recent molecular data suggesting that the organism is more closely related to fungi than to protozoa. A reservoir outside of the human host has never been determined, and there is some epidemiologic evidence to suggest person-to-person transmission. It remains unclear whether patients with *Pneumocystis* pneumonia represent primary or reactivation infections, as there is no reliable skin test or serologic assay to determine prior exposure status. Dummer and colleagues[135] reported six cases of *Pneumocystis* pneumonia in 14 heart/lung recipients 3–19 months after transplant. In contrast, patients who receive only heart trans-

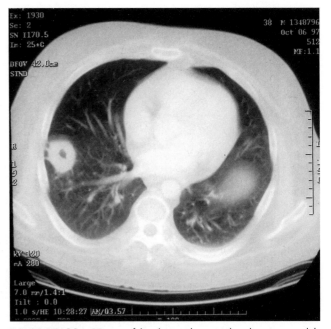

FIGURE **15–22.** CT scan of the chest with a peripheral cavitary nodule in the right lung due to *Aspergillus fumigatus.*

plantation have an incidence of *Pneumocystis* pneumonia of 5% or less in most series even without prophylactic trimethoprim/sulfamethoxazole (TMP/SMX). A recent study[228] in pediatric cardiac transplant patients reported *Pneumocystis* pneumonia in 10 (7%) of 152 recipients. Patients are at greatest risk for *Pneumocystis* pneumonia for the first 6 months following transplantation and the risk appears greatest in patients receiving cytolytic induction and among patients with frequent rejection episodes. Symptoms of acute disease include fever; nonproductive cough; dyspnea; and occasionally headache, confusion, and cutaneous lesions.

The diagnosis of *Pneumocystis* pneumonia is suggested in the cardiac transplant patient with fever, nonproductive cough, dyspnea, and progressive hypoxemia with a chest x-ray demonstrating diffuse interstitial infiltrates. Alveolar infiltrates and cavitary lesions, as seen among patients with AIDS, may be present. The diagnosis is confirmed by the demonstration of characteristic helmet-shaped organisms on lung biopsy (Fig. 15–23) or bronchoalveolar lavage. Foamy intra-alveolar infiltrates are often described. Special stains such as Gomori's methenamine silver, Wright-Giemsa, and Papanicolaou are essential to demonstrate the organism in histopathologic specimens.

The treatment of *Pneumocystis* pneumonia is TMP/SMX (20 mg/kg and 100 mg/kg daily) parenterally or orally in four divided doses for at least 3 weeks (Table 15–5). Patients who cannot tolerate TMP/SMX due to adverse events (e.g., fever, rash, leukopenia, renal dysfunction) may receive pentamidine 3–4 mg/kg paren-

terally. Other regimens have not been extensively reviewed in non-AIDS patients, but include dapsone/trimethoprim, clindamycin-primaquine, and atovaquone. These compounds may be useful alternative agents for *Pneumocystis* pneumonia.

Primary prevention of *Pneumocystis* pneumonia is widely practiced and has all but eliminated *Pneumocystis* pneumonia in adult transplant recipients. TMP/SMX DS given daily or three times weekly is extremely effective prophylaxis in patients with AIDS and in transplant recipients when given for 6 months after transplant. Other regimens including monthly inhaled pentamidine and daily dapsone are unproven in transplant recipients. TMP/SMX prophylaxis also affords some protection against nocardiosis, listeriosis, and toxoplasmosis, as well as against some bacterial agents of respiratory and urinary tract infection. In a study from the Cleveland Clinic,[184] the incidence of *Pneumocystis* pneumonia after organ transplantation declined after the first year except in lung transplant patients, prompting the authors to recommend indefinite prophylaxis in these patients.

Cryptococcus Neoformans

C. neoformans infection usually occurs more than 6 months after transplantation. The principal organs involved by *C. neoformans* are the lungs (Fig. 15–24), which serve as the portal of entry, and the central nervous system (Fig. 15–25). Central nervous system involvement usually produces clinically apparent meningitis, and the diagnosis is established by direct tissue exami-

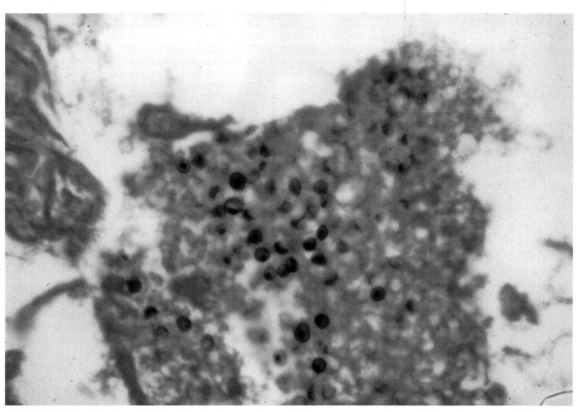

FIGURE **15–23.** Transbronchial lung biopsy demonstrating multiple organisms consistent with *Pneumocystis carinii* (Gomori's methenamine silver stain).

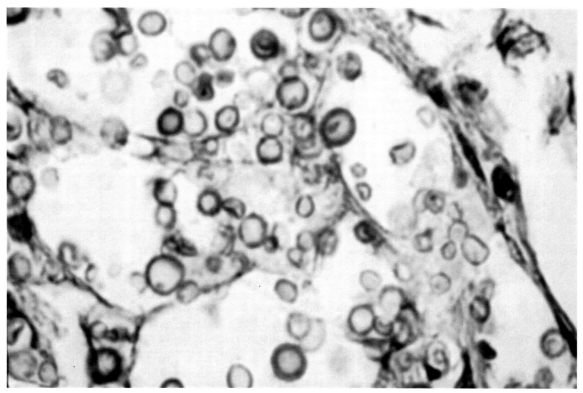

FIGURE **15–24.** Periodic acid–Schiff stain from lung tissue demonstrating multiple encapsulated yeast consistent with *Cryptococcus neoformans.*

nation, culture, and/or assay for cryptococcal antigen of the cerebrospinal fluid. Cryptococcemia alone may be seen[299, 335, 341] among immunocompromised patients without obvious localizing signs. Cutaneous involvement is also common among immunocompromised pa-

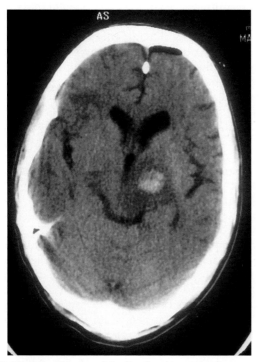

FIGURE **15–25.** CT scan of the head with contrast demonstrating a left periventricular cryptococcoma with surrounding edema.

tients with disseminated cryptococcosis. The rash may take on many forms, but a molluscum contagiosum-like umbilicated nodular rash is strongly suggestive of *C. neoformans.*[366] Cellulitis[395] and myositis[34] are not uncommon presentations of disseminated disease in cardiac transplant patients. Focal involvement of bone,[65, 226] joint,[38, 313] eye,[364] kidney,[359] peritoneum,[350] or the prostate[207] may occur. Induction therapy with amphotericin B with or without 5-flucytosine followed by fluconazole therapy for at least 6 months is appropriate therapy for most patients (Table 15–5). Lifelong suppression with fluconazole is generally not necessary.

Zygomycosis (Mucormycosis)

Zygomycosis, which is most commonly due to *Rhizopus* spp., is increasingly recognized as being caused by other members of the class such as *Cunninghamella, Absidia corymbifera, Bertholletiae, Rhizomucor pusillus,* and *Saksenaea vasiformis.* The portal of entry appears to be the respiratory tract; less often, the infection follows ingestion or traumatic inoculation of organisms into the skin. Diabetes mellitus is a known predisposing factor to zygomycosis. The clinical hallmark of mucormycosis is the rapid onset of symptoms and fever. Different clinical spectrums have been recognized, but the most important is rhinocerebral mucormycosis. Other forms are pulmonary, gastrointestinal, cutaneous, isolated mucormycotic brain lesions, endocarditis, and disseminated mucormycosis (as an isolated form or as a consequence of the other forms). Metastatic lesions can be found in the brain, spleen, kidney, heart, liver, pancreas, stomach, and omentum. The successful treatment of a heart transplant recipient with pulmonary cavitary zygomycosis has been reported.[420] Surgical excision of involved tissues and aggressive therapy with lipid formulations of amphotericin B (Tables 15–5 and 15–6) provide the only hope of successful outcome in these cases, although rhinocerebral zygomycosis has a dismal prognosis.

Histoplasma Capsulatum

H. capsulatum infection has been described in renal transplant patients,[472] but all solid organ transplant recipients are at risk for this infection, particularly those residing in the midwestern United States. While infection due to *H. capsulatum* can take many forms,[181–183, 467] the disseminated forms of this infection are most likely. Acute disseminated histoplasmosis is usually seen in infants and severely immunocompromised adults.[183] The hallmark of this form of histoplasmosis is massive infection of the cells of the reticuloendothelial system by the organism, with hepatosplenomegaly, lymphadenopathy, and marked bone marrow abnormalities. Clinically, these patients may appear acutely ill with high fever and relentless progression of symptoms. Diffuse interstitial involvement of the lung is also common.

The diagnosis of disseminated histoplasmosis can be made by histopathology and/or culture of the blood, bone marrow, or other involved organs. In acute disseminated histoplasmosis, examination of a peripheral blood smear may demonstrate the organism in leukocytes. While antibody-based tests (especially if done for both the H and M precipitins) are sometimes positive in disseminated histoplasmosis,[470, 471] measurement of *H. capsulatum* antigen is more likely to be diagnostic.[158, 468, 471] The antigen is present in low or undetectable amounts in patients with self-limited pulmonary histoplasmosis, but can be detected in a variety of body fluids of patients with disseminated disease. Measurement of antigen in the urine is the most useful general test and has a sensitivity of greater than 90%.[468, 471] The antigen is detectable in the blood in only 50–80% of patients, and the high sensitivity of urine testing presumably results from concentration of the antigen in the urine.[468, 471] With involvement of the central nervous system, the antigen can be detected in the cerebrospinal fluid approximately 40% of the time.[467] The antigen can also be detected in bronchoalveolar lavage fluid in 70% of patients with AIDS and histoplasmosis, and the urine antigen is also positive in more than 90% of such cases.[469] Induction therapy with amphotericin B for 10–14 days followed by lifelong therapy with itraconazole is the standard approach to therapy (Tables 15–5 and 15–6).

Blastomyces Dermatitidis

Primary infection with *B. dermatitidis* usually occurs through inhalation of infectious spores and can result in an acute self-limited pneumonia or may develop into a chronic pulmonary process. Patients with chronic pulmonary disease typically present with fever, weight loss, and productive cough. Asymptomatic pulmonary blastomycosis may also occur and is detected as a nodule or mass lesion on chest radiograph. Extrapulmonary involvement occurs, and verrucous or ulcerative skin lesions, osteomyelitis, and prostatitis or epididymoorchitis are common.[55] Meningitis occurs in up to 10% of patients with disseminated disease.[55] Blastomycosis has been reported rarely in solid organ transplant patients, but may produce aggressive multiorgan disease.[329] As in normal hosts, pulmonary findings are most common, but diffuse interstitial and/or alveolar changes with respiratory failure are more commonly seen in immunocompromised patients than in the normal host. Skin lesions are also frequent in these patients. Disseminated blastomycosis can progress rapidly to death.

The diagnosis of blastomycosis is usually made by visualizing the characteristic organism on direct examination of tissue or sputum. Culture is usually positive, but may require up to 4 weeks of incubation. Several serologic tests are commercially available, with the best current results being obtained with an enzyme immunoassay for antibody to the *B. dermatitidis* A antigen.[56, 240] However, available serologic assays lack sufficient sensitivity and specificity to be very useful in the detection and management of patients with blastomycosis. Treatment with induction amphotericin B followed by itraconazole or fluconazole for prolonged periods (6–12 months), possibly lifelong, is recommended.

Coccidioides Immitis

C. immitis is known primarily as a cause of acute undifferentiated fever, acute atypical pneumonia, and chronic pneumonia among patients from endemic areas of the southwest United States.[13] Disease outside of the lungs is evidence for hematogenous dissemination, but patients with extrapulmonary spread often present in a subacute fashion with minimal systemic symptoms. Bone pain, skin lesions, or signs of meningitis are typical, but immunosuppressed patients in general may present with aggressive multiorgan involvement.[120, 380] While the chest radiograph may be normal, a diffuse reticulonodular infiltrate on chest radiograph is often seen in the immunocompromised patient. Involvement of the spleen, liver, heart, kidney, bone marrow, prostate, and pancreas by *C. immitis* have all been documented at autopsy.[13, 60, 120, 249, 266]

Coccidioidomycosis has been reported in cardiac transplant recipients,[196, 449] and in the series of Hall[196] (11 episodes of coccidioidomycosis in nine heart transplant recipients), two patients had disseminated disease and the others had disease confined to the lungs.

In immunosuppressed patients who develop disseminated coccidioidomycosis, the usual complement fixation serologic tests may not provide evidence to support the diagnosis.[120, 155] Biopsy and culture of involved sites should thus always be pursued to confirm a diagnosis. Initial therapy with amphotericin B is appropriate for most cardiac transplant recipients with coccidioidomycosis, followed by long-term suppression with either fluconazole or itraconazole (Tables 15–5 and 15–6). With the appropriate therapy, death is uncommon.[196]

Other Fungi

Two members of the *Scedosporium* genus, namely, *Scedosporium apiospermum* (*Pseudallescheria boydii*) and *Scedosporium inflatum* (*S. prolificans*) have been associated with a highly aggressive deep-seated infection in immunocompromised patients. The infections caused by these organisms include sinusitis, endophthalmitis, otitis, endocarditis and pneumonia, with disseminated disease and occasional central nervous system, bone, and joint involvement.[369] The high incidence of sinusitis, pneumonia or both, point towards a respiratory route as the main portal of infection entry, although traumatic inoculation of the fungus through the skin is possible. The diagnosis rests on the isolation of the fungus from clinical specimens.

Phaeohyphomycosis is a fungal infection caused by a group of a darkly pigmented (dematiaceous) fungi that form in tissue either as solitary or short chains of yeast-like cells or as hyphae. Phaeohyphomycosis are an increasingly prevalent group of opportunistic fungal diseases. The five genera most frequently recognized are *Curvularia, Bipolaris, Exserohilum, Alternaria,* and *Cladosporium.*[254] Infection in the immunocompromised host can be divided into three distinct clinical syndromes: subcutaneous, paranasal, and cerebral infection. Dissemination may follow any of the three mentioned forms.

Histological examination and culture of tissue specimens obtained at biopsy achieve diagnosis of phaeohyphomycosis infections. Treatment consists of resection of localized lesions (most useful when the central nervous system is involved). Amphotericin B has been reported to be of limited activity. Oral treatment with itraconazole appears promising. Relapse is common, and overall prognosis is poor for the immunocompromised host.

PROTOZOAL INFECTIONS

Toxoplasma

Toxoplasma gondii is a ubiquitous intracellular protozoal parasite which infects humans, domesticated animals, and birds. Cats are the definitive host, and all other infected animals are secondary hosts. Human infection occurs either by ingestion of contaminated food products, transplacentally from infected mother to fetus, or from transplantation of organs from an infected donor to an uninfected recipient. In humans, the organism exists in two forms—the invasive form, or tachyzoite, and the latent form, or tissue cyst. The tachyzoite is an obligatory intracellular parasite and is capable of reproduction in virtually all mammalian cells. The tachyzoite is seen during acute infection. Tissue cysts are seen in chronically infected hosts, and may occur in any organ, but have a predilection for brain, skeletal muscle, and myocardium. Thus, among solid organ transplant recipients, previously unexposed cardiac transplant patients are at greatest risk for acute infection when exposed to an organ from a previously infected donor.[251]

Two forms of toxoplasmosis occur in transplant patients—acute and reactivation disease.[268] Acute infection occurs in previously uninfected patients from the donor organ or from ingestion of oocysts in cat feces or tissue cysts in undercooked meat.[268, 381, 481] Acute infection was first described among renal transplant recipients, but was subsequently recognized among cardiac transplant recipients.[16, 212, 288, 296, 462, 480] Symptomatic toxoplasmosis in donor-recipient mismatches occurs in as many as 70% of cases, and asymptomatic seroconversion occurs in the majority, though not all, of the remaining patients. Onset of illness may occur between 12 and 300 days after transplant, with most cases occurring before 80 days. Undifferentiated fever is the most common presenting physical finding. Pneumonitis, myocarditis, and encephalitis are the commonest clinical syndromes, though any organ system may be involved. Acute myocarditis, which can clinically and histologically resemble acute rejection, can occur, and tragic cases of fatal disseminated toxoplasmosis have been probably precipitated by the use of high-dose corticosteroids for treatment of presumed graft rejection in *T. gondii* mismatched patients. Unrecognized and untreated, acute symptomatic toxoplasmosis in the transplant recipient is often a rapidly fatal illness.

Reactivation disease in previously infected patients is less common than acute disease and may present with chorioretinitis, encephalitis, myocarditis, or disseminated disease with pneumonitis. Onset of disease is typically greater than 6 months after transplant and tends to be more focal than acute disease, affecting one organ system (e.g., eye, brain) more often than producing disseminated disease. While the disease is important to recognize because of its preventable nature and devastating consequences if untreated, it is fortunately rare, occurring in fewer than 1% of transplanted patients.[166, 212, 296, 325]

The definitive diagnosis of acute or reactivation toxoplasmosis depends on demonstration of the organism in histopathologic specimens.[455] While acute *Toxoplasma* myocarditis may resemble acute rejection, the presence of eosinophilia in an endomyocardial biopsy specimen should alert the clinician to the possibility of toxoplasmosis, although tachyzoites and cysts may be seen[193, 455] (Fig. 15–26). Special stains, especially the immunoperoxidase stain, are extremely useful in identifying *T. gondii* in tissue specimens. In lieu of definitive demonstration of organisms in tissue, serologic assays are useful in supporting a diagnosis of toxoplasmosis. Measurement of IgG and IgM antibodies by ELISA has become the standard methodology, replacing the older dye test.[480] Demonstration of a fourfold rise in IgG titers and/or IgM titers, or seroconversion form seronegative to seropositive in conjunction with a clinically compatible illness provides presumptive evidence of toxoplasmosis. Newer techniques, including PCR of serum and urine, are not standardized and remain investigational. Culture techniques for *T. gondii* are not generally available.

Untreated symptomatic toxoplasmosis in cardiac transplant recipients is usually fatal. At least two thirds of treated patients improve with specific therapy. While there are no controlled therapeutic trials in the treatment

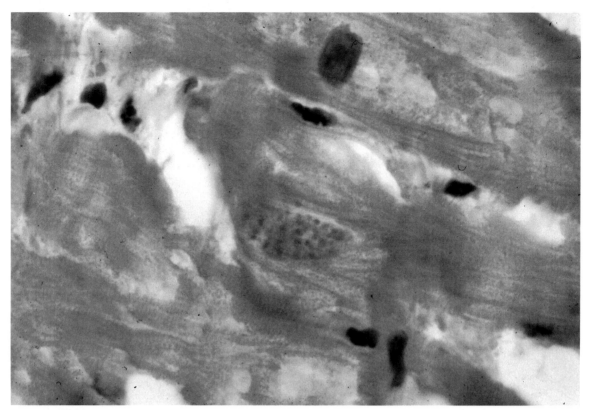

FIGURE 15–26. Hematoxylin and eosin stain of a myocardial biopsy following recent cardiac transplantation demonstrating the tachyzoite of a *Toxoplasma gondii.*

of toxoplasmosis in non-AIDS patients, much has been learned from the AIDS experience. The combination of sulfadiazine (4–6 g/day) and pyrimethamine (100–200 mg loading dose followed by 50–75 mg/day) appears to be the best regimen for acute or reactivation toxoplasmosis. Folinic acid (leucovorin) (5–10 mg/day) must be given in conjunction with this regimen to diminish hematotoxicity. Alternatives to this regimen include pyrimethamine-clindamycin (sulfa-allergic patients) and TMP/SMX, although no data regarding efficacy of these regimens exists in the transplant population. Therapy should be continued until all signs and symptoms of acute disease have resolved, but usually no less than 4–6 weeks. The need for chronic suppressive therapy is not clear, but the immunosuppression regimen should be minimized when possible.

In heart transplant recipients who are at high risk for acute disease (positive donor to negative recipient), prophylaxis consists of pyrimethamine 25 mg qd together with leucovorin 10 mg qd for 6 months.

Chagas' Disease

Chagas' disease is caused by the protozoan *Trypanosoma cruzi.* This is a disease that is endemic in Latin American countries and can rarely occur in the United States, since insects and mammals in the south and southwest of the United States may be infected. Human transmission occurs by the bite of the reduviid bug (the intermediate hosts being wild and domestic mammals), by blood transfusion, or congenitally. The acute phase results

from extensive dissemination and reproduction throughout the body. Acute infection typically presents as fever, myocarditis, and hepatosplenomegaly.[232] Patients with myocarditis present with heart failure which may either resolve or run a fulminant course. The parasites can be seen within the cardiac myocytes with a surrounding cellular infiltrate. Between 10 and 30 years after the acute infection,[232] chronic Chagas' disease may develop, presenting with a dilated cardiomyopathy. Other manifestations of the infection include megacolon, megaesophagus, and dilatation of the stomach, duodenum, ureters, or bronchi.[232] Cardiac transplantation has been performed for Chagas' disease.[48, 419]

There appears to be a high incidence of reactivation of Chagas' disease after transplantation, and although there may be a response to benzimidazole or nifurtimox, the disease may relapse off treatment.[234] In view of this, there is some opinion that transplantation should not be performed for end-stage Chagas cardiomyopathy.[234]

NEMATODE INFECTIONS

Strongyloides Stercoralis

Strongyloides is a disease caused by the intestinal nematode *Strongyloides stercoralis.* This parasite is endemic in certain parts of the world including Latin America, Southeast Asia, and the southern United States. In the normal host, *S. stercoralis* resides in the gastrointestinal tract and may be completely asymptomatic. In the immunosuppressed patient, two patterns of infection may occur.[375] The first is a disseminated infection which is the result of invasion of a number of tissues throughout the body by the organism, often accompanied by normal gut flora. The clinical presentation is that of a Gram-negative bacteremia that appears to be unresponsive to antibacterial therapy alone, since therapy against *S. stercoralis* is also required. The second pattern is a hyper-infestation syndrome which may present as a hemorrhagic pneumonia or enterocolitis representing an exaggeration of the usual process of *S. stercoralis* infection. Both of these syndromes have a mortality that is greater than 50%. The treatment of *S. stercoralis* infection is thiabendazole or ivermectin. However, ideally these syndromes can be prevented by screening of potential transplant recipients from endemic areas. There is a sensitive ELISA test for the antibody to this organism and seropositive individuals should be treated prior to transplantation with thiabendazole or ivermectin.

APPROACH TO INFECTION SYNDROMES AND SPECIFIC INFECTIONS

FEVER

Apart from the usual fever that occurs in the postoperative period and transient fever following bronchoscopy and bronchoalveolar lavage in heart/lung transplant recipients, a fever, for all practical purposes, represents a manifestation of infection. Unless dictated by the clinical situation, the use of empiric broad-spectrum antibiotic coverage should be resisted because of the possibility of predisposing these patients to fungal infections and promoting antibiotic resistance.

Uncomplicated fever in the cardiac transplant recipient should always be considered in the context of timing of the transplant, history of rejections, immunosuppressive regimen, epidemiologic exposure history, and donor history. An approach to evaluation of fever is presented in Table 15–12.

PULMONARY INFILTRATE

There is considerable opportunity for a number of defense mechanisms of the lung to be breached following heart and heart/lung transplantation, predisposing these patient to a variety of pulmonary infections. After heart/lung transplantation, the probability of breaching the pulmonary defense mechanisms is even greater than after heart transplantation, and may result from acute graft dysfunction, airway complications (dehiscence, stricture, and malacia), impairment of mucociliary transport, donor mucosal loss associated with the surgical procedure, loss of the cough reflex, and the long-term complication of obliterative bronchiolitis. Impaired alveolar macrophage function (loss of chemotaxis and phagocytosis) and alterations in surfactant contribute. The differential diagnosis of a pulmonary infiltrate in

TABLE 15–12	Important Considerations in the Evaluation of Fever in Cardiac Transplant Recipients
FACTOR	COMMENT
Timing of transplant	≤30 days: consider nosocomial sources—wound infection, UTI, pneumonia, venous catheter-associated bacteremia. Except for candidemia, fungal and other "classic" opportunistic infections are rare.
	1–6 mo: the period of maximum immunosuppression and classic transplant-associated infections such as CMV.
	>6 mo: community acquired infections are likely (pneumonia, gastroenteritis); typically the time when mycobacterial (e.g. *M. tuberculosis*) and endemic fungal infections (e.g., cryptococcosis, histoplasmosis) occur. CMV retinitis and herpes zoster are also "late" viral complications.
Donor	Review donor serology for HIV, VDRL *T. gondii*, CMV, hepatitis B and C; evidence of active granulomatous disease (e.g., TB or histoplasmosis) in donor. Symptomatic infection occurs within 6 mo in most cases (except HIV).
Recipient	Review CMV, *T. gondii* serology and look for evidence of mismatch (D+ R–). Consider reactivation tuberculosis or fungal disease (especially >6 mo following transplant).
Immunosuppressive regimen	Use of OKT3 and other antilymphocyte globulins substantially increases risk of CMV. Higher doses of glucocorticosteroids increase the risk of invasive fungal disease, especially molds.
History of rejection	Recent (i.e., within 6 mo) rejection therapy "resets the clock" such that CMV and other opportunistic pathogens are again seen commonly as in the 1- to 6-mo posttransplant interval.
Recent exposure history	Review recent occupational, recreational, and travel history. Review potential exposure to tuberculosis or potentially transmissible agents.

these immunosuppressed patients include the entire spectrum of potential bacterial, viral, fungal, protozoan, and mycobacterial pathogens, but must be distinguished from noninfectious causes of a pulmonary infiltrate including pulmonary edema, acute respiratory distress syndrome, posttransplant lymphoproliferative disorder, primary pulmonary neoplasia, and after heart/lung transplantation conditions such as primary graft failure, atelectasis and sputum retention associated with airway complications, reimplantation response, and acute pulmonary rejection. Important elements in the history include the timing of the appearance of pulmonary infiltrate in relation to the transplant or treatment of rejection, travel or environmental exposure, pretransplant serology of the donor and recipient (CMV and *Toxoplasma*), and for patients undergoing heart/lung transplantation the native lung disease (particularly pretransplant sputum cultures for patients with cystic fibrosis). Another clinical clue comes from the onset of symptoms (acute onset suggesting bacterial or viral infection and a slow onset suggesting fungal or parasitic infection). As in all immunosuppressed patients, symptoms of pneumonic illness, such as fever, cough, and sputum, may not develop. Hypoxemia out of proportion to the clinical and radiological findings suggests *Pneumocystis carinii* pneumonia.

A good quality **chest x-ray** is critical, but this may prove difficult if the patient is on a ventilator. The pneumonic process may present radiologically as focal, multifocal, or diffuse lesions with interstitial, alveolar, or a mixed pattern,[99] and rarely do the radiological findings suggest a specific organism. When a chest x-ray shows clear lung fields in the presence of signs and symptoms that suggest a pneumonic process, a **CT scan** should be performed. CT scans are also useful for localizing lesions, particularly where biopsy is contemplated. **Isolating the organism** is the most important investigation. Blood cultures are unlikely to be useful, and sputum cultures are only helpful if organisms that are not normally present in the pharynx are isolated, such as *Legionella*, mycobacteria, and fungi.[99] The diagnosis of pulmonary infection is based on **fiberoptic bronchoscopy, bronchoalveolar lavage** (BAL), and **transbronchial lung biopsy.** In the case of heart/lung transplant recipients, transbronchial lung biopsy is required to exclude noninfectious causes of the pulmonary infiltrate such as acute pulmonary rejection.

Following BAL, the infiltrate in the chest x-ray may worsen, and fever may occur in up to 50% of patients.[450] The BAL fluid brushing sample and transbronchial lung biopsy require investigation as outlined in Table 15–13.[99] A bacteria is considered likely causative of the pneumonic illness if on culture of the BAL fluid the bacterial concentration is equal to or greater than 10^4 or 10^5 colony-forming units (CFUs) per milliliter.[11, 191] Other investigations that may be considered (either because of the nature of the pulmonary lesion or failure of bronchoalveolar lavage to reveal the causative organism) include CT scan guided transthoracic needle biopsy or open lung biopsy (either by an open procedure or video-assisted thoracoscopy).

In the setting of a life-threatening pneumonic process, empiric antibiotic therapy is required before isolation of the organism occurs. If the process is indolent, delaying antimicrobial therapy is desirable to prevent complicating isolation of the organism.

WOUND INFECTION

Wound infections among cardiac transplant recipients are generally limited to the first 30 days following transplantation. Mediastinal infection is a serious complication after heart transplantation just as it is after nontransplant cardiac surgery. The incidence of mediastinal infection after cardiac transplantation is between 2 and 4.5%[25, 32, 211, 230] and is higher than after nontransplant cardiac surgical procedures. Factors associated with mediastinal infection include patients undergoing cardiac transplantation for ischemic cardiomyopathy versus dilated cardiomyopathy (perhaps reflecting previous sternotomy), patients who were UNOS status 1 prior to transplantation (perhaps reflecting the deleterious effect of a prolonged stay in the intensive care unit prior to transplantation with loss of physical reserves), and reexploration for bleeding. A group of patients at potential risk for wound infection after cardiac transplantation are patients that have been bridged with mechanial circulatory support, since infection is an important complication with these devices.[204, 284] However, the experience at UAB of patients being bridged to transplantation by an assist device who have a device infection suggests that the risk of mediastinal infection is low.

In patients after cardiac transplantation, the organisms most frequently involved are *Staphylococcus aureus* and coagulase-negative staphylococci, but other organisms have been implicated, including *Serratia* spp., *Klebsiella* spp., *Acinetobacter* spp., and *E. coli*. Unusual organisms such as *Mycoplasma*, an organism commonly found in the respiratory and genital tracts of healthy young adults, have been responsible for mediastinal infection after heart and heart/lung transplantation.[53, 414] The presentation of mediastinal infection in cardiac transplant recipients appears to be no different from that in patients after nontransplant cardiac surgery. Fever, drainage, and sternal instability are clues to the diagnosis. If unrecognized and untreated, mediastinal infection in cardiac transplant recipients carries a high mortality.

Management of mediastinal infection after cardiac transplantation tends to be as controversial as it is after conventional cardiac surgery. One of a number of approaches have been used, including debridement, sternal closure, and antibiotic irrigation,[316, 435] sternal and mediastinal debridement and rewiring,[32] and debridement and closure with muscle flaps (bilateral pectoralis major advancement flaps).[25, 118, 230] Our preference is the use of vascularized muscle flaps (pectoralis or rectus muscle) after sternal debridement. This therapy is highly effective, with greater than 90% chance of cure following a single procedure. Long-term survival of patients after heart transplantation who have successful treatment of mediastinal infection is no different than that of recipients without mediastinal infection.[25, 230]

CENTRAL NERVOUS SYSTEM INFECTION

CNS infection is rare, accounting for 1–2% of infection episodes following cardiac transplantation.[297] There is a considerable range of infectious and noninfectious conditions in the differential diagnosis of CNS disease after heart and heart/lung transplantation. Noninfectious conditions include cerebrovascular disease (including ischemic stroke and intracranial hemorrhage), drug-induced side effects (including cyclosporine- and tacrolimus-associated seizures and leukoencephalopathy), and CNS malignancies (primary cerebral lymphoma and spread from systemic lymphoma).

There are three patterns of infection: meningitis, focal lesions, and encephalitis. Although certain symptoms and signs tend to cluster with each pattern, there is

TABLE 15-13	Investigations on Bronchoscopic Samples in Transplant Patients		

| | LABORATORY INVESTIGATIONS | |
SAMPLE	Essential	Optional
Protected bacteriologic sample (brush or catheter)	Gram stain	Search for bacteria in neutrophils
Aspiration	Quantitative culture Legionella (IFA/DFA stains, culture on BCYE* medium) Mycobacteria and nocardia (AFB stain, culture) Fungi (wet mount, culture)	India ink

Lavage fluid	Cytologic exam of lavage fluid on smear and after cytocentrifugation: direct examination, differential count, viral inclusions, pathogens	Stains:
		  Papanicolaou
		  Periodic acid–Schiff
		  Perls' Prussian blue (hemosiderin-laden macrophages)

	Stains:
	  May-Grünwald-Giemsa
	  Gomori's methenamine silver (or alternative stain for P. carinii)
		Immunodetermination of CD4/CD8 alveolar lymphocytes

	Microbiologic processing:
	  Gram stain, culture
	  Legionella (IFA/DFA, culture on BCYE medium)
	  Mycobacteria
	  Fungi (wet mount stain, culture)
	Virus
	  All possible viruses, particularly the herpes family: centrifugation culture, antigen detection
		Toxoplasmosis: IFA
		Aspergillus antigen
		
		Adeno- and respiratory viruses: IFA/DFA, culture

Transbronchial biopsy†	Histology	

*BCYE, buffered charcoal yeast extract; IFA, indirect immunofluorescence; DFA, direct immunofluorescence.
†Transbronchial biopsy is essential for noninfectious processes and less contributive than BAL for infectious pneumonia.

considerable clinical overlap. CNS infection should always be considered in heart and heart/lung transplant recipients who develop headache, altered mental state, confusion, unexplained fever, seizures, and neurological focal symptoms and signs. Patients with meningitis tend to present with headache, fever, and a stiff neck, although in transplant recipients, absence of these findings does not exclude meningitis. Focal CNS infection may present in many different ways including hemiparesis, cortical sensory loss, aphasia, visual deficits, and

ataxia when the process involves the cerebellum, and cranial nerve deficits if the brain stem is involved. An encephalopathic picture due to infection ususally presents as disorientation, altered mental state, and coma.

A clue to the potential organism resulting in CNS infection can be gained from the timing of the infection in relationship to the transplant procedure (Table 15–14). Although there is considerable overlap, a rapidly developing CNS syndrome suggests either a bacterial

TABLE 15-14	Temporal Relationship of the Neurological Syndrome to the Date of Transplant	

	FOCAL PARENCHYMAL DISEASE	DIFFUSE MENINGOENCEPHALITIS

Early (≤ 1 month after transplant)	Bacterial brain abscess
	  Staphylococcus abscess
	  Gram-negative abscess
	  Anaerobe abscess
	Aspergillus brain abscess
	Candida brain abscess
		Candida meningitis
		Bacterial meningitis
		  Gram-positive meningitis
		    (Streptococcus or Staphylococcus)
		  Gram-negative meningitis
		Herpes simplex meningoencephalitis

Late (>1 month after transplant)	Progressive multifocal leukoencephalopathy (PML) Aspergillus brain abscess Nocardia brain abscess Mucor/Rhizopus encephalitis	Listeria meningitis Cryptococcal meningitis Listeria meningitis Varicella-zoster meningoencephalitis Human herpesvirus-6 (HHV-6) meningoencephalitis CMV encephalitis

Adapted from Aksumit AJ: Central nervous system. In Bowden RA, Ljungman P, Paya CV (eds): Transplant Infections. Philadelphia; Lippincott-Raven Publishers, 1998.

abscess or an organism with vascular invasion such as *Aspergillus,* while a more slowly developing deficit over days to weeks suggests an indolent opportunistic infection such as *Cryptococcus.* CNS infections occurring early after transplantation are likely to be bacterial, usually from an extra-CNS source. Other sites should be examined including the lungs, sinuses, wound, and invasive monitoring line sites. Other clues to the causative organism of CNS infection may come from investigation of the lungs (*Aspergillus, Nocardia, Cryptococcus*); skin (varicella-zoster); and nasal, oral, or sinus mucus membrane (mucormycosis). Candida CNS infection is likely to have obvious extra-CNS sites, as it is almost always part of a disseminated infection.

Imaging of the brain is an important diagnostic test, not only to determine if there is a mass effect that would contraindicate spinal tap, but to determine the nature of the CNS infection. In bacterial meningitis, CT scanning is usually normal. Cerebritis and early abscess formation is more likely to be evident on an MRI scan (particularly with gadolinium enhancement) than CT scan.[5] CT scan with contrast will show ring enhancement around a brain abscess. *Listeria* meningitis will usually not demonstrate CT scan or MRI scan abnormalities unless there is abscess formation or brain stem invasion.[5] MRI and CT scanning will reveal abscesses associated with *Candida* infection, *Aspergillus* infection, and nocardial infection, although MRI scanning is usually better able to detect small abscesses than CT scanning.

Examination of the CSF in patients with bacterial infection usually demonstrates low CSF glucose, but Gram stain in patients with meningitis is positive in only 50–60% of patients, and the cerebrospinal fluid is usually sterile in patients with brain abscess.[5] In patients with *Listeria* meningitis, there is usually an acute purulent response in the CSF (for acute meningitis mostly neutrophils as opposed to lymphocytes if the picture is subacute), elevated CSF protein, and decreased CSF glucose. Gram stain of the CSF is usually negative, but cultures are positive in 70–90% of patients. With positive blood cultures but negative CSF culture, *Listeria* can be assumed to be the cause of the meningitis.[5] Cryptococcal meningitis may result in organisms being identified from spinal fluid, but examination for cryptococcal antigen is much more sensitive.[5] Identification of *Candida* in the CSF by fungal stains has a low yield.

Rarely, the diagnosis of mass lesions can only be made by brain biopsy, which can be performed precisely using stereotactic techniques.

A rare but important neurological infection is progressive multifocal leukoencephalopathy (PML). This infection is due to JC virus, which is a slow virus that destroys oligodendrocytes, leading to multifocal demyelination of the brain.[5] The process may involve the cerebral cortex, brain stem, or cerebellum, and the clinical picture is one of focal cortical syndromes (involving visual deficits, hemiparesis, aphasia), frontal lobe dementia (disinhibited behavior, apathy, slowing of cognitive function), brain stem involvement (hemiparesis or hemisensory deficits associated with unilateral cranial nerve deficits), and/or cerebellar syndromes (clumsiness, imbalance, disturbances of gait).[5] MRI is very sensitive and specific

for PML.[5] Demonstration of JC virus in the urine or blood by PCR is insensitive, since viral shedding may occur in the absence of PML.[5] The findings on CSF examination are usually normal and virus is not able to be cultured from the spinal fluid.[5] The presence of viral DNA by PCR in the spinal fluid is specific for the diagnosis of PML.[5] The disease is progressive and no therapy is available, although cidofovir has been proposed as possible therapy.

BACTEREMIA

As with other immunocompromised individuals, bacteremia from any microbial agent is potentially life threatening. In the early posttransplant period, virtually all septicemia is caused by nosocomial pathogens, most especially aerobic Gram-positive cocci, Gram-negative rods, and fungi (especially *Candida* spp.). The source of infection in the early phase after transplantation is almost always related to intravenous catheters, wound infection, pneumonia, or urinary tract infection. Blood cultures will be positive in patients with clinical "sepsis" in only about 50–60% of episodes, such that an empiric approach to therapy is usually warranted.

In the later time frame after transplantation, community-acquired organisms predominate among patients who do not have chronic indwelling central venous catheters. Bacteremia may particularly occur due to *S. pneumoniae, K. pneumoniae, P. aeruginosa,* group A *Streptococcus,* and *S. aureus.* Fungal septicemia due to *Candida* spp. is rare in the absence of a central venous catheter and a recent history of systemic antibacterial therapy.

URINARY TRACT INFECTION

Urinary infections (UTIs) among transplant recipients are etiologically and epidemiologically similar to UTIs among other hospitalized patients. Most are associated with instrumentation and urinary catheter use. There are no data to suggest that upper urinary tract infections are more common among cardiac transplant recipients, but among those with upper urinary tract infections, complications are more likely to occur. This is true of diabetic patients, and one can easily extrapolate this to cardiac transplant recipients. Thus, bacteremic UTIs are very likely more common in these patients along with other complications such as intrarenal and perinephric abscess. Etiologic organisms include predominantly aerobic gram-negative bacilli, *Enterococcus* spp., and *Candida* spp.

SKIN AND SOFT TISSUE

There are a number of infectious and noninfectious (such as malignancies and drug-related dermatoses) conditions that can cause a diagnostic dilemma in heart and heart/lung transplant recipients. Skin and soft tissue infections may not have the typical presentation that is seen in immunocompetent individuals because of the altered inflammatory response, and what appears to be a usual skin infection may be caused by an unusual organism.[107] Organisms may reflect dissemination of a systemic infection or may reflect the susceptibility of skin and soft tissue to organisms from intravenous lines, drug-related dermatoses (e.g., steroid-induced thinning of the skin), and alteration in the normal flora of the skin.[107]

Skin and soft tissue infections in the early posttransplant period are almost always due to intravenous catheter site and wound infections. Thus, the organisms commonly seen in wound infections described above apply here as well. The form of infection may be either cellulitis, folliculitis, or abscess formation.

In the mid and late posttransplant period, Grampositive organisms, especially β-hemolytic streptococci and *S. aureus* are the principal pathogens causing spontaneous or posttraumatic skin and soft tissue infections. Rarely, aerobic Gram-negative rods are associated with this syndrome. Atypical organisms, including *Nocardia* spp., nontuberculous mycobacteria (especially *M. chelonae*) and *C. neoformans* must be considered among patients who do not respond to conventional antibacterial therapy and/or who present with atypical clinical findings such as nodular or ulcerative lesions or multifocal lesions. A skin biopsy should be performed early in the course of a patient with atypical or poorly responsive skin and soft tissue infection to confirm the presence of atypical pathogens, and routine, fungal, and mycobacterial cultures performed on biopsy specimens.

GASTROINTESTINAL AND HEPATOBILIARY INFECTIONS

The gastrointestinal and hepatobiliary systems are of particular importance as target organs for opportunistic infection in the cardiac transplant recipient. Symptoms such as abdominal pain, gastrointestinal bleeding, dyspepsia, and diarrhea can present significant diagnostic dilemmas, and infectious complications must be distinguished from noninfectious problems such as peptic ulceration, pancreatitis, cholelithiasis, lymphoma, and immunosuppression-related toxicity. Gastrointestinal CMV may cause esophagitis, gastritis, duodenitis, colitis, hepatitis, pancreatitis, cholecystitis, and cholangitis (see section Viral Infections). Patients with symptoms of esophagitis, gastritis, and colitis should undergo endoscopy and biopsy. Herpes simplex virus esophagitis may be diagnosed by the finding of discrete vesicles and ulceration, and biopsy of these ulcers may demonstrate typical inclusions or multinucleate epithelial cells. CMV infection is diagnosed by the typical finding of "owl's eye" intranuclear inclusions in the mucosal epithelium. Other opportunistic infections of the gastrointestinal and hepatobiliary system are uncommon, though rarely *Aspergillus* colitis or cholecystitis has occurred in solid organ transplant recipients.

C. difficile and the common bacterial agents of enteritis are not known to be more common among transplant recipients. However, immunosuppressed patients may be at greater risk for complications. In the case of *C. difficile*, these include colonic dilatation, ileus, perforation, secondary bacteremia with colonic flora, and possibly predisposition to subsequent infection with VRE.

DONOR HEART INFECTION

Aortic Suture Line Infection

Aortic infection after heart and heart/lung transplantation is a rare but potentially lethal complication. Although a number of reports have appeared in the literature on this complication and its successful and unsuccessful management, its true incidence is unknown. From these reports of aortic infection after heart[2, 42, 286, 318, 327, 404] and heart/lung transplantation[2, 7, 30, 130, 431] it is possible to make some general inferences about the pathology, presentation, and management of this important condition. Although it may be quite difficult to determine the site of origin within the aorta because of the destructive nature of this infection, sites that have been considered include the aortic suture line, aortic cannulation site, aortic vent site, or arising within the donor or recipient aorta. The process may result in a localized false aneurysm or may destroy the ascending aorta (Fig. 15–27). The organisms most frequently involved include *Pseudomonas aeruginosa*, *Staphylococcus aureus*, and *Candida* spp. Aortic infection with *Candida* spp. seems to be a particular problem after heart/lung transplantation.[130] This may be in part related to the open airway so close to the aorta during the performance of heart/lung transplantation, as well as the predisposition to fungal infection because of the use of broadspectrum perioperative antibiotics. In an autopsy study of heart/lung transplant recipients,[427] 3 of 20 recipients were found to have *Candida* at the aortic anastomosis, of which two had a *Candida* infection of the tracheal anastomosis. The source of the *Candida* after heart/lung transplantation is likely to be donor in origin. The presentation of aortic infection has included the following: rupture, sepsis, and compression from the expanding false aneurysm. A variety of methods have confirmed the diagnosis, including echocardiography, angiography, radionuclide angiography, magnetic resonance imaging, and computerized tomography. Two reports[286, 327] made comment of the fact that echocardiography did not detect the false aneurysm, presumably because of the position of the false aneurysm, so that echocardiography should probably not be completely relied upon to exclude ascending aortic infection.

The principles of the management of this condition are clear. In the event of rupture, which invariably results in cardiopulmonary collapse, the only chance of survival is immediate operation. Whether the false aneurysm is ruptured or unruptured cardiopulmonary bypass should probably be established by groin cannulation. The false aneurysm may be adherent to the back of the sternum and consequently deep hypothermia prior to opening the sternum is advisable. Although a variety of materials have been used to repair the aorta (Dacron, autologous pericardium, bovine pericardium, and allograft tissue), the use of autologous tissue or allograft

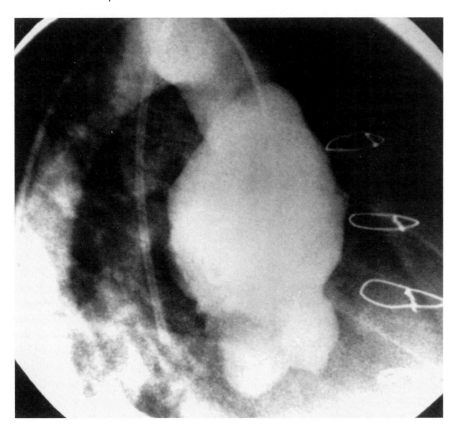

FIGURE **15-27.** Ascending aortogram demonstrating a false aneurysm involving most of the ascending aorta. (From McGiffin DC, Galbraith AJ, McCarthy JB, Tesar PJ: Mycotic false aneurysm of the aoritic suture line after transplantation. J Heart Lung Transplant 1994;13:926–928. Copyright 1994, Elsevier Science, with permission.)

aortic tissue is probably preferable. Because of the lethality of this condition, a number of other adjunctive procedures should be considered, including omental or muscle flaps to increase blood supply and obliterate dead space around the aorta, and mediastinal antibiotic irrigation. A prolonged course (at least 6 weeks and perhaps longer) of the appropriate antimicrobial agent based on culture data from the false aneurysm wall should be administered. The chances of survival after attempted repair of a ruptured aortic false aneurysm is low, but nevertheless, survival has been achieved.[286]

Endocarditis

Endocarditis after heart transplantation is a rare event. A number of sites of intracardiac infections after trans-

TABLE 15-15	Prophylactic Regimens for Dental, Oral, Respiratory Tract, or Esophageal Procedures	
SITUATION	AGENTS	REGIMEN
Standard general prophylaxis	Amoxicillin*	Adults, 2 g (children, 50 mg/kg[†]) PO 1 hr before procedure
Unable to take oral medications	Ampicillin	Adults, 2 g IM/IV (children 50 mg/kg[†] IM/IV) within 30 min before procedure
Allergic to penicillin	Clindamycin	Adults, 600 mg (children 20 mg/kg[†]) PO 1 hr before procedure
	Cephalexin or cefadroxil[‡] OR	Adults, 2 g (children 50 mg/kg[†]) PO 1 hr before procedure
	Azithromycin or clarithromycin	Adults, 500 mg (children 15 mg/kg[†]) IV within 30 min before procedure
Allergic to penicillin and unable to take oral medications	Clindamycin OR	Adults, 600 mg (children 20 mg/kg[†]) IV within 30 min before procedure
	Cefazolin[‡]	Adults, 1 g (children 25 mg/kg[†]) IM/IV within 30 min before procedure

*Amoxicillin is preferred over penicillin because it has better gastrointestinal absorption and higher and more sustained serum inhibitory levels against oral streptococci.
[†]Total children's dose should not exceed adult dose.
[‡]Cephalosporins should not be used in individuals with immediate-type hypersensitivity reaction (urticaria, angioedema, or anaphylaxis) to penicillins.
From American Heart Association.

TABLE 15–16	Prophylactic Regimens for Genitourinary/Gastrointestinal (Excluding Esophageal) Procedures	
SITUATION	**AGENTS**	**REGIMEN**
High-risk patients	Ampicillin plus gentamicin	Adults: ampicillin 2 g IM/IV plus gentamicin 1.5 mg/kg (not to exceed 120 mg) within 30 min of starting the procedure; 6 hr later, ampicillin 1 g IM/IV or amoxicillin 1 g PO
		Children: ampicillin 50 mg/kg* IM/IV (not to exceed 2 g) plus gentamicin 1.5 mg/kg* within 30 min of starting the procedure; 6 hr later, ampicillin 25 mg/kg IM/IV or amoxicillin 25 mg/kg* PO
High-risk patients allergic to ampicillin/amoxicillin	Vancomycin plus gentamicin	Adults: vancomycin 1 g IV over 1–2 hr plus gentamicin 1.5 mg/kg (not to exceed 120 mg); complete infusion within 30 min of starting the procedure
		Children: vancomycin 20 mg/kg* IV over 1–2 hr plus gentamicin 1.5 mg/kg* IM/IV within 30 min of starting the procedure
Moderate-risk patients	Amoxicillin or ampicillin	Adults: amoxicillin 2 g PO 1 hr before procedure, or ampicillin 2 g IM/IV within 30 min of starting the procedure
		Children: amoxicillin 50 mg/kg* PO 1 hr before procedure, or ampicillin 50 mg/kg* IM/IV within 30 min of starting the procedure
Moderate-risk patients allergic to ampicillin/amoxicillin	Vancomycin	Adults: vancomycin 1 g IV over 1–2 hr; complete infusion within 30 min of starting the procedure
		Children: vancomycin 20 mg/kg* IV over 1–2 hr; complete infusion within 30 min of starting the procedure

*Total children's dose should not exceed adult dose
From American Heart Association.

plantation have been described, including the mitral valve,[104] tricuspid valve,[417] left ventricular wall,[200] intra-atrial septum,[433] pulmonary artery conduit in a heterotopic heart,[361] and a mechanical aortic valve prosthesis in the native heart of a heterotopic transplant.[233] In refractory cases of recurrent endocarditis in the transplanted heart, retransplantation and prolonged antibiotic therapy has been curative.[165] The same general principles that are used for the treatment of endocarditis in nontransplant patients should be applied in patients with endocarditis after heart or heart/lung transplantation.

Although the risk of endocarditis in heart transplants following invasive procedures is very low, endocarditis prophylaxis is probably justified, and the recommendations of the American Heart Association for the prevention of bacterial endocarditis should be used[106] (Tables 15–15 and 15–16).

PREVENTION OF INFECTION

PROPHYLAXIS

Antimicrobial prophylaxis after heart and heart/lung transplantation is an integral part of prevention of infection, and the benefits clearly outweigh the disadvantages, which include toxicity, antimicrobial resistance, colonization resistance, and predisposition to fungal in-

fection (in the case of antibacterial agents). A recommended antimicrobial prophylaxis regimen for heart and heart/lung transplantation is outlined in Table 15–9.

ACTIVE IMMUNIZATION

Prevention of infection by active immunization in solid organ transplant recipients must take into account six basic principles. First, prevention of infection is far better than treatment, especially for patients with impaired host defenses. Second, the need for preventive efforts should be determined by circumstances specific to each patient. Third, the likelihood of acquiring and preventing infection is closely related to the patient's underlying net state of immunosuppression. Fourth, vaccine efficacy is often diminished in immunocompromised patients. As an example, fewer than 20% of renal transplant recipients of hepatitis B vaccine have detectable antibody 12 months following vaccination. Because of the poor immunologic response to vaccines among many transplant recipients, necessary vaccinations should be administered prior to transplantation whenever possible. Fifth, the potential exists for a vaccine-associated nonspecific immunologic response which leads to allograft rejection or increased autoimmune activity. While this has not been reported among recipients of hepatitis B, pneumococcal, or influenza vaccination, anecdotal reports of allograft rejection following tetanus toxoid exist. Sixth, live vaccines should generally be avoided among this population. A possible exception is the newly released varicella vaccine, though data on its safety in transplant recipients is incomplete. A summary of current vaccination recommendations in solid organ transplant recipients is included in Table 15–17. Immunization recommendations in pediatric patients are also discussed in Chapter 20.

INFECTION CONTROL

One of the more important and controversial areas surrounding solid organ transplantation concerns measures to prevent nosocomial infection in transplant recipients. Few data are available from prospective studies in solid organ transplantation to guide the formulation of infection control practices specific to thoracic transplantation. Recently, the CDC has issued a draft statement for guidelines to prevent opportunistic infections in bone marrow transplant recipients, and the basic principles of this statement should apply to many immunocompromised patients, in particular solid organ transplant recipients.[79] The guidelines for prevention of opportunistic infections in HIV-positive patients (Table 15–18) are useful for heart and heart/lung transplant recipients.

Room Ventilation

The goal of proper room ventilation is to reduce the number of fungal spores and other pathogens in the ambient air, thereby potentially reducing the number of opportunistic pneumonias. This is usually accomplished by high-volume air exchange (at least 10 exchanges per hour) in a positive-pressure setting, and is usually used in conjunction with high-efficacy particulate air (HEPA) filtration. HEPA filters remove 99.9% of particles larger than 0.3 μm. Patient rooms should be tightly sealed to prevent outdoor contamination, and the doors should be closed to maintain positive pressurization.

A modification of HEPA filtration and positive pressurization is the laminar air flow (LAF) room. In the LAF room, air moves in parallel, entering from one wall through HEPA filters and exiting through the opposite

wall. It is often used in conjunction with patient decontamination and has been studied extensively in bone marrow transplant (BMT) recipients. LAF rooms are expensive and their benefit limited to a few studies among BMT patients. Their routine use in solid organ transplantation is sporadic and the benefits unproven. However, use of positive-pressure room ventilation is advisable in severely leukopenic patients (to minimize entry of airborne pathogens from outside the room). Conversely, infected patients with highly contagious airborne infections should be kept in "negative-pressure" rooms to protect other transplant patients.

Isolation and Barrier Precautions, Hand Washing

Routine protective isolation for patients after cardiac transplantation is not necessary, since it offers no demonstrable protection against infection.[167, 459] Nonetheless, published guidelines for universal precautions should be followed closely in this patient group. Hand washing is the *single* most important and effective procedure for preventing nosocomial infection. All health care workers should wash their hands before and after entering the patient's room. If gloves are worn, health care workers should wash their hands before gloves are put on and again after removal of gloves. Although hand washing with an antimicrobial soap and water is preferred, hygienic hand rubs may be used as adjuncts and not replacements to hand washing.[258]

Plants

Although exposure to flowers and plants is not a proven cause of nosocomial fungal or bacterial infections, many experts strongly recommend avoidance of potted plants and fresh dried flowers because of the potential inhalation of aspergillus or other fungal spores.[458, 459] In general, these items should be avoided in the early posttransplant period.

Health Care Workers

All health care workers with diseases transmissible by air, droplet, and/or direct contact (e.g., VZV, gastroen-

TABLE 15–17	Immunizations for Heart and Heart/Lung Transplant Recipients			
VACCINE	BEFORE	AFTER	COMMENTS	
Tetanus/diphtheria	++	++	Revaccination every 10 yr after primary series and booster	
Hepatitis B	++	+/-	Immunogenecity of HBV vaccine only 5–15% in organ transplant recipients	
Hepatitis A	++	+/-	Especially indicated for liver transplants and international travelers	
Haemophilus influenzae Type B	++	+	Especially indicated for children ≤ 6 yr	
Pneumococcus (multivalent)	++	+	Indication after transplant is not established	
Influenza A and B	+/-	++	Seasonal vaccination	
Varicella zoster virus (attenuated-live)	++	-	Only for seronegative patients; posttransplant use not approved	
Measles-mumps-rubella (live-attenuated)	++	Contraindicated	Primary pediatric series	
Oral polio vaccine	++	Contraindicated	Primary pediatric series	
Inactivated polio vaccine	-	+	Indicated for unvaccinated post-transplant patients	

TABLE 15-18	U.S. Public Health Service/Infectious Diseases Society of America Guidelines for the Prevention of Opportunistic Infections*

Environmental and Occupational Exposure

- Increased risk of exposure to tuberculosis with employment in health care facilities, correctional institutions, homeless shelters
- Child care—increased risk of CMV, cryptosporidiosis, hepatitis A, and giardiasis (risk diminished by handwashing after fecal contact)
- Occupations with animal contact (veterinary work, pet stores, farms, slaughterhouses)—risk of cryptosporidiosis, toxoplasmosis, salmonellosis, campylobacteriosis or *Bartonella* infection (current data do not support advising against work in these environments)
- Avoid contact with young farm animals (especially with diarrhea)
- Handwashing after gardening and other soil contact
- In areas endemic for histoplasmosis, insufficient evidence to recommend avoiding activities such as cave exploring, cleaning chicken coops, disturbing soil beneath bird-roosting sites

Pet-Related Exposures

- Avoid contact with pets with diarrhea and have the animal examined by a veterinarian
- When obtaining a new pet, avoid animals <6 mo of age, expecially if they have diarrhea
- Avoid stray animals
- Wash hands after handling pets
- Avoid contact with pet feces to reduce the risk of cryptosporidiosis, salmonellosis, and campylobacteriosis
- Avoid contact with reptiles (e.g., snakes, lizards, iguanas, and turtles) because of the risk of salmonellosis
- Gloves should be used during the cleaning of aquariums
- Cat ownership—consider increased risk of toxoplasmosis, *Bartonella* infection, and enteric infections
    - Obtain cat >1 yr in good health
    - Clean litter boxes daily and wash hands
    - Keep cats indoors, don't allow to hunt and should not be fed raw or undercooked meat
    - Avoid cat scratches (declawing not generally advised)
    - Don't allow cats to lick cuts
- Bird ownership—not necessary to screen healthy birds for *Cryptococcus neoformans*, *Mycobacterium avium* or *Histoplasma capsulatum*

Food Exposure

- Avoid raw or undercooked eggs and egg products; avoid raw or undercooked poultry, meat or seafood; avoid unpasteurized dairy products
- Poultry and meat should be well cooked and not pink in the middle
- Produce should be washed thoroughly before being eaten
- Avoid cross-contamination of foods via hand and utensils during food preparation
- Reheat "ready-to-eat" foods such as cold cuts until they are steaming hot before eating
- Don't drink water directly from lakes and rivers (increased risk of giardiasis and cryptosporidiosis)
- Avoid swimming in water contaminated by human or animal waste
- In a community with a "boil water advisory," boil water for 1 min

Travel Related Exposure

- During travel to developing countries, avoid food and beverages that may be contaminated, especially raw fruits and vegetables, raw or undercooked seafood or meat, tap water or ice made with tap water, unpasteurized milk or dairy products, and items sold by street vendors
- Antimicrobial prophylaxis for traveler's diarrhea not recommended routinely in developing countries (if risk of infection is very high and period of travel brief, prophylaxis may be warranted—ciprofloxacin 500 mg daily or trimethoprim/sulfamethoxazole 1 double-strength tablet daily)
- If traveler's diarrhea develops, take ciprofloxacin 500 mg bid for 3–7 days
- Travelers should be aware of preventive measures such as chemoprophylaxis for malaria, protection against arthropod vectors, protective clothing, and shoes where fecal contamination of soil or sand likely
- Updating of vaccinations

*These recommendations for prevention of exposure to opportunistic infections were compiled for HIV-positive patients but seem prudent for transplant recipients.
Modified from Centers for Disease Control: 1997 USPHS/IDSA guidelines for the prevention of opportunistic infections in persons infected with human immunodeficiency virus. Morb Mortal Wkly Rep 1997;46;1–47.

teritis, HSV lesions of fingers or lips, and upper respiratory infections such as influenza and RSV) should be restricted from direct patient contact and temporarily reassigned. Health care workers with sexually transmitted diseases or blood-borne infections such as HIV and HBV should not be restricted from patient contact, provided they follow appropriate guidelines for prevention of accidental patient exposure.[81]

Visitors

Visitors with upper respiratory infection, flu-like illness, or recent exposure to either VZV or oral polio vaccine (within 6 weeks) should not be allowed to have direct patient contact. There is no absolute age limitation on visitation, but all visitors must be able to comply with hand-washing and appropriate isolation precautions.

Masks

Because of frequent hospital construction and potential exposure to fungal spores, patients who have recently undergone transplantation should wear masks when they are required to go off the transplant floor.

INFECTION CONTROL SURVEILLANCE

Routine surveillance of solid organ transplant recipients and the environment are not warranted outside of epidemiologic clustering of cases. Some experts recommend routine sampling of air, ventilation ducts, and filters for mold during periods of construction or when surveillance indicates a possible increase in invasive mold disease.[461]

References

1. Abraham SN, Beachey EH: Host defenses against adhesion of bacteria to mucosal surfaces. *In* Gallin JI, Fauci AS (eds): Advances in Host Defense Mechanisms, Vol 4. New York: Raven Press, 1985; pp 63–89.
2. Adams BK, Fataar A, Boniaszczuk J, Kahn D: Equilibrium radionuclide angiocardiography in the detection of unsuspected mycotic aneurysms in cardiac transplantation. Transplantation 1992;53:681–683.
3. Aebischer MC, Zala LB, Braathen LR: Kaposi's sarcoma as manifestation of immunosuppression in organ transplant recipients. Dermatology 1997;195:91.
4. AHFS Drug Information©. 1999;518–539.
5. Aksumit AJ: Central nervous system. *In* Bowden RA, Ljungman P, Paya CV (eds): Transplant Infections. Philadelphia: Lippincott-Raven Publishers, 1998.
6. Alain S, Honderlick P, Grenet D, Stern M, Vadam C, Sanson-LePors MJ, Mazeron MC: Failure of ganciclovir treatment associated with selection of a ganciclovir-resistant cytomegalovirus strain in a lung transplant recipient. Transplantation 1997;63:1533–1536.
7. Albes J, Haverich A, Freihorst J, von der Hardt H, Manthey-Stiers F: Management of mycotic rupture of the ascending aorta after heart-lung transplantation. Ann Thorac Surg 1990;50:982–983.
8. Ali A, Mehra MR, Stapleton DD, Kemmerly SA, Ramireddy K, Smart FW, Augustine S, Ventura HO: *Vibrio vulnificus* sepsis in solid organ transplantation: a medical nemesis. J Heart Lung Transplant 1995;14:598.
9. Alpern RJ, Dowell VR Jr: Clostridium septicum: infections and malignancy. JAMA 1969;209:385–388.
10. Amber IJ, Gilbert EM, Schiffman G, Jacobson JA: Increased risk of pneumococcal infections in cardiac transplant recipients. Transplantation 1990;49:122–125.
11. American Thoracic Society: Hospital-acquired pneumonia in adults: diagnosis, assessment of severity, initial antimicrobial therapy, and preventive strategies. A consensus statement. Am J Respir Crit Care Med 1995;153:1711–1725.
12. Amiot L, Langanay T, Drénou B, Lelong B, Le Prise PY, Logeais Y, Colimon R, Fauchet R: Spontaneous recovery from severe parvovirus B19 pure red cell aplasia, in a heart transplant recipient, as demonstrated by marrow culture. Hematol Cell Ther 1998;40:71–73.
13. Ampel NM, Wieden MA, Galgiani JN: Coccidioidomycosis. Clinical update. Rev Infect Dis 1989;11:897.
14. Anand BS, Yoffe B, Young JB: Ganciclovir treatment of active hepatitis B virus infection in a heart transplant patient. J Clin Gastroenterol 1996;22:144.
15. Anderson CB, Haid SD, Hruska KA, Etheredge EA: Significance of microbial contamination of stored cadaver kidneys. Arch Surg 1978;113:269–271.
16. Andersson R, Sandberg T, Berglin E, Jeansson S: Cytomegalovirus infections and toxoplasmosis in heart transplant recipients in Sweden. Scand J Infect Dis 1992;24:411–417.
17. Andreone PA, Olivari MT, Elick B, Arentzen CE, Sibley RK, Bolman RM, Simmons RL, Ring WS: Reduction of infectious complications following heart transplantation with triple-drug immunotherapy. J Heart Transplant 1986;5:13–19.
18. Anthuber M, Kemkes BM, Heiss MM, Schuetz A, Kugler C: HIV infection after heart transplantation: a case report. J Heart Transplant 1991;10:611–613.
19. Apalsch AM, Green M, Ledesma-Medina J, Nour B, Wald ER: Parainfluenza and influenza virus infections in pediatric organ transplant recipients. Clin Infect Dis 1995;20:394–399.
20. Apalsch AM, Nour B, Jaffe R: Systemic cat-scratch disease in a pediatric liver transplant recipient and review of the literature. Pediatr Infect Dis J 1993;12:769–774.
21. Arabia FA, Rosado LJ, Huston CL, Sethi GK, Copeland JG III: Incidence and recurrence of gastrointestinal cytomegalovirus infection in heart transplantation. Ann Thorac Surg 1993;55:8–11.
22. Arbustini E, Grasso M, Diegoli M, Percivalle E, Grossi P, Bramero M, Campana C, Goggi C, Gavazzi A, Vigano M: Histopathologic and molecular profile of human cytomegalovirus infections in patients with heart transplants. Am J Clin Pathol 1992;98:205–213.
23. Arduino RC, Johnson PC, Miranda AG: Nocardiosis in renal transplant recipients undergoing immunosuppression with cyclosporine. Clin Infect Dis 1993;16:505–512.
24. Arnow PM, Andersen RL, Mainous PD, Smith EJ: Pulmonary aspergillosis during hospital renovation. Am Rev Respir Dis 1978;118:49–53.
25. Ascherman JA, Hugo NE, Sultan MR, Patsis MC, Smith CR, Rose EA: Single-stage treatment of sternal wound complications in heart transplant recipients in whom pectoralis major myocutaneous advancement flaps were used. J Thorac Cardiovasc Surg 1995;110:1030–1036.
26. Asher DM, Gibbs CJ Jr, Gajdusek DC: Pathogenesis of subacute spongiform encephalopathies. Ann Clin Lab Sci 1976;6:84–103.
27. Assan R, Feutren G, Debray-Sachs M, Quiniou-Debrie MC, Laborie C, Thomas G, Chatenoud L, Bach JF: Metabolic and immunological effects of cyclosporin in recently diagnosed type I diabetes mellitus. Lancet 1985;1:67.
28. Avery RK: Prevention and treatment of cytomegalovirus infection and disease in heart transplant recipients. Curr Opin Cardiol 1998;13:112–129.
29. Bailey TC, Ettinger NA, Storch GA, Trulock EP, Hanto DW, Dunagan WC, Jendrisak MD, McCullough CS, Kenzora JL, Powderly WG: Failure of high-dose oral acyclovir with or without immune globulin to prevent primary cytomegalovirus disease in recipients of solid organ transplants. Am J Med 1993;95:273–278.
30. Balaji S, Whitehead B, Elliott MJ, de Leval MR: Pseudoaneurysm of the aorta after heart-lung transplantation: diagnosis by color flow Doppler mapping. J Heart Lung Transplant 1992;11:160–163.
31. Baldanti F, Simoncini L, Sarasini A, Zavattoni M, Grossi P, Revello MG, Gema G: Ganciclovir resistance as a result of oral ganciclovir in a heart transplant recipient with multiple human cytomegalovirus strains in blood. Transplantation 1998;66:324–329.
32. Baldwin RT, Radovancevic B, Sweeney MS, Duncan JM, Frazier OH: Bacterial mediastinitis after heart transplantation. J Heart Lung Transplant 1992;11:545–547.
33. Balfour HH Jr, Welo PK, Sachs GW: Cytomegalovirus vaccine trial in 400 renal transplant candidates. Transplant Proc 1985;17:81–83.
34. Barber BA, Crotty JM, Washburn RG, Pegram PS: *Cryptococcus neoformans* myositis in a patient with AIDS. Clin Infect Dis 1995;21:1510–1511.
35. Barnhart GR, Hastillo A, Goldman MH, Szentpetery S, Wolfgang TC, Mohanakumar T, Katz MR, Rider S, Zhanrahan J, Lower RR, Hess ML: A prospective randomized trial of pretransfusion/azathioprine/prednisone versus cyclosporine/prednisone immunosuppression in cardiac transplant recipients: preliminary results. Circulation 1985;72(suppl II):II-227–II-230.
36. Basgoz N, Preiksaitis JK: Post-transplant lymphoproliferative disorder. Infect Dis Clin North Am 1995;9:901–923.
37. Bass JW, Vincent JM, Person DA: The expanding spectrum of *Bartonella* infections: I. Bartonellosis and trench fever. Pediatr Infect Dis J 1997;16:2–10.
38. Bayer AS, Choi C, Tillman DB, Guze LB: Fungal arthritis. V. Cryptococcal and histoplasmal arthritis. Semin Arthritis Rheum 1980;9:218–227.
39. Beachey EH: Bacterial adherence: adhesin-receptor interactions mediating the attachment of bacteria to mucosal surfaces. J Infect Dis 1981;143:325–345.
40. Benedetti E, Gruessner AC, Troppmann C, Papalois BE, Sutherland DER, Dunn DL, Gruessner RWG: Intra-abdominal fungal infections after pancreatic transplantation: incidence, treatment, and outcome. J Am Coll Surg 1996;183:307–316.
41. Bergen GA, Sakalosky PE, Sinnott JT: Transient aplastic anemia caused by parvovirus B19 infection in a heart transplant recipient. J Heart Lung Transplant 1996;15:843–845.
42. Berggren H, Berglin E, Kjellman U, Mantovani V, Nilsson B: Successful outcome after massive bleeding in a heart transplant recipient with mycotic aortitis. Scand J Thorac Cardiovasc Surg 1994;28:45–47.
43. Bertoni E, Rosati A, Zanazzi M, Azzi A, Zakrzewfka K, Guidi S, Salvadori M: Severe aplastic anaemia due to B19 parvovirus infection in renal transplant recipient. Nephrol Dial Transplant 1995;10:1462–1463.
44. Bieber E, Quinn JP, Venezio FR, Miller JB, Loyola University Cardiac Transplantation Team: Salmonellal empyema in a heart transplant recipient. J Heart Transplant 1989;8:262–263.

45. Bijnen AB, Weimar W, Dik P, Oberop H, Jeekel J: The hazard of transplanting contaminated kidneys. Transplant Proc 1984;16:27–28.

46. Bizollon T, Palazzo U, Chevallier M, Ducert C, Trepo C: HCV recurrence after OLT: a pilot study of ribavirin therapy following initial combination with IFN. Hepatology 1996;24:293A.

47. Black JR, Herrington DA, Hadfield TL, Wear DJ, Margileth AM, Shigekawa B: Life-threatening cat-scratch disease in an immunocompromised host. Arch Intern Med 1986;146:394–396.

48. Bocchi EA, Bellotti G, Uip D, Kalil J, deLourdes Higuchi M, Fiorelli A, Stolf N, Jatene A, Pilleggi F: Long-term follow-up after heart transplantation in Chagas' disease. Transplant Proc 1993;25:1329–1330.

49. Böker KHW, Ringe B, Krüger M, Pichlmayr R, Manns MP: Prostaglandin E plus famciclovir—a new concept for the treatment of severe hepatitis B after liver transplantation. Transplantation 1994;57:1706–1708.

50. Boley TJ, Popek EJ: Parvovirus infection in pregnancy. Semin Perinatol 1993;17:410–419.

51. Bourge RC, Kirklin JK, White-Williams C, Naftel DC, George JF, Morrow R, Tarkka M, Welborn JM: Methotrexate pulse therapy in the treatment of recurrent acute heart rejection. J Heart Lung Transplant 1992;11:1116–1124.

52. Bowen PA, Lobel SA, Caruana RJ, Leffell MS, House MA, Rissing JP, Humphries AL: Transmission of human immunodeficiency virus (HIV) by transplantation: clinical aspects and time course analysis of viral antigenemia and antibody production. Ann Intern Med 1988;108:46–48.

53. Boyle EM, Burdine J, Bolman RM III: Successful treatment of mycoplasma mediastinitis after heart-lung transplantation. J Heart Lung Transplant 1993;12:508–512.

54. Boyle J, Briggs JD, Mackie RM, Junor BJR, Aitchison TC: Cancer, warts, and sunshine in renal transplant patients: a case-control study. Lancet 1984;1:702–705.

55. Bradsher RW: Clinical considerations in blastomycosis. Infect Dis Clin Pract 1992;1:97–104.

56. Bradsher RW, Pappas PG: Detection of specific antibodies in human blastomycosis by enzyme immunoassay. South Med J 1995;88:1256–1259.

57. Bramwell NH, Davies RA, Koshal A, Keon WJ, Walley VM: Fatal gastrointestinal hemorrhage caused by cytomegalovirus duodenitis and ulceration after heart transplantation. J Heart Transplant 1987;6:303–306.

58. Bridges ND, Spray TL, Collins MH, Bowles NE, Towbin JA: Adenovirus infection in the lung results in graft failure after lung transplantation. J Thorac Cardiovasc Surg 1998;116:617.

59. Britt RH, Enzmann DR, Remington JS: Intracranial infection in cardiac transplant recipients. Ann Neurol 1981;9:107–119.

60. Bronnimann DA, Adam RD, Galgiani JN, Habib MP, Petersen EA, Porter B, Bloom JW: Coccidioidomycosis in the acquired immunodeficiency syndrome. Ann Intern Med 1987;106:372–379.

61. Brooks RG: Prospective study of Candida endophthalmitis in hospitalized patients with candidemia. Arch Intern Med 1989;149:2226–2228.

62. Brooks RG, Hofflin JM, Jamieson SW, Stinson EB, Remington JS: Infectious complications in heart-lung transplant recipients. Am J Med 1985;79:412–422.

63. Brown KE, Anderson SM, Young NS: Erythrocyte P antigen: cellular receptor for B19 parvovirus. Science 1993;262:114–117.

64. Brown P, Gajdusek DC, Gibbs CJ Jr, Asher DM: Potential epidemic of Creutzfeldt-Jakob disease from human growth hormone therapy. N Engl J Med 1985;313:728–738.

65. Burch KH, Fine G, Quinn EL, Eisses JF: Cryptococcus neoformans as a cause of lytic bone lesions. JAMA 1975;231:1057–1059.

66. Cadranel J, Grippon P, Lunel F, Desruennes M, Leger P, Azar N, Moussalli J, Pauwells A, Cabrol A, Salmon P, LeCharpentier Y, Cabrol C, Huraux JM, Opolon P: Chronic liver dysfunction in heart transplant patients, with special reference to viral B, C, and non-A, non-B, non-C hepatitis. A retrospective study in 80 patients with follow-up of 60 months. Transplantation 1991;52:645–650.

67. Caillot D, Bernard A, Couaillier J, Casanovas P, Durand C, Cuisenier B, Solary E, Bonnin A, Mailard M, Boscarolo F, Kara-Bumme F, Favre JP, Guy H: Interest of CT-scan in the strategy for early diagnosis and surgery in neutropenic patients with invasive pulmonary aspergillosis. 36th Interscience Conference on Antimicrobial Agents and Chemotherapy, 1996, Abstract No. J50, p 227.

68. Caillot D, Durand C, Casasnovas O, Couaillier JF, Bernard A, Buisson M, Solary E, Brachet A, Cuisenier B, Bonnin A, Debuche V, De Montaignac A, Magnin G, Arnould L, Petrella T, Guy H: Aspergillose pulmonaire invasive des patients neutropéniques. Analyse d'une série de 36 cas: apport du scanner thoracique et de l'itraconazole. Ann Med Interne 1995;146:84–90.

69. Canver CC, Patel AK, Kosolcharoen P, Voytovich MC: Fungal purulent constrictive pericarditis in a heart transplant patient. Ann Thorac Surg 1998;65:1792.

70. Canadian Multicentre Transplant Study Group: A randomized clinical trial of cyclosporine in cadaveric renal transplantation. N Engl J Med 1983;309:809–815.

71. Canadian Multicentre Transplant Study Group: A randomized clinical trial of cyclosporine in cadaveric renal transplantation: analysis at three years. N Engl J Med 1986;314:1219–1225.

72. Carrigan DR, Drobyski WR, Russler SK, Tapper MA, Knox KK, Ash RC: Interstitial pneumonitis associated with human herpesvirus-6 infection after marrow transplantation. Lancet 1991;338:147–149.

73. Cassinotti P, Weitz M, Siegl G: Human parvovirus B19 infection: routine diagnosis by a new nested polymerase chain reaction assay. J Med Virol 1993;40:228–234.

74. Centers for Disease Control: Human-to-human transmission of rabies via a corneal transplant—France. MMWR 1980;29:25.

75. Centers for Disease Control: Human-to-Human transmission of rabies via corneal transplant—Thailand. MMWR 1981;30:473–474.

76. Centers for Disease Control and Prevention: Rapidly progressive dementia in a patient who received a cadaveric dura mater graft. JAMA 1987;257:1036–1037.

77. Centers for Disease Control and Prevention: Clarification of human immunodeficiency virus screening practices for organ donors. Fed Register 1996;61:56548–56549.

78. Centers for Disease Control: 1997 USPHS/IDSA guidelines for the prevention of opportunistic infections in persons infected with human immunodeficiency virus. Morb Mortal Wkly Rep 1997;46:1–47.

79. Centers for Disease Control: Guidelines for preventing opportunistic infections among hematopoietic stem cell transplant recipients. Morb Mortal Wkly Rep 2000;49:1–125.

80. Centers for Disease Control: Guidelines for preventing transmission of human immunodeficiency virus through transplantation of human tissue and organs. Morb Mortal Wkly Rep 1994;43:1.

81. Centers for Disease Control: Public health service inter-agency guidelines for screening donors of blood, plasma, organs, tissues and semen for evidence of hepatitis B and hepatitis C. Morb Mortal Wkly Rep 1991;40:1–17.

82. Centers for Disease Control: Recommendations for preventing transmission of human immunodeficiency virus and hepatitis B virus to patients during exposure-prone invasive procedures. Morb Mortal Wkly Rep 1991;10(RR No.8):1–8.

83. Centers for Disease Control: U.S. Public Health Service guidelines for testing and counseling blood and plasma donors for human immunodeficiency virus type 1 antigen. Morb Mortal Wkly Rep 1996;45:1–9.

84. Centers for Disease Control and Prevention: Intravascular Device-related infections prevention. Fed Register 1995;60:49978.

85. Centers for Disease Control and Prevention: Recommendations for prevention and control of hepatitis C virus (HCV) infection and HCV related chronic disease. Morb Mortal Wkly Rep 1998;47(RR-19):1–39.

86. Chan MK, Chang WK: Renal transplantation from HBsAg positive donors to HBsAg negative recipients. BMJ 1988;297:522–523.

87. Chan TK, Wu PC, Lau JYN, Lai CL, Lok ASF, Cheng IKP: Clinicopathologic features of hepatitis C virus infection in renal allograft recipients. Transplantation 1994;58:996–1000.

88. Chang FY, Singh N, Gayowski T, Marino IR: Parvovirus B19 infection in a liver transplant recipient. Case report and review in organ transplant recipients. Clin Transplant 1996;10:243–247.

89. Chang FY, Singh N, Gayowski T, Wagener MM, Marino IR: Fever in liver transplant recipients: changing spectrum of etiologic agents. Clin Infect Dis 1998;26:59–65.

90. Chatis PA, Crumpacker CS: Resistance of herpes viruses to antiviral drugs. Antimicrob Agents Chemother 1992;36:1589–1595.

91. Choucino C, Goodman SA, Greer JP, Stein RS, Wolff SN, Dummer JS: Nocardial infections in bone marrow transplant recipients. Clin Infect Dis 1996;23:1012–1019.

92. Chou S: Cytomegalovirus infection and reinfection transmitted by heart transplantation. J Infect Dis 1987;155:1054–1056.

93. Chow JW, Yu VL: Staphylococcus aureus nasal carriage in hemodialysis patients. Arch Intern Med 1989;149:1258–1262.

94. Ciulli F, Tamm M, Dennis B, Biocina B, Mullins P, Wells FC, Large SR, Wallwork J: Donor-transmitted bacterial infection in heart-lung transplantation. Transplant Proc 1993;25:1155–1156.

95. Cobian L, Houston S, Greene J, Sinnott JT: Parainfluenza virus respiratory infection after heart transplantation: successful treatment with ribavirin. Clin Infect Dis 1995;21:1040–1041.

96. Cohen BJ, Buckley MM: The prevalence of antibody to human parvovirus B19 in England and Wales. J Med Microbiol 1988;25:151–153.

97. Collins LA, Samore MH, Roberts MS, Luzzati R, Jenkins RL, Lewis WD, Karchmer AW: Risk factors for invasive fungal infections complicating orthotopic liver transplantation. J Infect Dis 1994;170:644–652.

98. Cone RW, Hackman RC, Huang ML, Bowden RA, Meyers JD, Metcalf M, Zeh J, Ashley R, Corey L: Human herpesvirus-6 in lung tissue from patients with pneumonitis after bone marrow transplantation. N Engl J Med 1993;329:156–161.

99. Cordonnier C, Cunningham I: Pneumonia. In Bowden RA, Ljungman P, Paya CV (eds): Transplant Infection. Philadelphia: Lippincott-Raven Publishers, 1998, pp 105–120.

100. Corey L, Spear PG: Infections with herpes simplex viruses (part 1). N Engl J Med 1986;314:686–691.

101. Corral DA, Darras FS, Jensen CWB, Hakala TR, Naides SJ, Krause JR, Starzl TE, Jordan ML: Parvovirus B19 infection causing pure red cell aplasia in a recipient of pediatric donor kidneys. Transplantation 1993;55:427–430.

102. Costanzo-Nordin MR, Swinnen LJ, Fisher SG: Cytomegalovirus infections in heart transplant recipients: relationship to immunosuppression. J Heart Lung Transplant 1992;11:837–846.

103. Couchoud C, Cucherat M, Haugh M, Pouteil-Noble C: Cytomegalovirus prophylaxis with antiviral agents in solid organ transplantation. Transplantation 1998;65:641.

104. Couniham PJ, Yelland A, de Belder MA, Pepper JR: Infective endocarditis in a heart transplant recipient. J Heart Lung Transplant 1991;10:275–279.

105. Crespo MG, Arnal FM, Gomez M, Monserrat L, Suarez F, Rodriguez JA, Paniagua MJ, Cuesta M, Juffe A, Castro-Beiras A: Cytomegalovirus colitis mimicking a colonic neoplasm or ischemic colitis 4 years after heart transplantation. Transplantation 1998;66:1562–1565.

106. Dajani AS, Taubert KA, Wilson W, Bolger AF, Bayer A, Ferrieri P, Gewitz MH, Shulman ST, Nouri S, Newburger JW, Hutto C, Pallasch TJ, Gage TW, Levison ME, Peter G, Zuccar G Jr: Prevention of bacterial endocarditis: recommendations by the American Heart Association. JAMA 1997;277:1794–1801.

107. Daoud MS, Gibson LE, Su WPD: Skin infections. In Bowden RA, Ljungman P, Paya CV (eds): Transplant Infections. Philadelphia: Lippincott-Raven Publishers, 1998.

108. Darenkov IA, Marcarelli MA, Basadonna GP, Friedman AL, Lorber KM, Howe JG, Crouch J, Bia MJ, Kliger AS, Lorber MI: Reduced incidence of Epstein-Barr virus-associated post-transplant lymphoproliferative disorder using preemptive antiviral therapy. Transplantation 1997;64:848–852.

109. Dauber JH, Paradis IL, Dummer JS: Infectious complications in pulmonary allograft recipients. Clin Chest Med 1990;11:291–308.

110. Davis CL, Harrison KL, McVicar JP, Forg P, Bronner MP, Marsh CL: Antiviral prophylaxis and the Epstein-Barr virus-related post-transplant lymphoproliferative disorder. Clin Transplant 1995;9:53–59.

111. Decker LL, Klaman LD, Thorley-Lawson DA: Detection of the latent form of Epstein-Barr virus DNA in the peripheral blood of healthy individuals. J Virol 1996;70:3286–3289.

112. Delgado R, Lumbreras C, Alba C, Pedraza MA, Otero JR, Gomez R, Moren E, Noriega AR, Paya CV: Low predictive value of polymerase chain reaction for diagnosis of CMV disease in liver transplant recipients. J Clin Microbiol 1992;30:1876–1878.

113. Delmonico FL, Snydman DR: Organ donor screening for infectious diseases. Transplantation 1998;65:603–610.

114. deMan RA, Balk AHHM, Jonkman FAM, Niesters HGM, Osterhaus ADME, Verbrugh HA, Drescher J, Wagner D, Borst HG, Haverich A, Flik J, Stachan-Kunstyr R, Verhagen W, Lunel F, Rosenheim M, Dorent R, Huraux JM, Gandjbakhch I, Brucker G: Letter to the Editor: patient to patient hepatitis B transmission during heart biopsy procedures. A report of the European Working Party on viral hepatitis in heart transplant recipients. J Hosp Infect 1996;34:71–72.

115. Demeter LM: JC, BK and other polyomaviruses; progressive multifocal leukoencephalopathy. In Mandell GL, Bennett JE, Dolin R (eds): Principles and Practice of Infectious Diseases. 4th ed. New York: Churchill Livingstone, 1995, p 1400.

116. Demmler GJ, Six HR, Hurst SM, Yow MD: Enzyme-linked immunosorbent assay for the detection of IgM-class antibodies to cytomegalovirus. J Infect Dis 1986;153:1152.

117. Denning DW: Diagnosis and management of invasive aspergillosis. Curr Clin Top Infect Dis 1996;16:277–299.

118. DePinto D, Park S, Houck J, Pifarre R: Letter to the Editor: successful treatment of mediastinitis and empyema in a heart transplant patient: one-stage procedure. J Heart Lung Transplant 1993;12:883–884.

119. De Repentigny L, Kaufman L, Cole GT, Kruse D, Latge JP, Matthews RC: Immunodiagnosis of invasive fungal infections. J Med Vet Mycol 1994;32(suppl 1):239–252.

120. Deresinski SC, Stevens DA: Coccidioidomycosis in compromised hosts: experience at Stanford University Hospital. Medicine 1974;54:377–395.

121. DesJardin JA, Gibbons L, Cho E, Supran SE, Falagas ME, Werner BG, Snydman DR: Human herpesvirus 6 reactivation is associated with cytomegalovirus infection and syndromes in kidney transplant recipients at risk for primary cytomegalovirus infection. J Infect Dis 1998;178:1783–1786.

122. Diagnostic tests for HIV. Med Lett 1997;39:81–83.

123. Diaz-Gonzalez VM, Altemose GT, Ogorek C, Palazzo I, Piña IL: Cytomegalovirus infection presenting as an apple-core lesion of the colon. J Heart Lung Transplant 1997;16:1171.

124. Dockrell DH, Mendez JC, Jones M, Harmsen WS, Ilstrup DM, Smith TF, Wiesner RH, Krom RAF, Paya CV: Human herpesvirus 6 seronegativity before transplantation predicts the occurrence of fungal infection in liver transplant recipients. Transplantation 1999;67:399–403.

125. Dockrell DH, Prada J, Jones MF, Patel R, Bradley AD, Harmsen WS, Ilstrup DM, Wiesner RH, Krom RAF, Smith TF, Paya CV: Seroconversion to human herpesvirus-6 following liver transplantation is a marker of cytomegalovirus disease. J Infect Dis 1997;176:1135–1140.

126. Dodd RY: The risk of transfusion transmitted infection. N Engl J Med 1992;327:419.

127. Doig RL, Boyd PJR, Eykyn S: Staphylococcus aureus transmitted in transplanted kidneys. Lancet 1975;2:243–245.

128. Domen RE, Nelson KA: Results of a survey of infectious disease testing practices by organ procurement organizations in the United States. Transplantation 1997;63:1790.

129. Douglas DD, Rakela J, Mamish D, Wright TL, Krom RAF, Wiesner RH: Transmission of hepatitis B virus (HBV) infection from orthotopic donor livers. Hepatology 1992;16:49A.

130. Dowling RD, Baladi N, Zenati M: Disruption of the aortic anastomosis after heart-lung transplantation. Ann Thorac Surg 1990;49:118–122.

131. Dresdale AR, Drusin RE, Lamb J, Smith CR, Reemtsma K, Rose EA: Reduced infection in cardiac transplant recipients. Circulation 1985;72(suppl II):II-237–II-240.

132. Duffy P, Wolf J, Collins G, DeVoe AG, Streeten R, Cowen D: Possible person-to-person transmission of Creutzfeldt-Jakob disease [letter]. N Engl J Med 1974;290:692–693.

133. Dummer JS, Armstrong J, Somers J, Kusne S, Carpenter BJ, Rosenthal JT, Ho M: Transmission of infection with herpes simplex virus by renal transplantation. J Infect Dis 1987;155:202–206.

134. Dummer JS, Erb S, Breinig MK, Ho M, Rinaldo CR, Gupta P, Ragni MV, Tzakis A, Makowa L, Van Thiel D: Infection with human immunodeficiency virus in the Pittsburgh transplant population: a study of 583 donors and 1043 recipients, 1981–1986. Transplantation 1989;47:134.

135. Dummer JS, Montero CG, Griffith BP, Hardesty RL, Paradis IL, Ho M: Infections in heart-lung transplant recipients. Transplantation 1986;41:725–729.

136. Dummer JS, White L, Ho M, Griffith BP, Hardesty RL, Bahnson HT: Morbidity of cytomegalovirus infection in recipients of heart or heart/lung transplants who received cyclosporin. J Infect Dis 1985;152:1182–1191.

137. Edelstein PH: Antimicrobial chemotherapy for Legionnaires' disease: a review. Clin Infect Dis 1995;21(suppl 3):S265–S276.

138. Edelstein PH: Legionnaires' disease. Clin Infect Dis 1993;16: 741–749.

139. Egan JJ, Lomax J, Barber L, Lok SS, Martyszczuk R, Yonan N, Fox A, Deiraniya AK, Turner AJ, Woodcock AA: Preemptive treatment for the prevention of cytomegalovirus disease in lung and heart transplant recipients. Transplantation 1998;65:747–752.

140. Elkins CC, Frist WH, Dummer JS, Stewart JR, Merrill WH, Carden KA, Bender HW: Cytomegalovirus disease after heart transplantation: is acyclovir prophylaxis indicated? Ann Thorac Surg 1993;56:1267–1273.

141. Enders G, Dotsch J, Bauer J, Nutzchadel W, Hengel H, Haffner D, Schalasta G, Searle K, Brown KE: Life-threatening parvovirus B19—associated myocarditis and cardiac transplantation as possible therapy: two case reports. Clin Infect Dis 1998;26:355–358.

142. Engelhard D, Elishoov H, Strauss N, Naparstek E, Nagler A, Simhon A, Raveh D, Slavin S, Or R: Nosocomial coagulase-negative staphylococcal infections in bone marrow transplantation recipients with central vein catheter—a 5-year prospective study. Transplantation 1996;61:430–434.

143. Engelhard D, Geller N: Gram-positive bacterial infections. In Bowden RA, Ljungman P, Paya CV (eds): Transplant Infections. Philadelphia: Lippincott-Raven Publishers 1998, p 167.

144. Erice A, Rhame FS, Heussner RC, Dunn DL, Balfour HH Jr: Human immunodeficiency virus infection in patients with solid-organ transplants: report of five cases and review. Rev Infect Dis 1991;13:537–547.

145. Escudero-Fabre A, Cummings O, Kirklin JK, Bourge RC, Aldrete JS: Cytomegalovirus colitis presenting as hematochezia and requiring resection. Arch Surg 1992;127:102.

146. Ettinger NA: Immunocompromised patients: solid organ and bone marrow transplantation. In Niederman MS, Sarosi GA, Glassroth J (eds): Respiratory Infections. Philadelphia: WB Saunders Company 1994, pp 181–198.

147. European Multicentre Trial Group: Cyclosporine in cadaveric renal transplantation: one-year follow-up of a multicentre trial. Lancet 1983;2:986.

148. Farrugia E, Schwab TR: Management and prevention of cytomegalovirus infection after renal transplantation. Mayo Clin Proc 1992;67:879–890.

149. Faulds D, Heel RC: Ganciclovir: a review of its antiviral activity, pharmacokinetiac properties and therapeutic efficacy in cytomegalovirus infections. Drugs 1990;39:597–638.

150. Feldhoff CM, Balfour HH, Simmons RL, Najarian JS, Mauer SM: Varicella in children with renal transplants. J Pediatr 1981;98: 25–31.

151. Feldman S, Hughes WT, Daniel CB: Varicella in children with cancer: seventy seven cases. Pediatrics 1975;56:388–397.

152. Ferguson RM, Rynasiewicz JJ, Sutherland DER, Simmons RL, Najarian JS: Cyclosporin A in renal transplantation: a prospective randomized trial. Surgery 1982;92:175–182.

153. Fietze E, Prosch S, Reinke P, Stein J, Docke WD, Staffa G, Loning S, Devaux S, Emmrich F, von Baehr R: Cytomegalovirus infection in transplant recipients. The role of tumor necrosis factor. Transplantation 1994;58:675–680.

154. Filice GA: Nocardiosis. In Niederman MS, Sarosi GA, Glassroth J (eds): Respiratory Infections. Philadelphia: WB Saunders Company, 1994.

155. Fish DG, Ampel NM, Galgiani JN, Dols CL, Kelly PC, Johnson CH, Pappagianis D, Edwards JE, Wasserman RB, Clark RJ, Antoniskis D, Larsen RA, Englender SJ, Petersen EA: Coccidioidomycosis during human immunodeficiency virus infection. A review of 77 patients. Medicine 1990;69:384–391.

156. Fishman JA, Rubin RH: Infection in organ-transplant recipients. Med Prog 1998;338:1741–1751.

157. Flomenbaum MA, Jarcho JA, Schoen FJ: Progressive multifocal leukoencephalopathy fifty-seven months after heart transplantation. J Heart Lung Transplant 1991;10:888–893.

158. Fojtasek MF, Kleiman MB, Connolly-Stringfield P, Blair R, Wheat LJ: The *Histoplasma capsulatum* antigen assay in disseminated histoplasmosis in children. Pediatr Infect Dis J 1994;13:801–805.

159. Fornairon S, Pol S, Legendre C, Carnot F, Mamzer-Bruneel MF, Brechot C, Kreis H: The long-term virologic and pathologic impact of renal transplantation on chronic hepatitis B virus infection. Transplantation 1996;62:297–299.

160. Foster RS Jr, Winn WC Jr, Marshall W, Gump DW: Legionnaires' disease following renal transplantation. Transplant Prc 1979;11: 93–95.

161. Freeman RB, Giatras I, Falagas ME, Supran S, O'Connor K, Bradley J, Snydman DR, Delmonico FL: Outcome of transplantation of organs procured from bacteremic donors. Transplantation 1999;68:1107–1111.

162. Friedlaender MM, Kaspa RT, Rubinger D, Silver J, Popovtzer MM: Renal transplantation is not contraindicated in asymptomatic carriers of hepatitis B surface antigen. Am J Med 1989; 14:204–210.

163. Fuller J, Levinson MM, Kline JR, Copeland J: Legionnaires' disease after heart transplantation. Ann Thorac Surg 1985;39: 308–311.

164. Gajdusek DC, Gibbs CJ Jr, Asher DM, Brown P, Diwan A, Hoffman P, Nemo G, Rohwer R, White L: Precautions in medical care of, and in handling materials from, patients with transmissible virus dementia (Creutzfeldt-Jakob 'disease). N Engl J Med 1977;297:1253–1258.

165. Galbraith AJ, McCarthy J, Tesar PJ, McGiffin DC: Letter to the Editor: cardiac transplantation for prosthetic valve endocarditis in a previously transplanted heart. J Heart Lung Transplant 1999;18:805.

166. Gallino A, Maggiorini M, Kiowski W, Martin X, Wunderli W, Schneider J, Turina M, Follath F: Toxoplasmosis in heart transplant recipients. Eur J Clin Microbiol Infect Dis 1996;15:389–393.

167. Gamberg P, Miller JL, Lough ME: Impact of protection isolation on the incidence of infection after heart transplantation. J Heart Transplant 1987;6:147.

168. Gane E, Saliba F, Valdecasas GJ, O'Grady J, Pescovitz MD, Lyman S, Robinson CA: Randomized trial of efficacy and safety of oral ganciclovir in the prevention of cytomegalovirus disease in liver transplant recipients. The Oral Ganciclovir International Transplantation Study Group. Lancet 1997;350:1729–1733.

169. Gangahar DM, Liggett SP, Casey J, Carveth SV, Reese HE, Buchman RJ, Breiner MA: Case report: two episodes of cytomegalovirus-associated colon perforation after heart transplantation with successful result. J Heart Transplant 1988;7:377–379.

170. Gassenmaier A, Fuchs P, Schell H, Pfister H: Papillomavirus DNA in warts of immunosuppressed renal allograft recipients. Arch Dermatol Res 1986;278:219–223.

171. Gentry LO: Cardiac transplantation and related infections. Semin Respir Infect 1993;8:199–206.

172. George MJ, Snydman DR, Werner BG, Griffith J, Falagas ME, Dougherty NN, Rubin RH: The independent role of cytomegalovirus as a risk factor for invasive fungal disease in orthotopic liver transplant recipients. Am J Med 1997;103:106–113.

173. Gerna G, Zavattoni M, Baldantı F, Sarasini A, Chezzi L, Grossi P, Revello MG: Human cytomegalovirus (HCMV) leukoDNAemia correlates more closely with clinical symptoms than antigenemia and viremia in heart and heart/lung transplant recipients with primary HCMV infection. Transplantation 1998;65:1378–1385.

174. Gerna G, Zipeto D, Percivalle E, Parea M, Revello MG, Maccario R, Peri G, Milanesi G: Human cytomegalovirus infection of the major leukocyte subpopulations and evidence for initial viral replication in polymorphonuclear leukocytes from viremic patients. J Infect Dis 1992;166:1236–1244.

175. Gibel LJ, Sterling W, Hoy W, Harford A: Is serological evidence of infection with syphilis a contraindication to kidney donation? Case report and review of the literature. J Urol 1987;138:1226–1227.

176. Gill VJ, Zierdt CH, Wu TC, Stock F, Pizzo PA, MacLowry JD: Comparison of lysis-centrifugation with lysis-filtration and a conventional unvented bottle for blood cultures. J Clin Microbiol 1984;20:927–932.

177. Gish R, Lau JYN, Brooks L, Fang JWS, Steady SL, Imperial JC, Garcia-Kennedy R, Esquivel CO, Keeffe EB: Ganciclovir treat-

ment of hepatitis B virus infection in liver transplant recipients. Hepatology 1996;23:1–7.

178. Glenn J: Cytomegalovirus infections following renal transplantation. Rev Infect Dis 1981;3:1151–1178.

179. Glezen WP, Frank AL, Taber LH, Kasel JA: Parainfluenza virus type 3: seasonality and risk of infection and reinfection in young children. J Infect Dis 1984;150:851–857.

180. Gnann JW Jr: Other herpesviruses: herpes simplex virus, varicella-zoster virus, human herpesvirus types 6, 7, and 8. In Bowden RA, Ljungman P, Paya CV (eds): Transplant Infections. Philadelphia: Lippincott-Raven Publishers, 1998.

181. Goodwin RA, Loyd JE, Des Prez RM: Histoplasmosis in normal hosts. Medicine 1981;60:231–266.

182. Goodwin RA Jr, Owens FT, Snell JD, Hubbard WW, Buchanan RD, Terry RT, Des Prez RM: Chronic pulmonary histoplasmosis. Medicine 1976;55:413–452.

183. Goodwin RA, Shapiro JL, Thurman GH, Thurman SS, Des Prez RM: Disseminated histoplasmosis: clinical and pathologic correlations. Medicine 1980;59:1.

184. Gordon SM, La Rosa SP, Kalmadi S, Arroliga AC, Avery RK, Truesdell-LaRosa L, Longworth DL: Should prophylaxis for Pneumocystis carinii pneumonia in solid organ transplant recipients ever be discontinued? Clin Infect Dis 1999;28:240–246.

185. Gorensek MJ, Stewart RW, Keys TF, McHenry MC, Babiak T, Goormastic M: Symptomatic cytomegalovirus infection as a significant risk factor for major infections after cardiac transplantation. J Infect Dis 1988;158:884–887.

186. Gorensek MJ, Stewart RW, Keys TF, McHenry M, Longworth DL, Rehm SJ, Babiak T: Decreased infections in cardiac transplant recipients on cyclosporine with reduced corticosteroid use. Cleve Clin J Med 1989;56:690–687.

187. Gray J, Wreghitt TG, Pavel P, Smyth RL, Parameshwar J, Stewart S, Cary N, Large S, Wallwork J: Epstein-Barr virus infection in heart and heart/lung transplant recipients: incidence and clinical impact. J Heart Lung Transplant 1995;14:640.

188. Green M, Cacciarelli TV, Mazariegos GV, Sigurdsson L, Qu L, Rowe DT, Reyes J: Serial measurement of Epstein-Barr viral load in peripheral blood in pediatric liver transplant recipients during treatment for posttransplant lymphoproliferative disease. Transplantation 1998;66:1641–1644.

189. Greenberg SB: Viral pneumonia. Infect Dis Clin North Am 1991;5:603–621.

190. Grefte A, Van der Giessen M, Van Son W, The TH: Circulating cytomegalovirus (CMV)-infected endothelial cells in patients with an active CMV infection. J Infect Dis 1993;167:270–277.

191. Griffin J, Meduri G: New approaches in the diagnosis of nosocomial pneumonia. Med Clin North Am 1994;78:1091–1122.

192. Grose C: Variation on a theme by Fenner: the pathogenesis of chickenpox. Pediatrics 1981;68:735–737.

193. Grossi P, De Maria R, Caroli A, Zaina MS, Minoli L: Infections in heart transplant recipients: the experience of the Italian Heart Transplant Program. J Heart Lung Transplant 1992;11:847–866.

194. Grossi P, Revello MG, Minoli L, Percivalle E, Zavattoni M, Poma G, Martinelli L, Gerna G: Three-year experience with human cytomegalovirus infections in heart transplant recipients. J Heart Transplant 1990;9:712–719.

195. Guiot HFL: Role of competition for substrate in bacterial antagonism in the gut. Infect Immun 1982;38:887–892.

196. Hall KA, Sethi GK, Rosado LJ, Martinez JD, Huston CL, Copeland JG: Coccidioidomycosis and heart transplantation. J Heart Lung Transplant 1993;12:525–526.

197. Hall WA, Martinez AJ, Dummer JS: Progressive multifocal leukoencephalopathy after cardiac transplantation. Neurology 1988;38:995–996.

198. Hall WA, Martinez AJ, Dummer JS, Griffith BP, Hardesty RL, Bahnson HT, Lunsford LD: Central nervous system infections in heart and heart-lung transplant recipients. Arch Neurol 1989;46:173–177.

199. Hanto DW, Frizzera G, Gajl-Peczalska J, Purtilo DT, Klein G, Simmons RL, Najarian JS: The Epstein-Barr virus (EBV) in the pathogenosis of post-transplant lymphoma. Transplant Proc 1981;13:756–760.

200. Hasan A, Hamilton JRL, Au J, Gascoigne A, Corris PA, Freeman R, Dark JH: Surgical management of infective endocarditis after

heart-lung transplantation. J Heart Lung Transplant 1993;12:330–332.

201. Hatton MP, Duker JS, Reichel E, Morley MG, Puliafito CA: Treatment of relapsed cytomegalovirus retinitis with the sustained-release ganciclovir implant. Retina 1998;18:50.

202. Herberman RB: Natural killer cells. Annu Rev Med 1986;37:347–352.

203. Heilman CA: Respiratory syncytial and parainfluenza viruses. J Infect Dis 1990;161:402–406.

204. Herrmann M, Weyand M, Greshake B, von Eiff C, Proctor RA, Scheld HH, Peters G: Left ventricular assist device infection is associated with increased mortality but is not a contraindication to transplantation. Circulation 1997;95:814–817.

205. Hibberd PL, Tolkoff-Rubin NE, Cosimi AB, Schooley RT, Isaacson D, Doran M, Delvecchio A, Delmonico FL, Auchincloss H, Rubin RH: Symptomatic cytomegalovirus disease in the cytomegalovirus antibody seropositive renal transplant recipient treated with OKT3. Transplantation 1992;53:68–72.

206. Hibberd PL, Tolkoff-Rubin NE, Conti D, Stuart F, Thistlethwaite JR, Neylan JF, Snydman DR, Freeman R, Lorber MI, Rubin RH: Preemptive ganciclovir therapy to prevent cytomegalovirus disease in cytomegalovirus antibody-positive renal transplant recipients: a randomized controlled trial. Ann Intern Med 1995;123:18–26.

207. Hinchey WW, Someren A: Cryptococcal prostatitis. Am J Clin Pathol 1981;75:257–260.

208. Hirsch MS: Herpes simplex virus. In Mandell GL, Bennett JE, Dolin R (eds): Principles and Practice of Infectious Diseases. 4th ed. New York: Churchill Livingstone, 1995, pp 1336–1345.

209. Hobbs JR, Milner RDG, Watt PJ: Gamma-M deficiency predisposing to meningococcal septicaemia. BMJ 1967;4:583–586.

210. Hoesley CJ, Dismukes WE: New antifungal agents: emphasis on lipid formulations of amphotericin B. Clin Updates Fungal Infect 1999;2:1–5.

211. Hofflin JM, Potasman I, Baldwin JC, Oyer PE, Stinson EB, Remington JS: Infectious complications in heart transplant recipients receiving cyclosporine and corticosteroids. Ann Intern Med 1987;106:209–216.

212. Holliman RE, Johnson JD, Adams S, Pepper JR: Toxoplasmosis and heart transplantation. J Heart Transplant 1991;10:608–610.

213. Hoofnagle JH, Di Bisceglie AM: The treatment of chronic viral hepatitis. N Engl J Med 1997;336:347–356.

214. Hoofnagle JH, Di Bisceglie AM: Serologic diagnosis of acute and chronic viral hepatitis. Semin Liver Dis 1991;11:73–83.

215. Horbach I, Fehrenbach FJ: Legionellosis in heart transplant recipients. Infection 1990;18:361.

216. Hosenpud JD, Hershberger RE, Pantely GA, Norman DJ, Hovaguimian H, Cobanoglu A, Starr A: Late infection in cardiac allograft recipients: profiles, incidence, and outcome. J Heart Lung Transplant 1991;10:380–386.

217. Houff SA, Burton RC, Wilson RW, Henson TE, London WT, Baer GM, Anderson LJ, Winkler WG, Madden DL, Sever JL: Human-to-human transmission of rabies virus by corneal transplant. N Engl J Med 1979;300:603–604.

218. Hoxtell EO, Mandel JS, Murray SS, Schuman LM, Goltz RW: Incidence of skin carcinoma after renal transplantation. Arch Dermatol 1977;113:436–438.

219. Hsu J, Griffith BP, Dowling RD, Kormos RL, Dummer JS, Armitage JM, Zenati M, Hardesty RL: Infections in mortally ill cardiac transplant recipients. J Thorac Cardiovasc Surg 1989;98:506–509.

220. Humar A, Gregson D, Caliendo AM, McGeer A, Malkan G, Krajden M, Corey P, Greig P, Walmsley S, Levy G, Mazzulli T: Clinical utility of quantitative cytomegalovirus viral load determination for predicting cytomegalovirus disease in liver transplant recipients. Transplantation 1999;68:1305–1311.

221. Hummel M, Schüler S, Weber U, Schwertlick G, Hempel S, Theiss D, Rees W, Mueller J, Hetzer R: Aspergillosis with Aspergillus osteomyelitis and diskitis after heart transplantation: surgical and medical management. J Heart Lung Transplant 1993;12:599.

222. Husni RN, Gordon SM, Longworth DL, Arroliga A, Stillwell PC, Avery RK, Maurer JR, Mehta A, Kirby T: Cytomegalovirus infection is a risk factor for invasive aspergillosis in lung transplant recipients. Clin Infect Dis 1998;26:753–755.

223. Hutter JA, Scott J, Wreghitt T, Higenbottam T, Wallwork J: The importance of cytomegalovirus in heart-lung transplant recipients. Chest 1989;95:627–631.

224. Iberer F, Tscheliessnigg K, Halwachs G: Letter to the Editor: cytomegalovirus antigenemia as a marker for antiviral therapy after heart transplantation. J Heart Lung Transplant 1996;15:314.

225. Irving WL, Ratnamohan VM, Hueston LC, Chapman JR, Cunningham AL: Dual antibody rises to cytomegalovirus and human herpesvirus type 6: frequency of occurrence in CMV infections and evidence for genuine reactivity to both viruses. J Infect Dis 1990;161:910–916.

226. Jamil S, Brennessel D, Pessah M, Hilton E: Fluconazole treatment of cryptococcal osteomyelitis. Infect Dis Clin Pract 1992;1: 115–117.

227. Janner D, Bork J, Baum M, Chinnock R: Severe pneumonia after heart transplantation as a result of human parvovirus B19. J Heart Lung Transplant 1994;13:336–338.

228. Janner D, Bork J, Baum M, Chinnock R: Pneumocystis carinii pneumonia in infants after heart transplantation. J Heart Lung Transplant 1996;15:758–763.

229. Kadian M, Hawkins L, Nespral J, Schwartz M, Miller C: Use of hepatitis B core antibody positive multiorgan donors. Presented at the Second International Congress of the Society for Organ Sharing Vancouver, British Columbia, 1993.

230. Karwande SV, Renlund DG, Olsen SL, Gay WA, Richenbacher WE, Hawkins JA, Millar RC, Marks JD: Mediastinitis in heart transplantation. Ann Thorac Surg 1992;54:1039.

231. Kemper CA, Lombard CM, Deresinski SC, Tompkins LS: Visceral bacillary epithelioid angiomatosis: possible manifestations of disseminated cat scratch disease in the immunocompromised host: a report of two cases. Am J Med 1990;89:216.

232. Keogh AM: Recurrence of myocardial disease in the transplanted heart. In Cooper DKC, Miller LW, Patterson GA (eds): The Transplantation and Replacement of Thoracic Organs. Hingham, MA: Kluwer Academic Publishers, 1996.

233. Khoo DE, Zebro TJ, English TAH: Bacterial endocarditis in a transplanted heart. Pathol Res Pract 1989;185:445–447.

234. Kirchhoff LV: American trypanosomiasis (Chagas' disease)—a tropical disease now in the United States. N Engl J Med 1993;329:639.

235. Kirklin JK, Bourge RC, Naftel DC, Morrow WR, Deierhoi MH, Kauffman RS, White-Williams C, Nomberg RI, Holman WL, Smith DC Jr: Treatment of recurrent heart rejection with mycophenolate mofetil (RS-61443) initial clinical experience. J Heart Lung Transplant 1994;3:444–450.

236. Kirklin JK, Bourge RC, White-Williams C, Naftel DC, Thomas FT, Thomas JM, Phillips MG: Prophylactic therapy for rejection after cardiac transplantation. J Thorac Cardiovasc Surg 1990;99:716–724.

237. Kirklin JK, Holm A, Aldrete JS, White C, Bourge RC: Gastrointestinal complications after cardiac transplantation. Ann Surg 1990;211:538–542.

238. Kirklin JK, Naftel DC, Levine TB, Bourge RC, Pelletier GB, O'Donnell J, Miller LW, Pritzker MR, and the Cardiac Transplant Research Database Group: Cytomegalovirus after heart transplantation. Risk factors for infection and death: a multiinstitutional study. J Heart Lung Transplant 1994;13:394–404.

239. Kleim V, Ringe B, Holhorst K, Frei U: Kidney transplantation in hepatitis B surface antigen carriers. Clin Invest 1994;72:1000–1006.

240. Klein BS, Vergeront JM, Kaufman L, Bradsher RW, Kumar UN, Mathai G, Varkey B, Davis JP: Serological tests for blastomycosis: assessments during a large point-source outbreak in Wisconsin. J Infect Dis 1987;155:262–268.

241. Klein RS, Recco RA, Catalano MT, Edberg SC, Casey JI, Steigbigel NH: Association of streptococcus bovis with carcinoma of the colon. N Engl J Med 1977;297:800–802.

242. Knox KK, Carrigan DR: HHV-6 and CMV pneumonitis in immunocompromised patients. Lancet 1994;343:1647.

243. Knudsen PJ, Dinarello CA, Strom TB: Glucocorticoids inhibit transcriptional and posttranscriptional expression of interleukin-1 in U937 cells. J Immunol 1987;139:4129.

244. Kobashigawa J, Miller L, Renlund D, Mentzer R, Alderman E, Bourge R, Costanzo M, Eisen H, Dureau G, Ratkovec R, Hummel M, Ipe D, Johnson J, Keogh A, Mamelok R, Mancini D, Smart F, Valantine H: A randomized active-controlled trial of mycophenolate mofetil in heart transplant recipients. Transplantation 1998;66:507–515.

245. Koneru B, Tzakis AG, Depuydt LE, Demetris AJ, Armstrong JA, Dummer JS, Starzl TE: Transmission of fatal herpes simplex infection through renal transplantation. Transplantation 1988;45: 653–656.

246. Koskinen PK, Krogerus LA, Nieminen MS, Mattila SP, Häyry PJ, Lautenschlager IT: Quantitation of cytomegalovirus infection-associated histologic findings in endomyocardial biopsies of heart allografts. J Heart Lung Transplant 1993;12:343–354.

247. Koskinen PK, Nieminen MS, Mattila SP, Häyry PJ, Lautenschlager IT: The correlation between symptomatic CMV infection and CMV antigenemia in heart allograft recipients. Transplantation 1993;55:547–551.

248. Krahenbuhl O, Tschopp J: Perforin-induced pore formation. Immunol Today 1991;12:399–402.

249. Kramer MR, Marshall SE, Starnes VA, Gamberg P, Amitai Z, Theodore J: Infectious complications in heart-lung transplantation. Arch Intern Med 1993;153:2010–2016.

250. Krech U: Complement-fixing antibodies against cytomegalovirus in different parts of the world. Bull WHO 1973;49:103–105.

251. Krick JA, Remington JS: Current concepts in parasitology: toxoplasmosis in the adult—an overview. N Engl J Med 1978;298:550.

252. Kruger RM, Shannon WD, Arens MQ, Lynch JP, Storch GA, Trulock EP: The impact of ganciclovir-resistant cytomegalovirus infection after lung transplantation. Transplantation 1999;68: 1272–1279.

253. Kuppermann BD: Therapeutic options for resistant cytomegalovirus retinitis. J Acquir Immune Defic Syndr Hum Retrovirol 1997;14:S13–S21.

254. Kwon-Chung KJ, Bennett JE (eds): Medical Mycology. Philadelphia: Lea & Febiger, 1992.

255. Lake K, Anderson D, Milfred S, Love K, Pritzker M, Emery R: The incidence of cytomegalovirus disease is not increased after OKT3 induction therapy. J Heart Lung Transplant 1993;12: 537–538.

256. Lake KD, Smith CI, LaForest SKM, Pritzker MR, Emery RW: Outcomes of hepatitis C positive (HCV+) heart transplant recipients. Transplant Proc 1997;29:581–582.

257. Lammermeier DE, Sweeney MS, Haupt HE, Radovancevic B, Duncan JM, Frazier OH: Use of potentially infected donor hearts for cardiac transplantation. Ann Thorac Surg 1990;50:222–225.

258. Larson EL: APIC guideline for hand washing and hand antisepsis in health care settings. Am J Infect Control 1995;23:251–269.

259. Leigh IM, Glover MT: Skin cancer and warts in immunosuppressed renal transplant recipients. Recent Results Cancer Res 1995;139:69–86.

260. Lentino JR, Rosenkranz MA, Michaels JA, Kurup VP, Rose HD, Rytel MW: Nosocomial aspergillosis: a retrospective review of airborne disease secondary to road construction and contaminated air conditioners. Am J Epidemiol 1982;116:430–437.

261. Lerner PI: Nocardiosis. Clin Infect Dis 1996;22:891–905.

262. Linder J: Infection as a complication of heart transplantation. J Heart Transplant 1988;7:390–394.

263. Linnemann CC Jr, First MR: Risk of pneumococcal infections in renal transplant patients. JAMA 1979;241:2619–2621.

264. Ljungman P, Lonnqvist B, Ringden O, Skinhoj P, Gahrton G, for the Nordic Bone Marrow Transplant Group: A randomized trial of oral versus intravenous acyclovir for treatment of herpes zoster in bone marrow transplant recipients. Bone Marrow Transplant 1989;4:613–615.

265. Locksley RM, Flournoy N, Sullivan KM, Meyers J: Infection with varicella zoster virus after marrow transplantation. J Infect Dis 1985;152:1172–1181.

266. Lopez AM, Williams PL, Ampel NM: Acute pulmonary coccidioidomycosis mimicking bacterial pneumonia and septic shock: a report of two cases. Am J Med 1993;95:236–239.

267. Lowance D, Neumayer HH, Legendre CM, Squifflet JP, Kovarik J, Brennan PJ, Norman D, Mendez R, Keating MR, Coggon GL, Crisp A, Lee IC: Valacyclovir for the prevention of cytomegalovirus disease after renal transplantation. N Engl J Med 1999; 340:1462.

268. Luft BJ, Naot Y, Araujo FG, Stinson EB, Remington JS: Primary and reactivated toxoplasma infection in patients with cardiac transplants. Ann Intern Med 1983;99:27–31.

269. Lurain NS, Ammons HC, Kapell KS, Yeldandi VV, Garrity ER, O'Keefe JP: Molecular analysis of human cytomegalovirus strains

from two lung transplant recipients with the same donor. Transplantation 1996;62:497–502.

270. Lynfield R, Herrin JT, Rubin RH: Varicella in pediatric renal transplant recipients. Pediatrics 1992;90:216–220.

271. Macdonald PS, Keogh AM, Marshman D, Richens D, Harvison A, Kaan AM, Spratt PM: A double-blind placebo-controlled trial of low-dose ganciclovir to prevent cytomegalovirus disease after heart transplantation. J Heart Lung Transplant 1995;14:32.

272. Mackowiak PA, Martin RM, Smith JW: The role of bacterial interference in the increased prevalence of oropharyngeal gram negative bacilli among alcoholics and diabetics. Am Rev Respir Dis 1979;120:589–593.

273. MacLean LD, Dossetor JB, Gault MH, Oliver JA, Inglis FG, MacKinnon KJ: Renal homotransplantation using cadaver donors. Arch Surg 1965;91:288–306.

274. Madayag RM, Johnson LB, Bartlett ST, Schweitzer EJ, Constantine NT, McCarter RJ, Kuo PC, Keay S, Oldach DW: Use of renal allografts from donors positive for hepatitis B core antibody confers minimal risk for subsequent development of clinical hepatitis B virus disease. Transplantation 1997;64:1781.

275. Mañez R, Breinig MC, Linden P, Wilson J, Torre-Cisneros J, Kusne S, Dummer S, Ho M: Posttransplant lymphoproliferative disease in primary Epstein-Barr virus infection after liver transplantation: the role of cytomegalovirus disease. J Infect Dis 1997;176:1462.

276. Marsh RF, Hanson RP: Transmissible mink encephalopathy: infectivity of corneal epithelium. Science 1975;187:656.

277. Marshall W, Foster RS Jr, Winn W: Legionnaires' disease in renal transplant patients. Am J Surg 1981;141:423–429.

278. Martin-Santos JM, Alonso-Pulpon L, Pradas G, Cuervas-Mons V, Anguita M, Mulero-Mendoza J, Escribano E, Martinez-Beltran J, Figuera-Aymerich D: Septic arthritis by Salmonella enteritidis after heart transplantation. J Heart Transplant 1987;6:177–179.

279. Martino P, Raccah R, Gentile G, Venditti M, Girmenia C, Mandelli F: Aspergillus colonization of the nose and pulmonary aspergillosis in neutropenic patients: a retrospective study. Haematologica 1989;74:263–265.

280. Massin E, Zeluff BJ, Carrol CL, Radovancevic B, Benjamin RS, Ewer MS, Bransford TL, Buja LM: Cardiac transplantation and aspergillosis. Circulation 1994;90:1552–1556.

281. Matthews RC: Comparative assessment of the detection of candidal antigens as a diagnostic tool. J Med Vet Mycol 1996;34:1–10.

282. Mauch TJ, Bratton S, Myers T, Krane E, Gentry SR, Kashtan CE: Influenza B virus infection in pediatric solid organ transplant recipients. Pediatrics 1994;94:225–229.

283. Mazzulli T, Drew LW, Yen-Lieberman B, Jekic-McMullen D, Kohn DJ, Isada C, Moussa G, Chua R, Walmsley S: Multicenter comparison of the Digene Hybrid Capture CMV DNA Assay (version 2.0), the pp65 antigenemia assay and cell culture for detection of cytomegalovirus viremia. J Clin Microbiol 1999; 37:958–963.

284. McCarthy PM, Schmitt SK, Vargo RL, Gordon S, Keys TF, Hobbs RE: Implantable LVAD infections: implications for permanent use of the device. Ann Thorac Surg 1996;61:359–365.

285. McDiarmid SV, Jordan S, Lee GS, Toyoda M, Goss JA, Vargas JH, Martin MG, Bahar R, Maxfield AL, Ament ME, Busuttil RW: Prevention and preemptive therapy of posttransplant lymphoproliferative disease in pediatric liver recipients. Transplantation 1998;66:1604–1611.

286. McGiffin DC, Galbraith AJ, McCarthy JB, Tesar PJ: Mycotic false aneurysm of the aortic suture line after heart transplantation. J Heart Lung Transplant 1994;13:926–928.

287. McGiffin DC, Kirklin JK, Naftel DC, Bourge RC: Competing outcomes after heart transplantation: a comparison of eras and outcomes. J Heart Lung Transplant 1997;16:190–198.

288. McGregor CG, Fleck DG, Nagington J, Stovin PGI, Cory-Pearce R, English TAH: Disseminated toxoplasmosis in cardiac transplantation. J Clin Pathol 1984;37:74–77.

289. McGregor RS, Zitelli BJ, Urbach AH, Malatack JJ, Gartner JC Jr: Varicella in pediatric orthotopic liver transplant recipients. Pediatrics 1989;83:256–261.

290. McLelland J, Rees A, Williams G, Chu T: The incidence of immunosuppression-related skin disease in long-term transplant patients. Transplantation 1988;46:871–873.

291. McMaster P, Haynes IG, Michael J, Adu D, Vlassis T, Roger S, Turney J, Stock S, Buckels J, Mackintosh P, Ezzibdeh M: Cyclosporine in cadaveric renal transplantation: a prospective randomized trial. Transplant Proc 1983;15(suppl I):2523–2527.

292. McOmish F, Yap PL, Jordan A, Hart H, Cohen BJ, Simmonds P: Detection of parvovirus B19 in donated blood: a model system for screening by polymerase chain reaction. J Clin Microbiol 1993;31:323–328.

293. Mendez J, Espy M, Smith TF, Wilson J, Wiesner R, Paya CV: Clinical significance of viral load in the diagnosis of cytomegalovirus disease after liver transplantation. Transplantation 1998; 65:1477–1481.

294. Mendez JC, Sia IG, Tau KR, Espy MJ, Smith TF, Chou S, Paya CV: Novel mutation in the CMV UL97 gene associated with resistance to ganciclovir therapy. Transplantation 1999;67: 755–757.

295. Merigan TC, Renlund DG, Keay S, Bristow MR, Starnes V, O'Connell JB, Resta S, Dunn D, Gamberg P, Ratkovec RM, Richenbacher WE, Millar RC, DuMond C, DeAmond B, Sullivan V, Cheney T, Buhles W, Stinson EB: A controlled trial of ganciclovir to prevent cytomegalovirus disease after heart transplantation. N Engl J Med 1992;326:1182.

296. Michaels MG, Wald ER, Fricker FJ, del Nido PJ, Armitage J: Toxoplasmosis in pediatric recipients of heart transplants. Clin Infect Dis 1992;14:847–851.

297. Miller LW, Naftel DC, Bourge RC, Kirklin JK, Brozena SC, Jaracho J, Hobbs RE, Mills RM, and the Cardiac Transplant Research Database Group: Infection after heart transplantation: a multiinstitutional study. J Heart Lung Transplant 1994;13:381–393.

298. Min KW, Wickemeyer WJ, Chandran P, Shadur CA, Gervich D, Phillips SJ, Zeff RH, Song J: Fatal cytomegalovirus infection and coronary arterial thromboses after heart transplantation: a case report. J Heart Transplant 1987;6:100–105.

299. Mitchell TG, Perfect JR: Cryptococcosis in the era of AIDS—100 years after the discovery of Cryptococcus neoformans. Clin Microbiol Rev 1995;8:515–540.

300. Miyashita EM, Yang B, Babcock GJ, Thorley-Lawson DA: Identification of the site of Epstein-Barr virus persistence in vivo as a resting B cell. J Virol 1997;17:4882–4891.

301. Montoya JG, Giraldo LF, Stinson EB, Gamberg P, Hunt S, Giannetti N, Miller J, Remington JS: Infectious complications in 620 heart transplant patients at Stanford University Medical Center [abstract 236]. Program and Abstracts of the 37th Annual Infectious Diseases Society of America, Philadelphia, PA, November 18–21, 1999, p 80.

302. Mossad SB, Avery RK, Goormastic M, Hobbs RE, Stewart RW: Significance of positive cultures from donor left atrium and postpreservation fluid in heart transplantation. Transplantation 1997;64:1209–1210.

303. Muñoz P, Palomo J, Muñoz R, Rodríquez-Creixéms M, Pelaez T, Bouza E: Tuberculosis in heart transplant recipients. Clin Infect Dis 1995;21:398–402.

304. Murray HW: Interferon-gamma: the activated macrophage and host defense against microbial challenge. Ann Intern Med 1988;108:595–608.

305. Musch DC, Martin DF, Gordon JF, Davis MD, Kuppermann BD, and the Ganciclovir Implant Study Group: Treatment of cytomegalovirus retinitis with a sustained-release ganciclovir implant. N Engl J Med 1997;337:83–90.

306. Musher DM: Streptococcus pneumoniae. In Mandell GL, Bennett JE, Dolin R (eds): Principles and practice of Infectious Diseases. 4th ed. New York: Churchill Livingstone, 1995, pp 1811–1826.

307. Naides SJ: Parvovirus B19 infection. Rheum Dis Clin North Am 1993;19:457–475.

308. Naides SJ, Weiner CP: Antenatal diagnosis and palliative treatment of non-immune hydrops fetalis secondary to fetal parvovirus B19 infection. Prenat Diagn 1989;9:105–114.

309. Najarian JS, Strand M, Fryd DS, Ferguson RM, Simmons RL, Ascher NL, Sutherland DER: Comparison of cyclosporine versus azathioprine-antilymphocyte globulin in renal transplantation. Transplant Proc 1983;15(suppl I):2463–2468.

310. Navari RM, Sullivan KM, Springmeyer SC, Siegel MS, Meyers JD, Buckner CD, Sanders JE, Stewart PS, Clift RA, Fefer A: Mycobacterial infections in marrow transplant patients. Transplantation 1983;36:509–513.

311. Neild G, Anderson M, Hawes S, Colvin BT: Parvovirus infection after renal transplant [letter]. Lancet 1986;2:1226–1227.

312. Nelson PW, Delmonico FL, Tolkoff-Rubin NE, Cosimi AB, Fang LST, Russell PS, Rubin RH: Unsuspected donor Pseudomonas infection causing arterial disruption after renal transplantation. Transplantation 1984;37:313–314.

313. Newton JA Jr, Anderson MD, Kennedy CA, Oldfield EC III: Septic arthritis due to Cryptococcus neoformans without associated osteomyelitis: case report and review. Infect Dis Clin Pract 1994;3:295.

314. Noble WC: Carriage of Staphylococcus aureus and beta-haemolytic streptococci in relation to race. Acta Dermatol Venereol 1974;54:403–405.

315. Nour B, Green M, Michaels M, Reyes J, Tzakis A, Gartner JC, McLoughlin L, Starzl TE: Parvovirus B19 infection in pediatric transplant patients. Transplantation 1993;56:835–838.

316. Novick RJ: In discussion of Karwande SV, Renlund DG, Olsen SL: Mediastinitis in heart transplantation. Ann Thorac Surg 1992;54:1039–1045.

317. Novick RJ, Moreno-Cabral CE, Stinson EB, Oyer PE, Starnes VA, Hunt SA, Shumway NE: Nontuberculous mycobacterial infections in heart transplant recipients: a seventeen-year experience. J Heart Transplant 1990;9:357–363.

318. Oaks TE, Pae WE, Pennock JL, Myers JL, Pierce WS: Aortic rupture caused by fungal aortitis: successful management after heart transplantation. J Heart Transplant 1988;7:162–164.

319. Ochs HD, Ament ME, Davis SD: Giardiasis with malabsorption in X-linked agammaglobulinemia. N Engl J Med 1972;287:341–342.

320. Odenheimer DB, Matas AJ, Tellis VA: Donor cultures reported positive after transplantation: a clinical dilemma. Transplant Proc 1986;18:465–466.

321. Ong JP, Barnes DS, Younossi ZM, Gramlich T, Yen-Lieberman B, Goormastic M, Sheffield C, Hoercher K, Starling R, Young J, Smedira N, McCarthy P: Outcome of de novo hepatitis C virus infection in heart transplant recipients. Hepatology 1999;30:1293–1298.

322. Ooi BS, Chen BTM, Lim CH, Khoo OT, Chan KT: Survival of a patient transplanted with a kidney infected with Cryptococcus neoformans. Transplantation 1971;11:428–429.

323. Oren I, Sobel JD: Human herpes virus type 6: review. Clin Infect Dis 1992;14:741–746.

324. Organ donation for transplantation. Med Lett 1995;37:60–62.

325. Orr KE, Gould FK, Short G, Dark JH, Hilton CJ, Corris PA, Freeman R: Outcome of Toxoplasma gondii mismatches in heart transplant recipients over a period of 8 years. J Infect 1994;29:249–253.

326. Osterhaus ADME, Vos MC, Balk AHMM, de Man RA, Mouton JW, Rothbarth PH, Schalm SW, Tomaello AM, Niesters HG, Verbrugh HA: Transmission of hepatitis B virus among heart transplant recipients during endomyocardial biopsy procedures. J Heart Lung Transplant 1998;17:158–166.

327. Palac RT, Strausbaugh LJ, Antonovic R, Floten HS: An unusual complication of cardiac transplantation—infected aortic pseudoaneurysm. Ann Thorac Surg 1991;51:479–481.

328. Palestine AG, Nussenblatt RB, Chan C-C: Side effects of cyclosporin A on the course of infection with Giardia muris in mice. Am J Trop Med Hyg 1986;35:496.

329. Pappas PG, Threlkeld MG, Bedsole GD, Cleveland KO, Gelfand MS, Dismukes WE: Blastomycosis in immunocompromised patients. Medicine 1993;72:311–325.

330. Parfrey PS, Forbes RDC, Hutchinson TA, Kenick S, Farge D, Dauphinee WD, Seely JF, Guttmann RD: The impact of renal transplantation on the course of hepatitis B liver disease. Transplantation 1985;39:610–615.

331. Patel R, Paya CV: Cytomegalovirus infection and disease in solid organ transplant recipients. In Bowden RA, Ljungman P, Paya CV (eds): Transplant infections. Philadelphia: Lippincott-Raven Publishers, 1998, pp 229–244.

332. Patel R, Roberts GD, Keating MR, Paya CV: Infections due to nontuberculous mycobacteria in kidney, heart, and liver transplant recipients. Clin Infect Dis 1994;19:263–273.

333. Patel R, Smith TF, Espy M, Wiesner RH, Krom RAF, Portela D, Paya CV: Detection of cytomegalovirus (CMV) in sera of liver transplant recipients. J Clin Microbiol 1994;32:1431.

334. Patel R, Snydman DR, Rubin RH, Ho M, Pescovitz M, Martin M, Paya CV: Cytomegalovirus prophylaxis in solid organ transplant recipients. Transplantation 1996;61:1279–1289.

335. Patterson TF, Andriole VT: Current concepts in cryptococcosis. Eur J Clin Microbiol Infect Dis 1989;8:457–465.

336. Pattison JR, Jones SE, Hodgson J, Davis LR, White JM: Parvovirus infections and hypoplastic crisis in sickle-cell anemia [letter]. Lancet 1981;1:664–665.

337. Paya CV, Fung JJ, Nalesnik MA, Kieff E, Green M, Gores G, Habermann TM, Wiesner RH, Swinnen LJ, Woodle ES, Bromberg JS: Epstein-Barr virus-induced post-transplant lymphoproliferative disorders. ASTS/ASTP EBV-PTLD Task Force and The Mayo Clinic Organized International Consensus Development Meeting. Transplantation 1999;68:1517.

338. Pepose JS, Holland GN: Cytomegalovirus infections of the retina. In Schachat AP, Murphy RB (eds): Retina. 2nd ed, vol 2. St. Louis: Mosby, 1994, pp 1559–1570.

339. Pereira B, Milford E, Kirkman R, Levey A: Transmission of hepatitis C virus by organ transplantation. N Engl J Med 1991;325:454–460.

340. Pereira BJG, Wright TL, Schmid CH, Bryan CF, Cheung RC, Cooper ES, Hsu H, Heyn-Lamb R, Light JA, Norman DJ: Screening and confirmatory testing of cadaver organ donors for hepatitis C virus infection—A U.S. national collaborative study. Kidney Int 1994;46:886–892.

341. Perfect JR, Durack DT, Gallis HA: Cryptococcemia. Medicine 1983;62:98–109.

342. Peters TG, Reiter C, Boswell R: Transmission of tuberculosis by kidney transplantation. Transplantation 1984;38:514–516.

343. Petri WA Jr: Infections in heart transplant recipients. Clin Infect Dis 1994;18:141–148.

344. Pfaff WW, Blanton JW: Hepatitis antigenemia and survival after renal transplantation. Clin Transplant 1997;11:476–479.

345. Pillay D, Ali AA, Liu SF, Kops E, Sweny P, Griffiths PD: The prognostic significance of positive CMV cultures during surveillance of renal transplant recipients. Transplantation 1993;56:103–108.

346. Pirsch J, Belzer F: Transmission of HCV by organ transplantation. N Engl J Med 1992;326:412.

347. Pittet D, Monod M, Suter PM, Frenk E, Auckenthaler R: Candida colonization and subsequent infections in critically ill surgical patients. Ann Surg 1994;220:751–758.

348. Plotkin SA, Drew WL, Felsenstein D, Hirsch MS: Sensitivity of clinical isolates of human cytomegalovirus to 9-(1,3-dihydroxy-2-propoxymethl) guanine. J Infect Dis 1985;152:833–834.

349. Plotkin SA, Starr SE, Friedman HM, Brayman K, Harris S, Jackson S, Tustin NB, Grossman R, Dafoe D, Barker C: Effect of Towne live virus vaccine on cytomegalovirus disease after renal transplant. Ann Intern Med 1991;114:525–531.

350. Poblete RB, Kirby BD: Cryptococcal peritonitis. Am J Med 1987;82:665–667.

351. Police MA, Henry M: Promising new treatments for cytomegalovirus retinitis. JAMA 1995;273:1457–1459.

352. Porter HJ, Quantrill AM, Fleming KA: B19 parvovirus infection of myocardial cells. Lancet 1988;1:535–536.

353. Portela D, Patel R, Larson-Keller J, Ilstrup DM, Wiesner RH, Steers JL, Krom RA, Paya CV: OKT3 treatment for allograft rejection is a risk factor for cytomegalovirus disease in liver transplantation. J Infect Dis 1995;171:1014–1018.

354. Preiksaitis JK, Cockfield SM: Epstein-Barr Virus and lymphoproliferative disorders after transplantation. In Bowden RA, Ljungman P, Paya CV (eds): Transplant Infections. Philadelphia: Lippincott-Raven Publishers, 1998, pp 245–263.

355. Pucci A, Ghisetti V, Donegani E, Barbio A, David E, Fortunato M, Papandrea C, Pansini S, Zattera G, di Summa M: Histologic and molecular diagnosis of myocardial human cytomegalovirus infection after heart transplantation. J Heart Lung Transplant 1994;13:1072–1080.

356. Quagliarello VJ, Scheld WM: Drug therapy: treatment of bacterial meningitis. N Engl J Med 1997;336:708–716.

357. Ragozzino MW, Melton LJ III, Kurland LT, Chu CP, Perry HO: Population based study of herpes zoster and its sequelae. Medicine (Baltimore) 1982;61:310–316.

358. Ramage JK, Hale A, Gane E, Cohen B, Boyle M, Mufti G, Williams R: Parvovirus B19-induced red cell aplasia treated with plasmapheresis and immunoglobulin. Lancet 1994;343:667–668.

359. Randall RE Jr, Stacy WK, Toone EC, Prout GR, Madge GE, Shadomy HJ, Shadomy S, Utz JP: Cryptococcal pyelonephritis. N Engl J Med 1968;279:60–65.

360. Ratnamohan VM, Chapman J, Howse H, Bovington K, Robertson P, Byth K, Allen R, Cunningham AL: Cytomegalovirus and human herpesvirus 6 both cause viral disease after renal transplantation. Transplantation 1998;66:877–882.

361. Reddy SC, Katz WE, Medich GE: Infective endocarditis of the pulmonary artery conduit in a recipient with heterotopic heart transplant: diagnosis by transesophageal echocardiography. J Heart Lung Transplant 1994;13:139–141.

362. Rees W, Schüler S, Hummel M, Hempel S, Möller J, Hetzer R: Primary cutaneous *Nocardia farcinica* infection after heart transplantation: a case report. J Thorac Cardiovasc Surg 1995;109: 181–183.

363. Reid KR, Menkis AH, Novick RJ, Pflugfelder PW, Kostuk WJ, Reid J, Whitby JL, Powell AM, McKenzie FN: Reduced incidence of severe infection after heart transplantation with low intensity immunosuppression. J Heart Lung Transplant 1991;10:894–900.

364. Rex JH, Larsen RA, Dismukes WE, Cloud GA, Bennett JE: Catastrophic visual loss due to Cryptococcus neoformans meningitis. Medicine (Baltimore) 1993;72:207–224.

365. Rex JH, Walsh TJ, Anaissie EA: Fungal infections in iatrogenically compromised hosts. Adv Intern Med 1998;43:321–371.

366. Rico MJ, Penneys NS: Cutaneous cryptococcosis resembling molluscum contagiosum in a patient with AIDS. Arch Dermatol 1985;121:901–902.

367. Ridgeway AL, Warner GS, Phillips P, Forshag MS, McGiffin DC, Harden JW, Harris RH, Benjamin WH, Zorn G, Dunlap NE: Transmission of *Mycobacterium tuberculosis* to recipients of single lung transplants from the same donor. Am J Respir Crit Care Med 1996;153:1166–1168.

368. Rinehart JJ, Balcerzak SP, Sagone AL, LoBuglio AF: Effects of corticosteroids on human onocyte function. J Clin Invest 1974; 54:1337–1343.

369. Rippon JW: Medical Mycology. The Pathogenic Fungi and the Pathogenic Actinomycetes. 3rd ed. Philadelphia: WB Saunders Company, 1988.

370. Rogers TR, Barnes RA: Prevention of airborne fungal infection in immunocompromised patients. J Hosp Infect 1988;11:15–20.

371. Rosen FS, Cooper MD, Wedgwood RJP: The primary immunodeficiencies. N Engl J Med 1984;311:300–310.

372. Rosen HR, Benner KG, Flora KD, Rabkin JM, Orloff SL, Olyaei A, Chou S: Development of ganciclovir resistance during treatment of primary cytomegalovirus infection after liver transplantation. Transplantation 1997;63:476–478.

373. Rostaing L, Izopet J, Sandres K, Cisterne JM, Puel J, Durand D: Changes in hepatitis C virus RNA viremia concentrations in long-term renal transplant patients after introduction of mycophenolate mofetil. Transplantation 2000;69:991–994.

374. Rubin RH: Infection in the organ transplant recipient. *In* Rubin R, Young L (eds): Clinical Approach to Infection in the Compromised Host. 3rd ed. New York: Plenum Medical Book Company, 1994, pp 629–705.

375. Rubin RH: Foreword. *In* Bowden RA, Ljungman P, Paya CV (eds): Transplant Infections. Philadelphia: Lippincott-Raven Publishers, 1998.

376. Rubin RH, Cosimi AB, Hirsch MS, Herrin JT, Russell PS, Tolkoff-Rubin NE: Effects of antithymocyte globulin on cytomegalovirus infection in renal transplant recipients. Transplantation 1981;31:143–145.

377. Rubin RH, Fishman JA: Infection in the organ transplant recipient. *In* Ginns LC, Cosimi B, Morris PJ (eds): Transplantation. Malden, MA: Blackwell Science, 1999, pp 747–769.

378. Rudin JE, Wing EJ: A comparative study of Legionella micdadei and other nosocomial acquired pneumonia. Chest 1984;86: 675–680.

379. Rüdlinger R, Smith IW, Bunney MH, Hunter JAA: Human papillomavirus infections in a group of renal transplant recipients. Br J Dermatol 1986;115:681–692.

380. Rutala PJ, Smith JW: Coccidioidomycosis in potentially compromised hosts: the effect of immunosuppressive therapy in dissemination. Am J Med Sci 1978;275:283–295.

381. Ryning FW, McLeod R, Maddox JC, Hunt S, Remington JS: Probable transmission of Toxoplasma gondii by organ transplantation. Ann Intern Med 1979;90:47–49.

382. Samuelson J: *In* Cotran RS, Kumar V, Collins T (eds): Robbins Pathologic Basis of Disease. 6th ed., Chapter 14. Philadelphia: WB Saunders Company, 1999.

383. Sarubbi FA, Kopf HB, Wilson MB, McGinnis MR, Rutala WA: Increased recovery of Aspergillus flavus from respiratory specimens during hospital construction. Am Rev Respir Dis 1982;125:33–38.

384. Sastry V, Brennan PJ, Levy MM, Fishman N, Friedman AL, Naji A, Barker CF, Brayman KL: Vancomycin-resistant enterococci: an emerging pathogen in immunosuppressed transplant recipients. Transplant Proc 1995;27:954–955.

385. Saulsbury FT, Winkelstein JA, Yolken RH: Chronic rotavirus infection in immunodeficiency. J Pediatr 1980;97:61–65.

386. Savage DC: Colonization by and survival of pathogenic bacteria on intestinal mucosal surfaces. *In* Britton G, Marschall KC (eds): Adsorption of Microorganisms to Surfaces. New York: John Wiley, 1980, pp 175–206.

387. Sayers MH, Anderson KC, Goodnough LT, Kurtz SR, Lane TA, Pisciotto P, Silberstein LE: Reducing the risk for transfusion-transmitted cytomegalovirus infections. Ann Intern Med 1992; 116:55–62.

388. Schowengerdt KO, Ni J, Denfield SW, Gajarski RJ, Bowles NE, Rosenthal G, Kearney DL, Price JK, Rogers BB, Schauer GM, Chinnock RE, Towbin JA: Association of parvovirus B19 genome in children with myocarditis and cardiac allograft rejection. Diagnosis using the polymerase chain reaction. Circulation 1997;96: 3549.

389. Schowengerdt KO, Ni J, Denfield SW, Gajarski RJ, Radovancevic B, Frazier OH, Demmler GJ, Kearney D, Bricker JT, Towbin JA: Diagnosis, surveillance and epidemiologic evaluation of viral infections in pediatric cardiac transplant recipients with use of polymerase chain reaction. J Heart Lung Transplant 1995;15: 111–123.

390. Schrier RD, Nelson JA, Oldstone MBA: Detection of human cytomegalovirus in peripheral blood lymphocytes in a natural infection. Science 1985;230:1048–1051.

391. Schwarz TF, Wiersbitzky S, Pambor M: Case report: detection of parvovirus B19 in a skin biopsy of a patient with erythema infectiosum. J Med Virol 1994;43:171–174.

392. Segovia J, Pulpón LA, Crespo MG, Daza R, Rodriguez JC, Rubio A, Serrano S, Carreno MC, Varela A, Aranguena R, Yebra M: *Rhodococcus equi:* first case in a heart transplant recipient. J Heart Lung Transplant 1994;13:332–335.

393. Shepherd FA, Maher E, Cardella C, Cole E, Greig P, Wade JA, Levy G: Treatment of Kaposi's sarcoma after solid organ transplantation. J Clin Oncol 1997;15:2371–2377.

394. Shepp DH, Dandliker PS, Meyers JD: Treatment of varicella zoster virus infection in severely immunocompromised patients: a randomized comparison of acyclovir and vidarabine. N Engl J Med 1986;314:208–212.

395. Shrader SK, Watts JC, Dancik JA, Band JD: Disseminated cryptococcosis presenting as cellulitis with necrotizing vasculitis. J Clin Microbiol 1986;24:860–862.

396. Sia IG, Wilson JA, Groettum CM, Espy MJ, Smith TF, Paya CV: Cytomegalovirus (CMV) DNA load predicts relapsing CMV infection after solid organ transplantation. J Infect Dis 2000;181: 717–720.

397. Siber GR, Schur PH, Aisenberg AC, Weitzman SA, Schiffman G: Correlation between serum IgG2-concentrations and the antibody response to bacterial polysaccharide antigens. N Engl J Med 1980;303:178–182.

398. Simmons BP, Gelfand MS, Roberts GD: Nocardia otitidiscaviarum (Caviae) infection in a heart transplant patient presented as having a thigh abscess (madura thigh). J Heart Lung Transplant 1992;11:824–826.

399. Simonds RJ, Holmberg SD, Hurwitz RL, Coleman TR, Bottenfield S, Conley LJ, Kohlenberg SH, Castro KG, Dahan BA, Schable CA, Rayfield MA, Rogers MF: Transmission of human immunodeficiency virus type 1 from a seronegative organ and tissue donor. N Engl J Med 1992;326:726–732.

400. Simpson GL, Stinson EB, Egger MJ, Remington JS: Nocardial infections in the immunocompromised host: a detailed study in a defined population. Rev Infect Dis 1981;3:492–507.

401. Singh N, Paterson DL, Chang FY, Gayowski T, Squier C, Wagner MM, Marino IR: Methicillin-resistant *Staphylococcus aureus:* the other emerging resistant gram-positive coccus among liver transplant recipients. Clin Infect Dis 2000;30:322–327.

402. Singh N, Yu VL, Mieles L, Wagener MM, Miner RC, Gayowski T: High-dose acyclovir compared with short-course preemptive ganciclovir therapy to prevent cytomegalovirus disease in liver transplant recipients. A randomized trial. Ann Intern Med 1994;120:375–327.

403. Sinnott JT, Cullison JP, Rogers K: Treatment of cytomegalovirus gastrointestinal ulceration in a heart transplant patient. J Heart Transplant 1987;6:186–188.

404. Slater AD, Ganzel BL, Keller M, Tobin GR II, Gray LA Jr: Repair of infected pseudoaneurysm with aortic arch replacement after orthotopic heart transplantation. J Heart Transplant 1990;9:230–235.

405. Smart FW, Naftel DC, Costanzo MR, Levine TB, Pelletier GB, Yancy CW, Hobbs RE, Kirklin JK, Bourge RC: Risk factors for early, cumulative, and fatal infections after heart transplantation: a multiinstitutional study. J Heart Lung Transplant 1996;15:329–341.

406. Smyth RL, Higenbottam TW, Scott JP, Stewart S, Fradet G, Wallwork J: Experience of cytomegalovirus infection in heart-lung transplant recipients. Am Rev Respir Dis 1990;141:A410.

407. Snydman DR, Werner BG, Heinze-Lacey B, Berardi VP, Tilney NL, Kirkman RL, Milford EL, Cho SI, Bush HL, Levey AS, Strom TB, Carpenter CB, Levey RH, Harmon WE, Zimmerman CE, Shapiro ME, Steinman T, LoGerfo F, Idelson B, Schroter GPJ, Levin MJ, McIver J, Leszczynski J, Grady GF: Use of cytomegalovirus immune globulin to prevent cytomegalovirus disease in renal-transplant recipients. N Engl J Med 1987;317:1049–1054.

408. Soderberg C, Larsson S, Bergstedt-Lindqvist S, Moller E: Definition of a subset of human peripheral blood mononuclear cells that are permissive to human cytomegalovirus infection. J Virol 1993;67:3166–3175.

409. Spees EK, Light JA, Oakes DD, Reinmuth B: Experiences with cadaver renal allograft contamination before transplantation. Br J Surg 1982;69:482–485.

410. Stagno S, Tinker MK, Elrod C, Fuccillo DA, Cloud G, O'Beirne AJ: Immunoglobulin M antibodies detected by enzyme-linked immunosorbent assay and radioimmunoassay in the diagnosis of cytomegalovirus infections in pregnant women and newborn infants. J Clin Microbiol 1985;21:930–935.

411. Stamm AM, Dismukes WE, Simmons BP, Cobbs CG, Elliott A, Budrich P, Harmon J: Listeriosis in renal transplant recipients: report of an outbreak and review of 102 cases. Rev Infect Dis 1982;4:665–682.

412. Stamm AM, Smith SH, Kirklin JK, McGiffin DC: Listerial myocarditis in cardiac transplantation. Rev Infect Dis 1990;12:820–823.

413. Standaert SM, Dummer JS: Other bacterial infections. In Bowden RA, Ljungman P, Paya CV (eds): Transplant Infections. Philadelphia: Lippincott-Raven Publishers, 1998, pp 203–214.

414. Steffenson DO, Dummer JS, Granick MS: Sternotomy infections with mycoplasma hominis. Ann Intern Med 1987;106:204–208.

415. Steinbach S, Sun L, Jiang RZ, Flume P, Gilligan P, Egan TM, Goldstein R: Transmissibility of Pseudomonas cepacia infection in clinic patients and lung-transplant recipients with cystic fibrosis. N Engl J Med 1994;331:981–987.

416. Stempel CA, Lake J, Kuo G, Vincenti F: Hepatitis C—its prevalence in end-stage renal failure patients and clinical course after kidney transplantation. Transplantation 1993;55:273–276.

417. Stewart MJ, Huwez F, Richens D, Naik S, Wheatley DJ: Infective endocarditis of the tricuspid valve in an orthotopic heart transplant recipient. J Heart Lung Transplant 1996;15:646–649.

418. Stinson EB, Bieber CP, Griepp RB, Clark DA, Shumway NE, Remington JS: Infectious complications after cardiac transplantation in man. Ann Intern Med 1971;74:22–23.

419. Stolf NA, Higushi L, Bocchi E, Bellotti G, Auler JO, Uip D, Amato Neto V, Pileggi F, Jatene AD: Heart transplantation in patients with Chagas' disease cardiomyopathy. J Heart Transplant 1987;6:307–312.

420. Studemeister AE, Kozak K, Garrity E, Venezio FR, Loyola University Cardiac Transplant Team: Survival of a heart transplant recipient after pulmonary cavitary mucormycosis. J Heart Transplant 1988;7:159–161.

421. Sturm I, Watschinger B, Geissler K, Guber SE, Popow-Kraupp T, Horl WH, Pohanka E: Chronic parvovirus B19 infection-associated pure red cell anemia in a kidney transplant recipient. Nephrol Dial Transplant 1996;11:1367–1370.

422. Sullivan MT, Williams AE, Fang CT, Grandinetti T, Polesz BJ, Ehrlich GD: Transmission of human T-lymphotropic virus types I and II by blood transfusion. Arch Intern Med 1991;151:2043–2048.

423. Swinnen LJ, Costanzo-Nordin MR, Fisher SG, O'Sullivan EJ, Johnson MR, Heroux AL, Dizikes GJ, Pifarre R, Fisher RI: Increased incidence of lymphoproliferative disorder after immunosuppression with the monoclonal antibody OKT3 in cardiactransplant recipients. N Engl J Med 1990;323:1723–1728.

424. Taege AJ: Listeriosis: recognizing it, treating it, preventing it. Cleve Clin J Med 1999;66:375–380.

425. Tamkun JW, Hynes RO: Plasma fibronectin is synthesized and secreted by hepatocytes. J Biol Chem 1983;258:4641–4647.

426. Tanabe K, Tokumoto T, Ishikawa N, Koyama I, Takahashi K, Fuchinoue S, Kawai T, Koga S, Yagisawa T, Toma H, Ota K, Nakajima H: Comparative study of cytomegalovirus (CMV) antigenemia assay, polymerase chain reaction, serology, and shell vial assay in the early diagnosis and monitoring of CMV infection after renal transplantation. Transplantation 1997;64:1721–1725.

427. Tazelaar HD, Yousem SA: The pathology of combined heartlung transplantation: an autopsy study. Hum Pathol 1988;19:1403–1416.

428. Terrault N, Holland C, Ferrell L, Hahn JA, Lake JR, Roberts JP, Ascher NL, Wright TL: Interferon alpha for recurrent hepatitis B infection after liver transplantation. Liver Transplant Surg 1996;2:132–135.

429. Thadepalli H, Chan WH, Maidman JE, Davidson EC Jr: Microflora of the cervix during normal labor and the puerperium. J Infect Dis 1978;137:568–572.

430. The TH, van der Ploeg M, van den Berg AP, Vlieger AM, van der Giessen M, van Son WJ: Direct detection of cytomegalovirus in peripheral blood leukocytes: a review of the antigenemia assay and polymerase chain reaction. Transplantation 1992;54:193–198.

431. Thomson D, Menkis A, Pflugfelder P, Kostuk W, Ahmad D, McKenzie FN: Mycotic aortic aneurysm after heart-lung transplantation. Transplantation 1989;47:195–197.

432. Tindall RSA, Rollins JA, Phillips JT, Greenlee RG, Wells L, Belendiuk G: Preliminary results of a double-blind, randomized, placebo-controlled trial of cyclosporine in myasthenia gravis. N Engl J Med 1987;316:719–724.

433. Toporoff B, Rosado LJ, Appleton CP, Sethi GK, Copeland JG: Successful treatment of early infective endocarditis and mediastinitis in a heart transplant recipient. J Heart Lung Transplant 1994;13:546–548.

434. Torok TJ: Parvovirus B19 and human disease. Adv Intern Med 1992;37:431–455.

435. Trento A, Dummer JS, Hardesty RL, Bahnson HT, Griffith BP: Mediastinitis following heart transplantation: incidence, treatment and results. Heart Transplant 1984;3:336–340.

436. Tuder RM, Weinberg A, Panajotopoulos N, Kalil J: Cytomegalovirus infection amplifies class I major histocompatibility complex expression on cultured human endothelial cells. J Heart Lung Transplant 1994;13:129–138.

437. Turik MA, Markowitz SM: A successful regimen for the prevention of seroconversion after transplantation of a heart positive for hepatitis B surface antigen. J Heart Lung Transplant 1992;11:781–783.

438. Turkmen A, Sever MS, Ecder T, Yildiz A, Aydin AE, Erkoc R, Eraksoy H, Eldegez U, Ark E: Posttransplant malaria. Transplantation 1996;62:1521–1523.

439. Tyrrell DLJ, Mitchell MC, DeMan RA, Schalm SW, Main J, Thomas HC, Fevery K, Nevens F, Beranek P, Vicary C: Phase II trial of lamivudine for chronic hepatitis B. Hepatology 1993;18:112A.

440. Uemura N, Ozawa K, Tani K, Nishikawa M, Inoue S, Nagao T, Uchida H, Matsunaga Y, Asano S: Pure red cell aplasia caused by parvovirus B19 infection in a renal transplant recipient [letter]. Eur J Haematol 1995;54:68–69.

441. Ustinov JA, Loginov RJ, Bruggeman CA, van der Meide PH, Häyry PJ, Lautenschlager IT: Cytomegalovirus induces class II expression in rat heart endothelial cells. J Heart Lung Transplant 1993;12:644–651.

442. Valantine HA: Prevention and treatment of cytomegalovirus disease in thoracic organ transplant patients: evidence for a beneficial effect of hyperimmune globulin. Transplant Proc 1995;27:49–57.

443. Valantine HA, Luikart H, Doyle RL, Theodore J, Hunt SA, Robbins RC, Reitz BA: CMVIG favorably affects long-term outcome after heart, heart-lung and lung transplantation. J Heart Lung Transplant 1999;18:193.

444. Valantine-von Kaeppler HA, Poirier CD, Doyle R, Theodore J, Woodley S, Luikart H, Hunt SA, Stinson EB, Reitz BA: CMV hyperimmune globulin and ganciclovir is more effective than ganciclovir alone for CMV prophylaxis after cardiothoracic transplantation. Circulation 1997;96:350.

445. van der Bij W, van Son WJ, van den Berg APM, Tegzess AM, Torensma R, The TH: Cytomegalovirus (CMV) antigenemia: rapid diagnosis and relationship with CMV-associated clinical syndromes in renal allograft recipients. Transplant Proc 1989;21:2061–2064.

446. van der Meer JWM: Defects in host defense mechanisms. In Rubin R, Young L (eds): Clinical Approach to Infection in the Compromised Host. 3rd ed. New York: Plenum Medical Book Company, 1994.

447. van der Waay D, Berghuis-de Vries JM, Lekkerkerk-van der Wees JEC: Colonization resistance of the digestive tract and the spread of bacteria to the lymphatic organs in mice. J Hyg (Cambridge) 1972;70:335–342.

448. Van Etta LL, Filice GS, Ferguson RM, Gerding DN: Corynebacterium equi: a review of twelve cases of human infection. Rev Infect Dis 1983;5:1012–1018.

449. Vartivarian SE, Coudron PE, Markowitz SM: Disseminated coccidioidomycosis. Unusual manifestations in a cardiac transplantation patient. Am J Med 1987;83:949–52.

450. Verra F, Hmouda H, Rauss A, Lebargy F, Cordonnier C, Bignon J, Lemaire F, Brochard L: Bronchoalveolar lavage in immunocompromised patients: clinical and functional consequences. Chest 1992;101:1215–1220.

451. von Eiff M, Roos N, Schulten R, Hesse M, Zuhlsdorf M, van de Loo J: Pulmonary aspergillosis: early diagnosis improves survival. Respiration 1995;62:341–347.

452. Wachs ME, Amend WJ, Ascher NL, Bretan PN, Emond J, Lake JR, Melzer JS, Roberts JP, Tomlanovich SJ, Vincenti F, Stock P: The risk of transmission of hepatitis B from HBsAg(−), HBcAb(+), HBIgM(−) organ donors. Transplantation 1995;59:230–234.

453. Wade JJ, Rolando N, Hayllar K, Philpott-Howard J, Casewell MW, Williams R: Bacterial and fungal infections after liver transplantation: an analysis of 284 patients. Hepatology 1995;21:1328–1336.

454. Wadowsky RM, Yee RB, Mezmar L, Wing EJ, Dowling JN: Hot water systems as sources of Legionella pneumophila in hospital and nonhospital plumbing fixtures. Appl Environ Microbiol 1982;43:1104–1110.

455. Wagner FM, Reichenspurner H, Überfuhr P, Weiss M, Fingerle V, Reichart B: Toxoplasmosis after heart transplantation: diagnosis by endomyocardial biopsy. J Heart Lung Transplant 1994;13:916–918.

456. Walker RC: Gram-negative infections. In Bowden RA, Ljungman P, Paya CV (eds): Transplant Infections. Philadelphia: Lippincott-Raven Publishers, 1998, pp 181–194.

457. Walker RG, d'Apice AJF, Mathew TH, Jacob C, Hardie IR, Menzies BO, Miach PJ: Long-term follow-up of a prospective trial of low-dose versus high-dose steroids in cadaveric renal transplantation. Transplant Proc 1987;19:2825–2828.

458. Walsh TJ: Trichosporonosis. Infect Dis Clin North Am 1989;3:43–53.

459. Walsh TJ, Dixon DM: Nosocomial aspergillosis: environmental microbiology, hospital epidemiology, diagnosis and treatment. Eur J Epidemiol 1989;5:131–142.

460. Walsh TJ, Hier DB, Caplan LR: Aspergillosis of the central nervous system: clinicopathological analysis of 17 patients. Ann Neurol 1985;18:574–582.

461. Walsh TR, Guttendorf J, Dummer S, Hardesty RL, Armitage JM, Kormos RL, Griffith BP: The value of protective isolation procedures in cardiac allograft recipients. Ann Thorac Surg 1989;47:539–545.

462. Waser M, Leonardi L, Mohacsi P, Laske A, Turina M, Gallino A: Toxoplasmosis in the heart transplant patient. Ther Umsch 1990;47:152–156.

463. Weber TR, Freier DT, Turcotte JG: Transplantation of infected kidneys. Transplantation 1979;27:63–65.

464. Wedemeyer H, Pethig K, Wagner D, Flemming P, Oppelt P, Petzold DR, Haverich A, Manns MP, Boeker KHW: Long-term outcome of chronic hepatitis B in heart transplant recipients. Transplantation 1998;66:1347–1353.

465. Wendt CH, Fox JMK, Hertz MI: Paramyxovirus infection in lung transplant recipients. J Heart Lung Transplant 1995;14:479–485.

466. Wendt CH, Weisdorf DJ, Jordan MC, Balfour HH Jr, Hertz MI: Parainfluenza virus respiratory infection after bone marrow transplantation. N Engl J Med 1992;326:921–926.

467. Wheat LJ, Batteiger BE, Sathapatayavongs B: Histoplasma capsulatum infections of the central nervous system. A clinical review. Medicine 1990;69:244–260.

468. Wheat LJ, Connolly-Stringfield PO, Kohler RB, Frame PT, Gupta MR: Histoplasma capsulatum polysaccharide antigen detection in diagnosis and management of disseminated histoplasmosis in patients with acquired immunodeficiency syndrome. Am J Med 1989;87:396–400.

469. Wheat LJ, Connolly-Stringfield P, Williams B, Connolly K, Blair R, Bartlett M, Durkin M: Diagnosis of histoplasmosis in patients with the acquired immunodeficiency syndrome by detection of Histoplasma capsulatum polysaccharide antigen in bronchoalveolar lavage fluid. Am Rev Respir Dis 1992;145:1421–1424.

470. Wheat LJ, Kohler RB, French MLV, Garten M, Kleiman M, Zimmerman SE, Schlech W, Ho J, White A, Brahmi Z: Immunoglobulin M and G histoplasmal antibody response in histoplasmosis. Am Rev Respir Dis 1983;128:65–70.

471. Wheat LJ, Kohler RB, Tewari RP: Diagnosis of disseminated histoplasmosis by detection of Histoplasma capsulatum antigen in serum and urine specimens. N Engl J Med 1986;314:83–88.

472. Wheat LJ, Smith EJ, Sathapatayavongs B, Batteiger B, Filo RS, Leapman SB, French MV: Histoplasmosis in renal allograft recipients: two large urban outbreaks. Arch Intern Med 1983;143:703–707.

473. Whimbey EE, Englund JA: Community respiratory virus infections in transplant recipients. In Bowden RA, Ljungman P, Paya CV (eds): Transplant Infections; Philadelphia: Lippincott Raven Publishers, 1994, pp 295–308.

474. Wicki J, Samii K, Cassinotti P, Voegeli J, Rochat T, Beris P: Parvovirus B19-induced red cell aplasia in solid-organ transplant recipients. Two case reports and review of the literature. Hematol Cell Ther 1997;39:199–204.

475. Wiener SL, Wiener R, Urivetzky M, Shafer S, Isenberg HD, Janov C, Meilman E: The mechanism of action of a single dose of methylprednisolone on acute inflammation in vivo. J Clin Invest 1975;56:679–689.

476. Wilkinson HW, Thacker WL, Benson RF, Polt SS, Brookings E, Mayberry WR, Brenner DJ, Gilley RG, Kirklin JK: Legionella birminghamensis species novum isolated from a cardiac transplant recipient. J Clin Microbiol 1987;25:2120–2122.

477. Wilson ML, Davis TE, Mirrett S, Reynolds J, Fuller D, Allen SD, Flint KK, Koontz F, Reller LB: Controlled comparison of the BACTEC high-blood-volume fungal medium, BACTEC plus 26 aerobic blood culture bottle and 10-milliliter isolator blood culture system for detection of fungemia and bacteremia. J Clin Microbiol 1993;31:865–871.

478. Wilson JP, Turner HR, Kirchner DA, Chapman SW: Nocardial infections in renal transplant recipients. Medicine 1989;68:38–57.

479. Winkelstein A: The effects of azathioprine and 6 MP on immunity [review]. J Immunol Pharmacol 1979;1:429–454.

480. Wreghitt TG, Gray JJ, Balfour AH: Problems with serological diagnosis of Toxoplasma gondii infections in heart transplant recipients. J Clin Pathol 1986;39:1135–1139.

481. Wreghitt TG, Hakim M, Gray JJ, Balfour AH, Stovin PGI, Stewart S, Scott J, English TAH, Wallwork J: Toxoplasmosis in heart and heart and lung transplant recipients. J Clin Pathol 1989;42:194–199.

482. Wright PF, Hatch MH, Kasselberg AG, Lowry SP, Wadlington WB, Karzon DT: Vaccine-associated poliomyelitis in a child with sex-linked agammaglobulinemia. J Pediatr 1977;91:408–412.

483. Young LS, Rubin RH: Introduction. In Rubin R, Young L (eds): Clinical Approach to Infection in the Compromised Host. 3rd ed. New York: Plenum Medical Book Company, 1994.

484. Young RC, Bennett JE, Vogel CL, Carbone PP, DeVita VT: Aspergillosis: the spectrum of the disease in 98 patients. Medicine 1970;49:147–173.

485. Younossi ZM, Braun WE, Protiva DA, Gifford RW, Straffon RA: Chronic viral hepatitis in renal transplant recipients with allografts functioning for more than 20 years. Transplantation 1999;67:272.

486. Zangwill SD, Hsu DT, Kichuk MR, Garvin JH, Stolar CJH, Haddad J, Stylianos S, Michler RE, Chadburn A, Knowles DM, Addonizio LJ: Incidence and outcome of primary Epstein-Barr virus infection and lymphoproliferative disease in pediatric heart transplant recipients. J Heart Lung Transplant 1998;17:1161–1166.

487. Zein NN, McGregor CGA, Wendt NK, Schwab K, Mitchell S, Persing DH, Rakela J: Prevalence and outcome of hepatitis C infection among heart transplant recipients. J Heart Lung Transplant 1995;14:865–869.

488. Zenati M, Milano A, Livi U, Cattelan A, Casarotto D: Successful treatment of disseminated infection with Listeria monocytogenes in a heart transplant recipient [letter]. J Heart Lung Transplant 1994;13:345–346.

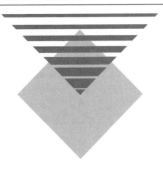

Long-Term Outcome After Heart Transplantation

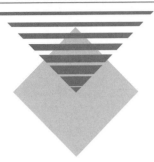

CHAPTER SIXTEEN

Survival After Heart Transplantation

with the collaboration of
DAVID C. NAFTEL, Ph.D. AND ROBERT N. BROWN, B.S., Ch.E.

Survival following orthotopic cardiac transplantation has seen tremendous improvement since the initial foray into heart transplantation in the late 1960s (see Chapter 1). This chapter will deal with the evolution of the changing outcomes and focus on survival, causes of death, and risk factors for mortality during the current era. This information is of critical importance, since survival is the ultimate yardstick for determining the long-term success of this therapy. After all, it is life expectancy which will be the primary determinant of the place of transplantation among other medical and surgical therapies for advanced heart failure. The ability to predict the short- and long-term outcome for individual patients (patient-specific predictions) (see Chapter 3) will play a fundamental role in matching therapies to specific patients. Of note, many survival analyses are considered in detail in other chapters. Survival after pediatric heart transplantation is discussed in detail in Chapter 20. Survival after combined heart/lung and heart/kidney transplantation is considered in Chapter 21. Survival after heterotopic transplantation is discussed in Chapter 10, and survival after cardiac retransplantation in Chapter 22. These specific areas will not be discussed in this chapter.

In the process of advancing knowledge and improving outcome after transplantation, considerable attention has been directed at determining **causes of death.** This carries major importance because numerous preventive, surveillance, and therapeutic opportunities are available to reduce the incidence of each major cause of death if targeted research investigates their risk factors, impact, and prevention at varying time periods after transplantation. The major cases of death after cardiac transplantation in the current era are depicted in Table 16–1. Our understanding of these causes of death and their risk factors is complicated by the close relationship between such things as rejection and infection (see Chapters 14 and 15), early graft failure and infections during the first few months after transplant (see Chapters 9 and 15), and recurrent rejection and subsequent malignancies (see Chapter 18) in leading to a fatal outcome. Thus, the assignment of a specific **cause of death** by physicians caring for the patient is nearly always somewhat subjective and should indicate the process which most directly produced the fatal outcome. It is recognized that the opinions of different physicians and other transplant experts may occasionally differ as to the underlying cause of death in a specific patient. The analysis of causes of death is further confounded by the number and variety of "other" causes of death (Table 16–2) in addition to those causes most commonly examined (graft failure, rejection, infection, allograft vasculopathy, and malignancy). These "other" causes of death account for approximately 30% of all posttransplant mortality.

The reader should note that some causes of death and risk factor analyses are also discussed in some detail in other chapters, such as cardiac allograft rejection (Chapter 14), allograft coronary artery disease (Chapter 17), recipient evaluation and selection (Chapter 6), and other long-term complications (Chapter 18). A major source of information for this chapter is derived from analyses from the 10-year experience of the Cardiac Transplant Research Database (CTRD), which includes 7,283 patients who underwent cardiac transplantation at 42 United States and Canadian transplant centers between 1990 and 2000.

The identification of **risk factors** deserves special comment. A major thrust of outcomes research in cardiac transplantation focuses on the identification of risk fac-

TABLE 16-1	Causes of Death After Cardiac Transplantation (CTRD: 1990-1999, N = 7, 283)									
	INTERVAL TO DEATH									
PRIMARY CAUSES OF GRAFT DEATH	<1 yr		1-3 yr		3-5 yr		5-10 yr		Total	
	N	%*	N	%	N	%	N	%	N	%
Early graft failure[1]	241	23%	0	0%	0	0%	0	0%	241	13%
Infection	257	24%	40	12%	11	6%	17	9%	325	18%
Rejection[2]	175	17%	49	14%	15	8%	5	3%	227	13%
Allograft CAD[3]	52	5%	78	22%	58	29%	52	27%	240	13%
Malignancy	27	3%	49	14%	49	25%	63	33%	188	11%
Other[4]	302	29%	133	38%	66	33%	56	29%	557	31%
Total	1054	100%	349	100%	199	100%	193	100%	1,795	100%
Unknown	42		31		9		17		99	
Total	1,096		380		208		210		1,894	

CTRD, Cardiac Transplant Research Database; CAD, coronary artery disease.
1. Death and retransplantation for early graft failure were both considered the same event. 2. Death and retransplantation for rejection were both considered the same event. 3. Death and retransplantation for allograft CAD were both considered the same event. 4. Other causes of death are listed in Table 16-2.
* Refers to % of total deaths during that time interval.
From Bourge RC, Naftel DC, Hill JA, Boehmer JP, Waggoner L, Kasper EK, Lee F, Czerska B, Thomas K, Kirklin JK: The emergence of co-morbid diseases impacting survival after cardiac transplantation: a ten year multi-institutional experience [abstract]. J Heart Lung Transplant 2001;20:167.

tors for specific events or outcomes before or after the procedure. The statistical basis of this process is extensively discussed in Chapter 3. It is of great importance to understand and acknowledge that analyses to identify risk factors for the various causes of death represent an attempt, based on rigorous clinical outcome studies, to uncover or approximate the **real factors** which contribute to the specific outcome. In a field such as heart transplantation, sufficient patient numbers for proper analysis nearly always, of necessity, requires multi-institutional data. In that process, despite the rigor of our efforts, true risk factors may be missed and inaccurate ones identified for a variety of reasons: proper data variables may not be collected in the study, patients with the risk factor in question may have been excluded from transplantation because of changing practice patterns (thereby eliminating the possibility of statistically "identifying" the risk factor), some variables may be closely related to or surrogates of the actual biological risk factor, and some spurious risk factors which defy common sense or existing knowledge may be identified

"by chance" in the analysis (see again Chapter 3). Thus, any such analysis of risk factors for causes of death must be viewed as an approximation of the **true** risk factors, the proximity to truth being a function of the number (sample size) and variety of patients analyzed, the selection of variables to be collected and analyzed, and the expertise, thoughtfulness, and interaction of the investigators performing the analysis.

CHANGING SURVIVAL OVER TIME

The evolution of cardiac transplantation from an experimental procedure to an accepted procedure to a highly successful therapy can be chronicled by the actuarial survival curves of different eras. After Christiaan Barnard's historic first transplant, and following the initial foray into and subsequent abandonment of cardiac transplantation by a number of centers, there was a small group of heart transplant units that continued this

TABLE 16-2	Causes of Death After Cardiac Transplantation (CTRD: 1990-1999, N = 7,283)									
	INTERVAL TO DEATH									
PRIMARY CAUSES OF DEATH: Category "Other"	<1 yr		1-3 yr		3-5 yr		5-10 yr		Total	
	N	%	N	%	N	%	N	%	N	%
Miscellaneous	111	11%*	25	7%	20	10%	15	8%	170	10%
Nonspecific cardiac death	50	5%	34	10%	10	5%	3	2%	98	6%
Neurologic	46	4%	12	3%	8	4%	8	4%	74	4%
Sudden cardiac death	35	3%	35	10%	17	8%	14	7%	101	6%
Multisystem failure	25	2%	7	2%	2	1%	6	3%	40	2%
Respiratory failure	16	2%	3	0.9%	4	2%	2	1%	25	1%
Pulmonary embolism	9	0.9%	8	2%	0	0%	2	1%	19	1%
Hepatic failure	6	0.6%	2	0.6%	1	0.5%	2	1%	11	0.6%
Renal failure	4	0.4%	6	0.2%	4	2%	4	2%	18	1%

CTRD, Cardiac Transplant Research Database.
* Refers to % of total deaths during that interval.
From Bourge RC, Naftel DC, Hill JA, Boehmer JP, Waggoner L, Kasper EK, Lee F, Czerska B, Thomas K, Kirklin JK: The emergence of co-morbid diseases impacting survival after cardiac transplantation: a ten year multi-institutional experience [abstract]. J Heart Lung Transplant 2001;20:167.

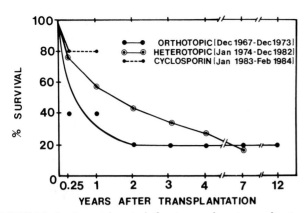

FIGURE **16–1.** Actuarial survival of patients undergoing cardiac transplantation at Groote Schuur Hospital, Cape Town: 1967–1983. (From Cooper DKC, Lanza RP: Heart Transplantation. Boston: Kluwer Academic Publishers, 1984.)

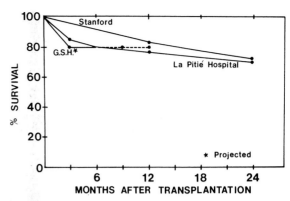

FIGURE **16–3.** Actuarial survival of patients undergoing cardiac transplantation using cyclosporine A immunosuppression at Stanford Medical Center, La Pitie Hospital (Paris) and Groote Schuur Hospital (Cape Town). (From Cooper DKC, Lanza RP: Heart Transplantation. Boston: Kluwer Academic Publishers, 1984.)

clinical experiment through the 1970s. The discouraging midterm survival following cardiac transplantation during the era of 1967 through 1973 is depicted in Figure 16–1, indicating an actuarial survival of approximately 30% at 1 year and 20% at 2 years following orthotopic cardiac transplantation. With the ongoing commitment of several institutions despite inadequate immunosuppressive agents, the 1-year survival increased to about 60% during the 1970s, as documented by the experience at Stanford, Cape Town, and LaPitie Hospital in Paris (Fig. 16–2).

It is generally acknowledged that the availability of cyclosporine provided the immunologic environment necessary for routine survival following cardiac transplantation. Prior to the cyclosporine era, cardiac transplantation was like ''Russian roulette'': approximately one third of the patients would die early from overwhelming rejection or infection (secondary to excessive immunosuppression with antithymoycyte globulin), about one third of the patients would do very well for the long term, and one third of the patients would struggle with recurrent early infection or rejection and survive for months or years with a generally poor quality of life. The improvement in survival following the introduction of cyclosporine is immediately apparent by examining early survival curves with cyclosporine therapy (Fig. 16–3). Undoubtedly, other factors played a role in this major increment in survival, including the introduction of endomyocardial biopsy for the diagnosis of rejection (1972) and many other advancements. The excitement about cyclosporine (after preliminary experimental trials) and the despair concerning the results with azathioprine and prednisone stimulated many programs (including the University of Alabama at Birmingham [UAB]) to temporarily discontinue transplantation for about 6 months until cyclosporine became commercially available.

Cyclosporine was initially utilized with prednisone in a two-drug maintenance immunosuppressive regimen,

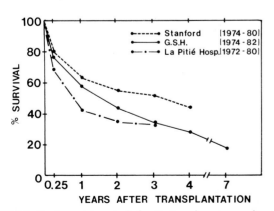

FIGURE **16–2.** Actuarial survival of patients undergoing cardiac transplantation using conventional immunosuppression at Stanford Medical Center, La Pitie Hospital (Paris) and Groote Schuur Hospital (Cape Town). (From Cooper DKC, Lanza RP: Heart Transplantation. Boston: Kluwer Academic Publishers, 1984.)

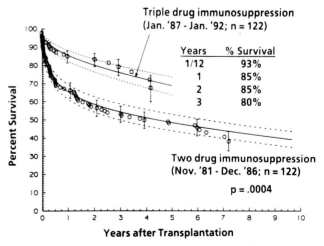

FIGURE **16–4.** Actuarial and parametric analyses of survival using azathioprine and steroids for immunosuppression (UAB, November 1981–1987, 122 patients) and when triple-drug immunosuppression including cyclosporine was used (UAB, 1987–December 1991, 121 patients). (From Kirklin JW, Barratt-Boyes BG: Cardiac Surgery. New York: Churchill Livingstone, 1992.)

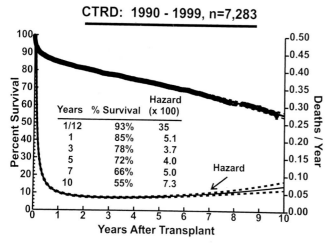

FIGURE 16-5. Actuarial and parametric survival (upper curve) and hazard function (lower curve) for patients undergoing primary cardiac transplantation in the Cardiac Transplant Research Database (CTRD) between 1990 and 1999 (n = 7,283).

but there was a further increment in survival when cyclosporine was utilized with both azathioprine and prednisone, as evidenced by the superb results at the University of Minnesota[4] with routine use of "triple - drug" immunosuppression (cyclosporine, prednisone, and azathioprine). This further increment in survival is reflected by actuarial survival curves at UAB during the decade of the 1980s, comparing two-drug immunosuppression with a triple-drug protocol (Fig. 16-4).[31] A similar trend toward improved survival during the decade of the 1990s compared to the 1980s is documented in the ISHLT Registry[20] and the United Network of Organ Sharing.[45]

During the decade of the 1990s, cardiac transplantation evolved into a well-developed and mature therapy with generally similar survival outcomes at experienced institutions. The practice of cardiac transplantation during this decade was characterized by increasing waiting times, an increasing proportion of recipients undergoing transplantation from an urgent status, longer donor ischemic times, and an increasing use of donors on pressor support.[39] Despite these changes, the 1-year survival improved or remained similar at most institutions.[25, 39] This is reflected by the experience of the CTRD in the United States, which gathered extensive outcome data from more than 40 experienced heart transplant centers. The overall early and mid-term survival of the CTRD over the past 10 years is displayed in Figure 16-5.[6]

OVERVIEW OF CAUSES OF DEATH

When evaluating the success of cardiac transplantation (and other surgical interventions), survival is typically measured in terms of short-term and long-term outcome. Although the great improvement in survival over the past 25 years has been most dramatic during the first 3 posttransplant months (with decreased death

from early graft failure, rejection, and infection), the standard benchmark for early success has been **1-year survival.** Until recently (when attention has increasingly focused on 3-year, 5-year, and even longer term survival) heart transplant programs world-wide were judged, to a great extent, by their 1-year survival rates. Thus, examination of causes of death during the first year takes on considerable importance. Also, the distribution of causes of death and their likelihood is quite different during the first year compared to later years. For example, early graft failure (during the first month), rejection, and infection account for over 60% of deaths during the first year (Table 16-1), whereas after the first year they account for less than 25% of primary causes of death. In their place, allograft coronary artery disease and malignancy become increasingly prominent causes of death (about 10% during the first year compared to nearly 50% after that). For these reasons, we will divide the discussion of causes of death and their risk factors into mortality during the first year and mortality after the first year.

It should be remembered that the time period for **early phase** risk factors is determined by the **hazard function** (instantaneous risk) analysis (see Chapter 3), but for convenience we will discuss those risk factors in the section on **first year mortality.** In contrast, **constant phase** risk factors exert their effect throughout the posttransplant period, and the time period for **late phase** risk factors is determined by the hazard function equations. These two phases will be discussed under the section **Mortality After the First Year.** The changing risk over time is reflected by the hazard function for each cause of death. The risk of death from early graft failure, rejection, infection, and neurological causes is greatest early after transplantation (Fig. 16-6)[6] and decreases rapidly

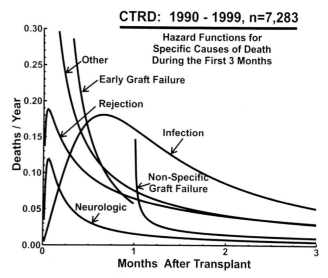

FIGURE 16-6. Hazard functions for specific causes of death during the first 3 months after primary cardiac transplantation in the CTRD, 1990-1999 (n = 7,283). (From Bourge RC, Naftel DC, Hill JA, Boehmer JP, Waggoner L, Kasper EK, Lee F, Czerska B, Thomas K, Kirklin JK: The emergence of co-morbid diseases impacting survival after cardiac transplantation: a ten year multi-institutional experience [abstract]. J Heart Lung Transplant 2001;20:167.)

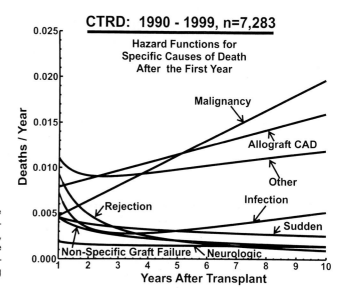

FIGURE **16-7.** Hazard functions for specific causes of death after the first year following primary cardiac transplantation in the CTRD, 1990–1999 (n = 7,283). (From Bourge RC, Naftel DC, Hill JA, Boehmer JP, Waggoner L, Kasper EK, Lee F, Czerska B, Thomas K, Kirklin JK: The emergence of co-morbid diseases impacting survival after cardiac transplantation: a ten year multi-institutional experience [abstract]. J Heart Lung Transplant 2001;20:167.)

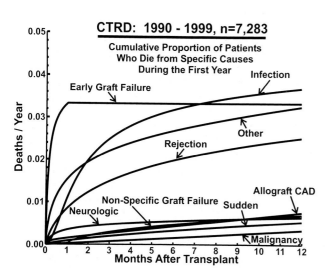

FIGURE **16-8.** Competing outcomes analysis of specific causes of death during the first year after transplantation in the CTRD. (From Young JB, Hauptman PJ, Naftel DC, Ewald G, Aaronson K, Dec GW, Taylor DO, Higgins R, Platt L, Kirklin JK: Determinants of early graft failure following cardiac transplantation, a 10 year multi-institutional, multi-variable analysis [abstract]. J Heart Lung Transplant 2001;20:212.)

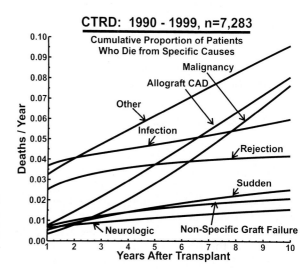

FIGURE **16-9.** Competing outcomes analysis of specific causes of death during the first 10 years after transplantation (CTRD). (From Costanzo MR, Eisen HJ, Brown RN, Mehra M, Benza RL, Torre G, Yancy CW, Davis S, McCloud M, Kirklin JK: Are there specific risk factors for fatal allograft vasculopathy? An analysis of over 7,000 cardiac transplant patients [abstract]. J Heart Lung Transplant 2001;20:152.)

TABLE 16-3	Annual Probabilities of Death Due to Specific Causes (CTRD: 1990–1999, N = 7,283)										
	PROBABILITY (%) OF DEATH DURING THE YEAR IF ALIVE AT THE BEGINNING OF THE YEAR										ENTIRE 10 YR
CAUSE OF DEATH	1	2	3	4	5	6	7	8	9	10	
Early graft failure	3.3	0	0	0	0	0	0	0	0	0	3.3
Rejection	2.5	0.6	0.4	0.3	0.2	0.2	0.1	0.1	0.1	0.1	4.2
Infection	3.7	0.5	0.3	0.3	0.3	0.3	0.4	0.4	0.4	0.5	6.0
Allograft CAD	0.8	0.8	0.9	1.0	1.1	1.2	1.3	1.3	1.4	1.5	8.1
Malignancy	0.3	0.5	0.7	0.8	1.0	1.1	1.4	1.5	1.7	1.8	7.7
Nonspecific graft failure	0.7	0.3	0.3	0.2	0.2	0.2	0.2	0.2	0.1	0.1	2.1
Neurologic	0.7	0.2	0.1	0.1	0.1	0.1	0.1	0.1	0.1	0.1	1.6
Sudden cardiac death	0.5	0.4	0.3	0.3	0.3	0.3	0.3	0.3	0.3	0.3	2.5
Other	3.2	0.9	0.9	0.9	0.9	1.0	1.0	1.0	1.1	1.1	9.6
Total	15.7	4.2	3.9	3.9	4.1	4.4	4.8	4.9	5.2	5.5	45.1

CAD, coronary artery disease.

over the ensuing months. The major late causes of death, allograft coronary artery disease and malignancy, have a gradually increasing risk over time, as indicated by the hazard function in Figure 16–7.[6]

The cumulative impact of each cause of death is best illustrated in a **competing outcomes depiction** (see again Chapter 3). Figure 16–8 depicts the cumulative proportion of patients dying from the most common causes of death during the first year.[47] Once again, we see the major impact of early graft failure, rejection, and infection as causes of death during the first year. The progressive impact of allograft coronary artery disease and malignancy as causes of death in later years is evident from the competing outcomes depiction after the first year (Fig. 16–9).[8] The total mortality at any time after transplant is the sum of the individual cause-of-death curves (Figs. 16–8 and 16–9). Using the same competing outcomes methods, the actual probability of death from the various causes during any given time interval is shown in Table 16–3.

Subsequent sections will discuss risk factors for overall and specific causes of death during early and later time periods after cardiac transplantation. Although many single and multi-institutional studies have examined predictive factors for death, the most detailed analysis to date of these risk factors comes from a 10-year multi-institution analysis from the CTRD. Table 16–4 summarizes the risk factors identified for the major causes of death.[6]

MORTALITY DURING THE FIRST YEAR

DEATH FROM ALL CAUSES

Impact

In the current era, the 1-month, 3-month and 1-year survival in experienced heart transplant centers is reflected in the CTRD experience between 1990 and 2000 (Fig. 16–5). The accompanying hazard function indicates that the risk is highest early after transplant and rapidly falls thereafter, merging with a constant hazard at about 1 year. A slowly increasing late hazard (risk)

is evident after about 7 years. The major causes of death during the first year are listed in Table 16–1 and are discussed below.

Risk Factors

The comprehensive risk factor analysis by the CTRD reflects our current understanding of those factors which are predictive of mortality (Table 16–5). There are some additional risk factors which were not identified in this analysis, such as a positive prospective, cytotoxic crossmatch (see Chapter 7). However, this and certain other risk factors do not appear by multivariable analyses because either no or very few patients (or donors) with these risk factors are selected for transplantation, thereby eliminating the possibility of detecting them by statistical analysis (see Chapter 3). An earlier multi-institution analysis identified similar pretransplant risk factors for mortality.[5]

A few of the risk factors will be illustrated by nomograms from the multivariable analysis. The interaction between **longer ischemic time, older donor age,** and **recipient ventilator support** is depicted in Figure 16–10.[47] When considering all causes of death, it is important to remember, as shown in this depiction, that the deleterious effects of older donor age (in this case, 50 years of age) and/or very prolonged ischemic times are particularly pronounced in patients who are already debilitated and critically ill (indicated by ventilator support).

Figure 16–11 illustrates an interesting finding in this 10-year study regarding the **duration of ventricular assist device (VAD) support.** Patients who underwent transplantation after a very short period (< 14 days) of VAD support had a worse outcome than those who were supported for longer periods. The two abbreviated curves to the left of the nomogram, indicating support time of less than 14 days, revealed a higher risk for the same ischemic time than when devices were left in place for longer periods. It is now widely appreciated that a major value of ventricular assist devices is to allow reversibly injured noncardiac organs to recover normal function before proceeding with cardiac transplantation (see Chapter 8). This invariably takes at least 14–30 days, and the identification of very short VAD times as a

TABLE 16-4   Risk Factors for Death (CTRD: 1990–1999, N = 7,283)

RISK FACTOR	Overall	EGF	Infection	Rejection	CAD	Malignancy
				p VALUE		
RECIPIENT						
Older age	.008		<.0001			<.0001
Younger age	.0002			<.0001	<.0001	.003
White male						.0003
Black	<.0001			<.0001	<.0001	
Hispanic				.03		
Obese	.005		.0003	<.0001		
Cachectic	.01		.0008			
Congenital etiology	.002	.0003				
Noncongenital etiology	.03					
Ischemic etiology					.0001	
Insulin-dependent diabetes	.0004					
Any diabetes			.03			
Pulmonary disease	.03		.02			
Peripheral vascular disease	.03					
Herpes-negative	.03			.01		
Cigarette use within 6 mo	.0005				.01	.003
Any cigarette use			.04			
Gout					.001	
Cocaine use	.003	.02				
Lower creatinine clearence at listing	.0006		.0004			
Higher serum creatinine at transplant	<.0001	.0005	.0001			
PAs-PCWP	.0005	.005		.03		
Mean RAP	.01	.02	.02			
PRA > 10	<.0001	.005				.005
Previous sternotomy	<.0001	.0002	.002			
> 1 previous sternotomy	.03	.03				
Ventilator	<.0001	<.0001	.008			
IABP	.01		.03			
VAD, 14 days or less	.005		.0008			
Days on VAD	.04	.01				
Earlier date of transplant	<.0001			<.0001	<.0001	
DONOR						
Older donor age	<.0001	<.0001	<.0001	.001	<.0001	
Female	.0001					
Male	.03					
Hepatitis C positive				.02		
Abnormal echo	.01	.03				
Diabetes	.01	.02				
CMV positive					.04	
Longer ischemic time	<.0001	.0001	<.0001			
MISMATCH						
Recipient BMI-donor BMI (higher)	.004	.02				
CMV-negative recipient, CMV-positive donor				.008		
Total HLA mismatch (4–6)				.009		

EGF, early graft failure; CAD, coronary artery disease; PAs, pulmonary artery systolic pressure; PCWP, mean pulmonary capillary wedge pressure; RAP, right atrial pressure; PRA, panel reative antibody; IABP, intra-aortic balloon pump; VAD, ventricular assist device; CMV, cytomegalovirus; BMI, body mass index; HLA, human leukocyte antigen.
From Bourge RC, Naftel DC, Hill JA, Boehmer JP, Waggoner L, Kasper EK, Lee F, Czerska B, Thomas K, Kirklin JK: The emergence of co-morbid diseases impacting survival after cardiac transplantation: a ten year multi-institutional experience [abstract]. J Heart Lung Transplant 2001;20:167.

TABLE 16-5   Risk Factors for Death (Any Cause) (CTRD: 1990–1999, N = 7,283)

RISK FACTOR	EARLY PHASE		CONSTANT PHASE		LATE PHASE	
	Relative Risk	p Value	Relative Risk	p Value	Relative Risk	p Value
RECIPIENT						
Older age[1]	1.13	.008	1.41	.008		
Younger age[2]			1.94	.0002		
Black			2.02	<.0001		
Obese recipient[3]	2.35	.005				
Cachectic recipient[4]	2.5	.01				
Congenital etiology	1.89	.002				
Noncongenital etiology			3.76	.03		
Insulin-dependent diabetes			1.66	.0004		
Pulmonary disease	1.35	.03				
Peripheral vascular disease					11.3	.03
Herpes-negative	1.29	.03				
Cigarette use within 6 mo			1.49	.0005		
Cocaine use			3	.003		
Lower creatinine clearance at listing[5]	1.28	.0006				
Higher serum creatinine at transplant[6]	1.43	<.0001	1.23	.01		
PAs-PCWP[7]	1.4	.0005				
Mean RAP[8]	1.22	.01				
PRA > 10	1.71	<.0001				
Previous sternotomy	1.44	<.0001				
>1 previous sternotomy	1.77	.03				
Ventilator	2.18	<.0001				
IABP	1.36	.01				
VAD, 14 days or less	1.86	.005				
Days on VAD[9]	1.29	.04				
Earlier date of transplant[10]			1.91	<.0001		
DONOR						
Older donor age[11]	1.24	<.0001	1.23	<.0001		
Female	1.36	.0001				
Male			1.23	.03		
Abnormal echo	1.7	.01				
Diabetes			2.06	.01		
Longer ischemic time[12]	1.7	<.0001				
MISMATCH						
Recipient BMI–donor BMI (smaller donor, larger recipient)[13]	1.49	.004				

PAs, pulmonary artery systolic pressure; PCWP, mean pulmonary capillary wedge pressure; RAP, right atrial pressure; PRA, panel reactive antibody; IABP, intra-aortic balloon pump; VAD, ventricular assist device; BMI, body mass index.
1. Relative risk compares age 50–60. 2. Relative risk compares age 30–20. 3. Relative risk compares body mass index of 25–30. 4. Relative risk compares body mass index of 25–15. 5. Relative risk compares creatine clearance of 100–50. 6. Relative risk compares serum creatinine of 1.0–2.0. 7. Relative risk compares systolic pulmonary gradient of 15–40. 8. Relative risk compares right atrial pressure of 5–20. 9. Relative risk compares days on VAD of 30–180. 10. Relative risk compares transplant year of 1999–1992. 11. Relative risk compares donor age of 25–40. 12. Relative risk compares ischemic time of 180–300 minutes. 13. Relative risk compares BMI difference of 10–20.
From Bourge RC, Naftel DC, Hill JA, Boehmer JP, Waggoner L, Kasper EK, Lee F, Czerska B, Thomas K, Kirklin JK: The emergence of co-morbid diseases impacting survival after cardiac transplantation: a ten year multi-institutional experience [abstract]. J Heart Lung Transplant 2001;20:167.

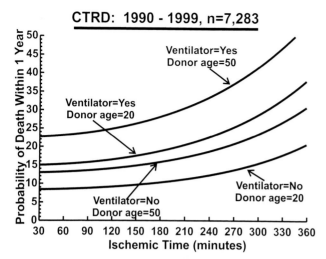

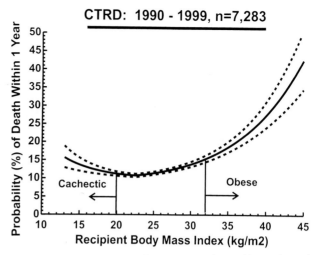

FIGURE **16–10.** Nomogram from CTRD multivariable analysis depicting the effect of recipient ventilator support, donor age, and ischemic time on death during first year. Other significant risk factors (see Table 15–5) are set at their mean value. (From Young JB, Hauptman PJ, Naftel DC, Ewald G, Aaronson K, Dec GW, Taylor DO, Higgins R, Platt L, Kirklin JK: Determinants of early graft failure following cardiac transplantation, a 10 year multi-institutional, multi-variable analysis [abstract]. J Heart Lung Transplant 2001;20:212.)

FIGURE **16–12.** Nomogram from CTRD multivariable analysis depicting the effect of recipient body mass index on death within 1 year.

risk factor for poorer outcome (see again Table 16–5) supports this notion. On the other hand, extremely long duration of VAD support appears to gradually increase the risk of transplantation (Table 16–5 and Fig. 16–11), perhaps due to an increased risk of VAD complications over time.

Marked **obesity** and, to a lesser extent **cachexia,** are also risk factors for death (Fig. 16–12). Marked obesity has a particularly adverse affect, which supports the policy of, whenever possible, requiring weight reduction in very obese heart failure patients prior to listing. Similar conclusions were reached in a study by Grady

and colleagues,[17] in which male patients whose weight was greater than 140% of ideal body weight had significantly worse early and intermediate term survival (Fig. 16–13).

It is widely appreciated that preexisting **renal dysfunction** importantly increases the risk of transplantation unless combined heart and kidney transplantation is performed (see Chapter 21). In addition to the possibility of dialysis with prolonged instrumentation and the potential for infection, depressed renal reserves forces a prolonged delay in achieving therapeutic cyclosporine levels during the critical first weeks after transplantation, and this likely increases the chance of troublesome rejection. Furthermore, maintenance of a euvolemic state is hampered by reduced urine output, increasing the

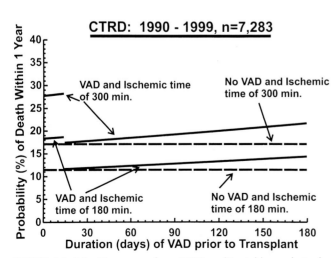

FIGURE **16–11.** Nomogram from CTRD multivariable analysis depicting the effect of ventricular assist device (VAD) use, VAD duration, and ischemic time on death in first year.

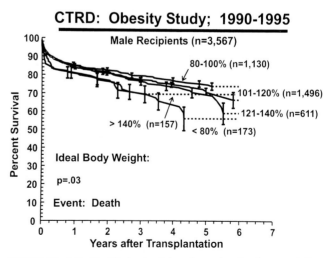

FIGURE **16–13.** Stratified actuarial analyses showing the association between percent ideal body weight and survival after heart transplant in males. (From Grady KL, White-Williams C, Naftel DC, Costanzo M, Pitts D, Rayburn B, VanBakel A, Jaski B, Bourge RC: Are preoperative obesity and cachexia risk factors for post heart transplant morbidity and mortality: a multi-institutional study of preoperative weight-height indices. J Heart Lung Transplant 1999;18:763.)

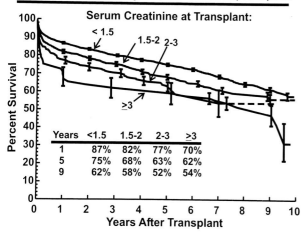

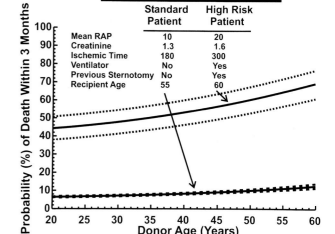

FIGURE **16–14.** Actuarial survival in CTRD stratified by creatinine at transplant. (From Bourge RC, Naftel DC, Hill JA, Boehmer JP, Waggoner L, Kasper EK, Lee F, Czerska B, Thomas K, Kirklin JK: The emergence of co-morbid diseases impacting survival after cardiac transplantation: a ten year multi-institutional experience [abstract]. J Heart Lung Transplant 2001;20:167.)

FIGURE **16–16.** Nomogram (with 70% confidence intervals) from CTRD multivariable analysis contrasting a standard versus high-risk patient profile.

likelihood of high filling pressures. The sequelae of these interrelated developments combine to decrease the overall reserves of the patient in the event of important early graft dysfunction, infection, or rejection. The risk-unadjusted impact of a higher serum creatinine in transplantation is depicted in Figure 16–14 and by nomogram in Figure 16–15.[6] Currently, few transplant centers would proceed with transplantation in the face of a creatinine exceeding 2.5 unless combined heart and kidney transplant was planned.

The impact of **transplant center volume** as a risk factor for survival has been contentious. However, multi-institutional data from the International Society for Heart and Lung Transplantation (ISHLT) Registry has consistently identified low center volume (< about 10 heart transplants per year) as a predictor of 1-year[20, 22, 23] and 5-year mortality.[20]

From the 10-year CTRD experience, combinations of risk factors which generate unacceptably high risk can be examined. Figure 16–16 illustrates the very high risk when a debilitated recipient with previous surgery who is ventilator dependent receives a suboptimal donor heart with very prolonged ischemic time.[6]

DEATH FROM EARLY GRAFT FAILURE

Impact

The importance of early graft failure is evident from Table 16–1, which indicates that it is the most common cause of death during the first 3 months after transplant. However, the actual mortality from acute graft failure during the 10-year CTRD experience was only 2.7%,[47] indicating that donor selection and methods of myocardial preservation (see Chapter 9) have been generally effective during the past decade (see Chapter 9). Of note, however, is the finding that fatal graft failure has **not decreased** in frequency over the past decade, supporting the belief that we await major breakthroughs in donor heart preservation to further decrease the incidence of this event.

Risk Factors

The major risk factors for early graft failure are reflected in both donor and recipient characteristics (Table 16–6). Risk factors for early graft failure undoubtedly relate

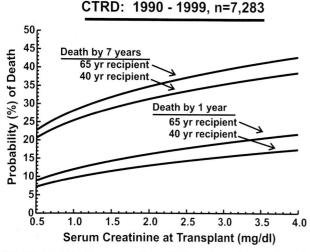

FIGURE **16–15.** Nomogram from CTRD multivariable analysis depicting the effect of serum creatinine and recipient age on death by 1 and 7 years after transplant. (From Bourge RC, Naftel DC, Hill JA, Boehmer JP, Waggoner L, Kasper EK, Lee F, Czerska B, Thomas K, Kirklin JK: The emergence of co-morbid diseases impacting survival after cardiac transplantation: a ten year multi-institutional experience [abstract]. J Heart Lung Transplant 2001;20:167.)

TABLE 16-6	Risk Factors for Early Graft Failure (CTRD: 1990-1999, N = 7,283)		

| | EARLY PHASE | | |
RISK FACTOR	Relative Risk	p Value
RECIPIENT		
Congenital etiology	2.66	.0003
Higher serum creatinine at transplant*	1.49	.0005
PAs-PCWP*	1.61	.005
Mean RAP*	1.39	.02
PRA > 10	1.78	.005
Previous sternotomy	1.79	.0002
>1 previous sternotomy	2.59	.03
Ventilator	3.13	<.0001
Days on VAD*	1.6	.01
DONOR		
Older donor age*	1.51	<.0001
Abnormal echo	1.59	.03
Diabetes	2.17	.02
Longer ischemic time*	1.63	.0001
MISMATCH		
Recipient BMI–donor BMI (smaller donor, larger recipient)*	1.54	.02

PAs, pulmonary artery systolic pressure; PCWP, mean pulmonary capillary wedge pressure; RAP, right atrial pressure; PRA, panel reactive antibody; VAD, ventricular assist device; BMI, body mass index (kilograms per meters of height).
* See Table 16–5 for relative risk comparisons.
From Young JB, Hauptman PJ, Naftel DC, Ewald G, Aaronson K, Dec GW, Taylor DO, Higgins R, Platt L, Kirklin JK: Determinants of early graft failure following cardiac transplantation, a 10 year multi-institutional, multi-variable analysis [abstract]. J Heart Lung Transplant 2001;20:212.

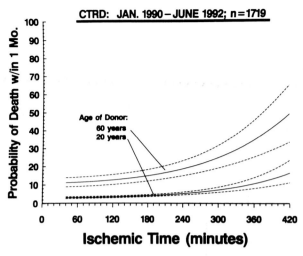

FIGURE 16-17. Nomogram from CTRD multivariable analysis depicting varying ischemic time for two donors, aged 20 and 60 years. Equation is solved for 50-year-old male recipient who is not on ventilator, not on ventricular assist device, has not undergone previous sternotomy, and has pulmonary vascular resistance of 2.2 Wood units; and male donor who is not diabetic, not receiving inotropic support, did not die of cardiac arrest, and has no diffuse wall motion abnormalities. Dashed lines represent 70% confidence limits around parametric curves. (From Young JB, Naftel DC, Bourge RC, Kirklin JK, Clemson BS, Porter CB, Rodeheffer RJ, Kenzora JL: Matching the heart donor and heart transplant recipient. Clues for successful expansion of the donor pool: a multivariable, multiinstitutional report. J Heart Lung Transplant 1994;13:365.)

myocardial function or reduced peripheral vascular resistance, in which case high-dose inotropic support may induce subendocardial ischemia and potential necrosis (see Chapter 9). In the study by Young and colleagues, increasing inotropic support, particularly dopamine or

to conditions in the donor which decrease myocardial reserves and conditions in the recipient which provide increased stress to the newly transplanted heart. Many of these risk factors are intimately interrelated, and these relationships can often be depicted to examine the magnitude of these risk interactions.

Many studies have demonstrated an increased risk of early death with prolonged **donor ischemic time.** A multi-institutional analysis by Young and colleagues indicated by multivariable analysis that longer ischemic times represents a risk factor for hospital mortality, particularly with older donor age (Fig. 16–17).[48] Other studies[5] have also suggested that, with current methods of heart preservation (see Chapter 9), the risk of prolonged ischemic time becomes most evident after about 5 hours. It should be appreciated that the accurate interpretation of longer ischemic time as a risk factor is confounded by the fact that long ischemic time may occasionally be a surrogate for situations such as long distance procurement in a desperate situation, unusually complex recipient reoperations, and other situations which are not readily amenable to analysis.

Extensive clinical experience indicates that **high doses of donor inotropic support** indicate either depressed

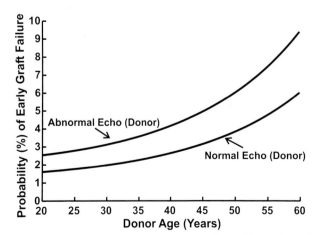

FIGURE 16-18. Nomogram from CTRD multivariable analysis depicting the effect of donor age and left ventricular function by echocardiography (echo) on fatal early graft failure. (From Young JB, Hauptman PJ, Naftel DC, Ewald G, Aaronson K, Dec GW, Taylor DO, Higgins R, Platt L, Kirklin JK: Determinants of early graft failure following cardiac transplantation, a 10 year multi-institutional, multi-variable analysis [abstract]. J Heart Lung Transplant 2001;20:212.)

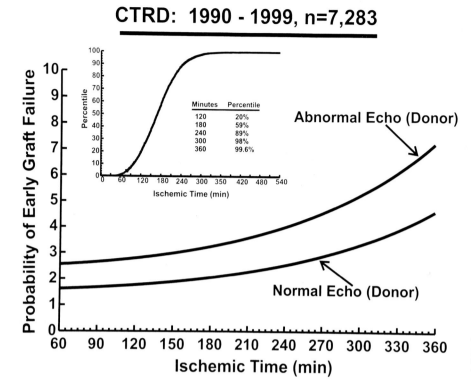

CTRD: 1990 - 1999, n=7,283

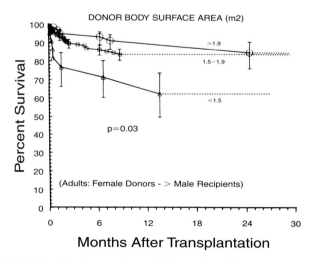

FIGURE 16-19. Nomogram from CTRD multivariable analysis depicting the effect of left ventricular function (by echo) and ischemic time on fatal early graft failure. Insert depicts the frequency distribution of ischemic times. (From Young JB, Hauptman PJ, Naftel DC, Ewald G, Aaronson K, Dec GW, Taylor DO, Higgins R, Platt L, Kirklin JK: Determinants of early graft failure following cardiac transplantation, a 10 year multi-institutional, multivariable analysis [abstract]. J Heart Lung Transplant 2001;20:212.)

dobutamine greater than 20 μg/kg/min with or without additional inotropic agents was an independent risk factor for acute cardiac failure and early mortality.[48]

Depressed systolic function in a donor heart is widely recognized as an indicator of severely reduced reserves and possible subendocardial ischemia or infarction, presumably secondary to catecholamine storm following brain death (see Chapter 9). Echocardiographic wall motion abnormalities have been identified as an independent risk factor in a multi-institutional study.[48] Our own experience and that of others suggest that the presence of an initial mild or moderate depression of left ventricular function does not necessarily contraindicate use of the heart. In practice, moderate increases in dopamine or dobutamine support (if initial doses are low), or reduction in afterload if the donor is severely hypertensive, can frequently normalize ventricular systolic function (by echocardiography). Although formal studies are lacking, clinical use of hearts with an initial ejection fraction of 40% or more, particularly if inotropic support is only moderate and filling pressures are within normal limits, is usually consistent with good cardiac function after implantation. However, the effect of **wall motion abnormalities** on the donor echocardiogram is particularly predictive of poor outcome (early graft failure) with increasing donor age (Fig. 16–18) and prolonged ischemic time (Fig. 16–19).[48]

The adverse impact of **older donor age** likely relates to the general decline in myocardial reserves with advancing age.[3, 48] Older donor age augments the deleterious effects of other risk factors (see again Figs. 16–17 and 16–18).

Size difference between the donor and recipient is generally well tolerated except when these differences are extreme. Young and colleagues demonstrated that **small female donors** (particularly with body surface area < about 1.5 m²) had an important risk of early graft failure when transplanted into **larger male recipients** (Fig. 16–20).[48] In the 10-year CTRD analysis, increasing

FIGURE 16-20. Actuarial survival (Kaplan-Meier) for recipient more than 16 years of age stratified by donor body surface area (BSA > 1.9 m², n = 62; BSA 1.5–1.9 m², n = 170; BSA < 1.5 m², n = 22). (From Young JB, Naftel DC, Bourge RC, Kirklin JK, Clemson BS, Porter CB, Rodeheffer RJ, Kenzora JL: Matching the heart donor and heart transplant recipient. Clues for successful expansion of the donor pool: a multivariable, multiinstitutional report. J Heart Lung Transplant 1994;13:365.)

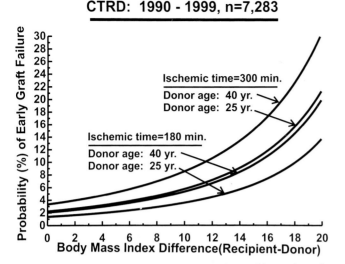

FIGURE **16-21.** Nomogram from CTRD multivariable analysis depicting the effect of body mass index (see Table 16–6 for definition) difference between a larger recipient and a smaller donor, ischemic time, and donor age on fatal early graft failure. (From Young JB, Hauptman PJ, Naftel DC, Ewald G, Aaronson K, Dec GW, Taylor DO, Higgins R, Platt L, Kirklin JK: Determinants of early graft failure following cardiac transplantation, a 10 year multi-institutional, multi-variable analysis [abstract]. J Heart Lung Transplant 2001;20:212.)

size (body mass index) difference between the recipient and donor (when the donor was smaller) progressively increased the risk of early graft failure irrespective of gender (Table 16–6). Not surprisingly, the tolerance for considerably smaller donors transplanted into larger recipients is quite well tolerated with younger donors and shorter ischemic times, but the size difference is less well tolerated with older donors and longer ischemic times (Fig. 16–21).[47]

The traditional guidelines for donor recipient size matching held that a donor who weighed more than 20% less than recipient weight increased the risk of acute cardiac failure. With increasing experience, most centers have broadened these criteria, although the limits of size differential have never been clearly established. For a number of years, our own practice has been to accept an adult male donor heart weighing 160 pounds or more for any size recipient (no matter how large) as long as the donor heart function is normal, the donor age is relatively young, and the projected ischemic time is less than about 3½ hours.

Although formal analyses are lacking, caution is advisable in utilizing a larger donor heart compared to that of the recipient, particularly if the heart appears "athletic" or hypertrophied and the recipient pericardial space is restricted or fibrosed, as is often seen with prior operations and/or a previously placed ventricular assist device. Use of an "oversized" donor heart in this setting may lead to physiologic "tamponade" of the new heart, producing restrictive physiology following transplantation. In addition, an oversized heart in a constricted pericardial space has been noted on rare occasion to produce compression of the main and left pulmonary

artery because of the mass effect of the heart in a limited space.

Predictably, patients with **previous operations** (with a slightly increased risk of destabilizing bleeding or acute hemodynamic deterioration with sternotomy) and those with **congenital heart disease** (potentially complicating the technical aspects of the transplant procedure) are at slightly higher risk for early graft failure.[5,48] Figure 16–22 shows the increasing risk of prior sternotomies with very prolonged ischemic times.

Many studies, from the earliest era of cardiac transplantation, have identified **higher pulmonary vascular resistance** as a risk factor for early graft failure (Fig. 16–23).[29,48] The effect of increasing pulmonary vascular resistance in adult patients is a continuous relationship rather than a sharp increase in risk at any given pulmonary vascular resistance level.[29] With the evolution of understanding of reactive versus fixed pulmonary vascular resistance, as discussed in Chapters 6 and 20, it became clear that the actual value of pulmonary vascular resistance was less important than its reactivity. Increasingly, for patients with pulmonary vascular resistance more than about 4 Wood units, or pulmonary systolic blood pressure above 55 mm Hg, prolonged efforts are initiated to demonstrate reversibility, including nitric oxide, milrinone, nitroglycerin infusions, and even left ventricular assist device support in order to reduce the reactive component of pulmonary vascular resistance. In many instances, these measures have neutralized the incremental risk of initially elevated pulmonary vascular resistance. It is of interest that, in the 10-year CTRD analysis, the notion of elevated pulmonary vascular resistance as a risk factor for early graft failure was most accurately represented by the **systolic transpulmonary**

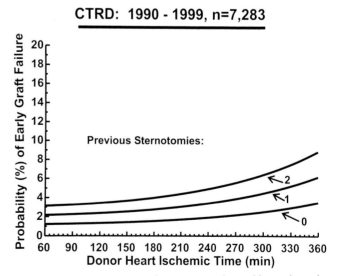

FIGURE **16-22.** Nomogram from CTRD multivariable analysis depicting the effect of donor ischemic time, and number of prior sternotomies on fatal early graft failure. (From Young JB, Hauptman PJ, Naftel DC, Ewald G, Aaronson K, Dec GW, Taylor DO, Higgins R, Platt L, Kirklin JK: Determinants of early graft failure following cardiac transplantation, a 10 year multi-institutional, multi-variable analysis [abstract]. J Heart Lung Transplant 2001;20:212.)

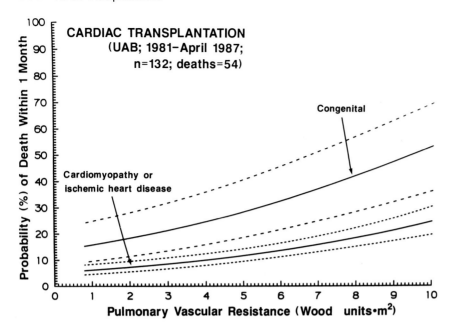

FIGURE **16–23.** Nomogram from multivariable equation depicting the effect of pulmonary vascular resistance and cardiac diagnosis on 1-month mortality. Dashed lines enclose 70% confidence limits. (From Kirklin JK, Naftel DC, Kirklin JW, Blackstone EH, White-Williams C, Bourge R: Pulmonary vascular resistance and the risk of heart transplantation. J Heart Transplant 1988;7:331–336.)

gradient (the difference between the pulmonary artery systolic pressure and pulmonary capillary wedge pressure). This relationship makes intuitive sense because it is the pulmonary capillary wedge pressure which is usually the stimulus for reactive increases in pulmonary vascular resistance, and the systolic pulmonary artery pressure is most reflective of the afterload against which the right ventricle must contract. The decreased tolerance of the right ventricle for destabilizing bleeding following transplantation, with the need for multiple trans-

fusions, is particularly problematic in the setting of prior elevation of pulmonary vascular resistance (Fig. 16–24). Some studies suggest that the adverse effects on survival of increased pulmonary vascular resistance (or transpulmonary gradient) extend to the first 6–12 months after transplant, perhaps related to decreased cardiac reserves in the face of persistent elevation of pulmonary vascular resistance.[12]

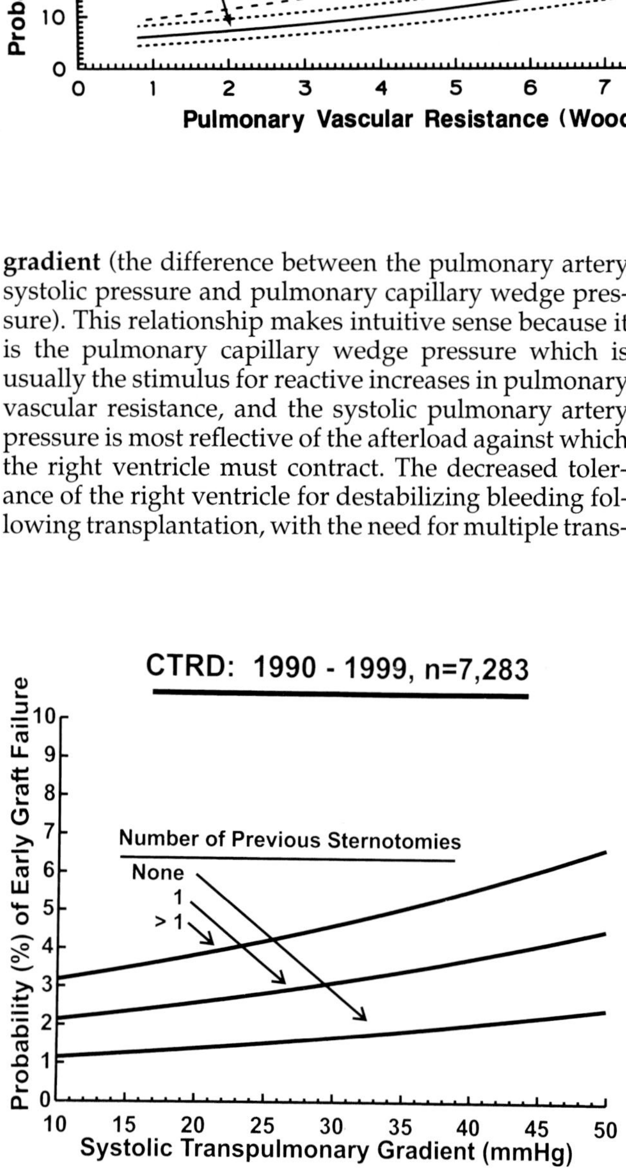

Attempts to expand the donor pool with the use of "marginal" donors (i.e., donor hearts with predicted reduction of myocardial reserves) may increase the probability of early graft failure in an attempt to increase the number of patients for whom transplantation is available[1] (see Chapter 9). Young and colleagues[48] used multi-institutional data to generate expected 1-month survival profiles for various donor risk factors (Fig. 16–25). The balance between extending the donor pool (e.g. with older aged donors) in order to increase the availability of transplantation (and decrease the likelihood of death while waiting) and the likely increased associated early mortality (with less optimal donors) challenges the decision-making abilities of even the most experienced transplant surgeons and physicians.[3] However, as depicted in Figure 16–26, when donors with decreased myocardial reserves (such as a 50-year-old donor with ischemic time exceeding 5 hours) are utilized in recipients who are critically ill (ventilator support) with decreased reserves, the likelihood of early graft failure is importantly increased, supporting the notion that "margin donors into marginal recipients yield marginal outcomes."

DEATH FROM REJECTION

Impact

Mortality within the first 30 days caused by rejection usually occurs from two causes, hyperacute rejection or

FIGURE **16–24.** Nomogram from CTRD multivariable analysis depicting the effect of number of prior sternotomies and systolic transpulmonary gradient on fatal early graft failure. (From Young JB, Hauptman PJ, Naftel DC, Ewald G, Aaronson K, Dec GW, Taylor DO, Higgins R, Platt L, Kirklin JK: Determinants of early graft failure following cardiac transplantation, a 10 year multi-institutional, multi-variable analysis [abstract]. J Heart Lung Transplant 2001;20:212.)

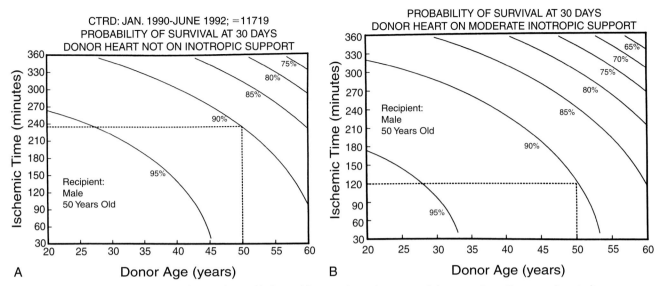

FIGURE 16-25. Nomogram from multivariable hazard function donor/recipient risk factor analysis. Concentric lines indicate predicted 30-day mortality rate as function of donor age and ischemic time in presence of no inotropic support before donor harvesting (*A*) and moderate inotropic support (*B*). Other risk factors set for depiction include no ventilator support, no donor diabetes, no wall motion abnormalities, recipient age 50 years, pulmonary vascular resistance 2.2 Wood units, male donor into male recipient, and donor death not from cardiac arrest. (From Young JB, Naftel DC, Bourge RC, Kirklin JK, Clemson BS, Porter CB, Rodeheffer RJ, Kenzora JL: Matching the heart donor and heart transplant recipient. Clues for successful expansion of the donor pool: a multivariable, multiinstitutional report. J Heart Lung Transplant 1994;13:365.)

accelerated acute rejection. Although hyperacute rejection has occurred rarely after cardiac transplantation, the precise diagnosis is often problematic (see Chapter 14) and, with the current sophisticated immunologic evaluation prior to and at the time of donor selection (see Chapter 7), this nearly uniformly fatal complication should be extremely rare. We have not identified hyperacute rejection in the past 15 years of clinical transplanta-

CTRD: 1990 - 1999, n=7,283

At time of transplant:

Ventilator, 50 y.o. Donor

Ventilator, 25 y.o. Donor

No Ventilator, 50 y.o. Donor

No ventilator, 25 y.o. Donor

Probability (%) of Early Graft Failure vs. **Donor Heart Ischemic Time (min)**

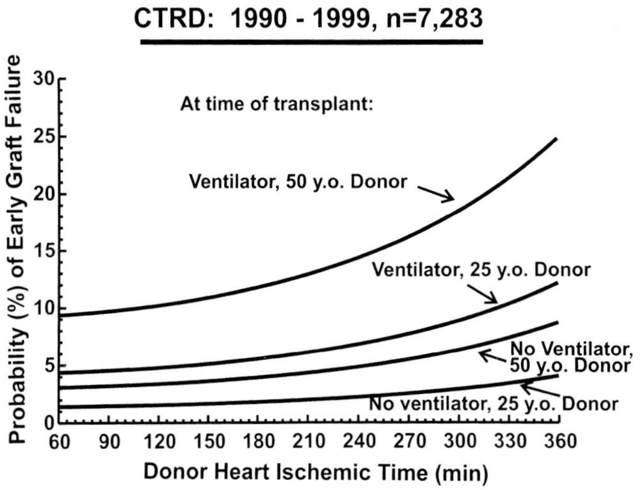

FIGURE 16-26. Nomogram from CTRD multivariable analysis depicting the effect of donor ischemic time, recipient ventilator support, and donor age on fatal early graft failure. (From Young JB, Hauptman PJ, Naftel DC, Ewald G, Aaronson K, Dec GW, Taylor DO, Higgins R, Platt L, Kirklin JK: Determinants of early graft failure following cardiac transplantation, a 10 year multi-institutional, multi-variable analysis [abstract]. J Heart Lung Transplant 2001;20:212.)

tion. Acute cellular rejection, however, is an important cause of early mortality, accounting for about 20% of mortality during the first year[48] (see Chapter 14). The likelihood of death from rejection is highest during the first month and rapidly decreases thereafter (Fig. 16–6). The risk of fatal rejection never disappears, but it is an unusual occurrence after the first year.

Risk Factors

The risk factors for rejection death identified from the 10-year CTRD analysis are depicted in Table 16–7. **Younger age** may reflect a more vigorous immune response, and **black race** is known to have greater diversity of HLA antigens[24, 33] (see Chapter 14) (Fig. 16–27). The relationship between **higher preoperative pulmonary artery systolic gradient** (pulmonary artery systolic pressure minus capillary wedge pressure) and rejection death may reflect lower tolerance for hemodynamically compromising rejection, which could result in higher capillary wedge pressure, reappearance of reactive pulmonary artery hypertension, and right ventricular failure. Similarly, **older donor age** may reflect less cardiac reserves in the face of hemodynamically compromising rejection.

Cytomegalovirus (CMV) status has been implicated as a risk factor for recurrent rejection, and this analysis showed CMV mismatch (CMV-negative recipient and CMV-positive donor) to be a risk factor for rejection death. CMV has previously been implicated in rejection, possibly secondary to crossreactivity of viral and HLA antigens (see Chapter 14) (Fig. 16–28).

High degrees of **HLA mismatch** also slightly increase the risk of fatal rejection, as seen in Figure 16–29 and

TABLE 16–7	Risk Factors for Rejection Death (CTRD: 1990–1999, N = 7,283)	
	DECLINING PHASE	
RISK FACTOR	Relative Risk 1	p Value
RECIPIENT		
Younger age*	1.65	<.0001
Black	2.03	<.0001
Hispanic	1.75	.03
Obese recipient*	1.21	<.0001
Negative herpes serology	1.86	.01
PAs-PCWP*	1.44	.03
Earlier date of transplant*	2.53	<.0001
DONOR		
Older donor age*	1.28	.001
MISMATCH		
CMV-negative recipient, CMV-positive donor	1.52	.008
Total HLA mismatch (4–6)	1.77	.009

PAs, pulmonary artery systolic pressure; PCWP, mean pulmonary capillary wedge pressure; CMV, cytomegalovirus; HLA, human leukocyte antigen.
* See Table 16–5 for relative risk comparisons.
From Bourge RC, Naftel DC, Hill JA, Boehmer JP, Waggoner L, Kasper EK, Lee F, Czerska B, Thomas K, Kirklin JK: The emergence of co-morbid diseases impacting survival after cardiac transplantation: a ten year multi-institutional experience [abstract]. J Heart Lung Transplant 2001;20:167.

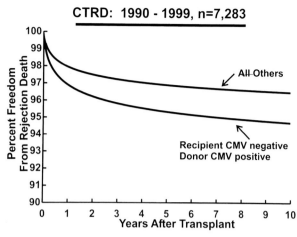

FIGURE **16–28.** Nomogram from CTRD multivariable analysis depicting the effect of cytomegalovirus (CMV) mismatch on freedom from rejection death.

suggested by earlier studies.[14, 36] De Mattos and colleagues, in a univariate analysis, identified two DR mismatches (compared to 0 or 1 mismatch) as a predictor of decreased survival at 1 year.[10]

Although **panel reactive antibody** (PRA) percent was not identified as a risk factor for rejection death in this analysis and others,[26] increasing levels of PRA were identified in the study by Lavee and colleagues[32] as a predictor of posttransplant death from acute or chronic rejection (allograft vasculopathy). Similar findings have been reported in renal transplantation.[36]

Perhaps of greatest interest has been the progressive **decrease** in the likelihood of fatal rejection over the 10 years of the CTRD study (Fig. 16–30). This likely reflects improvements in immunosuppressive modalities and management during the past decade (see Chapters 13 and 14).

DEATH FROM INFECTION

Impact

In the current era, infection accounts for approximately 10–15% of mortality during the first posttransplant month[48] and is the leading cause of mortality during the

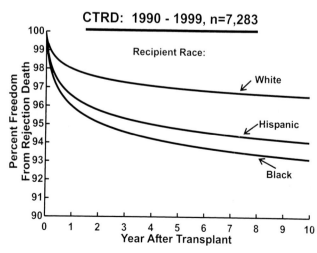

FIGURE **16–27.** Nomogram from CTRD multivariable analysis depicting the effect of recipient race on the freedom from rejection death.

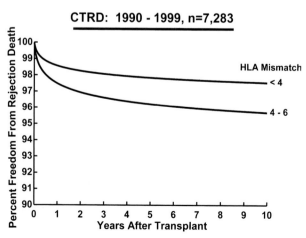

FIGURE **16–29.** Nomogram from CTRD multivariable analysis depicting the effect of HLA mismatch on freedom from rejection death.

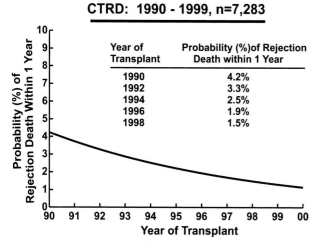

CTRD: 1990 - 1999, n=7,283

Year of Transplant	Probability (%)of Rejection Death within 1 Year
1990	4.2%
1992	3.3%
1994	2.5%
1996	1.9%
1998	1.5%

FIGURE **16–30.** Nomogram from CTRD multivariable analysis depicting the effect of year of transplantation on the probability of rejection death within 1 year.

first year (Table 16–1). The risk factors for infection and the posttransplant environment which increases the susceptibility to infection are discussed extensively in Chapter 15. Despite the important current risk of death from infection early after transplantation, multiple stud-

ies have documented the decrease in the incidence of fatal infections over the past decade compared to earlier eras.[2, 5, 16, 19, 21, 34, 37, 44]

Risk Factors

The risk factors for fatal infection in the current era (by multivariable analysis from the CTRD) are listed in Table 16–8. The recipient and donor risk factors in this table undoubtedly reflect factors which contribute to **decreased resistance to infection** (older recipient age, obese or cachectic recipient, preexisting pulmonary disease, and ventilator dependency at transplant), a more critically ill recipient with **less general reserves** (depressed renal function, higher mean right atrial pressure, intra-aortic balloon support, and recent VAD placement), and surgical conditions associated with greater general risk of a **complicated postoperative course** (previous sternotomy). The donor risk factors (older donor age and longer ischemic time) similarly reflect factors which are associated with **less donor heart reserves** and a greater likelihood of postoperative depressed cardiac function.

The magnitude of interactions between several of these variables is depicted in the nomogram in Figure 16–31. Similar risk factors have been identified in other multi-institutional studies.[42] As discussed in Chapter 15, the mortality is highest for fungal infections (23% mor-

TABLE 16-8	Risk Factors for Infection Death (CTRD: 1990–1999, N = 7,283)			
	EARLY PHASE		**CONSTANT PHASE**	
RISK FACTOR	Relative Risk	p Value	Relative Risk	p Value
RECIPIENT				
Older age*	1.46	<.0001		
Obese recipient*	5.67	.0003		
Cachectic recipient*	7.51	.0008		
Any diabetes			1.99	.03
Pulmonary disease	1.73	.02		
Any cigarette use			1.81	.04
Lower creatinine clearance at listing*	1.56	.0004		
Higher serum creatinine at transplant*	1.61	.0001		
Mean RAP*	1.42	.02		
Previous sternotomy	1.53	.002		
Ventilator	2.37	.008		
IABP	1.58	.03		
VAD, 14 days or less	3.32	.0008		
DONOR				
Older donor age*	1.29	<.0001		
Hepatitis C positive			5.14	.02
Longer ischemic time*	1.88	<.0001		

RAP, right atrial pressure; IABP, intra-aortic balloon pump; VAD, ventricular assist device.
* See Table 16–5 for relative risk comparisons.
From Bourge RC, Naftel DC, Hill JA, Boehmer JP, Waggoner L, Kasper EK, Lee F, Czerska B, Thomas K, Kirklin JK: The emergence of co-morbid diseases impacting survival after cardiac transplantation: a ten year multi-institutional experience [abstract]. J Heart Lung Transplant 2001;20:167.

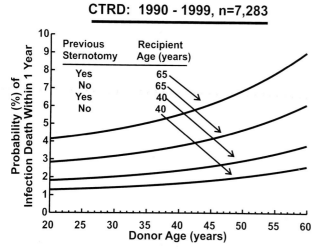

FIGURE **16-31.** Nomogram from CTRD multivariable analysis depicting the effect of previous sternotomy, recipient age, and donor age on infection death within 1 year.

tality in the study by Smart and colleagues),[42] followed by protozoal, bacterial, and viral infections. Risk factors for death in specific infections are discussed in Chapter 15. In a multi-institutional CTRD study[30] the major risk factor for fatal CMV infection was a higher number of infections (of any type) during the first month after transplantation.

The adverse effect of donor or recipient risk factors for fatal infections is especially high in the debilitated elderly patient, particularly those requiring pretransplant ventilator support who receive a heart from an older donor with a prolonged ischemic time (Fig. 16–32).

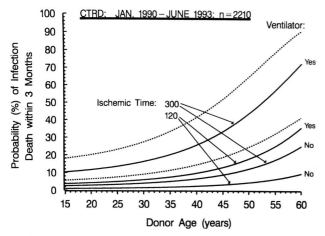

FIGURE **16-32.** Nomogram of the solution for the multivariate equation for death caused by infection. The variables in the equation are set such that recipient is a 55-year-old man and donor ischemic times of 120 and 300 minutes are displayed. The 70% confidence limits are shown only for the patient with ventilator support with 300 minutes of donor ischemic time (upper curve). (From Smart F, Naftel DC, Costanzo M, Levine T, Pelletier G, Yancy C, Hobbs R, Kirklin J, Bourge R: Risk factors for early, cumulative and fatal infections after heart transplantation: a multiinstitutional study. J Heart Lung Transplant 1996;15:329–341.)

The very high expected mortality from infection (and other causes) argues strongly against proceeding with transplantation in that situation. The high frequency of potentially fatal bacterial pneumonias and bacteremias in this subset of patients likely relates to colonization of the tracheobronchial tree during pretransplantation intubation, prolonged indwelling lines, and repeated instrumentation of the patient, all occurring in a state of generalized debilitation.

MORTALITY AFTER THE FIRST YEAR

DEATH FROM ALL CAUSES

Impact

As the long-term efficacy of cardiac transplantation continues to be rigorously examined, the causes and cause-specific risk factors for late mortality are increasingly important. It is well known that the risk of death from specific causes differs depending on the time elapsed since the transplant operation. The hazard functions for various causes of death vary greatly between the first year (Fig. 16–6) and later years (Fig. 16–7). This is also reflected in the cumulative proportion of patients dying from specific causes early versus late after cardiac transplantation (Figs. 16–8 and 16–9). Examination of these figures underscores the fact that early graft failure, rejection, and infection as major causes of death during the first year are replaced in later years by allograft coronary artery disease, malignancy, and a host of miscellaneous causes of late mortality. After the first 5 years, malignancy and allograft coronary artery disease account for more than 50% of the mortality (Table 16–1). It is noteworthy that patients who have survived 5 years following transplantation have a gradually increasing likelihood of fatal malignancy or allograft coronary artery disease events in the ensuing years.

Risk Factors

The reader will notice that the risk factors identified for mortality during the first year are all factors identifiable at the time of transplantation. In contrast, risk factors examined in this section include a multivariable analysis not only of **pretransplant variables,** but also **events** occurring **during the first year** following transplantation. The risk factor analysis presented here for the 10-year CTRD study is *conditional*, indicating that only patients surviving the first year after transplantation are examined.

The risk factors identified for overall mortality (death from any cause) after the first year are listed in Table 16–9. **Older age** at transplant has been shown in this analysis and other studies (particularly for patients > 60 years of age)[38] to be a risk factor for late death. As depicted in the non-risk-adjusted stratified actuarial (Fig. 16–33), a history of insulin-dependent **diabetes** prior to transplantation exerts a small but significant adverse effect on late survival.[6] Evidence of **chronic allograft dysfunction,** as evidenced by depressed ejection

TABLE 16-9	Risk Factors for Death (Any Cause) After 1 Year (CTRD: 1990–1999, N = 5,357)	

	CONSTANT PHASE	
RISK FACTOR	Relative Risk	p Value
RECIPIENT		
Older age[1]	1.51	.001
Younger age[1]	2.19	<.0001
Black	1.7	<.0001
Noncongenital etiology	2.36	.04
Insulin-dependent diabetes	1.51	.004
Cigarette use within 6 mo	1.54	.0002
Higher serum creatinine at transplant[1]	1.33	.0004
PRA > 10	1.4	.04
Earlier date of transplant[1]	1.34	.03
DONOR		
Older donor age[1]	1.13	.01
MEDICAL HISTORY IN FIRST POSTTRANSPLANT YEAR		
Mild CAD	1.29	.02
Moderate and severe CAD	2.99	<.0001
Lymphoma	4.37	.0004
Other nonskin malignancy	4.74	<.0001
Lower LV ejection fraction[2]	2.05	<.0001
Rejection	1.36[3]	<.0001
Less time since last rejection[4]	1.99	<.0001
Rejection with hemodynamic compromise	1.77	.0004
Infection	1.11[5]	.006
Less time since last infection[6]	1.95	.002
Greater number of infections[7]	1.55	.007
Higher serum cholesterol[8]	2.14	.003

PRA, panel reactive antibody; CAD, coronary artery disease; LV, left ventricular. 1. See Table 15–5 for relative risk comparisons. 2. Relative risk compares ejection fraction of 60–40. 3. Rejection without hemodynamic compromise at 3 mo after transplant. 4. Relative risk compares time since last rejection of 0–30 days. 5. Infection at 6 mo after transplant. 6. Relative risk compares time since last infection of 0–30 days. 7. Relative risk compares 1–4 infections. 8. Relative risk compares serum cholesterol of 200–300.
From Bourge RC, Naftel DC, Hill JA, Boehmer JP, Waggoner L, Kasper EK, Lee F, Czerska B, Thomas K, Kirklin JK: The emergence of co-morbid diseases impacting survival after cardiac transplantation: a ten year multi-institutional experience [abstract]. J Heart Lung Transplant 2001;20:167.

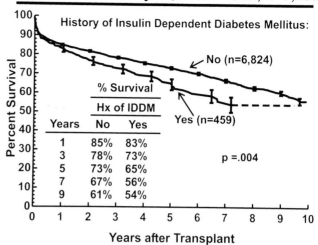

CTRD: Death Analysis, 1990 - 1999, n=7,283

FIGURE **16–33.** Actuarial survival in the CTRD analysis stratified by history of insulin-dependent diabetes mellitus. (From Bourge RC, Naftel DC, Hill JA, Boehmer JP, Waggoner L, Kasper EK, Lee F, Czerska B, Thomas K, Kirklin JK: The emergence of co-morbid diseases impacting survival after cardiac transplantation: a ten year multi-institutional experience [abstract]. J Heart Lung Transplant 2001;20:167.)

rejection markers which are risk factors for subsequent mortality include vasculitis on endomyocardial biopsy[18, 43] and the demonstration of circulating anti-donor HLA antibodies after transplant.[15, 40]

There is evidence that **late survival is gradually improving,** even within the last decade, as indicated by the identification of earlier date of transplantation as a

fraction at the end of the first year, predicts a worse outcome late after transplantation. This effect is especially pronounced when, as evidenced by a history of rejection with hemodynamic compromise, the depressed function likely results from **repeated** episodes of cellular or humoral **rejection** (Fig. 16–34). Rejection with hemodynamic compromise is discussed in detail in Chapter 14. As shown by Mills and colleagues,[35] rejection associated with marked depression of left ventricular function and the use of inotropic support carries a poor intermediate prognosis, with a mortality rate of as much as 40% within the following 12 months. Other

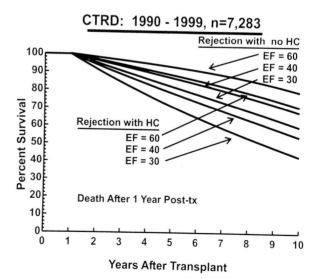

FIGURE **16–34.** Nomogram from CTRD multivariable analysis depicting the effect of ejection fraction and rejection with or without hemodynamic compromise (HC) on survival among patients who have survived the first posttransplantation year.

risk factor for late mortality in the 10-year CTRD study (Fig. 16–35).

DEATH FROM ALLOGRAFT VASCULOPATHY

Impact

Allograft vasculopathy is often cited as the major limitation of truly long-term survival following transplantation. From this discussion, this statement is obviously a gross oversimplification, but it is true that the risk of fatal allograft coronary artery disease gradually increases during the years following cardiac transplantation (see again Table 16–3 and Fig. 16–7). Similar findings were reported by Yancy and colleagues.[46]

Risk Factors

The major risk factors for late mortality from allograft coronary artery disease are listed in Table 16–10. Not surprisingly, the most important predictor of late mortality from allograft vasculopathy is the **development of coronary artery disease** during the first posttransplant year, particularly when it is severe (Fig. 16–36).[9] The incremental effect of **older donor age** on the development of allograft vasculopathy is discussed at length in Chapter 17, and increasing donor age also produces a slightly higher risk of fatal coronary artery events.[8]

Ischemic etiology of advanced heart failure has been identified in some studies as a risk factor for the development of late allograft vasculopathy (see Chapter 17). In this 10-year analysis, ischemic etiology of advanced heart failure was associated with a small but highly significant increase in the risk of fatal coronary artery events in the midterm following transplantation (Fig. 16–37).

A surprising finding in this 10-year multi-institutional study was the identification of **younger recipient age**

TABLE 16-10	Risk Factors for Allograft CAD Death After 1 Year (CTRD: 1990–1999, N = 5,357)

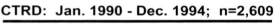

RISK FACTOR	RELATIVE RISK	p VALUE
Recipient		
Younger age[1]	1.44	<.0001
Black	2.07	.0002
Ischemic etiology	1.84	.0003
Cigarette use within 6 mo of listing	1.72	.008
Earlier date of transplant[1]	2.5	.0004
Donor		
Older donor age[1]	1.25	.02
Medical history in first posttransplant year		
Mild CAD	2.08	.0002
Moderate and severe CAD	6	<.0001
Lower LV ejection fraction[2]	3.53	.001
Greater time in rejection[2]	1.17	.0002

CAD, coronary artery disease; LV, left ventricular.
1. See Table 16–5 for relative risk comparisons. 2. See Table 16–6 for relative risk comparisons.
From Costanzo MR, Elsen HJ, Brown RN, Mehra M, Benza RL, Torre G, Yancy CW, Davis S, McCloud M, Kirklin JK: Are there specific risk factors for fatal allograft vasculopathy? An analysis of over 7,000 cardiac transplant patients [abstract]. J Heart Lung Transplant 2001;20;152.

(down to 20 years of age, but excluding children) as a risk factor for fatal allograft coronary artery disease events. The finding of younger adult age as a risk factor for fatal allograft coronary disease is not unique to this study. A multivariable analysis from Papworth[41] identified both younger age (age 20–30 years) and older age (> 50 years) as strong risk factors for graft loss due to

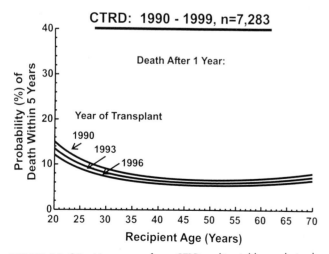

FIGURE **16–35.** Nomogram from CTRD multivariable analysis depicting the effect of year of transplantation and recipient age on the likelihood of death within 5 years among patients who have survived the first posttransplantation year.

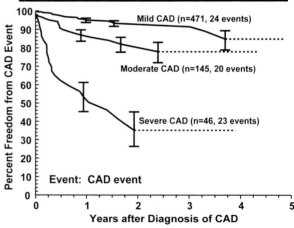

FIGURE **16–36.** Actuarial (Kaplan-Meier) freedom from occurrence of CAD event according to degree of CAD present at time when CAD was first detected by coronary angiography. *Top line,* Mild CAD. *Middle line.* Moderate CAD. *Bottom line,* Severe CAD. Error bars indicate 70% confidence limits. (From Costanzo MR, Naftel DC, Pritzker MR, Heilman JK, Boehmer JP, Brozena SC, Dec GW, Ventura HO, Kirklin JK, Bourge RC, Miller LW, and the Cardiac Transplant Research Database: Heart transplant coronary artery disease detected by coronary angiography: a multiinstitutional study of preoperative donor and recipient risk factors. J Heart Lung Transplant 1998;17:744–753.)

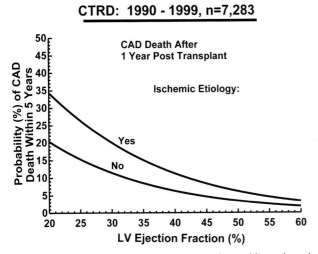

CTRD: 1990 - 1999, n=7,283

FIGURE **16-37.** Nomogram from the CTRD multivariable analysis depicting the effect of ischemic etiology and left ventricular ejection fraction at the end of the first year on the probability of death from allograft coronary artery disease (CAD) within 5 years, examined among patients who have survived the first year following cardiac transplantation. (From Costanzo MR, Eisen HJ, Brown RN, Mehra M, Benza RL, Torre G, Yancy CW, Davis S, McCloud M, Kirklin JK: Are there specific risk factors for fatal allograft vasculopathy? An analysis of over 7,000 cardiac transplant patients [abstract]. J Heart Lung Transplant 2001;20:152.)

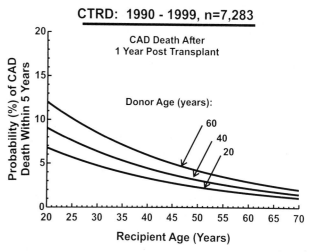

CTRD: 1990 - 1999, n=7,283

FIGURE **16-38.** Nomogram from the CTRD multivariable analysis depicting the effect of donor age and recipient age on the probability of death from allograft coronary artery disease (CAD) within 5 years, examined among patients who have survived the first year following cardiac transplantation. (From Costanzo MR, Eisen HJ, Brown RN, Mehra M, Benza RL, Torre G, Yancy CW, Davis S, McCloud M, Kirklin JK: Are there specific risk factors for fatal allograft vasculopathy? An analysis of over 7,000 cardiac transplant patients [abstract]. J Heart Lung Transplant 2001;20:152.)

coronary occlusive disease. These findings provide further supporting evidence for the notion that allograft vasculopathy is a complex interplay between immunologic phenomena related to the transplanted heart and an accelerated form of atherosclerosis. The pathophysiology for these complex interactions is discussed in detail in Chapter 17. We presume that a more aggressive immune response of the younger adult contributes to a small but significant increase in the risk of fatal coronary artery events. This finding has particular importance in relationship to donor age. While the magnitude of the effect of younger recipient age on the likelihood of fatal coronary artery disease remains quite small (approximately a 4% increase in the likelihood of fatal coronary artery disease within 5 years in a 20-year-old vs. a 60-year-old recipient), this effect is magnified considerably in older donors (Fig. 16–38).[8] Although not specifically examined in this study, it seems likely that a similar risk profile for coronary artery mortality would occur in teenagers and adolescents. These data provide further argument against allocating older donor hearts to adolescents, teenagers, and very young adults unless no other option is available.

It is widely believed that **cigarette smoking** is an important risk factor for allograft vasculopathy, a concept which is supported by this analysis. Cigarette smoking within the months prior to transplantation likely identifies the patients likely to continue smoking following transplantation (posttransplant cigarette use was not specifically examined in this study), and that was found to be a small but important risk factor for subsequent fatal coronary artery events (Fig. 16–39).

Thus careful screening of patients for cigarette use, and the requirement for prolonged cigarette abstinence, is a defendable policy in terms of promoting long-term survival.

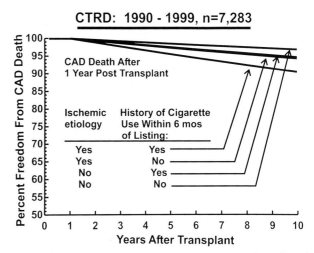

CTRD: 1990 - 1999, n=7,283

FIGURE **16-39.** Nomogram from the CTRD multivariable analysis depicting the effect of ischemic etiology and history of cigarette use within 6 months of listing on the freedom from fatal allograft coronary artery disease (CAD), examined in patients who have survived the first year following transplantation. (From Costanzo MR, Eisen HJ, Brown RN, Mehra M, Benza RL, Torre G, Yancy CW, Davis S, McCloud M, Kirklin JK: Are there specific risk factors for fatal allograft vasculopathy? An analysis of over 7,000 cardiac transplant patients [abstract]. J Heart Lung Transplant 2001;20:152.)

DEATH FROM MALIGNANCY

Impact

As noted in Figures 16–7 and 16–9, the risk of fatal malignancy progressively increases in the years following transplantation. It is well established that the probability of malignancy is substantially higher in immunosuppressed patients compared to the normal population. The time-related risk of various malignancies is discussed in Chapter 18 (see Fig. 18–6), and the differing hazard function for death with posttransplant lymphomas versus other malignancies is depicted in Figures 18–7 and 18–10. In the multi-institutional study by De Salvo and colleagues, malignancy was the primary or contributing cause of death in 8% of patients after transplant. Posttransplant lymphoproliferative disease and lung cancer were the most common fatal malignancies.[11] An important reduction in late fatal malignancy can only be achieved with the availability of more targeted baseline immunosuppression, the induction of partial tolerance, and more intensive posttransplant surveillance for the development of early malignancies.

Risk Factors

The risk factors for late malignancy death are summarized in Table 16–11. As expected, the presence of a **malignancy during the first year** is a strong prognostic indicator for subsequent fatal malignancy (Fig. 16–40). De Salvo and colleagues also identified the history of a pretransplant malignancy as a risk factor for posttransplant death from malignancy.[11] **Advanced age** at transplant, particularly in patients over age 60,[38] is a risk factor for malignancy death. The very important adverse effect of continued cigarette use (approximated by cigarette use within 6 months of listing), is most

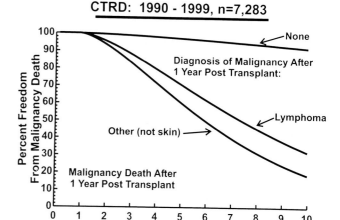

FIGURE 16–40. Nomogram from the CTRD multivariable analysis depicting the effect of malignancy (lymphoma or other) during the first posttransplantation year on the freedom from subsequent malignancy death.

pronounced in older, white, male recipients (Fig. 16–41). This highlights the importance of close surveillance to detect occult malignancies related to cigarette smoking, especially lung cancer. This relationship further supports the strict policy of abstinence from cigarette use during the months before and permanently after transplantation.

TABLE 16–11	Risk Factors for Malignancy Death After 1 Year (CTRD: 1990–1999, N = 5,357)

RISK FACTOR	RELATIVE RISK	p VALUE
Recipient		
Older age*	1.63	<.0001
White male	1.96	.002
Cigarette use within 6 mo of listing	2.28	.0001
PRA > 10 (pretransplant)	3.01	<.0001
Medical history in first posttransplant year		
Lymphoma	13.8	<.0001
Other nonskin malignancy	20.3	<.0001

PRA, panel reactive antibody.
* See Table 16–5 for relative risk comparison.
From Costanzo MR, Elsen HJ, Brown RN, Mehra M, Benza RL, Torre G, Yancy CW, Davis S, McCloud M, Kirklin JK: Are there specific risk factors for fatal allograft vasculopathy? An analysis of over 7,000 cardiac transplant patients [abstract]. J Heart Lung Transplant 2001;20:152.

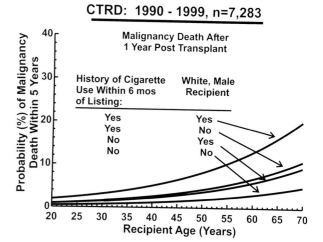

FIGURE 16–41. Nomogram from the CTRD multivariable analysis depicting the effect of recipient age, white male, and the history of cigarette use on the likelihood of malignancy death within 5 years, examined in patients who have survived the first year following heart transplantation. (From Bourge RC, Naftel DC, Hill JA, Boehmer JP, Waggoner L, Kasper EK, Lee F, Czerska B, Thomas K, Kirklin JK: The emergence of co-morbid diseases impacting survival after cardiac transplantation: a ten year multi-institutional experience [abstract]. J Heart Lung Transplant 2001;20: 167.)

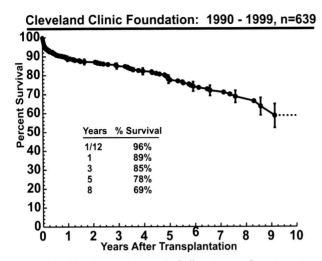

Cleveland Clinic Foundation: 1990 - 1999, n=639

Years	% Survival
1/12	96%
1	89%
3	85%
5	78%
8	69%

FIGURE **16–42.** Actuarial survival of all patients undergoing primary orthotopic cardiac transplantation, Cleveland Clinic Foundation: 1990–1999 (n = 639).

CURRENT SURVIVAL EXPECTATIONS

INSTITUTIONAL SURVIVAL

The major improvements in cardiac transplantation over the past 20 years have been most dramatic in the early months after transplant. A simple glance at any actuarial curve underscores the profound impact that early mortality has on late survival. In the current era, the 1-month survival should approach 95% in most institutions, with a 1-year survival exceeding 85%. The previous extensive discussion of risk factors underscores the notion that this survival target is heavily dependent upon multiple recipient risk factors which can be identified prior to transplantation.

The results of cardiac transplantation at the Cleveland Clinic over the past 10 years are displayed in Figure 16–42, in which the 1-year survival for all patients undergoing cardiac transplantation approaches 90%, with 5-year survival of 78%. The overall experience at UAB

since 1981 is portrayed in Figure 16–43. It is of interest that over three different eras of transplantation, the survival has progressively improved. During the past 5 years (upper actuarial curve), the overall 1-year survival (including all transplanted patients from neonates to elderly adults) is 90%. The impact of reduced early mortality on late survival is evident in this depiction.

As noted in this chapter, predictors of mid- and long-term survival following cardiac transplantation are more difficult to identify prior to transplantation and are heavily dependent upon events such as rejection, infection, allograft coronary artery disease, and malignancies which develop after the transplant procedure. However, for patients transplanted during the last 15 years, 10-year survival is typically about 50–60% in most institutions[13] (see again Fig. 16–5). For transplantation to be a truly effective long-term therapy for advanced heart failure, a 10-year survival of 70–75% would be an appropriate goal. This would require a low early mortality as well as appropriate long-term patient surveillance to reduce mid and late deaths from rejection, infection, allograft vasculopathy, and malignancies. Of critical importance will undoubtedly be the introduction of new immunosuppressive therapies and the refinement of therapeutic options to induce the state of partial tolerance which may have an important impact on the frequency of rejection-related events and the level of chronic immunosuppression necessary for long-term graft function. In Figure 16–43, the parametric curve which generates a 75% 10-year survival is superimposed on the most recent actuarial survival curve. From this depiction, it is evident that early and midterm survival in many institutions has improved to the point where 75% 10-year survival may be achievable.

PATIENT-SPECIFIC PREDICTIONS

As the field of heart transplantation evolves and advances, there will be increasing interest (and pressure) to more accurately predict the results of heart transplantation for a given individual and to modify or "tai-

FIGURE **16–43.** Actuarial survival following primary cardiac transplantation in 3 eras at the University of Alabama at Birmingham (UAB). The top actuarial curve depicts the years 1994–1999 (n = 229); the second curve 1987–1993 (n = 182); and the lower actuarial depiction is 1981–1986 (n = 122). The solid line superimposed over the upper actuarial curve represents the parametric depiction of survival which generates 75% survival at 10 years.

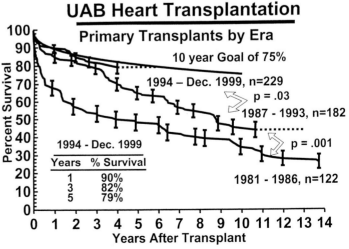

UAB Heart Transplantation
Primary Transplants by Era

10 year Goal of 75%
1994 – Dec. 1999, n=229
p = .03
1987 - 1993, n=182
p = .001
1981 - 1986, n=122

1994 - Dec. 1999	
Years	% Survival
1	90%
3	82%
5	79%

TABLE 16-12	Risk Stratification for Long-Term Survival (CTRD: 1990-1999, N = 7,283)

HIGH SURVIVAL PATIENTS (N = 1,156)	LOW SURVIVAL PATIENTS (N = 462)
All of the following conditions must be true: Recipient age: <65 yr Donor age: <40 yr Ischemic time: <240 min Other risk factors*: 0 Year of transplant ≥1994	At least one of the following conditions must be true: Donor age: >55 yr Ischemic time >360 min On ventilator at time of transplant History of cocaine use Other risk factors*: ≥4

* Other risk factors: history of insulin-dependent diabetes, history of alcohol abuse, history of peripheral vascular disease, history of pulmonary disease, congenital etiology, history of cigarette smoking (within 6 mo), abnormal septal wall motion (donor), and gender mismatch.
From Kirklin JK, Miller LW, Brown RN, Alvarez RJ, Porter CB, Van Bakel AB, Jaski BE, Wannenburg T, White-Williams C, Bourge RC: Who is most likely to enjoy long term survival after cardiac transplantation? Risk stratification in a year multi-institutional experience [abstract]. J Heart Lung Transplant 2001;20:168.

lor" the treatment of patients following transplantation depending on their risk profile for future events.

Selection of Therapy for Patients with Advanced Heart Failure

As alternative long-term therapies such as chronic mechanical circulatory support become available, the proper "triage of patients" into various therapeutic options will gain increasing importance. Given that the availability of donor hearts will always be limited, there is a strong impetus to identify patients who have a suboptimal long-term result from cardiac transplantation and who, therefore, might be initially selected for long-term mechanical support trials. Equally important is the identification of patients with advanced heart failure whose survival after heart transplantation is particularly good, so that when other less-proven therapies are available, cardiac transplantation is preferentially offered to those patients with high long-term expected survival.

An opportunity for such patient- or group-specific risk factor analyses is available from the 10-year CTRD study. Among the more than 7,000 patients entered into the study, a group of more than 1,000 patients with high long-term survival (80% at 6 years) were identified (Table 16–12).[28] In contrast, patients with many comorbid conditions experienced low midterm survival. The actuarial survival from the CTRD study for the high survival and low survival groups of Table 16–12 are depicted in Table 16–13.

Refinement of Therapy and Surveillance Based on Expected Outcome Events

Reliable patient-specific predictive models could have a valuable role in predicting for specific patients the most likely adverse or fatal outcomes in the coming months or years, based on their own characteristics and their medical experiences following transplantation. If physicians knew the specific causes of death that were most likely for a given patient, specific efforts to increase surveillance or alter treatment strategies could be considered.

Consider three patients with separate risk profiles, but each of whom have a predicted 1-year survival of 80% (based on the 10-year CTRS study) (Table 16–14). A patient-specific simulation of likely causes of death can be constructed from the 10-year multi-variable analysis for each risk profile (Table 16–15). Note that in profile 1, a rather standard patient was exposed to a higher than usual risk of death from early graft failure with a suboptimal donor. Profile 2 indicates a hypothetical patient with characteristics which increase the probability of death from rejection, and profile 3 has an increased probability of infection mortality. These simulations can be depicted graphically in a patient-specific competing outcomes simulation (Figs. 16–44 to 16–46).

Similar patient-specific modeling could be used to evaluate possible adjustments in surveillance and therapy at, for example, the first annual posttransplant evaluation. Physician confidence in such simulations, of course, relates directly to the confidence in the data and the analysis which generated the simulation model. The development of such patient-specific models (Fig. 16–47) will likely form a critical component of future outcomes research in cardiac transplantation and other therapies for advanced heart failure.

TABLE 16-13	Risk Stratification for Long-Term Survival (CTRD: 1990-1999, N = 7,283)

	PERCENT SURVIVAL*		
YEARS AFTER TRANSPLANT	High Survival (N = 1,156)	Average Survival (N = 5,665)	Low Survival (N = 462)
1/12	95%	93%	85%
1/2	91%	88%	76%
1	89%	85%	72%
3	84%	78%	65%
6	80%	70%	55%
10	—	55%	44%

* Actuarial survival at indicated time interval.
From Kirklin JK, Miller LW, Brown RN, Alvarez RJ, Porter CB, Van Bakel AB, Jaski BE, Wannenburg T, White-Williams C, Bourge RC: Who is most likely to enjoy long term survival after cardiac transplantation? Risk stratification in a year multi-institutional experience [abstract]. J Heart Lung Transplant 2001;20:168.

TABLE 16-14	**Pretransplant Profiles of Three Patients and Donors**		
	PATIENT PROFILE 1	PATIENT PROFILE 2	PATIENT PROFILE 3
Recipient			
Age (yr)	35	**26**	**65**
Gender/ethnicity	Male/white	**Black**	Male/white
BMI	24	32	29
Etiology	Idiopathic	Idiopathic	Ischemic
Comorbidity	None	None	**Ventilator**
CM	+	–	+
Creatinine clearance	100	68	68
Serum creatinine	1.4	1.2	**2.0**
Sternotomies	**2**	0	0
PRA	0	0	0
RAP	9	7	7
PAs-PCWP	23	35	10
Tx date	1999	1999	1999
Donor			
Age	**44**	**40**	35
Gender	Male	Male	Male
Weight	74 kg	74 kg	74 kg
BMI	**20**	22.5	22.5
CMV	+	+	+
Ischemic time	**300**	150	180
Echo	Normal	Normal	Normal
Mismatch			
Total HLA mismatch (basic)	4	**5**	6

BMI, body mass index; CMV, cytomegalovirus; PRA, panel reactive antibodies; RAP, right atrial pressure; PAs, pulmonary atrial systolic pressure; PCWP, mean pulmonary capillary wedge pressure; HLA, human leukocyte antigen.

TABLE 16-15	**Patient-Specific Simulation for 1-Year Mortality**		
	PROBABILITY (%) OF DEATH DURING FIRST YEAR		
CAUSES OF DEATH	Patient Profile 1*	Patient Profile 2	Patient Profile 3
Early graft failure	10.0%	2.7%	5.7%
Rejection	1.8%	10.8%	0.6%
Infection	2.7%	0.9%	9.0%
Allograft CAD	0.6%	1.3%	0.3%
Malignancy	0.1%	0.0%	0.4%
Other	5.5%	5.1%	4.5%
Total	20.7%	20.8%	20.5%

* See Table 16–14 for details of each patient profile.

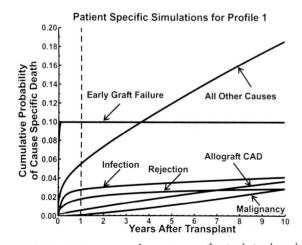

FIGURE **16-44.** Nomogram of a patient-specific simulation based on the CTRD multivariable analysis for the patient profile 1 depicted in Table 16–14. The separate causes of death are depicted in a competing outcomes analysis.

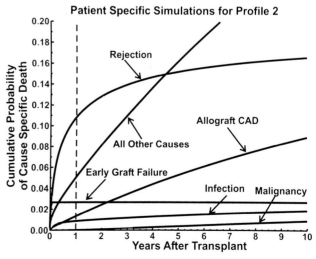

FIGURE **16-45.** Nomogram of a patient-specific simulation for patient profile 2 (Table 16–14), based on the CTRD multivariable analysis. The separate causes of death are depicted in a competing outcomes analysis.

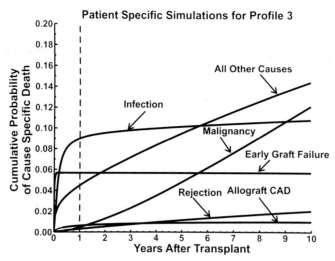

FIGURE **16–46.** Nomogram of a patient-specific simulation for patient profile 3 (Table 16–14), based on the CTRD multivariable analysis. The separate causes of death are depicted in a competing outcomes analysis.

FUTURE USE OF PATIENT SPECIFIC PREDICTIVE MODELS IN ALLOCATION OF THERAPY AND POST TRANSPLANT MANAGEMEMNT

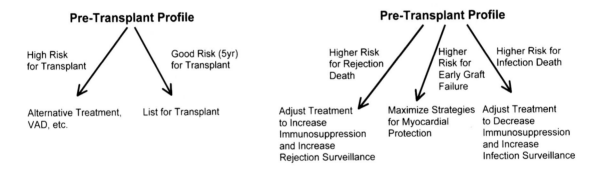

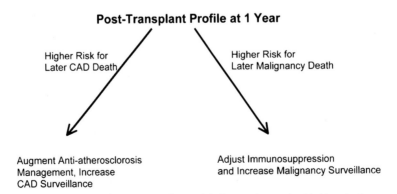

FIGURE **16–47.** Possible applications of patient-specific models for predicting the likelihood of separate causes of death following cardiac transplantation, based on multivariable analysis.

References

1. Anyanwu AC, Rogers CA, Murday AJ: Should recipient risk be a factor in choosing recipients for suboptimal donor hearts: a multi-institutional study. Transplant Proc 1999;31:1399–1400.

2. Baumgartner WA: Infection in cardiac transplantation [abstract]. Heart Transplantation 1983;3:75–80.

3. Bennett LE, Edwards EB, Jaski B: Transplantation with older donor hearts for presumed stable recipients: an analysis of the joint international society for heart and lung transplantation/United network for organ sharing thoracic registry. J Heart Lung Transplant 1998;17:901–905.

4. Bolman RM, Elick B, Olivari MT, Ring WS, Arentzen CE: Improved immunosuppression for heart transplantation. Heart Transplantation 1985;4:315–318.

5. Bourge RC, Naftel DC, Costanzo-Nordin M, Kirklin JK, Young JB, Kubo SH, Olivari MT, Kasper EK: Pretransplantation risk factors for death after heart transplantation: a multiinstitutional study. J Heart Lung Transplant 1993;12:549–562.

6. Bourge RC, Naftel DC, Hill JA, Boehmer JP, Waggoner L, Kasper EK, Lee F, Czerska B, Thomas K, Kirklin JK: The emergence of co-morbid diseases impacting survival after cardiac transplantation: a ten year multi-institutional experience [abstract]. J Heart Lung Transplant 2001;20:167.

7. Cooper DKC, Lanza RP: Heart Transplantation. Boston: Kluwer Academic Publishers, 1984.

8. Costanzo MR, Eisen HJ, Brown RN, Mehra M, Benza RL, Torre G, Yancy CW, Davis S, McCloud M, Kirklin JK: Are there specific risk factors for fatal allograft vasculopathy? An analysis of over 7,000 cardiac transplant patients [abstract]. J Heart Lung Transplant 2001;20:152.

9. Costanzo MR, Naftel DC, Pritzker MR, Heilman JK, Boehmer JP, Brozena SC, Dec GW, Ventura HO, Kirklin JK, Bourge RC, Miller LW, and the Cardiac Transplant Research Database: Heart transplant coronary artery disease detected by coronary angiography: a multiinstitutional study of preoperative donor and recipient risk factors. J Heart Lung Transplant 1998;17:744–753.

10. De Mattos AM, Head MA, Everett J, Hosenpud J, Hershberger R, Cobanoglu A, Ott G, Ratkovec R, Norman DJ: HLA-DR mismatching correlates with early cardiac allograft rejection, incidence, and graft survival when high-confidence-level serological DR typing is used. Transplantation 1994;57:626–630.

11. De Salvo TG, Naftel DC, Kasper EK: The differing hazard of lymphoma vs. other malignancies in the current era [abstract]. J Heart Lung Transplant 1998;17:7.

12. Erickson KW, Costanzo-Nordin MR, O'Sullivan J, Johnson MR, Zucker MJ, Pifarre R, Lawless CE, Robinson JA, Scanlon PJ: Influence of preoperative transpulmonary gradient on late mortality after orthotopic heart transplantation. J Heart Lung Transplant 1990;9:526–537.

13. Fraund S, Pethig K, Franke U, Wahlers T, Harringer W, Cremer J, Fieguth HG, Oppelt P, Haverich A: Ten year survival after heart transplantation: palliative procedure or successful long term treatment? Heart 1999;82:47–51.

14. Frist WH, Oyer PE, Baldwin JC, Stinson EB, Shumway N: HLA compatibility and cardiac transplant recipient survival [abstract]. Ann Thorac Surg 1987;44:242–246.

15. George JF, Kirklin JK, Shroyer TW, Naftel DC, Bourge RC, McGiffin DC: Utility of posttransplantation panel reactive antibody measurements for the prediction of rejection frequency and survival of heart transplant recipients. J Heart Lung Transplant 1995;14:856–864.

16. Gorensek MJ, Stewart RW, Keys TF: Decreased infections in cardiac transplant recipients on cyclosporine with reduced corticosteroid use. Cleve Clin J Med 1989;56:690–695.

17. Grady KL, White-Williams C, Naftel DC, Costanzo M, Pitts D, Rayburn B, VanBakel A, Jaski B, Bourge RC: Are preoperative obesity and cachexia risk factors for post heart transplant morbidity and mortality: a multi-institutional study of preoperative weight-height indices. J Heart Lung Transplant 1999;18:763.

18. Herskowitz A, Soule LM, Ueda K, Tamura F, Baumgartner WA, Borkon AM: Arteriolar vasculitis on endomyocardial biopsy: a histologic predictor of poor outcome in cyclosporine-treated heart transplant recipients. J Heart Lung Transplant 1987;6:127–136.

19. Hofflin JM, Potasman I, Baldwin JC, Oyer PE: Infectious complications in heart transplant recipients receiving cyclosporine and corticosteroids. Ann Intern Med 1987;106:209–216.

20. Hosenpud JD, Bennett LE, Keck BM, Fiol B, Boucek MM, Novick RJ: The registry of the International Society for Heart and Lung Transplantation: 15th official report. J Heart Lung Transplant 1998;17:656–668.

21. Hosenpud JD, Hershberger RE, Pantely GA: Late infection in cardiac allograft recipients: profiles, incidence, and outcome. J Heart Lung Transplant 1991;10:380–386.

22. Hosenpud JD, Novick RJ, Bennett LE, Keck BM, Fiol B, Daily P: The registry of the International Society for Heart and Lung Transplantation: 13th official report 1996. J Heart Lung Transplant 1996;15:655–674.

23. Hosenpud JD, Novick RJ, Breen TJ, Keck BM, Daily P: The registry of the International Society for Heart and Lung Transplantation: 12th official report 1995. J Heart Lung Transplant 1995;14:805–815.

24. Jarcho J, Naftel DC, Shroyer TW, Kirklin JK, Bourge RC, Barr ML, Pitts D, Starling RC: Influence of HLA mismatch on rejection after heart transplantation: a multi-institutional study. J Heart Lung Transplant 1994;13:583.

25. John R, Rajasinghe H, Chen JM, Weinberg AD, Sinha P, Itescu S, Lietz K, Mancini D, Oz MC, Smith CR, Rose EA, Edwards NM: Impact of current management practices early and late death in more than 500 consecutive cardiac transplant recipients. Ann Surg 2000;232:302–311.

26. Kerman RH, Kimball P, Scheinen S, Radovancevic B, Van Buren CT, Kahan BD, Frazier OH: The relationship among donor-recipient HLA mismatches, rejection, and death from coronary artery disease in cardiac transplant recipients. Transplantation 1994;57:884–888.

27. Kirklin JW, Barratt-Boyes BG: Cardiac Surgery. New York: Churchill Livingstone, 1992.

28. Kirklin JK, Miller LW, Brown RN, Alvarez RJ, Porter CB, Van Bakel AB, Jaski BE, Wannenburg T, White-Williams C, Bourge RC: Who is most likely to enjoy long term survival after cardiac transplantation? Risk stratification in a year multi-institutional experience [abstract]. J Heart Lung Transplant 2001;20:168.

29. Kirklin JK, Naftel DC, Kirklin JW, Blackstone EH, White-Williams C, Bourge R: Pulmonary vascular resistance and the risk of heart transplantation. J Heart Lung Transplant 1988;7:331–336.

30. Kirklin JK, Naftel DC, Levine TB, Bourge RC, Pelletier G, O'Donnell J, Miller LW, Pritzker MH: Cytomegalovirus after heart transplantation. Risk factors for infection and death: a multi-institutional study. J Heart Lung Transplant 1994;13:394–404.

31. Kobashigawa J, Kirklin JK, Naftel DC, Bourge RC, White-Williams C, Mohanty P, Clintron GB, Bhat G: Pretransplantation risk factors for acute rejection after heart transplantation: a multiinstitution study. J Heart Lung Transplant 1993;12:355–366.

32. Lavee J, Kormos RL, Duquesnoy RJ, Zerbe TR, Armitage JM, Vanek M, Hardesty RL, Griffith BP: Influence of panel-reactive antibody and lymphocytotoxic crossmatch on survival after heart transplantation. J Heart Lung Transplant 1991;10:921–930.

33. Lazda VA: The impact of HLA frequency differences in races on the access to optimally HLA-matched cadaver renal transplants. Transplantation 1992;53:352–357.

34. Miller LW, Naftel DC, Bourge RC: Infection after heart transplantation: a multiinstitutional study. J Heart Lung Transplant 1994;13:381–393.

35. Mills RM, Naftel DC, Kirklin JK, Van Bakel AB, Jaski BE, Massin EK, Eisen HJ, Lee FA, Fishbein DP, Bourge RC: Heart transplant rejection with hemodynamic compromise: a multiinstitutional study of the role of endomyocardial cellular infiltrate. J Heart Lung Transplant 1997;16:813–821.

36. Opelz G: Effect of HLA matching in heart transplantation. Collaborative Heart Transplant Study [abstract]. Transplant Proc 1989;21:794–796.

37. Pennington DG, Kanter KR, McBride LR: Seven years experience with the Pierce-Donachy ventricular assist device. J Thorac Cardiovasc Surg 1988;96:901–911.

38. Robin J, Ninet J, Trone F, Bonnefoy E, Neidecker J, Boissonat P, Champsaur G: Long term results of heart transplantation deteriorate more rapidly in patients over 60 years of age. Eur J Cardiothorac Surg 1996;10:259–263.

39. Rodeheffer RJ, Naftel DC, Stevenson LW, Porter CB, Young JB, Millee LW, Kenzora JL, Haas GJ, Kirklin JK, Bourge RC: Secular trends in cardiac transplant recipient and donor management in the united states 1990 to 1994. Circulation 1996;94:2883–2889.

40. Rose EA, Smith CR, Petrossian GA, Barr ML, Reemitsma K: Humoral immune responses after cardiac transplantation: correlation with fatal rejection and graft atherosclerosis. Surgery 1989;106:203–208.

41. Sharples LD, Caine N, Mullins P, Scott JP, Solis E, English TAH, Large SR, Schofield PM, Wallwork J: Risk factor analysis for the major hazards following heart transplantation—rejection, infection, and coronary occlusive disease. Transplantation 1991;52:244–252.

42. Smart F, Naftel DC, Costanzo M, Levine T, Pelletier G, Yancy C, Hobbs R, Kirklin J, Bourge R: Risk factors for early, cumulative and fatal infections after heart transplantation: a multiinstitutional study. J Heart Lung Transplant 1996;15:329–341.

43. Smith SH, Kirklin JK, Geer JC, Caulfield JB, McGiffin DC: Arteritis in cardiac rejection after transplantation. Am J Cardiol 1987;59:1171–1173.

44. Stinson EB, Bieber CP, Griepp RB, Clark DA, Shumway NE: Infectious complications after cardiac transplantation in man. Ann Intern Med 1971;74:22–36.

45. UNOS United Netwoork for Organ Sharing—Annual Report. Annual Report 2000.

46. Yancy CW, Naftel DC, Foley BA, Kobashigawa JA, Pitts D, Rodeheffer RJ, Renlund DG, Kaiser EG, McGiffin DC: Death after heart transplantation: a competing outcomes analysis. J Heart Lung Transplant 2000;19:52.

47. Young JB, Hauptman PJ, Naftel DC, Ewald G, Aaronson K, Dec GW, Taylor DO, Higgins R, Platt L, Kirklin JK: Determinants of early graft failure following cardiac transplantation, a 10 year multi-institutional, multi-variable analysis [abstract]. J Heart Lung Transplant 2001;20:212.

48. Young JB, Naftel DC, Bourge RC, Kirklin JK, Clemson BS, Porter CB, Rodeheffer RJ, Kenzora JL: Matching the heart donor and heart transplant recipient. Clues for successful expansion of the donor pool: a multivariable, multiinstitutional report. J Heart Lung Transplant 1994;13:365.

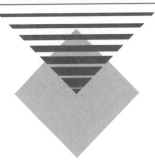

CHAPTER SEVENTEEN

Cardiac Allograft Vasculopathy (Chronic Rejection)

with the collaboration of
RAYMOND L. BENZA, M.D. AND JOSE TALLAJ, M.D.

Chronic rejection of the cardiac allograft, also called allograft vasculopathy, refers to the concentric narrowing or focal obstruction of the coronary arteries (and sometimes veins) of the transplanted heart. Though more often occurring late after transplantation, it sometimes can represent a fulminant process seen several months following surgery. Importantly, allograft arteriopathy with subsequent ischemia and myocardial dysfunction appears to be a leading cause of death during long-term follow-up of heart transplant recipients. The use of the term *rejection* for this process implies an immunologic basis which will be discussed in this chapter. However, the term chronic rejection must be clearly differentiated from the term humoral rejection, which is discussed in Chapter 14 and implies an acute antibody-mediated process with microvascular involvement. This disease should also be distinguished from "native vessel" atherosclerosis, which is present *de novo* in the donor heart and transferred as a passive passenger into the allograft recipient. Though this passenger atherosclerosis can have important consequences and sequelae, its pathophysiology, tendency to progress, and response to therapy can be quite different than the arteriopathy characterized as chronic rejection. Our understanding of chronic rejection has been further complicated by the pathophysiology of its development and progression, which undoubtedly includes components of passenger "native vessel" atherosclerosis, immune-mediated endothelial damage, and atherosclerosis which develops and progresses after transplantation.

TABLE 17–1	**Chronic Cardiac Allograft Rejection Terms**

Cardiac allograft vasculopathy
Allograft arteriopathy
Allograft vascular disease
Transplant coronary artery disease
Accelerated graft atherosclerosis
Graft vascular disease
Posttransplant vascular occlusive disease
Secondary atheromatous disease
Obliterative arteritis
Intimal proliferative disease
Vascular immuno-obliterative disease

Many terms have been used to describe this potentially devastating process (Table 17–1). In order to distinguish chronic rejection and allograft vascular disease from native coronary artery disease, we will use the term **cardiac allograft vasculopathy,** allograft vascular disease, allograft arteriopathy, or allograft coronary artery disease. These are broad enough characterizations that include both arterial and venous processes.

HISTORICAL PERSPECTIVE

Pathologic processes associated with transplantation of arterial conduits and organs have been observed for many decades. Indeed, in a landmark series of experiments dealing with arterial vessel preservation and transplantation, Alexis Carrel in 1910 reported the fact that canine carotid artery allografts in place for 90 days demonstrated an abnormally thickened intima, degenerated muscle fibers of the media, and muscle cells invading the intima more often than not. Carrel also noted that, in one transplant experiment, the carotid artery was yellow in color only over the segment that had been transplanted.[37] Carrel was wise enough to hypothesize that gaining insight into this transplanted vessel process might contribute to understanding the pathogenesis of atherosclerosis more generally. Remember that atherosclerotic disease was an enigma at that time (as it still in large part is), with the term "atherosclerosis" just coming into use to characterize obliterative arterial disease in the first decade of the 1900s. Indeed, the pathophysiology of atherosclerosis was outlined by J. G. Adami in 1909, with his thesis stating that atherosclerosis was a response to injury.[1] Carrel hypothesized that implantation of the carotid artery from one animal into another prompted an initial injury characterized by disintegration of tissues and autolytic fermentations with subsequent metabolic arrest and suspension of vital cellular activities. These notations were coupled with Carrel's observations of basic biologic incompatibility associated more generally with solid organ transplant experiments (see Chapter 1). Hume in 1955[146] described widespread atherosclerosis in the large- and medium-sized vessels of cadaveric renal allografts when anastomosed to the profunda artery and femoral vein. This atherosclerosis was quite distinct from that seen in the native vessels. In Hume's early report, renal graft function for over 5 months was noted, with no immunosuppression other than 2 months of testosterone administration. Though Hume's manuscript mentioned the possibility of antibodies and individuality precipitating the disease, the patient had been severely hypertensive, and it was this difficulty that was ultimately blamed for the atherosclerotic process.

As experience with renal transplantation grew, the presence of renal artery allograft vasculopathy became more evident and did not appear to correlate with either radiation or drug immunosuppressive therapy. In the early era of solid organ transplantation, total lymphoid irradiation, azathioprine, 6-mercaptopurine, actinomycin, chlorambucil, cyclophosphamide, or hydrocortisone was used with varying frequency and regimens, and patients sometimes developed renal allograft arteriopathy which characterizes allograft vascular disease in general. Porter in 1963[243] suggested that allograft vascular disease was present in well over one third of renal grafts that survived longer than 32 days. The disease was unresponsive to intensification of immunosuppression, and these investigators believed that the pathologic process was likely a manifestation of "rejection" in its late stages. Porter also suggested that allograft vascular disease could be precipitated by systemic hypertension or graft ischemia.

Cardiac allograft vasculopathy was first highlighted by Lower in 1968 when he and his team reported that intimal proliferative and obliterative coronary artery changes characteristic of chronic vascular rejection were noted in the epicardial coronary arteries of long-term canine heart transplant recipients.

Allograft vascular disease in a human heart transplant was first reported in an early short-term post–heart transplant survivor from Christiaan Barnard's Cape Town experience. Thompson[304] detailed the anatomic findings of an autopsy performed on Barnard's longest surviving heart transplant recipient at the time. The patient was a 58-year-old gentleman who had lived almost 19 months after his surgery. Thompson characterized the coronary arteries as having broad, yellow, uniformly atheromatous lesions. He noted that every coronary artery from the main trunk of the epicardial vessels to the smallest intramuscular branches seemed affected. The diffuseness and rapid progression of this obliterative arteriopathy in the absence of clinical signs of ischemic heart disease were notable to Thompson. In fact, he commented on his amazement at the findings by noting the atheroma had a higher intensity and wider distribution than any he had seen in 40 years of performing autopsies. Interestingly, these dramatic findings led Thompson to suggest that patients with ischemic heart disease and high cholesterol levels should not undergo cardiac transplantation. Shortly after Thompson's observations came to fore, the longest living heart transplant survivor amongst Stanford University's cohort died of an acute myocardial infarction 21 months after surgery. Necropsy findings in this individual, and six other early heart transplant recipients surviving greater than 1 month, included obliterative vasculitis of the coronary arteries.[23]

All of these observations prompted Griepp and colleagues to introduce the practice of routine posttransplant surveillance annual coronary arteriography in 1972.[116] Subsequently, this group reported on the natural history of the process with recommendations regarding control of the problem after human heart transplant.[115] The Stanford group suggested treating heart transplant patients postoperatively with prophylactic warfarin and dipyridamole in conjunction with weight control and a low-cholesterol and low-saturated-fat diet. The pioneers of transplantation did not know what a dramatic and difficult long-term problem allograft vasculopathy would turn out to be.

PATHOLOGY OF CARDIAC ALLOGRAFT VASCULOPATHY

The basic pathologic lesion of transplant vasculopathy is a diffuse and progressive thickening of the arterial intima that develops in both the epicardial and intramyocardial arteries of the transplanted heart. The anatomic layers of the arterial wall are shown in Figure 17–1. There are many similarities between the pathological findings in ordinary atherosclerosis and allograft vasculopathy. Perhaps most importantly, both processes involve primarily the arterial intima, with relative sparing of the underlying media.

MACROSCOPIC APPEARANCE

When hearts with chronic rejection are studied at autopsy, a variety of gross macroscopic changes can be noted. The anastomotic sites at the great vessels are generally completely healed, and this occurs within a

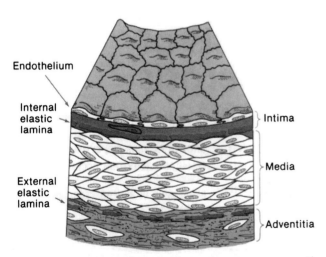

Endothelium

Internal elastic lamina

Intima

Media

External elastic lamina

Adventitia

FIGURE **17-1.** Structure of a normal muscular coronary artery. The intima is lined by endothelial cells on its inner (luminal) aspect and bounded by the internal elastic lamina on its outer aspect. The media is the muscular portion of the arterial wall, bounded by the internal elastic lamina and external elastic lamina. The adventitia forms the outer layer of the arterial wall. (From Ross R, Glomset J: The pathogenesis of atherosclerosis [abstract]. N Engl J Med 1976;295:369. Copyright 1976 Massachusetts Medical Society, with permission.)

few weeks. Suture lines are buried in connective tissue, with smooth endocardial surfaces overlying the region of the anastomoses. Atherosclerotic changes can be noted in the proximal donor aorta, with striking demarcation between the native recipient aorta distal to the anastomoses and atheroma present more proximally. Thrombus formation and infection foci are generally not reported. In patients dying of chronic rejection, the gross appearance of the myocardium is most generally characterized by profound hypertrophy with variable extent of scarring.

Figure 17–2 is a transverse section of an autopsy heart specimen taken from a 28-year-old male dying 8 months after transplant of sudden onset cardiogenic shock (without prior angina pectoris). Shortly after transplantation, baseline coronary angiography revealed normal coronary anatomy and did not suggest the presence of significant donor-derived coronary artery disease. The specimen shows extensive areas of scarring throughout the left ventricle. Many aspects of the scars suggested healed myocardial infarctions.

Occasional patients dying of sudden cardiac death syndrome after long-term heart transplant have been noted to have relatively little diffuse disease. Rarely, a discrete location of occlusion may be particularly obvious, such as in the artery supplying the atrioventricular node. In arteries demonstrating superimposed thrombus, this coronary obstruction is typically more extensive and not as clearly associated with plaque rupture as is native vessel coronary artery disease. Sometimes, old occlusive thrombus is noted that has undergone fibrous replacement and recanalization.

In some hearts, evidence of old scar suggesting remote myocardial infarction is coupled with an acute infarct caused by superimposed thrombotic obstruction of allograft coronary arteries. Macroscopic inspection of the coronary arteries will generally demonstrate them to be quite abnormal. The major trunks of the epicardial coronary arteries are diffusely thickened, and a yellowish hue due to lipid deposition in the vessel wall can often be appreciated. On transverse section of the epicardial arteries, marked reduction in luminal cross-sectional area is frequently seen with generally symmetric enlargement of the intima and media. Occasionally, superimposed thrombosis, as alluded to above, can be seen. The epicardial surface of the heart is not infrequently bound by dense fibrous adhesions to adjacent mediastinum, while the native portions of the pulmonary arteries and aorta generally appear grossly unremarkable.

DISTRIBUTION OF DISEASE

The distribution of intimal proliferation in allograft vascular disease can extend to almost every segment of the coronary arterial tree. Large and small epicardial and some penetrating intramyocardial arteries with a well-defined muscular layer are frequently involved.[23, 24, 26, 53, 57, 155, 311] Involvement of these smaller intramyocardial arteries is seen more frequently in longer term survi-

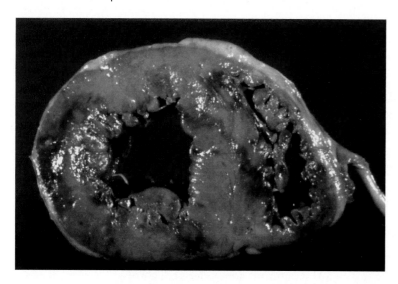

FIGURE **17–2.** Cross-section of heart of a patient who died with allograft arteriopathy. The multiple areas of infarcted tissue are noted to be both chronic and acute.

vors.[53] Smaller vessels less than 40 μm which lack an organized muscular layer are generally spared.[57,155] Arterioles with a muscular media between 50 and 100 μm are variably involved, and those larger than 100–150 μm are nearly universally affected.[23,53,57] Although the degree of intimal proliferation is thought to increase in the distal, smaller arteries, in actuality it is fairly uniform between the proximal and distal portions of these vessels. This "obliterative" appearance commonly referred to on angiogram most likely results from the naturally smaller distal luminal areas, which may be occluded by less intimal thickening than would be required proximally.

Despite the diffuse nature of the general disease process, many aspects suggest a heterogeneous involvement of the coronary arterial tree. It is common to find both concentric and eccentric areas of intima plaque, more pronounced intimal thickening at branch points, and multiple areas of focal epicardial stenosis. These features suggest a pathogenesis similar to conventional atherosclerosis.[210]

MICROSCOPIC APPEARANCE

Microscopic changes of allograft vasculopathy can be seen as early as 30 days after transplant. However, it is important to distinguish allograft vasculopathy from passenger atherosclerosis that is donor derived. A careful epicardial artery cross-sectional analysis may demonstrate focal coronary atherosclerosis more typical of native vessel disease during autopsy evaluation.

Depending upon the survival time of the recipient and cause of death, a variety of coronary changes can be noted. Many findings are related to myocardial vessels, while others characterize the immunologic status (degree of inflammatory cellular infiltrate) of the patient at the time of death. Patients surviving long term after heart transplantation still may show evidence of concomitant acute cellular rejection or microvascular rejection (see Chapter 14). Focal lymphocytic infiltration may also be seen in perimeter zones of myocardial infarction.

Intima

Marked proliferation of myointimal cells is the most striking and significant component of allograft vascular disease (Figs. 17–3 and 17–4). It is this process which leads to the progressive obliteration of the lumen of epicardial branches of the main coronary arteries. This process extends down through the penetrating branches as well as many intracardiac small coronary branches. This diffuse and prominent intramyocardial coronary artery involvement with concentric intimal fibrosis of marked degree is one overriding characteristic of the pathology of cardiac allograft vasculopathy. However, the intimal thickening in the epicardial coronary arteries may be quite eccentric. Lipid deposits are common in the epicardial vessels but are generally not seen in the thickened intima of the intramyocardial vessels.

The arterial pathologic changes in chronic rejection are typically an **accelerated form of arteriosclerosis.** Indeed, the lesions of allograft vascular disease mature over time, producing a spectrum of coronary vessel pathology, but that period is extraordinarily compressed compared to native vessel atherosclerosis. Microscopically, the **intima of the allograft coronary artery is thickened by the proliferation of smooth muscle cells.** Sometimes, clusters of lipid-filled macrophages or foam cells can be seen to lie adjacent to the internal elastic lamina, but the lamina is largely intact, with only occasional areas of fragmentation or reduplication through which smooth muscle cells migrate.

Occasionally, lymphocytes (generally cytotoxic lymphocytes) are noted to be infiltrating the subendothelial layer, producing a so-called "endothelialitis." There is controversy over whether this term accurately characterizes the immunobiology of allograft atherosclerotic disease, since the relationship of the lymphocytes to subsequent development of graft arteriopathy is not clearly delineated.

The **intimal morphological features** of allograft vasculopathy have been classified into four general categories based on the prominence of fibrous intimal thickening versus atheromatous degeneration, the distribu-

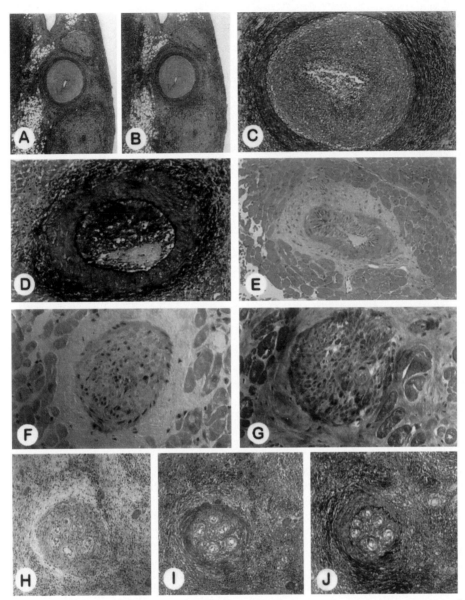

FIGURE **17–3.** Vasculopathy, light microscopy. *A,* Light micrograph showing an epicardial coronary artery with severe narrowing of its lumen by intimal proliferation of cells and deposition of connective tissue (red-blue). The smooth muscle of the media is stained red. The adventitia is fibrotic and stains blue. The myocaradium also stains red (left). There are two large foci of lymphocytic infiltrate flanking the coronary artery (Masson's trichrome, 1.25X). *B,* A section adjacent to *A* is shown. This section shows the delimitation of the media and the intima with more clarity (darker red media and light pink-red intima) (Verhoeff-Van Gieson elastic stain, 1.25X). *C,* Higher magnification showing the intima, media, and adventitia. The intima shows marked proliferation of cells which almost completely narrow its lumen. There is conspicuous vacuolation of the cells indicating that there is intracellular lipid accumulation. Note that the elastic laminae are intact (Verhoeff-Van Gieson elastic stain, 4X). *D,* A smaller intracardiac coronary artery shows an eccentric lesion in the intima that partially occludes its lumen (>60%). There is a small thrombus with entrapped erythrocytes (yellow cells) in the lower part of the arterial lumen (Verhoeff-Van Gieson elastic stain, 10X). *E,* Small intracardiac coronary artery shows early proliferative disease in the intima and abundant proteoglycan accumulation (light blue discoloration subjacent to the endothelial cells). Note the abundant fibrosis of the adventitia, hematoxylin & eosin [H&E], (20X). *F,* Occlusive proliferation of smooth muscle cells in a small intramural coronary artery (H&E, 40X). *G,* This stain proves that most of the luminal narrowing is secondary to smooth muscle proliferation (red staining cells) and little accumulation of collagen (Masson's trichrome, 40X). *H,* Recanalized intramural coronary artery secondary to healed vasculitis (H&E, 20X). *I,* The same artery as *H* shows marked adventitial and intraluminal accumulation of collagen (Masson's trichrome, 20X). *J,* The elastic stain shows a fragmented elastic lamina suggestive of earlier vasculitis (Verhoeff-Van Gieson elastic stain, 20X).

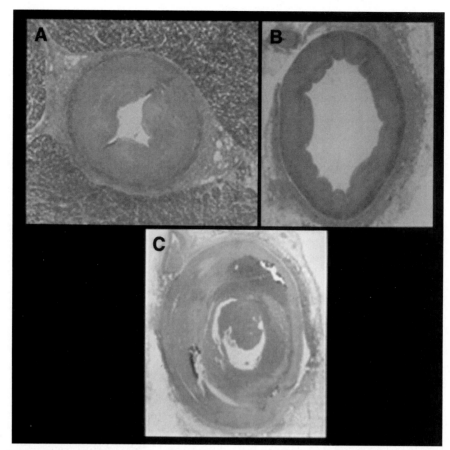

FIGURE **17-4.** Cross-section of a coronary artery with severe allograft vasculopathy (*A*) and native vessel coronary artery disease (*B* and *C*) in a patient with a heterotopic heart transplant who died with severe vasculopathy of the transplanted heart (*A*) and acute infarction of the native heart (*C*). A more normal native coronary artery is seen in *B*.

tion of disease, and elapsed time since transplantation.[155] Although there are exceptions to these descriptions, they provide a useful framework for categorizing the intimal morphology.

Coronary Arteries with No to Mild Intimal Thickening

In the absence of important passenger (transmitted) allograft coronary artery disease, the intima in allograft coronaries within 6 months of transplant generally shows mild intimal thickening and/or fibrosis, with a mild increase in myointimal cells and extracellular matrix.[23]

Fibrous Intimal Thickening Confined to Proximal and Midcoronary Arteries

During the first posttransplant year, the most common lesion is hyperplasia of the large- to medium-sized epicardial arteries, with sparing of the smallest epicardial branches and the intramyocardial branches.[155] Intimal thickening is due primarily to an increased extracellular matrix and proliferation of cells with prominent myofilaments (myointimal cells).[25, 53, 57] The extracellular space contains a mixture of fibrous tissue or collagen, a myxoid basophilic ground substance, and deposits of fibrin intermixed with intact and fragmented red blood

cells and nuclear debris, probably because of a breach of the endothelial integrity. Monoclonal antibody (MAb) markers specific for smooth muscle performed on explanted hearts confirms that these myointimal cells are transformed smooth muscle cells.[24] The degree of luminal compromise is usually mild to moderate in this category, although significant narrowing can be present in some instances.[25, 155] This type of fibrous intimal thickening limited to the large epicardial vessels can be observed as early as 1 week and as late as 4–5 years after transplantation.[155]

Fibrofatty Atheromatous Plaques of Proximal to Mid Regions of Epicardial Arteries Only

Hearts surviving more than 1 year often develop fibrofatty atheromatous plaques localized to the large- and medium-sized epicardial coronary arteries, with relatively normal small arterial segments. These plaques are composed of a dense fibrous layer overlying a lipid-rich pool of extracellular cholesterol clefts, vacuolated lipoproteinaceous material, and foam cells.[23–25, 82, 155, 311] Spindle-shaped intimal smooth muscle cells are common in the collagenous zones overlying the fatty deposits. These plaques closely resemble native vessel coronary atherosclerosis and in some cases, when discovered early after transplant, may represent donor disease. In-

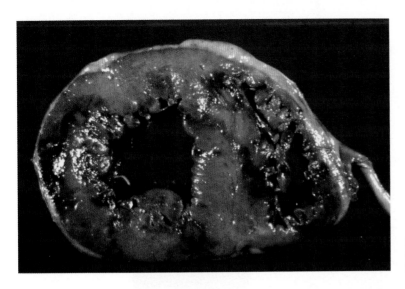

FIGURE **17–2.** Cross-section of heart of a patient who died with allograft arteriopathy. The multiple areas of infarcted tissue are noted to be both chronic and acute.

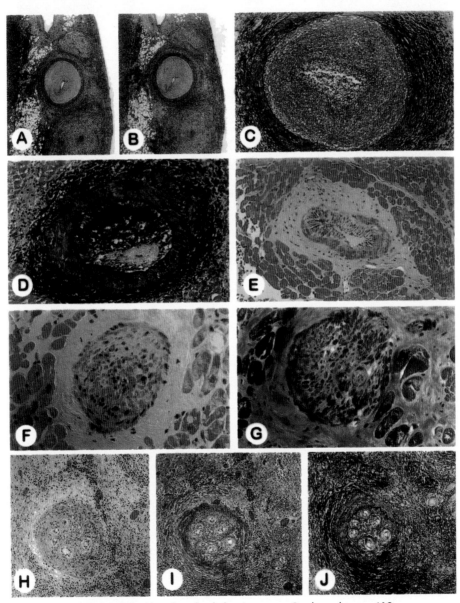

FIGURE **17–3.** Vasculopathy, light microscopy. See legend, page 619.

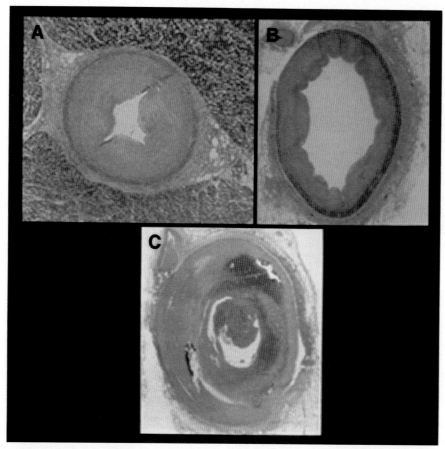

FIGURE **17-4.** Cross-section of a coronary artery with severe allograft vasculopathy (*A*) and native vessel coronary artery disease (*B* and *C*) in a patient with a heterotopic heart transplant who died with severe vasculopathy of the transplanted heart (*A*) and acute infarction of the native heart (*C*). A more normal native coronary artery is seen in *B*.

terestingly, some of these fatty lesions called "intermediate" lesions possess only sheets of lipid-laden foam cells (transformed smooth muscle cells or macrophages) present in the interface between the elastic interna and fibrotic intima but no well-defined extracellular lipid core.[23, 25, 26, 155, 311] Sex chromatin determinations in cross-sex transplants indicate that these cells are of donor origin.[23]

The distribution of lipid and therefore the ultimate morphologic appearance of these lesions depends in general on the relative amount of time that has passed since transplant. The intermediate concentric lesions are more common earlier after transplant and are rare if the graft has survived more than 5 years. The classic appearing eccentric atheromas (fibrofatty lesions) become much more common in grafts surviving longer than 6 years. Eccentricity of these lesions also appears to be time dependent and varies with the relative amount of extracellular lipid. Many of these eccentric lesions represent focal stenoses and contain a large extracellular lipid component. Plaque calcification is frequently present in hearts older than 5 years and in those with a more atheromatous appearance.[155]

Diffuse Fibrous Intimal Thickening with or without Atheromatous Plaques

This last category is often referred to in descriptions of allograft coronary artery disese. This category is distinguished from the earlier described "fibrous intimal thickening category" primarily by the widespread and diffuse nature of the intimal proliferation. Grafts with this severe form of intimal proliferation typically range from 2–11 years after implantation. This manifestation of allograft vascular disease involves not only the large and small epicardial arteries, but now also the intramyocardial coronary arteries as well. It is limited to coronary arteries with a muscular media and most strikingly narrows the first portions of the intramyocardial branches. The smallest vessels, which lack an organized muscular coat, are spared.[23, 26, 155] Because the small branches of the coronary circulation are involved, it produces a "pruning effect" on coronary angiogram.[26] Progressive proliferation of intimal cells results in considerable narrowing of terminal coronary artery lumens to the point of almost complete occlusion.[25, 26, 311] In light of the diffuse nature of this form of the disease and because small vessels are involved, multiple small infarcts may be observed in the myocardium.[155, 311] This morphologic subset of allograft vasculopathy is usually not seen in isolation, but rather in conjunction with atheromatous plaques.[25, 26, 155]

Elastic Lamina

The internal elastic lamina is a collagenous band within the vessel wall that serves as a physical barrier between the intima and media (see again Fig. 17–1). The changes that occur to this structure are often used to distinguish allograft vasculopathy from native atherosclerosis. It is commonly stated that the elastic lamina remains virtually intact except for small breaks in allograft vasculopathy, as opposed to native atherosclerosis, where it is commonly disrupted.[23, 24, 26, 57] Although generally true, it is well documented that allograft vasculopathy late after transplant (>5 years) has a greater similarity to native vessel atherosclerosis, with a fibrofatty appearance and more frequent disruption of the internal elastic lamina.[53]

Media

The changes described for the media are distinctly different from the intima. In arteries with little or no intimal proliferation, the thickness of the media is usually within normal limits and appears unaffected by graft coronary disease.[24, 25] Attenuation and focal fibrous or fatty replacement of the media is seen in hearts with fibrofatty atheromatous plaques.[155] In patients with diffuse fibrous intimal thickening with or without atheromatous plaques, complete fibrous replacement of the media is common.[23, 26, 57, 155]

Veins

Though the term "cardiac allograft vasculopathy" is frequently used to include changes noted in the intramyocardial veins, in reality veins are seldom affected by this process. When it is noted, only very modest intimal fibrous thickening is usually apparent.

DIFFERENCES BETWEEN NATIVE VESSEL ATHEROSCLEROSIS AND ALLOGRAFT VASCULOPATHY

The morphologic characteristics and histological features of allograft vascular disease compared with native vessel coronary artery disease are listed in Table 17–2. It should be remembered that coronary lesions in transplanted hearts may be remnants of native vessel atherosclerosis that are transported as passengers when the heart is moved from donor to recipient. Also important is the fact that new lesions occurring after transplantation can resemble typical atherosclerotic lesions noted in vessels of hearts not transplanted. Though many vessels affected by allograft vascular disease are indistinguishable from native vessel and more ordinary atherosclerosis, the most often cited characteristics of allograft vasculopathy from a microscopic viewpoint which differentiate it from ordinary atherosclerosis are the presence of an active or healed vasculitis in the affected vessels, a prominence of outer medial defects due to foam cell transformation in the epicardial coronary arteries, the diffuse nature of the atherosclerosis, the obliterative narrowing of intramyocardial coronary arteries, calcification being observed less frequently in graft arteriopathy, an intact internal elastic lamina, and a different deposition pattern. As will subsequently be discussed, native vessel coronary artery disease, unlike allograft vasculopathy, rarely is associated with up-regulation of major histocompatibility receptor complexes on the endothelial surfaces. Ordinary atherosclerosis has a predilection for arterial branch points, whereas second- and third-order arterial branches and penetrating intramyo-

TABLE 17–2	Typical Differences Between Allograft Vascular Disease and Native Vessel Coronary Artery Disease	
PATHOLOGIC CHARACTERISTIC	ALLOGRAFT VASCULAR DISEASE	NATIVE CORONARY ARTERY DISEASE
Lesion morphology	Diffuse, concentric, but variable	Focal, proximal, eccentric
Vessels involved	Intramyocardial, epicardial branches	Epicardial, spares intramyocardial branches
Veins involved	Yes	No
Collateral vessels	Minimal	Often extensive
Initial lesion	Smooth muscle cell proliferation	Fatty streaks
Internal elastic lamina	Intact	Disrupted
Endothelial lymphocytes	Sometimes	Absent
T-cell location	Subendothelial	Edge of plaque
Endothelial MHC class II	Present	Absent
Calcium deposition	Rare	Common
Inflammation	Present	Rare

MHC, major histocompatibility.

cardial arteries tend to be spared. In contrast, allograft vasculopathy typically has diffuse involvement of all arterial levels, although focal lesions are also commonly observed.

PATHOPHYSIOLOGY AND IMMUNOBIOLOGY OF ALLOGRAFT VASCULAR DISEASE

OVERVIEW

Endothelial cells line the luminal aspect of the intima and, in the cardiac allograft, provide the barrier between the blood elements of the recipient and the myocardial cells of donor origin. Furthermore, endothelial cells represent the site which is initially and constantly presented to host immune cells and molecules. Endothelial cell injury is the seminal event which triggers the cellular and metabolic sequences leading to allograft vasculopathy. Many direct and indirect sources of information suggest that the basic sequence of cellular events which generate and propagate the lesions of allograft vascular disease are qualitatively similar to those of ordinary atherosclerosis. For example, although the process is characteristically diffuse, nearly half of affected patients also have focal areas of stenosis in epicardial arteries, more typical of nontransplant atherosclerosis.[162, 211]

Much of the knowledge about the pathophysiology of transplant allograft vascular disease in humans has been derived from animal models, mostly from studies in rats,[2, 48, 128] rabbits,[6, 177] and mice.[267, 278] There is general agreement from these studies that in both processes there is an early inflammatory infiltration of the arterial intima by T-lymphocytes and monocytes/macrophages which precedes the subsequent expansion of the intima with smooth muscle cells and extracellular matrix proteins, promoted by a variety of cytokines and growth factors (Fig. 17–5). The causes of allograft injury have been categorized as alloantigen independent (including the basic atherosclerotic mechanisms, endothelial dam-

age at the time of transplant, and infection) and alloantigen dependent (including the immunologic response to the new graft) mechanisms (Fig. 17–6). Cardiac allograft vasculopathy, then, is the end result of this chronic inflammatory process that elicits a repair response which induces the proliferation of vascular wall smooth muscle cells and the production of a connective tissue matrix that eventually compromises the vascular lumen.[65] The components and details of this pathophysiologic process following cardiac transplantation are discussed in the following sections.

THE ATHEROSCLEROTIC COMPONENT

Response-to-Injury Hypothesis

Current theories about the pathogenesis of atherosclerotic lesions date back to the studies of Virchow,[320] von Rokitansky,[321] Duguid,[62] and others. In 1973, Ross and Glomset[264, 266] proposed the *Response-to-Injury Hypothesis* in the pathogenesis of atherosclerosis. This hypothesis states that an initial "**injury**" to the endothelium results in a variety of manifestations of **endothelial dysfunction**. This dysfunctional state is characterized by "activation" of the endothelium in which a cascade of molecular and cellular events occur (see subsequent sections) which culminate in intimal thickening and ultimately luminal narrowing or obliteration.

In native vessel atherosclerosis, the exact causative factor (source of injury) which leads to endothelial injury and activation is unknown, and a variety of mechanisms have been proposed. Among possible inciting factors, it is now well accepted that oxidized low-density lipoprotein is atherogenic.[295, 296] Lipids are essential for maintaining homeostasis of the endothelium-blood barrier and produce antioxidants.[206] When the low-density lipoprotein component of cholesterol is oxidized, it becomes chemotactic for monocytes and macrophages, which become foam cells and are incorporated into the atherosclerotic plaque.[248] Oxidized low-density lipoprotein is directly cytotoxic to arterial endothelium, induces the release of cytokines from macrophages, and these cyto-

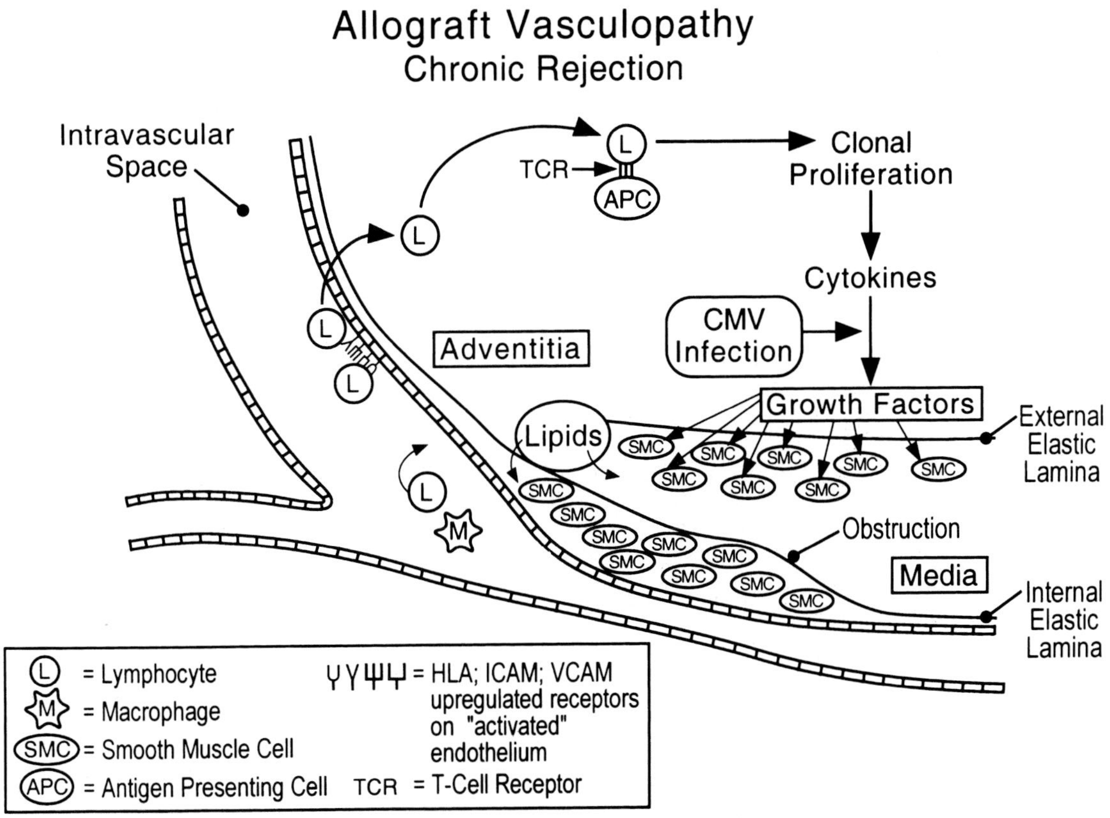

Allograft Vasculopathy
Chronic Rejection

FIGURE **17-5.** A unifying concept of the development of allograft arteriopathy. Coronary obstructive lesions in the allograft develop after endothelial injury, followed by a typical reparative response that is inflammatory cell driven. T-lymphocytes, macrophages, and neutrophils migrate to the subendothelial spaces by interacting with a variety of adhesion molecules and HLA receptors that are expressed after the endothelial cells become "activated." T-cell clones are up-regulated, and in the process, a variety of cytokines and growth factors become elaborated. In addition to their effects on the myocyte, these agents stimulate smooth muscle cell proliferation which leads to coronary atherosclerosis and lumen obstruction. Lipid perturbation and CMV infection as well as other nonimmune factors play a significicant role in the process.

kines impair arteriolar dilatation (normally modulated by endothelium-derived relaxing factor).[34, 172] The link between dyslipidemia after cardiac transplantation and allograft vascular disease is supported by observations that allograft vascular disease in animal models develops more rapidly when hyperlipemic conditions are created.[214]

In **allograft vascular disease,** the exact molecular mechanisms have not been elucidated, but there is considerable evidence that several powerful sources of endothelial injury are presented to the transplanted heart, including the initial ischemia/reperfusion injury, episodes of acute cellular rejection, antibody-mediated (humoral) rejection, possibly infections such as cytomegalovirus, and chronic exposure of the allograft endothelial surface to the activated host immune system; all occurring in the face of (and likely contributing to) the variety of factors operative in the basic atherosclerotic process.

Although the details of precisely how the transplant-specific immunologic and nonimmunologic factors interact and amplify the atherogenic factors to produce the pathologic picture of allograft vasculopathy have not been proven, several conceptual aspects seem clear. Whereas the standard atherosclerotic disease process is usually focal/segmental, most prominent at vessel branching points where there is greater rheologic shear stresses, and occurring over many years; allograft vasculopathy can be conceptualized as an accelerated form of native coronary artery disease in which the local slow burning "brushfires" of coronary atherosclerosis are intensified and spread by pouring "gasoline" (the immunologic component of host-allograft interaction) on the process, igniting the "fire" (endothelial injury/activation) to greater intensity, spreading it rapidly throughout the coronary arterial system, and compressing the time frame for the pathologic process.

Endothelial Cell Activation

When the endothelium is injured, as described above, endothelial cells may play a pivotal role in the development of atherosclerosis and allograft vascular disease by becoming "activated." Endothelial activation may lead to the induction of genes which are normally suppressed and the inhibition of "beneficial" genes. This endothelial dysfunction (endothelial activation) is likely the initial inciting event of allograft vasculopathy (and atherosclerosis). A summary of the major functions of the endothelial cell relevant to atherogenesis is depicted in Figure 17-7. Endothelial cells contain surface receptors for a wide variety of molecules including growth

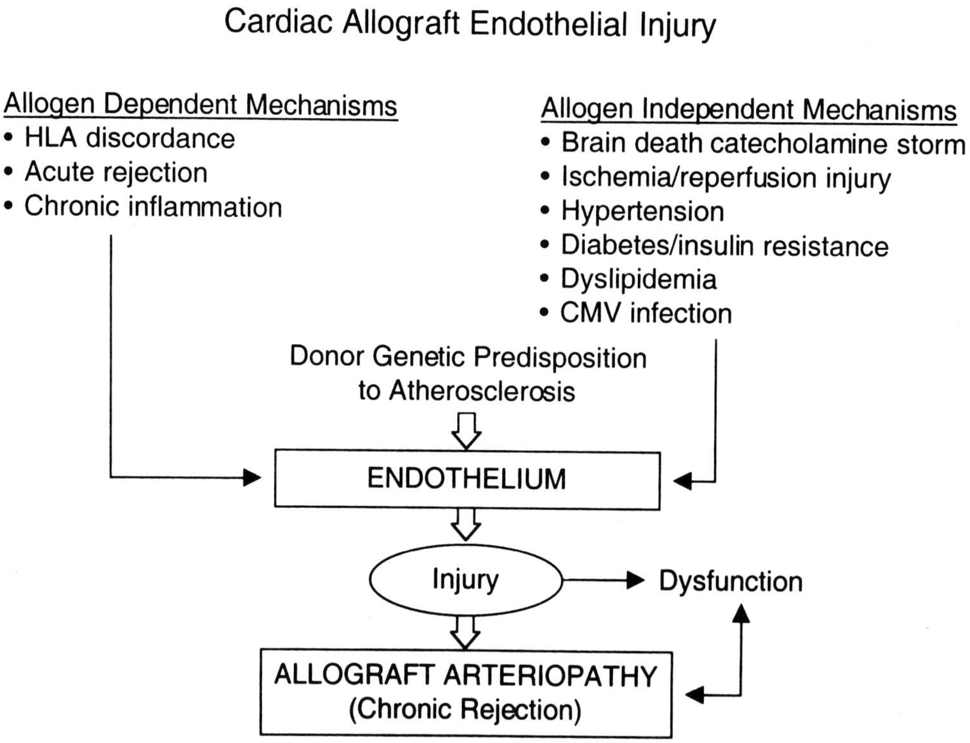

Cardiac Allograft Endothelial Injury

Allogen Dependent Mechanisms
- HLA discordance
- Acute rejection
- Chronic inflammation

Allogen Independent Mechanisms
- Brain death catecholamine storm
- Ischemia/reperfusion injury
- Hypertension
- Diabetes/insulin resistance
- Dyslipidemia
- CMV infection

Donor Genetic Predisposition
to Atherosclerosis

ENDOTHELIUM

Injury → Dysfunction

ALLOGRAFT ARTERIOPATHY
(Chronic Rejection)

FIGURE **17–6.** Integration of alloantigen-dependent (immune) and alloantigen-independent (nonimmune) mechanisms of endothelial injury that likely work in synergy to promote the development of allograft arteriopathy (chronic rejection).

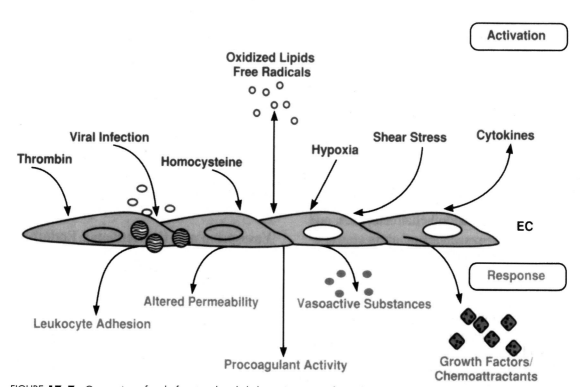

FIGURE **17–7.** Generation of a dysfunctional endothelium. A variety of stimulatory or "injury-provoking" agents have been implicated in the process of endothelial cell (EC) activation. Many of the responses of the endothelium are associated with the progression of vascular disease. (From DiCorleto PE, Gimbrone MA: Vascular endothelium. *In* Fuster V, Ross R, Topol EJ [eds]: Atherosclerosis and Coronary Artery Disease. Philadelphia: Lippincott-Raven, 1996, pp 387–399, with permission.)

factors, vasoactive substances, low-density lipoproteins, and molecules from the immune system. The activated endothelial cell can also have critical interactions with smooth muscle cells, macrophages, and platelets, all of which play a critical role in the atherosclerotic and allograft vasculopathic process. Whatever the inciting factor, **endothelial injury and subsequent activation** initiates a cascade of molecular and cellular events which are largely independent of the specific noxious stimulus and **lie at the core of allograft vasculopathy.** A number of cytokines and growth factors (see later section) can be released by endothelial cells which influence the behavior of adjacent vascular cells and blood elements (Fig. 17–8).

Injury to the endothelial layer can take several forms depending on the overall integrity of this layer, and is classified as denuding or nondenuding injury. **Denuding injury** involves the loss of a substantial area of endothelial coverage. It may occur during significant episodes of cellular rejection or vasculitis, or possibly during the period of ischemia/reperfusion at the time of transplantation. **Nondenuding injury** does not involve a significant loss of endothelial coverage at any one particular time, but rather is manifested by relatively rapid replacement of individual endothelial cells that are injured and lost, and it is principally reflected in endothelial dysfunction. This injury may result from immunologic factors as well as nonimmunologic factors such as modified lipoproteins (as in native coronary atherosclerosis), viruses, ischemia, abnormal shear stress and flow, as well as other metabolic factors. Both forms of injury may coexist and recur. Whatever the form of injury, however, the ensuing cascade of events is very similar. It has been hypothesized that a common transcription factor, **nuclear factor-kappa B** (NF-κB),[44] and possibly other signaling pathways[108, 195] induce the inappropriate and ultimately damaging gene expression by activated endothelial cells.

Large areas of denuded endothelium allow interactions to occur between the cellular (platelets, monocytes, T-lymphocytes) and noncellular elements (lipoproteins, fibrin) of the blood and the wall of the artery. Monocyte

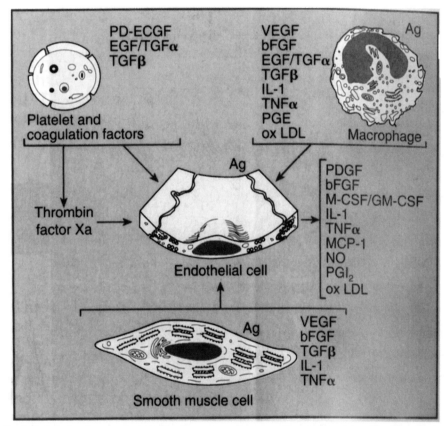

FIGURE **17–8.** Endothelial cells interact with platelets, macrophages, and smooth muscle cells. The principal products of platelets, macrophages, and smooth muscle cells that may affect the endothelium are shown in this figure. Endothelial mitogens that can be produced by macrophages include vascular endothelial growth factor (VEGF), fibroblast growth factor (FGF), and transforming growth factor-α (TGF-α). Transforming growth factor-β (TGF-β), as well as interleukin-1 (IL-1) and tumor necrosis factor-α (TNF-α), is capable of inhibiting endothelial proliferation and can also induce secondary gene expression of other growth regulatory molecules by the endothelium. TGF-β is a potent inducer of connective tissue matrix synthesis. Endothelial cells also produce numerous vasoactive substances, such as prostacyclin (PG1₂) and nitric oxide (NO). Oxidized LDL (oxLDL), produced by endothelium, macrophages, or smooth muscle cells, can profoundly injure neighboring endothelial and smooth muscle cells. Platelets can provide a host of vasoactive substances, coagulation factors, and mitogens. Thrombin and factor Xa from plasma may also stimulate the endothelium to a procoagulant state. Endothelial cells can also synthesize a number of growth-regulatory molecules, as noted to the right of the endothelial cell, that can induce proliferation of neighboring cells and their formation of connective tissue. (From Ross R: The pathogenesis of atherosclerosis: a perspective for the 1990s. Nature 1993;362:801–809. Copyright 1993 Macmillan Magazines Limited, with permission.)

or platelet adhesion is frequent, as is microthrombi formation.[125, 219, 277, 298, 300] These cells and clots serve as a rich source of growth factor and cytokine expression which then influence the development of intimal proliferation.

The nondenuding form of endothelial injury is probably the more common after transplantation and is likely a chronic ongoing process. This form of injury is similar to that which underlies early atherosclerosis and may account for both the fibrous intimal thickening and atheromatous generation of some forms of allograft vasculopathy. Rapid turnover of injured endothelial cells from this form of injury results in dysfunctional cellular activities manifested as alterations in endothelial permeability, loss of antithrombogenic characteristics with microthrombi formation, increased adhesions of leukocytes, and release of vasoactive substances and growth factors. Abnormal small vessel **flow characteristics** resulting from endothelial dysfunction are common after transplant and further damage the endothelium by inciting retraction of endothelial cells and their detachment from adjoining cells. These areas then serve as potential sites for monocyte or platelet adhesion and/or microthrombi formation.[125, 219, 277, 298] Alterations in the **permeability characteristics** of the endothelial layer also allow interactions to occur between the cellular and noncellular elements of the blood and the wall of the artery. The result of these interactions, as noted above for denuding injury, leads to the initiation and perpetuation of vascular injury. The **thromboresistent character** of the endothelial layer is also affected by endothelial injury. This protective feature is due to the presence of cell surface proteoglycans (see Box) that form the surface coat and to the expression of PGI_2, nitric oxide, and various plasminogen activators. Dysfunction of endothelial cells, leading to the underexpression of these factors, will promote vasoconstriction, abnormal flow characteristics, platelet interactions, and thrombi development. All of these consequences further promote the development of atherosclerosis and allograft vasculopathy.

Proteoglycans

Proteoglycans are a relatively diverse group of hydrophilic protein polysaccharides that have one or more glycosaminoglycan chains covalently bonded to a core glycoprotein backbone. These proteins provide the vascular wall with turgor and viscoelasticity and interact with vascular cell cytokines and growth factors to modify vascular cell adhesion, proliferation, and migration.[335] They play an important role in the regulation of vascular permeability, hemostasis, thrombosis, and lipid metabolism.[34, 251, 335, 336] Proteoglycans have been classified according to the predominant type of glycosaminoglycan attached to a specific core glycoprotein, and include chondroitin sulfate, dermatan sulfate, heparan sulfate, and keratan sulfate. A variety of core proteins have been identified, giving rise to great structural diversity. Vascular proteoglycans are prominently identified in the interstitial extracellular matrix, in basement membranes, in cell membranes, and within cells.[339] Within the interstitial extracellular matrix, these protein complexes in conjunction with collagen fibrils create a compressible compartment which allows the resistance of the deformity imposed by the pulsatile nature of blood flow.

Proteoglycans present on the surface of (and synthesized by) endothelial cells contribute to the maintenance of a local anticoagulant environment that resists fibrin formation and microvascular thrombosis. Some forms of heparin (synthesized by mast cells within the vascular wall), heparan sulfate, and dermatan sulfate are powerful anticoagulants because of their ability to interact with serine protease inhibitors (serpins) such as antithrombin-III and heparin cofactor II, which potentiate the inactivation of specific clotting enzymes. Proteoglycans such as thrombomodulin bind thrombin and interact with protein C to inactivate thrombin.

Altered proteoglycans are implicated in a number of pathologic states, including altered permeability of the vascular wall, lipoprotein accumulation within atheromatous lesions, and intimal thickening in vascular disease.[51]

Smooth Muscle Cells

Smooth muscle cells derived from the media that accumulate in the intimal layer are the fundamental cell of the fibroproliferative intimal lesion in atherosclerosis and allograft vasculopathy. In addition to their role in maintaining arterial wall tone, the smooth muscle cells (like fibroblasts) play a major role in synthesizing and secreting collagen and other connective tissue substances. They contain receptors for a number of ligands that can influence the atherosclerotic (and allograft vasculopathic) process, including low-density lipoprotein[39] (a principal cholesterol–carrying plasma lipoprotein), growth stimulators (such as platelet-derived growth factor), and growth inhibitors (such as transforming growth factor β [TGF-β]). The endothelium normally provides a barrier to the passage of plasma proteins and growth factors into the media,[266] but in the presence of endothelial injury, proteins pass through the endothelial layer (increased permeability) and accumulate in the media. Growth factors then stimulate smooth muscle cells to migrate into the intima and proliferate.

A characteristic of smooth muscle cells which is central to their role in atherosclerosis and allograft arteriopathy is their ability to display a spectrum of phenotypes ranging from the highly synthetic **proliferative** smooth muscle cell to the highly **contractible** smooth muscle cell. The primary function of the vascular smooth muscle cell is contraction, for which this cell type has evolved a complex repertoire of receptors, signaling molecules, and contractile apparatus. Of great importance is that smooth muscle cells are also capable of numerous other functions during development, during vascular generation and repair, and in vascular disease.[54] Depending on local mechanical forces, humoral factors, and response to local injury, a smooth muscle cell can exhibit a broad spectrum of differing phenotypes. This remarkable flexibility of smooth muscle cells allows such cells in mature blood vessels to express a contractile phenotype in which they proliferate very slowly and

Coronary Artery Remodeling

The remodeling process in atherosclerosis and allograft vasculopathy refers to a compensatory change in vessel size in the presence of an atherosclerotic lesion. The process of compensatory vessel enlargement is an adaptive mechanism to maintain a normal lumen diameter despite an internally expanding atherosclerotic plaque.[109] The changes in vessel architecture appear to be mediated by four basic cellular events: cell growth, programmed cell death, cell migration, and matrix modulation.[109] Favorable remodeling (vessel dilatation) appears to be at least partly mediated by release of nitric oxide (NO) and prostacyclin from endothelial cells. Physiologic factors promoting favorable remodeling include increased flow and shear stress. Remodeling is impaired by excessive production of vasoconstrictors such as endothelin-1 (ET-1). Excessive accumulation of extracellular matrix in the intima and adventitia (promoted by various cytokines and growth factors) impairs the ability of the vessel to expand outward, thereby impeding remodeling.[79]

Coronary blood flow in response to acetylcholine is impaired in transplant patients secondary to endothelial dysfunction and thus may contribute to the impairment of compensatory dilation in vessels with allograft vascular disease. Impaired nitric oxide production and elevated ET-1 levels are common after transplant. This imbalance leads to unfavorable remodeling through chronic vasoconstriction and impaired flow. In addition, the balance of cytokines and growth factors that favors impaired or unfavorable remodeling predominates in the expanding intima of vessels with developing vasculopathy. Thus, unfavorable flow and vasconstriction resulting from endothelial dysfunction and excessive matrix deposition in the intima and adventitia are likely the underlying factors preventing favorable remodeling in allograft vasculopathy.[98, 99]

composite of collagen and elastic fibers embedded in a viscoelastic gel comprised of proteoglycans, glycoproteins, hyaluronan (a hydrophilic polysacchride that exists as helical structures with pronounced viscoelasticity), and water.[334] **Collagens** are proteins that provide tensile strength to the vascular wall and, through their interactions with other molecules in the extracellular matrix, participate in a number of functions critical to blood vessel integrity. These proteins consist of a triple helix of polypeptide chains, and six different types of collagens have been identified in blood vessels. Type I and Type III collagen comprise about 80% of the total blood vessel wall collagens and they are organized into "nests" which surround smooth muscle cells in the media of muscular arteries.[41, 328] The principal source of collagen in the arterial intima and media is smooth muscle cells. Cytokines and growth factors generally enhance collagen synthesis by smooth muscle cells. TGF-β1 has the most potent effect, and this synthetic effect is inhibited by interferon-γ (IFN-γ).[7] Excessive synthesis and accumulation of extracellular matrix proteins within the intima is a primary cause of unfavorable coronary artery remodeling (see Box) in the presence of allograft vasculopathy. More than 50% of the intimal proliferative lesion is composed of extracellular matrix, of which the principal protein is collagen.[79]

Fibronectin is a principal glycoprotein synthesized by vascular cells. This and other vascular glycoproteins regulate vascular extracellular matrix integrity. Fibronectin is a major attachment protein for vascular cells and acts as a substrate for vascular cell migration.[334] This protein is present throughout all layers of the vascular wall, and it accumulates in areas of intimal thickening in allograft coronary artery disease.[42, 217, 250] Fibronectin is thought to facilitate lymphocyte trafficking and smooth muscle cell migration in the atherosclerotic process.

produce small amounts of extracellular matrix proteins. However, if an artery is injured, some smooth muscle cells must adopt a synthetic phenotype for the reparative process while others must maintain the contractile phenotype in order to maintain normal vessel function.

Following endothelial injury, smooth muscle cells which have migrated from the media to the intima change from a contractile phenotype to a synthetic phenotype.[262] Once in the damaged area, they proliferate and secrete extracellular matrix proteins. Smooth muscle cells in the synthetic phenotype can respond in an autocrine manner with secretion of and response to platelet-derived growth factor and other growth stimulators. Damaged smooth muscle cells release fibroblast growth factor, which can stimulate other smooth muscle cells and endothelial cells and also produce a number of other growth factors and cytokines capable of amplifying the stimulation-proliferation process.[107, 188, 189, 193]

Vascular Extracellular Matrix

Within the media, smooth muscle cells are intimately related to the vascular extracellular matrix, which is a

Critical Cytokines and Growth Factors

The elaboration of cytokine growth factors and other cytokines from endothelial cells (Table 17–3) and by infiltrating cells and donor cells represents a key event in the proliferative response which underlies the development of allograft arteriopathy.[7, 322] These factors can act in a paracrine (acting on neighbor cells) and autocrine (acting on the secreting cell) manner to induce and amplify the proliferative process. Many of these factors act synergistically[55] and serially (one factor stimulating the release of other factors) to promote migration and entrance of inflammatory cells into the vascular wall

TABLE 17–3	Endothelial-Derived Cytokines and Growth Factors in Allograft Vasculopathy	
CYTOKINES		GROWTH FACTORS
Interleukin-1		Platelet-derived growth factor
Interleukin-6		Fibroblast growth factors
Interleukin-8		Insulin-like growth factor
Monocyte chemotactic protein		Transforming growth factor-β
Colony-stimulating factors		
Tumor necrosis factor-α		

and to stimulate smooth muscle cell migration and proliferation, matrix deposition, and ultimately intimal thickening, which is characteristic of the disease.

Platelet-Derived Growth Factor

Platelet-derived growth factor (PDGF) is an extremely potent mitogen (a substance that induces proliferation of other cells) that binds tightly to responsive cells. It also is chemotactic to the same cells for which it is a mitogen.[31, 117] This cytokine is produced by macrophages, endothelial cells, and smooth muscle cells, and is likely produced within the intima itself.[58, 97] Because of its chemotactic and mitogenic effects on smooth muscle cells, PDGF is thought to play an integral role in the pathogenesis of atherosclerosis and allograft vasculopathy.[55, 81, 140, 348, 349] Interleukin-1 (IL-1) stimulates the expression of PDGF-α in cultured fibroblasts, and tumor necrosis factor (TNF) stimulates endothelial cell release of PDGF.[119, 187, 252] Increased levels of mRNA for PDGF-α have correlated with the subsequent development of allograft vascular disease.

Fibroblast Growth Factor

Fibroblast growth factor (FGF) is a cytokine integral to the initiation and perpetuation of the developing intima, and like PDGF, is likely important in the pathogenesis of allograft vasculopathy. As with PDGF, several forms exist for FGF, including acidic FGF (aFGF) and basic FGF (bFGF). aFGF is also known as heparin-binding growth factor-1 (HBGF). FGF is a potent mitogen and chemoattractant for vascular smooth muscle cells as well as a potent angiogenesis factor in vivo.[329] aFGF has been shown in animal models to induce striking smooth muscle hyperplasia in myocardial vessels in areas of ischemic injury but has no effect on vessels in adjacent normal areas.[19] In a study of allograft rejection and vasculopathy, Zhao and colleagues demonstrated that the aFGF gene was expressed in the majority of biopsies (86%) they studied, and its presence was not correlated with rejection.[350] The source of aFGF mRNA in these allografts is likely from infiltrating T-cells, myocytes, or smooth muscle cells within the media or intima.[350] aFGF may play a role in the pathogenesis of vasculopathy both through its proliferative and chemoattractant properties for smooth muscle cells and by enhancing the expression of PDGF.[107, 135]

Insulin-like Growth Factor

Insulin-like growth factor-1 (IGF-1) appears to be a convergent point for multiple growth factors that may be involved in allograft vasculopathy and atherosclerosis.[55] IGF-1 release from the vascular wall may serve both as a primary mitogen and also act in concert with other mitogens such as PDGF and FGF to induce smooth muscle proliferation.[140] In addition, multiple other growth factors seem to induce the expression of IGF-1 and its receptor. TGF-β as well as bFGF and PDGF induce IGF release, while TGF-α and aFGF induce up-regulation of the IGF-1 receptor. IGF-1 has been shown to accelerate

development of transplant atherosclerosis in a rat orthotopic aortic transplantation model.[161] Inhibition of IGF by angiopeptin has been shown to reduce vascular smooth muscle proliferation.[86–88] A clinical trial using angiopeptin for prevention of allograft vasculopathy has been reported[326] (see later section, Treatment of Allograft Arteriopathy).

Transforming Growth Factor-β

TGF-β is a polypeptide cytokine produced by a variety of cells that can modulate cellular differentiation and proliferation, including the production of extracellular matrix.[29] TGF-β has seemingly paradoxical effects on the development of the atherosclerotic plaque, in that it can both promote as well as attenuate lesion development.[197, 222, 253, 279] It appears to have immunologic, proatherosclerotic, antiatherosclerotic, as well as procoagulant properties. TGF-β can inhibit the migration and proliferation of smooth muscle cells in vitro, but at the same time can promote extracellular matrix expansion due to stimulation of matrix formation and suppression of matrix degradation.[66, 147, 257] TGF-β prothrombotic activity likely stems from its ability to stimulate production of plasminogen activator inhibitor-1 (see subsequent section).[254]

Tumor Necrosis Factor-α

TNF-α has several biological effects which may promote the development of allograft vasculopathy. These biological activities include endothelial activation, increased expression of adhesion molecules, induction of other cytokines (including PDGF), angiogenesis, and matrix development.[269] The presence of TNF-α in cardiac allografts is well documented.[10, 148]

Role of the Coagulation/Fibrinolytic Systems

As noted above, the normal endothelial surface presents a nonthrombotic surface to blood cells. However, under certain abnormal conditions, the damaged (activated) endothelial cells produce a thrombogenic state.[148] The existence of a local prothrombotic or antithrombotic state is determined by the balance achieved between factors elaborated by the endothelium (Fig. 17–9).

Multiple endothelial mechanisms exist to maintain an **antithrombotic state.** Endothelial cells synthesize prostacyclin (PGI_2), an arachidonic acid metabolite which is an extremely potent inhibitor of platelet aggregation.[331] In addition, there are two principal natural anticoagulant pathways which inhibit thrombin generation and the conversion of fibrinogen to fibrin. The **heparin sulfate–antithrombin III pathway** targets inactivation of thrombin by the interaction (binding) of heparin and heparan sulfate with antithrombin III (AT-III).[71, 131, 136, 303] Heparin and heparan sulfate are related molecules formed from the same monosaccharides.[30, 198] Heparin is synthesized only by mast cells within the vascular wall, and heparan sulfates are synthesized by all vascular wall cells. The second major natural anticoagulant pathway is

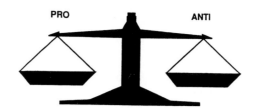

FIGURE **17–9.** The vascular endothelial hemostatic-thrombotic balance. Various endothelial-associated factors and functions contribute to a dynamic physiologic antagonism or "balance" between local prothrombotic activity and antithrombotic effects. (Adapted from DiCorleto PE, Gimbrone MA: Vascular endothelium. *In* Fuster V, Ross R, Topol EJ [eds]: Atherosclerosis and Coronary Artery Disease. Philadelphia: Lipincott-Raven, 1996, pp 387–399.)

PRO

- **Platelet-activating factor**
- **Tissue factor**
- **Von Willebrand factor**
- **Plasminogen activator Inhibitor-1**
- **Fibronectin**
- **Thrombospondin**
- **Factor V**
- **Other coagulation factors**

ANTI

- **Prostacyclin**
- **Heparin-like molecules**
- **Thrombomodulin**
- **Tissue plasminogen activator**
- **Urokinase plasminogen activator**

the **thrombomodulin-protein C pathway.** Thrombomodulin, a proteoglycan produced by endothelial cells, binds thrombin and also interacts with protein C to inactivate thrombin through an AT-III–independent pathway.[30] The **tissue plasminogen activator** mechanism of the fibrinolytic system is also endothelial associated.

In contrast to these antithrombotic functions, the endothelium is also capable of **prothrombotic activity.** Endothelial cells can synthesize adhesive cofactors of platelets, such as von Willebrand factor, fibronectin, and thrombospondin; and also procoagulant components such as factor V and tissue factor, a trigger for the coagulation cascade, culminating in fibrin generation. Importantly, endothelium also generates an inhibitor of the fibrinolytic pathway, **plasminogen activator inhibitor-1 (PAI-1)**, which can inhibit fibrin breakdown.

Impaired fibrinolytic activity and/or **enhanced thrombogenicity** associated with endothelial cell injury likely play a critical role in the development of allograft vascular disease. Considerable evidence supports a unifying hypothesis suggesting that arterial and arteriolar endothelial activation,[173] with up-regulation of intercellular adhesion molecule-1 (ICAM-1) (see later section, Leukocyte Adhesion Molecules) and HLA-DR (see later section, Immunologic Component), promotes subsequent allograft coronary artery disease because of perturbation of hemostasis,[77] fibrinolysis,[175, 176] and anticoagulation.[174]

Enhanced thrombogenicity has been demonstrated in transplanted hearts. Endothelial thrombomodulin is down-regulated by cytokines such as IL-1 and TNF released by activated macrophages,[47, 174, 242] and its reactivity and expression on endothelial cells recover after successful immunosuppressive therapy for cellular rejection. Enhanced thrombogenicity may also be integrally linked to **humoral rejection.**[78] The role of antibodies and complement in the development of allograft vasculopathy may be mediated through endothelial activation which in turn leads to up-regulation of tissue factor and down-regulation of thrombomodulin and AT-III promoting thrombogenicity and fibrin deposition.[27] Fibrinogen, the precursor to fibrin, circulates in significantly greater concentrations in cardiac transplant patients when compared with control patients and also

tends to be higher in heart transplant patients with accelerated vasculopathies than those without.[283] Normal vascular and perivascular spaces should not contain fibrin, and its presence is indicative of vascular damage.[75, 237] Examination of hearts removed for retransplantation and at autopsy have demonstrated diffuse deposits of fibrin in the microcirculation, interstitium, and within myocardial cells.[175]

Similar to the coagulant/anticoagulant systems, the **fibrinolytic** balance within the graft and in the recipient's plasma is perturbed after transplant. Impaired fibrinolysis is a known risk factor for native atherosclerosis and atherosclerosis-related events[17, 157] and the posttransplant situation is very similar. Impaired fibrinolysis results from an imbalance in the relative levels of the plasminogen activators, **tissue plasminogen activator** (t-PA) or **urokinase plasminogen activator** (u-PA),[82] and the physiologic inhibitor of t-PA and u-PA, **PAI-1.** This imbalance may influence the development of allograft vasculopathy via several distinct mechanisms. Underexpression of t-PA and u-PA, or overexpression of PAI-1 within the lumen of the vessel or within the vessel wall impedes plasmin generation.[22] This favors the accumulation of fibrin and thrombus formation and provides a stimulus for the development of vasculopathy. Depletion of t-PA from arterial and arteriolar smooth muscle cells in the first 3 months after cardiac transplantation has been associated with development and severity of transplant coronary artery disease.[176]

Vasoconstriction/Vasodilation Balance

Although smooth muscle cells in the media of muscular arteries regulates vascular tone, endothelial cells also play a powerful role in the local regulation of vascular tone (Fig. 17–10). Nitric oxide (endothelial-derived relaxing factor) and prostacyclin, acting via a different mechanism, are potent local vasodilators elaborated by endothelial cells. These local vasodilators are balanced by endothelial-derived vasoconstrictor substances, including angiotensin II (generated at the endothelial luminal surface by angiotensin-converting enzyme), PDGF factor (which can induce smooth muscle contraction), vasoconstrictor prostaglandins, and endothelin-1 (the most potent vasoconstrictor known).

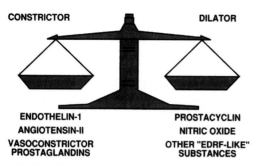

FIGURE 17-10. The vascular endothelial vasoconstrictor-vasodilator balance. Various endothelial products contribute to the local regulation of vascular tone through their effects on smooth muscle contractility. EDRF, endothelium-derived relaxation factor.

In the generation of atherosclerosis, oxidized low-density lipoprotein inhibits endothelium-dependent arterial relaxation.[38, 100] Hypoxia induces an abnormal vasoconstrictive response in animal models, possibly through reduced nitric oxide production.[280]

Leukocyte Adhesion Molecules

In the presence of endothelial dysfunction or regenerating endothelium after a denuding injury (caused by oxidized low-density lipoproteins in atherosclerosis and possibly immune-related events after cardiac transplantation), leukocyte adhesion molecules such as vascular cell adhesion molecule-1 (VCAM-1) and ICAM-1 are up-regulated,[74] promoting monocyte adhesion and subsequent diapedesis into the subendothelial space. Very-low-density lipoprotein hydrolyzed by lipoprotein lipase has been shown to induce monocyte adhesion to cultured endothelial cells.[270]

VCAM-1 is a mononuclear leukocyte-selective adhesion molecule that is expressed on monocytes, lymphocytes, eosinophils, and basophils but not neutrophils[11] and can be induced by IFN-γ and TNF. The coexpression of VCAM-1 with MHC antigens on endothelial cells and medial smooth muscle cells suggests that VCAM-1 may participate in mononuclear cell recruitment. In experimental, diet-induced atherosclerosis, endothelial cell VCAM-1 induction precedes monocyte attachment and migration,[186] suggesting a possible role in native coronary artery disease. This process may also play a role in the development of allograft vasculopathy. The combination of VCAM-1 expression along with MHC antigens induces the vascular endothelium of the allograft to mediate adhesion and activation of host T-cells that culminate in the release of inflammatory mediators which may promote allograft vasculopathy.[11, 315]

Expression of the **ICAM-1** receptor has been documented to occur immediately (< 24 hours) and/or in delayed (> 30 days) fashion after transplantation.[245] Early activation likely promotes rejection and may additionally, in the case of ICAM-1, allow the release of toxic intermediates from neutrophils, leading to endothelial injury.[68, 69] Clinical and animal models of heart transplantation point to a second, later phase of ICAM-1 expression that coincides with the histologic onset of allograft arteriopathy.[245] This later phase, which occurs more than 30 days after transplant, is noted by the up-regulation of perivascular ICAM-1 accompanied by HLA-DR expression.[173] Increased ICAM-1/HLA-DR arterial/arteriolar expression in the first 3 months after transplantation is associated with both an increased risk and earlier development of allograft vascular disease.

The exact mechanism responsible for this link between ICAM-1 and allograft vasculopathy is unknown, but the binding of ligand to endothelial ICAM-1 may activate the endothelium and lead to late, nondenuding form of vascular injury.[173] Experimental animal models suggest that donor ICAM-1 and P-selectin may play a pivotal role in leukocyte trafficking, facilitating the onset of parenchymal rejection and possibly the development of transplant atherosclerosis.[59]

Role of Macrophages

Macrophages are derived from circulating monocytes and generally act as scavenger cells to remove foreign substances by phagocytosis and intracellular hydrolysis. The monocyte-derived macrophage plays a critical role in the inflammatory process that initiates allograft vasculopathy (and atherosclerosis). Macrophages act as scavengers for oxidized low-density lipoproteins, ingesting lipid to form foam cells. They also are a source of vasoactive substances, chemotactic molecules, growth-inhibitory and growth-stimulating factors, and lytic enzymes.[263] At least six growth factors are known to be synthesized and secreted by macrophages: PDGF, FGF, epidermal growth factor (EGF), IL-1 (a cytokine that induces expression of PDGF genes in fibroblasts), TGF-β, and monocyte colony-stimulating factor (M-CSF). Macrophages of recipient origin also process donor antigen and can act as antigen-presenting cells to adjacent T-cells, promoting localized inflammatory injury to the vessel endothelium.

Platelets

Platelets facilitate the atherosclerotic process not only through their role in the development of thrombus, but also through elaboration of vasoactive substances and multiple growth factors. The growth factors include PDGF, FGF, EGF, and TGF-β (all of which are also formed by activated macrophages).[14, 227, 265] At sites of endothelial injury and disruption, platelets adhere, aggregate, and release their granules, providing growth factors which stimulate a vasoconstrictive and proliferative response.

ROLE OF THE TRANSPLANT IMMUNE RESPONSE IN ALLOGRAFT VASCULOPATHY

Endothelium

It is logical to assume that immunologic mechanisms play the most significant role in development of allograft arteriopathy. Given the position of the endothelium as the interface between the host blood-borne immunologic elements and the allograft, the **vascular endothelium** is the likely immune target in allograft vasculopathy.

Endothelial cells express both MHC **class I** (HLA-A and HLA-B) and **class II** (HLA-DR) antigens *in vivo* and *in vitro*,[126, 129, 249, 324] and they can also serve **as antigen presenting cells,** capable of presenting both donor antigens (direct presentation) and antigens from other sources such as microorganisms.[137, 138, 215, 226, 323, 325] Furthermore, endothelial cells, under conditions of activation, can be induced to express a variety of **adhesion molecules** (as described above), including ICAM-1 and VCAM-1, which are necessary for adherence of leukocytes in the immune response.[32, 36]

That being said, it has been difficult to demonstrate an association between acute cell-mediated or immunoglobin-mediated vascular cardiac allograft rejection and subsequent allograft vascular disease. The strongest circumstantial evidence for an allograft-specific (and therefore immunologic) mechanism for allograft vasculopathy is the involvement of the great vessels (in addition to the coronary arterial tree and coronary veins)[231] up to but not beyond the suture lines.[191]

Endothelial cells exposed to allogeneic lymphocytes up-regulate mRNA that codes for a panel of mesenchymal growth factors including bFGF, TGF-α, TGF-β, PDGF, and heparin-binding EGF.[140] Of course, there may be many other receptor sites important in the immunopathogenesis of allograft arteriopathy. Obviously, cytokines, particularly IL-2, are released in large quantities by allogeneic activated T-cells. Also, posttransplant arterial and arteriolar endothelial ICAM-1/HLA-DR expression has been linked to the development of allograft vascular disease.[173]

Role of Humoral Immunity

The traditional view of chronic allograft rejection (allograft vasculopathy) has included a primary role of humoral mechanisms, with deposition of antigen-antibody complexes along the allograft endothelial surface leading to endothelial injury, fibromuscular proliferation, and intimal thickening. To date, however, there is insufficient direct evidence to prove a primary role of humoral (antibody-mediated) rejection in the development of allograft vasculopathy. Several human studies provide indirect evidence which suggests a link between the two phenomena (humoral rejection and allograft arteriopathy). Hammond and colleagues found an increased incidence of transplant coronary artery disease among patients who had prior demonstration of antibody deposition in the cardiac allograft by immunofluorescence studies.[124] The degree of posttransplant anti-HLA antibody formation in the recipient (as judged by panel-reactive antibody) has correlated with the development of allograft vasculopathy,[182] but other studies have failed to identify a relationship between antigraft antibodies and this process.[139, 286, 319] Also, antibodies specific for a polypeptide called vimentin (possibly exposed following endothelial injury) are rarely identified except in patients with progressive allograft vasculopathy.[50, 261]

Additional supporting information is available from immunodeficient mice experiments. In a heterotopic mouse model, alloantibody formation is associated with more severe allograft coronary disease.[267] In mice deficient of T- and B-cell function who receive heterotopic heart transplants, allograft coronary artery disease does not develop until they are exposed to antibodies against transplantation antigens of the donor strain. Furthermore, allograft arteriopathy is not noted in recipients that fail to produce donor-specific antibody, but does develop in those who can produce antibodies to the endothelial cell receptors.[267] Several additional animal experiments[140] have demonstrated with MHC mismatch models, that strain combinations which result in alloantibody formation have greater intimal proliferation than those combinations where alloantibody is not noted. All of these observations point toward an antibody-mediated component of allograft arteriopathy.

The Role of Cellular Immunity

Although unproven, there is increasing indirect evidence that acute cellular rejection may play an important role in the development of allograft vasculopathy. Several animal studies have reinforced the potential for cell-mediated immunity to produce allograft arteriopathy. Experiments using heterotopic models of heart and aortic transplantation have demonstrated the ability to reliably produce vascular changes characteristic of allograft arteriopathy when extensive mononuclear cell infiltration was present and associated with smooth muscle cell proliferation and intimal thickening. Heterotopic heart transplantation in rat strains which match for MHC and differ for non-MHC antigens often develop acute rejection within 3 weeks, and rejected allografts show intense mononuclear cell infiltrate with later lesions demonstrating fibrotic intimal thickening.[3] Futhermore, acute rejection in animal models is associated with enhanced endothelial expression of leukocyte adhesion molecules and HLA antigens.[127, 130, 302]

Experiments using rat strain combinations selected for various mismatches in class I, class II, or minor non-MHC antigens have demonstrated that allograft arteriopathy can be reproduced in many different strain combinations, that the severity of intimal proliferation could be enhanced by an intraperitoneal injection of donor lymphocytes, and that the first cell line to appear is the macrophage, followed by T-cells, natural killer cells, and to a lesser extent, B-cells.[49] In models of mouse carotid artery transplants,[278] the allograft arteriopathy process starts with an inflammatory infiltrate containing activated T-cells and macrophages followed by progressively worsening intimal thickening, which is driven primarily by smooth muscle cell proliferation and accumulation.

Evidence for cell-mediated immunity playing a major role in human cardiac arteriopathy generally relates to the relationship some have observed between multiple episodes of cellular rejection and later development of allograft arteriopathy (see later section, Immunologic Risk Factors). Numerous human transplantation studies on explanted or autopsied hearts provide supportive evidence for a link between cellular rejection and allograft vasculopathy. The demonstration of cellular infiltrates containing T-cells and macrophages in the media and adventitia of vessels involved with allograft arteriopathy,[191] the finding of lymphocytic endothelialitis in affected vessels,[144] and the demonstration of lymphocytes and macrophages below the endothelial layer[269] all establish the frequent presence of the cellular components of acute rejection in vessels affected by allograft arteriopathy.

In clinical heart transplant studies, recipient lymphocyte responses to donor-specific human aortic endothelial cells have been examined sequentially after transplant.[139] An increased lymphocyte proliferative response to donor endothelial cells was associated with the development of transplant coronary artery disease during the first year.[139] Increased levels of aFGF along with PDGF-α have been noted in allografts during rejection. Myocytes and vascular structures may be an important source for these growth factors which are known to participate in atherogenesis.[349]

All things considered, it is likely that a combination of cell-mediated and antibody-mediated immune responses coupled to the more traditional mechanisms for atherosclerosis all contribute to endothelial injury, with subsequent perivascular inflammation and smooth muscle cell proliferative responses resulting in subsequent obliterative arteriopathy.

OTHER TRANSPLANT-RELATED FACTORS

Infection as an Etiology for Cardiac Allograft Vasculopathy

Several pathogens which can cause persistent or latent chronic infections have been implicated as cofactors in the development of atherosclerosis and subsequent cardiovascular events as well as allograft vasculopathy.[60] It is an important issue generally because of the frequency of these infections and the fact that some of them can be treated by antibiotics or prevented with vaccines. Serologic and epidemiologic data demonstrate an association between several pathogens and clinical events related to atherosclerosis but do not distinguish between causal relations and simple secondary infection.[208] Antigens, genetic material, or cultivatable infectious agents, especially those that replicate in macrophages, have been demonstrated by pathologic examination to be associated with inflammatory lesions of atherosclerosis, but it is unclear whether the infectious agents exert their pathologic effects directly or through immune responses to microbial antigens that cross-react with normal human antigens. Most agree, however, that infectious agents are not sufficient causes of atherosclerosis (or allograft vasculopathy) alone, but rather act in concert with known risk factors such as genetic predisposition, cigarette smoking, diabetes, lipid perturbation, hypertension, and, in the case of transplant patients, the immunologic milieu.

Though a large number of pathogens have been associated with atherosclerosis, Chlamydia pneumoniae and viruses of the herpes group, such as cytomegalovirus, have received the most attention. Chlamydia pneumoniae is the pathogen with the most evidence of a causal association with atherosclerosis, and preliminary data have suggested that macrolide/azalide therapy of patients

with atherosclerosis is beneficial in the secondary prevention of coronary heart disease. Large-scale studies are ongoing to explore this issue in the general population, but no data exist in heart transplant patients regarding this tactic.

Because of the chronic immunosuppression required to control cardiac allograft rejection, heart transplant recipients are particularly susceptible to **cytomegalovirus (CMV) infection.** Experimental data show that the herpesvirus can infect endothelial cells and that specific viral antigens can up-regulate inflammatory cytokines that lead to increases in adhesion molecules and thrombotic factors. Inhibition of apoptosis of smooth muscle cells may also contribute to the disease process.

Koskinen and coworkers[170] demonstrated that cardiac biopsy specimens showed significant capillary and arteriolar changes after CMV infection that related to serial changes in coronary angiograms. Allograft explants demonstrating significant arteriopathy at the time of autopsy have a higher incidence of positive in situ hybridization for CMV nucleic acid in the vascular intima than explants without allograft arteriopathy.[341] In an experimental model of rat aorta transplantation, CMV infection enhanced vascular inflammation and increased the degree of intimal proliferation compared to uninfected controls.[185]

It has been speculated that an interaction exists between CMV and the allogeneic response. Presumably, an infection of one or more cell types occurs within the vascular wall. Leukocytes are a cytomegalovirus reservoir, and their activation and involvement in the inflammatory response may increase viral replication. There appears to be a unique relationship between CMV, the endothelium, and CD4$^+$ lymphocytes.[274] MHC class I antigens are up-regulated in CMV-infected endothelial cells.[306, 314, 327] Although most studies have not identified up-regulation of HLA class II antigen expression with CMV infection, CMV-infected heart endothelial cells in rat heart models have shown increased class II expression.[310] CMV also increases procoagulant activity of cultured endothelial cells[260] and expression of VCAMs. Given the fact that CMV infection is very common in heart transplant recipients and that this infection appears to influence detrimental endothelial activities, this virus probably does play a role in allograft vasculopathy pathophysiology. Clinical studies which identify cytomegalovirus infection as a risk factor for allograft vasculopathy are discussed in the later section, Risk Factors for Allograft Vasculopathy. Whether or not other pathogens such as Chlamydia pneumoniae are also important in this process is much less clear.

Ischemia and Reperfusion Injury

Ischemia and reperfusion injury likely contribute to early endothelial damage after transplantation, and this can set the stage for development of allograft arteriopathy (see also Chapter 9). One hypothesis is that ischemia, thermal, and reperfusion injury of the endothelial layer induces a process within the microvasculature that is oxygen free radical based and leads to complement activation, with recruitment and activation of passing leukocytes and macrophages during reperfusion. Extensive myocardial necrosis (as measured by troponin I levels) early after cardiac transplantation has correlated with subsequent development of allograft vasculopathy.[297] Injured endothelial cells are known to release oxygen radicals and other mediators of injury such as proteases, cytokines, and eicosanoids, which all are chemoattractants to leukocytes. Postischemic reperfusion injury could set the stage for additional endothelial injury and subsequent dysfunction that is then transferred to interstitial injury with subsequent stimulus of smooth muscle cell proliferation.

Ischemic injury may also intensify the immune response to the allograft. Endothelial expression of HLA antigens is up-regulated by even short periods of ischemia.[54, 143, 171] Release of donor endothelial antigens is precipitated by graft ischemia, which may promote the formation of anti-endothelial antibodies.[123, 124, 133] These events may promote acute cellular and humoral rejection, potentially stimulating events leading to allograft vasculopathy.[54] Thus, in the complex setting of the post-transplant inflammatory milieu coupled to subsequent nonimmunologic risk factors, this initial injury may be important in setting the stage for, or actually triggering, long-term endothelial damage and vasculopathy.

DIAGNOSIS OF CARDIAC ALLOGRAFT VASCULOPATHY

Cardiac allograft vasculopathy (or resultant myocardial ischemia) can be diagnosed in many different ways in the heart transplant patient, but the discovery of characteristic coronary lesions is generally made at the time of routine surveillance angiography or intravascular ultrasound, or after noninvasive tests have been done to clarify the etiology of left ventricular systolic or diastolic dysfunction (particularly when there is no evidence of myocardial cellular infiltrate characteristic of acute rejection), or during autopsy. Because the development of allograft vasculopathy is generally slow and insidious, documentation of the presence of disease well before significant physiologic sequelae arise may potentially allow for intervention at its earliest manifestation. Furthermore, rapid progression of disease to a life-threatening degree can also occur (usually without symptoms), and detection may allow treatment, which could include retransplantation (see later sections). Therefore, most heart transplant programs perform routine surveillance studies at fixed, predefined intervals, in an attempt to determine presence, extent, significance, and progression of this coronary disease.

CORONARY ANGIOGRAPHY

Since the introduction of routine yearly surveillance angiography by the Stanford group in 1972, it has been the "gold standard" for detection and follow-up of allograft vasculopathy. The angiographic details demonstrate the usual heterogeneity of the disease process. Accelerated graft atherosclerosis is typically characterized angiographically by diffuse concentric narrowing that is particularly prominent in middle to distal coronary vessels with occasional sudden distal vessel obliteration.[102, 103] Distal vessels are, furthermore, generally smaller than proximal vessels with a characteristic abrupt distal vessel tapering or sudden occlusion of distal branches creating a pruned tree effect in secondary branches (Fig. 17–11).

Angiographic Classification of Allograft Vasculopathy

A classification scheme developed at Stanford University[101] provides a "morphologic" description of angiographic arterial lesions. This classification recognized that allograft vasculopathy represents a continuum of pathologic changes ranging from concentric intimal proliferation to the more eccentric "atheromatous" disease characteristic of native coronary disease and sought to represent this phenomena in detailed angiographic representation (Fig. 17–12). According to this A through C classification scheme, type A lesions are focal, discrete, tubular, or multiple areas of stenosis in large epicardial vessels. These lesions may reflect passenger atherosclerosis (if the status of donor coronary artery disease at the time of transplant is unknown) or acquired atherosclerosis. Type B1 and B2 lesions demonstrate a transition from more normal proximal vessels with long smooth narrowings that are either abrupt or gradually occurring with concentrically narrowed and obliterated distal vessels. Type C lesions are narrowed irregular distal vessels that terminate abruptly, creating the pruned tree effect. Histologic correlation with these angiographic findings demonstrates that Type A lesions typically represent atheromatous plaque closely resembling natural atherosclerosis, whereas type B and C lesions usually represent areas of extensive fibrointimal thickening/proliferation with or without some atheromatous features (intermediate lesions).[154]

Though the angiographic features of allograft vascular disease generally are different from the angiographic findings noted in patients with nontransplant coronary artery disease, it should be stressed that the more typical discrete proximal epicardial stenoses seen in native vessel coronary disease also occur in the transplanted heart (either at a site of passenger atherosclerosis or "typical" atherosclerosis superimposed on diffuse allograft arterial disease).[101]

An alternative angiographic classification was proposed by Costanzo and colleagues[46] in which disease was categorized as mild, moderate, or severe based on the number, location, and severity of stenoses (Table 17–4). Other more complex scoring systems have also been reported.[202]

Collateral coronary blood supply generally does not develop with much frequency in allograft recipients. When it does occur, the collaterals typically develop a "blush pattern" on the angiogram. The usual paucity of collaterals possibly relates to the rapidity of development of this disease.

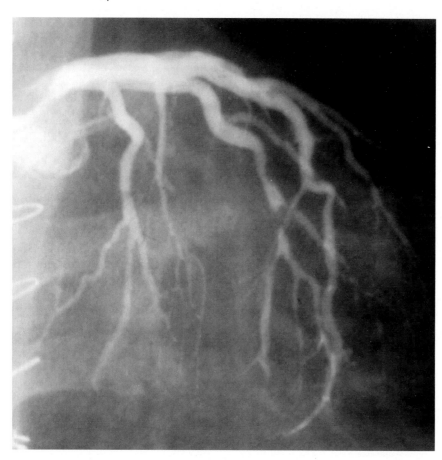

FIGURE **17–11.** Coronary angiogram demonstrating severe allograft arteriopathy of large epicardial, smaller secondary branches, and distal vessels (note the abrupt cutoff of several arteries) in a patient who was 5 years posttransplant and died suddenly.

Allograft Vascular Disease

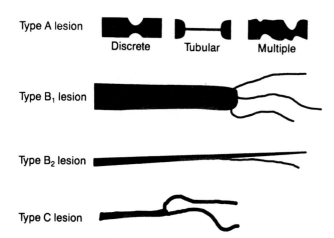

FIGURE **17–12.** Anatomic abnormalities in transplant coronary vascular disease. Type A lesion: discrete, tubular or multiple stenoses. Type B₁ lesion: abrupt onset with distal diffuse concentric narrowing and obliterated vessels. Type B₂ lesion: gradual, concentric tapering with distal portion having some residual lumen. Type C lesion: narrowed irregular distal branches with terminations that are often nontapered and squared off, ending abruptly. (From Gao S-Z, Alderman E, Schroeder J, Silverman JF: Accelerated coronary vascular disease in the heart transplant patient: coronary arteriographic findings. J Am Coll Cardiol 1988;12:334–340. Reprinted with permission from the American College of Cardiology.)

Interpretation of Angiograms

Because the progression of disease can be subtle, insidious, and concentric, casual visual inspection of the arteriogram may miss significant stenoses. Serial coronary angiography is advisable to define the extent and progression of vascular allograft arteriopathy. Serial angiograms should be compared by side-to-side analysis and, in some cases, the performance of quantitative angiographic study. Interpretation of angiograms should take into account the more symmetrical nature of allograft arteriopathy which may make identification of significant narrowing quite difficult without side-by-side comparison techniques. In addition to the usual description of focal obstructive lesions, the angiographer should search for and describe pruned tree patterns as well as plaque or nonsignificant arterial narrowing without focal obstructive lesions.[33]

Disadvantages of Coronary Angiography

Despite the tremendous advantages of coronary angiography in detecting and following the course of allograft coronary artery disease and planning timing of certain interventions, important disadvantages are also apparent. Perhaps most importantly, its invasive nature means that frequent, ongoing interrogation of the coronary arterial tree is not feasible.

Of even greater concern is the relative **insensitivity of angiography** in identifying potentially severe allograft vasculopathy. This deficiency of angiography was first

TABLE 17–4	Angiographic Categorization of Allograft Vascular Disease		
CAD CLASS*	LEFT MAIN	PRIMARY VESSELS	BRANCHES
Mild	<50%	Maximum lesion <70%	Isolated single-branch stenosis >70% or any branch stenosis <70% (including diffuse narrowing)
Moderate	50–70%	One vessel >70%	Isolated branch stenosis >70% in branches of 2 systems
Severe	>70%	Two or more vessels >70%	Isolated branch stenosis >70% in all 3 systems

CAD, coronary artery disease.
*The maximum level of involvement in any category determines the class.
Adapted from Costanzo MR, Naftel DC, Pritzker MR, Heilman JK, Boehmer JP, Brozena SC, Dec GW, Ventura HO, Kirklin JK, Bourge RC, Miller LW, The Cardiac Transplant Research Database: Heart transplant coronary artery disease detected by coronary angiography: a multiinstitutional study of preoperative donor and recipient risk factors. J Heart Lung Transplant 1998;17:744–753.

widely appreciated when many transplant programs noted the findings of extensive allograft vasculopathy on autopsy of patients dying days or weeks following a reportedly "normal" coronary angiogram.[93, 225, 258, 285, 342] Pathologic correlation with routine qualitative angiography underscores its insensitivity in detecting the early changes characteristic of allograft coronary disease. This relative insensitivity in part relates to the nature of the disease process. The often symmetrical concentric distribution of allograft coronary disease and the reliance on "normal" adjacent vessels or the proximal position of an involved artery for comparison makes interpretation difficult, since these areas and adjacent vessels may themselves have a uniform reduction in luminal cross-sectional area.[61] Thus, apparently mild stenoses may, in fact, represent a major reduction in actual lumen cross-sectional area. Luminal reductions up to 25–50% will often go undetected by this means.[154] Direct comparisons of quantitative angiography with routine angiography clearly demonstrate the enhanced sensitivity of the quantitative technique because of its ability to detect small changes in vessel diameter.[230]

Another limitation is the level of resolution, which is about 500 μm, making small- and mid-sized penetrating intramural arteries too small to examine.[33] Although careful side-by-side examination of serial angiograms can identify the loss of secondary and tertiary branching vessels, diffuse small-vessel disease may go largely undetected. Since small-vessel disease can occur independent of significant epicardial disease, patients with a normal angiogram can still have a significant plaque burden.

Timing of Angiography

Though there are certain clinical characteristics that suggest the presence of substantive occlusive coronary disease, the difficulty is most often noted during routine surveillance coronary angiography. Often, a baseline study is performed early after the transplant procedure in order to discover passenger atherosclerosis which is becoming more common as donor age increases. Early angiography provides a baseline mark that can be used as a comparison for subsequent surveillance studies that allows more precise estimation of disease progression. Subsequent coronary angiography is generally recom-

mended on an annual basis, or more frequently if important, new allograft vasculopathy is identified. Some adult patients many years after transplantation are followed with noninvasive method (such as stress dobutamine echocardiography), but this should be the exception, since the onset and rate of progression of allograft vascular disease is unpredictable, even late after transplantation, and palliative interventions such as angioplasty may be appropriate.

Considerations During Angiography Procedures

There are a few special considerations to remember when performing angiography after heart transplantation. Likely the most serious consideration will be the integrity of renal function and whether or not ionic or nonionic media will be used. In a similar vein, decisions regarding performance of contrast left ventriculography will be governed by the degree of renal impairment. Echocardiography is likely a better test for assessment of ventricular function during follow-up of the heart transplant recipient because, in addition to quantifying the degree of left ventricular systolic and diastolic dysfunction, this test will give insight into right ventricular performance, valve integrity, status of the pericardium, and will allow the clinician to estimate systolic right ventricular pressure. Also, insight regarding acute cell-mediated rejection can emerge after echocardiography (see Chapter 14).

Other considerations during catheterization of the transplanted heart include the fact that occasionally cannulation of the right coronary ostium with preformed catheters passed from the groin is difficult because of a downward location and counterclockwise rotation of the heart after transplantation. The usual risks associated with coronary angiography are present during catheterization of the cardiac allograft with respect to mechanical trauma of the arteries, aortic root, or valve structures. Significant arrhythmias, on the other hand, may be less frequently seen. This likely relates to the fact that most of the studies are done in patients with reasonable coronary flows despite the presence of allograft arteriopathy, and a denervated heart may be protected from problematic ventricular arrhythmias.[28] Furthermore, in the denervated allograft, vagal nerve-mediated bradycardia is not seen. One should remember that heart transplant recipients undergoing cardiac catheterization can still have "vasovagal" or "vasoregulatory" hypotensive episodes due to vasodilation during the procedure, since only the heart has been denervated. Also important is the fact that hemodynamic instability can be precipitated during cardiac allograft angiography when severe disease is present. Transient ischemia to the sinoatrial or atrioventricular nodes can cause sudden heart block which should not be treated with atropine (ineffective due to the denervated state of the heart), but generally responds to isoproterenol infusion.

Intracoronary nitroglycerin should be routinely used during posttransplant coronary angiography to maximally dilate the vessels, minimize and reverse spasm, and improve visualization of collaterals.[28] Electrocardiographic ST segments will sometimes be noted to rise in precipitous and concerning fashion, indicating the sluggish nature of coronary flow in some patients with severe allograft arteriopathy.

INTRAVASCULAR ULTRASONOGRAPHY

The insertion of small intravascular ultrasound probes capable of rapidly rotating such that two-dimensional imaging of the coronary artery can be observed has provided valuable insight into atherosclerotic processes in general, as well as the reasons for angiographic inaccuracy. Whereas angiography visualizes the coronary artery as a planar silhouette of the contrast-filled lumen, intravascular ultrasonography (IVUS) enables visualization of the entire circumference of the vessel. The intravascular ultrasound catheter employs a small ultrasound probe mounted on the catheter tip which can be advanced over a small angioplasty guidewire down the coronary artery and during slow pullback provides a 360-degree, real-time, cross-sectional view of the entire length of the vessel. This allows observation of lesions and calculation of intimal thickening. The catheter is approximately 3.0 Fr, or less than 1 mm in diameter, and this allows it to be advanced to the most distal portion of all three major coronary arteries. High frequencies of ultrasound (20–50 MHz) are employed, which enable high spatial resolution. Particularly important is the fact that several reports have documented the safety of this procedure, particularly in heart transplant patients.[54, 206, 240, 241]

IVUS Images

Real-time visualization of the coronary artery allows the operator to immediately detect substantive luminal narrowing and avoid unnecessary traumatic probing. The cross-sectional coronary artery image is a circle with a central black hole which is catheter artifact. A bright spot next to the black hole is artifact generated by the guidewire. The remainder of the lumen is either dark black or has a grainy appearance. Coronary arteries in posttransplant patients typically have a trilaminar appearance, with a bright inner layer (intima), an echofine middle layer (media), and a bright, dense outer layer (adventitia).[210] There usually is a distinct line of demarcation for the intima, media, and surrounding tissue. The presence of three distinct layers generally indicates an intimal thickness of more than 0.16 mm.[290, 319] The **lumen area** is determined by tracing the circumference of the leading edge of the blood-intima surface (Fig. 17–13). **Lumen diameter, lumen cross-sectional area, intimal cross-sectional area, maximal intimal thickness,** and calculation of **intimal index**[156] are depicted in Figure 17–14. The measurement of intimal (plaque) thickness by ultrasound has been validated by autopsy studies.[8, 305]

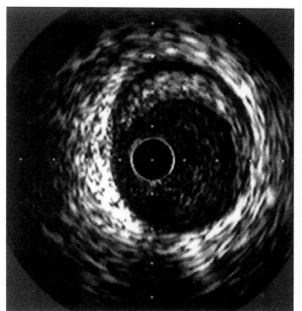
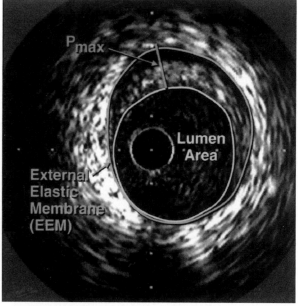

FIGURE **17–13.** Typical appearance of coronary artery by intravascular ultrasound. The circle within the lumen area is catheter artifact. Planimetry tracings indicate the boundaries between layers. See text for details.

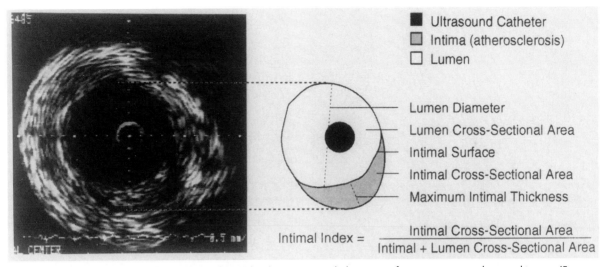

FIGURE **17-14.** Standard measurements obtained with computerized planimeter of an intracoronary ultrasound image. (From Johnson JA, Kobashigawa JA: Quantitative analysis of transplant coronary artery disease with use of intracoronary ultrasound. J Heart Lung Transplant 1995;14:S198–S202. Copyright 1995, Elsevier Science, with permission.)

Comparison with Angiography

Experience has clearly demonstrated that IVUS is much more sensitive than coronary angiography for the detection of allograft vascular disease.[238, 290] Several studies have indicated that over 50% of transplant patients with normal coronary angiograms have significant intimal thickening on IVUS.[290, 318] Furthermore, patients with abnormal coronary angiograms can also be noted to have moderate or severe intimal thickening in areas felt to be normal by angiography.[209]

Information Provided by IVUS

Of considerable importance is the finding that the greatest percentage of eccentric intracoronary stenoses occur at vessel branch points and that plaque distribution in cardiac transplant patients is **heterogeneous,** which is much more like atherosclerosis in native coronary arteries.[213, 223] Despite the fact that typical pathologic descriptions of coronary arteries from heart transplant recipients suggest allograft arteriopathy is of a uniform concentric appearance, IVUS demonstrates that these lesions are often nonuniform eccentric lesions (Fig. 17–15).[84, 224, 259, 290, 307] Many of the observations made at the time of IVUS have raised questions about the pathophysiology of this process. If it is entirely an immunogenic difficulty, focal lesions should be less common. Other studies have provided information which supports the role of local sheer stresses in the location and extent of intimal thickening.[179] Thus, IVUS studies support the notion that allograft vascular disease is an accelerated form of atherosclerosis with both immune- and non–immune-mediated endothelial injury.

One important point when comparing year-to-year changes of IVUS is to precisely identify regions of interest and comparison. The normal or least diseased site and most diseased site at 1 year or thereafter can be selected for measurement and quantification. Alternatively, multiple sites can be analyzed. The lumen and media-adventitial border of areas of interest can be manually traced with direct measurements of cross-sectional area, circumference, minimum diameter, and maximum diameter taken. Manual measurements of the minimum and maximum plaque thickness can also be made. Although measurements are generally taken using a single frame, the operator retains the ability to resort to a full motion sequence to assist in optimal border delineation in measurement.

The enhanced sensitivity of this technique over standard angiographic methods relies on its unique ability to detect intimal thickening. Although allograft vascular disease represents a continuum of pathologic changes in the transplanted vasculature, most will agree that fibrointimal proliferation is the hallmark and unique feature of the disease. Both IVUS and autopsy findings have confirmed the high prevalence of early post transplantation fibrointimal proliferation and its nearly universal appearance later in transplant recipients.

Grading the Severity of Allograft Vasculopathy with IVUS

The threshold is somewhat arbitrary for determining the degree of new intimal thickening (compared to early posttransplant baseline studies) which is indicative of allograft vasculopathy. However, several useful studies have helped clarify the limits of "normal." From autopsy studies, most young adults have a coronary intima which is at least 0.12 mm thick, but normal thickness may range between about 0.10 and 0.30 mm in normal adults between 20 and 40 years of age.[114, 281, 316] Intimal thickness in normal adults increases with age and varies with gender.[114, 281, 316]

Normal, nondiseased coronary arteries imaged with IVUS should produce an ultrasound image with a homogeneous wall appearance without layering. Mild to moderate intimal thickening as detected by IVUS characteristically demonstrates a "three-layer appearance."[114, 281, 316] This appearance is due to a relatively

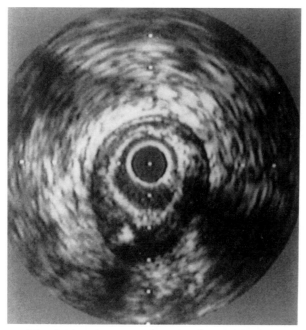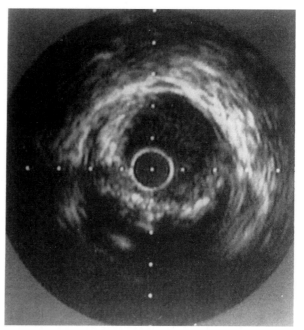

FIGURE **17–15.** Intravascular images from distal and proximal segments of left anterior descending coronary artery in a patient who received a transplant 4 years previously. *Left panel,* disease involving the entire circumference of the vessel in the distal left anterior descending coronary artery (circumferential). *Right panel,* eccentric plaque occupying two thirds of the circumference, leaving a quarter of the vessel wall free of disease in the proximal segment (noncircumferential). (From Tuzcu EM, DeFranco AC, Hobbs R, Rincon G, Bott-Silverman C, McCarthy P, Stewart R, Nissen SE: Prevalence and distribution of transplant coronary artery disease: Insights from intravascular ultrasound imaging. J Heart Lung Transplant 1995;14:202–207. Copyright 1995, Elsevier Science, with permisson.)

bright intimal and adventitial signal separated by a hypoecho region corresponding to the medial layer.[114, 281, 316] A classification scheme proposed by the Stanford group is illustrated in Table 17–5. As noted in this scheme, intimal thickness less than 0.3 mm is considered minimal to mild disease and could be reflective of preexisting donor intimal proliferation.

The thickness of the media generally is unchanged or decreases with the development of allograft vasculopathy, and the media is usually about 0.20–0.23 mm. The thickness of normal intima plus media in young and middle-aged individuals is about 0.45–0.50 mm.[309] Thus, a frequently used **criteria by IVUS** which indicates a lesion with abnormal intimal thickening (evidence of allograft vascular disease) is an **intimal thickness greater than 0.3 mm** or an **intima plus media thickness greater than 0.5 mm.**[160, 164, 256, 308]

These general guidelines can be used to help compare studies utilizing different classification schemes and aid in understanding the true prevalence and time course of allograft vasculopathy. In view of the previously dis-

cussed ability of IVUS to diagnose and quantify allograft arteriopathy and the limitations of coronary angiography, it is common to see the two procedures combined, particularly during initial studies early after transplant when severe or advanced arteriopathy is not suspected and early diagnosis of nonobstructive coronary artery lesions desired.

Limitations of IVUS

Despite the immense value of IVUS in the detection and characterization of allograft coronary artery disease, several theoretic shortcomings of this technique currently exist. First, although some common classification systems exist, the transplant community has not yet adopted any single grading system. This makes direct comparisons between different studies difficult. Second, the use of various ultrasound probes of different resolving power (20–40 MHz) can lead to varying levels of detection, with the more sensitive 30- or 40-MHz systems having higher sensitivities. With current catheters,

TABLE 17–5	**Ultrasound Classification of Allograft Vascular Disease**			
GRADE/SEVERITY	I/MINIMAL	II/MILD	III/MODERATE	IV/SEVERE
Intimal thickness and extent of plaque	<0.3 mm	<0.3 mm	0.3–0.5 mm *or*	>1.0 mm *or*
	<180 degrees	>180 degrees	>0.5 mm, <180 degrees	>0.5 mm, >180 degrees

Adapted from St Goar FG, Pinto FJ, Alderman EL, Valantine HA, Schroder JS, Gao SZ, Stinson EB, Popp RL: Intracoronary ultrasound in cardiac transplant recipients: in vivo evidence of "angiographically silent" intimal thickening. Circulation 1992;85:979–987.

only vessels with a diameter of about 1.5 mm or greater can be imaged. Third, most studies have selectively visualized the left anterior descending artery, making the assumption that allograft vascular disease occurs uniformly throughout the coronary tree, a finding we now know from autopsy and other IVUS studies not to be true.[255] Fourth, most current studies have been cross-sectional in nature and not serial assessments of the same recipients, making true estimations of progression difficult. Finally, no true initial estimate of donor intimal thickness before or immediately after transplantation exists, and therefore the true incidence of new intimal proliferation after transplantation is not known. Since intimal thickening is a normal consequence of aging, older donors may have a greater degree of intimal thickening, which may be normal.

CORONARY ANGIOSCOPY

Another emerging coronary imaging technique is angioscopy. Percutaneous coronary angioscopy can characterize plaque color and surface morphologic features of allograft arteriopathy. Still, however, this requires coronary angiography and the passage of a catheter down the coronary arteries to image the endothelium of these vessels. Neither the significance of yellow lipid-laden lesions, similar to those of native coronary artery disease, nor the significance of white nonpigmented and fibrotic lesions, similar to those noted with post-percutaneous angioplasty restenosis, has been helpful for defining severity and progression of allograft arteriopathy.

DETERMINATION OF CORONARY FLOW RESERVE

Coronary flow reserve is defined as the ratio of coronary blood flow at maximal hyperemia to baseline blood flow. In practice, measurements of blood flow *velocity* are used. By the nature of the calculation, changes in baseline flow may significantly affect coronary flow reserve. Determination of coronary flow reserves is based on the Doppler principle, which states that the change in frequency of sound waves is related either to the velocity of the transmitter or, if the transmitter is stationary, to the velocity of the receiver (in this case, red blood cells).

In normal patients without coronary artery disease, calculated coronary flow reserve is typically greater than 3:1, with considerable individual variability. In post-transplant patients, a predictable change in coronary flow reserve has been detected over time,[340] with a peak value at 2–4 years followed by a gradual decrease thereafter. The early decrease in flow reserves has been attributed to endothelial dysfunction secondary to preservation plus relative anemia and/or increased filling pressures early after transplant.[210]

Coronary flow reserve quantification has been studied in cardiac allograft recipients in order to characterize more precisely endothelial function and link coronary injury to allograft arteriopathy development and long-

term outcome. Furchgott and colleagues reported in 1980 that intact and properly functioning vascular endothelium was required to mediate normal acetylcholine vasodilation.[94] This observation promulgated the concept that an endothelium-derived relaxing factor (EDRF) was responsible for this dilatory response. EDRF is actually nitric oxide, which is synthesized by the endothelium constitutive nitric oxide synthase pathway. Nitric oxide appears to be an important mediator of vasodilation in healthy arteries and also likely inhibits platelet aggregation and adhesion as well as smooth muscle cell proliferation and leukocyte adhesion.[218] Thus, finding abnormal endothelial responses implies that these factors are perturbed, and it is likely that they relate to the atherogenic process. Nitric oxide appears to be released from vascular endothelium in response to acetylcholine administration, as well as physiologic stimuli, including blood-endothelium sheer stress.

In healthy subjects without coronary atherosclerosis, intracoronary acetylcholine results in coronary vasodilation. In contradistinction, patients with angiographic plaque detected at the time of coronary angiography, or frank coronary stenosis, demonstrate coronary vasoconstriction angiographically with the same concentrations of acetylcholine. The observed effect of acetylcholine *in vivo* is a balance of acetylcholine's direct vasoconstricting effects mediated through smooth muscle muscarinic receptors and its vasodilating action resulting from the release of endothelium-derived nitric oxide. In uninjured endothelium, vasodilation is the predominant response, whereas injured endothelium incapable of producing nitric oxide appropriately vasoconstricts after exposure to this agent. This endothelial dysfunction is noted in patients with atherosclerosis or even simply risk factors for atherosclerosis. Importantly, intravascular ultrasound studies have noted that abnormal vasoconstrictor responses actually precede intimal thickening and are, therefore, felt to be an early marker of endothelial dysfunction with subsequent atherosclerosis progression (Fig. 17–16).[169]

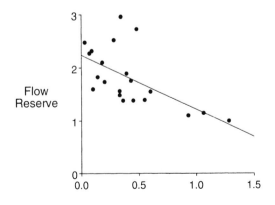

Average Maximal Intimal Thickness

FIGURE **17–16.** Myocardial flow reserve (y axis) as a function of average maximal intimal thickness (mm; x axis) in the territory of the LAD. Increases in intimal thickness were associated with decreases in myocardial flow reserve. The relation was Y = –1.03x + 2.25 (r = .62, SEE = 0.3, P < .005). (From Kofoed KF, Czernin J, Johnson J, Kobashigawa J, Phelps ME, Laks H, Schelbert HR: Effects of cardiac allograft vasculopathy on myocardial blood flow, vasodilatory capacity, and coronary vasomotion. Circulation 1997;95:600–606.)

Fish and colleagues[83] initially described coronary response to acetylcholine infusion in patients after cardiac transplantation. They reported vasoconstriction in all segments of arteries with angiographic evidence of allograft arteriopathy. They also, however, reported vasoconstriction in most of the coronary segments without angiographic evidence of disease. This disturbing finding was speculated to be predictive of subsequent atherosclerosis development.

ENDOMYOCARDIAL BIOPSY DIAGNOSIS OF ALLOGRAFT ARTERIOPATHY

On occasion, the obliterative vascular lesions of allograft arteriopathy are seen on routinely performed surveillance endomyocardial biopsy.[221, 233] Also, there are a few reports of myocardial infarction or ischemic myocardial damage being noted on endomyocardial biopsy.[106, 221] Though these findings are quite specific, endomyocardial biopsy is too insensitive to be of much utility in diagnosing allograft arteriopathy, since samples are, for the most part, removed from the right ventricle, and most significant vascular disease involves the left coronary system and left ventricle. It should be pointed out, however, that if obliterative arteriolar lesions are seen on endomyocardial biopsy, the pathologic process is likely widespread and severe, and the long-term prognosis is poor.

SERUM MARKERS OF ALLOGRAFT VASCULOPATHY

Measurements of IL-2 receptor levels, cardiac isoenzymes, and troponin levels have been employed as screening tools to detect allograft arteriopathy. Thus far, they have been somewhat nonspecific.[96, 178] Soluble IL-2 receptor levels greater than 1,000 U/mL have correlated with occlusive lesions greater than 50%,[343] but measurement of plasma cytokine levels in general has not been helpful. Also, lipoprotein-A, endothelin, platelet factor 4, and albumin levels have not been useful during screening evaluation of patients. On the other hand, Dunn et al.[63] and Crisp et al.[50] noted that donor nonspecific anti-endothelial antibodies had a sensitivity of 71% and a specificity of 95% in detecting 25% luminal stenosis at the time of coronary angiography.

In a study by Faulk and colleagues, elevation of troponin T levels appeared to correlate with future development of allograft arteriopathy.[77] Patients with persistent troponin T values of 0.10 ng/mL or greater were found to develop the disease at a mean follow-up of about 9 months, whereas patients who had initial troponin T levels less than 0.10 ng/mL did not develop disease during 40 months of follow-up. Higher levels of troponin I in the first weeks after transplantation, indicating important myocardial necrosis, have been associated with the development of allograft arteriography.[297]

IMAGING AND PERFUSION STUDIES

Noninvasive screening tests for myocardial ischemia and infarction frequently useful during evaluation of native coronary artery disease and its sequelae have generally proved unreliable in detecting cardiac allograft arteriopathy, particularly when used in a routine surveillance screening fashion.[284, 285] Smart and colleagues reported a 5-year evaluation of a battery of noninvasive studies for detection of allograft vasculopathy, including gated radionuclide wall motion exercise studies, 24-hour ambulatory Holter monitoring, two-dimensional echocardiograms with Doppler imaging at rest, and routine exercise electrocardiograms. Though the studies had negative predictive values of greater than 75%, sensitivity and positive predictive values ranged only from 21–53%. Interestingly, abnormal Holter monitor recordings consisting of bradyarrhythmias had the highest positive predictive value.

In another study of multiple yearly noninvasive tests over a 5-year period, no test had greater than 75% sensitivity for detecting allograft coronary artery disease by angiography.[72] Most noninvasive diagnostic tests rely on the induction of ischemia with stress manifested by regional abnormalities of wall motion or radionuclide uptake. Lack of sensitivity with nuclear perfusion studies has been thought due to the diffuse nature of the disease, particularly in small vessels, which produces relatively homogeneous rather than regional flow disturbances. Use of more sophisticated spectrographic thallium imaging rather than conventional tomographic imaging has been suggested to improve diagnostic accuracy, but the use of newer agents such as sestamibi has not resulted in a high enough sensitivity and positive predictive value to be employed during routine yearly screening evaluation.

More recently, interest has focused on the use of **dobutamine stress echocardiography** as a means to diagnose occult allograft arteriopathy.[4, 132, 200] When properly performed, the sensitivity for detecting significant allograft arteriopathy by dobutamine stress echocardiography can be as high as 80%, with up to 100% specificity. In a study by Spes and colleagues,[289] dobutamine stress echo had a specificity of 88% and a sensitivity of 72% for detection of allograft coronary artery disease as defined by IVUS and angiography. Perhaps more important was the finding that cardiac events occurred in only 1.9% of patients who had a normal stress test, compared with 6.3% of patients with normal resting studies. Serial worsening of abnormalities noted by dobutamine stress echocardiography identified a group with higher risk of subsequent adverse events. Compared to patients without such findings, the risk ratio increased to 7.26. Based on available studies, dobutamine echocardiography may be better than radionuclide scintigraphy even when coronary artery disease definition is liberalized to include angiographic stenosis less than 50%, diffuse distal tapering, or intimal thickening by intravascular ultrasonography.[345] However, it should be remembered that considerable experience and expertise is required to obtain consistent results with dobutamine stress echo compared with resting echocardiography.[239, 289]

Ultrafast computerized tomographic (CT) imaging and positron emission tomography (PET) have also been used with variable results. These tests, however, are expensive and have limited accessibility. In cardiac allograft recipients, PET imaging shows a significantly higher resting myocardial perfusion than in normal subjects because the transplant recipients have denervation-induced reflex tachycardia and cyclosporine-induced hypertension. Large myocardial perfusion deficits are not therefore secondary to a decreased vasodilatory capacity.[275] Because myocardial perfusion reserve increases over time in heart transplant recipients and even normalizes several years after transplantation, and transplanted ventricles hypertrophy significantly, interpretation of the PET scan can be quite difficult. Finally, both spectrographic radionuclide scanning and positron emission tomography rely on differences between normal and abnormal areas to detect allograft vasculopathy, and the distal disease may be misinterpreted as normal tissue if the disease is local and affects an area at risk that is too small to detect, or, if it is too diffuse and produces a balanced ischemia pattern without regional differences in perfusion, will go unnoticed.

CURRENT RECOMMENDATIONS FOR SURVEILLANCE STUDIES

For patients with known allograft vasculopathy, intermittent angiography is mandatory, usually every 6–12 months depending on rapidity of change and severity of disease on previous studies. The major interventions of percutaneous transluminal coronary angioplasty (PTCA), coronary bypass surgery, and retransplantation all require angiography for final decision-making.

In patients without known allograft coronary artery disease, yearly angiography with or without IVUS should remain the standard method of surveillance. As other additional therapies (see later section, Treatment of Allograft Arteriopathy) demonstrate efficacy, the value of very early detection by IVUS gains greater importance, providing the maximal opportunity for initiating or changing therapy based on subtle appearance or progression of disease. The use of noninvasive techniques such as dobutamine stress echocardiography in experienced centers may be helpful in patients at greater risk for invasive procedures (depressed renal function, difficult vascular access) or patients with stable angiographic/IVUS studies who are approaching 10 or more years after transplantation. However, the reported sensitivity of less than 75% for dobutamine stress echo is not adequate for its routine replacement of IVUS/angiography.

CLINICAL PRESENTATION

The clinical presentation of allograft vasculopathy (aside from that discovered in asymptomatic patients undergoing surveillance coronary angiography or IVUS) may be acute with new-onset heart failure, arrhythmia (particularly ventricular arrhythmias), transmural or non–Q-wave infarction, syncope, or sudden cardiac death syndrome. It is important to remember that any arrhythmia, particularly atrial arrhythmias and those occurring in the early posttransplant period, may be due to acute

cellular rejection and, therefore, whenever presented with clinical findings that suggest ischemic processes due to allograft arteriopathy, consideration of acute rejection is also important. Though acute cell-mediated rejection has been noted at any time point after heart transplantation, it is less likely during long-term follow-up, and clinical changes, therefore, are more likely related to allograft arteriopathy (chronic rejection). Thus, it is of paramount importance to consider allograft arteriopathy late after transplantation to explain ventricular dysfunction, chest and abdominal pain syndromes, unexplained dyspnea, rhythm disturbances, and electrocardiographic changes. New onset of ventricular tachycardia or fibrillation as a heralding manifestation of advanced allograft vasculopathy is less common than bradyarrhythmias and heart block. Indeed, syncope and sudden cardiac death syndrome in the setting of allograft arteriopathy have been noted due to heart block and excessive bradycardia.

The development of new-onset right heart failure (jugular venous distention, hepatomegaly, and peripheral edema) likely represents acute rejection, but it also can be caused by an acute myocardial infarction in the face of allograft arteriopathy. Indeed, patients several years after transplantation who develop acute right upper quadrant pain (reflecting hepatic capsule distention from sudden liver congestion) must be vigorously evaluated for both acute rejection and myocardial infarction or chronic ischemic syndrome caused by allograft vasculopathy.

Typically, acute ischemic syndromes are not accompanied by anginal-like chest pains because of cardiac denervation occurring during transplant (see also Chapter 11). This absence of angina or chest pain with an acute myocardial infarction often results in the delay of diagnosis or actual misdiagnosis when heart transplant patients are being evaluated. Unfortunately, acute myocardial infarction is associated with high mortality (> 25%), and this is likely due to the absence of sufficient collateral blood flow.[103] Some heart transplant patients can have angina, which likely reflects cardiac reinnervation. In patients surviving longer after transplantation (> about 5 years), reinnervation can occasionally be detected by norepinephrine release into the coronary sinus after intracoronary tyramine challenge (see also Chapter 11).[292, 332, 337] Though the extent of reinnervation and its timing are unpredictable, its presence would allow the patient to have anginal symptoms. Thus, any patient several years after heart transplantation who develops chest pain should be evaluated for allograft arteriopathy. One should also consider this possibility whenever an electrocardiographic change occurs or a patient's functional status deteriorates.

NATURAL HISTORY OF ALLOGRAFT VASCULOPATHY

DONOR DISEASE

This issue of "passenger" coronary artery disease present in the donor heart at time of transplant has been difficult to distinguish from early *de novo* onset of allograft vasculopathy because of the elapsed interval between transplant and the first angiographic or IVUS study. Clearly, however, the incidence of donor disease is highly variable and dependent on age, sex, and other factors in the donor. Judging by early angiography (within the first 6 months after transplantation), only about 2% of donor hearts have important coronary artery disese at the time of transplant.[46] By IVUS studies, about 15–25% of donor hearts have abnormal (Stanford class III–IV) intimal thickening.[169, 255] The issue of true "donor" disease present at the time of transplant has some importance, since serial IVUS studies indicate that the progression of donor disease and the development of *de novo* allograft vasculopathy may often be independent of each other.[158]

INCIDENCE

Determining the incidence of allograft vasculopathy is difficult because of heterogeneity in surveillance intervals and evaluation technique. Furthermore, "passenger" or native coronary artery disease in the donor heart confounds these determinations. One clear and overriding notion, however, is that this problem is frighteningly common and leads to important morbidity and mortality during long-term follow-up. In any discussion of allograft vasculopathy incidence, the method of detection (usually angiography or IVUS) must be clearly stated, since the greater sensitivity of IVUS will provide a higher estimate of incidence than angiography.

By **angiographic assessment,** the incidence of allograft coronary artery disease has been estimated at 10–15% per year, with a prevalence of nearly 50% by 5 years after transplantation.[103] The largest analysis of posttransplant coronary angiography was reported from the Cardiac Transplant Research Database (CTRD) project, with evaluation of nearly 6,000 postoperative angiograms performed in over 2,600 heart transplant recipients who underwent transplantation between 1990 and 1994.[46] Angiographic diagnosis of allograft arteriography was classified as mild, moderate, or severe based on the degree of left main involvement, primary vessel stenosis, or branch vessel stenosis (see again Table 17–4) (see earlier section, Diagnosis of Cardiac Allograft Vasculopathy). Based on angiographic analysis, the actuarial freedom from **any coronary artery disease** (allograft vasculopathy) was 90% at 1 year and 53% at 5 years (Fig. 17–17). From this large, current database, the best estimate of the incidence of any degree of allograft vasculopathy detected by angiography is approximately **10% during the first year,** 20% by the second year, and **nearly 50% by the fifth posttransplant year.** Thus, the likelihood of angiographically apparent disease appears to increase about 10% per year during the first 5 posttransplant years. The early peaked hazard curve (Fig. 17–17), indicating very early appearance of coronary disease by angiography, likely reflects donor disease.

Although the high incidence of any coronary artery disease is striking (nearly half of surviving patients by 5 years), the likelihood of more severe forms of allograft vasculopathy is much lower (Fig. 17–18). Thus, only about 10% of patients develop severe disease (see Table 17–6) or experience a graft-losing event due to coronary artery disease within 5 years.

It is of interest to compare these estimates with those obtained by the much more sensitive technique of **coronary intravascular ultrasound** (IVUS). Although single-vessel IVUS protocols are commonly employed, there is considerable evidence to suggest that this provides an inadequate representation of the coronary arterial tree. Intimal proliferation is frequently heterogeneous and may occur in only one or two vessels.[165, 255] The striking impact of multivessel IVUS compared to a single-vessel study was reported by Kapadia and colleagues from the Cleveland Clinic[160] (Fig. 17–19). The limitations of single-vessel IVUS are illustrated in Figure 17–20. Thus, increasing the IVUS study from one vessel to three vessels nearly doubles the percentage of patients

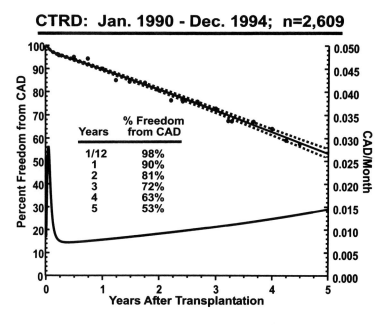

CTRD: Jan. 1990 - Dec. 1994; n=2,609

Years	% Freedom from CAD
1/12	98%
1	90%
2	81%
3	72%
4	63%
5	53%

FIGURE **17–17.** Actuarial (Kaplan-Meier) freedom from the presence of CAD detected by coronary angiography after heart transplantation (top line). Hazard function (bottom line) for appearance of any coronary artery disease on angiograms after heart transplantation is represented on vertical axis as number of patients per month in whom any CAD is detected. (From Costanzo MR, Naftel DC, Pritzker MR, Heilman JK, Boehmer JP, Brozena SC, Dec GW, Ventura HO, Kirklin JK, Bourge RC, Miller LW, The Cardiac Transplant Research Database: Heart transplant coronary artery disease detected by coronary angiography: a multiinstitutional study of preoperative donor and recipient risk factors. J Heart Lung Transplant 1998;17:744–753.)

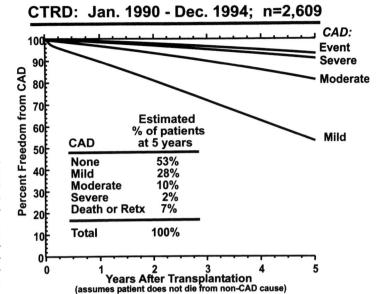

FIGURE **17–18.** Actuarial (Kaplan-Meier) freedom from presence of mild (bottom line), moderate (middle line), or severe (top line) CAD detected by coronary angiography performed later than 6 months after heart transplantation. A CAD event was defined as death or retransplantation due to coronary vasculopathy. (From Costanzo MR, Naftel DC, Pritzker MR, Heilman JK, Boehmer JP, Brozena SC, Dec GW, Ventura HO, Kirklin JK, Bourge RC, Miller LW, The Cardiac Transplant Research Database: Heart transplant coronary artery disease detected by coronary angiography: a multiinstitutional study of preoperative donor and recipient risk factors. J Heart Lung Transplant 1998; 17:744–753.)

TABLE 17-6	Angiographic Progression of Allograft Vasculopathy (CTRD, 1990–1994, N = 2,609)				
	INTERVAL AFTER TRANSPLANT (MO)				
CAD CLASS	0–6 (n = 1,293)	7–18 (n = 2,080)	19–30 (n = 1,327)	31–42 (n = 749)	43–54 (n = 336)
None	90.0%	85.7%	81.5%	77.8%	71.1%
Mild	8.0%	9.2%	12.4%	15.8%	19.9%
Moderate	1.1%	3.2%	3.8%	3.5%	6.0%
Severe	0.9%	1.9%	2.3%	2.9%	3.0%

CTRD, Cardiac Transplant Research Database; CAD, coronary artery disease; N, the number of patients with coronary angiograms in each specific interval.
Adapted from Costanzo MR, Naftel DC, Pritzker MR, Heilman JK, Boehmer JP, Brozena SC, Dec GW, Ventura HO, Kirklin JK, Bourge RC, Miller LW, The Cardiac Transplant Research Database: Heart transplant coronary artery disease detected by coronary angiography: a multiinstitutional study of preoperative donor and recipient risk factors. J Heart Lung Transplant 1998;17:744–753.

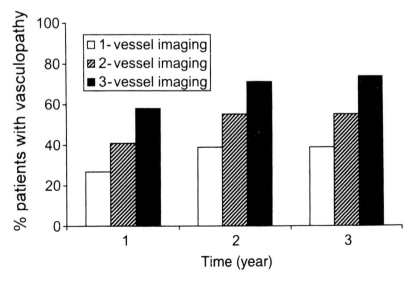

FIGURE **17–19.** Prevalence of transplant vasculopathy in patients studied at 1, 2 and 3 years after transplantation. For each time point, the prevalence of transplant vasculopathy lesions is higher when all three vessels are imaged with intravascular ultrasound compared to a single vessel imaging. The prevalence is 27%, 40%, and 58% at 1 year, 40%, 58%, and 71% at 2 years; and 40%, 58%, and 74% at 3 years for patients with one-, two-, and three-vessel imaging, respectively. (From Kapadia SR, Ziada KM, L'Allier PL, Crowe TD, Rincon G, Hobbs RE, Bott-Silverman C, Young JB, Nissen SE, Tuzcu EM: Intravascular ultrasound imaging after cardiac transplantation: advantage of multivessel imaging. J Heart Lung Transplant 2000;19:167–172.)

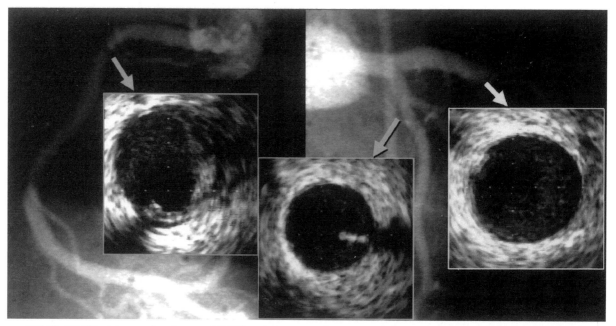

FIGURE **17–20.** Intravascular ultrasound (IVUS) study in a transplant patient with a normal coronary angiogram. By IVUS, this patient had no evidence of transplant vasculopathy lesions in the LAD or the LCX, but had an eccentric plaque in RCA. Therefore, if only the LAD or LCX were imaged, this patient could be labeled potentially as disease free. The arrows indicate the sites from which ultrasound images were obtained. (From Kapadia SR, Ziada KM, L'Allier PL, Crowe TD, Rincon G, Hobbs RE, Bott-Silverman C, Young JB, Nissen SE, Tuzcu EM: Intravascular ultrasound imaging after cardiac transplantation: advantage of multivessel imaging. J Heart Lung Transplant 2000;19:167–172. Copyright 2000, Elsevier Science, with permission.)

identified with allograft coronary artery disease at 1, 2, and 3 years after transplant. Furthermore, only a minority of patients have involvement of all three epicardial vessels, emphasizing the fact that a minority of transplant patients develop vasculopathy simultaneously in all three vessels. Still, multivessel imaging is difficult, time consuming, and more costly. These limitations must be balanced against the potential benefits provided by adequate sampling of transplant vasculopathy lesions.

Summarizing these angiographic and IVUS studies, the **incidence of allograft arteriopathy by 1 year** is about **10% by angiography,** about **25% by single-vessel IVUS,** and nearly **60% by three-vessel IVUS. By 3 years,** the incidence of any allograft arteriopathy is about **30% by angiography,** about **40% by single-vessel IVUS,** and nearly **75% by three-vessel IVUS.** Despite the high incidence of allograft vasculopathy by IVUS, its development is not inescapable. A significant number of patients have been studied at 10 years after transplant and found to have little or no intimal thickening by IVUS.[210]

Also of interest is a recent report suggesting that allograft arteriopathy is infrequent in some populations. The reported incidence of coronary artery disease in Chinese heart transplant recipients was only 2% (evaluated by angiography) at 4 years after transplant.[145] The hypothesized explanation for this striking difference from other reports was a low percentage of recipients with ischemic heart disease, low occurrence of active CMV infection, few rejection episodes, less donor-recipient racial disparity, and lower HLA mismatches.

DISEASE PROGRESSION

Progression of allograft arteriopathy is highly variable and relates in part to whether the lesions are passenger atherosclerosis transferred with the donor heart at the time of transplant or *de novo* lesions. Also important with respect to progression is the immunologic and non-immunologic milieu related to allograft arteriopathy pathophysiology. Some patients have a remarkably accelerated progression of disease, with substantial arteriopathy noted within the first year. Others may have an isolated single-vessel lesion which remains unchanged for long periods of time. Once patients develop at least a 70% stenosis by angiography in one vessel, they have a worse prognosis, with important mortality reported within the following year.[104, 163]

Thus, in many respects knowledge about the **progression** of allograft vasculopathy (and its variability and determinants) is as important as information about the disease process itself. Unfortunately, secure knowledge in this regard is difficult to come by, since most studies generate inferences on disease progression in *individuals* by examing (either by angiography or IVUS) many patients at various time points after transplantation (cross sectional studies) (Table 17–7),[255] with few well-studied sequential longitudinal studies on individual patients.

McGiffin and colleagues[202] examined *angiographic* progression of allograft vascular disease by employing a scoring system based on angiographic severity of coronary artery disease in epicardial arteries and the amount of myocardium in jeopardy. In general, a score of 15 or

TABLE 17-7	Progression of Allograft Vasculopathy by IVUS				
YEARS AFTER TRANSPLANTATION	NO. OF PATIENTS	INTIMAL THICKNESS (mm)	INTIMAL INDEX	ECC	CALC
Baseline (<2 mo)	50	0.09 ± 0.02*	0.07 ± 0.01	18%	9%
1	52	0.16 ± 0.02*	0.14 ± 0.02	44%	2%
2	47	0.23 ± 0.03	0.17 ± 0.02	43%	9%
3	33	0.26 ± 0.04	0.20 ± 0.03	39%	6%
4	34	0.27 ± 0.03	0.21 ± 0.03	35%	12%
5	35	0.33 ± 0.04	0.24 ± 0.03	51%	6%
6–10	42	0.33 ± 0.04	0.25 ± 0.03	38%	24%
11–15	11	0.30 ± 0.06	0.27 ± 0.05	27%	46%

IVUS, intravascular ultrasound; CALC, studies showing calcification; ECC, studies showing eccentric lesions.
* $p < .05$ versus value in succeeding year.
Data are expressed as mean value = SEM or percent of studies.
Adapted from Rickenbacher PR, Pinto FJ, Lewis NP, Hunt SA, Aldermann EL, Schroeder JS, Stinson EB, Brown BW, Valantine HA: Prognostic importance of intimal thickness as measured by intracoronary ultrasound after cardiac transplantation. Circulation 1995;92:3452.

more indicated severe three-vessel disease. From this study, although there was considerable variability, once allograft vasculopathy was identified, the rate of progression of disease was similar irrespective of the time after transplant when coronary artery disese was first identified (Fig. 17–21). It is of interest that earlier detected coronary artery disease was not, on average associated with an accelerated rate of progression compared to disease first detected years later. However, the seriousness of progression to severe allograft vasculopathy is underscored in the large multicenter analysis by Costanzo and colleagues[46] (Fig. 17–22), in which the probability of graft loss (death or retransplant) due to allograft vasculopathy was greater than 60% within 2 years after diagnosing **severe disease** (see Table 17–5) by angiography. In contrast, the likelihood of death or retransplant for vasculopathy was less than 20% within 2 years for milder forms of diseases. Allograft vasculopathy as a cause of posttransplant mortality is further discussed in Chapter 16.

IVUS studies have given greater insight into allograft arteriopathy progression and prognosis, demonstrating distinct heterogeneity of transplant coronary disease. A cross-sectional study from Stanford[255] (limited by the lack of serial studies in individual patients) provides some useful insights into the progression of intimal thickening. The severity of allograft vasculopathy, as judged by the degree of intimal thickening, tends to progress with time after transplantation, but there is considerable variability between arterial sites within the same individual and between individuals. Based on a multiinstitutional study, on the average, the most striking progression of disease occurs during the first posttransplant year, with slow progression thereafter. Several studies have identified rapid progression of intimal thickening by IVUS as a risk factor for adverse outcome

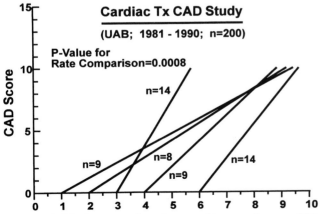

FIGURE **17–21.** Regression lines for rate of increase in mean CAD score according to the year of first angiographic detection of CAD. (From McGiffin DC, Savunen T, Kirklin JK, Naftel DC, Bourge RC, Paine TD, White-Williams C, Sisto T, Early L: Cardiac transplant coronary artery disease: a multivariable analysis of pretransplantation risk factors for disease development and morbid events. J Thorac Cardiovasc Surg 1995;109:1081–1089.)

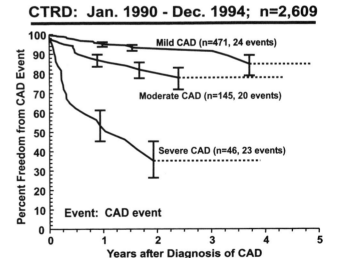

FIGURE **17–22.** Actuarial (Kaplan-Meier) freedom from occurrence of allograft coronary artery disease (CAD) event (death or retransplantation caused by CAD) according to degree of CAD present at time when CAD was first detected by coronary angiography. Top line, mild CAD. Middle line, moderate CAD. Bottom line, severe CAD. Error bars indicate 70% confidence limits. (From Costanzo MR, Naftel DC, Pritzker MR, Heilman JK, Boehmer JP, Brozena SC, Dec GW, Ventura HO, Kirklin JK, Bourge RC, Miller LW, The Cardiac Transplant Research Database: Heart transplant coronary artery disease detected by coronary angiography: a multiinstitutional study of preoperative donor and recipient risk factors. J Heart Lung Transplant 1998;17:744–753.)

(see later section, Prediction of Adverse Outcome by Intravascular Ultrasound).

It is important to note that in doing serial IVUS studies, many confounding variables must be taken into consideration. Possibly most important is ensuring that initial ultrasound examination is done within a few weeks of transplantation to document baseline status of the artery. This is the only way to identify passenger atherosclerosis, and it is now known that these lesions often have a different natural history, with less progression or lumen area reduction. Subsequent serial examination of identical matched sites enables quantification of specific lesion progression and avoids the statistical hazard of pooling data from many different sites, since each site serves as its own control. With this approach, an observed change in dimensions over time can be attributed to disease progression and/or remodeling.

RISK FACTORS FOR ALLOGRAFT VASCULAR DISEASE

The previous section Pathophysiology and Immunobiology of Allograft Vascular Disease summarizes the evidence linking atherosclerosis, acute cellular and humoral rejection, infection, and events surrounding the transplant operation to endothelial injury and the subsequent cascade of events leading to allograft vasculopathy. In view of the variety of pathogenic factors which contribute to allograft vascular disease, the imprecision in making the diagnosis of acute cellular and humoral rejection (see Chapter 14), and the reliance on the rather imprecise method of angiography for the detection of allograft coronary artery disease in most clinical studies, it is not surprising that specific risk factors for the development of allograft vasculopathy have been difficult to demonstrate. However, information from a number of clinical studies has provided important insight into the multitude of risk factors which interact to promote allograft vasculopathy.

IMMUNOLOGIC RISK FACTORS

Although many studies have failed to identify specific immunologic risk factors for allograft vasculopathy, several important reports have linked immunologic disparity between donor and recipient, acute cellular rejection, and humoral rejection with the subsequent development of allograft vasculopathy.

Donor/Recipient Immunologic Disparity

Several clinical studies have identified a correlation between the degree of HLA mismatch and the development of allograft vasculopathy. Cocanaugher and colleagues demonstrated the additive effects of lipid perturbation (particularly triglyceride elevation) and the degree of HLA mismatch on worsening allograft arteriopathy.[43] This study and that of Costanzo[45] indicate that complete HLA-B and HLA-DR mismatch is associated with a higher incidence of allograft arteriopathy. The HLA-DR mismatch is particularly important in these analyses.

Endothelial Activation

Although endothelial activation is considered the sentinal event in allograft vascular disease, few clinical studies have examined this relationship. In an eloquent set of studies, Labarrere and colleagues examined markers of endothelial activation (ICAM-1 and HLA-DR) on arteries and arterioles in endomyocardial biopsies and correlated the findings with evidence of coronary artery disease on angiography.[173] Endothelial activation was common following transplantation and, importantly, the proportion of biopsies during the first 3 months which showed activation (expression of endothelial cell **ICAM-1 and HLA-DR**) was significantly related to the **risk of any coronary artery** disease (Fig. 17–23), time required to develop coronary disease, progression of disease, and the likelihood of graft failure.

Humoral Rejection

Hammond and colleagues[123] reported an association between antibody deposition in the cardiac allograft (by immunofluorescence), acute rejection, and reduced survival. This group also suggested that an increased incidence of allograft arteriopathy was noted in patients with positive immunofluorescence staining of endomyocardial biopsies said to be diagnostic of "vascular" rejection.[124] In a large retrospective study,[182] the degree of panel reactive antibody (PRA) responsiveness correlated with both acute cellular rejection developing within the first 3 posttransplant months and subsequent development of allograft arteriopathy. Other studies have also suggested that the development of antibody to donor endothelium predicted development of arteriopathy.[122, 123, 141, 150, 204, 286]

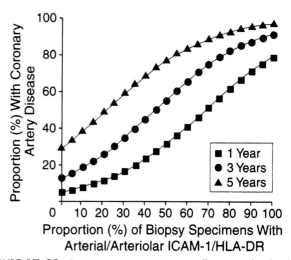

FIGURE **17–23.** Logistic regression estimates illustrating the development of coronary artery disease in allograft recipients with different percentages of biopsy specimens positive for arterial/arteriolar endothelial ICAM-1/HLA-DR during the first 3 months after transplantation. ICAM-1 indicates intercellular adhesion molecule-1. (From Labarrere CA, Nelson DR, Faulk WP: Endothelial activation and development of coronary artery disease in transplanted human hearts. JAMA 1997;276:1169–1175.)

Acute Cellular Rejection

Although many clinical studies have failed to identify acute rejection phenomena as a risk factor for allograft vasculopathy,[76, 299] several studies have suggested a link between indices of acute rejection and subsequent allograft coronary disease. Uretsky and colleagues[309] reported that the occurrence of two or more major rejection episodes were statistically correlated with the prevalence and severity of allograft vasculopathy. Early elevation of plasma soluble IL-2 receptor levels (a marker for activation of the lymphocytic immune system) has shown significant correlation with the subsequent development of allograft arteriopathy.[343] A positive correlation between higher rejection scores and allograft arteriopathy was also identified by Schutz and colleagues[273] The notion that increasing severity of rejection increases the risk and severity of allograft vasculopathy is further supported by an intravascular ultrasound study by Mehra and colleagues, in which a first-year mean biopsy score greater than 1 (a measure of rejection severity and frequency of insidious rejection) was an independent predictor (along with donor age >35 years and hypertriglyceridemia) of severe intimal hyperplasia.[203]

Because of the multifactorial nature of allograft vasculopathy and the relative insensitivity of angiography as a detection method, large cohorts of patients are likely necessary to unveil true relationships between acute rejection and subsequent allograft vasculopathy. That opportunity became available with a detailed analysis of the Cardiac Transplant Research Database, in which Ventura and colleagues examined pretransplant variables as well as multiple rejection and infection variables during the first 6 months after transplant for their effect on the development of allograft vasculopathy by angiography.[317] The study group consisted of 2,134 patients (with over 7,000 angiograms) from 38 institutions who underwent cardiac transplantation between 1990 and 1996 and had no angiographic evidence of allograft vasculopathy on the first annual coronary angiogram. The risk factors (identified by multivariable hazard function analysis) for subsequent allograft coronary artery disease are listed in Table 17–8. The recipient and donor pretransplant risk factors were similar to those identified by Costanzo and coworkers[46] (see later section, Nonimmunologic Risk Factors). Of particular interest was the

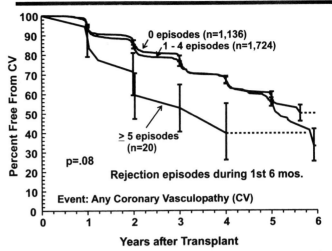

FIGURE **17–24.** Actuarial (Kaplan-Meier) freedom from occurrence of any coronary vasculopathy (CV) stratified by the number of rejection episodes during the first 6 months after transplant. Error bars indicate 70% confidence limits. CTRD, Cardiac Transplant Research Database. (From Ventura H, Kirklin JK, Eisen H, Michler R, Clemson B: The combined impact of pretransplant risk factors and rejection frequency and severity on the prevalence of post transplant coronary vasculopathy [abstract]. J Heart Lung Transplant 1997;16:66.)

strong correlation between rejection frequency during the first 6 months (Fig. 17–24) and subsequent allograft vasculopathy. The interaction between rejection frequency and donor age as risk factors for allograft coronary disease is depicted in Figure 17–25. Based on the multivariable analysis, high- and low-risk groups for subsequent allograft vasculopathy were identified (Fig. 17–26).

These authors also analyzed risk factors for **severe allograft vasculopathy** (Fig. 17–27), defined either ac-

TABLE 17-8	Risk Factors for Any Allograft Vasculopathy by Angiography (CTRD, 1990–1995, N = 2,134)
RISK FACTOR	p VALUE
Recipient:	
Age (older)	.02
Black	.008
Donor:	
Age (older)	<.0001
Male	<.0001
Rejections during first 6 mo:	
Number of episodes	.001

CTRD, Cardiac Transplant Researach Database.
Adapted from Ventura H, Kirklin JK, Eisen H, Michler R, Clemson B: The combined impact of pretransplant risk factors and rejection frequency and severity on the prevalence of post transplant coronary vasculopathy [abstract]. J Heart Lung Transplant 1997;16:66.

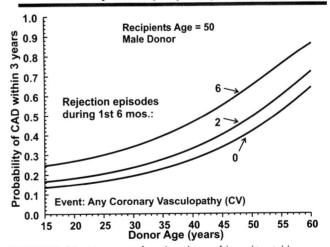

FIGURE **17–25.** Nomogram from the solution of the multivariable equation for allograft vasculopathy, depicting the effect of increasing rejection episodes on the development of allograft coronary artery disease (CAD). CTRD, Cardiac Transplant Research Database. (From Ventura H, Kirklin JK, Eisen H, Michler R, Clemson B: The combined impact of pretransplant risk factors and rejection frequency and severity on the prevalence of post transplant coronary vasculopathy [abstract]. J Heart Lung Transplant 1997;16:66.)

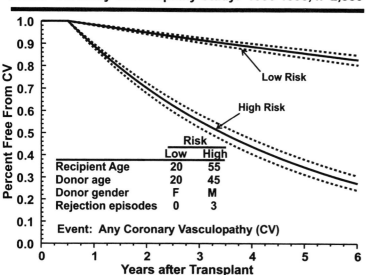

CTRD: Coronary Vasculopathy Study: 1990-1995, n=2,880

FIGURE **17-26.** Solution from the multivariable equation (as in Fig. 17-25) depicting high- and low-risk patients for the event allograft vasculopathy. Dashed lines indicate 70% confidence limits. CTRD, Cardiac Transplant Research Database. (From Ventura H, Kirklin JK, Eisen H, Michler R, Clemson B: The combined impact of pretransplant risk factors and rejection frequency and severity on the prevalence of post transplant coronary vasculopathy [abstract]. J Heart Lung Transplant 1997; 16:66.)

cording to angiographic criteria in Table 17-4[46] or allograft vasculopathy causing death or retransplantation. The risk factors identified for this event are listed in Table 17-9. Thus, as suggested in prior studies,[204, 273] this analysis provides substantial clinical evidence that more frequent and severe forms (rejection with hemodynamic compromise) of rejection contribute to more severe forms of allograft vasculopathy (Fig. 17-28).

NONIMMUNOLOGIC RISK FACTORS

In addition to risk factors for immune-mediated components of allograft vasculopathy, many nonimmune factors contribute to the development of the disease (Table 17-10).

Donor Atherosclerosis Risk Factors

Early "passenger" coronary artery disease and/or general risk factors for atherosclerosis in the **donor** play an important contributing role to the development of allograft vasculopathy. Since the early Stanford experience, **older donor age** has long been suspected as a risk factor for allograft coronary disease. This finding has been supported by multivariable analysis in a single center study[202] and in recent multi-institutional studies[46, 317] (Table 17-8). Additional donor risk factors include donor male gender (Fig. 17-29) and a history of hypertension (Fig. 17-30).[46] These donor risk factors are consistent with existing knowledge about atherosclerosis risk factors in the general population.[105]

The adverse effect of older donor age on the later development of angiographically detectable allograft

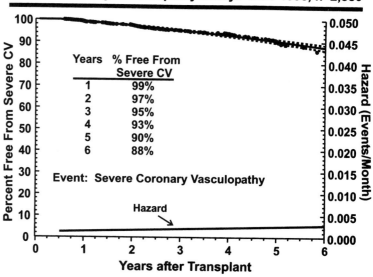

CTRD: Coronary Vasculopathy Study: 1990-1995, n=2,880

FIGURE **17-27.** Actuarial (Kaplan-Meier) freedom from severe (see text for definition) allograft coronary vasculopathy (CV). The dashed lines indicate the 70% confidence limits. The lower line is the hazard function. (From Ventura H, Kirklin JK, Eisen H, Michler R, Clemson B: The combined impact of pretransplant risk factors and rejection frequency and severity on the prevalence of post transplant coronary vasculopathy [abstract]. J Heart Lung Transplant 1997;16:66.)

TABLE 17-9	**Risk Factors for Severe Allograft Vasculopathy by Angiography (CTRD: 1990–1995, N = 2,134)**

RISK FACTOR	*p* VALUE
Recipient:	
Black	.002
Donor:	
Age (older)	<.0001
Rejections during first 6 mo:	
Number of episodes	.0007
Number of episodes with hemodynamic compromise	.003

CTRD, Cardiac Transplant Researach Database.
Adapted from Ventura H, Kirklin JK, Eisen H, Michler R, Clemson B: The combined impact of pretransplant risk factors and rejection frequency and severity on the prevalence of post transplant coronary vasculopathy [abstract]. J Heart Lung Transplant 1997;16:66.

TABLE 17-10	**Potential Nonimmunologic Risk Factors for Allograft Arteriopathy**

- Donor atherosclerosis risk factors
- Presence of passenger atherosclerosis
- Recipient age and gender
- Recipient cardiac diagnosis
- Cytomegalovirus infection
- Lipid abnormalities
- Hypertension
- Diabetes mellitus
- Obesity
- Cigarette smoking
- Markers for impaired fibrinolysis
- Homocysteine levels
- Immunosuppressive drugs
- Ischemic time
- Reperfusion injury

coronary artery disese is most pronounced for donors above about 40 years of age (Fig. 17–31). However, the effect of older donor age on the development of *severe* allograft vasculopathy is less pronounced (Fig. 17–32). Older donor age has also been identified as a risk factor for earlier severe intimal hyperplasia by intravascular ultrasound.[203]

Risk factors for "passenger" coronary artery disease present at transplant have been indirectly explored by Costanzo and colleagues.[46] In a multivariable analysis of angiographic coronary artery disease identified within the first 6 months after transplant (approximating donor coronary disease), older donor age ($p < .0001$) and donor history of hypertension ($p < .0002$) were risk factors for early coronary artery disease. As noted in an earlier section, this has some importance, since that rate of disease progression may differ from allograft vasculopathy which appears after transplant.[158]

Recipient Age and Gender

Older age and male gender are recognized risk factors for atherosclerosis in the general population. In large multi-institutional studies, older recipient age (Table 17–8)[317] and, in some analyses, male gender (Fig. 17–29) appear to increase the risk of developing allograft vasculopathy. However, the gender and age of the donor appear to be more significant predictors of disease development than recipient demographics. A multivariable analysis of patients transplanted in the 1980s suggested that male recipients of female donor hearts were at increased risk of graft loss from allograft vasculopathy,[276] but this finding was not substantiated in more recent multi-institutional studies.[46, 317]

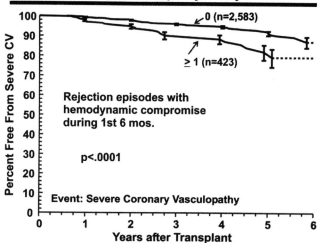

FIGURE **17–28.** Actuarial (Kaplan-Meier) freedom from allograft vasculopathy stratified by the number of hemodynamically compromising rejection episodes. (From Ventura H, Kirklin JK, Eisen H, Michler R, Clemson B: The combined impact of pretransplant risk factors and rejection frequency and severity on the prevalence of post transplant coronary vasculopathy [abstract]. J Heart Lung Transplant 1997;16:66.)

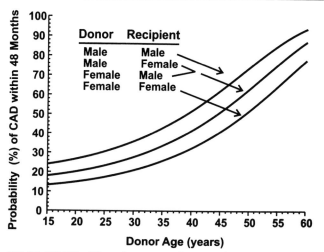

FIGURE **17–29.** Effect of interaction between donor age and donor recipient sex on probability of CAD within 48 months after heart transplantation. CTRD, Cardiac Transplant Research Database. (From Costanzo MR, Naftel DC, Pritzker MR, Heilman JK, Boehmer JP, Brozena SC, Dec GW, Ventura HO, Kirklin JK, Bourge RC, Miller LW, The Cardiac Transplant Research Database: Heart transplant coronary artery disease detected by coronary angiography: a multiinstitutional study of preoperative donor and recipient risk factors. J Heart Lung Transplant 1998; 17:744–753.)

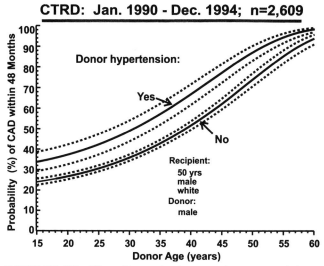

FIGURE **17–30.** Effect of interaction between donor age and donor history of hypertension on probability of CAD within 48 months after heart transplantation. CTRD, Cardiac Transplant Research Database. (From Costanzo MR, Naftel DC, Pritzker MR, Heilman JK, Boehmer JP, Brozena SC, Dec GW, Ventura HO, Kirklin JK, Bourge RC, Miller LW, The Cardiac Transplant Research Database: Heart transplant coronary artery disease detected by coronary angiography: a multiinstitutional study of preoperative donor and recipient risk factors. J Heart Lung Transplant 1998;17:744–753.)

Cytomegalovirus Infection

The evidence for cytomegalovirus contributing to the genesis of allograft vasculopathy is reviewed in the earlier section, Infection as an Etiology for Cardiac Allograft Vasculopathy. Grattan and colleagues[112] reported the

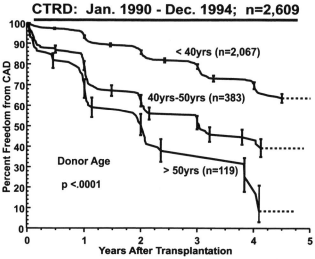

FIGURE **17–31.** Actuarial (Kaplan-Meier) freedom from appearance of any CAD on angiograms performed later than 6 months after heart transplant stratified by donor age. Top line, Donors younger than 40 years of age. Middle line, Donors 40–50 years of age. Bottom line, Donor older than 50 years of age. Error bars indicate 70% confidence limits. CTRD, Cardiac Transplant Research Database. (From Costanzo MR, Naftel DC, Pritzker MR, Heilman JK, Boehmer JP, Brozena SC, Dec GW, Ventura HO, Kirklin JK, Bourge RC, Miller LW, The Cardiac Transplant Research Database: Heart transplant coronary artery disease detected by coronary angiography: a multiinstitutional study of preoperative donor and recipient risk factors. J Heart Lung Transplant 1998;17:744–753.)

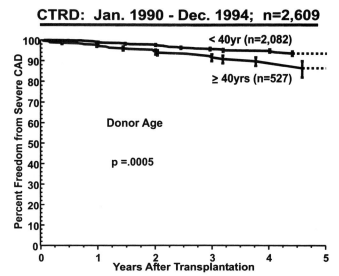

FIGURE **17–32.** Actuarial (Kaplan-Meier) freedom from appearance of severe CAD on angiograms performed later than 6 months after heart transplant stratified by donor age. Top line, Donors younger than 40 years of age. Bottom line, Donors older than 40 years of age. CTRD, Cardiac Transplant Research Database. (From Costanzo MR, Naftel DC, Pritzker MR, Heilman JK, Boehmer JP, Brozena SC, Dec GW, Ventura HO, Kirklin JK, Bourge RC, Miller LW, The Cardiac Transplant Research Database: Heart transplant coronary artery disease detected by coronary angiography: a multiinstitutional study of preoperative donor and recipient risk factors. J Heart Lung Transplant 1998;17:744–753.)

clinical association between CMV and allograft arteriopathy in 1989, noting that 28% of CMV-infected patients developed severe coronary obstructive lesions, but only 10% of patients not infected with CMV exhibited the same degree of allograft arteriopathy by the fifth posttransplant year ($p < .05$). Also, death or graft loss from allograft vasculopathy was more common among patients with CMV infections. Other studies pointing to CMV as a risk factor for allograft vasculopathy have been reported by Lobe et al.[192] and McDonald et al.[201] By multivariable analysis, a pretransplant positive CMV serology in the recipient has also been identified as a risk factor for subsequent allograft arteriopathy by angiogram.[202] One study[70] found that only those patients who had evidence of prolonged CMV infection, defined as a persistently positive blood buffy coat culture of CMV over a 4-month period, had a significant increase in the incidence of allograft vasculopathy.

Thus, although not all studies have identified a relationship,[18] the preponderance of evidence supports an interaction of CMV infection with other nonimmunologic and immunologic factors that contributes to the development of allograft vasculopathy.

Impaired Fibrinolysis

Impaired fibrinolysis in the donor heart could lead to increased fibrin deposition and earlier onset of allograft vasculopathy. Of the three genotypes for PAI-1, the **2/2 PAI-1 donor genotype** has been associated (by multivariable analysis) with earlier onset of posttransplant allograft coronary artery disease.[22] The authors hypothesize that genotype-specific overexpression of PAI-1 may lead to localized depletion of t-PA.

Other evidence supports deficiencies in fibrinolysis as a risk factor for allograft vasculopathy. Allografts with persistent **depletion of t-PA** in coronary arteriolar smooth-muscle cells on endomyocardial biopsies during the first 3 months after transplant had earlier onset of allograft vasculopathy.[176]

Posttransplant Lipid Disorders

A predictive model to assess risks for cardiac allograft vasculopathy based on intravascular ultrasonography was developed by Mehra and colleagues.[203] Significant independent predictors of severe intimal hyperplasia in their model included donor age greater than 35 years, a first posttransplant year mean biopsy score greater than 1, and hypertriglyceridemia at two incremental levels of risk (150–250 mg/dL and > 250 mg/dL). Based on the absence or presence of these factors, 12 individual categories of risk were ascertained with increasing relative risks and predicted probabilities for severe intimal hyperplasia. Additionally, subjects with severe intimal thickening had a fourfold higher cardiac event rate than those without this finding. Among patients with documented allograft vasculopathy, average triglyceride levels tend to be higher in those who suffer fatal ischemic events.[43] A 2-year cardiac transplant IVUS study by Valantine and colleagues found a significant correlation between higher LDL/HDL ratio and maximum intimal thickness.[312]

Perhaps the most compelling link, however, between dyslipidemia and allograft vasculopathy with subsequent cardiac events is the favorable effect of pravastatin on survival and freedom from allograft vasculopathy identified in a randomized trial[167] (see later section, Treatment of Allograft Arteriopathy).

Homocysteine Levels

A high homocysteine level is a risk factor for atherosclerosis and thrombosis in general populations.[199] Plasma homocyteine levels are generally higher in transplant patients than in the general population, which may in part be caused by low levels of folate and vitamin B$_6$.[118] In a study of heart transplant recipients, hyperhomocysteinemia (defined as a plasma level > 14.6 mmol/L) was (by univariate analysis) more common in patients who suffered vascular complications, including coronary artery disease, compared to other patients.[118]

The mechanisms of vascular disease development in the setting of hyperhomocysteinemia are likely complex but may relate to increased oxidant stress.[194] Vitamin B$_6$ deficiency probably contributes to atherosclerotic complications in these patients, as this deficiency is a risk factor for coronary artery disease, stroke, and peripheral vascular disease. This vitamin plays an important role in the metabolism of homocysteine and has an antithrombotic effect on platelets. Vitamin replacement with folic acid and vitamin B$_6$ can correct these nutritional deficiencies[12] in renal and heart transplant patients. Whether or not this translates into reduction of the incidence of allograft arteriopathy is currently unknown.

Recipient Cardiac Diagnosis

The effect of cardiac diagnosis prior to transplant on the development of allograft arteriopathy is controversial. A multivariable analysis by Sharples and colleagues identified patients transplanted for ischemic heart disease to be at greater risk for allograft vasculopathy.[276] Several large recent studies, however, have failed to confirm this finding.[46, 202, 316]

Other General Risk Factors for Atherosclerosis

Although not easily demonstrated by formal statistical analyses of transplant patient populations, many of the other risk factors for atherosclerosis in the general population likely contribute to the development of allograft vasculopathy. Hypertension, diabetes mellitus, and obesity all promote the development of atherosclerosis in the general population and probably also in the transplant recipient. The heart transplant patient is not immune to any of these problems and, indeed, immunosuppressive medications may aggravate these conditions.

Diabetes mellitus or insulin resistance and glucose intolerance is common in patients after cardiac transplantation. Steroids may contribute to this problem as well as hypertension. In the nontransplant patient there is a clear association of atherosclerotic cardiovascular disease with diabetes, but only a weak association exists, if at all, between diabetes and transplant allograft vascular disease.

Hypertension is common after cardiac transplantation and likely relates to pretransplant risk of this problem as well the posttransplant use of cyclosporine and steroids. Cyclosporine clearly causes hypertension as does tacrolimus. There has not, however, been a clearcut relationship demonstrated between hypertension and the development of allograft arteriopathy.[67, 228, 232, 276, 309, 338]

In a similar vein, **cigarette smoking** has not been proven to be a factor in the development of allograft vasculopathy after cardiac transplantation, although common sense suggests a detrimental effect.[67, 228, 232, 276, 309, 338] Cigarette smoking has been implicated as a risk factor for fatal allograft vasculopathy (see Chapter 16).

Prediction of Adverse Outcome by Intravascular Ultrasound

As noted in earlier discussions of coronary angiography and intravascular ultrasound (see earlier section, Diagnosis of Cardiac Allograft Vasculopathy), the likelihood of detecting early forms of allograft vasculopathy is greatly increased by the use of IVUS. In an IVUS study of patients 1–10 years (mean, 3.1 years) after transplantation, Rickenbauer and colleagues[255] demonstrated (by multivariable analysis) that intimal thickening of the left anterior descending artery (measured in up to four locations) greater than 0.3 mm was a significant predictor of both the subsequent development of angiographic coronary disease and, more importantly, subsequent death or retransplantation due to allograft vasculopathy.

In another univariate (risk unadjusted) analysis of IVUS at varying posttransplant times, Mehra and coauthors[204] found a significant association between a severe grade of intimal thickness and the subsequent development of cardiac events (sudden death, acute myocardial infarction, or the need for angioplasty).

Kapadia and colleagues from the Cleveland Clinic evaluated the utility of IVUS to predict clinical outcome after heart transplantation.[159] In 100 patients undergoing early multivessel IVUS after transplant which was then repeated about 1 year later, sites of disease (defined as a lesion with an intimal thickness > 0.5 mm) were identified and related to adverse outcome (defined as death, new congestive heart failure, myocardial infarction, and depressed left ventricular function or wall motion abnormalities on resting two-dimensional echocardiography). Among patients who showed new lesions of allograft arteriopathy (defined as an increase in intimal thickness > 0.5 mm at one or more paired sites), composite adverse clinical outcome rate was 25% during 43 months of follow-up. In contradistinction, patients without rapid progression had an adverse outcome rate of only 11% ($p = .03$). By multivariable analysis, patients with rapidly progressive intimal thickening suffered a worse clinical outcome (relative risk, 3.1; 95% confidence interval, 1.1–8.8; $p = .03$). It appears that rapidly progressive intimal thickening in the first year after cardiac transplantation is a powerful predictor of significant adverse events (death, myocardial infarction, and heart failure) in subsequent years. It has been suggested that these patients may be an appropriate group for more aggressive anti-atherosclerotic and immunosuppressive therapy.

Based on these and other IVUS studies, the sensitivity of this technique may provide valuable information through scheduled, routine studies that could stimulate more intensive risk-factor modification and/or more frequent angiographic evaluation (to allow for angioplasty therapy or relisting for cardiac retransplantation) (see later sections).

TREATMENT OF ALLOGRAFT ARTERIOPATHY

The treatment of established cardiac allograft vasculopathy has been largely ineffective, and current therapeutic strategies have focused on prevention. Based on identified pathogenic mechanisms and characterization of immune and nonimmune risk factors, multiple approaches have been evaluated (Table 17–11), with some proving moderately successful. Although several immunosuppressive modalities will be discussed which ameliorate allograft vasculopathy in experimental models and have some clinical evidence which suggests benefit, none has yet proven to be clearly efficacious in clinical heart transplant vasculopathy. Much of the therapeutic strategy is derived from approaches for risk reduction used in patients with nontransplant atherosclerosis, specifically control of hypertension, treatment of hyperlipidemia, control of diabetes, reduction of obesity, abstinence from

TABLE 17–11	Treating Allograft Arteriopathy: Potential Tactics to Prevent or Treat

Antihypertensive agents
  Calcium channel blockers
  Angiotensin converting enzyme inhibitors
Lipid-lowering agents
  HMG-CoA reductase inhibitors
Reduced endothelial injury at time of transplant
  Prevention of myocardial injury at brain death
  Improved myocardial preservation
  Prevention of reperfusion injury
Newer immunosuppressive agents
  Mycophenolate mofetil
  Rapamycin
  Anticytokine/adhesion molecule monoclonal antibodies as induction
  Leflunomide
  Gusperimus
Older immunosuppressive strategies
  Methotrexate
  Cyclophosphamide
  Induction lymphocytolytic strategies (monoclonal/polyclonal antibodies)
Prophylactic antimicrobial therapy
  Ganciclovir infusions
  Chronic prophylactic antimicrobial administration
Antiproliferative agents
  Angiopeptin
  Low-molecular-weight heparin (enoxaparin)
  Estrogen therapy
Antiplatelet agents
Antioxidants/vitamins
  Fish oil
  Omega-3 fatty acids
  Vitamin E
  Vitamin B$_6$
  Folic acid
Photophoresis
Lipoprotein aphoresis
Coronary revascularization
  Percutaneous transluminal coronary angioplasty/stent placement
  Percutaneous rotablator/atherectomy
  Coronary artery bypass
Transmyocardial laser revascularization
Cardiac retransplantation

cigarette smoking, and exercise. Modification of these risk factors in patients with native vessel coronary disease has been helpful; however, only limited information is available with respect to the heart transplant population. The following discussion will review the major available and theoretical approaches for prevention and control of allograft vasculopathy.

CALCIUM CHANNEL BLOCKERS

Calcium channel blocking agents have anti-atherosclerotic properties which are independent of their antihypertensive effect. Schroeder and colleagues[272] evaluated **diltiazem** in a clinical trial of 116 heart transplant patients. The drug was dispensed early after transplant and patients were evaluated with quantitative coronary angiographic studies at 1 and 2 years. Compared to control patients, the patients treated with diltiazem had less intimal thickening and were less likely to develop significant reduction in coronary artery luminal diameter compared with their baseline values.

Whether or not other drugs of this class provide similar effects is not clear. Atkinson and colleagues[15] evaluated amlodipine in a rat heterotopic transplant model and demonstrated that coronary narrowing was attenuated. Furthermore, this study suggested that smooth muscle cell migration and proliferation involved calcium-dependent mechanisms that were blocked at least partially by amlodipine.

Information from the International Nifedipine Trial on Anti-atherosclerotic Therapy (INTACT) (a multicenter randomized, double-blind study in established atherosclerosis) suggests a beneficial role of calcium channel blockers in inhibiting the development of coronary atherosclerotic lesions.[203, 333] Calcium channel blocker attenuation of atherosclerosis has been a longstanding and controversial issue,[271] with some suggesting that these drugs may also stabilize endothelial function and inhibit platelet aggregation with subsequent decrease in the release of platelet-derived growth factors. Use of calcium channel blockers may then result in attenuation of intimal thickening both directly and secondarily due to controlling systemic hypertension which is extraordinarily common after cardiac transplantation. It should also be pointed out that diltiazem increases cyclosporine levels by about 15–20% when concomitantly administered to patients receiving this drug. It is difficult to tell if this, as well, contributes to attenuation of intimal thickening and allograft arteriopathy seen by the Stanford group. **Diltiazem is currently routinely prescribed for most patients following cardiac transplantation.**

ANGIOTENSIN CONVERTING ENZYME INHIBITORS

There has been a great deal of interest in using angiotensin converting enzyme (ACE) inhibitors to prevent cardiac events in patients with atherosclerosis. Studies of Left Ventricular Dysfunction (SOLVD) demonstrated that patients with heart failure given enalapril had a significant reduction in atherosclerotic related cardiac events.[347] More recently, the Heart Outcomes Prevention Evaluation (HOPE) proved that ramipril routinely given in patients with prior myocardial infarction, known coronary artery disease, past stroke or carotid artery disease, and diabetics with risk factors for atherosclerosis, had dramatic reduction in the incidence of myocardial infarction, stroke, manifest heart failure, and progression of diabetes.[91, 347] Importantly, in a HOPE substudy that evaluated progression of carotid artery disease with B-mode ultrasound, patients allocated to the angiotensin converting enzyme inhibitor group had less advancement of atherosclerotic disease.

No similar studies have been done with this class of drugs in heart transplant patients, but there is reason to suspect that a benefit would be seen. Furthermore, in a rat heterotopic heart transplant model,[168] captopril was associated with a lower incidence of cellular and vascular rejection, minimal intimal proliferation, and reduced smooth muscle cell proliferation. Captopril and angiotensin converting enzyme inhibitors in general may inhibit endothelial damage and prevent atherosclerosis and their subsequent events through a paracrine renin-angiotensin mechanism or a suppressive effect on platelet activating factor.[246]

LIPID-LOWERING AGENTS

Hyperlipidemia is common after cardiac transplantation, and there is increasing evidence to suggest that lipid reduction therapy is an important intervention in transplant recipients.[9, 80] A randomized trial[167] demonstrated that patients taking pravastatin (started within 2 weeks of transplantation) during the first year after transplantation had significantly lower mean cholesterol levels (193 ± 36 vs. 248 ± 49 mg/dL, $p < 0.001$), with less frequent rejection episodes of hemodynamic significance (3 vs. 14 patients, $p = .005$), better survival (94% vs. 78%, $p = .925$), and a lower incidence of allograft arteriopathy at the time of either angiography or autopsy ($p = .049$). Some of these patients had undergone IVUS at both baseline and 1 year, and those patients in the pravastatin group had significantly less progression of coronary intimal thickness ($p = .002$) and intimal index ($p = .031$). It has been suggested that pravastatin has immunosuppressant as well as lipid-lowering effects. Interestingly, the cytotoxicity of natural killer cells in the pravastatin treatment group was substantially lower than in the control group (about 10% vs. 22% specific lysis, $p = .014$). Natural killer cell activity and growth factor–induced cell proliferation have also been inhibited by other lipid-lowering drugs of this class. On the basis of this and other studies, it has become common to **routinely prescribe pravastatin** immediately after transplantation irrespective of what the lipid profile is. The use of other lipid-lowering agents is discussed in Chapter 18.

ANTIPLATELET THERAPY

Aspirin has been shown to reduce platelet aggregation and is associated with a reduction in cardiac events in nontransplant patients with coronary artery disease.[95, 294] Despite the lack of evidence that it prevents allograft vasculopathy,[142, 220] aspirin therapy has become a standard part of posttransplant management (although the recommended dose remains controversial).

IMMUNOSUPPRESSIVE DRUGS

Given the fact that allograft arteriopathy is, at least in part, related to inflammation as part of T and B-cell–mediated rejection, newer immunosuppressive strategies have the potential to decrease the incidence, intensity, and progression of allograft arteriopathy (see also Chapter 13).[113, 207, 216, 293] Although no available immunosuppressive agents have a proven effect on the development of clinical allograft arteriopathy, both mycophenolate mofetil and sirolimus have been shown experimentally to attenuate smooth muscle cell proliferation.

Mycophenolate mofetil, as discussed in Chapter 13, is being evaluated in a multicenter clinical trial.[166] One-year follow-up data from this double-blind randomized trial of 650 heart transplant patients demonstrated survival and rejection benefit in patients randomized to mycophenolate mofetil compared to azathioprine. Intravascular ultrasound evaluation of allograft coronary arteries demonstrated a significant ($p = .007$) benefit of mycophenolate compared to azathioprine in the mean change in lumen area from baseline to 12 months after transplant.

Sirolimus has been observed to reverse chronic graft vascular disease in a rodent model of heart transplantation.[244] Sirolimus was able to substantially limit myocardial cellular infiltrate and attenuate intimal proliferation. This suggests that sirolimus, given early after transplantation, may attenuate allograft arteriopathy by a mechanism which inhibits smooth muscle cell proliferation (see also Chapter 13).

Antimetabolites such as methotrexate and cyclophosphamide have been used in an ad hoc fashion directed at a possible immune-mediated component of CAV. There have, however, been no randomized trials using methotrexate or cyclophosphamide for this purpose, and their effectiveness on established allograft vasculopathy is dubious.

Newer immunosuppressive agents, such as leflunomide and gusperimus, interfere with signals transduced by cytokines and growth factors and interrupt the proliferation of fibroblasts and smooth muscle cells (see Chapter 13). These drugs may thus have a future role in prevention of allograft vascular disease.

PHOTOPHERESIS

The technique of photopheresis is described in detail in Chapter 13. Barr and colleagues reported a reduction in the progression of intimal thickening over time by IVUS in a group of patients receiving prophylactic monthly photopheresis, compared to controls.[21] Although the precise mechanism is unknown, the observed decrease in circulating anti-HLA antibodies after treatment suggests the development of anti-idiotypic antibodies which could reduce humoral-mediated endothelial damage. Though this approach is presently being explored, it is a time-consuming and costly therapy.

APHORESIS STRATEGIES

Extracorporeal low-density lipoprotein precipitation during aphoresis therapy[181, 234, 235] has shown some effect in nontransplant patients with progressive coronary artery obstructive disease not controlled by lipid-lowering drugs alone. This approach has also been suggested for allograft arteriopathy, but the major drawback is the cost, inconvenience, and technical requirements of the treatment protocol.

ANTICYTOMEGALOVIRUS THERAPY

In view of the considerable evidence that CMV infection contributes to the development of allograft vasculopa-

thy, strategies to prevent development of this infection have been explored. Valantine and colleagues[313] analyzed a large cohort of patients who were randomized to receive either ganciclovir or placebo during the initial month after heart transplantation in an attempt to prevent development of CMV infection. Immunosuppression consisted of OKT3 prophylaxis initially and then maintenance therapy with cyclosporine, prednisone, and azathioprine. During a mean follow-up of nearly 5 years, for patients not receiving a calcium channel blocker, the actuarial incidence of allograft coronary artery disease in ganciclovir-treated patients was 43% versus 60% in patients randomized to placebo ($p < .03$). In the subset on calcium channel blocker therapy, the incidence of allograft disease was also less in the ganciclovir group, but the differences were not significant. By Cox multivariate analysis, independent predictors of allograft arteriopathy were donor age greater than 40 years ($p < .01$) and not receiving ganciclovir ($p = .04$). This observation suggests that prophylactic ganciclovir initiated immediately and routinely after heart transplantation, irrespective of CMV serology or development of subsequent infections, reduces the incidence of allograft arteriopathy.

The protective effect of ganciclovir against allograft vasculopathy is consistent with experimental studies in rat aortic allograft models.[184] In these experiments in which recipient animals were inoculated with CMV 1 day after transplantation, ganciclovir initiated on the day of transplant and then maintained for 2 weeks abolished the enhancing effect of CMV on allograft arteriopathy, blocked early adventitial inflammation and medial necrosis, and reduced smooth muscle cell proliferation. Importantly, later initiation of ganciclovir was ineffective in preventing allograft arterial disease.

Thus, early administration of ganciclovir seems important in preventing infection with CMV as well as the long-term adverse effects of CMV on transplant coronary artery disease. Whether or not ganciclovir is additive to calcium channel blocker use in reducing the likelihood of allograft vasculopathy has not been clarified.

ANTICOAGULANTS

An impaired anticoagulant pathway has been associated with the development of allograft vasculopathy (see earlier section, Pathophysiology and Immunobiology of Allograft Vascular Disease), and experimental evidence suggests that **heparin** is effective in blunting the allograft vasculopathy process. In addition to its anticoagulant effects, endogenous heparin (produced by mast cells within the vascular wall) is involved in the repair of injured vascular endothelium.[288] In nontransplant models of vascular injury, heparin has been shown to impede vascular smooth muscle cell migration and proliferation and decrease intimal thickening.[120, 247] Heparin binds to tissue thrombospondin and prevents its incorporation into the membranes of smooth muscle cells (an essential step in smooth muscle cell proliferation).[196] In addition, experimental transplant studies suggests that heparin has an immune-modulating capacity which, in conjunction with immunosuppressive therapy, delays immune cellular infiltration of the allograft and the onset of cellular rejection.[111, 190]

Low-molecular-weight heparins are depolymerized heparins usually constructed by chemical or enzymatic digestion of heparin, with molecular weight of about 5,000. They have the advantage over standard heparin of longer half-life, improved bioavailability, and lower incidence of thrombocytopenia.[73] In a rat heterotopic heart transplant model,[16] low-molecular-weight heparin added to a cyclosporine regimen diminished the incidence and severity of allograft arteriopathy as well as graft rejection. This and other evidence has given support to design of trials with antithrombotic agents such as enoxaparin.

INHIBITION OF MONOCYTE ADHESION AND MIGRATION

Adhesion of monocytes to injured endothelial surfaces is one of the early events in allograft vasculopathy. Inhibition of adhesion molecules such as ICAM-1, VCAM-1, fibronectin, E-selectin, P-selectin, and monocyte chemotactic protein could have an important impact on the allograft vasculopathy process.[52] Treatment with antibodies against leukocyte function-associated antigen-1 (LFA-1) and ICAM-1 receptor-ligand pairs for 1 week prolongs survival of mouse cardiac allografts.[149] Antibodies against LFA-1 are also effective in preventing experimental graft arteritis.[268]

GROWTH FACTOR INHIBITION

Angiopeptin, an analog of somatostatin (an inhibitor of growth hormone), has an inhibitory effect on vascular smooth muscle cell proliferation, possibly by inhibiting the release of insulin-like growth factors which promote myointimal hyperplasia. A preliminary study has indicated the safety of angiopectin in cardiac transplant patients,[326] but its efficacy in preventing allograft vascular disease remains to be established. The potential role of heparin and ACE inhibitors in the inhibition of growth factors has been discussed earlier.

REDUCTION OF HOMOCYSTEINE

As previously noted, Gupta and colleagues[118] studied homocysteine, folate, and vitamin B$_6$ concentrations in heart transplant patients, noting that high plasma homocysteine concentration is a risk factor for atherosclerosis and thrombosis in nontransplant patients. Administration of folic acid can easily reverse hyperhomocysteinemia, but whether this will translate into a decrement of vascular events after transplant is not known.

ANTIOXIDANTS AND FISH OIL

Considerable evidence supports the concept that antioxidants might reduce atherosclerosis and its subsequent

adverse events in both transplanted and nontransplanted patients. As noted previously (see earlier section, Pathophysiology and Immunobiology of Allograft Vascular Disease), oxidized low-density lipoprotein is atherogenic.[344] The antioxidants **vitamin E** and **probucol** reduce native atherosclerosis in animals.[35, 287, 339] In another study,[282] **ascorbic acid** (vitamin C) and **alpha-tocopherol** in combination with low-dose cyclosporine prolonged allograft survival in a rat heterotopic heart transplant model.

Although randomized clinical trials with vitamin E (400 units daily) have not produced conclusive evidence of its benefit on atherosclerosis,[56, 110] several retrospective studies have suggested an important reduction in coronary events with vitamin E.[256, 291] An attractive but unproven hypothesis states that oxygen-derived free radicals are involved in allograft vascular disease, and chronic antioxident therapy would reduce allograft arteriopathy.

Omega-3 fatty acids, the likely beneficial component of **fish oil,** may benefit the allograft coronary endothelium by induction of favorable changes in lipoproteins, inhibition of platelet aggregation, reduction of serum thromboxane, altered plasma membrane fluidity, and reduction in growth factor production.[183, 205, 344] Although the concept is intriguing, experimental results have not been striking. Yun and coauthors[346] failed to demonstrate a beneficial effect of fish oil on allograft vascular disease in a rat heterotopic transplant model.

However, Fleischhauer and colleagues[85] reported a fascinating clinical study designed to determine whether dietary fish oil supplementation enhanced endothelium-mediated vasodilator response during routine coronary angiography. Interestingly, the patients treated with fish oil demonstrated a normal vasodilator response to acetylcholine compared with control patients, who demonstrated vasoconstrictor responses at the same doses. There were no differences in response to nitroglycerin between control and treated patients. The authors concluded that dietary supplementation with fish oil significantly altered endothelium-dependent coronary vasodilation after heart transplant without altering the responses to endothelium-independent vasodilation. Whether this effect could translate into alteration of the natural history of allograft arteriopathy remains to be determined.

Barbir and coworkers[20] studied the effect of therapy with fish oil versus fibric acid in heart transplant patients with lipid perturbation. Therapy with fish oil (maxepa) (10 g/day) for 3 months was compared to a fibric acid derivative (bezafibrate) (400 mg/day), which has lipid-lowering effects,[229] enhances anticoagulation,[351] decreases plasma viscosity, and reduces fibrinogen levels.[5, 13] After 1 month, bezafibrate reduced total cholesterol levels by 13%, low-density lipoprotein cholesterol levels by 20%, and apolipoprotein B levels by 13% with an increase in apolipoprotein A1 and high-density lipoprotein cholesterol. Maxepa had no effect on these lipids but was as effective as bezafibrate in reducing triglycerides (36% and 31%, respectively). Potential effects on the incidence of subsequent allograft arteriopathy or cardiac event rates were not reported.

Thus, the clinical and experimental studies of antioxidant therapy and fish oil administration have suggested that this therapy is not fraught with substantial toxicity, and adverse side effects are generally minimal. The hypothesis that antioxidants and fish oil preparations can be used to attenuate allograft arteriopathy is appealing, but convincing clinical trial data are still lacking to support its effectiveness in attenuating allograft vasculopathy.

ESTROGEN THERAPY

The administration of estrogens in experimental models of rabbit heart and aortic allografts produces an attenuating effect on the progression of allograft vasculopathy.[89, 90, 151] Clinically, estrogen therapy retards the development and progression of coronary artery disease in postmenopausal women,[301] possibly through a cytoprotective effect on endothelial and smooth muscle cells.[90] The favorable effect of estrogens on experimental allograft vascular disease may relate to inhibition of smooth muscle cell proliferation and macrophage migration, preservation of endothelium, and modulation of serum lipoproteins. Its effect on clinical cardiac allograft vasculopathy is currently unknown.

REDUCTION OF ENDOTHELIAL INJURY AT TRANSPLANT

As discussed in Chapter 9, ischemic and reperfusion injury at the time of donor heart harvesting and implantation initiates a cascade of cellular and molecular events involving anoxic cellular injury, release of and injury induced by oxygen free radicals, and leukocyte-mediated injury initiated by the humoral amplification system. All of these forces act to initiate and/or aggrevate endothelial injury (see Fig. 12–23). The available and potential methods of reducing endothelial injury at the time of transplantation are discussed in Chapters 9 and 10.

PERCUTANEOUS TRANSLUMINAL CORONARY ANGIOPLASTY

As might be anticipated, revascularization strategies in patients with allograft arteriopathy have not been pursued aggressively because of the diffuse and distal vessel nature of the disease often noted. Nonetheless, because many patients do develop focal obstructive disease in more proximal coronary arteries, or have anatomically significant passenger atherosclerosis, percutaneous coronary revascularization and coronary artery bypass graft surgery have been attempted.

With the realization that focal proximal and midcoronary artery stenoses are a common manifestation of allograft vasculopathy, PTCA has been increasingly applied as palliative therapy for specific forms of allograft arteriopathy with discreet areas of stenosis. From multiple studies it is clear that PTCA is highly effective (nearly 95%) in achieving angiographic success (<50% residual stenosis) of focal lesions.[40, 121] The initial and late results are similar to or somewhat less than those in nontransplanted vessels,[40] which suggest that balloon-induced arterial trauma does not incite rapid progression of arterial narrowing. Allograft survival rates after angioplasty are highly variable (60–70% at 1–2 years[121, 153]) most likely reflecting the overall severity of the allograft vasculopathy. More recently, coronary stenting has shown some incremental improvement in outcome among cardiac transplant recipients.[134, 152] In a study of heart transplant recipients, conventional percutaneous angioplasty yielded mild and mostly inadequate gain in vessel luminal area (3.17 ± 0.92 mm^2 to 3.70 ± 1.21 mm^2). Coronary stenting led to greater luminal gain (3.70 ± 1.21 mm^2 to 5.86 ± 1.76 mm^2). After treatment with aspirin and ticlopidine only, all patients were clinically event free after a mean follow-up of 7.72 ± 5.45 months. At the mean follow-up, significant restenosis (> 50%) was found by intravascular ultrasound or by angiography 6 months after stent placement in 6 of 24 stented vessels (25%) in 16 patients.[134]

In our own experience, PTCA with stenting is the standard procedure for focal coronary stenoses after cardiac transplantation. For example, at UAB, more than 20 patients have received angioplasty therapy (up to five angioplasties/patient) from 2–12 years after transplantation. We have found it to be highly effective palliation, but close angiographic surveillance (every 4–6 months) is advisable in order to identify restenosis and, more importantly, new areas of focal stenosis in the accelerated atherosclerotic process which might be amenable to further PTCA procedures. However, there is no secure evidence that this procedure importantly alters the natural history of the disease.

Failed attempts at angioplasty are associated with substantial complications, including occasional periprocedure myocardial infarction with death. Angiographic **diffuse distal arteriopathy** is the major factor adversely affecting short- and intermediate-term allograft survival following PTCA.[121]

Directional **coronary atherectomy** has been reported in a small number of patients, with angiographic success noted in about 80 percent of lesions addressed.[121, 153, 300]

CORONARY ARTERY BYPASS SURGERY

Coronary artery bypass surgery has been infrequently applied as a palliative therapy for allograft vasculopathy.[64, 121] Because of the greater myocardial stress compared to PTCA and the generally diffuse nature of allograft vasculopathy, it is not surprising that the reported mortality has been high. In a multi-institutional survey, perioperative mortality was 33% (4 of 12 patients).[121] As in PTCA, diffuse and severe distal disease is an important risk factor for postoperative mortality. The likelihood of progressive disease and the important perioperative mortality make this aggressive therapy unattractive except in the small subset of patients who are not candidates for retransplantation, do not have diffuse distal angiographic disease, and have focal proximal disease (such as left main or ostial coronary stenoses) which is not amenable to safe PTCA/stenting.

TRANSMYOCARDIAL LASER REVASCULARIZATION

With the advent of transmyocardial laser revascularization, interest in applying this technology to allograft arteriopathy patients arose. A few anecdotes exist, with some suggesting benefit and others indicating rather high risk and adverse outcome after the procedure.[92, 212, 236] The procedure is designed to create channeling through the myocardium such that blood flow will occur from communication with the endoventricular surface of the left ventricle. Though the operation has been performed in non–heart transplant recipients, controversy exists about its effectiveness. It is uncertain if this procedure will palliate the difficulties associated with allograft arteriopathy, but some remain hopeful.[180, 330]

REPEAT TRANSPLANTATION

Because little effective therapy exists for allograft arteriopathy and morbidity and mortality rates are high in patients who become symptomatic because of this complication, cardiac retransplantation is often advised when the disease is severe. A detailed discussion of cardiac retransplantation is found in Chapter 22.

References

1. Adami JG: The nature of the arteriosclerotic process. Am J Med Sci 1909;138:485.
2. Adams DH, Russell ME, Hancock WW, Sayegh MH, Wyner LR, Karnovsky MJ: Chronic rejection in experimental cardiac transplantation: studies in the Lewis-F344 model. Immunol Rev 1993;5:19.
3. Adams DH, Tilney NL, Collins JJ: Experimental graft arteriosclerosis. Transplantation 1992;53:1115.
4. Akosah KO, Mohanty PK, Funai JT, Jesse RL, Minisi AJ, Crandall CW, Kirchberg D, Guerraty A, Salter D: Noninvasive detection of transplant coronary artery disease by dobutamine stress echocardiography. J Heart Lung Transplant 1994;13:1024–1038.
5. Almer LO, Kjellstrom T: The fibrinolytic system and coagulation during bezafibrate treatment of hypertriglyceridemia. Atherosclerosis 1986;61:81–85.
6. Alonso DR, Starek PK, Minick CR: Studies on the pathogenesis of atheroarteriosclerosis induced in rabbit cardiac allografts by the synergy of graft rejection and hypercholesterolemia. Am J Pathol 1977;87:415–422.
7. Amento EP, Ehsani N, Palmer H, Libby P: Cytokines and growth factors positively and negatively regulate interstitial collagen gene expression in human vascular smooth muscle cells. Arterioscler Thromb 1991;11:1223–1230.
8. Anderson M, Simpson I, Katritsis D, Davies MJ, Ward DE: Intravascular ultrasound imaging of the coronary arteries: an in vitro evaluation of measurement of area of the lumen and atheroma characterization. Br Heart J 1992;48:276.
9. Anguita M, Alonso-Pulpon L, Arizon J, Cavero MA, Valles F, Segovia J, Perez-Jimenez F, Crespo M, Concha M: Comparison of the effectiveness of lovastatin therapy for hypercholesterolemia after heart transplantation between patients with and without pretransplant atherosclerotic coronary artery disease. Am J Cardiol 1994;74:776–779.
10. Arbustini E, Grasso M, Diegoli M, Bramerio M, Foglieni AS, Albertario M, Martinelli L, Gavazzi A, Goggi C, Campana C:
11. Expression of tumor necrosis factor in human acute cardiac rejection. An immunohistochemical and immunoblotting study. Am J Pathol 1991;139:709–715.
11. Ardehali A, Laks H, Drinkwater DC, Ziv E, Drake TA: Vascular cell adhesion molecule-1 is induced on vascular endothelial and medial smooth muscle cells in experimental cardiac allograft vasculopathy. Circulation 1995;92:450–456.
12. Arnadottir M, Hultberg B: Treatment with high dose folic acid effectively lowers plasma homocysteine concentration in cyclosporin treated renal transplant recipients. Transplantation 1997;64:1087–1095.
13. Arntz HR, Leohardt H, Lang PD, Vollmar J: Effects of bezafibrate and clofibrate on blood rheology and lipoproteins in primary hyperlipoproteinaemia. J Clin Trials 1981;18:280–286.
14. Assoian RK, Komoriya A, Meyers CA: Transforming growth factor-β in human platelets: identification of a major storage site, purification, characterization. J Biol Chem 1983;258:7155.
15. Atkinson JB, Wudel JH, Hoff SJ, Stewart JR, Frist WH: Amlodipine reduces graft coronary artery disease in rat heterotopic cardiac allografts. J Heart Lung Transplant 1993;12:1036–1043.
16. Aziz S, Yoshikazu T, Gordon D, McDonald TO, Fareed J, Verrier ED: A reduction in accelerated graft coronary disease and an improvement in cardiac allograft survival using low molecular weight heparin in combination with cyclosporine. J Heart Lung Transplant 1993;12:634–643.
17. Aznar J, Estelles A, Tormo G, Sapena P, Tormo V, Blanch S, Espana F: Plasminogen activator inhibitor activity and other fibrinolytic variables in patients with coronary artery disease. Br Heart J 1988;59:535–541.
18. Balk A, Linden M, Meeter K: Is there a relation between transplant coronary artery disease and the occurrence of CMV infection? [abstract]. Am J Cardiol 1991;10:188.
19. Banai S, Jaklitsch MT, Casscells W, Shou M, Shrivastav S, Correa R, Epstein SE: Effects of acidic fibroblast growth factor on normal and ischemic myocardium. Circ Res 1991;69:76–85.
20. Barbir M, Hunt B, Kushwaha S, Kehely A, Prescot R, Thompson GR, Mitchell A, Yacoub M: Maxepa versus bezafibrate in hyperlipidemic cardiac transplant recipients. Am J Cardiol 1992;70:1596–1601.
21. Barr ML, Berger CL, Wiederman JG, Murphy MP, Jorgensen BA, McLaughlin SN, Schenkel FA, Papino P, He X, Marobe CC, Rose EA: Photochemotherapy for the prevention of graft atherosclerosis in cardiac transplantation. J Heart Lung Transplant 1993;12:585.
22. Benza RL, Grenett HE, Bourge RC, Kirklin JK, Naftel DC, Castro PF, McGiffin DC, George JF, Booyse FM: Gene polymorphisms for plasminogen activator inhibitor-1/tissue plasminogen activator and development of allograft coronary artery disease [abstract]. Circulation 1998;98:2248–2254.
23. Bieber CP, Stinson EB, Shumway NE, Payne R, Kosek J: Cardiac transplantation in man. VII. Cardiac allograft pathology. Circulation 1970;61:753–772.
24. Billingham ME: Cardiac transplant atherosclerosis. Transplant Proc 1987;19:19–25.
25. Billingham ME: Histopathology of graft coronary disease. J Heart Lung Transplant 1992;11:538–544.
26. Billingham ME: Pathology of graft vascular disease after heart and heart-lung transplantation and its relationship to obliterative bronchiolitis. Transplant Proc 1995;27:2013–2016.
27. Blakely ML, Van Der Werf WJ, Berndt MC, Dalmasso AP, Bach FH, Hancock WW: Activation of intragraft endothelial and mononuclear cells during discordant xenograft rejection. Transplantation 1994;58:1059–1066.
28. Boffa G, Faggian G, Buja G: Coronary artery spasm in heart transplant recipients. J Heart Lung Transplant 1989;8:154–158.
29. Border WA, Ruoslahti E: Transforming growth factor-beta in disease: the dark side of tissue repair. J Clin Invest 1992;90:1–7.
30. Bourin MC, Lindahl U: Glycosaminoglycans and the regulation of blood coagulation. Biochem J 1993;289:313–330.
31. Bowen-Pope DF, Ross R: Platelet-derived growth factor. II. Specific binding to cultured cells. J Biol Chem 1982;257:5161.
32. Briscoe DM, Schoen FJ, Rice GE: Vascular adhesion molecule-1 is induced on endothelium during acute rejection in human cardiac allografts. Transplantation 1991;51:537.

33. Bruschke AV, Padmos I, Buis B, Van Benthem A: Arteriographic evaluation of small coronary arteries. J Am Coll Cardiol 1990; 15:784.

34. Camejo G, Camejo EH, Olsson U, Bondjers G: Proteoglycans and lipoproteins in atherosclerosis. Curr Opin Lipidol 1993;4: 385–391.

35. Carew TE, Schwenke DC, Steinberg D: Atherogenic effect of probucol unrelated to its hypocholesterolemic effect: evidence that antioxidants in vivo can selectively inhibit low density lipoprotein degradation in macrophage-rich fatty streaks and slow progression of atherosclerosis in the Watanabe heritable hyperlipidemic rabbit. Proc Natl Acad Sci USA 1987;84:7725–7729.

36. Carlos T, Gordon D, Fishbien D: Vascular adhesion molecule-1 is induced on endothelium during acute rejection in human cardiac allografts. J Heart Lung Transplant 1992;11:1103.

37. Carrel A: Latent life of arteries. J Exp Med 1910;12:460.

38. Casino PR, Kilcoyne CM, Quyyumi AA, Hoeg JM: The role of nitric oxide in endothelium-dependent vasodilation of hypercholesterolemic patients. Circulation 1993;88:2541.

39. Chait A, Ross R, Albers JJ, Bierman EL: Platelet-derived growth factor stimulates activity of low density lipoprotein receptors. Proc Natl Acad Sci USA 1980;77:4084.

40. Christensen BV, Meyer SM, Iacarella CL, Kub SH, Wilson RF: Coronary angioplasty in heart transplant recipients: a quantitaive angiographic long term followup study. J Heart Lung Transplant 1994;13:212–220.

41. Clark JM, Glagov S: Transmural organization of the arterial media. The lamellar unit revisited. Arteriosclerosis 1985;5:19–34.

42. Clausell N, Rabinovitch M: Upregulation of fibronectin synthesis by interleukin-1 beta in coronary artery smooth muscle cells is associated with the development of the post-cardiac transplant arteriopathy in piglets. J Clin Invest 1993;92:1850–1858.

43. Cocanougher B, Ballantyne CM, Pollack MS: Degree of HLA mismatch as a predictor of death from allograft arteriopathy after heart transplantation. Transplant Proc 1993;25:233.

44. Collins T: Endothelial nuclear factor-kappa B and the initiation of the atherosclerotic lesion. Lab Invest 1993;68:499–508.

45. Costanzo-Nordin MR: Cardiac allograft vasculopathy: relationship with acute cellular rejection and histocompatibility [review]. J Heart Lung Transplant 1992;11:S90.

46. Costanzo MR, Naftel DC, Pritzker MR, Heilman JK, Boehmer JP, Brozena SC, Dec GW, Ventura HO, Kirklin JK, Bourge RC, Miller LW, The Cardiac Transplant Research Database: Heart transplant coronary artery disease detected by coronary angiography: a multiinstitutional study of preoperative donor and recipient risk factors. J Heart Lung Transplant 1998;17:744–753.

47. Cotran RS: New roles for the endothelium in inflammation and immunity. Am J Pathol 1987;129:407–413.

48. Cramer DV, Chapman FA, Wu GD: Cardiac transplantation in the rat. II. Alteration of the severity of donor graft arteriosclerosis by modulation of the host immune response. Transplantation 1990;50:554.

49. Cramer DV, Wu G, Chapman FA, Cajulis E, Wang H, Makowka L: Lymphocytic subsets and histopathologic changes associated with the development of heart transplant arteriosclerosis. J Heart Lung Transplant 1992;11:458–466.

50. Crisp SJ, Dunn MJ, Rose ML, Barbir M, Yacoub MH: Antiendothelial antibodies after heart transplantation: the accelerating factor in transplant-associated coronary artery disease. J Heart Lung Transplant 1994;13:81.

51. Curwen KD, Smith SC: Aortic glycosaminoglycans in atherosclerosis susceptible and resistant pigeons. Exp Mol Pathol 1977; 27:121–133.

52. Cybulsky MI, Gimbrone MA Jr: Endothelial expression of a mononuclear leukocyte adhesion molecule during atherogenesis. Science 1991;251:788–791.

53. Davies H, Al-Tikriti S: Coronary arterial pathology in the transplanted human heart. Int J Cardiol 1989;25:99–118.

54. Day JD, Rayburn BK, Gaudin PB, Baldwin WM, Lowenstein CJ, Kasper EK, Baughman KL, Baumgartner WA, Hutchins GM, Hruban RH: Cardiac allograft vasculopathy: the central pathogenetic role of ischemia in endothelial cell injury. J Heart Lung Transplant 1995;14:785–790.

55. Delafontaine P, Brin M, Anwar A, Hayry P, Okura Y: Growth factors and receptors in allograft arteriosclerosis. Transplant Proc 1999;31:111–114.

56. DeMaio SJ, King SB, Lembo JN, Roubin GS, Hearn JA, Bhagavan HN, Sgoutas DS: Vitamin E supplementation, plasma lipids and incidence of restenosis after percutaneous transluminal coronary angioplasty (PTCA). J Am Coll Nutr 1992;11:68–73.

57. Demetris AJ, Zerbe T, Banner B: Morphology of solid organ allograft arteriopathy: identification of proliferating intimal cell populations. Transplant Proc 1989;21:3667–3669.

58. DiCorleto PE, Gimbrone MA: Vascular endothelium. In Fuster V, Ross R, Topol EJ (eds): Atherosclerosis and Coronary Artery Disease. Philadelphia: Lippincott-Raven, 1996, pp 387–399.

59. Dietrich H, Hu Y, Zou Y, Dirnhofer S, Kleindienst R, Wick G, Xu Q: Mouse model of transplant arteriosclerosis: role of intercellular adhesion molecule-1. Arterioscler Thromb Vasc Biol 2000;20: 343–352.

60. Dodet B, Plotkin S: Infection and atherosclerosis. Am Heart J 1999;138:S417–S418.

61. Dressler FA, Miller LW: Necropsy versus angiography: how accurate is angiography? J Heart Lung Transplant 1992;11(suppl):S56.

62. Duguid JB: Thrombosis as a factor in the pathogenesis of coronary atherosclerosis. J Pathol Bacteriol 1946;58:207.

63. Dunn MJ, Crisp SJ, Rose ML, Taylor PM, Yacoub MH: Antiendothelial antibodies and coronary artery disease after cardiac transplantation. Lancet 1992;339:1566.

64. Dunning JJ, Kendall SWH, Mullins PA, Chauhan A, Graham TR, Biocina B, Schofield PM, Large SR: Coronary artery bypass grafting nine years after cardiac transplantation. Ann Thorac Surg 1992;54:571–572.

65. Duquesnoy RJ, Demetris AJ: Immunopathology of cardiac transplant rejection. Curr Opin Cardiol 1995;10:193–206.

66. Edwards DR, Murphy G, Reynolds JJ, Whitham SE, Docherty AJ, Angel P, Heath JK: Transforming growth factor beta modulates the expression of collagenase and metalloproteinase inhibitor. EMBO J 1987;6:1899–1904.

67. Eich D, Thompson JA, Ko DJ, Hastillo A, Lower R, Katz S, Katz M, Hess ML: Hypercholesterolemia in long-term survivors of heart transplantation: an early marker of accelerated coronary artery disease. J Heart Lung Transplant 1991;10:45–49.

68. Entman ML, Youker K, Shappell SB, Siegel C, Rothlein R, Dreyer WJ, Schmalstieg FC, Smith CW: Neutrophil adherence to isolated adult canine myocytes. Evidence for a CD18-dependent mechanism. J Clin Invest 1990;85:1497–1506.

69. Entman ML, Youker K, Shoji T, Kukielka G, Shappell SB, Taylor AA, Smith CW: Neutrophil induced oxidative injury of cardiac myocytes: a compartmented system requiring CD11b/CD18-ICAM-1 adherence. J Clin Invest 1992;90:1335–1345.

70. Everett JP, Hersberger RE, Norman DJ: Prolonged cytomegalovirus infection with viremia is associated with development of cardiac allograft vasculopathy. J Heart Lung Transplant 1992; 11:S133.

71. Falk E: Why do plaques ruture? Circulation 1992;86:III-30–III-40.

72. Fang JC, Rocco T, Jarcho J, Ganz P, Mudge JH: Noninvasive assessment of transplant associated arterial sclerosis [abstract]. Am Heart J 1998;135:980–987.

73. Fareed J, Kumar A, Walenga JM, Emanuele RM, Williamson K, Hoppensteadt D: Antithrombotic actions and pharmacokinetics of heparin fragments. Nouv Rev Fr Hematol 1984;26:267–275.

74. Faruqi RM, DiCorleto PE: Mechanisms of monocyte recruitment and accumulation. Br Heart J 1993;69:S19–S20.

75. Faulk WP, Labarrere CA, Pitts D, Halbrook H: Anticoagulant and fibrinolytic pathways in normal and transplanted human hearts. J Heart Lung Transplant 1992;11:211.

76. Faulk WP, Labarrere CA, Pitts D, Halbrook H: Laboratory-clinical correlates of time-associated lesions in the vascular immunopathology of human cardiac allografts. J Heart Lung Transplant 1993;12:S125–S134.

77. Faulk WP, Labarrere CA, Torry RJ, Nelson DR: Serum cardiac troponin-T concentrations predict development of coronary artery disease in heart transplant patients. Transplantation 1998; 66:1335–1339.

78. Faulk WP, Rose M, Meroni PL: Association of anti-endothelial antibodies with cellular rejection, vascular damage and coronary artery disease in cardiac allograft recipients [abstract]. J Heart Lung Transplant 1997;16:65.

79. Faxon DP, Coats W, Currier J: Remodeling of the coronary artery after vascular injury. Prog Cardiovasc Dis 1997;40:129–140.

80. Fay L: Cytomegalovirus and coronary artery disease in heart transplant patients accelerated low density lipoprotein and lipoprotein (A) modification as a proposed factor. J Heart Lung Transplant 1994;12:155.

81. Fellstrom B, Deimeny E, Larsson E, Klareskog L, Tufveson G, Rubin K: Importance of PDGF receptor expression in accelerated atherosclerosis-chronic rejection. Transplant Proc 1989;21:3689–3691.

82. Fibbi G, Magnelli L, Pucci M, delRosso M: Interaction of urokinase A chain with receptor of human keratinocytes stimulates release of urokinase-like plasminogen activator. Exp Cell Res 1990;187:33–38.

83. Fish RD, Nabel EG, Selwyn AP, Ludmer PL, Mudge GH, Kirshenbaum JM, Schoen FJ, Alexander RW, Ganz P: Responses of coronary arteries of cardiac transplant patients to acetylcholine. J Clin Invest 1988;81:21.

84. Fitzgerald PJ, St Goar FG, Connolly AJ, Pinto FJ, Billingham ME, Popp RL, Yock PG: Intravascular ultrasound imaging of coronary arteries: is three layers the norm? Circulation 1992;86:154–158.

85. Fleischhauer FJ, Yan W, Fischell TA: Fish oil improves endothelium-dependent coronary vasodilation in heart transplant recipients. J Am Coll Cardiol 1993;21:982–989.

86. Foegh ML: A treatment for accelerated myointimal hyperplasia? J Heart Lung Transplant 1992;11:28–31.

87. Foegh ML: Transplant atherosclerosis/chronic rejection in rabbits: inhibition by angiopeptine. Transplant Proc 1993;25:2095–2097.

88. Foegh ML, Khirabadi BS, Chambers E, Amamoo S, Ramwell PW: Inhibition of coronary artery transplant atherosclerosis in rabbits with angiopeptine, an octapeptide. Atherosclerosis 1989;78:229–236.

89. Foegh ML, Khirabadi BS, Nakasnishi T, Vargas R, Ramwell PW: Estradiol protects against experimental cardiac transplant atherosclerosis [abstract]. Transplant Proc 1987;19:90–95.

90. Foegh ML, Zhao Y, Lou H, Katz NM, Ramwell PW: Estrogen and prevention of transplant atherosclerosis [abstract]. J Heart Lung Transplant 1995;14:S170–S172.

91. Francis GS: ACE inhibition in cardiovascular disease. N Engl J Med 2000;342:201–202.

92. Frazier OH, Kadipasaoglu K, Radovancevic B, Cichan H, March R, Miroseini M, Cooley D: Transmyocardial laser revascularization in allograft coronary artery disease. Ann Thorac Surg 1998;65:1138–1141.

93. Frazier OH, McAllister HA, Jammal CT, Van Buren CT, Okereke OU, Radovancevic B, Cooley D: Occlusive coronary arteries: a cause of early death in a cardiac transplant patient. Ann Thorac Surg 1987;43:554.

94. Furchgott RF, Zawadzki VJ: The obligatory role of endothelial cells in the relaxation of arterial smooth muscle by acetylcholine. Nature 1980;288:373.

95. Fuster V, Cohen M, Halperin J: Aspirin in the prevention of coronary disease. N Engl J Med 1989;321:183–185.

96. Fyfe A, Daly P, Galligan L, Pirc L, Feindel C, Cardell C: Coronary sinus sampling of cytokines after heart transplantation: evidence for macrophage activation and interleukin-4 production within the graft. J Am Coll Cardiol 1993;21:171–176.

97. Gajdusek CM: Release of endothelial cell derived growth factor (ECDGF) by heparin. J Cell Physiol 1984;121:13–21.

98. Galis ZS, Myszynski M, Sukhova GK, Simon-Morrissey E, Unemori EN, Lark MW, Amento E, Libby P: Cytokine-stimulated human vascular smooth muscle cells synthesize a complement of enzymes required for extracellular matrix digestion. Circ Res 1994;75:181–189.

99. Galis ZS, Sukhova GK, Lark MW, Libby P: Increased expression of matrix metalloproteinases and matrix degrading activity in the vulnerable regions of human atherosclerotic plaque. J Clin Invest 1994;94:2493–2503.

100. Galle J, Schenck I, Schollmeyer P, Wanner C: Cyclosporine and oxidized lipoproteins affect vascular reactivity influence of the endothelium. Hypertension 1993;21:315–321.

101. Gao S-Z, Alderman E, Schroeder J, Silverman JF: Accelerated coronary vascular disease in the heart transplant patient: coronary arteriographic findings. J Am Coll Cardiol 1988;12:334–340.

102. Gao S-Z, Alderman EL, Schroeder JS, Hunt SA, Wiederhold V, Stinson EB: Progressive coronary luminal narrowing after cardiac transplantation. Circulation 1990;82:269–275.

103. Gao S-Z, Schroeder JS, Alderman EL: Prevalence of accelerated coronary artery disease in heart transplant survivors: comparison of cyclosporin and azathioprine regimens. Circulation 1989; 80(suppl III):100.

104. Gao S, Hunt S, Schroeder J, Alderman E, Hill IR, Stinson EB: Does rapidity of development of transplant coronary artery disease portend a worse prognosis? J Heart Lung Transplant 1994; 13:1119–1124.

105. Gao SZ, Schroeder JS, Alderman EL, Hunt SA, Silverman JF, Wiederhold V, Stinson EB: Clinical and laboratory correlates of accelerated coronary artery disease in the cardiac transplant patients [abstract]. Circulation 1987;76(suppl):V56–V61.

106. Gaudin P, Rayburn B, Hutchins G: Peritransplant injury to the myocardium associated with the development of accelerated arteriosclerosis in heart transplant recipients. Am J Surg Pathol 1994;18:338–346.

107. Gay CG, Winkles JA: Interleukin 1 regulates heparin-binding growth factor 2 gene expression in vascular smooth muscle cells. Proc Natl Acad Sci USA 1991;88:296.

108. Gerritsen ME, Bloor CM: Endothelial cell gene expression in response to injury. FASEB J 1993;7:523–532.

109. Gibbons GH: The pathogenesis of graft vascular disease: implications of vascular remodeling [abstract]. J Heart Lung Transplant 1995;14:S149–S158.

110. Gillilan MJ, Mondell B, Warbasse JR: Quantitative evaluation of vitamin E in treatment of angina pectoris. Am Heart J 1977;93:444–449.

111. Gorski A: Immunomodulating activity of heparin. FASEB J 1991;5:2287–2291.

112. Grattan MT, Moreno-Cabral CE, Stannes VA, Oyer PE, Shumway NE: Cytomegalovirus infection is associated with cardiac allograft rejection and atherosclerosis. JAMA 1989;261:3561–3566.

113. Gregory CR, Pratt RE, Shorthouse R, Dzau VJ, Billingham M, Morris R: Effects of treatment with cyclosporine, FK506, rapamycin, mycophenolic acid, or deoxyspergualin on vascular muscle proliferation in vitro and in vivo. Transplant Proc 1993; 25:770–771.

114. Greshman GA: Atherosclerosis: its origins and development in man. In Peeters H, Gresham GA, Paoletti R (eds): Arterial Pollution and Integrated View on Atherosclerosis. New York: Plenum Press, 1983, pp 7–21.

115. Griepp RB, Stinson E, Bieber CP, Reitz BA, Copeland JG, Oyer P, Shumway NE: Control of graft arteriosclerosis in human heart transplant recipients. Surgery 1977;81:262.

116. Griepp RB, Wexler L, Stinson EB, Dong E, Shumway NE: Coronary arteriography following cardiac transplantation. JAMA 1972;21:147.

117. Grotendorst G, Seppa HEJ, Kleinman HK, Martin G: Attachment of smooth muscle cells to collagen and their migration toward platelet-derived growth factor. Proc Natl Acad Sci USA 1981; 78:2669.

118. Gupta A, Moustapha A, Jacobsen D, Goormastic E, Tuzcu E, Hobbs R, Young J, James K, McCarthy P, VanLente F, Green R, Robinson K: High homocysteine, low folate, and low vitamin B6 concentrations: prevalent risk factors for vascular disease in heart transplant recipients. Transplantation 1998;65:544–550.

119. Hajjar KA, Hajjar DP, Silverstein RL: Tumor necrosis factor-mediated release of platelet-derived growth factor from cultured endothelial cells. J Exp Med 1987;166:235.

120. Hales CA, Kradin RL, Brandstetter RD, Zhu YJ: Impairment of hypoxic pulmonary artery remodeling by heparin in mice. Am Rev Respir Dis 1983;128:747–751.

121. Halle AA, DiSciascio G, Massin EK, Wilson RF, Johnson MR, Sullivan HJ, Bourge RC: Coronary angioplasty, atherectomy and bypass surgery in cardiac transplant recipients. J Am Coll Cardiol 1995;26:120–128.

122. Halloran PF, Schlaut J, Solez K: The significance of anti-class I response. II. Clinical and pathologic features of renal transplants with anti-class I like antibody. Transplantation 1992;53:550.

123. Hammond EH, Yowell RL, Nunoda S: Vascular (humoral) rejection in heart transplantation: pathologic observations and clinical interpretations. J Heart Transplant 1989;8:430–443.

124. Hammond EH, Yowell RL, Price GD: Vascular rejection and its relationship to allograft coronary artery disease. J Heart Lung Transplant 1992;11:S111.

125. Harker LA, Slichter SJ, Scott CR, Ross R: Homocysteine induced arteriosclerosis. The role of endothelial cell injury and platelet response in its genesis. J Clin Invest 1976;58:731–741.

126. Hart DNJ, Fuggle SV, Williams KA: Localization of HLA-ABC and DR antigens in human kidney. Transplantation 1981;31:428.

127. Hauptman PJ, Davis SF, Miller L, Yeung AC: The role of nonimmune risk factors in the development and progression of graft arteriosclerosis: preliminary insights from a multicenter intravascular ultrasound study. J Heart Lung Transplant 1995;14:S238.

128. Hayry P, Isoneimi H, Yilmaz S, Mennander A, Lemstrom K, Raisanen-Sokolowski A, Koskinen P, Ustinov J, Lautenschlager I, Taskinen E: Chronic allograft rejection. Immunol Rev 1993; 134:33–81.

129. Hayry P, von Willebrand E, Anderson LC: Expression of HLA-ABC and -DR locus antigens on human kidney endothelial tubular and glomerular cells. Scand J Immunol 1980;11:303.

130. Heemann UW, Schmid C, Azuma H, Tilney NL: The role of leukocyte adhesion molecules in acute transplant rejection [abstract]. Curr Opin Nephrol Hypertens 1994;3:459–464.

131. Heller-Harrison RA, Carter WG: Pepsin-generated type VI collagen is a degradation product of GP 140. J Biol Chem 1984; 259:6858–6864.

132. Herregods MC, Anastassious I, van Cleemput J, Bijens B, de Geest H, Daenen W: Dobutamine stress echocardiography after heart transplantation. J Heart Lung Transplant 1994;13:1039–1044.

133. Hess ML, Hastillo A, Mohanakumar T, Cowley MJ, Vetrovac G, Szentpetery S, Wolfgang TC, Lower RR: Accelerated atherosclerosis in cardiac transplantation: role of cytotoxic B-cell antibodies and hyperlipidemia. Circulation 1983;68:94–101.

134. Heublein B, Pethig K, Maas C, Wahlers T, Haverlich A: Coronary artery stenting in cardiac allograft vascular disease. J Am Coll Cardiol 1997;32:1636–40.

135. Higgy NA, Davidoff AW, Grothman GT, Hollenberg MD, Benediktsson H, Paul LC: Expression of platelet-derived growth factor receptor in rat heart allografts. J Heart Lung Transplant 1991; 10:1012–1025.

136. Hinek A, Boyle J, Rabinovitch M: Vascular smooth muscle cell detachment from elastin and migration through elastic laminae is promoted by chondroitin sulfate-induced shedding of the 67-kDa cell surface elastin binding protein. Exp Cell Res 1992; 203:344–353.

137. Hirschberg H: Accessory cell function of human endothelial cells. I. A sub-population of Ia positive cells is required for antigen presentation. Hum Immunol 1981;2:235.

138. Hirschberg H: Presentation of viral antigens by vascular endothelial cells in vitro. Hum Immunol 1981;2:235.

139. Hosenpud JD, Everett JP, Morris TE, Mauck KA, Shipley GD, Wagner CR: Cardiac allograft vasculopathy: association with cell-mediated but not humoral alloiummunity to donor-specific vascular endothelium. Circulation 1995;92:205–211.

140. Hosenpud JD, Morris TE, Shipley GD, Mauck KA, Mauck KA, Wagner CR: Cardiac allograft vasculopathy: preferential regulation of endothelial cell-derived mesenchymal growth factors in response to a donor-specific cell-mediated allogeneic response. Transplantation 1996;61:939–948.

141. Hosenpud JD, Shipley GD, Mauck KA, Morris TE, Wagner CR: The temporal reduction in acute rejection following cardiac transplantation is not associated with a reduction in cell-mediated responses to donor-specific vascular endothelium. J Heart Lung Transplant 1995;14:926–937.

142. Hoyt G, Gollin G, Billingham M, Miller DC, Jamieson SW: Effects of anti-platelet regimens in combination with cyclosporine on heart allograft vessel disease. Heart Transplant 1984;4:54–56.

143. Hruban RH, Beschorner WE, Baumgartner HR, Augustine SM, Ren H, Reitz BA, Hutchins GM: Accelerated arteriosclerosis in heart transplant recipients is associated with a T-lymphocyte-mediated endothelialitis [abstract]. Am J Pathol 1990;263:871–882.

144. Hruban RH, Beschorner WE, Baumgartner WA: Accelerated arteriosclerosis in heart transplant recipients: an immunopathology study of 22 transplanted hearts. Transplant Proc 1991;23:1230.

145. Hsu RB, Chu SH, Wang SS, Ko W, Chou N, Lee C, Chen M, Lee Y: Low incidence of transplant coronary artery disease in Chinese heart recipients. J Am Coll Cardiol 1999;33:1573–1577.

146. Hume DM, Merrill JP, Miller BF, Thorn GW: Experiences with renal homotransplantation in the human: report of nine cases. J Clin Invest 1955;34:327.

147. Ignotz RA, Massague J: Transforming growth factor-beta stimulates the expression of fibronectin and collagen and their incorporation into the extracellular matrix. J Biol Chem 1986;261:4337–4345.

148. Imagawa D, Millis J, Seu P, Olthoff K, Hart J, Wasef E, Dempsey R, Stephens S, Busuttil R: The role of tumor necrosis factor in allograft rejection: III. evidence that anti-TNF antibody prolongs allograft survival in rats with acute rejection. Transplantation 1991;51:57–62.

149. Isobe M, Yagita H, Okumura K, Ihara A: A specific acceptance of cardiac allograft after treatment with antibodies to ICAM-1 and LFA-1. Science 1992;255:1125.

150. Iwasaki Y, Talmage D, Stazl TE: Humoral antibodies in patients after renal homotransplantation. Transplantation 1967;5:191.

151. Jacobsson J, Cheng L, Lyke K, Kuwahara M, Kagan E, Ramwell PW, Foegh ML: Effect of estradiol on accelerated atherosclerosis in rabbit heterotopic aortic allografts. J Heart Lung Transplant 1992;11:1188.

152. Jain SP, Ramee SR, White CJ, Mehra MR, Ventura HO, Zhang S, Jenkins JS, Collins TJ: Coronary stenting in cardiac allograft vasculopathy. J Am Coll Cardiol 1998;32:1636–1640.

153. Jain SP, Ventura HO, Ramee SR, Collins TJ, Isner JM, White CJ: Directional coronary atherectomy in heart transplant recipients. J Heart Lung Transplant 1993;12:819–823.

154. Johnson DE, Alderman EL, Schroeder JS, Gao SZ, Hunt S, DeCampli WM, Stinson EB, Billingham ME: Transplant coronary artery disease: histopathologic correlations with angiographic morphology. J Am Coll Cardiol 1991;17:449–457.

155. Johnson DE, Gao SZ, Schroeder JS, DeCampli WM, Billingham ME: The spectrum of coronary artery pathologic findings in human cardiac allografts. J Heart Lung Transplant 1989;8:349–359.

156. Johnson JA, Kobashigawa JA: Quantitative analysis of transplant coronary artery disease with use of intracoronary ultrasound. J Heart Lung Transplant 1995;14:S198–S202.

157. Juhan-Vague I, Alessi MC: Plasminogen activator inhibitor 1 and atherothrombosis. Thromb Haemost 1993;70:138–143.

158. Kapadia SR, Nissen SE, Ziada KM, Guetta V, Crowe TD, Hobbs RE, Starling RC, Young JB, Tuzcu EM: Development of transplantation vasculopathy and progression of donor-transmitted atherosclerosis. Circulation 1998;98:2672–2678.

159. Kapadia SR, Ziada KM, Boparai N, Platt L: Coronary artery intimal thickening during the first year of cardiac transplantation predicts late clinical outcome: a serial IVUS study [abstract]. J Am Coll Cardiol 1999;33:A218.

160. Kapadia SR, Ziada KM, L'Allier PL, Crowe TD, Rincon G, Hobbs RE, Bott-Silverman C, Young JB, Nissen SE, Tuzcu EM: Intravascular ultrasound imaging after cardiac transplantation: advantage of multivessel imaging. J Heart Lung Transplant 2000;19:167–172.

161. Kemna MS, Valantine HAHSA, Schroeder JS, Chen YD, Reaven GM: Metabolic risk factors for atherosclerosis in heart transplant recipients [abstract]. Am Heart J 1994;128:68–72.

162. Keogh A, Valantine H, Hunt S: Predictors of proximal epicardial artery disease after heart transplantation [abstract]. J Heart Lung Transplant 1991;10:188.

163. Keogh A, Valantine H, Hunt S, Schroeder JS, McIntosh N, Oyer PE, Stinson EB: Impact of proximal or midvessel discrete coronary artery stenosis on survival after heart transplantation. J Heart Lung Transplant 1992;11:892–901.

164. Kerber S, Rahmel A, Heinemann-Vechtel O, Budde T, Deng M, Scheld HH, Breithardt G: Angiographic, intravascular ultrasound and functional findings early after orthotopic heart transplantation. Int J Cardiol 1995;49:119–129.

165. Klauss V, Mudra H, Uberfuhr P, Theisen K: Intraindividual vaiability of cardiac allograft vasculopathy as assessed by intravascular ultrasound. Am J Cardiol 1995;76:463–466.

166. Kobashigawa J, Miller L, Renlund D, Mentzer R, Alderman E, Bourge R, Costanzo M, Eisen H, Dureau G, Ratkovec R, Hummel M, Ipe D, Johnson J, Keogh A, Mamelok R, Mancini D, Smart F, Valantine H: A randomized active-controlled trial of mycophenolate mofetil in heart transplant recipients. Transplantation 1998;66:507–515.

167. Kobashigawa JA, Katznelson S, Laks H, Johnson JA, Yeatman L, Wang XM, Chia D, Terasaki PI, Sabad A, Cogert GA: Effect of pravastatin on outcomes after cardiac transplantation. N Engl J Med 1995;333:621–627.

168. Kobayashi J, Crawford SE, Backer CL, Zales VR, Takami H, Hsueh C, Huang L, Mavroudis C: Captopril reduces graft coronary artery disease in a rat heterotopic transplant model. Circulation 1993;88:II-286–II-290.

169. Kofoed KF, Czernin J, Johnson J, Kobashigawa J, Phelps ME, Laks H, Schelbert HR: Effects of cardiac allograft vasculopathy on myocardial blood flow, vasodilatory capacity, and coronary vasomotion. Circulation 1997;95:600–606.

170. Koskinen PK, Nieminen MS, Krogerus LA: Cytomegalovirus infection and accelerated cardiac allograft vasculopathy in human cardiac allografts. J Heart Lung Transplant 1993;12:724.

171. Kovacsovics TJ, Peitsch MC, Kress A, Isliker H: Antibody independent activation of C1: differences in the mechanism of C1 activation by nonimmune activators and by immune complexes; C1r-independent activation of C1as by cardiolipin vesicles [abstract]. J Immunol 1987;138:1864–1870.

172. Kugiyama K, Kerns SA, Morrisett JD, Roberts R, Henry PD: Impairment of endothelium-dependent arterial relaxation by lysolecithin in modified low-density lipoproteins. Nature 1990; 344:160–162.

173. Labarrere CA, Nelson DR, Faulk WP: Endothelial activation and development of coronary artery disease in transplanted human hearts. JAMA 1997;276:1169–1175.

174. Labarrere CA, Pitts D, Halbrook H, Faulk WP: Natural anticoagulant pathways in normal and transplanted human hearts. J Heart Lung Transplant 1992;11:342–347.

175. Labarrere CA, Pitts D, Halbrook H, Faulk WP: Tissue plasminogen activator, plasminogen activator inhibitor-1, and fibrin as indexes of clinical course in cardiac allograft recipients: an immunocytochemical study. Circulation 1994;89:1599–1608.

176. Labarrere CA, Pitts D, Nelson DR, Faulk WP: Vascular tissue plasminogen activator and the development of coronary artery disease in heart transplant recipients. N Engl J Med 1995; 333:1111–1116.

177. Laden AMK: Experimental atherosclerosis in rat and rabbit cardiac allografts. Arch Pathol 1972;93:240–245.

178. Ladowski JS, Sullivan M, Schatzlein MH, Peterson AC, Underhill DJ, Scheeringa RA: Cardiac isoenzymes following heart transplantation. Chest 1992;102:1520.

179. Laks H: Only optimal donors should be accepted for heart transplantation: Antagonist. J Heart Lung Transplant 1995;14:1043–1046.

180. Lancet TMR, March R, Gurnn T: Cardiac allograft vasculopathy: the potential role for transmyocardial laser revascularization. J Heart Lung Transplant 1995;14:S242–S246.

181. Lang DM, Schuff-Warner P: Cardiac allograft vasculopathy and HELP therapy. Am J Cardiol 1998;82:1000–1001.

182. Lavee J, Kormos RL, Duquesnoy RJ: Influence of panel reactive antibody and lymphocytotoxic crossmatch on survival after heart transplantation. J Heart Lung Transplant 1991;10:921.

183. Leaf A, Weber PC: Cardiovascular effects of omega 3 fatty acids. N Engl J Med 1988;318:57.

184. Lemstrom KB, Bruning JH, Bruggeman CA, Koskinen PK, Aho PT, Yilmaz S, Lautenschlager IT, Hayry PJ: Cytomegalovirus infection enhanced allograft arteriosclerosis is prevented by DHPG prophylaxis in the rat. Circulation 1994;90:1969–1978.

185. Lemstrom KB, Bruning JH, Bruggeman CA, Lautenschlager IT, Hayry PJ: Cytomegalovirus infection enhances smooth muscle cell proliferation and intimal thickening of rat aortic allografts. J Clin Invest 1993;92:549–558.

186. Li H, Cybulsky MI, Gimbrone MA Jr, Libby P: An atherogenic diet rapidly induces VCAM-1, a cytokine-regulatable mononuclear leukocyte adhesion molecule, in rabbit aortic endothelium. Arteriorscler Thromb 1993;13:197–204.

187. Libby P, Janicka MW, Dinarello CA: Interleukin-1 (IL-1) promotes production by human endothelial cells of activity that stimulates the growth of arterial smooth muscle cells. Fed Proc 1985;44:737.

188. Libby P, Ordovas JM, Birinyi LK: Inducible interleukin 1 gene expression in human vascular smooth muscle cells. J Clin Invest 1986;78:1432.

189. Libby P, Warner SJC, Salomon RN: Production of platelet-derived growth factor-like mitogen by smooth muscle cells from human atheroma. N Engl J Med 1988;318:1493.

190. Lider O, Mekori YO, Miller T: Inhibition of T lymphocyte heparanase by heparin prevents T cell migration and T cell mediated immunity. Eur J Immunol 1990;20:493–499.

191. Liu G, Butany J: Morphology of graft arteriosclerosis in cardiac transplant recipients. Hum Pathol 1992;23:768–773.

192. Loebe M, Schuler S, Zais O: Role of cytomegalovirus infection in the development of coronary artery disease in the transplanted heart. J Heart Lung Transplant 1990;9:707.

193. Loppnow H, Libby P: Proliferating or interleukin 1 activated human vascular smooth muscle cells secrete copious interleukin 6. J Clin Invest 1990;85:731.

194. Loscalzo J: The oxident stress of hyperhomocysteinemia. J Clin Invest 1996;98:5–15.

195. Luscher TF, Tanner FC, Tschudi MR, Noll G: Endothelial dysfunction in coronary artery disease. Annu Rev Med 1993;68:499–508.

196. Majack RA, Goodman LV, Dixit VM: Cell surface thrombospondin is functionally essential for vascular smooth cell proliferation. J Cell Biol 1988;106:415–422.

197. Majesky MW, Lindner V, Twardzik DR, Schwartz SM, Reidy MA: Production of transforming growth factor β_1 during repair of arterial injury. J Clin Invest 1991;88:904–910.

198. Marcum JA, Rosenberg RD: Anticoagulantly active heparin sulfate proteoglycan and the vascular endothelium. Semin Thromb Hemost 1987;13:464–467.

199. Mayer E, Jacobsen D, Robinson K: Homocysteine and coronary atherosclerosis. J Am Coll Cardiol 1996;27:517–521.

200. Mazeika P, Nadazdin A, Oakley C: Dobutamine stress echocardiography for detection and assessment of coronary artery disease. J Am Coll Cardiol 1992;90:1203–1211.

201. McDonald K, Rector TS, Braunlin EA, Kubo SH, Olivari MT: Association of coronary artery disease in cardiac transplant recipients with cytomegalovirus infection. Am J Cardiol 1989; 64:359–362.

202. McGiffin DC, Savunen T, Kirklin JK, Naftel DC, Bourge RC, Paine TD, White-Williams C, Sisto T, Early L: Cardiac transplant coronary artery disease: a multivariable analysis of pretransplantation risk factors for disease development and morbid events. J Thorac Cardiovasc Surg 1995;109:1081–1089.

203. Mehra MR, Ventura HO, Chambers R, Collins TJ, Ramee SR, Kates MA, Smart FW, Stapleton DD: Predictive model to assess risk for cardiac allograft vasculopathy: predictive model to assess risk for cardiac allograft vasculopathy: an intravascular ultrasound study. J Am Coll Cardiol 1995;26:1537–1544.

204. Mehra MR, Ventura HO, Smart FW: Clinical relevance of vascular endothelial cell antigens in the genesis of cardiac allograft vasculopathy: an intravascular ultrasound study. Presented at the American Society of Transplant Physicians Chicago, IL, 1995.

205. Mehta J, Lopez LM, Wargovich T: Eicosapentaenoic acid: its relevance in atherosclerosis and coronary artery disease. Am J Cardiol 1987;59:155–159.

206. Meilahn EN, Ferrell RE: Naturally occurring low blood cholesterol and excess mortality. Coronary Artery Dis 1993;4:843.

207. Meiser BM, Billingham ME, Morris RE: Graft vessel disease: the role of rejection and the effect of cyclosporine, FK506, and rapamycin. Lancet 1991;13:1297–1298.

208. Merieux M: International symposium on infection and atherosclerosis. Am Heart J 1999;138:S417–S560.

209. Miller L: The role of intracoronary ultrasound for the diagnosis of cardiac allograft vasculopathy. Transplant Proc 1995;27:1989–1992..

210. Miller L, Wolford T, Donohue T: Cardiac allograft vasculopathy; new insights from intravascular ultrasound and coronary flow measurements. Transplant Rev 1995;9:77–96.

211. Miller LW: Transplant coronary artery disease [editorial]. J Heart Lung Transplant 1992;11:S1.

212. Miller LW, Wolford T: The surgical management of allograft coronary disease: a paradigm shift. Semin Thorac Cardiovasc Surg 1996;8:133–138.

213. Mills RM, Hill JA, Theron HD, Gonzales JI, Pepine CJ, Conti CR: Serial quantitative coronary angiography in the assessment of coronary disease in the transplanted heart. J Heart Lung Transplant 1992;11:S52–S55.

214. Minick CR, Murphy GE: Experimental induction of atheroarteriosclerosis by the synergy of allergic injury to arteries and lipid-rich diet. Am J Pathol 1973;73:265.

215. Moen T, Moen M, Thorsby E: HLA D region products are expressed in endothelial cells. Tissue Antigens 1980;15:112.

216. Mohacsi PJ, Tuller D, Hulliger B, Wijngaard PLJ: Different inhibitory effects of immunosuppressive drugs on human and rat aortic smooth muscle and endothelial cell proliferation stimulated by platelet-derived growth factor or endothelial cell growth factor. J Heart Lung Transplant 1997;16:484–492.

217. Molossi S, Clausell N, Rabinovitch M: Coronary artery endothelial interleukin-1 beta mediates enhanced fibronectin production related to post-cardiac transplant arteriopathy in piglets. Circulation 1993;88:II-248–II-256.

218. Moncada S, Higgs A: A mechanism of disease: the L-arginine nitric oxide pathway. N Engl J Med 1993;329:2002–2012.

219. More S: Thromboatherosclerosis in normolipemic rabbits: a result of continued endothelial damage. Lab Invest 1973;29:478–487.

220. Muskett A, Burton NA, Eiuchwald EJ, Shelby J, Hendrickson M, Sullivan JJ: The effect of antiplatelet drugs on graft atherosclerosis in rat heterotopic cardiac allografts. Transplant Proc 1987;4:74–75.

221. Neish AS, Loh E, Schoen FJ: Myocardial changes in cardiac transplant-associated coronary arteriosclerosis: potential for timely diagnosis. J Am Coll Cardiol 1992;19:586–592.

222. Nikol S, Isner JM, Pickering JG, Kearney M, Leclerc G, Weir L: Expression of transforming growth factor-beta 1 is increased in human vascular restenosis lesions. J Clin Invest 1992;90:1582–1592.

223. Nissen SE, Tuczu M, DeFranco A: Predominances of coronary disease in proximal segments with sparing of distal sites. Evidence from intravascular ultrasound [abstract]. J Heart Lung Transplant 1994;13(suppl):S59.

224. Nissen SE, Tuzcu M, DeFranco AC: Predominances of coronary disease in proximal segments with sparing of distal sites: evidence from intravascular ultrasound. J Heart Lung Transplant 1994;13:S59.

225. Nitkin RS, Hunt SA, Schroeder JS: Accelerated atherosclerosis in a cardiac transplant patients. J Am Coll Cardiol 1985;6:243.

226. Nunez G, Ball EJ, Stasny P: Accessory cell function of human endothelial cells. J Immunol 1983;131:666.

227. Oka Y, Orth DN: Human plasma epidermal growth factor/beta urogastrone is associated with blood platelets. J Clin Invest 1983;72:249.

228. Olivari MT, Homans DC, Wilson RF, Kubo SH, Ring WS: Coronary artery disease in cardiac transplant patients receiving triple-drug immunosuppressive therapy [abstract]. Circulation 1989;80:III-111–III-115.

229. Olsson AG, Lang PD, Vollmar J: Effect of bezafibrate during 4.5 years of treatment of hyperlipoproteinemia. Atherosclerosis 1985;55:195–203.

230. ONeill BJ, Pflugfelder PW, Singh NR, Menkis AH, McKenzie FN, Kostuk WJ: Frequency of angiographic detection and quantitative assessment of coronary arterial disease one and three years after cardiac transplantation. Am J Cardiol 1989;63:1221–1226.

231. Oni AA, Ray J, Hosenpud JD: Coronary venous intimal thickening in explanted cardiac allografts. Transplantation 1992;53:1247–1251.

232. Pahl E, Fricker FJ, Armitage J: Coronary arteriosclerosis in pediatric heart transplant survivors: limitation of long-term survival. J Pediatr 1990;116:177.

233. Palmer D, Tsai C, Roodman S: Heart graft arteriosclerosis. An ominous finding on endomyocardial biopsy. Transplantation 1985;39:384–388.

234. Park JW, Merz M, Braun P: Regression of transplant coronary artery disease during chronic low density lipoprotein aphoresis. Transplant 1997;16:290–297.

235. Park JW, Vermeltfoort M, Braun P, May E, Merz M: Regression of transplant coronary artery disease during chronic HELP therapy: a case study. Atherosclerosis 2000;115:118.

236. Patel V, Radovansevic B, Springer W, Frazier O, Massin E, Benrey J, Kadipasaoglu K, Cooley D: Revascularization procedures in patients with transplant coronary artery disease. Eur J Cardiothorac Surg 1997;11:895–901.

237. Patrassi GM, Sartori MT, Viero ML, Scarano L, Boscaro M, Girolami A: The fibrinolytic potential in patients with Cushing's dis-

238. Pflugfelder PW, Boughner DR, Rudas L, Kostuk WJ: Enhanced detection of cardiac allograft arterial disease with intracoronary ultrasonographic imaging. Am Heart J 1993;126:1583–1591.

239. Picano E, Lattazini F, Orlanini A, Marini C, L'Abbate A: Stress echocardiography and the human factor; the importance of being expert [abstract]. J Am Coll Cardiol 1990;17:666–669.

240. Pinto F, Chenzbraun A, Botas J: Feasibility of serial intracoronary ultrasound imaging for assessment of progression of intimal proliferation in cardiac transplant recipients. Circulation 1994;90:2348–2355.

241. Pinto F, St Goard F, Gao SZ: Immediate and one-year safety of intracoronary ultrasonic imaging. Evaluation with serial quantitative angiography. Circulation 1993;88:1709–1714.

242. Pober JS: Cytokine-mediated activation of vascular endothelium: physiology and pathology. Am J Pathol 1988;133:426–433.

243. Porter KA, Thompson WB, Owen K, Kenyon JR, Mowbray JF, Peart WS: Obliterative vascular changes in four human kidney homotransplants. Br Med J 1963;2:639–645.

244. Poston RS, Billingham ME, Hyot E, Pollard J, Shorthouse R, Morris R, Robbins R: Rapamycan reverses chronic graft vascular disease in a novel cardiac allograft model. Circulation 1999;100:67–74.

245. Poston RS, Hoyt EG, Robbins RC: Effects of increased ICAM-1 on reperfusion injury and chronic graft vascular disease. Ann Thorac Surg 1997;64:1004–1012.

246. Powell JS, Clozel JP, Muller RK: Inhibition of angiotensin converting enzyme prevents myointimal proliferation after vascular injury. Science 1989;245:186.

247. Pukac L, Hirsch GM, Lormeau JC, Karnovsky MJ: Antiproliferative effects of novel, nonanticoagulant heparin derivatives on vascular smooth muscle cells in vitro and in vivo. Am J Pathol 1991;139:1501–1509.

248. Quinn MT: Endothelial cell-derived chemotactic activity for mouse peritoneal macrophages and the effects of modified forms of low-density lipoproteins. Proc Natl Acad Sci USA 1985;82:5949–5953.

249. Rabin BS, Griffith BP, Hardesty RL: Vascular endothelial cell HLA-DR antigen and myocyte necrosis in human allograft rejection. J Heart Lung Transplant 1985; 4:293.

250. Rabinovitch M, Molossi S, Clausell N: Cytokine-mediated fibronectin production and transendothelial migration of lymphocytes in the mechanism of cardiac allograft vascular disease: efficacy of novel therapeutic approaches [abstract]. J Heart Lung Transplant 1995;14:S116–S123.

251. Radhakrishnamurthy B, Srinivasan P, Vijayagopal P, Berenson GS: Arterial wall proteoglycans-biological properties related to the pathogenesis of atherosclerosis. Eur Heart J 1990;11:148–157.

252. Raines EW, Dower SK, Ross R: Interleukin-1 mitogenic activity for fibroblasts and smooth muscle cells is due to PDGF-AA. Science 1989;243:393–396.

253. Reidy MA, Fingerle J, Lindner V: Factors controlling the development of arterial lesions after injury. Circulation 1992;86:III-43–III-46.

254. Reilly CF, McFall RC: Platelet-derived growth factor and transforming growth factor-beta regulate plasminogen activator inhibitor-1 synthesis in vascular smooth muscle cells. J Biol Chem 1991;266:9419–9427.

255. Rickenbacher PR, Pinto FJ, Lewis NP, Hunt SA, Aldermann EL, Schroeder JS, Stinson EB, Brown BW, Valantine HA: Prognostic importance of intimal thickness as measured by intracoronary ultrasound after cardiac transplantation. Circulation 1995;92:3452.

256. Rimm EB, Stampfer MJ, Ascherio A, Giovannucci E, Colditz GA, Willett WC: Vitamin E consumption and the risk of coronary heart disease in men. N Engl J Med 1993;328:1450–1456.

257. Roberts AB, Sporn MB, Assoian RK, Smith JM, Roche NS, Wakefield LM, Heine UI, Liotta LA, Falanga V, Kehrl JH: Transforming growth factor type beta: rapid induction of fibrosis and angiogenesis in vivo and stimulation of collagen formation in vitro. Proc Natl Acad Sci U S A 1986;83:4167–4171.

258. Rodney RA, Johnson LL: Myocardial perfusion scintigraphy to assess heart transplant vasculopathy. J Heart Lung Transplant 1992;11(suppl):S74.

ease: a clue to their hypercoagulable state. Blood Coagul Fibrinolysis 1992;3:789–793.

259. Roelandt J, diMario C, Pandian N: Three-dimensional reconstruction of intracoronary ultrasound images. Rationale, approaches, problems, and directions. Circulation 1994;90:1044–1055.

260. Rose EA, Pepino P, Barr ML, Smith GR, Ratner AJ, Ho E, Berger C: Relation of HLA antibodies and graft atherosclerosis in human cardiac allograft recipients. J Heart Lung Transplant 1992;11: S120–S123.

261. Rose ML, Dunn MJ, Wheeler C: Identification of antiendothelial antibodies associated with accelerated coronary artery disease following cardiac transplantation [abstract]. J Heart Lung Transplant 1995;14:S49.

262. Ross R: The pathogenesis of atherosclerosis: a perspective for the 1990s. Nature 1993;362:801–809.

263. Ross R, Fuster V: The pathogenesis of atherosclerosis. In Fuster V, Ross R, Topol EJ (eds): Atherosclerosis and Coronary Artery Disease. Philadelphia: Lippincott-Raven, 1996, pp 441–460.

264. Ross R, Glomset J: The pathogenesis of atherosclerosis [abstract]. N Engl J Med 1976;295:369.

265. Ross R, Glomset J, Kariya B, Harker L: A platelet-dependent serum factor that stimulates the proliferation of arterial smooth muscle cells in vitro. Proc Natl Acad Sci USA 1974;71:1207.

266. Ross R, Glomset JA: Atherosclerosis and the arterial smooth muscle cell. Science 1973;180:1332.

267. Russell PS, Chase CM, Winn HJ, Colvin RB: Coronary atherosclerosis in transplanted mouse hearts: III. Effects of recipient treatment with a monoclonal antibody to the interferon-γ. Transplant 1994;57:1367–1371.

268. Sadahiro M, McDonald TO, Thomas R, Allen MD: Leukocyte receptors are a better target than endothelial adhesion, molecule ligands for reducing cellular and vascular rejection. J Heart Lung Transplant 1993;12(1 pt 2):S71.

269. Salomon RN, Hughes CCW, Schoen FJ, Payne DD, Pober JS, Libby P: Human coronary transplantation-associated arteriosclerosis: evidence for a chronic immune reaction to activated graft endothelial cells. Am J Pathol 1991;138:791–798.

270. Saxena U, Kulkarni NMM, Ferguson E, Newton RS: Lipoprotein lipase mediated lipolysis of very low density lipoproteins increases monocyte adhesion to aortic endothelial cells. Biochem Biophys Res Commun 1992;189:1653–1658.

271. Schmitz G, Hankowitz J, Kovacs EM: Cellular processes in atherogenesis: potential targets of calcium channel blockers. Atherosclerosis 1991;88:109.

272. Schroeder JS, Gao SZ, Alderman EL, Hunt SA, Johnstone I, Boothroyd DB, Wiederhold V, Stinson EB: A preliminary study of diltiazem in the prevention of coronary artery disease in heart transplant recipients. N Engl J Med 1993;328:164–170.

273. Schutz A, Kemkes BM, Kugler C, Angermann C, Schad N, Rienmuller R, Fritsch S, Anthuber M, Neumaier P, Gokel JM: The influence of rejection episodes on the development of coronary artery disease after heart transplantation. Eur J Cardiothorac Surg 1990;4:300–307.

274. Sedmak DD, Roberts WH, Stephens RE: Inability of cytomegalovirus infection of cultured endothelial cells to induce HLA class II antigen expression. Transplantation 1990;49:458.

275. Senneff MJ, Hartman J, Sobel BE, Geltman EM, Bergmann SR: Persistence of coronary vasodilator responsivity after cardiac transplantation. Am J Cardiol 1993;71:333.

276. Sharples LD, Caine N, Mullins P, Scott JP, Solis E, English TA, Large SR, Schofield PM, Wallwork J: Risk factor analysis for the major hazards following heart transplantation—rejection, infection, and coronary occlusive disease. Transplantation 1991; 52:244–252.

277. Shepard BL, French JE: Platelet adhesion in the rabbit abdominal aorta following the removal of the endothelium: a scanning and transmission electron microscopial study. Proc Soc Exp Biol Med 1971;176:427–432.

278. Shi C, Russell ME, Bianchi C, Newell JB, Haber E: Murine model of accelerated transplant arteriosclerosis. Circ Res 1994;75: 199–207.

279. Shi Y, O'Brien JE Jr, Fard A, Zalewski A: Transforming growth factor-beta 1 expression and myofibroblast formation during arterial repair. Arterioscler Thromb Vasc Biol 1996;16:1298–1305.

280. Simonet S, De Bailliencourt JP, Descombes JJ, Mennecier P, Laubie M, Verbeuren TJ: Hypoxia causes an abnormal contractile response in the atherosclerotic rabbit aorta: implication of reduced nitric oxide and cGMP production. Circ Res 1993;72:616–630.

281. Sims FH, Gavin JB: The early development of intimal thickening of human coronary arteries. Coron Artery Dis 1990;1:205–213.

282. Slakey DP, Roza AM, Pieper GM, Johnson CP, Adams MB: Delayed cardiac allograft rejection due to combined cyclosporine and antioxidant therapy. Transplantation 1993;56:1305–1309.

283. Small M, Lowe GD, Beattie JM, Hutton I, Lorimer AR, Forbes CD: Severity of coronary artery disease and basal fibrinolysis. Haemostasis 1987;17:305–311.

284. Smart F, Grinstead WC, Cocanougher B, Smart FW, Minor ST, Raizner AE, Henry PD, Roberts R, Pratt CM, Young JB: Detection of transplant arteriopathy: does exercise thallium scintigraphy improve noninvasive diagnostic capabilities? Transplant Proc 1991;23:1189.

285. Smart FW, Ballantyne CM, Cocanougher B, Farmer JA, Sekela ME, Noon GP, Young JB: Insensitivity of noninvasive tests to detect coronary artery vasculopathy after heart transplant. Am J Cardiol 1991;67:243.

286. Smith JD, Danskine AJ, Rose ML, Yacoub MH: Specificity of lymphocytotoxic antibodies formed after cardiac transplantation and correlation with rejection episodes. Transplantation 1992; 53:1358–1362.

287. Smith TL, Kummerow FA: Effect of dietary vitamin E on plasma lipids and atherogenesis in restricted ovulator chickens. Atherosclerosis 1989;75:105–109.

288. Snow AD, Bolender RP, Wight TN, Clowes AW: Heparin modulates the composition of the extracellular matrix domain surrounding arterial smooth muscle cells. Am J Pathol 1990;137: 313–330.

289. Spes CH, Klauss V, Mudra H, Schnaack SD, Tammen AR, Rieber J, Siebert U, Henneke K, Uberfuhr P, Reichart B, Theisen K, Angermann CE: Diagnostic and prognostic value of serial dobutamine stress echocardiography for noninvasive assessment of cardiac allograft vasculopathy. Circulation 1999;100:509–515.

290. St Goar FG, Pinto FJ, Alderman EL, Valantine HA, Schroder JS, Gao SZ, Stinson EB, Popp RL: Intracoronary ultrasound in cardiac transplant recipients: in vivo evidence of "angiographically silent" intimal thickening. Circulation 1992;85:979–987.

291. Stampfer MJ, Hennekens CH, Manson JE, Colditz GA, Rosner B, Willett WC: Vitamin E consumption and the risk of coronary disease in women. N Engl J Med 1993;328:1444–1449.

292. Stark R, McGinn A, Wilson R: Chest pain in cardiac transplant recipients. Evidence of sensory reinnervation after cardiac transplantation. N Engl J Med 1991;324:1791–1807.

293. Steele DM, Hullett DA, Bechstein WO, Kowalski J, Smith LS, Kennedy E, Allison AC, Sollinger HW: Effects of immunosuppressive therapy on the rat aortic allograft model. Transplant Proc 1993;25:754.

294. Steering C: Steering Committee of the Physicians' Health Study Research Group. Final report on the aspirin component of the ongoing physicians' health study. N Engl J Med 1989;321: 129–135.

295. Steinberg D: Antioxidants and atherogenesis; a current assessment. Circulation 1991;84:1420–1425.

296. Steinberg D, Wirtzturm JL: Lipoproteins and atherogenesis: current concepts. JAMA 1990;264:3047–3052.

297. Steinhuble SR, VanLente F, Anzlovar N, Young JB: Immediate post transplant myocyte necrosis detected by elevated serum levels of troponin I is associated with an adverse long-term graft outcome. Scientific Proceedings of the 17th Annual Meeting of the American Society of Transplant Physicians 1998;407:180.

298. Stemerman MB, Ross R: Experimental arteriosclerosis. I. Fibrous plaque formation in primates, an electron microscope study. J Exp Med 1972;136:769–789.

299. Stovin PG, Sharples LD, Schofield PM, Cary NR, Mullins PA, English TA, Wallwork J, Large SR: Lack of association between endomyocardial evidence of rejection in the first six months and the later development of transplant-related coronary artery disease. J Heart Lung Transplant 1993;12:110–116.

300. Strikwerda S, Umans V, van der Linden MM, van Suylen RJ, Balk AH, de Feyter PJ, Serruys PW: Percutaneous directional atherectomy for discrete coronary lesions in cardiac transplant patients. Am Heart J 1992;123:1686–1690.

301. Sullivan JM, Vander Zwaag R, Lemp GF, Hughes JP, Maddock V, Kroetz FW, Ramanthan KB, Mirvis DM: Post menopausal estrogen use and coronary atherosclerosis. Ann Intern Med 1988;108:358.

302. Tanaka H, Sukhova GK, Swanson SJ, Cybulsky MI, Schoen FJ, Libby P: Endothelial and smooth muscle cells express leukocyte adhesion molecules heterogeneously during acute rejection of rabbit cardiac allografts. Am J Pathol 1994;144:938–951.

303. Thie M, Harrach B, Schonherr E, Kresse H, Robenek H, Rauterbert J: Responsiveness of aortic smooth muscle cells to soluble growth mediators is influenced by cell matrix contact. Arterioscler Thromb 1993;13:994–1004.

304. Thompson JG: Production of severe atheroma in a transplanted human heart. Lancet 1969;2:1088.

305. Tobis JM, Mallery J, Mahon D: Intravascular ultrasound imaging of human coronary arteries in vivo: analysis of tissue characterization with comparison to in vitro histological specimens. Circulation 1991;83:913–926.

306. Tuder RM, Weinberg A, Panajotopoulos N, Kalil J: Cytomegalovirus infection amplifies class I major histocompatibility complex expression on cultured human endothelial cells. J Heart Lung Transplant 1994;13:129–138.

307. Tuzcu EM, DeFranco AC, Hobbs R, Rincon G, Bott-Silverman C, McCarthy P, Stewart R, Nissen SE: Prevalence and distribution of transplant coronary artery disease: Insights from intravascular ultrasound imaging. J Heart Lung Transplant 1995;14:202–207.

308. Tuzcu E, Hobbs R, Rincon G, Bott-Silverman C, De Franco AC, Robinson K, McCarthy PM, Stewart RW, Guyer S, Nissen SE: Occult and frequent transmission of atherosclerotic coronary disease with cardiac transplantation. Insights from intravascular ultrasound. Circulation 1995;91:1706–1713.

309. Uretsky BF, Murali S, Reddy GSR: Development of coronary atery disease in cardiac transplant patients receiving immunosuppressive therapy with cyclosporin and prednisone. Circulation 1987;76:244.

310. Ustinov JA, Loginov RJ, Bruggeman CA, van der Meide PH, Hayry PJ, Lautenschlager IT: Cytomegalovirus induces class II expression in rat heart endothelial cells. J Heart Lung Transplant 1993;12:644–651.

311. Uys CJ, Rose AG: Pathologic findings in long-term cardiac transplants. Arch Pathol Lab Med 1984;108:112–116.

312. Valantine H: Role of lipids in allograft vascular disease: a multicenter study of intimal thickening detected by intravascular ultrasound [abstract]. J Heart Lung Transplant 1995;14:S234–S237.

313. Valantine H, Gao S-Z, Menon S, Renlund D, Hunt S, Oyer P, Stinson EB, Brown BW, Merigan TC, Schroeder JS: Impact of prophylactic immediate posttransplant ganciclovir on development of transplant atherosclerosis. Circulation 1999;100:61–66.

314. Van Dorp WT, Johns E, Buggeman CA: Direct induction of MHC class I, but not class II expression on endothelial cells by cytomegalovirus. Transplantation 1989;48:469.

315. van Seventer GA, Newman W, Shimizu Y, Nutman TB, Tanaka Y, Horgan KJ, Gopal TV, Ennis E, O'Sullivan D, Grey H: Analysis of T cell stimulation by superantigen plus major histocompatibility complex class II molecules or by CD3 monoclonal antibody: costimulation by purified adhesion ligands VCAM-1, ICAM-1, but not ELAM-1. J Exp Med 1991;174:901–913.

316. Velican D, Velican C: Comparative study of age related changes and atherosclerotic involvement of the coronary arteries of male and female subjects up to forty years of age. Atherosclerosis 1981;38:39–50.

317. Ventura H, Kirklin JK, Eisen H, Michler R, Clemson B: The combined impact of pretransplant risk factors and rejection frequency and severity on the prevalence of post transplant coronary vasculopathy [abstract]. J Heart Lung Transplant 1997;16:66.

318. Ventura HO: Coronary artery imaging with intravascular ultrasound in patients following cardiac transplantation. Transplantation 1992;53:216.

319. Ventura HO, Ramee SR, Jain A, White CJ, Collins TJ, Mesa JE, Murgo JP: Coronary artery imaging with intravascular ultrasound in patients following cardiac transplantation. Transplantation 1992;53:216.

320. Virchow R: Phlogose und thrombose in gefassystem. In Virchow R (ed): Gesammelte Abhandlungen zur Wissenschaftlichen Medicin. Berlin: Meidinger Sohn, 1856, 458.

321. vonRokitansky C: A Manual of Pathological Anatomy Translated by Day. The Sydenham Society 4. 1852.

322. Wagner CR, Morris TE, Shipley GD, Hosenpud JD: Regulation of human aortic endothelial cell-derived mesenchymal growth factors by allogeneic lymphocytes in vitro. A potential mechanism for cardiac allograft vasculopathy. J Clin Invest 1993;92:1269–1277.

323. Wagner CR, Vetto RM, Burger DR: The mechanism of antigen presentation by endothelial cells. Immunobiology 1984;168:453.

324. Wagner CR, Vetto RM, Burger DR: Expression of I-region-associated antigen (Ia) and interleukin 1 by subcultured human endothelial cells. Cell Immunol 1985;93:91–104.

325. Wagner CR, Vetto RM, Burger DR: Subcultured endothelial cells can function independently as fully competent antigen-presenting cells. Hum Immunol 1985;2:235.

326. Wahlers T, Mugge A, Oppelt P, Heublein B, Fieguth HG, Jurmann MJ, Uthoff K, Haverich A, Albes JM, Foegh M: Preventive treatment of coronary vasculopathy in heart transplantation by inhibition of smooth muscle cell proliferation with angiopeptin. J Heart Lung Transplant 1995;14:143–150.

327. Waldman WJ, Adams PW, Orosz CG: T lymphocyte activation by cytomegalovirus-infected, allogeneic cultured human endothelial cells. Transplantation 1992;54:887.

328. Walker-Caprioglio HM, Trotter JA, Little SA, McGuffee LJ: Organization of cells and extracellular matrix in mesenteric arteries of spontaneously hypertensive rats. Cell Tissue Res 1992;269:141–149.

329. Weich HA, Iberg N, Kagsbrun M, Folkman J: Expression of acidic and basic fibroblast growth factors in human and bovine vascular smooth muscle cells. Growth Factors 1990;2:313–320.

330. Weis M, vonScheidt W: Cardiac allograft vasculopathy: a review. Circulation 1997;96:2069–2077.

331. Weksler BB, Marcus AJ, Jaffe EA: Synthesis of prostaglandin I2 (prostacyclin) by cultured human and bovine endothelial cells. Proc Natl Acad Sci U S A 1977;74:3922–3928.

332. Wharton J, Polak J, Gordon L, Banner NR, Springall DR, Rose M, Khagani A, Wallwork J, Yacoub MH: Immunohistochemical demonstration of human cardiac innervation before and after transplantation. Circ Res 1990;66:900–912.

333. Wiedermann JG, Wasserman HS, Weinberger JZ: Severe intimal thickening by intracoronary ultrasound predicts early death in cardiac transplant recipients. Circulation 1994;90:I–93.

334. Wight TN: The vascular extracellular matrix. In Fuster V, Ross R, Topol EJ (eds): Atherosclerosis and Coronary Artery Disease. Philadelphia: Lippincott-Raven, 1996, pp 421–440.

335. Wight TN, Kinsella MG: The role of proteoglycans in cell adhesion, migration and proliferation. Curr Opin Cell Biol 1992;4:793–801.

336. Williams KJ, Tabas I: The response to retention hypothesis of early atherogenesis. Arterioscler Thromb Vasc Biol 1995;15:551–561.

337. Wilson R, Christenson B, Olivari M, Simon A, White CW, Laxson DD: Evidence for structural sympathetic reinnervation after orthotopic cardiac transplantation in humans. Circulation 1991;83:1210–1220.

338. Winters GL, Kendall TJ, Radio SJ, Wilson JE, Costanzo-Nordin MR, Switzer BL, Remmenga JA, McManus BM: Posttransplant obesity and hyperlipidemia: major predictors of severity of coronary arteriopathy in failed human heart allografts. J Heart Lung Transplant 1990;9:364–371.

339. Wojcicki J, Rozewicka L, Barcew-Wiszniewska B, Samochowiec L, Juzwiak S, Kadlubowska D, Tustanowski S, Juzyszyn Z: Effect of selenium and vitamin E on the development of experimental atherosclerosis in rabbits. Atherosclerosis 1991;87:9–16.

340. Wolford T, Donohue T, Bach R: Coronary flow reserve in angiographically normal coronary arteries varies with time post transplantation. Eur Heart J 1994;15:3237.

341. Wu TC, Hruban RH, Ambinder RF, Pizzorno M, Cameron DE, Baumgartner WA, Reitz BA, Hayward GS, Hutchins GM: Demonstration of cytomegalovirus nucleic acid in the coronary arteries of transplanted hearts. Am J Pathol 1992;140:739–747.

342. Young J: An ischemic burden of a different sort. Am J Cardiol 1992;70(suppl):9F.

343. Young J, Windsor N, Kleiman N, Lowry R, Cocanougher B, Lawrence EC: The relationship of soluble interleukin-2 receptor levels

to allograft arteriopathy after heart transplantation. J Heart Lung Transplant 1992;11:S79–S82.

344. Young JB: Fish oil and antioxidants after heart transplantation: future strategies or eye of newt and wing of bat revisited? J Heart Lung Transplant 1995;14:S250–S254.

345. Young JB: Allograft vasculopathy: diagnosising the nemesis of heart transplantation [abstract]. Circulation 1999;100:458–460.

346. Yun KL, Michie SA, Fann JI, Billingham ME, Miller DC: Effects of fish oil on graft arteriosclerosis and MHC class II antigen expression in rat heterotopic cardiac allografts. J Heart Lung Transplant 1991;10:1004–1011.

347. Yusuf S, Sleight P, Pogue J, Bosch J, Davies R, Dagenais G: Effects of an angiotensin-converting-enzyme inhibitor, ramipril, on cardiovascular events in high-risk patients. The heart outcomes prevention evaluation study investigators. N Engl J Med 2000;342:145–153.

348. Zhao XM, Frist WH, Yeoh TK, Miller GG: Confirmation of alternatively spliced platelet-derived growth factor-A chain and correlation with expression of PDGF receptor α in human cardiac allografts. Transplantation 1995;59:605–611.

349. Zhao XM, Yeoh TK, Frist WH, Porterfield DL, Miller GG: Induction of acidic fibroblast growth factor and full-length platelet-derived growth factor expression in human cardiac allografts: analysis by PCR, in situ hybridization, and immunohistochemistry. Circulation 1994;90:677–685.

350. Zhao XM, Yeoh TK, Hiebert M, Frist WH, Miller GG: The expression of acidic fibroblast growth factor (heparin-binding growth factor-1) and cytokine genes in human cardiac allografts and T cells. Transplantation 1993;56:1177–1182.

351. Zimmerman R, Ehlers W, Walter E, Hoffrichter A, Lang PD, Andrassy K, Schlierf G: The effect of bezafibrate on the fibrinolytic enzyme system and the drug interaction with racemic phenprocoumon. Atherosclerosis 1978;29:477–485.

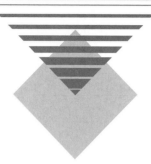

CHAPTER EIGHTEEN

Other Long-Term Complications

with the collaboration of
BARRY K. RAYBURN, M.D.

Although early graft failure, rejection, infection, and allograft vasculopathy are the major complications which limit survival during the first several years after cardiac transplantation, numerous other complications contribute to late morbidity and mortality. This chapter discusses those prominent complications which result from or are facilitated by chronic immunosuppression or some other aspect of the "transplant experience."

HYPERTENSION

INCIDENCE

Arterial hypertension is among the most predictable and at times frustrating complications of heart transplantation. It is of both historical and practical interest that the incidence of posttransplant hypertension in the pre-cyclosporine era was approximately 20%. While this figure is still significantly higher than the general population, it is not surprising in a population with preexisting heart disease who likely had hypertension as a contributing risk factor. In the cyclosporine era, the incidence of hypertension has been reported to range from 40% to more than 90%[180, 236, 254] of heart transplant recipients. In one study of heart transplant patients receiving cyclosporine, azathioprine, and prednisone immunosuppression, no patient had hypertension before transplantation, whereas 68% of the patients were hypertensive within 2 weeks, and 93% met the criteria for hypertension at 6 months.[180]

MECHANISMS

General Risk Factors

The same risk factors for hypertension which are operative in the general population also affect transplant recipients. Male gender, a family history of hypertension, and recipient age above 20 years were identified in one study as predictors of posttransplant hypertension.[186] However, the lack of powerful demographic predictors of hypertension is underscored by another study which found no correlation between age, sex, race, body weight and family history, and the subsequent development of hypertension.[255] Several authors[180, 186] noted the lack of an association between pre- or posttransplant serum creatinine levels and the development of hypertension. Farge and colleagues, however, found that a faster rise in creatinine early after transplantation did correlate with the subsequent development of hypertension, suggesting that nephrotoxicity may play a role in its development.[81] Perhaps the most dominant reason that demographic variables are poor independent predictors of hypertension is that the **use of cyclosporine is directly linked to the development of posttransplant hypertension.** The temporal relationship between the introduction of cyclosporine and the increase in the incidence of hypertension transplantation has implicated cyclosporine in a directly causative role.

Cyclosporine

The mechanism by which **cyclosporine** induces systemic hypertension has been extensively studied (see also Chapter 13), and proposed mechanisms fall into three broad categories: direct sympathetic stimulation, neurohormonal activation, and direct vascular effects. The relative contribution of these three mechanisms remains controversial, and our understanding has been hampered by the complexities of studying them independently in humans. Each has the common end point of vasoconstriction of the renal vasculature, resulting in retention of sodium and an elevated plasma volume. Although the mechanisms of tacrolimus and cyclosporine are similar (calcineurin blockade), the prevalence of hypertension may be somewhat less in patients receiving tacrolimus than cyclosporine immunosuppression.[199]

Evidence for **sympathetic stimulation** leading to renal vasoconstriction with subsequent sodium and fluid retention comes from both animal and human data. Studies in anesthetized rats have demonstrated a cyclosporine dose-dependent increase in vascular resistance, arterial blood pressure, and renal and lumbar sympathetic nerve activity.[166] Administration of an alpha-adrenergic blocking agent markedly attenuates this effect. Human studies in heart transplant recipients as well as patients with myasthenia gravis being treated with cyclosporine supports a similar mechanism[220] (see Chapter 11). Recordings of muscle sympathetic nerve traffic demonstrated increased sympathetic firings in both of these populations, prompting the conclusion that increased sympathetic activity was responsible for cyclosporine-induced hypertension. However, other studies utilizing different techniques[123, 152, 240] have failed to demonstrate increased sympathetic activity in human transplant recipients. The explanation for these discrepant findings is unclear, but the complexities of studying the sympathetic nervous system in isolation may account for some of the differences.

Neurohormonal activation also appears to contribute to cyclosporine-induced hypertension. Although circulating levels of vasoconstricting neurohormones have been shown to return to normal after transplantation,[148, 180] there remains an increased responsiveness of blood vessels to these neurohormones.[47, 143] This suggests that even in the face of normal circulating levels of norepinephrine or vasopressin, vasoconstriction may occur. Studies of the renin-angiotensin system have also demonstrated variable results, with some authors finding at least modest elevations in plasma renin activity,[67, 120] while other studies note no abnormalities in resting levels.[20, 33, 223]

The **direct vascular effects** of cyclosporine are likely of substantial importance in posttransplant hypertension. Experimental studies have shown that cyclosporine induces vasoconstriction of isolated arteries in the presence of alpha-adrenergic blockade, sympathectomy, thromboxane receptor blockade, or acetylcholine.[42] Calcium channel antagonists did inhibit this response, suggesting a role for increased intracellular calcium. This behavior is highly suggestive of the effects of **endothelin-1.** Cyclosporine stimulates endothelin release from cultured endothelial[38, 182] and renal epithelial cells. Other studies implicate endothelin directly in cyclosporine-induced nephrotoxicity, which is likely strongly related to its hypertensive effects.[136] Cyclosporine also increases the production of renal thromboxane A_2, further promoting renal vasoconstriction.[53] Although the relative contribution of each of these mechanisms is unknown, the aggregate effect is a substantial vasoconstriction, particularly in the renal vasculature, which directly contributes to hypertension in this population. Few studies are available delineating the role of tacrolimus, but it is likely that the same or similar mechanisms are at work with that agent. The hypothesized mechanisms for posttransplant hypertension are summarized in Figure 18–1.[232]

Steroids

Corticosteroids may play a minor role due to an intrinsic mineralocorticoid effect leading directly to sodium retention, but steroid-sparing regimens seem to have little effect on the hypertension in this population.[236]

Cardiac Denervation

The integrated cardiorenal system is unable to respond normally to acute changes in volume status in cardiac, but not hepatic, transplant recipients[33] (see also Chapter 11). This and other studies point to a role for cardiac denervation in the salt sensitivity demonstrated in post–heart transplant hypertension. The normal **diurnal variation** of blood pressure is lost following cardiac transplantation[208, 232, 271] (Fig. 18–2). The absence of the normal 10% decline in blood pressure during sleep may contribute to the tendency for cyclosporine-induced hypertension.

EFFECTS OF HYPERTENSION ON THE TRANSPLANTED HEART

The transplanted, denervated heart may also exhibit an abnormal inotropic response to marked hypertension.

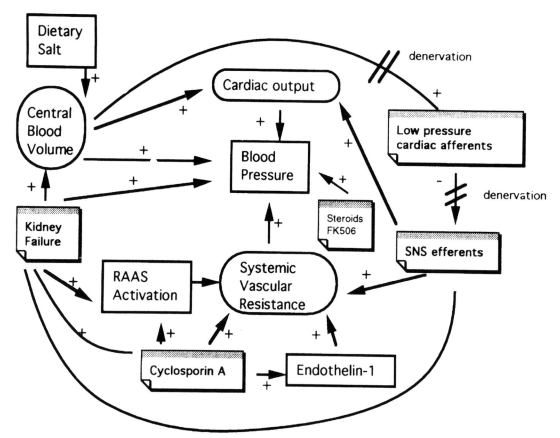

FIGURE 18-1. Simplified hypothesis for mechanisms contributing to *de novo* hypertension in transplant patients. (+) indicates mechanisms which act to increase BP; (−) those which decrease BP. RAAS, renin-aldosterone-angiotensin system; SNS, sympathetic nervous system. (From Singer DR, Jenkins GH: Hypertension in transplant recipients. J Hum Hypertens 1996;10:395–402, with permission.)

Ventricular/vascular mismatch refers to an abnormal relationship between peripheral vascular resistance and the ventricular inotropic state normally mediated by sympathetic innervation.[236] Because of cardiac denervation, the heart does not respond to the increased impedance imposed by hypertension by increasing the inotropic state of the ventricle via sympathetic innervation. Since the transplanted heart adapts poorly to elevated afterload, persistent marked hypertension can cause left ventricular systolic dysfunction.[236]

In the presence of hypertension, the loss of normal nocturnal decline in blood pressue in the transplant patient (see again Fig. 18–2) further promotes secondary left ventricular hypertrophy by increasing the "hypertensive burden" in a given 24-hour period.[156, 232, 236, 263]

TREATMENT

The goals for the treatment of posttransplant hypertension generally mirror those for essential hypertension. Treatment of hypertension can lead to regression of posttransplant left ventricular hypertrophy,[9] and certain agents may also help preserve renal function.[126] In view of the known tendency for loss of diurnal variation of blood pressure (see above), ambulatory blood pressure monitoring has been suggested as a useful way to assess the efficacy of therapy in this population.[115]

The treatment of posttransplant hypertension is further complicated by the tendency for wide blood pressure fluctuations. Because of inadequate circulatory compensation for hypovolemia and/or acute vasodilation (see Chapter 11), the development of acute infection with fever or dehydration may precipitate an abrupt fall in blood pressure, particularly in the setting of vasodilator therapy for hypertension. Ventricular dysfunction secondary to allograft rejection or allograft vasculopathy (with silent myocardial infarction) must always be considered when **sudden normalization of blood pressure** occurs in a previously hypertensive heart transplant patient. A prompt electrocardiogram and echocardiogram are advisable, with further investigations as indicated to evaluate possible rejection or allograft coronary artery disease (see Chapters 14 and 17).

Sodium Restriction

As in essential hypertension, therapy can be divided broadly into nonpharmacologic and pharmacologic categories. Among the most important nonpharmacologic strategies is sodium restriction. Significant reduction in systemic blood pressure has been observed in response to a short-term reduction in dietary sodium,[231] but sodium restriction alone is usually insufficient to fully control posttransplant hypertension.

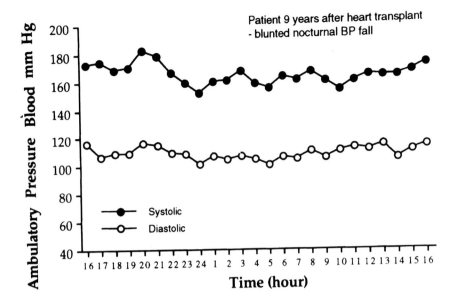

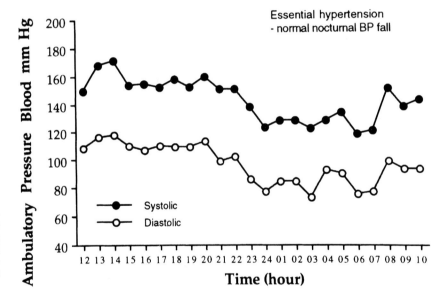

FIGURE **18-2.** Ambulatory blood pressure monitoring (Spacelabs 90207 device) in a patient with untreated essential hypertension and in a cardiac transplant recipient never treated for high blood pressure. (From Singer DR, Jenkins GH: Hypertension in transplant recipients. J Hum Hypertens 1996;10:395–402.)

Pharmacologic Strategies

The pharmacologic strategies are generally based on a background of sodium restriction. Although reduction of cyclosporine or corticosteroid dose has been suggested as a mechanism for controlling hypertension, such dose reductions are generally ineffective in reducing hypertension and potentially dangerous in terms of acute rejection. Pharmacologic therapy for hypertension after transplantation could potentially include almost any agent used for essential hypertension. However, **monotherapy is effective in less than 50% of patients,** and multiple agents in a tailored regimen are frequently needed to achieve adequate control of hypertension.

The **calcium channel blocking agents** are usually the first line of therapy for hypertension in cyclosporine-treated patients. **Diltiazem** has the advantage of decreasing the cyclosporine dose (see discussion in Chapter 13) and therefore decreasing immunosuppression costs. A retrospective study of posttransplant hypertension treated with either prazosin or **nifedipine** concluded that both agents produced comparable blood pressure control, but improved creatinine clearance was observed with nifedipine, suggesting a nephroprotective effect from this calcium channel blocker.[126]

Angiotensin converting enzyme (ACE) inhibitors are effective agents for posttransplant hypertension and are also first-line drugs. **Enalapril** and furosemide[9] alone or in combination with verapamil were reported to normalize blood pressure within 3 months. A reduction in left ventricular mass correlated with the degree of blood pressure reduction. The ACE inhibitor fosinopril also has been effective in heart transplant recipients with hypertension.[5] A randomized trial from the Cardiac Transplant Research Database compared **diltiazem** and **lisinopril**[37] in patients within 1 year of transplantation. Thirty-eight percent of the diltiazem group and 46% of the lisinopril group (the differences were not significant) responded with adequate blood pressure control. There were no differences in dropout rates, side effects limiting therapy, or mortality. The authors concluded that either regimen was safe but that monotherapy was unlikely to be sufficient for the majority of patients with posttransplant hypertension. The combination of a calcium channel blocker with an ACE inhibitor is a commonly employed strategy.

Diuretic therapy has been discussed as part of an overall treatment strategy, and some have suggested its role given the increase in plasma volume demonstrated following heart transplantation. Concerns exist, however, because of the potential danger of exacerbating renal toxicity from other agents.[236] If renal function is normal, a diuretic is probably advisable in the antihypertensive regimen of patients not controlled with one or two drugs.

Alpha-adrenergic blocking agents and other centrally acting vasodilators may also play a role in the treatment of posttransplant hypertension in some patients. Clonidine is a useful adjunct in patients poorly responsive to the agents discussed above. Doxazosin is also frequently effective. Hydralazine and minoxidil are rarely used because they may produce sodium and water retention.

Beta blocking agents have historically been avoided in posttransplant patients because of their relative chronotropic incompetence and the concern regarding inadequate heart rate response to exercise. Although no studies currently have confirmed this strategy, we have utilized the vasodilating beta blocker carvedilol with some success in posttransplant patients.

Omega-3 fatty acids promote endothelial-dependent vasodilation.[229, 266] A randomized trial in heart transplant patients showed omega-3 fatty acids to be effective in controlling hypertension.[264] Another study also demonstrated efficacy of omega-3 fatty acid therapy beginning 4 days after transplantation.[7] Omega-3 fatty acids prevented an elevation in systolic blood pressure and blunted the rise in diastolic blood pressure over a 6-month period. Despite this reported efficacy, the use of omega-3 fatty acids has not become commonplace, perhaps in part because of gastrointestinal side effects in many patients.

In summary, based on available studies and clinical experience, a strategy of aggressive sodium restriction combined with a calcium channel blocking agent or an ACE inhibitor is **recommended initial therapy for hypertension.** A combination of these two classes is often effective since multiple drugs are usually required. If renal function is normal, a diuretic may be a useful adjunct. Additional agents are added as needed to achieve effective control. Recommended doses for commonly employed antihypertensive agents are listed in Tables 5–6 and 5–7.

CHRONIC RENAL DYSFUNCTION

Renal complications of heart transplantation include both acute and chronic renal failure. Acute renal failure following heart transplantation is discussed in Chapter 12. This discussion will focus on chronic renal dysfunction.

INCIDENCE AND TIME-RELATED RENAL DETERIORATION

Studies early in the cyclosporine experience suggested a high incidence of end-stage renal disease with chronic cyclosporine therapy,[173, 174] but this occurred in an era when the chronic dose of cyclosporine was higher than is currently recommended. In the current era of cyclosporine-based immunosuppression, data from the International Society for Heart and Lung Transplantation (ISHLT) registry indicate that about 20% of patients have some form of renal dysfunction at 1 year following transplant and 24% by 4 years.[112] At 4 years, about 7% of patients have a serum creatinine greater than 2.5 mg/dL and about 2% of patients are on chronic dialysis.[258] Some centers have reported the incidence of end-stage renal disease to be 3% to 8%,[100, 190, 261] with nearly a third of patients having a stable creatinine exceeding 2 mg/dL at 5 years.[280]

The rate of progression of renal dysfunction is highly variable, not surprising given the variety of risk factors in addition to cyclosporine immunosuppression. It does seem clear that early renal dysfunction immediately following cardiac transplantation (usually in the setting of cyclosporine administration) is not predictive of late, progressive renal failure, assuming that renal function normalizes after the initial insult. If early postoperative renal dysfunction reflects important pretransplant reduction in glomerular filtration rate, there probably is an increased likelihood of progressive late renal dysfunction.[224] Although there is considerable variability, the major decline in renal function among cyclosporine-treated patients tends to occur during the first 6–12 months following transplantation after which there is often gradual further decline.[58, 149, 258]

RISK FACTORS

Clearly, the major risk factor for late renal dysfunction is chronic administration of a calcineurin inhibitor immunosuppressive agent (cyclosporine or tacrolimus). Several studies have examined other possible risk factors for the development of chronic renal insufficiency, with somewhat conflicting results. One study found that patients with chronic posttransplant renal insufficiency were older, had a lower glomerular filtration rate at the time of transplant, and were treated with more antihypertensive medications.[224] Thus, although cyclosporine or tacrolimus is likely the major determinant of late renal dysfunction following transplantation, other major contributing factors are present in this patient population, including preexisting renal dysfunction from chronic heart failure, diabetes, hypertension, and generalized atherosclerosis. A lack of association between the development of nephrotoxicity and the dose or duration of cyclosporine therapy has been noted in several studies.[101, 280]

PATHOPHYSIOLOGY OF NEPHROTOXICITY FROM CALCINEURIN INHIBITION

Considerable experimental evidence indicates that both the immunosuppressive as well as the nephrotoxic effects of cyclosporine depend on the ability of cyclosporine to inhibit calcineurin, a calcium-dependent serine-threonine phosphatase with important regulatory effects on various genes (see Chapter 13). Although more is known about the renal effects of cyclosporine than tacrolimus, both are calcineurin blocking agents and the nephrotoxic effects are likely similar for both.[40] The renal toxicity of calcineurin inhibitors appears in two basic forms (early functional nephrotoxicity and later structural nephrotoxicity), and the manifestations of each are partially interrelated.

Mechanisms of Functional (Early) Nephrotoxicity

The initial administration of cyclosporine can cause a rapid and intense **vasoconstriction of preglomerular (afferent) arterioles** which is thought to be mediated by an increase in sympathetic tone, activation of the renin angiotensin system, decreased production of vasodilator molecules, and increased production of vasoconstrictor molecules.[6, 75] In animal studies, cyclosporine has a known direct toxic effect on vascular endothelial cells which leads to release of vasoactive compounds that can induce vasoconstriction and cause endothelial cell damage.[282] The effect of this initial vasoconstriction is a decrease in renal blood flow and decrease in glomerular filtration rate, both of which are dose related and reversible.[6, 181] Considerable indirect experimental evidence implicates **endothelin-1** in this process. Also, cyclosporine stimulates endothelin-1 production via calcium-dependent mechanisms in cultured human vascular endothelial cells.[155] Also, cyclosporine-induced endothelial cell damage causes release of endothelin-1 from these cells,[269] and the sequelae of experimental cyclosporine-induced renal arteriolar vasoconstriction is prevented by administration of an endothelin receptor antagonist.[28, 36, 44]

The mechanisms of cyclosporine-induced nephrotoxicity are multifactorial and likely involve circulating as well as local mediators. In addition to endothelin,[253] other mediators include thromboxane[205] and the renin-angiotensin system.[20] Cyclosporine-induced increase in renal sympathetic nerve activity may promote renal vasoconstriction, particularly afferent arteriolar tone.[217] The physiologic sequelae of these changes is a fall in glomerular rate and renal plasma flow. The nephrotoxic interaction of cyclosporine with nonsteroidal anti-inflammatory agents (such as indomethicin) which selectively reduce prostaglandin synthesis suggests that urinary prostaglandins may have a protective effect against cyclosporine nephrotoxicity.[172] The nephrotoxic effects of cyclosporine are also discussed in Chapter 13.

Mechanisms of Structural (Chronic) Nephrotoxicity

It has been hypothesized that the combination of recurring or sustained cyclosporine-induced acute renovascular effects coupled with direct cyclosporine toxicity on renal tubular epithelial cells sets the stage for chronic structural damage. Sustained functional nephrotoxicity induces glomerular ischemia, promoting chronic glomerular injury. Proximal tubular cells are particularly susceptible to cyclosporine - mediated injury, induced by either sustained ischemia secondary to cyclosporine-related vasoconstriction or by direct toxic effects of cyclosporine on tubular cells.[40, 183] Cyclosporine has been shown experimentally to cause apoptosis in tubular and interstitial cells, potentially inducing tubular atrophy and subsequent fibrosis. These effects of cyclosporine also promote the influx of inflammatory cells into the interstitium, with resultant fibroblast proliferation and matrix synthesis.[183]

The functional result of these structural changes that occur in the kidney with chronic cyclosporine therapy[173] differs from the effects of chronic azathioprine therapy (without cyclosporine or tacrolimus). Myers and colleagues[173] found that mean glomerular filtration rate (GFR) was significantly reduced in cyclosporine-treated patients versus azathioprine-treated controls. This occurred in the setting of similar cardiac output, elevated blood pressure in the cyclosporine patients, and comparably reduced renal plasma flow. A calculation of apparent renal vascular resistance demonstrated a twofold increase in the cyclosporine-treated patients. Additional physiologic studies demonstrated a mild impairment of both proximal and distal tubular function in cyclosporine-treated patients. Compared to non-cyclosporine (and nontacrolimus) transplant recipients, patients on cyclosporine have high renal vascular resistance, more proteinuria, and evidence of greater renal microvascular injury.[174]

PATHOLOGY

In considering the pathology of chronic renal dysfunction following cardiac transplantation, it should be emphasized that many patients with end-stage heart failure who undergo heart transplantation have intrinsically abnormal kidneys secondary to processes such as chronic low cardiac output, atherosclerotic kidney disease, and diabetes. All of these can contribute to chronic posttransplant renal dysfunction and its pathologic picture. In this discussion we will focus on the histologic findings of **calcineurin inhibitor-induced nephrotoxicity.** As discussed above, the early *functional* form of renal dysfunction can be associated with severe (but usually reversible) renal dysfunction with few histologic abnormalities. In contrast, chronic structural changes in the kidney may be apparent histologically with clinical renal function which ranges from essentially normal to end-stage renal disease. Calcineurin inhibitor-induced nephrotoxicity can produce structural renal abnormalities involving the renal arterioles, glomeruli, tubules, and interstitium.

Arteriolar Abnormalities

The **afferent arteriolar lesions** are perhaps the most important cyclosporine-related injury, which affect not only the glomeruli, but also tubules and interstitum.[27,79,162] Following the initial vasoconstriction induced by cyclosporine, progressive damage to the vascular endothelium and arteriolar smooth muscle may occur, resulting in vacuolization, cell necrosis, and subsequent deposition of fibrin and platelet thrombi over a denuded basement membrane.[62] Intimal thickening contributes to progressive luminal narrowing which is further aggravated by nodular protein deposits in the vascular wall.[11,24,62,162,163] In its severe form, a thrombotic microangiopathy develops.

Glomerular Changes

Glomerular lesions induced by cyclosporine are generally considered an extension of the arteriopathy into the glomerulus,[62,162] with the frequency of glomerular lesions reflecting the severity of the arteriopathy.[168] The degree of glomerular pathology ranges from subtle changes in the basement membrane to focal **glomerular sclerosis,** with deposition of fibrin thrombi and, rarely, global glomerular sclerosis.[162,163]

Tubular Changes

The **proximal tubules** are especially susceptible to cyclosporine injury. The tubular pathology includes vacuolization, necrosis, giant mitochondria in tubular epithelial cells, microcalification, and most prominently, **tubular atrophy.**[80,101,128,163,233]

Interstitial Lesions

The typical renal interstitial changes consist of irregular foci of fibrosis which accompany areas of tubular atrophy.[23] The location of atrophied tubules and associated fibrosis adjacent to areas of normal-appearing tubules gives the appearance of **strips of interstitial fibrosis,** which tend to become progressive lesions.[161,163,230,247]

This pattern of pathologic changes, combined with the consistent physiologic findings of decreased GFR and elevated renal vascular resistance, suggests that **glomerular ischemia in the setting of afferent arteriolopathy** plays an important role in progressive renal failure in cyclosporine-treated patients, perhaps combined with direct tubular toxicity.[23] Clinical and experimental data suggest a combined effect of hemodynamic changes and an interaction between cyclosporine and various endogenous systems such as the renin angiotensin system and cytokines such as transforming growth factor β (TGF-β). These endogenous agents are capable of inducing fibrosis and causing the scarring seen pathologically.

Limited information is available regarding the role of **tacrolimus** in the development of renal failure following heart transplantation. However, tacrolimus appears to increase renal endothelin production,[141,201,244] and the mechanisms involved in acute and chronic tacrolimus renal toxicity appear to be very similar to those of cyclosporine.[141,201,244]

TREATMENT

The management of chronic renal insufficiency following cardiac transplantation generally involves supportive care and consideration of reduced cyclosporine (or tacrolimus) dosing. As noted above, however, reduction in cyclosporine dosing does not always stop the progression of either the functional or pathologic changes seen in posttransplant nephrotoxicity. Nevertheless, every effort should be made to aggressively reduce cyclosporine or tacrolimus doses at the earliest signs of persistent moderate elevation of serum creatinine (≥ 2 mg/dL).

Calcium channel blockers have been proposed as an intervention to reduce cyclosporine-induced nephrotoxicity by reduction of afferent arteriolar tone.[165] In addition, verapamil competes with cyclosporine for inhibition of a p-glycoprotein transporter which is expressed on renal tubular epithelial cells. Theoretically, the administration of verapamil along with cyclosporine may reduce the accumulation of cyclosporine within the tubular cells.[23] However, clinical trials have failed to substantiate these hypotheses,[37,280] and the benefits of these agents are more likely secondary to control of hypertension than to specific renal effects.[280] The ACE inhibitor captopril demonstrated some benefit in ameliorating the deleterious renal effects of cyclosporine,[17] at least in the short term, by decreasing renal vascular resistance and increasing renal plasma flow. Similarly, enalapril has been reported in a small group of patients to stabilize renal function and control hypertension.[73]

Rigorous monitoring of cyclosporine levels, aggressive treatment of hypertension, reduction of cyclosporine dose with decreased renal function, and avoidance of other nephrotoxic agents is advisable, but few data are available to provide more precise guidance in the treatment or prevention of chronic renal changes following heart transplantation. Drug interactions which promote posttransplant cyclosporine nephrotoxicity are listed in Table 13–11.

Although limited experience is available in heart transplant patients, preliminary studies in renal transplantation indicate that switching from cyclosporine- or tacrolimus-based immunotherapy to **sirolimus-based** immunosuppression may have a renal-sparing effect if initiated before renal dysfunction is progressive[154] (see also Chapter 13). Sirolimus can be used with mycophenolate and prednisone or combined with low-dose cyclosporine or tacrolimus. When this therapeutic change is initiated within 1–2 months after transplantation, a prompt improvement in serum creatinine by about 15% has been reported.[154] Proper monitoring of sirolimus levels has been recommended during the transition period.

One consistent finding of clinical relevance is that after a certain point, the pathologic and physiologic changes of cyclosporine nephrotoxicity are capable of progressing, despite a reduction in cyclosporine dose.[280] Thus, late drastic reduction in cyclosporine dosage (and levels) after renal damage is established may increase the risk of rejection without providing relief from progressive renal dysfunction. Progression to the need for chronic dialysis appears to convey a poor outcome, as might be expected.[261] If the heart transplant allograft function is good and other nonrenal subsystems are intact, consideration for renal transplantation is advisable.

HYPERLIPIDEMIA

Because of the well-known relationship between hyperlipidemia and atherosclerosis in nontransplant patients, it is logical to hypothesize that transplant recipients with lipid perterbations would also be at higher risk for developing atherosclerosis (see Chapter 17) and subsequent cardiovascular events after heart transplantation.

INCIDENCE AND PATTERNS OF HYPERLIPIDEMIA

Lipid perturbation has been reported in 60–80% of heart transplant patients receiving standard triple-drug immunosuppressant regimens consisting of cyclosporine, azathioprine, and prednisone. Characteristic patterns of dyslipidemia develop following cardiac transplantation. Beginning at about 3 months, heart transplant recipients frequently demonstrate increases in total cholesterol, low-density lipoprotein (LDL) cholesterol, apolipoprotein B, and triglyceride levels.[16] As the interval increases between transplantation and follow-up, increased lipid levels may slowly fall but often do not return to normal levels. Reports vary regarding levels of high-density lipoprotein (HDL) cholesterol.[82, 95] Interestingly, lipoprotein A levels may decrease by nearly 40% after cardiac transplantation,[95] and this is a strong predictor of atherosclerosis in the general population.

Ballantyne and colleagues[16] reported that mean total cholesterol values in 100 sequential cardiac transplant recipients surviving at least 3 months increased from a pretransplant level of 168 ± 7 mg/dL to 234 ± 7 mg/dL 3 months after transplantation. The low pretransplant cholesterol level for the group likely reflects the severity of their heart failure. Indeed, low total cholesterol and

LDL levels correlate with severe heart failure. In the Ballantyne study, the LDL cholesterol rose from 111 ± 6 mg/dL to 148 ± 6 mg/dL and triglyceride levels from 106 ± 6 mg/dL to 195 ± 10 mg/dL after transplantation. Significant further increases were not observed after the 3 month evaluation, but low-density lipoprotein cholesterol and triglyceride levels were elevated in 64% and 41% of the patients, respectively, at the 6-month follow-up point despite aggressive dietary intervention.

CAUSES OF HYPERLIPIDEMIA

Causes of dyslipidemia in heart transplant patients include high-fat diets, genetic predisposition to hyperlipemia, and immunosuppressive medications. Though most patients undergoing heart transplantation are below ideal body weight before transplant because of their severe heart failure, they become ponderous after the procedure, with steroids frequently blamed for this morphogenesis.[102] Several studies have demonstrated that transplant patients are likely to **gain weight** during the first year following transplantation.[13] By multivariable analysis, a correlation exists between the amount of weight gain and the serum cholesterol level after transplantation. This study suggests an independent effect of dietary factors and weight gain in the development of posttransplant hypercholesterolemia. Some patients with ischemic heart disease undergoing cardiac transplantation have **familial hyperlipidemia,** and this genetic state will continue to contribute to the posttransplant lipid abnormalities.[252]

Corticosteroids and **cyclosporine** are important core immunomodulating drugs used after heart transplantation, and they both contribute to the development of hyperlipidemia.[133] **Cyclosporine** decreases bile acid synthesis from cholesterol, thus increasing serum cholesterol levels. Cyclosporine is also reported to bind to the LDL receptor which increases serum levels of LDL cholesterol.[65] Decreased lipoprotein lipase activity is also noted with cyclosporine therapy, and this results in impaired clearance of both very-low-density and low-density lipoprotein. Triglyceride levels are also generally elevated with cyclosporine immunosuppression. Cyclosporine blood levels have been shown to correlate directly with total and LDL cholesterol, and inversely with HDL cholesterol.[142]

Tacrolimus appears to have similar though perhaps less pronounced effects on lipid metabolism than cyclosporine. One randomized study of heart transplant patients receiving either cyclosporine or tacrolimus as part of triple-drug therapy[251] found lower levels of serum cholesterol, LDL, and triglycerides at 3, 6, and 12 months in patients treated with tacrolimus.

Prednisone increases acetyl coenzyme A (CoA) carboxylase activity and free fatty acid synthesis. Additionally, prednisone increases hepatic synthesis of very-low-density lipoprotein, down-regulates low-density lipoprotein receptor activity, increases the activity of 3-hydroxy 3-methylglutaryl coenzyme A (HMG-CoA) reductase, and inhibits lipoprotein lipase. These effects contribute to increased levels of very-low-density lipo-

TABLE 18-1 HMG-CoA Reductase Inhibitors*

STATINS	INITIAL DOSE†	INCREMENTAL DOSE INCREASE	MAXIMUM DOSE/DAY	SIDE EFFECTS
Lovastatin (Mevacor)	10 mg (17%) give with meals in evening	20 (25%)→40 (32%)	40 mg	Muscle, hepatic enzyme changes, memory loss, sleeplessness, muscle inflammation (CPK elevation)
Pravastatin (Pravachol)	10 mg (17%) give with meals in evening	20 (25%)→40 (32%)	40 mg	CPK, hepatic enzyme abnormalities
Fluvastatin (Lescol)	20 mg (15%)	40 (25%)	40 mg	CPK, hepatic enzyme abnormalities
Simvastatin (Zocor)	20 mg (32%)	40 (40%)→80 (50%)	80 mg	CPK, hepatic enzyme abnormalities
Atorvastatin (Lipitor)	10 mg (40%)	20 (40%)→40 (52%)→80 (60%)	80 mg	CPK, hepatic enzyme abnormalities
Cerivastatin (Baycol)	0.2 mg (25%)	0.3 (28%)	0.4 mg	CPK, hepatic enzyme abnormalities

CPK, creatinine phosphokinase.
*Exercise caution when using HMG-CoA reductase inhibitors in patients on cyclosporine because of the increased risk of rhabdomyolysis.
†Approximate % lowering of LDL value in parentheses next to doses. Triglycerides are usually lowered by 10–20%, and HDL cholesterol is usually increased by 5–15%.

protein, total cholesterol, and triglycerides while decreasing high-density lipoprotein levels.

THERAPY

Most of the current lipid-lowering agents fall into one of these drug classes: HMG-CoA reductase inhibitors, bile acid sequestrants, fibric acid derivatives, and nicotinic acid.

HMG-CoA Reductase Inhibitors

HMG-CoA reductase is a key rate-limiting enzyme in the biosynthesis of cholesterol. HMG-CoA reductase inhibitor drugs ("-statins") inhibit this enzyme and reduce LDL cholesterol levels. The major drugs in this category are listed in Table 18–1. **Pravastatin** has proven to be effective in reducing cholesterol levels after transplant. In a randomized trial in heart transplant patients (see also Chapter 17), pravastatin produced significant reduction in cholesterol levels at 3, 6, 9, and 12 months after transplantation.[134] Somewhat surprising was the additional apparent benefit in reduced incidence of rejection with hemodynamic compromise, decreased transplant coronary artery disease, and improved 1-year survival. Another randomized trial in heart transplant patients demonstrated that **simvastatin** (dose, 5–20 mg/day) compared to no lipid therapy was effective in reducing LDL cholesterol levels (110 mg/dL vs. 150 mg/dL, $p = .001$).[270] **Rhabdomyolysis** has occurred in patients receiving both cyclosporine and an HMG-CoA reductase inhibitor, particularly if they are also taking gemfibrozil or niacin.[82, 116] This problem appears to be rare if low doses of HMG-CoA inhibitors are prescribed for patients on cyclosporine.

In view of the pervasiveness of lipid disorders after cardiac transplantation coupled with the favorable impact of pravastatin in transplant patients (see previous discussion),[134] it is currently advisable to **routinely prescribe pravastatin, beginning early after transplantation, to all patients, irrespective of their lipid levels** as long as their liver function remains normal (Table 18–2). Adjustment of dose and specific lipid-lowering agents is then undertaken to control specific lipid abnormalities. Potential adverse effects of the various classes of lipid-lowering agents in heart transplant recipients are listed in Table 18–3.

Bile Acid Sequestrants

These agents bind with bile acids, thus interrupting bile acid recirculation. However, because these drugs may interfere with cyclosporine absorption, cyclosporine levels should be closely monitored during therapy. Two common drugs in this class are **cholestyramine** and **colestipol.**

Fibric Acid Derivatives

These lipid-regulating agents are especially useful as treatment for markedly elevated triglyceride levels. They effectively decrease triglycerides and very-low-density lipoprotein (VLDL) cholesterol, and increase HDL cholesterol. LDL levels are only moderately reduced. The two major drugs in this class are gemfibrozil and clofibrate.[102] The mechanism of action of these drugs

TABLE 18-2 Pravastatin Protocol After Heart Transplantation*

- Pravastatin (Pravachol) is recommended for all adult patients with a normal liver profile
- Begin pravastatin during transplant hospitalization if possible, at starting dose of **10 mg** PO qd (if LFTs are normal)
- Assess LFTs in 6 wk; if LFTs are normal, increase dose to 20 mg qd
- Assess LFTs in 6 wk; if normal, increase dose to 40 mg qd
- After 3 mo on 40 mg pravastatin, if triglycerides >200 mg/dL or LDL > 130 mg/dL, change to **atorvastatin** (Lipitor) 40 mg qd (maximum atorvastatin dose, 80 mg qd, with normal LFTs)
- Lipid profiles are obtained at 6 wk, 3 mo, 6 mo, and 1 yr after transplant, then yearly
- Lipid profile target: triglycerides < 200 mg/dL, LDL < 100 mg/dL, HDL > 40 mg/dL

LFTs, liver function tests; LDL, low-density lipoprotein; HDL, high-density lipoprotein.
*UAB protocol; other statin agents are appropriate if so desired.

TABLE 18-3 Potential Adverse Effects of Lipid-Lowering Drugs in Heart Transplant Recipients

CLASS OF LIPID-LOWERING AGENT*	POSSIBLE ADVERSE EFFECTS	COMMENTS
Bile acid resin (cholestyramine)	May prevent absorption of fat-soluble vitamins; poor compliance because of constipation and bloating	May inhibit absorption of cyclosporine and absorption of other fat-soluble drugs; space dose by 2 hr with interacting drug; may increase triglyceride concentrations
Nicotinic acid	Flushing, pruitus, increase in liver enzymes, increased uric acid concentrations, altered glucose tolerance, and exacerbation of peptic ulcer	Concomitant cyclosporine and prednisone use may exacerbate adverse effects
Fibric acid derivative (gemfibrozil)	Gallstones, myositis (especially in patients with decreased renal function), nausea, gastrointestinal upset	Increased risk of myositis with concomitant HMG-CoA reductase inhibitors and immunosuppressive drugs
Antioxidant (Probucol)	Flatulence, loose stools, prolonged QT interval on electrocardiogram, decreased HDL	May interact with cyclosporine and cause fluctuation in cyclosporine concentrations
HMG-CoA reductase inhibitor	Abdominal pain, flatulence, increase in transaminase concentration, myositis, sleep disturbances	May increase liver function enzymes; increased risk of myositis with high-dose HMG-CoA reductase inhibitor and/or fibric acid derivatives with cyclosporine

HDL, high-density lipoprotein cholesterol; HMG-CoA, 3-hydroxy-3-methylglutaryl coenzyme A.[16]
*Common examples are listed in parentheses.

is not definitely established, but gemfibrozil (lopid) has been shown to decrease hepatic extraction of free fatty acids, thereby reducing hepatic triglyceride production. It also inhibits the synthesis of and increases clearance of VLDL carrier apolipoprotein B, decreasing production of VLDL. Furthermore, these drugs decrease the incorporation of long-chain fatty acids into newly formed triglycerides and increase excretion of cholesterol in the feces.

Gemfibrozil is generally used when there is isolated, marked elevation of triglycerides. The starting dose is 300 mg daily with gradual increase to a maximum dose of 600 mg bid. The major side effects are rash and gastrointestinal upset (rare). It is **advisable to avoid the combination of fibric acid derivatives and HMG-CoA reductase inhibitors** together for the treatment of hyperlipidemias following transplantation because of the important risk of rhabdomyolysis.

Other Lipid-Lowering Therapies

Limited information is available on the use of nicotinic acid, probucol, and LDL cholesterol apheresis in heart transplant patients.[188, 246]

Alterations in Immunosuppression

Because of the potential contribution of corticosteroids and cyclosporine to hyperlipidemia, patients with this condition who respond poorly to lipid-lowering agents should be considered for tapering off steroids and/or conversion from cyclosporine to tacrolimus. For example, among pediatric heart transplant recipients, significant reduction in serum lipid levels has been documented with conversion from a regimen of cyclosporine, azathioprine, and prednisone to the two-drug combination of tacrolimus and azathioprine.[248]

BONE COMPLICATIONS

OSTEOPOROSIS

With the requirement for corticosteroids as part of the immunosuppressive program for many transplant patients, osteoporosis becomes a major source of morbidity, particularly in older men and postmenopausal women.

Definition and Diagnosis

Osteoporosis is defined as an abnormally low bone volume for age, race, and sex.[147, 170, 171, 227] Inherent in the definition is a reduction in the mass of bone per unit volume, which results in a degree of skeletal fragility sufficient to increase the risk of fracture. The diagnosis of osteopenia and osteoporosis is based on **bone mineral density** (BMD) criteria developed by the World Health Organization. The measurement of bone mineral density was developed because of the inaccuracy of subjectively assessing bone mineralization from conventional radiographs. Techniques for measuring BMD include quantitative computerized tomography, single photon and dual-photon absorptiometry, and dual-energy x-ray absorptiometry (DEXA). DEXA is the method of choice for measuring BMD, which is assessed in the lumbar spine (L1–4), the proximal end of the femur (neck, trochanter, and total hip), and Ward's triangle. The DEXA measurement is an integral of both cortical and cancellous bone mineral content normalized to the size of the projected bone area. The BMD score is usually reported as a T-score and Z-score. The **T-score** represents the number of standard deviations that a BMD measurement is above or below the mean peak bone mass of a young normal population which is matched to sex and race. The **Z-score** expresses the number of standard deviations that a patient differs from the mean value for an age-, sex-, and race-matched population. The T-score is generally preferred for identification and grading of osteoporosis because the Z-score is influenced by the increased prevalence of osteoporotic disease in older patients. The World Health Organization criteria is based on the T-score (Table 18–4).

Incidence and Clinical Sequelae

Most heart transplant patients tend to have some degree of bone density loss, as indicated by the reported average posttransplant bone density of approximately 1 standard deviation below the normal expected for age- and sex-matched controls.[177] In a cross-sectional study[227] at 2 years after cardiac transplantation, severe osteoporosis was detected in the lumbar spine in 28% of patients and in the femoral neck in 20% of patients.

BMD tends to progressively decline after transplantation, with most of the loss of bone density occurring during the first 6 months after transplant[25, 216] (Fig. 18–3). Bone loss is most prominent in the lumbar spine.[216] In several studies, there was little further decline noted between 6 and 12 months after transplantation, suggesting that the rate of bone loss slows somewhat after the early posttransplant period.

Ultimately, the major concern regarding osteoporosis is the development of **fractures** and their morbid consequences. Vertebral fractures have been reported in 10–30% of patients,[147, 160, 171, 210] with an important ongoing risk in patients with osteoporosis.[179, 216, 260] However, the correlation is poor between vertebral bone marrow density and the incidence of vertebral compression fractures.[147, 177, 216, 227]

Pathophysiology

Osteoporosis results from an abnormality in the **remodeling of bone** (its formation and resorption), which is a continuous process. The remodeling process is dependent, among other things, on an adequate supply of calcium. Proper calcium homeostasis depends on the efficiency of intestinal absorption, most of which occurs in the proximal small intestine. Both active transport

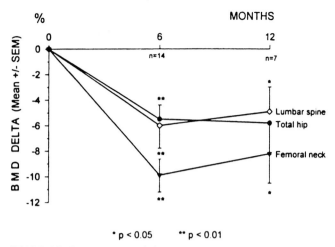

FIGURE 18–3. Bone mineral density percent change (BMD delta) at the lumbar spine, femoral neck, and total hip before and after transplantation in 14 patients. (From Berguer DG, Krieg MA, Thiebaud D: Osteoporosis in heart transplant recipients: a longitudinal study. Transplant Proc 1994;26:2649–2651.)

and diffusion-limited absorption are involved, and both processes are facilitated by vitamin D. A deficiency of vitamin D, intestinal disease, or severe dietary calcium deprivation may prevent adequate intestinal absorption of calcium and promote the development of osteoporosis.

Osteoporosis is characterized by a decrease in cortical bone thickness and in the number and size of trabeculae of cancellous bone. The formation of cancellous bone tends to be less in osteoporosis, and the rate of bone loss is greater in the metacarpals, the femoral neck, and vertebral bodies compared to the midshaft of the femur, the tibia, and the skull.[140]

Glucocorticoids have long been known to cause accelerated bone loss and a higher than normal incidence of vertebral fractures.[153] The most rapid bone loss occurs in the first 12–18 months of therapy, which is similar to that observed in transplant patients. Glucocorticoids reduce bone density by **direct inhibition of osteoblast function and impairment of collagen and new bone formation.**[41] The biochemical effect is reduction in serum **osteocalcin,** which serves as a marker of bone turnover.[138, 204] Additional effects of glucocorticoids include impaired absorption of calcium, increased renal loss of calcium and, particularly in males, decreased production of gonadal hormones.[153]

Despite these well known effects of glucocorticoids, several observations suggest that steroids alone do not explain the bone loss seen in transplant recipients. Several studies of bone loss in transplant patients have noted an elevation rather than a reduction in serum osteocalcin levels,[177, 210, 227] suggesting increased turnover and reformation of bone, rather than a suppression of osteoblast activity. Furthermore, classic steroid-induced osteopenia demonstrates a high degree of correlation between osteopenia and the occurrence of vertebral fractures. As noted above, the incidence of fractures does not correlate with the degree of bone density change in posttransplant patients.

TABLE 18–4	Definitions of Osteoporosis Based on BMD or BMC Values
Normal	A BMD/BMC value > 1 SD below the average value of a young adult (T > −1)
Low bone mass (osteopenia)	A BMD/BMC value > 1 SD below the young adult average but not more than 2.5 SD below (−2.5 < T < −1)
Osteoporosis	A BMD/BMC value > 2.5 SD below the young adult average value (T < −2.5)
Severe (established) osteoporosis	A BMD/BMC value > 2.5 SD below the young adult average with one or more osteoporotic fractures

BMC, bone mineral content; BMD, bone mineral density; SD, standard deviation; T, T-score (see text for definition).
Adapted from World Health Organization: Assessment of Fracture Risk and Its Application to Screening for Postmenopausal Osteoporosis. WHO technical report series 843. Geneva: WHO, 1994.

Cyclosporine has also been implicated in the development of osteoporosis.[76] The data examining the effect of cyclosporine on bone metabolism is somewhat controversial and mostly based on animal studies. Unfortunately, little information is available in human subjects, in part because of the rarity of isolated cyclosporine administration. Although *in vitro* data suggest that cyclosporine inhibits bone resorption,[129] rodent experiments indicate that cyclosporine causes a marked increase in bone turnover with elevation of serum osteocalcin and a decrease in bone density.[169, 222] Cyclosporine may also decrease testosterone levels in male patients, further contributing to osteopenia.[226]

The accelerated bone loss (and increased remodeling activity) in postmenopausal women suggests that **estrogens** play an important role in the prevention of bone loss. Excessive alcohol consumption promotes osteoporosis by decreasing bone formation.

Finally, many patients following heart transplantation have some degree of **renal insufficiency** which may also play a role in the development of osteoporosis. Impaired renal clearance of parathormone[177] and abnormalities in vitamin D metabolism have been reported.[226]

Thus, the cause of bone loss in the posttransplant population is almost certainly multifactorial. Futhermore, there is compelling evidence that the process typically begins well **before** transplantation.[147, 170, 171, 226] Several factors contribute to bone loss in patients with heart failure, including advanced age, tobacco use, immobility, loop diuretics, and poor nutritional status (cardiac cachexia). Heart failure patients prior to transplantation have demonstrated bone mineral density approximately 20% below normal. This preexisting decrease in bone mineral density sets the stage for events following transplantation. As noted above, bone loss is most rapid during the first 6 months following transplantation, which coincides with the period of most aggressive immunosuppression. This finding, coupled with the potent adverse effects of corticosteroids and the lesser effects of cyclosporine on bone metabolism, strongly implicates immunosuppressive agents as the direct cause of accelerated bone loss in this population.

Management

The approach to the management of osteoporosis is outlined in Table 18–5. We recommended **routine screening** of all posttransplant patients with measurements of

TABLE 18-5	**Management of Osteoporosis After Heart Transplantation***

- Posttransplant yearly DEXA
- Elimination or minimization of corticosteroids
- Calcium supplementation
- Estrogen in postmenopausal or hypogonadal women
- Testosterone in hypogonadal men
- Bisphosphonates (treatment and evidence of ongoing bone loss)
- Calcitonin (if bisphosphonates not tolerated)
- Vitamin D (probably not necessary with normal renal function)
- Resistance exercise training
- Daily walking

DEXA, dual-energy x-ray absorptiometry.
*UAB protocol.

bone mineral density,[170] directing additional therapy at those patients who demonstrate significant decrement in bone density. Treatment for osteoporosis following transplantation has mostly focused on **prevention of ongoing bone loss.** Despite the prevalence of bone loss seen in heart failure patients undergoing transplantation, no studies to date have examined the effects of an aggressive program of treatment *prior* to transplantation. A recent study confirmed the presence of osteopenia or osteoporosis in nearly 50% of patients referred for transplant evaluation.[226] Given the time course of posttransplant bone loss, a strategy focusing on initiation of therapy at the time of transplant evaluation or listing is a potentially important area for future research.

The majority of studies on bone density and metabolism in posttransplant patients include background therapy with **elemental calcium.** Such supplementation is a standard part of the therapy of osteoporosis in nontransplant patients and is probably advisable in all posttransplant patients without specific contraindications. The daily intake of elemental calcium should be 15,000 mg/day (diet and/or supplementation). Beyond supplementation of elemental calcium, **measurement of gonadal hormones** with consideration of appropriate replacement therapy is advisable. The administration of **estrogens** in postmenopausal women produces a decrease in urinary excretion of calcium and other markers of bone resorption, but bone formation does not increase. The major effect on the use of estrogens is in preventing osteoporosis rather than treating clinical disease.

Vitamin D preparations increase calcium absorption, and may be effective in osteoporosis, since serum levels of vitamin D are typically mildly depressed. The combination of low-dose vitamin D combined with calcium supplementation is frequently effective in maintaining bone mass and decreasing the incidence of hip fracture in elderly women with osteoporosis.[140] Oral administration of **calcitriol** may also improve intestinal calcium absorption,[35, 130, 216] suppress bone resorption, stimulate osteoblastic new bone formation,[119] and decrease bone loss. In a nontransplant study, prophylactic calcitriol was associated with a marked reduction in lumbar spine bone loss during corticosteroid therapy.[215] However, vitamin D supplementation is probably not necessary in recipients with normal renal function.

Bisphosphonates are potent inhibitors of bone resorption and appear to be effective in glucocorticoid-induced osteoporosis. They are typically administered cyclically in alternation with calcium and vitamin D supplements. This regimen typically causes an increase in the density of spinal bone and may decrease the incidence of fractures.

Calcitonin decreases osteoclastic bone resorption. The salmon calcitonin (intranasal preparation) as opposed to the human calcitonin preparation may be more potent and is preferred when bisphosphonates are not tolerated.

The choice of supplemental therapy in patients who exhibit significant bone loss or who are at high risk for osteoporosis (elderly, postmenopausal, and/or a significantly decreased baseline bone density) is guided somewhat by two randomized trials in post–heart transplant patients. Garcia-Delgado and colleagues randomized patients following transplantation to one of three treatment strategies: oral bisphosphonate in cyclical therapy, nasal salmon calcitonin, or vitamin D supplementation.[96] All patients received 1 g of elemental calcium. Patients treated with vitamin D supplementation had an increase in bone mineral density at 6 months after transplantation that was maintained at 12 and 18 months. Patients treated with either the bisphosphonate regimen or with salmon calcitonin were noted to have less bone loss at 12 and 18 months than they had at 6 months, but they were still below their baseline values. In another study, patients were randomly assigned to receive bisphosphonate therapy or a vitamin D derivative along with 1.25 g of supplemental calcium.[259] Both groups had significant bone loss at 6, 12, and 24 months following transplantation; however, the group treated with the vitamin D derivative had less bone loss at each time point.

The effect of resistance exercise training in patients following heart transplantation has also been examined.[32] In one study, male transplant patients were randomly assigned to a specific program of resistance exercise focused at the lumbar spine or to routine care. After 6 months of exercise training, the treatment group had bone mineral density values substantially higher than the control group and not statistically different from their pretransplant values (Fig. 18–4). Based on the available data, a regimen of **elemental calcium, vitamin D supplementation, and proper exercise training,** perhaps beginning as early as time of listing for transplantation, seems warranted.

AVASCULAR NECROSIS

Avascular necrosis is a condition characterized by interruption of the blood supply to the bone with ischemia and ultimately death of bone and cartilage. Following cardiac transplantation, the major predisposing factor is the use of long-term corticosteroid therapy. The prevalence of avascular necrosis in cardiac transplant recipients is between 3 and 6%,[31, 147, 216] most frequently involving **the femoral head.** The mechanism of avascular necrosis in transplant recipients has not been elucidated, but the impairment of blood supply may be related to replacement of marrow with fat (reducing marrow blood flow), and osteoporosis may be an important predisposing condition. Loss of blood flow to the femoral head is not necessarily followed by necrosis as bone reabsorption and the laying down of new bone can occur. The rate of progression of avascular necrosis before subchondral collapse occurs is high, and after subchondral collapse and loss of joint space, there is progressive osteoarthritis. The symptoms of avascular necrosis depend on the bone involved. Avascular necrosis of the femoral head results in pain that is relentless, is frequently problematic at night, and may occur even without weight bearing.

The diagnosis is confirmed by imaging studies. Plain radiographs of the bone are usually not helpful in the early diagnosis, whereas magnetic resonance imaging (MRI) is a sensitive means of diagnosing early avascular

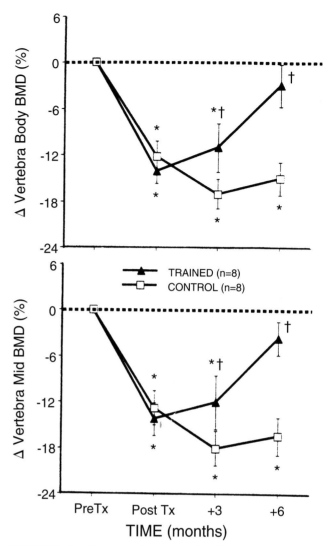

FIGURE 18–4. Changes in lumbar vertebral body and middle bone mineral density (BMD) at 2 months after heart transplantation and after 3 and 6 months of a resistance exercise program or a control period. Data are mean value ± SEM. *$p \le .05$ versus pretransplantation value $^+p \le .05$ training versus control group. (From Braith RW, Mills RM, Welsch MA, Keller JW, Pollock ML: Resistance exercise training restores bone mineral density in heart transplant recipients. J Am Coll Cardiol 1996;28:1471–1477.)

necrosis. Treatment depends on the severity of symptoms and the bone involved. Avascular necrosis of the femoral head ultimately results in the destruction of the joint, and the only effective therapy is total hip replacement.

MALIGNANCIES

SOURCES OF POSTTRANSPLANT MALIGNANCIES

Neoplastic disorders after cardiac transplantation arise from three major causes: (1) transplantation in patients with preexisting malignancies, (2) transmission of a malignancy from donor to recipient, and (3) *de novo* malig-

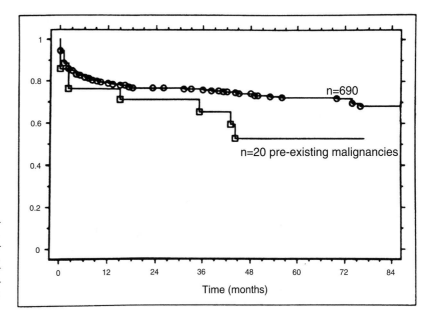

FIGURE **18–5.** One- and 5-year survival in heart recipients with and without preexisting malignancies. (From Koerner MM, Tenderich G, Minami K, Mannebach H, Koertke H, zuKnyphausen E, El-Banayosy A, Baller D, Kleesiek K, Gleichmann U, Meyer H, Koerfer R: Results of heart transplantation in patients with preexisting malignancies. Am J Cardiol 1997;79: 988–991.)

nancy arising in the recipient following cardiac transplantation.

Recurrence of Preexisting Malignancies

In considering potential recipients for cardiac transplantation, a history of previous malignancy is an important issue because of the risk of subsequent recurrence after transplantation (see Chapter 6). The problem of preexisting malignancies has been studied in renal transplant patients, and in over 900 renal transplant patients with preexisting malignancies, there was a 22% rate of recurrence, 13% of the recurrences occurring despite treatment of the primary malignancy 5 or more years prior to transplantation.[194, 195] Considerably less information is available in heart and heart/lung transplant patients. In a compilation[197] of nearly 150 heart and heart/lung transplant recipients with preexisting malignancies treated an average of 7 years prior to transplantation, persistence or recurrence of the malignancy occurred in 19% of patients. In selected patients undergoing cardiac transplantation with previously treated malignancy, the reported recurrence rate has been low.[39, 71, 135] Long-term survival of patients undergoing cardiac transplantation with a previous malignancy is similar (but not identical) to that of patients without previous malignancy (Fig. 18–5). Prior malignancy as a risk factor for mortality after cardiac transplantation (Table 18–6) is discussed in Chapter 16.

Defining a mandatory waiting period from treatment for any type of malignancy to cardiac transplantation that is associated with a low risk of recurrence after transplantation has not been possible. Furthermore, an excessively long mandatory waiting period may not be possible for an individual patient because of a poor natural history with heart failure. However, information from Penn[197] has demonstrated that tumors most likely to recur in heart, lung, and heart/lung transplant recipients are carcinomas of the lung, nonmelanoma skin cancers, lymphomas, carcinomas of the bladder, and pancreatic cancer.

Transplantation of a Donor Malignancy

Transplantation of a donor malignancy to a recipient has been described in heart transplantation.[159] In the Cincinnati Transplant Tumor Registry (CTTR) through 1995, four of nine thoracic transplant recipients who received organs from donors with an unrecognized malignancy subsequently died from metastatic carcinoma of the bronchus, medulloblastoma, melanoma, and nephroblastoma.[197] Obviously, an intensive search for unsuspected malignant disease in the donor by history, during workup of the donor, and during the procurement is mandatory. In a report from the United Network for Organ Sharing (UNOS) Scientific Registry which recorded the outcome of solid organ transplant recipients (including heart transplant recipients) whose donors had a past history of a malignancy, no donor transmitted recipient malignancy was identified.[122] These findings can be attributed in part to the fact that the majority of donor malignancies were nonmelanoma skin cancers or central nervous system (CNS) tumors, and the majority of those donors with nonskin and non-CNS cancers had

TABLE 18–6	Risk Factors for Death Due to Malignancy (CTRD: July 1993–1996, N = 3,158)	
	p VALUE	
RISK FACTOR	Early	Late
Age (older)	—	<.0001
Pretransplant malignancy	—	.02

From DeSalvo TG, Naftel DC, Kasper EK, Rayburn BK, Leier CV, Massin EK, Cintron GB, Yancy CW, Keck S, Aaronson K, Kirklin JK, and the Cardiac Transplant Research Database: The differing hazard of lymphoma vs. other malignancies in the current era [abstract]. J Heart Lung Transplant 1998;17:70.

a cancer-free interval of greater than 5 years (including cancers of the genitourinary tract, breast, thyroid, lymphoma, and throat/tongue). Transplantation of organs from donors with primary central nervous system malignancies is generally considered an acceptable risk even though there have been rare instances of extraneural spread of astrocytomas, glioblastomas,[189] and medulloblastomas,[131] and transmission of CNS tumors to recipients of solid organ transplants.[56, 91, 117, 167, 214] It is important to note that in the UNOS study, no cardiac transplant recipient whose donor had a history of a primary cerebral malignancy developed donor-transmitted CNS cancer (in 73% of the donors with a primary CNS malignancy, the histology of the tumor was not specified), suggesting the relative safety of using organs from donors with primary cerebral malignancies. The question of whether donors with primary CNS tumors who have undergone ventriculoperitoneal or ventriculoatrial shunts should be used as organ donors is currently unresolved.

In the case of transplantation of tumors from donor to recipient, theoretically one would expect that if the immunosuppression was stopped (only practical with renal transplant recipients), the recipient immune system would destroy the transplanted tumor cells. However, from the CTTR[193] only half of the renal transplant recipients with a transplanted malignancy experienced complete regression of the tumor with withdrawal of immunosuppression, the remainder dying of transplanted malignant disease following withdrawal of immunosuppression and therapy for the tumor. Withdrawal of immunosuppression is not, of course, possible after the discovery of a transplanted tumor to a cardiac transplant recipient, but it seems prudent to recommend reduction of immunosuppression to the lowest possible level.

De Novo *Recipient Malignancy*

The development of *de novo* recipient malignancy as a result of immunosuppression associated with heart and heart/lung transplantation is a major long-term complication. There are important differences, however, between malignancy arising in transplant patients and those arising in the normal population. The incidence of malignancy in solid organ transplant recipients is approximately three to four times that of the general population, although the incidence of certain malignancies appears to be particularly high following transplantation.[198] Numerically, cutaneous malignancies, posttransplant lymphoproliferative disorder (PTLD), and carcinoma of the lung constitute the most important malignancies after cardiac transplantation (Tables 18–7 and 18–8).[68] It is interesting to note that the time-related appearance of cutaneous malignancy, like PTLD, shows an early (within the first 12–18 months) risk, as opposed to lung cancer and other types of malignancy (Fig. 18–6).

TABLE 18-8	Noncutaneous Malignancies After Heart Transplantation (CTRD: 1990–1996, N = 5,379)	
NONCUTANEOUS MALIGNANCY (INITIAL DIAGNOSIS)	N	% OF 156 MALIGNANCIES
PTLD	43	28
Lung	32	21
Prostate	11	7
Sarcoma	8	5
Colon	7	4
Stomach	7	4
Kidney	4	3
Breast	2	1
Cervix	2	1
Other	40	26
Total	156	100

PTLD, posttransplant lymphoproliferative disease.
From DeSalvo TG, Naftel DC, Kasper EK, Rayburn BK, Leier CV, Massin EK, Cintron GB, Yancy CW, Keck S, Aaronson K, Kirklin JK, and the Cardiac Transplant Research Database: The differing hazard of lymphoma vs. other malignancies in the current era [abstract]. J Heart Lung Transplant 1998;17:70.

TABLE 18-7	Malignancy Following Cardiac Transplantation (CTRD: July 1993–1996, N = 3,158)	
	PATIENTS	
TYPE OF MALIGNANCY	N	% of 3,158
Noncutaneous	67	2.1%
PTLD	21	0.7%
Lung	9	0.3%
Other	37	1.2%
Cutaneous	54	1.7%
Squamous	31	1.0%
Basal	24	0.8%
Melanoma	3	0.1%
Any malignancy	112*	3.5%

* A patient may be in more than one subcategory.
From DeSalvo TG, Naftel DC, Kasper EK, Rayburn BK, Leier CV, Massin EK, Cintron GB, Yancy CW, Keck S, Aaronson K, Kirklin JK, and the Cardiac Transplant Research Database: The differing hazard of lymphoma vs. other malignancies in the current era [abstract]. J Heart Lung Transplant 1998;17:70.

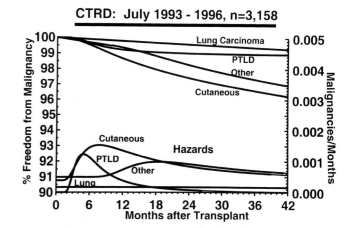

FIGURE **18–6.** Parametric estimate of freedom from malignancy after heart transplantation for various malignancies and the respective hazard function. (From DeSalvo TG, Naftel DC, Kasper EK, Rayburn BK, Leier CV, Massin EK, Cintron GB, Yancy CW, Keck S, Aaronson K, Kirklin JK, and the Cardiac Transplant Research Database: The differing hazard of lymphoma vs. other malignancies in the current era [abstract]. J Heart Lung Transplant 1998;17:70.)

TABLE 18-9	Time of Appearance of Neoplasms Following Transplantation		
TYPE OF MALIGNANCY	RANGE (mo)	AVERAGE (mo)	MEDIAN (mo)
Lymphomas	0.25–305.5	33	12
Kaposi's sarcoma	1–225.5	21	12.5
Carcinomas of kidney	1–213.5	55	41
Sarcomas (excluding Kaposi's)	2–239.5	70	43.5
Carcinomas of cervix	1.5–250	59	46
Hepatobiliary carcinomas	1–289.5	82	67.5
Skin cancers	1–313	83	69
Carcinomas of vulva/perineum	1.5–285.5	114	113.5
All cancers	0.25–324	62	46

From Penn I: Neoplastic complications of organ transplantation. In Ginns CM (ed): Transplantation. Malden, MA: Blackwell Science, 1999.

The interval of time from transplantation to the appearance of a malignancy may be quite short, particularly in the case of lymphomas and lymphoproliferative disorders (Table 18–9).[198] Information from the Cardiac Transplant Research Database (CTRD) also indicates a difference in the time course of the death due to malignancy for lymphoma and lymphoproliferative disorders as opposed to other nonlymphoma malignancies with an early (within the first year) peaking phase of risk of fatality from lymphoma or lymphoproliferative disorders (Fig. 18–7).

MECHANISMS INVOLVED IN INDUCTION OF NEOPLASIA

The development of neoplasia after transplantation, just as in the normal population, is the result of the interaction of multiple factors. However, in patients after transplantation there are additional factors involved, including the presence of a graft of different histocompatability to the host, immunosuppressive agents, and the use

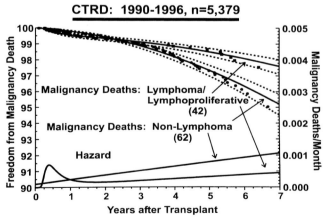

FIGURE **18-7.** Parametric estimate of freedom from lymphoma/lymphoproliferative and nonlymphoma (solid line) malignancy deaths surrounded by 70% confidence limits (dashed lines) with deaths placed actuarially. Hazard function for each type of malignancy death is indicated by the solid line. (From DeSalvo TG, Naftel DC, Kasper EK, Rayburn BK, Leier CV, Massin EK, Cintron GB, Yancy CW, Keck S, Aaronson K, Kirklin JK, and the Cardiac Transplant Research Database: The differing hazard of lymphoma vs. other malignancies in the current era [abstract]. J Heart Lung Transplant 1998;17:70.)

from time to time of potentially carcinogenic drugs. All these factors produce a complex milieu from which malignant disease may arise. The situation is further complicated by genetic factors which play a role in determining an individual's susceptibility to the effects of potentially carcinogenic agents. For example, HLA antigens partially determine the susceptibility to virus-induced neoplasia. In renal transplant recipients, HLA-A11 is associated with a lower incidence of cutaneous cancer,[86] although in Queensland, Australia, the reverse is true.[19] Patients with HLA-B27 and HLA-DR7 appear to have an increased risk of cutaneous cancer. HLA-DR homozygosity was found in heart transplant recipients to be associated with an increased risk of skin cancer.[184] The most important factors influencing the development of neoplasia after transplantation are disturbances in immune function and oncogenic viruses.[198]

Disturbances in Immune Function

The immune surveillance theory hypothesizes that with the enormous turnover of cells on a daily basis, potentially malignant mutations may occur which are recognized and destroyed by the immune system. **Disordered immune surveillance**[198] involves failure of the immune system to detect and destroy a mutated cell, resulting in the development of a malignancy. With impaired immunity associated with immunosuppression, this failure of immune surveillance may be one of the mechanisms of neoplastic development.

Chronic antigenic stimulation due to foreign antigens may play a role in neoplastic development after transplantation, but this currently has not been substantiated in humans. Experimentally, animals that have chronic antigenic stimulation through rejection of skin grafts may develop lymphomas.[110] Kaposi's sarcoma, which is seen after transplantation with an incidence many times that of the normal population, may possibly arise because of chronic stimulation of the endothelial cells from which this malignancy may arise. This chronic stimulation could come from a number of sources including the immune response, prolonged exposure to foreign histocompatibility antigens, and repeated infections.[198] The higher incidence of malignant disease after cardiac transplantation for chronic Chagas' disease may be, in part, the result of chronic antigenic stimulation of the lymphoreticular system by *Trypanosoma cruzi* infection.[29]

Impaired Immunoregulation

It has been hypothesized that because of immunosuppression, **impaired immunoregulation** (the cellular and humoral feedback mechanisms that are required to prevent uncontrolled proliferation of immune cells) may participate in the development of lymphoid tumors.[198]

The high incidence of epithelial tumors following transplantation may be explained by the **synergistic action of immunosuppressive agents with other carcinogens.** For example, metabolites of azathioprine can cause chemical photosensitization which may promote skin cancer.[108] Ultraviolet light radiation is carcinogenic, but it also has a direct toxic and suppressive effect on immunoregulatory cells of the epidermis such as the cells of Langhans. In combination with immunosuppression, this provides a milieu for cutaneous carcinogenesis. Experimental evidence suggests that immunosuppressive agents such as cyclosporine and azathioprine are themselves **carcinogenic.** However, experimentally, their carcinogenicity appears to be related to their role as a facilitator of experimentally induced tumors.

The **burden of immunosuppression** may also have a role in the development of neoplasia. The use of OKT3 as either an induction agent or for treatment of rejection is associated with an increase in the incidence of PTLD.[250] Furthermore, there was an inverse relationship between the dose of OKT3 and the length of time to the appearance of PTLD. The higher immunosuppression maintenance doses in heart transplantation as opposed to renal transplantation may in part explain the higher incidence of non-Hodgkin's lymphoma occurring in heart transplant recipients[185] (Fig. 18–8).

Oncogenic Viruses

Epstein-Barr virus (EBV) infection in the normal population is associated with Hodgkin's disease, rare T-cell lymphomas, Burkitt's lymphoma, and nasopharyngeal carcinoma. Primary EBV infection after transplantation nearly always results from an EBV-seronegative recipient receiving a seropositive donor organ which results in latent infection of B-cells (see Chapter 15). One of the key steps in the transformation of B-cells with EBV infection is circularization of the linear genome to form an episome (an extrachromosomal circular structure in the cell nucleus) (Fig. 18–9).[203] These transformed B-cells are then able to proliferate indefinitely. Two EBV proteins (EBV nuclear protein 1 and latent membrane protein) have been identified in B-lymphocytes which proliferate in response to EBV. Identification of these proteins with monoclonal antibodies may facilitate earlier detection of PTLD. A critical part of the process of immortalization of B-cells is the production of growth factors including interleukin-6 (IL-6) as well as other regulatory cytokines such as IL-4, interferon-α (IFN-α), and interferon-γ (INF-γ). The initial proliferation of EBV-infected B-cells is polyclonal, but eventually oligoclonal or monoclonal lines may develop, ultimately resulting in transformation to a malignant state.

B-cells may not be the only target of EBV, as EBV-associated smooth muscle tumors have been described after cardiac transplantation (hepatic smooth muscle neoplasm)[61] and neoplasms arising in the cardiac allograft.[10]

In the normal population, **human papillomaviruses** (HPV) have been identified as being involved in the genesis of anogenital and uterine cervical cancer. The risk of lower genital tract carcinoma *in situ* is substantially greater in renal transplant recipients than that in the normal population, and is associated with a marked increase in the incidence of HPV infection.[202]

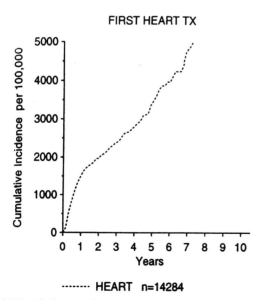
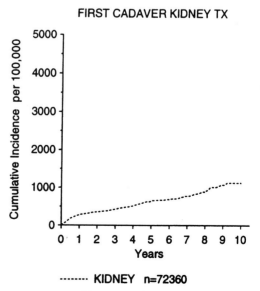

FIGURE **18–8.** Cumulative incidence of non-Hodgkin's lymphomas in recipients of heart transplants (left) or cadaver kidney transplants (right). The numbers of patients studied are indicated at the bottom of each graph. (From Opelz G: Are post transplant lymphomas inevitable? Nephrol Dial Transplant 1996;11:1952–1955.)

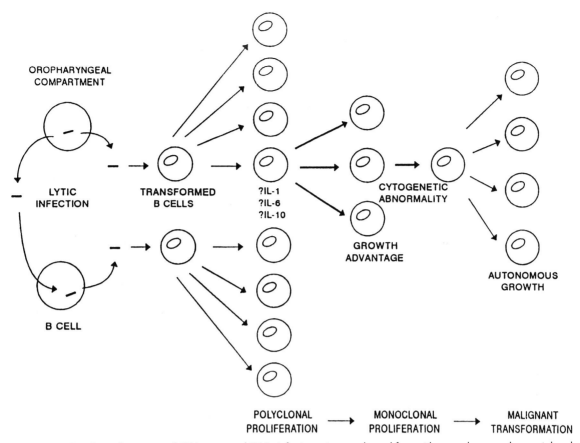

FIGURE **18-9.** The pathogenesis of EBV-associated PTLD. Infectious viruses released from either oropharyngeal or peripheral blood B-cells infects resting B-cells resulting in B-cell transformation and polyclonal proliferation. Certain transformed B-cells may have a selective growth advantage leading to clonal components of the lymphoproliferative process. Malignant transformation may occur as a consequence of the development of cytogenetic abnormalities. (–) represents linear viral genome in lytic cycle. (0) represents circular episomal virus in latently infected B-cell. (From Preiksaitis JK, Cockfield SM: Epstein Barr virus and lymphoproliferative disorders after transplantation. In Bowden RA, Ljungman P, Paya CV (eds): Transplant Infections. Philadelphia: Lippincott-Raven, 1998, with permission.)

It is also possible that **herpes simplex virus** (HSV) may be involved in the genesis of carcinoma of the lip (HSV-1) and carcinoma of the uterine cervix (HSV-2), but at the moment this is speculative.

SURVIVAL AFTER POSTTRANSPLANT MALIGNANCY

The probability of dying from a malignancy by 7 years after cardiac transplantation, from the Cardiac Transplant Research Database, is 8% (Fig. 18–10).[68] The hazard function for death due to malignancy demonstrates a small early peak followed by a progressively rising late risk (Fig. 18–10). The risk factors for death due to malignancy were only present in the late phase and included older age at operation and pretransplant malignancy (Table 18–6).[68] The important impact of pretransplant malignancy on the probability of death due to malignancy after transplantation is illustrated in Figure 18–11.[68] A detailed discussion of malignancy as a cause of death after cardiac transplantation is found in Chapter 16.

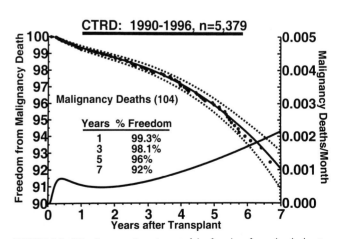

FIGURE **18-10.** Parametric estimate of the freedom from death due to malignancy (solid line) including the 70% confidence limits (dashed lines), with the deaths placed actuarially. Also included is the hazard function (solid line). (From DeSalvo TG, Naftel DC, Kasper EK, Rayburn BK, Leier CV, Massin EK, Cintron GB, Yancy CW, Keck S, Aaronson K, Kirklin JK, and the Cardiac Transplant Research Database: The differing hazard of lymphoma vs. other malignancies in the current era [abstract]. J Heart Lung Transplant 1998;17:70.)

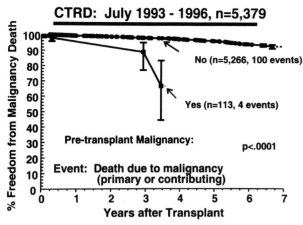

FIGURE 18–11. Actuarial freedom from malignancy death stratified by presence or absence of a pretransplant malignancy (the standard error is indicated by the vertical bars). (From DeSalvo TG, Naftel DC, Kasper EK, Rayburn BK, Leier CV, Massin EK, Cintron GB, Yancy CW, Keck S, Aaronson K, Kirklin JK, and the Cardiac Transplant Research Database: The differing hazard of lymphoma vs. other malignancies in the current era [abstract]. J Heart Lung Transplant 1998;17:70.)

POSTTRANSPLANT LYMPHOPROLIFERATIVE DISORDER

Epstein-Barr virus-induced posttransplant lymphoproliferative disorder (PTLD) is defined as **the presence of an abnormal proliferation of lymphoid cells,**[18] induced by the Epstein-Barr virus (EBV). The term PTLD includes a broad spectrum of lymphoproliferative disease, including both hyperplastic (including posttransplant infectious mononucleosis and plasma cell hyperplasia) and neoplastic processes. In this section, we will restrict the definiton of PTLD to **neoplastic** forms of lymphoproliferative disease. This heterogeneous group of lymphoproliferative diseases was first described in 1968 when they were called "reticulum cell sarcomas." A number of cardiac transplant centers described PTLD, and these descriptions indicated the heterogeneous nature of the condition, with descriptions of its multiclonality[51] and in some cases monoclonality,[50] the potential reversibility of PTLD in some cases with reduction of immunosuppression,[237] and the progressive and usually lethal course of monoclonal lymphoproliferative disorders.[139, 225]

Pathogenesis

In solid organ transplantation, PTLD is believed to originate from EBV infection of the recipient's B-lymphocytes.[111, 175, 234] The EBV most commonly originates from a transplanted organ (from an EBV serologically positive donor) when the recipient is EBV serologically negative. EBV could also be acquired through blood transfusions or community contacts. Alternatively, lytic replication of latent EBV disease can occur in the presence of chronic immunosuppression. The abnormal EBV-specific immune surveillance induced by the transplant state of immunosuppression allows the increased burden of EBV to infect recipient B-cells and induce their transformation into expanding B-cell clones which can become neoplastic.[191]

Risk Factors

A number of risk factors have been identified for the development of PTLD (Table 18–10). The risk of **a pretransplant EBV-seronegative** recipient developing PTLD is 24 to 33 times greater than in patients who were seropositive prior to transplantation.[52, 209, 267, 268] The risk of developing PTLD in pretransplant seropositive recipients who develop reactivation of EBV infection is currently unknown. The risk of PTLD is clearly increased by the prolonged use of **cytolytic therapy** such as OKT3. Although the precise link between T-cell cytolytic agents such as OKT3 and the development of PTLD is not yet established, it has been hypothesized that OKT3 results in the generation of inflammatory cytokines such as tumor necrosis factor (TNF) that may promote EBV transcription and reactivation from a latent state.[265] The increased risk of PTLD with prolonged OKT3 administration has also been identified after cardiac transplantation, particularly when the total dose exceeds 75 mg.[57]

The risk of PTLD appears to be increased by the development of **cytomegalovirus (CMV) disease,** particularly the high-risk group of CMV donor positive to recipient negative serologic mismatch. Although there is no evidence that CMV directly participates in the genesis of PTLD, it augments the risk associated with the use of OKT3 and pretransplant EBV seronegativity. In fact, the synergistic effect of a CMV mismatch combined with pretransplant recipient seronegativity for EBV and the use of OKT3 increases the risk of PTLD more than 500 times the risk in a patient without these three risk factors after nonrenal transplantation[267] (Fig. 18–12).

The observation has been made of an increased incidence of PTLD in pediatric recipients of liver transplantation[60] and renal transplantation[219] who received FK506-based immunosuppression.

Pathology of PTLD

A number of histological classifications of PTLD exist, but a major shortcoming is that the usual pathological features which suggest a malignant process (cellular atypia, necrosis and invasiveness) are not predictive of the clinical course of the disease. For example, even nontransplant patients with acute infectious mononucle-

TABLE 18–10	**Risk Factors for the Development of PTLD**

- Strong link with EBV infection
- Risk of PTLD related to type of organ grafted (heart and heart/lung recipients at greater risk than renal or liver recipients)
- Chronic antigenic stimulation may increase the risk of PTLD
- PTLD associated with increased intensity of immunosuppression
- Risk of PTLD increased in the presence of CMV infection

From Preiksaitis JK, Cockfield SM: Epstein Barr virus and lymphoproliferative disorders after transplantation. In Bowden RA, Ljungman P, Paya CV (eds): Transplant Infections. Philadelphia: Lippincott-Raven, 1998, with permission.

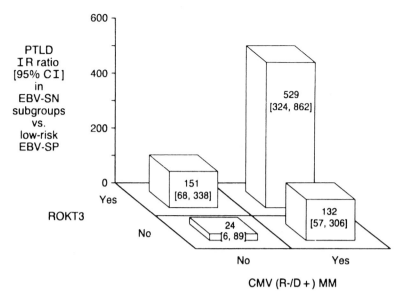

FIGURE **18–12.** The incidence rate (IR) ratio of posttransplantation lymphoproliferative disorder (PTLD) in Epstein-Barr virus seronegative (EBV-SN) subgroups versus low-risk EBV-seropositive (EBV-SP) recipients without identifiable risk factors. Cytomegalovirus (CMV) recipient negative/donor positive (R–/D+) seromismatch (MM) increased the IR ratio for PTLD by four- to fivefold whether or not severe rejection requiring OKT3 (ROKT3) occurred. Conversely, ROKT3 increased the IR ratio for PTLD by four- to sixfold whether or not a CMV (R–/D+) MM had occurred. (From Walker RC, Marshall WF, Strickler JG, Wiesner RH, Velosa JA, Habermann TM, McGregor CG, Paya CV: Pretransplantation assessment of the risk of lymphoproliferative disorder. Clin Infect Dis 1995;20:1346–1353.)

osis may have on lymph node biopsy atypical immunoblasts, necrosis and distortion of the underlying architecture, and Reed-Sternberg cells that would suggest a malignant process.[94, 256] The terms "polymorphic hyperplasia" and "polymorphic lymphoma" do not predict the clinical course or response to therapy such as reduction in immunosuppression or antiviral therapy.[203] The inadequacies of the current histological classifications have been summarized in a consensus meeting on EBV-induced PTLD[191] and include (1) the use of incompletely defined descriptions such as "polymorphism" versus "monomorphism" which are subject to individual interpretation, (2) lack of differentiation between EBV-positive and EBV-negative PTLD, (3) lack of uniformity in the incorporation of features such as monoclonality or other nonmorphological features such as oncogene rearrangements or mutations that may have prognostic importance, and (4) inconsistency in providing information about the donor versus host origin of tumor which may have prognostic significance.

Despite these limitations, the histological classifications do serve a role (Table 18–11).[203] Within this classi-

fication, there is a spectrum of disease. At one end is a plasmacytic hyperplasia that is similar to that seen in infectious mononucleosis where the architecture of the lymph node is preserved, and the response is polyclonal with evidence of EBV infection and without oncogene or tumor suppressor gene alterations.[132] This process is relatively benign. At the other end of the spectrum are lesions that have features consistent with monoclonal non-Hodgkin's lymphoma which have a monoclonal population of cells and cytogenic abnormalities which result in activation of one or more proto-oncogenes (c-myc, N-ras) or mutations involving the p53 tumor suppressor gene (bcl-2 or bcl-6),[45, 66] a process that is more likely to have the course of a malignancy. In the consensus meeting on EBV-induced PTLD,[191] it was recommended that posttransplant infectious mononucleosis and plasma cell hyperplasia be included under the heading of PTLD, but be segregated as reactive hyperplasias. It was also recommended that the term "PTLD" without such a qualification be used in reference to neoplastic forms of PTLD that are currently termed "polymorphic PTLD" (which include polymorphic lymphoma and

TABLE 18–11 Classification of the Histologic Lesions Found in PTLD

CATEGORY		PLASMACYTIC DIFFERENTIATION	IMMUNOBLASTS	CYTOLOGIC ATYPIA	NECROSIS	CLONALITY	ACTIVATION OF ONCOGENES/ TUMOR SUPPRESSOR GENES
Polymorphic							
I	Plasmacytic hyperplasia	++	+/++	—	—	Polyclonal	No
	Polymorphic	++	++/+++	—	—	Usually monoclonal	No
II	B-cell hyperplasia Polymorphic B-cell lymphoma	+	++/+++	+/+++	+++	Monoclonal	No
Monomorphic							
III	Immunoblastic lymphoma	+	+++	+/+++	+	Monoclonal	Yes
IV	Multiple myeloma	+	—	+++	+	Monoclonal	Yes

Data from Frizzera et al., 1981[92]; Knowles et al., 1995[132], Nalesnik et al., 1997,[176] and Preiksaitis et al., 1998.[203]

TABLE 18-12	**Clinical Presentation of PTLD**

- Infectious mononucleous-like illness
- Organ system involvement
  - Allograft
  - Gastrointestinal tract
  - Central nervous system
  - Lungs
  - Other
- Disseminated disease

polymorphic B-cell hyperplasia which can also be a monoclonal lesion) or "lymphomatous" PTLD (which includes monomorphic PTLD).

Diagnosis

The diagnosis of PTLD rests on a tissue biopsy, and adequate tissue is required for assessment of cell type, clonality, biological studies, and architectural background.[191] Needle biopsies should only be used if excisional biopsy or larger tissue biopsies are not possible, and specimens obtained by cytology have only a limited role in the diagnosis of PTLD.[191]

Criteria for diagnosis of the neoplastic forms of EBV-positive PTLD should include (1) disruption of the underlying architecture by a lymphoproliferative process, (2) monoclonal or oligoclonal cell populations as demonstrated by cellular and/or viral markers, and (3) evidence of EBV infection in many of the cells. A diagnosis can be made in the presence of one or two criteria alone in the proper clinical setting.

Molecular and immunologic diagnostic advances offer the opportunity for further refinement in diagnosis. Immunoglobulin or T-cell receptor gene rearrangement studies enhance the determination of tumor clonality, monoclonal antibodies may allow identification of lymphocyte subset phenotypes, and detection of EBV may be facilitated by more sensitive virologic techniques.[191] Quantitative EBV polymerase chain reaction (PCR) technology may allow earlier detection of circulating EBV and quantification of viral load, both of which may promote earlier identification of PTLD.

Clinical Presentation

There is a wide spectrum of clinical presentations of PTLD (Table 18–12). Within the first year after transplantation, especially among younger patients after heart and heart/lung transplantation, an **infectious mononucleosis-like illness** may occur, characterized by fever, myalgia, sore throat, and lymphadenopathy (in particular, cervical adenopathy and tonsillar hypertrophy).[203] This illness is usually a polyclonal B-cell proliferation. The adenotonsillar enlargement can be so dramatic as to result in rapid airway obstruction.[78, 104]

PTLD may present with **allograft involvement**, particularly in heart/lung transplant recipients (nearly always just the lung) and intestinal transplant recipients, less frequently liver and renal transplant recipients, and rarely cardiac transplant recipients. PTLD involving a cardiac allograft has been rarely described,[1, 12, 72, 249, 276]

and in virtually all cases the cardiac involvement was part of a multiorgan process. PTLD has been detected in routine endomyocardial biopsy,[72, 105] with the identification of EBV-positive lymphocytes in the cardiac biopsy infiltrates. This raises the issue of possible confusion between acute cardiac rejection and a PTLD involving the heart, and the finding of an atypical myocardial lymphocyte infiltration on an endomyocardial biopsy should prompt a search for other sites that may be involved with PTLD (see further discussion in Chapter 14). Although *in situ* hybridization for EBV can be used to detect EBV-positive lymphocytes in the endomyocardial biopsy specimens, the yield rate even in patients with known PTLD is low[105] and appears not to be a useful screening test.

The **gastrointestinal tract** may be involved in PTLD,[46, 85, 103, 245, 275, 281] and may result in necrosis, bleeding, perforation, and obstruction. The survival of patients with gastrointestinal PTLD may be better than PTLD involving other sites possibly because gastrointestinal tract PTLD may be amenable to surgical resection.[46]

The **central nervous system** may be involved either in association with disseminated disease, or disease can be confined to the central nervous system. The usual presentations are change in mental status or the development of a focal neurological deficit. The diagnosis is made by an imaging study, and the lesion enhances with contrast (Fig. 18–13). **Lungs** may be involved in patients with PTLD, particularly in heart/lung transplant recipients.[277] The typical presentation is respiratory dysfunction, and the imaging study demonstrates multi-

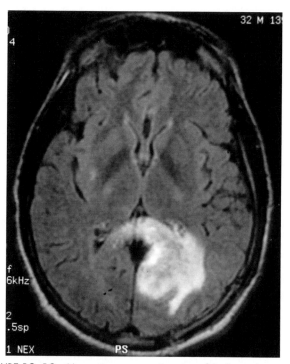

FIGURE **18-13.** Magnetic resonance imaging of the brain demonstrating a left parieto-occipital mass also involving the corpus callosum which enhances with contrast, typical of cerebral PTLD. There were also changes due to a recent brain biopsy.

ple pulmonary nodules (Fig. 18–14). Many other sites can be involved with PTLD, including liver, bone marrow, lymph nodes, kidney, soft tissue, thyroid, adrenal, and genital tracts. **Disseminated PTLD** is associated with poor survival.

EBV-negative PTLD has been described after solid organ transplantation including heart and heart/lung transplantation,[145] but it is considerably less common than EBV-positive PTLD. Although the number of reported cases is small, some general comments can be made. EBV-negative B-cell PTLD demonstrates the same range of pathology as does EBV-positive B-cell PTLD, including polyclonal and monoclonal morphology. EBV-negative PTLDs appear to present later after transplantation, and survival is significantly poorer than patients with EBV-positive PTLDs (Fig. 18–15). **T-cell PTLD** has rarely been reported after heart transplantation.[84, 125, 262, 272] T-cell PTLDs may be EBV-positive or EBV-negative. Based on the small number of cases described in heart transplant patients and the somewhat larger number of cases described after renal transplantation,[106] it appears that presentation is usually late after transplantation with an aggressive course and very poor survival.

Multiple myeloma is a rare form of PTLD that has been described in cardiac transplant recipients.[49, 88] The role of EBV in the genesis of myeloma is uncertain, but these myelomas may be either EBV-positive or EBV-negative. Myeloma in renal transplant recipients and the much smaller number of cardiac transplant recipients is associated with poor survival.

Treatment of PTLD

The optimal treatment of PTLD remains a contentious issue because of the lack of consensus in defining the

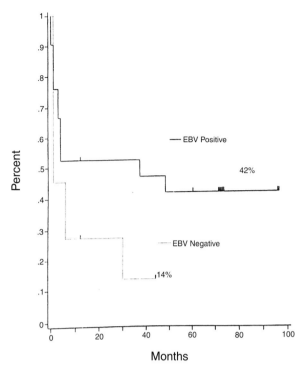

FIGURE **18–15.** Overall survival rate of patients with PTLD not associated with EBV (.....) and associated with EBV (—). Information is from patients undergoing renal, heart and liver transplantation ($p < .01$). (From Leblond V, Davi F, Charlotte F, Dorent R, Bitker MO, Sutton L, Gandjbakhch I, Binet JL, Raphael M: post transplant lymphoproliferative disorders not associated with Epstein-Barr virus: a distinct entity? J Clin Oncol 1998;16:2052–2059.)

pathology of PTLD, the absence of a clear relationship between morphological features such as clonality and cytogenetic abnormalities and clinical course, absence of large treatment trials, and a lack of agreement between therapeutic protocols. A number of therapies have been employed or are under investigation (Table 18–13). The basic options for treatment of PTLD include (1) reduction of immunosuppression, (2) surgical extirpation, (3) chemotherapy, (4) antiviral agents, (5) anti–B-cell monoclonal antibodies, and (6) cell-based therapies. The treatment of pediatric PTLD is discussed in Chapter 20.

All patients with PTLD should, as the primary therapy, undergo **reduction in immunosuppression.** The extent to which immunosuppression should be reduced and the duration of reduction is currently unknown. The response rate is difficult to assess in part due to the frequency of concomitant therapy. The likelihood of regression of PTLD (both polyclonal and monoclonal) following reduction of immunosuppression (after solid organ transplantation) has been estimated to be between 20 and 50%.[21, 175, 191] Composite figures after solid organ transplantation indicate that patients with polyclonal PTLD undergoing a reduction in immunosuppression have a response rate of 50–65%. In patients with a monoclonal PTLD, the reported response rate is much lower.[218] A general approach to the treatment of PTLD is presented in Table 18–14.

The current approach recommended by the collaborative Southwest Oncology Group/Eastern Cooperative Oncology Group for the treatment of PTLD[191] after any solid organ transplant begins with reduction of immu-

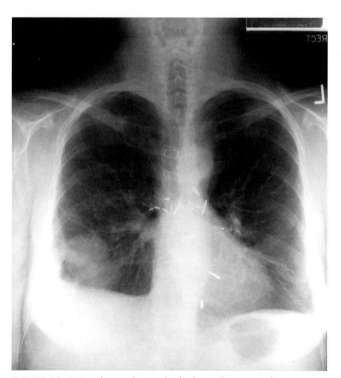

FIGURE **18–14.** Chest radiograph of a heart/lung transplant recipient with PTLD demonstrating multiple pulmonary nodules.

TABLE 18-13	Management of PTLD After Heart Transplantation: Suggested Guidelines

Recommended treatment
  Limited disease
    Surgical extirpation or localized radiation therapy
    Minor/moderate (e.g., 25%) immunosuppression reduction
  Extensive disease
    Critically ill: stop all immunosuppression; prednisone at 7.5–10 mg/day; frequent biopsies; treat with bolus of corticosteroids if required
    Not critically ill: decrease cyclosporine tacrolimus by 50%, discontinue azathioprine/mycophenolate mofetil, and maintain prednisone at 7.5–10 mg/day
  If recent EBV serologic conversion or evidence of circulating virus (by PCR)
    Ganciclovir 5 mg/kg IV bid for 3 mo, followed by oral cytovene for 1 yr
    Further therapy based on serial quantitation of viral load
Alternative/complementary measures
  Recombinant interferon-α (not as a single agent):
    3×10^6 U/m²/day SC daily for up to 3 mo
    Standard dose modifications for toxicities
    6 mo of 3 times/wk as maintenance treatment if clinical response observed at 3 mo
  If the previous measures fail to control the disease:
    Chemotherapy, anthracycline-based regimens: CHOP, ProMACE-CytaBOM for two cycles beyond a clinical response
  Investigational approaches:
    Anti-IL-6 antibody
    Infusion of HLA-matched peripheral blood mononuclear cells with anti-EBV cytotoxic activity
    Dendritic cell therapy
    Anti-CD20, -CD21, -CD24, or anti-CD40 antibodies
    Remove episomes—low-dose hydroxyurea

Modified from Paya CV, Fung JJ, Nalesnik MA, Kieff E, Green M, Gores G, Habermann TM, Wiesner RH, Swinnen LJ, Woodle ES, Bromberg JS: Epstein-Barr virus induced post transplant lymphoproliferative disorders. Transplantation 1999;68:1517–1525.

nosuppression. Patients who are critically ill with extensive disease have the prednisone decreased to a maintenance dose of 7.5–10 mg/day and all other immunosuppression discontinued. If there is no objective reduction in tumor mass within 10–20 days, other alternatives/complementary measures are used (Table 18–13). For patients who are less critically ill with limited disease, cyclosporine (or tacrolimus) and prednisone are reduced by at least 50% and azathioprine (or mycophenolate mofetil) is discontinued. After 14 days of decreased immunosuppression, a further decrease of 50% is then considered. It is of course imperative in patients after heart or heart/lung transplantation that intensive monitoring for rejection (including serial endomyocardial or transbronchial lung biopsies) occurs during a period of significant reduction in immunosuppression. It must be remembered that these recommendations are based largely on renal transplant experience, and this degree of reduction in immunosuppression in heart transplant patients may not be safe.

Surgical extirpation or debulking of PTLD increases the likelihood of a cure.[54, 175] Tonsillectomy and adenoidectomy for pediatric patients with PTLD after heart transplant without concomitant reduction in immunosuppression (localized disease to the tonsils and adenoids) appears to be effective.[279] The effectiveness of surgical excision may in part be explained by the fact

that gastrointestinal PTLD, for example, may present earlier than other sites of extranodal involvement because of mechanical complications. In the current state of knowledge, however, it is impossible to separate the effects of surgical therapy and immunosuppression reduction, as they are likely to occur contemporaneously.

Antiviral agents such as acyclovir and ganciclovir have been used, but the efficacy of this therapy in PTLD has not been substantiated. Acyclovir and ganciclovir block EBV DNA replication by interfering with EBV-associated DNA polymerase. Both drugs are only effective against the replicative or lytic phase of EBV infection and therefore may not be effective in PTLD, since both drugs are likely ineffective against transformed B-cells. *In vitro* data indicate that **ganciclovir** is a more effective antiviral agent against EBV than acyclovir, with considerably greater inhibition of EBV-associated polypeptides.[151] Antiviral therapy may be effective in the early stages of PTLD before a large population of infected polyclonal B-cells has emerged, but currently this is unproven. The use of hydroxyurea may be effective as antiviral therapy by targeting latent infected B-cells.[48]

Localized radiation therapy has been used mainly as an adjuvant therapy for cytotoxic chemotherapy and has had some success, particularly with central nervous system PTLD.[54] Central nervous system involvement has a particularly poor prognosis and requires special therapeutic considerations. In addition to reduction in immunosuppression, the most effective therapy for central nervous system PTLD is radiation therapy.[191, 196] Systemic chemotherapy is mandatory, usually with high-dose methotrexate, often with additional cytosine arabinoside.

For patients in whom reduction in immunosuppression and local therapy has been ineffective, a number of alternative systemic measures are available. **IFN-α** has antiviral and antiproliferative effects, and regression of PTLD after therapy with IFN-α has been reported[63, 83, 114] after isolated therapy and in combination with chemotherapy.[178] In a double lung transplant recipient with PTLD,[83] a reduction in IL-4 and IL-10 mRNA

TABLE 18-14	General Approach to PTLD*

Prevention
- High-risk group (recipient negative–donor positive)
    Monitoring for seroconversion
    At conversion, acyclovir or cytovene for 6 mo (see Table 15–9)
    Avoidance of cytolytic therapy

Treatment
- Localized disease
    Immunosuppression reduction
    Surgical resection if possible
    Ganciclovir†
    Chemotherapy‡ if unresponsive to above measures or if not surgically removable
- Disease in more than one anatomic site
    Immunosuppression reduction
    Ganciclovir†
    Chemotherapy‡

*UAB protocol.
†If evidence of circulating EBV.
‡Chemotherapy should be used cautiously, since this therapy is discretionary and its aggressive use in the setting of immunosuppression is potentially fatal.

levels in bronchoalveolar lavage was found in association with IFN-α therapy, suggesting that INF-α led to a down-regulation of helper T-cell cytokines which could provide growth factors for the proliferation of B-cells. There is a potential risk of precipitating rejection with IFN-α therapy because of the possibility of up-regulation of HLA expression in the allograft.[203]

Cytotoxic chemotherapy is another alternative therapy that has been used with some success after solid organ transplantation including heart transplantation,[26, 46, 97, 150, 207, 249] and the regimens that appear to have been effective are anthracycline-based (CHOP, ProMACE-CytaBOM). For B-cell PTLD, these cytotoxic chemotherapy regimens appear to be reasonably effective, but for T-cell PTLD, based on a very small number of patients, the response rate is extremely poor.[106, 262]

Anti–B-cell monoclonal antibodies directed against CD21 and CD24 appear to be effective therapy in some patients with PTLD.[22, 87, 146] In one multicenter trial, anti-CD21 and anti-CD24 antibodies showed an overall response rate of 61% (80% in oligoclonal types and 46% in monoclonal disorders).[191] In the multicenter study by Fischer and colleagues,[87] 14 bone marrow transplant patients and 12 solid organ transplant recipients (four heart, one heart/lung transplant recipient) received CD21- and CD24-specific antibodies for the treatment of B-cell PTLD that had not responded to reduction in immunosuppression and/or had unfavorable features such as multiple organ involvement, rapid progression, or histologic markers associated with poor prognosis. Complete remission occurred in 16 of the 26 patients, but only in patients with oligoclonal B-cell PTLD and did not occur in patients with central nervous system involvement. A case of EBV-positive B-cell PTLD of the central nervous system has been reported in an infant after cardiac transplantation. Treatment with a combination of CD21- and CD24-specific anti–B-cell antibodies and recombitant IFN-α-2b intravenously was ineffective, but anti-CD21 antibody infused intrathecally resulted in high local concentrations of monoclonal antibodies and produced dramatic clinical improvement with clearance of the parenchymal lesions.[241] **Anti-CD20 antibody** in pediatric and adult transplant recipients with PTLD refractory to reduction of immunosuppression is currently under trial.[191] Use of **anti–IL-6 monoclonal antibodies**[70] has been considered.

TABLE 18-15	Prophylaxis Against EBV-PTLD in Heart and Heart/Lung Transplantation

• Pretransplant EBV seronegativity
  EBV antiviral prophylaxis
  EBV vaccine development
  EBV viral load surveillance in peripheral blood
  Prophylactic adoptive immunotherapy (cloned T-cell lines)
  Elimination of cytolytic therapy in patients at high risk for EBV PTLD
• CMV disease and/or CMV D+/R−
  CMV antiviral prophylaxis
  CMV hyperimmune globulin

EBV, Epstein-Barr virus; CMV, cytomegalovirus.

TABLE 18-16	Protocol* for Epstein-Barr Virus/PTLD Surveillance and Prophylaxis for EBV-Negative Recipient and EBV-Positive Donor†

• Obtain EBV IgM and IgG serologies 6 wk after transplantation, then every 3 mo for 1 yr or until seroconversion
• At time of seroconversion, begin ganciclovir 5 mg/kg IV bid for 2 mo, then oral ganciclovir 1 g 3 times daily for 1 yr
• At time of seroconversion, schedule abdomen and chest CT scan every 3 mo for 1 yr, then yearly for 2 yr

EBV, Epstein-Barr virus; CT, computerized tomography.
*UAB protocol.
†Serology negative for EBV in recipient and positive in donor

Cell-based therapy has been used to treat PTLD after bone marrow transplantation. Since EBV-positive PTLD usually arises in donor B-lymphocytes in bone marrow transplant recipients, EBV-specific donor T-cells may be effective in limiting donor PTLD in the recipient.[30, 74, 187, 212] Other cell-based therapies under investigation include the infusion of HLA-matched T-cells from an EBV-positive donor and the use of *ex vivo* activated natural killer and T-lymphocytes.[176]

Prophylaxis

Neutralization of three important risk factors (pretransplant EBV seronegativity, CMV disease and/or CMV mismatch (D+/R−), and cytolytic therapy) could result in a substantial reduction in the incidence of PTLD (Tables 18–15 and 18–16). There are a number of potential approaches to prophylaxis in the setting of pretransplant EBV seronegativity. **Antiviral drugs** (see Chapter 15) have not been proven to decrease the incidence of EBV PTLD. Part of the uncertainty with current antiviral agents against EBV is the fact that effective prophylaxis requires presence of drug at the time of transmission of lytic-replicative EBV from the donor to the recipient. An **EBV vaccine** administered before transplant to EBV-negative individuals is under investigation but not yet clinically available.

The **monitoring of EBV viral load** in peripheral blood and possibly in oropharyngeal secretions may have a role in detecting recipients at risk for PTLD. The preliminary information suggests that patients with at least 200 EBV genomes per 10^5 peripheral blood lymphocytes is predictive of subsequent PTLD with a sensitivity and specificity of 92.8% and 100%, respectively[213] (healthy seropositive individuals have 0.1–2 EBV genomes per 10^5 peripheral blood lymphocytes). This approach may be valuable in preemptively targeting at-risk recipients. Exposing EBV-negative individuals to EBV-positive blood prior to transplantation has been suggested,[191] but is not currently recommended prophylaxis. Use of prophylactic adoptive immunotherapy with cloned EBV-specific T-cells is an investigative approach.

Prophylaxis against **CMV** disease and, in the high-risk situation of a CMV-positive donor to CMV-negative recipient, preemptive antiviral therapy with ganciclovir and hyperimmune globulin is recommended and may be important in reducing the incidence of PTLD (see

Chapter 15). The use of aggressive immunosuppression including **cytolytic therapy**, particularly for the treatment of acute rejection, is an important risk factor for the development of subsequent PTLD, which may be neutralized by newer, more targeted immunosuppressive modalities.

Survival

Survival is difficult to ascertain, since some reports calculate survival of a PTLD "group" (i.e., development of PTLD anytime during follow-up) from the time of transplant rather than the time of diagnosis of PTLD. Survival of heart transplant recipients after the diagnosis of lymphoma or lymphoproliferative disease ranges from approximately 45–80% at 2 years (Fig. 18–16). Although not rigorously studied, there are morphological features (polyclonality, lack of cytogenetic abnormalities) and clinical features (localized PTLD, gastrointestinal and pulmonary PTLD) that are associated with better survival in heart transplant recipients.[46] Multivisceral disease, late PTLD, and CNS involvement are associated with worse outcome.[22] Survival after PTLD in pediatric heart transplant recipients is discussed in Chapter 20.

LUNG CANCER

Lung cancer is the most common noncutaneous malignancy after cardiac transplantation, and PTLD and lung cancer are the most common fatal malignancies.[68] Lung cancer usually occurs in patients with a substantial pretransplant smoking history.[89, 99, 200] Despite the fact that these patients after transplantation are closely followed, the diagnosis of lung cancer is often made when it has reached an advanced stage with metastatic disease (Table 18–17).[68] Successful surgical resection of stage I lung cancers[89, 200] is associated with good intermediate-term survival. However, for the majority of patients, survival after the diagnosis of lung cancer is poor (Fig. 18–17), and a feature of all reports[59, 89, 99, 200] is the rapid demise

TABLE 18-17	Lung Carcinoma After Heart Transplantation (CTRD: 1990–1996, N = 5,379)

SITES OF INVOLVEMENT AT INITIAL DIAGNOSIS (MULTIPLE SITES ARE POSSIBLE)	N	% of 32*
CNS	1	3
Pulmonary (lung)	31	97
Bone	6	22
Hepatic	4	13
GI, large bowel	1	3
Lymph nodes, subcutaneous	2	6
Lymph nodes, deep	4	13
Other	3	9

CNS, central nervous system; GI, gastrointestinal.
*32 patients developed lung cancer.
From DeSalvo TG, Naftel DC, Kasper EK, Rayburn BK, Leier CV, Massin EK, Cintron GB, Yancy CW, Keck S, Aaronson K, Kirklin JK, and the Cardiac Transplant Research Database: The differing hazard of lymphoma vs. other malignancies in the current era [abstract]. J Heart Lung Transplant 1998;17:70.

of these patients and the ineffectiveness of therapy when the diagnosis of metastatic lung cancer is made.

CANCER OF SKIN AND LIPS

Cutaneous premalignant and malignant epithelial lesions are the most commonly seen tumors after heart transplantation, accounting for nearly 40% of *de novo* cancers.[59] They are frequently associated with precancerous keratoses, Bowen's disease, and keratoacanthomas. In the general population, the ratio of squamous cell carcinoma (SCC) to basal cell carcinoma (BCC) is 1:2 to 1:5.[195, 211] However, following cardiac transplantation, not only is the incidence of SCC and BCC increased over the normal population, but the ratio of SCC to BCC is reversed[144] (Fig. 18–18). Risk factors for the development of cutaneous cancer include exposure to ultraviolet radiation (particularly applies to SCC's), older age, male sex, fair skin, and blue eyes.[144] The incidence of malignant melanomas and Merkel's cell tumor is also higher in

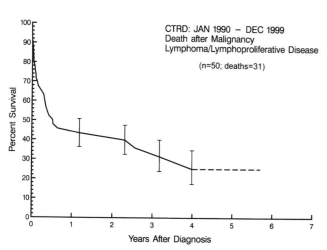

FIGURE **18–16.** Actuarial survival of heart transplant recipients from the time of diagnosis of lymphoma/lymphoproliferative disease. (From the Cardiac Transplant Research Database.)

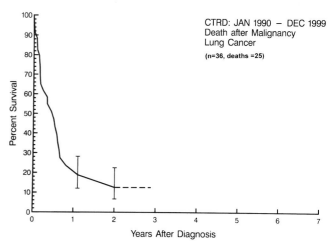

FIGURE **18–17.** Actuarial survival of heart transplant recipients from the time of diagnosis of lung cancer. (From the Cardiac Transplant Research Database.)

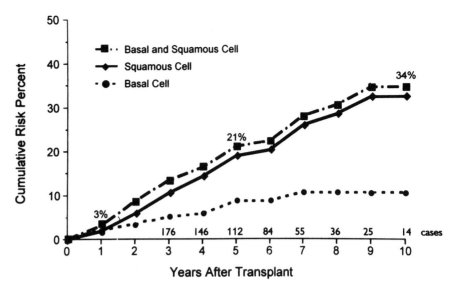

FIGURE **18-18.** Comparison of cumulative risk in development of squamous cell carcinoma and basal cell carcinoma after cardiac transplantation. (From Lampros TD, Cobanoglu A, Parker F, Ratkovec R, Norman DJ, Hershberger R: Squamous and basal cell carcinoma in heart transplant recipients. J Heart Lung Transplant 1998;17:586–591.)

transplant recipients. Compared to renal transplant recipients, heart transplant patients are about twice as likely to develop a cutaneous malignancy, are less likely to have extracephalic lesions, and, on average, develop the first premalignant or malignant epithelial lesions earlier following transplantation.[77] The differences may relate to the fact that cardiac transplant patients are usually older than renal transplant recipients and possibly to a higher intensity of immunosuppression in cardiac transplant recipients.

Reduction of immunosuppression (particularly discontinuation of azathioprine) should be considered in any patient with cutaneous malignancies even though it does not cause regression of existing tumors. Premalignant skin lesions can be treated with a 6-week course of topical 5-fluorouracil cream applied twice daily or with topical 0.05% tretinoin cream. Other means of treating cutaneous malignancies include surgical excision and cryosurgery. The probability of death from a cutaneous BCC or SCC is low (Fig. 18–19), with fatality usually secondary to distant metastases.

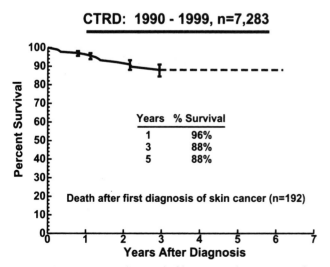

FIGURE **18-19.** Actuarial survival of heart transplant recipients from the time of diagnosis of cutaneous basal and squamous cell carcinomas. (From the Cardiac Transplant Research Database.)

KAPOSI'S SARCOMA

Kaposi's sarcoma is a rare multifocal vascular tumor whose incidence is many times that occurring in the normal population. The incidence of Kaposi's sarcoma is greatly increased in patients with acquired immunodeficiency syndrome (AIDS). This tumor has a male predominance and most frequently occurs in patients of Mediterranean, Jewish, and African extraction. In the CTTR, 59% of patients with Kaposi's sarcoma had nonvisceral involvement (skin, conjunctiva, or oropharyngolaryngeal mucosa), and 41% had visceral disease (mainly involving the gastrointestinal tract, lungs, and lymph nodes).[196] Kaposi's sarcoma may be associated with human herpesvirus-8 (HHV-8) infection.[4, 124] Kaposi's sarcoma has been rarely described after cardiac transplantation.[2, 90, 118, 278] Initial therapy is substantial reduction in immunosuppression, and in the CTTR this therapy alone produced approximately 30% remission rate for nonvisceral disease and 16% remission rate for visceral disease.[197] A variety of other therapies have been employed, including cytotoxic chemotherapy, surgery, radiation therapy and INF-α.

CARCINOMA OF THE FEMALE GENITAL TRACT

Carcinoma of the cervix has a substantially increased incidence in transplant patients (as do all epithelial tumors), and in the CTTR, 72% of patients had *in situ* lesions. In renal transplant patients with carcinomas of the vulva and perineum, one third had in situ lesions.[192] There is often multicentric involvement, including the vulva, vagina, cervix, and anus. These cancers may be preceded by condyloma acuminatum caused by human papillomavirus, which should be regarded as a premalignant condition. It is important that all postadolescent female heart and heart/lung transplant patients undergo regular pelvic examination with cervical smears and aggressive treatment of *in situ* lesions to prevent progression to invasive carcinomas.

TABLE 18-18	Routine Surveillance for Post–Heart Transplant Complications (Other than Rejection, Infection, and Allograft Vasculopathy)*

TEST	FREQUENCY
• Stool for occult blood	Yearly (patients >50 yr of age)
• Colonoscopy alternating with flexible sigmoidoscopy	Every 3 yr (> 50 yr of age)
• Digital rectal exam	Yearly (males > 50 yr of age)
• Prostate specific antigen testing	Every 2 yr (males > 50 yr of age)
• Mammogram	Yearly (females >35 yr of age)
• Pelvic exam and Pap smear	Yearly (females > 35 yr of age)
• Chest x-ray	With each routine clinic vist (at least every 6 mo)
• Dermatology	Yearly
• Lipid profile	Every 6–12 mo
• Bone density screening	Yearly
• Ophthalmology exam	Yearly
• Dental exam	Every 6 mo

*Adapted from protocols at Cleveland Clinic and UAB for detection of malignancy, hyperlipidemia, osteoporosis, and ocular complications. Surveillance protocols for rejection, infection, and allograft vasculopathy are contained in Chapters 14, 15, and 17.

MALIGNANCY SCREENING AND DETECTION

Given the ongoing and likely increasing risks of malignancy following transplantation, an important part of long-term transplant care involves selective screening for certain malignancies. A recommended protocol is listed in Table 18–18. When seen by physicians, transplant patients should undergo careful examination of the skin (including the scalp and lips), the oral pharynx, and lymph nodes. A chest x-ray should be a standard part of each clinic visit during the first year following transplantation, and should be obtained every 6 months thereafter. The detailed list of surveillance examinations and studies listed in Table 18–18 should be performed by physicians who are expert in the detection of malignancies in these areas.

A high index of suspicion is necessary for the early detection of posttransplant malignancies. This is especially true of PTLD, which can present with a variety of symptoms. Neurologic or cognitive abnormalities may be the presenting symptoms for PTLD, other CNS malignancies, infection, or drug toxicities. Unexplained fever, particularly when accompanied by malaise and weight loss, should prompt a thorough evaluation for possible PTLD and other malignancies. A thorough physical examination and chest x-ray should be followed by computerized tomographic (CT) scans of the abdomen and chest if a diagnosis is not evident. Chronic bone pain may signify PTLD or metastatic bone lesions as well as steroid-induced compression fractures or avascular necrosis. Any lesion should be biopsied to exclude possible malignancy/PTLD.

GASTROINTESTINAL COMPLICATIONS

Numerous minor and some major potentially life-threatening gastrointestinal (GI) complications may occur after heart transplantation that require urgent recognition and institution of therapy. In addition to disorders which occur in the general population, GI complications following cardiac transplantation may occur as complications of preexisting diseases, transplant medications, or the transplant condition. This section will discuss gastrointestinal complications occurring after the initial transplant hospitalization. Complications occurring during the early postoperatiave period are also discussed in Chapter 12.

PREEXISTING GASTROINTESTINAL DISORDERS

In the assessment of patient candidacy for heart and heart/lung transplantation, it is important to detect gastrointestinal conditions that may lead to serious posttransplant complications, including peptic ulcer disease, diverticular disease, and cholelithiasis. If there is suspicion of **peptic ulcer disease,** upper gastrointestinal endoscopy can be safely performed in patients with heart failure, and healing should be demonstrated before a patient is listed for cardiac transplantation. The finding of **diverticular disease** does not necessarily contraindicate transplantation, and the usual strategies to manage diverticular disease should be employed following cardiac transplantation. Patients with known diverticular disease who develop abdominal pain after transplantation must be evaluated for possible diverticular complications such as diverticulitis, abscess formation, or perforation. **Cholelithiasis** has been reported in up to 30%[98, 238] of heart transplant recipients, perhaps reflecting the predominance of coronary artery disease as a cause for heart failure in transplantation and the associated hyperlipidemia. Patients with symptomatic cholelithiasis ideally should undergo laparoscopic cholecystectomy prior to transplantation, if possible, to avoid the possibility of early postoperative cholecystitis. In patients who have asymptomatic cholelithiasis prior to transplantation, laparoscopic cholecystectomy is probably not necessary unless symptoms develop. **Inflammatory bowel disease** clearly increases the risk of posttransplant intestinal complications, but there is insufficient data to allow firm recommendations regarding the advisability of transplantation. The majority of patients with ulcerative colitis who undergo liver transplantation for the development of primary sclerosing cholangitis do experience improvement in their symptoms of inflammatory bowel disease,[242] presumably due to immunosuppression. In patients with ulcerative colitis who undergo cardiac transplantation, heightened postoperative surveillance by colonoscopic examinations is necessary for early detection of colorectal cancer.

PREVALENCE AND PREDISPOSING FACTORS

Minor complications (abdominal pain, nausea and vomiting, diarrhea, constipation, stomatitis, and gastroesophageal reflux) will affect approximately two thirds of patients.[43] An identifiable cause is found in less than half of patients with minor gastrointestinal complaints, most of which result from the effects of medications. Approximately 15–30% of transplant recipients develop major GI complications during the first 3–5 years.[14, 55, 228] These complications appear to be most common within the first 30 days after transplantation, 50% occurring within 2 months of transplantation and 70% by 1 year.

Corticosteroids have been associated with an increased risk of peptic ulceration, bowel perforation, gastrointestinal bleeding, and pancreatitis.[64, 109, 158, 243] A temporal relationship has been observed between pulse corticosteroid therapy and the onset of abdominal complications, including most cases of acute bowel perforation. Some reports have cited up to one third of all major abdominal complications occurring in this setting. Given the increased frequency of acute allograft rejection (and therefore pulse steroid administration) in the first 3 months following cardiac transplantation, it is not surprising that major GI complications are concentrated within this time frame.[157] Other immunosuppressive agents also contribute to the development of GI complications (Table 18–19).

The distribution of major gastrointestinal complications will likely vary from center to center, but a number of important complications may occur (Table 18–19). The most common conditions (or complications) are peptic ulcer disease, cholelithiasis, diverticular disease, pancreatitis, and gastrointestinal invasive CMV disease.

UPPER GASTROINTESTINAL DISEASE

In heart and heart/lung transplant patients, the etiology of **peptic ulcer disease** has not been clearly elucidated, whereas in the normal population the most common cause is *Helicobacter pylori* infection. *Helicobacter pylori* infection almost certainly does play a role in peptic ulcer

disease in transplant recipients, but there are other possible causes including invasive CMV disease, herpes (HSV) infection, and ulcer disease either caused or contributed to by the use of corticosteroids.

The incidence of peptic ulcer disease is likely higher in patients receiving corticosteroids, probably due to disruption of mucosal integrity. Injury to the vagus nerve after heart/lung transplantation may also contribute to ulcer disease because of delayed gastric emptying. Esophagitis may result from *Candida albicans*, invasive CMV disease, or HSV infection. The symptoms of upper gastrointestinal disease include dysphagia, epigastric pain, nausea, vomiting, bloating, and odynophagia. The investigation of choice is upper gastrointestinal endoscopy. Ulcerative lesions should be biopsied for the detection of invasive CMV disease. The **treatment** of esophageal candidiasis, invasive gastrointestinal CMV disease, and HSV infection is outlined in Chapter 15. For patients with *H. pylori*, treatments incorporate both antisecretory therapy (H$_2$-receptor antagonist or proton pump inhibitor) and antimicrobial therapy (such as combination therapy including bismuth, metronidazole, and tetracycline).

CHOLELITHIASIS

Cholelithiasis may present with the typical symptoms of biliary colic, acute cholecystitis and, rarely, cholangitis. Acalculous cholecystitis has been described after cardiac transplantation[228] and is associated with bile stasis and gallbladder ischemia. Cyclosporine has been implicated in the genesis of gallstones.[121] Ursodeoxycholic acid has been used to dissolve noncalcified gallstones, but there is little information about its efficacy. Treatment of symptomatic cholelithiasis is laparoscopic cholecystectomy, but the role of this procedure for asymptomatic cholelithiasis has not been clarified.

DIVERTICULAR DISEASE

Diverticular disease is common in heart transplant recipients (incidence is similar to the general population), but complications of diverticular disease (diverticulitis, abscess formation, and perforation) are unusual. Diverticulitis should be treated by intravenous antibiotics with consideration for elective colon resection if more than one episode occurs. Perforation of a diverticulum usually requires prompt surgical therapy. Other rare causes of large bowel perforation are Ogilvie's syndrome (usually occurs in the right colon as opposed to diverticular disease in the left colon) and toxic megacolon, both occurring in patients who are very ill following transplantation. The probability of perforation of the colon is probably increased by the use of corticosteroids.

TABLE 18-19	Gastrointestinal Complications After Cardiac Transplantation
CAUSATIVE OR PREDISPOSING FACTOR	**COMPLICATIONS**
Immunosuppression	
Corticosteroids	Peptic ulceration, bleeding, perforation, toxic megacolon, intestinal perforation, pancreatitis
Cyclosporine	Hepatocellular injury, cholelithiasis
Azathioprine	Cholestatic/hepatocellular injury, pancreatitis
Mycophenolate mofetil	Diarrhea
Infection	
CMV	Esophagitis, gastritis with gastric bleeding or ulceration, colitis, hepatitis
HSV	Oral ulceration, esophagitis, colitis
Adenovirus	Colitis
Clostridium difficile	Pseudomembranous colitis
Salmonella	Diarrhea
Candida albicans	Pharyngitis, esophagitis
PTLD	Bowel obstruction, perforation

CMV, cytomegalovirus; HSV, herpes simplex virus; PTLD, posttransplant lymphoproliferative disorder.

PANCREATITIS

Cholelithiasis, hyperlipidemia, invasive CMV disease, and drug toxicity (such as azathioprine) may cause pancreatitis. The incidence of pancreatitis after cardiac transplantation is low (approximately 5–10%), but autopsy evidence of unsuspected pancreatitis may be found in patients dying from other causes, so the real incidence is probably unknown. The management of acute pancreatitis should be aggressive, in line with that of pancreatitis in nontransplant patients.

GENERAL THERAPEUTIC CONSIDERATIONS

Given the variety of organs and disease processes which are included under gastrointestinal complications, mortality figures differ widely among reports and provide only general indications of the seriousness of these conditions and the success of therapeutic interventions. Operative interventions for either diagnosis or treatment are necessary in about half of major gastrointestinal complications. Hospital mortality after major gastrointestinal complications, often requiring operations, varies from under 10% to as high as 30% or more.[55, 69, 127, 157, 239] Truly elective gastrointestinal surgical procedures carry a very low mortality, which in most experiences approaches zero.[127, 228] However, in the presence of acute gastrointestinal complications,[127, 157] aggressive investigation and intervention are necessary to optimize survival rates. This relates in part to the difficulty of diagnosis due to chronic steroid administration as well as other conditions mimicking the symptoms of these serious complications. Furthermore, the immunosuppressed state of these patients allows rapid progression of intraabdominal infection and its sequelae.

Urgent abdominal surgery is frequently necessary for such gastrointestinal complications as perforation due to peptic ulcer disease or diverticular disease, gastrointestinal bleeding, complications of cholelithiasis and complications of pancreatitis. The mortality associated with urgent gastrointestinal surgery is substantially increased by a delay in surgical intervention. For example, in a study of renal transplant recipients with colonic perforation, patient survival was 86% if the surgery was performed within 24 hours of perforation, but if surgery was delayed for more than 24 hours following perforation, survival was only 25%.[137] Similar excellent survival has been reported with surgical therapy for gastrointestinal complications after cardiac transplantation when the interval between symptom onset and surgery was less than 3 days.[127]

HYPERGLYCEMIA

Glucocorticoids induce persistent hyperglycemia in approximately 5–10% of nondiabetic patients undergoing cardiac transplantation.[93] Among patients with diabetes mellitus, chronic glucocorticoids exacerbate their hyperglycemic tendencies. Glucocorticoids stimulate hepatic synthesis of glucose from amino acids and glycerol, stimulate the deposition of glucose in the liver as glycogen, diminish glucose utilization, increase protein breakdown, and activate lipolysis. The net effect of these physiologic alterations is to increase blood glucose levels.[221] Cyclosporine and, to a greater extent, tacrolimus may also induce glucose intolerance, but their effect is considerably less than that of glucocorticoids. In general, withdrawal of chronic steroids is associated with a high rate of resolution of hyperglycemia (with discontinuation of insulin or oral agents) in transplant patients treated with either cyclosporine or tacrolimus maintenance immunosuppression. Long-term effects of persistent hyperglycemia are likely the same as from diabetes resulting from other causes.

OCULAR COMPLICATIONS

A number of eye conditions may result from immunosuppression drugs. The most frequent immunosuppressive complications are related to systemic corticosteroids. Corticosteroid-induced **cataracts** are usually posterior subcapsular opacities that do not interfere with vision, but they may progress to the stage of visual impairment that requires surgery. The relationship between steroid dose and the development of cataracts remains contentious, but it appears that a daily dose of over 15 mg of prednisone for a year is usually required to produce cataracts. However, detectable posterior subcapsular changes may occur in less than a year. Systemic corticosteroids have induced intraocular pressure elevation or aggravated chronic open-angle **glaucoma,** but this complication is rare.

A number of rare ocular complications have been associated with systemic **cyclosporine** therapy including optic disc edema (probably a direct toxic effect of the drug on the optic nerve) and other rare complications such as papilledema and cortical blindness due to increased intracranial pressure. Severe ocular pain has been rarely described without evidence of ocular abnormalities.

A number of infections may affect the eye including CMV, herpes zoster, and *Candida;* their treatment is outlined in Chapter 15.

LATE PACEMAKER IMPLANTATION

Implantation of permanent pacing systems for bradyarrhythmias during the transplant hospitalization is discussed in Chapters 11 and 12. Early pacemaker implantation is usually prompted by persistent sinus node dysfunction or, less commonly, intermittent or continuous atrioventricular block. It is well known that pacemakers implanted for sinus node dysfunction occurring early are usually not utilized after the first 6 months due to spontaneous recovery of sinus node function (see again Chapter 12). However, whenever atrioventricular block is the indication for permanent pacing, patients generally remain pacer dependent during long-term follow-up.[206]

Late bradycardias (beyond 5 months after transplant) are rare, reported in about 1.5% of patients.[164] The atrial contribution to ventricular contraction is particularly important in heart transplant patients (see Chapter 11), and pacing systems should be selected which preserve this function. Approximately half the reported incidences of late bradycardia are related to acute allograft rejection, and these generally respond to antirejection therapy. However, symptomatic bradycardia or episodes of complete heart block should be considered dangerous arrhythmias when they present months or years following transplantation, in that they may be a harbinger of serious rejection or allograft vasculopathy. Documented bradycardic episodes or complete heart block late after transplantation represent an indication for pacemaker implantation. Likewise, recurrent syncope without clear etiology should also prompt consideration for pacemaker implantation. It is extremely important, however, that prompt evaluation for rejection and allograft vasculopathy is undertaken when a bradyarrhythmic event is identified. Such patients should undergo prompt echocardiographic assessment, endomyocardial biopsy, and coronary angiography (if not recently obtained). Even if no rejection is identified by endomyocardial biopsy, the possibility of humoral rejection may exist, and close surveillance with echocardiography and repeat endomyocardial biopsy is strongly advised in such patients, even after pacemaker placement. We and others have observed rapid deterioration and sudden death secondary to allograft vasculopathy or hemodynamically compromised rejection within weeks after pacemaker implantation for complete heart block which developed years after transplantation.

LATE TRICUSPID REGURGITATION

INCIDENCE

With the availability of frequent echocardiographic assessment of heart function and atrioventricular valve function, detection of mild degrees of tricuspid and mitral valve insufficiency is common in the months and years following cardiac transplantation. Whereas severe and symptomatic mitral valve insufficiency is extremely rare, progressive tricuspid insufficiency is a well-recognized complication of transplantation, likely related to repeated endomyocardial biopsies.[34, 107, 113, 235, 257] The incidence of moderately severe or worse tricuspid insufficiency has been reported to increase from about 5% at 1 year to nearly 50% at 4 years after transplantation.[107] Severe, symptomatic tricuspid insufficiency, however, is much less common, occurring in about 1–5% of patients 5 or more years following transplantation.[113, 235]

MECHANISMS

Tricuspid valve insufficiency appearing after cardiac transplantation has been variously attributed to disturbed right atrial geometry created by the right atrial anastomosis in the standard orthotopic technique,[15] torsion of the atria during ventricular systole and diastole,[8] asynchronous contraction of the donor and recipient atrial compartments,[8] papillary muscle dysfunction,[3] postoperative dilatation secondary to pulmonary hypertension, and biopsy-induced tricuspid valve insufficiency. Several reports do suggest that the bicaval technique of implantation provides superior freedom from tricuspid regurgitation compared to the traditional orthotopic technique (see also Chapter 10).[15]

In the small subset of patients who exhibit sufficiently severe and symptomatic tricuspid insufficiency to require operation, the overwhelming major cause of tricuspid valve injury appears to be repeated endomyocardial biopsies.[107, 257, 273] Extensive injury to multiple chordae may result in a flail tricuspid leaflet, worsening the symptoms of tricuspid insufficiency. The risk of this injury appears to increase with greater numbers of endomyocardial biopsies.[15, 107]

INDICATIONS FOR OPERATION

Surgical intervention is **rarely** necessary for post transplant tricuspid insufficiency. However, occasional patients will develop signs of abdominal ascites, hepatic congestion, and fatigue, which are associated with elevated mean right atrial pressure (usually 15 mm Hg or more with prominent V-waves) and are not responsive to salt and fluid restriction and diuretic therapy. Such patients should be considered for tricuspid valve surgery as long as their general condition is good and chronic renal insufficiency is absent. It is important to perform coronary angiography and a routine endomyocardial biopsy close to the time of proposed operation to exclude active rejection or allograft vasculopathy, both of which could importantly increase the risk of operation.

SURGICAL TECHNIQUES

The operation is performed using standard techniques of cardiopulmonary bypass with a beating, perfused heart at normothermia. Standard precautions (femoral vessel exposure or catheter cannulation) for transplant reoperations are advisable, since the right atrium may often be large and immediately under the sternum. In children, standard annuloplasty techniques are performed whenever possible. In adult patients, annuloplasty techniques are sometimes appropriate, but tricuspid valve replacement with a bioprosthesis may be advisable in patients who are many years following transplantation and in whom there is extensive chordal damage with one or more flail leaflets.

RESULTS OF OPERATION

In the absence of important coronary artery disease, acute rejection, renal dysfunction, and other comorbidities, the operative mortality is low (< 5%), and the symptomatic outcome is usually excellent.

References

1. Abu-Farsakh H, Cagle PT, Buffone GJ, Bruner JM, Weilbaecher D, Greenberg SD: Heart allograft involvement with Epstein-Barr virus-associated posttransplant lymphoproliferative disorder. Arch Pathol Lab Med 1992;116:93–95.

2. Aebischer MC, Zala LB, Braathen LR: Kaposi's sarcoma as manifestation of immunosuppression in organ transplant recipients. Dermatology 1997;195:91–92.

3. Akasaka T, Lythall DA, Kushawaha SS, Yoshida K, Yoshikawa J, Yacoub MH: Valvular regurgitation in heart-lung transplant recipients. A Doppler color flow study. J Am Coll Cardiol 1990;15:576–581.

4. Alkan S, Karcher DS, Ortiz A, Khalil S, Akhtar M, Ali MA: Human herpesvirus-8/Kaposi's saracoma-associated herpesvirus in organ transplant patients with immunosuppression. Br J Haematol 1997;96:412–414.

5. Almenar L, Osa A, Palencia M, Flores A, Sanchez E: Effects of fosinopril on the blood pressure and lipid profile of patients undergoing heart transplantation. J Heart Lung Transplant 1997;16:454–459.

6. Andoh TF, Burdmann EA, Bennett WM: Nephrotoxicity of immunosuppressive drugs: experimental and clinical observations. Semin Nephrol 1997;17:34–45.

7. Andreassen AK, Hartmann A, Offstad J, Geiran O: Hypertension prophylaxis with omega-3 fatty acids in heart transplant recipients. J Am Coll Card 1997;29:1324–1331.

8. Angerman CE, Spes CH, Tammen A: Anatomic characteristics and valvular function of the transplanted heart: transthoracic versus transesophageal echocardiographic findings. J Heart Lung Transplant 1990;9:331–338.

9. Angermann CE, Spes CH, Willems S, Dominiak P, Kemkes BM, Theisen K: Regression of left ventricular hypertrophy in hypertensive heart transplant recipients treated with enalapril, furosemide, and verapamil. Circulation 1991;84:583–593.

10. Anguita J, Rico ML, Palomo J, Munoz P, Preciado V, Menarguez J: Myocardial Epstein-Barr virus-associated cardiac smooth-muscle neoplasm arising in a cardiac transplant recipient. Transplantation 1998;66:400–401.

11. Antonovych TT, Sabnis SG, Austin HA, Palestine AG, Balow JE, Nussenblatt RB, Helfrich GB, Foegh ML, Alijani MR: Cyclosporine A induced arteriolopathy. Transplant Proc 1988;2(suppl 3):951–958.

12. Armitage JM, Kormos RL, Stuart RS, Fricker FJ, Griffith BP, Nalesnik M, Hardesty RL, Dummer JS: Post transplant lymphoproliferative disease in thoracic organ transplant patients: ten years of cyclosporine-based immunosuppression. J Heart Lung Transplant 1991;10:877–887.

13. Augustine SM, Baumgartner WA, Kasper EK: Obesity and hypercholesterolemia following heart transplantation. J Transplant Coord 1998;8:179–187.

14. Augustine SM, Yeo CJ, Buchman TG, Achuff SC, Baumgartner WA: Gastrointestinal complications in heart and in heart/lung transplant patients. J Heart Lung Transplant 1991;10:547–555.

15. Aziz TM, Burgess MI, Rahman AN, Campbell CS, Deiraniya AK, Yonan NA: Risk factors for tricuspid valve regurgitation after orthotopic heart transplantation. Ann Thorac Surg 1999;68:1247–1251.

16. Ballantyne CM, Radovancevic B, Farmer JA, Frazier OH, Chandler L, Payton-Ross C, Cocanougher B, Jones PH, Young JB, Gotto AM: Hyperlipidemia after heart transplantation: report of a 6-year experience with treatment recommendations. J Am Coll Card 1992;19:1315.

17. Bantle JP, Paller MS, Boudreau RJ, Olivari MT, Ferris TF: Long term effects of cyclosporine on renal function in organ transplant recipients. J Lab Clin Med 1990;115:233–240.

18. Basgoz N, Preiksaitis JK: posttransplant lymphoproliferative disorder. Infect Dis Clin North Am 1995;9:901–923.

19. Bavinck JNB, Claas FHJ, Hardie DR, Green A, Vermeer BJ, Hardie IR: Relation between HLA antigens and skin cancer in renal transplant recipients in Queensland, Australia. J Invest Dermatol 1997;108:708–711.

20. Bellet M, Cabrol C, Sassano P, Leger P, Corvol P, Menard J: Systemic hypertension after cardiac transplantation: effect of cyclosporine on the renin-angiotensin-aldosterone system. Am J Cardiol 1985;56:927–931.

21. Benkerrou M, Durandy A, Fischer A: Therapy for transplant-related lymphoproliferative diseases. Hemat Oncol Clin North Am 1993;7:467–475.

22. Benkerrou M, Jais JP, Leblond V, Durandy A, Sutton L, Bordigoni P, Garnier JL, LeBidois J, LeDeist F, Blanche S, Fischer A: Anti-B-cell monoclonal antibody treatment of severe posttransplant B-lymphoproliferative disorder: prognostic factors and long-term outcomes. Blood 1998;92:3137–3147.

23. Bennett WM, DeMattos A, Meyer MM, Andoh T, Barry JM: Chronic cyclosporine nephropathy: The Achilles' heel of immunosuppressive therapy. Kidney Int 1996;50:1089–1100.

24. Bergstrand A, Bohman SO, Farnsworth A, Gokel JM, Krause PH, Lang W, Hihatsch MJ, Oppedal B, Sell S, Sibley RK, Thiru S, Verani R, Wallace AC, Zollinger HU, Ryffel B, Thiel G, Wonigeit K: Renal histopathology in kidney transplant recipients immunosuppressed with cyclosporine A: results of an international workshop. Clin Nephrol 1985;24:107–119.

25. Berguer DG, Krieg MA, Thiebaud D: Osteoporosis in heart transplant recipients: a longitudinal study. Transplant Proc 1994;26:2649–2651.

26. Bernstein D, Baum D, Berry G, Dahl G, Weiss L, Starnes VA, Gamberg P, Stinson EB: Neoplastic disorders after pediatric heart transplantation. Circulation 1993;88:230–237.

27. Bertani T, Ferrazzi P, Schieppati A, Ruggenenti P, Gamba A, Parenzan L, Mecca G, Perico N, Imberti O, Remuzzi A: Nature and extent of glomerular injury induced by cyclosporine in heart transplant patients. Kidney Int 1991;40:243–250.

28. Bloom ITM, Bentley FR, Garrison RN: Acute cyclosporine-induced renal vasoconstriction is mediated by endothelin-1. Surgery 1993;114:480–488.

29. Bocchi EA, Higuchi M, Vieira MLC, Stolf N, Bellotti G, Fiorelli A, Uip D, Jatene A, Pileggi F: Higher incidence of malignant neoplasms after heart transplantation for treatment of chronic Chagas' heart disease. J Heart Lung Transplant 1998;17:399–405.

30. Boyle TJ, Berend KR, DiMaio JM, Coles RE, Via DF, Lyerly HK: Adoptive transfer cytotoxic T lymphocytes for the treatment of transplant associated lymphoma. Surgery 1993;114:218–226.

31. Bradbury G, Benjamin J, Thompson J, Klees E, Copeland JG: Avascular necrosis of bone after cardiac transplantation. Prevalence and relationship to administration and dosage of steroids. J Bone Joint Surg Am 1994;76:1385–1388.

32. Braith RW, Mills RM, Welsch MA, Keller JW, Pollock ML: Resistance exercise training restores bone mineral density in heart transplant recipients. J Am Coll Cardiol 1996;28:1471–1477.

33. Braith RW, Mills RMJ, Wilcox CS, Davis GL, Wood CE: Breakdown of blood pressure and body fluid homeostasis in heart transplant recipients. J Am Coll Cardiol 1996;27:375–383.

34. Braverman AC, Coplen SE, Mudge GH, Lee RT: Ruptured chordae tendineae of the tricuspid valve as a complication of endomyocardial biopsy in heart transplant patients. Am J Cardiol 1990;66:111–113.

35. Bressot C, Meunier PJ, Chapuy MC, Lejune E, Edouard C, Darby AJ: Histomorphometric profile, pathophysiology and reversibility of corticosteroid induced osteoporosis. Metab Bone Rel Res 1979;1:303–319.

36. Brooks DP, Contino LC: Prevention of cyclosporine A induced renal vasoconstriction by the endothelin receptor antagonist SB 209670. Eur J Pharmacol 1995;294:571–576.

37. Brozena SC, Johnson MR, Ventura HO, Hobbs R, Miller L, Olivari MT, Clemson B, Bourge RC, Quigg R, Mills RM, Naftel DC: Effectiveness and safety of diltiazem or lisinopril in treatment of hypertension after heart transplantation. J Am Coll Cardiol 1996;27:1707–1712.

38. Bunchman TE, Brookshire CA: Cyclosporine-induced synthesis of endothelin by cultured human endothelial cells. J Clin Invest 1988;88:310–314.

39. Caforio ALP, Tursi V, Brombin M, Feltrin G, Anmgelini A, Livi U: Heart transplantation in patients with neoplastic disease. Transplant Proc 1998;30:1928.

40. Campistol JM, Sacks SH: Mechanisms of nephrotoxicity. Transplantation 2000;69:5–10

41. Canalis E: Effects of glucocorticoids on type I collagen synthesis, alkaline phosphatase activity, and deoxyribonucleic acid content in cultured rat calvariae. Endocrinology 1983;112:931–939.

42. Carrier M, Tronc F, Stewart D, Pelletier LC: Dose-dependent effect of cyclosporin on renal artery resistance of dogs. Am J Physiol 1991;261:H1791-H1796.

43. Cates J, Chavez M, Laks H: Gastrointestinal complications after cardiac transplantation: a spectrum of diseases. Am J Gastroenterol 1991;86:412-416.

44. Cavarape A, Endlich K, Feletto F: Contribution of endothelin receptors in renal microvessels in acute cyclosporine-mediated vasoconstriction-mediated vasoconstriction in rats. Kidney Int 1998;53:963-969.

45. Chadburn A, Cesarman E, Knowles DM: Molecular pathology of post transplantation lymphoproliferative disorders. Semin Diagn Pathol 1997;14:15-26.

46. Chen JM, Barr ML, Chadburn A, Frizzera G, Schenkel FA, Sciacca RR, Reison DS, Addonizio LJ, Rose EA, Knowles DM, Michler RE: Management of lymphoproliferative disorders after cardiac transplantation. Ann Thorac Surg 1993;56:527-538.

47. Chervu I, Karubian F, Campese V: The role of endothelial factors; cyclosporin and erythropoietin in hypertension in chronic renal failure. Curr Opin Cardiol 1992;7:776-781.

48. Chodosh J, Holder VP, Gan Y, Belgaumi A, Sample J, Sixbey J: Eradication of latent Epstein-Barr virus by hydroxyurea alters the growth-transformed cell phenotype. J Infect Dis 1998;177:1194.

49. Chucrallah AE, Crow MK, Rice LE, Rajagopalan S, Hudnall SD: Multiple myeloma after cardiac transplantation: an unusual form of post transplant lymphoproliferative disorder. Hum Pathol 1994;25:541-545.

50. Cleary ML, Sklar J: Lymphoproliferative disorders in cardiac transplant recipients are multiclonal lymphomas. Lancet 1984;8401:541-545.

51. Cleary ML, Warnke R, Sklar J: Monoclonality of lymphoproliferative lesions in cardiac-transplant recipients: clonal analysis based on immunoglobulin-gene rearrangements. N Engl J Med 1984;310:477-482.

52. Cockfield SM, Preiksaitis JK, Jewell LD, Parfrey NA: post transplant lymphoproliferative disorder in renal allograft recipients: clinical experience and risk factor analysis in a single center. Transplantation 1993;56:88-96.

53. Coffman TM, Carr DR, Yarger WE, Klotman PE: Evidence that renal prostaglandin and thromboxane production is stimulated in chronic cyclosporine nephrotoxicity. Transplantation 1987;43:282-285.

54. Cohen JI: Epstein-Barr virus lymphoproliferative disease associated with acquired immunodeficiency. Medicine 1991;70:137-160.

55. Colon R, Frazier OH, Kahan BD, Radovancevic B, Duncan JM, Lorber MI, Van Buren CT: Complications in cardiac transplant patients requiring general surgery. Surgery 1988;103:32-38.

56. Colquhoun SD, Robert ME, Shaked A, Rosenthal JT, Millis TM, Farmer DG, Jurim O, Busuttil RW: Transmission of CNS malignancy by organ transplantation. Transplantation 1994;57:970-974.

57. Costanzo-Nordin MR, O'Sullivan EV, Hubbel EA, Zucker MJ, Pifarre R, McManus BM, Winters GL, Scanlon PJ, Robinson JA: Long term followup of heart transplant recipients treated with murine anti-human mature T cell monoclonal antibody (OKT3): the Loyola experience. J Heart Lung Transplant 1989;8:288-295.

58. Costanzo MR, Beto JA, Potempa LD, Bansal VK, Heroux AL, Kao WG, Pifarre R, Johnson MR: Longitudinal effects of cyclosporine administration at 0 to 60 months after heart transplantation. Transplant Proc 1994;26:2704-2709.

59. Couetil JP, McGoldrick JP, Wallwork J, English TAH: Malignant tumors after heart transplantation. J Heart Lung Transplant 1990;9:622-626.

60. Cox KL, Lawrence-Miyasaki LS, Garcia-Kennedy R, Lennette ET, Martinez OM, Krams SM, Berquist WE, So SKS, Esquivel CO: An increased incidence of Epstein-Barr virus infection and lymphoproliferative disorder in young children on FK506 after liver transplantation. Transplantation 1995;59:524-529.

61. Davidoff A, Hebra A, Clark BJ, Tomaszewski JE, Montone KT, Ruchelli E, Lau HT: Epstein-Barr virus-associated hepatic smooth muscle neoplasm in a cardiac transplant recipient. Transplantation 1996;61:515-517.

62. Davies DR, Bittman I, Pardo J: Histopathology of calcineurin inhibitor-induced nephrotoxicity. Transplantation 2000;69:SS11-SS12.

63. Davis CL, Wood BL, Sabath DE, Joseph JS, Stehman-Breen C, Broudy VC: Interferon-α treatment of post transplant lymphoproliferative disorder in recipients of solid organ transplants. Transplantation 1998;66:1770-1779.

64. Dayton MT, Kleckner SC, Brown DK: Peptic ulcer perforation associated with steroid use. Arch Surg 1987;122:376-380.

65. de Groen PC: Cyclosporine; low density lipoprotein and cholesterol. Mayo Clin Proc 1988;63:1012.

66. Delecluse HJ, Rouault JP, French M, Dureau G, Magaud JP, Berger F: post transplant lymphoproliferative disorders with genetic abnormalities commonly found in malignant tumors. Br J Haematol 1995;89:90-97.

67. Deray G: Effects of cyclosporin on plasma renin activity, catecholamines and prostaglandins in patients with idiopathic uveitis. Am J Nephrol 1988;8:298-304.

68. DeSalvo TG, Naftel DC, Kasper EK, Rayburn BK, Leier CV, Massin EK, Cintron GB, Yancy CW, Keck S, Aaronson K, Kirklin JK, and the Cardiac Transplant Research Database: The differing hazard of lymphoma vs. other malignancies in the current era [abstract]. J Heart Lung Transplant 1998;17:70.

69. DiSesa VJ, Kirkman RL, Tilney NL, Mudge GH, Collins JJ, Cohn LH: Management of general surgical complications following cardiac transplantation. Arch Surg 1989;124:539-541.

70. Durandy A, Emilie D, Peuchmaur M, Forveille M, Clement C, Wijdenes J, Fischer A: Role of IL-6 in promoting growth of human EBV-induced B-cell tumors in severe combined immunodeficient mice. J Immunol 1994;152:5361-5367.

71. Edwards BS, Hunt SA, Fowler MB, Valantine HA, Stinson EB, Schroeder JS: Cardiac transplantation in patients with preexisting neoplastic diseases. Am J Cardiol 1990;65:501-504.

72. Eisen HJ, Hicks D, Kant JA, Montone KT, Mull R, Pigott J, Tomaszewski JE: Diagnosis of post transplantation lymphoproliferative disorder by endomyocardial biopsy in a cardiac allograft recipient. J Heart Lung Transplant 1994;13:241-245.

73. Elliott WJ, Murphy MB, Karp R: Long term preservation of renal function in hypertensive heart transplant recipients treated with enalapril and a diuretic. J Heart Lung Transplant 1991;10:373-379.

74. Emanuel DJ, Lucas KG, Mallory GB, Edwards-Brown MK, Pollock KE, Conrad PD, Robertson KA, Smith FO: Treatment of posttransplant lymphoproliferative disease in the central nervous system of a lung transplant recipient using allogeneic leukocytes. Transplantation 1997;63:1691-1694.

75. English J, Evan A, Houghton DC, Bennett WM: Cyclosporine induced acute renal dysfunction in the rat. Evidence of arteriolar vasoconstriction with preservation of tubular function. Transplantation 1987;44:135-141.

76. Epstein S, Shane E: Transplantation osteoporosis In Feldman MR: Kelsey JX (eds): Osteoporosis. New York: Academic Press, 1996, pp 947-957.

77. Euvrard S, Kanitakis J, Pouteil-Noble C, Disant F, Dureau G, Finaz D, Villaine J, Claudy A, Thivolet J: Comparative epidemiologic study of premalignant and malignant epithelial cutaneous lesions developing after kidney and heart transplantation. J Am Acad Dermatol 1995;33:222-229.

78. Fairley JW, Hunt BJ, Glover GW, Radley-Smith RC, Yacoub MH: Unusual lymphoproliferative oropharyngeal lesions in heart and heart/lung transplant recipients. J Laryngol Otol 1990;104:720-724.

79. Falkenhain ME, Cosio FG: Cyclosporine (CsA) causes progressive glomerular sclerosis (GS) and arteriolar hyalinosis (AH) in kidneys of heart (HTx) and liver (LTx) transplant recipients. J Am Soc Nephrol 1994;5:1003.

80. Falkenhain ME, Cosio FG, Sedmak DD: Progressive histologic injury in kidneys from heart and liver transplant recipients receiving cyclosporine. Transplantation 1996;62:364-370.

81. Farge D, Julien J, Amrein C, Guillemain R, Vulser C, Mihaileanu S, Dreyfus G, Carpentier A: Effect of systemic hypertension on renal function and left ventricular hypertrophy in heart transplant recipients. J Am Coll Cardiol 1990;15:1095-1101.

82. Farmer JA, Ballantyne CM, Frazier OH, Radovancevic B, Payton-Ross C, Patsch W, Morrisett JD, Gotto AM, Young JB: Lipoprotein and apolipoprotein changes after cardiac transplantation. J Am Coll Cardiol 1991;18:926.

83. Faro A, Kurland G, Michaels MG, Dickman PS, Greally PG, Spichty KJ, Noyes BB, Boas SR, Fricker FJ, Armitage JM, Zeevi A:

Interferon-alpha affects the immune response in post-transplant lymphoproliferative disorder. Am J Respir Crit Care Med 1996;153:1442–1447.

84. Fatio R, Sutsch G, Mayer K: Post-transplant lymphoproliferative disorders in cardiac transplant patients. Transplant Proc 1998; 30:1118–1120.

85. Fatio R, Sutsch G, Mayer K, Kurrer MO, Follath F, Kiowski W: Unusual course of T-cell lymphoproliferative disorder in a cardiac transplant patient. Transplant Proc 1998;30:1121.

86. Festenstein H, Garrido F: MHC antigens and malignancy. Nature 1986;322:502–503.

87. Fischer A, Blanche S, LeBidois J, Bordigoni P, Garnier JL, Niaudet P, Morinet F, LeDeist F, Fischer AM, Griscelli C: Anti-B-cell monoclonal antibodies in the treatment of severe B-cell lymphoproliferative syndrome following bone marrow and organ transplantation. N Engl J Med 1991;324:1451–1456.

88. Fischer T, Miller M, Bott-Silverman C, Lichtin A: Posttransplant lymphoproliferative disease after cardiac transplantation. Transplantation 1996;63:1687–1690.

89. Fleming RH, Jennison SH, Naunheim KS: Primary bronchogenic carcinoma in the heart transplant recipient. Ann Thorac Surg 1994;57:1300–1301.

90. Frances C, Farge D, Boisnic S: Kaposi's syndrome following transplantation. J Mal Vasc 1991;16:163–165.

91. Frank S, Muller J, Bonk C, Haroske G, Schackert HK, Schackert G: Transmission of glioblastoma multiforme through liver transplantation. Lancet 1998;352:31.

92. Frizzera G, Hanto DW, Gajl-Peczalska KJ, Rosai J, McKenna RW, Sibley RK, Holahan KP, Lindquist LL: Polymorphic diffuse B-cell hyperplasias and lymphomas in renal transplant recipients. Cancer Res 1981;41:4262–4279.

93. Fryer JP, Granger DK, Leventhal JR, Gillingham K, Najarian JS, Matas AJ: Steroid related complications in the cyclosporine era. Clin Transplant 1994;8:224–229.

94. Gall EA, Stout HA: The histological lesions in lymph nodes in infectious mononucleosis. Am J Pathol 1940;16:433–453.

95. Gao SZ, Schroeder JS, Hunt SA, Billingham ME, Valantine HA, Stinson EB: Acute myocardial infarction in cardiac transplant recipients. Am J Cardiol 1989;64:1093–1097.

96. Garcia-Delgado I, Prieto S, Gil-Fraguas L, Robles E, Rufilanchas JJ, Hawkins F: Calcitonin, etidronate, and calcidiol treatment in bone loss after cardiac transplantation. Calcif Tissue 1997; 60:155–159.

97. Garrett TJ, Chadburn A, Barr ML: Post transplantation lymphoproliferative disorders treated with cyclophosphamide-doxorubicin-vincristine-prednisone chemotherapy. Cancer 1993;72: 2782–2785.

98. Girardet RR, Rosenbloom P, DeWeese BM, Masri ZH, Attum AA, Barbie RN, Yared SF, Lusk RA, Lansing AM: Significance of asymptomatic biliary tract disease in heart transplant recipients. J Heart Lung Transplant 1989;8:391–399.

99. Goldstein DJ, Williams DL, Oz MC, Weinberg AD, Rose EA, Michler RE: De novo solid malignancies after cardiac transplantation. Ann Thorac Surg 1995;60:1783–1789.

100. Goldstein DJ, Zuech N, Sehgal V, Weinberg AD, Drusin R, Cohen D: Cyclosporine-associated end-stage nephropathy after cardiac transplantation. Transplantation 1997;63:664–668.

101. Griffiths MH, Crowe AV, Papadaki NR, Banner MH, Yacoub MH, Thompson FD, Neild GH: Cyclosporin nephrotoxicity in heart and lung transplant patients. Q J Med 1996;89:751–763.

102. Grundy SM: National cholesterol education program. Second report of the expert panel on detection, evaluation and treatment of high blood cholesterol in adults. Circulation 1994;89:1329.

103. Guettier C, Hamilton-Dutoit S, Guillemain R, Farge D, Amrein C, Vulser C, Hofman P, Carpentier A, Diebold J: Primary gastrointestinal malignant lymphomas associated with Epstein-Barr after heart transplantation. Histopathology 1992;20:21–28.

104. Hague K, Catalano P, Rothschild M, Strauchen J, Fyfe B: Post transplant lymphoproliferative disease presenting as sudden respiratory arrest in a three year old child. Ann Otol Rhinol Laryngol 1997;106:244–247.

105. Hanasono MM, Kamel OW, Chang PP, Rizeq MN, Billingham ME, van de Rijn M: Detection of Epstein-Barr virus in cardiac biopsies of heart transplant patients with lymphoproliferative disorders. Transplantation 1995;60:471–473.

106. Hanson MN, Morrison VA, Peterson BA, Stieglbauer KT, Kubic VL, McCormick SR, McGlennen RC, Manivel JC, Brunning RD, Litz CE: Posttransplant T-cell lymphoproliferative disorders—an aggressive, late complication of solid-organ transplantation. Blood 1996;88:3626–3633.

107. Hausen B, Albes JM, Rohde R, Demertzis S, Mugge A, Schafers HJ: Tricuspid valve regurgitation attributable to endomyocardial biopsies and rejection in heart transplantation. Ann Thorac Surg 1995;59:1134–1140.

108. Hemmens VJ, Moore DE: Photochemical sensitization by azathioprine and its metabolites: II. Azathioprine and nitroimidazole metabolites. Photochem Photobiol 1986;43:257–262.

109. Henry DA, Johnston A, Dobson A, Duggan J: Fatal peptic ulcer complications and the use of non-steroidal anti-inflammatory drugs, aspirin, and corticosteroids. BMJ 1987;295:1227–1229.

110. Hirsch MS, Proffitt MR, Black PH: Autoimmunity, oncornaviruses and lymphomagenesis. Contemp Top Immunobiol 1997;6:209–227.

111. Ho M, Breinig MK, Dummer JS, Miller G, Atchison RW, Andiman W, Starzl TE, Eastman R, Griffith BP, Hardesty RL: Epstein-Barr, virus infections and DNA hybridization studies in posttransplantation lymphoma and lymphoproliferative lesions: the role of primary infection. J Infect Dis 1985;152:876.

112. Hosenpud JD, Bennett LE, Keck BM, Fiol B, Boucek MM, Novick RJ: The registry of the international society for heart and lung transplantation: sixteenth official report—1999. J Heart Lung Transplant 1999;18:611–626.

113. Huddleston CB, Rosenbloom M, Goldstein JA, Pasque MK: Biopsy-induced tricuspid regurgitation after cardiac transplantation. Ann Thorac Surg 1994;57:832–837.

114. Ippoliti G, Martinelli L, Lorenzutti F, Incardona S, Negri M, Balduzzi P, Rovati B, Ascari E, Vigano M: Posttransplant lymphoproliferative disease after heart transplantation on sandimmune therapy: treatment with interferon alfa-2b and intravenous immunoglobulin. Transplant Proc 1994;26:2660–2661.

115. Jenkins GH, Singer DR: Hypertension in thoracic transplant recipients. J Hum Hyperten 1998;12:813–823.

116. Johns MR: Transplant coronary disease: nonimmunologic risk factors. J Heart Lung Transplant 1992;11:S124.

117. Jonas S, Bechstein WO, Rayes N, Neuhaus R, Guckelberger O, Tullius SG, Schmidt G, Riess H, Lobeck H, Vogl T, Neuhaus P: Posttransplant malignancy and newer immunosuppressive protocols after liver transplantation. Transplant Proc 1996;28:3246–3247.

118. Jones D, Ballestas ME, Kaye KM, Gulizia JM, Winders GL, Fletcher J, Scadden DT, Aster JC: Primary-effusion lymphoma and Kaposi's sarcoma in a cardiac transplant recipient. N Engl J Med 1998;339:444–449.

119. Jowell PS, Epstein S, Fallon MD, Reinhardt TA, Ismail F: 1,25 Dihydroxyvitamin D3 modulates glucocorticoid induced alteration in serum bone Gla protein and bone histomorphometry. Endocrinology 1987;120:531–536.

120. Julien J: Cyclosporin induced stimulation of the renin-angiotensin system after liver and heart transplantation. Transplantation 1993;56:885–891.

121. Kahan BD, VanBuren CT, Flechners S, Jarowenko M, Yasummura T, Rogers AJ, Yoshimura N, LeGrue S, Drath D, Kerman RH: Clinical and experimental studies using cyclosporine. Surgery 1985;97:125.

122. Kauffman HM, McBride MA, Delmonico FL: First report of the united network for organ sharing transplant tumor registry: donors with a history of cancer. Transplantation 2000;70:1747–1751.

123. Kaye D, Thompson J, Jennings G, Esler M: Cyclosporine therapy after cardiac transplantation causes hypertension and renal vasoconstriction without sympathetic activation. Circulation 1993;88:1101–1109.

124. Kedda MA, Margolius L, Kew MC, Swanepoel C, Pearson D: Kaposi's sarcoma associated herpesvirus in Kaposi's sarcoma occurring in immunosuppressed renal transplant recipients. Clin Transplant 1996;10:429–431.

125. Kemnitz J, Cremer J, Gebel M, Uysal A, Haverich A, Georgii A: T-cell lymphoma after heart transplantation. Am J Clin Pathol 1990;94:95–101.

126. Kirk AJB, Omar I, Bateman DN: Cyclosporine associated hypertension in cardiopulmonary transplantation. Transplantation 1989;48:428–430.

127. Kirklin JK, Holm A, Aldrete JS, White C, Bourge RC: Gastrointestinal complications after cardiac transplantation. Ann Surg 1989;211:538–542.

128. Kirwan PD: Giant mitochondria and multiple cilia in proximal convoluted tubules of renal transplant patients receiving cyclosporine-A immunosuppression. Micron 1982;13:353–354.

129. Klaushofer K, Hoffmann O, Stewart PJ, Czerwenka E, Koller K, Peterlik M, Stern PH: Cyclosporine A inhibits bone resorption in cultured neonatal mouse calvaria. J Pharmacol Exp Ther 1987;243:584–590.

130. Klein RG, Arnaud SB, Gallagher JC, DeLuca HF, Riggs BL: Intestinal calcium absorption in exogenous hypercortisolism, role of 25-hydroxyvitamin D and corticosteroid dose. J Clin Invest 1977;60:253–259.

131. Kleinman GM, Hochberg FH, Richardson EP: Systemic metastases of medulloblastoma: report of two cases and review of the literature. Cancer 1981;48:2296–309.

132. Knowles DM, Cesarman E, Chadburn A, Frizzera G, Chen J, Rose EA, Michler RE: Correlative morphologic and molecular genetic analysis demonstrates three distinct categories of post transplantation lymphoproliferative disorders. Blood 1995; 85:552–565.

133. Kobashigawa J, Kasiake BL: Hyperlipidemia in solid organ transplantation. Transplantation 1997;63:331–338.

134. Kobashigawa J, Katznelson S, Laks H, Johnson JA, Yeatman L, Wang XM, Chia D, Terasaki PI, Sabad A, Cogert GA: Effect of pravastatin on outcomes after cardiac transplantation. N Engl J Med 1995;333:621.

135. Koerner MM, Tenderich G, Minami K, Mannebach H, Koertke H, zuKnyphausen E, El-Banayosy A, Baller D, Kleesiek K, Gleichmann U, Meyer H, Koerfer R: Results of heart transplantation in patients with preexisting malignancies. Am J Cardiol 1997;79:988–991.

136. Kon U, Sugiura M, Inagami T, Haruie BR, Ichikawa I, Hoover RC: Role of endothelin in cyclosporine-induced glomerular dysfunction. Kidney Int 1990;37:1487–1491.

137. Koneru B, Selby R, OHair DP, Tzakis A, Hakala TR, Starzl TE: Nonobstructing colonic dilation and colon perforations following renal transplantation. Arch Surg 1990;125:610.

138. Kotowicz MA, Hall S, Hunder GC, Cedel SL, Mann KG, Riggs BL: Relationship of glucocorticoid dosage to serum bone Gla-protein concentration in patients with rheumatologic disorders. Arthritis Rheum 1990;33:1487–1492.

139. Kowal-Vern A, Swinnen L, Pyle J, Radvany R, Dizikes G, Michalov M, Molnar Z: Characterization of post cardiac transplant lymphomas: histology, immunophenotyping, immunohistochemistry, and gene rearrangement. Arch Pathol Lab Med 1996;120:41–48.

140. Krane SM, Holick MF: Metabolic bone disease. In: Fauci AS, Braunwald E, Isselbacher KJ, Wilson JD, Martin JB, Kasper DL, Hauser SL, Longo DL (eds): Harrison's Principles of Internal Medicine. New York: McGraw Hill, 1998, pp 2247–2259.

141. Kumano K, Chen J, He M, Endo T, Masaki Y: Role of endothelin in FK 506-induced renal hypoperfusion in rats. Transplant Proc 1995;17:550–553.

142. Kuster GM, Drexel H, Bleisch JA, Rentsch K, Pei P, Binswanger U, Amann FW: Relation of cyclosporine blood levels to adverse effects on lipoproteins. Transplantation 1994;57:1479–1483.

143. Lamb FS, Webb RC: Cyclosporine augments reactivity of isolated blood vessels. Life Sci 1987;40:2571–2578.

144. Lampros TD, Cobanoglu A, Parker F, Ratkovec R, Norman DJ, Hershberger R: Squamous and basal cell carcinoma in heart transplant recipients. J Heart Lung Transplant 1998;17:586–591.

145. Leblond V, Davi F, Charlotte F, Dorent R, Bitker MO, Sutton L, Gandjbakhch I, Binet JL, Raphael M: Post transplant lymphoproliferative disorders not associated with Epstein-Barr virus: a distinct entity? J Clin Oncol 1998;16:2052–2059.

146. Leblond V, Sutton L, Dorent R, Davi F, Bitker MO, Gabarre J, Charlotte F, Ghoussoub JJ, Fourcade C, Fischer A: Lymphoproliferative disorders after organ transplantation: a report of 24 cases observed in a single center. J Clin Oncol 1995;13:961–968.

147. Lee A, Mull R, Keenan GF, Callegari PE, Dalinka MK, Eisen HJ, Mancini DM, DiSesa VJ, Attie MF: Osteoporosis and bone morbidity in cardiac transplant recipients. Am J Med 1994; 96:35–41.

148. Levine TB, Olivari MT, Cohn JN: Effects of orthotopic heart transplantation on sympathetic control mechanisms in congestive heart failure. Am J Med 1986;58:1035–1040.

149. Lewis RM, VanBuren CT, Radovancevic B, Frazier OH, Janney RP, Powers PL, Golden DL, Giannakis JG, Macris MP, Kerman RH: Impact of long term cyclosporine immunosuppressive therapy in native kidneys versus renal allografts: serial renal function in heart and kidney transplant recipients. J Heart Lung Transplant 1991;10:63–70.

150. Lien YH, Schroter GPJ, Weil R, Robinson WA: Complete remission and possible immune tolerance after multidrug combination chemotherapy for cyclosporine-related lymphoma in a renal transplant patient with acute pancreatitis. Transplantation 1991;52:739–742.

151. Lin JC, Smith MC, Pagano JS: Comparative efficacy and selectivity of some nucleoside analogs against Epstein-Barr virus. Antimicrob Agents Chemother 1985;27:971.

152. Lucini D, Milani RV, Ventura HO, Mehra MR, Messerli FH, Murgo JP, Regenstein F, Copley B, Malliani A, Pagani M: Cyclosporine-induced hypertension: evidence for maintained baroreflex circulatory control. J Heart Lung Transplant 1997;16:615–620.

153. Lukert BP: Glucocorticoid-induced osteoporosis. In Feldman F, Marcus R, Kelsey J (eds): Osteoporosis. New York: Academic Press, 1996, pp 801–820.

154. Macdonald AS: Management strategies for nephrotoxicity. Transplantation 2000;S69:SS31–SS36.

155. Marsen TA, Weber F, Egink G, Suckau G, Baldamus CA: Cyclosporine A induces prepro endothelin-1 gene transcription in human endothelial cells. Eur J Pharmacol 1999;379:97–106.

156. McKoy RC, Uretsky BF, Kormos R, Hardesty RI, Griffith BP, Salerni R: Left ventricular hypertrophy in cyclosporin induced systemic hypertension after cardiac transplantation. Am J Cardiol 1988;62:1140–1142.

157. Merrell SW, Ames SA, Nelson EW, Renlund DG, Karwande SV, Burton NA, Sullivan JJ, Jones KW, Gay WA Jr: Major abdominal complications following cardiac transplantation. Arch Surg 1989;124:889–894.

158. Messer J, Reitman D, Sacks HS, Smith H, Chalmers TC: Association of adrenocorticoid therapy and peptic ulcer disease. N Engl J Med 1983;309:21–24.

159. Meyding-Lamade U, Krieger D, Schnabel P: Cerebral metastases of an allogenic renal cell carcinoma in a heart recipient without renal cell carcinoma. J Neurol 1996; 243:425–427.

160. Meys E, Terreaux-Duvert F, Beaume-Six T, Dureau G, Meunier PJ: Bone loss after cardiac transplantation: effects of calcium, calcidiol and monofluorophosphate. Osteoporos Int 1993; 3:329–332.

161. Mihatsch MJ, Basler V, Curschellas E, Kyo M, Duerig M, Huser B, Landmann J, Thiel G: Giant mitochondria in "zero-hour" transplant biopsies. Ultrastruct Pathol 1992;16:277–282.

162. Mihatsch MJ, Ryffel B, Gudat F: The differential diagnosis between rejection and cyclosporine toxicity. Kidney Int 1995;48:S63–S69.

163. Mihatsch MJ, Thiel G, Ryffel B: Histopathology of cyclosporine nephrotoxicity. Transplant Proc 1988;20(suppl 3):759–771.

164. Miyamoto Y, Curtiss EI, Kormos RL, Armitage JM, Hardesty RL, Griffith BP: Bradyarrhythmia after heart transplantation: incidence, time course, and outcome. Circulation 1990;82(suppl):IV-313–IV-317.

165. Morales JM, Rodriguez-Paternina E, Araque A, Andres A, Hernandez E, Ruilope LM, Rodicio JL: Long-term protective effect of a calcium antagonist on renal function in hypertensive renal transplant patients on cyclosporine therapy: a 5 year prospective randomized study. Transplant Proc 1994;26:2598–2599.

166. Morgan BJ, Lyson T, Scherrer U, Victor RG: Cyclosporin causes sympathetically mediated elevations in arterial pressure in rats. Hypertension 1991;18:458–466.

167. Morse DL, Pickard LK, Guzewich JJ, Devine BD, Shayegani M: Development of a malignant tumor in a liver transplant graft procured from donor with a cerebral neoplasm. Transplantation 1990;50:875–877.

168. Moruzumi K, Gudat F, Thiel G: Is cyclosporine associated glomerulopathy a new glomerular lesion in renal allografts using CSA? 14th International Congress of the Transplantation Society, 1992.

169. Movsowitz C, Epstein S, Fallon M, Ismail F, Thomas S: Cyclosporin A in vivo produces severe osteopenia in the rat: effect of dose and duration of administration. Endocrinology 1988;123:2571–2577.

170. Muchmore JS, Cooper DK, Ye Y, Schlegel VT, Pribil A, Zuhdi N: Prevention of loss of vertebral bone density in heart transplant patients. J Heart Lung Transplant 1992;11:959–963.

171. Muchmore JS, Cooper DK, Ye Y, Schlegel VT, Zuhdi N: Loss of vertebral bone density in heart transplant patients. Transplant Proc 1991;23:1184–1185.

172. Murray BM, Paller MS, Ferris TF: Effect of cyclosporine on renal hemodynamics in conscious rats. Kidney Int 1985;28:767–774.

173. Myers BD, Ross J, Newton L, Luetscher J, Perlroth M: Cyclosporine-associated chronic nephropathy. N Engl J Med 1984;311:699–705.

174. Myers BD, Sibley R, Newton L, Tomlanovich SJ, Boshkos C, Stinson E, Luetscher JA, Whitney DJ, Krasny D, Coplon NS: The long term course of cyclosporine associated chronic nephropathy. Kidney Int 1988;33:590–600.

175. Nalesnik MA, Jaffe R, Starzl TE, Demetris AJ, Porter K, Burnham JA, Makowka L, Ho M, Locker J: The pathology of posttransplant lymphoproliferative disorders occurring in the setting of cyclosporine A-prednisone immunosuppression. Am J Pathol 1988;133:173–192.

176. Nalesnik MA, Rao AS, Furukawa H, Pham SM, Zeevi A, Fung JJ, Klein G, Gritsch HA, Elder E, Whiteside TL, Starzl TE: Autologous lymphokine-activated killer cell therapy of Epstein-Barr virus-positive and -negative lymphoproliferative disorders arising in organ transplant recipients. Transplantattion 1997;63:1200–1205.

177. Negri AL, Perrone S, Gallo R, Bogado CE, Zanchetta JR: Osteoporosis following heart transplantation. Transplant Proc 1996;28:3321–3324.

178. OBrien S, Bernert RA, Logan JL, Lien YH: Remission of posttransplant lymphoproliferative disorder after interferon alpha therapy. J Am Soc Nephrol 1997;8:1483–1490.

179. Olivari MT, Antolick A, Kaye MP, Jamieson SW, Ring WS: Heart transplantation in elderly patients. J Heart Lung Transplant 1988;7:258–264.

180. Olivari MT, Antolick A, Ring WS: Arterial hypertension in heart transplant recipients treated with triple-drug immunosuppressive therapy. J Heart Lung Transplant 1989;8:34–39.

181. Olyaei AJ, deMattos AM, Bennett WM: A practical guide to the management of hypertension in renal transplant recipients. Drugs 1999;58:1011–1027.

182. Ong AC: Effect of cyclosporin A on endothelin synthesis by cultured human renal cortical epithelial cells. Transplantation 1993;8:748–753.

183. Ong ACM, Fine LG: Tubular-derived growth factors and cytokines in the pathogenesis of tubulointerstitial fibrosis; implications for human renal disease progression. Am J Kidney Dis 1994;23:205–209.

184. Ong CS, Keogh AM, Kossard S, Macdonald PS, Spratt PM: Skin cancer in Australian heart transplant recipients. J Am Acad Dermatol 1999;40:27–34.

185. Opelz G: Are post transplant lymphomas inevitable? Nephrol Dial Transplant 1996;11:1952–1955.

186. Ozdogan E, Banner N, Fitzgerald M, Musumeci F, Khaghani A, Yacoub M: Factors influencing the development of hypertension after heart transplantation: J Heart Lung Transplant 1990;9:548–553.

187. Papadopoulos EB, Ladanyi M, Emanuel D, Mackinnon S, Boulad F, Carabasi MH, Castro-Malaspina H, Childs BH, Gillio AP, Small TN: Infusion of donor leukocytes to treat Epstein-Barr virus-associated lymphoproliferative disorders after allogeneic bone marrow transplantation. N Engl J Med 1994;330:1185–1191.

188. Park JW, Vermeltfoort M, Braun P, May E, Merz M: Regression of transplant coronary artery disease during chronic HELP therapy. A case study. Atherosclerosis 1995;115:1.

189. Pasquier B, Pasquier D, N'Golet A, Panh MH, Couetil J: Extraneural metastases of astrocytomas and glioblastomas: clinicopathologic study of two cases and review of literature. Cancer 1980;45:112–125.

190. Pattison JM, Petersen J, Kuo P, Valantine V, Robbins RC, Theodore J: The incidence of renal failure in one hundred consecutive

191. Paya CV, Fung JJ, Nalesnik MA, Kieff E, Green M, Gores G, Habermann TM, Wiesner RH, Swinnen LJ, Woodle ES, Bromberg JS: Epstein-Barr virus induced post transplant lymphoproliferative disorders. Transplantation 1999;68:1517–1525.

192. Penn I: Cancers of the anogenital region in renal transplant recipients. Cancer 1986;58:611–616.

193. Penn I: Transmission of cancer with donor organs. Transplant Proc 1988;20:739–740.

194. Penn I: The effect of renal transplantation in patients with a history of curative cancer therapy. In Stewart W (ed): Cellular Immune Mechanisms and Tumor Dormancy. Boca Raton, FL: CRC Press, 1992.

195. Penn I: The effect of immunosuppression on preexisting cancers. Transplantation 1993;55:742–747.

196. Penn I: Sarcomas in organ allograft recipients. Transplantation 1995;60:1485–1491.

197. Penn I: Malignant neoplasia in the immunocompromised patient. In Cooper DKC, Miller LW, Pattersen GA (eds): The Transplantation and Replacement of Thoracic Organs. Hingham, MA: Kluwer Academic, 1996.

198. Penn I: Neoplastic complications of organ transplantation. In Ginns LC, Cosimi AB, Morris PJ (eds): Transplantation. Malden, MA: Blackwell Science, 1999.

199. Pham SM, Kormos RL, Hattler BG, Kawai A, Tsamandas AC, Demetris AJ, Murali S, Fricker FJ, Chang HC, Jain AB, Starzl TE, Hardesty RI, Griffith BP: A prospective trial of tacrolimus (FK506) in clinical heart transplantation: intermediate term results. J Thorac Cardiovasc Surg 1996;111:762–764.

200. Pham SM, Kormos RL, Landreneau RJ: Solid tumors after heart transplantation: lethality of lung cancer. Ann Thorac Surg 1995;60:1623–1626.

201. Porayko MK, Textor SC, Krom RA, Hay JE, Gores GJ, Richards TM, Crotty PH, Beaver SJ, Steers JL, Wiesner RH: Nephrotoxic effects of primary immunosuppression with FK 506 and cyclosporine regimens after liver transplantation. Transplant Proc 1994;69:105–111.

202. Porreco R, Penn I, Droegemueller W: Gynecologic malignancies in immunosuppressed organ homograft recipients. Obstet Gynecol 1975;45:359–364.

203. Preiksaitis JK, Cockfield SM: Epstein Barr virus and lymphoproliferative disorders after transplantation. In Raleigh BLP (ed): Transplant Infections. Philadelphia: Lippincott-Raven, 1998.

204. Prummel MF, Wiersinga WM, Lips P, Sanders GTP, Sauerwein HP: The course of biochemical parameters of bone turnover during treatment with corticosteroids. J Clin Endocrin 1991;72:382–386.

205. Quereda C, Sabater J, Villafruela J, Revalderia JG, Marcen R: Urinary thromboxane B2 and cyclic AMP in cyclosporine-A treated kidney transplantation. Transplant Proc 1994;26:2604–2605.

206. Raghavan C, Maloney JD, Nitta J, Lowry RW, Saliba WI, Cocanougher B, Zhu WX, Young JB: Long-term followup of heart transplant recipients requiring permanent pacemakers. J Heart Lung Transplant 1995;14:1081–1089.

207. Raymond E, Tricottet V, Samuel D, Reynes M, Bismuth H, Misset JL: Epstein Barr virus related lymphoproliferative disorders treated with cyclophosphamide doxorubicin vincristine prednisone chemotherapy. Cancer 1995;72:1344.

208. Reeves RA, Shapiro AP, Thompson ME, Johnsen AM: Loss of nocturnal decline in blood pressure after cardiac transplantation. Circulation 1986;73:401–408.

209. Renard TH, Andrews WS, Foster ME: Relationship between OKT3 administration, EBV seroconversion, and the lymphoproliferative syndrome in pediatric liver transplant recipients. Transplant Proc 1991;23:1473–1476.

210. Rich GM, Mudge GH, Laffel GL, LeBoff MS: Cyclosporine A and prednisone-associated osteoporosis in heart transplant recipients. J Heart Lung Transplant 1992;11:950–958.

211. Roenigk K, Roenigk H: Dermatologic Surgery Principles and Practice. New York: Marcel Dekker, 1996.

212. Rooney CM, Smith CA, Ng CYC, Loftin S, Li C, Krance RA, Brenner MK, Heslop HE: Use of gene modified virus specific T

[at top of column:] heart lung transplant recipients. Am J Kidney Dis 1995; 26:643–648.

lymphocytes to control Epstein Barr virus related lymphoproliferation. Lancet 1995;345:9–13.

213. Rowe DT, Qu L, Reyes J, Jabbour N, Yunis E, Putnam P, Todo S, Green M: Use of quantitative competitive PCR to measure Epstein Barr virus genome load in the peripheral blood of pediatric transplant patients with lymphoproliferative disorders. J Clin Microbiol 1997;35:1612–1615.

214. Ruiz JC, Cotorruelo JG, Tudela V, Ullate PG, Val-Bernal F, deFrancisco AL, Zubimendi JA, Prieto M, Canga E, Arias M: Transmission of glioblastoma multiforme to two kidney transplant recipients from the same donor in the absence of ventricular shunt. Transplantation 1993;55:682–683.

215. Sambrook PN, Birmingham J, Kempler S, Kelly PJ, Pocock N, Eisman JA: Prevention of corticosteroid osteoporosis; a comparison of calcium, calcitriol and calcitonin. N Engl J Med 1993;328:52.

216. Sambrook PN, Kelly PJ, Keogh AM, Macdonald P, Spratt P, Freund J, Eisman JA: Bone loss after heort transplantation: a prospective study. J Heart Lung Transplant 1994;13:116–120.

217. Sander M, Lyson T, Thomas S, Victor RG: Renal hemodynamics, urinary eicosanoids, and endothelin after liver transplantation. Am J Hypertens 1996;9:1215–1385.

218. Savage P, Waxman A: Post transplantation lymphoproliferative disese. Q J Med 1997;90:497–503.

219. Scantlebury VP, Shapiro R, Tzakis A, Jordan ML, Vivas C, Ellis D, Gilboa N, Hopp L, Irish W, Mitchell S: Pediatric kidney transplantation at the University of Pittsburgh. Transplant Proc 1994;26:46–47.

220. Scherrer U, Vissing SF, Morgan BJ, Rollins JA, Tindall RS, Ring S, Hanson P, Mohanty PK, Victor RG: Cyclosporine induced sympathetic activation and hypertension after heart transplantation. N Engl J Med 1990;323:693–699.

221. Schimmer BP, Parker KL: Adrenocorticotropic hormone; adrenocortical steroids and their synthetic analogs; inhibitors of the synthesis and actions of adrenocortical hormones. *In* Hardman JG, Limbird LE, Molinoff PB, Ruddon RW, Gilman AG (eds): Goodman & Gilman's The Pharmacologic Basis of Therapeutics. New York: McGraw-Hill, 1996, pp 1459–1485.

222. Schlosberg M, Movsowitz C, Epstein S, Ismail F, Fallon M, Thomas S: The effect of cyclosporin A administration and its withdrawal on bone mineral metabolism in the rat. Endocrinology 1989;124:2179–2185.

223. Sehested J: Effects of acute administration of cyclosporin on levels of cardiovascular hormones in heart transplant recipients. Am J Cardiol 1993;72:484–486.

224. Sehgal V, Radhakrishan J, Appel GB, Valeri A, Cohen DJ: Progressive renal insufficiency following cardiac transplantation: cyclosporine, lipids and hypertension. Am J Kidney Dis 1995;26:193–201.

225. Selleslag DL, Boongaerts MA, Daenen W, De Wolf-Peeters C, Janssens L, Vanhaecke J: Occurrence of lymphoproliferative disorders in heart transplant recipients. Acta Clin Belg 1991; 46:68–74.

226. Shane E, Rivas M, McMahon DJ: Bone loss and turnover after cardiac transplantation. J Clin Endocrinol 1997;82:1497–1506.

227. Shane E, Rivas MC, Silverberg SJ, Kim TS, Staron RB, Bilezikian JP: Osteoporosis and bone morbidity in cardiac transplant recipients. Am J Med 1993;94:257–264.

228. Sharma S, Reddy V, Ott G, Sheppard B, Ratkovec R, Hershberger R, Norman D, Hosenpub J, Cobanoglu A: Gastrointestinal complications after orthotopic cardiac transplantation. Eur J Cardiothorac Surg 1996;10:616–620.

229. Shimokawa H, Lam JYT, Chesebro JH, Bowie EJW, Vanhoutte PM: Effects of dietary supplementation with cod-liver oil on endothelium-dependent response in porcine coronary arteries. Circulation 1987;76:898–905.

230. Shulman H, Striker G, Deeg HJ, Kennedy M, Storb R, Thomas ED: Nephrotoxicity of cyclosporine A after allogeneic marrow transplantation. N Engl J Med 1981;305:1392–1395.

231. Singer DR, Markandu ND, Buckley MG, Miller MA, Sagnella GA, Lachno DR, Cappuccio FP, Murday A, Yacoub MH, MacGregor GA: Blood pressure and endocrine responses to changes in dietary sodium intake following cardiac transplantation. Circulation 1994;89:1153–1189.

232. Singer DR, Jenkins GH: Hypertension in transplant recipients. J Hum Hypertens 1996;10:395–402.

233. Solez K, Racusen LC, Marcussen N, Slatnik I, Keown P, Burdick JF, Olsen S: Morphology of ischemic acute renal failure, normal function and cyclosporine toxicity in cyclosporine-treated renal allograft recipients. Kidney Int 1993;43:1058–1067.

234. Spiro IJ, Yandell DW, Li C, Saini S, Ferry J, Powelson J, Katkov WN, Cosimi AB: Brief report: lymphoma of donor origin occurring in the porta hepatis of a transplanted liver. N Engl J Med 1993;329:27.

235. Stahl RD, Karwande SV, Olsen SL, Taylor DO, Hawkins JA, Renlund DG: Tricuspid valve dysfunction in the transplanted heart. Ann Thorac Surg 1995;59:477–480.

236. Starling RC, Cody RJ: Cardiac transplant hypertension. J Heart Lung Transplant 1990;65:106–111.

237. Starzl TE, Nalesnik MA, Porter B: Reversibility of lymphomas and lymphoproliferative lesions developing under cyclosporin-steroid therapy. Lancet 1984;1:583–587.

238. Steck TB, Costanzo-Nordin MR, Keshavarzian A: Prevalence and management of cholelithiasis in heart transplant patients. J Heart Lung Transplant 1991;10:1029–1032.

239. Steed DL, Brown B, Reilly JJ, Peitzman AB, Griffith BP, Hardesty RL, Webster MW: General surgical complications in heart and heart-lung transplantation. Surgery 1985;98:739–744.

240. Stein CM, He H, Pincus T, Wood AJ: Cyclosporine impairs vasodilatation without increased sympathetic activity in humans. Hypertension 1995;26:705–710.

241. Stephan JL, LeDeist F, Blanche S, LeBidois J, Peuchmaur M, Lellouch-Tubiana A, Hirn M, Griscelli C, Fischer A: Treatment of central nervous system B lymphoproliferative syndrome by local infusion of B cell-specific monoclonal antibody. Transplantation 1992;54:246–249.

242. Stephens J, Goldstein R, Crippin J, Husberg B, Holman M, Gonwa TA, Klintmalm G: Effects of orthotopic liver transplantation and immunosuppression on inflammatory bowel disease in primary sclerosing cholangitis patients. Transplant Proc 1993;25:1122–1123.

243. Sterioff S, Orringer MB, Cameron JL: Colon perforations associated with steroid therapy. Surgery 1974;75:56–58.

244. Stillman IE, Andoh TF, Burdmann EA, Bennett WM, Rosen S: FK506 nephrotoxicity: morphologic and physiologic characterization of a rat model. Lab Invest 1995;73:794–803.

245. Stylianos S, Chen MHM, Treat MR, LoGerfo P, Rose EA: Colonic lymphoma as a cause of massive bleeding in a cardiac transplant recipient. J Cardiovasc Surg 1990;31:315–317.

246. Sundararajan V, Cooper DKC, Muchmore J, Liguori C, Zuhdi N, Novizky D, Chen PN, Bourne DW, Corder CN: Interaction of cyclosporine and probucol in heart transplant patients. Transplant Proc 1991;23:2028.

247. Suzuku T, Furusato M, Takasaki S: Giant mitochondria in the epithelial cells of the proximal convoluted tubules of diseased human kidneys. Lab Invest 1975;33:578–590.

248. Swenson JM, Frickery FJ, Armitage JM: Immunosuppression switch in pediatric heart transplant recipients: cyclosporine to FK506. J Am Coll Cardiol 1995;25:1183–1188.

249. Swinnen L, Mullen GM, Carr TJ, Costanzo MR, Fisher RI: Aggressive treatment for postcardiac transplant lymphoproliferation. Blood 1995;86:3333–3340.

250. Swinnen LJ, Costanzo-Nordin MR, Fisher SG, O'Sullivan EJ, Johnson MR, Heroux AL, Dizikes GJ, Pifarre R, Fisher RJ: Increased incidence of lymphoproliferative disorder after immunosuppression with the monoclonal antibody OKT3 in cardiac transplant recipients. N Engl J Med 1990;323:1723–1728.

251. Taylor DO, Barr ML, Radovancevic B, Renlund DG, Mentzer RM, Smart FW, Tolman DE, Frazier OH, Young JB, VanVeldhuisen P: A randomized, multicenter comparison of tacrolimus and cyclosporine immunosuppressive regimens in cardiac transplantation: decreased hyperlipidemia and hypertension with tacrolimus. J Heart Lung Transplant 1999;18:336–345.

252. Taylor DO, Thompson JA, Hastillow A, Barnhart G, Rider S, Lower RR, Hess ML: Hyperlipidemia after clinical heart transplantation. J Heart Lung Transplant 1989;8:209.

253. Textor SC, Wilson DJ, Lerman A, Romero JC, Burnett JC, Wiesner R, Dickson ER, Krom RAA: Renal hemodynamics, urinary eicosanoids, and endothelin after liver transplantation. Transplantation 1992;54:74–80.

254. Thompson ME, Shapiro AP, Johnsen AM: New onset hypertension following cardiac transplantation: a preliminary report and analysis. Transplant Proc 1983;2573–2577.

255. Thompson ME, Shapiro AP, Johnsen AM, Itzkoff JM, Hardesty RL, Griffith BP, Bahnson HT, McDonald RH, Hastillo A, Hess M: The contrasting effects of cyclosporine A and azathioprine on arterial blood pressure and renal function following cardiac transplantation. Int J Cardiol 1986;11:219–229.

256. Tindle BH, Parker JW, Lukes RJ: "Reed-Sternberg cells" in infectious mononucleosis. Am J Clin Pathol 1972;58:607–617.

257. Tucker PA, Jin BS, Gaos CM, Radovancevic B, Frazier OH, Wilansky S: Flail tricuspid leaflet after multiple biopsies following orthotopic heart transplantation: echocardiographic and hemodynamic correlation. J Heart Lung Transplant 1994;13:466–472.

258. VanBuren CT, Burke JF, Lewis RM: Renal function in patients receiving long-term cyclosporine therapy. J Am Soc Nephrol 1994;4:17–22.

259. VanCleemput J, Daenen W, Geusens P, Dequeker P, VanDeWerf F, Vanhaecke J: Calcitonin, etidronate, and calcidiol treatment in bone loss after cardiac transplantation. Transplantation 1996; 61:1495–1499.

260. VanCleemput J, Daenen W, Nijs J, Geusens P, Dequeker J, Vanhacke J: Timing and quantification of bone loss in cardiac transplant recipients. Transplant Int 1995;8:196–200.

261. vanGelder T, Balk AHMM, Zietse R, Hesse C, Mochtar B, Weimer W: Survival of heart transplant recipients with cyclosporine-induced renal insufficiency. Transplant Proc 1998;30:1122–1123.

262. vanGorp J, Doomewaard H, Verdonck LF, Kopping C, Vos PF, vandenTweel JG: Posttransplant T-cell lymphoma. Cancer 1994;73:3064–3072.

263. Ventura HO, Mehra MR, Stapleton DD, Smart FW: Cyclosporine induced hypertension in cardiac transplantation. Med Clin North Am 1997;81:1347–1357.

264. Ventura HO, Milani RV, Lavie CJ, Smart FW, Stapleton DD, Toups TS, Price HL: Cyclosporine-induced hypertension. Efficacy of omega-3 fatty acids in patients after cardiac transplantation. Circulation 1993;88:II-281–II-285.

265. Vincenti F, Danovitch GM, Neylan JF, Steiner RW, Everson MP, Gaston RS: Pentoxifylline does not prevent the cytokine-induced first dose reaction following OKT3—a randomized, double-blind placebo-controlled study. Transplantation 1996;61:573.

266. vonSchacky C, Fischer S, Weber PC: Long term effects of dietary marine ω-3 fatty acids upon plasma and cellular lipids, platelet function and eicosanoid formation in humans. J Clin Invest 1985;76:1626–1631.

267. Walker RC, Marshall WF, Strickler JG, Wiesner RH, Velosa JA, Habermann TM, McGregor CG, Paya CV: Pretransplantation assessment of the risk of lymphoproliferative disorder. Clin Infect Dis 1995;20:1346–1353.

268. Walker RC, Paya CV, Marshall WF, Strickler JG, Wiesner RH, Velosa JA, Habermann TM, Daly RC, McGregory CG: Pretransplantation seronegataive Epstein-Barr virus status is the primary risk factor for posttransplantation lymphoproliferative disorder in adult heart, lung and other solid organ transplantation. J Heart Lung Transplant 1995;14:214–221.

269. Watschinger B, Sayegh MH: Endothelin in organ transplantation. Am J Kidney Dis 1996;27:151–161.

270. Wenke K, Thiery J, Meiser B, Arndtz N, Seidel D, Reichart B: Long term simvastatin therapy for hypercholesterolemia in heart transplant patients. Z Kardiol 1995;84:130.

271. Wenting GJ, van den Meiracker AH, Simoons ML, Bos E, Ritsema v Eck HJ, Manin'tVeld AJ, Weimar W, Schalekamp MA: Circadian variation of heart rate but not blood pressure after heart transplantation. Transplant Proc 1987;19:2554–2555.

272. Wiles HB, Laver J, Baum D: T-cell lymphoma in a child after heart transplantation. J Heart Lung Transplant 1994;13:1019–1023.

273. Williams MJA, Lee MY, DiSalvo TG, Dec GW, Picard MH, Palacios IF, Semigran MJ: Biopsy-induced flail tricuspid leaflet and tricuspid regurgitation following orthotopic cardiac transplantation. Am J Cardiol 1996;77:1339–1344.

274. World Health Organization: Assessment of Fracture Risk and Its Application to Screening for Postmenopausal Osteoporosis. WHO technical report series 843. Geneva: WHO, 1994.

275. Wotherspoon AC, Diss TC, Pan L, Singh N, Whelan J, Isaacson PG: Low grade gastric B-cell lymphoma of mucosa associated lymphoid tissue in immunocompromised patients. Histopathology 1996;28:128–134.

276. Ying AJ, Myerowitz PD, Marsh WL: post transplantation lymphoproliferative disorder in cardiac transplant allografts. Ann Thorac Surg 1997;64:1822–1824.

277. Yousem SA, Randhawa P, Locker J, Paradis IL, Dauber JA, Griffith BP, Nalesnik M: posttransplant lymphoproliferative disorders in heart/lung transplant recipients: primary presentation in the allograft. Hum Pathol 1989;20:361–369.

278. Zahger D, Lotan C, Admon D, Klapholz L, Kaufman B, Shimon D, Woolfson N, Gotsman MS: Very early appearance of Kaposi's sarcoma after cardiac transplantation in Sephardic Jews. Am Heart J 1993;126:999–1000.

279. Zangwill SD, Hsu DT, Kichuk MR, Garvin JH, Stolar CJ, Haddad J, Stylianos S, Michler RE, Chadburn A, Knowles DM, Addonizio LJ: Incidence and outcome of primary Epstein Barr virus infection and lymphoproliferataive disease in pediatric heart transplant recipients. J Heart Lung Transplant 1998;17:1161–1166.

280. Ziestse R, Balk AH, Dorpel MA, Meeter K, Bos E, Weimer W: Time course of the decline in renal function in cyclosporine-treated heart transplant recipients. Am J Nephrol 1994;14:1–5.

281. Zimmerman KA, Dabezies MA, Schnall SF, Maurer AH, Dempsey DT: Acute gastrointestinal hemorrhage from non-Hodgkin's lymphoma of the jejunum after orthotopic heart transplantation. Am J Gastroenterol 1993;88:1449–1450.

282. Zoja C, Furci L, Ghilardi F, Zilio P, Benigni A, Remuzzi G: Cyclosporin-induced endothelial cell injury. Lab Invest 1986; 55:455–462.

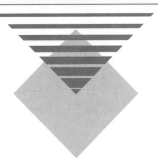

CHAPTER NINETEEN

Quality of Life After Heart Transplantation

with the collaboration of
CONNIE WHITE-WILLIAMS, R.N., M.S.N.

Success after cardiac transplantation has focused prominently on survival, which is an endpoint conducive to documentation, analysis, and risk-factor stratification (see Chapter 16). Using survival as the overwhelming indicator of benefit was appropriate in an era when cardiac transplantation was reserved for those patients who had less than 50% likelihood of survival at 1 year. However, transplantation today is often considered for patients with a survival likelihood in excess of 50% at 24 months, especially if they are very symptomatic with a poor "quality of life."[82, 84] It is apparent that the improvement not only in survival but also in quality of life can be dramatic for the patient suffering from the ravages of end-stage heart failure who is transformed (by transplantation) into a person with nearly normal heart function and returns to a productive working environment with a stable, supportive family unit. Unfortunately, many patients following heart transplantation are unable to realize this ideal outcome. Their long-term satisfaction with their life can be tarnished by the permanent demands of a complex medical regimen, an altered body image secondary to immunosuppressive medications, emotional stresses about the pos-

sibility of rejection and infection, and the long-term uncertainty about other potential complications. Thus, it becomes increasingly important to devise reproducible methods which can be analyzed and which offer accurate insight into the benefit of cardiac transplantation in these more subjective areas.

The physiologic sequelae of the failing heart inflict profound alterations on many aspects of life that cannot be directly predicted or quantified by physiologic parameters. These aspects of life that, in their aggregate, constitute happiness or life satisfaction, and that may be affected by disease states and their therapies, are often described as **quality of life** indices. There is universal agreement that an important determinant and description of the success of a therapeutic intervention for the failing heart is its impact, qualitatively and quantitatively, on the patient's quality of life, compared both to the preintervention disease state (natural history) and to other interventions. The assessment of quality of life outcome following transplantation, therefore, becomes increasingly important when comparing the physiologic, functional, and "life satisfaction" outcomes compared to similar indicators of success with other strategies such as aggressive pharmacologic management of heart failure[84, 85] or, eventually, permanent mechanical circulatory support devices. Thus, in making the decision to proceed with cardiac transplantation instead of another present or future therapeutic option for "end-stage" heart disease, outcome measures of survival, morbidity, physiologic response, and quality-of-life benefits will all factor into the final therapeutic recommendation.

THE STUDY OF QUALITY OF LIFE

DEFINITION

In 1993, the World Health Organization defined quality of life as "the individual's perception of their position in life in the context of the culture and value systems in which they live and in relation to their goals, expectations, standards, and concerns.''[96] In the assessment of cardiac transplantation, quality of life may be generally defined as *the patient's perception of the effect of the heart failure state and its therapy (cardiac transplantation or other treatment strategies) on his or her ability to live a meaningful and satisfying life.*

THE DOMAINS OF QUALITY OF LIFE

Using this definition, it is apparent that isolated descriptions of morbidity and mortality are insufficient to characterize quality of life. In the attempt to provide the most accurate characterization of this complex, subjective, and multifaceted outcome variable called "quality of life," there will necessarily be both **objective** and **subjective** components. Although the components which contribute to this assessment have been categorized in many ways,[22, 86] we will discuss quality of life in four general domains (Table 19–1). The selection of outcome variables and their assignment to specific domains is somewhat subjective, since there is considerable overlap in many of these terms, and their subjective nature does not permit categorizations which are all mutually exclusive.

Physical/Mental Status

This domain of quality of life includes many components which can be assessed in an objective, semiquantitative or graded fashion that is familiar to health care providers. **Functional class** prior to heart transplantation and in a time-related fashion after transplantation is often assessed with the standard New York Heart Association (NYHA) classification system. **Disease symptoms** or somatic complaints such as dyspnea, chest pain, joint pain, leg weakness, and so forth can be objectively graded and recorded. **Exercise capacity** can be quantified through formal exercise testing (see Chapters 6 and 11) in a time-related fashion following transplantation and compared to pretransplant values. **Cognitive function** can be formally analyzed using intelligent quotients and short-term memory tests.

Functional Ability

The patient's ability to perform normal tasks (activities of daily living), assessment of his or her general endurance or energy level, and the ability to perform domestic tasks in the household are important aspects of this domain. Particularly important in the posttransplant patient is assessment of his or her ability to return to previous employment and the resultant financial stability for the family unit. Sexual function may also be discussed within this domain.

Psychological Well-Being

This domain clearly encompasses the essence of "quality of life." Accurate information must be provided about complex subjective perceptions of the patient at various times following transplantation regarding his or her emotional state, satisfaction with his or her life after transplantation, and the ability to cope with the limitations and potential complications of life with a transplanted heart (see again Table 19–1). This very subjective domain is also perhaps the most important area in which the patient judges the "happiness" benefit of additional survival conferred by the transplant experience.

Social Interactions

The social domain includes the components of spousal, family, and community support systems and interactions, which also are complex and multifactorial. In addition to these subjective aspects, objective information is gathered about social actions which are potentially harmful to long-term patient and graft survival, such as smoking, alcohol consumption, and drug abuse. Objective data can also be gathered on the socioeconomic impact of transplantation on the patient and his or her family.

METHODOLOGY FOR THE ASSESSMENT OF QUALITY OF LIFE

The methodology for quality of life studies includes the **instruments** (or tools) for measuring quality of life variables, the study design for testing quality of life hypotheses, and methods of data analysis. The specific data gathering methods or instruments used for quality of life assessment include a wide variety of psychosocial testing and information-gathering tools (Table 19–2).[4, 23, 30–32, 33, 36, 40, 41, 93–95]

These instruments can be generally categorized as those **generic** to overall quality of life assessment, **dis-**

TABLE 19–1	Major Domains and Outcome Variables in Quality of Life Analyses
DOMAINS	OUTCOME VARIABLES
Physical/mental status	Functional class (NYHA) Symptoms of disease Exercise capacity Cognitive function Sleep patterns
Functional ability	Activities of daily living Domestic function Energy Employment Financial stability Sexual function
Psychological well-being	Life satisfaction Perceived quality of life Self-esteem Depression/hostility Ability to cope with illness Anxiety Body image Stress
Social interactions	Family relationships Marital/partner relationship Recreational activities Substance abuse

NYHA, New York Heart Association.

TABLE 19–2	Common Tools Employed in Heart Transplant Quality of Life Studies

DOMAIN	TOOL
Physical/mental status	Dyspnea and fatigue scale QOL index[23] Lough's QOL questionnaire Nottingham health profile SF-36 Living with heart failure questionnaire Heart transplant symptom checklist Heart transplant rating scale
Functional ability	Sickness impact profile[22] QOL index[23] Lough's QOL questionnaire SF-36 Living with heart failure questionnaire Work history Heart transplant rating scale
Psychological well-being	Psychosocial adjustment to illness QOL index[23] Profile of mood states Lough's QOL questionnaire Beck depression inventory Multiple affect adjustive checklist Nottingham health profile SF-36 Positive and negative affect schedule[93–95] Living with heart failure questionnaire Spielberger state trait anxiety inventory Heart transplant stressor scale[41] Heart transplant compliance questionnaire Jalowic coping scale[40] Global adjustment to illness scale Cardiac depression scale[36] Heart transplant rating scale Rating question form[30, 33] Heart transplant intervention scale[32]
Social interactions	QOL index Lough's QOL questionnaire Nottingham health profile Heart transplant rating scale SF-36 Living with heart failure Heart transplant social support index Heart transplant work history tool[32]

ease or therapy-specific instruments, those which are specific for a certain domain, and items which are specific for a given study that addresses a specific issue in quality of life.

By the nature of these studies, the specific instruments measure variables which may be objective or subjective. Objective measurements include most variables in the domain of physical/mental status, assessment of vocational status, documentation of substance abuse, and financial impact of transplantation. Subjective measurements deal with the patient's perceptions and expectations of how satisfied he or she is with many subjective aspects of his or her life as a result of the disease process (in this case, advanced heart failure) and the therapeutic intervention (in this case, heart transplantation).

The main source of information relating to each outcome variable is the patient, usually through some type of focused questionnaire administered either by the patient to him or herself or by a quality of life investigator.

Other respondents include relatives and caregivers for the patient. The setting of quality of life surveys can focus on either an in-hospital or out-of-hospital setting.

A major difficulty in the interpretation of quality of life studies lies in the effectiveness of a given tool to approximate truth and its ability to reflect wide variability of responses among patients. In the world of statistics (see Chapter 3), data analysis can be subjected to mathematical scrutiny and to tests which indicate the likelihood that chance alone could produce such a result. Complex mathematical models can be used to examine risk factors for specific outcomes and their significance as well as the magnitude of their effect. Such "checks and balances" in the methods for and the conclusions drawn from quality of life studies are inherently more problematic because of the largely subjective nature of the endpoints under study. Nevertheless, because of the extreme importance of quality of life issues in transplantation and health care in general, formal methods of statistical analysis have been increasingly applied to quality of life instruments and studies. The specific tools or instruments utilized in such studies are evaluated for their **reliability** (the ability to generate a similar set of responses from a given patient on multiple administrations of the same test), **validity** (the ability of the given test to generate a result which reflects the outcome variable under study), and **sensitivity** (the likelihood of detecting an outcome which actually exists).

Another important challenge in quality of life studies is ascertaining whether the patients responding to a given questionnaire are actually representative of the transplant population under study. In fact, two of the most common reasons for not responding are patients being "too sick" (likely to provide negative responses) or "too busy" (likely to be enjoying a more positive quality of life). Thus, nonresponders are not a random sample of posttransplant patients and, therefore, jeopardize the accuracy of inferences generated from the analysis. There are two general approaches to minimize, or at least quantify, this problem. First, every effort should be made to generate a high response rate. A clear strategy and well-defined protocol for identifying, contacting, and following the patients is necessary. One barrier to a high response rate is the length and complexity of the typical quality of life questionnaire. If the instrument has been written for a 12th grade education level, patients with lower educational levels would be unable to answer a self-administered questionnaire. Second, careful records should be kept and summarized on patients who do not respond. In some studies, investigators can examine the outcome of nonresponders according to the reason for no response.

Techniques of **multivariable analysis** (see Chapter 3) are applied to many quality of life studies. Since many of the outcome variables are subjective, distinguishing between dependent (outcome) variables and independent risk factors (predictors) becomes problematic. When subjective variables are related, the timing of occurrence of each variable becomes critically important in determining whether it can be a potential risk factor for another variable. Consider the outcome "depression at 5 years" and the risk factor "unemployed at 5 years."

These variables are probably associated but one is not necessarily a function of the other. Was the patient depressed first and then became unemployed or was he or she unemployed first and subsequently became depressed?

SPECIFIC ASPECTS OF QUALITY OF LIFE AFTER CARDIAC TRANSPLANTATION

OVERVIEW OF QUALITY OF LIFE

Early Outcome

There is general agreement that cardiac transplantation produces prompt and sustained improvement in the health status and perception of general well-being among patients with advanced heart failure (Table 19–3). The most dramatic and prompt improvement occurs in exertional activities. This benefit in physical performance along with general health perception and overall quality of life are the areas most consistently changed in a positive way following transplantation.[2] Other indices of productive living, however, are often

| TABLE 19–3 | Impact of Heart Transplantation on Quality of Life Variables During First 5 Years* |

DOMAIN	VARIABLES	IMPROVED	NO CHANGE OR WORSE
Physical/ mental status	Functional class	X	
	Symptoms of disease	X	
	Exercise capacity	X	
	Cognitive function	X	
	Sleep patterns		X
Functional ability	Activities of daily living	X	
	Domestic function	X	
	Energy	X	
	Employment		X
	Financial stability		X
	Sexual function		X
	Life satisfaction	X	
	Perceived quality of life	X	
	Self-esteem	X	
Psychological well-being	Depression/ hostility	X	
	Ability to cope with illness		X
	Anxiety	X	
	Body image	X	
	Stress	X	
	Family relationships	X	
Social interactions	Marital/partner relations	X	
	Substance abuse	X	

*Based on responses from quality of life questionnaires.

not realized during the first year. The potential complications and complex medical regimen (with its inherent side effects) increase the stresses, fears, anxieties and depression which are common after this massive intervention. It is noteworthy that patients who were sickest prior to transplantation are less satisfied during the first year with many aspects of their life (as judged by quality of life indictors) than patients who are less ill at time of transplantation.[29] Concerns about financial status and the ability to sustain income are ongoing problems for many patients and detract from the quality of life benefit. Sexual function is often importantly impaired, further contributing to depression and anxiety.[11] The multitude of studies in this area support the general conclusion that heart transplantation is extremely effective in increasing duration and quality of life as well as hope for the future, but early and sustained assistance by members of the transplant team, spouse, and other friends and family members are necessary to help the heart transplant recipient maximize the quality of life benefits.

Comparison with Other Interventions

Comparisons between patients 6 months after heart transplantation and patients receiving 6 months of intensive medical therapy for heart failure have revealed better physical and social functioning in heart transplant patients but persistent high levels of anxiety and depression, with poor adjustment to illness in both groups.[61]

When quality of life indices in heart transplant recipients are compared to other solid organ transplant patients, subtle differences have been reported. Although some quality of life indicators are worse in heart transplant patients than after either renal or liver transplantation, functional improvement frequently occurs earlier after heart transplantation despite greater pretransplant physical disability.[73]

Long-Term Outcome

In general, there appears to be progressive improvement in the level of anxiety,[43] depression,[24, 43] general well-being,[43] emotional functioning,[59] social functioning,[9] sleep,[9] perceived quality of life,[24, 48, 59] and general health status[9] as the years pass following cardiac transplantation.[68] Few studies have examined the long-term (10 years or more) quality of life outcome following cardiac transplantation. Among patients surviving out to 14 years after transplant, there appears to be sustained good to excellent quality of life outcomes, with improvement in perceived health, physical condition, and endurance as well as self-accomplishment, interpersonal relationships, and social activities.[49]

Unfortunately, an important segment of patients continues to experience negative life changes with respect to finances,[49] sexual function,[49, 75] physical appearance related to immunosuppression medications,[75] sleep patterns, and domestic functioning.[75] These negative life perceptions are not associated with the duration of time since transplantation, indicating that these perceptions do not worsen over the years following initial transplantation.[75]

In a German study of patients 9 to 13 years after transplantation, 91% were in NYHA functional class I or II and 79% viewed their overall health as good to excellent.[49] This superb long-term functional outcome among survivors of transplantation must be put in the context of heart transplantation as a palliative rather than a curative operation. Thus, it is not surprising that the majority of these long-term patients still viewed their health-related quality of life as inferior to a healthy population, with persistent disability in the area of work and recreation and an important incidence of distress from sleep disorders, pain, suboptimal energy level, sexual dysfunction, and the long-term complications associated with steroids and other immunosuppressive agents.[15, 49]

PHYSICAL/MENTAL STATUS

As noted above, a universal finding in transplant studies is a major increase in functional status secondary to replacement of the heart failure state with a more normally functioning human allograft. Whereas nearly all pretransplant patients suffer NYHA class III or IV symptoms of heart failure, the posttransplant NYHA class is I or II in the vast majority of recipients. In a study by Bunzel and colleagues, patients reported greatest improvement in physical status among the quality of life indices.[6] **Exercise capacity** is generally remarkably improved, although in most cases it does not return to normal (see Chapter 11). In fact, some studies have failed to demonstrate appreciable improvement in such indices as 6-minute walk, maximum work load, oxygen uptake, and anerobic threshold during the early months following cardiac transplantation.[91] Objective measures of exercise capacity[34, 54, 64, 71] indicate that the majority of improvement occurs during the first posttransplant year. However, because of the physiologic derangement of the transplanted heart and persisting physiologic impairment induced by the heart failure state (see Chapter 11), formal exercise capacity generally remains less than would be expected in healthy subjects.[34, 54, 71] However, a further increment in posttransplant exercise capacity is generally achieved with a gradual, individualized exercise protocol. Thus, it appears that focused training is an important ingredient for the achievement of fitness after transplantation.[63]

Disease symptoms are usually dramatically improved by the transplant procedure, with nearly 90% of patients reporting no or minimal symptoms of heart disease.[20] In the National Transplant Study (based on information from 85% of all U.S. transplant programs), heart, kidney, and liver transplant patients reported a similar and high sense of well-being. Only 7% of heart transplant patients rated their health status as poor.

Thus, transplantation is clearly effective in improving the physical and mental status domain of patients with end-stage heart failure, both early after transplant and at 5 years.[6, 24, 28, 52, 65] Functional status, disease symptoms and symptom distress,[28, 29, 65] exercise capacity, and cognitive function[9] are generally improved. Sleep patterns, however, often remain abnormal following transplantation,[8] particularly compared to the normal population.

FUNCTIONAL ABILITY

Activities of Daily Living

The National Transplant Study concluded that physical activity level and functional rehabilitation were generally satisfactory in 80–85% of surviving patients.[20] General indicators of functional ability are usually improved over heart failure patients on optimal medical therapy within 6 months of transplantation[91] and equivalent to renal transplant recipients.[21]

Longitudinal studies[42] have documented that functional activities and leisure function are generally greatly improved at 5 years after transplant compared to the pretransplant state. This includes domestic function,[5, 24] activities of daily living,[6, 24] and energy. Despite marked improvements, some degree of functional impairment often persists. Evans reported[20] that 66% of patients were limited in some activity they desired; 52% were unable to perform some aspects of physical labor, housework, or schoolwork; 43% had trouble bending, stooping or lifting; 34% had difficulty walking several blocks or climbing stairs; 9% needed assistance in travel within their community; and 7% were largely restricted to bed or home. Later after transplantation, long-term complications of steroid immunosuppression, such as muscular weakness, myalgias, osteopenia, or aseptic necrosis of weight-bearing joints, may seriously impair activities of daily living.

The United Kingdom Heart Transplant Study[7, 8] found that heart transplant patients reported consistent improvement in a variety of functional areas compared to their pretransplant heart failure state. The general quality of life was rated as "high" in only 8% of patients before transplantation compared to 67% within 3 months after transplantation. In functional areas, 84% of patients had difficulties at their job before transplantation compared to 50% afterwards; and 94% had problems taking care of their home before transplant compared to 20% after transplantation.

Suboptimal Areas of Functional Ability

There are several areas of the functional domain which often remain unsatisfactory, even years after transplantation. **Sexual function** has been reported as improved in some studies[5, 6, 28] and worse in others.[61] Sexual concerns in patients after transplantation are often multifaceted and relate to the psychological impact of body image concerns, loss of self-esteem, the impact of altered roles and responsibilities, and the effects of medications.[87] Avoidance of sexual activity due to anxiety is reported in up to 50% of recipients.[81] Despite persistent sexual problems for many patients, sexual function is often greatly improved compared to that during advanced heart failure. The United Kingdom Heart Transplant Study reported that 84% of patients surveyed had problems with sexual function before transplant compared to 29% afterwards.[7, 8] However, another study concluded that only about 50% of transplanted patients are satisfied with their sexual life.[37]

A critical component of an acceptable quality of life is **financial stability.** Many transplant patients consider this the most important requirement for an acceptable quality of life,[58, 66] which underscores the importance of returning to gainful employment if at all possible. **Vocational functioning and employment** are variably reported as persistently impaired[5, 60] or worse[24] after transplantation. Not surprisingly, the **financial situation** is nearly uniformly worse[6, 28] 5 years after transplant.

Employment after Cardiac Transplantation

Return to work after cardiac transplantation should be an important goal from both a patient and family standpoint as well as the societal perspective. When the cost/benefit ratio of cardiac transplantation is examined dispassionately, leaving aside the obvious benefits in terms of extension of life, the question of the economic burden on society of transplantation has raised concerns as to the advisability of this procedure. The withdrawal of Medicaid funding for solid organ transplantation by Oregon in 1987 is representative of this type of cost/benefit examination. Therefore, it is incumbent on the cardiac transplant community to be proactive in encouraging potential recipients to return to work, not only to enhance the quality of life of recipients,[37, 49, 75] but also to provide a tractable argument to counter the economic concern that the cost of cardiac transplantation outweighs the benefit.

Return to work rates range from 32% up to 86%[19, 37, 42, 58, 62, 67, 77, 79, 92] and are obviously influenced by a number of factors including the demographics of the area served by the transplant center, the methods used to conduct an employment survey (in one study,[66] the response rate to a mailed questionnaire was 55%), and the country surveyed. In the United States, it would appear that approximately 30–45% of cardiac transplant recipients are employed,[66] similar to employment estimates after kidney and liver transplantation.[20] A study by Meister and colleagues[58] found that 32% of patients studied returned to work, 25% were retired, and only 7.5% were medically disabled. However, another 36% were termed "insurance disabled"; that is, patients who could have returned to work but did not because health insurance would have been lost in the absence of employment. Cardiac transplant recipients most likely to return to work are women (including homemaking) and younger and better educated recipients.[66]

There are a number of reasons why cardiac transplant recipients do not return to work.

1) **The loss of health insurance and disability** is a major deterrent to reemployment. In the United States, the laws regarding disability and Medicare health insurance limit successful return to employment after cardiac transplantation. The current laws are not structured to respond to the possibility of a patient being chronically disabled and then subsequently no longer being disabled after a successful heart transplant. Particularly problematic is the patient who was receiving disability and Medicare health insurance prior to a heart transplant and wishes to return to work after recovering from the transplant procedure. Unless this patient has secondary full-coverage health insurance or is successful in securing health insurance which does not have a preexisting condition clause with a mandatory waiting period, resuming employment will trigger loss of Medicare health insurance, which is likely to impose a very significant financial burden on the patient and his or her family. Furthermore, the Social Security Administration may also conduct a review, find a patient after a heart transplant no longer disabled, and the patient would then lose both disability insurance and Medicare. These regulations are, unfortunately, significant disincentives for patients after cardiac transplantation to resume employment. These barriers to employment are likely to persist until legislative reform improves the access of transplant recipients to employment without risking their access to health care.[77]

2) A critical factor in a large number of patients who remain unemployed and those that do not plan to seek employment is the **self-perception of an inability to work** which is at odds with their transplant physician's assessment of their functional abilities. In the study by Paris,[66] 61% of cardiac transplant recipients who were unemployed believed that they were incapable of work, whereas only 13% were considered medically disabled by their physicians.

3) **The length of medical disability prior to transplantation** negatively impacts the likelihood of employment after transplantation. This in part results from an adaptation to life without employment, but also may reflect the possibility that these patients with long-term disability are less likely to have their previous job available after transplantation.

4) **The length of disability after transplantation** is equally important. If patients are successful in returning to work after cardiac transplantation, they usually do so within the first year. Following the first year, successful return to employment is considerably less likely.

In some occupations, resuming former employment may not be possible because of health requirements of the job. For example, airplane pilots are required to have both a pilot's license and a medical certificate. Pilots with heart disease are required to report this to the Federal Aviation Administration (FAA), and disease severe enough to require cardiac transplantation would automatically result in loss of a medical certificate. The reissuance of a pilot's medical certificate after successful heart transplantation has been an issue faced by a number of heart transplant centers. The FAA's major concern regarding reissuance of a medical certificate to a cardiac transplant recipient revolves around the problem of coronary allograft vasculopathy and the associated risk of sudden death or unexpected incapacitation. In situations such as this, appropriate studies and detailed risk-adjusted analyses allow some transplant patients to return to their prior job if the predicted risk is low enough.[57]

The return to employment rate after cardiac transplantation is disappointing, but there are certainly a number of avenues open to improve the situation, including changing the disability and health insurance laws, using vocational-rehabilitation evaluation, and, if necessary, pursuing legal options to ensure the rights of patients who are willing and able to work but are denied employment unfairly.

PSYCHOLOGICAL WELL-BEING

Although the physical benefits of cardiac transplantation are realized almost immediately and the functional benefits usually are apparent within months, the psychological adjustments are often greatly delayed.[47] Patient anxiety and emotional liability may initially worsen following hospital discharge; one study found that over 50% of patients suffered emotional instability and mood lability and were generally more anxious at 4 and 12 months than immediately following transplantation.[80] In a multicenter study of psychological problems related to the transplant procedure, the most significant psychological difficulties noted prior to transplantation were depression and increased stress within the family unit.[56] The frequency of anxiety and depression in patients with advanced heart failure has been confirmed in other studies.[17, 52] Following transplantation, denial, abnormal euphoria, guilt, anxiety, and a feeling of changed body image are often reported.[38, 80, 87]

Overt psychiatric difficulties are rather common, with disorders of affect, mood, irritability, and grandiosity present at some time in nearly 50% of patients.[80] Anxiety disorders are common but usually short lived, and frank delirium is rare. Acute delirum, organic mood disorders, and acute anxiety may result from neurologic complications of the transplant procedure, reactions to initial immunosuppressive therapy, or acute psychologic stresses related to the transplant procedure. Psychiatric dysfunction usually improves during the first postoperative year, but patients needing psychiatric therapy before transplantation are likely to need it afterwards.[55]

Corticosteroids, particularly at the high doses common early after transplantation, can produce irritability, anxiety, and mood swings.[44, 80] Transplant patients generally report deterioration in self-image secondary to physical effects of steroids and cyclosporine.[2]

Frustration, resentment, and anger are frequently reported if the outcome of transplantation does not meet the expectations of patient and family.[55] These difficulties, often stemming from postoperative complications, may cause dysfunction in family and social relationships. Despite the frequency of important problems with psychological adjustment early after transplant, these indices typically improve during the first posttransplant year, particularly when there is better compliance with the transplant regimen, fewer medical complications experienced, and development of more effective coping strategies.[31] Not surprisingly, perceived quality of life during the first year is also closely related to the patient's general perception about life satisfaction, health status following transplantation, and employment status.[59] Psychological benefit during the first 6 months is generally worse for patients who were sicker before transplant compared to less-ill patients.[29]

In general, over the intermediate term, cardiac transplantation has a favorable effect on most areas of psychological well-being. During the first 5 posttransplant years, patients generally experience improved well-being and life satisfaction; improved body image, quality of life perception, and emotional stability; and less anxiety and depression.[5, 6, 9, 24, 28, 42, 43, 52, 59, 65] When quality of life measures from before transplantation have been compared to 5 years after transplant, patients report less anxiety,[42, 43, 52] greater life satisfaction,[28] less or no depression,[24, 43] better perceived quality of life,[6, 28, 65] and improved body image.[42] The psychological areas generally not improved are the amount of stress and effectiveness of coping with stress.[9, 24, 28, 42, 43, 59]

SOCIAL INTERACTIONS

Despite the improvement in many quality of life areas, social interactions often initially suffer, undoubtedly related to stress, anxiety, and other issues in the psychological domain. Family relationships (including spouses, significant others, children, extended family, and friends) are notably strained in many quality of life studies.[2] During the first 5 years after transplant, however, many indices of socialization are improved from the serious heart failure state.[13, 42, 91] The improvement in social functioning may favorably impact other outcome variables. Harvison[37] found a positive link between social satisfaction and productivity. Another study found a significant association between marriage and less rejection as well as fewer hospitalizations.[83] Patients who are able to form strong relationships with the transplant team are more likely to be compliant with long-term follow-up.[5, 6, 9, 24, 28, 52, 59, 65]

SPECIAL ISSUES

THE INFLUENCE OF AGE AND GENDER ON QUALITY OF LIFE OUTCOMES

Age

It is not surprising that older patients (> about 55 years of age) who are robust enough (except for their advanced heart failure) to undergo cardiac transplantation might have less anxiety and greater appreciation for the additional years of life generated by the transplant operation. Indeed, Coffman and colleagues[12, 42, 72] reported less anxiety, better perceived quality of life, improved domestic environment, improved family relationships, and less psychological distress in patients over 55 years compared to younger patients.

Gender

Several studies have suggested that women experience a higher overall rate of symptom frequency compared to men,[50] have greater stress and dissatisfaction about changes in appearance, yet cope with general stresses, on the average, more effectively than men.[27, 50] Male recipients, as a group, are more distressed by changes in sexual function and inability to return to work.[27] In one study, no significant differences between gender groups were noted with respect to functional status, overall satisfaction with transplantation, or overall quality of life.[27] The major issue of *pregnancy* is discussed in a subsequent section.

COMPLIANCE

Patient compliance to medications and medical instructions is routinely evaluated prior to listing patients for cardiac transplantation in the belief that this is predictive of posttransplant compliance. The importance of compliance in posttransplant survival is obvious, and lack of compliance has been linked to rejection-related morbidity and mortality.[78] In general, patients understand the critical importance of consistently taking their medications at the appropriate time and are more compliant in this area than, for example, following a diet, exercising, and taking their vital signs.[30] Studies of the frequency and predictors of noncompliance after cardiac transplantation are confounded by variability among studies in the definition and magnitude of noncompliance examined as well as the individuals responding to inquiries. However, certain psychosocial traits have been shown to increase the likelihood of noncompliant behavior (Table 19–4).[16] Recipients with high anxiety levels, a high anger/hostility level, and/or avoidance coping strategies are more prone to noncompliance.[16] The likelihood of noncompliance increases in the setting of poor social support from friends and family, poor caregiver support, and/or substance abuse before or after transplant.[81] Lower levels of educational background, particularly with inadequate social support, also decrease compliance.[55]

REHABILITATION OF THE TRANSPLANT PATIENT

With evidence of deficits in multiple quality of life domains, it should be emphasized that rehabilitation after cardiac transplantation requires multidisciplinary efforts. In addition to a formal exercise and physical training program, rehabilitation should include collaboration between transplant physicians, home health care providers, and family members, with the goal of optimizing physical, psychological, social, and vocational function.

The need for exercise training is apparent when considering the chronically debilitated state of most heart failure patients. Rapid deterioration of hemodynamic performance in hospitalized patients is underscored by the reported 25% decline in maximal oxygen uptake within 3 weeks of sustained bed rest.[76] Despite increasing blood supply to exercise muscles after transplantation, deconditioning is often severe as evidenced by muscle atrophy and a reduction in mitochondrial volume and density.[18] One study reported that cross-sectional area of the thigh was reduced by about 15% in patients with advanced heart failure before transplantation.[53] When initiated early after transplantation, formal exercise training has been shown to increase physical work capacity.[46] Thus, rehabilitation of leg strength may be of particular importance, particularly since proximal leg muscle weakness is exacerbated by steroid immunosuppression.

PREGNANCY AND PATERNITY FOLLOWING HEART TRANSPLANTATION

With the progressive improvement in long-term survival of patients after heart and heart/lung transplantation, the issue of the advisability of pregnancy in a transplant recipient is becoming increasingly important. Clearly, there are important issues involving maternal and fetal risks as well as the realization that survival after heart and heart/lung transplantation is less than that of the normal population, and therefore a significant proportion of these children, by the time they are teenagers, will have lost their natural mothers.

There have been isolated reports of successful pregnancy with either vaginal[51] or cesarean[10, 45] delivery following cardiac transplantation. Registries of pregnancies after heart,[88, 90] heart/lung,[88] and lung[3] transplantation provide useful information, but suffer from the fact that these surveys may not have been inclusive.

Thirty weeks after gestation, the blood volume of the mother has increased an average of 40% above prepregnancy levels.[70] However, there is every expectation that the normally functioning denervated allograft will respond successfully to the increased hemodynamic demand through increased stroke volume (which also occurs in the innervated heart of a nontransplant pregnant patient), increased heart rate, and augmented contractility.[39]

Maternal Risks

There have been reports of successful pregnancies in renal transplant patients treated with cyclosporine where deterioration of **renal function** did not occur with or following pregnancy.[69] Although the glomerular filtration rate increases during pregnancy, heart transplant

TABLE 19–4	Psychosocial Risk Factors for Noncompliance After Cardiac Transplantation

- High anxiety level
- High anger-hostility level
- Use of avoidance coping strategies
- Poor support from friends and family
- Poor caregiver support
- Substance abuse
- Low education level

recipients with prepregnancy normal renal function will probably not experience deterioration in renal function during pregnancy. The more difficult situation is in patients with cyclosporine-induced nephrotoxicity, where renal function may deteriorate with pregnancy, which may also be complicated by difficult hypertension. Although insufficient data are available, pregnancy in heart transplant recipients with significant cyclosporine-induced nephrotoxicity is probably not advisable.

There are insufficient data to determine whether or not the likelihood of **rejection** of the heart (or lungs in the case of heart/lung transplantation) is higher during pregnancy. Because of the higher likelihood of acute rejection of the heart (and lungs) during the first 6–12 months, pregnancy should be deferred to beyond 12 months after transplantation. Because of the ongoing concern regarding cardiac rejection during pregnancy, the usual schedule of biopsies should be performed, but under echocardiographic rather than fluoroscopic guidance. In an international survey of children born to heart and heart/lung transplant recipients, about 20% of pregnant recipients developed rejection during pregnancy.[90] In a registry[26] of lung transplant recipients (which is likely of relevance to heart/lung transplant recipients), three of eight patients experienced pulmonary rejection during pregnancy and all three patients subsequently died, two of obliterative bronchiolitis and one of fungal infection. Thus, the risk of rejection of the heart (and lung in heart/lung recipients) during pregnancy is clearly of concern.

The risk of **infection** during pregnancy appears to be no higher than that experienced by nonpregnant patients.

Hypertension is common during pregnancy and frequently requires additional therapy.[88] Angiotensin-converting enzyme inhibitor drugs should be discontinued during pregnancy to avoid possible fetal effects, including oligohydramnios, pulmonary hypoplasia, and neonatal renal dysfunction.[35] Preeclampsia has a significantly higher incidence than in the normal population, possibly as high as 20%.[90]

The most frequent **alteration to immunosuppression** is an increase in the dose of cyclosporine during pregnancy, required in 41% of patients in one series.[90] In this same report, 22% of patients underwent empiric lowering of the cyclosporine dose (presumably to decrease the risk of nephrotoxicity), and several patients experienced rejection episodes.

Premature delivery was reported in 30% of patients,[90] and the cesarean section rate was 33%.[90]

Maternal **mortality** during pregnancy appears to be rare, but late maternal deaths have occurred, reflecting the ongoing risks of transplantation and immunosuppression. Although the limited information currently supports the relative safety of pregnancy after heart and heart/lung transplantation, the pregnancy should be regarded as high risk and managed as a collaborative effort between transplant physicians, obstetricians, and neonatologists. Although the information available does not suggest that transplant physicians categorically dissuade heart and heart/lung transplant recipients from pregnancy, there are maternal and fetal risks that need to

be clearly explained to the potential parents. Obviously, there will be situations where, because of serious ongoing complications (such as recurrent cardiac rejection, important allograft vasculopathy, or severe cyclosporine-induced nephrotoxicity), women should be counseled against pregnancy.

Fetal Risks

Risks to the fetus are probably more significant than the maternal risks and are certainly higher than in the general population. There does not appear to be an increased risk of **fetal abnormalities** as a result of immunosuppressive drugs. Although cyclosporine crosses the placenta and is detectable in the blood stream of newborn babies, it does not appear to result in immunosuppression of the infant, since the lymphocyte profile of these babies is not suggestive of chronic immunosuppression.[74]

Small-for-gestational age does appear to have a significantly higher incidence than in the general population, and in one series[88] 50% of the infants had a birth weight of less than the tenth percentile (mothers having undergone heart or heart/lung transplantation). Data on long-term development of babies born to heart transplant recipients are not available, but based on babies born to renal transplant recipients, it is likely normal. Most series have not reported intrauterine or neonatal deaths,[88, 90] but in the much larger series of patients undergoing pregnancy after renal transplantation, the spontaneous abortion rate was 16%, similar to the general population.[14]

Although not reported in heart transplant patients undergoing pregnancies, **Rh incompatibility** (Rh-negative patients receiving an Rh-positive heart) could result in isoimmunization.

Breast-Feeding

Cyclosporine and azathioprine can both be detected in mother's milk, although at low concentrations. It is probably prudent to avoid breast-feeding in these mothers.

Paternity

Because of the concern of teratogenic effects of immunosuppressive agents, the issue of male heart and heart/lung transplant recipients fathering children has been of concern. In renal transplant recipients,[1] the incidence of male-mediated teratogenicity is no higher than in the general population. Limited information is available regarding paternity following cardiac transplantation, but, as with renal transplantation, there is no evidence that the incidence of fetal abnormalities is any higher than in the general population.[89] This is despite the significant incidence of chromosomal abnormalities (chromatid aberrations such as gaps and breaks, ring chromosomes and translocations) noted in renal transplant recipients receiving azathioprine (62%) and cyclosporine (68%) compared with normal healthy individuals (0%).[25]

References

1. Ahlswede KM, Ahlswede BA, Jarrell BE, Moritz MJ, Armenti VT: National Transplantation Pregnancy Registry: outcomes of Pregnancies Fathered by Male Transplant Recipients. New York: Plenum Press, 1994.
2. Angermann CE, Bullinger M, Spes CF, Zellner M, Kemke BM, Theisen K: Quality of life in long-term survivors of orthotopic heart transplantation. Kardiologie 1992;81:411–417.
3. Armenti VT, Gertner GS, Eisenberg JA, McGrory CH, Moritz MJ: National transplantation pregnancy registry: outcomes of pregnancies in lung recipients. Transplant Proc 1998;30:1528–1530.
4. Bergner M, Bobbitt RA, Carter WB, Gilson BS: The sickness impact profile: development and final revision of a health status measure. Med Care 1981;14:787–806.
5. Bohachick P, Anton BB, Wooldridge PJ, Kormos RL, Armitage JM, Hardesty RL, Griffith BP: Psychosocial outcome six months after heart transplant surgery: a preliminary report. Res Nurs Health 1992;15:165–173.
6. Bunzel B, Grundbock A, Laczkovics A, Holzinger C, Teufelsobaver H: Quality of life after orthotopic heart transplantation. J Heart Lung Transplant 1991;10:455–459.
7. Buxton MJ, Acheson R, Caine N, Gibson S, O'Brien BJ: Costs and benefits of the heart transplant programmes at Harefield and Papworth Hospitals. DHSS Res Report No. 12 1985;12.
8. Caine N, O'Brien B: Quality of life and psychological aspects of heart transplantation. In Wallwork J (ed): Heart and Heart-Lung Transplantation. Philadelphia: WB Saunders Company, 1989, pp 389–422.
9. Caine N, Sharples LD, English TAH, Wallwork J: Prospective study comparing quality of life before and after heart transplantation. Transplant Proc 1990;22:1437–1439.
10. Camann WR, Goldman GA, Johnson MD, Moore J, Greene M: Cesarean delivery in a patient with a transplanted heart. Anesthesiology 1989;71:618–620.
11. Christopherson LK, Griepp RB, Stinson EB: Rehabilitation after cardiac transplantation. JAMA 1976;236:2082–2084.
12. Coffman KL, Valenza M, Czer LSC, Friemark D, Aleksic I, Hardsty D, Queral C, Admon D, Barath P, Blanche C, Trento A: An update on transplantation in the geriatric heart transplant patient. Psychosomatics 1997;38:487–496.
13. Collins EG, White-Williams C, Jalowiec A: Spouse quality of life before and 1 year after heart transplantation. Crit Care Nurs Clin North Am 2000;12:103–110.
14. Davison JM: Renal transplantation and pregnancy. Am J Kidney Dis 1987;9:374–380.
15. DeCampli WM, Liukart H, Hunt S, Stinson EB: Characteristics of patients surviving more than ten years after cardiac transplantation. J Cardiovasc Surg 1995;108:240–252.
16. Dew MA, Roth LH, Thompson ME, Kormos RL, Griffith BP: Medical compliance and its predictors in the first year after heart transplantation. J Heart Lung Transplant 1996;15:631–645.
17. Dracup K, Walden JA, Stevenson LW, Brecht ML: Quality of life in patients with advanced heart failure. J Heart Lung Transplant 1992;11:273–279.
18. Drexler H, Reide U, Munzel T, Konig H, Funke E, Just H: Alterations of skeletal muscle in chronic heart failure. Circulation 1992;85:1751–1759.
19. Evans RW: The economics of heart transplantation. Circulation 1987;75:63–76.
20. Evans RW: Executive summary: the national cooperative transplanation study: BHARC-100-91-020. Battelle-Seattle Research Center, 1991.
21. Evans RW, Manninen DL, Maier A, Garrison LP: The quality of life of kidney and heart transplant recipients. Transplant Proc 1985;17:1579–1582.
22. Ferrans CE: Development of a quality of life index for patients with cancer. Oncol Nurs Forum 1990;17(suppl):15–21.
23. Ferrans CE, Powers MJ: Quality of life index: development and psychometric properties. Adv Nurs Sci 1985;8:15–24.
24. Fisher DC, Lake KD, Reutzel TJ, Emery RW: Changes in health-related quality of life and depression in heart transplant recipients. J Heart Lung Transplant 1995;14:373–381.
25. Fukuda M, Aikawa I, Ohmori Y, Yoshimura N, Nakai I, Matui S, Oka T: Chromosome aberrations in kidney transplant recipients. Transplant Proc 1987;1:2245–2247.
26. Gertner G, Coscia L, McGrory C, Moritz M, Armenti VT: Pregnancy in lung transplant recipients. Progr Transplant 2000;10:109–112.
27. Grady KL, Jalowiec A, Costanzo MR, Pifarre R, White-Williams C, Bourge RC, Kirklin JK: Differences in quality of life indicators based on UNOS status, age, and gender after heart transplantation [abstract]. J Heart Lung Transplant 1994;13:S45.
28. Grady KL, Jalowiec A, White-Williams C: Improvement in quality of life in patients with heart failure who undergo transplantation. J Heart Lung Transplant 1996;15:749–757.
29. Grady KL, Jalowiec A, White-Williams C: Differences in quality of life by pretransplant indicators of illness severity at 6 months after heart transplantation. J Heart Lung Transplant 1997;16:102.
30. Grady KL, Jalowiec A, White-Williams C: Patient compliance at one year and two years after heart transplantation. J Heart Lung Transplant 1998;17:383–394.
31. Grady KL, Jalowiec A, White-Williams C: Predictors of quality of life in patients at 1 year after heart transplantation. J Heart Lung Transplant 1999;18:202–210.
32. Grady KL, Jalowiec A, White-Williams C, Hetfleisch M, Penicook J, Blood M: Heart transplant candidates' perception of helpfulness of health care provider interventions. Cardiovas Nurs 1993;29:33–37.
33. Grady KL, Jalowiec A, White-Williams C, Pifarre R, Kirklin JK, Bourge RC, Costanzo MR: Predictors of quality of life in patients with advanced heart failure awaiting transplantation. J Heart Lung Transplant 1995;14:2–10.
34. Gullestad L, Haywood G, Ross H, Bjornerheim R, Geiran O, Kjekshus J, Simonsen S, Fowler M: Exercise capacity of heart transplant recipients. The importance of chronotropic incompetence. J Heart Lung Transplant 1996;15:1075–1083.
35. Hanssens M, Keirse MJNC, Vankelecom F, VanAssche FA: Fetal and neonatal effects of treatment with angiotensin-converting enzyme inhibitors in pregnancy. Obstet Gynecol 1991;78:128–135.
36. Hare DL, Davis CR: Validation of a new depression scale for cardiac patients. J Psychosom Res 1996;40:379–386.
37. Harvison A, Jones BM, McBride M, Taylor F, Wright O, Chang VP: Rehabilitation after heart transplantation: the Australian experience. J Heart Lung Transplant 1988;7:337–341.
38. Helmberger PS: Unwrapping the second gift of life. The Inside Story of Transplants As Told By Recipients and their Families, Donor Familes and Health Professionals. Minneapolis: Chronimed Publishing, 1992.
39. Hunt SA: Pregnancy in heart transplant recipients: a good idea? J Heart Lung Transplant 1991;100:499–503.
40. Jalowiec A: Confirmatory factory analysis of the Jalowiec Coping Scale. In Waltz CF, Strickland OL (eds): Measurement of Nursing Outcomes. New York: Springer, 1988, pp 287–305.
41. Jalowiec A, Grady KL, White-Williams C: Stressors in patients awaiting a heart transplant. Behav Med 1994;19:145–154.
42. Jones BM, Change VP, Esmore D, Spratt P, Shanahan MX, Farnsworth AE, Keogh A, Downs K: Psychological adjustment after cardiac transplantation. Med J Aust 1988;149:118–122.
43. Jones BM, Taylor F, Downs K, Spratt P: Longitudinal study of quality of life and psychological adjustment after cardiac transplantation. Med J Aust 1992;157:24–26.
44. Jones BM, Taylor FJ, Wright OM, Spratt P, Shanahan MX, Farnsworth AE, Keogh A, Downs K: Quality of life after heart transplantation in patients assigned to double or triple drug therapy. J Heart Lung Transplant 1990;9:392.
45. Key TC, Resnik R, Dittrich HC, Reisner LC: Successful pregnancy after cardiac transplantation. Am J Obstet Gynecol 1989;160:367–371.
46. Kobashigawa J, Leaf DA, Lee N, Gleeson MP, Liu HH, Hamilton MA, Moriguchi JD, Kawata N, Einhorn K, Herlihy E, Laks H: A controlled trial of exercise rehabilitation after heart transplantation. N Engl J Med 1999;340:272–277.
47. Kuhn WF, Davis MH, Lippman SB: Emotional adjustment to cardiac transplantation. Gen Hosp Psychiatry 1988;10:108.
48. Littlefield C, Abbey S, Fiducia D, Cardella C, Greig P, Levy G, Maurer J, Winton T: Quality of life following transplantation of the heart, liver, and lungs. Gen Hosp Psychiatry 1996;18:36S–47S.

49. Lough ME, Lindsey AM, Shian JA, Stotts NA: Life satisfaction following heart transplant. J Heart Lung Transplant 1985;4:446–449.
50. Lough ME, Lindsey AM, Shinn JA, Stotts NA: Impact of symptom frequency and symptom distress on self-reported quality of life in heart transplant recipients. Heart Lung 1987;16:193–200.
51. Lowenstein BR, Vain NW, Perrone SV, Wright DR, Boullon FJ, Favaloro RG: Successful pregnancy and vaginal delivery after heart transplantation. Am J Obstet Gynecol 1988;158:589–590.
52. Mai FM, McKenzie FN, Kostuk WJ: Psychosocial adjustment and quality of life following heart transplantation. Can J Psychiatry 1990;35:223–227.
53. Mancini DM, Walter G, Reichek N, Lenkinski R, McCully KK, Mullen JL, Wilson JR: Contribution of skeletal muscle atrophy to exercise intolerance and altered muscle metabolism in heart failure. Circulation 1992;85:1364–1373.
54. Mandak JS, Aaronson KD, Mancini DM: Serial assessment of exercise capacity after heart transplantation. J Heart Lung Transplant 1995;14:468–478.
55. Maricle RA, Hosenpud JD, Norman DJ, Woodbury A, Pantley GA, Cobanoglu AM, Starr A: Depression in patients being evaluated for heart transplantation. Gen Hosp Psychiatry 1989;11:418.
56. McAlear MJ, Copeland J, Fuller J, Copeland J: Psychological aspects of heart transplantation. J Heart Lung Transplant 1991;10:125–128.
57. McGiffin DC, Naftel DC, Spann JL, Kirklin JK, Young JB, Bourge RC, Mills RM: Risk of death or incapacitation after heart transplantation, with particular reference to pilots. J Heart Lung Transplant 1998;17:497–504.
58. Meister ND, McAleer MJ, Meister JS: Returning to work after heart transplantation. J Heart Lung Transplant 1986;5:154–161.
59. Molzahn AE, Burton JR, McCormick P, Modry DC, Soetaert P, Taylor P: Quality of life of candidates for and recipients of heart transplants. Can J Cardiol 1997;13:141–146.
60. Mulcahy D, Fitzgerald M, Wright C, Sparrow J, Pepper J, Yacoub M, Fox KM: Long term followup of severely ill patients who underwent urgent cardiac transplantation. BMJ 1993;306:98–101.
61. Mulligan T, Sheehan H, Hanrahan J: Sexual function after heart transplantation. J Heart Lung Transplant 1991;10:125–128.
62. Niset G, Coustry-Degre C, Degre S: Psychosocial and physical rehabilitation after heart transplantation: 1 year followup. Cardiology 1988;75:311–317.
63. Olivari MT, Yancy CW, Rosenblatt RL: An individualized protocol is more accurate than a standard protocol for assessing exercise capacity after heart transplantation. J Heart Lung Transplant 1996;15:1069–1074.
64. Osada N, Chaitman BR, Donohue TJ, Wolford TL, Stelken AM, Miller LW: Long term cardiopulmonary exercise performance after heart transplantation. Am J Cardiol 1997;79:451–456.
65. Packa D: Quality of life of adults after heart transplant. J Cardiovasc Nurs 1989;3:12–22.
66. Paris W, Woodbury A, Thompson S, Levick M, Nothegger S, Hutkin-Slade L, Arbuckle P, Cooper DK: Social rehabilitation and return to work after cardiac transplantation—a multi center survey. Transplantation 1992;53:433–438.
67. Paris W, Woodbury A, Thompson S, Levick M, Nothegger S, Hutkin-Slade L, Arbuckle P, Cooper DK: Returning to work after heart transplantation. J Heart Lung Transplant 1993;12:45–54.
68. Pennock JL, Oyer PE, Reitz BA, Jamieson SW, Bieber CP, Wallwork J, Stinson EB, Shumway NE: Cardiac transplantation in perspective for the future. J Thorac Cardiovasc Surg 1982;83:168–177.
69. Prieto C, Errasti P, Olaizola J, Morales JM, Andres A, Medina C, Ortuno B, Purroy A, Rodicio JL: Successful twin pregnancies in renal transplant recipients taking cyclosporine. Transplantation 1989;48:1065–1067.
70. Pritchard JA: Changes in the blood volume during pregnancy and delivery. Anesthesiology 1965;26:393–399.
71. Renlund DG, Taylor DO, Ensley RD, OConnell JB, Gilbert EM, Bristow MR, Ma H, Yanowitz FG: Exercise capacity after heart transplantation: influence of donor and recipient characteristics. J Heart Lung Transplant 1996;15:16–24.
72. Rickenbacher PR, Lewis NP, Valantine HA, Luikart H, Stinson EB, Hunt S: Heart transplantation in patients over 54 years of age. Eur Heart J 1997;18:870–878.
73. Riether AM, Smith SL, Lewison BJ, Cotsonis GA, Epstein CM: Quality of life changes and psychiatric and neurocognitive outcome after heart and liver transplantation. Transplantation 1992;54:444–450.
74. Rose ML, Dominguez M, Leaver N, Lachno R, Yacoub MH: Analysis of T cell subpopulations and cyclosporine levels in the blood of two neonates born to immunosuppressed heart/lung transplant recipients. Transplantation 1989;48:224–226.
75. Rosenblum DS, Rosen ML, Pine ZM, Rosen SH, Borg-Stein J: Health status and quality of life following cardiac transplantation. Arch Phys Med Rehabil 1993;74:490–493.
76. Saltin B, Blomqvist G, Mitchell J, Johnson RL, Wildenthal K, Chapman CB: Response to exercise after bed rest and after training. Circulation 1968;37(suppl):1–87.
77. Samuelsson RG, Hunt SA, Schroeder JS: Functional and social rehabilitation of heart transplant recipients under age thirty. Scand J Thorac Cardiovasc Surg 1984;18:97–103.
78. Schweizer RT, Rovelli M, Palmeri D, Vossler E, Hull D, Bartus S: Noncompliance in organ transplant recipients. Transplantation 1990;49:374–377.
79. Shapiro PA: Life after heart transplantation. Prog Cardiovasc Dis 1990;32:405–418.
80. Shapiro PA, Kornfeld DS: Psychiatric outcome of heart transplantation. Gen Hosp Psychiatry 1989;11:352–357.
81. Shapiro PA, Williams DL, Foray AT, Gelman IS, Wukich N, Sciacca R: Psychosocial evaluation and prediction of compliance problems and morbidity after heart transplantation. Transplantation 1995;12:1462–1466.
82. Skotzko CE: Quality of life after heart transplantation. In Cooper DK, Miller LW, Patterson GA (eds): The Transplantation and Replacement of Thoracic Organs. Hingham, MA: Kluwer Academic Publishers, 1996, pp 405–407.
83. Skotzko CE, Brownfield E, Kobashigawa J: Nonpsychotic psychiatric disorders and outcome after cardiac transplantation. Psychosomatics 1994;35:200.
84. Stevenson LW, Dracup KA, Tilliach JH: Efficacy of medical therapy tailored for severe congestive heart failure in patients transferred for urgent cardiac transplantation. Am J Cardiol 1988;58:1046–1050.
85. Stevenson LW, Sietsema K, Tilliach JH, Lem V, Walden J, Kobashigawa J: Exercise capacity for survivors of cardiac transplantation or sustained medical therapy for heart failure. Circulation 1990;81:78–85.
86. Stewart AL: Conceptual and methodologic issues in defining quality of life: state of the art. Prog Cardiovasc Nurs 1992;7:3–11.
87. Tabler JB, Frierson RL: Sexual concerns after heart transplantation. J Heart Lung Transplant 1990;9:397–403.
88. Troche V, Ville Y, Fernandez H: Pregnancy after heart or heart/lung transplantation: a series of 10 pregnancies. Br J Obstet Gynecol 1998;105:454–458.
89. Wagoner LE, Taylor DO, Olsen SL: Immunosuppressive therapy, management, and outcome of heart transplant recipients during pregnancy. J Heart Lung Transplant 1994;13:993–1000.
90. Wagoner LE, Taylor DO, Olsen SL, Price GD, Rasmussen LG, Larsen CB, Scott JR: Immunosuppressive therapy, management and outcome of heart transplant recipients during pregnancy. J Heart Lung Transplant 1993;26:993–1000.
91. Walden JA, Stevenson LW, Dracup K, Wilmarth J, Kobashigawa J, Moriguchi J: Heart transplantation may not improve quality of life for patients with stable heart failure. J Heart Lung Transplant 1989;18:497–506.
92. Wallwork J, Caine N: A comparison of the quality of life of cardiac transplant patients and coronary artery bypass graft patients before and after surgery. Qual Life Cardiovasc Care 1985;317:331.
93. Watson D: Intraindividual and interindividual analyses of positive and negative affect: their relation to health compliance, perceived stress, and daily activities. J Pers Soc Psychol 1988;54:1020–1030.
94. Watson D: The vicissitudes of mood measurement: effects of varying descriptors, time frames, and response formats on measures of positive and negative affect. J Pers Soc Psychol 1988;55:128–141.
95. Watson D, Clark LA. The PANAS-X: preliminary manual for the positive and negative affect schedule—expanded form. Southern Methodist University 1991;2:35.
96. World Health Organization: Measurement of Quality of Life in Children. Geneva: World Health Organization, 1993.

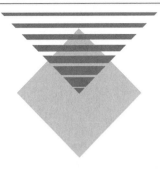

Special Situations in Heart Transplantation

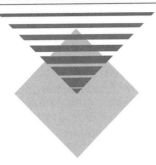

CHAPTER TWENTY

Pediatric Heart Transplantation

with the collaboration of
RICHARD E. CHINNOCK, M.D. AND F. BENNETT PEARCE, M.D.

Many aspects of the application of cardiac transplantation to infants and children follow directly from the principles practiced in adult cardiac transplantation. However, with the evolution and maturation of the field, many aspects of recipient selection, management of the patient prior to transplantation, techniques of cardiac transplantation, immunosuppressive strategies, and long-term management of pediatric patients have required a fund of information and a level of expertise which differs in many respects from adult cardiac transplantation. A few of the unique issues in pediatric transplantation have been highlighted in Table 20–1. Indeed, many experienced institutions have a completely separate pediatric heart transplant team which focuses on pediatric heart transplantation, just as with congenital heart disease in general. This chapter

TABLE 20-1	Pediatric Versus Adult Heart Transplantation—Issues of Distinction

- Congenital heart disease (technical challenges)
    Anatomic limitations
    Small patient size
- Maturity/immaturity of the immune system
- Greater likelihood of needing retransplantation
- Difficulty with suitable ventricular assist devices
- Unusual underlying diseases mandating transplantation
- More challenging psychosocial issues by nature of patient/family dependence
- Greater likelihood of neurologic defects

will discuss those unique aspects of pediatric transplantation.

The application of heart transplantation to children and infants seems almost preordained when we recall its historical development. Although routine successful cardiac transplantation in neonates and infants would await the pioneering efforts of Bailey and his colleagues at Loma Linda in the mid-1980s,[14] the first attempt at neonatal heart transplantation occurred nearly 20 years before, when Adrian Kantrowitz performed the world's second human heart transplant in an 18-day-old infant with Ebstein's malformation and refractory congestive heart failure. The patient received the heart of an anencephalic infant, but died 5 hours after the transplant procedure.[144] The first successful neonatal heart transplant for hypoplastic left heart syndrome was performed by Bailey in 1985.[75]

In the current era, approximately 3,500–4,000 heart transplants are performed per year according to data from the International Society of Heart and Lung Transplantation (ISHLT) Registry.[126] Worldwide, approximately 350–400 pediatric heart transplants are currently performed annually in a limited number of centers, constituting about 10% of the overall heart transplant experience.[30, 35] The ISHLT registry has identified fewer than 90 centers worldwide in this activity since 1993.[35]

CONDITIONS CONSIDERED FOR CARDIAC TRANSPLANTION

The optimal selection of pediatric recipients for cardiac transplantation is in a state of evolution, since knowledge of the natural history of many of the pediatric conditions for which cardiac transplantation is recommended is currently incomplete, and the long-term results (>10 years) of pediatric transplantation are currently unknown. The issue is further complicated by a somewhat different definition of "successful therapy" for an infant or child undergoing cardiac transplantation compared to most adults. Ten years of additional survival with transplantation would allow many young adults with end-stage heart disease the chance to see their children grow to adulthood and provide older adults a decade of additional quality survival; such would be considered successful therapy for an adult suffering from advanced symptoms of heart failure with limited life expectancy. However, "successful" trans-

plantation for the pediatric patient must provide a high likelihood of survival into adulthood and potentially beyond, thus requiring survival of 20 years or more, with the expectation of retransplantation for some or most of the survivors.

For the patient with profound systemic ventricular dysfunction and advanced symptoms of heart failure after previous corrective or palliative cardiac surgery, the decision for cardiac transplantation is readily made, since the quality and predicted duration of life without such therapy are particularly poor. In many other conditions for which cardiac transplantation is currently employed, the decision-making process is more complex, since sufficient information is not available to predict which therapy or combination of therapies will provide the best opportunity for truly long-term survival.

There are currently five general categories of disease processes for which cardiac transplantation is considered as a therapeutic option. These categories include (1) cardiomyopathic processes, (2) anatomically uncorrectable congenital heart disease, (3) congenital heart disease at high risk for repair, (4) refractory heart failure after previous surgery for congenital heart disease, and (5) rare indications such as unresectable cardiac tumors and/or intractable arrhythmias (Table 20–2). Among infants (<1 year of age), congenital heart disease accounts for 75–80% of diagnoses (of which two thirds currently are hypoplastic left heart syndrome), and cardiomyopathies account for only about 10% of diagnoses.[35, 49] In contrast, cardiomyopathy is the principal diagnosis in patients aged 1–10 and 11–17 years. The distribution of diagnoses for infants and children under 18 years of age undergoing cardiac transplantation in the multi-institutional Pediatric Heart Transplant Study (PHTS) (1993–1997) is listed in Table 20–3. One third of the patient population was less than 1 month of age at listing, nearly all carrying a diagnosis of hypoplastic left heart syndrome (Table 20–4).[188]

CARDIOMYOPATHY

The primary disorders of heart muscle (cardiomyopathy) in infants and children (which exclude congenital

TABLE 20-2	Conditions Considered for Pediatric Cardiac Transplantation

Cardiomyopathy
    Dilated
    Hypertrophic
    Restrictive
Anatomically uncorrectable congenital heart disease
    Hypoplastic left heart syndrome
    Pulmonary atresia, intact ventricular septum plus sinusoids
    Severely unbalanced atrioventricular (AV) septal defects with AV valve insufficiency
    Other forms of "single ventricle" poorly suited for Fontan pathway
Congenital heart disease at high risk for repair
    Severe Shone's complex
    Interrupted aortic arch and severe subaortic stenosis
    Critical aortic stenosis with severe endocardial fibroelastosis
    Ebstein's anomaly in a symptomatic newborn
Refractory heart failure after previous cardiac surgery
Unresectable symptomatic cardiac neoplasms

TABLE 20-3	Recipient Diagnosis: Pediatric Heart Transplant Study; Patients Listed for Cardiac Transplantation from 1993–1998 (N = 1,235)		
DIAGNOSIS		**N**	**% of 1,235**
Hypoplastic left heart syndrome*		337	27%
Other forms of complex congenital heart disease		402	33%
Idiopathic dilated cardiomyopathy		296	24%
Myocarditis		61	4.9%
Hypertropic cardiomyopathy		29	2.3%
Restrictive cardiomyopathy		50	4.0%
Adriamycin cardiac toxicity		19	1.5%
Ischemic cardiomyopathy		16	1.3%
Cardiomyopathy secondary to acquired valvular disease		3	0.2%
Postpartum cardiomyopathy		3	0.2%
Becker's muscular dystrophy		6	0.5%
Glycogen storage disease		2	0.2%
Carnitine deficiency		1	0.1%
Metabolic disease		1	0.1%
Familial cardiomyopathy		1	0.1%
Cardiac tumor		4	0.3%
Left ventricular fibroma		1	0.1%
Maternal systemic lupus erythematosis		1	0.1%
Unknown		2	0.2%
Total		1,235	100%

*Includes 91 patients who had a Norwood, bidirectional Glenn, or Fontan procedure prior to listing.

cardiac malformations or acquired cardiac disorders in which heart muscle is *not primarily* affected) occur in three basic patterns: dilated cardiomyopathy, hypertrophic cardiomyopathy, and restrictive cardiomyopathy.[41] Right ventricular dysplasia (arrhythmogenic right ventricular cardiomyopathy[71] and isolated left ventricular (myocardial) non-compaction[59] are additional rare cardiomyopathies seen in children. Although most cases are considered "idiopathic," molecular genetic techniques have uncovered differing etiologies for many of the common clinical and echocardiographic patterns. Most current clinical therapy involves the treatment of the phenotype that is the end-result of these various etiologies, but improved understanding of the etiologies and the mechanisms by which the heart is affected may allow for therapies that modify the course of myocardial damage. Cardiomyopathies occur in all pediatric age groups, even small infants. Among newborn infants, the incidence of cardiomyopathy is approximately 1 in 10,000 live births.[38]

TABLE 20-4	Pediatric Patients Listed for Cardiac Transplantation: Pediatric Heart Transplant Study, 1993–1998 (N = 1,235)	
AGE AT LISTING	**NO.**	**%**
<0	23	2%
0–1 mo	368	30%
1 mo–6 mo	153	12%
6 mo–12 mo	81	7%
1 yr–6 yr	199	16%
6 yr–12 yr	166	13%
12 yr–18 yr	245	20%
Total	1,235	100%

Adapted from McGiffin DC, Naftel DC, Kirklin JK, Morrow WR, Towbin J, Shaddy R, Alejos R, Rossi A: Predicting outcome following listing for cardiac transplantation in children: comparison of Kaplan-Meier and parametric competing risk analysis. J Heart Lung Transplant 1997;16:713–722.

Dilated Cardiomyopathy

Dilated cardiomyopathy is characterized by left or biventricular systolic dysfunction with increased ventricular cavity size without a commensurate increase in left ventricular wall thickness. Dilated cardiomyopathy is the most common form of cardiomyopathy to present with symptoms in childhood and adolescence.

Etiologies

Acute myocarditis as a cause of subsequent cardiomyopathy is documented in a minority of cases and requires endomyocardial biopsy to establish the diagnosis. In general, the pathological diagnosis is based on the finding of myocardial cell injury with degeneration or necrosis and an inflammatory infiltrate which is not secondary to ischemia.[183] Pathological criteria have been established for myocarditis which is "active," "borderline," "persistent," and "resolving."[183] In infants, the finding of acute inflammation by biopsy has been a favorable prognostic sign for subsequent recovery.[185] Viral nucleic acid has been isolated from autopsy, pathologic, and endomyocardial biopsy specimens,[183] but even with multiple biopsies, evidence of viral infection accompanying (and potentially causing) the episode of myocarditis is documented in less than 50% of cases, related partly to the focal nature of viral myocarditis[63] and partly to the intensity of investigative efforts. The use of polymerase chain reaction (PCR) and in situ hybridization techniques have increased the yield of virus from endomyocardial biopsies to about 65% of biopsied myocarditis cases.[183]

The viruses most commonly implicated are enteroviruses (especially Coxsackie B virus) and adenovirus. The virus is presumed to exert a pathologic effect through direct cytopathic and subsequent autoimmune mechanisms. Considerable evidence from animal models indicates myofiber necrosis within 3 days of myocardial viral infection, followed by infiltrating macrophages, natural killer cells, and protective antiviral antibodies 3–12 days after inoculation.[172, 184, 223, 234] Cell-mediated immune mechanisms have been implicated in the chronic phase of tissue injury after acute viral infection which ultimately leads to dilated cardiomyopathy. Using PCR and other molecular detection techniques, persisting viral RNA is often identified in areas of chronic myocardial injury. Possible mechanisms of viral participation in the transition between acute myocarditis and dilated cardiomyopathy include continuous triggering of the immune inflammatory response or recurrence of acute infection and exacerbation of the inflammatory response.[184] The presence of costimulatory molecules B7-1, B7-2, and CD-40 on cardiac myocytes in patients with myocarditis may potentiate myocyte attack by infiltrating T-cells and provides additional support for an autoimmune mechanism.[247]

Therapy for myocarditis involves immune modulation in addition to symptomatic treatment for the associated congestive heart failure. Intravenous gamma globulin has been shown to decrease the mortality and hasten the recovery of ventricular function in children presenting with acute onset left ventricular dysfunction.[82] In an uncontrolled study, prednisone appeared to improve outcome in some children with biopsy-proven myocarditis.[54] However, animal studies indicate that administration of steroids early during the viral replication phase can actually enhance myocardial damage, whereas later administration may be beneficial.[269] Recently, the use of dual therapy immunosuppression (cyclosporine and prednisolone) was shown to benefit children with biopsy-proven myocarditis.[157] Controlled clinical trials have not yet produced secure information that such therapy affects the natural history of acute myocarditis.

Familial dilated cardiomyopathy, in which a familial pattern of inheritance can be identified, may account for 20% or more of pediatric cases of dilated cardiomyopathy.[15] The mode of inheritance is frequently autosomal dominant. Baig and colleagues found echocardiographic abnormalities in 30% of asymptomatic relatives, of which more than one fourth progressed to develop overt dilated cardiomyopathy.[15] Genetic studies have localized the genetic defect to the long arm of chromosome 1 (1q32) in at least one large familial group.[85] Abnormalities in cytoskeletal proteins (in contrast to contractile proteins) have been linked to dilated cardiomyopathy.[147]

Anthracycline cardiomyopathy results from anthracycline compounds, which have been used to treat leukemias and solid tumors in children for nearly 30 years. Doxorubicin (Adriamycin), a cytotoxic anthracycline antibiotic isolated from a streptomyces species, is a common chemotherapeutic agent with cardiac toxicity as a major side effect. The cytotoxic effect on malignant cells results from inhibition of nucleotide replication and inhibition of DNA and RNA polymerases. The mechanism of cardiac toxicity is probably different, and oxygen free radical formation[255] with reduction of copper and iron has been implicated in the induction of cardiac myocyte apoptosis.[299] Early acute toxicity can occur during ther-

apy, is associated with lymphocyte infiltration and myocardial cell necrosis on biopsy, and is usually reversible if the anthracycline is discontinued.

Late cardiac failure and subclinical abnormalities of cardiac function can occur as well, and the most powerful predictor of late heart failure is the cumulative anthracycline dose. The likelihood of developing heart failure after doxorubicin therapy is estimated to be 1.5% at a cumulative dose of 300 mg/m², 5% at 400 mg/m², nearly 8% at 450 mg/m², and 20% at 500 mg/m². Additional risk factors for development of cardiomyopathy include prior mediastinal irradiation, concurrent administration of cyclophosphamide, and younger patient age (<4 years).

Although many patients who develop cardiomyopathy develop symptoms of heart failure within the first year, occasional patients may recover and then relapse or progress to worsening heart failure years later.[171] Particularly in children, the interval between anthracycline therapy and the development of severe heart failure may be as long as 6–10 years.[106] Anthracyclines appear to impair myocardial growth, and progression of somatic growth without appropriate increases in ventricular wall thickness may be one of the mechanisms responsible for the delayed development of cardiac abnormalities and congestive heart failure.[171] Thus, children may be at particular risk for delayed cardiac toxicity, and progressive congestive heart failure may not develop until adolescence or early adulthood.

In order to limit toxicity, monitoring of echocardiographic shortening fraction or ejection fraction by multiple gated acquisition scanning (MUGA) has become a standard part of most chemotherapeutic protocols, instituting dose reduction or drug discontinuation at the earliest signs of ventricular dysfunction. In addition to cardiac imaging techniques, newer biochemical markers of cardiac injury such as troponin T may play a role in the future.[212] The effectiveness of specific monitoring techniques for the purpose of chemotherapy dose reduction in the prevention of myocardial injury remains controversial.[171]

At present, the only effective therapy for end-stage anthracycline cardiomyopathy is transplantation. This may produce an important demand on the available donor pool when one considers estimates that by the year 2010, 1 out of 250 adults age 15–45 will be a survivor of childhood cancer.[29]

Cardiomyopathy secondary to inherited systemic disease processes can be grouped into three broad categories: inborn errors of metabolism (including storage diseases and disorders that produce toxic metabolites), muscular dystrophies, and mitochondrial cardiomyopathies. Identification of systemic disease etiologies in cases of cardiomyopathy is important for several reasons: (1) these inherited disorders may account for as much as 20% of dilated cardiomyopathies; (2) this may eventually allow for etiology-specific therapy; (3) the natural history of the underlying disorder may make transplantation an unwise option; and (4) genetic counseling may be provided for the family once the systemic disorder and the inheritance pattern are known. Because there are so many diagnostic tests available to the practitioner, an approach which is guided by historical data, extracardiac features on physical exam, and basic biochemical patterns of presentation has been advocated. This should eliminate the "shotgun" approach to these evaluations and help ensure more complete workups in specific categories. A detailed categorization and diagnostic approach has been provided by Schwartz and Towbin.[245, 272] Because of the frequency of associated malformations or dysfunction involving multiple organ systems, children with these inherited systemic disease processes are rarely referred for cardiac transplantation. Particular interest has focused on the role of carnitine (see Box) in the development and treatment of inherited infant and childhood cardiomyopathy.

Origin of the left coronary artery from the pulmonary artery can present at any time in the first year of life with congestive heart failure, left ventricular dilation, and systolic dysfunction.[284] This condition is mentioned here since it can mimic other forms of cardiomyopathy and responds to corrective surgical therapy (without transplantation) if the diagnosis is made promptly. The physical exam and history may not pro-vide any clue to the etiology at the time of presentation. The electrocardiogram (ECG) may distinguish between anomalous left coronary and acute myocarditis.[140] Use of three variables (Q-wave width in lead I, Q-wave depth and ST amplitude in lead aVL) yielded a sensitivity of 100% and specificity of 96%. The diagnosis may be confirmed with color Doppler findings of a typical retrograde diastolic signal in the pulmonary artery (which is distinct in location from the typical signal produced by a patent ductus arteriosus)[145, 243] or with angiographic aortic root injection. In addition to important left ventricular dysfunction, patients may have significant mitral regurgitation. The untreated mortality is in excess of 90%.[284] Surgical connection of the anomalous coronary artery to the aorta is the therapy of choice, often producing partial or complete recovery of left ventricular systolic function.[246] Concomitant surgical maneuvers to reduce mitral valve incompetence may be necessary.

Incessant supraventricular tachycardia may induce dilated cardiomyopathy and is important to consider, since it is reversible with proper therapy.[252] The finding of a heart rate consistent with sinus tachycardia may delay diagnosis. A 12-lead electrocardiogram (ECG) is needed to assess the p-wave axis, as the rhythm may be mistaken for sinus tachycardia on a single monitor lead. Identification and therapy of the tachycardia may reverse the ventricular dysfunction. Chronic ventricular tachycardia may produce a similar picture, but is less likely to be confused with sinus tachycardia on ECG.[101]

Carnitine

L-Carnitine is levocarnitine, which is 3-hydroxy-44-N-trimethylaminobutyric acid. Carnitine is present in all tissues and is an essential cofactor in mitochondrial energy metabolism, facilitating the transport of long-chain fatty acids across the inner mitochondrial membrane. The initial step in this transport process is the activation of fatty acid with coenzyme A (CoA) in the cytosol to form fatty acyl-CoA. The activated fatty acyl-CoA requires carnitine for its transport into the mitrochondria via the enzyme carnitine acyltransferase I. Since the heart is chiefly dependent on aerobic breakdown of fat for its energy supply, insufficient availability of carnitine can produce progressive myocardial dysfunction. This insufficiency of carnitine can result from inborn areas of metabolism, poor dietary intake or malabsorbation of carnitine, and excessive losses of carnitine in the urine secondary to altered renal tubular function.[264] An autosomal recessive disorder of carnitine membrane transport has been described which results in low muscle carnitine levels and low plasma levels.[271] Secondary carnitine deficiency states have also been described in which acyl-CoA builds up within the mitochondria secondary to inborn areas of metabolism (many of the organic acidurias), resulting in low levels of free carnitine and increased levels of acylcarnitines.

Carnitine levels are considered insufficient if the plasma free carnitine level is less than 20 mmol/L or the ratio of plasma acylcarnitine to free carnitine is greater than 0.4. Chronic carnitine administration (15–450 mg/kg/day) has been reported to produce improvement in the systolic cardiac function in some children with suspected carnitine deficiency.[290] When improvement occurs, it usually begins within days of initiating carnitine therapy but maximal improvement in ventricular size and function may require months or years.[290] Unfortunately, the mortality remains high (as much as 40%), even among patients with documented deficiency who receive carnitine replacement therapy.[290]

Clinical Course

The initial presentation may occur at any age, usually with the abrupt onset of congestive heart failure or with more chronic failure to thrive,[290] decreased appetite, and lethargy. Occasionally, there is an identifiable preceding viral illness. Atrial and ventricular dysrrhythmias are common.

Because of the relatively small number of patients at any one institution, the variety of possible etiologies, and the lack of uniform therapy, the true natural history and predictors of poor outcome have not been established with confidence. Marked differences in survival following diagnosis have been reported, with a first year mortality ranging from 20–40%[57, 95, 114, 185, 264] and 5-year mortality of 40–70%.[57, 185] Few reports have duplicated the very favorable survival of 84% at 10 years reported by Friedman and colleagues.[95]

Despite the lack of large patient cohorts for analysis, a number of **risk factors** for poor outcome have been suggested by a number of single-institution reports. Prognosis appears to differ somewhat according to age at onset, with a more favorable outcome in infants compared to children over about 5 years of age.[57, 95, 114] Familial cardiomyopathy and endocardial fibroelastosis portend a poor prognosis. Hemodynamic features associated with poor survival include severe persistent depression of left ventricular systolic function (shortening fraction ≤0.12 and ejection fraction <0.20),[57, 185] severe mitral regurgitation,[264] and persistent left ventricular end-diastolic pressure greater than or equal to 20 mm Hg.[45] However, in the case of myocarditis with hemodynamic compromise, patients with acute onset of high fever and shock (fulminant myocarditis) may paradoxically have a more favorable prognosis than other forms of acute myocarditis.[186] Other factors associated with worse outcome include mural thrombus on echocardiography,[264] globular (rather than elliptical) left ventricular shape,[57, 185] and presence of complex atrial and ventricular arrhythmias.[95, 114]

Indications for Cardiac Transplantation

There are currently no established guidelines about specific hemodynamic, echocardiographic, and clinical criteria which indicate the advisability of cardiac transplantation. However, the risk of death is highest during the first 3 months after presentation, so decisions regarding transplantation should be made relatively soon after intense medical therapy is initiated. When any of the risk factors listed above are present and there is persistence of severe hemodynamic derangement, poor systolic function and/or symptoms of severe congestive heart failure despite aggressive medical therapy, early referral for cardiac transplantation is recommended.

Hypertrophic Cardiomyopathy

Hypertrophic cardiomyopathy (HCM) is characterized by inappropriate left ventricular and occasionally right ventricular hypertrophy with preserved systolic function, with or without left ventricular outflow obstruction. The hypertrophic response occurs in the absence of an intracardiac or systemic stimulus for hypertrophy and is associated with microscopic evidence of myocardial fiber disarray.[105, 178, 287] The prevalence of HCM in adolescents has been estimated at 2 per 1,000 based on echocardiographic data,[177] and it is the most common cardiac cause of sudden death in teenagers and young adults.

The basic pathophysiologic manifestation of hypertrophic cardiomyopathy is impaired diastolic relaxation resulting in decreased ventricular compliance,[42, 286–288] possibly related to increased myocyte cytoplasmic calcium[115, 285] which interferes with the reuptake of calcium by the sarcoplasmic reticulum at the initiation of diastolic relaxation. Hypertrophic cardiomyopathy is divided into two subsets: those with obstruction (at either the subaortic or midventricular level) and those without obstruction. In nonobstructive HCM, systolic function is usually normal or supernormal until the disease reaches advanced stages, at which time impaired systolic function may develop.

Etiologies

The most well-defined form is familial hypertrophic cardiomyopathy, which has an autosomal dominant pattern of inheritance in over 75% of affected families.[180, 245] Chromosomal mutations have been found in the genes for B-myosin heavy chain, cardiac troponin-T, and α-tropomyosin.[134, 150, 286] Rare causes of hypertrophic cardiomyopathy include multiple inborn errors of metabolism and a variety of congenital malformation syndromes, especially Noonan's syndrome.[245]

Clinical Course

The clinical presentation is characterized by dyspnea, chest pain, syncope, and arrhythmias. Initial symptoms of congestive heart failure are rare. The natural history after diagnosis is highly variable. In patients with the **obstructive** form, the initial presentation may be sudden death in affected adolescents and young adults (who may be athletic). When left ventricular outflow obstruction is progressive, particularly with subaortic obstruction, recommended therapy includes dual chamber pacing or transaortic myectomy.

In the **nonobstructed** form, the annual mortality in pediatric patients is about 4–6% per year.[287] Long-term survival is importantly reduced when there is presentation in infancy, syncopal symptoms, a family history of progressive HCM,[179] myocardial ischemia,[78] progressive posterior left ventricular hypertrophy,[263] sustained ventricular tachycardia,[181, 191] mitral regurgitation, and development of atrial fibrillation.[286]

Indications for Cardiac Transplantation

Cardiac transplantation is generally reserved for symptomatic patients with multiple risk factors for poor survival or when impaired systolic function marks the onset of advanced stages of the disease.

Restrictive Cardiomyopathy

Restrictive cardiomyopathy is the rarest form of childhood cardiomyopathy, accounting for only about 5% of reported cases.[169] The hallmark is severe biventricular diastolic dysfunction with marked atrial enlargement. The ventricular size and systolic function are normal, but the atrial pressures are markedly elevated.

Etiologies

Most cases of restrictive cardiomyopathy in children are idiopathic.[76, 122, 146, 253] Other rare causes include infiltrative diseases of the myocardium such as amyloidosis, sarcoidosis, scleroderma, endomyocardial fibroelastosis, mucopolysaccharidoses, and glycogen storage disease.[76, 169] Some cases may be familial.

Clinical Course

Symptoms result from progressive systemic and pulmonary venous congestion. Embolic events may occur in up to one third of patients; anticoagulation is therefore advisable.[76] The natural history is not well known, but survival is generally poor, with reported 1- and 5-year survival of approximately 50% and 25%,[76, 169] respectively, with a median time from presentation to death of about 1 year.[52] This contrasts with the more favorable survival with adult forms of idiopathic restrictive cardiomyopathy, in whom the average life expectancy is 8 to 10 years.[8, 122, 146, 253]

Indications for Cardiac Transplantation

In view of the very poor natural history and the tendency for progressive increase in pulmonary vascular resistance, cardiac transplantation is advisable when the diagnosis is secure, hemodynamics are severely abnormal, and signs of systemic and pulmonary venous congestion are present.

ANATOMICALLY UNCORRECTABLE CONGENITAL HEART DISEASE

The term "anatomically uncorrectable congenital heart disease" includes any cardiac malformation for which a two-ventricle repair is not possible or advisable. For such patients, palliative operations including the modified Fontan procedure (creation of separation of the pulmonary and systemic circulations by using the ventricular mass as the systemic pump and creating a connection between the inferior and superior venae cavae and the pulmonary arteries, either directly or through the right atrium, without a ventricular pump in the pulmonary circuit) have been traditionally recommended. Cardiac transplantation is recommended for certain subsets with poor short-term or intermediate survival.

Hypoplastic left heart syndrome (HLHS) (see Box) currently represents the largest infant group undergoing cardiac transplantation.[198] Among 118 infants under 6

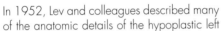

Hypoplastic Left Heart Syndrome

In 1952, Lev and colleagues described many of the anatomic details of the hypoplastic left heart syndrome as a pathologic complex which they called "hypoplasia of the aortic tract."[168] The term "hypoplastic left heart syndrome" was used by Noonan and Nadis in 1958 to describe this pathologic entity.[208] During the next decade, several publications emphasized atresia of the aortic valve as the critical component of hypoplastic left heart syndrome.[142, 274, 277] However, as palliative operations for this condition gained some success, the entity of "hypoplastic left heart syndrome" became less precise and in some reports included patients with variable degrees of aortic stenosis and hypoplasia of the left ventricle in which a two-ventricle repair may be possible. In the pure form of hypoplastic left heart syndrome, the features include atresia of the aortic valve and severe hypoplasia of the entire ascending aorta and arch up to the level of a large patent ductus arteriosus. The interventricular septum is intact, there is severe mitral valve hypoplasia or atresia, and a variable sized interatrial communication is present.

With current fetal echocardiographic technology, the diagnosis of hypoplastic left heart syndrome can be made *in utero* at 16–20 weeks of gestation. This provides adequate time for counseling the parents about the natural history of the disease and treatment options.

After birth, the systemic circulation is totally dependent upon patency of the ductus arteriosus. Without prostaglandin E_1 infusion, death occurs rapidly from systemic hypoperfusion when the ductus closes. With ductal patency, administration of oxygen usually aggravates the baby's condition by reducing the pulmonary vascular resistance and increasing pulmonary blood flow at the expense of systemic blood flow.

months of age listed for cardiac transplantation in the Pediatric Heart Transplant Study, 57% of patients carried a primary diagnosis of HLHS.[199]

The current recommended therapeutic options[221] are (1) an initial series of palliative operations leading to a later Fontan procedure or (2) cardiac transplantation. Treatment with a series of palliative reconstructive operations leading to the modified Fontan procedure has produced variable results. A few institutions have reported good early and intermediate-term survival,[88, 129, 132, 210] but many centers continue to experience a high early and midterm mortality.[132] The excellent early and intermediate-term survival after primary infant cardiac transplantation reported by Bailey and colleagues at Loma Linda,[13, 14] as well as other institutions (see later section, Survival), have encouraged a number of institutions to adopt infant cardiac transplantation as the treatment of choice for this condition. However, the shortage of available donors in the infant age group coupled with the mortality during extended prostaglandin support has yielded a 15–20% mortality prior to transplantation.[132, 199] When added to a 10% or greater hospital mortality for transplantation, the overall expected mortality at 6 months may approach 30–40% in experienced institutions.[132] Several institutions have reported improved results in first-stage palliation for HLHS which approach 70% 3-month survival,[129, 210] but at least two additional procedures are necessary for chronic palliation. Thus, there is currently no clear advantage of one strategy over the other (Fig. 20–1). In the report of a 21-institution experience with surgery for aortic atresia, Jacobs and colleagues concluded that either strategy (primary transplantation or Fontan pathway) could yield comparable 2- to 3-year survival at experienced centers with a strong institutional commitment to *one* of the two surgical management protocols.[132]

The long-term advantage of a strategy of initial Norwood procedure (reconstruction of the ascending aorta and arch using the main pulmonary artery and additional patch material plus construction of a central shunt) in preparation for a later Fontan procedure, versus initial transplantation must await years of follow-up, perhaps best accomplished through multi-institutional studies. It is likely that transplantation (or retransplantation) may eventually play an important role in both treatment strategies, either as primary therapy or as secondary therapy for some patients unable to undergo completion of the Fontan, some who experience a failed Fontan, and for some who experience important allograft vascular disease following initial transplantation.

Although secure long-term information is not yet available, the survival 5 or more years after neonatal or infant heart transplantation is superb if the patient survives to receive a donor heart and survives the initial transplant hospitalization. Thus, if the therapy is available, it is our opinion that cardiac transplantation will likely produce the best long-term survival. However, since at least 20% of such babies will die awaiting transplantation, we recommend that each institution adopt one of three primary policies (until more secure information is available) based on their experience and available expertise: (1) initial cardiac transplantation as primary

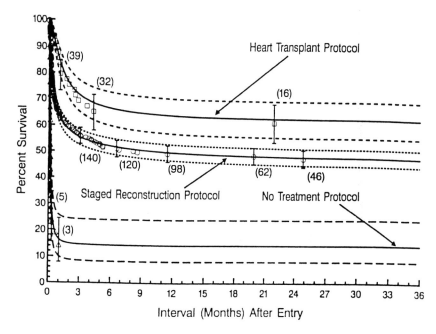

FIGURE **20-1.** Actuarial survival of neonates (n = 323) at 21 institutions in the Congenital Heart Surgeon's Study, entered into one of three treatment protocols for aortic atresia (hypoplastic left heart syndrome) between January 1, 1994, and January 1, 1997. Survival curves include all deaths from time of entry into the protocol. For the heart transplantation protocol, this includes deaths while awaiting transplant. The staged reconstruction protocol included an initial Norwood procedure in preparation for a later Fontan procedure. The vertical bars indicate ± 1 standard error. The numbers in parentheses indicate the number of patients remaining at the designated time in follow-up. The solid lines are the parametric estimates of survival, and the dashed lines enclose the 70% confidence limits. (From Jacobs ML, Blackstone EH, Bailey LL, The Congenital Heart Surgeons Society: Surgery for congenital heart disease (intermediate survival in neonates with aortic atresia: a multi-institutional study). J Thorac Cardiovasc Surg 1998;116:417–431.)

therapy, (2) initial Norwood procedure as a neonate with subsequent planned transplantation (unless right ventricular function remains normal), or (3) initial Norwood procedure with planned Fontan later (reserving transplantation for clinical failures before or after the Fontan). We prefer option 1 when possible.

Pulmonary atresia with intact ventricular septum is generally treated with the Fontan pathway. However, the subset with marked sinusoidal connections between the coronary arteries and the right ventricle (particularly if the distal coronary arterial tree fills from a right ventricular injection) has a particularly poor survival. Although a recent report suggests improved results with the Fontan pathway,[133] we currently recommend cardiac transplantation for this condition.

Complete atrioventricular septal defects with severe right or left ventricular dominance carry a high mortality with attempted correction. Patients with this malformation are generally considered for the Fontan pathway. In the presence of severe atrioventricular (AV) valve insufficiency, cardiac transplantation is advisable.

Other forms of **single-ventricle with severe left ventricular outflow tract obstruction** have been selected for cardiac transplantation by some groups.[34] However, when the ventricular morphology is suitable for a Damus procedure (use of the main pulmonary artery to establish a connection to the ascending aorta which "bypasses" an area of subaortic stenosis)[174] followed by a bidirectional Glenn shunt (connection of the superior vena cava to the right, or left, pulmonary artery), such patients can usually be effectively palliated with the Fontan approach.

It remains controversial whether **complex single ventricle with asplenia** is better treated by cardiac transplantation[34] or the Fontan approach. If such malformations are associated with specific risk factors for the Fontan operation, such as AV valve insufficiency or depressed systemic ventricular systolic function, cardiac transplantation is clearly advisable.

For all patients evaluated for the **Fontan pathway**, cardiac transplantation should be considered as the desired therapy, either initially or after a bidirectional Glenn procedure, when sufficient risk factors for death after the Fontan procedure are present to predict an early post-Fontan mortality of perhaps 20% or higher. These include such factors as important systemic AV valve insufficiency, moderate (but not severe) elevation of pulmonary vascular resistance, and depressed systemic ventricular function.

In the future, the options of palliative operations leading to the modified Fontan procedure and cardiac transplantation will become more complementary than competitive. Such an integrated approach will require much more complete information about the "extended-term" (20 years or more) results of pediatric cardiac transplantation, the benefit, if any, of cardiac transplantation within the first few months of life rather than later in childhood, the long-term results of the Fontan operation with a systemic ventricle of right ventricular morphology as in hypoplastic left heart syndrome, and the results of infant xenotransplantation. Eventually, sufficient knowledge about these issues will allow the development of an individual "therapeutic profile" for the patient with anatomically uncorrectable congenital heart disease in which primary cardiac transplantation or a series of palliative operations with or without subsequent cardiac transplantation can be rationally planned in a way that maximizes the probability of "extended-term" survival with good quality of life.

CONDITIONS AT HIGH RISK FOR CORRECTIVE OPERATION

Patients with potentially correctable congenital heart disease but at greatly increased operative risk can also be considered for cardiac transplantation. Differences in experience and surgical results at individual institutions compared to transplantation would influence the decision regarding cardiac transplantation versus attempted surgical correction in certain malformations such as complex truncus arteriosus (with severe truncal valve insufficiency, interrupted aortic arch, or coronary artery anomalies), some severe forms of Shone's syndrome, complex interrupted aortic arch, and certain other malformations. For example, interrupted aortic arch with severe or multiple levels of left ventricular outflow tract obstruction is associated with high early mortality with complete repair or palliation.[141] Although controversy exists regarding the anatomic definition of "severe left ventricular outflow tract obstruction," studies from the Congenital Heart Surgeon's Society[141] indicate a high mortality (40% or higher) with operations which include an initial procedure to enlarge the left ventricular outflow tract. Six-month mortality exceeded 40% when the left ventricular–aortic junction diameter was less than or equal to 4.0 mm (Z-value ≤ -7), and was even higher (approximately 75%) with multiple levels of obstruction.[141] These high-risk subsets should be considered for initial cardiac transplantation.

SEVERE HEART FAILURE AFTER PREVIOUS SURGERY FOR CONGENITAL HEART DISEASE

Following surgery for complex congenital heart disease, the two most common indications for cardiac transplantation are refractory systemic ventricular failure following a two-ventricle repair and a failed Fontan operation. Pediatric patients with advanced systemic ventricular failure following corrective surgery follow essentially the same medical treatment protocols and selection criteria for cardiac transplantation as for adult patients. A detailed discussion of these issues can be found in Chapters 5 and 6.

There continues to be uncertainty about **the long-term outcome after the Fontan procedure,** particularly with respect to the number of years of expected good quality

of life. Predictions are complicated by the continued evolution of surgical techniques and the variety of cardiac malformation for which the Fontan operation is utilized. Some useful insights into the long-term outcome after an optimal Fontan procedure is supplied by Fontan and colleagues.[89] From their analysis, it appears that the likelihood of deterioration to New York Heart Association (NYHA) Class III symptoms of heart failure increases after 12–14 years (Fig. 20–2) as does the hazard function for cardiac failure as a cause of late death (Fig. 20–3). When heart failure progresses to the development of recurrent ascites, generalized fluid retention, low systemic cardiac output, and occasionally progressive cyanosis without intracardiac shunting, the prognosis for even intermediate-term survival is poor. In the absence of mechanical obstruction between the right atrium and pulmonary arteries (which would require surgical revision), medical therapy is largely ineffective. Systemic ventricular systolic and diastolic function is usually reduced, and the situation is worse if there is moderate elevation of pulmonary vascular resistance. The central venous pressure is nearly always 20 mm Hg or higher. The limited survival coupled with the profound reduction in quality of life justifies cardiac transplantation for such patients. The development of progressive heart failure can be subtle, especially when the patient instinctively limits his or her activities to compensate. Patients who clearly are developing worsening heart failure post-Fontan should be referred for transplant evaluation early, since cardiac decompensation and the need for inotropic support is a sign of imminent death. In a multi-institutional study from the Pediatric Heart Transplant Study, Bernstein and colleagues found that among post-Fontan patients who are dependent on intravenous inotropes at the time of listing for transplantation, over one third die before a heart transplant can be performed.[26]

Some controversy exists regarding the safety of cardiac transplantation in the presence of extensive **pulmo-**

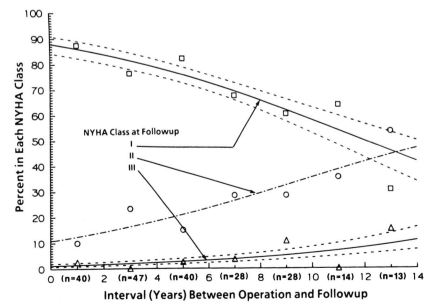

FIGURE **20–2.** Graph of nomogram of specific solution of logistic regression equation depicting time-related functional status of surviving patients after the Fontan operation. Along horizontal axis is interval between surgery and last follow-up; at each odd-numbered interval along horizontal axis is the number of patients (in parentheses) with that interval between surgery and last follow-up. Vertical axis indicates percentage of patients in New York Heart Association (NYHA) functional class at follow-up intervals. The dashed lines indicate the 70% confidence intervals. The symbols indicate actual percentages (NYHA Classes I, II, and III, respectively). (From Fontan F, Kirklin JW, Fernandez G, Costa F, Naftel DC, Tritto F, Blackstone EH: Outcome after a "perfect" Fontan operation. Circulation 1990;81:1520–1536.)

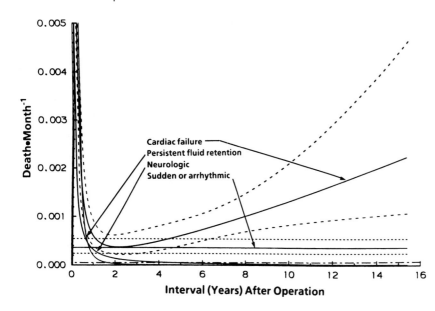

FIGURE **20-3.** Graph showing hazard function (instantaneous risk of death at each moment in time after surgery) of the most prevalent modes of death following the Fontan operation. The dashed lines indicate the 70% confidence limits. (From Fontan F, Kirklin JW, Fernandez G, Costa F, Naftel DC, Tritto F, Blackstone EH: Outcome after a "perfect" Fontan operation. Circulation 1990;81:1520–1536.)

nary arteriovenous malformations which occasionally occur in Fontan patients who have undergone a prior Glenn procedure. The potential exists for persistent desaturation following cardiac transplantation which could increase early morbidity and mortality. Lamour and colleagues reported three patients with extensive pulmonary arteriovenous malformations, a failed Fontan procedure, and an average arterial saturation of 67% (without intracardiac shunting). All three underwent successful cardiac transplantation and reconstruction of systemic venous connections, with early and late (2–40 months) systemic saturation greater than 95% on room air.[163] Graham and colleagues also reported prompt resolution of pulmonary arteriovenous malformations following heart transplantation.[108]

CARDIAC TUMORS

Unresectable cardiac tumors represent a rare indication for cardiac transplantation. Since primary cardiac tumors rarely metastasize, cardiac transplantation may be advised if there are no major associated congenital anomalies and the tumor is confined to the portion of the heart removed at transplantation. The most common tumor of infancy and childhood is rhabdomyoma, often with associated tuberous sclerosis. Although spontaneous tumor regression is common in tumors associated with tuberous sclerosis, heart transplantation may be indicated when there is severe left ventricular outflow obstruction, hemodynamic compromise, or serious ventricular arrhythmias.[257] In a 2-year experience reported by the multi-institution Pediatric Heart Transplant Study (1993–1994), cardiac transplant operations for a cardiac tumor represented less than 1% of transplants in children between the ages of 1 and 18 years.

RECIPIENT EVALUATION

Each potential recipient must undergo an evaluation which examines potential anatomic and physiologic de-

rangements as well as other organ system dysfunction, systemic illness, and social factors which may preclude transplantation as a therapeutic option.[93] A typical evaluation protocol for pediatric patients is provided in Table 20–5.[48] The general contraindications to pediatric cardiac transplantaton are listed in Table 20–6.

ANATOMIC CONSIDERATIONS

The major anatomic contraindication is **small pulmonary arteries** which cannot be satisfactorily enlarged surgically. Specific studies have not been performed to identify the lower limit of pulmonary artery size suitable for cardiac transplantation, but inferences can be drawn from studies in tetralogy of Fallot. Postrepair right ventricular systolic pressure in the presence of a normal pulmonary annulus (as in the case of cardiac transplantation) can be predicted as a function of right and left pulmonary artery size in the absence of anomalies of distribution and size of the peripheral pulmonary arteries[153] using the ratio of the angiographic diameter of the right pulmonary artery plus the left pulmonary artery divided by the descending aorta at the diaphragm (McGoon ratio).[28] A McGoon ratio of greater than about 2.0 predicts a right ventricular systolic pressure less than about 50 mm Hg, and a ratio less than 1.5 predicts a right ventricular systolic pressure greater than 60 mm Hg (assuming a left ventricular systolic pressure of 100 mm Hg) after repair of tetralogy. Experimental studies predict acute right ventricular failure after cardiac transplantation when the normal right ventricle must generate systolic pressures in excess of about 50 mm Hg to achieve adequate cardiac output. Our own clinical experiences among patients with elevated pulmonary vascular resistance supports the inference that the probability of acute right ventricular failure increases progressively when right ventricular systolic pressure exceeds approximately 50 mm Hg immediately following cardiac transplantation. Therefore, extrapolating from the McGoon ratio for tetralogy of Fallot, the risk of acute

TABLE 20-5	Pediatric Cardiac Transplantation Evaluation Protocol
Cardiology	Chest x-ray
	ECG
	Echocardiogram
	Exercise stress test including maximal oxygen consumption*
	May include endomyocardial biopsy
	May include drug studies to manipulate cardiac index and pulmonary vascular resistance
Hematology	Complete blood count and differential
	Prothrombin and partial thromboplastin time
Blood chemistry	Serum electrolytes, magnesium, calcium, phosphorus
	Serum transaminases, bilirubin, albumin, total protein, alkaline phosphatase, cholesterol, triglycerides, uric acid, lactic dehydrogenase, creatine phosphokinase, carnitine
Renal	Urinalysis
	Serum blood urea nitrogen and creatinine
	24-h urine collection for creatinine clearance
Pulmonary	Pulmonary function tests
Serology	CMV, EBV, varicella, herpes, hepatitis, HIV titers
Cultures	Blood, throat, urine, stool, sputum for bacterial viral, parasites, fungus†
Immunology	HLA typing
	Panel reactive antibody (titer and type of anti-HLA antibodies)
Neurology	CT or MRI scan†
	EEG†
Consultations	Neurology (also to exclude associated skeletal muscle disease)†
	Genetic†
	Psychology†
	Physical/occupational therapy†
	Dietetics†
	Social worker
	Financial/health insurance coordinatory

ECG, electrocardiogram; CMV, cytomegalovirus; EBV, Epstein-Barr virus; HIV, human immunodeficiency virus; HLA, human leukocyte antigen; CT, computerized tomographic; MRI, magnetic resonance imaging; EEG, electroencephalogram.
*When feasible.
†If medically indicated.

cardiac failure (and likely mortality) after cardiac transplantation would appear to increase progressively if the McGoon ratio by angiography is less than 2.0 and particularly if it is less than 1.5, unless the native pulmonary arteries can be augmented at the time of transplantation. To date, insufficient data are available to refine these predictions.

Other anatomic features which would preclude safe cardiac transplantation include subsets of anomalous pulmonary venous connection without a suitable pulmonary venous confluence for direct anastomosis to the donor left atrium (unless they connect directly to the coronary sinus or right atrium) or with pulmonary vein stenosis, important pulmonary artery hypoplasia or stenosis at or distal to the hilum, and ectopia cordis. Abnormalities of body situs, systemic venous return, and malpositions of the great vessels can be managed surgically at the time of cardiac transplantation[67, 79, 279] (see later section, Surgical Techniques).

PULMONARY VASCULAR RESISTANCE

As in adult cardiac transplantation, the major risk from elevated pulmonary vascular resistance (PVR) is acute right ventricular failure early following transplantation. When considering transplantation in **neonates and small infants** in the first few months of life, if the main and branch pulmonary arteries are normal in size and distribution, the elevated pulmonary vascular resistance of the newborn period usually rapidly normalizes after transplantation and is not associated with an increased incidence of right ventricular failure. An important exception may be persistence of **pulmonary venous obstruction** for weeks or months while awaiting cardiac transplantation which may produce marked elevation of pulmonary artery pressure that may not normalize promptly after cardiac transplantation and represents an important risk factor for early donor right ventricular failure. Physiologic pulmonary venous obstruction may occur with anomalous pulmonary venous connection with unrecognized obstruction, congenital pulmonary venous stenosis, or hypoplastic left heart syndrome with an atrial septal defect which is restrictive soon after birth. In general, cardiac catheterization is not necessary for the transplant evaluation of small infants less than about 3 months of age unless some type of pulmonary venous obstruction is suspected by echocardiography.

In older children and teenagers with cardiomyopathy, the hemodynamic evaluation is similar to that for adult recipients (see Chapter 6). As discusssed in the previous section, most well-preserved transplanted hearts can generate systolic pressures up to 50 mm Hg with adequate cardiac output. When the pulmonary artery and right ventricular systolic pressure immediately after transplantation exceed about 50 mm Hg, however, the probability of acute right ventricular distention, elevated right atrial pressure, and right ventricular failure with low systemic output increases. Although not proven, donor right ventricular reserves may be greater in a well-preserved donor heart, in donor hearts from neonates or small infants with elevated pulmonary vascular resistance of the newborn period, and possibly from donor hearts taken from larger donors (compared

TABLE 20-6	Contraindications to Pediatric Heart Transplantation

Irreversible elevated pulmonary vascular resistance (≥ 6 Wood units $\cdot$ m^2)
Diffuse hypoplasia of right and left pulmonary arteries
Total anomalous pulmonary venous connection without pulmonary venous confluence
Ectopia cordis
Active systemic infection
Infection with HIV or chronic active hepatitis B or C
Malignancy without cure or of recent onset
Severe primary renal or hepatic dysfunction
Multiorgan system failure
Major central nervous system abnormality
Severe dysmorphism
Marked prematurity (< 36 weeks)
Low birth weight (< 2 kg)
Positive drug screen
Lack of family support

to the recipient) as long as cardiac compression or right ventricular outflow obstruction does not occur secondary to a constricted recipient pericardial space.

The relationship between calculated PVR and the likelihood of acute posttransplant right ventricular failure and death remains controversial. In children, both indexed and nonindexed (Table 20–7) calculations of pulmonary vascular resistance have been used. Although theoretically a specific level or "cut-off" of PVR should be identifiable above which the probability of death becomes prohibitive, in practice that has not been possible. Several studies have identified higher pulmonary vascular resistance (treated as a continuous variable) as a risk factor for early mortality.[155] Traditionally, a resistance calculation of 6–7 indexed Wood units (WU · m²) has been suggested as a level above which transplantation is not recommended, but there are other factors which complicate this calculation. Perhaps the most important factor is **reactivity** of the pulmonary vascular bed in response to lowering of the left atrial (or pulmonary capillary wedge) pressure and/or to the administration of pulmonary vasodilator agents.[56] Thus, a **fixed resistance** of 6 WU · m² or more or a pulmonary artery systolic pressure exceeding about 55 mm Hg in the presence of left atrial pressure less than or equal to 20 mm Hg or a transpulmonary gradient (mean pulmonary artery pressure minus pulmonary capillary wedge pressure) exceeding about 15 mm Hg (which is unresponsive to vasodilator therapy) represent a clear contraindication to cardiac transplantation. When there is excessive pulmonary blood flow secondary to a patent ductus arteriosus (such as in hypoplastic left heart syndrome), patent systemic to pulmonary artery shunts, or aortopulmonary collateral flow, accurate calculation of pulmonary vascular resistance may be difficult or impossible. In patients with longstanding increased pulmonary blood flow who have pulmonary hypertension and normal or mildly increased left atrial pressure, there may be important fixed elevation of pulmonary vascular resistance with little or no reactive component to their disease. When this is identified, cardiac transplantation is contraindicated.

When the pulmonary artery systolic pressure is "reactive" to a high pulmonary capillary wedge pressure, intravenous vasodilator therapy may produce a reduction in pulmonary artery pressure (and resistance) either through direct pulmonary vasodilation or through reduction of left atrial pressure. Since most acutely transplanted hearts will maintain a left atrial pressure less than about 18 mm Hg in the early transplant period, a measured pulmonary artery pressure of less than 50 mm Hg with a wedge pressure of 20 or more in the face of normal or low normal cardiac output usually indicates pulmonary vascular resistance suitable for cardiac transplantation.

Vasodilator testing may involve acute testing in the catheterization laboratory (cath lab) or periodic reevaluation following longer duration therapy with infusions of inotropic or vasodilator agents for days or weeks in the hospital setting. Patients with poor left ventricular function and left atrial hypertension may have a dramatic fall in vascular resistance following periods of inotropic support and intensive heart failure management. Unfortunately, small studies in pediatric populations, lack of standardization of vasodilator protocols, and the heterogeneity of pediatric pulmonary hypertension conditions have made it difficult to recommend a standard approach for evaluation in the catheterization laboratory.

Vasodilator testing in the catheterization laboratory setting has historically been based on intravenous vasodilators. Some of these vasodilators include intravenous nitroprusside,[68] tolazoline,[46] acetylcholine,[1] isoproterenol,[193] adenosine,[209] prostaglandin E₁,[102, 152] prostacyclin, inhaled oxygen, and inhaled nitric oxide (NO). Undesirable effects of most intravenous vasodilators include systemic hypotension, changes in cardiac output, and worsening ventilation/perfusion mismatch. These effects can endanger the patient as well as negatively affect the quality of the data obtained at the time of vasodilator testing. In addition, cardiopulmonary bypass (at the time of transplantation) may result in reversible postoperative endothelial dysfunction. Thus, a favorable preoperative response with an endothelium-dependent agent may not be predictive of a similar postoperative response.

These problems with intravenous vasodilators and the early favorable reports of nitric oxide administration have led to the increased investigation of nitric oxide (see Box) as a vasodilator in the catheterization laboratory setting in children.[1, 24, 70, 161, 232] Based on its selective pulmonary properties, nitric oxide more closely approximates the "ideal" pulmonary vasodilator agent.[239] Further discussion of the use of nitric oxide following heart/lung transplantation is found in Chapter 21.

Many patients being evaluated for transplantation have compromised circulation and are potentially at risk for decompensation in the catheterization laboratory. For these reasons, the **conduct of the catheterization** is deliberate with a plan that is developed prior to the procedure in order to minimize catheter manipulation and duration of the catheterization. Meticulous supportive care can help prevent hemodynamic decompensation as well as variations which may adversely affect the quality of the data which forms the basis for decision-making. It is our practice (University of Alabama at Birmingham [UAB]) to have a cardiac anesthesia team present and participating in the procedure, since many patients are intubated and managed with neuromuscu-

---

TABLE 20–7 **Calculation of Indices of Pulmonary Vascular Resistance**

$$PVR \text{ (absolute units)} = \frac{80 \, (PA \, mean - LA)}{CO} \, dynes \cdot sec^{-1} \cdot cm^{-5}$$

$$PVR \, (WU) = \frac{PA \, mean - LA}{CO}$$

$$PVRI \, (WU \cdot m^2) = \frac{(PA \, mean - LA)}{CI}$$

$$TPG \text{ (mm Hg)} = PA \, mean - LA$$

PVR, pulmonary vascular resistance; WU, Wood units; PA mean, mean pulmonary pressure (mm Hg); LA, left atrial mean pressure (mm Hg), often approximated by capillary wedge pressure; CO, cardiac output; PVRI, pulmonary vascular resistance indexed to body surface area; CI, cardiac index (L/min/m²); TPG, transpulmonary gradient.

Nitric Oxide

The endothelial cell is important in the maintenance of resting pulmonary and systemic vascular tone. Nitric oxide (NO) was identified in 1987 as endothelium-derived relaxing factor, the product of endothelial cells that stimulates relaxation of adjacent vascular smooth muscle and produces vasodilation.[131, 216] Nitric oxide is produced in the endothelial cell from l-arginine by the enzyme nitric oxide synthase (NOS). Nitric oxide passes by diffusion from the endothelial cell to the vascular smooth muscle cell where it stimulates the production of intracellular cyclic guanosine monophosphate via the enzyme guanylate cyclase,[47] which in turn stimultes smooth muscle relaxation.

The healthy endothelial cell produces nitric oxide in response to acetylcholine infusion through its action on muscarinic receptors on the cell surface.[100] This "endothelium-dependant" vasodilator response is an indicator of the health of the endothelial cell. When the endothelial response is abnormal, vasodilator testing may not produce a response despite a large component of reversible vasoconstriction. Inhaled NO reaches the vascular smooth muscle cells directly and thus does not depend upon the health of the endothelium. It may produce a strong vasodilator response despite endothelial dysfunction (as demonstrated by the lack of vasodilation in response to an endothelium-dependant agent).[1]

Once the inhaled NO diffuses from the alveoli into the circulation, it is inactivated by hemoglobin as it enters the vessel lumen,[230] with a half-life of about 30 seconds. Because of these properties, NO is administered as a gas and is a selective pulmonary vasodilator. The breakdown of NO is accomplished by its rapid binding to hemoglobin to form methemoglobin. Since methemoglobin is incapable of binding with oxygen, the methemoglobin level must be monitored during NO therapy and maintained at a safe level of less than 5 g/dL. The concentration of NO as an inhalation agent is 5–80 parts per million (ppm). Higher concentrations are dangerous because of the rapid conversion of NO to highly toxic nitrogen dioxide (NO_2) in the presence of oxygen, which can produce pneumonitis and pulmonary edema.

NO is administered from a regulated cyclinder containing medical grade 400 ppm NO in pure N_2. Concentrations of inspired NO and NO_2 are monitored with an electrochemical analyzer. Inspired O_2 is monitored as well, and air/oxygen carrier gas flows are maintained in excess of 5 L/min to minimize transit time in the ventilation system. Excess gas flow from the ventilation system and the gas analyzer are scavenged to prevent environmental contamination. Stainless steel fittings are used in place of rubber connectors to prevent corrosion. Recently, we have used the Inovent (Ohmeda) system which has simplified the procedure and conforms to the above protocol for NO administration. Further details of nitric oxide chemistry, metabolism and clinical use are provided in Chapter 21.

tion or pulmonary vascular resistance are avoided. Oxygen saturation, end-tidal CO_2, heart rate, and blood pressure are monitored continuously. Samples for oximetery under baseline conditions and following medication administration are collected as closely together in time as is practical.

The calculation of pulmonary/systemic vascular resistance is standard (Table 20–7) and requires measurement of these pressures: pulmonary artery mean, systemic artery mean, right atrial mean, and left atrial mean (pulmonary capillary wedge may be used if the waveform appears physiologic). Systemic and pulmonary blood flow can be determined using thermodilution or oximetry. The pitfalls of thermodilution calculation of cardiac output are discussed in Chapter 6. The obtained value is indexed to the patient's body surface area. Oxygen samples are obtained from mixed venous, systemic arterial, pulmonary venous, and pulmonary arterial blood. Sampling from these sites will allow the calculation (estimation) of the magnitude and direction of any intracardiac shunt. The oxygen consumption can be measured using the polarographic technique with the Waters device[161] or can be estimated using the patient's age, sex, and heart rate according to standard tables.[283] When NO is used to assess pulmonary reactivity, it is administered with 100% O_2. The concentration of NO is monitored and not allowed to exceed 80 ppm and that of NO_2 is kept below 3 ppm. Hemodynamic measurements are obtained 10 minutes after initial NO exposure and after 10 minutes following each dose change.

GENETIC AND METABOLIC

As noted earlier in this chapter, cardiomyopathies in infants and children may have a genetic or metabolic etiology.[245] Inborn errors of metabolism may initially present with hypoketotic hypoglycemia, metabolic acidosis, hyperammonemia, acute or chronic encephalopathy, generalized hypotonia or muscle weakness, gross retardation, generalized failure to thrive, and/or coarse facial features. The presence of these findings in association with echocardiographic evidence of cardiomyopathy should stimulate a specific investigation for possible genetic inborn errors of metabolism. Because skeletal muscle abnormalities often coexist with genetic or metabolic cardiomyopathies, specific evaluation of muscle tone and strength is an important part of the evaluation. If abnormalities are detected, muscle biopsy may be indicated as well as consultation for neurologic and genetic evaluation.

NEUROLOGIC

Any patient with suspected neurologic disease or dysfunction should be evaluated by a pediatric neurologist. Specific neurologic evaluation is of particular importance in infants with ductal dependent circulation, who may have suffered a neurologic insult prior to recognition of their cardiac disease. In addition, poor cardiac function with its attendant poor perfusion of end organs may lead to compromise of neurologic function.

lar blockade in addition to anesthetic agents. The anesthetic agent used most frequently in our laboratory is Diprivan by continuous infusion. A combination of intravenous midazolam and a narcotic agent is also effective.[1] Inhalational agents which can affect cardiac func-

A pretransplant electroencephalogram is indicated for any child with an abnormal neurologic exam, since seizures from multiple causes may occur in the perioperative period. Muscle tone and feeding ability are often underdeveloped, especially in infants waiting prolonged periods for their donor organ. Occupational and physical therapy are useful if the child's clinical status will allow it. Full discussion with the parents of the severity, etiology, and prognosis of any neurologic deficit is important so that a truly informed decision can be made about the option for transplantation. Severe and probable irreversible neurologic defects may be a contraindication to transplantation. Mental retardation is not a contraindication to cardiac transplantation. In fact, these patients can get along very well for many years, provided the family support system is strong. However, in very severe forms of mental retardation with essentially no ability for self-care, cardiac transplantation is probably not advisable.

GASTROINTESTINAL

Low cardiac output can also reduce gastrointestinal perfusion with diminished absorptive capacity and decreased appetite. Infants and children can often benefit from small-volume, constant infusion enteral nutrition delivered via a transpyloric tube. If this is not possible, then parenteral nutrition must be aggressively pursued. Posttransplant outcome is in part related to pretransplant nutritional management. The child with a "failed" Fontan, with associated ascites and malabsorption, may be at particular risk if nutrition is neglected. Patients with protein-losing enteropathy (usually secondary to a failed Fontan) can experience complete reversal of that condition within several months after cardiac transplantation.

RENAL

Assessment of renal function is problematic in the critically ill child awaiting transplantation, in whom decreased urine output and elevated blood urea nitrogen and creatinine may result from renal dysfunction and/ or overly aggressive diuretic management. Even in the face of apparently serious renal dysfunction, if the heart can be replaced and perfusion to the kidneys restored, remarkable improvement of renal function can occur. In the setting of chronic renal failure with superimposed cardiac failure, combined heart and kidney transplantation has been applied in children as young as 8 years old. In infants and small children, irreversible renal failure is a contraindication to transplantation.

INFECTIOUS DISEASE

Culture and serologic screening are similar for the pediatric and adult patient, and are discussed in Chapter 6. In the newborn, especially with microcephaly or hepatomegaly, congenital "TORCH" infections (toxoplasma,

other organisms [parvovirus, human immunodeficiency virus, Epstein-Barr virus, herpes virus, varicella, syphilis, enteroviruses], rubella, cytomegalovirus, and hepatitis)[205] should be considered.

HLA SENSITIZATION

As in adults, each potential pediatric recipient should be screened for the presence of antibodies against HLA antigens. The general evaluation and management of pediatric patients with elevated panel reactive antibody (PRA) titers is similar to that for adults and is discussed in Chapter 7. Sensitization is particularly relevant for patients with congenital heart disease and previous cardiac operations, in that prior transfusions, or possibly the use of fresh or cryopreserved homografts in the repair,[261] may induce the formation of anti-HLA antibodies. As discussed in Chapters 7 and 14, sensitized pediatric patients may benefit from intravenous gamma globulin (applicable to all ages) and/or plasmapheresis (for patients about 15 kg or larger) in the postoperative period, particularly if the crossmatch is positive.[80, 130, 233] In smaller patients, plasma volume exchange procedures have been utilized.

The importance of elevated PRA levels in the newborn awaiting cardiac transplantation remains controversial, since these antibodies may be of maternal origin. It is unclear whether a positive PRA in this situation increases the likelihood of hyperacute or accelerated acute rejection and should therefore mandate a prospective crossmatch at the time of transplantation. Given the frequency of long-distance procurement (and the resultant inability to perform a pretransplant crossmatch) in neonatal cardiac transplantation, some centers have disregarded an elevated PRA in this particular situation without apparent ill effects.

MALIGNANCY

As with adults, the presence of prior malignancy in a child undergoing cadiac transplantation increases the probability of recurrence in the setting of chronic immunosuppression. Specific time-related (years between "cure" of malignancy and transplantation) and cancer-specific probabilities of recurrence after transplant are unavailable, but general guidelines have been useful. For most childhood malignancies, a disease-free interval of 5 years coupled with a prognosis of "likely cure" by pediatric oncologic consultants indicates an "acceptable" risk for transplantation. For children with less than 5 years since malignancy "cure" who have a short predicted life expectancy without transplantation, individual decisions are made after consultation with pediatric oncology experts.[104] In all cases of prior malignancy, the family should be fully informed of the potential risk of tumor recurrences.

PSYCHOSOCIAL

Psychosocial issues have a major impact on successful transplantation. In the pediatric patient, family support is critical for long-term survival. A detailed family evaluation should be performed, not only so the medical team can assess the family, but also so the family can make an informed decision as to whether transplantation is in the family's best interest. Some have argued that transplantation for children is an established therapy and that families should not have the option of deciding against this potentially life-saving modality. However, there is still enough uncertainty about long-term issues that this decision should not be taken out of the hands of the family. In addition, in a resource-scarce donor organ environment, insisting on transplantation would deny an organ to a patient whose family is fully supportive of transplantation. The psychosocial evaluation should include assessment of family support systems, access to reliable transportation and telephone, any history of noncompliance, ability to understand written or spoken resource materials, and ability to work with the transplant team. This evaluation is not intended to document reasons to deny transplantation, but rather to identify strengths and weaknesses so that appropriate resources can be made available to the family. However, cardiac transplantation is ill-advised if the family, because of drugs, neglect, or other circumstances, cannot comply with the medical and follow-up requirements of transplantation.

MANAGEMENT OF PATIENTS AWAITING TRANSPLANTATION

Most pediatric patients awaiting heart transplantation can be managed medically out of hospital. The protocols for patients with advanced heart failure, including those in need of inotropic support or intravenous vasodilator therapy, are similar to those utilized in adults with advanced heart failure, and details of these therapeutic strategies and protocols are discussed in Chapter 5.

CONDITIONS WITH DUCTAL DEPENDENCE

The principle of pharmacologic therapy for hypoplastic left heart syndrome (and other ductal dependent conditions) while awaiting transplantation is maintenance of ductal patency with continuous prostaglandin E_1 (PGE_1) infusion. However, the prolonged (weeks or months) administration of standard doses of intravenous PGE_1 has resulted in a clinical state often not conducive to survival. When the standard dose of approximately 0.1 $\mu g/kg/min$ is administered for weeks or months, there is an important incidence of apnea spells and the need for mechanical ventilation; marked tissue edema, which complicates the transplant operation; severe hyperostosis, which complicates recovery from transplantation; and uncontrolled pulmonary overcirculation, which increases pulmonary resistance, induces heart failure, and compromises systemic circulation. Over the past several years, however, several alterations in medical management have greatly improved survival and reduced morbidity among neonates with hypoplas-

tic left heart syndrome awaiting cardiac transplantation. It is now known that low-dose prostaglandin (as low a dose as is necessary to maintain ductal patency) importantly decreases the adverse effects of PGE_1. Most neonates are able to maintain ductal patency with PGE_1 doses as low as 0.01–0.02 $\mu g/kg/min$, with a low incidence of apnea, less subcutaneous edema, and markedly reduced hyperostosis. This allows most babies awaiting transplantation to be extubated and receive oral feedings. Pulmonary vascular resistance is further adjusted by reducing the inspired O_2 concentration below 21% (as low as 18%) with the addition of nitrogen to inspired oxygen gas mixture, delivered through nasal cannulae. A systemic oxygen saturation by pulse oximetry of 70–75% is considered adequate oxygenation. Thus, in the current era, most neonates and infants awaiting cardiac transplantation for hypoplastic left heart syndrome receive continuous low-dose PGE_1 therapy through a small peripheral intravenous catheter or a Broviac central venous catheter and are extubated and maintained on feedings orally or through a feeding catheter while awaiting cardiac transplantation. In this setting, infections are rare and the clinical condition generally remains good for up to several months while awaiting a suitable donor.

Periodic echocardiographic assessment of the interatrial communication is important in order to identify restriction of the patent foramen ovale. Although some controversy exists as to whether mild to moderate restriction of the patent foramen is deleterious (worsening pulmonary hypertension and hyoxemia) or beneficial (reduction in pulmonary blood flow), the development of severe restriction (atrial gradient of 15 mm Hg or more) of the interatrial communication is a poor prognostic sign and an important risk factor for fatality following cardiac transplantation. When severe restriction is identified, attempts at balloon dilation in the catheterization laboratory are advisable.[50, 160, 226] If these are unsuccessful and the gradient between right and left atrium remains high, surgical enlargement of the patent foramen should be considered.

OUTCOME AFTER LISTING FOR CARDIAC TRANSPLANTATION

Despite more than 100 deaths per day among infants less than 1 year of age in the United States alone, donor availability continues to be the major obstacle to successful pediatric cardiac transplantations. Among all listed infants and children, the mortality prior to transplantation is approximately 15–20%.[198]

The outcome after listing for various risk categories can be examined using a competing outcomes analysis (see Chapter 3), such as the analysis of the multi-institutional PHTS from 1993–1996.[188] Figure 20–4 illustrates such an analysis for status 1 patients over 6 months of age, which includes all patients supported with inotropic agents or mechanical circulatory support systems. By 6 months after listing, approximately 70% of patients had undergone cardiac transplantation, and nearly 20% had died while waiting.[187] By multivariable analysis, the

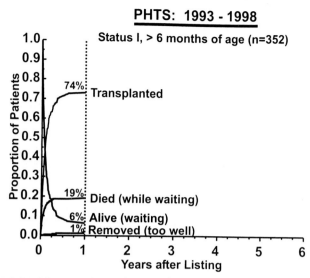

FIGURE **20–4.** Outcome of 352 pediatric patients >6 months of age listed for cardiac transplantation as Status 1 (see text for definition) in the Pediatric Heart Transplant Study (PHTS) between 1993 and 1998. The competing outcomes model depicts the actual probability of transplantation, death while waiting, remaining on the list while awaiting transplantation, or removal from the list. Time 0 is the time of listing. At any time point, the sum of the probabilities of each event totals 100%.

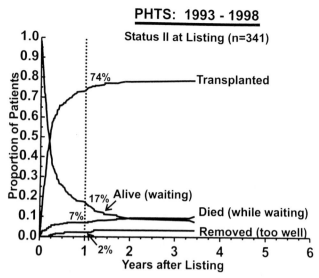

FIGURE **20–5.** Outcome of 341 pediatric patients >6 months of age listed for cardiac transplantation as Status 2 (see text for definiton) in the Pediatric Heart Transplant Study (PHTS) between 1993 and 1998. The depiction is as in Figure 20–4 also.

need for ventilator support was an independent predictor of death before transplantation (Table 20–8).

In the group of less critically ill children (Status 2) who are not supported in an intensive care unit, the time course for events following listing is much more protracted (Fig. 20–5). Thus, by 6 months only about 65% of patients had undergone transplantation and by 12 months 75%. About 10% of patients had died without a transplant by 12 months.

A similar analysis for infants less than 6 months of age is depicted in Figure 20–6. This group is noteworthy because the primary diagnosis for such patients listed in the current era is hypoplastic left heart syndrome in nearly 60% of patients.[199] By 6 months after listing, most patients have either undergone transplantation or died. Factors which increase the risk of death while waiting are depicted in Table 20–8. Smaller infants have a longer waiting time. Among patients with HLHS, blood group O was a risk factor for both waiting time and death prior to transplant due to the distribution of some type

O donor hearts to non–type O recipients during that time period.

These analyses illustrate the high risk of death during the first several months after listing for the most seriously ill patients (Status 1). In fact, for this group of patients, the risk of death prior to transplantation is greater than the combined risks for death during the first 2 years following transplantation. Unless organ donation increases, improvement in overall survival must await better predictors of cardiac deterioration, improved support for infants dependent on PGE_1, improved methods of mechanical circulatory assistance for critically ill children awaiting transplantation, or alter-

TABLE 20–8	Risk Factors* for Outcomes After Listing	
	LONGER TIME TO TRANSPLANTATION	DEATH WHILE WAITING
Infants < 6 mo[†]	Smaller size Blood type O (If HLHS)	Inotropic support Smaller size Blood type O
Infants and children > 6 mo	Status 2 Blood type O	Status 1 Ventilator

HLHS, hypoplastic left heart syndrome.
*$p < .05$ by multivariable analysis, pediatric heart transplant study.[188]
[†]During this era, all infants under 6 mo of age were automatically considered as Status 1.

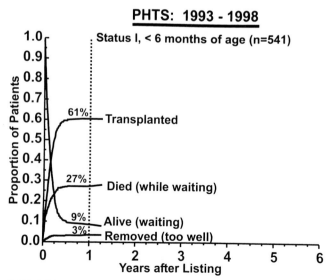

FIGURE **20–6.** Outcome of 541 infants under 6 months of age in the Pediatric Heart Transplant Study (PHTS) listed for heart transplantation between 1993 and 1998. All patients were considered Status 1. The depiction is as in Figure 20–4 also.

TABLE 20-9	**Revised UNOS Transplant List Status Categories**

Status 1A meets at least one of these criteria:
- Requires assistance with a ventilator, balloon pump, or mechanical assist device including ECMO
- Requires infusion of high dose (e.g., dobutamine >7.5 μg/kg/min or milrinone > 0.5 μg/kg/min) or multiple inotropes
- A patient < 6 mo old exhibiting reactive pulmonary hypertension > 50% of systemic levels
- Any patient whose life expectancy is judged to be < 14 days, such as patient with refractory arrhythmia

Status 1B meets at least one of these criteria:
- Requires infusion of low-dose (less than Status 1A dose) single inotrope
- Less than 6 mo old not meeting Status 1A criteria
- Growth failure (<5th percentile for weight and/or height, or loss of 1.5 SD of expected growth) due to heart disease

Status 2 covers all other active patients

SD, standard deviation; ECMO, extracorporeal membrane oxygenator.
From Canter CE: Preoperative assessment and management of pediatric heart transplantation. Prog Pediatr Cardiol 2000;11:91–97.

native donor sources (such as xenotransplantation; see Chapter 23).

PEDIATRIC ORGAN ALLOCATION

As in adult heart transplantation, great variability exists among countries regarding the allocation algorithms. In the United States, allocation of donor hearts is based on the severity of the patient's cardiac illness, duration of time on the waiting list, the distance of the patient from the donor, and ABO blood types. The shortage of organs for pediatric recipients and the risk factor analyses noted above have prompted a revision in the United Network for Organ Sharing (UNOS) allocation criteria. In January 1999, the allocation rules were modified to increase the likelihood of donor hearts being available for the sickest pediatric recipients. The highest priority (most severely ill) status has been subdivided into status 1A and status 1B[48] (Table 20-9). Patients with blood group O receive priority for donor blood group O hearts within each urgency status. Hearts from adolescent donors (ages 11–18 years) are allocated preferentially to adolescent or child recipients within each status category.

THE PEDIATRIC HEART DONOR

DIAGNOSIS AND CAUSES OF BRAIN DEATH

The diagnosis of brain death in infants and children was historically controversial, and a complete discussion of the development of and current guidelines for the diagnosis of pediatric brain death is found in Chapter 9. A historical summary of the concepts of brain death is also found in Chapter 1. Despite the concerns discussed in Chapter 9, the diagnosis of brain death in preterm and term infants can usually be made clinically, and current guidelines include a period of observation because of these confounding factors.[10]

The major causes of brain death in infant donors are birth asphyxia, sudden infant death syndrome, metabolic causes, intracranial hemorrhage, infection, and child abuse.[33] The most common cause of brain death in children is trauma (penetrating and nonpenetrating); other causes such as intracranial hemorrhage and smoke inhalation occur rarely.[11]

CONTRAINDICATIONS TO INFANT HEART DONATION

The general contraindications to infant heart donation are (1) complex cardiac malformation, (2) overwhelming untreated sepsis, (3) suspected hepatitis or retrovirus infection, (4) positive serology for human immunodeficiency virus (HIV) or hepatitis C, and (5) marked reduction in myocardial contractility despite appropriate volume loading and inotropic support (with a fractional shortening of less than 20% and/or major wall motion abnormalities).[33] Left ventricular dysfunction is only a relative contraindication, since depressed contractility is frequently reversible[33] and consistent with normal posttransplant graft function. Infant donor hearts have functioned normally even after extended external chest compressions (up to an hour or more), as long as the ejection fraction exceeds about 0.40 and the inotropic support is not excessive.[149]

PRESERVATION OF THE INFANT DONOR HEART

For children and adolescent donors, the principles of myocardial protection, donor management, and harvesting techniques are essentially the same as for the adult donor and are described in detail in Chapter 9. However, the neonatal and small infant donor present special challenges to the transplant surgeon, as evidenced by the higher incidence of death from acute cardiac failure early after cardiac transplantation in infants under 6 months of age compared to older recipients.[49] Thus, management of the neonatal myocardium during harvest and implantation deserves special comment.

There is considerable evidence that the "immature" neonatal myocardium is structurally, functionally, and biochemically different from "mature" myocardium.[96] However, these inferences are largely derived from experiments using nonhuman tissue. It is well known that considerable differences exist in the ultrastructure of the myocardium between different species,[17] and these ultrastructural differences have biochemical correlates. For example, there is considerable variability in the mechanism of the regulation of intracellular calcium between species. Also, some experimental models (e.g., an isolated canine heart model) demonstrate considerably greater accumulation of myocardial edema under the conditions of ischemia and reperfusion than is typically seen in the human myocardium.[236, 259] In addition, certain methodological limitations of isolated perfused heart models (such as asanguinous vs. blood-perfused models) complicate their interpretation.[276] All these problems contribute to the uncertainty surrounding the transferability of experimentally derived information to the human situation. Thus, despite considerable information available from animal models in a variety of species, the structural differences between the neonatal and adult human myocardium have not been fully characterized. Furthermore, the exact age at which "immature" neonatal myocardium transitions to "mature" myocardium is unknown.

However, from available studies, several inferences can be drawn about the structural characteristics of the "immature" neonatal myocardium. Contractile and relaxation properties of the heart are known to be closely linked to calcium regulation in the sarcoplasmic reticulum (SR). Myofiber contraction is initiated by the increase in myofibrillar calcium following calcium release from the sarcoplasmic reticulum.[289] Myofiber relaxation results from calcium reuptake by the SR (and decreasing myofibrillar calcium).[289] Calcium handling in the neonatal myocardium is probably different from the adult, in that the sarcolemma of "immature" myocardium is able to bind calcium to a greater degree than "mature" myocardium.[35, 91] This suggests that the sarcolemma of immature hearts may be less vulnerable to the influx of calcium into the cell during ischemia.[37, 175] However, once calcium has entered the cell during ischemia or reperfusion, calcium-mediated injury may be worse in the immature myocardium,[37] since the neonatal sarcoplasmic reticulum is not able to reuptake calcium as efficiently. Myocardial edema per se does not appear to play a role in the differences in the age-related response to ischemia.[16]

The biochemistry of energy production may also have important differences. Although both the mature and immature myocardium depend principally on fatty acids for energy production, the neonatal heart appears to have greater glycogen stores,[175] suggesting that anaerobic glycolysis may have a greater role in the immature myocardium. These biochemical observations combined with studies demonstrating better ventricular function after 90 minutes of hypothermic arrest in normal immature versus mature myocardium[40] lend support to the notion that the normal immature myocardium is less vulnerable to hypothermic ischemia and hypoxemia than mature myocardium.[16, 40, 72, 113, 135, 206, 218] Indirect evidence from porcine models also suggests that neonatal cardiac function may be better maintained after brain death than older hearts in terms of left ventricular systolic function, preload recruitable stroke work,[73, 218] and beta-adrenergic receptor density and function.[72, 73, 217]

Whether these inferences regarding neonatal myocardial response to brain death and prolonged ischemia are clinically relevant remains controversial. The reported experience from Loma Linda suggests a low incidence of primary graft failure in infant cardiac transplantation, even with ischemic times out to nearly 10 hours.[13] This contrasts, however, with a multicenter pediatric transplant analysis, in which death from acute graft failure accounted for 75% of the first month mortality in infants under 6 months of age.[49] In older children and teenagers, a similar multicenter analysis indicated less than 3%

early mortality from graft failure, accounting for 35% of deaths in the first month.[248] This implies that, although the immature heart may be more tolerant of ischemia than adult hearts, there may be less myocardial reserves to effectively overcome moderate degrees of reversible dysfunction, less margin of error in the techniques of myocardial protection, and/or greater potential for damage during the period of reperfusion after prolonged ischemia.

As in adult cardiac transplantation, controversy exists regarding the optimal **solutions for myocardial preservation** in the neonate and infant. The general principles of myocardial preservation techniques and solutions are discussed in Chapter 9. Given the important incidence of fatal early graft dysfunction in neonates and small infants, the strategies for myocardial preservation and reperfusion become especially relevant. Current strategies have focused on methods to reproducibly extend the safe period of cold ischemia. The superiority of solutions mimicking the extracellular versus intracellular milieu remains contentious. University of Wisconsin (UW) solution (an intracellular solution initially developed for pancreas preservation)[5, 23, 275] has provided excellent preservation of neonatal and older pediatric hearts in clinical cardiac transplantation (up to about 6 hours), and its efficacy is supported by many experimental studies (see also Chapter 9). In neonatal porcine models using an isolated working left heart preparation, UW solution at 4°C provided better preservation of high-energy phosphates and immediate left ventricular work potential than a standard extracellular (Stanford) solution.[43] The components of UW solution and their effects are discussed in Chapter 9.

However, an acalcemic solution with a high glucose concentration (Roe's solution) has provided excellent preservation for neonatal cardiac transplantation with ischemic times exceeding 8 hours[138, 149, 151] (Table 20–10). Some experimental studies suggest that UW solution may not be as effective for extended preservation of the neonatal heart (out to 20 hours), resulting in inferior protection compared to a solution providing proton buffering with histidine and exogenous glucose and insulin.[190]

Thus, although a variety of solutions appear to provide adequate myocardial preservation of the infant heart, considerable evidence suggests that the optimal solution has not yet been identified.

SURGICAL TECHNIQUES

For infants and children with cardiomyopathy and some forms of congenital heart disease, the transplant procedure is carried out essentially as described in Chapter 10, with the exception that we have generally utilized the standard orthotopic technique (rather than the bicaval technique) in younger patients to avoid the possibility of stenosis at the superior vena caval anastomosis. However, for patients with complex congenital heart disease, special modifications of both the donor and recipient operation are necessary to accommodate a variety of

TABLE 20-10	Composition of University of Wisconsin and Roe's Cardioplegic Solutions

University of Wisconsin	
Hydroxyethyl starch (pentafraction)	50 g/L
Lactobionic acid	100 mmol/L
Phosphate	25 mmol/L
Magnesium sulfate	5 mmol/L
Raffinose	30 mmol/L
Adenosine	5 mmol/L
Allopurinol	1 mmol/L
Glutathione reduced	3 mmol/L
Dexamethasone	16 mg/L
Insulin	40 U/L
Potassium	120 mEq/L
Sodium	30 mEq/L
Total osmolarity	323
PH	7.4
Roe's	
NaCl	27 mEq
KCL	20 mEq
MgSO	3 mEq
Methylprednisolone (Solu-Medrol)	250 mg
5% dextrose in water	1,000 mL
Adjusted to pH 7.4 with NaHCO₃	
Important: Store at 4°C	

Adapted from Jeevanandam V: Myocardial preservation for pediatric cardiac transplantation. *In* Franco KL (ed): Pediatric Cardiopulmonary Transplantation. Armonk, NY: Futura Publishing Company, Inc, 1997.

anatomic malformations. For purposes of surgical planning, five categories of anatomic abnormalities must be considered: (1) aortic arch hypoplasia or interruption, (2) anomalies of systemic venous return, (3) anomalies of pulmonary venous connection, (4) congenital or acquired stenoses or interruption of the central pulmonary arteries, and (5) cardiac situs malformations.

DONOR OPERATION

The general details of donor preparation, management, and intraoperative techniques are discussed in Chapter 9. In the presence of recipient congenital heart disease, the donor operation must be tailored to the anatomic needs of the recipient. The details of anatomic parts required must be carefully communicated to the donor harvesting team (Fig. 20–7). It is important to remember that harvesting lungs for transplantation could affect the ability to harvest sufficient cardiac tissue for some recipient conditions (see following discussion), and this must be realized prior to procurement. The other principles of donor management are the same as discussed for adults in Chapter 9. The pediatric cardioplegia solution currently utilized at UAB is UW solution as a single dose of 25 to 50 mL/kg (up to a maximum of 1 L) by gravity infusion. At Loma Linda, Roe's solution is administered by gravity infusion. Profound topical cooling with iced saline solution provides additional cooling prior to storage in UW solution (UAB) or Roe's solution (Loma Linda) at about 4°C for transport.

In the case of **hypoplastic left heart syndrome** or aortic arch interruption, the aortic arch is extensively mobilized after administration of cardioplegia and excision of the heart and right and left pulmonary arteries. A long stump of innominate artery is harvested to allow access for reinserting the aortic cannula after completion of the arch reconstruction in the recipient operation. The proximal stumps of left carotid and left subclavian arteries are also harvested as well as the upper half of the descending thoracic aorta (well past the ligamentum arteriosum) (Figure 20–8).

With recipient **anomalies of systemic venous return,** extended removal of the superior vena cava, left innominate vein, and inferior vena cava may be required (Fig. 20–7). Anomalies of recipient inferior vena cava (IVC) position (such as situs inversus) may require some additional length of inferior vena cava (down to the level of the diaphragm), but this is not possible with concomitant harvesting for liver transplantation. In that situation, the recipient IVC can be lengthened with adjacent atrial tissue to accommodate the standard donor IVC orifice. Additional length of superior vena cava is neces-

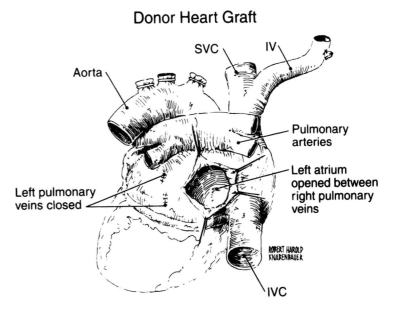

Donor Heart Graft

FIGURE **20-7.** Posterior view of extended harvesting of donor cardiac parts to facilitate cardiac transplantation for various cardiac malformation. Note additional length of aorta, superior and inferior venae cavae (SVC and IVC), innominate vein (IV), and pulmonary arteries which can be obtained. The entire left atrium and proximal pulmonary veins can also be harvested. In this depiction, the left pulmonary venous orifices have been oversewn and the right orifices enlarged for transplantation in a recipient with anomalous pulmonary venous connection. (From del Rio MJ: Transplantation in complex congenital heart disease. Prog Pediat Cardiol 2000;11:107–113. Copyright 2000, Excerpta Medical Inc, with permission.)

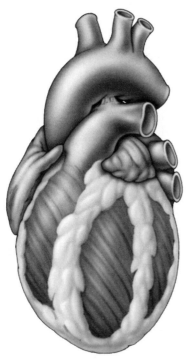

FIGURE **20-8.** Donor heart for hypoplastic left heart syndrome, with additional length of aortic arch and head vessels.

sary with a previous recipient bidirectional Glenn procedure, and a long segment of the left innominate vein is necessary for reconstruction of a donor left superior vena cava.

Anomalies of pulmonary venous connection may require complete resection of the donor left atrium, dividing each donor pulmonary vein separately. Management of **central pulmonary artery anomalies** frequently requires harvesting of the donor main and central pulmonary arteries out to the takeoff of the upper lobe branch. This would not be possible if one or both lungs were being harvested for lung transplantation. **Abnormalities of cardiac situs** and positional anomalies of the great vessels may require various modifications of the donor harvest as described above (Fig. 20–7).[75]

RECIPIENT OPERATION

Hypoplastic Left Heart Syndrome

Cardiac transplantation for hypoplastic left heart syndrome includes reconstruction of the aortic arch in addition to cardiac replacement. This requires an obligatory period of circulatory arrest. Particularly in the presence of other complex associated anomalies, a strategy for repair is necessary which limits the total period of circulatory arrest to a safe duration. Although the "safe" period of total circulatory arrest has not been clearly established, clinical and experimental studies suggest that at a nasopharyngeal temperature of 15°–18°C with appropriate cooling techniques, 30 minutes of circulatory arrest is nearly always associated with absence of functional or structural neurological damage. Circula-

tory arrest duration of 45 minutes is usually safe, and periods exceeding 60 minutes are associated with a progressive increase in the likelihood of permanent neurological damage.[44, 65, 77, 260, 270, 292] A strategy of transplantation for hypoplastic left heart syndrome which utilizes cardiopulmonary bypass for the cardiac replacement and limits circulatory arrest to the period of arch reconstruction provides near routine circulatory arrest times under 40 minutes.[75]

When a suitable donor is identified, the recipient with hypoplastic left heart syndrome is intubated and a double-lumen 5-Fr 2.5-cm catheter (Cook) is inserted into the femoral vein. A 22-gauge catheter (Medicut) is inserted into the radial artery for pressure monitoring, and a 20-gauge catheter is inserted via cut-down into a superficial vein at the wrist for infusion of blood products. A bladder catheter with an indwelling temperature probe is inserted. These procedures can be performed either in the neonatal intensive care unit or in the operating room at the time of transplantation.

Pretransplant immunotherapy is ordered and administered (see Chapter 12). For infants, all platelets and packed red cells to be infused are cytomegalovirus (CMV) negative and leukoreduced.

The heart is exposed through a median sternotomy. Exposure of the aortic arch is facilitated with a slight extension of the incision into the right or left side of the base of the neck (Fig. 20–9). The thymus is excised, taking care to avoid injury to the phrenic nerves with the cautery. Before establishing cardiopulmonary bypass, the innominate artery, left carotid artery, aortic arch, and ductus arteriosus can be completely mobilized. Manipulation of the heart is completely avoided to prevent ventricular fibrillation. Arterial cannulation (10- to 12-Fr perfusion cannula) is accomplished via the main pulmonary artery by advancing the cannula well into

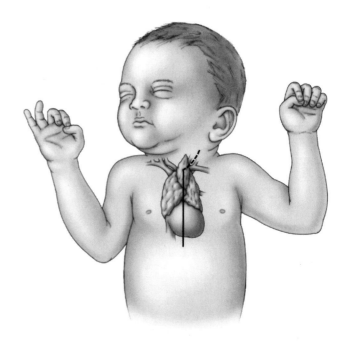

FIGURE **20-9.** Incision for recipient operation in cardiac transplantation for hypoplastic left heart syndrome. The dashed lines indicate extension of the incision to facilitate exposure of the aortic arch.

the ductus arteriosus (Fig. 20–10). Upon commencing bypass at 2.5 L/min/m², a tourniquet placed around the ductus arteriosus is snugged around the proximal ductus and cannula to exclude the pulmonary circulation. The right atrium is initially cannulated for venous return with a 20-Fr angled metal cannula. Cooling is continued until the nasopharyngeal temperature is 16°C. At that time, profound hypothermic perfusion at 15°–16°C is established at a flow rate of about 1.0 L/min/m² to continue profound cerebral cooling. During the cooling phase, silk string tourniquets are placed around the superior and inferior venae cavae. A left atrial catheter is inserted. The ascending aorta is ligated just proximal to the take-off of the innominate artery.

When the nasopharyngeal temperature is 18°C or less, the pulmonary artery is cross-clamped proximal to the arterial cannula. A brief period of circulatory arrest is established while the venous cannula is removed and the native heart is excised. The superior and inferior venae cavae are now cannulated through the open right atrium, and the cannulae are secured in position with the tourniquets. Cardiopulmonary bypass is again commenced and profound cooling is continued.

The donor atrial anastomoses are constructed as in a standard orthotopic heart transplant procedure (see Chapter 10) using continuous 5.0 polypropylene for the left atrial anastomosis followed by the right atrial anastomosis. With the right atrial anastomosis nearly completed, total circulatory arrest is established. The caval cannulae are removed, and the right atrial suture line is completed. The innominate and left carotid arteries

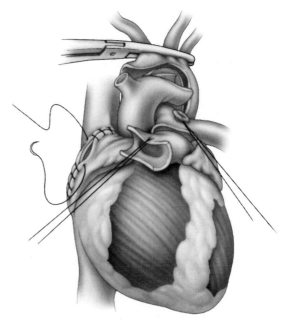

FIGURE **20–11.** Cardiac transplantation for hypoplastic left heart syndrome: beginning of arch reconstruction. The right atrial anastomosis has been completed. The donor pulmonary artery and the recipient ductal sump are retracted with stay sutures to expose the aortic arch. An incision is made in the recipient arch and extended past the level of the ductus. The donor arch is contoured and trimmed in preparation for arch reconstruction. See text for further details.

are clamped, the arterial cannula is removed, and the ductus is ligated and divided distally. Exposure of the arch is facilitated by retracting the ductal stump inferiorly with the ligature and retracting the donor pulmonary artery with a stay suture (Fig. 20–11). The entire arch is opened and all ductal tissue is excised. The incision is extended distally until normal descending aorta is visualized.

The donor aorta is prepared by excising the superior aspect of the donor aorta including the left subclavian and left carotid arteries (Fig. 20–12). The innominate artery is preserved for later cannulation. Enough donor

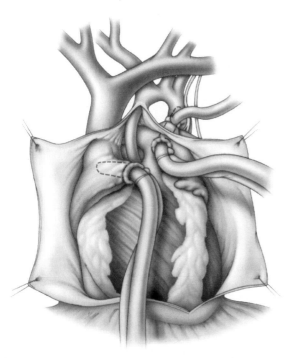

FIGURE **20–10.** Cannulation for cardiopulmonary bypass in transplantation for hypoplastic left heart syndrome. The inflow cannula is inserted into the proximal main pulmonary artery and passed through the ductus into the aortic arch. The tourniquet is tightened around the ductus after initiation of cardiopulmonary bypass to exclude the lungs from perfusion. A single venous cannula is positioned in the right atrium.

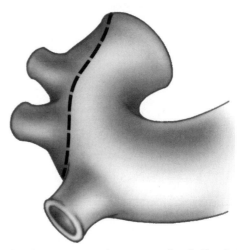

FIGURE **20–12.** Donor ascending aorta and arch. The dashed lines indicate the area of incision to excise the stump of left carotid and left subclavian arteries in preparation for arch reconstruction.

aorta is preserved to produce a widely patent arch reconstruction with continuous 6.0 polypropylene (Fig. 20–13). The innominate artery is cannulated for re-establishment of cardiopulmonary bypass and air is evacuated through the suture line before securing it. A single venous cannula is positioned though the right atrial appendage, and cardiopulmonary bypass is recommenced (Fig. 20–14). The donor heart is "gently" reperfused with a mean arterial pressure of 30–40 mm Hg and low-flow perfusion for several minutes before gradually establishing "full flow." When effective contraction is present, the pulmonary artery anastomosis is constructed with 6.0 polypropylene. The remainder of the operation is completed and cardiopulmonary bypass discontinued as for other heart transplant and congenital cardiac procedures.

The **excision of ductal tissue** at its entrance into the distal arch is important in providing secure aortic tissue for the anastomosis and to minimize the likelihood of a posttransplant stenosis ("coarctation") in this area. In the weeks and months following transplantation, diminished pedal pulses offer a clue to the development of a coarctation if the echocardiogram shows normal cardiac function and rejection is excluded. If a **coarctation** develops, it can usually be effectively treated with balloon dilation. Sherali and colleagues from Loma Linda reported a 16% incidence of coarctation after transplantation for HLHS.[251] Balloon dilatation was successful in alleviating the coarctation in all cases at a mean of 6.2 months after transplantation.

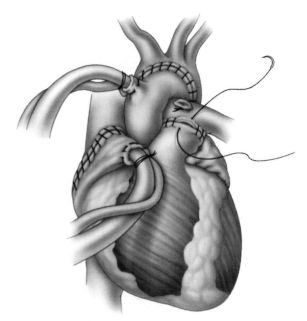

FIGURE **20–14.** After completion of the arch anastomosis, the arterial cannula is inserted into the stump of donor innominate artery, and de-airing of the aortic arch is carried out through the suture line before removing the clamp on the head vessels. An angled venous cannula is inserted through the right atrial appendage. The right atrial and arch suture lines are shown completed, and the final sutures are being placed on the pulmonary artery anastomosis.

Left-Sided Superior Vena Cava (without Drainage to Coronary Sinus)

Although tunneling techniques have been described,[55] our preference is to circumferentially mobilize the left superior vena cava (LSVC) and transect it with a rim of left atrial wall attached, much as in the preparation of the right superior vena cava (RSVC) in the standard bicaval technique. The maximal possible length of donor SVC and innominate vein are harvested and a direct anastomosis to the LSVC is made, above the level of the pulmonary artery anastomosis and anterior to the ascending aorta (Fig. 20–15). If there is a large RSVC present, a cuff of native right atrium (larger than usual) is maintained with the right SVC, and this can be connected to the donor SVC or to the donor right atrium, taking care to preserve the sinus node.

Left Superior Vena Cava Draining to Coronary Sinus

The same technique can be used here for reconstruction of the LSVC. Alternatively, the native heart excision can be performed by incising the left atrio-ventricular groove such that the coronary sinus is left undisturbed (Fig. 20–16). The standard orthotopic technique can then be employed, taking care not to disturb the coronary sinus with the left atrial anastomosis. The disadvantage of this method is the complexity (and possible prevention) of endomyocardial biopsy by way of the superior vena cava (unless there is also an adequate sized RSVC) due to the sharp angulation of the bioptome necessary to biopsy the right ventricular septum.

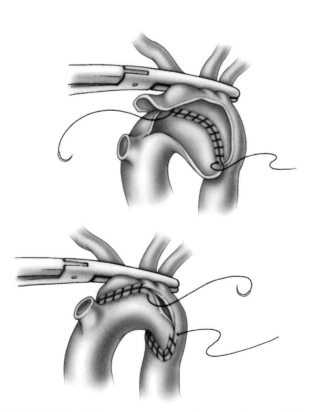

FIGURE **20–13.** Arch reconstruction in cardiac transplantation for hypoplastic left heart syndrome.

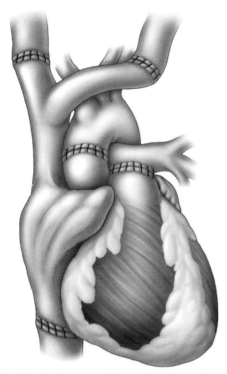

FIGURE **20–15.** Cardiac transplantation in the setting of persistent bilateral superior vena cavae. Excess donor superior vena cava and left innominate vein are harvested for the reconstruction. This method of reconstruction is particularly suited for the recipient with previous bilateral bidirectional Glenn anastomoses.

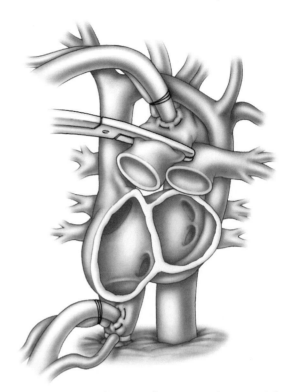

FIGURE **20–16.** Surgical option in the presence of persistent left superior vena cava draining into the coronary sinus. The recipient atrial remnants are fashioned such that the entire course of the left superior vena cava and coronary sinus are preserved by leaving a small remnant of left ventricle over the area of coronary sinus for subsequent construction of the left atrial anastomosis. For clarity, the superior vena caval cannula has been removed.

Anomalous Pulmonary Venous Connection

In most varieties of total anomalous pulmonary venous connection, a standard cardiac repair can be performed to connect the posterior common pulmonary venous sinus to the native left atrial chamber, after which the standard bicaval or orthotopic technique is employed.[226] Alternatively, the donor left atrium can be utilized to fashion a patulous direct connection to the common pulmonary venous sinus. When the anomalous connections are of the mixed type without a separate common pulmonary venous sinus, transplantation may be facilitated by excising any atrial septum and incorporating the common posterior atrial mass into the left atrial anastomosis, followed by a bicaval technique for systemic venous connections. Long-term surveillance is necessary for possible late pulmonary venous obstruction.[226] To facilitate management of the variety of anatomic arrangements, it is often useful to have the entire donor left atrium harvested.

Severe Hypoplasia of Recipient Left Atrium

If necessary, the native left atrium can be enlarged by incising between the left superior and inferior pulmonary veins (Fig. 20–17). The donor left atrium is harvested so the individual pulmonary veins are dissected circumferentially, mobilized for a short distance and then individually divided. Prior to implantation, a flap of left atrium can be created from donor left atrial wall, or if necessary, by anastomosing the remnants of pulmo-

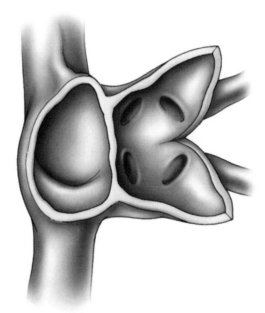

FIGURE **20–17.** Enlargement of hypoplastic recipient left atrium by incising between the left superior and inferior pulmonary veins.

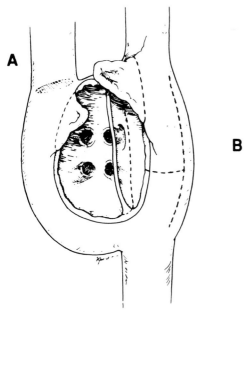

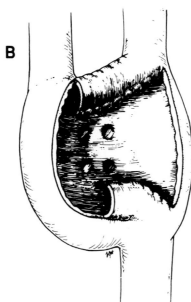

FIGURE **20–18.** Situs inversus of the viscera and atria. *A,* Dotted lines show intended lines of incision for excision of the atrial septum and creation of caval baffles from the recipient left atrium. *B,* Intracardiac baffles fashioned from left-sided atrial tissue reroute systemic venous return from the left superior vena cava (SVC) and inferior vena cava (IVC) to the right of the pulmonary vein orifices. (From Francko KL: Pediatric Cardiopulmonary Transplantation. Armonk, NY: Futura Publishing Company, Inc, 1997, with permission.)

nary veins together. The leading edge of the flap can be fashioned into the enlarged incision in the native left atrium.

Pulmonary Artery Bifurcation Stenosis

Sufficient length of donor right and left pulmonary artery is harvested to allow a direct anastomosis or onlay graft onto the native pulmonary arteries. The donor pulmonary arteries must be anastomosed without distortion or angulation to avoid important gradients.

Situs Inversus and Dextrocardia

In entities where the heart is in a dextrocardia position and the apex points rightward, there may be insufficient space within the left side of the pericardium to accommodate the new heart. A flap of pericardium above the phrenic nerve can be created on the left side to support the transplanted heart much as with heterotopic transplantation on the right and allow it to extend into the left pleural space. When there is also situs inversus of the viscera and atria, the cavae and morphologic right atrium are left-sided. In order to move the orifices of the IVC and SVC to a right-sided position (for anastomosis to the donor right atrium), a tunnel can be created with recipient atrial tissue after excising the atrial septum (Fig. 20–18).[90] The donor left atrium can then be sutured around the recipient pulmonary veins, incorporating them into the donor left atrium (Fig. 20–19). Alternatively, recipient right atrial tissue can be utilized to extend the length of both cavae, moving the orifices into a position that can accommodate a bicaval anastomotic technique.

Transposition of the Great Arteries

The transplant procedure is modified only with respect to the great vessel anastomoses.[119, 137] Additional length of donor aorta is harvested, usually including the entire

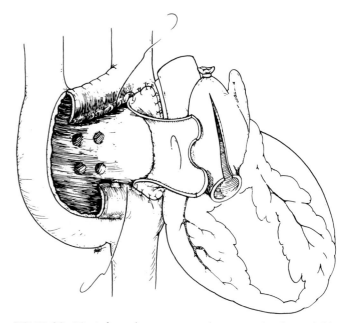

FIGURE **20–19.** Left atrial anastomosis is being completed in a child with situs inversus. The donor left atrium is sutured to the recipients free left margin and the intracardiac baffles. The remaining atrial cuff is anastomosed to the recipient atrium to the right of the pulmonary veins. (From Franco KL: Pediatric Cardiopulmonary Transplantation. Armonk, NY: Futura Publishing Company, Inc, 1997, with permission.)

aortic arch. In the recipient, the ascending aorta, arch, and arch vessels are mobilized to allow the native aorta to move rightward for its connection with the donor aorta. The native right pulmonary artery is dissected free from the aorta. The proximal right and left pulmonary arteries are retained in the donor and then trimmed as necessary. Usually, a direct anastomosis can be made to the open end of the native main pulmonary artery. If not, the opening can be extended onto the proximal left native pulmonary artery and the rightward extent of the opening in the native main pulmonary artery partially closed.

Interatrial Septal Anomalies

Although multiple techniques have been described to reconstruct the atrial septum (such as after prior Mustard or Senning procedures), these are usually unnecessary in older children and adolescents in the presence of right-sided cavae. The standard techniques of bicaval cardiac transplantation are utilized after excising the right atrial mass.

POSTOPERATIVE MANAGEMENT

Many details of pediatric postoperative management are similar to those in adult patients (see Chaper 12). Aspects unique to pediatric cardiac transplantation are discussed in this section.

INOTROPIC SUPPORT

The standard inotropic agents and doses employed after pediatric cardiac transplantation are covered in Chapter 12.

PROSTAGLANDIN THERAPY

In patients with ductal-dependent circulation maintained on PGE_1 infusion prior to transplant, it is advisable to continue the PGE_1 at approximately 0.02 μg/kg/min for 24–48 hours and then gradually taper it over 1–2 days. Although controlled studies are lacking, patients on PGE_1 for weeks may have an increased propensity for reactive pulmonary hypertension if it is abruptly discontinued.

PGE_1 may also have beneficial immunosuppressive properties separate from its ductal effects. PGE_1 impairs the ability of cytotoxic T-cells to lyse target cells[262] and may have a synergistic effect with cyclosporine mediated through inhibition of interleukin(IL)-2.[238, 262] A study from Loma Linda found less frequent and less severe rejection during the first year (univariate analysis) in a group of infants treated with PGE_1 (0.02–0.05 μg/kg/min) for 5–10 days after transplant compared to no PGE_1.[9]

TREATMENT OF POSTOPERATIVE PULMONARY HYPERTENSION

Pulmonary hypertension immediately following cardiac transplantation is a serious event if associated with right ventricular dysfunction. Particularly when the pulmonary arterial systolic pressure exceeds about 50 mm Hg, the likelihood of acute right ventricular failure increases rapidly. The likelihood of acute right ventricular dysfunction is further increased when donor right ventricular function is abnormal at the time of procurement and with prolonged donor ischemic times (possibly greater than about 6 hours).[97]

Optimal therapy for postoperative pulmonary hypertension is discussed in Chapter 12, and generally includes PGE_1 or inhaled nitric oxide, combined with alkalinization through hyperventilation, infusion of vasodilator therapy, and selection of inotropic agents with minimal pulmonary vasoconstrictive effects.[18]

PULMONARY MANAGEMENT

Most aspects of ventilator and postextubation pulmonary care are the same as those practiced after standard cardiac surgery for infants and children. However, airway and parenchymal lung compression may occur if the donor heart is considerably larger than the recipient heart. Aggressive pulmonary toilet and close observation for respiratory dysfunction are recommended for the first several days following extubation.

IMMUNOSUPPRESSION IN THE PEDIATRIC PATIENT

The pharmacology, metabolism, mechanism of action, and dosing of immunosuppressive agents is discussed in Chapter 13. A number of different immunosuppression protocols are in use and, to date, any differences in survival cannot be attributed to differences in immunosuppression.

Cyclosporine

Maintenance immunosuppression is usually based on cyclosporine, either as double therapy with azathioprine or triple therapy with azathioprine and steroids. The management of cyclosporine differs in infants and children compared with adults because of the more rapid hepatic metabolism of the drug, and hence higher doses given more frequently (3 times per day) are required. In contrast to the frequency of renal impairment with chronic cyclosporine in adults, children may be more resistant to the deleterious effects. Laine and colleagues noted that cyclosporine in pediatric patients is generally compatible with normal glomerular function, often with only minor tubular abnormalities.[162] The bioavailability of Neoral is greater than Sandimmune in children, as in adults (see Chapter 13), and many pediatric protocols preferentially utilize Neoral for this reason.

Tacrolimus

Another basic immunosuppressive strategy in children includes tacrolimus instead of cyclosporine, as monotherapy or as part of a double- or triple-drug regimen.[7] The experience at the University of Pittsburgh indicates that tacrolimus is a very effective primary immunosuppressive agent, and that 80% of pediatric patients can be weaned off steroids with tacrolimus as monotherapy.[6] Using this strategy, Armitage and colleagues reported 82% survival at 3 years.[6] Tacrolimus has the important advantage over cyclosporine that hirsutism, gingival hyperplasia, and abnormal facial bone growth are avoided and hypertension is uncommon. An extensive discussion of side effects of tacrolimus is found in Chapter 13.

Steroid Protocols

Steroids are known to provide effective immunosuppression as part of a three-drug immunosuppressive regimen, and recurrent rejection is often effectively treated by increasing the daily prednisone (or prednisolone) dose. However, chronic steroid therapy is known to retard growth and skeletal development in children and has many other undesirable long-term effects (see Chapter 13). Therefore, most pediatric cardiac transplant programs either use no steroids as maintenance immunosuppression[13] or taper steroids off over the first 3–12 months after transplant.[51] The details of steroid dosing and tapering schedules vary by transplant center, in large part due to incomplete information about their effect on the immune response in children. As discussed in Chapter 13, steroids have an inhibitory effect on the expression of cytokines (derived from T-cells and antigen presenting cells) such as IL-1, IL-2, IL-3, IL-6, tumor necrosis factor-α and interferon-γ.[127] Further support for the antirejection "benefit" of corticosteroids is derived from multiple studies in pediatric renal and liver transplantation which indicate a higher risk of acute rejection and graft loss following steroid withdrawal.[84, 176, 228, 231] However, the superb survival reported after pediatric heart transplantation with steroid-free immunosuppression[13, 87] indicates that prednisone is not a critical component of the immunosuppressive regimen for most patients, as long as cyclosporine levels are therapeutic and azathioprine or mycophenolate is well tolerated. In the case of tacrolimus-based immunosuppression, monotherapy with tacrolimus alone is often effective in children.[7] Some have argued that the use of steroids for weeks or months after transplant may promote upregulation of cytokine receptors and thereby "set the stage" for increased rejection upon abrupt steroid withdrawal.[127] Withdrawal of steroids, even from low doses, is often associated with an increased frequency of rejection during the weeks or months after withdrawal. This increased risk may exist for 6 months or more following discontinuation of steroids.[51] This observation has led some to speculate that it may be safer to never use chronic steroids rather than using a protocol of gradual withdrawal over weeks or months.[220]

From a practical standpoint, the specific tapering schedule for children receiving prednisone must be determined by the patient's rejection history. For example, a child with an uncomplicated rejection history who has one isolated rejection episode can have a more rapid taper of steroids. Another child who is having recurrent or persistent rejection should have a very slow taper while periodically assessing the graft by biopsy for possible rejection. In general, rejection surveillance with echocardiograms or cardiac biopsies should be intensified during steroid tapering.

An immunosuppressive dose of prednisone is considered to be 0.1–0.5 mg/kg/day. Physiologic replacement is about 5 mg/m²/day. After bolus steroid therapy for rejection, the patient is generally placed on approximately 0.5 mg/kg/day given once in the morning. This is weaned (the rapidity of the wean is dependent on rejection history as noted above), if possible, to a dose which approximates physiologic replacement, or to the level at which the patient was last rejection free. In the child with a complicated rejection history or in whom rejection is only found on biopsy, many would insist on an acceptable biopsy prior to weaning steroids. While the goal should always be to wean completely off steroids, most children do quite well with minimal side effects if they can be weaned to a dose of prednisone equal to physiologic replacement (about 0.1–0.2 mg/kg) given on an every-other-day schedule. One should always remember that the child on chronic steroids will need additional amounts in the face of illness or surgery.

Induction Therapy

The mechanism, pharmacology, and dosing of various "induction" therapeutic agents are discussed in Chapter 13. Induction therapy is a common feature of many pediatric immunosuppressive protocols, with considerable variation in the type of induction therapy and age groups selected for induction. Polyclonal anti–T-cell antibody preparations, including equine (Atgam) and rabbit (antithymocyte globulin or serum), and monoclonal preparations (OKT3) have been utilized.[36, 136, 167] Although no clear advantage of induction therapy has been demonstrated, one study suggested a reduction in late deaths among infants with antithymocyte serum, which appeared to be superior to OKT3.[36]

Immunosuppression Strategy at UAB

The pediatric immunosuppressive strategy utilized at UAB consists of preoperative cyclosporine, methylprednisolone, and azathioprine (or mycophenolate mofetil); intraoperative methylprednisolone; and postoperative maintenance therapy with cyclosporine, azathioprine (or mycophenolate mofetil), and prednisolone (Table 20–11). This is the same general strategy as employed in adults, and the specific dosages are discussed in Chapter 13. Prednisolone is started at a dose of 1 mg/kg/day immediately after transplantation and tapering is initiated 21 days after transplantation or 14 days after the last dose of OKT3. The dose is decreased by 0.05 mg/kg every 3 days to a dose of 0.1 mg/kg/day, and then tapered off over the first 3–6 months unless recurrent rejection occurs. Induction therapy with OKT3 (0.1–0.2 mg/kg/dose) for 7 days is utilized for infants under

TABLE 20-11	**Immunosuppression Protocol (UAB)**

Pretransplant
   Cyclosporine 1–3 mg/kg PO
   Methylprednisolone 15 mg/kg IV 4–6 hr before surgery, 10 mg/
    kg IV 1–2 hr before surgery
   Azathioprine 4 mg/kg IV or PO
Intraoperative
   Methylprednisolone 10 mg/kg IV postbypass
Posttransplant
   Methylprednisolone 2.5 mg/kg IV q 8 hr × 3 doses
   OKT3* 0.1–0.2 mg/kg/day IV × 7–10 days (adjust with T-cell
    markers to achieve an absolute count of CD3$^+$ lymphocytes of
    <20/mL and <10% of total lymphocytes CD3$^+$).
   Prednisolone 1 mg/kg/day, tapered to 0.1 mg/kg/day by 2 mo
    and off by 6 mo unless recurrent rejection
   Cyclosporine: aim for whole blood target level of 350–450 ng/
    mL for first 6 mo, 250–350 at 6–12 mo, and 150–250 thereafter
    (reduce level with renal dysfunction)
   Azathioprine: 1–3 mg/kg/day PO, adjust to keep WBC > 3,000

WBC, white blood cell count.
*Prophylactic OKT3 is used for infants < 6 mo of age who are positive for
Epstein-Barr serology or if renal dysfunction delays use of cyclosporine.

6 months of age or for any patient with renal dysfunction
that prevents administration of cyclosporine during the
first few days after transplantation.

Loma Linda Immunosuppression Strategy

The Loma Linda immunosuppression protocol differs
in many respects and is outlined in Table 20–12.
Cyclosporine is initiated intravenously at 0.1 mg/kg/h
when a donor is identified and then withheld during
the transplant operation. It is restarted at the same infusion rate in the intensive care unit at 0.1–0.2 mg/kg/h.
Following extubation, cyclosporine is switched to an
oral dose of 10–20 mg/kg/day in divided doses every
8–12 hours, adjusted to achieve whole blood target levels (monoclonal antibody assay) of 250–300 ng/mL.
Children less than 4 years of age generally require tid
dosing because of more rapid cyclosporine metabolism
in younger children. *Azathioprine* is administered in a
dose of 3 mg/kg intravenously (IV) or orally (PO) once
daily, beginning on the first postoperative day. The dose
is adjusted to maintain the white blood count greater

TABLE 20-12	**Immunosuppression Protocol (Loma Linda)**

Pretransplant
   Cyclosporine 0.1 mg/kg/hr IV when donor identified
Intraoperative
   None
Posttransplant
   Cyclosporine 0.1 mg/kg/hr, switch to PO dose following
    extubation, aim for whole blood target dose of 250–300 ng/mL
   Methylprednisolone 20–25 mg/kg IV q 12 hr × 4 doses
   Azathioprine 3 mg/kg/day IV or PO; adjust dose for WBC >
    4,000
   Antithymocyte globulin (thymoglobulin) 1.5 mg/kg/day IV for
    first 5 days in infants >1 mo of age

WBC, white blood cell count.

than 4,000/mL. *Methylprednisolone* is administered every
12 hours at a dose of 20–25 mg/kg IV for the first 2 days
after transplant, then discontinued. Oral prednisone is
not routinely employed after transplant unless recurrent
rejection occurs. *Antithymocyte globulin (thymoglobulin)*
is generally used as induction therapy (1.5 mg/kg IV
once daily) for the first 5 days after transplant in infants
more than 30 days of age.

OTHER ROUTINE POSTTRANSPLANT MEDICATIONS

A variety of other routine nonimmunosuppressive medications are employed by most pediatric transplant programs. The standard protocol for UAB is listed in Table
20–13 and that for Loma Linda in Table 20–14. Commonly used antihypertensive medictions are listed in
Table 20–15. A more complete list of therapies for infection prophylaxis is found in Chapter 15, Table 15–9.

VACCINATION PROTOCOLS

Protecting the transplanted child from vaccine preventable diseases is an important part of posttransplant care.
In the pretransplant period, vaccines are deferred while

TABLE 20-13	**Routine Nonimmunosuppressive Medications (UAB)**

MEDICATION	DOSE	PURPOSE
Verapamil	4–6 mg/kg/day PO in 3 divided doses	Increase cyclosporine levels, treat hypertension
Trimethoprim/ sulfamethoxazole	10 mg/kg/day in 2 doses on Mon, Wed, Fri for 1 yr	Prophylaxis against *Pneumocystis carinii*
Acyclovir	4 mg/kg/day in 2 doses for 1 yr	Prophylaxis against CMV and herpes simplex (should be stopped when taking ganciclovir)
Bicitra	2–3 mEq/kg/day PO	Treatment of cyclosporine-induced renal tubular acidosis if serum bicarbonate level <20 mEq/L
Nystatin	<5 kg: 1 mL PO tid 5–10 kg: 2 mL PO tid 11–20 kg: 3 mL PO tid 21–50 kg: 4 mL PO tid for 1 yr	Prophylaxis against *Candida* infections (thrush)

TABLE 20-14	**Routine Nonimmunosuppressive Medications (Loma Linda)**

- Intravenous immune globulin (Sandoglobulin): a 9–12% solution in a dose of 2 g/kg is generally administered over 24 hr starting right after transplant and repeated at times of increased immunosuppression.
- Ranitidine: administered while taking Solu-Medrol; 1–2 mg/kg/day IV in 3 or 4 divided doses or 2–4 mg/kg/day PO in 2 divided doses.
- Aspirin: 3–5 mg/kg/day (1/2 baby aspirin for infants) when platelet count is chronically >500,000/mL.
- Ganciclovir: 10 mg/kg/day IV in 2 divided doses while hospitalized as prophylaxis against CMV in CMV-negative recipients who receive CMV-positive hearts.
- Acyclovir: 30 mg/kg/day PO in 3 divided doses for 3 mo as prophylaxis against CMV (not used if patient received ganciclovir).

awaiting a donor organ, since the vaccination process stimulates the immune system and could possibly potentiate early graft rejection.

After transplantation, immunizations are given at the routine times, using **killed vaccine** only. Diphtheria, pertussis, tetanus (DPT) and Salk inactivated injectable polio vaccine are given at the usual age of childhood immunizations (2, 4, 6, 18 months, and 5 years of age) unless contraindicated. *Haemophilus influenzae* type B (HIB) vaccine can be administered at the same time as DPT and polio. Pneumococcal vaccine (Pneumovac) is recommended at 2 years of age with a booster 6 years later, since transplant recipients (especially those with asplenia syndromes) are at increased risk for pneumococcal infection. Immunization should be delayed in the presence of an acute febrile illness, acute rejection episodes, seizures, adverse reactions, or immunoglobulin therapy. The administration of all vaccines should be deferred until at least 6 weeks after the administration of intravenous gammaglobulin. It is advisable to avoid tapering of immunosuppression at the time of immunizations.

Until further information is available regarding their safety in immunocompromised patients, vaccines with **attenuated** viruses, such as measles, mumps, rubella (MMR) should be avoided. However, it should be noted that the MMR vaccine has been given successfully in the pediatric acquired immunodeficiency syndrome (AIDS) population,[192] where the level of immunosuppression is

TABLE 20-15	**Common Drugs for Treatment of Hypertension After Pediatric Cardiac Transplantation**

DRUG	DOSE
Hydralazine	0.75–3 mg/kg/day PO in 2–4 doses
Nifedipine	0.6–0.9 mg/kg/day PO in 3–4 doses
Verapamil	2–7 mg/kg/day PO in 3 doses
Diltiazem	1.5–2 mg/kg/day in 3–4 doses
Minoxidil	0.2–1.0 mg/kg/day PO in 1–2 doses
Enalapril	0.1–0.5 mg/kg/day PO in 1–2 doses
Captopril	Infants: 0.25–0.6 mg/kg/dose titrated to maximum of 4 mg/kg/day in 2–4 doses
	Children: 0.5–4 mg/kg/day PO in 2–3 doses

greater than most transplanted children, and it could probably be used safely after transplantation. In fact, it has been used at Loma Linda during an outbreak of native measles with no complications. Children after transplant who are exposed to **measles or mumps** are generally treated with immune serum globulin. Transplant children exposed to chickenpox (**varicella**) may receive passive immunization with varicella zoster immune globulin (VZIG). In the school-aged child, multiple exposures require repeated doses of VZIG if passive protection is offered with each exposure. Children who are beyond the first transplant year and who are not on routine steroids generally handle varicella disease quite well if acyclovir (80 mg/kg/day divided qid) is begun early in the course of varicella. MMR and varicella vaccines can probably be safely administered to children more than 1 year after transplant, but their routine use cannot be officially recommended until prospective controlled studies are performed.

SURVIVAL

OVERVIEW

Early and late survival after cardiac transplantation in older children and adolescents has paralleled the experience in adults (see Chapter 16). Among children and adolescents undergoing cardiac transplantation in the late 1970s and early 1980s, the late survival has been unfavorably influenced by higher early mortality, with 1-, 5-, and 10-year survivals in the range of 75%, 60%, and 50% respectively.[240] Since about 1985, most transplant programs have employed cyclosporine- and azathioprine-based immunosuppression with or without steroid maintenance. In the current era in experienced institutions, expected 1-year survival is 80–90%,[198] 2-year survival 80–85%,[143, 248, 256] and 5-year survival approximately 70–80%.[143] The survival after pediatric cardiac transplantation in the current era is reflected by the PHTS multi-institutional experience between 1993 and 1998, including 683 pediatric patients (Fig. 20–20). The ISHLT registry has reported an overall pediatric survival of 75% at 1 year and 64% at 5 years over the past 13 years,[36] but the more recent data reviewed here indicate a more realistic (and more favorable) early and intermediate survival at experienced centers. Multiple studies have indicated improving results in pediatric cardiac transplantation, even over the past 5 years.[98, 198, 278]

The experience with neonatal and infant cardiac transplantation dates only back to 1985, and meaningful long-term survival is only now exceeding 10 years. The major determinant of survival out to 5 years or more after infant cardiac transplantation is the initial hospital mortality after transplant. When early mortality is reduced to a low level, the intermediate survival after neonatal and infant cardiac transplantation is particularly good. The superb early results in cardiac transplantation among neonates and young infants coupled with the paucity of deaths between 1 and 5 years at Loma Linda[13] and other institutions suggests the possibility of more

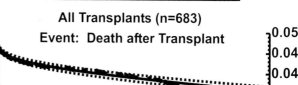

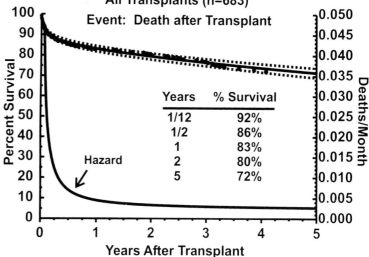

FIGURE **20–20.** Survival after cardiac transplantation, Pediatric Heart Transplant Study (1993–1997, n = 683). The upper curve is the parametric survival curve with the 70% confidence limits (dashed lines). The actuarial point estimates are displayed as closed circles. The lower curve is the hazard function (instantaneous risk) for death. The units for the hazard function are along the right-sided vertical axis.

effective induction of partial immunologic tolerance after cardiac transplantation in this age group compared to children and adults. The unique experience at Loma Linda now shows significant survival advantage at 10 years in patients transplanted as neonates versus other infants. The actuarial survival at Loma Linda for the overall neonatal experience (transplantation in the first month of life) is 80% at 5 years and 77% at 10 years. For all other infants (transplantation at age 1 month to 1 year), the actuarial survival is 68% at 5 years and 60% at 10 years.[62]

In many institutions, however, the results of cardiac transplantation for HLHS (which comprise the vast majority of neonatal transplants) have been less good than for other conditions. At UAB, the actuarial survival at 5 years for cardiac transplantation as primary therapy for HLHS is 63% (1994 to July 2000, n = 14), compared to 80% for all other pediatric conditions (1994 to July 2000, n = 19). The difference is totally accounted for by early mortality, as there have been no deaths after 6 months in the HLHS group and two deaths at 2 years (from allograft vasculopathy and sudden unexplained death) in the non-HLHS group. The increased early mortality for cardiac transplantation in HLHS is reflected in the overall PHTS experience for patients undergoing transplantation between 1993 and 1997 (Fig. 20–21).

CAUSES OF DEATH

When examining or discussing causes of death after pediatric cardiac transplantation, one must specify the time period after transplant, the diagnosis, and the age group, since these three variables directly affect ob-

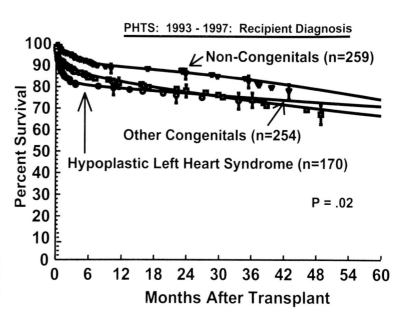

FIGURE **20–21.** Actuarial survival after transplant stratified by recipient diagnosis. Pediatric Heart Transplant Study (PHTS: 1993–1997, n = 683). The symbols represent the actuarial point estimates. Time 0 is the time of transplant.

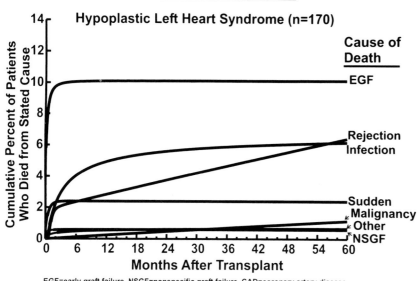

FIGURE **20–22.** Competing outcomes depiction for causes of death following cardiac transplantation for hypoplastic left heart syndrome in the Pediatric Heart Transplant Study (PHTS: 1993–1997, n = 170). The solid lines indicate the parametrically determined cumulative percent of patients who died from the stated cause at any given time after transplant (out to 60 months). EGF, early graft failure; NSGF, nonspecific graft failure.

served causes of death. Frazier and colleagues performed a competing outcomes analysis (see Chapter 3) for the first 5 years of the multi-institutional PHTS.[92] The important impact of early mortality is partly related to diagnosis, as shown in a competing outcomes analyses for hypoplastic left heart syndrome (Fig. 20–22), other forms of congenital heart disease (Fig. 20–23), and noncongenital heart disease (which is mainly cardiomyopathy) (Fig. 20–24). Comparing all causes of death over a 5-year period, the major difference between the three groups is **early graft failure** (EGF). Whereas only 1% of patients in the noncongenital group died from EGF, the EGF mortality increased to 5% for non-HLH congenitals and 10% for HLH. This dramatic difference is displayed in Figure 20–25. The reasons for such differences at most institutions likely relate to the smaller ''margin

of error'' in properly preserving neonatal and small infant hearts and the increased complexity of transplantation for complex congenital heart disease (often with multiple prior operations) compared to cardiomyopathies.

Allograft rejection is the leading cause of death during the first 5 years after transplantation for the overall pediatric population (Fig. 20–26),[92] producing a rejection-related mortality of about 7% over 5 years. The hazard function (instantaneous risk) for fatal rejections has an early peak at about 1 month, followed by a low constant risk over the next 5 years. Thus, fatal rejection is most likely to occur in the first month after transplant, but it continues to contribute a small ongoing risk for as long as these patients have been followed. Data from the PHTS suggests that fatality is more likely after rejec-

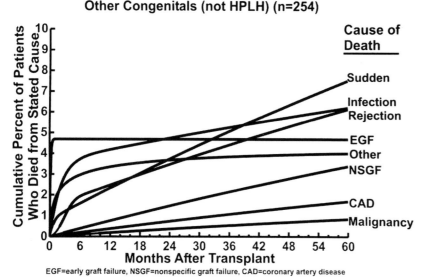

FIGURE **20–23.** Competing outcomes depiction for causes of death following cardiac transplantation for patients with congenital heart disease other than hypoplastic left heart syndrome in the Pediatric Heart Transplant Study (PHTS: 1993–1997, n = 254). The depiction is as in Figure 20–22. HPLH, hypoplastic left heart syndrome; EGF, early graft failure; CAD, coronary artery disease.

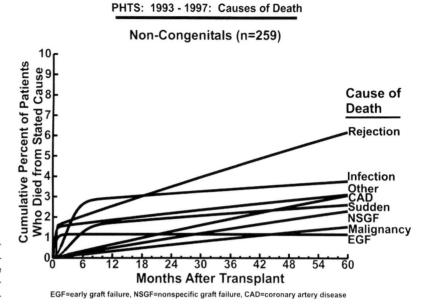

PHTS: 1993 - 1997: Causes of Death

Non-Congenitals (n=259)

FIGURE **20-24.** Competing outcomes depiction for causes of death following cardic transplantation for patients with a diagnosis other than congenital heart disese in the Pediatric Heart Transplant Study (PHTS: 1993–1997, n = 259). The depiction is as in Figure 20–22.

EGF=early graft failure, NSGF=nonspecific graft failure, CAD=coronary artery disease

tion with hemodynamic compromise (see section on rejection and Chapter 14) and after late rejection.[198]

Among all pediatric patients, **infection** is the second most common cause of mortality during the first 5 years after transplant (Fig. 20–26). Approximately 5% of patients die from infection by 5 years.[92] A detailed discussion of infections after cardiac transplantation is found in Chapter 15.

The risk of death from documented **allograft vasculopathy** remains low (<2%) over the first 5 years (Fig. 20–26). However, the possibility exists that at least some of the deaths from nonspecific graft failure[32] and sudden unexplained deaths may have resulted from unidentified coronary artery disease or from unrecognized rejection.[92]

Malignancy accounts for few deaths during the first 5 years, the risk of fatal malignancy being about 1%.

RISK FACTORS FOR EARLY MORTALITY

Elevated Pulmonary Vascular Resistance

Elevation of pulmonary vascular resistance clearly increases the risk of acute right ventricular failure early after transplant, particularly if there is an important element of donor heart dysfunction. Chen and colleagues have demonstrated a progressive increase in risk from "normal" pulmonary vascular resistance to "abnormal but reactive" to "abnormal and poorly reac-

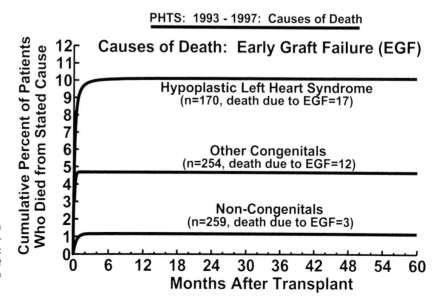

PHTS: 1993 - 1997: Causes of Death

FIGURE **20-25.** Competing outcomes depiction for death from early graft failure (EGF) in three diagnostic categories of patients undergoing cardiac transplantation in the Pediatric Heart Transplant Study (PHTS: 1993–1997, n = 683). The depiction is as in Figure 20–22.

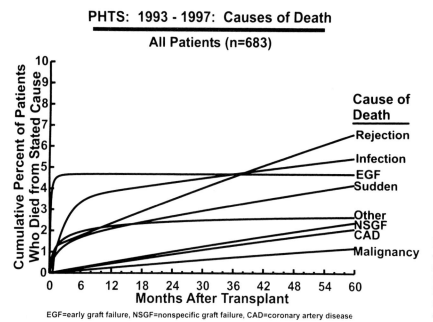

PHTS: 1993 - 1997: Causes of Death

All Patients (n=683)

EGF=early graft failure, NSGF=nonspecific graft failure, CAD=coronary artery disease

FIGURE **20-26.** Competing outcomes depiction for causes of death following cardiac transplantation for all patients in the Pediatric Heart Transplant Study (PHTS: 1993–1997, n = 683). The depiction is as in Figure 20–22. EGF, early graft failure; NSGF, nonspecific graft failure; CAD, coronary artery disease.

tive.''[56] Further discussion of PVR is found earlier in this chapter.

Donor Ischemic Time

The safe duration of ischemic time in infant cardiac transplantation remains controversial. Extrapolating from the adult experience,[39] many groups have considered a total ischemic time exceeding 4–5 hours to be associated with a progressive increase in early acute cardiac failure and mortality. Because of the limited donor pool for neonatal and infant cardiac transplantation, widespread application of this therapy requires utilization of donors from great geographic distances. During the first decade of infant cardiac transplantation at Loma Linda, they challenged the accepted "safe" ischemic time by occasionally accepting donors from distances which resulted in ischemic times of 6–9 hours. Using an intracellular based myocardial preservation solution (Roe's solution), they were not able to identify longer ischemic time as a risk factor for early mortality.[33] Similarly, a recent multi-institutional study[48] did not identify ischemic time as a predictor of early mortality after infant heart transplantation. Among children greater than 1 year of age, longer ischemic time was also not identified as a risk factor by multivariable analysis in a recent multi-institutional pediatric heart transplant study.[248] It is noteworthy that by univariate analysis longer ischemic times were associated with a higher mortality, but they occurred more frequently in the setting of left ventricular assist devices which are known to be a risk factor for early death. Only about 10% of patients had an ischemic time longer than 5½ hours. Thus, with current methods of donor heart preservation, the actual safe ischemic time for infant and pediatric heart transplantation remains unknown, but an ischemic time of up to 6 hours and possibly as much as 8 hours can probably be endured by a normal pediatric donor heart without an increased likelihood of posttransplant acute cardiac failure.[74]

Donor/Recipient Size Ratio

The extension of cardiac transplantation into infancy necessitated a redefinition of acceptable donor/recipient size ratios in order to utilize available donors. In the infant age group, a donor/recipient weight ratio of 0.7–3.0 is considered safe,[99] but lobar or complete lung collapse in the first week after transplantation is more common (up to 75% of patients) when the donor/recipient ratio exceeds about 1.6. In a multi-institutional study,[248] donor/recipient ratio was not a risk factor for early mortality. The distribution of donor/recipient weights and body surface area observed in the multi-institutional PHTS experience are displayed in Figure 20–27. Larger ratios are the most suitable for recipients with a large cardiac silhouette. In a recipient with normal heart size, a ratio exceeding 2 is probably more likely to result

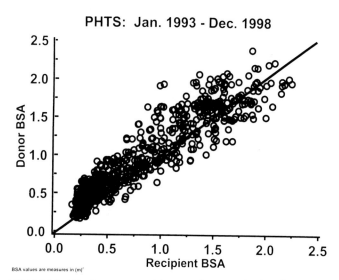

PHTS: Jan. 1993 - Dec. 1998

BSA values are measures in (m)'

FIGURE **20-27.** Scattergram of donor and recipient body surface areas (BSA) for patients undergoing cardiac transplantation in the Pediatric Heart Transplant Study, January 1993 to December 1998 (n = 383). The solid line is the line of identical donor and recipient BSA.

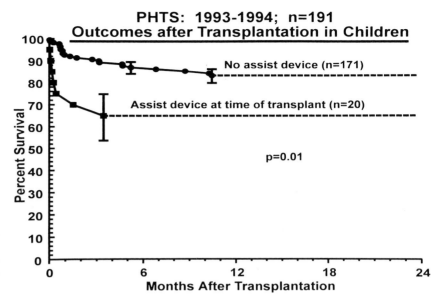

FIGURE **20–28.** Actuarial survival (Kaplan-Meier) for patients requiring an assist device at the time of transplantation (lower line, n = 20) vs. all other patients (upper line, n = 171). Pediatric Heart Transplant Study (PHTS: 1993–1994, n = 191). (From Shaddy RE, Naftel DC, Kirklin JK, Boyle G, McGiffin DC, Towbin JA, Ring WS, Pearce B, Addonizio L, Morrow WR, and the Pediatric Heart Transplant Study Group: Outcome of cardiac transplantation in children: survival in a contemporary multi-institutional experience. Circulation 1996;94[suppl II]:II-69–II-73.)

in primary nonclosure of the sternum following cardiac transplantation, particularly if important donor cardiac dysfunction is present. Less information is available about the safety of using a heart from a much smaller donor, such that the donor-recipient weight ratio is less than 0.7. Caution is advisable in transplantation with a very small donor/recipient size ratio. A limited experience suggests that as the ratio falls below 1.0, the risk of acute graft failure may increase.[265]

Mechanical Circulatory Support

There seems little doubt that critically ill children requiring mechanical circulatory support are at increased risk for death following cardiac transplantation (Fig. 20–28).[248] This relates in part to the lack of effective long-term ventricular assist systems for children compared to adults and the increased risk of infection with less adequate organ system support using extracorporeal membrane oxygenator (ECMO) or pediatric intra-aortic balloon support compared to left ventricular support devices or biventricular support available in adults. In a multi-institutional pediatric study, the 1-month mortality following transplantation for patients supported with mechanical assistance was 25% versus 5% with no assist device.[248]

Younger Age

As discussed earlier, differing survival rates have been reported when patients are stratified by age. Controversy exists regarding the effect of younger age in children undergoing cardiac transplantation. By multivariable analysis, Shaddy and colleagues identified younger age as a possible risk factor ($p = .1$) for children over 1 year of age undergoing cardiac transplantation in a multi-institutional study,[248] and the 1-year survival in infants less than 1 year of age at transplant (most of whom were HLHS) was significantly less than in children over 1 year.[49] However, others with extensive experience in neonatal transplantation have reported an in-

verse relationship between pediatric age and survival, with the greatest intermediate term survival in neonates and infants, and the lowest survival in children and adolescents.[61] A more recent depiction of survival in the PHTS, stratified by age (Fig. 20–29), reflects current results in experienced centers. In this recent 6-year PHTS experience, age at transplantation was not a significant risk factor for death ($p = .3$) by univariate analysis.[198] The 1-year survival for patients under 2 years of age (with *no* increased risk in infants under 6 months) was about 80% at 1 year, compared to about 86% for pediatric patients over 2 years of age.[198] As discussed earlier, note the paucity of deaths after the first 6 months in patients undergoing transplantation in the first 6 months of life.

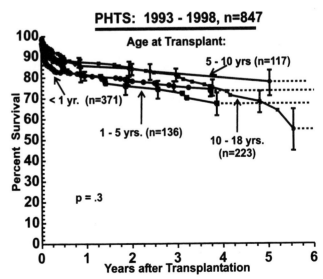

FIGURE **20–29.** Stratified actuarial survival after primary cardiac transplantation in PHTS infants and children. There was no significant difference in survival rates between age groups as analyzed by univariate analysis (p = 0.3, log rank test). (From Morrow WR, Frazier E, Naftel DC: Survival after listing for cardiac transplantation in children. Prog Pediatr Cardiol 2000;11:99–105.)

Diagnosis

The cardiac diagnosis has been examined as a possible risk factor for early mortality with differing conclusions. With the possible exception of HLHS, most analyses support the conclusion that in transplant centers experienced in the surgery of complex congenital heart disease, diagnosis per se (e.g., cardiomyopathy vs. complex uncorrectable congenital heart disease) is not an independent risk factor, unless there have been multiple prior sternotomies (see below).[49, 249] As discussed earlier in this chapter, the diagnosis of HLHS is a risk factor for early mortality in many institutions, and may be a surrogate for younger age, since the vast majority of infants transplanted in the first year of life have HLHS. The clear exception to this finding is the experience of a few centers, with a concentrated experience in HLHS, in which the late mortality after transplantation for this condition is actually lower than for other conditions.[61]

Prior Cardiac Operations

Controversy exists as to whether prior cardiac surgery, and more specifically a previous sternotomy, increases the risks of death early after pediatric cardiac transplantation. In experienced centers, most surgeons and analyses support the notion that cardiac transplantation in a reoperative setting does not increase the risk of early mortality (although it does increase the degree of difficulty of the operation). This conclusion is supported by several analyses.[50, 75, 240] It is of interest that a multi-institutional (PHTS) study by Canter and colleagues identified a history of previous sternotomy as the significant risk factor for early mortality ($p = .0003$) among infants undergoing cardiac transplantation (Fig. 20–30).[49] However, in this very young age group, previ-

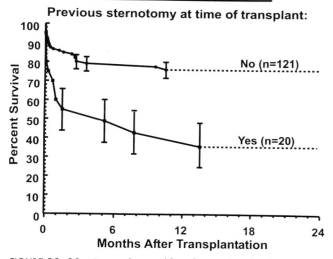

PHTS: 1993-1994; n=141 Infants

Previous sternotomy at time of transplant:

FIGURE **20–30.** Actuarial survival for infants with and without a previous sternotomy at the time of transplantation. Pediatric Heart Transplant Study (PHTS: 1993–1994, n = 141). (From Canter C, Naftel D, Caldwell R, Chinnock R, Pahl E, Frazier E, kirklin JK, Boucek M, Morrow R, and the Pediatric Heart Transplant Study Group: Survival and risk factors for death after cardiac transplantation in infants: a multi-institutional study. Circulation 1997;96:227-231.)

ous sternotomy usually indicated a very recent attempt at surgical repair with poor outcome (and thus the need for cardiac transplantation), representing a particularly high-risk group of patients. Thus, it was likely the patient's condition rather than the prior sternotomy itself which portended a poor outcome.

Donor Cause of Death

A recent multi-institutional study identified donor death from causes other than closed head trauma as a risk factor for death after infant cardiac transplantation.[49] The precise explanation is unclear but could relate to other factors such as blood loss at time of some injuries or the effect of prolonged hypoxia in some settings prior to death. The cause of death may correlate with the degree of donor cardiac injury, as reflected by cardiac troponin I levels.[109]

LATE SURVIVAL

Limited information is available regarding late survival (10 years or more) following pediatric cardiac transplantation. Such data are of particular importance in the pediatric population, since routine survival for 15–20 years or more is necessary for this therapy to provide effective long-term palliation and quality of life. Since late survival is heavily influenced by early mortality, every effort must be made to minimize hospital mortality after pediatric cardiac transplantation. Examination of the competing outcomes analyses in Figures 20–22 through 20–26 indicate the ongoing risks of death from rejection, infection, allograft vasculopathy, and malignancy out to at least 5 years after transplantation.[92] Extrapolation from these and other data suggests that the risk of late death from malignancy and allograft vasculopathy may further increase as follow-up is extended. Analysis of late survival from an earlier era of cardiac transplantation indicated an important decrement of survival between 10 and 15 years after transplant,[254] primarily due to rejection and allograft vasculopathy. Judging from current trends in adult cardiac transplantation (see Chapter 16), current expectations of 75% survival at 10 years seem realistic with current hospital mortality and available immunosuppressive strategies. As noted earlier, examination of the survival curves in Figure 20–28 and data from Loma Linda[62] suggest that there may be a long-term (>10 years) survival advantage for infants undergoing cardiac transplantation in the first month of life. Among 97 infants undergoing cardiac transplantation in the first month of life, the actuarial survival at 13 years was 77%.[62]

ACUTE ALLOGRAFT REJECTION

The basic immune response to the event of cardiac transplantation is discussed in Chapter 2, and the pathophysiology and clinical aspects of rejection, which are similar in pediatric and adult transplantation, are discussed in

Chapter 14. There continues to be controversy about the effect of age on the immunologic response to transplantation, with only indirect evidence that the transplant immune response in infants and neonates (see Box) responds differently from older children and adults.[250] The possibility exists that if cardiac transplantation is performed within the first few days or weeks of postnatal life, then the probability of acute cardiac rejection may be less than in older infants ("window of opportunity" of neonatal cardiac transplantation).[12] The clinical experience at Loma Linda suggests that patients undergoing transplantation in the first month or so of life experience less rejection with less immunosuppression than older infants and children.[12] Neonatal hyporesponsiveness has been demonstrated in animals, but amelioration of the immune response to a cardiac allograft in human neonates has not been clearly established.

The effect of thymectomy (routinely performed by many cardiac surgeons at the time of infant cardiac surgery or transplantation) on the baby's immune response is unknown, but any immunologic effect of thymectomy appears mild and short-lived. There does appear to be some reduction in circulating CD3+ and CD4+ T-cells, which persists out to a year, but indices of lymphocyte proliferation are normal within 1 year. Thus, a neonatal thymectomy appears to cause only a modest decrease in T-lymphocyte levels without a demonstrable decrease in immune function.[282]

METHODS OF DIAGNOSIS

The diagnosis of acute rejection in infants and children is most commonly ascertained by three modalities: clinical evidence, echocardiography, and endomyocardial biopsy. **Biopsy** criteria are identical to those utilized in adult cardiac transplantation (see Chapter 14), and the procedure is associated with few complications in experienced pediatric centers.[222] The major disadvantage of endomyocardial biopsy relates to the frequent need for general anesthesia, the expense of hospitalization, and the potential loss of venous access with repeated biopsies in infants and children.

Clinical clues to the presence of acute rejection include alterations in the child's activity level, listlessness, irritability, poor feeding, fever, atrial and ventricular ectopy, S3 gallop, persistent resting tachycardia, tachypnea, dyspnea, hepatic congestion, ileus, and other evidence of heart failure or low cardiac output (Table 20–16). However, there is no clinical constellation of symptoms or signs which is specific for rejection. Antirejection therapy would rarely be initiated for clinical signs alone in the absence of echocardiographic or biopsy confirmation except with clinical evidence of low cardiac output.

Diagnosis of acute rejection by two-dimensional transthoracic **echocardiography** has been controversial. While nearly all transplant physicians would initiate antirejection therapy when there is echocardiographic evidence of depressed systolic function in the absence of another clear explanation (such as early graft dysfunction in the first few days after transplantation or in the presence of extensive allograft vasculopathy), other echocardiographic criteria for rejection have not yet been reproducible, and therefore accepted, in all institutions. However, several of the most successful pediatric heart transplant programs (including most notably the experience generated by the transplant team at Loma Linda) have relied almost exclusively on echocardiography for the diagnosis of acute rejection in infants. A number of echocardiographic changes that reflect an increase in left ventricular mass, impairment of systolic and diastolic function, new pericardial effusion, and/or new mitral

TABLE 20–16	**Clinical Signs and Symptoms of Possible Graft Rejection**

1. Nonspecific symptoms
    Irritability
    Malaise
    Poor feeding
    Change in sleeping pattern
2. Alterations in cardiac rhythm
    New-onset tachycardia
    New-onset bradycardia
    Presence of third heart sound
    Decreasing ECG voltage
    New-onset atrial or ventricular arrhythmias or conduction changes
3. Signs of congestive heart failure or low cardiac output
    Presence of third heart sound
    Rales
    Tachypnea
    Pulmonary edema
    Hepatosplenomegaly
    Diapheresis
    Cool and mottled extremities
    Oliguria

TABLE 20-17	Threshold Values For Echocardiographic Rejection Parameters In Children	

PARAMETERS	THRESHOLD	WEIGHTED SCORE
Interventricular septal thickening fraction	<25%	1
Left ventricular posterior wall thickening fraction	<70%	2
Left ventricular volume (LVV)*	<65%	2
Left ventricular mass (LVM)*	>130%	1
LVV/LVM	<45%	1
Maximum velocity of posterior wall thinning	<11 (−1/sec)†	1
Average velocity of left ventricular wall thinning	<25 mm/sec	1
Average velocity of left ventricular enlargement	<60 mm/sec	1
Mitral insufficiency	>1+/4	1
Total		11

*Percent of predicted normal for body surface area.
†Corrected for dimension at maximum velocity.
Adapted from Boucek MM, Mathis CM, Boucek RJ, Hodgkin DD, Kanakriyeh MS, McCormack J, Gundry SR, Baley LL: Prospective evaluation of echocardiography for primary rejection surveillance after infant heart transplantation: comparison with endomyocardial biopsy. J Heart Lung Transplant 1994;13:66–73.

TABLE 20-18	Echocardiographic Rejection Grade in Children	

FINDINGS	ECHO GRADE	INTERPRETATION
Score of 0	1	Normal
Score of 1–3	2	Probably normal
Score of 4–6 or new pericardial effusion or new mitral regurgitation (≥2+)	3	Probable rejection
Score of 7–11 or LVSF <28%	4	Rejection

LVSF, left ventricular shortening fraction.
Adapted from Boucek MM, Mathis CM, Boucek RJ, Hodgkin DD, Kanakriyeh MS, McCormack J, Gundry SR, Baley LL: Prospective evaluation of echocardiography for primary rejection surveillance after infant heart transplantation: comparison with endomyocardial biopsy. J Heart Lung Transplant 1994;13:66–73.

insufficiency (Tables 20–17 and 20–18) have been reported to correlate with histologic evidence of acute cardiac rejection.[31, 61, 173, 266] With experience, the reported sensitivity and specificity of echocardiography at predicting rejection by biopsy is as high as 92% and 98%, respectively.[31]

Regardless of which method of detection is predominantly used, it would seem prudent to incorporate all three modalities into a strategy of surveillance for acute cardiac rejection. The utilization of these modalities in various age groups was examined in a multi-institutional study and is shown in Figure 20–31.[237]

Another promising method which has not yet been widely applied in children is telemetric monitoring of **intramyocardial electrogram recordings,** which is also discussed in Chapter 14. This technique requires the implantation of a dual-chamber telemetry pacemaker with left and right ventricle screw-in electrodes. Daily

distant telemetric monitoring of changes in QRS amplitude have been reported to reliably predict rejection.[202]

ROUTINE LONG-TERM SURVEILLANCE FOR REJECTION

There is considerable variability among transplant programs regarding protocols for long-term rejection surveillance. In programs such as at UAB that utilize endomyocardial biopsies, biopsies during the first year are generally performed in children every 2 weeks for the first 2 months, then monthly for the next 2 months, then every 3 months for the remainder of the first year. In infants, a routine endomyocardial biopsy is scheduled at 3 weeks, 6 weeks, 10 weeks, and every 3 months thereafter for the first year. An echocardiogram is generally performed weekly for the first 2 months, then at gradually increasing intervals thereafter during the first year. If clinical or echocardiographic signs suggest rejection, a prompt cardiac biopsy is performed.

In programs which utilize primarily echocardiography for the diagnosis of rejection, endomyocardial biopsies, particularly in infants and small children, are only performed when there is echocardiographic evidence of rejection.

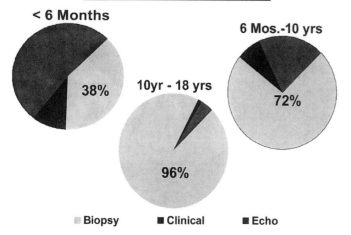

FIGURE 20–31. Pie chart of proportion of rejection episodes diagnosed by biopsy, clinical criteria alone, and echo. Pediatric Heart Transplant Study (PHTS: 1993–1994, n = 332).

Longer term surveillance is also highly varible. At UAB, during the second year after transplant, routine clinic visits with an echocardiogram are scheduled every 3 months, with a biopsy every 6 months. During years 3–5, a clinic visit is scheduled every 4 months (usually with an echocardiogram) and a biopsy once yearly. After 5 years, routine clinic visits are every 6 months with a yearly biopsy. The precise biopsy and echocardiogram schedule are tailored to the rejection history of the patient, with more frequent biopsies in the presence of recent or frequent rejection or tapering of immunosuppression. It is always understood, however, that clinical signs or symptoms suggestive of rejection should prompt an immediate clinic visit and echocardiogram, with biopsy if indicated.

TREATMENT OF ACUTE REJECTION

As in adult cardiac transplantation, the standard therapeutic options for acute rejection include pulse therapy with intravenous or oral steroids, antilymphocyte globulin, OKT3, conversion from azathioprine to mycophenolate, conversion from cyclosporine to tacrolimus, plasmapheresis, photopheresis, total lymphoid irradiation, methotrexate, and alteration of maintenance immunosuppression. The details of these immunotherapeutic modalities are discussed in Chapter 13, and the strategies for rejection therapy are discussed in Chapter 14. Specific features of antirejection therapy in infants and children are discussed here.

Asymptomatic or minimally symptomatic infants and children with echocardiographic or endomyocardial biopsy evidence of rejection, but with preserved hemodynamics, usually receive intravenous methylprednisolone during the first 3 months after transplant and outpatient intravenous or oral steroids for isolated rejection after 3 months. At **UAB**, infants less than 7 kg receive either 100 mg of intravenous methylprednisolone or 100 mg of oral prednisolone daily for 3 days and patients 7 kg or more receive 15 mg/kg/dose of intravenous methylprednisolone or oral prednisolone for 3 days. At **Loma Linda**, methylprednisolone 20–25 mg/kg IV to a maximum dose of 100 mg is given every 12 hours for eight doses. Ranitidine prophylaxis is administered during the steroid therapy. Furosemide and antihypertensive therapy are administered as necessary.

Patients with moderate to severe symptoms and/or evidence of hemodynamic compromise are hospitalized and receive intravenous steroid therapy as outlined above plus additional immunosuppressive therapy and inotropic support as needed. A detailed discussion of recurrent or persistent rejection is found in Chapter 14. The additional immunosuppressive therapy for infants and children usually includes one or more of the following:

1. Antithymocyte globulin (thymoglobulin) (rabbit) 1.5 mg/kg/day IV for 7–10 days in an intensive care setting.

2. Antithymocyte globulin (Atgam) (equine) 15 mg/kg/day IV for 7–10 days in an intensive care setting.

3. OKT3—the dose is usually 0.1–0.2 mg/kg up to a maximum of 5 mg IV for 5–10 days. Benadryl 1 mg/kg IV is administered before each OKT3 dose. The effectiveness of antibody preparations (OKT3 and ATG) should be verified by T-cell markers (see Table 20–11) on about day 3 of therapy. OKT3 is rarely used in young children at Loma Linda (but employed in infants and children at UAB).

4. Conversion from azathioprine to mycophenolate mofetil.

5. Conversion from cyclosporine to tacrolimus.

6. Methotrexate, usually in dose of 10 mg/m²/wk (maximum dose of 7.5 mg) administered as three divided doses 12 hours apart (or as a single dose once per week). Dosage adjusted to avoid severe leukopenia.

Further dosing and other details of these immunosuppressive modalities are discussed in Chapter 13.

TIME-RELATED NATURE OF REJECTION

The precise definition of acute rejection has been especially problematic in pediatric heart transplantation because of the considerable interinstitutional variability in the method of diagnosis and the uncertain correlation between echocardiography and biopsy. In this discussion and in most published analyses, acute rejection is defined as intensification of immunosuppression based on either biopsy, echocardiographic, or clinical diagnosis of rejection. Despite more variability in the method of diagnosing rejection in pediatric patients, the time-related nature of rejection is similar to that observed in adults, with the highest incidence of acute rejection occurring in the first 2 months after transplantation. In a multi-institutional study of pediatric patients undergoing cardiac transplantation between 1993 and 1995, 60% of patients experienced one or more rejection episodes in the first 3 months (Fig. 20–32).[237] This mirrors the experience observed in adult recipients.[158] The associated hazard function for first rejection is highest between 1 and 2 months after transplant. The cumulative rejection frequency (Fig. 20–33)[237] is similar to that observed in the adult population.[158]

RISK FACTORS FOR EARLY REJECTION

Less information is available regarding the factors which predispose to rejection in infants and children compared to adults (see Chapter 14). It is likely, though, that risk factors for rejection are similar for all ages.

Controversy exists as to whether **recipient age** is a risk factor for rejection. Younger age has been identified by single- as well as multi-institutional studies as a predictor of earlier rejection,[154, 158, 159] but the number of pediatric patients was small compared to adults in these

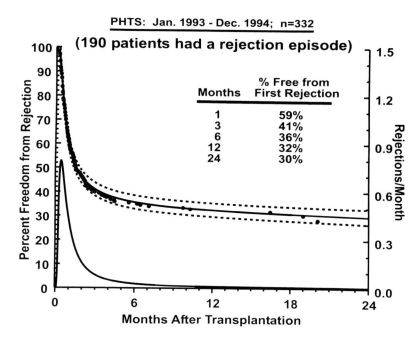

FIGURE **20–32.** Freedom from rejection. Pediatric Heart Transplant Study (PHTS: 1993–1994, n = 332). The upper curve is the parametric freedom from first rejection. The dashed lines enclose the 70% confidence limits. The closed circles represent the actuarial point estimates. The lower curve is the hazard function (instantaneous risk) for first rejection.

studies. Furthermore, these studies could not examine the possibility that neonates and infants may actually have a lower rejection tendency than older children. The notion that neonates and young infants may exhibit partial tolerance was first suggested clinically by reports from Loma Linda regarding neonatal cardiac transplantation.[58]

When pure pediatric heart transplant populations which include an important neonatal component have been analyzed, older age at transplant has been identified as a risk factor for earlier and more frequent rejection.[61, 237] A multivariable analysis from the PHTS identified older age among pediatric patients as a risk factor for first rejection ($p = .02$) and cumulative rejection ($p = .002$) in the first 6 months. The risk-unadjusted age-stratified actuarial freedom from rejection is depicted

in Figure 20–34 and the cumulative rejection in Figure 20–35.[237] The interpretation of these analyses is confounded by the differing methods of rejection detection in the various age groups, but from all available information it appears likely that neonates and young infants as a group have a lower rejection tendency than children, and that children are slightly less prone to rejection than teenagers and young adults, after which the rejection tendency very slightly decreases as adult age advances.

With current methods of immunosuppression, rejection as a primary cause of death is relatively uncommon among the overall pediatric population, the actuarial freedom from *fatal* rejection being 95% at 2 years in the PHTS analysis. Rotondo and colleagues found that fatal rejection accounted for a smaller proportion of overall mortality in infants compared to children and adolescents (6% in patients less than 6 months of age at transplant, 30% in patients 6 months to 10 years, and 23% in children over 10 years).[237]

Other risk factors noted in adults (see Chapter 14) have been less securely identified in pediatric studies. The effect of HLA mismatches has not been well studied. Donor/recipient gender mismatch was identified as a probable risk factor ($p = .07$) for rejection in a multi-institutional multivariate analysis,[237] but not in another single-institution study.[61] Although limited information is available, cytomegalovirus infection after transplant may predispose to rejection.[110] Recipient black race may also predispose to increased rejection.[237]

HUMORAL REJECTION

Humoral rejection after cardiac transplantation is discussed in detail in Chapter 14. Few studies have examined humoral rejection in pediatric transplant patients. In a study by Zales and colleagues,[295] 8 out of 131 biopsy specimens (processed for light microscopy and immu-

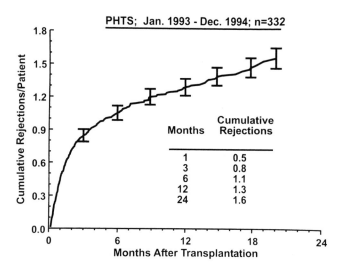

FIGURE **20–33.** Average cumulative rejection following cardiac transplantation. Pediatric Heart Transplant Study (PHTS: 1993–1994, n = 332). The error bars represent 70% confidence limits.

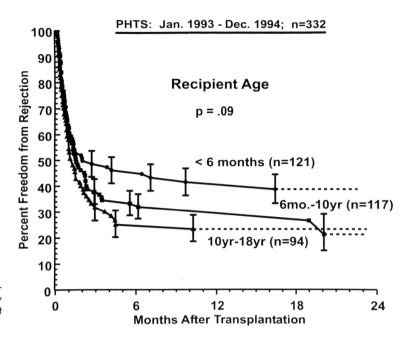

FIGURE **20–34.** Actuarial freedom from first rejection, stratified by age at transplant. Pediatric Heart Transplant Study (PHTS: 1993–1994, n = 332). The error bars represent 70% confidence limits.

nofluorescence) from 30 patients revealed evidence of immunoglobulin and complement C3 deposition in the myocardium (hallmarks of antibody-mediated rejection), often with accompanying evidence of cellular rejection. In this study, no relationship was noted between the presence of positive pretransplant panel reactive antibodies or B-cell crossmatch at the time of transplantation and subsequent humoral rejection. Several studies suggest a possible correlation between demonstrated humoral rejection (immunoglobulin and complement deposition by immunofluorescence) and the subsequent development of allograft vasculopathy.[4, 103, 116–118, 120, 121, 170, 235, 294] When humoral rejection is suspected or identified, specific anti–B-cell immunotherapy seems advisable (see Chapter 14).

LATE REJECTION

Rejection after the first year occurs in about 25% of surviving patients. In a multi-institutional study, Webber and colleagues examined rejection after the first year in 431 pediatric patients.[281] Risk factors for late rejection included more than one episode of rejection in the first year ($p = .009$), recipient black race ($p = .0002$), and older age at transplant (p = .0003). The occurrence of late rejection was associated with 25% subsequent mortality, often within several months, and most often caused by rejection, unexplained sudden death, or coronary vasculopathy. In the absence of late rejection, mortality between years 1 and 4 was only 1.2% ($p < .0001$). Thus, late rejection appears to identify a higher risk group

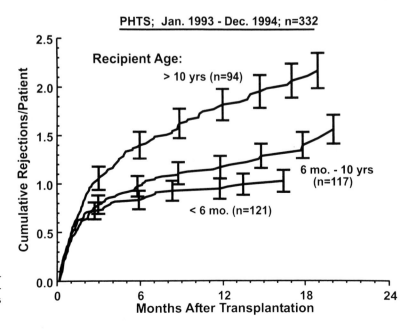

FIGURE **20–35.** Average cumulataive rejections per patient, stratified by age at transplant. Pediatric Heart Transplant Study (PHTS: 1993–1994, n = 332). The error bars represent 70% confidence limits.

for subsequent mortality. This group of patients should receive increased rejection surveillance, augmented immunosuppression, and consideration for coronary angiography.

REJECTION WITH HEMODYNAMIC COMPROMISE

Rejection with hemodynamic compromise (HC) appears to hold the same ominous prognosis in pediatric recipients as it does in adults.[197] Pahl and colleagues in the PHTS noted severe hemodynamic compromise in about 10% of rejection episodes, with no important differences by age group.[214] Rejection with HC was a serious event, portending greater than 50% mortality within 6 months. Thus, rejection with HC should prompt aggressive initial therapy accompanied by an increase in maintenance immunosuppression with very close rejection surveillance for at least 6 months.

INFECTION

The diagnosis, treatment, and prognosis of infections common to both pediatric and adult patients are discussed in Chapter 15. This section will cover aspects of posttransplant infection which are unique to the pediatric population.

TYPES AND TIME-RELATED NATURE OF INFECTION

With the evolution of pediatric heart transplantation, there has been a gradual decrease in the incidence of serious infection[3, 81, 83, 107, 166, 196, 227] and a change in the pattern of infections. Fungal and protozoal infections

were more common in the early years of pediatric transplantation,[3, 83, 196] but these are uncommon in the current era in which bacterial and viral infections predominate.

In the current era, the risk of posttransplant infection is highest during the first posttransplant month and rapidly declines thereafter.[244] About 25% of patients experience one or more infections during the first month, and nearly 50% suffer infectious complications during the first year (Fig. 20–36). Approximately half the patients who have one infection also suffer a subsequent infection.

About 60% of all infections are bacterial, 30% are viral, 7% are fungal, and less than 3% are protozoal.[244] Although most types of bacterial infections have been observed after pediatric heart transplantation, staphylococcal species, *Pseudomonas*, and *Enterobacter cloacae* are particularly common (Table 20–19). Cytomegalovirus accounts for the majority of viral infections and is the most common single infectious agent. Respiratory infection with respiratory syncytial virus is most common in children less than 6 months of age, with the potential long-term sequelae of significant reactive airway disease. As in adult cardiac transplantation, the most common sites of posttransplant infection are blood and lung (Table 20–20). The greatest period of risk differs somewhat among infection types. The risk or hazard of bacterial and fungal infections is highest during the first month, whereas the peak risk for viral infection occurs during the second month (Fig. 20–37).

RISK FACTORS FOR INFECTION

In a multi-institutional analysis of 276 infections during the first 2 years following pediatric heart transplantation,[244] risk factors predicting earlier onset of infection included younger recipient age ($p = .05$), ventilator support at time of transplant ($p = .002$), positive donor

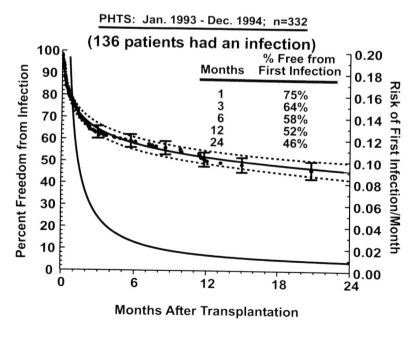

FIGURE **20–36.** Freedom from infection. Upper curve represents parametric freedom from infection with its 70% confidence limits (dotted lines). The closed circles represent the actuarial point estimates (Kaplan-Meier) and their 70% confidence limits (error bars). The lower curve represents the hazard function (instantaneous risk) for first infection after heart transplantation. The risk of first infection/month is indicated on the right-sided vertical axis. PHTS, Pediatric Heart Transplant Study. (From Schowengerdt KO, Naftel DC, Seib PM, Pearce FB, Addonizio LJ, Kirklin JK, Morrow WR, Pediatric Heart Transplant Study Group: Infection after pediatric heart transplantation: results of a multi-institutional study. J Heart Lung Transplant 1997;16:1207–1216.)

Within the figure:

PHTS: Jan. 1993 - Dec. 1994; n=332
(136 patients had an infection)

Months	% Free from First Infection
1	75%
3	64%
6	58%
12	52%
24	46%

Y-axis (left): Percent Freedom from Infection
Y-axis (right): Risk of First Infection/Month
X-axis: Months After Transplantation

TABLE 20-19 List of Infections by Class and Organism During the First 2 Years Following Pediatric Cardiac Transplantation (PHTS, N = 332 Patients)

	NO.
Bacterial (n = 164)	
Staphylococcus epidermidis	25
Staphylococcus aureus	11
Staphylococcus (other)	4
Streptococcus viridans	4
Streptococcus pneumoniae	2
Enterococcus	13
Pseudomonas aeruginosa	16
Pseudomonas (other)	11
Enterobacter cloacae	17
Enterobacter (other)	4
Clostridium difficile	11
Klebsiella pneumoniae	3
Klebsiella (other)	3
Escherichia coli	3
Serratia marcescens	2
Pseudomonas maltophilia	3
Unspecified	18
Other (single isolates)	14
Viral (n = 86)	
Cytomegalovirus	51
Viral, noncytomegalovirus (n = 35)	
Varicella zoster	11
Respiratory syncycial virus	10
Herpes simplex virus	6
Adenovirus	1
Epstein-Barr virus	1
Rotavirus	1
Unspecified	5
Fungal (n = 19)	
Candida spp.	12
Aspergillus spp.	2
Cryptococcus spp.	1
Rhizopus spp.	1
Rhizomucor spp.	1
Unspecified	2
Protozoal (n = 7)	
Pneumocystis	7

Adapted from Schowengerdt KO, Naftel DC, Seib PM, Pearce FB, Addonizio LJ, Kirklin JK, Morrow WR, Pediatric Heart Transplant Study Group: Infection after pediatric heart transplantation: results of a multi-institutional study. J Heart Lung Transplant 1997;16:1207–1216.

CMV serology with negative recipient serology (p = .04), and longer donor ischemic time (p = .03).

Although speculative, the increased risk of infection in **young infants** (especially less than about 6 months of age) may relate to the relative immaturity of their immune system and possibly to their longer intensive care unit (ICU) stay, with potentially longer duration of invasive monitoring. The transplant infant is also more likely than older children or adults to have increased susceptibility to pulmonary infection from encapsulated organisms such as *Haemophilus influenzae*, *Neisseria meningitides*, and streptococcal pneumonia.[112] **Ventilator support** at time of transplant identifies patients who are critically ill and suggests a greater susceptibility not only to pneumonia, but to all types of early bacterial infections. **Longer donor ischemic time** may identify a subset with a somewhat greater chance of donor heart dysfunction and therefore a longer ICU stay.

The increased infection tendency (particularly CMV infection) when a **CMV-negative recipient** receives a **CMV-positive organ** (Fig. 20–38)[244] mirrors the well-documented adult experience.[156, 196] Controversy exists regarding the relationship between induction therapy with OKT3 or some form of antithymocyte serum (ATS) and the subsequent development of infection, particularly with CMV. Although a general perception exists that the risk of CMV infection is heightened by a course of OKT3 or ATS, this relationship has proven difficult to establish in the current era.[49, 196] This may relate to the frequent use of ganciclovir for CMV prophylaxis in patients who receive OKT3 or ATS therapy. Although the effectiveness of CMV prophylaxis following pediatric heart transplantation has not been proven, several studies have suggested efficacy of CMV prophylaxis after solid organ transplantation with ganciclovir[49, 66, 165, 194] or CMV immunoglobulin.[258]

OUTCOME AFTER INFECTION

Most infections after pediatric heart transplantation can be successfully treated, and mortality is highly related

TABLE 20-20 Sites of Infections During the First 2 Years Following Pediatric Cardiac Transplantation (PHTS: 1993-1994, n = 332 Patients)

	CLASS OF INFECTION				
LOCATION*	Bacterial	Cytomegalovirus	Viral (Noncytomegalovirus)	Fungal	Protozoal
Blood	60	35	2	3	—
Lung	56	13	15	7	7
Gastrointestinal	17	6	3	1	—
Urine	16	17	1	6	—
Skin	3	—	11	3	—
Wound, surgical	8	—	—	2	—
Peritoneal	7	—	—	1	—
Soft tissue	3	1	1	2	—
Bone	3	—	—	—	—
Central nervous system	2	—	—	—	—
Other	11	5	6	2	—

PHTS, Pediatric Heart Transplant Study.
*Some infections occurred in more than one location.
From Schowengerdt KO, Naftel DC, Seib PM, Pearce FB, Addonizio LJ, Kirklin JK, Morrow WR, Pediatric Heart Transplant Study Group: Infection after pediatric heart transplantation: results of a multi-institutional study. J Heart Lung Transplant 1997;16:1207–1216.

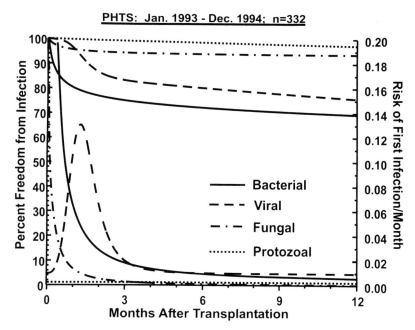

PHTS: Jan. 1993 - Dec. 1994; n=332

FIGURE **20-37.** Freedom from infection according to causative agent. Upper family of curves depicts parametric freedom from infection caused by indicated infectious agent. Lower family of curves represents associated hazard function (instaneous risk). PHTS, Pediatric Heart Transplant Study. (From Schowengerdt KO, Naftel DC, Seib PM, Pearce FB, Addonizio LJ, Kirklin JK, Morrow WR, Pediatric Heart Transplant Study Group: Infection after pediatric heart transplantation: results of a multi-institutional study. J Heart Lung Transplant 1997;16: 1207–1216.)

to the type of infection. With current available therapy, the mortality associated with a CMV infection is only about 5% and the mortality of bacterial and non-CMV viral infections 10–15%, but the mortality of fungal infection remains high, at about 50%.[244] Favorable outcome in all infections is highly dependent upon an aggressive surveillance program as well as prompt diagnosis and early initiation of appropriate antibiotic therapy (see Chapter 15 for details of therapy).

The incidence and mortality of posttransplant infections has steadily declined over the past decade. Some of the factors which may contribute to the lower incidence of serious or fatal infections in the current era include increased surgical experience with complex re-operative congenital heart surgery[112]; the introduction of cyclosporine combined with azathioprine and low dose or no corticosteroids[3, 125, 203]; the use of tacrolimus without steroids[111, 268]; the avoidance of prolonged indwelling venous catheters; identification of measures to prevent or decrease transfusion-associated pathogens such as hepatitis B, hepatitis C, and CMV; and strict avoidance of structural construction near the hospital transplant unit with its known risk of *Aspergillus* innoculation.

PHTS: Jan. 1993 - Dec. 1994; n=332

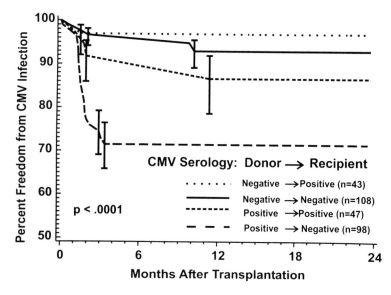

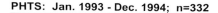

FIGURE **20-38.** Actuarial (Kaplan-Meier) freedom from cytomegalovirus infection, stratified by donor and recipient cytomegalovirus serologic status. PHTS, Pediatric Heart Transplant Study; CMV, cytomegalovirus. (From Schowengerdt KO, Naftel DC, Seib PM, Pearce FB, Addonizio LJ, Kirklin JK, Morrow WR, Pediatric Heart Transplant Study Group: Infection after pediatric heart transplantation: results of a multi-institutional study. J Heart Lung Transplant 1997;16:1207–1216.)

ALLOGRAFT CORONARY ARTERY DISEASE

Coronary artery disease (CAD) is a major limitation to long-term survival after pediatric heart transplantation, just as in adults. The pathology of the allograft vasculopathy is the same as that observed in adult heart transplant recipients[27] and is discussed in detail in Chapter 17.

DIAGNOSIS

Coronary allograft vasculopathy in adults is detected in more than 80% of long-term survivors by 8 years after cardiac transplantation and is frequently progressive.[189] The traditional method of detection by coronary angiography importantly underestimates the incidence and severity of the disease.[139, 211] A multicenter national survey in 1994 concluded that the incidence of coronary allograft vasculopathy in children is similar to that in adult transplant recipients,[215] and a significant number of children who die late after cardiac transplantation of coronary allograft vasculopathy have a recent normal coronary angiogram.[201, 215]

Despite these limitations, the diagnosis of allograft CAD in the pediatric population has relied primarily on selective **coronary angiography,** with the same criteria as applied in adults (see Chapter 17). Intravascular ultrasound has not yet been widely utilized in pediatric patients.

Dobutamine stress echocardiography (DSE) is a promising noninvasive technique for the surveillance of pediatric cardiac transplant recipients to detect the development of CAD.[164, 213] The technique requires sedation (usually chloral hydrate and midazolam or droperidol/fentanyl); transthoracic echocardiographic imaging (both two-dimensional and M-mode) with digital analysis of images; electrocardiographic analysis; and monitoring of heart rate, blood pressure, and oxygen saturation with pulse oximetry. The dobutamine infusion protocol usually begins with an infusion dose of 5 μg/kg/min with 5–10 μg/kg/min increments every 3–6 minutes to a maximum dose of 50 μg/kg/min. The study is terminated before the maximum infusion dose if (1) 75% of age-predicted maximal heart rate (220 minus age in years) is achieved, (2) patient becomes hypotensive with systolic blood pressure less than 80 mm Hg, (3) patient becomes hypertensive with systolic blood pressure greater than 180 mm Hg or diastolic pressure greater than 100 mm Hg, (4) new wall motion abnormalities develop on echocardiography, (5) sustained supraventricular or ventricular arrhythmias occur, or (6) ischemic changes develop on ECG.[164]

An abnormal response to dobutamine, indicating possible ischemia, is defined as (1) reduction in myocardial wall thickness or wall motion (segmental or global), (2) failure of resting wall motion abnormality to improve during dobutamine infusion, (3) failure of ejection fraction to increase, (4) left ventricular chamber dilatation, (5) evidence of diastolic dysfunction, or (6) increased mitral insufficiency.

Larsen and colleagues from Loma Linda[164] noted a sensitivity of 72% and specificity of 80% with DSE in comparison to coronary angiography in a group of 70 pediatric patients. Ten of 14 abnormal angiographic studies were predicted by a positive DSE study. The four patients with an abnormal angiogram and a normal DSE had subsequent normal angiograms, suggesting arterial spasm at the initial study. If these are considered "normal," the sensitivity increases to 100%. In a similar study by Pahl and colleagues,[213] all five patients with allograft CAD by angiography or autopsy were identified by an abnormal DSE. In both studies, a positive DSE was strongly predictive of subsequent cardiac events (death or retransplantation) due to CAD (Fig. 20–39). In the Loma Linda study, at last follow-up 4% of the 50 patients with a normal DSE, compared with 27% of 21 patients with an abnormal DSE, had late cardiac events.

Based on these studies, dobutamine stress echocardiography is a promising surveillance technique for allograft CAD in pediatric recipients. In view of issues of cost, radiation exposure, patient discomfort, and limitations of vascular access in children, an attractive protocol based on current information is coronary angiography at the first annual follow-up and every other year thereafter with dobutamine stress echocardiography in the intervening years. A positive DSE or angiogram would indicate the need for more frequent angiographic evaluation.

RISK FACTORS

More frequent rejection during the first 6 months after transplantation[201, 215] and rejection with hemodynamic compromise after the first year[201] have been identified as predictors of subsequent development of CAD. Additional atherogenic and immunologic risk factors for CAD in adult transplant recipients are discussed in

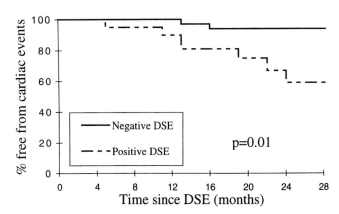

FIGURE 20–39. Actuarial (Kaplan-Meier) freedom from posttransplant coronary artery disease - related events, including death, retransplantation, and the new development of angiographic coronary artery disease according to positive or negative dobutamine stress echocardiography (DSE). (From Larsen RL, Applegate PM, Dyar DA, Ribeiro PA, Fritzsche SD, Mulla NF, Shirali GS, Kuhn MA, Chinnock RE, Shah PM: Dobutamine stress echocardiography for assessing coronary artery disease after transplantation in children. J Am Col Cardiol 1998;32:515–520.)

Chapter 17, and these likely also apply to the pediatric patient.

PROGNOSIS

The prognosis for disease progression and death after identification of allograft CAD in infants and children has not been clearly delineated, but several studies suggest that angiographic identification of allograft coronary artery disease in children may portend a more ominous outcome than similar findings in adults.[201, 213, 224] Thus, in many pediatric cardiac transplant centers, the identification of important coronary artery disease is an indication for retransplantation (the only effective therapy available). Despite its ominous natural history, coronary artery disease in children and adolescents has not been a major cause of mortality during the first 5 years following transplantation. In the PHTS analysis, death with documented coronary disease (by cath or autopsy), accounted for less mortality over 5 years than did rejection, infection, or early graft failure (see again Fig. 20–26).

THERAPY

Therapy for allograft CAD is extensively discussed in Chapter 17. Theoretically, the same pharmacologic and immunologic interventions should produce a similar benefit in children as in adults. Unfortunately, few such studies have specifically examined the pediatric transplant population. One exception to the adult experience may be the utility of percutaneous angioplasty in children, where size of coronary arteries and limited vascular access have severely restricted its application.

Currently, the only effective therapy for pediatric allograft CAD is retransplantation. Razzouk and colleagues reported a similar operative mortality (8.3% vs. 9.0%, $p = .9$) and late survival (83.3% vs. 74.4% at 4 years, $p = .85$) for children undergoing retransplantation for allograft CAD compared to pediatric patients undergoing primary cardiac transplantation.[224] In an earlier experience, Michler and colleagues reported a similar time-related incidence of infection and rejection after the second transplant as occurred after the original transplant.[195]

An important future challenge in pediatric heart transplantation is to minimize the incidence and consequences of this serious problem by decreasing the immunological insult to the endothelium, improving detection of coronary artery disease, and developing strategies for prevention and treatment by modification of traditional atherogenic risk factors and reduction of allograft rejection.

OTHER OUTCOME INDICATORS

MALIGNANCY

The available information on malignancies after pediatric heart transplantation focuses heavily on posttransplant lymphoproliferative disease (PTLD). A complete discussion of PTLD can be found in Chapter 18, and additional information relevant to pediatric patients is presented here.

Numerous studies in pediatric solid organ transplantation have concluded that the major risk factor for the development of PTLD is the new onset of Epstein-Barr virus (EBV) infection,[124, 280, 298] which appears to be the etiologic agent in over 80% of pediatric PTLD cases.[53] This is usually accompanied by the conversion of a negative EBV serology before transplant to a positive serology post-transplant, most commonly in the setting of an EBV-negative recipient receiving an organ from an EBV-positive donor. In the majority of pediatric PTLD cases, the EBV genome can be isolated from the tumor. In a study of 50 pediatric heart transplant recipients, Zangwill and colleagues reported that 63% (12 of 19) of EBV-negative patients who converted to EBV-positive after transplant developed PTLD a mean of 29 months (range, 3–72 months) after transplant compared to 0% (0 of 12) among EBV-negative patients who remained EBV-negative after transplant ($p = .001$) and 5% among patients who were EBV-positive before transplant ($p = .02$).[298]

The time to onset of PTLD also differs according to recipient EBV status. In "primary mismatch" patients (EBV-positive donor, EBV-negative recipient), Webber and colleagues noted a median time to onset of PTLD of 4 months after transplantation, with all cases occurring during the first year.[280] In contrast, seronegative recipients with seronegataive donors had a much more variable (4 months to 7 years) time to onset of disease. It now seems clear that the vast majority of PTLD cases in "primary EBV mismatch" settings are driven by EBV infection transmitted from the donor heart. In cases of EBV-induced PTLD with an EBV-negative donor, potential sources of EBV infection include perioperative use of blood products or a subsequent community-acquired EBV infection.[280]

Slightly over half the patients have disease localized to the tonsils and adenoids, with a histologic diagnosis of plasmacytic hyperplasia. The presenting symptoms are typically nasal congestion, sinusitis, or nasopharyngeal obstruction. Reduction of immunosuppression plus tonsillectomy and adenoidectomy with or without acyclovir is usually curative, with an occasional patient developing local recurrence. Nearly uniform survival is expected, and progression to a more aggressive form of PTLD is rare.[298] This underscores the importance of ear, nose, and throat examinations at intervals after conversion from EBV-negative, to EBV-positive after transplantation.

The more serious form of pediatric PTLD is B-cell lymphoma (polyclonal or monoclonal) or polymorphic B-cell hyperplasia. Initial presenting signs and symptoms include asymptomatic abnormal chest x-ray, unexplained anemia, unexplained gastrointestinal symptoms, central nervous system changes, respiratory symptoms, bone pain, asymptomatic lymphadenopathy, and fever of unknown origin. The diagnostic evaluation of patients with any suggestive symptoms is discussed in Chapter 18.

Currently, first line of therapy is reduction of immunosuppression (usually elimination of azathioprine and reduction or temporary elimination of cyclosporine or tacrolimus) in order to increase host immunologic surveillance. Some studies suggest an increased incidence of PTLD with tacrolimus-based immunosuppression,[64, 69] but other reports have not confirmed this.[25, 229, 278] Until more secure information is available, it may be appropriate to switch from tacrolimus to low-dose cyclosporine if PTLD occurs. Surgical extirpation is advocated when feasible. Multiple agent chemotherapy is an important component of therapy, but debate continues whether chemotherapy should routinely be part of initial therapy or reserved for treatment failure or recurrence after initial immunosuppression reduction, surgery (if feasible) and acyclovir. Other adjunctive antiviral agents which have been utilized include ganciclovir, interferon, and anti–B-cell antibodies. Using a multitude of therapies, the reported mortality related to posttransplant B-cell lymphoma is approximately 20–40%.[298]

In the UAB experience since 1990, three patients between 4 and 12 years of age have developed posttransplant lymphoma at 5–53 months following pediatric heart or heart/lung transplantation. We have adopted an aggressive strategy of discontinuation of azathioprine, reduction of cyclosporine dosage while maintaining oral prednisone, and treatment with aggressive chemotherapy combined with surgical extirpation whenever possible. All three patients have responded to this regimen with disappearance of tumor as evidenced by computerized tomographic (CT) scanning and recurrence-free survival at 1–5 years after therapy. It is noteworthy, however, that recurrent and sometimes severe rejection often accompanies reduction of immunosuppression, particularly following completion of chemotherapy (with its own immunosuppressive effects). Augmentation of immunosuppression and close rejection surveillance with echocardiography and biopsy may be necessary to control recurrent rejection.

In view of the association with Epstein-Barr virus, all recipients with negative EBV serology at the time of transplantation should undergo surveillance for EBV serologic conversion at frequent intervals during the first year following transplantation. Serologic conversion should be considered a possible harbinger of PTLD, and close surveillance measures (possibly including abdominal and chest CT scanning) for PTLD should be initiated during the subsequent year. Intermittent examination by an ear, nose, and throat specialist after conversion may also be advisable because of the abundance of lymphoid tissue in the posterior pharynx. The current UAB protocol for surveillance of EBV-negative recipients is provided in Table 20–21.

RENAL DYSFUNCTION

As in adult heart transplant patients, there is a predictable 10–30% decrease in renal function (as measured by serum creatinine or glomerular filtration rate) 1 or more years after cardiac transplantation with cyclosporine- or

TABLE 20–21	**Surveillance Protocol for EBV-Negative Recipient and EBV-Positive Donor (UAB)**

- EBV IgM and IgG serologies obtained after transplant at 1 mo, then every 2 mo for 1 yr, then every 6 mo until 3 yr after transplant (or until conversion).
- Obtain ENT evaluation every 3 mo after conversion for 2 yr, then every 6 mo for an additional yr.
- Consider CT scan of chest and abdomen 3, 6, 12, 18, and 24 mo after conversion.
- Treatment for conversion:
    1. Oral acyclovir (15 mg/kg/day) for 12 mo
    2. Reduce immunosuppression if rejection history appropriate

EBV, Epstein-Barr virus; ENT, ear, nose, and throat; CT, computerized tomographic.

tacrolimus-based immunosuppression. Renal function usually remains stable thereafter in most patients with appropriate adjustment of cyclosporine and tacrolimus doses. Late renal function in children 10 or more years after transplant is generally good, with essentially normal serum creatinine levels and low normal glomerular filtration rates in most patients.[62] An occasional patient will require dialysis and/or late renal transplantation.

NEUROPSYCHOLOGIC DEVELOPMENT FOLLOWING CARDIAC TRANSPLANTATION

Neurologic Injury Early Following Transplantation

Numerous neurologic abnormalities have been reported in infants and children following cardiac transplantation.[94, 182] However, precise information about the incidence, causes, and risk factors for neurologic dysfunction following cardiac transplantation are confounded by the critically ill condition of many patients prior to the transplant procedure. Neonates with ductal-dependent cardiac malformations are often markedly desaturated for weeks or months prior to transplantation and many have chronic reductions in systemic, and likely cerebral, perfusion due to their congenital heart disease. In older children and adolescents, early posttransplant neurologic injury is rare, occurring with similar frequency as in adults. In infants and children, early neurologic events most commonly include isolated seizures and temporary altered mental status.[182]

The most common setting for neurologic injury is infants undergoing cardiac transplantation for hypoplastic left heart syndrome, with its obligatory use of **deep hypothermic total circulatory arrest** in order to reconstruct the aortic arch. Cardiac transplantation for other congenital heart malformations and for cardiomyopathy rarely require circulatory arrest to accomplish the procedure. A large body of experimental and clinical information exists relating to the probability of temporary and permanent neurologic damage following a period of circulatory arrest. Experimental studies by Treasure and others suggest that irreversible structural damage is more likely when total circulatory arrest time exceeds 45–60 minutes with the brain at 18°C.[22, 44, 65, 77,]

[260, 270, 292] Postoperative seizures and choreoathetosis are more common after the use of total circulatory arrest than with conventional cardiopulmonary bypass using low-flow perfusion with or without brief periods of circulatory arrest.[204]

Unfortunately, reliable information about the safe limits of total circulatory arrest and the precise conditions which minimize the likelihood of cerebral damage have not been established, largely because of considerable interinstitutional differences in the methodology of inducing circulatory arrest, including the rapidity of cooling, brain temperature during the period of circulatory arrest, the degree of hemodilution (hematocrit during cooling), calcium concentration in the perfusate, and acid-base strategy during cooling (alpha-stat vs. pH-stat). It is of interest that Eke and colleagues from Loma Linda[86] reported favorable neurodevelopmental outcome in 38 infants undergoing cardiac transplantation using deep hypothermic circulatory arrest for 42–70 minutes (mean, 56 minutes). Using the techniques of profound hemodilution, low-calcium perfusate during cardiopulmonary bypass (ionized calcium level of approximately 0.4 mmol/L on bypass), core cooling, infusion of a calcium channel blocker, and an alpha-stat management of ventilation during cooling, no relationship was found between either the rate of cooling or the duration of total circulatory arrest and the neurodevelopmental outcome up to 2½ years following transplantation.[86]

Transient or persistent neurologic abnormalities have been reported in about 20% of infant transplant recipients.[20] In the Loma Linda experience, the most common abnormality early after transplantation was transient seizures. Four months after transplantation, generalized hypotonia was the most common neurologic abnormality, occurring in about 10% of survivors.[20] Late neurologic deficits are rare. Despite these findings, most would agree that whenever possible the transplant operation for hypoplastic left heart syndrome should be organized in a way that limits the period of circulatory arrest to less than about 40 minutes after profound cooling to 16°–18°C. Our recommended method of brain protection during this operation is discussed in the earlier section, Surgical Techniques.

Late Neuropsychological Development

Multiple studies in infants and children undergoing heart transplantation indicate that developmental, cognitive, and behavioral measures are usually within the normal range many years later.[20, 291] Approximately two thirds of patients followed for more than 10 years at Loma Linda were described as developmentally normal by their parents.[62] However, the group of heart transplant patients as well as other open-heart surgery pediatric patients typically score below a group of "healthy children" in IQ score and developmental indices.[291] Long-term studies from Loma Linda after infant transplantation indicate an approximate 10-point decrease in standardized testing when compared to a normal population.[20]

Baum and colleagues noted that infants undergoing cardiac transplantation (most with hypoplastic left heart syndrome) showed considerable variability in IQ testing, with more children than expected in the lower ranges 5 or more years after transplantation.[21] Visual motor and spatial skills often showed significant deficits. It is unknown whether such intellectual deficits result from hemodynamic derangement prior to transplant, from circulatory arrest required for the transplant procedure, or are brain abnormalities associated with hypoplastic left heart syndrome. Young children after transplant appear at particular risk for social isolation, while older children and adolescents are, as a group, prone to depression.[21]

Thus, although the vast majority of pediatric heart transplant patients have an excellent quality of life, full participation in school, and an adequate neuropsychological development, special educational, emotional, and behavioral support are often necessary and comprise an important part of their long-term care.

CARDIAC ALLOGRAFT GROWTH AND FUNCTION

Following cardiac transplantation in infants and children, the denervated heart undergoes relatively normal growth in terms of left ventricular volume and muscle mass in proportion to the body surface area (Fig. 20–40).[123, 296] Furthermore, in the absence of severe rejection or allograft vascular disease, left ventricular ejection fraction and resting cardiac index usually remain normal, although there is frequently evidence of restrictive physiology.[296, 297] This diastolic dysfunction and an inadequate chronotropic response to exercise may account for the usual finding of suboptimal cardiac output at peak exercise.[128, 207, 293] Despite this, the vast majority of pediat-

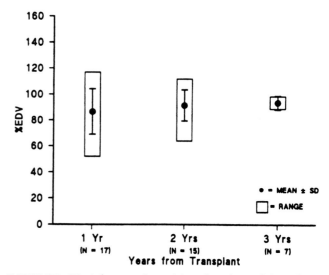

FIGURE **20–40.** Left ventricular end-diastolic volume of donor hearts plotted as percent of predicted normal end-diastolic volume (% EDV) for recipient body size at 1, 2, and 3 years after transplant. (From Zales VR, Wright KL, Muster AJ, Backer CL, Benson DW, Mavroudis C: Ventricular volume growth after cardiac transplantation in infants and children. Circulation 1992;86:II-272–II-275.)

ric heart transplant patients remain in NYHA Class I, without restrictions in activity or lifestyle.[254]

SOMATIC GROWTH

Most infants and children undergoing cardiac transplantation experience relatively normal growth. In general, their growth parameters are usually at the lower range of normal.[123] The causes for occasional mild persistent growth impairment are multifactorial, partly related to the growth retardation induced by chronic cardiac illness, partly related to the effects of chronic immunosuppression, and possibly related to the transplant procedure itself.

The reported growth after pediatric cardiac transplantation appears somewhat better than for children undergoing liver transplantation, in whom stature remains below normal,[59] and renal transplantation, which is associated with persistent reduction in height and weight.[267]

There has been considerable speculation about the potential benefit of heart transplantation in the neonatal period or during infancy in terms of subsequent somatic development. Baum and colleagues from Loma Linda found that normal growth patterns are observed sooner when cardic transplantation occurs in the first month of life compared to later in infancy, but no difference was discernible 6 months after transplant.[20] Beyond 5 years, nearly 90% of infants undergoing heart transplantation have height and weight in the normal range.[60] This rapid normalization of growth after infant transplantation contrasts with children and adolescents undergoing cardiac transplantation, in whom height and weight are more commonly below normal.[2, 19] Whether this difference relates to the impact of chronic cardiac disease or to the greater use of steroids in older children remains unresolved. It is of interest, however, that Hirsch and colleagues noted no difference in weight and stature among infants undergoing cardiac transplantation with no maintenance steroids versus low-dose maintenance steroids (0.1–0.2 mg/kg/day).[123]

FUTURE PROGRESS

Considerable progress has been made in the science and practice of pediatric cardiac transplantation, but many unresolved issues persist. Increasing the number of donor hearts is a pressing issue and the solution to this problem may possibly lie with xenotransplantation and the use of anencephalic donors as well as other novel strategies such as the use of hearts after resuscitation of asystolic donors. Improvements in immunosuppression and strategies to induce tolerance would significantly enhance long-term survival. When the results of pediatric cardiac transplantation become more predictable and the procedure becomes more generally available, the true role of this therapy in the management of complex congenital heart disease can be better defined.

References

1. Adatia I, Perry S, Landzberg ML, Moore P, Thompson JE, Wessel DL: Inhaled nitric oxide and hemodynamic evaluation of patients with pulmonary hypertension before transplantation. J Am Coll Cardiol 1995:25;1656–1664.
2. Addonizio LJ, Hsu DT, Rose EA, Gersony WM: Linear growth in pediatric cardiac transplant patients. J Am Coll Cardiol 1989;13:134A.
3. Andreone PA, Olivari MT, Elick B, Arentzen CE, Sibley RK, Bolman RM, Simmons RL, Ring WS: Reduction of infectious complications following heart transplantation with triple-drug immunotherapy. J Heart Transplant 1986;5:13–19.
4. Arbustini E, Grasso M, Diegoli M, Bramerio M, Foglieni AS, Albertario M, Martinelli L, Gavazzi A, Goggi C, Campana C: Expression of tumor necrosis factor in human acute cardiac rejection: an immunohistochemical and immunoblotting study. Am J Pathol 1991;139:709–715.
5. Arakawa T, Carpenter JF, Kita YA, Crowe JH: The basis for toxicity of certain cryoprotectants: a hypothesis. Cryobiology 1990;27:401–415.
6. Armitage JM, Fricker FJ, Kurland G: Pediatric lung transplantation. The years 1985 to 1992 and the clinical trial of FK 506. J Thorac Cardiovac Surg 1993;105:337–346.
7. Armitage JM, Fricker FJ, Nido PD, Starzl TE, Hardesty RL, Griffith BP: A decade (1982 to 1992) of pediatric cardiac transplantation and the impact of FK 506 immunosuppression. J Thorac Cardiovasc Surg 1993;105:464–473.
8. Ammash NM, Seward JB, Bailey KR: Clinical profile and outcome of idiopathic restrictive cardiomyopathy. Circulation 2000;101:2490–2496.
9. Assaad A: Posttransplantation management of the newborn and the immunosuppressive role of prostaglandin E₁. J Heart Lung Transplant 1993;12:S191–S194.
10. Ashwal S, Caplan AL, Cheatham WA, Evans RW, Peabody JL: Session IV: Social and ethical controversies in pediatric heart transplantation. J Heart Lung Transplant 1991;10:860–876.
11. Backer CL, Zales VR, Idriss FS, Lynch P, Crawford S, Benson DW, Mavroudis C: Heart transplantation in neonates and in children. J Heart Lung Transplant 1992;11:311–319.
12. Bailey L, Kahan B, Nehlsen-Cannarella S, Sprent J, Starnes V: Session V: The neonatal immune system: window of opportunity? J Heart Lung Transplant 1991;10:828–829.
13. Bailey LL, Gundry SR, Razzouk AJ, Wang N, Sciolaro CM, Chiavarelli M, Loma Linda University Pediatric Heart Transplant Group: Bless the babies: one hundred fifteen late survivors of heart transplantation during the first year of life. J Thorac Cardiovasc Surg 1993;105:805–815.
14. Bailey LL, Nehlson-Cannarella SL, Doroshow RW, Jacobson JG, Martin RD, Allard MW, Hyde MR, Dang Bui RH, Petry EL: Cardiac allograft transplantation in newborns and therapy for hypoplastic left heart syndrome. N Engl J Med 1986;315:949–951.
15. Baig MK, Goldman JH, Caforio ALP, Coonar AS, Keeling PJ, McKenna WJ: Familial dilated cardiomyopathy: cardiac abnormalities are common in asymptomatic relatives and may represent early disease. J Am Coll Cardiol 1998;31:195–201.
16. Baker JE, Boerboom LE, Olinger GN: Age-related changes in the ability of hypothermia and cardioplegia to protect ischemic rabbit myocardium. J Thorac Cardiovasc Surg 1988;96:717–724.
17. Baker JE, Boerboom LE, Olinger GN: Is protection of ischemic neonatal myocardium by cardioplegia species dependent? J Thorac Cardiovasc Surg 1990;99:280–287.
18. Bauer J, Dapper F, Demirakca S, Knothe C, Thul J, Hagel KJ: Perioperative management of pulmonary hypertension after heart transplantation in childhood. J Heart Lung Transplant 1997;16:1238–1247.
19. Baum D, Bernstein D, Starnes VA, Oyer P, Pitlick P, Stinson E, Shumway N: Pediatric heart transplantation at Stanford: results of a 15 year experience. Pediatrics 1991;88:203–214.
20. Baum M, Chinnock R, Ashwal S, Peverini R, Trimm F, Bailey L: Growth and neurodevelopmental outcome of infants undergoing heart transplantation. J Heart Lung Transplant 1993;12:S211–S217.
21. Baum M, Freier MC, Freeman KR, Chinnock RE: Developmental outcomes and cognitive functioning in infant and child heart transplant recipients. Prog Pediatr Cardiol 2000;11:159–163.

22. Bellinger DC, Wernovsky G, Rappaport LA: Cognitive development of children following early repair of transposition of the great arteries using deep hypothermic circulatory arrest. Pediatrics 1991;87:701–707.

23. Belzer FO: Principles of organ preservation. Transplant Proc 1988;20:925–927.

24. Berner M, Beghetti M, Sphar-Schopfer I: Inhaled nitric oxide to test the vasodilator capacity of the pulmonary vascular bed in children with long standing pulmonary hypertension and congenital heart disease. Am J Cardiol 1996;77:532–535.

25. Bernstein D, Baum D, Berry G, Dahl G, Weiss L, Starnes V, Gamberg P, Stinson EB: Neoplastic disorders after pediatric heart transplantation. Circulation 1993;88(pt2):230–237.

26. Bernstein D, Naftel DC, Hsu DT, Addonizio LJ, Blume ED, Gamberg PL, Kirklin JK, Morrow WR, and the Pediatric Heart Transplant Study: Outcome of listing for cardiac transplantation for failed Fontan: a multi-institutional study. J Heart Lung Transplant 1999;18:69.

27. Berry GJ, Rizeq MN, Weiss LM, Billingham ME: Graft coronary disease in pediatric heart and combined heart-lung transplant recipients: a study of fifteen cases. J Heart Lung Transplant 1993;12:S309–S319.

28. Blackstone EH, Kirklin JW, Bertranou EG, Labrosse CJ, Soto B, Bargeron LM Jr: Preoperative prediction from cineangiograms of postrepair right ventricular pressure in tetralogy of Fallot. J Thorac Cardiovasc Surg 1979;78:542.

29. Bleyer WA: The impact of childhood cancer on the United States and the world. CA Cancer J Clin 1990;40:355–367.

30. Boucek MM, Faro A, Novick RJ, Bennett LE, Fiol B, Keck BM, Hosenpud JD: The Registry of the International Society of Heart and Lung Transplantation: third official pediatric report—1999. J Heart Lung Transplant 1999;18:1151–1172.

31. Boucek MM, Mathis CM, Boucek RJ, Hodgkin DD, Kanakriyeh MS, McCormack J, Gundry SR, Bailey LL: Prospective evaluation of echocardiography for primary rejection surveillance after infant heart transplantation: comparison with endomyocardial biopsy. J Heart Lung Transplant 1994;13:66–73.

32. Boucek MM, Mathis CM, Kanakryeh MS, Gundry SR, Bailey LL: Late cardiac graft failure and hypertrophic ventricular outflow obstruction post infant heart transplantation [abstract]. J Heart Lung Transplant 1991;10:162.

33. Boucek MM, Mathis CM, Kanakriyeh MS, McCormack J, Razzouk A, Gundry SR, Bailey L: Donor shortage: use of the dysfunctional donor heart. J Heart Lung Transplant 1993;12:S186–S190.

34. Boucek MM, Mathis CM, Razzouk A, Gundry SR, Bailey LL, Fullerton DA, Campbell DN: Indications and contraindications for heart transplantation in infancy. J Heart Lung Transplant 1993;12:S154–S158.

35. Boucek MM, Novick R, Bennett LE, Fiol B, Keck BM, Hosenpud JD: The registry of the International Society of Heart and Lung Transplantation: second official pediatric report—1998. J Heart Lung Transplant 1998;17:1141–1160.

36. Boucek RJ Jr, Naftel D, Boucek MM, Chinnock R, Morrow RW, Pahl E, DiSano S: Induction immunotherapy in pediatric heart transplant recipients: a multi-center study. J Heart Lung Transplant 1999;18:460–469.

37. Boucek RJ, Shelton ME, Artman M, Landon E: Myocellular calcium regulation by the sarcolemmal membrane in the adult and immature rabbit heart. Basic Res Cardiol 1985;80:316–325.

38. Boudin G, Mikol J, Guillard A, Engel AG: Fatal systemic carnitine deficiency with lipid storage in skeletal muscle, heart, liver and kidney. J Neurol Sci 1976;30:313–326.

39. Bourge RC, Naftel DC, Costanzo-Nordin M, Kirklin JK, Young JB, Kubo SH, Olivari MT, Kasper EK, and The Transplant Cardiologists Research Database Group: Pre-transplant risk factors for death after cardiac transplantation: a multi-institutional study. J Heart Lung Transplant 1993;12:549–562.

40. Bove EL, Stammers S: Recovery of left ventricular function after hypothermic global ischemia: age-related differences in the isolated working rabbit heart. J Thorac Cardiovasc Surg 1986;91:115.

41. Brandenburg RO, Chazor E, Cherian G, Falase AO, Grosgogeat Y, Loogen CKF, Judez VM, Orinius E, Goodwin JF, Olsen EGJ, Oakley CM, Pisa Z: Report of the WHO/SFC task force on definition and classification of cardiomyopathies. Circulation 1981;64:437A–437B.

42. Braunwald E, Morrow AG, Cornell WP, Aygen MM, Hilbish TF: Idiopathic hypertrophic subaortic stenosis. Am J Med 1960;22:924–945.

43. Breda MA, Drinkwater DC, Laks H, Bhuta S, Ho B, Kaczer E, Sebastian JL, Chang P: Successful long term preservation of the neonatal heart with a modified intracellular solution. J Thorac Cardiovasc Surg 1992;104:139–150.

44. Brunberg JA, Reilly EL, Doty DB: Central nervous system consequences in infants of cardiac surgery using deep hypothermic and circulatory arrest. Circulation 1973;50(suppl2):60–68.

45. Burch M, Siddiqui SA, Celermajer DS, Scott C, Bull C, Deanfield JE: Dilated cardiomyopathy in children: determinants of outcome. Br Heart J 1994;72:246–250.

46. Bush A, Busst CM, Knight WB, Shinebourne EA: Cardiovascular effects of tolazoline and rantidine. Arch Dis Child 1987;62:241–246.

47. Busse R, Mulsch A, Fleming I, Hecker M: Mechanisms of nitric oxide release from the vascular endothelium. Circulation 1993;87:V-18–V-25.

48. Canter CE: Preoperative assessment and management of pediatric heart transplantation. Prog Pediatr Cardiol 2000;11:91–97.

49. Canter C, Naftel D, Caldwell R, Chinnock R, Pahl E, Frazier E, Kirklin JK, Boucek M, Morrow R, and the Pediatric Heart Transplant Study Group: Survival and risk factors for death after cardiac transplantation in infants: a multi institutional study. Circulation 1997;96:227–231.

50. Canter CE, Moorhead S, Huddleston CB, Spray TL: Restrictive atrial septal communication as a determinant of outcome of cardiac transplantation for hypoplastic left heart syndrome. Circulation 1993;88:456–460.

51. Canter CE, Moorhead S, Saffitz JE, Huddleston CB, Spray TL: Steroid withdrawal in the pediatric heart transplant recipient initially treated with triple immunosuppression. J Heart Lung Transplant 1994;13:74–80.

52. Cetta F, O'Leary PW, Seward JB, Driscoll DJ: Idiopathic restrictive cardiomyopathy in childhood: diagnostic features and clinical course. Mayo Clin Proc 1995;70:634–640.

53. Chadburn A, Cesarman E, Knowles DM: Molecular pathology of posttransplant lymphoproliferative disorders. Semin Diagn Pathol 1997;14:15–26.

54. Chan KY, Iwahara M, Benson LN, Wilson GJ, Freedom RM: Immunosuppressive therapy in the management of acute myocarditis in children: a clinical trial. J Am Coll Cardiol 1991;17:458–460.

55. Chartraud C, Guerin R, Kangah M, Stanley P: Pediatric heart transplantation: surgical considerations for congenital heart disease. J Heart Transplant 1990;9:608–617.

56. Chen JM, Levin HR, Michler RE, Prusmack CJ, Rose EA, Aaronson KD: Reevaluating the significance of pulmonary hypertension before cardiac transplantation: determination of optimal thresholds and quantification of the effect of reversibility on perioperative mortality. J Thorac Cardiovasc Surg 1997;114:627–634.

57. Chen SC, Nouri S, Balfour I, Jureidini S, Appleton RS: Clinical profile of congestive cardiomyopathy in children. J Am Coll Cardiol 1990;15:189–193.

58. Chiavarelli M, Boucek MM, Nehlsen-Cannarella SL, Gundry SR, Razzouk AJ, Bailey LL: Neonatal cardiac transplantation: intermediate term results and incidence of rejection. Arch Surg 1992;127:1072–1076.

59. Chin TK, Perloff JK, Williams RG, Jue K, Mohrmann R: Isolated noncompaction of left ventricular myocardium. Circulation 1990;82:507–513.

60. Chinnock RE, Baum M: Somatic growth in infant heart transplant recipients. Pediatr Transplant 1998;2:30–34.

61. Chinnock RE, Baum MF, Larsen R, Bailey L: Rejection management and long-term surveillance of the pediatric heart transplant recipient: the Loma Linda experience. J Heart Lung Transplant 1993;12:S255–S264.

62. Chinnock RE, Cutler D, Baum M: Clinical outcome 10 years after infant heart transplantation. Prog Pediatr Cardiol 2000;11:165–169.

63. Chow LH, Radio SJ, Sears TD, McManus BM: Insensitivity of right ventricular endomyocardial biopsy in the diagnosis of myocarditis. J Am Coll Cardiol 1989;14:915–920.

64. Ciancio G, Siquijor AP, Burke GW, Roth D, Cirocco R, Esquenazi V, Byrne GE, Miller J: Post-transplant lymphoproliferative disease in kidney transplant recipients in the new immunosuppressive era. Clin Transplant 1997;11:243–249.

65. Clarkson PM, MacArthur BA, Barratt-Boyes BG, Whitlock RM, Neutze JM: Developmental progress after cardiac surgery in infancy using hypothermia and circulatory arrest. Circulation 1980;62:855–861.

66. Cooper DKC, Novitzky D, Schlegel V, Muchmore JS, Cuchiara A, Zuhdi N: Successful management of symptomatic cytomegalovirus disease with ganciclovir after heart transplantation. J Heart Lung Transplant 1991;10:656–663.

67. Cooper MM, Fuzesi L, Addonizio LJ, Hsu DT, Smith CR, Rose EA: Pediatric heart transplantation after operations involving the pulmonary arteries. J Thorac Cardiovasc Surg 1991;102:386–395.

68. Costard-Jacckle A, Fowler MB: Influence of preoperative pulmonary artery pressure on mortality after heart transplantation: testing of potential reversibility of pulmonary hypertension with nitroprusside is useful in defining a high risk group. J Am Coll Cardiol 1992;19:48–54.

69. Cox KL, Lawrence-Miyasaki LS, Garcia-Kennedy R, Lennette ET, Martinez OM, Krams SM, Berquist WE, So SK, Esquivel CO: An increased incidence of Epstein-Barr virus infection and lymphoproliferative disease in young children on FK506 after liver transplantation. Transplantation 1995;59:524–529.

70. Curran RD, Mavroudis C, Backer C, Sautel M, Zales VR, Wessel DL: Inhaled nitric oxide for children with congenital heart disease and pulmonary hypertension. Ann Thorac Surg 1995;60:1765–1771.

71. Dalientao L, Turrini P, Nava A, Rizzoli G, Angelini A, Buja G, Scognamiglio R, Thiene G: Arrhythmogenic right ventricular cardiomyopathy in young versus adult patients: similarities and differences. J Am Coll Cardiol 1995;25:655–664.

72. D'Amico AT, Buchanon SA, Lucke JC, van Trigt P: The preservation of cardiac function after brain death: a myocardial pressure-dimension analysis. Surg Forum 1990;41:277–279.

73. D'Amico TA, Schwinn DA, Meyers CH, van Trigt P: Desensitization of myocardial beta receptors after brain death. Surg Forum 1992;43:249–251.

74. de Begona JA, Gundry SR, Razzouk AJ, Boucek MM, Bailey LL: Prolonged ischemic times in pediatric heart transplantation: early and late results. Transplant Proc 1993;25:1645–1648.

75. del Rio MJ: Transplantation in complex congenital heart disease. Prog Pediatr Cardiol 2000;11:107–113.

76. Denfield SW, Rosenthal G, Gajarski RJ, Bricker JT, Schowengerdt KO, Price JK, Towbin JA: Restrictive cardiomyopathies in childhood. Tex Heart Inst J 1997;24:38–44.

77. Dickinson D, Sambrooks JE: Intellectual performance in children after circulatory arrest with profound hypothermia in infancy. Arch Dis Child 1979;54:1–6.

78. Dilsizian V, Bonow RO, Epstein SE, Fananapazir L: Myocardial ischemia detected by thallium scintigraphy is frequently related to cardiac arrest and syncope in young patients with hypertrophic cardiomyopathy. J Am Coll Cardiol 1993;22:796–804.

79. Doty DB, Renlund DG, Caputo GR, Burton NA, Jones KW: Cardiac transplantation in situs inversus. J Thorac Cardiovasc Surg 1990;99:493–499.

80. Dowling RD, Jones JW, Carroll MS, Gray LA Jr: Use of intravenous immunoglobulin in sensitized LVAD recipients. Transplant 1998;30:1110–1111.

81. Dresdale AR, Drusin RE, Lamb J, Smith CR, Reemtsma K, Rose EA: Reduced infection in cardiac transplant recipients. Circulation 1985;72(suppl):II-237–II-240.

82. Drucker NA, Colan SD, Lewis AB, Beiser AS, Wessel DL, Takahashi M, Baker AL, Perez-Atayde AR, Newburger JW: Gamma globulin treatment of acute myocarditis in the pediatric population. Circulation 1994;89:252–257.

83. Dummer JS, White LT, Ho M, Griffith BP, Hardesty RL, Bahnson HT: Morbidity of cytomegalovirus infection in recipients of heart or heart–lung transplants who received cyclosporine. J Infect Dis 1985;152:1182–1191.

84. Dunn SP, Falkenstein K, Lawrence JP, Meyers R, Vinocur CD, Billmire DF, Weintraub WH: Monotherapy with cyclosporine for chronic immunosuppression in pediatric liver transplant recipients. Transplantation 1994;57:544.

85. Durand JB, Bachinski LL, Bieling LC, Czernuszewicz GZ, Abchee AB, Yu QT, Tapscott T, Hill R, Ifegwu J, Marian AJ, Brugada R, Daiger S, Gregoritch JM, Anderson JL, Quinones M, Towbin JA, Roberts R: Localization of a gene responsible for familial dilated cardiomyopathy to chromosome 1q32. Circulation 1995;92:3387–3389.

86. Eke CE, Gundry SR, Baum MF, Chinnock RE, Razzouk AJ, Bailey LL: Neurologic sequelae of deep hypothermic circulatory arrest in cardiac transplant infants. Ann Thorac Surg 1996;61:783–788.

87. Ferrazzi P, Fiocchi R, Gamba A, Mamprin F, Senni M, Glauber M, Troise G, Parenzan L: Pediatric heart transplantation without chronic maintenance steroids. J Heart Lung Transplant 1993;12:S241.

88. Ferrell PE Jr, Chang AC, Murdison KA, Baffa JM, Norwood WI, Murphy JD: Outcome and assessment after the modified Fontan procedure for hypoplastic left heart syndrome. Circulation 1992;85:116–122.

89. Fontan F, Kirklin JW, Fernandez G, Costa F, Naftel DC, Tritto F, Blackstone EH: Outcome after a "perfect" Fontan operation. Circulation 1990;81:1520–1536.

90. Franco KL: Pediatric Cardiopulmonary Transplantation. Armonk, NY: Futura Publishing Company, Inc, 1997.

91. Frank JS, Rich TL: Age-dependent changes in the ultrastructure of the neonatal rat heart after Ca depletion and repletion. Am J Physiol 1983;245:H343–H353.

92. Frazier EA, Naftel DC, Canter CE, Boucek MM, Kirklin JK, Morrow WR, and the Pediatric Heart Transplant Study (PHTS): Death after heart transplantation in children: who dies when and why. J Heart Lung Transplant 1999;18:69.

93. Fricker FJ, Addonizio L, Bernstein D, Boucek M, Boucek R, Canter C, Chinnock R, Chin C, Kichuk M, Lamour J, Pietra B, Morrow R, Rotundo K, Shaddy R, Schuette EP, Schowengerdt KO, Sondheimer H, Webber S: Heart transplantation in children. Indications. Pediatr Transplant 1999;3:333–342.

94. Fricker FJ, Griffith BP, Hardesty RL, Trento A, Gold LM, Schmeltz K, Beerman LB, Fischer DR, Mathews RA, Neches WH: Experience with heart transplantation in children. Pediatrics 1987;79:138–146.

95. Friedman RA, Moak JP, Garson A: Clinical course of idiopathic dilated cardiomyopathy in children. J Am Coll Cardiol 1991;18:152–156.

96. Friedman WF: The intrinsic physiologic properties of the developing heart. Prog Cardiovasc Dis 1972;15:87–111.

97. Fukushima N, Gundry SR, Razzouk AJ, Bailey LL: Risk factors for graft failure associated with pulmonary hypertension after pediatric heart transplantation. J Thorac Cardiovasc Surg 1994;107:985–989.

98. Fullerton DA, Campbell DN, Jones SD, Jaggers J, Brown JM, Wollmering MM, Grover FL, Mashburn C, Luna M, Sondheimer HM, Boucek MM: Heart transplantation in children and young adults: early and intermediate-term results. Ann Thorac Surg 1995;59:804–812.

99. Fullerton DA, Gundry SR, de Begona JA, Kawauchi M, Razzouk AJ, Bailey LL: The effects of donor-recipient size disparity in infant and pediatric heart transplantation. J Thorac Cardiovasc Surg 1992;104:1314–1319.

100. Furchgott RF, Zawadzki JV: The obligatory role of endothelial cells in the relaxation of arterial smooth muscle by acetylcholine. Nature 1980;288:373–376.

101. Fyfe DA, Gillette PC, Crawford FA, Kline CH: Resolution of dilated cardiomyopathy after surgical ablation of ventricular tachycardia in a child. J Am Coll Cardiol 1987;9:231–234.

102. Gajarski RJ, Towbin JA, Bricker JT, Radovancevic B, Frazier OH, Price JK, Schowengerdt KO, Denfield SW: Intermediate follow-up of pediatric heart transplant recipients with elevated pulmonary vascular resistance index. J Am Coll Cardiol 1994;23:1682–1687.

103. Gill EA, Borrego C, Bray BE, Renlund DG, Gilbert EM: Left ventricular mass increases during vascular rejection [abstract]. J Heart Lung Transplant 1992;11:204.

104. Goldstein DJ, Seldomridge JA, Addonizio LL, Rose EA, Oz MC, Michler RE: Orthotopic heart transplantation in patients with treated malignancies. Am J Cardiol 1995;75:968–971.

105. Goodwin JF: The frontiers of cardiomyopathy. Br Heart J 1982;48:1–18.

106. Goorin AM, Chauvenet AR, Perez-Atayde AR, Cruz J, McKone R, Lipshultz SE: Initial congestive heart failure, six to ten years after doxorubicin chemotherapy for childhood cancer. J Pediatr 1990;116:144–147.

107. Gorensek MJ, Stewart TW, Keys TF, McHenry MC, Longworth DL, Rehm SJ, Babiak T: Decreased infections in cardiac transplant recipients on cyclosporine with reduced corticosteroid use. Cleve Clin J Med 1989;56:690–695.

108. Graham K, Sondheimer H, Schaffer M: Resolution of cavopulmonary shunt-associated pulmonary arteriovenous malformation after heart transplantation. J Heart Lung Transplant 1997;16:1271–1274.

109. Grant JW, Canter CE, Spray TL, Landt Y, Saffitz JE, Ladenson JH, Jaffee AS: Elevated donor cardiac troponin I. A marker of acute graft failure in infant heart recipients. Circulation 1994;90:2618–2621.

110. Grattan MT, Moreno-Cabral CE, Stames VA, Oyer PE, Stinson EB, Shumway NE: Cytomegalovirus infection is associated with cardiac allograft rejection and atherosclerosis. JAMA 1989;261:3561–3566.

111. Green M, Tzakis A, Reyes J, Nour B, Todos, Starzl TE: Infectious complications of pediatric liver transplantation under FK506. Transplant Proc 1991;3:3038–3039.

112. Green PS, Cameron DE, Augustine S, Gardner TJ, Reitz BA, Baumgartner WA: Exploratory analysis of time dependent risk for infection, rejection and death after cardiac transplantation. Ann Thorac Surg 1989;47:650–654.

113. Grice WN, Konishi T, Apstein CS: Resistance of neonatal myocardium to injury during normothermic and hypothermic ischemic arrest and reperfusion. Circulation 1987;76:V-150–V-155.

114. Griffin ML, Hernandez A, Martin TC: Dilated cardiomyopathy in infants and children. J Am Coll Cardiol 1988;11:139–144.

115. Gwathmey JK, Warren SE, Briggs GM, Copelas L, Feldman MD, Phillips PJ, Callahan M, Schoen FJ, Grossman W, Morgan JP: Diastolic dysfunction in hypertrophic cardiomyopathy: effect on active force generation during systole. J Clin Invest 1991;87:1023–1031.

116. Hajjar KA, Hajjar DP, Silverstein RL, Nachman RL: Tumor necrosis factor-mediated release of platelet-derived growth factor from cultured endothelial cells. J Exp Med 1987;166:235–245.

117. Hammond EH, Ensley RD, Yowell RL, Craven CM, Bristow MR, Renlund DG, O'Connell JB: Vascular rejection of human cardiac allografts and the role of humoral immunity in chronic allograft rejection. Transplant Proc 1991;23(suppl 2):26–30.

118. Hammond EH, Yowell RL, Nunoda S, Menlove RL, Renlund DG, Bristow MR, Gay WA, Jones KW, O'Connell JB: Vascular (humoral) rejection in heart transplantation: pathologic observations and clinical implications. J Heart Transplant 1989;8:430–443.

119. Harjula ALJ, Heikkila LJ, Nieminen MS, Kupari M, Keto P, Mattila SP: Heart transplantation in repaired transposition of the great arteries. Ann Thorac Surg 1988;46:611–614.

120. Herskowitz A, Soule LM, Ueda K, Tamura F, Baumgartner WA, Borkon AM, Reitz BA, Achuff SC, Traill TA, Baughman KL: Arteriolar vasculitis on endomyocardial biopsy: a histologic predictor of poor outcome in cyclosporine-treated heart transplant recipients. J Heart Transplant 1987;6:127–136.

121. Hess ML, Hastillo A, Mohanakumar T, Cowley MJ, Vetrovac G, Szentpetery S, Wolfgang TC, Lower RR: Accelerated atherosclerosis in cardiac transplantation: role of cytotoxic B-cell antibodies and hyperlipidemia. Circulation 1983;68(suppl II):II-94–II-101.

122. Hirota Y, Shimizu G, Kita Y, Nakayama Y, Suwa M, Kawamura K, Nagata S, Sawayama T, Izumi T, Nakano T, Toshima H, Sekiguchi M: Spectrum of restrictive cardiomyopathy: report of the national survey in Japan. Am Heart J 1990;120:188–194.

123. Hirsch R, Huddleston CB, Mendeloff EN, Sekarski TJ, Canter CE: Infant and donor organ growth after heart transplantation in neonates with hypoplastic left heart syndrome. J Heart Lung Transplant 1996;15:1093–1100.

124. Ho M, Jaffe R, Miller G: The frequency of Epstein-Barr virus infection and associated lymphoproliferative syndrome after transplantation and its manifestations in children. Transplantation 1986;45:719–727.

125. Hofflin JM, Potasman I, Baldwin JC, Oyer PE, Stinson EB, Remington JS: Infectious complication in heart transplant recipients receiving cyclosporine and corticosteroids. Ann Intern Med 1987;106:209–216.

126. Hosenpud JD, Bennett LE, Keck BM, Fiol B, Novick RJ: The registry of the International Society for Heart and Lung Transplantation: sixteenth official report—1999. J Heart Lung Transplant 1999;18:611–626.

127. Hricik DE, Almawi WY, Stromm TB: Trends in the use of glucocorticoids in renal transplantation. Transplantation 1994;57:979.

128. Hsu DT, Garafano RP, Douglas JF, Michler RE, Quegebeur JM, Gersony WM, Addonizio LJ: Exercise performance after pediatric heart transplantation. Circulation 1993;88:II-238–II-242.

129. Iannettoni MD, Bove EL, Mosca RS, Lupinetti FM, Dorostkar PC, Ludomirsky A, Crowley DC, Kulik TJ, Rosenthal A: Improving results with first-stage palliation for hypoplastic left heart syndrome. J Thorac Cardiovasc Surg. 1994;107:934.

130. Ibrahim J, Blume E, Phelan D, Lublin D, Canter CE: Successful cardiac transplantation of pre–sensitized children without a prospective crossmatch—preliminary results [abstract]. J Heart Lung Transplant 1999;18:83.

131. Ignarro LJ, Buga GM, Wood KS, Byrns RE, Chaudhuri G: Endothelium-derived relaxing factor produced and released from artery and vein is nitric oxide. Proc Natl Acad Sci U S A 1987;84:9265–9269.

132. Jacobs ML, Blackstone EH, Bailey LL, The Congenital Heart Surgeons Society: Surgery for congenital heart disease (intermediate survival in neonates with aortic atresia: a multi-institutional study). J Thorac Cardiovasc Surg 1998;116:417–431.

133. Jahangiri M, Zurakowski D, Bichell D, Mayer JE, delNido PJ, Jonas RA: Improved results with selective management in pulmonary atresia with intact ventricular septum. J Thorac Cardiovasc Surg 1999;118:1046–1055.

134. Jarcho JA, McKenna W, Pare PJA, Solomon SD, Geisterfer-Lowrance A, Holcombe RF, Dickie S, Levi T, Donsi-Keller H, Seidman JG, Seidman CE: Mapping a gene for familial hypertrophic cardiomyopathy to chromosome 14q1. N Engl J Med 1989;321:1372–1378.

135. Jarmakani JM, Nagatomo M, Nakazana M, Langer GA: Effect of hypoxia on myocardial high-energy phosphates in the neonatal mammalian heart. Am J Physiol 1978;235:H475.

136. Jazzar A, Fagiuoli S, Sisson S, Zuhdi N, Cooper DK: Induction therapy with cyclosporine without cytolytic agents results in a low incidence of acute rejection without significant renal impairment in heart transplant patients. Clin Transplant 1995;9:334–339.

137. Jebara VA, Dreyfus G, Acar C, Deloche A, Couetil JP, Fabiani JN, Carpentier A: Heart transplantation for corrected transposition of the great vessels. J Card Surg 1990;5:102–105.

138. Jeevanandam V: Myocardial preservation for pediatric cardiac transplantation: In Franco KL (ed): Pediatric Cardiopulmonary Transplantation. Armonk, NY: Futura Publishing Company, Inc, 1997.

139. Johnson DE, Alderman EL, Schroeder JS, Gao SZ, Hunt S, DeCampli WM, Stinson E, Billingham M: Transplant coronary artery disease: histopathologic correlations with angiographic morphology. J Am Coll Cardiol 1991;17:449–457.

140. Johnsrude CL, Perry JC, Cecchin F, Smith EO, Fraley K, Friedman RA, Towbin JA: Differentiating anomalous left main coronary artery originating from the pulmonary artery in infants from myocarditis and dilated cardiomyopathy by electrocardiogram. Am J Cardiol 1995;75:71–74.

141. Jonas RA, Quaegebeur JM, Kirklin JW, Blackstone EH, Daicoff G, and the Congenital Heart Surgeons Society: Outcomes in patients with interrupted aortic arch and ventricular septal defect. J Thorac Cardiovasc Surg 1994;107:1099–1113.

142. Kanjuh VI, Elliot RS, Edwards JE: Coexistent mitral and aortic valvular atresia. A pathologic study of 14 cases. Am J Cardiol 1965;15:611.

143. Kanter KR, Vincent RN, Miller BE, McFadden C: Heart transplantation in children who have undergone previous heart surgery: is it safe? J Heart Lung Transplant 1993;12:S218–S224.

144. Kantrowitz A, Haller JD, Joos H, Cerruti MM, Carstensen HE: Transplantation of the heart in an infant and an adult. Am J Cardiol 1968;22:782–790.

145. Karr SS, Parness IA, Spevak PJ, van der Velde ME, Colan SD, Sanders SP: Diagnosis of anomalous left coronary artery by

Doppler color flow mapping: distinction from other causes of dilated cardiomyopathy. J Am Coll Cardiol 1992;19:1271–1275.

146. Katritsis D, Wilmshurst PT, Wendon JA, Davies MJ, Webb-Peploe MM: Primary restrictive cardiomyopathy: clinical and pathologic characteristics. J Am Coll Cardiol 1991;18:1230–1235.

147. Katz AM: Cytoskeletal abnormalities in the failing heart. Circulation 2000;101:2672–2673.

148. Kavelaars A, Cats B, Visser GH, Zegers BJ, Bakker JM, van Rees EP, Heunen CJ: Ontogeny of the responses of human peripheral blood T cells to glucocorticoids. Brain Behav Immun 1996;10: 288–297.

149. Kawauchi M, Gundry SR, deBegona JA, Fullerton DA, Razzouk AJ, Boucek M, Kanakriyeh M, Bailey LL: Prolonged preservation of human pediatric hearts for transplantation: correlation of ischemic time and subsequent function. J Heart Lung Transplant 1993;12:55–58.

150. Kelly DP, Strauss AW: Inherited cardiomyopathies. N Engl J Med 1994;330:913–919.

151. Kempsford RD, Hearse DJ: Protection of the immature myocardium during global ischemia: a comparison of four clinical cardioplegic solutions in the rabbit heart. J Thorac Cardiovasc Surg 1989;97:856–863.

152. Kermode J, Butt W, Shann F: Comparison between prostaglandin E$_1$ and eprostenol (prostacyclin) in infants after heart surgery. Br Heart J 1991;66:175–178.

153. Kirklin JW, Blackstone EH, Pacifico AD, Kirklin JK, Bargeron LM Jr: Risk factors for early and late failure after repair of tetralogy of fallot, and their neutralization. Thorac Cardiovasc Surg 1984;32:208–214.

154. Kirklin J, Naftel DC, Bourge RC, White-Williams C, Caufield JB, Tarkka MR, Holman WL, Zorn GL: Rejection after cardiac transplantation: a time related risk factor analysis. Circulation 1992;86(suppl II):II-236–II-241.

155. Kirklin JK, Naftel DC, Kirklin JW, Blackstone EH, White-Williams C, Bourge RC: Pulmonary vascular resistance and the risk of heart transplantation. J Heart Transplant 1988;7:331–336.

156. Kirklin JK, Naftel DC, Levine TB, Bourge RC, Pelletier GB, O'Donnell J, Miller LW, Pritzker MR, and the Transplant Cardiologists Research Database (TCRD) Group, UAB: Cytomegalovirus after heart transplantation: risk factors for infection and mortality: a multi-institutional study. J Heart Lung Transplant 1994;13: 394–404.

157. Klienert S, Weintraub RG, Wilkinson JL, Choe CW: Myocarditis in children with dilated cardiomyopathy: incidence and outcome after dual therapy immunosuppression. J Heart Lung Transplant 1997;16:1248–1254.

158. Kobashigawa JA, Naftel DC, Bourge RC, Kirklin JK, Ventura HO, Mohanty PK, Cintron GB, Bhat G: Pre-transplant risk factors for acute rejection after cardiac transplantation: a multi-institutional study. J Heart Lung Transplant 1993;12:355–366.

159. Kubo SH, Naftel DC, Mills RC, O'Donnell J, Rodeheffer RJ, Cintron GB, Kenzora JL, Bourge RC, Kirklin JK: Risk factors for late recurrent rejection after cardiac transplantation. A multi-institutional, multivariable analysis. J Heart Lung Transplant 1995;14:409–418.

160. Kuhn MA, Larsen RL, Khan MA, Johnston JK, Chinnock RE, Chinnock RE, Bailey LL: The outcome of infants with hypoplastic left heart syndrome requiring balloon atrial septostomy. J Heart Lung Transplant 1997;16:71.

161. Lafarge CG, Miettinen OS: The estimation of oxygen consumption. Cardiovasc Res 1970;4:23–30.

162. Laine J, Jalanko H, Leijala M, Sairanen H, Holmberg C: Kidney function in cyclosporine-treated pediatric heart transplant recipients. J Heart Lung Transplant 1997;16:1217–1224.

163. Lamour JM, Hsu DT, Kichuk MR, Quaegebeur JM, Galantowicz ME, Martin EC, Gersony WM, Addonizio LJ: Regression of pulmonary arteriovenous malformations following heart transplantation. J Heart Lung Transplant 1997;16:71.

164. Larsen RL, Applegate PM, Dyar DA, Ribeiro PA, Fritzsche SD, Mulla NF, Shirali GS, Kuhn MA, Chinnock RE, Shah PM: Dobutamine stress echocardiography for assessing coronary artery disease after transplantation in children. J Am Coll Cardiol 1998;32:515–520.

165. Laske A, Gallino A, Mohacsi P, Bauer EP, Carrel T, von Segesser LK, Turina MI: Prophylactic treatment with ganciclovir for cytomegalovirus infection in heart transplantation. Transplant Proc 1991;23:1170–1173.

166. Laufer G, Laczkovics A, Wollenek G, Buxbaum P, Graninger W, Holzinger C, Wolner E: Infectious complications in heart transplant recipients with combined low dose cyclosporine, azathioprine and prednisolone (triple drug) immunosuppression. Transplant Proc 1989;21:2508–2511.

167. Lebeck LK, Chang L, Lopez-McCormack C, Chinnock R, Boucek M: Polyclonal antithymocyte serum: immune prophylaxis and rejection therapy in pediatric heart transplantation patients. J Heart Lung Transplant 1993;12:S286–S292.

168. Lev M: Pathologic anatomy and interrelationship of hypoplasia of the aortic tract complexes. Lab Invest 1952;1:61.

169. Lewis AB: Clinical profile and outcome of restrictive cardiomyopathy in children. Am Heart J 1992;123:1589–1593.

170. Libby P, Salomon RN, Payne DD, Schoen FJ, Pober JS: Functions of vascular wall cells related to development of transplantation-associated coronary arteriosclerosis. Transplant Proc 1989;21: 3677–3684.

171. Lipshultz SE, Colan SD, Gelber RD, Perez-Atayde AR, Sallan SE, Sanders SP: Late cardiac effects of doxorubicin therapy for acute lymphoblastic leukemia in childhood. N Engl J Med 1991;324: 808–815.

172. Lodge PA, Herzum M, Olszewski J, Huber SA: Coxsackievirus B-3 myocarditis: acute and chronic forms of the disease caused by different immunopathogenic mechanisms. Am J Pathol 1987; 128:455–463.

173. Loker J, Darragh R, Ensing G, Caldwell R: Echocardiographic analysis of rejection in the infant heart transplant recipient. J Heart Lung Transplant 1994;13:1014–1018.

174. Lui RC, Williams WG, Trusler GA, Freedom RM, Coles JG, Rebeyka IM, Smallhorn J: Expereince with the Damus-Kaye-Stansel procedure for children with Taussig-Bing hearts or univentricular hearts with subaortic stenosis. Circulation 1993;88:170–176.

175. Magovern JA, Pae WE Jr, Miller CA, Waldhausen JA: The mature and immature heart: response to normothermic ischemia. J Surg Res 1989;46:366–369.

176. Margarit C, Martinez Ibanez V, Tormo R, Infante D, Iglesias H: Maintenance immunosuppression without steroids in pediatric liver transplantation. Transplant Proc 1989;21:2230.

177. Maron BJ: Right ventricular cardiomyopathy: another cause of sudden death in the young. N Engl J Med 1988;318:178–180.

178. Maron BJ, Bonow RO, Cannon RO, Leon MB, Epstein SE: Hypertrophic cardiomyopathy: interrelations of clinical manifestations, pathophysiology, and therapy. N Engl J Med 1987;316:780–789, 844–852.

179. Maron BJ, Lipson LC, Roberts WG, Epstein SE: "Malignant" hypertrophic cardiomyopathy: identification of a subgroup of families with unusually frequent premature death. Am J Cardiol 1978;41:1133–1140.

180. Maron BJ, Nichols PF, Pickle LW, Wesley YE, Mulvihill JJ: Patterns of inheritance in hypertrophic cardiomyopathy: assessment by M-mode and two dimensional echocardiography. Am J Cardiol 1984;53:1087–1094.

181. Maron BJ, Savage DD, Wolfson JK, Epstein SE: Prognostic significance of 24 hour ambulatory electrocardiographic monitoring in patients with hypertrophic cardiomyopathy: a prospective study. Am J Cardiol 1981;48:252–257.

182. Martin AB, Bricker JT, Fishman M, Frazier OH, Price JK, Radovancevic B, Louis PT, Cabalka AK, Gelb BD, Towbin JA: Neurologic complications of heart transplantation in children. J Heart Lung Transplant 1992;11:933–942.

183. Martin AB, Webber S, Fricker FJ, Jaffe R, Demmler G, Kearney D, Zhang YH, Bodurtha J, Gelb B, Ni J, Bricker JT, Towbin JA: Acute myocarditis: rapid diagnosis by PCR in children. Circulation 1994;90:330–339.

184. Martino TA, Liu P, Sole MJ: Viral infection and the pathogenesis of dilated cardiomyopathy. Circulation 1994;74:182–188.

185. Matitiau A, Perez-Atayde A, Sanders SP, Sluysmans T, Parness IA, Spevak PJ, Colan SD: Infantile dilated cardiomyopathy: relation of outcome to left ventricular mechanics, hemodynamics, and histology at the time of presentation. Circulation 1994; 90:1310–1318.

186. McCarthy RE III, Boehmer JP, Hruban RH, Hutchins GM, Kasper EK, Hare JM, Baughman KL: Long term outcome of fulminant

myocarditis as compared with acute (nonfulminant) myocarditis. N Engl J Med 2000;342:690–695.

187. McGiffin DC, Kirklin JK, Pearce FB: Pediatric cardiac transplantation. *In* Advances in Cardiac Surgery, St. Louis: Mosby-Year Book, Inc, 1997, pp 149–176.

188. McGiffin DC, Naftel DC, Kirklin JK, Morrow WR, Towbin J, Shaddy R, Alejos R, Rossi A: Predicting outcome following listing for cardiac transplantation in children: comparison of Kaplan-Meier and parametric competing risk analysis. J Heart Lung Transplant 1997;16:713–722.

189. McGiffin DC, Savunen T, Kirklin JK, Naftel DC, Bourge RC, Paine TD, White-Williams C, Sisto T, Early L: Cardiac transplant coronary artery disease: a multivariable analysis of pretransplantation risk factors for disease development and morbid events. J Thorac Cardiovasc Surg 1995;109:1081–1089.

190. McGowan FX, Cao-Danh H, Takeuchi K, Davis PJ, del Nido PJ: Prolonged neonatal myocardial preservation with a highly buffered low-calcium solution. J Thorac Cardiovasc Surg 1994; 108:772–779.

191. McKenna WJ, England D, Doi YL, Deanfield JE, Oakley CM, Goodwin JF: Arrhythmia in hypertrophic cardiomyopathy, I: influence on prognosis. Br Heart J 1981;46:168–172.

192. McLaughlin M, Thomas P, Onorato I, Rubinstein A, Oleske J, Nicholas S, Krasinski K, Guigli P, Orenstein W: Live virus vaccines in human immunodeficiency virus–infected children: a retrospective surgey. Pediatrics 1988;82:229–233.

193. Mentzer RM, Alegre CA, Nolan CP: The effects of dopamine and isoproterinol on the pulmonary circulation. J Thorac Cardiovasc Surg 1976;71:807–814.

194. Merigan TC, Renlund GD, Keay S, Bristow MR, Starnes V, O'Connell JB, Resta S, Dunn D, Gamberg P, Ratkovec RM: A controlled trial of ganciclovir to prevent cytomegalovirus disease after heart transplantation. N Engl J Med 1992;326:1182–1186.

195. Michler RE, Edwards NM, Hsu D, Bernstein D, Fricker FJ, Miller J, Copeland J, Kaye MP, Addonizio L: Pediatric retransplantation. J Heart Lung Transplant 1993;12:S319–S327.

196. Miller LW, Naftel DC, Bourge RC, Kirklin JK, Brozena SC, Jarcho J, Hobbs RE, Mills RM: Infection after heart transplantation: a multiinstitutional study. Cardiac Transplant Research Database Group. J Heart Lung Transplant 1994;13:381–392.

197. Mills RM Jr, Naftel DC, Kirklin JK, Van Bakel AB, Jaski B, Massin E, Lee FA, Fishbein DP, Bourge RC, and the Cardiac Translant Research Database Group: Cardiac transplant rejection with hemodynamic compromise: a multi-institutional study of risk factors and endomyocardial cellular infiltrate. J Heart Lung Transplant 1997;16:813–821.

198. Morrow WR, Frazier E, Naftel DC: Survival after listing for cardiac transplantation in children. Prog Pediatr Cardiol 2000; 11:99–105.

199. Morrow WR, Naftel D, Chinnock R, Canter C, Boucek M, Zales V, McGiffin DC, Kirklin JK, and the Pediatric Heart Transplantation Study (PHTS) Group: Outcome of listing for cardiac transplantation in infants under 6 months. Predictors of death and interval to transplantation. J Heart Lung Transplant 1997;16:1255–1266.

200. Mossman TR, Schuymacher JH, Street NF, Budd R, O'Garra A, Fong TA, Bond MW, Moore KW, Sher A, Fiorentino DF: Diversity of cytokine synthesis and function of mouse CD4$^+$ T cells. Immunol Rev 1991;123:209–229.

201. Mulla NF, Johnston J, VanderDussen L, Shirali G, Larsen R, Kuhn M, Khan A, Chinnock R, Bailey L: Early re-transplantation for post-transplant coronary artery disease in children. J Heart Lung Transplant 1997;16:71.

202. Muller J, Warnecke H, Spiegelsberger S, Hummel M, Cohnert T, Hetzer R: Reliable noninvasive rejection diagnosis after heart transplantation in childhood. J Heart Lung Transplant 1993;12: 189–198.

203. Najarian JS, Fryd DS, Strand M, Canafax DM, Ascher NL, Payne WD, Simmons RL, Sutherland DE: A single institution, randomized prospective trial of cyclosporine versus azathioprine-antilymphocyte globulin for immunosuppression in renal allograft recipients. Ann Surg 1985;201:142–157.

204. Newburger JW, Jonas RA, Wernovsky G, Wypij D, Hickey PR, Kuban KCK, Farrell DM, Holmes GL, Helmers SL, Constantinou J, Carrazana E, Barlow JK, Walsh AZ, Lucius KC, Share JC, Wessel DL, Hanley FL, Mayer JE Jr, Castaneda AR, Ware JH: A comparison of the perioperative neurologic effects of hypothermic circulatory arrest versus low-flow cardiopulmonary bypass in infant heart surgery. N Engl J Med 1993;329:1057–1064.

205. Newton ER: Diagnosis of perinatal TORCH infections. Clin Obstet Gynecol 1999;42:59–70.

206. Nishioka K, Jarmakani JM: Effects of ischemia on mechanical function and high-energy phosphates in rabbit myocardium. Am J Physiol 1982;242:H107.

207. Nixon PA, Fricker FJ, Noyes BE, Webber SA, Orenstein DM, Armitage JM: Exercise testing in pediatric heart, heart-lung and lung transplant recipients. Chest 1995;107:1328–1335.

208. Noonan JA, Nadas AS: The hypoplastic left heart syndrome. Pediatr Clin North Am 1958;5:1029.

209. Nootens M, Schrader B, Kaufman E, Vestal R, Long W, Rich S: Comparitive acute effects of adenosine and prostacyclin in primary pulmonary hypertension. Chest 1995;107:54–57.

210. Norwood WI: Hypoplastic left heart syndrome. Ann Thorac Surg 1991;52:688.

211. O'Neill BJ, Pflugfelder PW, Singh NR, Menkis AH, McKenzie FN, Kostuk WJ: Frequency of angiographic detection and quantitative assessment of coronary arterial disease one and three years after cardiac transplantation. Am J Cardiol 1989;63:1221–1226.

212. Ottlinger ME, Pearsall L, Lipshultz SE: New developments in the biochemical assessment of myocardial injury in children: troponins T and I as highly sensitive and specific markers of myocardial injury. Prog Pediatr Cardiol 1998;8:71–81.

213. Pahl E, Crawford SE, Swenson JM, Duffy CE, Fricker FJ, Backer CL, Mavroudis C, Chjaudhry FA: Dobutamine stress echocardiography: experience in pediatric heart transplant recipients. J Heart Lung Transplant 1999;18:725–732.

214. Pahl E, Naftel DC, Canter CE, Frazier EA, Kirklin JK: Death after rejection with severe hemodynamic compromise in pediatric recipients. J Heart Lung Transplant 1998;17:61.

215. Pahl E, Zales VR, Fricker FJ, Addonizio LJ: Posttransplant coronary artery disease in children: a multicenter national survey. Circulation 1994;90:II-56–II-60.

216. Palmer RMJ, Ferrige AG, Moncada S: Nitric oxide release accounts for the biological activity of endothelium-derived relaxing factor. Nature 1987;327:524–526.

217. Peterseim DS, Chestnut LC, Meyers CH, D'Amico TA, Van Trigt P, Schwinn DA: Stability of the β-adrenergic receptor/adenylyl cyclase pathway of pediatric myocardium after brain death. J Heart Lung Transplant 1994;13:635–640.

218. Peterseim DS, Meyers CH, Craig DM, Davis JW, Campbell KA, D'Amico TA, Van Trigt P: Improved tolerance of the pediatric myocardium to brain death. J Heart Lung Transplant 1983;12: S236–S240.

219. Phocas I, Sarandakou A, Giannaki G, Malamitsi-Puchner A, Rizos D, Zourlas PA: Soluble intercellular, adhesion molecule-1 in newborn infants. Eur J Pediatr 1998;157:153–156.

220. Pietra BA, Boucek MM: Immunosuppression for pediatriac cardiac transplantation in the modern era. Prog Pediatr Cardiol 2000;11:115–129.

221. Pigott JD, Murphy JD, Barber G, Norwood WI: Palliative reconstructive surgery for hypoplastic left heart syndrome. Ann Thorac Surg 1998;45:122–128.

222. Pophal SG, Sigfusson G, Booth KL, Bacanu SA, Webber SA, Ettedgui JA, Neches WH, Park SC: Complications of endomyocardial biopsy in children. J Am Coll Cardiol 1999;34:2105–2110.

223. Rager-Zisman B, Allison AC: The role of antibody and host cells in the resistance of mice against infection by coxsackie B-3 virus. J Gen Virol 1973;19:329–338.

224. Razzouk AJ, Chinnock RE, Dearani JA, Gundry SR, Bailey LL: Cardiac retransplantation for graft vasculopathy in children. Arch Surg 1998;133:881–885.

225. Razzouk AJ, Chinnock RE, Gundry SR, Johnston JK, Larsen RL, Baum MF, Mulla NF, Bailey LL: Transplantation as a primary treatment for hypoplastic left heart syndrome: intermediate term results. Ann Thorac Surg 1996;62:1–8.

226. Razzouk AJ, Gundry SR, Chinnock RE, Larsen RL, Ruiz C, Zuppan CW, Bailey LL: Orthotopic transplantation for total anomalous pulmonary venous connection associated with complex congenital heart disease. J Heart Lung Transplant 1995;14:713–717.

227. Reid KR, Menkis AH, Novick RJ, Pflugfelder PW, Kostuk WJ, Reid J, Whitby JL, Powell AM, McKenzie FN: Reduced incidence

of severe infection after heart transplantation with low intensity immunosuppression. J Heart Lung Transplant 1991;10:894–900.

228. Reisman L, Lieberman KV, Burrows L, Schanzer H: Followup of cyclosporine-treated pediatric renal allograft recipients after cessation of prednisone. Transplantation 1990;49:76.

229. Riddler SA, Breinig MC, McKnight JLC: Increased levels of circulating Epstein-Barr virus-infected lymphocytes and decreased EBV nuclear antigen antibody responses are associated with the development of posttransplant lymphoproliferative disease in solid-organ transplant recipients. Blood 1994;84:972–984.

230. Rimar S, Gillis CN: Selective pulmonary vasodilation by nitric oxide is due to hemoglobin inactivation. Circulation 1993;88: 2884–2887.

231. Roberti I, Reisman L, Lieberman KV, Burrows L: Risk of steroid withdrawal in pediatric renal allograft recipients (a 5 year followup). Clin Transplant 1994;8:405.

232. Roberts JD, Lang P, Bigatello LM, Vlahakes GJ, Zapol WM: Inhaled nitric oxide in congenital heart disese. Circulation 1993; 87:447–453.

233. Robinson JA, Radveany RM, Muller MG, Garrity ER: Plasmapheresis followed by intravenous immunoglobulin in presensitized patients awaiting heart transplantation. Ther Apher 1997; 1:147–151.

234. Robinson JA, O'Connell JB, Roeges LM, Major EO, Gunnar RM: Coxsackie B3 myocarditis in athymic mice (41028). Proc Soc Exp Biol Med 1981;166:80–91.

235. Rose EA, Smith CR, Petrossian GA, Barr ML, Reemtsma K: Humoral immune responses after cardiac transplantation: correlation with fatal rejection and graft atherosclerosis. Surgery 1989; 106:203–208.

236. Rosenblum HM, Haasler GB, Spotnitz WD, Lazar HL, Spotnitz HM: Effects of simulated clinical cardiopulmonary bypass and cardioplegia on mass of the canine left ventricle. Ann Thorac Surg 1985;39:139–148.

237. Rotondo KM, Naftel DC, Boucek R, Canter CE, McGiffin DC, Pahl E, Chinnock RE, Morrow R, Kirklin JK, and the Pediatric Heart Transplant Study Group: Allograft rejection following cardic transplantation in infants and children: a multi-institutional study [abstract]. J Heart Lung Transplant 1996;15:S80.

238. Rowls JR, Foegh ML, Khirabadi BS, Ramwell PW: The synergistic effect of cyclosporine and iloprost on survival of rat cardiac allografts. Transplantation 1986;42:94–96.

239. Rubin LJ: Primary pulmonary hypertension. Chest 1993;104: 236–250.

240. Sarris GE, Smith JA, Bernstein D, Griffin ML, Pitlick PT, Baum D, Billingham ME, Oyer PE, Stinson EB, Starnes VA: Pediatric cardiac transplantation: the Stanford experience. Circulation 1994;90:II-51–II-55.

241. Schelonka RL, Infante AJ: Neonatal immunology. Semin Perinatol 1998;22:2–14.

242. Schelonka RL, Raaphorst FM, Infante D, Kraig E, Teale JM, Infante AJ: T cell receptor repertoire diversity and clonal expansion in human neonates. Pediatr Res 1998;43:396–402.

243. Schmidt KG, Cooper MJ, Silverman NH, Stanger P: Pulmonary artery origin of the left coronary artery: diagnosis by two-dimensional echocardiography, pulsed Doppler ultrasound and color flow mapping. J Am Coll Cardiol 1988;11:396–402.

244. Schowengerdt KO, Naftel DC, Seib PM, Pearce FB, Addonizio LJ, Kirklin JK, Morrow WR, Pediatric Heart Transplant Study Group: Infection after pediatric heart transplantation: results of a multi-institutional study. J Heart Lung Transplant 1997;16: 1207–1216.

245. Schwartz ML, Cox GF, Lin AE, Korson MS, Perez-Atayde A, Lacro RV, Lipshultz SE: Clinical approach to genetic cardiomyopathy in children. Circulation 1996;94:2021–2038.

246. Schwartz ML, Jonas RA, Colan SD: Anomalous origin of the left coronary artery from pulmonary artery: recovery of left ventricular function after dual coronary repair. J Am Coll Cardiol 1997;30:547–553.

247. Seko Y, Takahashi N, Ishiyama S, Nishikawa T, Kasajima T, Hiroe M, Suzuki S, Ishiwata S, Kawai S, Azuma M, Yagita H, Okumura K, Yazaki Y: Expression of costimulatory molecules B7-1, B7-2, and CD40 in the heart of patients with acute myocarditis and dilated cardiomyopathy. Circulation 1998;97:637–639.

248. Shaddy RE, Naftel DC, Kirklin JK, Boyle G, McGiffin DC, Towbin JA, Ring WS, Pearce B, Addonizio L, Morrow WR, and the Pediatric Heart Transplant Study Group: Outcome of cardiac transplantation in children: survival in a contemporary multi-institutional experience. Circulation 1996;94(suppl II):II-69–II-73.

249. Shaffer KM, Denfield SW, Schowengerdt KO, Towbin JA, Radovancevic B, Frazier OH, Price JK, Gajarski RJ: Cardiac transplantation for pediatric patients. Tex Heart Inst J 1998;25:57–63.

250. Shah MB, Schroeder TJ, First MR: Guidelines for immunosuppression management and monitoring after transplantation in children. Transplant Rev 1999;13:83–97.

251. Sherali O, Cephus C, Dyar D, Lombano F, Mulla N, Kuhn M, Wood L, Chinnock R, Johnston J, Bailey L, Ali Khan M, Larson R: Coarctation of aorta following infant/pediatric cardiac transplantation. J Heart Lung Transplant 1996;15:S71.

252. Shinbane JS, Wood MA, Jensen N, Ellenbogen KA, Fitzpatrick AP, Scheinman MM: Tachycardia-induced cardiomyopathy: a review of animal models and clinical studies. J Am Coll Cardiol 1997;29:709–715.

253. Siegel RJ, Shah PK, Fishbein MC: Idiopathic restrictive cardiomyopathy. Circulation 1984;70:165–169.

254. Sigfusson G, Fricker FJ, Bernstein D, Addonizio LJ, Baum D, Hsu DT, Chin C, Miller SA, Boyle GJ, Miller J, Lawrence KS, Douglas JF, Griffith BP, Reitz BA, Michler RE, Rose EA, Webber SA: Long-term survivors of pediatric heart transplantation: a multicenter report of sixty-eight children who have survived longer than five years. J Pediatr 1997;130:862–871.

255. Siveski-Iliskovic N, Hill M, Chow DA, Singal PK: Probucol protects against Adriamycin cardiomyopathy without interfering with its antitumor effect. Circulation 1995;91:10–15.

256. Slaughter MS, Braunlin E, Bolman RMI, Molina JE, Shumway SJ: Pediatric heart transplantation: results of 2 and 5 year followup. J Heart Lung Transplant 1994;13:624–630.

257. Smythe JF, Dyck JD, Smallhorn JF, Freedom RM: Natural history of cardiac rhabdomyoma in infancy and childhood. Am J Cardiol 1990;66:1247–1249.

258. Snydman DR, Wener BG, Heinze-Lacey B, Berardi VP, Tilney NL, Kirklman AB, Milford EL, Cho SI, Bush HL, Levey AS: Use of cytomegalovirus immune globulin to prevent cytomegalovirus disease in renal transplant recipients. N Engl J Med 1987; 317:1045–1054.

259. Spotnitz WD, Clark MB, Rosenblum HM: Effect of cardiopulmonary bypass and global ischemia on human and canine left ventricular mass: evidence of interspecies differences. Surgery 1984; 96:230–238.

260. Stevenson JG, Stone F, Dillard DH, Morgan BC: Intellectual development of children subjected to prolonged circulatory arrest during hypothermic open heart surgery in infancy. Circulation 1974;49, 50(suppl 2):54–59.

261. Stringham JC, Bul DA, Fuller TC, Kfoury AG, Taylor DO, Renlund DG, Karwande SV: Avoidance of cellular blood product transfusions in LVAD recipients does not prevent HLA allosensitization. J Heart Lung Transplant 1999;18:160–165.

262. Strom TAB, Carpenter CB, Cragoe EJ Jr, Norris S, Devlin R, Perper RJ: Suppression of in vivo and in vitro alloimmunity by prostaglandins. Transplant Proc 1977;9:1075–1079.

263. Suda K, Kohl T, Kovalchin JP, Silverman NH: Echocardiographic predictors of poor outcome in infants with hypertrophic cardiomyopathy. Am J Cardiol 1997;80:595–600.

264. Taliercio CP, Seward JB, Driscoll DJ, Fisher LD, Gersh BJ, Tajik AJ: Idiopathic dilated cardiomyopathy in the young: clinical profile and natural history. J Am Coll Cardiol 1985;6:1126–1131.

265. Tamisier D, Vouche P, LeBidois J, Mauriat P, Khoury W, Leca F: Donor-recipient size matching in pediatric heart transplantation: a word of caution about small grafts. J Heart Lung Transplant 1996;15:190–195.

266. Tantengco MV, Dodd D, Frist WH, Boucek MM, Boucek RJ: Echocardiographic abnormalities with acute cardiac allograft rejection in children: correlation with endomyocardial biopsy. J Heart Lung Transplant 1993;12:S203–S210.

267. Tejani A, Sullivan K: Long-term follow-up of growth in children post-transplantation. Kidney Int 1993;44(suppl I):S56–S58.

268. Todo S, Fung JJ, Starzl TE, Tzakis A, Demetris AJ, Kormos R, Jain A, Alessiani M, Takaya S, Shapiro R: Liver, kidney, and

thoracic organ transplantation under FK 506. Ann Surg 1990; 212:295–307.

269. Tomioka N, Kishimoto C, Matsumori A, Kawai C: Effects of prednisolone on acute viral myocarditis in mice. J Am Coll Cardiol 1986;7:868–872.

270. Treasure T, Naftel DC, Conger KA, Garcia JH, Kirklin JW, Blackstone EH: The effect of hypothermic circulatory arrest time on cerebral function, morphology, and biochemistry. J Thorac Cardiovasc Surg 1983;86:761.

271. Treem WR, Stanley CA, Finegold DN, Hale DE, Coates PM: Primary carnitine deficiency due to a failure of carnitine transport in kidney, muscle, and fibroblasts. N Engl J Med 1988;319:1331–1336.

272. Towbin JA: Molecular genetic aspects of cardiomyopathy. Biochem Med Metab Biol 1993;49:285–320.

273. Vigano A, Esposito S, Arienti D, Zagliani A, Massironi E, Principi N, Clerici M: Differential development of type 1 and type 2 cytokines and beta-chemokines in the ontogeny of healthy newborns. Biol Neonate 1999;75:1–8.

274. Von Reuden TJ, Knight L, Moller JH, Edwards JE: Coarctation of the aorta associated with aortic valve atresia. Circulation 1975;52:951.

275. Wahlberg JA, Southard JH, Belzer FO: Development of a cold storage solution for pancreas preservation. Cryobiology 1986; 23:477–482.

276. Walters HL III, Digerness SB, Naftel DC, Waggoner JR, Blackstone EH, Kirklin JW: The response to ischemia in blood perfused vs. crystalloid perfused isolated rat heart preparations. J Mol Cell Cardiol 1992;24:1063–1077.

277. Watson DG, Rowe RD: Aortic-valve atresia: report of 43 cases. JAMA 1962;179:14.

278. Webber SA: 15 years of pediatric heart transplantation at the University of Pittsburgh: lessons learned and future prospects. Pediatr Transplant 1997;1:8–21.

279. Webber SA, Fricker FJ, Michaels M, Pickering RM, del Nido PJ, Griffith BP, Armitage JM: Orthotopic heart transplantation in children with congenital heart disease. Ann Thorac Surg 1994; 58:1664–1669.

280. Webber SA, Green M: Post-transplantation lymphoproliferative disorders: advances in diagnosis, prevention and management in children. Prog Pediatr Cardiol 2000;11:145–157.

281. Webber SA, Naftel DC, Paker J, Mulla N, Balfour I, Cipriani L, Kirklin JK, Morrow WR, and the Pediatric Heart Transplant Study: Late rejection greater than 1 year after pediatric heart transplantation: an ominous finding. J Heart Lung Transplant 1999;18:69.

282. Wells WJ, Parkman R, Smogorzewska E, Barr M: Neonatal thymectomy: does it affect immune function? J Thorac Cardiovasc Surg 1998;115:1041–1046.

283. Wessel DL, Adatia I, Giglia TM: Use of nitric oxide and acetylcholine in the evaluation of pulmonary hypertension and endothelial function after cardiopulmonary bypass. Circulation 1993;88: 2128–2138.

284. Wesselhoeft H, Fawcett JS, Johnson JL: Anomalous origin of the left coronary artery from the pulmonary trunk: its clinical spectrum, pathology, and pathophysiology, based on a review of 140 cases with 7 further cases. Circulation 1968;38:403–425.

285. Wigle ED, Heimbecker RO, Gunton RW: Idiopathic ventricular septal hypertrophy causing muscular subaortic stenosis. Circulation 1962;26:325–340.

286. Wigle ED, Rakowski H, Kimball BP, Williams WG: Hypertrophic cardiomyopathy. Circulation 1995;92:1680–1692.

287. Wigle ED, Sasson Z, Henderson MA, Ruddy TD, Fulop J, Rakowski H, Williams WG: Hypertrophic cardiomyopathy; the importance of the site and the extent of hypertrophy: a review. Prog Cardiovasc Dis 1985;28:1–83.

288. Wigle ED, Wilansky S: Diastolic dysfunction in hypertrophic cardiomyopathy. Heart Failure 1987;3:83–93.

289. Winegard S: Calcium release from cardiac sarcoplasmic reticulum. Annu Rev Physiol 1982;44:451–462.

290. Winter S, Jue K, Prochazaka J: The role of L-carnitine in pediatric cardiomyopathy. J Child Neurol 1995;Suppl2:S45–S51.

291. Wray J, Pot-Mees C, Zeitlin H, Radley-Smith R, Yacoub M: Cognitive function and behavioural status in paediatric heart and heart-lung transplant recipients: the Harefield experience. BMJ 1994:309:837–841.

292. Wright JS, Hicks RG, Newman DC: Deep hypothermic arrest. Observations on later development in children. J Thorac Cardiovasc Surg 1979;77:466–467.

293. Young JB, Leon CA, Short HD, Noon GP, Lawrence EC, Whisennand HH, Pratt CM, Goodman DA, Weilbaecher D, Quinones MA, DeBakey ME: Evolution of hemodynamics after orthotopic heart and heart-lung transplantation: early restrictive patterns persisting in occult fashion. J Heart Transplant 1987;6:34–43.

294. Yowell RL, Hammond EH, Bristow MR, Watson FS, Renlund DG, O'Connell JB: Acute vascular rejection involving the major coronary arteries of a cardiac allograft. J Heart Transplant 1988; 7:191–197.

295. Zales VR, Crawford S, Backer CL, Lynch P, Benson DW Jr, Mavroudis C: Spectrum of humoral rejection after pediatric heart transplantation. J Heart Lung Transplant 1993;12:563–572.

296. Zales VR, Wright KL, Muster AJ, Backer CL, Benson DW, Mavroudis C: Ventricular volume growth after cardiac transplantation in infants and children. Circulation 1992;86:II-272–II-275.

297. Zales VR, Wright KL, Paul E, Becke CL, Mavroudis C, Muster AJ, Benson DW Jr: Normal left ventricular muscle mass and mass/volume ratio after pediatric cardiac transplantation. Circulation 1994;90:61–65.

298. Zangwill SD, Hsu DT, Kichuk MR, Garvin JH, Stolar CJH, Haddad J Jr, Stylianos S, Michler RE, Chadburn A, Knowles DM, Addonizio LJ: Incidence and outcome of primary Epstein-Barr virus infection and lymphoproliferative disease in pediatric heart transplant recipients. J Heart Lung Transplant 1998;17:1161–1166.

299. Zhu W, Zou Y, Aikawa R, Harada K, Kudoh S, Uozumi H, Hayashi D, Gu Y, Yamazaki T, Nagai R, Yazaki Y, Komuro I: MAPK superfamily plays an important role in daunomycin-induced apoptosis of cardiac myocytes. Circulation 1999; 100:2100–2107.

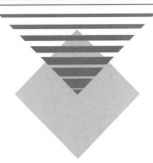

CHAPTER TWENTY-ONE

Combined Heart and Other Organ Transplantation

It was inevitable with the progressive improvement in the results of cardiac transplantation that transplantation of other organs together with the heart would eventually be considered. Numerically, the most important combined transplant is heart/lung transplantation. However, other combined transplants have been performed such as heart/kidney, heart/liver, and heart/lung/liver. This chapter will consider additional aspects involved in cardiac transplantation combined with other organs.

HISTORICAL BACKGROUND

Transplantation of the heart and lungs for end-stage lung disease with and without heart disease was a natural extension of cardiac transplantation. A number of separate threads of investigation converged to culminate in the successful application of heart/lung transplantation. As discussed in Chapter 1, the investigation of heart/lung transplantation in an experimental model can be traced back to the work of Carrel,[53] in which the heart/lung block was transplanted into the neck of the recipient animal. The work of Demikhov[75] was notable for his performance of an orthotopic heart/lung transplant in an experimental model using a technique not requiring cardiopulmonary bypass. Not surprisingly, there were only a few survivors of the many attempts, but the experiment at least proved that the concept was realistic. The next era of experimental investigation into heart/lung transplantation employed either hypothermia while the anastomoses were being completed[249] or the use of cardiopulmonary bypass, which was reported by Webb in 1957.[383, 384] A number of other investigators, including Lower,[118, 219] Longmire,[213] and Blanco,[40] carried out experiments involving a canine model of heart/lung transplantation, and each investigator observed substantial embarrassment of posttransplant ventilation manifesting either as failure to recover spontaneous respiration or an increased tidal volume but a markedly diminished respiratory rate and episodes of apnea. Lower's experiments involving heart/lung transplantation in dogs[219] also raised concern regarding the adequacy of posttransplant ventilatory mechanics, since all dogs died several days after the operation from pulmonary failure. This raised the very legitimate concern that cardiopulmonary transplantation might never be possible, presumably due to pulmonary denervation and loss of the Hering-Breuer reflex[44] (see Box). This view was supported by findings of similarly disturbed pulmonary ventilation after isolated denervation of the lungs,[23] and reinforced by the finding of inadequate ventilation fol-

Hering-Breuer Reflex

The Hering-Breuer inflation reflex has been widely studied in animals, in particular the cat and dog, but its role in human respiratory physiology is not certain. Stretch receptors which are myelinated nerve endings found in the smooth muscle of the conducting airways, respond to stretch by inhibiting sustained inspiration and prolonging expiratory time.[29] Rapid lung inflation inhibits inspiratory discharge from the respiratory center. In patients undergoing heart/lung transplantation the Hering-Breuer reflex is absent as demonstrated by a lack of expiratory prolongation with lung inflation. This is a test of vagal afferent traffic which is one of the limbs of the Hering-Breuer inflation reflex.[153]

lowing single-lung transplantation in the dog with either immediate contralateral pulmonary artery ligation[48] or contralateral pneumonectomy.[85] Furthermore, transplantation of the heart and one lung, leaving a native lung in place as a source of afferent stimuli for the respiratory center resulted in normal respiratory mechanics. When canine bilateral lung denervation or bilateral lung transplantation was done sequentially with an interval of 2–12 months between each side, surviving animals had normal respiratory mechanics,[203, 338, 339] although this was not a consistent finding.[10] Lung reinnervation could be demonstrated, but it was not accompanied by return of the Hering-Breuer reflex.[91] This suggested that other mechanisms were involved in the adaptive process of long-term surviving animals.

The serious disturbance of respiratory mechanics after heart/lung or bilateral lung transplantation in dogs appeared to be a major conceptual stumbling block for heart/lung transplantation until it was realized that in primates the Hering-Breuer reflex was not essential for normal respiratory mechanics.[54, 121, 247] The first clinical heart/lung transplant was performed by Cooley in 1968 in an infant with complete atrioventricular septal defect and pulmonary hypertension, but the patient died early postoperatively.[63] The second heart/lung transplant was performed by Lillehei in 1969. The patient died 8 days after the procedure, but breathed spontaneously from the third day.[206] The third heart/lung transplant was performed by Barnard[215] in 1971. This patient also breathed spontaneously and appeared to have good respiratory mechanics, but he died 23 days after the operation following a right pneumonectomy for a necrotic right donor bronchus (bilateral bronchial rather than a tracheal anastomosis was performed).

The history of heart/lung transplantation and lung transplantation are really intertwined. At the same time that the early experience in heart/lung transplantation was underway, clinical lung transplantation was making its first steps, but it was notable for its lack of success.[393] However, the successful heart/lung transplant by Reitz in 1981[301] restored enthusiasm for not only heart/lung transplantation but also for lung transplantation. Reitz's success was attributable to careful

and thorough preliminary experimental work in primates[299] and the use of cyclosporine as the primary immunosuppressive agent.

INDICATIONS FOR HEART/LUNG TRANSPLANTATION

The current indications for heart/lung transplantation are (1) Eisenmenger's syndrome with an uncorrected intracardiac defect, (2) uncorrectable congenital heart disease with atresia or diffuse severe hypoplasia of the pulmonary arteries and progressive heart failure, (3) coexistent severe cardiopulmonary disease with advanced heart or lung failure, and (4) primary and secondary pulmonary hypertension.

The medium and long-term results of lung transplantation (either single or bilateral) for diseases such as emphysema,[354, 356] idiopathic pulmonary fibrosis,[86] and suppurative lung diseases including cystic fibrosis[28] are as good and frequently superior to those of heart/lung transplantation.[11, 74, 76, 191] Therefore, heart/lung transplantation is not ordinarily indicated for these conditions in the absence of coexistent heart disease. The argument for bilateral sequential lung transplantation as opposed to heart/lung transplantation for primary lung disease includes the absence of the problem of coronary vasculopathy, a much lower incidence of serious bleeding and return to the operating room for control of bleeding, and the fact that the vagus nerves may be at a less risk of injury. However, it should be recognized that heart/lung transplantation continues to be used in some centers primarily for diseases such as cystic fibrosis because of an established record of good results with this technique. Centers that primarily use heart/lung transplantation for end-stage suppurative lung disease frequently maintain that heart/lung transplantation has certain advantages over bilateral sequential lung transplantation, since there is only one airway anastomosis required with the known lower likelihood of airway complications. Consequently, the use of heart/lung transplantation or double lung transplantation for, in particular, end-stage suppurative lung disease is at the discretion of the transplant center and there appears to be no compelling argument for one procedure or the other with the caveat that the heart from a heart/lung recipient is available as a domino-donor heart, invalidating the argument of wastage of the donor heart when heart/lung transplantation is used. Potential advantages of using the domino-donor heart when heart/lung transplantation is used is that the donor right ventricle has been potentially conditioned by elevated pulmonary vascular resistance and the heart from the recipient has not been subjected to the hostile environment of brain death.

Eisenmenger's Syndrome

Eisenmenger's syndrome is characterized by excessive muscularization of the pulmonary vasculature, resulting in marked irreversible elevation of pulmonary vascular resistance and reversal of a previously left-to-right shunt at the atrial, ventricular, or aortopulmonary level resulting in right-to-left shunting and cyanosis.

A distinction has been made in patients with Eisenmenger's syndrome between those with the nonrestrictive shunt at the atrial level (pretricuspid defect) and those with shunts below the tricuspid valve (posttricuspid defect). In patients with **nonrestrictive atrial defects,** following the maturation of the pulmonary circulation the pulmonary pressure falls to normal levels and when a significant left-to-right shunt develops (dictated by the relative compliance of the left and right ventricle), the pulmonary bed accommodates the shunt relatively easily. When patients with an atrial septal defect (ASD) develop the Eisenmenger response, the effect of the resultant pulmonary hypertension on right ventricular function is similar to that of primary pulmonary hypertension, with right ventricular dilatation and progressively worsening right ventricular contractility.[144, 396] In contrast, patients with **nonrestrictive posttricuspid defects** (such as ventricular septal defects) continue to have systemic right ventricular pressure after the neonatal period, and following the development of the Eisenmenger response, right ventricular function is usually preserved.[143, 145]

The **natural history** of Eisenmenger's syndrome has not been characterized well enough to allow transplant physicians to be entirely confident about the timing of listing for heart/lung transplantation. However, there are some clues to help make this decision. The study by Hopkins and colleagues[143] did find that in the short-term, patients with Eisenmenger's syndrome had superior survival to those with primary pulmonary hypertension (Fig. 21–1). Furthermore, the survival of patients with Eisenmenger's syndrome due to an ASD was no worse than that of patients with posttricuspid defects

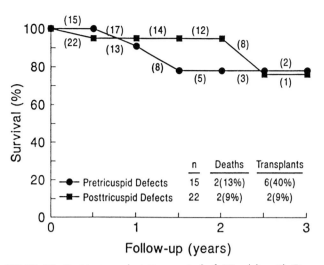

FIGURE **21-2.** Nontransplantation survival of 37 adults with Eisenmenger's syndrome. The group has been divided into those with pretricuspid defects and those with posttricuspid defects. The number of patients followed is shown for each follow-up interval. (From Hopkins WE, Ochoa LL, Richardson GW, Trulock EP: Medical management of heart failure and candidate selection: comparison of the hemodynamics and survival of adults with severe primary pulmonary hypertension or Eisenmenger syndrome. J Heart Lung Transplant 1996;15:100–105.)

(Fig. 21–2) despite the potentially greater right ventricular dysfunction associated with Eisenmenger's syndrome due to an ASD. This information needs to be interpreted with some caution, since in both Figures 21–1 and 21–2 patients were censored at the time of transplantation, and it is highly likely that this information is biased by informative censoring (see Chapter 3). In this study, none of the patients with Eisenmenger's syndrome had evidence of congestive heart failure either on physical examination or by hemodynamic measurements. The joint study on the Natural History of Congenital Heart Defects[182, 385] demonstrated a 25-year survival of 42%, most of these patients being enrolled before the age of 12 years, although from the information provided actuarial survival cannot be calculated.

In the absence of rigorously determined risk factors for death, it would appear then that the time course of deterioration in this condition is relatively slow and so the **timing of listing** for heart/lung transplantation is based on worsening cyanosis, the development of right ventricular failure (particularly when marked ascites and peripheral edema occur), right ventricular failure that is unresponsive to diuretic therapy, worsening oxygen saturation (particularly once it reaches 60% on exercise), and/or progressive symptoms of fatigue and breathlessness (particularly when associated with worsening polycythemia, especially if repeated phlebotomies are required).

Standard **therapy to prolong survival** prior to transplantation includes prevention of pregnancy, endocarditis prophylaxis, influenza vaccination, and avoiding dehydration.[143] There does not appear to be a role for prostacyclin infusion therapy in patients with Eisenmenger's syndrome.

An alternative to heart/lung transplantation is correction of the intracardiac defect associated with single-

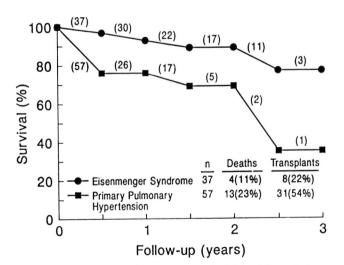

FIGURE **21-1.** Nontransplantation survival of 94 adults with Eisenmenger's syndrome or severe primary pulmonary hypertension. The number of patients followed is shown for each follow-up interval. It is important to note that patients were censored at time of transplantation, so this does not equate to a "natural history" study. (From Hopkins WE, Ochoa LL, Richardson GW, Trulock EP: Medical management of heart failure and candidate selection: comparison of the hemodynamics and survival of adults with severe primary pulmonary hypertension or Eisenmenger syndrome. J Heart Lung Transplant 1996;15:100–105.)

lung transplantation,[102, 220, 226, 349] although the intermediate-term results appear to be inferior to those of heart/lung transplantation[220] and currently it would not be considered the choice of therapy. However, there may be certain circumstances dictated by the anatomy or previous surgery where this option, although not ideal, may merit consideration.

Congenital Heart Disease with Atresia or Hypoplasia of the Pulmonary Arteries

Heart/lung transplantation is indicated in patients with progressive heart failure who have uncorrectable congenital heart disease and poor ventricular function with or without a previous cardiac procedure who have atresia or diffuse hypoplasia of the pulmonary arteries such that it is not feasible to make a connection between a donor pulmonary artery and the native pulmonary circulation. Under these unusual circumstances, however, even heart/lung transplantation may not be possible with a reasonable likelihood of success because of multiple previous shunt procedures.

Combined Cardiac and Pulmonary Disease

There are two circumstances under which heart/lung transplantation may be considered because of combined cardiopulmonary disease: (1) patients with end-stage heart disease and concomitant lung disease too severe for heart transplantation only, and (2) patients with end-stage lung disease with concomitant heart disease severe enough to preclude lung transplantation only. In the first instance, the indications for transplantation are dictated by the severity of the heart disease, and the decision to perform heart/lung transplantation versus cardiac transplantation alone will be determined by the severity of the lung disease, its natural history, and the likelihood of morbidity associated with retention of the native lungs (e.g., in patients with septic lung disease). No specific guidelines for this decision are currently available.

The more common situation would be patients with end-stage lung disease with concomitant heart disease, there being two groups of patients, one with heart disease secondary to pulmonary disease and a second group with unrelated cardiac disease. In the first group, the usual situation is a patient with end-stage parenchymal lung disease with severe right ventricular dysfunction due to pulmonary hypertension. This is quite uncommon except for primary pulmonary hypertension (see below). For diseases other than primary pulmonary hypertension, recovery of the severely dysfunctional right ventricle after single- or double-lung transplantation is not completely secure, and in this situation the choice of heart/lung transplantation or lung transplantation would be equally acceptable.

The most likely combination of unrelated pulmonary and cardiac disease is smoking-related emphysema and coronary artery disease. The timing of listing of patients with smoking-related emphysema for lung transplantation may be difficult because of the relatively slow progression of the disease. Transplantation should be con-

sidered when patients have marked limitations in activities of daily living, and the presence of any of the following are associated with poor survival: Forced expiratory volume in 1 second (FEV_1) below 30% of predicted (expected 3-year survival is 50–70%),[13] hypercapnia, PO_2 at rest less than 60 mm Hg, weight loss, life-threatening exacerbations (including mechanical ventilation), and accelerating decline both symptomatically and objectively. The decision to select heart/lung transplantation over single- or double-lung transplantation depends on the extensiveness of the coronary artery disease and presence of left ventricular dysfunction. The presence of more than mild left ventricular dysfunction and coronary artery disease that is not manageable by percutaneous transluminal coronary angioplasty is a contraindication to lung transplantation. Thus, under those circumstances, heart/lung transplantation is the preferable option.

Primary and Secondary Pulmonary Hypertension

There are three major pathological groups to consider:

1. Primary pulmonary hypertension.
2. Secondary pulmonary hypertension.
3. Pulmonary hypertension following a previously repaired congenital heart defect.

Available evidence suggests that for primary or secondary pulmonary hypertension, survival after bilateral lung transplantation is no different from that of heart/lung transplantation[24, 57] (Fig. 21–3). Consequently, the trend is now to use lung transplantation for these conditions, particularly since the donor heart would then become available for isolated heart transplant in another patient.

The area of controversy, however, is the choice of procedure for patients with primary or secondary pulmonary hypertension who have **severe right ventricular dysfunction.** The changes in the right ventricle with chronic pressure load include right ventricular hypertrophy, right ventricular dilatation, right ventricular systolic dysfunction, and displacement of the ventricular septum towards the left side creating a "D"-shaped left ventricle when viewed echocardiographically in the short axis. This abnormal left ventricular geometry directly impacts on left ventricular filling and stroke volume.[389] It is currently not possible to determine how much of the right ventricular dysfunction is due to afterload mismatch (which is reversible), and how much is the result of irreversible damage, and hence determine the likelihood of improvement in right ventricular function after transplantation. However, it has been clearly demonstrated that the relief of right ventricular afterload by single- or double-lung transplantation results in an immediate reduction in right ventricular size and a substantial improvement in right ventricular function in most patients in this category.[52, 166, 191, 273, 304, 325, 401] This improvement is sustained 3 months after transplantation[274] (Fig. 21–4). Furthermore, the left ventricular geometry is normalized by reversal of the leftward

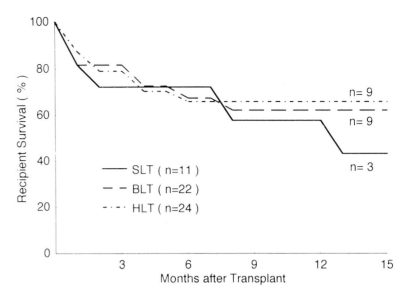

FIGURE 21-3. Actuarial survival of patients undergoing single-lung transplant (SLT), bilateral lung transplant (BLT), or heart/lung transplant (HLT) for primary or secondary pulmonary hypertension. (From Bando K, Armitage JM, Paradis IL, Keenan RJ, Hardesty RL, Konishi H, Komatsu K, Shah AN, Bahnson HT: Indications for and results of single, bilateral, and heart-lung transplantation for pulmonary hypertension. J Thorac Cardiovasc Surg 1994;108:1056–1065.)

displacement of the ventricular septum, resulting in improved ventricular filling through the amelioration of left ventricular diastolic dysfunction[201, 218] and improvement in left ventricular systolic function.[191] This same degree of improvement in right ventricular structure and function can also be seen in patients after thromboendarterectomy for pulmonary embolic disease[81] and is also similar to the remodeling of the right ventricle which is seen after cardiac transplantation in patients with secondary pulmonary hypertension.[34] However, this improvement in right ventricular structure and function is not universal[166] and hence the lower limit of right ventricular dysfunction which is still acceptable for lung transplantation is unknown and difficult to ascertain because of the inability to currently distinguish between afterload mismatch and fixed morphologic damage. It has been recommended that patients with a right ventricular ejection fraction of less than 0.2 should not be considered for lung transplantation. The current policy at the University of Alabama at Birmingham

(UAB) is to offer lung transplantation to patients with primary or secondary pulmonary hypertension irrespective of the degree of right ventricular dysfunction. Consequently, heart/lung transplantation in patients with primary or secondary pulmonary hypertension should probably be reserved for the few patients with associated significant left ventricular dysfunction.

SELECTION CRITERIA FOR HEART/LUNG TRANSPLANTATION

All of the general guidelines for listing for heart/lung transplantation are similar to those for isolated heart transplantation and are discussed in Chapter 6. It needs to be recognized that the natural history of conditions requiring heart/lung transplantation is not entirely predictable, and heart/lung donors are uncommon, particularly in the United States, resulting in a long waiting time. In order to have a high likelihood of success, heart/lung transplantation should not be performed as a procedure of desperation in patients whose physical and nutritional reserves have been unduly depleted. Several of the selection criteria are unique to heart/lung transplantation and require specific mention.

Age

Although the usual considerations of biological age versus chronological age must enter into the decision, 60 years is usually considered the upper age limit for heart/lung transplantation, in part due to the magnitude of the operation and the putative risks that accompany older age and in part due to the philosophical concerns of allocating organs to one patient when potentially three could benefit. A relationship between death after heart/lung transplantation and older age has not been formally demonstrated.

Previous Thoracic Surgery

Because postoperative bleeding has been such an important cause of mortality and morbidity after heart/lung

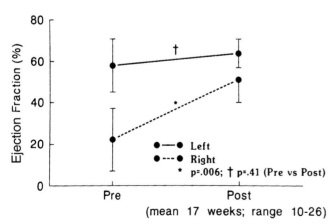

FIGURE 21-4. Changes in right ventricular ejection fraction measured by radionuclide ventriculography after single-lung transplantation for pulmonary hypertension (n = 7). (From Pasque MK, Trulock EP, Kaiser LR, Cooper JD: Single lung transplantation for pulmonary hypertension: three month hemodynamic follow-up. Circulation 1991;84:2275–2279.)

transplantation, and a major contributing factor to problems such as infection,[114, 315, 359] previous thoracic surgery has been regarded by some centers as a contraindication to heart/lung transplantation. The increased risk associated with prior operations (particularly thoracotomies) relates to two factors: first, the destabilizing effects of ongoing bleeding and significant transfusion requirement following transplantation; and second, the increased likelihood of damage to the phrenic nerve (with the subsequent deleterious effects on postoperative ventriculatory function) when visualization of the phrenic nerve is obscured by adhesions. However, with increasing experience and the use of such strategies as bilateral anterolateral transsternal thoracotomy (clam shell incision), argon beam coagulator, and perioperative high-dose antifibrinolytic therapy (ε-aminocaproic acid) and aprotonin, the risks of bleeding from vascular pleural and mediastinal adhesions and the subsequent coagulopathy should be reduced.[315] The use of heart and unilateral lung transplantation[167] has been reported as a method to avoid dissection in a particularly troublesome pleural space from previous surgery.

All prior thoracic surgical procedures do not carry the same risk of bleeding. For example, previous closure of an atrial septal defect through a sternotomy incision should not pose any particular difficulties for heart/lung transplantation. However, prior bilateral systemic pulmonary shunts in a patient with pulmonary atresia and multiple aortopulmonary collaterals is an entirely different proposition and the risk of heart/lung transplantation may be prohibitively high. Therefore, previous thoracic surgery should currently be regarded as a relative contraindication and the decision made on an individual patient basis.

Our policy at UAB is to consider patients for heart/lung transplantation who have prior sternotomies and/or thoracotomies if the patient is otherwise well preserved without nonthoracic organ dysfunction, is highly motivated, and is under 50 years of age.

Current Corticosteroid Therapy

Use of corticosteroid therapy at the time of heart/lung transplantation has been regarded as a contributing factor to poor tracheal anastomotic healing and subsequent dehiscence. Corticosteroids do clearly interfere with healing of the bronchus experimentally, and steroid use at the time of clinical lung and heart/lung transplantation has always been a major concern, but evidence from experimental lung transplantation[16] and clinical lung transplantation[236] does suggest that the importance of impaired bronchial healing by concurrent steroids may not be as significant as once thought. The satisfactory healing of the tracheal anastomosis in patients undergoing heart/lung transplantation with concurrent corticosteroid therapy[258] is further evidence that patients receiving corticosteroid therapy (prednisone of 20 mg/day or less) can safely undergo heart/lung transplantation.

EVALUATION FOR HEART/LUNG TRANSPLANTATION

The same evaluation process that is used for heart transplantation (as outlined in Chapter 6) is required for patients being considered for heart/lung transplantation. For patients with Eisenmenger's syndrome, it may be advisable, depending on the congenital malformation, to perform thoracic aortography to define aortopulmonary collaterals and to determine shunt patency, which, if present, must be controlled during the early phases of cardiopulmonary bypass. Patients with primary lung parenchymal disease will require, in addition to the evaluation process for their heart disease, assessment of their lung disease which would include comprehensive pulmonary function tests, computerized tomography (CT) scan of the chest (in ex-smokers with chronic obstructive lung disease), and evaluation of their exercise capacity through a 6-minute walk test.

For patients with pulmonary hypertension, hepatic function requires close scrutiny, since hyperbilirubinemia (particularly when it is >2.5 mg/dL) is a risk factor for death after heart/lung transplantation due in particular to bleeding and other consequences of hepatic dysfunction.[189] This no doubt reflects hepatic congestion and in time its progression to cardiac cirrhosis.

Heart/Lung Donor Evaluation

Unfortunately, only approximately 25% of organ donors have lungs that are usable for lung or heart/lung transplantation. This reflects the vulnerability of lungs in organ donors to a number of factors: concomitant lung injury (in the case of traumatic brain death), aspiration, prolonged ventilation, and neurogenic pulmonary edema as a consequence of brain death. The assessment of the heart/lung donor follows the same screening and assessment protocols as outlined in Chapter 9 except for the additional requirements to evaluate the lungs.

Donor History

Trauma, such as a motor vehicle accident as a cause of brain death, raises the possibility of lung injury due to contusion. A smoking history should not contraindicate use of the lungs, but the conventional criterion is less than a 20-pack-year history. A history of aspiration following the injury does contraindicate the use of the lungs. The heavy use of marijuana for many years by a potential heart/lung donor is not currently thought to be deleterious to lung function, although it perhaps should be considered as a marker for other high-risk activity which would contraindicate use of the heart/lung block.

Donor Age

An upper age limit for donor lungs for either lung transplantation or heart/lung transplantation has not been defined, but just as with donor heart criteria, age appears to interact with other variables such as ischemic time. In at least one study in lung transplantation, graft ischemic time was not itself identified as a risk factor for early death, but the interaction between older donor age and longer ischemic time was a significant predictor of 1-year mortality after lung transplantation[256] (Fig. 21–5). Although this information is obtained solely from a lung transplant experience, the important interaction of in-

1 Year Recipient Mortality

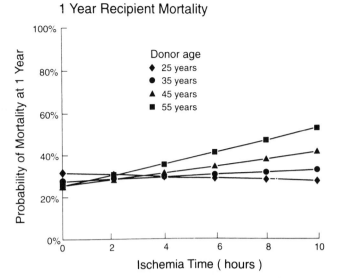

FIGURE **21-5.** Interaction between donor age, lung graft ischemia time, and probability of 1-year posttransplant mortality, according to data from the United Network of Organ Sharing. (From Novick RJ, Bennett LE, Meyer DM, Hosenpud JD: Influence of graft ischemic time and donor age on survival after lung transplantation. J Heart Lung Transplant 1999;18:425–431.)

creasing donor age and ischemic time is of clear relevance to heart/lung transplantation.

Donor Lung Function

A number of criteria for donor lung function have been established for both lung transplantation and heart/lung transplantation. By convention, acceptable gas exchange is indicated by a PaO_2 of 300 mm Hg or greater on a ventilatory setting of 5 cm of positive end-expiratory pressure (PEEP) with an FiO_2 of 1.0 for 5 minutes (oxygen challenge). There should be normal lung compliance with a peak airway of pressure of less than 30 mm Hg on the usual tidal volume settings.

In lung transplantation, in response to the increasing disparity between the number of patients requiring lung transplantation and the number of donor lungs available, donor lung criteria are being progressively liberalized, giving rise to the term "marginal donor." Donor criteria for lung transplantation have been liberalized by accepting lungs with radiologic evidence of contusion or an infiltrate, an oxygen challenge with a PO_2 of less than 300 mm Hg, and age older than 55 years. The use of these "marginal" donor lungs for single- or double-lung transplantation has not appeared to compromise survival. However, in heart/lung transplantation, the safety of using "marginal" donor lungs has not been satisfactorily demonstrated, although accepting donors up to the age of 60 years, with a smoking history, PO_2 of 100 mm Hg with an FiO_2 of 0.40, and a small pulmonary infiltrate appears to have been a safe extension of criteria in heart/lung transplantation.[335] However, given the fact that heart/lung transplantation frequently involves considerable bleeding, the administration of large amounts of blood and blood products and frequently prolonged cardiopulmonary bypass, it seems inadvisable to use donor lungs with anything more than relatively minor

deviations from currently accepted donor lung criteria to avoid important early graft dysfunction.

The classic lung donor criteria (for both lung and heart/lung transplantation) specify that there should not be any evidence of purulent secretions either by suction or on bronchoscopy. From a practical standpoint for both lung and heart/lung transplantation, this criterion is probably unrealistic. The majority of organ donors, particularly if they have been ventilated for more than 48 hours, will have purulent secretions and abundant white cells, and gram-negative organisms may be seen on the Gram stain of the sputum. This should not contraindicate use of the lungs. However, if on bronchoscopic inspection of the airway there is pus in all the segmental bronchi which continues to appear despite suctioning, these lungs should not be used. Evidence of aspiration should contraindicate use of the lungs, which should be suspected by history and tracheobronchial mucosal inflammation on bronchoscopic inspection. A polymicrobial sputum culture result is often used as *prima facie* evidence of aspiration, but this is at variance with the known unreliability of sputum cultures. Consequently, the diagnosis of aspiration should not rest solely on a sputum Gram stain, but must be supported by bronchoscopic findings. In the unlikely event of finding fungi in the sputum, lung donation is probably contraindicated.

Because of the vulnerability of donor lungs to injury, it is important that the oxygen challenge be repeated frequently up until the time of procurement (every 2–3 hours), and a final oxygen challenge should be performed just prior to procurement either in the intensive care unit or in the operating room. If there is any doubt about the suitability of the lungs or there has been a delay in commencing the procurement operation, repeating the chest x-ray just prior to moving the donor to the operating room may detect pulmonary infiltrates due to edema or infection that have not yet manifested on the oxygen challenge. The final assessment of the lungs for suitability for transplantation is made in the operating room by the procuring surgeon. The lungs should be palpated carefully and areas of firmness indicating either edema or infection should preclude use of the lungs for heart/lung transplantation.

There is currently interest in using lungs from non–heart-beating donors in an attempt to overcome the critical shortage of donor lungs for both lung and heart/lung transplantation. Experimental models of donor lungs undergoing periods of warm ischemia prior to blood perfusion[224] or transplantation in a recipient animal[88] have demonstrated satisfactory function in terms of gas exchange and pulmonary vascular resistance. The deleterious effects of warm ischemia of the donor lung with respect to catabolism of high-energy phosphates appears to be ameliorated by ventilation and cold crystalloid pulmonary flush.[376] However, there is an enormous gap to be bridged between these experimental models and the clinical reality of non–heart-beating donors for heart/lung transplantation, particularly when sobering experiments have demonstrated the highly deleterious effects of hypotension prior to warm ischemia on lung viability,[368] these experiments probably more accurately reflecting the clinical reality.

Donor/Recipient Matching

Donor/recipient matching for the cardiac portion of heart/lung transplantation is the same as for cardiac transplantation (see Chapter 9). Donor/recipient **lung size** matching needs to be separately considered. Patients undergoing heart/lung transplantation will usually have essentially normal thoracic volumes, the only exception being the unusual situation of heart/lung transplantation for patients with emphysema who have markedly increased thoracic volumes and the rare patient undergoing heart/lung transplantation for pulmonary fibrosis who will have smaller than normal thoracic volumes. Undersizing or oversizing of lungs for heart/lung transplantation can be accommodated to some extent by diaphragmatic movement, but significant undersizing will increase the risk of pleural space problems and significant oversizing may result in areas of pulmonary collapse predisposing to infection and compromise of venous return when the chest is closed. Numerous methods have been used to estimate the match between donor and recipient lung volumes, including height, weight, chest circumference, thoracic measurements on the chest x-ray, and matching the donor and recipient based on the predicted lung volume using a formula incorporating height, weight, sex, and age.[176]

Predicted Total Lung Capacity (L):

Male = (0.094 × height in cm)–(0.015 × age in years)–9.167

Female = (0.079 × height in cm)–(0.008 × age in years)–7.49

For most patients undergoing heart/lung transplantation who will have essentially normal thoracic volumes, a small amount of undersizing or oversizing (approximately 10–20% based on arteroposterior chest dimension and/or side–side chest dimensions) will be accommodated without difficulty, although considerable oversizing (up to 180% of predicted donor total lung capacity compared with actual recipient total lung capacity) has been reported with apparent adaptation of the lungs.[211] In the most unusual circumstance of a patient with smoking-related emphysema or α_1-antitrypsin deficiency emphysema undergoing heart/lung transplantation, considerable oversizing can be accommodated. When unacceptable oversizing appears to have occurred, some form of pneumoreduction can be used by either lung stapling[252] or an anatomical lung resection.[87]

Ischemic Time

Just as in heart transplantation (see Chapter 9), the ischemic time of the lungs is not a variable that should be viewed in isolation from other important factors such as donor lung function, projected duration of cardiopulmonary bypass time which is predicated upon the technical difficulty of the procedure, and the likely administration of large amounts of blood products in a patient with previous thoracic surgery. The relationship between increasing lung ischemic time and subsequent death has not been as rigorously studied as cardiac ischemic time, and the upper limit of safe lung ischemia is not known. A number of reports in lung transplantation have demonstrated that, within the limits of clinical lung transplantation, graft ischemic time alone is not a risk factor for early death after lung transplantation[109, 193, 256, 347, 394] (although as previously mentioned there is an important relationship between longer ischemic time and older donor age). Furthermore, perhaps somewhat surprisingly, the incidence of diffuse alveolar damage diagnosed by autopsy or biopsy specimens in patients undergoing clinical lung transplantation was no different, with ischemic times of less than 4 hours, or greater than 6 hours and there was no impact of ischemic times up to 9 hours on early graft function or survival.[106] However, a study by Snell and colleagues[346] in patients undergoing heart/lung and lung transplantation suggested that when using a single flush of Euro-Collins solution with prostacyclin and cold storage, lung ischemic time beyond 5 hours substantially increased mortality. At UAB, ischemic times of up to 6 hours on the second lung of a bilateral sequential lung transplant have been tolerated satisfactorily. There are some anecdotal reports of lung ischemic times out to 9 hours using a single flush method with satisfactory function, but for heart/lung transplantation it would seem that the current prudent limit of ischemia is probably up to 6 hours.

HEART/LUNG DONOR MANAGEMENT

The management of the cardiac donor is outlined in Chapter 9 and the management protocols are entirely applicable to the heart/lung donor. However, the vulnerability of the lungs to injury requires emphasis, and it is only by meticulous airway toilet and avoidance of excessive volume infusion that donor lung injury can be avoided. Based on the sputum Gram stain, a broad-spectrum antibiotic coverage, particularly to include gram-negative bacilli, is advisable. If radiological evidence of pulmonary edema does develop, this can usually be cleared with diuresis and minimization of volume infusion. Failure to clear should contraindicate the use of the lungs and may, in fact, represent the earliest manifestation of pulmonary infection.

LUNG PRESERVATION FOR HEART/LUNG TRANSPLANTATION

The goal of lung preservation in heart/lung transplantation, as in lung transplantation, is to maintain the physiological and biochemical integrity of the pulmonary graft during the period of time that the heart/lung block is transported and implanted into the recipient and to ensure satisfactory pulmonary graft function. As in heart transplantation, the pulmonary graft is required to function immediately, and a dysfunctional pulmonary graft can potentially have an important impact on mortality and morbidity after heart/lung transplantation. Clearly, the goals of lung preservation are not being fully met in clinical heart/lung transplantation, because of the small but important incidence of severe pulmonary graft dysfunction due to ischemia-reperfusion injury. Conversely, the current methods of lung preservation have contributed significantly to the success of heart/lung and lung transplantation by providing safe ischemic times up to approximately 6–7 hours, thus allowing long-distance heart/lung block procurement rather than transferring the donor to the transplant hospital[157] (as practiced in an earlier era of heart/lung transplantation).

Lung Metabolism

The metabolic requirements of lung tissue are met by intermediary metabolic pathways resulting in the generation of adenosine triphosphate (ATP), which is achieved by the utilization of oxygen through the mitochondrial cytochrome oxidase system, the major source of carbon being glucose. The lung as a whole utilizes approximately 25–50% less oxygen than metabolically active organs such as the brain cortex, cardiac muscle, liver, or renal cortex.[98] Other substrates can be used by the lung including fatty acids, lactate, glycerol, and fructose, but make a small contribution to the total carbon pool for lung intermediary metabolism.[98]

Ischemic-Reperfusion Injury of the Donor Lung

The process that underpins impaired pulmonary graft function after heart/lung transplantation is ischemic-reperfusion injury. Ischemic-reperfusion injury of the lung may manifest by abnormalities in a number of physiological measurements including gas exchange, pulmonary vascular resistance, airway resistance, and lung compliance, but arterial oxygenation is the most frequently used index of pulmonary graft function; **hypoxemia** is an invariable accompaniment of ischemic-reperfusion injury, most likely secondary to ventilation-perfusion inequality (or shunt).

Manifestations of ischemic-reperfusion injury are the result of a complex interplay between a number of processes including endothelial injury, production of oxygen-derived free radicals, cytokine release, leukocyte adherence and activation, complement cascade activation, and surfactant depletion.[377] As discussed in Chapter 9, the **vascular endothelium** is a highly active paracrine structure, and its vasomotor response to ischemia is an important determinant of the severity of reperfusion injury. The loss of vasomotor control on reperfusion of the pulmonary vessels is not simply a matter of an endothelial injury (damage to the nitric oxide [NO]-dependent vasoregulatory control mechanisms and endothelin receptor activity), but a more complex picture which includes the influx of leukocytes and the action of cytokines during reperfusion. All of these processes result in an increase in permeability of the endothelial-epithelial barrier, leading to pulmonary edema and an increase in pulmonary vascular resistance. Following reperfusion, generation of oxygen-derived free radicals, including superoxide, hydroxyl radical, and hydrogen peroxide, occurs quite rapidly through the xanthine oxidase pathway (particularly in the endothelial and alveo-

lar type II cells), iron catalyzed reactions, and adherent neutrophils. Unless there is a robust scavenger system in place there will be extensive protein degradation and lipid peroxidation in the endothelial cells, DNA strand breakage preventing synthesis of proteins required for cellular repair, and loss of cellular integrity.

Complement activation through the alternate pathway likely contributes to reperfusion injury by endothelial injury and increased permeability. **Leukocyte** adherence and activation is not only a part of ischemic reperfusion injury, but leukocyte trafficking is part of the processes of specific immune recognition and graft rejection (see Chapter 2). A number of **cytokines** are involved in the promotion of ischemic reperfusion injury in the lung, including tumor necrosis factor (TNF), interleukin (IL)-1, IL-8, and interferon-γ (IFN-γ). Platelet-activating factor (PAF) is a proinflammatory glycerophospholipid induced by the action of phosopholipase A_2 (from either leukocytes or endothelial cells), this activation occurring due to oxygen-derived free radicals, TNF, as well as other stimuli.[202, 378] There is clear alteration in both the function and composition of **surfactant** after hypothermic pulmonary preservation, but the role of surfactant depletion is uncertain.

Strategies for Pulmonary Preservation

A number of techniques have been used for preservation of the lungs for lung transplantation and heart/lung transplantation. Hypothermic immersion was a technique used in the early Toronto lung transplant experience,[366] although this method is no longer employed. The autoperfusing working heart/lung preparation has been a useful experimental model that has actually been used for clinical heart/lung transplantation.[127] However, autoperfusion has not provided the prolonged preservation that was anticipated and is a complicated technique that is no longer used. Donor core-cooling using a portable heart/lung machine involves cannulation of the donor ascending aorta and right atrium and cooling of the donor to approximately 10°C. This technique has proven to be an effective means of preserving donor lungs for heart/lung transplantation[126, 399] but does have the considerable disadvantage of lack of simplicity. The single flush-perfusion method with cold static storage, now the most widely practiced method of lung preservation, following from its use in renal, liver, and cardiac transplantation, was introduced for distant procurement in clinical heart/lung transplantation by the Stanford group.[22]

The use of **single flush perfusion** is clearly the most convenient method of lung preservation. There is a rapidly expanding literature on the subject of lung preservation using a number of experimental models, but this information has not yet translated into a clearly superior clinical strategy for lung and heart/lung transplantation. As in heart preservation (see Chapter 9), solutions for lung preservation can be grouped into either intracellular solutions, such as University of Wisconsin (UW) solution and Euro-Collins solution, or extracellular solutions such as low potassium-dextran solution (LPD) and Wallwork (which is a blood-based solution). ET-Kyoto solution is of the extracellular type and is under investigation. As of 1998, the most commonly used solution for lung and heart/lung transplantation was Euro-Collins solution.[146]

There have been a number of comparisons of preservation solutions performed using experimental models with both short-term and long-term (24 hours) preservation strategies. At least experimentally, these studies suggest (1) extracellular-based solutions provide preservation of pulmonary function that may be superior to intracellular solutions,[37, 303, 316] (2) UW solution provides superior preservation to Euro-Collins solution,[7] and (3) low potassium Euro-Collins solution is superior to standard Euro-Collins solution.[104] A new extracellular preservation solution, Celsior, which contains antioxidants and impermeant agents, has been demonstrated experimentally to promote excellent lung preservation.[296] In clinical practice, the evidence is lacking for superiority of one preservation method over all others. UW solution appears clinically to provide preservation that is comparable to that of Euro-Collins solutions.[125]

Preservation is considerably more complicated than just the preservation solution because there are other important considerations such as additional pharmacological additives and the conditions of storage and reperfusion. A large number of pharmacological adjunctive strategies have been tested experimentally, and there is some evidence for the effectiveness of some of these strategies. For example, use of high-dose steroid administration prior to procurement improved lung function at the time of organ recovery.[99] Use of prostaglandins either in the flush solution or by systemic administration prior to donor lung recovery is still a matter of controversy since there is not uniform experimental or clinical support.[194] The mechanism of benefit from prostaglandin E_1 or prostacyclin during lung harvest probably relates to improved distribution of the flush solution.[14, 139, 259]

Other pharmacological additives that have some experimental and/or clinical support include use of oxygen-derived free radical scavengers,[26, 79, 89, 90, 277, 306] calcium channel blockers,[120, 165] lazaroids (inhibitor of lipid peroxidation),[8, 131] pentoxifylline (which reduces neutrophil adhesion to the endothelium)[56, 265, 400] nitroglycerin (by modulating pulmonary vasomotor responses)[246] L-arginine (by enhancing the NO pathway),[333] surfactant,[47, 132] delta opioid (DADLE)[398] and the related hibernation trigger factors,[262] neutrophil inhibition molecules,[371] and inhaled nitric oxide.[266]

The conditions of storage and reperfusion of importance include storage of the lungs inflated,[352] storage temperature (10°C may be better than 4°C),[70] method of storage (cold air storage may be better than immersion in ice slush),[184] retrograde flush (may result in a better distribution of perfusion fluid than anterograde flush),[59] and controlled pressure reperfusion (reduced pressure initially).[147, 204]

Most of these strategies have not been validated clinically and are still investigational. Clearly, much more investigational work is required to improve lung preservation for lung and heart/lung transplantation in order to not only reduce the incidence of primary graft failure, but also to metabolically and physiologically optimize

donor lungs that would otherwise not be usable for transplantation.

TECHNIQUE OF COMBINED HEART AND LUNG TRANSPLANTATION

The basic technique of combined heart and lung transplantation has remained essentially unchanged since the early Stanford experience.[158] The major evolution in technique relates to methods of pulmonary preservation. Because of concerns about the limits of safe ischemic time, early experiences with combined heart and lung transplantation involved transport of the donor to the transplanting facility in order to minimize ischemic time. With the demonstration of clinical safety of isolated single-lung transplantation with long-distance procurement and longer ischemic times, similar procurement methods were applied to heart/lung transplantation.

The Donor Operation

The same preparations are made for procurement of the heart/lung block as they are for isolated heart and lung procurement (see Chapter 9). At UAB, 3 L of Euro-Collins solution are utilized for the pulmonary flush. Prostaglandin E_1 (500 μg) is injected into the superior vena cava just prior to harvest and the same amount is added to the flush solution. With commencement of the cardioplegic and pulmonary flush solutions, the left atrial appendage is amputated to allow egress of pulmonary flush from the left atrium. After completion of the cardioplegic solution flush and pulmonary flush, the cannulae are removed. The overriding consideration in removal of the heart/lung block is that absolute hemostasis behind the heart/lung block is required, since if bleeding occurs from the posterior mediastinal tissue after implantation, obtaining hemostasis may be very difficult. Throughout the excision of the heart/lung block the lungs are gently but fully ventilated on 100% oxygen. The transection of the inferior vena cava is completed and the superior vena cava is also transected at this point. The ascending aorta is divided. The pericardium anterior to the pulmonary veins is then excised on both sides using the electrocautery. The inferior pulmonary ligaments are then divided with the electrocautery and the cut edge of the excised pericardium is then joined by a transverse incision in the posterior pericardium to allow access to the posterior mediastinum. With the left hand underneath the left atrium pulling it forward, the pleural reflections posterior to the hilum of each lung and all small vessels crossing from the posterior mediastinum to the heart/lung block are divided with the electrocautery. The bronchial vessels (usually two on the left and one on the right) can be easily identified and secured with hemoclips. When the posterior mediastinal dissection from below is at the level of the hila of the lungs, the dissection is changed from above downwards. The lungs are inflated and the trachea then clamped with two straight Kocher clamps and the trachea divided between the clamps. Grasping the Kocher clamp on the heart/lung block and distracting it downwards and forwards, the esophagus is dissected from the back of the trachea by division with the electrocautery. The upper and lower dissection planes are then joined by dividing the pleural reflections. The heart/lung block is then removed from the thoracic cavity and placed in a plastic bag to which has been added cold UW solution. This bag is placed inside a further two bags, each being individually sealed and then in ice in a cooler for transportation.

Technique of Recipient Operation

Initial Preparation

Preoperative and intraoperative preparation for the heart/lung transplant operation is the same as for orthotopic cardiac transplantation. The heart and lungs of the recipient are exposed through a median sternotomy. The thymus is excised taking care to avoid phrenic injury, and both pleural spaces are widely open. A pericardial flap for later wrapping around the tracheal anastomosis is developed by incising the pericardium laterally and inferiorly, leaving about 5 cm of pericardium over the superior vena cava as the base for an autologous pericardial flap to be placed around the trachea. It is extremely important to avoid cautery at the superior extent of these dissections, since heat-transmitted injury to the phrenic nerves would be catastrophic to postoperative pulmonary function. The aorta is dissected free from the main pulmonary artery and the usual pursestrings are placed as for orthotopic cardiac transplantation.

Removal of Native Heart and Lungs

Cardiopulmonary bypass is established, the aorta is cross-clamped, and a standard cardiectomy is performed as for bicaval orthotopic cardiac transplantation. Pulmonary venous return to the left atrium is assessed, and if pulmonary venous return is excessive, appropriate reduction of perfusate temperature to profound hypothermic levels is instituted to allow intermittent low-flow perfusion to facilitate the dissection and avoid excessive blood loss. Otherwise, perfusate temperature is generally 25°C.

Beginning on the left side, an incision is made in the pericardium just anterior to the left pulmonary veins and as far below the phrenic nerve as possible. A pedicle of pericardium containing the phrenic nerve is then developed inferiorly almost to the diaphragm and superiorly just to the level of the pulmonary artery. Further dissection superiorly is avoided because of its proximity to the phrenic nerve. Cautery is avoided if at all possible during this dissection to preserve the phrenic nerve. The left atrium is divided posteriorly in its midportion and a cuff of left atrium along with the left pulmonary veins is dissected free and passed under the pericardial pedicle (Fig. 21–6). The left pulmonary artery is dissected circumferentially prior to its branches and divided. The lower lobe of the left lung is reflected superiorly and the inferior pulmonary ligament is divided with cautery. By gently reflecting the entire left lung anteriorly, the

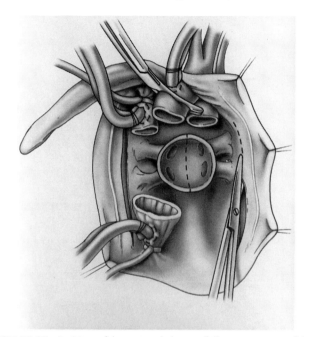

FIGURE **21–6.** View of the pericardial cavity following excision of the heart by standard cardiectomy (bicaval technique), development of the bilateral phrenic nerve pedicles, and division of the left atrium posteriorly in the midportion.

posterior attachments can be divided sharply and the lung mobilized away from the vagus nerve. The left main stem bronchus is then isolated by dividing lymphatic tissues around the bronchus with the cautery. A TA30 stapling device is used to staple the bronchus as proximally as is convenient. An antibiotic-soaked sponge is placed behind the bronchus and it is divided. The left lung is then passed off the field along with the instruments used to divide the bronchus.

On the right side, the pericardium is reflected leftward, and dissection to the pericardium is carried out immediately above the right pulmonary veins. A pericardial pedicle including the phrenic nerve is then mobilized to the level of the superior and inferior vena cavae. The pulmonary veins are mobilized and passed under the pericardial pedicle. As on the left side, the right pulmonary artery is dissected circumferentially and divided, the inferior pulmonary ligament is mobilized and divided, and the posterior pulmonary attachments are divided. The lung is gently freed from the area of the vagus nerve without cautery, and the right main stem bronchus is isolated. The TA30 stapling device is again used to staple the bronchus and it is then divided. After removing the right lung, the stumps of right and left pulmonary artery are mobilized and the pulmonary artery is excised, leaving a generous cuff around the area of the ligamentum arteriosum and left recurrent laryngeal nerve. The bronchial stumps are mobilized to the level of the carina with careful hemostasis of bronchial arteries (Fig. 21–7).

Approximately 30 minutes is reserved for gaining accurate and complete hemostasis in the posterior mediastinum, since later visualization of this area after implantation of the heart/lung block is not possible.

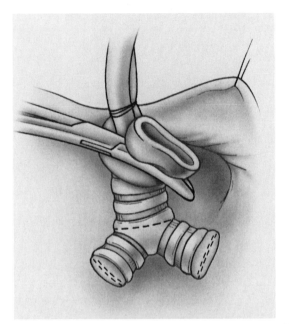

FIGURE 21-7. Bronchial stumps following excision of the right and left lungs. Each bronchial stump must be mobilized to allow access to the carina. The dashed line indicates the point of transection in preparation for the tracheal anastomosis. In order to preserve all possible blood supply to the native trachea, dissection *should not* be carried more than a few millimeters above the transection site. The aorta has been reflected superiorly to facilitate exposure.

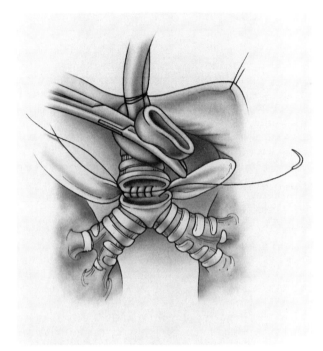

FIGURE 21-8. The heart/lung block has been placed in the pericardium cavity, the lungs have been passed below the pericardial pedicles (containing the phrenic nerves), and the anastomosis of the membranous floor of the trachea has been commenced. The pericardial flap for covering the tracheal suture line has been passed posterior to the trachea.

Implantation of the Heart/Lung Block

The heart/lung block is placed in the mediastinum by first passing the left lung under the left phrenic pedicle, followed by the right lung under the right phrenic pedicle. The two lungs are carefully examined to be certain no torsion has occurred in any of the lobes. The native trachea is divided just above the carina, taking care to avoid any dissection superior to the point of division in order to preserve all possible blood supply to the trachea. Two silk sutures are placed through the tracheal cartilage on each side to facilitate exposure with downward traction. The donor trachea is divided approximately 2 cm above the carina. In dividing the native trachea, it is important to leave the membranous portion slightly longer than the cartilagenous portion, since it tends to retract slightly after division. The anastomosis is constructed with continuous 3.0 polypropylene in adults and 4.0 polypropylene in children (Fig. 21–8). Care is taken to provide an air-tight anastomosis without necrosing the membranous portion and without turning excessive amounts of tissue into the trachea lumen. The pericardium is wrapped around the trachea and sutured to the thick lymphatic tissue anterior to the suture line.[133] Gentle inflation of the lungs with the tracheal anastomosis immersed in saline provides a check of the tracheal suture line.

The superior and inferior vena caval anastomoses and aortic anastomoses are constructed as in the bicaval orthotopic heart transplant procedure (Fig. 21–9). Typically, the superior vena caval anastomosis is constructed during the rewarming phase after removal of the cross-clamp. During the period of implantation, cold saline is used to irrigate the left pleural cavity, which also provides topical cardiac cooling. If the heart is displaced downward into the left thoracic cavity, a cradle for the heart is constructed by placing several sutures between the inferior aspect of the left pericardial pedicle and the posterior pericardium. The aortic cross-clamp is re-

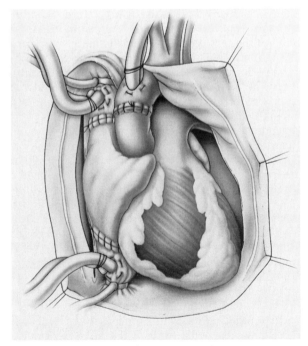

FIGURE 21-9. Completed inferior vena caval, superior vena caval, and aortic anastomoses.

moved after completion of the aortic anastomosis and de-airing the heart. The lungs are gently ventilated and cardiopulmonary bypass is discontinued as usual.

Special Considerations

Posterior mediastinal bleeding after implantation of the heart/lung block remains a major obstacle to an uncomplicated operation. Although we have routinely excised a cuff of left atrium around the right and left pulmonary veins and accurately dissected the hilar structures before dividing them, others have recommended bulk stapling at the hilar level after freeing up the posterior mediastinum from the vagus nerve.[380] We have in the past utilized the technique of covering the posterior mediastinum by suturing the posterior pericardium to the left parietal pleura[257] but currently prefer to leave it open for direct inspection. Icenogle and colleagues[154] and Lick and colleagues[205] have recommended placement of the lungs *anterior* to the phrenic nerves to facilitate displacing the lungs from the thoracic cavity to expose areas of posterior mediastinal bleeding after implantation.[154] We have not utilized this technique. Right and left main stem bronchial anastomosis rather than tracheal anastomosis has been recommended[112] as a means of minimizing dissection within the mediastinum and reducing the risk of hemorrhage. We would not recommend this technique.

Several maneuvers have been recommended to decrease the incidence of tracheal dehiscence. Almost certainly, the most important consideration is the preservation of blood supply to the distal native trachea by minimizing dissection superior to the site of transection. We routinely utilize a pericardial flap to wrap the anastomosis.[133] Others have recommended wrapping the tracheal anastomosis with a pedicle of greater omentum.

The technique of heart/lung transplantation needs to be modified for patients with situs inversus.[229] In this anomaly, the right atrium and superior and inferior vena cavae of the recipient are on the left side of the pericardial cavity. A technique has been described[238] to displace the atrial cuff for the right atrial anastomosis to the right by excising the recipient interatrial septum to create a large common atrium closing the pulmonary venous orifices, and closing the left anterior wall of the common atrium with right atrial tissue. The recipient right atrial wall is then on the right side of the pericardial cavity to which the donor right atrium can be anastomosed. A similar technique was described by Rabago[287] (Fig. 21–10). In an alternative technique for situs inversus (associated with separate left-sided inferior vena cava and hepatic vein entering the right atrium), Parry and colleagues fashioned superior and inferior vena caval conduits from autologous tissue (remnant of recipient right atrium for the inferior vena cava and spiral saphenous vein graft for the superior vena cava)[272] (Fig. 21–11). A heart/lung transplant was performed at UAB in a patient with right isomerism with dextrocardia and bilateral superior vena cava without an innominate vein. Continuity was achieved from the left superior vena cava to the right atrial anastomosis by creating a tube of residual left atrial wall, and a pericardial cradle for the transplanted heart was constructed from bovine pericardium.

Another surgical option that may rarely be available is heart and single-lung transplantation. This has been performed[95] in a patient with tricuspid and pulmonary atresia with a classic Glenn shunt to the right pulmonary artery and a Potts shunt to the left pulmonary artery. The "protected lung" on the right was retained and a heart/left lung transplant was performed using a left bronchial anastomosis. This procedure does have the putative advantage of retaining a native lung, perhaps limiting the consequences of obliterative bronchiolitis.

POSTOPERATIVE MANAGEMENT OF THE HEART/LUNG TRANSPLANT RECIPIENT

The management of the cardiac transplant recipient is outlined in Chapter 12 and the management of the heart/lung transplant recipient follows those guidelines except for the specific lung management. Heart/lung transplantation, however, is not usually associated with the management difficulties that may be associated with single-lung transplantation, for example, hyperinflation of the contralateral lung due to air trapping and hemodynamic instability in patients undergoing single-lung transplantation for primary pulmonary hypertension.

Hemodynamic Management

One of the critical aspects of hemodynamic management of patients after heart/lung transplantation is the minimization of pulmonary interstitial fluid accumulation. At this stage, the lungs are vulnerable to this phenomenon, and allowing the filling pressures to be as low as possible consistent with satisfactory circulation and treating hemodynamic instability with inotropic agents rather than excessive fluid administration are important strategies.

Pulmonary Management

Standard ventilatory methods are employed after heart/lung transplantation using a volume cycle ventilator, the goal being to ensure adequate oxygenation saturation 90% or greater with an FiO_2 as low as possible and peak pressure of less than 30 cm H_2O. PEEP of 5 cm H_2O is used, but higher levels of PEEP are only used if oxygenation is inadequate, usually in the setting of poor graft performance. Airway toilet is very important and this should be carried out every 2 hours (or more often if necessary) using saline instilled down the endotracheal tube and suctioned with a soft endotracheal suction catheter every 2 hours, but more frequently if required. During the period of mechanical ventilation, percussion and vibration to mobilize secretions should be performed every 4–6 hours. In the presence of satisfactory graft function, early weaning and extubation is highly desirable.

Fiberoptic bronchoscopy should be performed just prior to extubation to once again examine the anastomosis and donor mucosa for evidence of ischemic injury

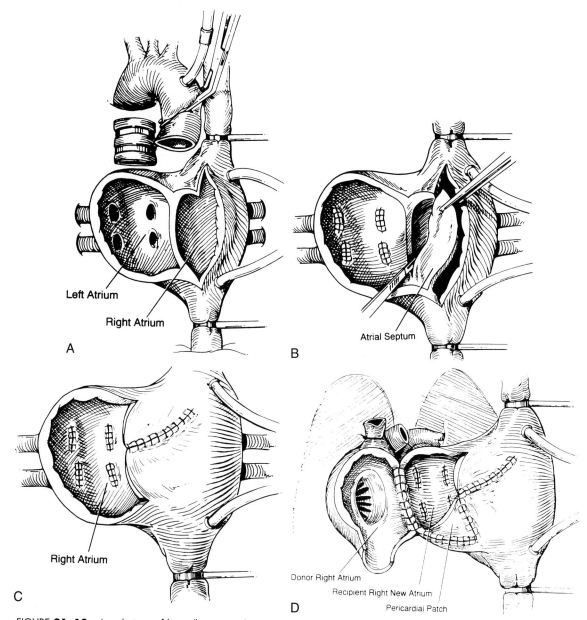

FIGURE 21–10. A technique of heart/lung transplantation in patients with situs inversus and dextracardia. *A*, After removal of both ventricles, a generous atrial cuff is left on both sides to be used in construction of the large right atrium. *B*, Resection of the atrial septum allowing blood flow from the right to the left atrium. Pulmonary veins on the right side are closed. *C*, Construction of the anterior wall of the recipient right atrium using part of the free wall of the right and left atrium. *D*, Completion of the transplantation anastomosing the donor right atrium with the mega-atrium of the recipient formed with both right and left atrium. If necessary, a pericardial patch can be used to enlarge this anastomosis and allow unrestricted blood flow. (From Rabago G, Copeland JG III, Rosapepe F: Heart-lung transplantation in situs inversus. Ann Thorac Surg 1996;62:296–298. Reprinted with permission from the Society of Thoracic Surgeons.)

and clear the airways of secretions. If ventilation is prolonged, fiberoptic bronchoscopy is performed as indicated.

Following extubation, patients should continue regular chest physical therapy, be encouraged to cough and deep breath (since airway secretions cannot be appreciated due to denervation), encouraged to use an incentive spirometer (as a guide, 10 minutes every hour while the patient is awake), and twice daily vibropercussion performed sitting and in the head-down, left, and right lateral recumbent positions. The latter two maneuvers should become incorporated into the patient's daily routine and continued lifelong.

Reimplantation Response

Reimplantation response is the term given to a process characterized by radiologic perihilar opacification of the graft, decreased lung compliance, and impairment of gas exchange commencing within 48 hours of lung transplantation. This constellation of findings should probably be considered within the spectrum of graft failure.

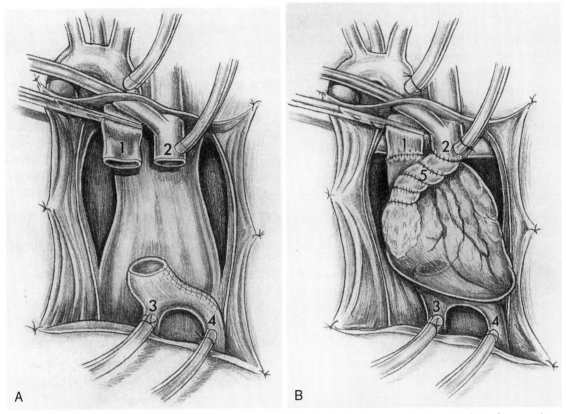

FIGURE **21–11.** An alternative technique of heart/lung transplantation for situs-inversus. *A,* The empty chest after cannulation of the great vessels and excision of the heart. The right atrium has been partially removed, and the remnant, comprising the insertion of both the inferior vena cava and the hepatic venous segment, has been rolled into a tube for connection to the donor right atrium. *B,* The chest after implantation of the heart/lung block. Continuity of the venous drainage of the upper body has been reestablished by anastomosing a spiral vein graft (5) from the right atrial appendage to the superior vena cava. (1 = aorta; 2 = superior vena cava; 3 = hepatic vein segment; 4 = inferior vena cava.) (From Parry AJ, O'Fiesh J, Wallwork J, Large SR: Heart-lung transplantation in situs inversus and chest wall deformity. Ann Thorac Surg 1994;58:1174–1176. Reprinted with permission from the Society of Thoracic Surgeons.)

This phenomenon was well known in early experimental and clinical lung transplantation, and its natural history is gradual resolution. The incidence of reimplantation response after heart/lung transplantation appears to be less than with single- or double-lung transplantation.[114] The cause of reimplantation response is unknown, but the likely possibilities include ischemic-reperfusion injury, surgical handling, lymphatic disruption, and denervation. With diuresis and fluid restriction, the process resolves in a matter of a few days. It is, however, important to distinguish this benign process from other important phenomena with quite different therapies, such as rejection and infection. Perihilar opacification of grafts occurring after 48 hours from transplantation strongly suggest a process other than reimplantation response.

Immunosuppression

The immunosuppression protocol outlined in Chapter 14 for heart transplantation is applicable to patients undergoing heart/lung transplantation. However, some programs, including that at UAB, have at some time used cytolytic therapy either with OKT3[351] or rabbit anti-thymocyte globulin (RATG) for 5–10 days coupled with initial prednisone maintenance therapy of 15 mg daily (in adults) rather than 1 mg/kg as used after heart transplantation. The benefits of this strategy have not been formally tested.

Immunosuppression trials in lung transplant patients have provided preliminary information that may eventually impact on immunosuppression protocols in heart/lung transplantation. A number of studies[264, 310, 412] suggest that mycophenolate mofetil may reduce the incidence of acute pulmonary rejection compared with azathioprine-based immunosuppression. Acute rejection in lung transplant recipients receiving tacrolimus may possibly have a lower incidence of acute pulmonary rejection compared to patients receiving cyclosporine-based immunosuppression.[170] Experimentally, sirolimus[214] in combination with cyclosporine appeared to strongly protect against acute pulmonary rejection. Leflunomide has also been demonstrated experimentally to prolong both pulmonary allograft and xenograft survival. In addition, because of its known ability to experimentally suppress obliterative airway disease, it will be an important immunosuppressant drug for future investigation in lung and heart/lung transplantation.[409] Aerosolized cyclosporine has been demonstrated experimentally to prevent acute pulmonary rejection with effective local cyclosporine concentrations in the lung[41, 82] and reduce the production of proinflammatory cytokines in lung tissue.[239]

Infection Prophylaxis

The infection prophylaxis protocol for heart/lung transplantation is the same as for heart transplantation and is outlined in Chapter 15.

Primary Graft Failure

Primary graft failure is a serious and potentially fatal complication after lung and heart/lung transplantation. The reported incidence of primary graft failure after heart/lung transplantation is approximately 2 to 7%,[315, 359] which appears to be less than with single- and double-lung transplantation. The ischemic-reperfusion phenomenon likely plays a major role in primary graft failure, although other contributing factors include donor lung injury such as contusion or infection and prolonged ischemic time. Ischemic reperfusion injury is characterized by an endothelial injury which is probably due to sequestration and activation of polymorphonuclear neutrophils which in turn results in the release of inflammatory cytokines and is intensified by the release of oxygen-derived free radicals. There is considerable experimental evidence regarding the deleterious effect of cardiopulmonary bypass on early pulmonary graft function[100] and on graft pulmonary vasomotor function,[105] no doubt contributing to the progression of the phenomena associated with primary graft failure through humoral amplification system activation and the systemic inflammatory response associated with cardiopulmonary bypass. The functional manifestations of the injury are increased pulmonary capillary permeability, pulmonary hypertension, decreased lung compliance, and increased airway resistance. As the time course of the lung injury continues, it is invariably complicated by infection, rejection, and perhaps airway anastomotic problems. However, in the lung transplant experience, if the patient survives, ultimately pulmonary function is usually good.[134]

A potentially important observation was made by Bridges and colleagues[45] regarding the role of adenovirus infection in graft failure in pediatric lung and heart/lung transplant recipients. These investigators performed prospective surveillance cultures for common respiratory viruses of childhood in lung and heart/lung transplant recipients and their donors. The identification of adenovirus was significantly associated with respiratory failure leading to death or graft loss (Fig. 21–12). What is of particular interest was the identification of adenovirus in two donors who were found to have adenovirus by polymerase chain reaction (PCR) in the donor lung before implantation, and both recipients developed early rapidly progressive pneumonitis and graft failure. If further investigation confirms these findings, testing for adenovirus in lung and heart/lung transplant donors as well as infection control measures to prevent the nosocomial spread of adenovirus to these recipients may be required.

When the capillary leak is of sufficient severity to seriously compromise oxygenation (arterial oxygen saturation less than about 90% despite inspired oxygen concentration of 90–100%) within the first 6–12 hours after transplantation, the tracheobronchial secretions are usually copious. This dangerous situation (which can proceed to fatal hypoxemia) requires intensive intervention with maneuvers designed to minimize transudation of fluid into the alveolar spaces and concomitantly reduce overall whole body oxygen demands. Reduction of oxygen demands is facilitated by sedation, paralysis, and moderate hypothermia (with a cooling blanket) to 35°–36°C if the situation is severe. The major elements of reducing transudation of fluid into alveoli include fluid restriction and diuresis to maintain the lowest possible left atrial pressure compatible with effective cardiac output and high PEEP at 15–20 cm H_2O, as long as the hemodynamics tolerate it. When the secretions

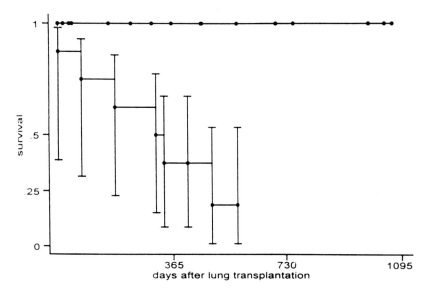

FIGURE **21-12.** Actuarial survival after pediatric lung transplantation, stratified by the presence or absence of adenovirus infection. Survival without adenovirus infection, shown in the upper curve, is taken as the interval from transplantation to last follow-up or to the date of identification of adenovirus infection, at which point patients were censored: survival after adenovirus infection (lower curve) is taken as the interval between identification of adenovirus infection and last follow-up or death. The difference in survival is significant ($p < .001$ by Wilcoxon-Gehan test). (From Bridges ND, Spray TL, Collins MH, Bowles NE, Towbin JA: Adenovirus infection in the lung results in graft failure after lung transplantation. J Thorac Cardiovasc Surg 1998;116:617–623.)

are particularly profuse, suctioning may seem necessary every 10–15 minutes to clear the endotracheal tube. At times, however, suctioning of this frequency may paradoxically worsen the oxygenation by transiently eliminating the PEEP during suctioning (with resultant worsening of fluid transudation into the alveolar spaces). In several instances, we have noted improvement in oxygenation with elimination of suctioning (which also carries the risk of inducing mucosal bleeding secondary to local trauma) for 6–8 hours so that high levels of PEEP can be continuously maintained.

Placement of a pulmonary artery catheter with continuous monitoring of cardiac output and mixed venous oxygen saturation provides initial information for management. If the pulmonary artery pressure is elevated (systolic pressure >40–45 mm Hg), interventions to lower it are advisable. Although not clearly established, there is sufficient experimental data and encouraging clinical experience to suggest that inhaled NO therapy (see Box) in the early postoperative period may be of benefit in the management of reimplantation response and primary graft failure[5, 221] in lung and heart/lung transplantation (the use of nitric oxide in pediatric heart transplantation is discussed in Chapter 20). In experimental transplant models, inhaled nitric oxide significantly attenuates reperfusion injury, the effect being im-

Inhaled Nitric Oxide Therapy

The biological effects of nitric oxide result from the molecule being small, having high lipid solubility, being able to rapidly traverse the cell membrane, having a short half-life of seconds, and having an affinity for the iron moiety of a number of molecules.[155] Nitric oxide is synthesized by the action of nitric oxide synthase (NOS) enzymes, which catalyzes the reaction of oxygen and the amino acid l-arginine to nitric oxide and l-citrulline.[281] There are endothelial, neuronal, and inducible[242] genes that code for NOS. The two functional forms of NOS are constitutive NOS (which is released from endothelial cells [eNOS] and neurons [nNOS])[140, 155] and inducible NOS (iNOS), which is expressed in smooth muscle cells and macrophages. Inducible NOS is not expressed under normal circumstances, but is up-regulated by such mediators as IL-1 and other cytokines as well as gram-negative endotoxin lipopolysaccharides (LPS).

The major physiologic action of NO is vasodilation occurring through the second messenger molecule, cyclic guanosine $-3'-5'$-monophosphate (cGMP). Nitric oxide binds to the iron moiety of guanylate cyclase, resulting in the synthesis of cGMP,[119] which activates a cGMP-dependent protein kinase which causes relaxation of smooth muscle. Nitric oxide has a number of other actions that are mediated by the nitric oxide–cGMP signal transduction system including platelet inhibition[15]; neurotransmission in the cerebellum, spinal cord, peripheral nervous system, and hippocampus[15]; and inhibition of the proliferation of vascular smooth muscle cells[307]; it also has a role in the immune system, contributing to macrophage cytotoxic activity.[320] Nitric oxide also has some actions that appear not to be mediated by the NO-cGMP transduction system including the scavenging of oxygen free radicals[61, 128, 163] and an inhibition of platelet and leukocyte aggregation.[142, 250, 285]

Although nitric oxide appears to have considerable beneficial actions, it is potentially injurious to a number of tissues because of its metabolic products. In the presence of oxygen, nitric oxide is oxidized to nitrogen dioxide[350] which is converted to nitric and nitrous acids.[151] In solution, nitric oxide reacts with superoxide (O^-_2) to form peroxynitrite $(OONO^-)$[101, 187] which, being a strong oxidant, catalyzes membrane liquid peroxidation[151] as well as having other potential toxic actions such as participating in myocardial ischemic reperfusion injury.[222] Because of its affinity for iron, nitric oxide combines with hemoglobin, resulting in a production of methemoglobin[17, 365] and by the same mechanism reacts with enzymes in the mitochondrial electron transport chain.

Inhaled nitric oxide therapy has not been fully established, but has been used in a variety of conditions such as adult respiratory distress syndrome (ARDS), primary pulmonary hypertension, persistent pulmonary hypertension of the newborn, congenital diaphragmatic hernia, high-altitude pulmonary edema, and graft dysfunction after lung and heart/lung transplantation. Clinical experience does suggest that in some patients this therapy is effective. The theoretical advantage of inhaled nitric oxide over other pulmonary vasodilators such as nitroprusside, nitroglycerin, or prostacyclin which nonselectively dilate the pulmonary vasculature including the nonventilated areas, is that inhaled nitric oxide preferentially dilates pulmonary vessels in well-ventilated areas of the lung to which the nitric oxide has been preferentially distributed, resulting in better matching of ventilation and perfusion.[151] Dosage must be maintained within certain limits because of the potential toxicity of methemoglobinemia and peroxynitrate formation, resulting in pulmonary edema and surfactant damage.[122]

At UAB, inhaled nitric oxide is delivered by the I-NOvent (Ohmeda) delivery system. This system delivers nitric oxide gas into the inspiratory limb of the ventilator circuit so that a constant concentration of nitric oxide is delivered throughout the inspired breath. This is achieved by tracking of the ventilator waveform so that the delivery of the nitric oxide can be synchronized and a proportional dose delivered. The nitric oxide gas is stored as a gas mixture of nitric oxide and nitrogen in an aluminum cylinder with a maximum pressure of 2,200 psi. The nitric oxide gas flows out of the cylinder into a high-pressure regulator, reducing the pressure to 65 psi. On entry into the delivery system, the low-pressure regulator reduces the pressure of the nitric oxide gas to 26 psi. The system has on-line monitoring of F_{IO_2}, nitric oxide (in ppm), and nitrogen dioxide (in ppm). Nitric oxide and nitrogen dioxide are measured by a chemiluminescent analyzer. The initial dose of nitric oxide is empiric, but it is not allowed to exceed 80 ppm. The usual practice is to continue inhaled nitric oxide until the mean pulmonary artery pressure falls below 20 mm Hg, maintaining the inspired concentration of nitric oxide below 80 ppm, the inspired concentration of nitrogen dioxide below 5% of nitric oxide concentration, and methemoglobin level less than 4 gm/dL. However, there may be other clinically useful effects of nitric oxide that are not mediated by the NO-cGMP transduction system as outlined earlier, and discontinuation of inhaled nitric oxide because of a lack of prompt pulmonary vasodilating effect may be premature.[151] Further details of nitric oxide physiology and clinical use are provided in Chapter 20.

provement in gas exchange, reduction of pulmonary vascular resistance,[18] as well as reduction of microvascular permeability.[27, 243] The degree of decrease in pulmonary vascular resistance associated with nitric oxide inhalation may reflect the severity of endothelial damage.[208] The optimal timing of administration of inhaled nitric oxide is controversial, with some studies suggesting that inhaled nitric oxide at the start of reperfusion may exacerbate the injury, while the greatest benefit is associated with initiation of NO within several hours of reperfusion, and less effect later.[19, 33, 130, 245, 266] Clinically, nitric oxide should probably be initiated as soon as important lung allograft dysfunction is suspected.

Postoperative Bleeding

Postoperative bleeding is a complication of particular concern with heart/lung transplantation. In an earlier era, two experienced centers reported fatal postoperative hemorrhage in 13–24% of patients undergoing heart/lung transplantation.[114, 227] Although the risk of dying from uncontrollable bleeding has been substantially reduced in the current era, postoperative bleeding still has an impact on mortality and morbidity, and in most hands, reoperation for bleeding after heart/lung transplantation is frequently required. For example, in the Papworth experience[326] total intraoperative blood loss was an independent risk factor for death in the first 3 months, no doubt reflecting the association of bleeding with other problems such as multisystem failure and infection. After retransplantation of heart/lung transplant recipients, not surprisingly, bleeding is an important early complication. Adams and colleagues from Harefield reported a 36% incidence of reexploration for bleeding with 32% of early deaths related to excessive hemorrhage.[4]

Meticulous and effective hemostasis is a critical factor in successful heart/lung transplantation. We believe that several aspects of intraoperative management have importantly reduced postoperative bleeding. After removal of the native heart and lungs, at least 30 minutes are dedicated to achieving complete hemostasis of the chest wall (if adhesions were present), pericardial edges, and the mediastinum. Bleeding points on the pericardial strips which contain the phrenic nerves or elsewhere near the nerves are controlled with 5.0 polypropylene sutures rather than diathermic coagulation to prevent inadvertent heat-induced nerve injury. The field should be quite "dry," with no identifiable active bleeding points before implanting the donor heart/lung block. The integrity of the coagulation system is reestablished as soon as possible after cardiopulmonary bypass with the routine use of aprotinin (during and after cardiopulmonary bypass) and infusion of platelets (through an appropriate leukocyte filter) and fresh frozen plasma immediately following the administration of protamine. For postoperative evacuation of blood, two chest tubes are placed in the mediastinum and each pleural space (six tubes total), with each set of two chest tubes attached to a separate drainage system. This facilitates identification of the area of bleeding and selection of incision

should reentry for bleeding be necessary. If reentry for bleeding is required because of excessive drainage in either pleural space, it is best to explore the pleural space through a right or left thoracotomy, which facilitates exposure of posterior mediastinal bleeding in these locations.

ACUTE REJECTION IN HEART/LUNG TRANSPLANT RECIPIENTS

The current understanding of acute pulmonary rejection is largely derived from lung transplantation and is directly transferable to heart/lung transplantation.

Classification of Lung Rejection

The classic view of graft rejection includes three relatively discrete forms based on the timing of onset—hyperacute, acute, and chronic (see Chapter 14).

Hyperacute rejection has been well described in kidney transplant recipients and has also been reported in cardiac transplant recipients, but its role in early rejection of a lung graft is less secure. The deleterious effect of a positive T-cell crossmatch on survival after heart/lung transplantation has been demonstrated,[342] but in this study no information was presented to suggest that hyperacute rejection was involved. A case report[103] of a patient undergoing single-lung transplantation who died of graft failure which commenced 1 hour after reperfusion of the lung does make a strong case for the role of hyperacute rejection, since the histological picture of severe diffuse alveolar damage, neutrophilic infiltrates, and IgG fluorescent staining within alveolar spaces was seen. It is possible that hyperacute rejection could be confused with diffuse alveolar damage due to ischemic-reperfusion injury. Chronic rejection is a process resulting in graft dysfunction and graft failure which is reflected in the **bronchiolitis obliterans syndrome** (BOS) and the pathological entity of bronchiolitis obliterans (see section later in this chapter). The process of acute rejection is a result of the recipient's immune response against the HLA antigens of the grafted lungs, and the fundamentals of the immunological process are likely the same for the lung as for the heart and are outlined in detail in Chapter 2.

Five years after heart/lung transplantation, approximately 40% of patients are free from acute pulmonary rejection[315] and approximately 50% of patients are free from acute cardiac rejection (Fig. 21–13).[315] This incidence of acute cardiac rejection is considerably less than that of patients undergoing isolated heart transplantation.[183] In the early years of heart/lung transplantation, the prevailing view was that rejection of the heart and lungs was concordant and therefore surveillance endomyocardial biopsy could monitor both cardiac and pulmonary rejection.[159, 300, 301] However, it soon became apparent that discordant rejection of the heart and lungs occurred clinically[115, 232, 324] and experimentally.[64, 261] Furthermore, acute rejection of the lungs was found to be not only more frequent but more severe than acute cardiac rejection, rendering the endomyocardial biopsy sur-

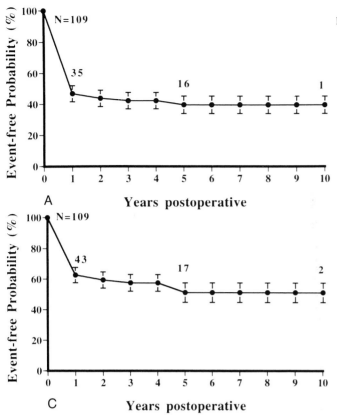

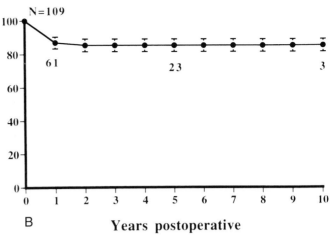

FIGURE **21–13.** Heart and lung rejection following heart/lung transplantation. *A,* Actuarial freedom from isolated pulmonary rejection after heart/lung transplantation. *B,* Actuarial freedom from simultaneous heart and lung rejection after heart/lung transplantation. *C,* Actuarial freedom from isolated cardiac rejection after heart/lung transplantation. (From Sarris GE, Smith JA, Shumway NE, Stinson EB, Oyer PE, Robbins RC, Billingham ME, Theodore J, Moore KA, Reitz BA: Long-term results of combined heart-lung transplantation: the Stanford experience. J Heart Lung Transplant 1994;13:940–949.)

veillance unreliable for the detection of acute pulmonary rejection. Clinically, asynchronous rejection can be appreciated by the rarity of observed simultaneous rejection of the heart and lung (Fig. 21–13). This phenomenon of asynchronous rejection is also known to occur in combined kidney/pancreas transplantation.[135] The mechanism of this differential rejection is unclear.

The phenomenon of **reduced cardiac rejection in combined heart/lung transplantation** compared with isolated heart transplantation has been referred to as the "combi-effect,"[386–388] and it was thought that the lymphoid tissue accompanying the lung provided a protective effect on the heart. On the other hand, it has been postulated that the bronchus-associated lymphoid tissue (BALT)[283] accompanying the lung may provoke a more vigorous pulmonary rejection response.[336] Another suggestion based on experimental information has hypothesized that there is an important difference in the expression of MHC antigens as well as non-MHC antigens that may account for the difference in rejection.[241] The frequency of acute pulmonary rejection appears to be less in patients receiving cytolytic therapy with RATG[113] after lung transplantation. Heart/lung transplant recipients appear to have less acute pulmonary rejection with less mismatching at the A locus and the DR locus, although this was not reflected in better survival.[175] This phenomenon has not been clearly demonstrated in lung transplant recipients.[395] Just as in heart transplantation and isolated lung transplantation, the greatest likelihood of acute rejection in heart/lung transplantation is in the first 3 months after transplantation.

Rejection of the lung involves a complex interplay of immune cells, cytokines, and soluble mediators, and the central pathological feature is a perivascular accumulation of T-lymphocytes which may be accompanied by an accumulation of T-lymphocytes around the bronchioles. In the severest forms of acute pulmonary rejection, the lymphocytic infiltrate involves not only blood vessels but alveolar pneumocyte damage, interstitial infiltrates, alveolar infiltrates, necrosis of the lung parenchyma, and necrotizing vasculitis. Not surprisingly, it has been demonstrated in experimentally rejecting lungs that the responsiveness of pulmonary arteries and veins to receptor-mediated processes is abnormal in both the endothelium and smooth muscle, a phenomenon which was reversible with resolution of acute rejection.[2]

The role of ischemic reperfusion injury in the subsequent development of acute pulmonary rejection is unclear. In an experimental model, Shiraishi and colleagues[332] found no relationship between ischemic injury and the subsequent development of acute pulmonary rejection, although another experimental study demonstrated up-regulation of MHC class II antigens on bronchial epithelium (but interestingly not on vascular endothelium) after lung transplantation, at least suggesting that the substrate for rejection may be induced.[6] Humoral rejection has been well described in heart, kidney, and liver transplant recipients, but has not been convincingly described in lung transplantation. A study by Saint Martin and colleagues[313] examining a large number of transbronchial and open lung biopsy specimens after lung transplantation could find no evidence by immunofluorescence suggesting humoral rejection. A response to plasmapheresis has been described[20] in the setting of acute rejection with histological features of pulmonary capillaritis resulting in diffuse alveolar hemorrhage. However, a humoral component was not documented in these cases.

Diagnosis

Acute pulmonary rejection must be differentiated from a number of other processes including diffuse alveolar damage from graft failure, pulmonary infection, bronchiolitis obliterans, organizing pneumonia, and the parenchymal consequences of airway injury. In the first few weeks after heart/lung transplantation, the diagnosis of acute pulmonary rejection is usually based on **clinical criteria.** A patient experiencing acute pulmonary rejection may report constitutional symptoms such as fatigue, malaise, decreasing exercise tolerance, shortness of breath, fever, and cough. There is likely to be desaturation on exercise and often increasing oxygen requirements at rest. Late after heart/lung transplantation, acute pulmonary rejection is frequently asymptomatic and detected on a routine surveillance transbronchial lung biopsy.

In the first few months after heart/lung transplantation, typical signs and symptoms of acute pulmonary rejection may be treated by pulse methylprednisolone (see next section) without histological confirmation. The diagnosis is confirmed by a rapid symptomatic and objective improvement.

The **chest x-ray** is insensitive and nonspecific for the diagnosis of acute pulmonary rejection. In the first few months after transplantation, diffuse shadowing may be perihilar or basal in location, with a homogeneous, inhomogeneous, or reticular pattern. In a study of radiological features of biopsy-proven acute pulmonary rejection after heart/lung transplantation in the first 3 months, the chest radiograph had a sensitivity of 78.5% for the diagnosis of acute pulmonary rejection, but after this period the sensitivity fell to 19%.[270] Radiological changes occurring in the setting of acute rejection may be unilateral and very similar to those seen in the presence of infection.[237] A number of other radiological techniques have been investigated to diagnose acute pulmonary rejection, but none has proven sensitive or specific enough for routine clinical use. The use of high-resolution computerized tomography[216] and conventional computerized tomography[233] does not add to the specificity of diagnosing acute pulmonary rejection. Other radiological methods have been investigated including clearance of ^{99m}Tc-DTPA, which is increased in pulmonary rejection,[137] and pulmonary lymphoscintigraphy, which experimentally has demonstrated decreased lymphatic drainage from the grafted lung in the presence of rejection[311] (which is based on the demonstration experimentally that lymphatic drainage is reestablished from the pulmonary allograft to the mediastinum in about 2 weeks after transplantation).[92, 312]

Hypoxemia is a nonspecific sign of acute pulmonary rejection, and this is most evident with rejection occurring in the first few weeks after transplantation.

Bronchoalveolar Lavage

The technique of bronchoalveolar lavage involves injecting 20 to 50 mL aliquots of non-bacteriostatic normal saline (up to 250 mL) through the suction channel of the bronchoscope, which is wedged in a segmental bronchus. Each aliquot is then aspirated and each specimen is quantitatively cultured and gram stained after centrifugation. A finding of greater than 10^5 colony forming units per mL indicates a significant parenchymal infection. Protected bronchoalveolar lavage may be even more effective in preventing contamination from proximal airways and involves inserting a protected balloon-tipped catheter into the distal airways for lavaging fluid from the segmental bronchi.

Bronchoalveolar lavage (see Box), which is routinely performed at the time of transbronchial lung biopsy for either surveillance or as part of the diagnostic work-up of pulmonary graft dysfunction, has as its major current role the exclusion of infection. Numerous studies have examined bronchoalveolar lavage fluid to distinguish between infection and rejection. The phenotypic expression of bronchoalveolar lavage cells (such as lymphocytes, monocytes, granulocytes)[330] and their functional changes have been correlated with rejection and infection in a number of animal models,[284, 331] but differences are too small for reliable diagnosis.[62] Increases in $CD8^+$ cells and an increase in the $CD4^+/CD8^+$ ratio has been demonstrated during acute pulmonary rejection, but these same changes were also seen during infection.[410] A number of other markers in bronchoalveolar lavage fluid and cells that may indicate acute pulmonary rejection have been investigated, including increases in endothelin-1 (experimentally[1] and clinically[319]), hyaluronic acid (clinically),[290] soluble HLA class I antigens (clinically),[305] and cytokines such as IL-6, IL-10, and IFN-γ,[152, 309] but none of these tests has sufficient sensitivity or specificity to be used in clinical practice.

Spirometry is one of the mainstays in the detection of graft dysfunction, an important cause being acute pulmonary rejection. Spirometry is not routinely performed during the transplant hospitalization because of the difficulty of interpreting changes in the presence of wound pain, early graft dysfunction, pulmonary infection, and atelectasis. However, following hospitalization, spirometry does become important in detecting graft dysfunction, although it is still not specific for acute pulmonary rejection. A fall in FEV_1 of greater than 10% is regarded as evidence of possible acute pulmonary rejection and is, at UAB, an indication for transbronchial lung biopsy. After approximately 6 months, a decline in FEV_1 and forced expiratory flow between 25% and 75% of the forced vital capacity (FEF_{25-75}) is predictive of acute rejection, but the probability that this fall is due to the development of bronchiolitis obliterans syndrome progressively rises. The value of changes in FEV_1 as a means of diagnosing acute rejection have been well demonstrated in heart/lung transplant recipients.[269] One of the advantages of spirometry is that it is not invasive, it is easy to perform, and home spirometric monitoring with telephonic transmission of the values to the transplant center can be a useful means of remotely monitoring graft function. Some of the devices that are available for home spirometric monitoring are quite sophisticated, and a number of different measurements of airflow can be determined, including flow-volume loops. However, only FEF_{25-75} has a known association with early graft dysfunction due to acute pulmonary rejection.

Transbronchial lung biopsy (see Box) has emerged as the mainstay of diagnosing acute pulmonary rejection after heart/lung transplantation. It is important not only for the diagnosis of acute pulmonary rejection but also for confirmation of the diagnosis of infections such as cytomegalovirus (CMV), *Pneumocystis carinii*, and herpes simplex.[344] It has also been important in detecting the presence of obliterative bronchiolitis, which may or may not be associated with bronchiolitis obliterans syndrome. Transbronchial lung biopsy in heart/lung transplantation has been reported to have a sensitivity for diagnosing acute pulmonary rejection of 94% with a specificity of 90%[321] based on the presence of histological changes on the biopsy specimen together with the consequent enhancement of immunosuppression based on a clinical diagnosis of rejection. The sensitivity of the technique, however, is likely not to be uniformly this good.[370]

Transbronchial Lung Biopsy

At UAB, the first transbronchial lung biopsy is performed by the surgical staff so that the airway can be inspected for evidence of anastmotic problems. All subsequent surveillance transbronchial lung biopsies are performed as an outpatient procedure by the pulmonary medicine transplant staff. Outpatient transbronchial lung biopsy is performed as an awake procedure using intravenous sedation with drugs such as midazolam or meperidine and topical lidocaine anesthesia of the upper airway. A transnasal approach is used and is performed under fluoroscopic control to allow alveolar sampling close to the pleural surface. This procedure has also been successful in children from 7–18 years of age.[195] The current recommendation of the lung rejection study group[402] is to obtain at least five pieces of alveolated lung parenchyma containing both bronchioles and more than 100 alveoli for the diagnosis and grading of acute pulmonary rejection. The unsatisfactory sampling rate appears to be approximately 20%.[177, 282] There is a small but appreciable complication rate from transbronchial lung biopsy including pneumothorax, hemoptysis (rarely severe), transient hypoxemia, and respiratory failure from oversedation.[55, 322, 370] Routine surveillance transbronchial lung biopsy following heart/lung transplantation is performed at 2, 4, 6, and 10 weeks, then every 3 months for the remainder of the first year, and then every 6 months indefinitely. The frequency of transbronchial lung biopsy is modified by the rejection pattern. At UAB, a follow-up transbronchial lung biopsy is performed 4 weeks after the treatment of an episode of acute pulmonary rejection.

All five transbronchial lung biopsy sections are fixed in formalin and standard paraffin sections are made with all biopsy specimens on the same slide. Three hematoxylin and eosin slides are made with cuts 1, 3, and 7, and cuts 2, 4, and 6 are stained for acid-fast bacilli, Gomori-methenamine-silver stain (for pneumocystis and fungi), and immunohistochemistry for CMV antigen.

A morphological grading system has been developed to be used not only as a guide for the treatment of acute pulmonary rejection, but also as a means of comparing severity of rejection between institutions (Table 21–1). The diagnosis of acute rejection is based on the presence of perivascular and interstitial mononuclear cell infiltrates and the grading system is determined by the intensity of the perivascular mononuclear cell cuffs which surround blood vessels (venules and arterioles) as well as extension of the mononuclear cell infiltrate beyond the vascular adventitia into the adjacent alveolar septa, indicating a higher grade of rejection. Although it is the presence of perivascular infiltrates that determines the grade of acute rejection, inflammation of the large and small airways is incorporated into the grading system as the "B" category to reflect the fact that airway inflammation may predispose to obliterative bronchiolitis (Fig. 21–14). If rejection is present it usually involves more than one vessel, but when interpreting a perivascular infiltrate, the presence of a solitary blood vessel with a mononuclear infiltrate is evaluated using the same criteria that are applied to multiple infiltrates. In the severest grade of rejection (grade A4) on a biopsy that was taken early after transplantation, there may be some confusion with the histological picture of diffuse alveolar damage that may occur from an acute lung injury, but it is usually possible to separate rejection from diffuse alveolar damage by the presence of perivascular and interstitial mononuclear cells which are not usually present in lung injury.

One of the difficulties in diagnosing acute pulmonary rejection on transbronchial lung biopsy is the interpretation of **perivascular infiltrates.** Perivascular infiltrates with mononuclear cells are often seen in patients who have CMV pneumonitis or pneumocystis pneumonia but have not undergone lung transplantation (but have depressed immunity),[363] indicating that there may be overlap between acute pulmonary rejection and infection. Of course, acute pulmonary infection and rejection may occur simultaneously. There are infections with perivascular mononuclear infiltrates that are unequivocally due to infection; for example, CMV pneumonitis may be associated with cytopathic changes and positive immunoperoxidase stain, and pneumocystis pneumonia may be confirmed by the presence of organisms. A large number of neutrophils together with perivascular mononuclear infiltrates may suggest infection rather than rejection.[403] A study by Sibley and colleagues[336] on the specificity of transbronchial lung biopsy after heart/lung and lung transplantation for infection and rejection, respectively, found considerable overlap between these two processes. Fifty percent of patients with perivascular infiltrates and evidence of infection who were treated only with antibiotics had disappearance of the infiltrates

TABLE 21–1	Working Formulation for Classification and Grading of Pulmonary Allograft Rejection	

GRADING	CLASSIFICATION	DESCRIPTION
A.	**Acute Rejection**	
A0	Normal pulmonary parenchyma	
A1	Minimal acute rejection	Scattered perivascular mononuclear infiltrates (2–3 cells in thickness); not obvious at low magnification (40× magnification)
A2	Mild acute rejection	Frequent perivascular mononuclear infiltrates; recognizable at low magnification; subendothelial infiltration by mononuclear cells ("endothelialitis"); no infiltration of mononuclear cells into adjacent alveolar septae or air spaces
A3	Moderate acute rejection	Dense perivascular mononuclear infiltrate; usually associated with endothelialitis; extension of the infiltrate into peribronchiolar alveolar septae and air spaces
A4	Severe acute rejection	Diffuse perivascular interstitial and air space infiltrate of mononuclear cells; prominent alveolar pneumocyte damage; hyaline membranes, macrophages, hemorrhage, and neutrophils
B.	**Acute Airway Damage**	
B0	No airway inflammation	
B1	Minimal airway inflammation	Rare scattered mononuclear cells in the submucosa of the bronchi or bronchioles
B2	Mild airway inflammation	Circumferential mononuclear cells and occasional eosinophils within the submucosa of bronchi and/or bronchioles; no significant transepithelial migration of lymphocytes
B3	Moderate airway inflammation	Dense band-like infiltrated mononuclear cells in the submucosa of bronchi and/or bronchioles; epithelial cell necrosis; marked lymphocyte transmigration through epithelium
B4	Severe airway inflammation	Dense band-like infiltrate of activated mononuclear cells in bronchi and/or bronchioles; dissociation of epithelium from basement membrane; epithelial ulceration; fibropurulent exudates with neutrophils; epithelial necrosis
BX	Ungradable because of sampling or infection	
C	**Chronic Airway Damage**	
C1	Active bronchiolitis obliterans	Intrabronchiolar and/or peribronchiolar submucosal mononuclear infiltrate; fibrosis; epithelial damage
C2	Inactive	Dense fibrous scarring without cellular infiltrates in the bronchioles
D	**Chronic Vascular Rejection**	Fibrointimal thickening of arteries and veins

Adapted from Yousem SA, Berry GJ, Cagle PT, Chamberlain D, Husain AN, Hruban RH, Marchevsky A, Ohori NP, Ritter J, Stewart S, Tazelaar HD: Revision of the 1990 working formulation for the classification of pulmonary allograft rejection: Lung rejection study group. J Heart Lung Transplant 1996;15:1–15.

on follow-up biopsies. Furthermore, a further confusing finding has been the apparent spontaneous disappearance of perivascular lymphocytic infiltrates in patients who are not given therapy for acute rejection.[336, 403] This study underscores the difficulty at times in distinguishing infection from rejection histologically, and the results of transbronchial lung biopsy should not be taken in isolation but considered as one piece of information in the clinical picture in an individual patient.

Open lung biopsy will occasionally be required after heart/lung transplantation for the diagnosis of graft dysfunction or when an infiltrate appears on chest x-ray. At UAB there is no hesitation in proceeding with open lung biopsy, particularly for the diagnosis of graft dysfunction when the transbronchial lung biopsy has been unsuccessful in demonstrating the cause.

Other methods have been investigated for diagnosing acute pulmonary rejection experimentally. Bronchial mucosal blood flow determined by a noninvasive laser Doppler flow meter is significantly reduced during acute rejection after single-lung transplantation[360, 361] and reverses after treatment of rejection.[358] An increase in blood eosinophil count was found to be an early marker of acute pulmonary or cardiac rejection after lung or heart transplantation, respectively.[369] Serum IL-2 levels were found to increase in the presence of acute pulmonary

rejection after lung transplantation, but similar findings occurred with pulmonary infection.[161] Increased level of exhaled nitric oxide[240] and inducible nitric oxide synthase (detected by mRNA lung tissue)[397] were found in experimental acute pulmonary rejection, suggesting that measurement of exhaled nitric oxide may represent a noninvasive way of detecting acute pulmonary rejection. None of these methods has yet been routinely incorporated into clinical practice after heart/lung or lung transplantation.

The diagnosis of acute cardiac rejection after heart/lung transplantation is made according to the endomyocardial biopsy protocol outlined in Chapter 14. However, after about 4 months, the diagnosis of acute cardiac rejection is rarely made after heart/lung transplantation,[108] and this information is confirmed by observing the relatively flat slope of the curve of freedom from acute cardiac rejection beyond 12 months after heart/lung transplantation (Fig. 21–13).

Treatment of Acute Rejection

The treatment of acute cardiac rejection after heart/lung transplantation follows the same protocols as for treatment of cardiac rejection after isolated heart transplantation and is outlined in Chapter 14.

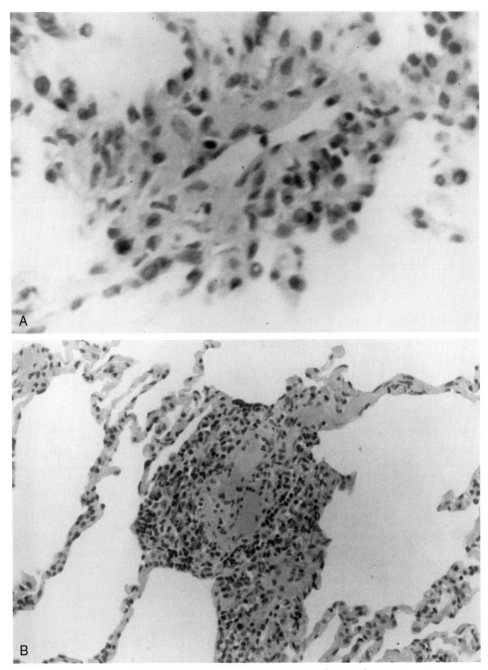

FIGURE **21–14.** *A,* Grade A1 pulmonary rejection. *B,* Grade A3 pulmonary rejection.
Illustration continued on following page

The great majority of heart/lung transplant patients experience at least one episode of acute pulmonary rejection.[169] There are a number of options for treating acute pulmonary rejection after heart/lung transplantation, and much of the experience has been derived from lung transplantation. The protocol for treatment of acute pulmonary rejection after heart/lung transplantation at UAB is outlined in Table 21–2. The initial two episodes are treated with pulse methylprednisolone, and these episodes are invariably early after transplantation. Acute pulmonary rejection occurring late (>6 months) after transplantation is still treated with pulse methylprednisolone, although other options may be used such as high-dose oral prednisone with a tapering schedule. Unresponsive rejection at UAB is treated by switching cyclosporine to tacrolimus and azathioprine to mycophenolate mofetil. Several studies suggest that tacrolimus is effective therapy for persistent and recurrent acute rejection after lung transplantation[148, 268] and may be as effective as OKT3.[234] OKT3 has been demonstrated to be effective therapy for reversing steroid-resistant and high-grade acute lung rejection during the first 6 months after transplantation[329] and may be effective therapy for patients with persistent rejection after heart/lung transplantation who have not received OKT3 as induction therapy. For patients with recalcitrant rejec-

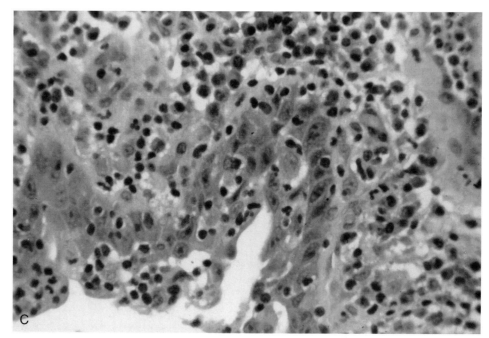

FIGURE **21-14.** *Continued* C, Grade B3 airway inflammation. See Table 21–1 for histologic features.

tion who have previously received OKT3, a number of options may be considered. Photopheresis[12] and total lymphoid irradiation are effective therapy for persistent and recurrent acute pulmonary rejection after heart/ lung and isolated lung transplantation.[373] Aerosolized cyclosporine has also been used after lung transplantation in patients with acute cellular rejection that was refractory to pulse steroids and cytolytic therapy.[171]

AIRWAY COMPLICATIONS

In the early days of lung transplantation, airway complications, particularly bronchial dehiscence, was a major cause of death. One of the important advances in lung transplantation has been the identification of factors contributing to airway complications, their prevention, and their management. In heart/lung transplantation, however, the incidence of airway problems is considerably

TABLE 21-2	Treatment of Acute Pulmonary Rejection in Heart/Lung Transplant Recipients (UAB)
INDICATION	TREATMENT
Initial episodes (2 episodes)	Methylprednisolone 1,000 mg daily IV (3 days)
Unresponsive rejection	Switch Cyclosporine to tacrolimus Azathioprine to mycophenolate mofetil *or* OKT3/Thymoglobulin
Recurrent rejection despite tacrolimus, mycophenolate, and/or OKT3/Thymoglobulin	Photopheresis

less than that of single and bilateral sequential lung transplantation, but the knowledge gained of this problem in lung transplantation is directly transferable to heart/lung transplantation.

Currently, the incidence of airway complications for single and bilateral sequential lung transplantation is between 4 and 14%,[72, 116, 318] with a risk of dying due to this complication of approximately 2%.[318] The risk of a major airway complication after heart/lung transplantation is approximately half that of single-lung transplantation.[334, 359]

The airway complications that may be seen after heart/lung transplantation are a spectrum of injury that invariably involve donor mucosal injury which may range from minor patchy loss to extensive denuding of the donor airway. If the injury involves more than just the mucosa, more serious complications are likely. Airway dehiscence (complete or partial) may be contained by mediastinal tissue or a perianastomotic wrap, or it may freely communicate with the mediastinum, producing mediastinal infection. The late sequela of partial dehiscence may be airway stricture formation, or, when extensive full-thickness airway injury occurs, tracheomalacia. Usually, multiple components contribute to the airway injury.

The fundamental etiologic factor in airway injury after heart/lung transplantation and lung transplantation is airway ischemia. The blood supply of the distal trachea and carina involves extensive extrapulmonary anastomoses between the bronchial arteries and vessels supplying other structures in the mediastinum, including esophageal, thymic, intercostal, thyrocervical, pericardiophrenic, and coronary arteries.[58, 69, 291] After single or bilateral sequential lung transplantation, without reimplantation of the bronchial arteries, the only source of blood supply to the donor bronchus is by retrograde perfusion from the pulmonary circulation until neovascularization of the donor bronchus occurs, which probably requires 3–4 weeks.[337] However, in heart/lung transplantation without reimplantation of the bronchial arteries, there is a potential source of oxygenated blood at a higher perfusion pressure to the donor airway through donor coronary-tracheal collateral vessels. Normally, these collateral vessels between the coronary and bronchial circulation are small and nonfunctional,[58] but they may increase substantially in the heart/lung donor block (Fig. 21–15) and also in certain nontransplant conditions.[38, 123, 379, 413] A further source of collateral blood supply from the pulmonary artery to the lower trachea has been demonstrated in the human.[196] This collateral blood supply of the donor airway in heart/lung transplantation contributes to the lower incidence of airway complications for this procedure as compared with lung transplantation that relies solely on a blood supply with poorly saturated blood at low perfusion pressure. The technique of en bloc double-lung transplantation which involved a tracheal anastomosis had a substantial incidence of airway complications,[275] likely related to the severing of the coronary-tracheal collaterals when the heart was removed from the heart/lung block. This incidence was substantially reduced when bronchial artery revascularization was performed in the en bloc double-lung transplant technique.[31, 278]

In addition to the blood supply of the donor airway, other factors contribute to airway ischemia. Phenomena which compromise an already tenuous blood supply to the donor airway include reperfusion-induced peribronchial edema, low cardiac output exacerbated by the use of alpha-adrenergic agents, acute pulmonary rejection which increases pulmonary vascular resistance (suggested by laser-Doppler measurements of submucosal blood flow in acute rejection),[358] and high-pressure ventilation reducing submucosal blood flow.

A number of measures can be taken to minimize the chances of an airway problem after heart/lung transplantation, including some important technical details. Keeping the **donor trachea** as short as possible (without impinging on the right or left main stem bronchus) will reduce the amount of donor airway that needs to be supplied by coronary-tracheal collateral vessels. Ensuring that preservation of the lungs is optimal will reduce the chances of primary graft dysfunction and airway edema. During excision of the heart/lung block from the donor, it is of utmost importance that the dissection does not involve areas that could compromise coronary-tracheal collateral vessels, specifically subcarinal dissection.

Bronchial artery revascularization has been performed in heart/lung transplantation by anastomosing the internal thoracic artery over the orifices of the bronchial arteries within the donor descending thoracic aorta[254] which, in a series of patients undergoing single- and double-lung transplantation and heart/lung transplantation had a patency at 2 years[253] of 100%. However, bronchial artery revascularization in heart/lung transplantation is unlikely to be widely applied because of the additional complexity that it entails. A number of anastomotic wraps have been used in heart/lung transplantation, but these are probably not essential for healing. The omental wrap does have the theoretical advantage of promoting neovascularization, but probably the major advantage of the wrap is to contain an anastomotic dehiscence. Other wraps that have been used include pericardial flaps, intercostal muscle flaps, and peritracheal adventitial wraps. Although the benefit is unproven, we routinely employ and recommend the use of a pericardial flap because of its simplicity and theoretical benefit in walling off a localized dehiscence.

Although the major source of tracheal anastomotic ischemia relates to the donor trachea, it is also important to remember that improper handling of the **native (recipient) tracheal end** can also produce an inadequate blood supply to that side of the anastomosis. The blood supply to the trachea comes in laterally, and it is known from the experience in tracheal resection that extensive "mobilization" of the proximal trachea by freeing up the lateral aspects of the trachea for several rings proximal to the anastomosis may compromise blood supply. Therefore, we expose only one ring of recipient trachea above the level of transection, use lateral silk stay sutures to facilitate its exposure, and incorporate surrounding peritracheal adventitial tissue with the anastomosis (taking care to avoid any intraluminal protrusion of such tissue).

In the postoperative period after heart/lung transplantation, avoidance of high-pressure ventilation, avoidance of high-dose alpha-adrenergic drug infusion, and prompt treatment of graft edema may help to preserve an already precarious blood supply to the donor airway.

In the unlikely event of a major dehiscence of the tracheal anastomosis, the only possibility of successful treatment is prompt reoperation, but the associated

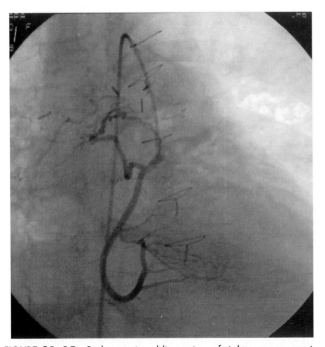

FIGURE **21–15.** Right anterior oblique view of right coronary angiogram in a patient following heart/lung transplantation. There is a markedly enlarged right atrial coronary branch that is providing collaterals to the carina.

spreading mediastinal sepsis usually has a fatal outcome. As previously mentioned, there is a wide spectrum of airway complications, and mucosal loss and small partial dehiscences that are contained will usually heal without long-term sequelae. However, more serious airway injuries, usually from a combination injury, may have important long-term sequelae. For example, a contained tracheal dehiscence associated with extensive mucosal loss can result in excessive granulation tissue around the dehiscence and tracheomalacia, which results in shortness of breath, wheezing, cough, retained secretions, and eventually respiratory failure. This type of problem may be evident as early as 2–4 weeks after transplantation and is best treated by restoring airway patency by laser photocoagulation to the granulation tissue and by insertion of airway stents. In the presence of malacia and granulation tissue, the expanding wire stent such as the Wall stent (Schneider) or the Gianturco stent (Cook, Inc.), which have been used in lung transplantation,[138] have proven useful. For an extensive injury of this type, bilateral expanding wire stents can be placed in the proximal main stem bronchi (Fig. 21–16) and for more chronic and cicatricial stenoses, laser resection and silicone stents may be useful.

Invasive fungal infection may be superimposed on airway complications after heart/lung and lung transplantation, and they may occur independently of airway and anastomotic injury. *Aspergillus* has been the most frequently described anastomotic infection, but candidal anastomotic infection also occurs.[46, 162, 188, 271] It is important that during transbronchial lung biopsy the anastomotic area is also biopsied in any patient with evidence of necrotic pseudomembranes to exclude invasive fungal infection. Morbidity and mortality associated with invasive anastomotic fungal infection is high, but successful treatment of candidal invasive anastomotic infection after lung transplantation has been reported[271] with

a combination of intravenous amphotericin B, inhaled amphotericin B, and oral fluconazole.

OBLITERATIVE BRONCHIOLITIS

Obliterative bronchiolitis was first described by Lange in 1901[198] and refers to a condition in nontransplant patients that is characterized by plugging of the small airways with granulation tissue and destruction of the small airways due to obliterative scarring. Obliterative bronchiolitis has been described in association with a number of precipitating factors including toxic fume exposure (such as sulfur dioxide, chlorine, phosgene, ozone, and ammonia), infectious agents such as mycoplasma and viral infections, and secondary to other causes such as hypersensitivity pneumonitis and eosinophilic pneumonia.

Obliterative bronchiolitis was first recognized as a complication of clinical lung transplantation by Burke and colleagues in 1984,[49] who described the condition after heart/lung transplantation, and it was subsequently recognized after single- and double-lung transplantation.[73, 212] Obliterative bronchiolitis is currently the major limiting factor to long-term survival after lung and, along with allograft coronary artery disease, after heart/lung transplantation. Even though the prevalence of obliterative bronchiolitis varies depending on the criteria used to make the diagnosis, there is no doubt regarding its frequent occurrence among recipients of heart/lung and lung transplants (Fig. 21–17) (actuarial freedom from obliterative bronchiolitis in survivors being 76% at 1 year and 37% at 3 years)[374] and its substantial impact on survival. The prevalence of obliterative bronchiolitis in children and adolescents surviving heart/lung transplantation appears to be at least as great as in adults.[390]

Although most series have not found a difference in the prevalence of obliterative bronchiolitis after heart/lung versus lung transplantation,[136, 174, 293] one report[391] (heart/lung transplantation for primary pulmonary hypertension) did suggest that the prevalence of obliterative bronchiolitis was lower than that usually seen after single- or double-lung transplantation.

Pathology of Obliterative Bronchiolitis

Obliterative bronchiolitis is a disease of the terminal and respiratory bronchioles (see Box). The earliest histologic finding in obliterative bronchiolitis is ulceration of the bronchial epithelium followed by an intraluminal accumulation of reactive inflammatory cells and necrotic epithelial cells which becomes organized into granulation tissue plugging the bronchiolar lumen. The bronchiolar wall develops submucosal fibrosis and as the organization process continues, the bronchiolar lumen is obliterated by scar tissue[364, 406] (Fig. 21–18). The process is not necessarily uniform, and in any one histological section normal bronchioles may be seen alongside bronchioles infiltrated by inflammatory cells. Vascular changes have been described in patients with obliterative bronchiolitis, and these are characterized by myofibrointimal pro-

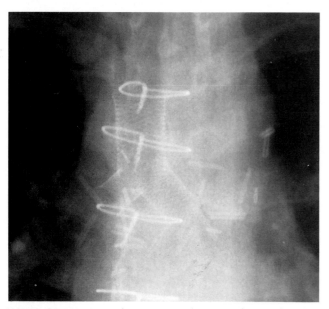

FIGURE **21–16.** X-ray demonstrating placement of expanding wire stents (Wall stents) in both main stem bronchi for an extensive airway injury after heart/lung transplantation.

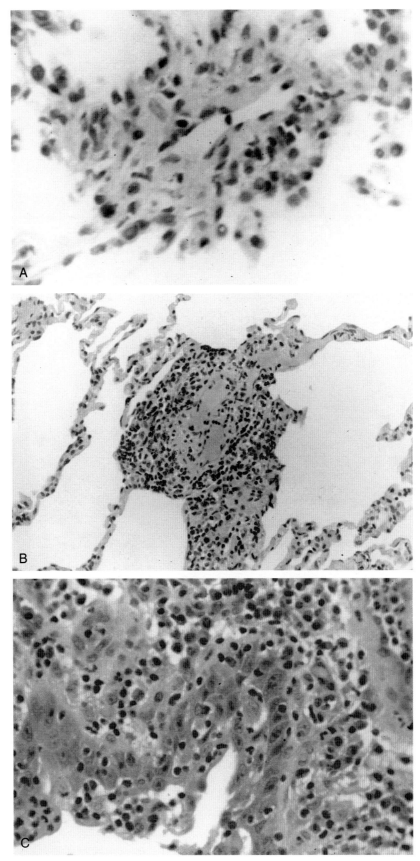

FIGURE **21–14.** *A*, Grade A1 pulmonary rejection. *B*, Grade A3 pulmonary rejection. *C*, Grade B3 airway inflammation. See Table 21–1 for histologic features.

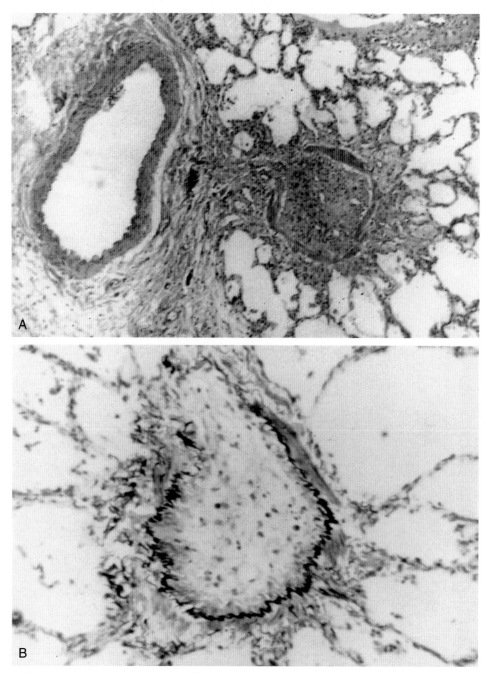

FIGURE **21–18.** *A,* Hematoxylin and eosin stain of bronchiole demonstrating active obliterative bronchiolitis. Note the normal alveoli surrounding the bronchiole. *B,* Trichrome stain of bronchiole demonstrating collagen deposition in obliterative bronchiolitis.

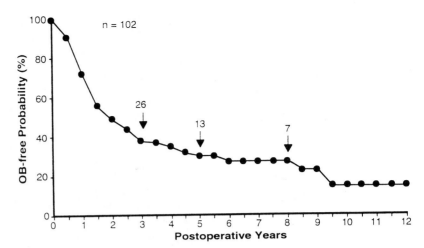

FIGURE **21-17.** Actuarial freedom from obliterative bronchiolitis (OB) in greater than 90-day survivors and recipients over 5 years of age after heart/lung and bilateral sequential lung transplantation (median onset, 689 days after transplantation). (From Valentine VG, Robbins RC, Wehner JH, Patel HR, Berry GJ, Theodore J: Total lymphoid irradiation for refractory acute rejection in heart/lung and lung allografts. Chest 1996;109:1184–1189.)

liferation with collagen deposition,[405] a process which may also affect the pulmonary veins. These vascular changes, however, may be seen in lung and heart/lung transplant recipients who do not have obliterative bronchiolitis.

Obliterative bronchiolitis must be distinguished from **bronchiolitis obliterans organizing pneumonia** (BOOP). Although the clinical and radiographic presentation may be similar, the histologic picture of BOOP is quite distinct and is characterized by intraluminal granulation tissue polyps which are attached to the bronchial wall and project into the alveolar ducts. This process is usually a reaction to a concomitant condition such as diffuse alveolar damage, infection, or rejection, and is also distinct from obliterative bronchiolitis in that BOOP is quite responsive to steroids.

Pathogenesis of Obliterative Bronchiolitis

The pathogenesis of obliterative bronchiolitis has not been fully elucidated. As the histology suggests, obliter-

Structure of the Bronchioles

In human lungs, the intrapulmonary bronchi ramify into the bronchioles, which consist of the terminal bronchioles and a transition area between the terminal bronchioles and the alveoli called the respiratory bronchioles.[280] The terminal bronchioles are between the 13th and 16th generations of airway branching[280] and are from 0.8–2.5 mm in length, with an average luminal diameter of 0.6 mm in the adult. Terminal bronchioles branch into two or three respiratory bronchioles, each on average having three generations.[60] Terminal bronchioles are lined by nonciliated columnar, ciliated columnar, and basal cells, whereas the respiratory bronchioles have a mixed population of cells, reflecting the fact that the respiratory bronchioles have the function not only of a conducting airway but also of gas exchange. The more proximal end of the respiratory bronchiole has a cell population similar to that of the terminal bronchiole, whereas the distal end of the respiratory bronchiole has the characteristics of alveolar epithelial lining with squamous cells and cuboidal cells with features of alveolar type II cells.

ative bronchiolitis is very likely related to airway injury, and there are a number of possible injurious processes that can be implicated. There is good reason to believe that obliterative bronchiolitis is primarily related to **immunologic injury.** A number of studies have demonstrated a relationship between the frequency (Fig. 21–19)[25] and severity (Fig. 21–20)[25] of acute cellular rejection after lung and heart/lung transplantation[25, 107, 192, 293, 322, 327, 381, 390] and the development of obliterative bronchiolitis. Furthermore, an experimental allograft model of transplantation of tracheal segments into the subcutaneous position in the rat demonstrated that lymphocytic infiltration was a precursor to fibrous obliteration of the allograft airway lumen,[42] and this did not occur in similarly implanted isografts. A number of other phenomena have been observed to indirectly suggest an immunologic etiology for obliterative bronchiolitis. In a small number of patients undergoing heart/lung transplantation Yousem and colleagues[407] demonstrated increased HLA class II antigen positive dendritic cells in the donor bronchial epithelium and submucosa in patients with obliterative bronchiolitis compared to those without it, although these increased dendritic cells also occurred in the recipient airways. Presumably, they could represent a source for antigen presentation as part of a chronic rejection process. Other indirect evidence suggesting the involvement of multiple immunological phenomena includes a demonstration that lymphocytes obtained from the lungs of patients with obliterative bronchiolitis recognize both class I and II donor HLA antigens,[288] the finding of CD8[+] lymphocytes with anti–class I HLA specificity in patients with obliterative bronchiolitis who rapidly succumbed to the process,[297] and the finding of donor antigen-specific lymphocyte hyporeactivity in patients without as compared to those with obliterative bronchiolitis.[298] This multiple immunological attack on the bronchial epithelium almost certainly includes a humoral component, which is suggested by the finding of anti-HLA antibodies in patients with obliterative bronchiolitis.[343, 355] Obliterative bronchiolitis has also been correlated with less microchimerism in blood, lymph node, and skin.[173]

A relationship between **cytomegalovirus** illness and subsequent development of obliterative bronchiolitis re-

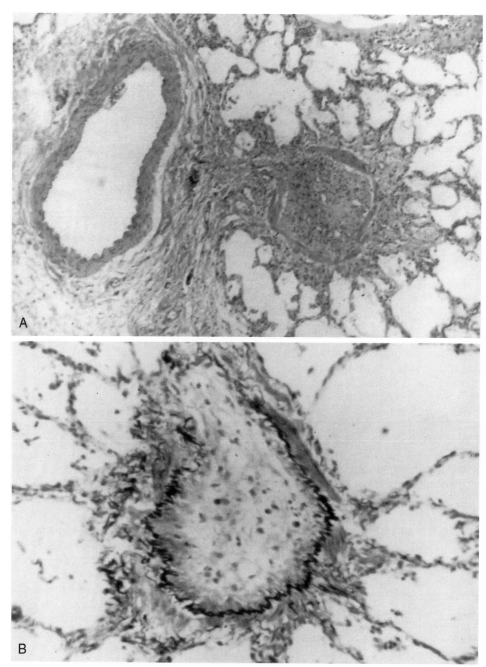

FIGURE **21–18.** *A,* Hematoxylin and eosin stain of bronchiole demonstrating active obliterative bronchiolitis. Note the normal alveoli surrounding the bronchiole. *B,* Trichrome stain of bronchiole demonstrating collagen deposition in obliterative bronchiolitis.

mains controversial. The inability to clearly establish this relationship may in part relate to the different criteria for CMV "involvement" such as CMV syndrome (positive CMV culture from any site with typical symptoms of CMV infection), CMV pneumonitis (pulmonary symptoms and signs with positive culture or typical CMV inclusions), asymptomatic pulmonary CMV infection (CMV isolation from BAL without symptoms or signs), CMV disease (positive CMV culture from any site with intracellular inclusions), and asymptomatic CMV infection (CMV culture from any site in the absence of symptoms of CMV infection). In a study by Kroshus, symptomatic CMV pulmonary infection was, by multivariable analysis, a risk factor for the subsequent

development of obliterative bronchiolitis, whereas asymptomatic CMV infection was not a risk factor.[192] The putative relationship between CMV and obliterative bronchiolitis has been also demonstrated by others,[25, 83, 172, 343] although it has not been a universal finding.[66, 381] The association is perhaps analogous to the development of coronary vasculopathy after cardiac transplantation and CMV infection[93, 111, 228, 231] and may represent a consequence of the known immunomodulating effect of viral infection. CMV infection is known to up-regulate the immune system by increasing the number and activity of antigen-presenting cells in lung[117] and kidney[367] allografts. During such infection, lymphocytes may be activated and release lymphokines that can augment the

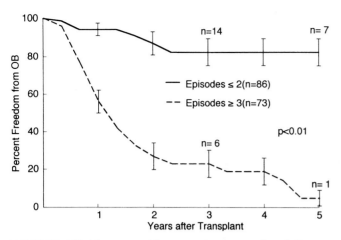

FIGURE **21–19.** The impact of three episodes or more of grade II acute rejection on development of obliterative bronchiolitis (OB). OB was more likely to develop in recipients with more frequent episodes of acute rejection than in those with fewer episodes of acute rejection (*p* < .01 by generalized Wilcoxon test). (From Bando K, Paradis IL, Similo S: Cardiac and pulmonary replacement: obliterative bronchiolitis after lung and heart-lung transplantation: an analysis of risk factors and management. J Thorac Cardiovasc Surg 1995;110:4–13.)

allogenic response. CMV-specific cells may up-regulate donor MHC antigens because of the release of cytokines such as IFN-γ.[411] An increased expression of MHC class II HLA antigens has previously been demonstrated in association with obliterative bronchiolitis.[362, 408] In an experimental model of obliterative bronchiolitis,[295] acute and chronic CMV infection increased the intensity of the immune response as well as the obliterative airway process, suggesting that the recipient immune response is up-regulated by CMV infection, which may also have a direct stimulatory effect on myofibroblast and smooth muscle cells. If this association were true, CMV prophylaxis at the time of transplantation and augmented immunosuppression would seem prudent.

Airway ischemia has been suggested[25] as a potential cause of obliterative bronchiolitis and could perhaps be responsible for or contribute to this process through the response to bronchiolar epithelial injury together with lymphatic disruption and pulmonary denervation (resulting in an impaired mucociliary function and secretion clearance).[294] Although these may not be the major factors, their contribution to the progression of the process seems likely.

Diagnosis

The term **bronchiolitis obliterans syndrome** (BOS) is used to describe the clinical deterioration of pulmonary graft function and is distinct from the term obliterative bronchiolitis, which describes the pathological features. This distinction recognizes the fact that BOS is not necessarily accompanied by its pathological counterpart and that the finding of obliterative bronchiolitis on a biopsy is not necessarily accompanied by clinical deterioration in graft function. The symptoms and signs of BOS after heart/lung transplantation may appear as early as 6 months after transplantation. Shortness of breath on exertion and a persistant cough are the earliest symptoms.

On clinical examination, expiration is prolonged and high-pitched squeaks are heard in late inspiration. As the process progresses, airway colonization, usually with *Pseudomonas,* may develop, and in the late stages hypoxemia and finally hypercapnia occur.

The physiological consequence of obliterative bronchiolitis is a **progressive fall in airflow** as measured by spirometric tests. The typical finding is a fall in both FVC and FEV_1, with the fall in FEV_1 usually being greater. The FEF_{25-75} is a more sensitive test for BOS, the fall in FEV_{25-75} usually occurring earlier and with a greater proportional decrease than FEV_1.[276] A typical pattern of decline in airflow after heart/lung transplantation is illustrated in Figure 21–21. Specific airway conductance (sGaw) measures dysfunction in small airways which, like FEV_{25-75}, is perhaps a more sensitive means of early detection of BOS.[30] The International Society for Heart and Lung Transplantation (ISHLT) has proposed a staging system for chronic dysfunction of lung allografts (largely reflecting BOS) (Table 21–3),[65] and this serves as a means of communicating the severity of graft dysfunction. Plain chest film features of obliterative bronchiolitis may be subtle and are usually nonspecific, but high-resolution computed tomography may demonstrate a number of features including air trapping, bronchiectasis, bronchial dilatation, and areas of consolidation.[124, 156, 217] On ventilation-perfusion scan a fall in ventilation can usually be detected.[124]

There is interest in identifying a sensitive biochemical marker of early obliterative bronchiolitis from bronchoalveolar lavage (BAL) fluid, since identification of obliterative bronchiolitis prior to loss of airflow may allow intervention at an early stage of this process. Fibroblast proliferative activity (an assay reflecting fibroblast-stimulating cytokines in BAL fluid),[160] and platelet-derived growth factor (PDGF) are examples of cytokines that may find a role in the early diagnosis of obliterative bronchiolitis. Hyaluronic acid has also been suggested

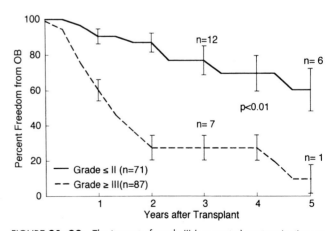

FIGURE **21–20.** The impact of grade III (or greater) acute rejection on freedom from the development of OB. OB was more likely to develop in recipients with one episode or more of grade III (or greater) acute rejection than in those with less severe (≤ grade II) acute rejection (*p* < .01 by generalized Wilcoxon test). (From Bando K, Paradis IL, Similo S: Cardiac and pulmonary replacement: obliterative bronchiolitis after lung and heart-lung transplantation: an analysis of risk factors and management. J Thorac Cardiovasc Surg 1995;110:4–13.)

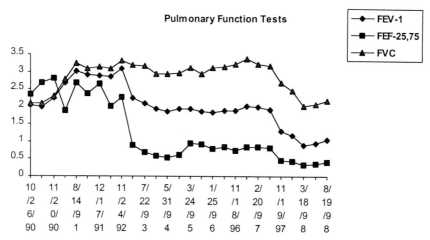

FIGURE 21-21. Typical pattern of declining airflow with the onset of bronchiolitis obliterans syndrome after heart/lung transplantation. See text for description of pulmonary function tests.

as a marker,[323] since it has been identified in BAL fluid from patients with fibrotic lung disease. Biochemical markers of granulocyte function from the peripheral blood[129] have been used to detect early obliterative bronchiolitis, but reliable early biochemical markers currently do not exist. The presence of obliterative bronchiolitis must be confirmed by histological examination of lung tissue. Biopsy is important not only to establish the diagnosis but also to exclude other causes of graft dysfunction, including acute rejection and infection. Unfortunately, the sensitivity of transbronchial lung biopsy in the diagnosis of obliterative bronchiolitis is variable,[190, 282, 404] likely due to the patchy nature of this condition. When the diagnosis is in doubt, open lung biopsy is probably more likely to confirm the diagnosis.

Treatment

Since the outlook for patients with BOS after lung and heart/lung transplantation is similar, the much greater lung transplant experience is an important source of information for describing the treatment of this condition. The results of treatment of established BOS have been poor, which is perhaps not surprising, since when the syndrome is clinically advanced there is extensive

and irreversible small airway scarring. The use of optimization of maintenance immunosuppression, high-dose steroids, cytolytic therapy,[71, 180] and methotrexate[84] have all been disappointing. Total lymphoid irradiation has also been used,[9, 80] with little favorable impact. There is preliminary evidence that photopheresis may be effective in stabilizing the progressive loss in airflow in established BOS.[3, 164, 263, 314, 340] Although not currently rigorously substantiated, the strategy of early detection and treatment of small airway immune injury may ameliorate BOS.

These histological lesions of obliterative bronchiolitis (active and inactive), acute cellular rejection (A_{0-4}, B_{0-4}) and lymphocytic bronchiolitis (A_0, B_{1-4}) are histologically distinct, and each may be found in an individual patient's biopsy. The strategy at UAB is currently to regard recalcitrant cellular rejection, late cellular rejection (>6 months),[179] lymphocytic bronchiolitis,[308] and active obliterative bronchiolitis as each being a part of an immune process that can potentially result in the progressive and irreversible scarring of obliterative bronchiolitis. When any of these clinical patterns or histological features are found, the immunosuppression is converted from cyclosporine to tacrolimus and from azathioprine to mycophenolate mofetil. The use of tacrolimus as either res-

TABLE 21-3	**Obliterative Bronchiolitis Staging System**
Stage 0:	No significant abnormality: FEV_1 80% or more of baseline value
	a. Without pathologic evidence of obliterative bronchiolitis
	b. With pathologic evidence of obliterative bronchiolitis
Stage 1:	Mild obliterative bronchiolitis syndrome: FEV_1 66–80% of baseline value
	a. Without pathologic evidence of obliterative bronchiolitis
	b. With pathologic evidence of obliterative bronchiolitis
Stage 2:	Moderate obliterative bronchiolitis syndrome: FEV_1 51–65% of baseline value
	a. Without pathologic evidence of obliterative bronchiolitis
	b. With pathologic evidence of obliterative bronchiolitis
Stage 3:	Severe obliterative bronchiolitis syndrome: FEV_1 50% or less of baseline value
	a. Without pathologic evidence of obliterative bronchiolitis
	b. With pathologic evidence of obliterative bronchiolitis

From Cooper JD, Billingham M, Egan T, Hertz MI, Higenbottam T, Lynch J, Mauer J, Paradis I, Patterson GA, Smith C, Trulock EP, Vreim C, Yousem S: A working formulation for the standardization of nomenclature and for clinical staging of chronic dysfunction in lung allografts. J Heart Lung Transplant 1993;12:713–716.

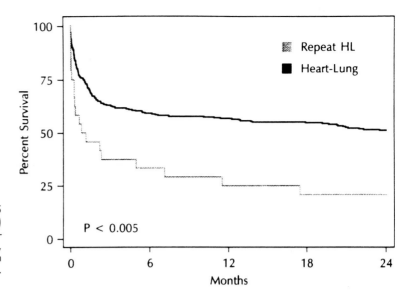

FIGURE **21–22.** Kaplan-Meier survival curve for the 25 patients undergoing repeat heart/lung transplantation (HL) compared with 290 first-time heart/lung recipients at Harefield Hospital ($p < .005$). (From Adams DH, Cochrane AD, Khaghani A, Smith JD, Yacoub MH: Retransplantation in heart-lung recipients with obliterative bronchiolitis. J Thorac Cardiovasc Surg 1994;107:450–459.)

cue therapy for BOS[178, 292] or as part of maintenance therapy, with a demonstrated reduction in the incidence of obliterative bronchiolitis[170] and delayed development of BOS[173] has been reported. The use of mycophenolate mofetil has been demonstrated[348, 392] to stabilize pulmonary function of patients with BOS. If the immune response has not been cleared by switching of maintenance immunosuppression, the patient is commenced on photopheresis. New immunologic agents such as sirolimus and leflunomide which have antiproliferative effects may find a role in lung and heart/lung transplantation because of these properties.

Once progressive BOS is established, at UAB these patients receive inhaled tobramycin (80 mg three times a day by a nebulizer) as prophylaxis against *Pseudomonas* airway infection, which would undoubtedly contribute to the airway injury. The results of retransplantation in heart/lung recipients with obliterative bronchiolitis are generally poor (Fig. 21–22), but the results of retransplantation will likely continue to improve. The type of retransplant procedure in heart/lung transplant recipients (single, double-lung, heart/lung) remains controversial. Obliterative bronchiolitis does not appear to recur in an accelerated fashion following retransplantation.[260]

CORONARY VASCULOPATHY

Although coronary vasculopathy occurs after heart/lung transplantation, its incidence is significantly less than that after heart transplantation.[341] In part, this may be due to the less frequent need for treatment of cardiac rejection in heart/lung transplant recipients and also the donor population, which is usually younger than cardiac transplant donors.[36, 315] A study by Whyte and colleagues[391] of the result of heart/lung transplantation in patients with primary pulmonary hypertension demonstrated 92% freedom from coronary vasculopathy at

5 years after transplantation (Fig. 21–23),[391] which is considerably lower than the reported incidence of coronary vasculopathy after heart transplantation. In an intracoronary ultrasound study[207] of matched heart and heart/lung transplant recipients, there was significantly less coronary vasculopathy in terms of incidence and severity in heart/lung transplant recipients. This lower incidence of coronary vasculopathy after heart/lung transplantation has also been observed in pediatric patients.[289] The development of obliterative bronchiolitis has been associated with the appearance of coronary vasculopathy.[36, 168]

LONG-TERM COMPLICATIONS OF IMMUNOSUPPRESSION

Long term complications of immunosuppression after heart/lung transplantation are identical to those after

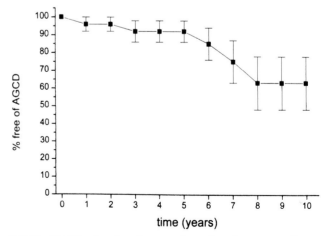

FIGURE **21–23.** Freedom from accelerated graft coronary disease (AGCD) after heart/lung transplantation for primary pulmonary hypertension. (From Whyte RI, Robbins RC, Altinger J, Barlow CW, Doyle R, Theodore J, Reitz BA: Heart-lung transplantation for primary pulmonary hypertension. Ann Thorac Surg 1999;67:937–941.)

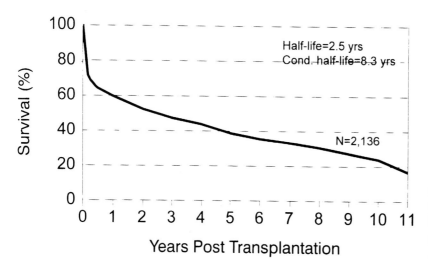

FIGURE **21–24.** Heart/lung transplantation actuarial survival based on data from the ISHLT registry. (From Hosenpud JD, Bennett LE, Keck BM, Fiol B, Novick RJ: The Registry of the International Society for Heart and Lung Transplantation: sixteenth official report—1999. J Heart Lung Transplant 1999;18:611–626.)

heart transplantation and are outlined in Chapters 13 and 18.

GRAFT-VERSUS-HOST DISEASE

Graft-versus-host disease (GVHD) is a very rare but lethal complication of heart/lung transplantation. A large quantity of lymphoid tissue is transplanted with the heart/lung block and GVHD has been reported in heart/lung transplant recipients.[150, 279, 359] The presentation of acute GVHD is similar to that which can occur after bone marrow transplantation and may include fever, maculopapular rash, diarrhea (due to colitis), hepatic dysfunction, pancytopenia, and pulmonary infiltrates. The diagnosis of GVHD is confirmed by immediate skin biopsy and by HLA typing of the peripheral lymphocytes. The only therapy which has a chance of being effective is aggressive cytolytic therapy to destroy donor lymphocytes, but the outcome is usually fatal.

SURVIVAL AFTER HEART/LUNG TRANSPLANTATION

Survival after heart/lung transplantation, although steadily improving, is still importantly less than that after heart transplantation. The ISHLT registry demonstrated a 1-year survival of approximately 60% and an 11-year survival of 21% (Fig. 21–24).[149] From the registry data, the causes of death (Fig. 21–25)[149] depend on the posttransplant time interval. Early after transplantation, the major causes of death include hemorrhage, nonspecific graft failure, and infection. During the remainder of the first year, the primary cause of death is infection, with a very large group of miscellaneous causes, and beyond 1 year the principal causes of death are obliterative bronchiolitis, infection, and miscellaneous causes. The multivariable analysis in the ISHLT registry demonstrated that risk factors for death during the first year after adult heart/lung transplantation include retransplantation, low center volume, and increasing donor age. The actuarial survival of patients undergoing

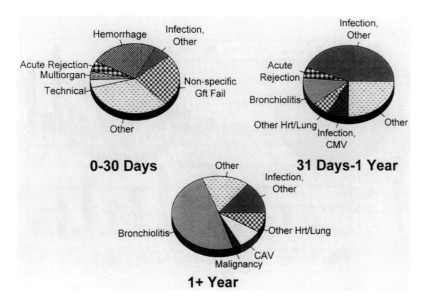

FIGURE **21–25.** Heart/lung transplantation cause of death by time after transplantation. CMV, cytomegalovirus; CAV, cardiac allograft vasculopathy. (From Hosenpud JD, Bennett LE, Keck BM, Fiol B, Novick RJ: The Registry of the International Society for Heart and Lung Transplantation: sixteenth official report—1999. J Heart Lung Transplant 1999;18:611–626.)

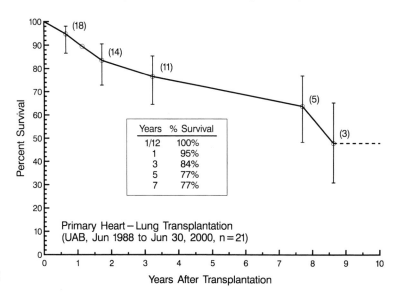

FIGURE **21–26.** Actuarial survival of patients undergoing heart/lung transplantation at UAB, 1988 to 2000.

heart/lung transplantation at UAB is 95% at 1 year, 84% at 3 years, and 77% at 7 years, which is comparable to that of isolated heart transplantation (Fig. 21–26).

COMBINED HEART/ KIDNEY TRANSPLANTATION

HISTORICAL BACKGROUND

Traditionally, the presence of severe coexistent renal disease (either associated or unassociated with the heart disease) in patients with end-stage heart disease has been an exclusionary criterion for cardiac transplantation because pretransplant renal dysfunction is believed to be a significant risk factor for increased morbidity and mortality. A serum creatinine greater than 2 mg/dL during the year prior to cardiac transplantation has been shown to be a risk factor for posttransplant acute renal failure in cyclosporine-treated patients.[230] A more recent analysis from the Cardiac Transplant Research Database (CTRD)[43] identified (by multivariable analysis) a higher creatinine in adult recipients at the time of transplantation as a possible risk factor for death after cardiac transplantation. The importance of higher creatinine at the time of transplantation as a risk factor for death would likely have been demonstrated convincingly if more patients with an abnormal creatinine had undergone cardiac transplantation (in this study, mean creatinine was 1.32 mg/dL; and only 6.3% of patients had a creatinine >2.0 mg/dL). McCaffrey and colleagues found that when the pretransplant creatinine was greater than 2.3 mg/dL, the 1-year and 5-year survival was 53% and 33%, respectively, compared with a 1- and 5-year survival of 89% and 81%, respectively, for patients without renal dysfunction.[225] Similarly, patients with end-stage renal disease with coexistent severe heart disease have not been considered for renal transplantation, because of the poor natural history of these patients. With the progressive improvement in the results

of cardiac transplantation and renal transplantation, it is not surprising that combined heart and kidney transplantation became a logical step. The first combined heart/kidney transplant was reported in 1978.[255] Since that time, there have been many reports of combined heart/kidney transplantation from the same donor in adults[32, 39, 51, 94, 110, 200, 209, 210, 317] and in a 12-year-old child.[223]

RECIPIENT SELECTION

There are three circumstances for which combined heart/kidney transplantation may be indicated: coexisting end-stage heart disease and intrinsic renal disease, severe renal dysfunction including acute tubular necrosis secondary to severe cardiac failure, and end-stage renal disease with secondary heart disease.

Combined End-Stage Heart Disease and Intrinsic Renal Disease

The most common indication for combined heart and kidney transplantation is coexisting combined end-stage heart and kidney disease. In a multicenter study[248] of 82 patients undergoing 84 combined heart and kidney transplant procedures, the most common pretransplant cardiac diagnoses were idiopathic dilated cardiomyopathy (38%) and end-stage ischemic heart disease (32%). Of the many causes of coexistent intrinsic renal disease, the most common diagnoses were diabetes mellitus (17%) and chronic glomerulonephritis (11%).

Although most patients with combined intrinsic end-stage renal disease and heart disease are on some form of dialysis,[110, 200, 317] the combined procedure may also be indicated in patients with end-stage heart disease and less severe intrinsic renal disease (worsened by heart failure) in whom cyclosporine-based immunosuppression after heart transplantation only would likely produce chronic renal failure. In patients with severe but not end-stage intrinsic renal disease with coexistent heart disease, the threshold of renal function below which the combined procedure would be recommended will vary from center to center, and the threshold cannot be defined with any precision. However, as a guide, combined heart and kidney transplantation in this particular group of patients should be considered when the creatinine clearance is less than 50 mL/min and/or the effective renal plasma flow (see Chapter 6) is less than 200 mL/min. An uncommon indication (but perhaps one that may increase in frequency) is patients requiring cardiac retransplantation due to coronary vasculopathy who have cyclosporine nephrotoxicity. This situation has previously been reported[32] and has been the indication for a combined heart/kidney transplant at UAB.

Severe Renal Dysfunction Secondary to Advanced Heart Failure

A more controversial indication for combined heart/kidney transplantation is renal failure, including acute tubular necrosis, which is secondary to severe heart failure. Although some argue that renal function will eventually recover in these patients and they can be successfully managed with postoperative dialysis, it would be highly unusual in the great majority of centers for heart transplantation to be performed in patients with acute renal failure secondary to low cardiac output. Thus, the results of the strategy of heart transplantation alone in these patients in most centers is unknown. A successful combined heart and kidney transplant has been performed at UAB in a patient with low cardiac output (due to primary graft failure) and renal failure due to acute tubular necrosis, the rationale being that survival of the patient was more likely with a working kidney as opposed to subjecting the patient to the risks of hemodialysis for an unknown period of time until renal function returned. Furthermore, if and when renal function does return if heart transplantation alone is performed, renal function would likely be abnormal due to some degree of permanent renal injury exacerbated by cyclosporine nephrotoxicity. A combined heart and kidney transplant was performed for this indication at The Prince Charles Hospital in Brisbane, Australia (A. Galbraith, personal communication).

End-Stage Renal Disease with Secondary Heart Disease

Combined heart and kidney transplantation should be rarely required for the group of patients with end-stage renal disease with secondary heart disease. There are a number of causes of cardiac failure in patients with end-stage renal disease, although the most frequent cause is coronary artery disease. However, there is a small group of patients in whom the end-stage renal disease is directly responsible for cardiac failure. Severe diastolic left ventricular dysfunction may result from chronic hypertension and systolic dysfunction may be induced by complications of end-stage renal disease such as overcirculation through a large fistula, anemia, and chronic volume overload.[186, 317] However, severe cardiac failure should be preventable in the majority of these patients

by careful attention to the treatment of hypertension and more frequent dialysis.[317] Uremic cardiomyopathy is a term used to describe a cardiomyopathic condition in patients with end-stage renal disease that cannot be attributed to hypertension, coronary artery disease, or overcirculation due to arteriovenous fistulas. Since this concept was suggested in 1944,[286] it remains controversial. There is some experimental evidence that uremia may be injurious to myofibers, but obtaining evidence for this process with end-stage renal disease remains difficult because of the invariably multiple reasons for heart failure in these patients. There are reports of patients with end-stage renal disease who have a cardiomyopathic process seemingly unrelated to hypertension or coronary artery disease whose left ventricular function improves after renal transplantation.[50, 197] A study by Larrson and colleagues[199] in patients with juvenile onset diabetes documented a reduction in left ventricular chamber size, decrease in left atrial size, decline in blood pressure, decrease in left ventricular wall thickness and mass, and improvement in diastolic function after renal transplantation. This improvement in cardiac function could be explained by altered loading conditions without necessarily invoking a uremic cardiomyopathic process. It would appear that patients with this type of cardiomyopathic process may be treatable by renal transplantation alone.

SURGICAL PROCEDURE

There are two approaches to the timing of combined heart and kidney transplantation: as a single combined procedure[200, 317] and as a staged operation. Our current preference at UAB is to complete the cardiac transplant procedure as the first stage and transfer the patient to the intensive care unit. The patient is returned to the operating room for renal transplantation several hours later when cardiac function has stabilized and mediastinal drainage is no longer of concern. Although this has the disadvantage of prolonging the renal ischemic time, it does have the advantage of ensuring good cardiac function (since the function of a transplanted kidney may be compromised by early dysfunction of the transplanted heart).[21] Since donor kidney ischemic time of up to 24 hours provides a 95% likelihood of immediate function, there seems to be considerable latitude for delaying the renal transplant procedure following the cardiac transplant.

IMMUNOSUPPRESSION

Most patients receive standard triple-drug immunosuppression.[248] Cytolytic therapy with either OKT3 or ATG is frequently employed as induction therapy,[39, 110, 200, 223, 317] a protocol which is also used at UAB. Cyclosporine is introduced as soon as cardiac function has stabilized, when there is good urine output, and when the serum creatinine normalizes (< about 1.7 mg/dL). The use of intravenous cyclosporine by continuous infusion in this

TABLE 21-4	Rejection Frequency in Isolated Heart Versus Heart/Kidney Transplant Recipients			
	HEART/KIDNEY RECIPIENTS		HEART RECIPIENTS[†]	
NO. OF REJECTION EPISODES*	N	%	N	%
0	35	62.5	416	45.7
1	11	19.6	244	26.8
≥2	10	17.9	251	27.6
Total reported	56	100.0	911	100.0

*Number of cardiac allograft rejection episodes in single and dual organ transplantation.
[†]$p = .02$ for group-to-group comparisons.
From Narula J, Bennett LE, DiSalvo T, Hosenpud JD, Semigran MJ, Dec GW: Outcomes in recipients of combined heart-kidney transplantation. Transplantation 1997;63:861–867, with permission.

circumstance does allow immediate discontinuation if renal function deteriorates (see Chapters 12 and 13).

INCIDENCE AND DIAGNOSIS OF ACUTE REJECTION

The multicenter report of Narula[248] demonstrated a lower incidence of acute cardiac and renal rejection than would have been expected after transplantation of each organ alone. Twenty-seven of 56 patients (48%) had no rejection of either organ. Renal allograft rejection occurred in 25% of patients. Cumulative cardiac rejection was lower in heart/kidney recipients than in patients undergoing heart transplantation alone (Table 21–4) and freedom from cardiac rejection was higher (Fig. 21–27),[248] although no formal statistical comparison was performed. Other reports have also noted reduction in renal allograft rejection, but the numbers of patients are too small for meaningful analysis.[39, 200] Other methodologic difficulties also confound the interpretation of these data. Renal allograft rejection is frequently diagnosed solely on biochemical markers, which are less sensitive than renal biopsy as a means of detecting acute renal rejection. However, this difference in the incidence of rejection of either organ in heart/kidney transplant recipients as compared with either organ transplanted alone may be a real phenomenon for which induction of partial tolerance has been proposed (see Chapter 2) as a mechanism.

A lack of concordance between rejection of the heart and rejection of the kidney has been reported,[110, 248] and underscores the necessity for simultaneous surveillance for rejection in both organs. Monitoring for renal rejection is usually by way of serum creatinine. Supplemental studies include isotope renal scans and ultrasound. Renal biopsy provides the most definitive diagnosis and is employed if the diagnosis of rejection is uncertain or if the patient fails to respond to an initial course of steroid therapy.

In the multicenter study by Narula and colleagues,[248] most episodes of rejection of both heart and kidney were treated with pulse methylprednisolone or oral prednisone. Patients with persistent rejection received cytolytic therapy with OKT3 or ATG and, in a small number of patients, total lymphoid irradiation or plasmapheresis.

SURVIVAL

The survival of patients after combined heart and kidney transplantation is not appreciably different from that of patients undergoing heart transplantation (Fig. 21–28),[248] and good survival is confirmed by other small reports.[39, 185, 225] At UAB, four patients have undergone combined heart/kidney transplantation; all patients are alive and well with good renal and cardiac allograft function 6 months to 5 years later. The intermediate-term results of combined heart and kidney transplantation suggest that this procedure is effective for the small

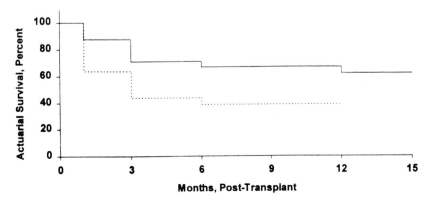

FIGURE **21–27.** Cardiac allograft rejection-free survival in combined heart/kidney and isolated heart allograft recipients. The data collected for 59 patients undergoing combined transplantation from 29 centers were compared to published data on 911 isolated heart recipients in the CTRD database. Solid line, combined heart-kidney transplant; dashed line, isolated heart transplant. (From Narula J, Bennett LE, DiSalvo T, Hosenpud JD, Semigran MJ, Dec GW: Outcomes in recipients of combined heart-kidney transplantation. Transplantation 1997;63:861–867.)

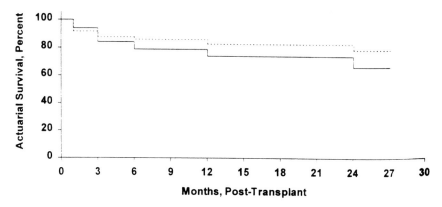

FIGURE **21–28.** Actuarial survival in combined heart/kidney and isolated heart allograft recipients. The data for 82 patients undergoing combined transplantation were compared with 14,340 patients registered with the UNOS database. There was no significant difference in the intermediate-term survival between the two groups ($p = .20$). Solid line, combined heart/kidney transplant; dashed line, isolated heart transplant. (From Narula J, Bennett LE, DiSalvo T, Hosenpud JD, Semigran MJ, Dec GW: Outcomes in recipients of combined heart-kidney transplantation. Transplantation 1997;63:861–867.)

group of patients with end-stage heart and renal disease, and cautious extension of this therapy to patients with end-stage heart disease complicated by acute severe renal dysfunction seems appropriate.

COMBINED HEART/LIVER AND HEART/ LUNG/LIVER TRANSPLANTATION

Combined heart and liver transplantation has been performed in a small number of patients with the unusual combination of end-stage heart and liver disease. Furthermore, combined transplantation of heart, lungs, and liver has been applied to patients with end-stage liver disease in association exclusively with end-stage lung disease, the most common disorder being cystic fibrosis. It could be argued that in this disease, combined lung and liver transplantation would produce equally as satisfactory results with the donor heart being available for another recipient. However, heart/lung transplantation is still performed in some centers for some patients with end-stage lung disease such as pulmonary hypertension and cystic fibrosis, so that combined heart/ lung/liver transplantation for patients with end-stage lung and liver disease should still be regarded as a contemporary transplant procedure. Furthermore, if the domino technique of heart transplantation is utilized (see Chapter 9), then the heart from the recipient would be available for cardiac transplantation.

RECIPIENT SELECTION

Combined Heart and Liver Transplantation

The world's experience with combined heart and liver transplantation is small. The United Network of Organ Sharing (UNOS) has recorded 15 combined heart/liver transplants performed in the United States between 1989 and 1997, although the number of combined heart/liver transplants that have been reported in the literature is considerably smaller. The indications for heart/liver transplant are (1) combined end-stage heart and liver disease due to unrelated causes, (2) combined end-stage heart and liver disease due to related causes, and (3) end-stage heart disease, the liver transplant be-

ing to correct an underlying metabolic disorder responsible for the end-stage heart disease.

Combined heart/liver transplantation has been performed for a small number of patients with unrelated end-stage heart and liver disease; the most common example is in patients with end-stage liver disease with severe ischemic heart disease for which no conventional therapy is possible.

Combined end-stage liver disease and severe heart disease from related causes provides the indication for heart/liver transplantation in several well-defined syndromes. Biliary atresia is often associated with cardiac abnormalities, which may require the combined procedure. Alagille syndrome may also be associated with cardiac anomalies, and the combined transplant may be indicated because of inferior survival following liver transplantation alone in patients with Alagille syndrome and significant cardiovascular anomalies. Another group of disorders where combined heart/liver transplantation has been reported is iron deposition disorders, such as a homozygous β-thalassemia[78, 267] (see Box)

 β-Thalassemia

Thalassemia is an inherited disorder resulting from mutation of genes of either the α- or β-globin moiety of the hemoglobin molecule which, depending on the extent to which either the quantity of α- or β-chain is reduced, produces a spectrum of hematological and clinical findings. The hallmark of the thalassemias is hypochromic and misshapened red cells. Homozygous β-thalassemia produces a chronic anemia and, untreated, the disease is fatal in childhood. Red cell transfusions prolong survival; however, the accumulation of iron may result in severe cardiac and hepatic failure. Patients who survive into adulthood have milder forms of the disease, termed β-thalassemia intermedia and, unless treated aggressively, may develop clinically significant hemosiderosis affecting liver, pancreas, and heart. Since the introduction of iron chelation therapy with deferoxamine, the incidence of cardiac and hepatic disease has been reduced. However, there are still some patients with severe thalassemia who present with iron-induced cardiac and hepatic failure for which there are no satisfactory therapeutic options except for combined heart/liver transplantation.

Hemochromatosis

Patients with genetic hemochromatosis have abnormal iron absorption from the gastrointestinal tract resulting in progressive iron accumulation. The disease has a recessive inheritance and is associated with HLA antigens A3, B14, and B7. Iron is deposited in multiple organs, in particular the liver and pancreas, leading to fibrosis and cirrhosis. The hepatic manifestations also include the development of hepatocellular carcinoma, which has become the primary cause of death in treated patients. Cardiac complications occur as the primary manifestation of genetic hemochromatosis in 15% of patients. A cardiomyopathy results from the deposition of iron in the myocardium leading to congestive heart failure. In addition, cardiac arrhythmias have been described as a result of the disease. The end-stage complications of genetic hemochromatosis can be prevented by phlebotomy to remove the excess iron present, but once end-stage disease is present, it is irreversible. Phlebotomy is required after transplantation to prevent recurrent disease.

Liver Disease in Cystic Fibrosis

The incidence of symptomatic liver disease in patients with cystic fibrosis ranges between 2.2%[353] and 16%,[375] encompassing the full age range of patients with this disease from neonates to adults. The peak onset of symptomatic liver disease appears to be in the first and second decades of life, progression to cirrhosis being rare after puberty. The natural history of the liver disease and the lung disease in these patients appears to run independent courses.[96] The etiology of liver disease in cystic fibrosis is uncertain, but is most likely multifactorial. Inspissated material obstructing the biliary ducts causing chronic inflammation and focal biliary cirrhosis is only part of the explanation, and other factors such as impaired nutrition may play a role. Ultimately, multilobular cirrhosis may result in portal hypertension, hypersplenism, and variceal bleeding.

and genetic hemochromatosis[357] (see Box). This combined procedure has also been performed for familial amyloidosis.[302]

Combined heart/liver transplantation may also be considered for patients with end-stage heart disease in whom liver transplantation is undertaken to reverse an underlying metabolic abnormality. The prototypic condition in which this strategy has been utilized is homozygous familial hypercholesterolemia[97, 244, 302, 328] (see Box). Using the combined procedure for this condition has the advantage of providing the liver as a source of low-density lipoprotein (LDL) receptors to remove LDL cholesterol from the circulation, since the amount of LDL cholesterol that could be removed by the donor heart alone with its very small concentration of LDL receptors would be insignificant. The efficacy of liver transplantation for this condition to provide a source of LDL receptors to lower plasma cholesterol has previously been demonstrated.[35, 141]

Familial Hypercholesterolemia

Familial hypercholesterolemia is a genetic disorder of the low density lipoproteins (LDL). The major function of LDL molecules is to distribute cholesterol to peripheral tissues, which occurs by the interaction of the LDL molecule with an LDL receptor on the cell surface and internalization of the LDL with its cholesterol into the interior of the cell. In the homozygous form of familial hypercholesterolemia, LDL receptors are absent, resulting in markedly elevated total cholesterol and LDL cholesterol, delayed LDL clearance, deposition of cholesterol over joints and pressure points (xanthomata), and in blood vessels. The manifestation of this is premature coronary atherosclerosis and sudden cardiac death, with many affected individuals dying before the age of 20 years.

Combined Heart/Lung and Liver Transplantation

There are a few conditions that could be considered for this procedure, although most centers contemplating transplantation in patients with end-stage lung and liver disease would primarily consider combined lung and liver transplantation. These conditions include cystic fibrosis with hepatic cirrhosis, primary biliary cirrhosis with pulmonary hypertension and α_1-antitrypsin deficiency emphysema with hepatic cirrhosis. The condition most frequently considered for the combined procedure is liver disease in cystic fibrosis (see Box).

An important issue in these patients is the indication for combined lung/liver or heart/lung/liver transplantation. Liver transplantation has been performed in patients with cystic fibrosis in whom lung transplantation was not indicated (mean FEV_1, 70%),[235, 251] and improvement in exercise tolerance and decreased sputum production has been reported.[251] The combined procedure should be reserved for patients with end-stage pulmonary disease associated with end-stage liver disease characterized by severe cirrhosis and portal hypertension. In a series of patients undergoing combined lung/liver and heart/lung/liver transplantation reported by Couetil,[68] all of their patients undergoing a combined procedure had end-stage pulmonary disease, and end-stage liver disease with severe cirrhosis, portal hypertension, and esophageal varices.

Heart/lung/liver transplantation has also been performed in a patient with combination of primary biliary cirrhosis and plexogenic pulmonary hypertension.[77]

TECHNIQUE OF COMBINED HEART/LIVER AND HEART/LUNG/LIVER TRANSPLANTATION

There are four different approaches that have been described for combined heart/liver and heart/lung/liver transplantation: (1) transplantation of the heart but maintaining the patient on cardiopulmonary bypass during the liver transplant; (2) transplantation of the entire heart/lung/liver en bloc; (3) transplantation of the heart with discontinuation of cardiopulmonary bypass, leaving the chest open followed by the liver transplantation; and (4) transplantation of the heart followed by transplantation of the liver from a second donor.

In the description of the first three cases of combined liver/heart transplantation, Shaw and colleagues[328] performed the cardiac transplant procedure first, reperfused the heart and established good cardiac function, and continued cardiopulmonary bypass during the liver transplant procedure. The portal vein was cannulated and drained into the pump oxygenator, which allowed the cardiopulmonary bypass circuit to serve as surrogate venovenous bypass to decompress the portal circulation during the anhepatic phase of the liver transplant. Cardiopulmonary bypass was discontinued after completion of the liver transplant. Not surprisingly, there was a substantial coagulopathy which took some hours to reverse.

An en bloc technique was described by Dennis and colleagues[77] whereby the donor heart, lung, and liver were removed without division of the inferior vena cava. In the recipient, prior to cardiopulmonary bypass, mobilization of the liver was completed followed by mobilization of the thoracic organs. After the establishment of cardiopulmonary bypass (venous drainage through the brachiocephalic and femoral veins), the heart, lungs, and liver were removed and the en bloc organs were implanted, the anastomoses being performed in the following order—trachea, ascending aorta, superior vena cava, infrahepatic inferior vena cava, portal vein, hepatic artery, and bile duct. This technique reduces the number of anastomoses but potentially increases the warm ischemic time of the hepatic allograft.

Another option described by Wallwork and colleagues[382] is a combined staged sequential procedure, the principles of which are the mobilization of the thoracic and abdominal organs, establishment of cardiopulmonary bypass, removal of the thoracic organs followed by implantation of the heart/lung block and continuation of partial cardiopulmonary bypass with a beating heart and ventilated lungs during the removal of the native liver, with implantation of the liver graft following discontinuation of cardiopulmonary bypass.

The technique that probably has the most appeal is a two-stage procedure with completion of the heart/lung transplant and discontinuation of cardiopulmonary bypass, leaving the thorax open for the liver transplantation followed by the liver transplant procedure in case portoatrial shunting is required.[67] One of the major advantages of this procedure is that the cardiac and liver transplant can be performed with minimal deviation from the standard procedures. Some patients may experience hemodynamic instability during the anhepatic phase due to decreased venous return as a result of clamping the inferior vena cava above and below the liver. Standard venovenous bypass (draining the inferior vena cava via the femoral vein and portal vein into the subclavian or internal jugular vein) during the liver transplant will help maintain venous return to the heart and minimize the hemodynamic changes associated with clamping the inferior vena cava. Detry and colleagues[78] have recommended the technique of liver transplantation during the combined procedure that involves partial inferior vena caval clamping, preserving inferior vena caval blood flow with a side-to-side anastomosis between donor and recipient inferior vena cava, only one caval anastomosis being required.

Figuera[97] reported a staged approach in which a patient suffering familial hypercholesterolemia underwent a heart transplant and 21 days later a liver transplant from a second donor. This procedure has been described on several occasions with excellent results and has the advantage of allowing the patient to recover from a heart transplant, preventing the hemodynamic destabilizing effects of clamping the inferior vena cava, and reducing the risk of contamination of the chest cavity from the liver transplant procedure. Unfortunately, sequential transplantation requires easy access to donor organs to minimize the time between transplants and would only be advisable for patients requiring liver transplantation to correct metabolic defects without end-stage liver disease. In addition, the protective immunologic effect of the transplanted liver on other organs transplanted from the same donor may be lost using this sequential method.

RESULTS

The intermediate survival after combined heart/liver transplantation is not available from the limited reports in the literature and will require longer follow-up in a larger cohort of patients. In homozygous familial hypercholesterolemia, liver transplantation is effective in reducing total plasma cholesterol by providing a liver with normal LDL receptors (Fig. 21–29).[372] The most

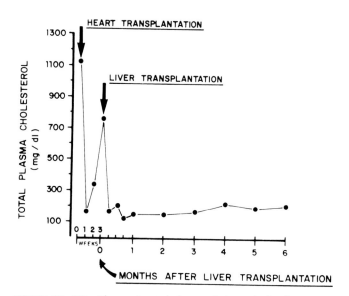

FIGURE **21–29.** Change in total plasma cholesterol after liver transplantation in a patient with homozygous familial hypercholesterolemia. (From Valdivielso P, Escolar JL, Cuervas-Mons V, Pulpon LA, Chaparro MA, Gonzalez-Santos P: Lipids and lipoprotein changes after heart and liver transplantation in a patient with homozygous familial hypercholesterolemia. Ann Intern Med 1988;108:24–26.)

experience for combined procedure of heart/lung/liver is in patients with cystic fibrosis. Couetil[68] reported seven children undergoing a combined heart/lung/liver (four patients), sequential double lung/liver (two patients), or bilateral lobar lung from a split left lung and reduced liver (one patient) with a combined actuarial survival of 85% at one year.

References

1. Aarnio P, Hämmäinen P, Fyhrquist F, Harjula A: Endothelin content of bronchoalveolar lavage fluid from allotransplanted pigs is increased during unmodified rejection. J Thorac Cardiovasc Surg 1994;107:216–219.

2. Aarnio P, Scherstén H, Tazelaar HD, Miller VM, McGregor CGA: Cardiac and pulmonary replacement: effects of acute rejection and antirejection therapy on arteries and veins from canine single lung allografts. J Thorac Cardiovasc Surg 1996;111:1219–1229.

3. Achkar A, Laaban JP, Andreau G: Extracorporeal photochemotherapy for bronchiolitis obliterans. Am J Respir Crit Care Med 1991;1:A2777.

4. Adams DH, Cochrane AD, Khaghani A, Smith JD, Yacoub MH: Retransplantation in heart-lung recipients with obliterative bronchiolitis. J Thorac Cardiovasc Surg 1994;107:450–459.

5. Adatia I, Lillehei C, Arnold JH, Thompson JE, Palazzo R, Fackler JC, Wessel DL: Inhaled nitric oxide in the treatment of postoperative graft dysfunction after lung transplantation. Ann Thorac Surg 1994;57:1311–1318.

6. Adoumie R, Serrick C, Giaid A, Shennib H: Early cellular events in the lung allograft. Ann Thorac Surg 1992;54:1071–1077.

7. Aeba R, Keenan RJ, Hardesty RL, Yousem SA, Hamamoto I, Griffith BP: University of Wisconsin solution for pulmonary preservation in a rat transplant model. Ann Thorac Surg 1992;53:240–246.

8. Aeba R, Killinger WA, Keenan RJ, Yousem SA, Hamamoto I, Hardesty RL, Griffith BP: Lazaroid U74500A as an additive to University of Wisconsin solution for pulmonary grafts in the rat transplant model. J Thorac Cardiovasc Surg 1992;104:1333–1339.

9. Afolabi OA, Parry G, Healy MD, Corris PA, Dark JH: The role of total lymphoid irradiation (TLI) in the treatment of obliterative bronchiolitis-2 years on [abstract]. J Heart Lung Transplant 1996;15:S102.

10. Alican F, Hardy JD: Lung reimplantation: effect on respiratory pattern and function. JAMA 1963;183:849–853.

11. Al-Kattan K, Tadjkarimi S, Cox A, Banner N, Khaghani A, Yacoub M: Clinical heart transplantation: evaluation of the long-term results of single lung versus heart-lung transplantation for emphysema. J Heart Lung Transplant 1995;14:824–831.

12. Andreu G, Achkar A, Couetil JP, Guillemain R, Heshmati F, Amrein C, Chevalier P, Dore ME, Capron F, Laaban JP, Carpentier A: Extracorporeal photochemotherapy treatment for acute lung rejection episode. J Heart Lung Transplant 1995;14:793–796.

13. Anthonisen NR: Prognosis in chronic obstructive pulmonary disease: results from multicenter clinical trials. Am Rev Respir Dis 1989;140:S95–S99.

14. Aoe M, Trachiotis GD, Okabayashi K, Manchester JK, Lowry OH, Cooper JD, Patterson GA: Administration of prostaglandin E$_1$ after lung transplantation improves early graft function. Ann Thorac Surg 1994;58:655–661.

15. Aranda M, Pearl RG: The pharmacology and physiology of nitric oxide: understanding its use in anesthesia and critical care medicine. Respir Anesth Pathophysiol Clin Update 1998;16:235–257.

16. Auteri JS, Jeevanandam V, Sanchez JA, Marboe CC, Kirby TJ, Smith CR: Normal bronchial healing without bronchial wrapping in canine lung transplantation. Ann Thorac Surg 1992;53:80–84.

17. Azoulay E, Lachia L, Blayo MC, Pocidalo JJ: Methemoglobinemia induced by nitric oxide in whole blood. Quantitative relationship. Toxicol Eur Res 1978;1:7–12.

18. Bacha EA, Hervé P, Murakami S, Chapelier A, Mazmanian GM, de Montpreville V, Libert JM, Dartevelle P: Lasting beneficial effect of short-term inhaled nitric oxide on graft function after lung transplantation. J Thorac Cardiovasc Surg 1996;112:590–598.

19. Bacha EA, Sellak H, Murakami S: Inhaled nitric oxide attenuates reperfusion injury in non-heartbeating-donor lung transplantation. Paris-Sud University Lung Transplantation Group. Transplantation 1997;63:1380–1386.

20. Badesch DB, Zamora M, Fullerton D, Weill D, Tuder R, Grover F, Schwarz MI: Pulmonary capillaritis: a possible histologic form of acute pulmonary allograft rejection. J Heart Lung Transplant 1998;17:415–422.

21. Bahnson HT, Gordon RD: Transplantation of other organs with the heart. Cardiovasc Clin 1990;20:237.

22. Baldwin JC, Frist WH, Starkey TD, Harjula A, Starnes VA, Stinson E, Oyer PE, Shumway NE: Distant graft procurement for combined heart and lung transplantation using pulmonary artery flush and simple topical hypothermia for graft preservation. Ann Thorac Surg 1987;43:670–673.

23. Ballinger WF II, Scicchitano LP, Baranski EJ, Camishion RC: The effects of cardiopulmonary denervation. Surgery 1964;55:574–580.

24. Bando K, Armitage JM, Paradis IL, Keenan RJ, Hardesty RL, Konishi H, Komatsu K, Shah AN, Bahnson HT: Indications for and results of single, bilateral, and heart-lung transplantation for pulmonary hypertension. J Thorac Cardiovasc Surg 1994;108:1056–1065.

25. Bando K, Paradis IL, Similo S: Cardiac and pulmonary replacement: obliterative bronchiolitis after lung and heart-lung transplantation: an analysis of risk factors and management. J Thorac Cardiovasc Surg 1995;110:4–13.

26. Bando K, Tago M, Teraoka H, Seno S, Senoo Y, Teramoto S: Extended cardiopulmonary preservation for heart/lung transplantation: a comparative study of superoxide dismutase. J Heart Transplant 1989;8:59–66.

27. Barbotin-Larrieu F, Mazmanian M, Baudet B, Detruit H, Chapelier A, Libert JM, Dartevell P, Herve P: Prevention of ischemia-reperfusion lung injury by inhaled nitric oxide in neonatal piglets. J Appl Physiol 1996;80:782–788.

28. Barlow CW, Robbins RC, Moon MR, Akindipe O, Theodore J, Reitz BA: Heart-lung versus double lung transplantation for suppurative lung disease. J Thorac Cardiovasc Surg 2000;119:466–476.

29. Barnes PJ: Neural control of airway smooth muscle. *In* Crystal RG, West JB (eds): The Lung: Scientific Foundation. New York: Raven Press, 1991, pp 903–916.

30. Bassiri AG, Girgis RE, Doyle RL, Thoedore J: Detection of small airway dysfunction using specific airway conductance. Chest 1997;111:1533–1535.

31. Baudet EM, Dromer C, Dubrez J, Jougon JB, Roques X, Velly JF, Deville C, Couraud L: Intermediate-term results after en bloc double-lung transplantation with bronchial arterial revascularization. J Thorac Cardiovasc Surg 1996;112:1292–1300.

32. Benvenuti C, Bourgeon B, Chopin D, Deleuze P, Aptecar E, Mourtada A, Baron C, Lebesneraie P, Remy P, Abbou C, Weil B, Cachera JP, Loisance D, Lang P: Combined heart and kidney transplantation. Transplant Proc 1995;27:1694.

33. Bhabra MS, Hopkinson DN, Shaw TE, Hooper TL: Low-dose nitric oxide inhalation during initial reperfusion enhances rat lung graft function. Ann Thorac Surg 1997;63:339–344.

34. Bhatia SJS, Kirshenbaum JM, Shemin RJ, Cohn LH, Collins JJ, Di Sesa VJ, Young PJ, Mudge GH, Sutton MG: Time course of resolution of pulmonary hypertension and right ventricular remodeling after orthotopic cardiac transplantation. Circulation 1987;76:819–826.

35. Bilheimer DW, Goldstein JL, Grundy SM, Starzl TE, Brown SM: Liver transplantation to provide low-density-lipoprotein receptors and lower plasma cholesterol in a child with homozygous familial hypercholesterolemia. N Engl J Med 1984;311:1658–1664.

36. Billingham ME: Pathology of graft vascular disease after heart and heart/lung transplantation and its relationship to obliterative bronchiolitis. Transplant Proc 1995;27:2013–2016.

37. Binns OAR, DeLima NF, Buchanan SA, Cope JT, King RC, Marek CA, Shockey KS, Tribble CG, Kron IL: Both blood and crystalloid-based extracellular solutions are superior to intracellular solutions for lung preservation. J Thorac Cardiovasc Surg 1996;112:1515–1521.

38. Bjork L: Anastomoses between the coronary and bronchial arteries. Acta Radiol Diagn 1966;4:93–96.

39. Blanche C, Valenza M, Czer LSC, Barath P, Admon D, Harasty D, Utley C, Trento A: Combined heart and kidney transplantation

with allografts from the same donor. Ann Thorac Surg 1994; 58:1135.

40. Blanco G, Adam A, Rodriguez-Perez D, Fernandez A: Complete homotransplantation of canine heart and lungs. AMA Arch Surg 1958;76:20–23.

41. Blot F, Tavakoli R, Sellam S, Epardeau B, Faurisson F, Bernard N, Becquemin MH, Frachon I, Stern M, Pocidalo JJ, Carbon C, Bisson A, Caubarrere I: Nebulized cyclosporine for prevention of acute pulmonary allograft rejection in the rat: pharmacokinetic and histologic study. J Heart Lung Transplant 1995;14:1162–1172.

42. Boehler A, Chamberlain D, Kesten S, Slutsky AS, Liu M, Keshavjee S: Lymphocytic airway infiltration as a precursor to fibrous obliteration in a rat model of bronchiolitis obliterans. Transplantation 1997;64:311–317.

43. Bourge RC, Naftel DC, Costanzo-Nordin MR, Kirklin JK, Young JB, Kubo SH, Olivari M, Kasper EK: Pretransplantation risk factors for death after heart transplantation: a multiinstitutional study. J Heart Lung Transplant 1993;12:549.

44. Breuer J, Hering E: Die Selbststeuerung Der Atmung Durch Den Nervus Vagus. Wein: SB Akad Wiss, 1868, pp 57–672.

45. Bridges ND, Spray TL, Collins MH, Bowles NE, Towbin JA: Adenovirus infection in the lung results in graft failure after lung transplantation. J Thorac Cardiovasc Surg 1998;116:617–623.

46. Brooks RG, Hofflin JM, Jamieson SW, Stinson EB, Remington JS: Infectious complications in heart/lung transplant recipients. Am J Med 1985;79:412–422.

47. Buchanan SA, Mauney MC, Parekh VI, DeLima NF, Binns OA, Cope JT, Shockey KS, Tri CG, Kron IL: Intratracheal surfactant administration preserves airway compliance during lung reperfusion. Ann Thorac Surg 1996;62:1617–1621.

48. Bücherl ES, Nasseri M, von Prondzynski B: Lung function studies after homotransplantation, autotransplantation, denervation of the left lung, and ligature of the right pulmonary artery. J Thorac Cardiovasc Surg 1964;47:455–465.

49. Burke CM, Theodore J, Dawkins KD, Blank N, Van Kessel A, Oyer PE, Stinson EB, Robin ED: Post-transplant obliterative bronchiolitis and other late lung sequelae in human heart/lung transplantation. Chest 1984;86:824–829.

50. Burt R, Gupta-Burt S, Suki W, Barcenas C, Ferguson J, Van Buren C: Reversal of left ventricular dysfunction after renal transplantation. Ann Intern Med 1989;111:635–640.

51. Cachera JP, Abbou C, Deleuze P, Hillion ML, Loisance D, Romano P, Laurent F, Touzani A, Tavolaro O, Hittenger L: Combined heart and kidney transplantation using the same donor. Eur J Cardiothorac Surg 1989;3:169–173.

52. Carere R, Patterson GA, Liu P, Williams T, Maurer J, Grossman R: Right and left ventricular performance after single and double lung transplantation. J Thorac Cardiovasc Surg 1991;102:115–123.

53. Carrel A: The surgery of blood vessels, etc. Johns Hopkins Hosp Bull 1907;18:18–28.

54. Castaneda AR, Zamora R, Schmidt-Habelmann P, Hornung J, Murphy W, Ponto D, Moller JH: Cardiopulmonary autotransplantation in primates (baboons). Late functional results. Surgery 1972;72:1064–1070.

55. Chan CC, Abi-Saleh WJ, Arroliga AC, Stillwell PC, Kirby TJ, Gordon SM, Petras RE, Mehta RE: Diagnostic yield and therapeutic impact of flexible bronchoscopy in lung transplant recipients. J Heart Lung Transplant 1996;15:196–205.

56. Chapelier A, Reignier J, Mazmanian M, Dulmet E, Libert JM, Dartevelle P, Barbotin F, Herve P, Brenot F, Lafont D, Simonneau G, Dartevelle P, Deslauriers J: Amelioration of reperfusion injury by pentoxifylline after lung transplantation. J Heart Lung Transplant 1995;14:676–683.

57. Chapelier A, Vouhé P, Macchiarini P: Comparative outcome of heart-lung and lung transplantation for pulmonary hypertension. J Thorac Cardiovasc Surg 1993;106:299–307.

58. Charan NB, Carvalho PG: Anatomy of the normal bronchial circulatory system in humans and animals. In Butler J (ed): Lung Biology in Health and Disease. Vol 57: The Bronchial Circulation. New York: Marcel Dekker, 1992.

59. Chen CZ, Gallagher RC, Ardery P, Dyckman W, Low HBC: Retrograde versus antegrade flush in canine left lung preservation for six hours. J Heart Lung Transplant 196;15:395–403.

60. Christie RV: Emphysema of the lungs. BMJ 1944;1:105.

61. Clancey RM, Leszczynska-Piziak J, Abramson SB: Nitric oxide, an endothelial cell relaxation factor, inhibits neutrophil superoxide anion production via a direct action on the NADPH oxidase. J Clin Invest 1992;90:1116–1121.

62. Clelland C, Higenbottam TW, Smyth RL: Lymphocyte counts in bronchoalveolar lavage (BAL) during acute rejection and infection in heart-lung transplantation (HLTx) [abstract]. Am Rev Respir Dis 1989;139:A242.

63. Cooley DA, Bloodwell RD, Hallman GL, Nora JJ, Harrison GM, Leachman RD: Organ transplantation for advanced cardiopulmonary disease. Ann Thorac Surg 1969;8:30–46.

64. Cooper DKC, Novitzky D, Rose AG, Reichart BA: Acute pulmonary rejection precedes cardiac rejection following heart-lung transplantation in a primate model. J Heart Transplant 1986; 5:29–32.

65. Cooper JD, Billingham M, Egan T, Hertz MI, Higenbottam T, Lynch J, Mauer J, Paradis I, Patterson GA, Smith C, Trulock EP, Vreim C, Yousem S: A working formulation for the standardization of nomenclature and for clinical staging of chronic dysfunction in lung allografts. J Heart Lung Transplant 1993;12:713–716.

66. Cooper JD, Patterson GA, Trulock EP, the Washington University Lung Transplant Group: Results of single and bilateral lung transplantation in 131 consecutive recipients. J Thorac Cardiovasc Surg 1994;107:460–470.

67. Couetil JPA, Houssin DP, Soubrane O, Chevalier PG, Dousset BE, Loulmet D, Achkar A, Tolan MJ, Amrein CI, Guinvarch A, Guillemain RJ, Birmbaum P, Carpentier AF: Combined lung and liver transplantation in patients with cystic fibrosis: a 4½-year experience. J Thorac Cardiovasc Surg 1995;110:1415–1422.

68. Couetil JPA, Soubrane O, Houssin DP, Dousset BE, Chevalier PG, Guinvarch A, Loulmet D, Achkar A, Carpentier AF: Combined heart/lung/liver, double lung/liver, and isolated liver transplantation for cystic fibrosis in children. Transplantation 1997; 10:33–39.

69. Daly RC, McGregor CGA: Postoperative management of the single lung transplant patient. In Cooper DKC, Miller LW, Patterson GA (eds): The Transplantation and Replacement of Thoracic Organs. Dordrecht, The Netherlands: Kluwer Academic Publishers, 1996.

70. Date H, Lima O, Matsumura A, Tsuji H, D'Avignon DA, Cooper JD: In a canine model, lung preservation at 10°C is superior to that at 4°C. J Thorac Cardiovasc Surg 1992;103:773–780.

71. Date H, Lynch JP, Sundareasan S, Patterson GA, Trulock EP: The impact of cytolytic therapy on bronchiolitis obliterans syndrome. J Heart Lung Transplant 1998;17:869–875.

72. Date H, Trulock EP, Arcidi JM, Sundaresan S, Cooper JD, Patterson GA: Improved airway healing after lung transplantation. An analysis of 348 bronchial anastomoses. J Thorac Cardiovasc Surg 1995;110:1424–1433.

73. de Hoyos AL, Patterson GA, Maurer JR, Ramirez JC, Miller JD, Winton TL: Pulmonary transplantation. Early and late results. The Toronto Lung Transplant Group. J Thorac Cardiovasc Surg 1992;103:295–306.

74. deLeval MR, Smyth R, Whitehead B, Scott JP, Elliott MJ, Sharples L, Caine N, Helms P, Martin IR, Higenbottam T, Wallwork J, Stark J: Heart and lung transplantation for terminal cystic fibrosis: a 4½ year experience. J Thorac Cardiovasc Surg 1991;101: 633–642.

75. Demikhov VP: Experimental transplantation of vital organs. Authorized translation from Russian by Haigh B. New York: Consultants Bureau, 1962.

76. Dennis C, Caine N, Sharples L, Smyth R, Higenbottam T, Stewart S, Wreghitt T, Large S, Wells FC, Wallwork J: Heart-lung transplantation for end-stage respiratory disease in patients with cystic fibrosis at Papworth Hospital. J Heart Lung Transplant 1993;12: 893–902.

77. Dennis CM, NcNeil KD, Dunning J, Stewart S, Friend PJ, Alexander G, Higenbottam TW, Calne RY, Wallwork J: Heart/lung/liver transplantation. J Heart Lung Transplant 1996;15:536–538.

78. Detry O, Honoré P, Meurisse M, Defraigne JO, Defechereux T, Sakalihasan N, Limet R, Jacquet N: Advantages of inferior vena caval flow preservation in combined transplantation of the liver and heart. Transplant Int 1997;10:150–151.

79. Detterbeck FC, Keagy BA, Paull DE, Wilcox BR: Oxygen free radical scavengers decrease reperfusion injury in lung transplantation. Ann Thorac Surg 1990;50:204–210.

80. Diamond DA, Michalski JM, Lynch JP, Trulock EP III: Efficacy of total lymphoid irradiation for chronic allograft rejection following bilateral lung transplantation. Int J Radiat Oncol Biol Phys 1998;41:795.

81. Dittrich HC, Chow LC, Nicod PH: Early improvement in left ventricular diastolic function after relief of chronic right ventricular pressure overload. Circulation 1989;80:823–830.

82. Dowling RD, Zenati M, Burckart GJ, Yousem SA, Schaper M, Simmons RL, Hardesty RL, Griffith BP: Aerosolized cyclosporine as single agent immunotherapy in canine lung allografts. Surgery 1990;108:198–204.

83. Duncan AJ, Duman JS, Paradis IL, Dauber JH, Yousem SA, Zenati MA, Kormos RL, Griffith BP: Cytomegalovirus infection and survival in lung transplant recipients. J Heart Lung Transplant 1992;10:638.

84. Dusmet M, Maurer J, Winton T, Kesten S: Methotrexate can halt the progression of bronchiolitis obliterans syndrome in lung transplant recipients. J Heart Lung Transplant 1996;15:948–954.

85. Duvoisin GE, Fowler WS, Payne WS, Ellis FH Jr: Reimplantation of the dog lung with survival after contralateral pneumonectomy. Surg Forum 1964;14:173–175.

86. Egan TM: Selection and management of the lung donor. In Patterson GA, Couraud L (eds): Lung Transplantation. Vol 3. Amsterdam: Elsevier Science, 1995, p 103.

87. Egan TM, Detterbeck FC, Mill MR, Paradowski LJ, Lackner RP, Ogden WD, Yankaskas JR, Westerman JH, Thompson JT, Weiner MA, Cairns EL, Wilcox BR: Improved results of lung transplantation for patients with cystic fibrosis. J Thorac Cardiovasc Surg 1995;109:224–235.

88. Egan TM, Lambert CJ, Reddick R, Ulicny KS, Keagy BA, Wilcox BR: A strategy to increase the donor pool: use of cadaver lungs for transplantation. Ann Thorac Surg 1991;52:1113–1121.

89. Egan TM, Ulicny KS, Lambert CJ, Wilcox BR: Effect of a free radical scavenger on cadaver lung transplantation. Ann Thorac Surg 1993;55:1453–1459.

90. Eppinger MJ, Ward PA, Jones ML, Bolling SF, Deeb GM: Disparate effects of nitric oxide on lung ischemia-reperfusion injury. Ann Thorac Surg 1995;60:1169–1175.

91. Eraslan S, Hardy JD, Elliott RL: Lung replantation: respiratory reflexes, vagal integrity, and lung function in chronic dogs. J Surg Res 1966;6:383–388.

92. Eraslan S, Turner MD, Hardy JD: Lymphatic regeneration following lung reimplantation in dogs. Surgery 1964;56:970.

93. Everett JP, Hershberger RE, Norman DJ, Chou S, Ratkovec RM, Cobanoglu A, Ott GY, Hosenpud JD: Prolonged cytomegalovirus infection with viremia is associated with development of cardiac allograft vasculopathy. J Heart Lung Transplant 1992;11:S133–S137.

94. Faggian G, Bortolotti U, Stellin G, Mazzucco A, Sorbara C, Tommaseo T, Gallucci V: Combined heart and kidney transplantation: a case report. J Heart Transplant 1986;5:480–483.

95. Fann JI, Wilson MK, Theodore J, Reitz BA: Combined heart and single-lung transplantation in complex congenital heart disease. Ann Thorac Surg 1998;65:823–825.

96. Feigelson J, Anagnostopoulos C, Poquet M, Pecau Y, Munck A, Navarro J: Liver cirrhosis in cystic fibrosis—therapeutic implications and long term follow up. Arch Dis Child 1993;68:653–657.

97. Figuera D, Ardaiz J, Martín-Júdez V, Pulpon LA, Pradas G, Cuervas-Mons V, Burgos R, Arcas M, Pardo F, Cienfuegos JA, Turrion VS, Tellez G, Sanz-Ortega E: Combined transplantation of heart and liver from two different donors in a patient with familial type IIa hypercholesterolemia. J Heart Transplant 1986; 5:327–329.

98. Fisher AB: Intermediary metabolism. In Crystal RG, West JB (eds): The Lung: Scientific Foundations. New York: Raven Press, 1991.

99. Follette DM, Rudich SM, Babcock WD: Improved oxygenation and increased lung donor recovery with high-dose steroid administration after brain death. J Heart Lung Transplant 1998; 17:423–429.

100. Francalancia NA, Aeba R, Yousem SA, Griffith BP, Marrone GC: Deleterious effects of cardiopulmonary bypass on early graft function after single lung allotransplantation: evaluation of a heparin-coated bypass circuit. J Heart Lung Trnasplant 1994;13: 498–507.

101. Freeman B: Free radical chemistry of nitric oxide: looking at the dark side. Chest 1994;105:79S–84S.

102. Fremes SE, Patterson GA, Williams WG, Goldman BS, Todd TR, Maurer J: Single lung transplantation and closure of patent ductus arteriosus for Eisenmenger's syndrome. J Thorac Cardiovasc Surg 1990;100:1–5.

103. Frost AE, Jammnal CT, Cagle PT: Hyperacute rejection following lung transplantation. Chest 1996;110:559–562.

104. Fukuse T, Albes JM, Brandes H, Takahashi Y, Demertzis S, Schäfers H-J: Comparison of low potassium Euro-Collins solution and standard Euro-Collins solution in an extracorporeal rat heart/lung model. Eur J Cardiothorac Surg 1996;10:621–627.

105. Fullerton DA, McIntyre RC Jr, Mitchell MB, Campbell DN, Grover FL: Lung transplantation with cardiopulmonary bypass exaggerates pulmonary vasomotor dysfunction in the transplanted lung. J Thorac Cardiovasc Surg 1995;109:212–217.

106. Gammie JS, Stukus DR, Pham SM, Hattler BG, McGrath MF, McCurry KR, Griffith BP, Keenan RJ: Effect of ischemic time on survival in clinical lung transplantation. Ann Thorac Surg 1999;68:2015–2020.

107. Girgis RE, Tu I, Berry GJ, Reichenspurner H, Valentine VG, Conte JV, Ting A, Johnstone I, Miller J, Robbins RC, Reitz BA, Theodore J: Risk factors for the development of obliterative bronchiolitis after lung transplantation. J Heart Lung Transplant 1996;15:1200–1208.

108. Glanville AR, Imoto E, Baldwin JC, Billingham ME, Theodore J, Robin ED: The role of right ventricular endomyocardial biopsy in the long-term management of heart/lung transplant recipients. J Heart Transplant 1987;6:357–361.

109. Glanville AR, Marshman D, Keogh A, Macdonald P, Larbalestier R, Kaan A, Bryant D, Spratt P: Outcome in paired recipients of single lung transplants from the same donor. J Heart Lung Transplant 1995;14:878–882.

110. Gonwa TA, Husberg BS, Klintmalm GB, Mai ML, Goldstein RM, Capehart JE, Miller AH, Johnston SB, Alivizatos PA: Simultaneous heart and kidney transplantation: a report of three cases and review of the literature. J Heart Lung Transplant 1992;11:152–155.

111. Grattan MT, Moreno-Cabral CE, Starnes VA, Oyer PE, Stinson EB, Shumway NE: Cytomegalovirus infection is associated with cardiac allograft rejection and atherosclerosis. JAMA 1989; 261:3561–3566.

112. Griffith BP: Discussion of "Technique of heart-lung transplantation" by Ph. Dartevelle. In Patterson GA, Couraud L (eds): Lung Transplantation. Vol 3. Amsterdam: Elsevier Science BV, 1995.

113. Griffith BP, Hardesty RL, Armitage JM, Kormos RL, Marrone GC, Duncan S, Paradis I, Dauber JH, Yousem SA, Williams P: Acute rejection of lung allografts with various immunosuppressive protocols. Ann Thorac Surg 1992;54:846–851.

114. Griffith BP, Hardesty RL, Trento A: Heart-lung transplantation: lessons learned and future hopes. Ann Thorac Surg 1987;43:6–16.

115. Griffith BP, Hardesty RL, Trento A, Bahnson HT: Asynchronous rejection of heart and lungs following cardiopulmonary transplantation. Ann Thorac Surg 1985;40:488–493.

116. Griffith BP, Magee MJ, Gonzalez IF, Houel R, Armitage JM, Hardesty RL, Hattler BG, Ferson PF, Landreneau RJ, Keenan RJ: Anastomotic pitfalls in lung transplantation. J Thorac Cardiovasc Surg 1994;107:743–754.

117. Griffith BP, Paradis IL, Zeevi A, Rabinowich H, Yousem SA, Duquesnoy RJ, Dauber JH, Hardesty RL: Immunologically mediated disease of the airways after pulmonary transplantation. Ann Surg 1988;208:371–378.

118. Grinnan GLB, Graham WH, Childs JW, Lower RR: Cardiopulmonary homotransplantation. J Thorac Cardiovasc Surg 1970;60: 609–615.

119. Gruetter CA, Barry BK, McNamara DB, Gruetter DY, Kadowitz PJ, Ignarro LJ: Relaxation of bovine coronary artery and activation of coronary arterial guanylate cyclase by nitric oxide, nitroprusside and a carcinogenic nitrosoamine. J Cyclic Nucleotide Res 1979;5:211–224.

120. Hachida M, Morton DL: The protection of ischemic lung with verapamil and hydralazine. J Thorac Cardiovasc Surg 1988;95: 178–183.

121. Haglin J, Telander RL, Muzzall RE, Kiser JC, Strobel CJ: Comparison of lung autotransplantation in the primate and dog. Surg Forum 1963;14:196–198.

122. Hallman M, Bry K, Lappalainen U: A mechanism of nitric oxide-induced surfactant dysfunction. J Appl Physiol 1996;80:2035–2043.

123. Halon DA, Turgeman Y, Merdler A, Hardoff R, Sharir T: Coronary artery to bronchial artery anastomosis in Takayasu's arteritis. Cardiology 1987;74:387–391.

124. Halvorsen RA Jr, DuCret RP, Kuni CC, Olivari MT, Tylen U, Hertz MI: Obliterative bronchiolitis following lung transplantation. Diagnostic utility of aerosol ventilation lung scanning and high resolution CT. Clin Nucl Med 1991;16:256–258.

125. Hardesty RL, Aeba R, Armitage JM, Kormos RL, Griffith BP: A clinical trial of University of Wisconsin solution for pulmonary preservation. J Thorac Cardiovasc Surg 1993;105:660–666.

126. Hardesty RL, Griffith BP: Procurement for combined heart/lung transplantation: Bilateral thoracotomy with sternal transection, cardiopulmonary bypass, and profound hypothermia. J Thorac Cardiovasc Surg 1985;89:795–799.

127. Hardesty RL, Griffith BP: Autoperfusion of the heart and lungs for preservation during distant procurement. J Thorac Cardiovasc Surg 1987;93:11–18.

128. Hassoun PM, Yu FS, Zulueta JJ, White AC, Lanzillo JJ: Effect of nitric oxide and cell redox status on the regulation of endothelial cell xanthine dehydrogenase. Am J Physiol 1995;268:L809–L817.

129. Hausen B, Dwenger A, Gohrbandt B, Niedermeyer J, Zink C, Demertzis S, Schafers HJ: Early biochemical indicators of the obliterative bronchiolitis syndrome in lung transplantation. J Heart Lung Transplant 1994;13:980–989.

130. Hausen B, Muller P, Bahra M, Ramsamooj R, Hewitt CW: Donor pretreatment with intravenous prostacyclin versus inhaled nitric oxide in experimental lung transplantation. Transplantation 1996;62:1714–1719.

131. Hausen B, Mueller P, Bahra M, Ramsamooj R, Morris RE, Hewitt CW: Donor treatment with the Lazeroid U74389G reduces ischemia-reperfusion injury in a rat lung transplant model. Ann Thorac Surg 1997;64:814–820.

132. Hausen B, Rohde R, Hewitt CW, Schroeder F, Beuke M, Ramsamooj R, Schafers HJ, Borst HG: Exogenous surfactant treatment before and after sixteen hours of ischemia in experimental lung transplantation. J Thorac Cardiovasc Surg 1997;113:1050–1058.

133. Haverich A, Frimpong-Boateng K, Wahlers T, Schafers HJ: Pericardial flap-plasty for protection of the tracheal anastomosis in heart-lung transplantation. J Card Surg 1989;4:136–139.

134. Haydock DA, Trulock EP, Kaiser LR, Knight SR, Pasque MK, Cooper JD: Management of dysfunction in the transplanted lung: experience with 7 clinical cases. Ann Thorac Surg 1992;53:635–641.

135. Hedman L, Frisk B, Brynger H, Frodin L, Tufveson G, Wahlberg J: Severe kidney graft rejection in combined kidney and pancreas transplantation. Transplant Proc 1987;19:3911–3912.

136. Heng D, Sharples LD, McNeil K, Stewart S, Wreghitt T, Wallwork J: Bronchiolitis obliterans syndrome: incidence, natural history, prognosis, and risk factors. J Heart Lung Transplant 1998;17:1255–1263.

137. Herve PA, Silbert D, Mensch J, Cerrina J, Ladurie FL, Rain B, Bavoux E, Chapelier A, Dartevelle P, Lafont D, Parquin F, Simonneau G, Duroux P: Increased lung clearance of [99m]TcDTPA in allograft lung rejection. Am Rev Respir Dis 1991;144:1333–1335.

138. Higgins R, McNeil K, Dennis C, Parry A, Large S, Nashef SA, Wells FC, Flower C, Wallwork J: Airway stenoses after lung transplantation: management with expanding metal stents. J Heart Lung Transplant 1994;13:774–778.

139. Higgins RSD, Letsou GV, Sanches JA, Eisen RN, Smith GJ, Franco KL, Hammond GL, Baldwin JC: Improved ultrastructural lung preservation with prostaglandin E₁ as donor pretreatment in a primate model of heart/lung transplantation. J Thorac Cardiovasc Surg 1993;105:965–971.

140. Hobbs AJ, Ignarro LJ: The nitric oxide-cyclic GMP signal transduction system. In Zapol WM, Bloch KD (eds): Nitric Oxide and the Lung [Lenfant C (ed): Lung Biology in Health and Disease] New York: Marcel Dekker, 1997, p 1; and Lamas S, Michel T: Molecular biological features of nitric oxide synthase isoforms. In Zapol WM, Bloch KD (eds): Nitric Oxide and the Lung [Lenfant C (ed): Lung Biology in Health and Disease.] New York: Marcel Dekker, 1997, p 59.

141. Hoeg JM, Starzl TE, Brewer HB Jr: Liver transplantation for treatment of cardiovascular disease: comparison with medication and plasma exchange in homozygous familial hypercholesterolemia. Am J Cardiol 1987;59:705–707.

142. Hogman M, Frostell C, Arnberg H, Sandhagen B, Hedenstierna G: Prolonged bleeding time during nitric oxide inhalation in the rabbit. Acta Physiol Scand 1994;151:125–129.

143. Hopkins WE, Ochoa LL, Richardson GW, Trulock EP: Medical management of heart failure and candidate selection: comparison of the hemodynamics and survival of adults with severe primary pulmonary hypertension or Eisenmenger syndrome. J Heart Lung Transplant 1996;15:100–105.

144. Hopkins WE, Waggoner AD: Right and left ventricular area and function determined by two-dimensional echocardiography in adults with the Eisenmenger syndrome from a variety of congenital anomalies. Am J Cardiol 1993;72:90–94.

145. Hopkins WE, Waggoner AD, Gussak H: Quantitative ultrasonic tissue characterization of myocardium in cyanotic adults with an unrepaired congenital heart defect. Am J Cardiol 1994;74:930–934.

146. Hopkinson DN, Bhabra MS, Hooper TL: Pulmonary graft preservation: a worldwide survey of current clinical practice. J Heart Lung Transplant 1998;17:525–531.

147. Hopkinson DN, Bhabra MS, Odom NJ, Bridgewater BJ, Van Doorn CA, Hooper TL: Controlled pressure reperfusion of rat pulmonary grafts yields improved function after twenty-four hours' cold storage in University of Wisconsin solution. J Heart Lung Transplant 1996;15:283–290.

148. Horning NR, Lynch JP, Sundaresa SR, Patterson GA, Trulock EP: Tacrolimus therapy for persistent or recurrent acute rejection after lung transplantation. J Heart Lung Transplant 1998;17:761–767.

149. Hosenpud JD, Bennett LE, Keck BM, Fiol B, Novick RJ: The Registry of the International Society for Heart and Lung Transplantation: sixteenth official report—1999. J Heart Lung Transplant 1999;18:611–626.

150. Hunt BJ: Graft versus host disease in heart and/or lung transplantation. In Rose ML, Yacoub MH (eds): Immunology of Heart and Lung Transplantation. London: Arnold, 1993, p 261.

151. Hurford WE: The biologic basis for inhaled nitric oxide. Respir Care Clin North Am 1997;3:357–369.

152. Iacono A, Dauber J, Keenan R, Spichty K, Cai J, Grgurich W, Burckart G, Smaldone G, Pham S, Ohori NP, Yousem S, Williams P, Griffith B, Zeevi A: Interleukin 6 and interferon-γ gene expression in lung transplant recipients with refractory acute cellular rejection. Transplantation 1997;64:263–269.

153. Iber C, Simon P, Skatrud JB, Mahowald MW, Dempsey JA: The Breuer-Hering reflex in humans: effects of pulmonary denervation and hyopcapnia. Am J Respir Crit Care Med 1995;152:217–224.

154. Icenogle TB, Copeland JG: A technique to simplify and improve exposure in heart-lung transplantation. J Thorac Cardiovasc Surg 1995;110:1590–1593.

155. Ignarro LJ, Buga GM, Wood KS, Byrns RE, Chaudhuri G: Endothelium-derived relaxing factor produced and released from artery and vein is nitric oxide. Proc Natl Acad Sci U S A 1987;84:9265–9269.

156. Ikonen T, Kivisaari L, Harjula ALJ, Lehtola A, Heikkila L, Kinnula VL, Kyosola K, Savola J, Sipponen J, Verkkala K, Mattila SP: Value of high-resolution computed tomography in routine evaluation of lung transplantation recipients during development of bronchiolitis obliterans syndrome. J Heart Lung Transplant 1996;15:587–595.

157. Jamieson SW, Baldwin J, Stinson EB, Reitz BA, Oyer PE, Hunt S, Billingham M, Theodore J, Modry D, Bieber CP, Shumway NE: Clinical heart-lung transplantation. Transplantation 1984;37:81–84.

158. Jamieson SW, Stinson EB, Oyer PE, Baldwin JC, Shumway NE: Operative technique for heart-lung transplantation. J Thorac Cardiovasc Surg 1984;87:930–935.

159. Jamieson SW, Stinson EB, Oyer PE, Reitz BA, Baldwin J, Modry D, Dawkins K, Theodore J, Hunt S, Shumway NE: Heart-lung transplantation for irreversible pulmonary hypertension. Ann Thorac Surg 1984;38:554–562.

160. Jonosono M, Fang KC, Keith FM, Turck CW, Blanc PD, Hall TS, Fukano AK, Rifkin CJ, Gold WM, Webb WR, Edinburgh KJ, Finkbeiner WE, Golden JA: Measurement of fibroblast proliferative activity in bronchoalveolar lavage fluid in the analysis of obliterative bronchiolitis among lung transplant recipients. J Heart Lung Transplant 1999;18:972–985.

161. Jordan SC, Marchevski A, Ross D, Toyoda M, Waters PF: Serum interleukin-2 levels in lung transplant recipients: correlation with findings on transbronchial biopsy. J Heart Lung Transplant 1992;11:1001–1004.

162. Kanj SS, Welty-Wolf K, Madden J, Tapson V, Baz MA, Davis RD, Perfect JR: Fungal infections in lung and heart/lung transplant recipients: report of 9 cases and review of the literature. Medicine 1996;75:142–156.

163. Kanner J, Harel S, Granit R: Nitric oxide as an antioxidant. Arch Biochem Biophys 1991;289:130–136.

164. Karamachandani K, McCabe M, Simpson K, Robinson J, Garrity E: Photopheresis in the management of bronchiolitis obliterans syndrome (BOS) following lung transplantation [abstract]. Am J Respir Crit Care Med 1997;155:A276.

165. Karck M, Schmid C, Siclari F, Dammenhayn L, Haverich A: Effects of calcium channel blockage in postischemic lung reperfusion. Transplant Proc 1990;22:2237.

166. Katz WE, Gasior TA, Quinlan JJ, Lazar JM, Firestone L, Griffith BP, Gorcsan J: Immediate effects of lung transplantation on right ventricular morphology and function in patients with variable degrees of pulmonary hypertension. J Am Coll Cardiol 1996;27:384–391.

167. Kawaguchi A, Gandjbakhch I, Pavie A, Bors V, Leger P, Cabrol A, Eugene M, Delcort A, Cabrol C: Heart and unilateral lung transplantation in patients with end-stage cardiopulmonary disease and previous thoracic operations. J Thorac Cardiovasc Surg 1989;98:343–349.

168. Kawai A, Paradis IL, Keenan RJ, Yamazaki K, Yousem SA, Ohori NP, Fricker FJ, Griffith BP: Chronic rejection in heart/lung transplant recipients: the relationship between obliterative bronchiolitis and coronary artery disease. Transplant Proc 1995;27:1288–1289.

169. Keenan RJ, Bruzzone P, Paradis IL, Yousem SA, Dauber JH, Stuart RS, Griffith BP: Similarity of pulmonary rejection among heart/lung and double-lung transplant recipients. Transplantation 1991;51:176–180.

170. Keenan RJ, Dauber JH, Iacono AT: Long-term follow-up clinical trial of tacrolimus versus cyclosporine for lung transplantation. J Heart Lung Transplant 1998;17:59A.

171. Keenan RJ, Dauber JH, Iacono A, Zeevi A, Yousem SA, Ohori NP, Burckart GJ, Kawai A, Smaldone GC, Griffith BP: Treatment of refractory acute allograft rejection with aerosolized cyclosporine in lung transplant recipients. J Thorac Cardiovasc Surg 1997;113:335–341.

172. Keenan RJ, Konishi H, Kawai A, Paradis IL, Nunley DR, Iacono AT, Hardesty RL, Weyant RJ, Griffith BP: Clinical trial of tacrolimus versus cyclosporine in lung transplantation. Ann Thorac Surg 1995;60:580–585.

173. Keenan B, Zeevi A, Banan R: Microchimerism is associated with a lower incidence of chronic rejection after lung transplantation [abstract]. J Heart Lung Transplant 1994;13:533.

174. Keller CA, Cagle PT, Brown RW, Noon G, Frost AE: Bronchiolitis obliterans in recipients of single, double, and heart/lung transplantation. Chest 1995;107:973–980.

175. Keogh A, Kaan A, Doran T, Macdonald P, Bryant D, Spratt P: HLA mismatching and outcome in heart, heart-lung, and single lung transplantation. J Heart Lung Transplant 1995;14:444–451.

176. Keshavjee S, Todd TR: Excision and storage of the donor lungs: In Cooper DKC, Miller LW, Patterson GA (eds): The Transplantation and Replacement of Thoracic Organs. Dordrecht, The Netherlands: Kluwer Academic Publishers, 1996, p 445.

177. Kesten S, Chamberlain D, Maurer J: Yield of surveillance transbronchial biopsies performed beyond two years after lung transplantation. J Heart Lung Transplant 1996;15:384–388.

178. Kesten S, Chaparro C, Scavuzzo M, Gutierrez C: Tacrolimus as rescue therapy for bronchiolitis obliterans syndrome. J Heart Lung Transplant 1997;16:905–912.

179. Kesten S, Maidenberg A, Winton T, Maurer J: Treatment of presumed and proven acute rejection following six months of lung transplant survival. Am J Respir Crit Care Med 1995;152:1321.

180. Kesten S, Rajagopalan N, Maurer J: Cytolytic therapy for the treatment of bronchiolitis obliterans syndrome following lung transplantation. Transplantation 1996;61:427–430.

181. Khaghani A, Banner N, Ozdogan E, Musumeci F, Theodoropoulos S, Aravot D, Fitzgerald M, Yacoub M: Medium-term results of combined heart and lung transplantation for emphysema. J Heart Lung Transplant 1991;10:15–21.

182. Kidd L, Driscoll DJ, Gersony WM, Hayes CJ, Keane JF, O'Fallon WM, Pieroni DR, Wolfe RR, Weidman WH: Second natural history study of congenital heart defects. Results of treatment of patients with ventricular septal defects. Circulation 1993;87(suppl I):I-38–I-51.

183. Kobashigawa JA, Kirklin JK, Naftel DC, Bourge RC, Ventura HO, Mohanty PK, Cintron GB, Bhat G: Pretransplantation risk factors for acute rejection after heart transplantation, a multi-institutional study. J Heart Lung Transplant 1993;12:355.

184. Kon ND, Hines MH, Harr CD, Miller LR, Taylor CL, Cordell AR, Mills SA: Improved lung preservation with cold air storage. Ann Thorac Surg 1991;51:557–562.

185. Kocher AA, Schlechta B, Kopp CW, Ehrlich M, Ankersmit J, Ofiner P, Langer F, Berlakovich GA, Grimm M, Wolner E, Laufer G: Combined heart and kidney transplantation using a single donor. Transplantation 1998;66:1760–1763.

186. Kooman JP, Leunissen KML: Cardiovascular aspects in renal disease. Curr Opin Nephrol Hypertens 1993;2:791.

187. Kooy NW, Royall JA: Agonist-induced peroxynitrite production from endothelial cells. Arch Biochem Biophys 1994;310:352–359.

188. Kramer MR, Denning DW, Marshall SE, Ross DJ, Berry G, Lewiston NJ, Stevens DA, Theodore J: Ulcerative tracheobronchitis after lung transplantation: a new form of invasive aspergillosis. Am Rev Respir Dis 1991;144:552–556.

189. Kramer MR, Marshall SE, Tiroke A, Lewiston NJ, Starnes VA, Theodore J: Clinical significance of hyperbilirubinemia in patients with pulmonary hypertension undergoing heart-lung transplantation. J Heart Lung Transplant 1991;10:317–321.

190. Kramer MR, Stoehr C, Whang JL, Berry GJ, Sibley R, Marshall SE, Patterson GM, Starnes VA, Theodore J: The diagnosis of obliterative bronchiolitis after heart-lung and lung transplantation: low yield of transbronchial lung biopsy. J Heart Lung Transplant 1993;12:675–681.

191. Kramer MR, Valantine HA, Marshall SE, Starnes VA, Theodore J: Recovery of the right ventricle after single-lung transplantation in pulmonary hypertension. Am J Cardiol 1994;73:494–500.

192. Kroshus TJ, Kshettry VR, Savik K, John R, Hertz MI, Bolman RM III: Risk factors for the development of bronchiolitis obliterans syndrome after lung transplantation. J Thorac Cardiovasc Surg 1997;114:195–202.

193. Kshettry VR, Kroshus TJ, Burdine J, Savik K, Bolman RM III: Does donor organ ischemia over 4 hours affect long-term survival after lung transplantation? J Heart Lung Transplant 1996;15:169–174.

194. Kukkonen S, Heikkilä LJ, Verkkala K, Mattila SP, Toivonen H: Prostaglandin E_1 or prostacyclin in Euro-Collins solution fails to improve lung preservation. Ann Thorac Surg 1995;60:1617–1622.

195. Kurland G, Noyes BE, Jaffe R, Atlas AB, Armitage J, Orenstein DM: Bronchoalveolar lavage and transbronchial biopsy in children following heart/lung and lung transplantation. Chest 1993;104:1043–1048.

196. Ladowski JS, Hardesty RL, Griffith BP: The pulmonary artery blood supply to the supracarinal trachea. J Heart Transplant 1984;4:40–42.

197. Lai K, Barnden L, Mathew T: Effect of renal transplantation on left ventricular function in hemodialysis patients. Clin Nephrol 1982;18:74–78.

198. Lange W: Ubert Eine Eigenthumliche: Erkrankung der kleinen bronchien und bronchiolen. Dtsch Arch Klin Med 1901;70:342.

199. Larrson O, Attman P-O, Beckman-Suurküla M, Wallentin I, Wikstrand J: Left ventricular function before and after kidney transplantation. A prospective study in patients with juvenile-onset diabetes mellitus. Eur Heart J 1986;7:779–791.

200. Laufer G, Kocher A, Grabenwöger M, Berlakovich GA, Zuckermann A, Ofiner P, Grimm M, Steininger R, Muhlbacher F: Simultaneous heart and kidney transplantation as treatment for end-stage heart and kidney failure. Transplantation 1997;64:1129–1134.

201. Lazar JM, Flores AR, Grandis DJ, Orie JE, Schulman DS: Effects of chronic right ventricular pressure overload on left ventricular diastolic function. Am J Cardiol 1993;72:1179–1182.

202. Lefer AM: Induction of tissue injury and altered cardiovascular performance by platelet-activating factor: relevance to multiple systems organ failure. Crit Care Clin 1989;5:331–352.

203. Lempert N, Blumenstock DA: Survival of dogs after bilateral reimplantation of the lungs. Surg Forum 1964;15:179–181.

204. Lick SD, Brown PS, Kurusz M, Vertrees RA, McQuitty CK, Johnston WE: Technique of controlled reperfusion of the transplanted lung in humans. Ann Thorac Surg 2000;69:910–912.

205. Lick SD, Copeland JG, Rosado LJ, Arabia FA, Sethi GK: Simplified technique of heart-lung transplantation. Ann Thorac Surg 1995; 59:1592–1593.

206. Lillehei CW: In discussion of: p. 515 of Wildevuur CRH, and Benfield JR: A review of 23 human lung transplantations by 20 surgeons. Ann Thorac Surg 1970;9:489–515.

207. Lim TT, Botas J, Ross H, Liang DH, Theodore J, Hunt SA, Oesterle SN, Yeung AC: Are heart-lung transplant recipients protected from developing transplant coronary artery disease? Circulation 1996;94:1573–1577.

208. Lindberg L, Kimblad PO, Sjoberg T, Ingemansson R, Steen S: Inhaled nitric oxide reveals and attenuates endothelial dysfunction after lung transplantation. Ann Thorac Surg 1996;62:1639–1643.

209. Livesay SA, Rolles K, Calne RY, Wallwork J, English TAH: Successful simultaneous heart and kidney transplantation using the same donor. Clin Transplant 1988;2:1.

210. Llorens R, Davalos G, Indaburu D, Gil O, Florez I, Berian JM, Cato J, Melero JM: Use of biventricular circulatory support as bridge to simultaneous heart and kidney transplantation. Eur J Cardiothorac Surg 1993;7:96–100.

211. Lloyd KS, Barnard P, Holland VA, Noon GP, Lawrence EC: Pulmonary function after heart-lung transplantation using larger donor organs. Am Rev Respir Dis 1990;142:1026–1029.

212. LoCicero J III, Robinson PG, Fisher M: Chronic rejection in single-lung transplantation manifested by obliterative bronchiolitis. J Thorac Cardiovasc Surg 1990;99:1059–1062.

213. Longmore DB, Cooper DKC, Hall RW, Sekabunga J, Welch W: Transplantation of the heart and both lungs. II. Experimental cardiopulmonary transplantation. Thorax 1969;24:391–398.

214. Longoria J, Roberts RE, Marboe CC, Stouch BC, Starnes VA, Barr ML: Sirolimus (Rapamycin) potentiates cyclosporine in prevention of acute lung rejection. J Thorac Cardiovasc Surg 1999;117:714–718.

215. Losman JG, Campbell CD, Replogle RL, Barnard CN: Joint transplantation of the heart and lungs. J Cardiovasc Surg 1982;23:440–452.

216. Loubeyre P, Revel D, Delignette A, Loire R, Mornex JF: High resolution computed tomographic findings associated with histologically diagnosed acute lung rejection in heart-lung transplant recipients. Chest 1995;107:132–138.

217. Loubeyre P, Revel D, Delignette A, Wiesendanger T, Philit F, Betocchi M, Loire R, Mornex JF: Bronchiectasis detected with thin-section CT as a predictor of chronic lung allograft rejection. Radiology 1995;194:213–216.

218. Louie EK, Rich S, Levitsky S, Brundage BH: Doppler echocardiographic demonstration of the differential effects of right ventricular pressure and volume overload on left ventricular geometry and filling. J Am Coll Cardiol 1992;19:84–90.

219. Lower RR, Stofer RC, Hurley EJ, Shumway NE: Complete homograft replacement of the heart and both lungs. Surgery 1961; 50:842–845.

220. Lupinetti FM, Bolling SF, Bove EL, Brunsting LA, Crowley DC, Lynch JP, Orringer MB, Whyte RI, Deeb GM: Selective lung or heart/lung transplantation for pulmonary hypertension associated with congenital cardiac anomalies. Ann Thorac Surg 1994; 57:1545–1549.

221. MacDonald P, Mundy J, Rogers P, Harrison G, Branch J, Glanville A, Keogh A, Spratt P: Successful treatment of life-threatening acute reperfusion injury after lung transplantation with inhaled nitric oxide. J Thorac Cardiovasc Surg 1995;110:861–863.

222. Matheis G, Sherman MP, Buckberg GD, Haybron DM, Young HH, Ignarro LJ: Role of L-arginine-nitric oxide pathway in myocardial reoxygenation injury. Am J Physiol 1992;262:H616–H620.

223. Matteucci MC, Strologo LD, Parisi F, Squitierei C, Caione P, Capozza N, Rizzoni G: Combined heart and kidney transplantation in a child. Will we need it more in the future? Transplantation 1997;63:1531–1533.

224. Mauney MC, Cope JT, Binns OA, King RC, Shockey KS, Buchanan SA, Wilson SW, Cogbill J, Kron IL, Tribble CG: Non-heart-beating donors: a model of thoracic allograft injury. Ann Thorac Surg 1996;62:54–62.

225. McCaffrey D, MacDonald P, Keogh A: Preoperative creatinine and prognosis following cardiac transplantation. Presentation at The Transplantation Society of Australia and New Zealand, Sixteenth Scientific Meeting, Canberra, April 1998.

226. McCarthy PM, Rosenkranz ER, White RC, Rice TW, Sterba R, Vargo R, Mehta AC: Single-lung transplantation with atrial septal defect repair for Eisenmenger's syndrome. Ann Thorac Surg 1991;52:300–303.

227. McCarthy PM, Starnes VA, Theodore J, Stinson EB, Oyer PE, Shumway NE: Improved survival after heart-lung transplantation. J Thorac Cardiovasc Surg 1990;99:54–60.

228. McDonald K, Rector TS, Braunlin EA, Kubo SH, Olivari MT: Association of coronary artery disease in cardiac transplant recipients with cytomegalovirus infection. Am J Cardiol 1989;64:359–362.

229. McGiffin DC, Karp RB: Cardiac transplantation in a patient with a persistent left superior vena cava and an absent right superior vena cava. Heart Transplant 1984;3:115–116.

230. McGiffin DC, Kirklin JK, Naftel DC: Acute renal failure after heart transplantation and cyclosporine therapy. Heart Transplant 1985;4:396.

231. McGiffin DC, Savunen T, Kirklin JK, Naftel DC, Bourge RC, Paine TD, White-Williams C, Sisto T, Early L: Cardiac transplant coronary artery disease: a multivariable analysis of pretransplantation risk factors for disease development and morbid events. J Thorac Cardiovasc Surg 1995;109:1081–1088.

232. McGregor CGA, Baldwin JC, Jamieson SW, Billingham ME, Yousem SA, Burke CM, Oyer PE, Stinson EB, Shumway NE: Isolated pulmonary rejection after combined heart-lung transplantation. J Thorac Cardiovasc Surg 1985;90:623–630.

233. Medina LS, Siegel MJ, Glazer HS, Anderson DJ, Semenkovich J, Bejarano PA, Mallory GB: Diagnosis of pulmonary complications associated with lung transplantation in children: value of CT vs histopathological studies. AJR Am J Roentgenol 1994;162:969–974.

234. Meiser BM, Überfuhr P, Fuchs A, Schulze C, Nollert G, Mair H, Martin S, Pfeiffer M, Reichenspurner H, Kreuzer E, Reichart B: Tacrolimus: a superior agent to OKT3 for treating cases of persistent rejection after intrathoracic transplantation. J Heart Lung Transplant 1997;16:795–800.

235. Mieles LA, Orenstein D, Teperman L, Podesta L, Koneru B, Starzl TE: Liver transplantation in cystic fibrosis. Lancet 1989;13:1073.

236. Miller JD, de Hoyos A, Patterson GA: An evaluation of the role of omentopexy and early postoperative corticosteroids in clinical lung transplantation. J Thorac Cardiovasc Surg 1993;105:247–252.

237. Millet B, Higenbottam TW, Flower CDR, Stewart S, Wallwork J: The radiographic appearances of infection and acute rejection of the lung after heart-lung transplantation. Am Rev Respir Dis 1989;140:62.

238. Miralles A, Muneretto C, Gandjbakhch I, Lecompte Y, Pavie A, Rabago G, Bracamonte L, Desruennes M, Cabrol A, Cabrol C: Heart-lung transplantation in situs inversus: a case report in a patient with Kartagener's syndrome. J Thorac Cardiovasc Surg 1992;103:307–313.

239. Mitruka SN, Pham SM, Zeevi A, Li S, Cai J, Burckart GJ, Yousem SA, Keenan RJ, Griffith BP: Aerosol cyclosporine prevents acute allograft rejection in experimental lung transplantation. J Thorac Cardiovasc Surg 1998;115:28–37.

240. Mizuta T, Fujii Y, Minami M, Tanaka S, Utsumi T, Kosaka H, Shirakura R, Matsuda H: Increased nitric oxide levels in exhaled air of rat lung allografts. J Thorac Cardiovasc Surg 1997;113:830–835.

241. Moller F, Hoyt G, Farfan F, Starnes VA, Clayberger C: Cellular mechanisms underlying differential rejection of sequential heart and lung allografts in rats. Transplantation 1993;55:650–655.

242. Moncada S, Higgs EA: Molecular mechanisms and therapeutic strategies related to nitric oxide. FASEB J 1995;9:1319–1330.

243. Moore TM, Khimenko PL, Wilson PS, Taylor AE: Role of nitric oxide in lung ischemia and reperfusion injury. Am J Physiol 1996;271:H1970–H1977.

244. Mora NP, Cienfuegos JA, Ardaiz J, Pardo F, Turrion VS, Pereira F, Herrera J, Castillo OJL, Figuera D: Special operative events in the first case of liver grafting after heart transplantation. Surgery 1988;103:264–267.

245. Murakami S, Bacha EA, Mazmanian GM, Detruit H, Chapelier A, Dartevelle P, Herve P: Effects of various timings and concentrations of inhaled nitric oxide in lung ischemia-reperfusion. The Paris-Sud University Lung Transplantation Group. Am J Respir Crit Care Med 1997;156:454–458.

246. Naka Y, Chowdhury NC, Oz MC, Smith CR, Yano OJ, Michler RE, Stern DM, Pinsky DJ: Nitroglycerin maintains graft vascular homeostasis and enhances preservation in an orthotopic rat lung transplant model. J Thorac Cardiovasc Surg 1995;109:206–211.

247. Nakae S, Webb WR, Theodorides T, Sugg WL: Respiratory function following cardiopulmonary denervation in dog, cat, and monkey. Surg Gynecol Obstet 1967;125:1285–1292.

248. Narula J, Bennett LE, DiSalvo T, Hosenpud JD, Semigran MJ, Dec GW: Outcomes in recipients of combined heart-kidney transplantation. Transplantation 1997;63:861–867.

249. Neptune WB, Cookson BA, Bailey C, Appler R, Rajkowski F: Complete homologous heart transplantation. AMA Arch Surg 1953;66:174–178.

250. Niu XF, Smith W, Kubes P: Intracellular oxidative stress induced by nitric oxide synthesis inhibition increases endothelial cell adhesion to neutrophils. Circ Res 1994;74:1133–1140.

251. Noble-Jamieson G, Valente J, Barnes ND, Friend PJ, Jamieson NV, Rasmussen A, Calne RY: Liver transplantation for hepatic cirrhosis in cystic fibrosis. Arch Dis Child 1994;71:349–352.

252. Noirclerc M, Shennib H, Giudicelli R, Latter D, Metras D, Colt HG, Mulder D: Size matching in lung transplantation. J Heart Lung Transplant 1992;11:S203–S208.

253. Norgaard MA, Efsen F, Andersen CB, Svendsen UG, Pettersson G: Medium-term patency and anatomic changes after direct bronchial artery revascularization in lung and heart/lung transplantation with the internal thoracic artery conduit. J Thorac Cardiovasc Surg 1997;114:326–331.

254. Norgaard MA, Efsen F, Arendrup H, Olsen PS, Svendsen UG, Pettersson G: Surgical and arteriographic results of bronchial artery revascularization in lung and heart/lung transplantation. J Heart Lung Transplant 1997;16:302–312.

255. Norman JC, Cooley DA, Kahan BD, Frazier OH, Keats AS, Hacker J, Massin EK, Duncan JM, Solis RT, Dacso CC, Luper WE, Winston DS, Reul GJ: Total support of the circulation of a patient with post-cardiotomy stone-heart syndrome by a partial artificial heart (ALVAD) for 5 days followed by heart and kidney transplantation. Lancet 1978;1:1125–1127.

256. Novick RJ, Bennett LE, Meyer DM, Hosenpud JD: Influence of graft ischemic time and donor age on survival after lung transplantation. J Heart Lung Transplant 1999;18:425–431.

257. Novick RJ, Menkis AH, McKenzie FN, Reid KR, Pflugfelder PW, Kostuk WJ, Ahmad D: Reduction in bleeding after heart-lung transplantation: the importance of posterior mediastinal hemostasis. Chest 1990;98:1383–1387.

258. Novick RJ, Menkis AH, McKenzie FN, Reid KR, Pflugfelder PW, Kostuk WJ, Ahmad D: The safety of low-dose prednisone before and immediately after heart-lung transplantation. Ann Thorac Surg 1991;51:642–645.

259. Novick RJ, Reid KR, Denning L, Duplan J, Menkis AH, McKenzie N: Prolonged preservation of canine lung allografts: the role of prostaglandins. Ann Thorac Surg 1991;51:853–859.

260. Novick RJ, Schäfers HJ, Stitt L, Andreassian B, Duchatele JP, Klepetko W, Hardesty RL, Frost A, Patterson GA: Recurrence of obliterative bronchiolitis and determinants of outcome in 139 pulmonary retransplant recipients. J Thorac Cardiovasc Surg 1995;110:1402–1413.

261. Novitsky D, Cooper DKC, Rose AG, Reichart B: Acute isolated pulmonary rejection following transplantation of the heart and both lungs: experimental and clinical observations. Ann Thorac Surg 1986;42:180–184.

262. Oeltgen PR, Horton ND, Bolling SF, Su TP: Extended lung preservation with the use of hibernation trigger factors. Ann Thorac Surg 1996;61:1488–1493.

263. O'Hagan A, Koo A, Stillwell P: Photopheresis (PP) for refractory bronchiolitis obliterans (OB) in lung transplantation. [abstract]. Chest 1996;110:37A.

264. O'Hair DP, Cantu E, McGregor C, Jorgensen B, Gerow-Smith R, Galantowicz ME, Schulman LL: Preliminary experience with mycophenolate mofetil used after lung transplantation. J Heart Lung Transplant 1998;17:864–868.

265. Okabayashi K, Aoe M, DeMeester SR, Cooper JD, Patterson GA: Pentoxifylline reduces lung allograft reperfusion injury. Ann Thorac Surg 1994;58:50–56.

266. Okabayashi K, Triantafillou AN, Yamashita M, Aoe M, DeMeester SR, Cooper JD, Patterson GA: Inhaled nitric oxide improves lung allograft function after prolonged storage. J Thorac Cardiovasc Surg 1996;112:293–299.

267. Olivieri NF, Liu PP, Sher GD, Daly PA, Greig PD, McCusker PJ, Collins AF, Francombe WH, Templeton DM: Brief report: combined liver and heart transplantation for end-stage iron-induced organ failure in an adult with homozygous beta-thalassemia. N Engl J Med 1994;330:1125–1127.

268. Onsager DR, Canver CC, Jahania MS, Welter D, Michalski M, Hoffman AM, Mentzer RM, Love RB: Efficacy of tacrolimus in the treatment of refractory rejection in heart and lung transplant recipients. J Heart Lung Transplant 1999;18:448–455.

269. Otulana BA, Higenbottam T, Hutter J, Wallwork J: Close monitoring of lung function allows detection of pulmonary rejection and infection in heart-lung transplantation. Am Rev Respir Dis 1988;137:A245.

270. Otulana BA, Higenbottam T, Scott J, Clelland C, Igboaka G, Wallwork J: Lung function associated with histologically diagnosed acute lung rejection and pulmonary infection in heart-lung transplant patients. Am Rev Respir Dis 1990;142:329–332.

271. Palmer SM, Perfect JR, Howell DN, Lawrence CM, Miralles AP, Davis RD, Tapson VF: Candidal anastomotic infection in lung transplant recipients: successful treatment with a combination of systemic and inhaled antifungal agents. J Heart Lung Transplant 1998;17:1029–1033.

272. Parry AJ, O'Fiesh J, Wallwork J, Large SR: Heart-lung transplantation in situs inversus and chest wall deformity. Ann Thorac Surg 1994;58:1174–1176.

273. Pasque MK, Kaiser LR, Dresler CM, Trulock EP, Triantafillou A, Cooper JD: Single-lung transplantation for pulmonary hypertension: technical aspects and immediate hemodynamic results. J Thorac Cardiovasc Surg 1992;103:475–482.

274. Pasque MK, Trulock EP, Kaiser LR, Cooper JD: Single lung transplantation for pulmonary hypertension: three month hemodynamic follow-up. Circulation 1991;84:2275–2279.

275. Patterson GA, Todd TR, Cooper JD, Pearson FG, Winton TL, Maurer J: Airway complications after double lung transplantation. J Thorac Cardiovasc Surg 1990;99:14–21.

276. Patterson GA, Wilson S, Whang JL, Harvey J, Agacki K, Patel H, Theodore J: Physiologic definitions of obliterative bronchiolitis in heart-lung and double lung transplantation: a comparison of the forced expiratory flow between 25% and 75% of the forced vital capacity and forced expiratory volume in one second. J Heart Lung Transplant 1996;15:175–181.

277. Paull DE, Keagy BA, Kron EJ, Wilcox BR: Reperfusion injury in the lung preserved for 24 hours. Ann Thorac Surg 1989;47:187–192.

278. Pettersson G, Norgaard MA, Arendrup H, Brandenhof P, Helvind M, Joyce F, Stentoft P, Olesen PS, Thiis JJ, Efsen F, Mortensen SA, Svendsen UG: Direct bronchial artery revascularization and en bloc double lung transplantation—surgical techniques and early outcome. J Heart Lung Transplant 1997;16:320–333.

279. Pfitzmann R, Hummel M, Grauhan O, Waurick P, Ewert R, Loebe M, Weng Y, Hetzer R: Acute graft-versus-host disease after human heart-lung transplantation: a case report. J Thorac Cardiovasc Surg 1997;114:285–287.

280. Plopper CG, Have-Opbroek AAWT: Anatomical and histological classification of the bronchioles. *In* Epler GR (ed): Diseases of the Bronchioles. New York: Raven Press, 1994.

281. Pollock JS, Forstermann U, Mitchell JA, Warner TD, Schmidt HH, Nakane M, Murad F: Purification and characterization of particulate endothelium-derived relaxing factor synthase from cultured and native bovine aortic endothelial cells. Proc Natl Acad Sci U S A 1991;88:10480–10484.

282. Pomerance A, Madden B, Burke MM, Yacob MH: Transbronchial biopsy in heart and lung transplantation: clinicopathologic correlations. J Heart Lung Transplant 1995;14:761–773.

283. Prop J, Kuijpers K, Petersen AH, Bartels HL, Nieuwenhuis P, Wildevuur CRH: Why are lung allografts more vigorously rejected than hearts? Heart Transplant 1985;4:433–436.

284. Prop J, Wagenaar-Hilbers JPA, Petersen AH, Wildevuur CRH: Characteristics of cells lavaged from rejecting lung allografts in rats. Transplant Proc 1988;20:217–218.

285. Provost P, Lam JYT, Lacoste L, Merhi Y, Waters D: Endothelium-derived nitric oxide attenuates neutrophil adhesion to endothelium under arterial flow conditions. Arterioscler Thromb 1994; 14:331–335.

286. Raab W: Cardiotoxic substances in the blood and heart muscle in uremia (their nature and action). J Lab Clin Med 1944;29:715.

287. Rabago G, Copeland JG III, Rosapepe F: Heart-lung transplantation in situs inversus. Ann Thorac Surg 1996;62:296–298.

288. Rabinowich H, Zeevi A, Yousem SA, Dauber JH, Kormos R, Hardesty RL, Griffith BP, Duquesnoy RJ: Alloreactivity of lung bioposy and bronchoalveolar lavage-derived lymphocytes from pulmonary transplant patients: correlations with acute rejection and bronchiolitis obliterans. Clin Transplant 1990;4:376.

289. Radley-Smith RC, Burke M, Pomerance A, Yacoub MH: Graft vessel disease and obliterative bronchiolitis after heart/lung transplantation in children. Transplant Proc 1995;27:2017–2018.

290. Rao PN, Zeevi A, Snyder J, Spichty K, Habrat T, Warty V, Dauber J, Paradis I, Duncan S, Pham S, Griffith B: Monitoring of acute lung rejection and infection by bronchoalveolar lavage and plasma levels of hyaluronic acid in clinical lung transplantation. J Heart Lung Transplant 1994;13:958–962.

291. Rees S: Arterial connections of the lung: the inaugural Keith Jefferson lecture. Clin Radiol 1981;32:1–15.

292. Reichenspurner H, Girgis RE, Robbins RC, Conte JV, Nair RV, Valentine V, Berry GJ, Morris RE, Theodore J, Reitz BA: Obliterative bronchiolitis after lung and heart/lung transplantation. Ann Thorac Surg 1995;60:1845–1853.

293. Reichenspurner H, Girgis RE, Robbins RC, Yun KL, Nitschke M, Berry GJ, Morris RE, Theodore J, Reitz BA: Stanford experience with obliterative bronchiolitis after lung and heart-lung transplantation. Ann Thorac Surg 1996;62:1467–1472.

294. Reichenspurner H, Meiser BM, Kur F, Wagner F, Welz A, Uberfuhr P, Briegel H, Reichart B: First experience with FK 506 for treatment of chronic pulmonary rejection. Transplant Proc 1995;27:2009.

295. Reichenspurner H, Soni V, Nitschke M, Berry GJ, Brazelton T, Shorthouse R, Huang X, Boname J, Girgis R, Raitz BA, Mocarski E, Sandford G, Morris RE: Enhancement of obliterative airway disease in rat tracheal allografts infected with recombinant rat cytomegalovirus. J Heart Lung Transplant 1998;17:439–451.

296. Reignier J, Mazmanian M, Chapelier A: Evaluation of a new preservation solution: Celsior in the isolated rat lung. J Heart Lung Transplant 1995;14:601–604.

297. Reinsmoen NL, Bolman RM, Savik K, Butters K, Hertz MI: Are multiple immunopathogenetic events occurring during the development of obliterative bronchiolitis and acute rejection? Transplantation 1993;55:1040–1044.

298. Reinsmoen NL, Bolman RM, Savik K, Butters K, Matas AJ, Hertz MI: Improved long-term graft outcome in lung transplant recipients who have donor antigen-specific hyporeactivity. J Heart Lung Transplant 1994;13:30–36.

299. Reitz BA, Burton NA, Jamieson SW, Bieber CP, Pennock JL, Stinson EB, Shumway NE: Heart and lung transplantation: autotransplantation and allotransplantation in primates with extended survival. J Thorac Cardiovasc Surg 1980;80:360–372.

300. Reitz BA, Guadiani VA, Hunt SA, Wallwork J, Billingham ME, Oyer PE, Baumgartner WA, Jamieson SW, Stinson EB, Shumway NE: Diagnosis and treatment of allograft rejection in heart-lung transplant recipients. J Thorac Cardiovasc Surg 1983;85:354–361.

301. Reitz BA, Wallwork JL, Hunt SA, Pennock JL, Billingham ME, Oyer PE, Stinson EB, Shumway NE: Heart-lung transplantation: successful therapy for patients with pulmonary vascular disease. N Engl J Med 1982;306:557–564.

302. Rela M, Muiesan P, Heaton ND, Corbaly M, Hajj H, Mowat AP, Williams R, Tan KC: Orthotopic liver transplantation for hepatic-based metabolic disorders. Transplant Int 1995;8:41–44.

303. Rinaldi M, Martinelli L, Volpato G, Minzioni G, Goggi C, Mantovani V, Vigano M: University of Wisconsin solution provides better lung preservation in human lung transplantation. Transplant Proc 1995;27:2869–2871.

304. Ritchie M, Waggoner AD, Dávila-Román VG, Barzilai B, Trulock EP, Eisenberg PR: Echocardiographic characterization of the improvement in right ventricular function in patients with severe pulmonary hypertension after single-lung transplantation. J Am Coll Cardiol 1993;22:1170–1174.

305. Rizzo M, Sundaresan S, Lynch J, Trulock EP, Cooper J, Patterson GA, Mohanakumar T: Increased concentration of soluble human leukocyte antigen class I levels in the bronchoalveolar lavage of human pulmonary allografts. J Heart Lung Transplant 1997;16: 1135–1140.

306. Roberts CS, Hennington MH, D'Armini AM, Griffith PK, Lemasters JJ, Egan TM: Donor lungs from ventilated cadavers: impact of a free radical scavenger. J Heart Lung Transplant 1996; 15:275–282.

307. Roberts JD, Roberts CT, Jones RC, Zapol WM, Bloch KD: Continuous nitric oxide inhalation reduces pulmonary arterial structural changes, right ventricular hypertrophy and growth retardation in the hypoxic newborn rat. Circ Res 1995;76:215–222.

308. Ross DJ, Marchevsky A, Kramer M, Kass RM: "Refractoriness" of airflow obstruction associated with isolated lymphocytic bronchiolitis/bronchitis in pulmonary allografts. J Heart Lung Transplant 1997;16:832–838.

309. Ross DJ, Moudgil A, Bagga A, Toyoda M, Marchevsky AM, Kass RM, Jordan SC: Lung allograft dysfunction correlates with γ-interferon gene expression in brochoalveolar lavage. J Heart Lung Transplant 1999;18:627–636.

310. Ross DJ, Waters PF, Levine M, Kramer M, Ruzevich S, Kass RM: Mycophenolate mofetil versus azathioprine immunosuppressive regimens after lung transplantation: preliminary experience. J Heart Lung Transplant 1998;17:768–774.

311. Ruggiero R, Fietsam R, Thomas GA, Muz J, Farris RH, Kowal TA, Myles JL, Stephenson LW, Baciewicz FA: Detection of canine allograft lung rejection by pulmonary lymphoscintigraphy. J Thorac Cardiovasc Surg 1994;108:253–258.

312. Ruggiero R, Muz J, Fietsam R Jr, Thomas GA, Welsh RJ, Miller JE, Stephenson LW, Bacjewicz FA: Reestablishment of lymphatic drainage after canine lung transplantation. J Thorac Cardiovasc Surg 1993;106:167–171.

313. Saint Martin GA, Reddy VB, Garrity ER, Simpson K, Robinson JA, Adent JK, Husain AN: Humoral (antibody-mediated) rejection in lung transplantation. J Heart Lung Transplant 1996;15:1217–1222.

314. Salerno CT, Park SJ, Kreykes NS, Kulick DM, Savik K, Hertz MI, Bolman RM: Adjuvant treatment of refractory lung transplant rejection with extracorporeal photopheresis. J Thorac Cardiovasc Surg 1999;117:1063–1069.

315. Sarris GE, Smith JA, Shumway NE, Stinson EB, Oyer PE, Robbins RC, Billingham ME, Theodore J, Moore KA, Reitz BA: Long-term results of combined heart-lung transplantation: the Stanford experience. J Heart Lung Transplant 1994;13:940–949.

316. Sasaki S, McCully DJ, Alessandrini F, LoCicero J III: Impact of initial flush potassium concentration on the adequacy of lung preservation. J Thorac Cardiovasc Surg 1995;109:1090–1096.

317. Savdie E, Keogh AM, Macdonald PS, Spratt PM, Graham AM, Golovsky D, Stricker PD, Spicer T, Hayes JM, Crozier J: Simultaneous transplantation of the heart and kidney. Aust N Z J Med 1994;24:554.

318. Schafers HJ, Haydock DA, Cooper JD: The prevalence and management of bronchial anastomotic complications in lung transplantation. J Thorac Cardiovasc Surg 1991;101:1044–1052.

319. Scherstén H, Hedner T, McGregor CGA, Miller VM, Martensson G, Riise GC, Nilsson FN: Increased levels of endothelin-1 in bronchoalveolar lavage fluid of patients with lung allografts. J Thorac Cardiovasc Surg 1996;111:253–258.

320. Schmidt HHW, Walter U: Nitric oxide at work. Cell 1994;78: 919–925.

321. Scott JP, Fradet G, Smyth RL, Mullins P, Pratt A, Clelland CA, Higenbottam T, Wallwork J: Prospective study of transbronchial biopsies in the management of heart-lung and single lung transplant patients. J Heart Lung Transplant 1991;10:626–637.

322. Scott JP, Higenbottam TW, Sharples L, Clelland CA, Smyth RL, Stewart S, Wallwork J: Risk factors for obliterative bronchiolitis

in heart-lung transplant recipients. Transplantation 1991;51: 813–817.

323. Scott JP, Peters SG, McDougall JC, Beck KC, Midthun DE: Post-transplantation physiologic features of the lung and obliterative bronchiolitis. Mayo Clin Proc 1997;72:170–174.

324. Scott WC, Haverich A, Billingham ME, Dawkins KD, Jamieson SW: Lethal rejection of the lung without significant cardiac rejection in primate heart-lung allotransplants. J Heart Transplant 1984;4:33–39.

325. Scuderi LJ, Bailey SR, Calhoon JH, Trinkle JK, Cronin TA, Zabalgoitia M: Echocardiographic assessment of right and left ventricular function after single lung transplantation. Am Heart J 1994; 127:636–642.

326. Sharples LD, Scott JP, Dennis C, Higenbottam TW, Stewart S, Wreghitt T, Large SR, Wells FC, Wallwork J: Risk factors for survival following combined heart/lung transplantation. Transplantation 1994;57:218–223.

327. Sharples LD, Tamm M, NcNeil K, Higenbottam TW, Stewart S, Wallwork J: Development of bronchiolitis obliterans syndrome in recipients of heart-lung transplantation—early risk factors. Transplantation 1996;61:560–566.

328. Shaw BW, Bahnson HT, Hardesty RL, Griffith BP, Starzl TE: Combined transplantation of the heart and liver. Ann Surg 1985;202:667–672.

329. Shennib H, Massard G, Reynaud M, Noirclerc M: Efficacy of OKT3 therapy for acute rejection in isolated lung transplantation. J Heart Lung Transplant 1994;13:514–519.

330. Shennib H, Nguyen D, Guttmann RD, Mulder DS: Phenotypic expression of bronchoalveolar lavage cells in lung rejection and infection. Ann Thorac Surg 1991;51:630–635.

331. Shionozaki F, Kondo T, Fijimura S, Nakada T: Technical establishment and detection of rejection in rat lung transplantation. Transplant Proc 1985;17:244.

332. Shiraishi T, Mizuta T, DeMeester SR, Ritter JH, Swanson PE, Wick MR, Cooper JD, Patterson GA: Effect of ischemic injury on subsequent rat lung allograft rejection. Ann Thorac Surg 1995; 60:947–951.

333. Shiraishi Y, Lee JR, Laks H, Waters PF, Meneshian A, Blitz A, Johnson K, Lam L, Chang PA: L-Arginine administration during reperfusion improves pulmonary function. Ann Thorac Surg 1996;62:1580–1587.

334. Shumway SJ, Hertz MI, Maynard R, Kshettry VR, Bolman RM III: Airway complications after lung and heart-lung transplantation. Transplant Proc 1993;25:1165–1166.

335. Shumway SJ, Hertz MI, Petty MG, Bolman RM: Liberalization of donor criteria in lung and heart-lung transplantation. Ann Thorac Surg 1994;57:92–95.

336. Sibley RK, Berry GJ, Tazelaar HD, Kraemer MR, Theodore J, Marshall SE, Billingham ME, Starnes VA: The role of transbronchial biopsies in the management of lung transplant recipients. J Heart Lung Transplant 1993;12:308–324.

337. Siegelman SS, Hagstrom JWC, Koerner SK, Veith FJ: Restoration of bronchial artery circulation after canine lung allotransplantation. J Thorac Cardiovasc Surg 1977;73:792–795.

338. Slim MS, Yacoubian HD, Simonian SJ, Sahyoun P: Bilateral reimplantation of canine lungs: anatomical and physiological observations in a long-term survivor. Ann Thorac Surg 1965;1:755–759.

339. Slim MS, Yacoubian HD, Wilson JL, Rubeiz GA, Ghandur-Manymneh L: Successful bilateral reimplantation of canine lungs. Surgery 1964;55:676–683.

340. Slovis B, Loyd J, King L: Photopheresis for chronic rejection of lung allografts. N Engl J Med 1995;332:962.

341. Smith JA, Stewart S, Roberts M, McNeil K, Schofield PM, Higenbottam TW, Nashef SA, Large SR, Wells FC, Wallwork J: Significance of graft coronary artery disease in heart/lung transplant recipients. Transplant Proc 1995;27:2019–2020.

342. Smith JD, Danskine AJ, Laylor RM, Rose ML, Yacoub MH: The effect of panel reactive antibodies and the donor-specific crossmatch on graft survival after heart and heart-lung transplantation. Transplant Immunol 1993;1:60–65.

343. Smith MA, Sundaresan S, Mohanakumar T, Trulock EP, Lynch JP, Phelan DL, Cooper JD, Patterson GA: Effect of development of antibodies to HLA and cytomegalovirus mismatch on lung transplantation survival and development of bronchiolitis obliterans syndrome. J Thorac Cardiovasc Surg 1998;116:812–820.

344. Smyth RL, Higenbottam TW, Scott JP, Wreighitt TG, Stewart S, Clelland CA, McGoldrick JP, Wallwork J: Herpes simplex virus infection in heart-lung transplant recipients. Transplantation 1990;49:735–739.

345. Snell GI, Esmore DS, Williams TJ: Cytolytic therapy for the bronchiolitis obliterans syndrome complicating lung transplantation. Chest 1996;109:874–878.

346. Snell GI, Rabinov M, Griffiths A, Williams T, Ugoni A, Salamonsson R, Esmore D: Lung and heart-lung transplantation: pulmonary allograft ischemic time: an important predictor of survival after lung transplantation. J Heart Lung Transplant 1996; 15:160–168.

347. Sommers KE, Griffith BP, Hardesty RL, Keenan RJ: Early lung allograft function in twin recipients from the same donor: risk factor analysis. Ann Thorac Surg 1996;62:784–790.

348. Speich R, Boehler A, Thurnheer R, Weder W: Salvage therapy with mycophenolate mofetil for lung transplant bronchiolitis obliterans. Transplantation 1997;64:533–535.

349. Spray TL, Mallory GB, Canter CE, Huddleston CB, Kaiser LR: Pediatric lung transplantation for pulmonary hypertension and congenital heart disease. Ann Thorac Surg 1992;54:216–225.

350. Stamler JS, Singel DJ, Loscalzo J: Biochemistry of nitric oxide and its redox-activated forms. Science 1992;258:1898–1902.

351. Starnes VA, Oyer PE, Bernstein D, Baum D, Gamberg P, Miller J, Shumway NE: Heart, heart-lung and lung transplantation in the first year of life. Ann Thorac Surg 1992;53:306–310.

352. Stevens GH, Sanchez MM, Chappell GL: Enhancement of lung preservation by prevention of lung collapse. J Surg Res 1973; 14:400–405.

353. Stern RC, Stevens DP, Boat TF, Doershuk CF, Izant RJ, Matthews LW: Symptomatic hepatic disease in cystic fibrosis: incidence, course, and outcome of portal systemic shunting. Gastroenterology 1976;70:645–649.

354. Sundaresan RS, Shiraishi Y, Trulock EP, Manley J, Lynch J, Cooper JD, Patterson GA: Cardiac and pulmonary replacement: single or bilateral lung transplantation for emphysema? J Thorac Cardiovasc Sur 1996;112:1485–1495.

355. Sundaresan S, Mohanakumar T, Phelan D: Development of cytotoxic antibodies post lung transplantation correlates with the development of bronchiolitis obliterans syndrome. Surg Forum 1994;45:447.

356. Sundaresan S, Semenkovich J, Ochoa L, Richardson G, Trulock EP, Cooper JD, Patterson GA: Cardiac and pulmonary replacement: successful outcome of lung transplantation is not compromised by the use of marginal donor lungs. J Thorac Cardiovasc Surg 1995;109:1075–1079.

357. Surakomol S, Olson LJ, Rastogi A, Steers JL, Sterioff S, Daly RC, McGregor CG: Combined orthotopic heart and liver transplantation for genetic hemochromatosis. J Heart Lung Transplant 1997;16:573–575.

358. Takao M, Katayama Y, Onoda K, Tanabe H, Hiraiwa T, Mizutani T, Yada I, Namikawa S, Yuasa H, Kusagawa M: Significance of bronchial mucosal blood flow for the monitoring of acute rejection in lung transplantation. J Heart Lung Transplant 1991; 10:956–967.

359. Tamm M, Wallwork J, Higenbottam T: Heart-lung transplantation: results. In Patterson GA, Couraud L (eds): Lung Transplantation. Vol 3. Amsterdam: Elsevier Science, 1995, pp 399–423.

360. Tanabe H: Diagnosis of lung transplant rejection by measurement of bronchial mucosal blood flow [in Japanese]. Mie Igaku 1989; 33:87.

361. Tanabe H, Takao M, Hiraiwa T, Mizutani T, Yada I, Namikawa S, Yuasa H, Kusagawa M: New diagnostic method for pulmonary allograft rejection by measurement of bronchial mucosal blood flow. J Heart Lung Transplant 1991;10:968–974.

362. Taylor P, Rose M, Yacoub M: Expression of MHC antigens in normal lungs and transplanted lungs with obliterative bronchiolitis. Transplantation 1989;48:506–510.

363. Tazelaar HD: Perivascular inflammation in pulmonary infections: implications for the diagnosis of lung rejection. J Heart Lung Transplant 1991;10:437–441.

364. Tazellar HD, Yousem SA: The pathology of combined heart-lung transplantation: an autopsy study. Hum Pathol 1988;19:1403–1416.

365. Toothill C: The chemistry of the in-vivo reaction between hemoglobin and various oxides of nitrogen. Br J Anaesth 1967;39:405–412.

366. The Toronto Lung Transplant Group: Unilateral lung transplantation for pulmonary fibrosis. N Engl J Med 1986;314:1140–1145.

367. Tourkantonis A, Lazardis A: Interaction between cytomegalovirus infection and renal transplant rejection. Kidney Int 1983;23:546.

368. Tremblay LN, Yamashiro T, DeCampos KN, Mestrinho BV, Slutsky AS, Todd TR, Keshavjee SH: Effect of hypotension preceding death on the function of lungs from donors with nonbeating hearts. J Heart Lung Transplant 1996;15:260–268.

369. Trull A, Steel L, Cornelissen J, Smith T, Sharples L, Cary N, Stewart S, Large S, Wallwork J: Association between blood eosinophil counts and acute cardiac and pulmonary allograft rejection. J Heart Lung Transplant 1998;17:517–524.

370. Trulock EP, Ettinger NA, Brunt EM, Pasque MK, Kaiser LR, Cooper JD: The role of transbronchial lung biopsy in the treatment of lung transplant recipients: an analysis of 200 consecutive procedures. Chest 1992;102:1049–1054.

371. Uthoff K, Zehr KJ, Lee PC, Low RA, Baumgartner WA, Cameron DE, Stuart RS: Neutrophil modulation results in improved pulmonary function after 12 and 24 hours of preservation. Ann Thorac Surg 1995;59:7–13.

372. Valdivielso P, Escolar JL, Cuervas-Mons V, Pulpon LA, Chaparro MA, Gonzalez-Santos P: Lipids and lipoprotein changes after heart and liver transplantation in a patient with homozygous familial hypercholesterolemia. Ann Intern Med 1988;108:204–206.

373. Valentine VG, Robbins RC, Berry GJ, Patel HR, Reichenspurner H, Reitz BA, Theodore J: Actuarial survival of heart/lung and bilateral sequential lung transplant recipients with obliterative bronchiolitis. J Heart Lung Transplant 1996;15:371–382.

374. Valentine VG, Robbins RC, Wehner JH, Patel HR, Berry GJ, Theodore J: Total lymphoid irradiation for refractory acute rejection in heart/lung and lung allografts. Chest 1996;109:1184–1189.

375. Valman HB, France NB, Wallis PG: Prolonged neonatal jaundice in cystic fibrosis. Arch Dis Child 1971;46:805–809.

376. vanRaemdonck DEM, Jannis NCP, Rega FRL, de Leyn PR, Flameng WJ, Lerut TE: Delay of adenosine triphosphate depletion and hypoxanthine formation in rabbit lung after death. Ann Thorac Surg 1996;62:233–241.

377. Veldhuizen RA, Lee J, Sandler D, Hull W, Whitsett JA, Lewis J, Possmayer F, Novick RJ: Alterations in pulmonary surfactant composition and activity after experimental lung transplantation. Am Rev Respir Dis 1993;148:208–215.

378. Vernon LP, Bell JD: Membrane structure, toxins and phospholipase A2 activity. Pharmacol Ther 1992;54:269–295.

379. Villar Do Valle P, Barcia A, Bargeron LM, Karp RB, Kirklin JW: Angiographic study of supravalvular aortic stenosis and associated lesions. Report of five cases and review of literature. Ann Radiol 1969;12:779–796.

380. Vouhe PA, Dartevelle PG: Heart-lung transplantation: technical modifications that may improve the early outcome. J Thorac Cardiovasc Surg 1989;97:906–910.

381. Wallwork J: Risk factors for chronic rejection in heart and lungs—why do heart and lungs rot? Clin Transplant 1994;8:341–344.

382. Wallwork J, Williams R, Calne RY: Transplantation of liver, heart and lungs for primary biliary cirrhosis and primary pulmonary hypertension. Lancet 1987;2:182–185.

383. Webb WR, Howard HS: Cardiopulmonary transplantation. Surg Forum 1957;8:313–317.

384. Webb WR, Howard HS, Neely WA: Practical methods of homologous cardiac transplantation. J Thorac Surg 1959;37:361–366.

385. Weidman WH, Blount SG Jr, DuShane JW, Gersony WM, Hayes CJ, Nadas AS: The Joint Study on the Natural History of Congenital Heart Defects. Clinical course in ventricular septal defect. Circulation 1975;56(suppl I):I-56–I-69.

386. Westra AL, Petersen AH, Caravati F, Wildevuur CRH, Prop J: The combi-effect: prolonged survival of heart grafts by combined transplantation of vascularized lymphoid tissue. Transplant Proc 1990;22:1963–1964.

387. Westra AL, Petersen AH, Prop J, Wildevuur CRH: The combi-effect—reduced rejection of the heart by combined transplantation with the lung or spleen. Transplantation 1991;52:952–955.

388. Westra AL, Peterson AH, Wildevuur CRH, Prop J: Factors determining prolongation of rat heart allograft survival by perioperative injection of donor spleen cells. Transplantation 1991;52:606–610.

389. Weyman AE, Wann S, Feigenbaum H, Dillon JC: Mechanism of abnormal septal motion in patients with right ventricular volume overload: a cross-sectional echocardiographic study. Circulation 1976;54:179–186.

390. Whitehead B, Rees P, Sorensen K, Bull C, Higenbottam TW, Wallwork J, Fabre J, Elliott M, de Leval M: Incidence of obliterative bronchiolitis after heart/lung transplantation in children. J Heart Lung Transplant 1994;13:903.

391. Whyte RI, Robbins RC, Altinger J, Barlow CW, Doyle R, Theodore J, Reitz BA: Heart-lung transplantation for primary pulmonary hypertension. Ann Thorac Surg 1999;67:937–941.

392. Whyte RI, Rossi SJ, Mulligan MS, Florn R, Baker L, Gupta S, Martinez FJ, Lynch JP: Mycophenolate mofetil for obliterative bronchiolitis syndrome after lung transplantation. Ann Thorac Surg 1997;64:945–948.

393. Wildevuur CR, Benfield JR: A review of 23 human lung transplantations by 20 surgeons. Ann Thorac Surg 1970;9:489–515.

394. Winton TL, Miller JD, deHoyos A, Snell G, Maurer J: Graft function, airway healing, rejection and survival in pulmonary transplantation are not affected by graft ischemia in excess of 5 hours. Transplant Proc 1993;25:1649–1650.

395. Wisser W, Wekerle T, Zlabinger G, Senbaclavaci O, Zuckermann A, Klepetko W, Wolner E: Influence of human leukocyte antigen matching on long-term outcome after lung transplantation. J Heart Lung Transplant 1996;15:1209–1216.

396. Wood P: The Eisenmenger syndrome or pulmonary hypertension with reversed central shunt. BMJ 1958;2:701–709, 755–762.

397. Worrall NK, Boasquevisque CH, Misko TP, Sullivan PM, Ferguson TB Jr, Patterson GA: Inducible nitric oxide synthase is expressed during experimental acute lung allograft rejection. J Heart Lung Transplant 1997;16:334–339.

398. Wu G, Zhang F, Salley RK, Diana JN, Su TP, Chien S: Delta opioid extends hypothermic preservation time of the lung. J Thorac Cardiovasc Surg 1996;111:259–267.

399. Yacoub MH, Khaghani A, Banner N, Tajkarimi S, Fitzgerald M: Distant organ procurement for heart and lung transplantation. Transplant Proc 1989;21:2548–2550.

400. Yamashita M, Schmid RA, Okabayashi K, Ando K, Kobayashi J, Cooper JD, Patterson GA: Pentoxifylline in flush solution improves early lung allograft function. Ann Thorac Surg 1996;61:1055–1061.

401. Yeoh TK, Kramer MR, Marshall S, Theodore J, Gibbons R, Valantine HA, Starnes VA: Changes in cardiac morphology and function following single lung transplantation. Transplant Proc 1991;23:1226–1227.

402. Yousem SA: Significance of clinically silent untreated mild acute cellular rejection in lung allograft recipients. Hum Pathol 1996;27:269–273.

403. Yousem SA, Berry G, Brunt E, Chamberlain D, Hruban R, Sibley R, Stewart S, Tazelaar H: A working formulation for the standardization of nomenclature in the diagnosis of heart and lung rejection. J Heart Transplant 1990;9:593.

404. Yousem SA, Berry GJ, Cagle PT, Chamberlain D, Husain AN, Hruban RH, Marchevsky A, Ohori NP, Ritter J, Stewart S, Tazelaar HD: Revision of the 1990 working formulation for the classification of pulmonary allograft rejection: Lung rejection study group. J Heart Lung Transplant 1996;15:1–15.

405. Yousem SA, Curley JM, Dauber JH, Paradis I, Rabinowich H, Zeevi A, Duquesnoy R, Dowling R, Zenati M, Hardesty R: HLA class II antigen expression in human heart/lung allografts. Transplantation 1990;49:991–995.

406. Yousem SA, Paradis IL, Dauber JH, Griffith BP: Efficacy of transbronchial lung biopsy in the diagnosis of bronchiolitis obliterans in heart lung transplant recipients. Transplantation 1989;47:893–895.

407. Yousem SA, Paradis IL, Dauber JH, Zeevi A, Duquesnoy RJ, Dal Col R, Armitage J, Hardesty RL, Griffith BP: Pulmonary arteriosclerosis in long-term human heart-lung transplant recipients. Transplantation 1989;47:564–569.

408. Yousem SA, Ray L, Paradis IL, Dauber JA, Griffith BP: Potential role of dendritic cells in bronchiolitis obliterans in heart-lung transplantation. Ann Thorac Surg 1990;49:424–428.

409. Yuh DD, Gandy KL, Morris RE, Hoyt G, Gutierrez J, Reitz BA, Robbins RC: Leflunomide prolongs pulmonary allograft and xenograft survival. J Heart Lung Transplant 1995;14:1136–1144.

410. Zeevi A, Rabinowich H, Paradis I, Gryzan S, Dauber JH, Hardesty RL, Kormos B, Griffith B, Duquesnoy RJ: Lymphocyte activation in bronchoalveolar lavages from heart-lung transplant recipients. Transplant Proc 1988;20:189–192.

411. Zeevi A, Uknis ME, Spichty KJ, Tector M, Keenan RJ, Rinaldo C, Yousem S, Duncan S, Paradis I, Dauber J, Griffith B, Duquesnoy RJ: Proliferation of cytomegalovirus primed lymphocytes in bronchoalveolar lavages from lung transplant patients. Transplantation 1992;54:635–639.

412. Zuckermann A, Klepetko W, Birsan T, Taghavi S, Artemiou O, Wisser W, Dekan G, Wolner E: Comparison between mycophenolate mofetil- and azathioprine-based immunosuppressions in clinical lung transplantation. J Heart Lung Transplant 1999;18:432–440.

413. Zureikat HY: Collateral vessels between the coronary and bronchial arteries in patients with cyanotic congenital heart disease. Am J Cardiol 1980;45:599–603.

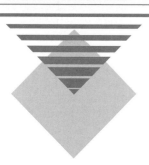

Cardiac Retransplantation

Since the earliest days of cardiac transplantation, it became apparent that cardiac retransplantation was going to be an inevitable consideration in a proportion of cardiac transplant recipients because of the appearance of graft failure due to a number of causes. Cardiac retransplantation was first reported in 1968 after orthotopic heart transplantation[3] and in 1980 following heterotopic transplantation.[13] According to data from the Registry for the International Society for Heart and Lung Transplantation (ISHLT), retransplantation accounts for about 2% of adult cardiac transplant procedures and nearly 3% of pediatric heart transplants.[6] In the Cardiac Transplant Research Database (CTRD), the actuarial freedom from retransplantation after a first cardiac transplant exceeds 95% at 10 years (Fig. 22–1).[15] As will be discussed in this chapter, cardiac retransplantation occurs under two very different settings with widely disparate outcomes: urgent or emergent retransplantation in a desperate situation and semi-elective retransplantation from an outpatient setting.

ETHICAL ISSUES

Like so many issues in transplantation, the ethical concerns regarding retransplantation are underpinned by the imbalance between the needs of cardiac transplan-

tation and the donor organs available. The ethical argument against allowing retransplantation revolves around the question of whether patients should be allowed a second cardiac transplant when there are patients waiting for (and in some cases dying before) their first transplant. Furthermore, the results of cardiac retransplantation have historically been clearly inferior to primary cardiac transplantation, and it is these concerns regarding the perceived unfairness of retransplantation that have prompted the position[2, 18] that it should not be allowed. On the other hand, the results of elective retransplantation, for example, for coronary allograft vasculopathy, have been progressively improving (Fig. 22–2), just as the results of primary cardiac transplantation were initially poor but progressively improved with time. An argument could be made that it is appropriate to continue retransplantation with the expectation that the results for all indications (and particularly elective retransplantation) will progressively improve. Also, infant and many childhood transplant procedures are predicated upon the availability of donor hearts for perhaps a series of heart transplants over a lifetime. Some have suggested that the allocation system should be altered so that patients waiting for their first heart would have higher priority than those awaiting cardiac retransplantation.[19] In the United States, cardiac retransplantation is permitted and patients awaiting retransplantation have the same chance (within the same status group) of receiving a heart as patients awaiting primary transplantation, and there is no evidence that this policy results in widespread inappropriate application of cardiac retransplantation.

CONDITIONS CONSIDERED FOR RETRANSPLANTATION

The causes of graft failure for which cardiac retransplantation has been considered include primary graft failure, intractable acute cardiac rejection, coronary allograft vasculopathy (numerically the most important indication), and early or late graft failure characterized by

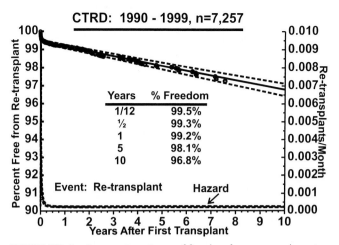

FIGURE **22–1.** Parametric estimate of freedom from retransplantation following a first heart transplant (solid line) and 70% confidence limits (dotted line). Each circle represents a retransplant procedure placed actuarially. Hazard function is indicated by the solid line surrounded by the 70% confidence limits (dashed line). CTRD, Cardiac Transplant Research Database. (From Radovancevic B, McGiffin DC, Kobashigawa JA, Cintron GB, Mullen GM, Pitts DE, O'Donnell J, Thomas C, Bourge RC, Naftel DC: A multi-institutional study of cardiac retransplantation: incidence, risk factors for mortality, and outcome [abstract]. J Heart Lung Transplant 2001;20:75.)

restrictive physiology or systolic dysfunction. The need for retransplantation can be grouped into two general situations: emergent retransplantation and elective retransplantation.

In reality, these two groups occur in two very different clinical settings. Patients undergoing **emergent retransplantation** are nearly always desperately ill with profound acute cardiac failure (often in overt shock) secondary to either acute graft failure at the time of transplantation or acute rejection with profound hemodynamic compromise, usually but not exclusively occurring within the first 6 months following transplantation. Such patients are on multiple inotropic agents in an intensive care unit, frequently with intra-aortic balloon pump support, often severely immunosuppressed, and usually with impending or overt multiorgan dysfunction. There are a number of reports of patients being managed by acute cardiac retransplantation with supportive measures such as prolonged cardiopulmonary bypass, intra-aortic balloon pumping,[20] and mechanical support of the circulation with ventricular assist devices[1, 8] or the artificial heart.[1, 10] In the current era of scarce donor supply, the likelihood of donor availability in a short period of time is poor in these very unstable situations.

In the **elective** retransplantation situation, the most common condition is chronic allograft vasculopathy in a stable patient who is functional, usually asymptomatic, and living at home. Retransplantation is recommended because of progressive and usually diffuse allograft coronary artery disease with preserved or depressed left ventricular function. Less common indications for elective retransplantation include progressive restrictive physiology and unexplained progressive systolic dysfunction.

In the 10-year experience of the CTRD, 105 out of 7,257 transplant recipients underwent retransplantation. The second transplant procedure was undertaken emergently for either early graft failure or acute rejection in 45 patients and semielectively for allograft vasculopathy or nonspecific graft failure in 49 patients. Miscellaneous causes accounted for the remainder.

SURVIVAL

There is general agreement that the overall results of retransplantation are inferior to those for primary cardiac transplantation. The evidence for inferior survival after retransplantation includes information from the ISHLT registry (Fig. 22–3)[4] and from the CTRD (Fig. 22–4).[15] It is noteworthy that the difference in survival is entirely accounted for by early mortality during the first 3–6 months. In a multivariable analysis of death after cardiac transplantation in the ISHLT data, cardiac retransplantation is a risk factor for mortality at both 1 year and 5 years after transplantation.[6] However, these results require closer scrutiny. There is persuasive evidence from multiple sources that the condition at the time of retransplantation (**emergent vs. elective**) is the major determinant of mortality. This is reflected in the CTRD experience (Fig. 22–5), in which retransplantation for early graft failure and acute rejection (nearly always an emergent procedure for seriously ill patients on inotropic support) is associated with poor survival. In contrast, patients transplanted for allograft vasculopathy (coronary artery disese) or nonspecific graft failure usually undergo retransplantation semielectively, and the survival is significantly better. Furthermore, the survival after retransplantation for allograft vasculopathy has progressively improved over the past

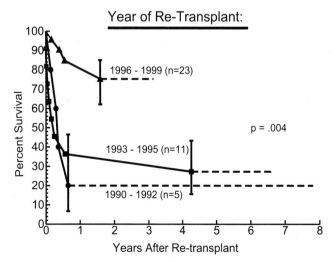

FIGURE **22–2.** Actuarial survival of patients undergoing retransplantation for coronary allograft vasculopathy stratified by era. CTRD, Cardiac Transplant Research Database. (From Radovancevic B, McGiffin DC, Kobashigawa JA, Cintron GB, Mullen GM, Pitts DE, O'Donnell J, Thomas C, Bourge RC, Naftel DC: A multi-institutional study of cardiac retransplantation: incidence, risk factors for mortality, and outcome [abstract]. J Heart Lung Transplant 2001;20:75.)

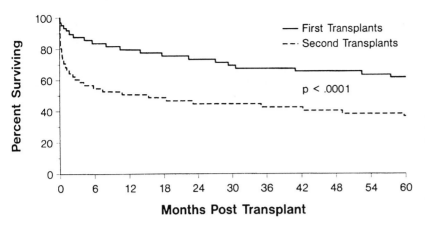

FIGURE **22-3.** Actuarial survival of recipients of second cardiac allografts and a matched group of primary transplant recipients, demonstrating markedly decreased survival in the repeat transplantation group. ISHLT registry data. (From Ensley RD, Hunt S, Taylor DO, Renlund DG , Menlove RL, Karwande SV, O'Connell JB, Barr ML, Michler RE, Copeland JG, Miller LW, Registry ISHLT: Predictors of survival after repeat heart transplantation. J Heart Lung Transplant 1992; 11S:142–158.)

decade (see again Fig. 22–2). These emergent indications for retransplantation appear as risk factors for death after retransplantation in a multivariable analysis from the CTRD (Table 22–1).

The difference in risk between emergent and semielective retransplantation is further reflected by the **interval of time** between first and second transplant procedures. Procedures during the first 6 months are usually performed emergently for severe hemodynamic compromise early after transplantation or for massive acute rejection. Retransplant procedures performed later are, for the most part, semielective for patients with allograft vasculopathy. Indeed, from the ISHLT data, the actuarial survival of patients with an intertransplant interval of greater than 9 months is superior to that of patients with an interval of less than 9 months (Fig. 22–6).[7] Once the intertransplant interval exceeds 2 years, the 1-year survival approximates that of primary transplantation (Fig. 22–7).

The reasons for poor survival after urgent or emergent retransplantation undoubtedly relate to the severely compromised condition of most patients in this situation. These patients suffer from profound low cardiac output and an impending shock-like state with its known sequelae on other organs. In earlier eras, patients in similar condition undergoing primary cardiac transplant as an emergent procedure suffered a high mortality. The advent of mechanical circulatory support allowed stabilization of such patients and provided time for reversal of organ dysfunction and patient rehabilitation, resulting in a well-compensated, hemodynamically robust patient several months later who could safely undergo cardiac transplantation after bridging with a chronic mechanical circulatory support device. Unfortunately, current left ventricular assist devices are poorly suited to support of the acutely rejecting heart, which,

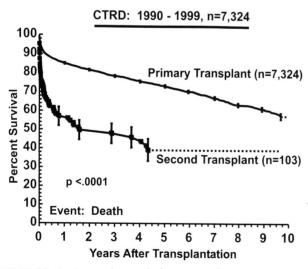

FIGURE **22-4.** Actuarial survival of patients undergoing primary and secondary cardiac transplantation. Vertical bars indicate the 70% confidence limits. CTRD, Cardiac Transplant Research Database. (From Radovancevic B, McGiffin DC, Kobashigawa JA, Cintron GB, Mullen GM, Pitts DE, O'Donnell J, Thomas C, Bourge RC, Naftel DC: A multi-institutional study of cardiac retransplantation: incidence, risk factors for mortality, and outcome [abstract]. J Heart Lung Transplant 2001;20:75.)

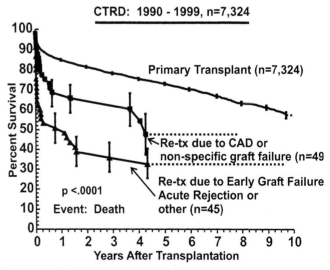

FIGURE **22-5.** Actuarial survival of patients undergoing primary cardiac transplantation, retransplantation due to coronary artery disease (CAD) or nonspecific graft failure, and retransplantation due to early graft failure, acute rejection, or other causes. The vertical bars are 70% confidence limits. CTRD, Cardiac Transplant Research Database. (From Radovancevic B, McGiffin DC, Kobashigawa JA, Cintron GB, Mullen GM, Pitts DE, O'Donnell J, Thomas C, Bourge RC, Naftel DC: A multi-institutional study of cardiac retransplantation: incidence, risk factors for mortality, and outcome [abstract]. J Heart Lung Transplant 2001;20:75.)

TABLE 22-1	Risk Factors for Death After Retransplantation (CTRD: 1990–1999, n = 7,259, with 106 retransplants)	
RISK FACTOR		*p* VALUE
Retx due to rejection		.0005
Retx due to early graft failure		.03
Female donor		.005

Retx, retransplantation.

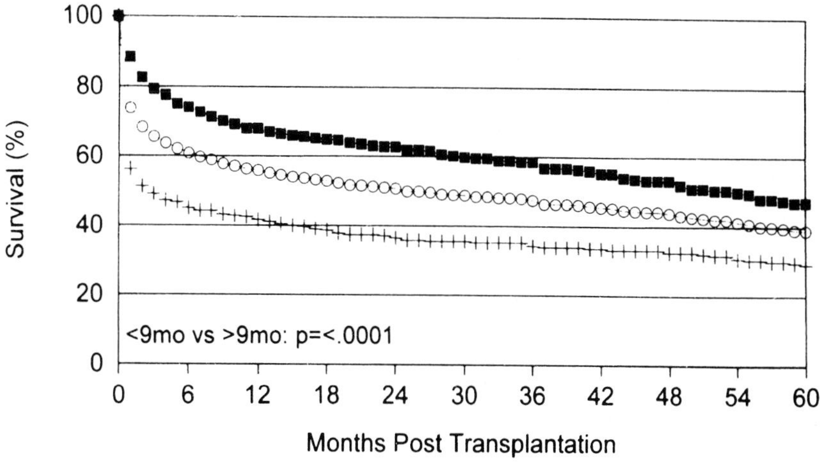

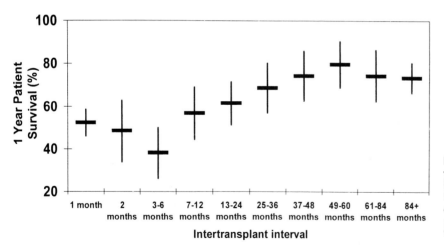

FIGURE **22-6.** Adult heart retransplantation actuarial survival, stratified by interval from original transplant. Open circle, overall retransplants (n = 899); cross (+), retransplants less than 9 months post-transplant; closed squares, retransplants more than 9 months post-transplant. (From Hosenpud JD, Bennett LE, Keck BM, Fiol B, Boucek MM, Novick RJ: The registry of the International Society for Heart and Lung Transplantation: 15th official report—1998. J Heart Lung Transplant 1998;17:656–668.)

FIGURE **22-7.** Adult heart retransplantation 1-year survival by interval from first transplant. (From Hosenpud JD, Bennett LE, Keck BM, Boucek MM, Novick RJ: The registry of the International Society of Heart and Lung Transplantation: 17th official report—2000. J Heart Lung Transplant 2000;19: 909–931.)

in the absence of adequate immunosuppression, undergoes progressive rejection with myocardial fibrosis and contraction (rather than dilatation) of the ventricular chambers. Ventricular assist device flows are then frequently compromised by poor inflow. If full immunosuppression is maintained, the risk of overwhelming infection is undoubtedly high in an already compromised host with the added complexity of a mechanical support system. Theoretically, replacement of the transplanted heart with a total artificial heart and discontinuation of immunosuppression may provide the most effective bridge to retransplantation, but there is insufficient experience with this strategy to make specific recommendations.

EVALUATION OF PATIENTS FOR RETRANSPLANTATION

Patients being considered for retransplantation should undergo a full reevaluation as for primary transplantation (see Chapter 6), but several issues are of particular importance. Sensitization (preformed antibodies) to donor antigens from the first transplant and/or to blood transfusions must be recognized and, if present, would necessitate a prospective crossmatch at the time of retransplantation (see Chapter 7). Chronic exposure to a calcineurin inhibitor drug (cyclosporine or tacrolimus) may have produced nephrotoxicity. The degree of renal impairment should be evaluated as for primary cardiac transplantation, and combined cardiac retransplantation and renal transplantation should be considered in patients with important renal dysfunction. It is important to exclude medical compliance issues as a contributing factor to the reasons for considering cardiac retransplantation, since not only may the same issues play a role in the loss of a second graft, but it does raise the important consideration of fairness and the appropriate use of scarce donor organs.

CARDIAC RETRANSPLANT PROCEDURE

In addition to the poor condition of the patient, an important contributing factor to the high mortality associated with retransplantation for acute rejection and primary graft failure is probably the tendency to use marginal donor hearts, given the desperateness of the situation. With "elective retransplantation" for chronic allograft vasculopathy, there should not be a sense of urgency, and the use of marginal donor hearts should be unnecessary. As with all cardiac transplant procedures that are performed in the setting of previous cardiac surgery, we recommend that a femoral artery and vein be either exposed or cannulated by a fine catheter (Angiocath) that would allow rapid institution of cardiopulmonary bypass if the heart or aorta were inadvertently entered during sternotomy (see further discussion in Chapter 10). The sternotomy should be performed with an oscillating saw. The use of aprotinin is advisable

in retransplant procedures as in cardiac transplant procedures following prior cardiac surgery. We recommend the bicaval technique of orthotopic cardiac transplantation (see Chapter 10). Patients who have previously undergone the biatrial technique can easily have a bicaval technique employed at the time of retransplantation.

IMMUNOSUPPRESSION

Preoperative loading of immunosuppressive drugs for retransplantation is unnecessary. Cytolytic therapy is not used with the exception of retransplantation in the setting of a positive B-cell crossmatch (a positive T-cell crossmatch should not occur because of prospective crossmatching). Intraoperative and immediate postoperative methylprednisolone boluses are given as for primary transplantation (see Chapter 12), and the pretransplant immunosuppressive drugs are continued after transplant.

REJECTION AND INFECTION

In a study from the CTRD, the time-related risk of initial **rejection** after cardiac retransplantation was the same as for primary transplantation (Fig. 22–8), and this finding has been previously observed.[9] Somewhat surprising is the finding from CTRD (Fig. 22–9)[15] and other studies that the time-related probability of **infection** is the same for retransplant as for primary transplant procedures.[9] A higher incidence of infection might be anticipated in patients undergoing retransplantation because

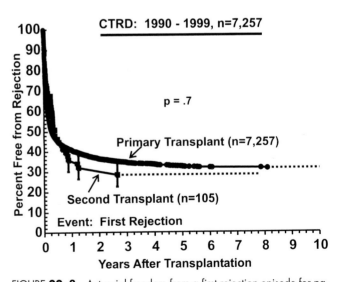

FIGURE 22–8. Actuarial freedom from a first rejection episode for patients undergoing primary transplantation and a retransplant procedure. Vertical bars indicate the 70% confidence limits. CTRD, Cardiac Transplant Research Database. (From Radovancevic B, McGiffin DC, Kobashigawa JA, Cintron GB, Mullen GM, Pitts DE, O'Donnell J, Thomas C, Bourge RC, Naftel DC: A multi-institutional study of cardiac retransplantation: incidence, risk factors for mortality, and outcome [abstract]. J Heart Lung Transplant 2001;20:75.)

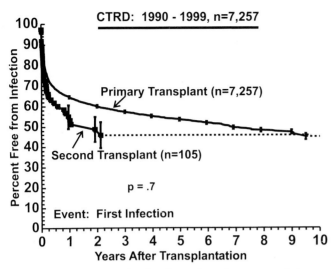

FIGURE 22-9. Actuarial freedom from a first infection episode for patients undergoing primary transplantation and a retransplant procedure. Vertical bars indicate the 70% confidence limits. CTRD, Cardiac Transplant Research Database. (From Radovancevic B, McGiffin DC, Kobashigawa JA, Cintron GB, Mullen GM, Pitts DE, O'Donnell J, Thomas C, Bourge RC, Naftel DC: A multi-institutional study of cardiac retransplantation: incidence, risk factors for mortality, and outcome [abstract]. J Heart Lung Transplant 2001;20:75.)

of their previous exposure to immunosuppression and likely impaired healing from long-term corticosteroids. Retransplantation for intractable rejection, however, probably does carry an increased risk of infection because of high-dose immunosuppression prior to retransplantation for the treatment of acute cardiac rejection.

ALLOGRAFT VASCULOPATHY AFTER RETRANSPLANTATION

When considering the use of scarce donor hearts for retransplantation in the patient with coronary allograft vasculopathy, an important concern is the likelihood of accelerated allograft vasculopathy in the second heart. Several reports[5, 17] suggest that the incidence of coronary vasculopathy in the second donor heart is no different than the primary transplant. Clearly, a high therapeutic priority in patients undergoing retransplantation for coronary allograft vasculopathy is the implementation of aggressive measures to reduce the incidence and progression of coronary artery disease in the new graft (see Chapter 17).

CURRENT INDICATIONS AND TIMING OF RELISTING

Based on available information regarding short- and long-term survival following retransplantation, we recommend that cardiac retransplantation **should be considered** as an **elective** procedure (i.e., for stable recipients living out of hospital) in patients whose expected

1-year survival is less than about 50% because of chronic allograft vasculopathy or ventricular dysfunction and/ or in patients who have cardiac dysfunction which is severe enough to produce chronic New York Heart Association (NYHA) Class III or IV heart failure symptoms unresponsive to medical therapy. Such patients must fulfill all the criteria for primary cardiac transplantation (see Chapter 6). The major cardiac abnormalities which constitute an indication for retransplantation are **coronary allograft vasculopathy,** severe symptomatic **diastolic dysfunction** secondary to restrictive physiology, and **progressive systolic dysfunction** secondary to recurrent acute rejection, allograft vasculopathy, or idiopathic. In the current era of donor shortages, cardiac retransplantation is **not advisable** as an emergent procedure for acute posttransplant graft failure or overwhelming acute rejection with shock, due to the high associated mortality.

The appropriate **timing of listing** for cardiac retransplantation is particularly problematic for coronary allograft vasculopathy, since it is dependent on transplant center-specific considerations such as the aggressiveness with which percutaneous transluminal coronary angioplasty (PTCA) or, rarely, coronary bypass surgery, are explored. At an earlier time, single-vessel coronary artery disease with a diameter reduction of greater than 70% was regarded as an indication for elective retransplantation[5] because coronary allograft vasculopathy was thought to have an unpredictable course with a high incidence of sudden death. It is now known that the progression of coronary allograft vasculopathy is inexorable but does occur at a rather predictable rate, and in patients with mild coronary allograft vasculopathy (essentially single-vessel coronary artery disease) the likelihood of death or retransplantation within 2 years of the diagnosis is low (see Chapter 17). In contrast, in patients with severe three-vessel coronary artery disease, the likelihood of death or retransplantation is considerably higher. As discussed in Chapter 17, PTCA appears to be effective palliative therapy for some patients with proximal and midcoronary artery lesions and may be useful in delaying the need for retransplantation. It remains to be determined whether additional tests to detect the presence of myocardial ischemia and quantify the ischemic burden can further refine the timing for listing. Our current policy is to consider patients for retransplantation when they have **severe three-vessel coronary artery disease** which is either not amendable to PTCA, stent placement, and/or atherectomy, or these measures are no longer effective.

PEDIATRIC RETRANSPLANTATION

One of the legacies of cardiac transplantation in children and neonates is the likelihood of several cardiac retransplant procedures being required over a lifetime because of the development of coronary allograft vasculopathy. Although the experience of cardiac retransplantation in children is small compared to that in adults, it appears

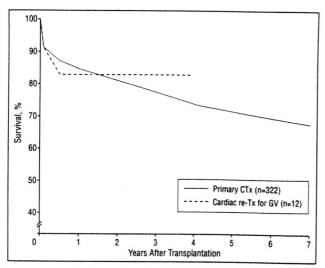

FIGURE 22-10. Actuarial survival of all children after primary cardiac transplantation (solid line) (n = 322) and children after cardiac retransplantation for graft vasculopathy (dashed line) (n = 12). (From Razzouk AJ, Chinnock RE, Dearani JA, Gundry SR, Bailey LL: Cardiac retransplantation for graft vasculopathy in children. Arch Surg 1998;133:881–885.)

that survival (Fig. 22–10), rejection, and infection after retransplantation mirror that of adult cardiac retransplantation.[11, 16] Some reports suggest that children may have a more rapid and unpredictable progression of allograft vascular disease than adults[12, 14, 16] (see Chapter 20). Accordingly, it has been suggested that listing for elective pediatric retransplantation should occur earlier in the course of coronary allograft vasculopathy,[16] perhaps with single-vessel disease.

References

1. Cabrol C, Gandjbakhch I, Pavie A, Bors V, Cabrol A, Leger P, Vaissier E, Levasseur JP, Petrie J, Simoneau JC, Copeland JG: Is the use of artificial hearts the future solution for interim treatment of patients awaiting retransplantation? Transplant Proc 1989;21: 3658–3659.
2. Collins EG, Mozdzierz GJ: Cardiac transplantation: determining limits. Heart Lung 1993;22:206–212.
3. Copeland JG, Griepp RB, Bieber CP, Billingham M, Schroeder JS, Hunt S, Mason J, Stinson EB, Shumway NE: Successful retransplantation of the human heart. J Thorac Cardiovasc Surg 1977;73: 242–247.
4. Ensley RD, Hunt S, Taylor DO, Renlund DG, Menlove RL, Karwande SV, O'Connell JB, Barr ML, Michler RE, Copeland JG, Miller LW, Registry ISHLT: Predictors of survival after repeat heart transplantation. J Heart Lung Transplant 1992;11S:142–158.
5. Gao SZ, Schroeder JS, Hunt S, Stinson EB: Retransplantation for severe accelerated coronary artery disease in heart transplant recipients. Am J Cardiol 1988;62:876–881.
6. Hosenpud JD, Bennett LE, Keck BM, Boucek MM, Novick RJ: The registry of the International Society of Heart and Lung Transplantation: 17th official report—2000. J Heart Lung Transplant 2000;19:909–931.
7. Hosenpud JD, Bennett LE, Keck BM, Fiol B, Boucek MM, Novick RJ: The registry of the International Society for Heart and Lung Transplantation: 15th official report—1998. J Heart Lung Transplant 1998;17:656–668.
8. Jurmann MJ, Wahlers T, Coppola R, Fieguth HG, Haverich A: Early graft failure after heart transplantation: management by extracorporeal circulatory assist and retransplantation. J Heart Lung Transplant 1989;8:474–478.
9. Karwande SV, Ensley RD, Renlund DG, Gay WA, Richenbacher WE, Doty DB, Hammond ME, Marks JD: Cardiac retransplantation: a viable option? Ann Thorac Surg 1992;54:840–845.
10. Loisance DY, Deleuze P, Kawasaki K, Hillion ML, Binhas M, Heurtematte P, Tavolaro O, Leandri J, Cachera JP: Total artificial heart as a bridge to retransplantation in acute cardiac rejection. J Heart Lung Transplant 1987;6:281–285.
11. Michler RE, Edwards NM, Hsu D, Bernstein D, Fricker FJ, Miller J, Copeland J, Kaye MP, Addonizio L: Pediatric retransplantation. J Heart Lung Transplant 1993;12S:319–327.
12. Mulla NF, Johnston J, VanderDussen L, Larsen R, Kuhn M, AliKhan MA, Chinnock R, Bailey L: Early retransplantation for post transplant coronary artery disease in children [abstract]. J Heart Lung Transplant 1997;16:71.
13. Novitzky D, Cooper DKC, Barnard CN: Orthotopic heart transplantation in a patient with a heterotopic heart transplant. Heart Transplant 1984;3:257.
14. Pahl E, Crawford SE, Swenson JM, Duffy CE, Fricker FJ, Backer CL, Mavroudis C, Chaudhry FA: Dobutamine stress echocardiography: experience in pediatric heart transplant recipients. J Heart Lung Transplant 1999;18:725–732.
15. Radovancevic B, McGiffin DC, Kobashigawa JA, Cintron GB, Mullen GM, Pitts DE, O'Donnell J, Thomas C, Bourge RC, Naftel DC: A multi-institutional study of cardiac retransplantation: incidence, risk factors for mortality, and outcome [abstract]. J Heart Lung Transplant 2001;20:75.
16. Razzouk AJ, Chinnock RE, Dearani JA, Gundry SR, Bailey LL: Cardiac retransplantation for graft vasculopathy in children. Arch Surg 1998;133:881–885.
17. Taniguchi S, Cooper DKC: Cardiac retransplantation—indications and results. *In* Cooper DKC, Miller LW, Patterson GA (eds): The Transplantation and Replacement of Thoracic Organs. Hingham, MA: Kluwer Academic Publishers, 1996, pp 347–351.
18. Tilney NL: A crisis in transplantation: too much demand for too few organs. Transplant Rev 1998;12:112–120.
19. Ubel PA, Arnold RM, Caplan AL: Rationing failure: the ethical lessons of the retransplantation of scarce vital organs. JAMA 1993;270:2469–2474.
20. Wahlers T, Frimpong-Boateng K, Haverich A, Schafers HJ, Coppola R, Jurmann M, Borst HG: Management of immediate graft failure after cardiac transplantation using cardiopulmonary bypass and intraaortic balloon-pumping followed by cardiac transplantation. Thorac Cardiovasc Surg 1986;34:389–390.

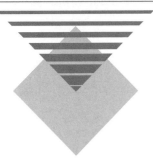

CHAPTER TWENTY-THREE

Xenotransplantation

with the collaboration of
JAMES F. GEORGE, Ph.D.

RATIONALE FOR XENOTRANSPLANTATION

The desire to use animals as a source of donor organs dates back to the earliest days in the history of transplantation, when the supply of human donor organs was known to be the major impediment to the widespread application of this therapy. However, xenotransplantation is not yet a clinically viable procedure because of strong nonspecific and specific antigraft immune responses that are apparently a function of the phylogenetic distance between donor and host. More recently, advances in understanding of the mechanisms and potential control of xenograft rejection have been used to achieve graft function with a much greater frequency and duration than previously observed.

If xenotransplantation can be safely implemented, there are compelling arguments for its use in clinical transplantation (Table 23–1). A steady and predictable source of donor organs could potentially result in improved outcome because transplant physicians would have more discretion as to when the transplant could be performed, possibly resulting in improved patient condition at the time of transplantation. Improved organ preservation with short ischemic times would also be likely. Furthermore, the potential for "elective" repeat heart transplantation would be enhanced by the ready availability of xenograft donor hearts.

The prospect that animals could be bred for use as organ donors also raises the possibility of genetic manipulation of the animals such that the donor organs would not elicit as strong an immune response. Pharmaceutical companies have recognized this possibility, and there are several well-financed efforts underway to produce such transgenic animals. These potential advantages of xenotransplantation must be weighed against important disadvantages (Table 23–1), which will be discussed in this chapter.

HISTORICAL NOTE

The modern era of xenotransplantation dates back to 1963, when Reemtsma, and subsequently Starzl and others, initiated a series of kidney and liver transplants from chimpanzees, baboons, and pigs.[40, 88] These efforts provided the background for Hardy and colleagues at the University of Mississippi to perform the first heart transplant in a human, utilizing a chimpanzee heart (1964)[39] (Table 23–2). A patient unable to wean from cardiopulmonary bypass after cardiac surgery received a chimpanzee heart as an orthotopic transplant. The patient died in the operating room approximately 1 hour after the conclusion of the procedure. The failure of the chimpanzee heart was attributed to the donor heart being too small to support the recipient. Hardy had

TABLE 23-1	Advantages and Disadvantages of Xenotransplantation

ADVANTAGES	DISADVANTAGES
• Inexhaustible supply of donor organs • Operations can be performed under less acute circumstances • Prevention of recurrences of certain diseases in the transplanted organ • Opportunity for genetic manipulation • Potential for performing repeat transplants electively	• Risk of zoonoses—unknown risk of the emergence of recombinant virus strains of unknown pathogenicity • Ethical objections by animal rights activists • Strong immunologic differences between donor and host • Physiologic incompatibilities between donor and host

wanted to perform a human-to-human transplant but turned to a xenograft when it became clear that it was not possible to obtain a human donor heart. The concept of "brain death" with organ retrieval from "heart beating cadavers" had not matured.

In 1968, Cooley and colleagues transplanted a sheep heart into a 48-year-old man suffering from cardiogenic shock following a myocardial infarction.[14] That same year, Ross and colleagues attempted to use a pig heart transplanted in the heterotopic position as a "bridge" to cardiac transplantation in a patient unable to be weaned from cardiopulmonary bypass following cardiac sur-

gery. Both grafts underwent fatal hyperacute rejection immediately after revascularization. Another unsuccessful attempt at xenotransplantation with a chimpanzee heart occurred in France in 1969, but few details are available.[60, 61]

Christiaan Barnard performed two unsuccessful heterotopic xenotransplants, one from a baboon and another from a chimpanzee. The chimpanzee heart functioned for 4 days, and the baboon heart failed within hours.[7]

Perhaps the most widely publicized experimental heart xenotransplantation was performed by Bailey and colleagues at Loma Linda in 1984. A baboon heart was transplanted into a baby (Baby Fae) with hypoplastic left heart syndrome. The recipient was treated with cyclosporine and other immunosuppressive agents, and the baby survived for 20 days without evidence of hyperacute rejection. Autopsy showed only mild evidence of cell-mediated rejection, and progressive graft failure was possibly related to a humoral mechanism based on blood group incompatibility.[6, 104] Other unsuccessful attempts are listed in Table 23–2.

IMMUNOLOGIC DISPARITY AMONG MAMMALIAN SPECIES

As discussed in Chapter 2, the immune response is a mechanism in which the primary function is self/non-

TABLE 23-2	World Experience in Clinical Heart Xenotransplantation

CASE	YEAR	SURGEON	INSTITUTION	DONOR	TYPE OF TRANSPLANT	OUTCOME	REFERENCE SOURCE
1	1964	Hardy	University of Mississippi, Jackson, Mississippi, USA	Chimpanzee	OHT	Functioned 2 hr; heart too small to support circulation	9
2	1968	Ross	National Heart Hospital, London, UK	Pig	HHT	Cessation of function within 4 min; probable hyperacute rejection	18, 95
3	1968	Ross	National Heart Hospital, London, UK	Pig	Perfused with human blood but not transplanted	Immediate cessation of function; probable hyperacute rejection	Unpublished
4	1968	Cooley	Texas Heart Institute, Houston, Texas, USA	Sheep	OHT	Immediate cessation of function; probable hyperacute rejection	13, 14
5	1969	Marion	Lyon, France	Chimpanzee	? OHT	Rapid failure, elevated pulmonary vascular resistance	60, 61
6	1977	Barnard	University of Cape Town, Cape Town, South Africa	Baboon	HHT	Functioned 5 hr; heart too small to support circulation	7
7	1977	Barnard	University of Cape Town, Cape Town, South Africa	Chimpanzee	HHT	Functioned 4 days; failed from probable vascular rejection	7
8	1984	Bailey	Loma Linda University, Loma Linda, California, USA	Baboon	OHT	Functioned 20 days; failed from probable vascular rejection	22
9	1991	Religa	Poland	Pig	OHT	Functioned <24 hr	24
10	1996	Baruah	India	Pig	OHT	Functioned <24 hr	Unpublished

OHT, orthotopic heart transplantation; HHT, heterotopic heart transplantation.
From Taniguchi S, Cooper DK: Clinical xenotransplantation: past, present and future [abstract]. Ann R Coll Surg Engl 1997;79:13–19.

self discrimination. This function maintains a defense against pathogenic organisms and also maintains self-integrity in an all-encompassing milieu of life on Earth. Developmental and comparative studies of immune responses in different organisms have generally found that, the greater the phylogenetic distance (see later section) between donor and host, the stronger the response towards the donor tissue, most likely due to the cumulative effect of multiple differences in protein sequences and basic physiology. This is certainly the case for vascularized organs exchanged between different mammalian species such as pig to primate, or rat to dog. Therefore, xenotransplants have been classified based on the kinetics of graft rejection.

DISCORDANT XENOGRAFTS

Organisms are classified in a hierarchical fashion based on similarities and differences in anatomy, biochemistry, and ultimately, the degree of genomic similarity. This classification, often called the phylogenetic tree, can be considered to be a rough approximation of the relative differences in time in which different species diverged during evolution. Therefore, humans and chimpanzees are said to be phylogenetically less distant from each other than pigs and humans. The relationship between rejection times and phylogenetic distance between donor and recipient was derived from some of the oldest and most spectacular observations in transplantation. Organs exchanged between highly dissimilar species are subject to hyperacute rejection, a phenomenon in which the transplanted organ is destroyed in minutes to hours after the vascular circulation is restored. In all instances, there are circulating natural antibodies in the recipient that lead to immediate antibody-mediated rejection. This is grossly visible as a nearly immediate loss of graft function associated with discoloration, blanching, and finally widespread hemorrhage within the organ. Combinations of donor and recipients that result in hyperacute rejection are said to be **discordant.**[11]

CONCORDANT XENOGRAFTS

In contrast to discordant donor and recipient pairs, concordant combinations do not result in hyperacute rejection. Such combinations are typically phylogenetically similar, such as chimpanzees and humans. Attempts to use concordant combinations clinically have been more successful (as defined by longer survival) than discordant combinations. Given the inherent advantages of concordant donor and recipient pairs, one would presume that these are the most likely to be clinically implemented. However, as discussed below, there are inherent problems with the use of concordant species for clinical transplantation.

CHOICE OF DONOR SPECIES FOR CLINICAL TRANSPLANTATION

While a number of different species combinations have been used in the laboratory, the choice of donor species for human use is necessarily limited because of size and anatomy. The implanted heart must be able to perform enough work to sustain life with nearly normal activities. Several early instances of xenograft failure can be attributed to this problem. From an immunological perspective, primates are the most compatible and obvious donors because of their close phylogenetic relationship with humans and attendant physiologic, molecular, and anatomic similarities. The phylogenetic distance between species has been quantified by biochemical data which indicate the degree of metabolic incompatibility between the two species. A scoring system has been developed which compares the evolutionary difference between humans (with an arbitrary score of 1) and other species, based on differences in the sequence of amino acids in albumin, which is known to change at a similar rate among species over evolutionary time. Evolutionary disparity between humans and higher nonhuman primates (relative score <3) is quite low compared to other mammals.[17] However, chimpanzees, the closest of nonhuman primate relatives (relative score 1.14), are an endangered species, as are gorillas and orangutans. They and other nonhuman primates, such as baboons, bear strong physical and behavioral resemblances to humans. Baboons would be a suitable size for infants and children but they are not adequate size for adult humans.

However, major limitations exist for the use of nonhuman primates as a source of donor hearts. From a medical standpoint, there is a potential risk of transfer of infections, particularly viral. Nonhuman primates may harbor hepatitis, Epstein-Barr virus, human immunodeficiency virus (HIV), and *Mycobacterium tuberculosis*. HIV appears to have originally been a simian immunodeficiency virus. Also, there is an increasing consensus that nonhuman primates, by virtue of their similarity to humans, are endowed with some of the same properties, which for the purposes of this discussion, are the capacity to feel pain, to suffer, and to experience emotion. The advantages and limitations of the baboon as a source of donor hearts are outlined in Table 23–3. Coupled with the fact that several nonhuman primate species are endangered, these similarities to man provide a strong impetus for public resistance that precludes their use for organ donation on the scale needed for a significant clinical impact.

The use of domestic animal species, such as pigs, has been widely considered as the most fruitful approach because of their large size and vascular anatomic similarities to humans (Table 23–3). However, their phylogenetic distance from humans is large (relative score >35) compared to nonhuman primates. The use of pigs as donors is much less likely to arouse strong opposition because they are available in large numbers and ethical

TABLE 23-3	Comparison of Baboons and Pigs as Sources of Organs and Tissues for Human Transplantation	
	BABOONS	PIGS
Breeding potential	Low • Only 1–2 offspring per pregnancy • 9 yr to maximum size • No experience in large scale farming	High • 5–12 offspring per pregnancy • Adequate size in 6 mo
Adequacy of heart size for adult humans	Inadequate	Adequate*
Anatomical similarity	Close	Moderately close
Knowledge of tissue typing	Limited, but improving	Extensive in selected herds
Necessity for blood type compatibility with humans	Important	Probably unimportant
Experience with genetic manipulation	None	Considerable
Availability of specific pathogen-free animals	No	Yes
Risk of zoonosis	High	Low

*Breeds of miniature swine are approximately 50% of the weight of domestic pigs at birth and reach a maximum weight of 200–300 lb (<130 kg).
Modified from Cooper DKC, Lanza RP: Xeno—The Promise of Transplanting Animal Organs into Humans. New York: Oxford University Press, 2000.

arguments against the use of such animals as a source of donor organs are difficult to sustain when millions are used every year as a source of food (see also later section, Ethical Considerations). Therefore, in the last 10 years, the bulk of developmental efforts in clinical xenotransplantation have been directed toward the use of pig organs. Other species combinations have been used in the laboratory to define the range of mechanisms that can potentially participate in xenograft rejection.

IMMUNOLOGIC BARRIERS

Experience has shown that the barriers to successful xenotransplantation are formidable. The most obvious and largest barriers in the current era are those posed by the immune system (Fig. 23–1). As shown below, the phylogenetic distance between donor and host gives rise to a number of antigenic and physiologic differences that are not present in allogeneic combinations, thereby presenting a number of unique immunologic targets. Xenograft rejection is classified according to the kinetics and mechanisms of antigraft responses that have been observed in a number of experimental systems as well as theoretical considerations (Table 23–4). There are four major immunologic barriers that are likely to threaten the success of xenotransplantation: hyperacute rejection, acute vascular rejection, acute cellular rejection (delayed xenograft rejection), and chronic rejection. With currently available techniques, hyperacute rejection can be prevented, acute vascular rejection can be delayed, and little is known about the other two.

HYPERACUTE REJECTION

The presence of natural anti–pig antibodies in humans and other primates directed against carbohydrate resi-

dues on pig vascular endothelium leads rapidly to antibody-mediated rejection (hyperacute rejection).[19, 34, 36, 75, 97] The primary components of this fatal process are antibody and complement, with secondary participation of coagulation factors and cellular inflammation. The primary target in vascularized organs is the vascular endothelium. Transplantation of hearts from pigs to pri-

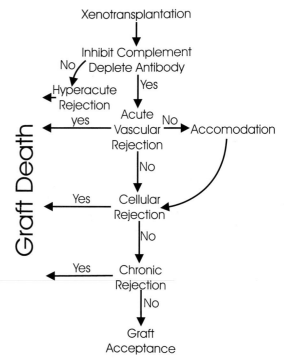

FIGURE **23–1.** An illustration of the sequence of barriers that must be overcome before clinical xenogeneic heart transplantation is a reality.

TABLE 23-4	**Comparison of Types of Xenograft Rejection**			
	HYPERACUTE REJECTION	ACUTE VASCULAR REJECTION	ACUTE CELLULAR REJECTION	CHRONIC REJECTION
Time Course Mechanism	Minutes to hours • Preformed anti-Gal antibodies • Failure of complement regulation • Type I endothelial cell activation	Hours to days • Xenoreactive antibodies • T cells, NK cells, monocytes macrophages activation	Days to weeks • T cells, NK cells (? similar to acute allograft rejection)	Weeks to years (?) • (?) Possibly similar to allograft vasculopathy; no animals have survived long enough for this to be observed

Gal, α-1,3 galactose.

mates results in cessation of function within minutes. The heart becomes swollen and distended with blood, with evidence of interstitial hemorrhage, edema, thrombus formation, and infiltration of neutrophils (Fig. 23–2). The normal pink color of the myocardium turns to a dusky hue.[91] In rhesus monkeys, diffuse deposition of IgM and classical complement pathway components, including C1q, C3, C4, and C5, can be found on the graft endothelial surfaces. A variety of experimental models show that the molecular and cellular basis of hyperacute rejection in the **pig to primate** combination can be attributed to three key components consisting of preformed antibodies, classical complement pathway activation, and vascular endothelial cells as shown in Figure 23–3.

Xenoreactive Antibodies

The hyperacute rejection of a pig heart by primates is almost soley determined by natural (preformed) antibodies directed against a single molecule, a carbohydrate disaccharide residue. This carbohydrate epitope is a terminal α-linked galactose residue called galactose-α-1,3-galactose (which will be abbreviated as **Gal** in this chapter). This carbohydrate residue is found on many cell types, but most importantly, on endothelial cells. These preformed xenoreactive antibodies are present in the circulation of all immunocompetent individuals without a prior history of immunization and strongly resemble antibodies against blood group antigens. Many studies have determined that Gal is the major xenoepitope on pigs that is recognized by these natural human and primate antibodies, and this relates to the evolutionary divergence of these species.

The evolution of pigs and primates apparently diverged approximately 64 million years ago. As a result of this evolutionary divergence, one major epitope of pigs, the carbohydrate Gal, is recognized by naturally occurring antibodies in humans and most primates. In pigs, this epitope is found on endothelial cells, erythrocytes, lymphocytes, and within the tissues of liver, heart, kidney, and lung.[97] It is of interest that essentially all endothelial cells have a high concentration of Gal except aorta.[66, 75] On endothelial cells, more than 20 glycoproteins have been identified which carry the Gal residue.[107]

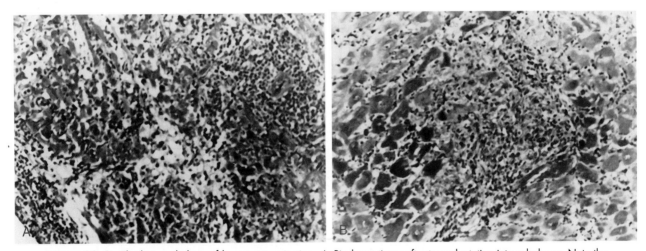

FIGURE **23–2.** The histopathology of hyperacute rejection. *A,* Pig heart tissue after transplantation into a baboon. Note the destruction of capillaries and massive interstitial edema. *B,* A high-powered view of capillary destruction in a vervet monkey heart transplanted into a baboon. (From Rose AG, Cooper DK, Human PA, Reichenspurner H, Reichart B: Histopathology of hyperacute rejection of the heart: experimental and clinical observations in allografts and xenografts. J Heart Lung Transplant 1991;10:223–224. Copyright 1991, Elsevier Science, with permission.)

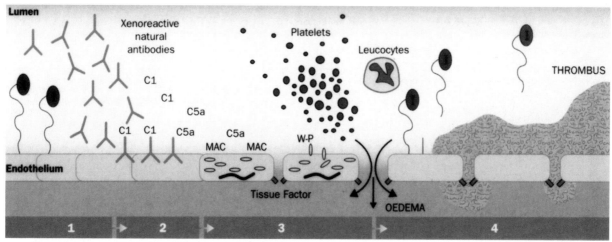

FIGURE **23-3.** Pathophysiology of hyperacute rejection. 1, Normal endothelium maintains an anticoagulant environment in which the contents of the vessels are prevented from leaking into the extravascular space. Tethering of factors such as antithrombin III and tissue factor inhibitor to glycosaminoglycan inhibits coagulation. 2, When the cross-clamp is removed from the donor heart, the recipient blood carries in preformed antigraft antibodies that immediately bind to the vascular endothelium and activate complement. The activation of complement liberates highly proinflammatory complement components, such as C5a, and results in the formation of membrane attack complexes that destroy membrane integrity. 3, At the same time, endothelial cells become activated, leading to retraction and leakage of serum into the interstitial space. Weibel-Palade bodies containing von Willebrand factor and P-selectin fuse with the cell membrane, resulting in the surface expression of their contents. 4, Circulating leukocytes and platelets adhere to the endothelial cell membrane, coagulation is initiated, and it proceeds in an uncontrolled fashion until the vessel is completely occluded. (From Dorling A, Riesbeck K, Warrens A, Lechler R: Clinical xenotransplantation of solid organs. Lancet 1997;349:867–871.)

The Gal epitope is synthesized by the enzyme α-**1,3-galactosyltransferase,** which catalyzes the addition of a terminal α-linked galactose to N-acetyl lactosamine (Fig. 23–4). Unlike pigs, Old World monkeys (see Box), apes, and humans do not have this enzyme. It is of importance to experts in the field of transgenic engineering that the Gal epitope shares some similarities with the human blood group B epitope. The final synthesis of blood group B antigen is catalyzed by the enzyme α-1,3-galactosyltransferase, which is a transferase that will only use fucosylated N-acetyl lactosamine (H substance) as substrate for the transfer of the terminal glucose. The genes for α-1,3-galactosyltransferase and the B blood group transferase are linked on chromosome 9,

indicating that they have a common evolutionary basis.[44, 98]

The natural antibodies to Gal are IgM molecules whose specificity is directed against carbohydrate epitopes in galactose and blood groups. In most species, there are also natural IgG and IgA antibodies directed against the same epitopes. Those species which do not express the Gal antigen are the species which have anti-Gal antibodies (humans and Old World monkeys). It is of interest that the anti-Gal antibodies can be induced in response to infectious agents, as Gal is expressed on certain bacteria (*Escherichia coli*, *Klebsiella*, and *Salmonella*) and some protozoa (*Plasmodium falciparum*, *Trypanosoma cruzi*, and *Leishmania mexicana*). These natural

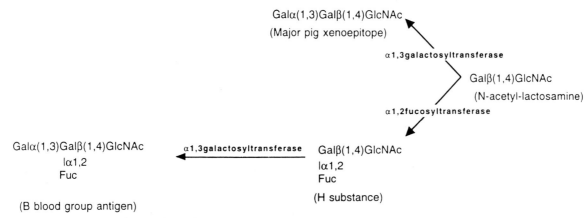

FIGURE **23-4.** Biosynthetic pathway for Galα(1,3)Gal and B blood group. The pathway begins with N-acetyl-lactosamine [Galβ(1,4)GlcNAc] and the α-1,3-galactosyltransferase adds galactose to form Galα(1,3)Gal. To synthesize B blood group by the B blood group transferase (also an α-1,3-galactosyltransferase), Galβ(1,4)GlcNac must first be converted to H substance by the α-1,2-fucosyltransferase. (From McKenzie IFC, Loveland BE, Fishman JA, Auchincloss H, Sandrin MS: Xenotransplantation. *In* Ginns LC, Cosimi AB, Morris PJ [eds]: Transplantation. Malden, MA: Blackwell Science, 1999, pp 827–874.)

Old World Monkeys

The common ancestor of the New and Old World monkeys appeared to have diverged approximately 40 million years ago. There is considerable controversy in the classification of New World monkeys and it has undergone several revisions, but one currently accepted view is that New World monkeys are comprised of marmosets and tamarins, sakis and uakaris, spider, woolly and howler monkeys, owl monkeys, and squirrel monkeys. A group of higher primates known as the Old World anthropoid primates are now represented by two superfamilies—the Old World monkeys (cheek-pouched monkeys and leaf monkeys) and Hominoidea (apes and humans).

antibodies are not present at birth, but rather develop weeks to months later, possibly after colonization of the gastrointestinal tract by microorganisms that contain the Gal epitope and sensitize the recipient.[65]

The xenoreactive antibodies against Gal serve as the activation point for the classical complement pathway and also may provide signals which activate porcine vascular endothelial cells.[106]

Complement and Regulators of Complement Activation

The formation of antibody complexes with the Gal epitopes leads to activation of the classical complement pathway, culminating in the formation of the membrane attack complex formed by the complement components C5a to C9.[16, 34, 36, 97] This results in damage to the cell membrane and liberation of chemotactic and proinflammatory complement fragments (see also Chapter 2). The generation of anaphylatoxins C3a, C4a, and C5a promotes rapid increases in vascular permeability, promotes chemotaxis and activation of macrophages and neutrophils, and facilitates the general amplification of an intense inflammatory response, including coagulation.

The activation of complement following xenotransplantation is also facilitated by species-specific differences in the regulators of complement activation (RCA) (see Box) on the cell surfaces of xenogeneic endothelial cells. From the perspective of xenotransplantation, these molecules are highly important because they inhibit the action of complement on the cell surface (Fig. 23–5). This regulatory system is of critical importance in hyperacute rejection, since RCAs normally act to hold the complement system "in check" by interfering with initiation and propagation of the complement cascade at critical points. One such molecule, called **decay accelerating factor (DAF)**, accelerates decay of the C3 convertases from the alternative and classical complement pathways and therefore inhibits the completion of the complement pathway on the cell surface. Other RCAs include membrane cofactor protein (MCP) which, like DAF, controls the C3 and C4 amplification steps; and CD59, which limits the polymerization of the membrane attack complex (Fig. 23–5). There are significant differences in the

structure of human and porcine DAF, such that pig DAF on the vascular endothelial cells of pig hearts cannot inhibit the human complement cascade that is initiated when the organ is perfused with human blood. Thus, in the absence of the normal regulatory process, the complement system erupts as a massively destructive force against the xenograft endothelium.

Endothelial Cell Activation

Platt and Bach noted that the transplantation of xenogeneic organs results in significant functional changes in vascular endothelial cells, a process termed "endothelial cell activation,"[83] in which the endothelium actively participates in the pathological changes that result in rapid graft destruction. One hypothesis states that acute xenograft vascular rejection is largely a result of endothelial cell activation of a specific type. Endothelial cell activation has been classified into two types (Table 23–5). Type I activation is independent of protein synthesis, can occur within minutes, and is believed to be a significant component of hyperacute rejection. The individual cells retract from one another, resulting in vascular leakage and expose carbohydrates, subendothelial collagen, and von Willebrand factor on the cell surface. In addition, P-selectin is translocated from cytoplasmic Weibel-Palade bodies in the cytoplasm[9, 21] and the cell membrane loses adenosine diphosphatase (ADPase),[83, 84, 89] resulting in the enhancement of platelet aggregation. These events collectively result in the loss of endothelial cell regula-

Regulators of Complement Activation

Of the known complement-regulating proteins, four of them have been investigated for a possible therapeutic role in xenotransplantation.

Decay accelerating factor (DAF) (CD55) is a 70-kDa protein with a phospholipid plasma membrane attachment and is widely distributed on human cells. It is structurally similar to MCP (see below), but its function is entirely different in that it accelerates the decay of the C3b/Bb and C4b/C2a C3 convertases from both the alternative and classical pathways.

Membrane cofactor protein (MCP) (CD46) is the most widespread complement regulator. This approximately 66-kDa protein acts as a cofactor for the serum protease, factor I, which cleaves C3b to C3bi and C3f. This highly efficient regulator also protects cells against lysis mediated by the classical pathway.

CD59 (protectin) is an approximately 70-kDa protein which has numerous functions involving complement and coagulation regulation as well as T-cell signaling.[28, 110] This molecule blocks polmerization of the terminal MAC by competitively interfering with C9 incorporation into the C5b-C8 complement complex.

CR1 (CD35) is a polymorphic cell surface protein of approximately 190–290 kDa which has binding sites for C3b and C4b. This molecule performs multiple functions of complement regulation, including decay acceleration of C3 and C5 convertases, proteolysis of C3b and C4b, and enhancement of phagocytosis.[114]

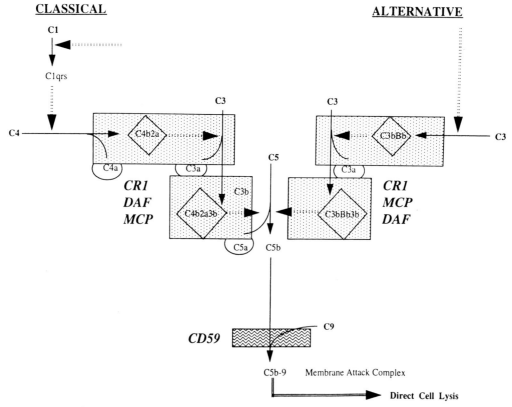

CLASSICAL

ALTERNATIVE

FIGURE 23-5. Sites of action of complement regulators, focusing on the proteins used in transplantation studies. Two sites, shown as shaded boxes, are controlled: the activation of C3 and 4 (but also impinging on C5) by the RCA molecules CR1, DAF, and MCP; and the regulation of the terminal (MAC) complex by CD59. CR1 and DAF accelerate the decay of the convertases, and CR1 and MCP are cofactors for the serum protease, factor 1, to cleave C3b and C4b. MCP and DAF differ in apparent regulatory efficiency for the two pathways, with CR1 probably most efficient. See text for abbreviations. (From McKenzie IFC, Loveland BE, Fishman JA, Auchincloss H, Sandrin MS: Xenotransplantation. *In* Ginns LC, Cosimi AB, Morris PJ [eds]: Transplantation. Malden, MA: Blackwell Science, 1999, pp 827–874, with permission.)

tion of vascular permeability, the loss of surface anticoagulant molecules, and the adoption of a proinflammatory stance by the cell (Fig. 23–6). The above events favor the deposition of coagulatory components such as thrombin on the cell surface, leading to fibrin deposition, which is associated with the activation and degranulation of platelets. The generation of coagulation rapidly

TABLE 23-5	**Endothelial Cell Activation**

Type I
- Independent of protein synthesis
- Occurs within minutes
- Associated with hyperacute rejection

Type II
- Up-regulation of:
    E-selectin
    ICAM-1
    P-selectin
    Genes that promote thrombosis
        Tissue factor
        Plasminogen activator inhibitor 1
    Activators of host cells
        IL-1
        IL-6
        IL-8
        MCP-1
        Others
    Thrombomodulin, heparan sulfate

ensues, promoting intravascular thrombosis and severe graft ischemia.[31]

ACUTE VASCULAR REJECTION

While there has been some controversy regarding the semantics of the immunological events that follow hyperacute rejection, it is accepted that the avoidance of hyperacute rejection is only a temporary reprieve from rapid graft destruction. **Delayed xenograft rejection** was a term originally used to describe rejection by rats of guinea pig hearts under conditions in which complement was depleted from the recipient. It is characterized by progressive infiltration by activated macrophages and natural killer (NK) cells.[38] Although some studies suggest that delayed xenograft rejection is a distinct entity,[38] we will consider it synonymous with **acute vascular rejection.** This form of rejection occurs as early as 24 hours after transplantation and can occur over days to weeks.[3, 5, 10, 108] It is characterized by endothelial swelling, focal ischemia, and diffuse microvascular thrombosis due to fibrin deposition.[55, 57, 85]

Acute vascular rejection is so named because of the histopathological resemblance to **presumed antibody-mediated rejection** of solid organ allografts. The role of antibodies in this process is supported by the observa-

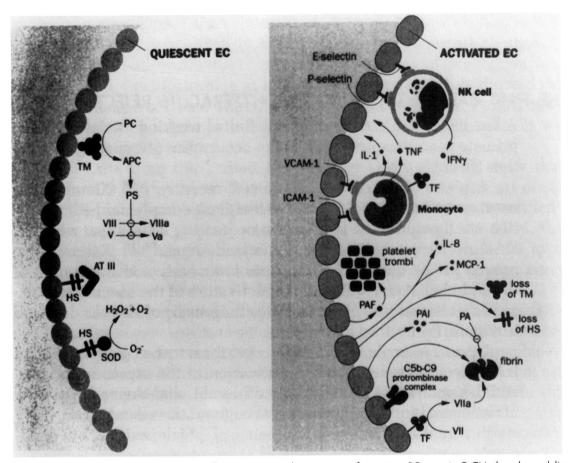

FIGURE 23-6. A schematic of endothelial cell (EC) activation during xenograft rejection. PC, protein C; TM, thrombomodulin; APC, activated protein C; PS, protein S; AT, antithrombin; HS, heparan sulfate; SOD, superoxide dismutase; NK, natural killer; IL-1, interleukin-1; TNF, tumor necrosis factor; IFN, interferon; VCAM-1, vascular cell adhesion molecule-1; ICAM-1, intercellular adhesion molecule-1; TF, tissue factor; MCP, membrane cofactor protein; PAI, plasminogen activator inhibitor; PA, plasminogen activator. (From Ferran C, Badrichani AZ, Cooper JT, Stroka DM, Bach FH: Xenotransplantation: progress toward clinical development. Adv Nephrol 1997;27:391–420.)

tions that there are detectable quantities of anti–donor antibodies in the circulation in animals that experience acute vascular rejection,[68] depletion of anti–donor antibodies delays rejection,[57] and administration of anti-donor antibodies leads to rejection.[80, 82] In the pig-to-primate combination, anti-Gal antibodies undoubtedly play an important role, with an[57, 126] interaction between vascular endothelial cells, antibodies, monocytes, NK cells,[42, 80, 82] complement, and neutrophils.[57, 112, 126] Endothelial activation (type II) (Table 23–5) may play a prominent role in acute vascular rejection, with a number of cell surface events promoting activation of genes and protein synthesis which can significantly potentiate immunologic events.

Regardless of the arguments concerning rejection after the initial "window" in which hyperacute rejection can occur, it is clear that humoral and cellular rejection mechanisms are not mutually exclusive and that both play a significant role. Importantly, in pig-to-baboon or pig-to-cynomolgus monkey models, evidence of acute vascular rejection has been identified in most transplanted hearts that do not succumb to hyperacute rejection.[100, 108, 125]

ACUTE CELLULAR REJECTION

Beyond hyperacute rejection (mediated by preexisting antibodies and/or complement) and acute vascular rejection (which appears to be mediated by elements of the innate immune system), it appears likely that acute cellular rejection will develop in a manner similar to that observed in allotransplantation.[71, 92, 121, 122] While this issue has only recently received significant study due to successes in preventing hyperacute rejection, it is generally thought that cell-mediated antigraft responses are likely to be very strong, and therefore less amenable to conventional immunosuppression protocols. Given the large number of antigenic proteins on xenogeneic cells, it is likely that the frequency of reactive T-cells will be high, since the frequency of reactive T-cell clones for allogeneic tissues is two to three orders of magnitude higher than that found for most antigens.[58] Also, complement and antibody binding serve to amplify immune responses by increased chemotaxis and by the liberation of factors that activate lymphocytes, macrophages, and neutrophils. Activation of NK cells could be a significant factor because it seems unlikely that they would be inhibited by xenogeneic MHC molecules. The major consequence of these activation mechanisms is that they may not be strongly inhibited by conventional immunosuppression.

CHRONIC REJECTION

Although little direct experimental evidence is available, it is anticipated that primates or humans who receive pig hearts and do not succumb to hyperacute or acute vascular rejection will be susceptible to chronic xenograft rejection of the nature seen in chronic allograft vasculopathy. This graft vasculopathy may well occur earlier and more aggressively than seen in allografts.

APPROACHES FOR THE PROMOTION OF XENOGRAFT ACCEPTANCE

As indicated previously, the majority of recent efforts have been directed towards pig-to-primate xenotransplantation. The success of allogeneic heart transplantation has been driven largely by the development of new immunosuppressive drugs. However, it has become ap-

parent that this strategy alone is unlikely to work for xenotransplantation because of the strength and rapidity of xenograft rejection.

HYPERACUTE REJECTION

Most of the efforts to prevent hyperacute rejection have centered around **antibody depletion** and **inhibition of the classical complement pathway.** The primary reason for this is that, as discussed in a previous section, hyperacute rejection of pig solid organ grafts appears to be almost entirely mediated by a few antibody specificities that bind to saccharide antigens such as Gal and subsequently activate the classical complement pathway.[25, 26] Using the methods described below, hyperacute rejection in the pig-to-primate model is currently preventable.

Genetic Approaches

In the last 10 years, a number of groups in academia and industry have sought to create strains of transgenic pigs that do not elicit hyperacute rejection in a human or nonhuman primate host. The rationale for this avenue of research is derived from the fact that the primary

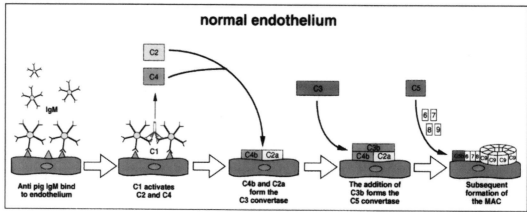

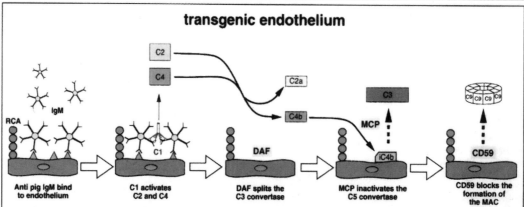

FIGURE **23–7.** Simplified schematic representation of the complement cascade activation on normal and transgenic pig endothelial cells. On normal pig endothelial cells, complement activation leads to the formation of the C3 and C5 convertases and ultimately to the membrane attack complex (MAC). The presence of the human regulators of complement activation, decay-accelerating factor (DAF), membrane cofactor protein (MCP), and CD59 on the surface of transgenic pig endothelial cells is expected to prevent the formation of or to inactivate the C3 and C5 convertases and the formation of the MAC, respectively. (From Cozzie E, White DJ: The generation of transgenic pigs as potential organ donors for humans. Nat Med 1995;1:964–966, with permission.)

effector mechanisms of hyperacute rejection are the complement cascades and the components that are generated by it. As discussed earlier in this chapter, the complement pathway is strongly regulated by RCAs. It was correctly hypothesized that the presence of human-specific RCAs present on porcine vascular endothelium would down-regulate the activation of human complement upon implantation of porcine organs and prevent hyperacute rejection (Fig. 23–7).[23] This was first demonstrated *in vitro*,[25, 73, 116] and subsequently *in vivo*.[23] The role of DAF in this context was demonstrated by Dalmasso and colleagues, who showed that the introduction of **human DAF** into porcine endothelial cells was effective in the prevention of complement-mediated lysis in the presence of human serum.[27] The strategy for the resolution of this problem has been to create transgenic pigs that express human DAF on the vascular endothelium.[12, 22, 33, 79, 93, 108, 111]

The development of transgenic species (see Box) will likely provide the cornerstone for translating xenotransplantation into a clinical reality. Considerable research efforts have been directed toward the creation of genetically modified pigs that contain human regulators of complement activation. Pigs transgenic for human CD59 and human complement regulatory protein have also been created. This approach has successfully prevented hyperacute rejection in the pig-to-primate experimental model.

Another transgenic approach which has been demonstrated in mice is the incorporation of a gene for human α-galactosidase, an enzyme that cleaves terminal α-linked galactosyl residues, thereby eliminating Galα(1,3)Gal and preventing antibody binding.[41, 75, 99] However, this is not a complete solution, since remaining N-acetyl lactosamine residues could also bind natural anti–pig antibodies.[76]

Perhaps the most promising approach to prevention of Gal synthesis would be the inactivation of α-1,3-galactosyl transferase by gene knockout technology. This has been accomplished in mice,[67, 105] but not yet in the pig.[67]

Depletion of Xenoreactive Antibodies and Complement

Given that hyperacute rejection of pig organs is mediated by antibody and the complement pathway, attempts have been made to circumvent the mechanism by depletion of xenoreactive antibodies or complement

---

Development of Transgenic Species

Transgenic animals are those in which the genome has been deliberately altered such that the expression of one or more genes is modified and that modification can be passed to subsequent progeny. This term was first coined by Gordon and Ruddle in 1981.[37] In mammals, fragments of linear DNA can be introduced into cells in which they are assembled into long tandem arrays by intracellular enzymes. These arrays can become integrated into the chromosome at an apparently random site. Fertilized mammalian eggs behave the same in this regard, so a fertilized mouse egg injected with a few hundred copies of linear DNA will integrate that DNA at some random site in a chromosome. Since the event has occurred in a germline cell, the integrated gene will be passed onto the progeny. Thus, animals modified in this manner are called *transgenic animals,* and the foreign genes that are introduced into such animals are called *transgenes.*

Prior to the development of transgenic animals, the only way to alter the genetic characteristics of an animal was through selective breeding based on the expression of a particular phenotype or trait. Selective breeding has long been used to produce animals bearing a desired trait (such as increased milk or beef production). For investigational purposes, it is even more desirable to be able to manipulate the expression of a specific gene in order to be able to answer questions about how the products of that gene are important in a particular molecular or cellular mechanism. For the purposes of xenotransplantation, investigators have produced pigs that bear the genes for human regulators of complement activation, including CD59 and decay accelerating factor.[22, 52] While there are differences in the details, in general transgenic pigs are produced in a manner similar to the production of transgenic mice.

Mice are most commonly used as transgenic animals because they are cheap, breed relatively quickly, and their genetics are very well characterized relative to other vertebrate species. However, transgenic technology has been applied to a number of species, including pigs, rabbits, sheep, birds, and fish. The most common means by which the genome of a particular individual is modified is through microinjection of DNA into the pronucleus of a fertilized ovum. The DNA usually consists of a *construct,* which is a piece of DNA that contains the gene of interest and a promotor that will confer the desired expression characteristics, such as expression of the gene in a particular tissue or group of cells. Once the DNA is inside the nucleus of the fertilized ovum, the DNA can become integrated into the chromosome, although the specific location of the integration appears to be largely random. The ovum is then transferred into the oviduct of a recipient female or foster mother that has been rendered "pseudopregnant" by mating with a vasectomized male in order to facilitate the implantation process.

Also important for investigational purposes and for xenotransplantation is the production of animals lacking a particular trait ("knockout animals"). The ability to achieve this relies on the fact that, while injected genes are usually inserted into a chromosome at random, about 1 in 1,000 times the injected gene will replace the normal gene by homologous recombination. Thus, by using an inactive gene in the injected construct, there will be a few events in which the normal gene is replaced with an inactive one, thus "knocking out" the normal gene. Thus, to produce knockout animals, the DNA is introduced into embryonic stem cells that grow in cell culture and are capable of growing into any cell in the body. Embryonic stem cells in which the desired gene has been integrated into the proper location are selected by drug resistance and sensitivity and then injected into an early mouse embryo at the blastocyst stage of development, ultimately producing a chimeric animal. By inbreeding for 10–20 generations, animals are then produced that have the trait in every cell.

components. This approach has utilized a variety of methods to deplete anti–Gal antibodies in recipient primates.[50, 120] The majority of studies were performed using extracorporeal immunoadsorption by routing blood through pig organs such as liver or kidney, or by passing the blood through immunoabsorption columns. The longest survival times were obtained when immunoabsorption was combined with other treatments. The addition of total lymphoid irradiation, cyclosporine, and corticosteroids resulted in survival times of 6, 8, and 15 days for pig hearts in a group of three baboons.[94] Somewhat longer survival times were obtained by treating three baboons with immunoadsorption, cyclosporine, total lymphoid irradiation, methotrexate, antithymocyte globulin, and splenic irradiation.[118, 119]

Inhibition of Xenoreactive Antibody Binding

Another approach is specific inhibition of xenoreactive antibody by infusing the recipient with materials that compete for the xenoreactive antibody binding sites. However, infusion of melibiose[123, 124] or α-Gal disaccharides and trisaccharides[90, 101] resulted in very limited survival benefit, with the longest survival of 18 hours for a single baboon.[90] These studies suggest that inhibition of anti–α-Gal antibodies was inefficient and/or that residual antibody, combined with the lack of functional regulators of complement activation, is enough to destroy a graft within several hours.

Depletion or Inhibition of Complement

This was one of the earliest and most successful methods for the inhibition of hyperacute rejection. Cobra venom factor (**CVF**)[46, 47, 54, 56] activates C3b systemically, resulting in the depletion of complement. Since hyperacute rejection in the pig-to-primate combination requires the presence of complement, the organ is protected from destruction. Soluble complement receptor 1 (**sCR1**) is a potent inhibitor of the classical and alternative complement pathways. The use of CVF has resulted in survival of pigs hearts in baboons for as long as 25 days when used in combination with other treatments such as cyclosporine, cyclophosphamide, splenectomy, corticosteroids, and methotrexate.[46, 47, 56] The results using sCR1 have been even more impressive. When given intermittently for 3 weeks in combination with cyclosporine, cyclophosphamide, and corticosteroids, survival times ranging from days to 6 weeks were obtained.[10, 29, 50, 56, 86, 87] Lastly, a method employing continuous infusion of IgG resulted in survival up to 10 days,[59] and the use of a chimeric protein combining DAF with human membrane cofactor protein (hCD46) reduced cardiac injury in an *ex vivo* perfusion model.[49]

ACUTE VASCULAR REJECTION

The amelioration of acute vascular rejection will likely require multiple approaches on an ongoing basis. Since antibody appears to be a significant component of this phenomenon, some of the measures taken for hyperacute rejection will probably be effective for acute vascular rejection as well. Trials using pigs transgenic for decay accelerating factor and CD59 plus high doses of cyclophosphamide have indicated that acute vascular rejection can be prevented, albeit at the cost of considerable toxicity.[112] The inhibition of neutrophil infiltration would be of additional help, possibly by the inhibition of adhesion receptors. Such mechanisms may also be of use in the inhibition of macrophages and NK cells.

Another approach which has been investigated to control or prevent acute vascular rejection is **accommodation,** which refers to the lack of injury to the porcine endothelial cells despite the presence of normal levels of anti–pig antibodies and complement.[2, 4, 17] Accommodation was described by Platt, Bach, and colleagues,[83] who showed that if anti–donor antibodies are temporarily depleted from the recipient, the organ can become established. Rejection does not occur even when anti–donor antibodies are restored to the circulation. The mechanism of accommodation is unknown, although some have speculated that blocking antibodies or anti-idiotypic antibodies may be operative.

Other potential approaches to prevent acute vascular rejection include monoclonal antibodies to suppress antibody production, immunotoxins directed against B-cell lines that produce Gal-specific antibodies, and induction of B-cell tolerance.[17]

ACUTE CELLULAR REJECTION

Little is known about the magnitude of this response to xenotransplantation, or whether current immunosuppressive agents for allotransplantation will be effective against it.

RESULTS OF PIG-TO-PRIMATE HEART XENOTRANSPLANTATION

The reported experience in pig-to-primate xenotransplantation of the heart is summarized in Table 23–6. The more recent experiments involve pigs transgenic for human regulatory proteins such as human complement DAF, human complement regulatory protein (CRP), and human CD59 (see previous discussion). **Heterotopically** transplanted hearts (non–life-supporting) from these animals have survived for as long as 99 days in nonhuman primates.[112] Results in heterotopic models which do not totally support the circulation have been generally better than life-supporting orthotopic models.

Pig-to-primate **orthotopic** xenotransplantation of transgenic pig hearts for human DAF have achieved to date a median survival of 12 days with a maximum of 39 days.[17] In one study, 5 of 10 animals survived for less than 18 hours.[100] Three of these animals contained unusually high titers of anti-Gal antibodies, but no grafts showed histological signs of hyperacute rejection. The five remaining animals died between 4 and 9 days after transplantation. Three hearts stopped beating due to

TABLE 23-6	Results of Pig-to-Primate Heart Xenotransplantation*					
RECIPIENT SPECIES	OUTCOME	NO. CASES	TREATMENT		YEAR	REFERENCE
Baboon (Newborn)	15, 81, 82, 82 hr	4	None		1995	45
Baboon (Newborn)	5–96 hr	7	None		1996	69
Baboon (Newborn)	<4 days	5	None		1997	70
	<6 days	2	Csa + MMF + CS			
Baboon (Newborn)	6 days	1	Csa + CPP + CS		1997	43
Baboon	10 min < 115 hr	2	EIA + Csa + CPP + CS		1996	15
Baboon	5 days (heterotopic) 30 hr (orthotopic)	2	EIA + SPx + Csa + CS + Mtx		1997	48 57
Baboon (Juvenile)	4–14 days	8	SPx + FUT175 ± FK506 ± Mtx ± ATG + EIA (lung) ± Csa ± DSG		1997	63
Baboon	<19 days	3	EIA + TLI + Csa + Mtx + ATG + SPI		1997	118
Cynomolgus	2 hr–7 days	4	Ig + SPx + Csa + AZA + CS		1995	59
Baboon	7–10 days	2	Ig + SPx + Csa + AZA + CS + EIA (kidney)		1995	59
Cynomolgus	48, 56, 73, 82, 90 hr	5	sCR1 Single Dose		1996	101
Cynomolgus	11 days	1	sCR1 (continuous) + CYA +CPP + CS		1996	86
Baboon	5, 6 days	2	CVF ± SPx		1996	47
Baboon	6–25 days	6	SPx + CVF + Csa ± CPP + CS ± Mtx		1997	46
Rhesus	<5 days	5	CAB-2.0		1997	96
Baboon	7, 15 days	2	EIA + WBI + TI + ATG + SPx + BM + Csa + MMF ± CVF		1998	51
Baboon	4, 11, 30 hr	3	**HDAF** + hCD59 + SPx + CPP + AZA + CS + EIA (kidney)		1995	64
Cynomolgus	5 days (mean)	8	**HDAF**		1995	115, 117
Baboon	<10 days	4	**hCD59** + EIA + SPx + Csa + CS + Mtx		1997	48, 57
Baboon	2, 13, 21 days	3	**HDAF**		1997	113
	5, 5, 9 days	3	**HDAF** + Csa + CPP + CS			
Baboon	< 29 days	6	**hCD59/hDAF** + EIA + Csa + CPP + CS		1997	57
	<5 days	5	**hCD59/hDAF** + Csa + CPP + CS			
Baboon	<9 days	10	**HDAF** + Csa + CPP + CS		1997	100
Baboon	<15 days	10	**HCRP** + Csa + CS + CPP ± MMF		1997	30
Baboon	39 days	1	**LDAF** + CPP + CS + MMF +Csa		2000	109

Csa, cyclosporine; CS, corticosteroids; SPx, splenectomy; FK506, tacrolimus; Mtx, methotrexate; CPP, cyclophosphamide; MMF, mycophenylate mofetil; AZA, azathioprine; PE, plasma exchange/pheresis; EIA, extracorporeal immunoadsorption (sometimes involving hemoperfusion through an isolated pig organ, as indicated); TLI, total lymphoid irradiation; FUT175, nafamstat mesilate; DSG, 15-deoxyspurgualin; SPI, splenic irradiation; Ig, human IgG given intravenously; sCR1, soluble complement receptor 1; CVF, cobra venom factor; CAB-2.0, recombinant soluble chimeric protein from human decay accelerating factor and human membrane cofactor protein; WBI, whole body irradiation; TI, thymic irradiation; BM, donor-specific bone marrow infusion; hDAF, pig transgenic for human decay accelerating factor; hCD59, pig transgenic for human CD59; hCRP, pig transgenic for human complement regulatory protein.
*Results include only those groups with survival times greater than 24 hr.
Modified from multiple tables in Lambrigts D, Sachs DH, Cooper DK: Discordant organ xenotransplantation in primates: world experience and current status. Transplantation 1998;66:547–561.

acute vascular rejection. The longest survivor was killed on day 9 with a beating histologically normal graft. In the reported orthotopically transplanted transgenic (DAF) porcine heart that survived for 39 days, the cause of death was not related to rejection.[108]

NONIMMUNOLOGIC BARRIERS

PHYSIOLOGIC BARRIERS

Most discussions regarding xenogeneic transplantation revolve around the interaction of the graft tissue with the host immune system. However, graft function, and therefore the maintenance of homeostasis, also involves a complex interplay between the donor organ and other host systems, which we shall call the "physiology" of the host. The word "physiology" encompasses gravitational influences (the donor animal may have a vertical or horizontal gait), blood pressure, response to hormones, pH, temperature, and receptors for soluble factors or hormones. It is not yet known what the relative importance of these factors would be under long-term circumstances. For example, blood clotting pathways are strongly regulated, yet among different species many of the tissue factors associated with blood clotting can vary in amino acid sequences by 50% or more. Many enzyme systems would be subject to similar problems.

Another physiologic difference relates to posture, which is upright in humans and horizontal in pigs. It is unknown, for example, whether the horizontal pig heart will function normally in an upright position in man.

The normal body temperature of pig is approximately 102.5°F (39°C). Whether a 3° to 4°F decrease in heart temperature following implantation into man adversely affects metabolic functions of the transplanted heart remains to be determined.

The growth of the porcine heart and eventual size disparity between it and the human recipient remains problematic. It is unknown whether, for example, human growth hormone will influence the growth of a transplanted pig organ or whether the pig organ will achieve the same size in man that it does in the pig. If the pig heart grew to a size which could not be accommodated by the pericardial space of the human thorax, a restrictive physiology may result. Such problems could theoretically be overcome by retransplantation, or possibly by the use of inbred miniature swine, which grow to a maximum size of 135 kg (in contrast to normal swine, which may grow to nearly 500 kg).

XENOZOONOSES

Infections transferred from xenotransplanted organs are termed xenozoonoses. Evidence seems to indicate that virtually all animal species (including humans) harbor clinically latent viruses, such as retroviruses. The potential risk of infection from nonhuman primates was discussed in the earlier section, Choice of Donor Species for Clinical Transplantation. The extent of the danger posed by the transfer of organisms has not been quantifiable. However, there is ample evidence that such species-to-species transfers can and do occur. Extremely dangerous hemorrhagic fever viruses such as the Ebola virus clearly have animal reservoirs. The influenza A virus, which was responsible for a large number of deaths early in the last century, undergoes a significant antigenic shift every few decades while it is harbored in pigs and birds. As many as 20% of slaughterhouse workers have serologic evidence of exposure to swine influenza.[41, 81]

Zoonotic infections may also include bacterial and parasitic infections that are occasionally transmitted from pigs to farmers, meat handlers, and people ingesting undercooked pork. These may include infections due to *Salmonella* species, *Brucella* and *Trichinella* species, rabies, anthrax, toxoplasmosis, leptospirosis, and listeriosis. Transgenic swine for transplantation would undergo extensive microbiologic screening to exclude pathogens likely to be transmitted to humans (Table 23–7).

Problems of latency and interspecies transfer also become more significant because the recipient of xenogeneic organs will be highly immunsuppressed, which could enhance the efficiency of transfer of potentially pathogenic organisms. Of perhaps greater concern than transmission of disease to the transplant recipient is the risk of transferring a porcine (or primate) infection to other members of the community.

Porcine endogenous retroviruses (PERV-A and B), which are similar to leukemia viruses in other species, can be found in all cell lines and normal tissues from pigs of a variety of different breeds. Given the ubiquitous nature of latent retroviruses in all species, it is unlikely that the production of virus-free animals is achievable. Transfer of PERVs into human cells has been demonstrated *in vitro*.[53, 62, 102] The possibility exists that elements of such viruses could undergo recombination with human retroviruses, potentially creating new retroviruses capable of inducing malignant changes or immunodeficiency states.[17] Since many retroviruses

TABLE 23–7	**Designated Pathogen-Free Miniature Swine for Xenotransplantation**

EXCLUDE ANIMALS WITH THE PRESENCE OF:

Ascaris summ	*Cryptosporidium parvum*
Brucella suis	Neospora
Leptospira	*Sarcocystis suihominis*
Listeria monocytogenes	*Trichinella spiralis*
Mycobacterium bovis	Adenovirus (porcine)
Mycobacterium tuberculosis	Cytomegalovirus (porcine)
Mycobacterium avium—	Encephalomyocarditis virus
intracellular complex	Influenza virus (porcine and human)
Mycoplasma hyopneumoniae	Porcine parvovirus
(lung transplant)	Porcine reproductive and respiratory
Salmonella typhi	syndrome virus
Salmonella typhimurium	Pseudorabies
Salmonella cholerasuis	Rabies
Shigella	Rotavirus
*Aspergillus**	
*Candida**	
Histoplasma capsulatum	
Toxoplasma gondii	
Strongyloides ransomi	

*Exclude animals with lesions.
From McKenzie IFC, Loveland BE, Fishman JA, Auchincloss H, Sandrin MS: Xenotransplantation. *In* Ginns LC, Cosimi AB, Morris PJ (eds): Transplantation. Malden, MA: Blackwell Science, 1999, pp 827–874.

have long latent periods, it may be years before the damaging effects are understood. However, there is some optimism from preliminary studies which have identified a pig genotype which contains a very small number of PERV copies per cell, such that transmission to man would be extremely unlikely.[78]

Thus, despite the many concerns, most experts conclude that, with proper breeding and housing conditions of transgenic pigs, the risk of transfer of known porcine infections to humans is small.[74]

MALIGNANCIES

The possible induction of malignancies is a major drawback to the aggressive immunosuppression protocols that have been utilized in pig-to-primate models. In kidney xenotransplantation from transgenic pig to cynomolgus monkey, the longest reported survival was 78 days with a regimen of splenectomy, cyclophosphamide, cyclosporine, and steroids. Of note, two of nine animals developed lymphoproliferative disease during the short period of survival.[8, 51] In another report, three of seven monkeys surviving up to 71 days developed lymphoproliferative disease despite five deaths from rejection.[77] These and other studies indicate that current immunosuppressive modalities provide inadequate control of xenotransplant rejection with excessive toxicity.

ETHICAL CONSIDERATIONS

Animal "Rights"

The first issue to be resolved is whether it is ethically responsible to use *any* animals as donors for human transplantation. There is a significant segment of society in the United States and Europe who believe that the killing of animals for medical purposes is wrong.[1, 35, 72] However, the current societal norm places a greater value on human life than on animal life and maintains that the use of animals for experimental and clinical research in xenotransplantation is permissible. If there were alternatives that would increase the supply of donor organs or that would provide other means of successfully treating end-stage organ failure for both children and adults, then it could be viewed as wrong to pursue xenotransplantation research. Such widespread alternatives do not currently exist. Therefore, under current standards, xenotransplantation has been allowed to continue.

The second major issue is which animal or animals are suitable for organ donation. The relative merits of pigs versus nonhuman primates has been discussed in the previous section, Choice of Donor Species for Clinical Transplantation. In contrast to the anthropomorphism of nonhuman primates, pigs carry a long history of domestication and breeding as a food source for man (see also earlier section, Choice of Donor Species for Clinical Transplantation). There have been few objections to the use of porcine cardiac valves or porcine-derived insulin for humans. The ready availability of pig organs would obviate the often long, expensive, and life-threatening wait for human organs. Thus, it appears that as long as standard compassionate care criteria are maintained, ethical issues will not be a major obstacle for the use of pigs, as it would be for nonhuman primates.

Informed Consent

It is clear that, like all experimental treatments or medications, experimental clinical transplantation with xenogeneic organs must be conducted according to the highest legal and ethical standards. The data concerning clinical xenotransplantation are sparse (see again Table 23–2). Although major scientific and technical advances have occurred in the field of xenotransplantation, major problems with adverse outcomes still exist. Initially, xenotransplantation will likely be reserved for patients who are terminally ill, and for whom allogeneic transplantation or other alternatives are not possible. Patients selected for this experimental therapy must be informed of the major uncertainties of rejection, the possibility of early malignancy, the unknown likelihood of infection transmission, and the length of survival in animal models. Terminally ill patients, especially children, are a uniquely vulnerable population in terms of truly informed consent. It is incumbent on the researchers performing the transplants that the subjects have complete and understandable information regarding the high probability of adverse events and their rights with regard to withdrawal. The latter issue is particularly important, because once a heart is transplanted there is no option for withdrawal from the procedure under study.

CRITERIA FOR CLINICAL TRIALS

No established guidelines exist for initiation for a clinical trial in cardiac xenotransplantation. Perhaps the most

logical initial indication would be as "bridging" therapy to allotransplantation. However, with the widespread availability of mechanical circulatory support systems, it is difficult to readily envision an adult group of patients who would not be suitable for mechanical circulatory support and yet would be suitable for xenotransplantation. Xenotransplantation could be reserved for patients in whom an assist device was not available, but that appears unlikely, since initial clinical trials in xenotransplantation will undoubtedly be restricted to those centers with established expertise in animal xenotransplantation, and such centers would almost certainly have well-developed clinical heart transplant and mechanical circulatory support programs.

Perhaps a more suitable initial group would be infants and children with rapidly failing cardiac performance who are on inotropic support and unlikely to survive until transplantation. Since the only generally available support device is the extracorporeal membrane oxygenator (ECMO), and since the results with ECMO are considerably inferior to other circulatory assist devices available for adults, xenotransplantation might be appropriate for some subsets of pediatric patients as a bridge to cardiac transplantation. However, the total number of such patients would be small, particularly at any one center. Furthermore, issues of informed consent would be complex. Another confounding aspect of any bridging trial of xenotransplantation to allotransplantation is the unknown interaction between antibodies and other immune elements directed against the xenograft and the MHC antigens expressed by the subsequent allograft.

For patients in whom xenotransplantation would be considered definitive therapy, it is also difficult to envision the appropriate group of patients for initial clinical trials. The rapid emergence of mechanical assist devices makes it unlikely that initial survival following xenotransplantation could compete with assist devices for patients unable to receive cardiac allotransplantation. In pediatric heart transplantation, the largest group of infants undergoing heart transplantation have hypoplastic left heart syndrome. With improving results of palliative operations leading to the Fontan pathway, it would be hard to justify the diversion of such patients toward a clinical trial in xenotransplantation.

Another approach would be to delay cardiac xenotransplantation until successful intermediate-term survival was demonstrated in a non–life-sustaining organ such as kidney, where removal of the porcine organ would be an option in the presence of excessive complications. If intermediate-term graft and patient survival without excessive complications could be established, extension of xenotransplantation to certain subsets of patients with advanced heart failure would be more readily justified.

Some experts in the field of xenotransplantation have suggested that clinical trials in heart transplantation should not be initiated until the median survival in a pig-to-primate model exceeded 3 months with demonstrated survival of at least 6 months.[17] Furthermore, there should be evidence of control of all aspects of rejection without excessive drug toxicity. Most experts are in agreement that governmental and international agencies should actively participate in the design of clinical trials, monitoring of outcome, and facilitating exchange of information obtained in such trials.

FUTURE DIRECTIONS

Based on available data, many believe that the likelihood of translating this technology into clinical reality with good long-term outcome in the foreseeable future looks bleak. After all, even with genetically manipulated pigs for DAF and other complement regulatory proteins, survival is still measured in weeks to months, and the development of early lymphoproliferative disease is of major concern regarding the toxicity of current immunosuppressive protocols.

Solving the problem of hyperacute rejection is a fantastic accomplishment, but there is little confidence that current strategies will solve the likely aggressive vascular rejection which is a prominent feature of animals surviving several weeks or more. Furthermore, very little is known about the nature or aggressiveness of acute cellular rejection and chronic rejection, which have not yet been examined since no primates with porcine hearts have survived long enough to enter this phase of the rejection cycle. It seems naive to suggest that these manifestations of allograft rejection will be less intense in a xenotransplant. Finally, many experts have suggested that current immunosuppressive agents are poorly suited for the control of rejection in xenotransplant models. The development of new immunosuppressive agents specifically suited for xenotransplantation will require expensive research and development efforts by industry, and such a financial commitment will likely not be embraced by pharmaceutical companies unless there is strong evidence for successful clinical xenotransplantation. Thus, in many ways, there seems relevance to a prediction attributed to Dr. Norman Shumway that "xenotransplantation will always be the future of transplantation."

However, there are reasons to believe there may be light at the end of this long and "provocative" tunnel. It appears nearly certain that if xenotransplantation of the heart is to become a viable therapeutic strategy for advanced heart failure with survival measured in years, its success will be inextricably linked to successful expansion of the principles of creating **transgenic porcine models.** Ultimately, these transgenic animals will contain not one but multiple (and perhaps many) human proteins which modify most aspects of the immune response mounted against the porcine vascular endothelium and myocytes. Thus, a porcine heart expressing human molecules for decay accelerating activity, membrane cofactor activity, and CD59-like activity might further increase the protection against complement-mediated or complement-enhanced forms of rejection.[23] One could envision transgenic hearts which expressed genes that down-regulate local immune responses through the deletion of adhesion receptors or the addition of receptors or ligands that inhibit cellular activation. Theoretically, transgenic pigs could express higher concentrations of human cytokines known to down-regulate immune responses, such as transforming growth factor-β. Adhesion molecules could be deleted which serve as sites for neutrophil or lymphocyte adhesion to endothelial surfaces following activation. Transgenic technology could be employed to produce "knock out" species of pigs which lack α-1,3-galactose or major histocompatibility complexes (perhaps with additional molecules that prevent attack of NK cells). Methods for induction of selective B-cell tolerance would also be critically important to avoid the toxicity associated with aggressive immunosuppressants to control natural anti–Gal antibody production.

If sufficient research funds and human resources were applied, construction of porcine colonies with many transgenic components could be established in a stepwise process analogous to the coordinated efforts which targeted the complete sequencing of the human genome. The years required to establish each new colony of transgenic pig coupled with the immense financial and scientific investment are formidable, but the end result could be quite incredible. The available technology in and the future possibilities of genetic engineering lend credence to the dream articulated by Cozzi and White[23] that ". . . not only will it be possible to produce pig organs to act as substitutes for human organs in transplantation but that with time such organs will be made less susceptible to rejection than their human counterparts."

References

1. Arundel M, McKenzie IFC: The acceptability of pig organ xenografts to patients awaiting a transplant. Xenotransplantation 1997;4:62–66.
2. Bach FH, Ferran D, Hechenleitner P: Accommodation of vascularized xenografts: expression of "protective genes" by donor endothelial cells in a host Th2 cytokine environment. Nat Med 1997;3:196–204.
3. Bach FH, Robson SC, Winkler H, Ferran C, Stuhlmeier KM, Wrighton CS, Hancock WW: Barriers to xenotransplantation. Nat Med 1995;1:869–873.
4. Bach FH, Turman MA, Vercellotti GM: Accommodation: a working paradigm for progressing toward clinical discordant xenografting. Transplant Proc 1991;23:205–207.
5. Bach FH, Winkler H, Ferran C, Hancock WW, Robson SC: Delayed xenograft rejection. Immunol Today 1996;17:379–384.
6. Bailey LL, Nehlsen-Cannarella SL, Concepcion W, Jolley WB: Baboon-to-human cardiac xenotransplantation in a neonate. JAMA 1985;254:3321–3329.
7. Barnard CN, Wolpowitz W, Losman JG: Heterotopic cardiac transplantation with a xenograft for assistance of the left heart in cardiogenic shock after cardiopulmonary bypass. S Afr Med J 1977;52:1035–1038.
8. Bhatti FNK, Zaidi A, Schoeckel M: Survival of life-supporting hDAF transgenic kidneys in primates is enhanced by splenectomy. Transplant Proc 1998;30:2467.
9. Blakely ML, Van der Werf WJ, Berndt MC, Dalmasso AP, Bach FH, Hancock WW: Activation of intragraft endothelial and mononuclear cells during discordant xenograft rejection. Transplantation 1994;58:1059–1066.
10. Bollinger RR: The potential of xenotransplants. Transplant Proc 1996;28:2024–2025.
11. Calne RY: Organ transplantation between widely disparate species. Transplant Proc 1970;2:550.
12. Carrington CA, Richards AC, Cozzi E, Langford G, Yannoutsos N, White DJ: Expression of human DAF and MCP on pig endothelial cells protects from human complement. Transplant Proc 1995;27:321–323.

13. Cooley DA: Experience with human heart transplantation. *In* Shapiro H (ed): Experience with Human Heart Transplantation. Durban: Butterworths, 1969, pp 203–208.

14. Cooley DA, Hallman GL, Bloodwell RD, Nora JJ, Leachman RD: Human heart transplantation: experience with 12 cases [abstract]. Am J Cardiol 1968;22:804.

15. Cooper DK, Cairns TDH, Taube DH: Extracorporeal immunoadsorption of anti-pig antibody in baboons using α Gal oligosaccharide immunoaffinity columns. Xenotransplantation 1996;4:27.

16. Cooper DK, Good AH, Koren E, Oriol R, Malcom AJ, Ippolito RM, Neethling FA, Romano E, Zuhdi N: Identification of alphagalactosyl and other carbohydrate epitopes that are bound by human anti-pig antibodies: relevance to discordant xenografting in man. Transplant Immunol 1993;1:198–205.

17. Cooper DK, Keogh AM, Brink J: Report of the xenotransplantation advisory committee of the international society for heart and lung transplantation. The present status of xenotransplantation and its potential role in the treatment of end-stage cardiac and pulmonary disease. J Heart Lung Transplant 2000;19:1125–1165.

18. Cooper DKC: The first heart transplants in the United Kingdom, 1968–1980. Guy's Hosp Gazette 1995;109:114–120.

19. Cooper DKC, Koren E, Oriol R: Oligosaccharides and discordant xenotransplantation. Immunol Rev 1994;141:31–58.

20. Cooper DKC, Lanza RP: Xeno—The Promise of Transplanting Animal Organs into Humans. New York: Oxford University Press, 2000.

21. Coughlan AF, Berndt MC, Dunlop LC, Hancock WW: In vivo studies of P-selectin and platelet activating factor during endotoxemia, accelerated allograft rejection, and discordant xenograft rejection. Transplant Proc 1993;25:2930–2931.

22. Cozzi E, Langford GA, Richards A, Elsome K, Lancaster R, Chen P, Yannoutsos N, White DJ: Expression of human decay accelerating factor in transgenic pigs. Transplant Proc 1994;26:1402–1403.

23. Cozzie E, White DJ: The generation of transgenic pigs as potential organ donors for humans. Nat Med 1995;1:964–966.

24. Czaplicki J, Blonska B, Religa Z: The lack of hyperacute xenogeneic heart transplant rejection in a human. J Heart Lung Transplant 1992;11:393–396.

25. Dalmasso AP, Platt JL, Bach FH: Reaction of complement with endothelial cells in a model of xenotransplantation. Clin Exp Immunol 1991;86(suppl):31–35.

26. Dalmasso AP, Vercellotti GM, Fischel RJ, Bolman RM, Bach FH, Platt JL: Mechanism of complement activation in the hyperacute rejection of porcine organs transplanted into primate recipients. Am J Pathol 1992;140:1157–1166.

27. Dalmasso AP, Vercellotti GM, Platt JL, Bach FH: Inhibition of complement-mediated endothelial cell cytotoxicity by decay-accelerating factor. Potential for prevention of xenograft hyperacute rejection. Transplantation 1991;52:530–533.

28. Davies A, Lachmann PJ: Membrane defence against complement lysis: the structure and biological properties of CD59. Immunol Res 1993;12:258–275.

29. Davis EA, Jakobs F, Pruitt SK, Greene PS, Qian Z, Lam TT, Tseng E, Levin JL, Baldwin WM, Sanfilippo F: Overcoming rejection in pig-to-primate cardiac xenotransplantation. Transplant Proc 1997;29:938–939.

30. Diamond LE, Martin MJ, Adams D, et al: Transgenic pig hearts and kidneys expressing human CD59,CD55, or CD46 are protected from hyperacute rejection upon transplantation into baboons. 4th International Congress for Xenogransplantation, 1997.

31. Dorling A, Riesbeck K, Warrens A, Lechler R: Clinical xenotransplantation of solid organs. Lancet 1997;349:867–871.

32. Ferran C, Badrichani AZ, Cooper JT, Stroka DM, Bach FH: Xenotransplantation: progress toward clinical development. Adv Nephrol Necker Hosp 1997;27:391–420.

33. Fodor WL, Williams BL, Matis LA: Expression of a human complement inhibitor in a transgenic pig as a model for the prevention of xenogeneic hyperacute rejection. Proc Natl Acad Sci USA 1994;91:11153–11157.

34. Galili U: Interaction of the natural anti-Gal antibody with alphagalactosyl epitopes: a major obstacle for xenotransplantation in humans. Immunol Today 1993;14:480–482.

35. Gallup: The American public attitudes towards organ donation and transplantation. Conducted for the Partnership for Organ Donations 1993. Partnership for Organ Donation, 1993.

36. Good AH, Cooper DK, Malcolm AJ, Ippolito RM, Koren E, Neethling FA, Ye Y, Zuhd N, Lamontage LR: Identification of carbohydrate structures that bind human antiporcine antibodies: implications for discordant xenografting in humans. Transplant Proc 1992;24:559–562.

37. Gordon JW, Ruddle RH: Integration and stable germ line transformation of genes injected into mouse pronuclei. Science 1981; 214:1244–1246.

38. Hancock WW: Delayed xenograft rejection. World J Surg 1997;21: 917–923.

39. Hardy JD, Kurrus FE, Chavez CM, Neely WA, Eraslan S, Turner MD, Fabian LW, Labecki TD: Heart transplantation in man: developmental studies and report of a case [abstract]. JAMA 1964;188:1132–1140.

40. Hitchcock CR, Kiser JC, Telander RL, Seljeskob EL: Baboon renal grafts. JAMA 1964;189:934.

41. Holzknecht ZE, Platt JL: Identification of porcine endothelial cell membrane antigens recognized by human xenoreactive natural antibodies. J Immunol 1995;154:4565–4575.

42. Itescu S, Kwiatkowski P, Artrip JH, Wang SF, Ankersmit J, Minanov DP, Michler RE: Role of natural killer cells, macrophages, and accessory molecule interactions in the rejection of pig-to-primate xenografts beyond the hyperacute period. Hum Immunol 1998;59:275–286.

43. Itescu S, Minanov O, Michler RE: Newborn pig-to-baboon cadiac xenotransplantation: a model of delayed xenograft rejection. *In* Cooper DK, Kemp E (eds): Xenotransplantation. Heidelberg: Springer, 1997, p 478.

44. Joziasse DH, Shaper JH, Jabs EW, Sharper NL: Characterisation of an α1,3-galactosyltransferase homologue on human chromosome 12 that is organized as a processed pseudogene. J Biol Chem 1991;266:6991–6998.

45. Kaplon RJ, Michler RE, Xu H, Kwiatkowski P, Edwards NM, Platt JL: Absence of hyperacute rejection in newborn pig-to-baboon cardiac xenografts. Transplantation 1995;59:1–6.

46. Kobayashi T, Taniguchi S, Neethling FA, Rose AG, Hancock WW, Ye Y, Niekrasz M, Kosanke S, Wright LJ, White DJ: Delayed xenograft rejection of pig-to-baboon cardiac transplants after cobra venom factor therapy. Transplantation 1997;64:1255–1261.

47. Kobayashi T, Taniguchi S, Ye Y: Delayed xenograft rejection in C3 depleted discordant (pig to baboon) cardiac xenografts treated with cobra venom factor. Transplant Proc 1996;28:560.

48. Kroshus TJ, Salerno CT, Dalmasso AP, Fodor WL, Bolman RM: Expression of human CD59 in transgenic pig hearts extends survival in an orthotopic pig-to-baboon model of heart transplantation. J Heart Lung Transplant 1997;16:111.

49. Kroshus TJ, Salerno CT, Dalmasso AP, Fodor WL, Bolman RM, Dalmasso AP: A recombinant soluble chimeric complement inhibitor composed of human CD46 and CD55 reduces acute cardiac tissue injury in models of pig-to-human heart transplantation. Transplantation 2000;69:2282–2289.

50. Lambrigts D, Sachs DH, Cooper DK: Discordant organ xenotransplantation in primates: world experience and current status. Transplantation 1998;66:547–561.

51. Lambrigts D, Van Calster P, Xu Y, Awwad M, Neethling FA, Kozlowski T, Foley A, Watts A, Chae SJ, Fishman J, Thall AD, White-Scharf ME, Sachs DH, Cooper DK: Pharmacologic immunosuppressive therapy and extracorporeal immunoadsorption in the suppression of anti-alphaGal antibody in the baboon. Xenotransplantation 1998;5:274–283.

52. Langford GA, Yannoutsos N, Cozzi E: Production of pigs transgenic for human decay accelerating factor. Transplant Proc 1994;26:1400–1401.

53. LeTissier P, Stoye J, Takeuchi Y, Patience C: Two sets of humantropic pig retrovirus. Nature 1997;389:681–682.

54. Leventhal JR, Dalmasso AP, Cromwell JW, Manivel CJ, Bolman RM, Matas AJ: Complement depletion prolongs discordant cardiac xenograft survival in rodents and non-human primates. Transplant Proc 1993;25:398–399.

55. Leventhal JR, Matas AJ, Sun LH, Bolman RM, Dalmasso AP, Platt JL: The immunopathology of cardiac xenograft rejection in the guinea pig-to-rat model. Transplantation 1993;56:1–8.

56. Leventhal JR, Sakiyalak P, Witson J, Simone P, Matas AJ, Bolman RM, Dalmasso AP: The synergistic effect of combined antibody

and complement depletion on discordant cardiac xenograft survival in nonhuman primates. Transplantation 1994;57:974–978.

57. Lin SS, Weidner BC, Byrne GW, Diamond LE, Lawson JH, Hoopes CW, Daniels LJ, Daggett CW, Parker W, Harland RC, Davis RD, Bollinger RR, Logan JS, Platt JL: The role of antibodies in acute vascular rejection of pig-to-baboon cardiac transplants. J Clin Invest 1998;101:1745–1756.

58. Liu Z, Sun YK, Xi YP, Maffei A, Reed E, Harris P, Suciu-Foca N: Contribution of direct and indirect recognition pathways to T-cell alloreactivity. J Exp Med 1993;177:1643–1650.

59. Magee JC, Collins BH, Harland RC, Lindman BJ, Bollinger RR, Frank MM, Platt JL: Immunoglobulin prevents complement mediated hyperacute rejection in swine-to-primate xenotransplantation. J Clin Invest 1995;96:2404–2412.

60. Marion P: Les transplantations caradiaques et les transplantations hepatiques [abstract]. Lyon Med 1969;222:585–608.

61. Marion P, Lapeyre D, Estanove S, Estanove JF, George M, Mikaeloff P, Vadot L: Clinical attempts at circulatory assistance [abstract]. Ann Chir Thorac Cardiovasc 1969;8:411–412.

62. Martin U, Kiessig V, Blusch JH: Expression of pig endogenous retrovirus by primary porcine endothelial cells and infection of human cells. Lancet 1998;352:692–694.

63. Matsumiya G, Gundry SR, Nehlsen-Cannarella S, Fagoaga OR, Morimoto T, Arai S, Fukushima N, Zuppan CW, Bailey LL: Serum interleukin-6 level after cardiac xenotransplantation in primates. Transplant Proc 1997;29:916–919.

64. McCurry KR, Kooyman DL, Alvarado CG: Human complement regulatory proteins protect swine-to-primate cardiac xenografts from humoral injury. Nat Med 1995;1:423–427.

65. McKenzie IF, Stocker J, Ting A, Morris PJ: Human lymphocytotoxic and haemagglutinating activity against sheep and pig cells. Lancet 1968;2:386–387.

66. McKenzie IF, Xing PX, Vaughan HA, Prenzoska J, Dabkowski PL, Sandrin MS: Distribution of the major xenoantigen (gal(α 1–3)gal) for pig to human xenografts. Transplant Immunol 1994;2:81–86.

67. McKenzie IFC, Loveland BE, Fishman JA, Auchincloss H, Sandrin MS: Xenotransplantation. In Ginns LC, Cosimi AB, Morris PJ (eds): Transplantation. Malden, MA: Blackwell Science, 1999, pp 827–874.

68. McPhaul JJ Jr, Stastney P, Freeman RB: Specificities of antibodies eluted from human cadaveric renal allografts. Multiple mechanisms of renal allograft injury. J Clin Invest 1981;67:1405–1414.

69. Michler RE, Xu H, O'Hair DP, Shah A, Kwiatkowski P, Minanov DP, Itescu S: Newborn discordant cardiac xenotransplantation in primates: a model of natural antibody depletion. Transplant Proc 1996;28:651–652.

70. Minanov OP, Artrip JH, Szabolcs M, Kwiatkowski P, Galili U, Itescu S, Michler RE: Triple immunosuppression reduces mononuclear cell infiltration and prolongs graft life in pig-to-newborn baboon cardiac xenotransplantation. J Thorac Cardiovasc Surg 1998;115:998–1006.

71. Moses RD, Auchincloss H Jr: Mechanism of cellular xenograft rejection. In Cooper DKC, Kemp E (eds): Xenotransplantation. Heidelberg: Springer, 1997, pp 140–174.

72. Nuffield Council on Bioethics: Animal-to-human transplants: the ethics of xenotransplantation. Council on Bioethics, 1996.

73. Oglesby TJ, Allen CJ, Liszewski MK, White DJ, Atkinson JP: Membrane cofactor protein (CD46) protects cells from complement mediated attack by an intrinsic mechanism. J Exp Med 1992;175:1547–1551.

74. Onions D, Cooper DKC, Alexander TJL: An approach to the control of disease transmission in pig-to-human xenotransplantation [abstract]. Xenotransplantation 2000;7:143–155.

75. Oriol R, Ye Y, Koren E, Cooper DKC: Carbohydrate antigens of pig tissues reacting with human antibodies as potential targets for hyperacute vascular rejection in pig-to-man organ xenotransplantation. Transplantation 1993;56:1433–1442.

76. Osman N, McKenzie IF, Ostenried K, Ioannou YA, Desnick RJ, Sandrin MS: Combined transgenic expression of α-galactosidase and α-1,2-fucosyl transferase leads to optimal reduction in the major xenoepitope Galα(1,3)Gal. Proc Natl Acad Sci USA 1997;94:14677–14821.

77. Ostlie DJ, Cozzi E, Vial CM: Improved renal function and fewer rejection episodes using SDZ RAD in life-supporting hDAF pig to primate renal xenotransplantation. Transplantation 1999;67:S118.

78. Patience C, Ericsson T, LaChance A, Oldmixon B, Andersson G: Pig endogenous retrovirus distribution in a MHC inbred herd of miniature swine [abstract]. Fifth Congress of the Internal Xenotransp Association, 1999.

79. Pelicci PG, Subar M, Weiss A, Dalla FR, Littman DR: Molecular diversity of the human T-gamma constant region genes. Science 1987;237:1051–1055.

80. Perper RJ, Najarian JS: Passive transfer transplantation immunity. Transplantation 1967;5:514–533.

81. Pirtle EC: Incidence of antibody to swine influenza virus in Iowa breeder and butcher pigs correlated with signs of influenza-like illness. Am J Vet Res 1973;34:83–85.

82. Platt JL, Lin SS: The future promises of xenotransplantation. Ann N Y Acad Sci 1998;862:5–18.

83. Platt JL, Vercellotti GM, Dalmasso AP, Matas AJ, Bolman RM, Najarian JS, Bach FH: Transplantation of discordant xenografts: a review of progress. Immunol Today 1990;11:450–457.

84. Platt JL, Vercellotti GM, Lindman BJ, Oegema TR Jr, Bach FH, Dalmasso AP: Release of heparan sulfate from endothelial cells. Implications for pathogenesis of hyperacute rejection. J Exp Med 1990;171:1363–1368.

85. Porter KA: Pathology of the Kidney. Boston: Little, Brown & Co, 1992.

86. Pruitt SK, Bollinger RR, Collins BH, Marsh HC, Levin JL, Rudolph AR, Baldwin WM, Sanfilippo F: Continuous complement (C) inhibition using soluble C receptor type 1 (sCR1): effect on hyperacute rejection (HAR) of pig-to-primate cardiac xenografts. Transplant Proc 1996;28:756.

87. Pruitt SK, Bollinger RR, Collins BH, Marsh HC, Levin JL, Rudolph AR, Baldwin WM, Sanfilippo F: Effect of continuous complement inhibition using soluble complement receptor type 1 on survival of pig-to-primate cardiac xenografts. Transplantation 1997;63:900–902.

88. Reemtsma K: Renal heterotransplantation from nonhuman primates to man. Ann N Y Acad Sci 1969;162:412–418.

89. Robson SC, Kaczmarek E, Siegel JB: Loss of ATP diphosphohydrolase activity with endothelial cell activation. J Exp Med 1997;185:153–163.

90. Romano E, Neethling FA, Nilsson K, Kosanke S, Shimizu A, Magnusson S, Svensson L, Samuelsson B, Cooper DK: Intravenous synthetic alphaGal saccharides delay hyperacute rejection following pig-to-baboon heart transplantation. Xenotransplantation 1999;6:36–42.

91. Rose AG, Cooper DK, Human PA, Reichenspurner H, Reichart B: Histopathology of hyperacute rejection of the heart: experimental and clinical observations in allografts and xenografts. J Heart Lung Transplant 1991;10:223–224.

92. Rose ML: Human T cell response to porcine tissues. In Cooper DKC, Kemp E, Platt JL (eds): Xenotransplantation. Heidelberg: Springer, 1997, pp 175–189.

93. Rosengard AM, Cary N, Horsley J, Belcher C, Langford G, Cozzi E, Wallwork J, White DJ: Endothelial expression of human decay accelerating factor in transgenic pig tissue: a potential approach for human complement inactivation in discordant xenografts. Transplant Proc 1995;27:326–327.

94. Roslin MS, Zisbrod Z, Burack JH, Tranbraugh RS, Strashun A, Jacobowitz IJ, Brewer RJ, Kim Y, Cunningham JN, Norin AJ: 15 day survival in pig to baboon heterotopic cardiac xenotransplantation. Transplant Proc 1992;24:572–573.

95. Ross DN: In: Shapiro H (ed): Experience with Human Heart Transplantation. Durban: Butterworths, 1969, p 227.

96. Salerno CT, Dalmasso AP, Kroshus TJ, Svendsen CA: A soluble chimeric complement inhibitor of C3- and C5-convertases prolongs xenograft survival in pig to primate cardiac transplantation [abstract]. 4th International Congress for Xenogransplantation, 1997.

97. Sandrin MS, Vaughan HA, Dabkowski PL, McKenzie IF: Antipig IgM antibodies in human serum reacts predominantly with Galα(1,3)Gal epitopes. Proc Natl Acad Sci USA 1993;90:11391–11395.

98. Sandrin MS, Vaughan HA, McKenzie IF: Identification of Galα(1,-3)Gal as the major epitope for pig-to-human vascularised xenografts. Transplant Rev 1994;8:134–149.

99. Satake M, Kawagishi N, Rydberg L, Kumagai-Braesch M, Samuelson BE, Tibell A, Andersson A, Korsgren O, Groth CG, Moller

E: Limited specificity of xenoantibodies in diabetic patients transplanted with fetal porcine islet cell clusters. Main antibody reactivity against α-linked galactose-containing epitopes. Xenotransplantation 1994;1:89–101.

100. Schmoeckel M, Bhatti FN, Zaidi A, Cozzi E, Waterworth PD, Tolan MJ, Pino-Chavez G, Goddard M, Warner RG, Langford GA, Dunning JJ, Wallwork J, White DJ: Orthotopic heart transplantation in a transgenic pig to primate model [published erratum appears in Transplantation 1998;66:943] [abstract]. Transplantation 1998;65:1570–1577.

101. Simon PM, Neethling FA, Taniguchi S, Goode PL, Zoph D, Hancock WW, Cooper DK: Intravenous infusion of Gal-alpha 1–3 Gal oligosaccharides in baboons delays hyperacute rejection of porcine heart xenografts [abstract]. Transplantation 1998;65:346–353.

102. Takeuchi Y, Patience C, Magre S, Weiss RA, Banerjee PT, LeTissier P, Stoye JP: Host range and interference studies of three classes of pig endogenous retrovirus. J Virol 1998;72:9986–9991.

103. Taniguchi S, Cooper DK: Clinical xenotransplantation: past, present and future [abstract]. Ann R Coll Surg Engl 1997;79:13–19.

104. Taniguchi S, Cooper DKC: Clinical Experience with Cardiac Xenotransplantation. *In* Cooper DK, Miller LW, Patterson GA (eds): The Transplantation and Replacement of Thoracic Organs. Lancaster: Kluwer, 1996, pp 743–747.

105. Tearle RG, Tange MJ, Zannettino ZL, Katerlos M, Shinkel TA, VanDenderen BJ, Lonie AJ, Lyons I, Nottle MB, Cox T, Becker C, Peura AM, Wigley PL, Crawford RJ, Robins AJ, Pearse MJ, d'Aprice AJ: The α-1,3-galactosyltransferase knockout mouse: implications for xenotransplantation. Transplantation 1996;61:13–19.

106. Vanohve B, deMartin R, Lipp J: Human xenoreactive natural antibodies of the IgM isotype activate pig endothelial cells [abstract]. Xenotransplantation 1994;1:17–23.

107. Vaughan HA, McKenzie IF, Sandrin MS: Biochemical studies of pig xenoantigens detected by naturally occurring human antibodies and the galactoseα(1–3)galactose reactive lectin. Transplantation 1995;59:102–109.

108. Vial CM, Bhatti FN, Ostlie DJ: Prolonged survival of orthotopic cardiac xenografts in an hDAF transgenic pig-to-baboon model. Transplantation 1999;67:117S.

109. Vial CM, Ostlie DJ, Bhatti FN, Cozzi E, Goddard M, Chavez GP, Wallwork J, White DJ, Dunning J: Life supporting function for over one month of a transgenic porcine heart in a baboon [abstract]. J Heart Lung Transplant 2000;19:224–229.

110. Walsh LA, Tone M, Thiru S, Waldmann H: The CD59 antigen multifunctional molecule. Tissue Antigens 1992;40:213–220.

111. Wang MW, Wright LJ, Sims MJ, White DJ: Presence of human chromosome 1 with expression of human decay-accelerating factor (DAF) prevents lysis of mouse/human hybrid cells by human complement [abstract]. Scand J Immunol 1991;34:771–778.

112. Waterworth PD, Cozzi E, Tolan MJ, Langford G, Braidley P, Chavez G, Dunning J, Wallwork J, White DJ: Pig to primate cardiac xenotransplantation and cyclophosphamide therapy [abstract]. Transplant Proc 1997;29:899–900.

113. Waterworth PD, Dunning J, Tolan MJ: Life-supporting pig-to-baboon heart [abstract]. J Heart Lung Transplant 1998;17:1201–1207.

114. Weiss L, Fischer E, Haeffner-Cavaillon N, Jouvin MH, Appay MD, Bariety J, Kazatchkine M: The human C3b receptor (CR1). Adv Nephrol 1989;18:249–270.

115. White DJ: hDAF transgenic pig organs: are they concordant for human transplantation [abstract]. Xenotransplantation 1996;4:50.

116. White DJ, Langford G, Cozzi E, Young VJ: Production of pigs transgenic for DAF: a strategy for xenotransplantation [abstract]. Xenotransplantation 1995;2:213.

117. White DJ, Oglesby T, Liszewski MK, Tedja I, Hourcade D, Wang MW, Wright L, Wallwork J, Atkinson JP: Expression of human decay accelerating factor or membrane cofactor protein genes on mouse cells inhibits lysis by human complement. Transplant Proc 1992;5:648–650.

118. Xu H, Gundry SR, Hancock WW: Prolonged discordant xenograft survival and delayed xenograft rejection in a pig-to-baboon orthotopic cardiac xenograft model [abstract]. J Thorac Cardiovasc Surg 1998;115:1342–1349.

119. Xu H, Gundry SR, Hancock WW, Izutani H, Zuppan CW, Bailey LL: Effects of immunosuppression and pretransplant splenectomy in newborn cardiac xenograft survival [abstract]. Transplant Proc 1998;30:1084.

120. Xu H, Gundry SR, Hancock WW, Zuppan C, Izutani H, Bailey LL: Effects of pretransplant splenectomy and immunosuppression of humoral immunity in a pig-to-newborn goat cardiac xenograft model. Transplant Proc 2000;32:1010–1014.

121. Yamada K, Auchincloss H Jr: Cell-mediated xenograft rejection. Curr Opin Organ Transplant 1999;4:90–94.

122. Yamada K, Sach DH, DerSimonian H: The human antiporcine xenogeneic T-cell response: evidence for allelic specificity of MLR and for both direct and indirect pathways of recognition. J Immunol 1995;155:5249–5256.

123. Ye Y, Neethling FA, Niekrasz M, Koren E, Richards SV, Martin M, Kosanke S, Oriol R, Cooper DK: Evidence that intravenously administered alphagalactosyl carbohydrates reduce baboon serum cytotoxicity to pig kidney cells (PK15) and transplanted pig hearts [abstract]. Transplantation 1994;58:330–337.

124. Ye Y, Neethling FA, Niekrasz M, Richards SV, Koren E, Merhav H, Kosanke S, Oriol R, Cooper DK: Intravenous administration of alpha-galactosyl carbohydrates reduces in vivo baboon serum cytotoxicity to pig kidney cells and transplanted pig hearts [abstract]. Transplant Proc 1994;26:1399.

125. Zaidi A, Schmoeckel M, Bhatti FN, Waterworth PD, Tolan MJ, Cozzi E, Chaves G, Langford G, Thiru S, Wallwork J, White DJ, Friend P: Life-supporting pig to primate renal xenotransplantation using genetically modified donors. Transplantation 1998;65:1584–1590.

126. Zehr KJ, Herskowitz A, Lee PC, Kuman P, Gillinov AM, Baumgartner WA: Neutrophil adhesion and complement inhibition prolongs survival of cardiac xenografts in discordant species [abstract]. Transplantation 1994;57:900–906.

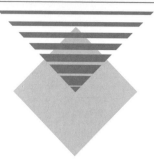

CHAPTER TWENTY-FOUR

Resource Allocation in Heart Transplantation

with the collaboration of
WALTER K. GRAHAM, J.D.

C ardiac transplantation is a highly labor-intensive therapy for advanced heart failure, requiring considerable human and institutional resources. As future therapies evolve for advanced heart failure, the allocation of available resources, both financial and therapeutic, will be increasingly challenging. This chapter will discuss details of the supply and demand for donors and resultant transplant activity, available information regarding the cost of this complex therapy, and the organization of these resources, both from an institutional and a national perspective. Eventually, complex analyses of demand, supply, and costs of specific therapies for end-stage heart disease will facilitate the decision-making process in the allocation of limited resources.

CARDIAC TRANSPLANTATION SUPPLY AND DEMAND

CADAVERIC DONOR AVAILABILITY

The number of cadaveric and living donors in the United States increased by almost 60% between 1990 and 1999, from 6,633 to 10,561 (Fig. 24–1).[20] This increase was particularly pronounced among living donor transplants (principally living-related renal transplants), which more than doubled from 2,124 in 1990 to 4,712 donors for transplantation in 1999, with cadaveric donor transplants increasing 30% during the same time period (Fig. 24–2). Nonetheless, the total number of donors appears to be plateauing, with the percentage increase in donors from 1998 to 1999 only 3% compared to an 8% increase in donors between 1997 and 1998. Fortunately, cadaveric donors often donate more than one organ. In 1999, the average was 3.6 organs per donor, with the number of transplants performed each year being nearly three times greater than the number of donors. Overall, the number of minority cadaveric donors increased from 18% of the total donors in 1990 to 24% in 1999. Among cadaveric donors in 1999, head trauma and cerebrovascular accidents/stroke accounted for 85% of all causes of brain death.

Despite overall gains in organ donors generally, cadaveric heart donors in the United States actually decreased from 2,449 in 1998 to 2,316 in 1999. In general, the number of hearts recovered for transplantation has been declining since the peak of 1995, when 2,526 hearts were recovered. In 1999, local transplants accounted for 65% of the total hearts recovered, and 31% were "shared" transplants with hearts being shipped out of the local procuring region. In 1999, hearts either not used for transplantation or used for research accounted for only 3% of the total. Poor organ function accounted for 61% of all donor organs consented but not recovered. Data from the International Society for Heart and Lung Transplantation (ISHLT) Registry indicate that the average heart donor's age is approximately 30 years. Numerous studies have examined the use of "marginal" or

Total Number of U.S. Donors Per Year
1988-1999

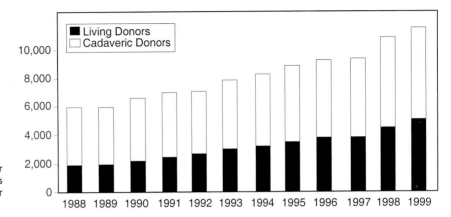

FIGURE **24-1.** Total number of U.S. donors per year, based on UNOS scientific registry data as of September 5, 2000. (From United Network for Organ Sharing: Annual Report, 2000.)

"extended" donors (see Chapter 9). If safe utilization of hearts from such donors could be implemented, the opportunity would exist for an important increase in donor supply.

HEART TRANSPLANT ACTIVITY

The worldwide experience in heart and heart/lung transplantation has been chronicled by the ISHLT Registry. Through 1999, the Registry has gathered data on 55,359 heart and 2,698 heart/lung transplant recipients since 1982.[11] Heart transplant activity increased progressively during the decade of the 1980s, with activity plateauing during the 1990s. Realizing that there is incomplete reporting of heart transplant activity to the ISHLT Registry, the peak year of recorded activity was 1995, during which 4,466 heart transplants were documented. There has been a gradual decrease in the number of documented heart transplants since that time, with 3,646 transplants documented worldwide during 1998. Similarly, with the increase in double-lung transplantation activity, there has been a progressive decrease in the number of heart/lung transplant procedures performed worldwide, reaching a peak of 237 reported procedures in 1989, with only 117 reported procedures in 1998.[11]

Data from the United Network of Organ Sharing (UNOS) in the United States indicates that the percentage of recipients on life support just prior to transplant decreased from 70% in 1998 to 61% in 1999. Those on

Total Number of Transplants Per Year
1988-1999

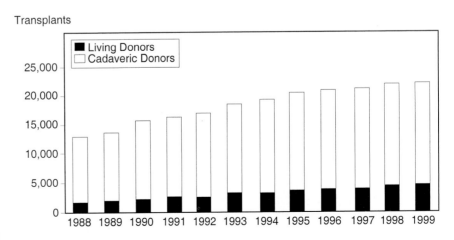

Based on UNOS Scientific registry data as of September 5, 2000

FIGURE **24-2.** Total number of U.S. transplants per year. (From United Network for Organ Sharing: Annual Report, 2000.)

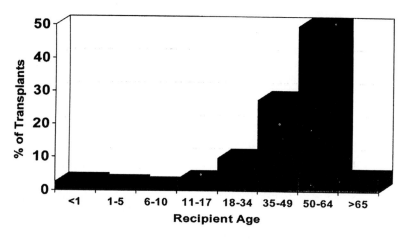

FIGURE **24–3.** Age distribution of heart transplant recipients. (From Hosenpud JD, Bennett LE, Keck BM, Boucek MM, Novick RJ: The Registry of the International Society for Heart and Lung Transplantation: 17th official report—2000. J Heart Lung Transplant 2000;19:909–931, with permission.)

life support in the intensive care unit (ICU) decreased by 21% between 1998 and 1999, while those on life support not in the ICU increased by 12%. The proportion of heart recipients not hospitalized just prior to transplantation increased over the last year, from 25% in 1998 to 34% in 1999. In 1999, 34% of heart recipients were in medical urgency Status 1A (highest medical urgency) at the time of transplant, 37% were in Status 1B, and 26% were in Status 2 (lowest medical urgency) (see Chapter 6). Worldwide, the age of recipients undergoing heart transplantation is heavily clustered between the ages of 35 and 65 years (Fig. 24–3).[11]

HEART WAITING LIST CHARACTERISTICS

The demand for transplanted organs has increased dramatically over the past decade. In the United States alone, more than 70,000 patients were registered for organ transplantation by the end of 1999 (Fig. 24–4).

The United States heart transplant waiting list more than doubled over the last 10 years, from 1,788 in 1990 to 4,121 registrants in 1999. However, the growth of the waiting list has slowed over the last few years and actually decreased last year from 4,185 registrants in 1998 to 4,121 registrants in 1999. While female registrants were only a small proportion of total heart wait list patients, the percentage grew from 15% in 1990 to 23% in 1999. At the end of 1990, only 8% of registrants had been on the waiting list for 2 years or more; however, by 1996 this group accounted for 27% of all heart transplant registrants, and by 1999 37% of registrants had been waiting 2 years or more.

In 1999, the median wait time for white registrants (217 days) was longer than the waiting times for Asians (67 days), blacks (184 days), and Hispanics (198 days). Due in part to the necessity of donor/recipient weight matching, the median wait time for males was longer (230 days in 1999) than for females (155 days in 1999), even though males consistently constitute approxi-

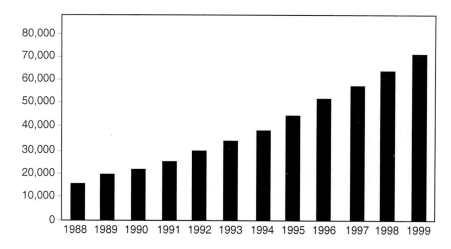

U.S. Organ Transplant Waiting List
Number of Patients Registered at Year's End
1988-1999

FIGURE **24–4.** U.S. organ transplant waiting list. (From United Network for Organ Sharing: Annual Report, 2000.)

mately 75% of the waiting list. In 1999, registrants with blood type O waited twice as long (363 days in 1999) as registrants with blood type A (158 days) and blood type B (162 days). Registrants with blood type AB had the shortest median waiting time (60 days in 1999). Fifty percent of registrants who had a beginning and ending status code of 1A (the most medically urgent) had an estimated waiting time of 30 days or less in 1999. Registrants with an ending status of 1A accounted for 30% of all active heart wait list registrants in 1999. As expected, the longest waiting times are for stable out-of-hospital patients.[20]

DEATH RATES ON THE HEART WAITING LIST

The death rate for the heart transplant waiting list has decreased dramatically over time, from 432.2 per 1,000 patient years in 1990 to 172.4 in 1999. The death rate in 1999 is the lowest of the last 10 years. As expected, registrants in the most medically urgent status category (i.e., Status 1A) had much higher death rates than did others. The death rate for Status 1A registrants in 1999 was 581.9 per 1,000 patient years, as compared with 202.7/1,000 patient years for Status 1B, and 130.7 for Status 2 registrants.

COSTS OF CARDIAC TRANSPLANTATION

OVERVIEW

Progress in treatments of major life-threatening illnesses comes at a significant toll. Organ transplantation is an excellent example of this difficulty. As patients progress through the varying stages of heart failure and approach advanced and end-stage disease, reversing the situation requires complicated and advanced therapeutics that are challenging to deliver and costly. The impact of overall health resources committed to the care of heart failure is quite staggering; in the United States alone, heart failure is the leading cause of hospitalization in adults over 65 years of age, requiring annual expenditures in excess of $20 billion.[17] In industrialized countries, the cost of treating heart failure accounts for 1–2% of total health care expenditures.[16] Because the practice of medicine and surgery does not conform to the usual free market economic principles controlling other commercial ventures, one must grapple independently with the dilemma of **resource allocation** for high-cost health care items. This is particularly problematic in environments such as Third World countries where resources are scarce. Barely being able to pay for life-saving routine vaccinations and medicines in these countries naturally limits sophisticated and expensive therapies such as organ transplantation. The lack of financial resources to create and maintain adequate (by developed nation standards) cardiac and cardiovascular treatment centers, pay for expensive machines and drugs, and subsidize training of individuals hoping to become skilled in transplant therapeutics is extremely problematic. Some

argue that the infrastructure necessary to support highly specialized and sophisticated programs such as organ transplantation will actually pull up standards throughout any given health care delivery system. Many less financially fortunate nations are grappling with the dilemma of paying for other expensive therapies designed to treat patients suffering from chronic, debilitating illnesses such as acquired immunodeficiency syndrome (AIDS).

A particularly negative view of the costs of heart transplantation has been put forth by noted social scientists Renee C. Fox and Judith P. Swazey,[9] who expressed their "deepening social and moral concern about the increase in zeal with which the procurement and transplantation of human organs and the quest to develop and implant artificial ones is being pursued," at the expense of more general public health needs. Of course, public health measures are necessary and important, but the Fox and Swazey stance ignores the fact that our prime purpose as health care providers is to help the suffering. Furthermore, ignoring the important field and therapeutic impact of organ replacement will simply deny humankind the benefits of important insight into immunologic mechanisms for many disease states, not to mention the extension of life for those with advanced heart failure.

One can argue that organ transplantation is most important for its role in promoting the study of biologic diversity and individuality. The legacy of insight into our immunologic characteristics is now considerable and has led to extraordinary progress throughout many fields seemingly unrelated to organ transplantation. The true cost of this is trivial. What could be more noble than pursuing scientific inquiry into means of more greatly unifying mankind's genetic diversity?

Nonetheless, heart transplantation is an expensive endeavor, and we struggle with providing it to as many ill heart failure patients as possible. Few individuals have contributed more to the understanding of the social and financial costs of organ transplantation than Roger W. Evans, Ph.D. His seminal work performed in the late 1980s during his tenure at the Battelle-Seattle Research Center gave us insight into these issues.[7, 8]

COMPONENTS OF HEART TRANSPLANT COSTS

Table 24–1 summarizes the major components of heart transplant costs along the lines of Evans' breakdown. Depending on how one defines inclusivity, the cost of

TABLE 24–1	Heart Transplant Cost Issues

- Patient evaluation
- Treatments while on wait list
- Surgical transplant costs
- Medical transplant costs
- Donor organ acquisition costs
- Long-term routine maintenance costs
- Costs of diagnosing and managing long-term morbidities

TABLE 24–2	Heart Transplant Versus Other Major Illness Treatment Expenses

	COSTS OF TREATMENT ($)	
Major psychiatric disorder (adolescent)	268,250	Per case (lifetime)*
Treatment of AIDS	27,550–213,150	Per case (lifetime)
Bone marrow transplant	159,950	Per case
Total parenteral nutrition	159,500	Per year per case
60% burn patient	145,000	Per case
Treatment of cancer	43,500	Per year per case
Maintenance hemodialysis	36,250	Per year per case
CABG	36,250	Per case
Heart transplant	34,075	Per year per case

CABG, coronary artery bypass graft; AIDS, acquired immunodeficiency syndrome.
*Dollars inflation adjusted from 1986 to 2000.
From Evans RW, Manninen DL, Dong FB: Costs, insurance coverage and reimbursement for heart transplantation. Final Report. 1991.

heart transplantation can include long-term care of the patient while trying to prevent the need for transplantation, care of the individual waiting for organ allocation, cost of the actual procedure itself, and long-term costs of posttransplant care until the patient dies. Specific components can include costs of patient evaluation, treatments while on the waiting list, surgical and medical transplant costs, donor organ acquisition costs, and long-term routine patient maintenance costs that include the costs of diagnosing and managing long-term morbidities. More succinctly put, the three primary elements of transplantation costs are hospital and clinic charges, professional fees, and donor organ acquisition costs. Obviously, it is difficult to sort through how much direct cardiac transplant-related expenses will be in any given cost center. Still, useful estimates have been developed using 1986 dollar analysis, and this allows comparisons with other major illness treatment expenses. Indeed, as Table 24–2 demonstrates, when per year per case costs are analyzed for a variety of common procedures, heart transplant compares quite favorably. Even when cost per year of life saved is considered (Table 24–3), heart transplantation falls in the middle of the pack. Because of the dramatic life-saving potential for cardiac transplantation, the initial cost when amortized over the many years of lives saved appears reasonable. One must remember that cardiac transplantation is not often per-

formed in patients with a life expectancy of more than 1 or 2 years without the procedure. This should be compared to a 40-year-old male with mild hypertension who requires many years of therapy while the likelihood of death is actually relatively low (yet greater than the "normal" population).

Evans and colleagues reported in 1991 that the median charge for a heart transplant was $91,570 with a hospital length of stay of 23 days. Total charges actually ranged between $67,234 and $142,079 for 50% of the cases studied. It must be remembered that these are dollar figures estimated in 1986, and this largely predates aggressive management of high-risk heart transplant candidates with ventricular assist device therapies and the more expensive posttransplant immunosuppressive drugs available today. Figure 24–5 compares the first year costs of various types of organ transplantation (in 1988 dollars) as presented by Evans and colleagues,[7] and notes that, though expensive, cardiac transplantation was not the most costly organ transplant procedure.

SOURCE OF PAYMENTS

In the National Cooperative Transplantation Study,[7] the analysis of payment sources for heart transplants in the United States suggested that 72% of the procedures were paid for by Blue Cross and Blue Shield or other private or commercial insurers. Medicare and Medicaid combined to pay for about 16% of the procedures, with only a few of the patients paying for heart transplantation "out-of-pocket" or through other sources (5.6% in this study). "Health maintenance organizations" paid for only 5.9% of procedures in this 1991 report. Clearly, this has changed, as vastly more managed care groups are paying for cardiac transplantation today, and Medicare is covering many more of these procedures.

Obviously, the level of reimbursement received by transplant hospitals is likely to be substantially less than billed charges or calculated costs. Interestingly, in 1991 reimbursement exceeded 80% of billed charges for 72% of the transplants analyzed in the Evans project. Currently, reimbursements are much lower than billed charges.

TABLE 24–3	Cost Per Year of Life Saved

THERAPY	COST/YEAR LIFE SAVED ($)
Hospital hemodialysis	95,410*
CAPD	83,085
Heart transplantation	38,938
Mild HTN (40-year-old male)	33,640
Severe HTN (40-year-old male)	16,530
CABG (three-vessel)	10,440
Neonatal ICU (1,000–1,500 g)	7,975

ICU, intensive care unit; CABG, coronary artery bypass graft; HTN, hypertension; CAPD, continuous ambulatory peritoneal dialysis.
*Dollars inflation adjusted from 1986 to 2000.
Modified from Drummond MF: Economic evaluation and the rational diffusion and use of health technology. Health Policy 1987;7:309–324.

Incurred First-Year Transplant Costs 1988

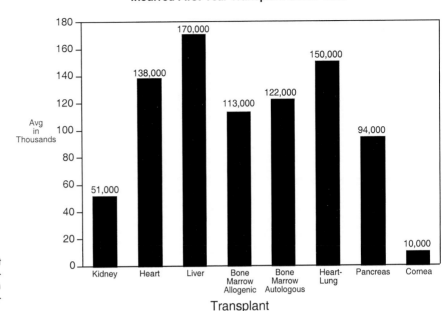

FIGURE **24–5.** Estimated first year transplant costs, 1988 U.S. dollars. (From Evans RW, Manninen DL, Dong FB: The National Transplantation Study: Final Report. Battelle-Seattle Research Center, 1991.)

COST EFFECTIVENESS

Health care treatment priorities can, obviously, be made on a political and public health stage. Certainly, individual institutions and providers must also make decisions about provision of such services. Cardiac transplantation is one of many "high-technology" therapies which society could consider too expensive in proportion to the number of patients receiving benefit. Indeed, within the United States, some state Medicaid programs have refused to pay for cardiac transplantation, arguing that it is in the best interest of public health not to use scarce resources to pay for expensive services focused on transplantation for only a few individuals. Instead, government health dollars could be shunted to other programs arguably having greater impact, such as maternal and child health care programs and "preventive" health care maintenance services.[10, 14, 22] Table 24–4 summarizes treatment priorities that 75 public health care directors in England and Wales ranked over a decade ago. Heart transplants were ranked 10th and liver transplants 11th on the list of a dozen treatments.[4] In this particular inquiry, advanced lung cancer treatments were the only therapeutic priority that ranked lower than transplantation.

However, this viewpoint ignores the massive impact of heart failure as a source of infirmity and death, affecting more than 4 million patients in the United States alone, with 400,000 new cases reported each year[1, 2] (see also Chapter 4). Heart failure is a leading cause of hospitalizations, which are one of the most expensive components of health care. Furthermore, the annual cost of heart failure care progressively rises with increasing severity (Table 24–5),[16] largely related to repeated hospitalizations. Heart transplantation clearly improves quality

and extends duration of life in advanced heart failure, and it is also generally cost-effective compared to medical therapy, considering the extended years of survival with less time spent hospitalized.[13] The cost per year of life saved by heart transplantation for this group of patients (see again Table 24–3) compares favorably with many other life-extending therapies. However, despite the unquestioned effectiveness of this therapy, this begs the question of who shall and can pay for these procedures? The demand for expensive heart failure therapy, including cardiac transplantation, clearly continues to increase, and this is attributed to our aging population with underlying cardiovascular disease risks which set the stage for the appearance of ventricular dysfunction as the disease progresses. The natural limits of donor

TABLE 24–4	Health Care Treatment Priorities
PRIORITY	THERAPY
1	Hip replacements
2	Cataract removal
3	CABG
4	Hemodialysis
5	Mammography
6	Hernia repair
7	AIDS treatment
8	Neonatal ICU (<800 g)
9	Parkinson's disease therapy
10	Heart transplants
11	Liver transplants
12	Advanced lung cancer therapy

CABG, coronary artery bypass graft; AIDS, acquired immunodeficiency syndrome; ICU, intensive care unit.
Modified from Dean M: Is your treatment economic, effective, efficient? Lancet 1991;337:480–481.

TABLE 24–5	Annual Cost of Heart Failure Related to New York Heart Association (NYHA) Class			
	COSTS*			
NYHA CLASS	France (FF)	The Netherlands (NLG)	Germany (DM)	Belgium (000 BeF)
I–II	5,760	700	2,580	32,000
III	22,126	1,200	4,428	7,800
IV	44,300	23,000	—	1,000,000

FF, French francs; NLG, Netherlands guilders; DM, German deutschmarks; BeF, Belgian francs.
*US$1 = FF5.00, NLG1.60, DM1.42, BeF38 (October 1995 exchange rates).
From Malek M: Health economics of heart failure. Heart 1999;82(suppl):11–13.

organ supply do hold cardiac transplantation costs in check, whereas use of chronic, "destination" mechanical circulatory assist will be far more problematic from a cost perspective.

PROGRAM ORGANIZATION

OVERVIEW

After considering the biological nuances of cardiac transplantation and demonstrating that outcomes are favorable and life saving, it becomes important to review the process of cardiac transplant service delivery. Clearly, successful transplantation of a heart from a brain-dead cadaveric organ donor into an ill patient with advanced heart failure is an extraordinarily complex multidisciplinary endeavor. Indeed, there may be no better example of "high tech" health care drama than the dynamic interaction between ill patients, skilled medical professionals, and the public in the process of transplantation in general and cardiac transplantation specifically. None of the advanced surgical technology commonly seen today can match the drama of organ transplantation, with its critical reliance on the loving good will of the public for success. This good will, of course, is the remarkably unselfish act of organ donation. Imagine the tragedy of brain death in a loved one, and then realize what is necessary to make organ transplantation happen.

Of course, without proper organization, this incredible medical miracle cannot succeed. The most skilled team of clinicians and surgeons will be unable to help their end-stage heart failure patients if no organized scheme is available to facilitate the organ donation process, identify and suitably manage candidates for transplant, and properly care for the patient after the operation. Obviously, cardiac transplant programs must be intimately linked to skilled and appropriately trained medical and surgical professionals, well-equipped and efficient inpatient and outpatient facilities, and a wide array of consultative support systems. These groups must interact with a national organ procurement and transplantation network as well as heart failure patient referral networks. Though many paradigms for cardiac transplant programs exist, it appears that the most suc-

cessful ventures are highly integrated services which exist in parallel to other solid organ transplant programs (specifically, liver, lung, and kidney transplant programs) in a single institution.

ELEMENTS OF CARDIAC TRANSPLANTATION SERVICES

Table 24–6 summarizes the critical elements of a heart transplant program. It seems logical that cardiac transplantation should be provided only by institutions having full-service cardiac surgery and cardiovascular medicine units and capable of supporting them to the fullest extent. Because of the great demands heart transplantation presents, teams having close working relationships between surgeons and cardiologists skilled in managing heart failure and transplant patients seem to be most successful. Seriously ill heart failure patients can wait long periods for heart donor allocation, and their care requires focused attention during this difficult period. Expert surgeons are necessary to ensure that donor or-

TABLE 24–6	Critical Elements of a Heart Transplant Program

- Full-service cardiovascular medicine and cardiac surgery
- Ventricular assist device access
- Cardiac transplant physicians
- Cardiac transplant surgeons
- Supportive consultative services
    Infectious diseases
    Immunology
    Critical care medicine
    Psychiatry
    Pathology
    Laboratory medicine
    Usual cadre of medical/surgical support consultation services
- Histocompatibility/immunology laboratory services
- Transplant social services
- Nursing service transplant coordinators
    Pretransplant evaluation
    Pretransplant patient management
    Posttransplant patient management
    Organ procurement
- Reimbursement specialists/counselors
- Affiliation with local/regional organ procurement organization
- Relationship with heart failure patient referral network

gan retrieval and cardiac allograft implantation occur with reproducible good early graft function, low early mortality, and minimal surgical morbidity. Programs providing cardiac transplantation must have access to ventricular assist devices and be skilled at their insertion and postoperative patient management. With the increasing need for patients to be bridged to transplantation in order to survive the pretransplant period, a substantial number of patients will require mechanical circulatory support, as detailed in Chapter 8.

A wide spectrum of supportive clinical and laboratory consultative services is mandatory. Most insurance providers will not allow patients to be referred for cardiac transplantation to centers not having well-documented and appropriately trained personnel to provide added expertise to the management of a heart transplant patient above that ordinarily required by day-to-day patient management routines.

Consultative personnel perhaps most important to organ transplant programs include infectious disease services, immunologists, critical care medicine specialists, pathologists, and laboratory medicine experts who can supervise a wide array of sophisticated immunologic and pharmacodynamic testing required for successful heart transplant patient management. Histocompatibility and immunology laboratories are essential for preoperative characterization of immunologic risks in heart transplant candidates. Experts skilled in evaluation of transplant candidates from a psychosocial standpoint are essential to exclude patients unlikely or incapable of following complex and taxing medication treatment protocols. Well-defined social and psychiatric risk factors for adverse outcome after transplantation have been identified and social service personnel trained and knowledgeable in the arena of solid organ transplantation are invaluable. Likewise, skilled nursing support services that can assist with the coordination of pretransplant patient evaluation as well as pretransplant and posttransplant patient management are essential to activating protocols designed to standardize practices in this patient population. Management of recurrent and recalcitrant rejection demands therapy in some situations with, for example, plasmapheresis and photopheresis protocols, and these services are critical to any successful cardiac transplant program. Strict adherence to prespecified treatment, follow-up, and surveillance protocols maximizes the likelihood of long-term survival after transplantation.

Organ procurement is essential to the success of cardiac transplantation, and nursing service personnel largely coordinate identification of potential cardiac donors, donor management, and organ retrieval. Reimbursement specialists and counselors play a prominent role in this age of limited resource allocation where many are uninsured or underinsured. It is a tragedy when a successful heart transplant recipient stops taking his medications several years out from the procedure because he cannot afford them or has no insurance coverage to help with the costs.

Another critical component of this complex therapy is affiliation with local and regional organ procurement organizations. Taking an active part in campaigning for organ donation ensures that heart transplant program personnel appreciate the difficulties associated with this endeavor and the limited supply of donor hearts. Programs should champion constructive relationships with local, regional, and national organ procurement organizations.

Finally, the development of close ties to heart failure patient referral networks ensures that proper heart transplant identification occurs. Creative interactions with referring physicians and groups will help to optimize pretransplant patient management schemes and assist with optimal patient follow-up after surgery. Having a "local" cardiologist and primary care physician actively involved with the care of the heart transplant recipient, in concert with the transplant center physicians, has been shown to improve outcomes.[18] In the absence of major transplant-related complications, patients who return home to the care of a local transplant physician have outcomes which are as good as those of patients followed at the transplant center.[15]

CARDIAC TRANSPLANT PHYSICIANS

The requirements for cardiac transplant physicians differ by country, but each country should establish competency and experience criteria for the medical physicians who assume the primary long-term care of these patients. In the United States, there are established criteria for a qualified transplant physician (see Box) as set forth by UNOS.

Equally important is the presence of a highly skilled heart failure cardiologist in cardiac transplant programs. The American College of Cardiology has defined general, specialized, and advanced training in heart failure medicine that defines these individuals.[12] For general training (Level I) in heart failure, the fundamental concepts involved in the pathophysiology of heart failure and its therapies must be well understood and taught as part of a core curriculum in a cardiology fellowship training program. Training in clinical management of heart failure should include supervised experience in both inpatient and outpatient settings and involve a spectrum of underlying etiologies of heart failure. Trainees should be well acquainted with all aspects of heart failure, particularly the different etiologies, and be particularly skilled at prescribing contemporary pharmacologic therapies to treat heart failure. Under optimal circumstances, the cardiology fellows will have rotated through dedicated heart failure/heart transplant clinical services, and this service should be incorporated during the trainee's clinical nonlaboratory experiences.

Specialized training (Level II) in heart failure and cardiac transplant medicine should be available to trainees who wish to have more advanced experiences in heart failure. Such programs will usually be found at institutions with active programs in cardiac transplantation and ventricular-assist device therapeutics. More advanced training will also include research efforts focused on the use of new or experimental treatment modalities (both drugs and devices), as well as cardiac transplantation.

Criteria for a Qualified Transplant Physician

UNOS requires that each heart transplant center must have on site a qualified transplant physician.[19] The cardiac transplant physician must be board certified or have achieved eligibility in adult or pediatric cardiology (or the subspecialty of his or her major area of interest) by the American Board of Internal Medicine (ABIM) or the American Board of Pediatrics (ABP). To qualify as a cardiac transplant physician, training experience requirements can be met if the following conditions are achieved. First, heart transplant training or experience during an individual's cardiology fellowship can qualify that individual as a cardiac transplant physician. This requires that the trainee will have been involved in 20 or more cardiac transplants under the direct supervision of a qualified cardiac transplant physician and in conjunction with a cardiac transplant surgeon at a UNOS-approved cardiac transplant center conducting 20 or more heart transplants each year. This individual has to document being involved with and having acquired a working knowledge of cardiac transplantation including the care of acute and chronic heart failure patients, donor selection, use of mechanical assist devices, recipient selection, pre- and postoperative hemodynamic care, postoperative immunosuppressive therapy, histological interpretation and grading of myocardial biopsies for rejection, and long-term outpatient follow-up. Additionally, it is required that the individual participate as an observer in five organ procurements and subsequent transplants. This training should be in addition to other clinical requirements for cardiology training. The individual must have a documenting letter sent directly to UNOS from the director of the individual fellowship training program, as well as the supervising qualified cardiac transplant physician verifying the fellow has met the above requirements and that he or she is qualified to become a medical director of a cardiac transplant program. The training must be performed at a hospital with an American Board of Internal Medicine certified fellowship training program in adult cardiology and/or an American Board of Pediatrics certified fellowship training program in pediatric cardiology.

When the training or experience requirements for the cardiac transplant physician have not been met during a cardiology fellowship, they can be met during a separate 12-month transplant medicine fellowship if the individual is a board-certified or eligible cardiologist and all of the following conditions are met: the applicant has been involved in 20 or more cardiac transplantations under the supervision of a qualified physician, the individual has acquired the same working knowledge outlined for cardiology trainees, and the individual has a letter sent directly to UNOS from the director of the individual fellowship training program as well as a supervising qualified cardiac transplant physician verifying that the fellow has met the above requirements and that he or she is qualified to become a medical director of a cardiac transplant program. Again, this experience must be obtained at a hospital with certified training programs in adult or pediatric cardiology. Expertise should be developed in the same above delineated areas.

If the cardiologist has not met the above requirements in a cardiology fellowship or specific cardiac transplant fellowship, requirements can be met by acquiring clinical experience if the same criteria as listed above are achieved. In some programs, cardiologists do not manage cardiac allograft patients. If the managing physician is not a cardiologist, he or she can qualify as the "cardiac transplant physician" to operate in conjunction with continuing involvement of a board-certified or eligible cardiologist if the same general criteria list above have been met. Support for this physician should be provided to UNOS by the heart transplant surgeon at the particular institution who has been directly involved with the individual and can certify his or her competence.

Advanced training (Level III) is characterized by a specialized training period of 12 months beyond the basic cardiovascular fellowship training, and focuses on clinical and basic science research in heart failure patients and in-depth cardiac transplant and ventricular-assist device therapy experience.

CARDIAC TRANSPLANT SURGEONS

In the United States, and increasingly in other countries, specific criteria have been established for a cardiac transplant surgeon. The criteria for a qualified heart transplant surgeon (see Box) established by UNOS[19] and the program criteria for training heart transplant surgeons set forth by the American Society of Transplantation provide standards for surgical expertise, training, and experience in this field. With the current focus on low surgical mortality and morbidity following often complex transplants in reoperative settings, standardized qualifications are a critical component of the judicious application of this scarce resource.

NATIONAL ORGANIZATION

A MODEL

The allocation of a limited resource like donor organs requires a national (or international) set of rules and guidelines for fair allocation and distribution. As an example of this process, we will discuss the **United Network of Organ Sharing.** Historical aspects of UNOS are discussed in Chapters 1 and 9 and the allocation algorithm is in Chapter 9. Since the 1960s when informal, voluntary sharing agreements between transplant programs began appearing across the country, a unique alternative to traditional government regulation has been evolving in the United States transplant community. Perhaps it is the nature of this science which depends as much on a surgeon's skill as on an organ donor family's selfless gift that galvanizes an entire sector of American medicine in this open, interactive, consensus-driven system for sharing scarce organs, refining professional standards, and increasing organ donations.

Criteria for a Qualified Heart Transplant Surgeon

Each heart transplant center must have on site a qualified heart transplant surgeon with current certification by the American Board of Thoracic Surgery or its equivalent. A qualified heart transplant surgeon may meet training/experience requirements by one of three pathways. (1) The individual may fulfill training/experience requirements during the applicant's cardiothoracic residency by performing as primary surgeon or first assistant 20 or more heart or heart/lung transplant procedures. The individual must demonstrate working knowledge of all aspects of heart transplantation and patient care including donor selection, donor procurement, recipient selection, postoperative hemodynamic care, postoperative immunosuppressive therapy, and outpatient follow-up. (2) If the requirements for heart transplant surgeon have not been met during the cardiothoracic residency program, they may be fulfilled during a subsequent 12-month cardiac transplantation fellowship, in which the Fellow performs as primary surgeon or first assistant 20 or more heart or heart/lung transplant procedures at a medical center with a cardiothoracic training program that is approved by the American Board of Thoracic Surgery. In addition, the Fellow must demonstrate working knowledge in all aspects of heart transplantation patient care as outlined above in pathway 1. (3) A board certified cardiothoracic surgeon may fulfill the requirements for a heart transplant surgeon by performing as primary surgeon, over a minimum of 2 or a maximum of 3 years, 20 or more heart or heart/lung transplant procedures at a UNOS-approved heart transplant program or its foreign equivalent. As indicated above, the surgeon must demonstrate a working knowledge of all aspects of heart transplantation and patient care. For all three pathways, the number of transplant procedures performed as primary surgeon or first assistant may be reduced to 10 if they are under the direct supervision of a UNOS-qualified heart transplant surgeon.

A crucial community activity in UNOS is the sharing of patient data among physicians who are also "sharing" donor organs among their respective patient populations and, in effect, practicing organ transplantation collectively. Organ transplantation clearly demonstrates Brennan's "moral interconnectedness of medical care" in which he describes how physician decisions about one patient affect all other patients.[3] Due to the inadequate organ supply, a surgeon's or physician's decision to accept a heart, liver, or lung for transplantation into a particular patient can mean the eventual death of another patient. The UNOS system is a product of transplantation's unique circumstances and challenges. The capacity for this community to work cooperatively is inherent to the success of transplantation.

The UNOS system preserves the leadership roles of physicians in the formation of public health care policy, while ensuring an effective and informed voice for patients and the public. Organ transplantation's success in "community self-determination" may well have far reaching social and political implications in governance matters, serving as a regulatory model for other medical fields. Perhaps more important is the fact that this interactive community affects continual quality improvement in health care delivery in the face of severely limited resources and does so on a national scale for an entire field.

THE TRANSPLANT COMMUNITY

The organ transplant "community" includes patients as well as transplant professionals, public members, organ donors, and donor family members. The commitment of UNOS to principles of professional self-regulation, together with the community's unique plan of providers and recipients, donors and beneficiaries, professionals and laity, are reflected in the organizational governance of UNOS. Half of the 40-member governing board of UNOS is composed of practicing transplant surgeons and physicians from whom the UNOS President and Vice President have been elected historically. One third of the board is a public group composed of transplant patients, organ donors, and family members, including a Vice President of Patient and Donor Family Affairs who is also a corporate officer of UNOS. The remaining board members and officers reflect community constituencies. An equally representative national committee system and a system of 11 geographic regions for organ distribution (Fig. 24–6) support the board.

On a national scale, the field is relatively small: in the United States, 276 transplant centers performed 21,506 solid organ transplants in 1999. However, this scale permits a very high level of participation with greater than 80% of all institutional members represented at each semiannual meeting of their UNOS region. This community, however, is not defined by geographical boundaries, but consists of stakeholders, that is, anyone having a "stake" in the community's decisions. Transplant patients have the most obvious stake; indeed, the entire expertise exists for their benefit. Family members who consented to the donation of a loved one's organs have a unique emotional stake in the integrity and effectiveness of the network. Individual practitioners within the institutions that are official UNOS "members" are community stakeholders by virtue of their professional interest in transplantation. Every member of the community is able to participate in community decisions through direct, personal involvement. This individual involvement distinguishes community self-determination from traditional American democracy, which relies on representational systems or agency regulation where direct personal participation is limited, if available at all. As such, the transplant community's move toward individual, personal involvement reflects a larger social shift in attitudes toward governance, a phenomenon that is, in large part, the result of advances in telecommunications and electronic information technology.

The UNOS system embraces traditional principles of professional self-regulation pioneered by the medical profession. Based upon philosophies that acknowledge the ethical importance of patient and physician autonomy, the UNOS model expands to embrace a broad and

UNOS Regional Map

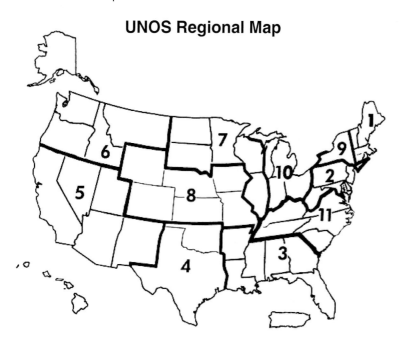

FIGURE **24-6.** UNOS regional map.

diverse community. Individual practitioners are deeply involved in all aspects of UNOS activities not only as representatives of their profession, but as advocates of their patients. While the depth and breadth of professional involvement is extraordinary, professional UNOS leadership serves as the foundation of a broader, collaborative community for policy development.

BACKGROUND OF AN ORGAN PROCUREMENT AND TRANSPLANTATION NETWORK

Transplantation's community self-determination in the United States arose out of the unprecedented public/private framework of the National Organ Transplant Act (NOTA) of 1984. This federal law directed the United States Department of Health and Human Services (DHHS) to establish a national Organ Procurement and Transplantation Network (OPTN) in the private sector by contract rather than traditional federal agency action regulation. It was clear to lawmakers that this complex and rapidly growing area of health care would benefit from a responsive rule-making system, and would flourish only with the knowledge, experience, and direct participation of transplantation's practitioners and beneficiaries.

Since 1986, UNOS, a private, not-for-profit membership corporation comprising all United States organ transplant organizations, has held the federal contract to operate the OPTN. As also discussed in Chapter 9, specific goals of the OPTN are to (1) maintain the nation's organ transplant waiting list; (2) coordinate the matching and distribution of donated organs to patients who need them; and (3) serve as the forum through which OPTN members develop the nation's transplant policies. The appropriate role of the federal government under the unique construct found in NOTA has been the focus of intense national debate, but the transplant

community interacting through the national network continue to form the core of the American organ transplant system. Political developments in organ transplantation during the latter part of the 1990s emphasize the difficulties such a system can encounter, and highlights the ability of reasoned individuals to reach compromise.

STRUCTURE FOR ORGAN DISTRIBUTION

At the beginning of 1998, 896 programs were in operation at 276 transplant centers across the United States. These programs obtained donated organs from within their own institutions and through the 63 organ procurement organizations (OPOs) designated by the federal government to conduct exclusive operations in their local areas across the United States. The OPO service areas and transplant programs are grouped into 11 UNOS regions for administrative purposes and, in some instances, organ sharing (Fig. 24–6).

OPOs serve as the integral link between the potential donor and recipient and are accountable for the **retrieval, preservation, allocation,** and **transportation** of organs for transplantation. OPOs are also primarily engaged in public and professional **education** on the critical need for organ donation. NOTA places responsibility for organ allocation expressly on OPOs and requires that OPO service areas be large enough to permit efficient organ procurement and equitable organ allocation. Therefore, UNOS policy has been based historically on a system in which organs procured by a given OPO are allocated first locally (i.e., to patients listed at transplant centers located in the OPO service area or an approved alternative area known as an "alternative local unit"). Certainly, inequities exist with this system, but it is a recognized fact that a tremendous incentive exists for local organ procurement if this process is followed. Generally, if a local match is not made, the organ is made available to centers within the region, and if a match is still not found, it is offered nationally. The reasons for this general algorithm in heart transplantation relate to the constraints of safe ischemic time (see Chapter 9 and 16). The full current UNOS algorithm for adult patients according to medical urgency is found in Chapter 9, and for pediatric patients in Chapter 20.

STRUCTURE FOR MAKING POLICY

UNOS builds consensus through direct stakeholder participation, but for efficiency UNOS employs some representational features such as constituent-based board and committees. However, all policy proposals are published for the entire community, and multiple opportunities are extended prior to adaptation. Written rationales are mailed directly to community members to encourage informed discussions about policy proposals. Individual comments can be voiced directly or via committee or board representation. Policy proposals are debated at public meetings in the 11 UNOS geographic regions, and national public hearings are conducted for most controversial issues. Because transplantation is so dynamic, the UNOS procedures are designed to be efficient, flexible, and timely, while also affording to all interested parties meaningful participation opportunities. The process routinely involves as many as 4,000 individuals across the country. Policy issues are examined using perspectives of ethics and legality, scientific data analysis, and personal experience and testimony of individuals in the transplant community and general public, including patients, patient families, donors, and donor families.

EQUITABLE ORGAN ALLOCATION

UNOS is guided by a set of basic principles in achieving and maintaining an equitable national organ allocation system. From these principles, specific measurable objectives have been derived. Equitable organ allocation policy is defined as those rules which, in balance with one another, enhance overall availability of transplantable organs, allocate organs based upon medical criteria, strive to give equal consideration to medical utility and justice, and provide transplant candidates reasonable opportunities to be considered for organ offers within comparable time periods. Equal consideration of medical utility is defined as the net medical benefit to all transplant patients as a group, and justice is defined as equity in distribution of both benefits and burdens among all transplant patients. Reasonable opportunities for organ offers must take into consideration similarities and dissimilarities in medical circumstances as well as technical and logistical factors in organ distribution. Equitable allocation of organs with specific reference to heart transplantation is further discussed in Chapters 6 and 9.

The goal of the UNOS organ allocation system is to achieve, in balance with one another, many well-defined objectives. These include efforts to maximize availability of transplantable organs by promoting consent for donation, enhancing procurement efficiency, minimizing organ discards, and promoting efficiency in organ distribution and allocation. Furthermore, goals include maximization of patient and graft survival and minimization of disparities in consistently measured waiting times until an offer of an organ for transplantation is made among patients with similar or comparable medical/demographic characteristics. Also important is minimizing fatalities while on the waiting list and maximizing the opportunity for patients with biological or medical disadvantages to receive a transplant. UNOS tries to minimize the effects related to geography although, by nature of the United States population and geographic makeup, this is difficult. Furthermore, UNOS is committed to allowing convenient access to transplantation, minimizing overall transplantation-related costs, providing flexibility for policy making, and providing accountability and public trust mechanisms.

FOSTERING THE PUBLIC'S TRUST

The field of organ transplantation has a singularly intensive need to continually merit the public's trust. The relationship between that trust and the altruistic gift of organ donation is delicate, and without it transplantation is not possible. Prospective donors are far more likely to say "yes" to donation if they believe their organs will be used in an equitable and efficient manner. This critical fact propels a community-wide commitment to scientific and ethical integrity and public accountability. Policy making consists of open and inclusive deliberations designed to permit the widest possible participation aimed at achieving authentic consensus. The public debate about transplant policy is informed and stimulated by extensive data analysis.

Since 1987, UNOS has collected data for all patients awaiting transplantation (Fig. 24–4), all organ donors (Fig. 24–2), and all transplant recipients, with annual follow-up data for more than 90% of all transplants. Data and analyses from those registries are regularly analyzed as part of the policy development process. Special data reports and analyses are routinely published for the public. For example, UNOS uses its extensive database to produce a report for the Department of Health and Human Services describing outcomes for each transplant program in the country. Centers' actual outcomes are compared to their risk-adjusted "expected" outcomes based upon national data for similar circumstances. In December of 1997, UNOS and DHHS issued the center-specific outcomes report for all transplants performed between 1988 and 1994.[21] By making data widely available and permitting mass participation in public policy, UNOS engenders an atmosphere of open collaboration and accountability.

GOVERNANCE, FLEXIBILITY, AND ACCOUNTABILITY

Authority is delegated to the OPTN from the Congress via UNOS' contract with DHHS as specified in NOTA, effecting substantial federal oversight and public accountability. The law sets the basis for the OPTN's decisions by establishing certain fundamental principles. It was the democratically elected members of Congress who determined that the procurement and allocation of organs would, with certain exceptions, occur initially within OPO services areas, as opposed to other geographic schemes, guided by a balance between duration of time waiting and medical urgency.

The approach of UNOS to community self-determination combines advantages of both government agency rule making and professional self-regulation. The public-private nature of the OPTN gives UNOS private sector efficiency and flexibility while enabling it to benefit from federal power and authority. The law's stipulation, for example, that DHHS establish the "private entity" OPTN "by contract," places the OPTN squarely in the private sector, but holds it to standards of openness, public accountability, and due process through contract oversight provided by the government. The model established by Congress in which DHHS is to act by contract rather than traditional agency action implies a collaborative approach between public and private sectors.

Like professional self-regulation, the self-determination process of UNOS produces policies through the direct participation of practicing physicians, which also minimizes costly gaps between what a policy may say "on paper" and the reality encountered at the patient/donor bedside. One of the most important benefits of OPTN policies is the ability of UNOS to expedite the development of procedures and standards and avoid the frustrating delay in policy revision that sometimes characterizes government regulations. The legislative directive of DHHS established the OPTN, but the contract reinforces the desire for a flexible approach. Community self-determination harnesses the powerful motivation of self-interest among participants while neutralizing the negative aspects of that self-interest through universal participation, consensus building, and peer pressure. As such, community self-determination is capable of achieving the highest levels of quality. Whereas government rule-making and professional self-regulation are proscriptive by nature and therefore constraining, community self-determination has the potential for generating a creative and productive environment. Considering the ever-broadening gap between supply and demand of precious transplantable organs, the proportional rise in waiting list fatalities, and the ethical and scientific complexities inherent in this field of health care, a creative and productive environment

is mandatory to the future success of organ transplantation.

References

1. American Heart Association: Heart and Stroke Facts: 1995 Statistical Supplement. Dallas. American Heart Association, 1994.
2. Bennett SJ, Saywell RM, Zollinger TW, Huster GA, Ford CE, Pressler ML: Cost of hospitalizations for heart failure: sodium retention versus other decompensating factors. Heart Lung 1999; 28:102–109.
3. Brennan TA: An ethical perspective on health care insurance reform. Am J Law Med 1993;19:37–74.
4. Dean M: Is your treatment economic, effective, efficient? Lancet 1991;337:480–481.
5. Drummond MF: Economic evaluation and the rational diffusion and use of health technology. Health Policy 1987;7:309–324.
6. Evans RW, Manninen DL, Dong FB: Costs, insurance coverage and reimbursement for heart transplantation. Final Report, 1991.
7. Evans RW, Manninen DL, Dong FB: The National Transplantation Study: Final Report. Battelle-Seattle Research Center, 1991.
8. Evans RW, Manninen DL, Dong FB: Costs, insurance coverage, and reimbursement for heart transplantation. In Shumway SJ, Shumway NE (eds): Thoracic Transplantation. Cambridge: Blackwell Science, 1995.
9. Fox RC, Swazey JP: Spare Parts: Organ Replacment in American Society. New York: Oxford University Press, 1992.
10. Goldsmith MF: Oregon pioneers "more ethical" Medicaid coverage with prioirty setting project. JAMA 1989;262:176–177.
11. Hosenpud JD, Bennett LE, Keck BM, Boucek MM, Novick RJ: The Registry of the International Society for Heart and Lung Transplantation: 17th official report—2000. J Heart Lung Transplant 2000;19:909–931.
12. Hunt SA, Bristow MR, Kubo SH, O'Connell JB, Young JB: Training in heart failure and transplantation. J Am Coll Cardiol 1995; 25:1–34.
13. Kirklin JK, Naftel DC, Boehmer JP, Kobashigawa JA, Kenzora JL, Mehra MR, Miller LW, Kubo SH, Stevenson LW, Bourge RC, and the Cardiac Transplant Research Database: Refining the criteria for heart transplant listing and status: a multi-institutional risk factor analysis for rehospitalization following listing [abstract]. J Heart Lung Transplant 1999;18:47.
14. Kitzhaber J: The Oregon health initiative. Lancet 1989;2:106.
15. Kushwaha S, Rodeheffer RJ, Weiss T, Jarcho J, Pritzker M, Smith AL, Heilman KJ, Clemson BS: Longer distance from transplant center is not associated with decreased suravival in post cardiac transplant patients [abstract]. J Heart Lung Transplant 2001;20:236.
16. Malek M: Health economics of heart failure. Heart 1999; 82(suppl):11–13.
17. Rick MW, Nease RF: Cost effectiveness analysis in clinical practice. Arch Intern Med 1999;159:1690–1700.
18. Rodkey SM, Hobbs RE, Goormastic M, Young JB: Does distance between home and transplant center adversely affect patient outcomes after heart transplant. J Heart Lung Transplant 1997;16: 496–503.
19. United Network for Organ Sharing: UNOS Bylaws; Appendix B; Section IIIC. UNOS Update 1991;7:11–3.
20. United Network for Organ Sharing: Annual Report, 2000.
21. United Network of Organ Sharing: Center Specific Report, 1999.
22. Welch HG, Larson EB: Dealing with limited resources: the Oregon decision to curtail funding for organ transplantation. N Engl J Med 1988;319:171–173.

Index

NOTE: Page numbers followed by f refer to figures; those followed by b refer to boxed material and those followed by t refer to tables.

ISBN 0-443-07655-3

90038